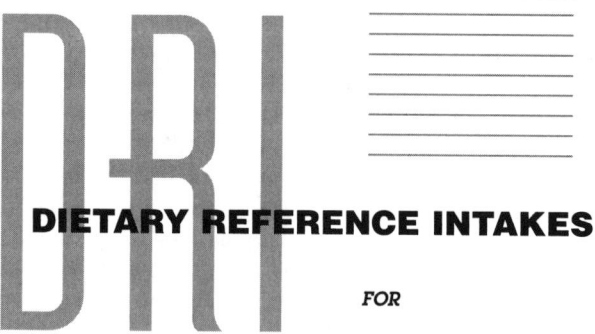

DIETARY REFERENCE INTAKES

FOR

Energy, Carbohydrate, Fiber, Fat, Fatty Acids, Cholesterol, Protein, and Amino Acids

Panel on Macronutrients, Panel on the Definition of Dietary Fiber, Subcommittee on Upper Reference Levels of Nutrients, Subcommittee on Interpretation and Uses of Dietary Reference Intakes, and the Standing Committee on the Scientific Evaluation of Dietary Reference Intakes

Food and Nutrition Board

INSTITUTE OF MEDICINE
OF THE NATIONAL ACADEMIES

THE NATIONAL ACADEMIES PRESS
Washington, D.C.
www.nap.edu

THE NATIONAL ACADEMIES PRESS   500 Fifth Street, N.W.   Washington, DC 20001

NOTICE: The project that is the subject of this report was approved by the Governing Board of the National Research Council, whose members are drawn from the councils of the National Academy of Sciences, the National Academy of Engineering, and the Institute of Medicine. The members of the committee responsible for the report were chosen for their special competences and with regard for appropriate balance.

This project was funded by the U.S. Department of Health and Human Services Office of Disease Prevention and Health Promotion, Contract No. 282-96-0033, TO #4; Health Canada; the U.S. Food and Drug Administration; the National Institutes of Health; the Centers for Disease Control and Prevention; the U.S. Department of Agriculture; the Department of Defense; the Institute of Medicine; the Dietary Reference Intakes Private Foundation Fund, including the Dannon Institute and the International Life Sciences Institute, North America; and the Dietary Reference Intakes Corporate Donors' Fund. Contributors to the Fund include Roche Vitamins Inc, Mead Johnson Nutrition Group, and M&M Mars. The views presented in this report are those of the Institute of Medicine Standing Committee on the Scientific Evaluation of Dietary Reference Intakes and its panels and subcommittes and are not necessarily those of the funding agencies.

Library of Congress Cataloging-in-Publication Data

Dietary reference intakes for energy, carbohydrate, fiber, fat, fatty acids, cholesterol, protein, and amino acids / Panel on Macronutrients, Panel on the Definition of Dietary Fiber, Subcommittee on Upper Reference Levels of Nutrients, Subcommittee on Interpretation and Uses of Dietary Reference Intakes, and the Standing Committee on the Scientific Evaluation of Dietary Reference Intakes, Food and Nutrition Board.
       p. ; cm.
    Includes bibliographical references and index.
    ISBN 0-309-08525-X (pbk.) — ISBN 0-309-08537-3 (hardcover)   1. Nutrition. 2. Reference values (Medicine)
    [DNLM: 1. Nutrition. 2. Diet. 3. Reference Values.] I. Institute of Medicine (U.S.). Panel on Macronutrients. II. Institute of Medicine (U.S.). Standing Committee on the Scientific Evaluation of Dietary Reference Intakes.
    QP141.D529 2005
    613.2—dc22
                                        2004031026

Additional copies of this report are available from the National Academies Press, 500 Fifth Street, N.W., Lockbox 285, Washington, DC 20055; (800) 624-6242 or (202) 334-3313 (in the Washington metropolitan area); Internet, http://www.nap.edu.

For more information about the Institute of Medicine, visit the IOM home page at: **www.iom.edu.**

The serpent has been a symbol of long life, healing, and knowledge among almost all cultures and religions since the beginning of recorded history. The serpent adopted as a logotype by the Institute of Medicine is a relief carving from ancient Greece, now held by the Staatliche Museen in Berlin.

"Knowing is not enough; we must apply.
Willing is not enough; we must do."
—Goethe

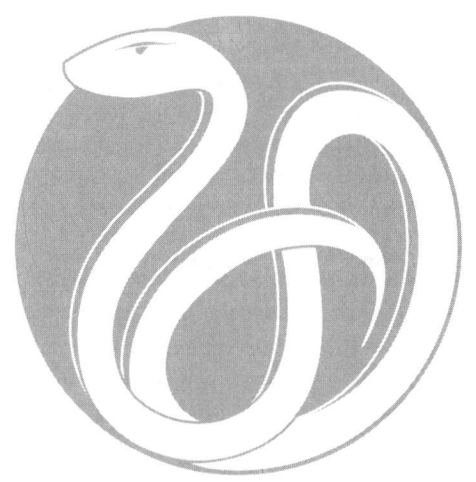

INSTITUTE OF MEDICINE
OF THE NATIONAL ACADEMIES

Advising the Nation. Improving Health.

THE NATIONAL ACADEMIES
Advisers to the Nation on Science, Engineering, and Medicine

The **National Academy of Sciences** is a private, nonprofit, self-perpetuating society of distinguished scholars engaged in scientific and engineering research, dedicated to the furtherance of science and technology and to their use for the general welfare. Upon the authority of the charter granted to it by the Congress in 1863, the Academy has a mandate that requires it to advise the federal government on scientific and technical matters. Dr. Ralph J. Cicerone is president of the National Academy of Sciences.

The **National Academy of Engineering** was established in 1964, under the charter of the National Academy of Sciences, as a parallel organization of outstanding engineers. It is autonomous in its administration and in the selection of its members, sharing with the National Academy of Sciences the responsibility for advising the federal government. The National Academy of Engineering also sponsors engineering programs aimed at meeting national needs, encourages education and research, and recognizes the superior achievements of engineers. Dr. Wm. A. Wulf is president of the National Academy of Engineering.

The **Institute of Medicine** was established in 1970 by the National Academy of Sciences to secure the services of eminent members of appropriate professions in the examination of policy matters pertaining to the health of the public. The Institute acts under the responsibility given to the National Academy of Sciences by its congressional charter to be an adviser to the federal government and, upon its own initiative, to identify issues of medical care, research, and education. Dr. Harvey V. Fineberg is president of the Institute of Medicine.

The **National Research Council** was organized by the National Academy of Sciences in 1916 to associate the broad community of science and technology with the Academy's purposes of furthering knowledge and advising the federal government. Functioning in accordance with general policies determined by the Academy, the Council has become the principal operating agency of both the National Academy of Sciences and the National Academy of Engineering in providing services to the government, the public, and the scientific and engineering communities. The Council is administered jointly by both Academies and the Institute of Medicine. Dr. Ralph J. Cicerone and Dr. Wm. A. Wulf are chair and vice chair, respectively, of the National Research Council.

www.national-academies.org

PANEL ON DIETARY REFERENCE INTAKES FOR MACRONUTRIENTS

JOANNE R. LUPTON (*Chair*), Faculty of Nutrition, Texas A&M University, College Station

GEORGE A. BROOKS, Department of Integrative Biology, University of California, Berkeley

NANCY F. BUTTE, Department of Pediatrics, U.S. Department of Agriculture/Agriculture Research Service Children's Nutrition Research Center, Baylor College of Medicine, Houston, Texas

BENJAMIN CABALLERO, Center for Human Nutrition, Johns Hopkins Bloomberg School of Public Health, Baltimore, Maryland

JEAN PIERRE FLATT, Department of Biochemistry and Molecular Biology, University of Massachusetts Medical Center, Worcester

SUSAN K. FRIED, Department of Nutritional Sciences, Rutgers University, New Brunswick, New Jersey

PETER J. GARLICK, Department of Surgery, State University of New York at Stony Brook

SCOTT M. GRUNDY, Center for Human Nutrition, University of Texas Southwestern Medical Center, Dallas

SHEILA M. INNIS, BC Research Institute for Children's and Women's Health, University of British Columbia, Vancouver

DAVID J.A. JENKINS, Department of Nutritional Sciences, University of Toronto, Ontario

RACHEL K. JOHNSON, Department of Nutrition and Food Sciences, University of Vermont, Burlington

RONALD M. KRAUSS, Department of Molecular Medicine, Lawrence Berkeley National Laboratory, University of California, Berkeley

PENNY KRIS-ETHERTON, Department of Nutrition, Pennsylvania State University, University Park

ALICE H. LICHTENSTEIN, Jean Mayer U.S. Department of Agriculture Human Nutrition Research Center on Aging, Tufts University, Boston, Massachusetts

FRANK Q. NUTTALL, Department of Medicine, University of Minnesota School of Medicine, Minneapolis

PAUL B. PENCHARZ, Departments of Pediatrics and Nutritional Sciences, University of Toronto, Ontario

F. XAVIER PI-SUNYER, Department of Medicine, Columbia University, New York

WILLIAM M. RAND, Department of Family Medicine and Community Health, Tufts University School of Medicine, Boston, Massachusetts

PETER J. REEDS (*deceased*), Department of Animal Sciences, University of Illinois at Urbana-Champaign

ERIC B. RIMM, Department of Nutrition, Harvard School of Public Health, Boston, Massachusetts

SUSAN B. ROBERTS, Jean Mayer U.S. Department of Agriculture Human Nutrition Research Center on Aging, Tufts University, Boston, Massachusetts

PANEL ON THE DEFINITION OF DIETARY FIBER

JOANNE R. LUPTON (*Chair*), Faculty of Nutrition, Texas A&M
University, College Station
GEORGE C. FAHEY, Department of Animal Sciences, University of
Illinois at Urbana-Champaign
DAVID J.A. JENKINS, Department of Nutritional Sciences, University of
Toronto, Ontario
JUDITH A. MARLETT, Department of Nutritional Science, University of
Wisconsin-Madison
JOANNE L. SLAVIN, Department of Food Science and Nutrition,
University of Minnesota, St. Paul
JON A. STORY, Department of Foods and Nutrition, Purdue University,
West Lafayette, Indiana
CHRISTINE L. WILLIAMS, Department of Pediatrics, Columbia
University, New York

Consultants

LEON PROSKY, Prosky Associates, Rockville, Maryland
ALISON STEPHEN, CanTox, Inc., Mississauga, Ontario

Staff

PAULA R. TRUMBO, Study Director
ALICE L. VOROSMARTI, Research Associate
KIMBERLY STITZEL, Research Assistant (until January 2001)
CARRIE L. HOLLOWAY, Research Assistant
GAIL E. SPEARS, Staff Editor
SANDRA AMAMOO-KAKRA, Senior Project Assistant
MICHELE RAMSEY, Senior Project Assistant (until June 2001)

SUBCOMMITTEE ON INTERPRETATION AND USES OF DIETARY REFERENCE INTAKES

SUSAN I. BARR (*Chair*), Department of Food, Nutrition, and Health, University of British Columbia, Vancouver

TANYA D. AGURS-COLLINS, Department of Oncology, Howard University Cancer Center, Washington, D.C.

ALICIA CARRIQUIRY, Department of Statistics, Iowa State University, Ames

ANN M. COULSTON, Hattner/Coulston Nutrition Associates, LLC., Palo Alto, California

BARBARA L. DEVANEY, Mathematica Policy Research, Princeton, New Jersey

JANET HUNT, U.S. Department of Agriculture/Agriculture Research Service, Grand Forks Human Nutrition Research Center, Grand Forks, North Dakota

SUZANNE MURPHY, Cancer Research Center of Hawaii, University of Hawaii, Honolulu

VALERIE TARASUK, Department of Nutritional Sciences, University of Toronto, Ontario

Staff

MARY POOS, Study Director
ALICE L. VOROSMARTI, Research Associate
HARLEEN SETHI, Project Assistant

Staff

ALLISON A. YATES, Study Director
MARY POOS, Senior Program Officer
SANDRA SCHLICKER, Senior Program Officer
PAULA R. TRUMBO, Senior Program Officer
ALICE L. VOROSMARTI, Research Associate
CARRIE L. HOLLOWAY, Research Assistant
GAIL E. SPEARS, Staff Editor
SANDRA AMAMOO-KAKRA, Senior Project Assistant

Dedication

The Panel on Macronutrients dedicates this report to the late Peter Reeds, a diligent and enthusiastic member of the panel who made significant contributions to this study. His expertise in protein and amino acid metabolism was a special asset to the panel's work, as well as a contribution to the understanding of protein and amino acid requirements.

Preface

This report is one in a series that presents a comprehensive set of reference values for nutrient intakes for healthy U.S. and Canadian individuals and populations. It is a product of the Food and Nutrition Board of the Institute of Medicine (IOM), working in cooperation with Canadian scientists.

The report establishes a set of reference values for dietary energy, carbohydrate, fiber, fat, fatty acids, cholesterol, protein, and amino acids to expand and replace previously published Recommended Dietary Allowances (RDAs) and Recommended Nutrient Intakes (RNIs) for the United States and Canada, respectively. Close attention was given throughout the report to the evidence relating macronutrient intakes to risk reduction of chronic disease and to amounts needed to maintain health. Thus, the report includes guidelines for partitioning energy sources (Acceptable Macronutrient Distribution Ranges) compatible with decreasing risks of various chronic diseases. It also provides a definition for dietary fiber.

The groups responsible for developing this report, the Panel on Macronutrients, the Panel on the Definition of Dietary Fiber, the Subcommittee on Upper Reference Levels of Nutrients (UL Subcommittee), the Subcommittee on Interpretation and Uses of Dietary Reference Intakes (Uses Subcommittee), and the Standing Committee on the Scientific Evaluation of Dietary Reference Intakes (DRI Committee), have analyzed the evidence on risks and beneficial effects of nutrients and other food components included in this review.

Although all reference values are based on data, available data were often sparse or drawn from studies with significant limitations in addressing various questions confronted by the panel and subcommittees. Thus, although governed by scientific rationales, informed judgments were often required in setting reference values. The reasoning used for each nutrient is described in Chapters 5 through 11. Chapter 13 addresses major conceptual issues related to the uses of the DRIs that were included in the early stages of the DRI process and have been developed further by the Uses Subcommittee.

The quality and quantity of information on overt deficiency diseases for protein, amino acids, and essential fatty acids available to the committee were substantial. Unfortunately, information regarding other nutrients for which their primary dietary importance relates to their roles as energy sources was limited most often to alterations in chronic disease biomarkers that follow dietary manipulations of energy sources.

Given the uniqueness of the nutrients considered in this report (i.e., they or their precursors serve as energy sources and, for this purpose, can substitute for each other in the diet), the inability to determine an Estimated Average Requirement (EAR) or a Tolerable Upper Intake Level (UL) in many cases is not surprising. Also, for most of the nutrients in this report (with a notable exception of protein and some amino acids), there is no direct information that permits estimating the amounts required by children, adolescents, the elderly, or pregnant and lactating women. Similarly, data were exceptionally sparse for setting ULs for the macronutrients. Dose–response studies were either not available or were suggestive of very low intake levels that could result in inadequate intakes of other nutrients. These information gaps and inconsistencies often precluded setting reliable estimates of upper intake levels that can be ingested safely.

The report's attention to energy would be incomplete without its substantial review of the role of daily physical activity in achieving and sustaining fitness and optimal health (Chapter 12). The report provides recommended levels of energy expenditure that are considered most compatible with minimizing risks of several chronic diseases and provides guidance for achieving recommended levels of energy expenditure. Inclusion of these recommendations avoids the tacit false assumption that light sedentary activity is the expected norm in the United States and Canada.

Readers are urged to recognize that the Dietary Reference Intakes (DRI) process is iterative in character. The Food and Nutrition Board and the DRI Committee and its subcommittees and panels fully expect that the DRI conceptual framework will evolve and be improved as novel information becomes available and is applied to an expanding list of nutrients and other food components. Thus, because the DRI activity is ongoing, comments were solicited widely and received on the published reports of this series. Refinements that resulted from this iterative process were included in the general information regarding approaches used (Chapters 1 through 4) and in the discussion of uses of DRIs (Chapter 13). With more experience, the proposed models for establishing reference intakes of nutrients and other food components that play significant roles in promoting and sustaining health and optimal functioning will be refined. Also, as new information or new methods of analysis are adopted, these reference values undoubtedly will be reassessed.

Many of the questions that were raised about requirements and recommended intakes could not be answered satisfactorily for the reasons given above. Thus, among the panel's major tasks was to outline a research agenda addressing information gaps uncovered in its review (Chapter 14). The research agenda is anticipated to help future policy decisions related to these and future recommendations. This agenda and the critical, comprehensive analyses of available information are intended to assist the private sector, foundations, universities, governmental and international agencies and laboratories, and other institutions in the development of their respective research priorities for the next decade.

This report has been reviewed in draft form by individuals chosen for their diverse perspectives and technical expertise, in accordance with procedures approved by the NRC's Report Review Committee. The purpose of this independent review is to provide candid and critical comments that will assist the institution in making its published report as sound as possible and to ensure that the report meets institutional standards for objectivity, evidence, and responsiveness to the study charge. The review comments and draft manuscript remain confidential to protect the integrity of the deliberative process. We wish to thank the following individuals for their review of this report:

Arne Astrup, The Royal Veterinary and Agricultural University; George Blackburn, Beth Israel Deaconess Medical Center; Elsworth Buskirk, Pennsylvania State University; William Connor, Oregon Health and Science University; John Hathcock, Council for Responsible Nutrition; Satish Kalhan, Case Western Reserve University School of Medicine; Martijn Katan, Wageningen Agricultural University; David Kritchevsky, The Wistar Institute; Shiriki Kumanyika, University of Pennsylvania School of Medicine; William Lands, National Institutes of Health; Geoffrey Livesey, Independent Nutrition Logic; Ross Prentice, Fred Hutchinson Cancer Research Center; Barbara Schneeman, University of California, Davis; Christopher Sempos, State University of New York, Buffalo; Virginia Stallings, Children's Hospital of Philadelphia; Steve Taylor, University of Nebraska; Daniel Tomé, Institut National Agronomique Paris-Grinon; and Walter Willett, Harvard School of Public Health.

Although the reviewers listed above have provided many constructive comments and suggestions, they were not asked to endorse the conclusions or recommendations nor did they see the final draft of the report before its release. The review of this report was overseen by Catherine Ross, Pennsylvania State University and Irwin Rosenberg, Tufts University, appointed by the Institute of Medicine, who were responsible for making certain that an independent examination of this report was carried out in accordance with institutional procedures and that all review comments were carefully considered. Responsibility for the final content of this report rests entirely with the authoring committee and the institution.

The Food and Nutrition Board gratefully acknowledges the Canadian government's support and Canadian scientists' participation in this initiative. This close collaboration represents a pioneering first step in the harmonization of nutrient reference intakes in North America. A description of the overall DRI project and of the panel's task is given in Appendix B.

The Food and Nutrition Board joins the DRI Committee, the Panel on Macronutrients, the Panel on the Definition of Dietary Fiber, the UL Subcommittee, and the Uses Subcommittee in extending sincere appreciation to the many experts who assisted with this report by giving presentations to the various groups charged with its development, providing written materials, participating in the groups' open discussions, analyzing data, and other means. Many, but far from all, of these individuals are named in Appendix C. Special gratitude is extended to the staff at ENVIRON International Corporation for providing national survey data.

The respective chairs and members of the Panel on Macronutrients and subcommittees performed their work under great time pressures. Their dedication made the report's timely completion possible. All gave their time and hard work willingly and without financial reward; the public and the science and practice of nutrition are among the major beneficiaries of their dedication. The Food and Nutrition Board thanks these individuals, and especially the staff responsible for its development—in particular, Paula Trumbo for coordinating this complex report, and Sandra Schlicker, who served as a program officer for the study. The intellectual and managerial contributions made by these individuals to the report's comprehensiveness and scientific base were critical to fulfilling the project's mandate. Sincere thanks also go to other FNB staff, including Alice Vorosmarti, Kimberly Stitzel, Carrie Holloway, Gail Spears, Sandra Amamoo-Kakra, and Michele Ramsey, all of whom labored over nearly three years of work to complete this document.

And last, but certainly not least, the Food and Nutrition Board wishes to extend special thanks to Sandy Miller, who initially served as chair of the Panel on Macronutrients; Joanne Lupton, who subsequently assumed the role of chair of the panel and continued in that role through the study's completion; and Vernon Young, who served as chair of the DRI Committee since the inception of the overall DRI activity. Professor Young's dedication to this and earlier DRI activities and his uncompromising standards for scientific rigor are most gratefully acknowledged.

Cutberto Garza
Chair, Food and Nutrition Board

Contents

---

*Appendixes A through M (pages 973-1257) are not printed in this book but are on the CD-ROM attached to the inside back cover.

Summary

This is one volume in a series of reports that presents dietary reference values for the intake of nutrients by Americans and Canadians. This report provides Dietary Reference Intakes (DRIs) for energy and the macronutrients carbohydrate, fiber, fat, fatty acids, cholesterol, protein, and amino acids. While the role of ethanol in macronutrient metabolism and energy is briefly discussed in this report, its role in chronic diseases will be reviewed in a future DRI report.

The development of DRIs expands and replaces the series of reports called *Recommended Dietary Allowances* (RDAs) published in the United States and *Recommended Nutrient Intakes* (RNIs) in Canada. A major impetus for the expansion of this review is the growing recognition of the many uses to which RDAs and RNIs have been applied and the growing awareness that many of these uses require the application of statistically valid methods that depend on reference values other than RDAs. This report includes a review of the roles that macronutrients are known to play in traditional deficiency diseases as well as chronic diseases.

The overall project is a comprehensive effort undertaken by the Standing Committee on the Scientific Evaluation of Dietary Reference Intakes of the Food and Nutrition Board, Institute of Medicine, the National Academies, in collaboration with Health Canada (see Appendix B for a description of the overall process and its origins). This study was requested by the Federal Steering Committee for Dietary Reference Intakes, which is coordinated by the Office of Disease Prevention and Health Promotion of the U.S. Department of Health and Human Services, in collaboration with Health Canada.

Major new approaches and findings in this report include the following:

• The establishment of Estimated Energy Requirements (EER) at four levels of energy expenditure (Chapter 5).

• Recommendations for levels of physical activity associated with a normal body mass index range (Chapter 12).

• The establishment of RDAs for dietary carbohydrate (Chapter 6) and protein (Chapter 10).

• The development of the definitions *Dietary Fiber, Functional Fiber,* and *Total Fiber* (Chapter 7).

• The establishment of Adequate Intakes (AI) for *Total Fiber* (Chapter 7).

• The establishment of AIs for linoleic and α-linolenic acids (Chapter 8).

• Acceptable Macronutrient Distribution Ranges as a percent of energy intake for fat, carbohydrate, linoleic and α-linolenic acids, and protein (Chapter 11).

• Research recommendations for information needed to advance the understanding of human energy and macronutrient requirements and the adverse effects associated with intake of higher amounts (Chapter 14).

APPROACH FOR SETTING DIETARY REFERENCE INTAKES

The scientific data used to develop Dietary Reference Intakes (DRIs) have come from observational and experimental studies. Studies published in peer-reviewed journals were the principal source of data. Life stage and gender were considered to the extent possible, but the data did not provide a basis for proposing different requirements for men, for pregnant and nonlactating women, and for nonpregnant and nonlactating women in different age groups for many of the macronutrients. Three of the categories of reference the values—the Estimated Average Requirement (EAR), Recommended Dietary Allowance (RDA), and Estimated Energy Requirement (EER)—are defined by specific criteria of nutrient adequacy; the third, the Tolerable Upper Intake Level (UL), is defined by a specific endpoint of adverse effect, when one is available (see Box S-1). In all cases, data were examined closely to determine whether a functional endpoint could be used as a criterion of adequacy. The quality of studies was examined by considering study design; methods used for measuring intake and indicators of adequacy; and biases, interactions, and confounding factors.

Although the reference values are based on data, the data were often scanty or drawn from studies that had limitations in addressing the various questions that confronted the panel. Therefore, many of the questions raised about the requirements for, and recommended intakes of, these macronutrients cannot be answered fully because of inadequacies in the present database. Apart from studies of overt deficiency diseases, there is a

BOX S-1
Dietary Reference Intakes

Recommended Dietary Allowance (RDA): *the average daily dietary nutrient intake level sufficient to meet the nutrient requirement of nearly all (97 to 98 percent) healthy individuals in a particular life stage and gender group.*

Adequate Intake (AI): *the recommended average daily intake level based on observed or experimentally determined approximations or estimates of nutrient intake by a group (or groups) of apparently healthy people that are assumed to be adequate—used when an RDA cannot be determined.*

Tolerable Upper Intake Level (UL): *the highest average daily nutrient intake level that is likely to pose no risk of adverse health effects to almost all individuals in the general population. As intake increases above the UL, the potential risk of adverse effects may increase.*

Estimated Average Requirement (EAR): *the average daily nutrient intake level estimated to meet the requirement of half the healthy individuals in a particular life stage and gender group.[a]*

[a] In the case of energy, an Estimated Energy Requirement (EER) is provided. The EER is the average dietary energy intake that is predicted to maintain energy balance in a healthy adult of a defined age, gender, weight, height, and level of physical activity consistent with good health. In children and pregnant and lactating women, the EER is taken to include the needs associated with the deposition of tissues or the secretion of milk at rates consistent with good health.

dearth of studies that address specific effects of inadequate intakes on specific indicators of health status, and a research agenda is proposed (see Chapter 14). The reasoning used to establish the values is described for each nutrient in Chapters 5 through 10. While the various recommendations are provided as single-rounded numbers for practical considerations, it is acknowledged that these values imply a precision not fully justified by the underlying data in the case of currently available human studies.

Except for fiber, the scientific evidence related to the prevention of chronic degenerative disease was judged to be too nonspecific to be used as the basis for setting any of the recommended levels of intake for the nutrients. The indicators used in deriving the EARs, and thus the RDAs, are described below.

NUTRIENT FUNCTIONS AND THE INDICATORS
USED TO ESTIMATE REQUIREMENTS

Energy is required to sustain the body's various functions, including respiration, circulation, physical work, and protein synthesis. This energy is supplied by carbohydrates, proteins, fats, and alcohol in the diet. The energy balance of an individual depends on his or her dietary energy intake and energy expenditure. The Estimated Energy Requirement (EER) is defined as the average dietary energy intake that is predicted to maintain energy balance in a healthy adult of a defined age, gender, weight, height, and level of physical activity, consistent with good health (Table S-1). In children and pregnant and lactating women, the EER is taken to include the needs associated with the deposition of tissues or the secretion of milk at rates consistent with good health. While EERs can be estimated for four levels of activity from the equations provided, the *active* physical activity level is recommended to maintain health.

Carbohydrates (sugars and starches) provide energy to cells in the body, particularly the brain, which is a carbohydrate-dependent organ. An Estimated Average Requirement (EAR) for carbohydrate is established based on the average amount of glucose utilized by the brain. The Recommended Dietary Allowance (RDA) for carbohydrate is set at 130 g/d for adults and children (Table S-2). There was insufficient evidence to set a daily intake of sugars or added sugars that individuals should aim for.

Dietary Fiber is defined as nondigestible carbohydrates and lignin that are intrinsic and intact in plants. *Functional Fiber* is defined as isolated, nondigestible carbohydrates that have been shown to have beneficial physiological effects in humans. *Total Fiber* is the sum of *Dietary Fiber* and *Functional Fiber*. Viscous fibers delay the gastric emptying of ingested foods into the small intestine, which can result in a sensation of fullness. This delayed emptying effect also results in reduced postprandial blood glucose concentrations. Viscous fibers can also interfere with the absorption of dietary fat and cholesterol, as well as the enterohepatic recirculation of cholesterol and bile acids, which may result in reduced blood cholesterol concentrations. An Adequate Intake (AI) for *Total Fiber* is set at 38 and 25 g/d for men and women ages 19 to 50, respectively (Table S-3).

Fat is a major source of fuel energy for the body and aids in the absorption of fat-soluble vitamins and other food components such as carotenoids. Because the percent of energy that is consumed as fat can vary greatly while still meeting daily energy needs, neither an AI nor EAR is set for adults (the AI for infants is given in Table S-4). *Saturated fatty acids, monounsaturated fatty acids,* and *cholesterol* are synthesized by the body and have no known beneficial role in preventing chronic diseases, and thus are not required in the diet. Therefore, no AI, EAR, or RDA is set. The *n-6*

TABLE S-1 Criteria and Dietary Reference Intake Values for Energy by Active Individuals by Life Stage Group[a]

Life Stage Group	Criterion	Active PAL EER[b] (kcal/d)	
		Male	Female
0 through 6 mo	Energy expenditure plus energy deposition	570	520 (3 mo)
7 through 12 mo	Energy expenditure plus energy deposition	743	676 (9 mo)
1 through 2 y	Energy expenditure plus energy deposition	1,046	992 (24 mo)
3 through 8 y	Energy expenditure plus energy deposition	1,742	1,642 (6 y)
9 through 13 y	Energy expenditure plus energy deposition	2,279	2,071 (11 y)
14 through 18 y	Energy expenditure plus energy deposition	3,152	2,368 (16 y)
> 18 y	Energy expenditure	3,067[c]	2,403[c] (19 y)
Pregnancy			
14 through 18 y	Adolescent female EER plus change		
1st trimester	in Total Energy Expenditure (TEE)		2,368 (16 y)
2nd trimester	plus pregnancy energy deposition		2,708 (16 y)
3rd trimester			2,820 (16 y)
19 through 50 y	Adult female EER plus change in		
1st trimester	TEE plus pregnancy energy		2,403[c] (19 y)
2nd trimester	deposition		2,743[c] (19 y)
3rd trimester			2,855[c] (19 y)
Lactation			
14 through 18 y	Adolescent female EER plus milk		
1st 6 mo	energy output minus weight loss		2,698 (16 y)
2nd 6 mo			2,768 (16 y)
19 through 50 y	Adult female EER plus milk energy		
1st 6 mo	output minus weight loss		2,733[c] (19 y)
2nd 6 mo			2,803[c] (19 y)

[a] For healthy active Americans and Canadians. Based on the cited age, an active physical activity level, and the reference heights and weights cited in Table 1-1. Individualized EERs can be determined by using the equations in Chapter 5.

[b] PAL = Physical Activity Level, EER = Estimated Energy Requirement. The intake that meets the average energy expenditure of individuals at the reference height, weight, and age (see Table 1-1).

[c] Subtract 10 kcal/d for males and 7 kcal/d for females for each year of age above 19 years.

polyunsaturated fatty acid, linoleic acid, is an essential fatty acid. A deficiency of *n*-6 polyunsaturated fatty acids is characterized by rough and scaly skin, dermatitis, and an elevated eicosatrienoic acid:arachidonic acid (triene:tetraene) ratio. The AI for linoleic acid is based on the median

TABLE S-2 Criteria and Dietary Reference Intake Values for Carbohydrate by Life Stage Group

Life Stage Group	Criterion	EAR[a] (g/d) Male	EAR[a] (g/d) Female	RDA[b] (g/d) Male	RDA[b] (g/d) Female	AI[c] (g/d)
0 through 6 mo	Average content of human milk					60
7 through 12 mo	Average intake from human milk plus complementary foods					95
1 through 3 y	Extrapolation from adult data	100	100	130	130	
4 through 8 y	Extrapolation from adult data	100	100	130	130	
9 through 13 y	Extrapolation from adult data	100	100	130	130	
14 through 18 y	Extrapolation from adult data	100	100	130	130	
> 18 y	Brain glucose utilization	100	100	130	130	
Pregnancy						
14 through 18 y	Adolescent female EAR plus fetal brain glucose utilization		135		175	
19 through 50 y	Adult female EAR plus fetal brain glucose utilization		135		175	
Lactation						
14 through 18 y	Adolescent female EAR plus average human milk content of carbohydrate		160		210	
19 through 50 y	Adult female EAR plus average human milk content of carbohydrate		160		210	

[a] EAR = Estimated Average Requirement. The intake that meets the estimated nutrient needs of half the individuals in a group.

[b] RDA = Recommended Dietary Allowance. The intake that meets the nutrient need of almost all (97–98 percent) individuals in a group.

[c] AI = Adequate Intake: the observed average or experimentally determined intake by a defined population or subgroup that appears to sustain a defined nutritional status, such as growth rate, normal circulating nutrient values, or other functional indicators of health. The AI is used if sufficient scientific evidence is not available to derive an EAR. For healthy infants receiving human milk, the AI is the mean intake. **The AI is not equivalent to an RDA.**

TABLE S-3 Criteria and Dietary Reference Intake Values for *Total Fiber* by Life Stage Group

Life Stage Group	Criterion	AI[a] (g/d) Male	AI[a] (g/d) Female
0 through 6 mo		ND[b]	ND
7 through 12 mo		ND	ND
1 through 3 y	Intake level shown to provide the greatest protection against coronary heart disease (14 g/1,000 kcal) × median energy intake level (kcal/1,000 kcal/d)	19	19
4 through 8 y	Intake level shown to provide the greatest protection against coronary heart disease (14 g/1,000 kcal) × median energy intake level (kcal/1,000 kcal/d)	25	25
9 through 13 y	Intake level shown to provide the greatest protection against coronary heart disease (14 g/1,000 kcal) × median energy intake level (kcal/1,000 kcal/d)	31	26
14 through 18 y		38	26
19 through 30 y	Intake level shown to provide the greatest protection against coronary heart disease (14 g/1,000 kcal) × median energy intake level (kcal/1,000 kcal/d)	38	25
31 through 50 y	Intake level shown to provide the greatest protection against coronary heart disease (14 g/1,000 kcal) × median energy intake level (kcal/1,000 kcal/d)	38	25
51 through 70 y	Intake level shown to provide the greatest protection against coronary heart disease (14 g/1,000 kcal) × median energy intake level (kcal/1,000 kcal/d)	30	21
> 70 y	Intake level shown to provide the greatest protection against coronary heart disease (14 g/1,000 kcal) × median energy intake level (kcal/1,000 kcal/d)	30	21

continued

TABLE S-3 Continued

Life Stage Group	Criterion	AI[a] (g/d)	
		Male	Female
Pregnancy			
14 through 18 y	Intake level shown to provide the greatest protection against coronary heart disease (14 g/1,000 kcal) × median energy intake level (kcal/1,000 kcal/d)		28
19 through 50 y	Intake level shown to provide the greatest protection against coronary heart disease (14 g/1,000 kcal) × median energy intake level (kcal/1,000 kcal/d)		28
Lactation			
14 through 18 y	Intake level shown to provide the greatest protection against coronary heart disease (14 g/1,000 kcal) × median energy intake level (kcal/1,000 kcal/d)		29
19 through 50 y	Intake level shown to provide the greatest protection against coronary heart disease (14 g/1,000 kcal) × median energy intake level (kcal/1,000 kcal/d)		29

[a] AI = Adequate Intake. Based on 14 g/1,000 kcal of required energy. The AI is the observed average or experimentally determined intake by a defined population or subgroup that appears to sustain a defined nutritional status, such as growth rate, normal circulating nutrient values, or other functional indicators of health. The AI is used if sufficient scientific evidence is not available to derive an Estimated Average Requirement (EAR). For healthy infants receiving human milk, the AI is the mean intake. **The AI is not equivalent to a Recommended Dietary Allowance (RDA).**
[b] ND = not determined.

intake of linoleic acid by different life stage and gender groups in the United States, where the presence of n-6 polyunsaturated fatty acid deficiency is nonexistent. The AI for linoleic acid is 17 and 12 g/d for men and women 19 through 50 years of age, respectively (Table S-5). *n-3 Polyunsaturated fatty acids* play an important role as structural membrane lipids, particularly in nerve tissue and the retina of the eye. These fatty acids also modulate the metabolism of n-6 polyunsaturated fatty acids and thereby influence the balance of n-6 and n-3 fatty acid-derived eicosanoids. The AI is based on the median intakes of α-linolenic acid in the United States

TABLE S-4 Criteria and Dietary Reference Intake Values for Total Fat by Life Stage Group

Life Stage Group	Criterion	AI^a (g/d)	
		Male	Female
0 through 6 mo	Average consumption of total fat from human milk	31	31
7 through 12 mo	Average consumption of total fat from human milk and complementary foods	30	30
1 through 3 y		ND^b	ND
4 through 8 y		ND	ND
9 through 13 y		ND	ND
14 through 18 y		ND	ND
> 18 y		ND	ND
Pregnancy		ND	ND
14 through 18 y		ND	ND
19 through 50 y		ND	ND
Lactation		ND	ND
14 through 18 y		ND	ND
19 through 50 y		ND	ND

[a] AI = Adequate Intake: the observed average or experimentally determined intake by a defined population or subgroup that appears to sustain a defined nutritional status, such as growth rate, normal circulating nutrient values, or other functional indicators of health. The AI is used if sufficient scientific evidence is not available to derive an Estimated Average Requirement (EAR). For healthy infants receiving human milk, the AI is the mean intake. **The AI is not equivalent to a Recommended Dietary Allowance (RDA).**
[b] ND = not determined.

where the presence of *n*-3 polyunsaturated fatty acid deficiency is non-existent. The AI for α-linolenic acid is 1.6 and 1.1 g/d for men and women, respectively (Table S-6). Eicosapentaenoic acid and docosahexaenoic acid contribute approximately 10 percent of the total *n*-3 fatty acid intake and therefore this percent contributes toward the AI for α-linolenic acid.

Proteins form the major structural components of all the cells of the body. Along with amino acids, they function as enzymes, membrane carriers, and hormones. The RDA for both men and women is 0.8 g/kg of body weight/d of protein and is based on meta-analysis of nitrogen balance studies (Table S-7). *Amino acids* are dietary components of protein; nine amino acids are considered indispensable and thus dietary sources must be provided. The relative ratio of indispensable amino acids in a food protein and its digestibility determines the quality of the dietary protein (see Table S-8).

TABLE S-5 Criteria and Dietary Reference Intake Values for *n*-6 Polyunsaturated Fatty Acids (Linoleic Acid) by Life Stage Group

Life Stage Group	Criterion	AI (g/d)[a] Male	Female
0 through 6 mo	Average consumption of total *n*-6 fatty acids from human milk	4.4	4.4
7 through 12 mo	Average consumption of total *n*-6 fatty acids from human milk and complementary foods	4.6	4.6
1 through 3 y	Median intake of linoleic acid from CSFII[b]	7	7
4 through 8 y	Median intake of linoleic acid from CSFII	10	10
9 through 13 y	Median intake of linoleic acid from CSFII	12	10
14 through 18 y	Median intake of linoleic acid from CSFII	16	11
19 through 30 y	Median intake of linoleic acid from CSFII	17	12
31 through 50 y	Median intake of linoleic acid from CSFII for 19 to 30 y group	17	12
51 through 70 y	Median intake of linoleic acid from CSFII	14	11
> 70 y	Median intake of linoleic acid from CSFII for 51 through 70 y group	14	11
Pregnancy			
14 through 18 y	Median intake of linoleic acid from CSFII for all pregnant women		13
19 through 50 y	Median intake of linoleic acid from CSFII for all pregnant women		13
Lactation			
14 through 18 y	Median intake of linoleic acid from CSFII for all lactating women		13
19 through 50 y	Median intake of linoleic acid from CSFII for all lactating women		13

[a] AI = Adequate Intake: the observed average or experimentally determined intake by a defined population or subgroup that appears to sustain a defined nutritional status, such as growth rate, normal circulating nutrient values, or other functional indicators of health. The AI is used if sufficient scientific evidence is not available to derive an Estimated Average Requirement (EAR). For healthy infants receiving human milk, the AI is the mean intake. **The AI is not equivalent to a Recommended Dietary Allowance (RDA).**

[b] CSFII = Continuing Survey of Food Intake by Individuals.

TABLE S-6 Criteria and Dietary Reference Intake Values for
n-3 Polyunsaturated Fatty Acids (α-Linolenic Acid) by Life
Stage Group

Life Stage Group	Criterion	AI[a] (g/d) Male	AI[a] (g/d) Female
0 through 6 mo	Average consumption of total *n*-3 fatty acids from human milk	0.5	0.5
7 through 12 mo	Average consumption of total *n*-3 fatty acids from human milk and complementary foods	0.5	0.5
1 through 3 y	Median intake of α-linolenic acid from CSFII[b]	0.7	0.7
4 through 8 y	Median intake of α-linolenic acid from CSFII	0.9	0.9
9 through 13 y	Median intake of α-linolenic acid from CSFII	1.2	1.0
14 through 18 y	Median intake of α-linolenic acid from CSFII	1.6	1.1
19 through 30 y	Highest median intake of α-linolenic acid from CSFII for all adult age groups	1.6	1.1
31 through 50 y	Highest median intake of α-linolenic acid from CSFII for all adult age groups	1.6	1.1
51 through 70 y	Highest median intake of α-linolenic acid from CSFII for all adult age groups	1.6	1.1
> 70 y	Highest median intake of α-linolenic acid from CSFII for all adult age groups	1.6	1.1
Pregnancy			
14 through 18 y	Median intake of α-linolenic acid from CSFII for all pregnant women		1.4
19 through 50 y	Median intake of α-linolenic acid from CSFII for all pregnant women		1.4
Lactation			
14 through 18 y	Median intake of α-linolenic acid from CSFII for all lactating women		1.3
19 through 50 y	Median intake of α-linolenic acid from CSFII for all lactating women		1.3

[a] AI = Adequate Intake: the observed average or experimentally determined intake by a defined population or subgroup that appears to sustain a defined nutritional status, such as growth rate, normal circulating nutrient values, or other functional indicators of health. The AI is used if sufficient scientific evidence is not available to derive an Estimated Average Requirement (EAR). For healthy infants receiving human milk, the AI is the mean intake. **The AI is not equivalent to a Recommended Dietary Allowance (RDA).**
[b] CSFII = Continuing Survey of Food Intake by Individuals.

TABLE S-7 Criteria and Dietary Reference Intake Values for Protein by Life Stage Group

Life Stage Group	Criterion
0 through 6 mo	Average consumption of protein from human milk
7 through 12 mo	Nitrogen equilibrium plus protein deposition
1 through 3 y	Nitrogen equilibrium plus protein deposition
4 through 8 y	Nitrogen equilibrium plus protein deposition
9 through 13 y	Nitrogen equilibrium plus protein deposition
14 through 18 y	Nitrogen equilibrium plus protein deposition
> 18 y	Nitrogen equilibrium
Pregnancy	
14 through 18 y	Nitrogen equilibrium plus protein deposition
19 through 50 y	Nitrogen equilibrium plus protein deposition
Lactation	
14 through 18 y	Nitrogen equilibrium plus milk nitrogen
19 through 50 y	Nitrogen equilibrium plus milk nitrogen

[a] AI = Adequate Intake, RDA = Recommended Dietary Allowance. The AI is the observed average or experimentally determined intake by a defined population or subgroup that appears to sustain a defined nutritional status, such as growth rate, normal circulating nutrient values, or other functional indicators of health. It is used if sufficient scientific evidence is not available to derive an EAR. For healthy infants receiving human milk, the AI is the mean intake. **The AI is not equivalent to an RDA.** The RDA is the intake that meets the nutrient need of almost all (97–98 percent) individuals in a group.

[b] EAR = Estimated Average Requirement. The intake that meets the estimated nutrient needs of half the individuals in a group.

CRITERIA AND PROPOSED VALUES FOR TOLERABLE UPPER INTAKE LEVELS

A risk assessment model is used to derive Tolerable Upper Intake Levels (ULs). The model consists of a systematic series of scientific considerations and judgments. The hallmark of the risk assessment model is the requirement to be explicit in all of the evaluations and judgments made.

There were insufficient data to use the model of risk assessment to set a UL for total fat, monounsaturated fatty acids, n-6 and n-3 polyunsaturated fatty acids, protein, or amino acids. While increased serum low density lipoprotein cholesterol concentrations, and therefore risk of coronary heart disease, may increase at high intakes of saturated fatty acids, *trans* fatty acids, or cholesterol, a UL is not set for these fats because the level at which risk begins to increase is very low and cannot be achieved by usual

AI or RDA for Reference Individual[a] (g/d)		EAR[b] (g/kg/d)		RDA (g/kg/d)		AI (g/kg/d)[c]
Males	Females	Males	Females	Males	Females	
9.1 (AI)	9.1 (AI)					1.52
11.0	11.0	1.0	1.0	1.2	1.2	
13	13	0.87	0.87	1.05	1.05	
19	19	0.76	0.76	0.95	0.95	
34	34	0.76	0.76	0.95	0.95	
52	46	0.73	0.71	0.85	0.85	
56	46	0.66	0.66	0.80	0.80	
	71[c]		0.88		1.1	
	71		0.88		1.1	
	71		1.05		1.3	
	71		1.05		1.3	

[c] The EAR and RDA for pregnancy are only for the second half of pregnancy. For the first half of pregnancy, the protein requirements are the same as those of the non-pregnant woman.

NOTE: Due to a calculation error in the prepublication copy, values are changed for: RDA for reference infants 7 through 12 mo from 13.5 g/d to 11.0 g/d; EAR for infants 7 through 12 mo from 1.1 g/kg/d to 1.0 g/kg/d; RDA for infants 7 through 12 mo from 1.5 g/kg/d to 1.2 g/kg/d; EAR for children 1 through 3 y from 0.88 g/kg/d to 0.87 g/kg/d; RDA for children 1 through 3 y from 1.10 g/kg/d to 1.05 g/kg/d; RDA for lactating women from 1.1 g/kg/d to 1.3 g/kg/d.

diets and still have adequate intakes of all other required nutrients. It is thus recommended that saturated fatty acid, *trans* fatty acid, and cholesterol consumption be as low as possible while consuming a nutritionally adequate diet. Although there were insufficient data to set a UL for added sugars, a maximal intake level of 25 percent or less of energy is suggested to prevent the displacement of foods that are major sources of essential micronutrients (see Chapter 11).

Although a specific UL was not set for any of the macronutrients, the absence of definitive data does not signify that people can tolerate chronic intakes of these substances at high levels. Like all chemical agents, nutrients and other food components can produce adverse effects if intakes are excessive. Therefore, when data are extremely limited or conflicting, extra caution may be warranted in consuming levels significantly above that found in typical food-based diets.

TABLE S-8 FNB/IOM Protein Quality Scoring Pattern (mg/g protein)

Indispensable Amino Acid	Recommended FNB/IOM Pattern[a]
Histidine	18
Isoleucine	25
Leucine	55
Lysine	51
Methionine + cysteine	25
Phenylalanine + tyrosine	47
Threonine	27
Tryptophan	7
Valine	32

[a] Based on Estimated Average Requirements for 1- to 3-year-old children for both indispensable amino acids and total protein.

ACCEPTABLE MACRONUTRIENT DISTRIBUTION RANGES FOR HEALTHY DIETS

Dietary Reference Intakes have been set for carbohydrate, n-6 and n-3 polyunsaturated fatty acids, protein, and amino acids based on controlled studies in which the actual amount of nutrient provided or utilized is known, or based on median intakes from national survey data. A growing body of evidence has shown that macronutrients, particularly fats and carbohydrate, play a role in the risk of chronic diseases.

Although various guidelines have been established that suggest a maximal intake level of fat and fatty acids (e.g., American Heart Association [Krauss et al., 1996], Dietary Guidelines for Americans [USDA/HHS, 2000]), the scientific evidence suggests that individuals can consume moderate levels without risk of adverse health effects, while increased risk may occur with the chronic consumption of diets that are too low or too high in these macronutrients. Much of this evidence is based on clinical endpoints (e.g., risk of coronary heart disease (CHD), diabetes, cancer, and obesity), which are associations rather than distinct endpoints. Furthermore, because there may be factors other than diet that may contribute to chronic diseases, it is not possible to determine a defined level of intake at which chronic diseases may be prevented or may develop.

Based on the evidence to suggest a role in chronic diseases, as well as information to ensure sufficient intakes of essential nutrients, Acceptable Macronutrient Distribution Ranges (AMDR) have been estimated for individuals (see Chapter 11). An AMDR is defined as a range of intakes for a particular energy source that is associated with reduced risk of chronic diseases while providing adequate intakes of essential nutrients. The AMDR is expressed as a percentage of total energy intake because its requirement, in a classical sense, is *not* independent of other energy fuel sources or of the total energy requirement of the individual. Each must be expressed in terms relative to each other. A key feature of each AMDR is that it has a lower and upper boundary, some determined mainly by the lowest or highest value judged to have an expected impact on health. If an individual consumes below or above this range, there is a potential for increasing the risk of chronic diseases shown to affect long-term health, as well as increasing the risk of insufficient intakes of essential nutrients.

When fat intakes are low and carbohydrate intakes are high, intervention studies, with the support of epidemiological studies, demonstrate a reduction in plasma high density lipoprotein (HDL) cholesterol concentration, an increase in the plasma total cholesterol:HDL cholesterol ratio, and an increase in plasma triacylglycerol concentration, all consistent with an increased risk of CHD. Conversely, interventional studies show that when fat intakes are high, many individuals gain additional weight. Weight gain on high fat diets can be detrimental to individuals already susceptible to obesity and will worsen the metabolic consequences of obesity, particularly risk of CHD. Moreover, high fat diets are usually accompanied by increased intakes of saturated fatty acids, which can raise plasma low density lipoprotein cholesterol concentrations and further heighten risk for CHD. Based on the apparent risk for CHD that may occur on both low and high fat diets, and the increased risk for CHD at higher carbohydrate intakes, an AMDR for fat and carbohydrate is estimated to be 20 to 35 and 45 to 65 percent of energy, respectively, for all adults. By consuming fat and carbohydrate within these ranges, the risk for CHD, as well as obesity and diabetes, may be kept at a minimum. Furthermore, these ranges allow for sufficient intakes of essential nutrients, while keeping the intake of saturated fat at moderate levels. To complement these ranges, the AMDR for protein is 10 to 35 percent of energy.

Based on usual median intakes of energy, it is estimated that a lower boundary level of 5 percent of energy will meet the Adequate Intake (AI) for linoleic acid (Chapter 8). An upper boundary for linoleic acid is set at 10 percent of energy for three reasons: (1) individual dietary intakes of linoleic acid in the North American population rarely exceed 10 percent of energy, (2) epidemiological evidence for safety of intakes greater than 10 percent of energy are generally lacking, and (3) high intakes of linoleic acid create a pro-oxidant state that may predispose to several chronic diseases, such as CHD and cancer. Therefore, an AMDR of 5 to 10 percent of energy is suggested for linoleic acid.

The AMDR for α-linolenic acid is set at 0.6 to 1.2 percent of energy. Ten percent of this range can be consumed as eicosapentaenoic acid

(EPA) and/or docosahexaenoic acid (DHA). The lower boundary of the range meets the AI for α-linolenic acid (Chapter 8). The upper boundary corresponds to the highest intakes from foods consumed by individuals in the United States and Canada. A growing body of literature suggests that diets higher in α-linolenic acid, EPA, and DHA may afford some degree of protection against CHD. Because the physiological potency of EPA and DHA is much greater than that for α-linolenic acid, it is not possible to estimate one AMDR for all n-3 fatty acids.

No more than 25 percent of energy from added sugars should be consumed. This maximal intake level is based on ensuring sufficient intakes of essential micronutrients that are, for the most part, present in relatively low amounts in foods and beverages that are major sources of added sugars in North American diets.

USING DIETARY REFERENCE INTAKES TO ASSESS NUTRIENT INTAKES OF GROUPS

Suggested uses of Dietary Reference Intakes (DRIs) appear in Box S-2. The transition from using previously published Recommended Dietary Allowances (RDAs) and Reference Nutrient Intakes (RNIs) to using each of the DRIs appropriately will require time and effort by health professionals and others.

For statistical reasons that are addressed briefly in Chapter 13 and in more detail in the report *Dietary Reference Intakes: Applications in Dietary Assessment* (IOM, 2000), the Estimated Average Requirement (EAR) is the appropriate reference intake to use in assessing the nutrient intake of groups, whereas the RDA is not. When assessing nutrient intakes of groups, it is important to consider the variation in intake in the same individuals from day to day, as well as underreporting. With these considerations, the prevalence of inadequacy for a given nutrient may be estimated by using national survey data and determining the percentage of the population below the EAR (see Chapter 13).

Assuming a normal distribution of requirements, the percentage of surveyed individuals whose intake is less than the EAR equals the percentage of individuals whose diets are considered inadequate based on the criteria of inadequacy chosen to determine the requirement. For example, intake data from the Continuing Survey of Food Intakes by Individuals (1994–1996, 1998), which collected 24-hour diet recalls for 1 or 2 days, indicate that:

• Less than 5 percent of adults at that time consumed dietary carbohydrate at a level less than the EAR.

BOX S-2
Uses of Dietary Reference Intakes for Healthy Individuals and Groups

Type of Use	For an Individual[a]	For a Group[b]
Assessment	**EAR:** use to examine the probability that usual intake is inadequate.	**EAR:** use to estimate the prevalence of inadequate intakes within a group.
	EER[d]**:** use to examine the probability that usual energy intake is inadequate.	**EER:** use to estimate the prevalence of inadequate energy intakes within a group.
	RDA: usual intake at or above this level has a low probability of inadequacy.	**RDA:** do not use to assess intakes of groups.
	AI[c]**:** usual intake at or above this level has a low probability of inadequacy.	**AI**[c]**:** mean usual intake at or above this level implies a low prevalence of inadequate intakes.
	UL: usual intake above this level may place an individual at risk of adverse effects from excessive nutrient intake.	**UL:** use to estimate the percentage of the population at potential risk of adverse effects from excess nutrient intake.
Planning	**RDA:** aim for this intake.	**EAR:** use to plan an intake distribution with a low prevalence of inadequate intakes.
		EER: use to plan an energy intake distribution with a low prevalence of inadequate intakes.
	AI[c]**:** aim for this intake.	**AI**[c]**:** use to plan mean intakes.
	UL: use as a guide to limit intake; chronic intake of higher amounts may increase the potential risk of adverse effects.	**UL:** use to plan intake distributions with a low prevalence of intakes potentially at risk of adverse effects.

RDA = Recommended Dietary Allowance
EER = Estimated Energy Requirement
EAR = Estimated Average Requirement
 AI = Adequate Intake
 UL = Tolerable Upper Level

[a] Evaluation of true status requires clinical, biochemical, and anthropometric data.

[b] Requires statistically valid approximation of distribution of usual intakes.

[c] For the nutrients in this report, AIs are set for infants for all nutrients, and for other age groups for fiber and n-6 and n-3 fatty acids. The AI may be used as a guide for infants as it reflects the average intake from human milk. Infants consuming formulas with the same nutrient composition as human milk are consuming an adequate amount after adjustments are made for differences in bioavailability. When the AI for a nutrient is not based on mean intakes of healthy populations, this assessment is made with less confidence.

[d] The EER may be used as the EAR for these applications.

- Less than 5 percent of children and adults consumed protein at levels less than the EAR.
- Less than 5 percent of adults consumed *Dietary Fiber* at levels greater than the AI.

RESEARCH RECOMMENDATIONS

Four major types of information gaps were noted: (1) a lack of data designed specifically to estimate average requirements for fiber and fat in presumably healthy humans, (2) a lack of data on the needs of macronutrients of infants, children, adolescents, the elderly, and pregnant women, (3) a lack of multidose, long-term studies to determine the role of specific macronutrients in reducing the risk of certain chronic diseases, and (4) a lack of studies designed to detect adverse effects of chronic high intakes of specific macronutrients.

Highest priority is thus given to studies that address the following research topics:

- long-term, dose–response studies to help identify the requirement of individual macronutrients that are essential in the diet (e.g., essential amino acids and *n*-6 and *n*-3 polyunsaturated fats) for all life stage and gender groups. It is recognized that it is not possible to identify a defined intake level of fat for maintaining health and decreasing risk of disease; however, it is recognized that further information is needed to identify acceptable ranges of intake for fat, as well as for protein and carbohydrate that are based on prevention of chronic diseases and maintaining health;
- studies to further understand the beneficial roles of *Dietary* and *Functional Fibers* in human health;
- studies during pregnancy designed to determine protein and energy needs;
- information on the form, frequency, intensity, and duration of exercise and physical activity that is successful in managing body weight in both children and adults;
- long-term studies on the role of glycemic response in preventing chronic diseases, such as diabetes and coronary heart disease, in healthy individuals, and;
- studies to investigate the levels at which adverse effects occur with chronic high intakes of specific macronutrients. For some nutrients, such as saturated fat and cholesterol, biochemical indicators of adverse effects can occur at very low intakes. Thus, more information is needed to ascertain defined levels of intakes at which onset of relevant health risks (e.g., obesity, coronary heart disease, and diabetes) occur.

REFERENCES

IOM (Institute of Medicine). 2000. *Dietary Reference Intakes: Applications in Dietary Assessment.* Washington, DC: National Academy Press.

Krauss RM, Deckelbaum RJ, Ernst N, Fisher E, Howard BV, Knopp RH, Kotchen T, Lichtenstein AH, McGill HC, Pearson TA, Prewitt TE, Stone NJ, Horn LV, Weinberg R. 1996. Dietary guidelines for healthy American adults. A statement for health professionals from the Nutrition Committee, American Heart Association. *Circulation* 94:1795–1800.

USDA/HHS (U.S. Department of Agriculture/Department of Health and Human Services). 2000. *Nutrition and Your Health: Dietary Guidelines for Americans.* Home and Garden Bulletin No. 232. Washington, DC: U.S. Government Printing Office.

1

Introduction to Dietary Reference Intakes

Dietary Reference Intakes (DRIs) comprise a set of reference values for specific nutrients, each category of which has special uses. The development of DRIs expands on the periodic reports called *Recommended Dietary Allowances,* published from 1941 to 1989 by the National Academy of Sciences, and *Recommended Nutrient Intakes,* published by the Canadian government. This comprehensive effort is being undertaken by the Standing Committee on the Scientific Evaluation of Dietary Reference Intakes of the Food and Nutrition Board, Institute of Medicine, the National Academies, in collaboration with Health Canada. See Appendix B for a description of the overall process, its origins, and other relevant issues that developed as a result of this new process.

WHAT ARE DIETARY REFERENCE INTAKES?

The reference values, collectively called the Dietary Reference Intakes (DRIs), include the Estimated Average Requirement (EAR), Recommended Dietary Allowance (RDA), Adequate Intake (AI), and Tolerable Upper Intake Level (UL) (Box 1-1). Establishment of these reference values requires that a criterion of nutritional adequacy be carefully chosen for each nutrient, and that the population for whom these values apply be carefully defined.

A requirement is defined as the lowest continuing intake level of a nutrient that, for a specific indicator of adequacy, will maintain a defined level of nutriture in an individual. The chosen criterion or indicator of nutritional adequacy upon which EARs and AIs are based is identified for each nutrient. The criterion may differ for individuals at different life stages. Particular attention is given throughout this report to the choice

21

BOX 1-1
Dietary Reference Intakes

Recommended Dietary Allowance (RDA): *the average daily dietary nutrient intake level sufficient to meet the nutrient requirement of nearly all (97 to 98 percent) healthy individuals in a particular life stage and gender group.*

Adequate Intake (AI): *the recommended average daily intake level based on observed or experimentally determined approximations or estimates of nutrient intake by a group (or groups) of apparently healthy people that are assumed to be adequate—used when an RDA cannot be determined.*

Tolerable Upper Intake Level (UL): *the highest average daily nutrient intake level that is likely to pose no risk of adverse health effects to almost all individuals in the general population. As intake increases above the UL, the potential risk of adverse effects may increase.*

Estimated Average Requirement (EAR): *the average daily nutrient intake level estimated to meet the requirement of half the healthy individuals in a particular life stage and gender group.*[a]

[a] In the case of energy, an Estimated Energy Requirement (EER) is provided. The EER is the average dietary energy intake that is predicted to maintain energy balance in a healthy adult of a defined age, gender, weight, height, and level of physical activity consistent with good health. In children and pregnant and lactating women, the EER is taken to include the needs associated with the deposition of tissues or the secretion of milk at rates consistent with good health.

---

and justification of the criterion used to establish requirement values and the intake levels beyond which the potential for increased risk of adverse effects may occur.

CATEGORIES OF DIETARY REFERENCE INTAKES

Estimated Average Requirement[1]

The *Estimated Average Requirement* (EAR) is the daily intake value that is estimated to meet the requirement, as defined by the specified indicator

---

[1] The definition of EAR implies a median as opposed to a mean, or average. The median and average would be the same if the distribution of requirements followed a symmetrical distribution and would diverge if a distribution were skewed.

or criterion of adequacy, in half of the apparently healthy individuals in a life stage or gender group (see Figure 1-1). A normal or symmetrical distribution (median and mean are similar) is usually assumed for setting the EAR. At an intake level equal to the EAR, half of a specified group would not have their nutritional needs met. This is equivalent to saying that randomly chosen individuals from the population would have a 50:50 chance of having their requirement met at this intake level. This use follows the precedent set by others who have used the term "Estimated Average Requirement" for reference values similarly derived but meant to be applied to population intakes (COMA, 1991).

The EAR's usefulness as a predictor of an individual's requirement depends on the appropriateness of the choice of the nutritional status indicator or criterion and the type and amount of data available. The general method used to set the EAR is the same for all nutrients. The specific approaches, which are provided in Chapters 5 through 10, differ since each nutrient has its own indicator(s) of adequacy, and different amounts and types of data are available for each.

The EAR serves three major functions: as the basis for the Recommended Dietary Allowance (RDA), as the primary reference point for

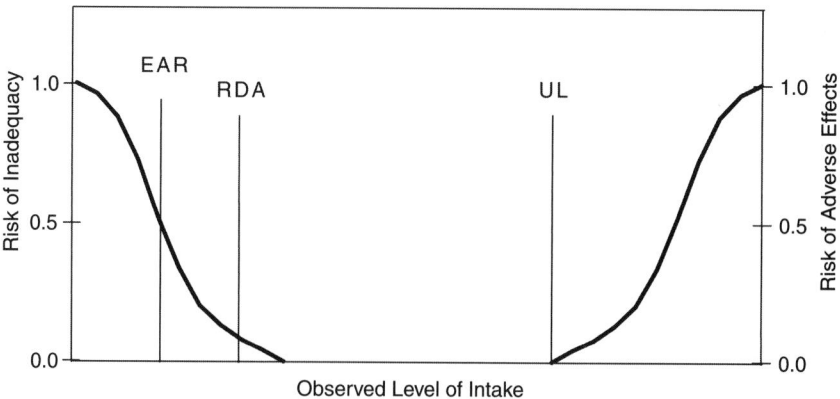

FIGURE 1-1 Dietary Reference Intakes. This figure shows that the Estimated Average Requirement (EAR) is the intake at which the risk of inadequacy is estimated to be 0.5 (50 percent) to an individual. The Recommended Dietary Allowance (RDA) is the intake at which the risk of inadequacy would be very small—only 0.02 to 0.03 (2 to 3 percent). At intakes between the RDA and the Tolerable Upper Intake Level (UL), the risk of inadequacy and of excess are both estimated to be close to 0.0. At intakes above the UL, the potential risk of adverse effects may increase.

assessing the adequacy of estimated nutrient intakes of groups (IOM, 2000a), and, together with estimates of the variance of intake, in planning for the intake of groups (see Chapter 13).

Recommended Dietary Allowance

The *Recommended Dietary Allowance* (RDA) is an estimate of the minimum daily average dietary intake level that meets the nutrient requirements of nearly all (97 to 98 percent) healthy individuals in a particular life stage and gender group (see Figure 1-1). The RDA is intended to be used as a goal for daily intake by individuals as this value estimates an intake level that has a high probability of meeting the requirement of a randomly chosen individual (about 97.5 percent). The process for setting the RDA is described below; it depends on being able to set an EAR and estimating the variance of the requirement itself. Note that if an EAR cannot be set due to limitations of the data available, no RDA will be set.

This approach differs somewhat from that used by the World Health Organization, Food and Agriculture Organization, and International Atomic Energy Agency (WHO/FAO/IAEA) Expert Consultation on *Trace Elements in Human Nutrition and Health* (WHO, 1996). That publication uses the term *basal requirement* to indicate the level of intake needed to prevent pathologically relevant and clinically detectable signs of a dietary inadequacy. The term *normative requirement* indicates the level of intake sufficient to maintain a desirable body store, or reserve. In developing an RDA (and Adequate Intake [AI], see below), emphasis is placed instead on the reasons underlying the choice of the criterion of nutritional adequacy used to establish the requirement. It is not designated as basal or normative.

Method for Setting the RDA When Nutrient Requirements Are Normally Distributed

When the distribution of a requirement among individuals in a group can be assumed to be approximately normal (or symmetrical), and a standard deviation (SD) of requirement ($SD_{requirement}$) can be determined, the EAR can be used to set the RDA as follows:

$$RDA = EAR + 2 \times SD_{requirement}.$$

If data about variability in requirements are insufficient to calculate an $SD_{requirement}$ for that specific nutrient in that population group, but normality or symmetry can be assumed, then a coefficient of variation (CV) of 10 percent will be assumed and the calculation becomes:

$$RDA = EAR + 2 \ (0.1 \times EAR) = 1.2 \times EAR.$$

The assumption of a 10 percent CV is based on extensive data on the variation in basal metabolic rate (FAO/WHO/UNA, 1985; Garby and Lammert, 1984) and the CV of 12.5 percent estimated for the protein requirements in adults (FAO/WHO/UNA, 1985). If there is evidence of greater variation, a larger CV will be used. In all cases, the method used to derive the RDA from the EAR is stated.

Since it is derived from the EAR, the RDA's usefulness as a goal depends on the choice of nutritional status indicator or criterion and the type and amount of data available. Its applicability also depends on the accuracy of the form of the requirement distribution and the estimate of the variance of requirements for the nutrient in the population subgroup for which it is developed.

For many of the macronutrients, there are few direct data on the requirements of children. In this case, EARs and RDAs for children are based on extrapolations from adult values. The methods for extrapolation are described in Chapter 2.

Method for Setting the RDA When Nutrient Requirements Are Not Normally Distributed

If the requirement of a nutrient is not normally distributed but can be transformed to normality, its EAR and RDA can be estimated by transforming the data, calculating the 50th (for the EAR) and the 97.5th percentiles (for the RDA), and transforming these percentiles back into the original units. In this case, the difference between the EAR and RDA cannot be used to obtain an estimate of the variance in the requirement (the SD or CV) since skewing is present.

Where factorial modeling is used to estimate the distribution of a requirement from the distributions of the individual components of the requirement (maintenance and growth), as was done in the case of protein and amino acid recommendations for children, it is necessary to add (termed *convolve*) the individual distributions. Estimating the convolution of two distributions in general is very difficult. However, this is easy to do with normal distributions since the average requirement is simply the sum of the averages of the individual component distributions, and an SD of the combined distribution can be estimated by standard statistical techniques. The 97.5th percentile can then be estimated. (For a discussion of the method, see Appendix B.)

Adequate Intake

If sufficient scientific evidence is not available to calculate an EAR, a reference intake called an *Adequate Intake* (AI) is provided instead of an RDA. The AI is a value based on experimentally determined approximations or estimates of observed median nutrient intakes by a group (or groups) of healthy people. In the judgment of the Standing Committee on the Scientific Evaluation of Dietary Reference Intakes, the AI is expected to meet or exceed the amount needed to maintain a defined nutritional state or criterion of adequacy in essentially all members of a specific, apparently healthy, population. Examples of defined nutritional states include normal growth, maintenance of normal circulating nutrient values, or other aspects of nutritional well-being or general health.

For young infants for whom human milk is the recommended sole source of food for most nutrients for the first 4 to 6 months of life, the AI is based on the daily mean nutrient intake of human milk in healthy, full-term infants who are exclusively fed human milk. The goal may be different for infants consuming infant formula for which the bioavailability of a nutrient may be different from that in human milk. For adults, the AI may be based on data from a single experiment, on estimated dietary intakes in apparently healthy population groups, or on a review of data from different approaches that, when considered alone, do not permit a reasonably confident estimate of an EAR.

Comparison of the Recommended Dietary Allowance and the Adequate Intake

There is much less certainty about an AI value than about an RDA value. Because AIs depend on a greater degree of judgment than is applied in estimating an EAR and subsequently an RDA, an AI may deviate significantly from, and may be numerically higher than, an RDA. For this reason, AIs must be used with greater care than is the case for RDAs. Also, an RDA is usually calculated from an EAR by using a formula that takes into account the expected variation in the requirement for the nutrient.

Both the AI and RDA are to be used as a goal for individual intake. In general, the values are intended to cover the needs of nearly all apparently healthy individuals in a life stage group. (For infants, the AI is the mean intake when infants in the age group are consuming human milk. Larger infants may have greater needs, which they meet by consuming more milk.) The AI for a nutrient is expected to exceed the RDA for that nutrient, and thus it should cover the needs of more than 97 to 98 percent of individuals. The degree to which the AI exceeds the RDA is likely to differ among nutrients and population groups. As with RDAs, AIs for children and adolescents may be extrapolated from adult values if no other usable data are available.

For people who have diseases that increase specific nutrient requirements or who have other special health needs, the RDA and AI each may serve as the basis for adjusting individual recommendations. Qualified health professionals should adapt the recommended intake to cover higher or lower needs.

Tolerable Upper Intake Level

The *Tolerable Upper Intake Level* (UL) is the highest level of daily nutrient intake that is likely to pose no risk of adverse health effects for almost all individuals in the specified life stage group (see Figure 1-1). As intake increases above the UL, there is the potential for an increased risk of adverse effects. The term *tolerable* was chosen to avoid implying a possible beneficial effect. Instead, the term is intended to connote a level of intake that can, with high probability, be tolerated biologically. The UL is not intended to be a recommended level of intake, as there is no established benefit for healthy individuals if they consume a nutrient in amounts exceeding the recommended intake (the RDA or AI).

The UL is based on an evaluation conducted by using the methodology for risk assessment of nutrients (see Chapter 4). The need for setting ULs has arisen as a result of the increased fortification of foods with nutrients and the use of dietary supplements by more people and in larger doses. The UL applies to chronic daily use and is usually based on the total intake of a nutrient from food, water, and supplements if adverse effects have been associated with total intake. However, if adverse effects have been associated with intake from supplements or food fortificants only, the UL is based on nutrient intake from one or both of those sources only, rather than on total intake. As in the case of applying AIs, professionals should avoid very rigid application of ULs and first assess the characteristics of the individual or group of concern (e.g., source of nutrient, physiological state of the individual, length of sustained high intakes, etc.).

For some nutrients, data may not be sufficient for developing a UL. This indicates the need for caution in consuming amounts greater than the recommended intake; it does not mean that high intake poses no potential risk of adverse effects.

The safety of routine, long-term intake above the UL is not well documented. Although members of the general population should be advised not to routinely exceed the UL, intake above the UL may be appropriate for investigation within well-controlled clinical trials. Clinical trials of doses above the UL should not be discouraged as long as subjects participating in these trials have signed informed consent documents regarding possible toxicity and as long as these trials employ appropriate, safe monitoring of trial subjects.

DETERMINATION OF ADEQUACY

Adequacy

In the derivation of Estimated Average Requirements (EARs) or Adequate Intakes (AIs), close attention has been paid to the determination of the most appropriate indicators of adequacy. A key question is, Adequate for what? In many cases, a continuum of benefits may be ascribed to various levels of intake of the same nutrient. One criterion may be deemed the most appropriate to determine the risk that an individual will become deficient in the nutrient, whereas another may relate to reducing the risk of a chronic degenerative disease, such as certain neurodegenerative diseases, cardiovascular disease, cancer, diabetes mellitus, or age-related macular degeneration.

Each EAR and AI is described in terms of the selected criterion or indicator of adequacy. The potential role of the macronutrients in the reduction of disease risk was considered in developing the EARs. With the acquisition of additional data relating intake more directly to chronic disease or disability, more sensitive and reliable indicators or criteria may be validated and thus the criterion for setting the EAR may change.

Role in Health

Unlike other nutrients, energy-yielding macronutrients can be used somewhat interchangeably (up to a point) to meet energy requirements of an individual. In this report, EARs or AIs have been provided for specific macronutrients or components of these classes of macronutrients where the data were adequate to establish a causal relationship between intake and a specific function or chosen criterion of adequacy. However, for the general classes of nutrients and some of their subunits, this was not always possible; the data do not support a specific number, but rather trends between intake and chronic disease identify a range. Given that energy needs vary with individuals, a specific number was not deemed appropriate to serve as the basis for developing diets that would be considered to decrease risk of disease, including chronic diseases, to the fullest extent possible. Thus Acceptable Macronutrient Distribution Ranges (AMDRs) have been established for macronutrients as percentages of total energy intake. These are ranges of macronutrient intakes that are associated with reduced risk of chronic disease, while providing recommended intakes of other essential nutrients.

Because much of this evidence is based on clinical endpoints (e.g., coronary heart disease, diabetes, cancer, and obesity), which point to trends rather than distinct endpoints, and because there may be factors other than diet that may contribute to chronic disease, it is not possible to determine a defined level of intake at which chronic disease may be prevented or may develop. Therefore, an AMDR is not considered to be a Dietary Reference Intake (DRI) that provides a defined intake level. An AMDR is provided to give guidance in dietary planning by taking into account the trends related to decreased risk of disease identified in epidemiological and clinical studies.

AMDRs are expressed as percentages of total energy intake because their requirements, in a classical sense, are *not* independent of each other or of the total energy requirement of the individual. Each must be expressed in terms relative to the others. A key feature of each AMDR is that it has a lower and upper boundary, some determined mainly by the lowest or highest value judged to have an expected impact on health. Above or below these boundaries there is a potential for increasing the risk of chronic diseases shown to effect long-term health. The macronutrients and their role in health are discussed in Chapter 3, as well as in Chapters 5 through 11.

PARAMETERS FOR DIETARY REFERENCE INTAKES

Nutrient Intakes

Each type of Dietary Reference Intake (DRI) refers to the average daily nutrient intake of individuals over time. The amount consumed may vary substantially from day-to-day without ill effects in most cases. Moreover, unless otherwise stated, all values given for Estimated Average Requirements (EARs), Recommended Dietary Allowances (RDAs), Adequate Intakes (AIs), or Acceptable Macronutrient Distribution Ranges (AMDRs) represent the quantity of the nutrient or food component to be supplied by foods from diets similar to those consumed in Canada and the United States. Healthy subgroups of the population often have different requirements, so special attention has been given to the differences due to gender and age, and often separate reference intakes are estimated for specified subgroups.

For some nutrients (e.g., trace elements), a higher intake may be needed for healthy people if the degree of absorption of the nutrient is unusually low on a chronic basis (e.g., because of very high fiber intake). If the primary source of a nutrient is a supplement, a higher or lower percentage may be absorbed and so a smaller or greater intake may be required, or an adverse effect may be demonstrated at a lower level of intake. When this is an issue, it is discussed for the specific nutrient in the section "Special Considerations."

The DRIs apply to the apparently healthy population, and while the RDAs and AIs are levels of intake recommended for individuals, meeting these levels would not necessarily be sufficient for individuals who are already malnourished. People with diseases that result in malabsorption syndrome or who are undergoing treatment such as hemo- or peritoneal dialysis may have increased requirements for some nutrients. Special guidance should be provided for those with greatly increased nutrient needs or for those with decreased needs such as energy due to disability or decreased mobility. Although the RDA or AI may serve as the basis for such guidance, qualified medical and nutrition personnel should make necessary adaptations for specific situations.

Life Stage Groups

The life stage groups described below were chosen while keeping in mind all the nutrients to be reviewed, not only those included in this report. Additional subdivisions within these groups may be added in later reports. If data are too sparse to distinguish differences in requirements by life stage or gender group, the analysis provided in establishing the DRI may be presented for a larger grouping.

Infancy

Infancy covers the period from birth through 12 months of age and is divided into two 6-month intervals. Except for energy, the first 6-month interval was not subdivided further because intake is relatively constant during this time. That is, as infants grow, they ingest more food; however, on a body-weight basis their intake remains nearly the same. During the second 6 months of life, growth velocity slows, and thus daily nutrient needs on a body-weight basis may be less than those during the first 6 months of life.

For protein, amino acids, carbohydrate, fat, and n-6 and n-3 poly-unsaturated fatty acids, the average intake by full-term infants who are born to healthy, well-nourished mothers and exclusively fed human milk has been adopted as the primary basis for deriving the AI during the first 6 months of life. This is the model used for other nutrients as well. The value established is thus not an EAR. The extent to which intake of human milk may result in exceeding the actual requirements of the infant is not known, and ethics of human experimentation preclude testing the levels known to be potentially inadequate. Therefore, the AI, while determined from the average composition of an average volume of milk consumed by this age group, is not an EAR in which only half of the group would be expected to have their needs met.

Using the infant fed human milk as a model is in keeping with the basis for estimating nutrient allowances of infants developed in the last revisions of the RDAs (NRC, 1989) and Recommended Nutrient Intakes (RNIs) (Health Canada, 1990). It also supports the recommendation that exclusive human-milk feeding is the preferred method of feeding for normal, full-term infants for the first 4 to 6 months of life. This recommendation has also been made by the Canadian Paediatric Society (Health Canada, 1990), the American Academy of Pediatrics (AAP, 1997), and in the Food and Nutrition Board report, *Nutrition During Lactation* (IOM, 1991).

In general, for this report, special consideration was not given to possible variations in physiological need during the first month after birth, or to the variations in intake of nutrients from human milk that result from differences in milk volume and nutrient concentration during early lactation. Specific DRIs to meet the needs of formula-fed infants are not proposed in this report. The previously published RDAs and RNIs for infants have led to much misinterpretation of the adequacy of human milk because of a lack of understanding about their derivation for young infants. Although they were based on human-milk composition and volume of intake, the previous RDA and RNI values allowed for lower bioavailability of nutrients from nonhuman milk. However, where warranted, information discussing specific changes in bioavailability or source of nutrients for use in developing formulations is included in the "Special Considerations" section of each chapter.

Ages 0 Through 6 Months. To determine the AI value for infants ages 0 through 6 months, the mean intake of a nutrient was calculated by multiplying the average concentration of the nutrient in human milk produced during the second through sixth month of lactation (derived from consensus values from several reported studies [Atkinson et al., 1995]) by the average volume of milk intake of 0.78 L/d as reported from studies of full-term infants by test weighing (Butte et al., 1984; Chandra, 1984; Hofvander et al., 1982; Neville et al., 1988). Because there is variation in both of these measures, the computed value represents the mean. It is assumed that infants will have adequate access to human milk and that they will consume increased volumes as needed to meet their requirements for maintenance and growth.

Ages 7 Through 12 Months. The reference body-weight method that has been used in previous DRI reports to extrapolate the AI for infants 0 through 6 months to an AI for older infants in the absence of direct data on older infants (IOM, 1997) is not appropriate for dietary fats or carbo-hydrates. This is because the amount of energy required on a body-weight basis is significantly lower during the second 6 months of life, due largely to the slower rate of weight gain/kg of body weight. Therefore, the basis of the AI values derived for this age category for dietary fats and carbo-hydrates was the sum of the specific nutrient provided by 0.6 L/d of human milk, which is the average volume of milk reported from studies in this age category (Heinig et al., 1993), and that provided by the usual intake of complementary weaning foods consumed by infants in this age category (Specker et al., 1997). This approach is in keeping with the current recom-mendations of the Canadian Paediatric Society (Health Canada, 1990), the American Academy of Pediatrics (AAP, 1997), and *Nutrition During Lactation* (IOM, 1991) for continued feeding of human milk to infants through 9 to 12 months of age with appropriate introduction of solid foods.

Toddlers: Ages 1 Through 3 Years

Two points were primary in dividing early childhood into two groups. First, the greater velocity of growth in height during ages 1 through 3 years compared with ages 4 through 5 years provides a biological basis for divid-ing this period of life. Second, because children in the United States and Canada begin to enter the public school system starting at age 4 years, ending this life stage prior to age 4 years seemed appropriate so that food and nutrition policy planners have appropriate targets and cutoffs for use in program planning.

Data are sparse for indicators of nutrient adequacy on which to derive DRIs for these early years of life. In these cases, extrapolation using the methods described in Chapter 2 has been employed.

Early Childhood: Ages 4 Through 8 Years

Major biological changes in velocity of growth and changing endo-crine status occur during ages 4 through 8 or 9 years (the latter depending on onset of puberty in each gender); therefore, the category of 4 through 8 years of age is appropriate. For many nutrients, a reasonable amount of data is available on nutrient intake and various criteria for adequacy (such as nutrient balance measured in children 5 through 7 years of age) that can be used as the basis for the EARs and AIs for this life stage group.

Puberty/Adolescence: Ages 9 Through 13 Years and 14 Through 18 Years

Because current data support younger ages for pubertal development, it was determined that the adolescent age group should begin at 9 years. The mean age of onset of breast development (Tanner Stage 2) for white girls in the United States is 10.0 ± 1.8 (standard deviation) years; this is a physical marker for the beginning of increased estrogen secretion (Herman-Giddens et al., 1997). In African-American girls, onset of breast development is earlier (mean 8.9 years ± 1.9). The reason for the observed racial differences in the age at which girls enter puberty is unknown. The onset of the growth spurt in girls begins before the onset of breast development (Tanner, 1990). The age group of 9 through 13 years allows for this early growth spurt of girls.

For boys, the mean age of initiation of testicular development is 10.5 to 11 years, and their growth spurt begins two years later (Tanner, 1990). Thus, to begin the second age category at 14 years and to have different EARs and AIs for girls and boys for some nutrients at this age seems biologically appropriate. All children continue to grow to some extent until as late as age 20 years; therefore, having these two age categories span the period of 9 through 18 years of age seems justified.

Young Adulthood and Middle-Aged Adults: Ages 19 Through 30 Years and 31 Through 50 Years

The recognition of the possible value of higher nutrient intakes during early adulthood on achieving optimal genetic potential for peak bone mass was the reason for dividing adulthood into ages 19 through 30 years and 31 through 50 years. Moreover, mean energy expenditure decreases during this 30-year period, and needs for nutrients related to energy metabolism may also decrease. For some nutrients, the DRIs may be the same for the two age groups. However, for other nutrients, especially those related to energy metabolism, EARs (and RDAs) are likely to differ for these two age groups.

Adulthood and Older Adults: Ages 51 Through 70 Years and Over 70 Years

The age period of 51 through 70 years spans the active work years for most adults. After age 70, people of the same age increasingly display variability in physiological functioning and physical activity. A comparison of people over age 70 who are the same chronological age may demonstrate as much as a 15- to 20-year age-related difference in level of reserve capacity and functioning. This is demonstrated by age-related declines in nutrient absorption and renal function. Because of the high variability in functional capacity of older adults, the EARs and AIs for this age group may reflect a greater variability in requirements for the older age categories. This variability may be most applicable to nutrients for which requirements are related to energy expenditure.

Pregnancy and Lactation

Recommendations for pregnancy and lactation may be subdivided because of the many physiological changes and changes in nutrient need that occur during these life stages. In setting EARs and AIs for these life stages, however, consideration is given to adaptations to increased nutrient demand, such as increased absorption and greater conservation of many nutrients. Moreover, nutrients may undergo net losses due to physiological mechanisms regardless of the nutrient intake. Thus, for some nutrients, there may not be a basis for EAR values that are different during these life stages than those for nonpregnant or nonlactating women of comparable age.

Reference Heights and Weights

Use of Reference Heights and Weights

Reference heights and weights are useful when more specificity about body size and nutrient requirements are needed than that provided by life stage categories. For example, while the EAR may be developed for the 4- to 8-year-old age group, a small 4-year-old child may be assumed to require less than the EAR for that age group, whereas a large 8-year-old may require more than the EAR. Based on the model for establishing RDAs, however, the RDA (and for that matter, an AI) should meet the needs of both.

In some cases, where data regarding nutrient requirements are reported on a body-weight basis, it is necessary to have reference heights and weights to transform the data for comparison purposes. Frequently, where data regarding adult requirements represent the only available data (e.g., on adverse effects of chronic high intakes for establishing Tolerable Upper Intake Levels [ULs]), extrapolating on the basis of body weight or size becomes a possible option to providing ULs for other age groups. Thus, for this and other reports, when data are not available, the EAR or UL for children or pregnant women may be established by extrapolation from adult values on the basis of body weight.

TABLE 1-1 New Reference Heights and Weights for Children and Adults in the United States

Sex	Age	Previous Median Body Mass Index[a] (kg/m²)	New Median Body Mass Index[b] (kg/m²)	New Median Reference Height,[b] cm (in)	New Reference Weight,[c] kg (lb)
Male, Female	2–6 mo	—	—	62 (24)	6 (13)
	7–12 mo	—	—	71 (28)	9 (20)
	1–3 y	—	—	86 (34)	12 (27)
	4–8 y	15.8	15.3	115 (45)	20 (44)
Male	9–13 y	18.5	17.2	144 (57)	36 (79)
	14–18 y	21.3	20.5	174 (68)	61 (134)
	19–30 y	24.4	22.5	177 (70)	70 (154)
Female	9–13 y	18.3	17.4	144 (57)	37 (81)
	14–18 y	21.3	20.4	163 (64)	54 (119)
	19–30 y	22.8	21.5	163 (64)	57 (126)

[a] Taken from male and female median body mass index and height-for-age data from the Third National Health and Nutrition Examination Survey (NHANES III), 1988–1994; used in earlier DRI reports (IOM, 1997, 1998, 2000a, 2000b, 2001).
[b] Taken from new data on male and female median body mass index and height-for-age data from the Centers for Disease Control and Prevention (CDC)/National Center for Health Statistics (NCHS) Growth Charts (Kuczmarski et al., 2000).
[c] Calculated from CDC/NCHS Growth Charts (Kuczmarski et al., 2000); median body mass index and median height for ages 4 through 19 years.

New Reference Heights and Weights

As is described in Appendix B, the DRI framework is an iterative process that was undertaken in 1994. At that time, reference heights and weights used in the DRI reports for the U.S. and Canadian populations were developed based on data from the Third National Health and Nutrition Examination Survey on body mass index (BMI) for children and young adults (IOM, 1997). With the recent publication of new U.S.-based growth charts for infants and children and the introduction of BMI recommendations for adults (Kuczmarski et al., 2000), reference heights and weights for adults and children have been updated. Besides being more current, these new reference heights and weights are more representative of the U.S. population. Table 1-1 provides these updated values. Appendix B includes information about the reference values that were used in the earlier DRI reports.

SUMMARY

Dietary Reference Intakes (DRIs) is a generic term for a set of nutrient reference values that include the Estimated Average Requirement, Recommended Dietary Allowance, Adequate Intake, and Tolerable Upper Intake Level. In addition, to provide guidance on the appropriate macronutrient distribution thought to decrease risk of disease, including chronic disease, Acceptable Macronutrient Distribution Ranges are established for the macronutrients. These reference values have been developed for life stage and gender groups in a joint U.S. and Canadian activity.

This report—one volume in a series—covers the DRIs for the dietary macronutrients: carbohydrate, fiber, fat, cholesterol, protein, and amino acids. It also provides recommendations for physical activity and energy expenditure to maintain health and decrease risk of disease.

REFERENCES

AAP (American Academy of Pediatrics). 1997. Breastfeeding and the use of human milk. *Pediatrics* 100:1035–1039.

Atkinson SA, Alston-Mills BP, Lonnerdal B, Neville MC, Thompson M. 1995. Major minerals and ionic constituents of human and bovine milk. In: Jensen RJ, ed. *Handbook of Milk Composition.* San Diego, CA: Academic Press. Pp. 593–619.

Butte NF, Garza C, Smith EO, Nichols BL. 1984. Human milk intake and growth in exclusively breast-fed infants. *J Pediatr* 104:187–195.

Chandra RK. 1984. Physical growth of exclusively breast-fed infants. *Nutr Res* 2:275–276.

COMA (Committee on Medical Aspects of Food Policy). 1991. *Dietary Reference Values for Food Energy and Nutrients in the United Kingdom.* Report on Health and Social Subjects, No. 41. London: HMSO.

FAO/WHO/UNA (Food and Agriculture Organization of the United Nations/ World Health Organization/United Nations Association). 1985. *Energy and Protein Requirements. Report of a Joint FAO/WHO/UNA Expert Consultation.* Technical Report Series. No. 724. Geneva: WHO.

Garby L, Lammert O. 1984. Within-subjects between-days-and-weeks variation in energy expenditure at rest. *Hum Nutr Clin Nutr* 38:395–397.

Health Canada. 1990. *Nutrition Recommendations. The Report of the Scientific Review Committee 1990.* Ottawa: Canadian Government Publishing Centre.

Heinig MJ, Nommsen LA, Peerson JM, Lonnerdal B, Dewey KG. 1993. Energy and protein intakes of breast-fed and formula-fed infants during the first year of life and their association with growth velocity: The DARLING Study. *Am J Clin Nutr* 58:152–161.

Herman-Giddens ME, Slora EJ, Wasserman RC, Bourdony CJ, Bhapkar MV, Koch GG, Hasemeier CM. 1997. Secondary sexual characteristics and menses in young girls seen in office practice: A study from the Pediatric Research in Office Settings Network. *Pediatrics* 99:505–512.

Hofvander Y, Hagman U, Hillervik C, Sjolin S. 1982. The amount of milk consumed by 1–3 months old breast- or bottle-fed infants. *Acta Paediatr Scand* 71:953–958.

IOM (Institute of Medicine). 1991. *Nutrition During Lactation.* Washington, DC: National Academy Press.

IOM. 1997. *Dietary Reference Intakes for Calcium, Phosphorus, Magnesium, Vitamin D, and Fluoride.* Washington, DC: National Academy Press.

IOM. 1998. *Dietary Reference Intakes for Thiamin, Riboflavin, Niacin, Vitamin B_6, Folate, Vitamin B_{12}, Pantothenic Acid, Biotin, and Choline.* Washington, DC: National Academy Press.

IOM. 2000a. *Dietary Reference Intakes: Applications in Dietary Assessment.* Washington, DC: National Academy Press.

IOM. 2000b. *Dietary Reference Intakes for Vitamin C, Vitamin E, Selenium, and Carotenoids.* Washington, DC: National Academy Press.

IOM. 2001. *Dietary Reference Intakes for Vitamin A, Vitamin K, Arsenic, Boron, Chromium, Copper, Iodine, Iron, Manganese, Molybdenum, Nickel, Silicon, Vanadium, and Zinc.* Washington, DC: National Academy Press.

Kuczmarski RJ, Ogden CL, Grummer-Strawn LM, Flegal KM, Guo SS, Wei R, Mei Z, Curtin LR, Roche AF, Johnson CL. 2000. CDC growth charts: United States. *Adv Data* 314:1–28.

Neville MC, Keller R, Seacat J, Lutes V, Neifert M, Casey C, Allen J, Archer P. 1988. Studies in human lactation: Milk volumes in lactating women during the onset of lactation and full lactation. *Am J Clin Nutr* 48:1375–1386.

NRC (National Research Council). 1989. *Recommended Dietary Allowances,* 10th ed. Washington, DC: National Academy Press.

Specker BL, Beck A, Kalkwarf H, Ho M. 1997. Randomized trial of varying mineral intake on total body bone mineral accretion during the first year of life. *Pediatrics* 99:E12.

Tanner JM. 1990. *Growth at Adolescence.* Oxford: Oxford University Press.

WHO (World Health Organization). 1996. *Trace Elements in Human Nutrition and Health.* Geneva: WHO.

2

Methods and Approaches Used

OVERVIEW

Carbohydrate, fat, and protein all have two major functions as classes of nutrients: they are required for many normal biological functions, and they serve as energy sources for body fuel. Physical activity can modulate the amount of energy required by the body. Specific subcomponents, such as some amino acids and fatty acids, are required for normal growth and development. Other subcomponents, such as fiber, play a role in decreasing risk of chronic disease.

Carbohydrate and fat are the primary fuel sources. For this purpose they can be largely utilized interchangeably. On the other hand, many metabolic processes favor one source over another. For example, under normal circumstances the brain functions almost exclusively on glucose (Dienel and Hertz, 2001). Conversely, membranes are composed of specific lipids. To a large extent, the body can synthesize de novo the lipids and carbohydrates it needs for these specialized functions. An exception is the requirement for small amounts of carbohydrate and n-6 and n-3 polyunsaturated fatty acids. Otherwise, there are no specific "dietary requirements"[1] for fat or carbohydrate for specific functions. Of course, some mixture of fat and carbohydrate is required as a source of fuel to meet the energy requirements of the body.

In order to apply the Dietary Reference Intake (DRI) process and approach to energy-yielding macronutrients, it was necessary to separate

---

[1]A requirement is defined as the lowest continuing intake level of a nutrient that, for a specific indicator of adequacy, will maintain a defined level of nutriture in an individual.

out the metabolic requirements for specific nutrients for which Estimated Average Requirements (EARs) or Adequate Intakes (AIs) have been derived. It was also necessary to provide quantitative guidance on proportions of specific sources of required energy based on evidence of decreased risk of disease (which, in most cases, is chronic disease).

Thus, a fundamental question to be addressed when reviewing the role of these nutrients in health is, What is the most desirable mix of energy sources that maximizes both health and longevity? Because individuals can live apparently healthy lives for long periods with a wide range of intakes of specific energy nutrients, it is not surprising that this optimal mix of such sources may be difficult to define. There are no clinical trials that compare various energy sources with longevity in humans. For this reason, recommendations about the desirable composition of energy sources must be based on either short-term trials that address specific health or disease endpoints, or surrogate markers (biomarkers) that correlate well with these endpoints. A large number of research studies have been carried out to examine the effects of the composition of energy sources on surrogate markers, and these have provided a basis for making recommendations.

Because diets with specific ratios of carbohydrate to fat, or specific ratios of subcomponents of each, have associations with the risk of various clinical endpoints (e.g., coronary heart disease, diabetes), Acceptable Macronutrient Distribution Ranges (AMDRs) have been proposed that consider these endpoints, as well as the need to consume diets that meet recommended intakes for micronutrients and essential fatty acids. These ranges are given as percentages of total energy intake. For any given diet consumed by an individual, the sum of the contribution to energy intake as a percentage of total intake for carbohydrate, fat, protein, and alcohol must equal 100 percent. The acceptable range of macronutrient intake is a range of intakes for a particular nutrient or class of nutrients that will confer decreased risk of disease and provide the most desirable long-term health benefits to apparently healthy individuals.

TYPES OF DATA USED

A number of disciplines have made key contributions to the evidence linking energy-yielding nutrients to outcomes that may relate to human health. Basic biological research, often involving animal models, provides critical information on mechanisms that may link nutrient consumption to beneficial or adverse health outcomes. While results from animal experiments are generally not used when establishing Dietary Reference Intakes (DRIs), selected animal studies are considered in the absence of human data.

Observational studies in humans include single-case and case-series reports and cross-sectional, cohort, and case-control studies. Experimental studies include randomized and nonrandomized therapeutic or prevention trials and controlled dose–response, balance, turnover, factorial, and depletion–repletion physiological studies. Clinical and epidemiological observational studies play a valuable role in generating hypotheses concerning the health risks and benefits of nutrient intake patterns. Randomized clinical trials in population groups of interest have the potential to provide definitive comparisons between selected nutrient intake patterns and subsequent health-related outcomes. Note, however, that randomized trials attempting to relate diet to disease states also have important limitations, which are elaborated in the discussion below.

Animal Models

Basic research using experimental animals affords considerable advantage in terms of control of nutrient exposures, environmental factors, and even genetics. In contrast, the relevance to free-living humans is often unclear. In addition, dose levels and routes of administration that are practical in animal experiments may differ greatly from those relevant to humans. Nevertheless, due to the opportunity to elaborate specific mechanisms of action, evidence from animal feeding experiments regarding protein, fat, and carbohydrate were included in the evidence reviewed when developing the decisions concerning the ability to specify the DRIs for these nutrients.

Human Feeding Studies

Controlled feeding studies, usually in a confined setting such as a metabolic unit, can yield valuable information on the relationship between nutrient consumption and health-related biomarkers. Much of the understanding of human nutrient requirements to prevent deficiencies is based on studies of this type. Studies in which the subjects are confined allow for close control of intake and activities and complete collection of nutrient or metabolite losses through urine and feces. Recurring sampling of biological materials, such as blood and skin sloughing, is also possible in this type of setting.

Nutrient balance studies measure nutrient status in relation to intake at various levels. Depletion–repletion studies, by contrast, measure nutrient status while subjects are maintained on diets containing marginally low or deficient levels of a nutrient; the deficit is then corrected with measured amounts of the nutrient under study over a period of time. However, these two types of studies have several limitations. Typically, due to resource constraints, they are limited in time to a few days or weeks, so longer-term outcomes cannot be measured with the same level of accuracy. In addition, since subjects are often confined, findings cannot necessarily be generalized to free-living individuals. Finally, the time and expense involved in such studies usually limit the number of subjects and the number of doses or intake levels that can be tested.

In spite of these limitations, feeding studies have played an important role in understanding nutrient needs and metabolism. Such data were considered in the DRI process and were given particular attention in the absence of reliable data to directly relate nutrient intake to disease risk in free-living individuals.

Observational Studies

In comparison to human feeding studies, observational epidemiological studies are frequently of direct relevance to free-living humans, but they lack the controlled setting. Hence, they are useful in establishing evidence of an association between the consumption of a nutrient and disease risk, but are limited in their ability to ascribe a causal relationship. A judgment of causality may be supported by a consistency of association among studies in diverse populations under various conditions, and it may be strengthened by the use of laboratory-based tools to measure exposures and confounding factors, rather than other means of data collection such as personal interviews.

In recent years, rapid advances in laboratory technology have made possible the increased use of biomarkers of exposure, susceptibility, and disease outcome in molecular epidemiological research. For example, one area of great potential in advancing current knowledge of the effects of diet on health is the study of genetic markers of disease susceptibility (especially polymorphisms in genes that encode metabolizing enzymes) in relation to dietary exposures. This development is expected to provide more accurate assessments of the risk associated with different levels of intake of nutrients and other food constituents.

While analytic epidemiological studies (studies that relate exposure to disease outcomes in individuals) have provided convincing evidence of an associative relationship between selected nondietary exposures and disease risk, there are a number of other factors that limit study reliability in research relating nutrient intakes to disease risk (Sempos et al., 1999). First, the variation in nutrient intake may be rather limited in the population selected for study. This feature alone may yield modest relative risk across intake categories in the population, even if the nutrient is an important factor in explaining large disease-rate variations among populations.

A second factor, one that gives rise to particular concerns about confounding, is the human diet's complex mixture of foods and nutrients that include many substances that may be highly correlated. Third, many cohort and case-control studies have relied on self-reports of diet, typically from food records, 24-hour recalls, or diet history questionnaires. Repeated application of such instruments to the same individuals shows considerable variation in nutrient consumption estimates from one time period to another with correlations often in the 0.3 to 0.8 range (Willett et al., 1985).

In addition, there may be systematic bias in nutrient consumption estimates from self-reports, as the reporting of food intakes and portion sizes may depend on individual characteristics such as body mass, ethnicity, and age. For example, some have demonstrated more pronounced and substantial underreporting of total energy consumption among obese persons than among lean persons (Heitmann and Lissner, 1995; Schoeller et al., 1990). Such systematic bias, in conjunction with random measurement error and limited intake range, has the potential to greatly impact analytical epidemiological studies based on self-reported dietary habits. Cohort studies using objective (biomarker) measures of nutrient intake may have an important advantage in the avoidance of systematic bias, though important sources of bias (e.g., confounding) may remain.

Finally, there can be the problem of multicollinearity, in which two independent variables are related to each other, resulting in a low p value for an association with a dependent variable, when in fact each of the independent variables have no relationship to the dependent variable (Sempos et al., 1999).

Randomized Clinical Trials

By randomly allocating subjects to the nutrient exposure level of interest, clinical trials eliminate the confounding that may be introduced in observational studies by self-selection. The unique strength of randomized trials is that, if the sample is large enough, the study groups will be similar not only with respect to those confounding variables known to the investigators, but also to other unknown factors that might be related to risk of the disease. Thus, randomized trials achieve a degree of control of confounding that is simply not possible with any observational design strategy, and thus they allow for the testing of small effects that are beyond the ability of observational studies to detect reliably.

Although randomized controlled trials represent the accepted standard for studies of nutrient consumption in relation to human health, they too possess important limitations. Specifically, individuals agreeing to be randomized may be a select subset of the population of interest, thus limiting the generalization of trial results. For practical reasons, only a small number of nutrients or nutrient combinations at a single intake level are generally studied in a randomized trial (although a few intervention trials to compare specific dietary patterns have been initiated in recent years). In addition, the follow-up period will typically be short relative to the preceding time period of nutrient consumption; the chronicity of intake may be relevant to the health outcomes under study, particularly if chronic disease endpoints are sought. Also, dietary intervention or supplementation trials tend to be costly and logistically difficult, and the maintenance of intervention adherence can be a particular challenge.

Many complexities arise in conducting studies among free-living human populations. The totality of the evidence from observational and intervention studies, appropriately weighted and corroborated by an understanding of the underlying mechanisms of action, must form the basis for conclusions about causal relationships between particular exposures and disease outcomes.

Weighing the Evidence

As a principle, only studies published in peer-reviewed journals have been used in this report. However, raw data or studies published in other scientific journals or readily available reports were considered if they appeared to provide important information not documented elsewhere.

For estimating requirements for energy, doubly labeled water data was collected from various investigators and subject to statistical analysis (see Appendix I). For other nutrients, to the extent possible, original scientific studies have been used to derive the DRIs. On the basis of a thorough review of the scientific literature, clinical, functional, and biochemical indicators of nutritional adequacy and excess were identified for each nutrient.

The quality of the studies was considered in weighing the evidence. The characteristics examined included the study design and the representativeness of the study population; the validity, reliability, and precision of the methods used for measuring intake and indicators of adequacy or excess; the control of biases and confounding factors; and the power of the study to demonstrate a given difference or correlation. Publications solely expressing opinions were not used in setting DRIs. Each assessment acknowledged the inherent reliability of each type of study design as described above, and standard criteria concerning the strength and dose–response and temporal pattern of estimated nutrient–disease or adverse effect associations, the consistency of associations among studies of various types, and the specificity and biological plausibility of the suggested relationships were applied (Hill, 1971). For example, biological plausibility would not be sufficient in the presence of a weak association and lack of evidence that exposure preceded the effect.

Data were examined to determine whether similar estimates of the requirement resulted from the use of different indicators and different types of studies. For a single nutrient, the criterion or indicator of adequacy for setting the Estimated Average Requirement (EAR) may differ from one life stage group to another because the critical function, the risk of a disease, or its biomarker may be different. When very poor or no data were available for a given life stage group, extrapolation was made from the EAR, Adequate Intake (AI), or Tolerable Upper Intake Level (UL) set for another group; explicit and logical assumptions on relative requirements or potential risk of adverse effects were made. Because EARs can be used for multiple purposes, they were established whenever sufficient supporting data were available.

Data Limitations

Although the reference values are based on data, the data were often scanty or drawn from studies that had limitations in addressing the various questions that arose in reviewing the data. Therefore, many of the questions raised about the requirements for, and recommended intakes of, these nutrients cannot be answered fully because of inadequacies in the present database. Apart from studies of overt deficiency diseases, there is a dearth of studies that address specific effects of inadequate intakes on specific indicators of health status, and thus a research agenda is proposed (see Chapter 14). For many of these nutrients, estimated requirements are based on balance, biochemical indicators, and clinical deficiency data because there is little information relating health status indicators to functional sufficiency or insufficiency.

Thus, after careful review and analysis of the evidence, including examination of the extent of congruent findings, scientific judgment was used to determine the basis for establishing the values. The reasoning used in developing the values is described for each nutrient in Chapters 5 through 11.

METHODS TO DETERMINE THE ADEQUATE INTAKE FOR INFANTS

As for other nutrients in previous Dietary Reference Intake (DRI) reports, the Adequate Intake (AI) for young infants (ages 0 through 6 months) is generally estimated to be the average intake by full-term infants who are born to healthy, well-nourished mothers and who are exclusively fed human milk. The extent to which intake of a nutrient from human milk may exceed the actual requirements of infants is not known, and ethics of human experimentation preclude the testing of levels known to be potentially inadequate. Using the infant exclusively fed human milk as a model is in keeping with the basis for earlier recommendations for intake (e.g., Health Canada, 1990; IOM, 1991). It also supports the recommendation that exclusive intake of human milk is the preferred method of feeding for normal, full-term infants for the first 4 to 6 months of life. This recommendation has been made by the Canadian Paediatric Society (Health Canada, 1990), the American Academy of Pediatrics (AAP, 1997), the Institute of Medicine (IOM, 1991), and many other expert groups, even though most infants in the United States no longer receive human milk by the age of 6 months.

In general, this report does not cover possible variations in physiological need during the first month after birth or the variations in intake of nutrients from human milk that result from differences in milk volume and nutrient concentration during early lactation. In keeping with the decision made by the Standing Committee on the Scientific Evaluation of Dietary Reference Intakes, specific DRIs to meet the needs of formula-fed infants have not been proposed in this report. The use of formula introduces a large number of complex issues, one of which is the bioavailability of different forms of the nutrient in different formula types. Where data are available regarding adjustments that should be made for various formulas, they are included in the "Special Considerations" sections of the nutrient chapters.

Ages 0 Through 6 Months

Except for energy, the AI for infants ages 0 through 6 months was based on: (1) the average concentration of the nutrient in human milk from mothers who had been lactating from 2 to 6 months (using consensus values from several reported studies, if possible), and (2) an average volume of milk intake of 0.78 L/d. This volume was reported from studies that used test weighing of full-term infants. In this procedure, the infant is weighed before and after each feeding (Allen et al., 1991; Hofvander et al., 1982; Michaelsen et al., 1994; Neville et al., 1988). Because there is variation in both the composition of milk and the volume consumed, the computed value represents the mean. It is assumed that infants will consume increased volumes of human milk during growth spurts to meet their needs for maintenance, as well as for growth.

Ages 7 Through 12 Months

There is evidence for different nutrient needs for energy, protein, and amino acids during the period of infant growth and gradual weaning to a mixed diet of human milk and solid foods from ages 7 through 12 months. There is little evidence, however, of markedly different needs for carbohydrate, fat, and n-6 and n-3 polyunsaturated fatty acids.

In previous DRI reports, some Estimated Average Requirements (EARs) for this age group were determined by extrapolating down from the EAR for young adults by adjusting for metabolic or total body size and growth. The AI was extrapolated up for infants ages 0 through 6 months by using the same type of adjustment (IOM, 2000). However, for the energy-yielding nutrients, these methods were not appropriate because the amount of energy required per body weight is significantly lower during the second 6 months, due largely to the slower rate of weight gain/kg of body weight.

Instead, the basis of the AIs derived for this age category for carbohydrate, fat, n-6 and n-3 polyunsaturated fatty acids, and protein was the sum of: (1) the content of the nutrient provided by 0.6 L/d of human milk, which is the average volume of milk reported from studies of infants receiving human milk in this age category (Dewey et al., 1984; Heinig et al., 1993), and (2) the content of the nutrient provided by the usual intakes of complementary weaning foods consumed by infants in this age category. Such an approach is in keeping with the current recommendations of the Canadian Paediatric Society (Health Canada, 1990), the American Academy of Pediatrics (AAP, 1997), and the Institute of Medicine (IOM, 1991) for continued feeding of infants with human milk through 9 to 12 months of age with appropriate introduction of solid foods. This method has also been used for some nutrients in previous DRI reports.

The amounts of fat and carbohydrate consumed from complementary foods were determined by using data from the Third National Health and Nutrition Examination Survey. One problem encountered in deriving intake data in infants was the lack of available data on total nutrient intake from a combination of human milk and solid foods in the second 6 months of life. Most intake survey data do not identify the milk source, but the published values indicate that cow milk and cow milk formula were most likely consumed. Thus, it is assumed in deriving the AIs for infants 7 through 12 months of age that complementary food intake is similar in both infants consuming human milk and formula-fed infants.

METHODS TO DETERMINE THE DIETARY REQUIREMENTS FOR CHILDREN AND ADULTS

Setting Estimated Average Requirements for Children and Adults

As described previously, various types of studies can be considered for estimating an average requirement. As discussed in Chapter 1, additional analysis of the data (e.g., transformation of data when nutrient requirements are not normally distributed) may be required. For determining estimated energy requirements using a doubly labeled water database, equations using stepwise multiple linear regressions were generated to predict total energy expenditure based on age, gender, height, and weight.

Extrapolating Data from Adults to Children

When data are lacking to set an Estimated Average Requirement (EAR) or Adequate Intake (AI) for children and adolescents, the EAR or AI can be extrapolated down by scaling requirements to the 0.75 power of body mass (IOM, 2001), which adjusts for metabolic differences demonstrated to be related to body weight, as described by Kleiber (1947) and explored further by West and coworkers (1997). Other approaches include extrapolating down based on the reference body weights, which has been done in developing Tolerable Upper Intake Levels (ULs) for some nutrients (IOM, 1997). Neither of these approaches, however, was used for setting an EAR or AI for the macronutrients under review as adequate data were available to develop Dietary Reference Intakes (DRIs) directly for the younger age groups.

Setting the Recommended Dietary Allowance for Children and Adults

To account for variability in requirements because of growth rates and other factors, a 10 percent coefficient of variation (CV) for the requirement is assumed unless data are available to support another value, as described in Chapter 1. For carbohydrate, protein, and the indispensable amino acids where EARs have been established, the CV was determined to be greater than 10 percent.

Methods to Determine Increased Needs for Pregnancy

It is known that the placenta actively transports certain nutrients from the mother to the fetus against a concentration gradient (Hay, 1994). However, for many nutrients, experimental data that could be used to set an EAR or AI for pregnancy are lacking. In these cases, the potential for increased need for these nutrients during pregnancy is based on theoretical considerations, including obligatory fetal transfer, if data are available, and on increased maternal needs related to increases in energy or protein metabolism, as applicable. Thus, in some cases, the EAR can be determined by the additional weight gained during pregnancy. Carmichael and colleagues (1997) reported that the median weight gain of women who had good pregnancy outcomes was approximately 16 kg. In six studies of U.S. women, no consistent relationship between maternal age and weight gain was observed (IOM, 1990). Therefore, as is the case for protein, 16 kg is added to the reference weight for nonpregnant adolescent girls and women for setting the EAR.

Methods to Determine Increased Needs for Lactation

For the nutrients under study, it is assumed that the total requirement of lactating women equals the requirement for the nonpregnant, nonlactating woman of similar age plus an increment to cover the amount needed for milk production. To allow for inefficiencies in use of certain nutrients, the increment may be greater than the amount of the nutrient contained in the milk produced. Details are provided in each nutrient chapter.

ESTIMATES OF NUTRIENT INTAKE

Reliable and valid methods of food composition analysis are crucial in determining the intake of a nutrient needed to meet a requirement. While data regarding total fat, cholesterol, protein, and amino acid content of various foods have been available for many years, data for individual fatty acids have only recently been available. For nutrients such as energy, fiber, and *trans* fatty acids, analytical methods to determine the content of the nutrient in food have serious limitations.

Methodological Considerations

The quality of nutrient intake data varies widely across studies. The most valid intake data are those collected from the metabolic study protocols in which all food is provided by the researchers, amounts consumed are measured accurately, and the nutrient composition of the food is determined by reliable and valid laboratory analyses. Such protocols are usually possible with only a few subjects. Thus, in many studies, intake data are self-reported (e.g., through 24-hour recalls of food intake, diet records, or food frequency questionnaires).

Potential sources of error in estimating intake from self-reported intake data include over- or underreporting of portion sizes and frequency of intake, omission of foods, and inaccuracies related to the use of food composition tables (IOM, 2000; Lichtman et al., 1992; Mertz et al., 1991). In addition, because a high percentage of the food consumed in the United States and Canada is not prepared from scratch in the home, errors can occur due to a lack of information on how a food was manufactured, prepared, and served. Therefore, the values reported by nationwide surveys or studies that rely on self-reporting are often inaccurate and possibly biased, with a greater tendency to underestimate actual intake (IOM, 2000).

It is well known that energy intake is underreported in national surveys (Cook et al., 2000; Mertz et al., 1991; Schoeller et al., 1990). Estimates of underreporting of energy intake in the Third National Health and Nutrition Examination Survey were 18 percent of the adult men and 28 percent of the adult women participating (Briefel et al., 1997). Underreporters indicated that their fat intake was approximately 30.5 percent calories, whereas "adequate" reporters indicated a fat intake of 35 percent of calories. In addition, alcohol intake, which accounted for approximately 4 percent of the total energy intake in men and 2 percent in women, is thought to be routinely underreported as well (McDowell et al., 1994).

Adjusting for Day-to-Day Variation

Because of day-to-day variation in dietary intakes, the distribution of 1-day (or 2-day) intakes for a group is wider than the distribution of usual intakes, even though the mean of the intakes may be the same (for further elaboration, see Chapter 13). To reduce this problem, statistical adjustments have been developed (NRC, 1986; Nusser et al., 1996) that require at least 2 days of dietary data from a representative subsample of the population of interest. However, no accepted method is available to adjust for the underreporting of intake, which may average as much as 18 to 28 percent for energy (Briefel et al., 1997; Mertz et al., 1991).

DIETARY INTAKES IN THE UNITED STATES AND CANADA

Sources of Dietary Intake Data

The major sources of current dietary intake data for the U.S. population include the Third National Health and Nutrition Examination Survey (NHANES III), which was conducted from 1988 to 1994 by the U.S. Department of Health and Human Services, and the Continuing Survey of Food Intakes by Individuals (CSFII), which was conducted by the U.S. Department of Agriculture (USDA) from 1994 to 1996. NHANES III examined 30,000 individuals aged 2 months and older. A single 24-hour diet recall was collected for all participants. A second recall was collected for a 5 percent nonrandom subsample to allow adjustment of intake estimates for day-to-day variation. The CSFII collected two nonconsecutive 24-hour recalls from approximately 16,000 individuals of all ages. Both surveys used the food composition database developed by USDA to calculate nutrient intakes (Perloff et al., 1990) and were adjusted by the method of Nusser and colleagues (1996).

Appendix D provides the mean and the 1st through 99th percentiles of intake for added sugars and amino acids from NHANES III, adjusted by methods described by the National Research Council (NRC, 1986) and by Feinleib and coworkers (1993) for persons aged 6 years and older. Appendix E provides similar data for energy, carbohydrate, dietary fiber, fat, fatty acids, cholesterol, protein, and alcohol by life stage group from the first phase of the CSFII, adjusted for day-to-day variation by the method of Nusser and colleagues (1996).

Survey data from 1990 to 1997 for several Canadian provinces are available for energy, carbohydrate, fat, saturated fat, and protein intake (Appendix F).

Food Sources

For some nutrients, two types of information are provided about food sources: identification of the foods that are the major contributors of the nutrients to diets in the United States, and the food sources that have the highest content of the nutrient. The determination of foods that are major contributors depends on both nutrient content of a food and the total consumption of the food (amount and frequency). Therefore, a food that has a relatively low concentration of a nutrient might still be a large contributor to total intake if that food is consumed in relatively large amounts.

SUMMARY

General methods for examining and interpreting the evidence for establishing reference intakes for macronutrients are presented in this chapter, with special attention given to infants, children, and pregnant and lactating women. Methodological problems and sources of dietary intake data are also discussed. Relevant details are provided in the nutrient chapters that follow.

REFERENCES

AAP (American Academy of Pediatrics). 1997. Breastfeeding and the use of human milk. *Pediatrics* 100:1035–1039.

Allen JC, Keller RP, Archer P, Neville MC. 1991. Studies in human lactation: Milk composition and daily secretion rates of macronutrients in the first year of lactation. *Am J Clin Nutr* 54:69–80.

Briefel RR, Sempos CT, McDowell MA, Chien S, Alaimo K. 1997. Dietary methods research in the Third National Health and Nutrition Examination Survey: Underreporting of energy intake. *Am J Clin Nutr* 65:1203S–1209S.

Carmichael S, Abrams B, Selvin S. 1997. The pattern of maternal weight gain in women with good pregnancy outcomes. *Am J Public Health* 87:1984–1988.

Cook A, Pryer J, Shetty P. 2000. The problem of accuracy in dietary surveys. Analysis of the over 65 UK National Diet and Nutrition Survey. *J Epidemiol Community Health* 54:611–616.

Dewey KG, Finley DA, Lönnerdal B. 1984. Breast milk volume and composition during late lactation (7–20 months). *J Pediatr Gastroenterol Nutr* 3:713–720.

Dienel GA, Hertz L. 2001. Glucose and lactate metabolism during brain activation. *J Neurosci Res* 66:824–838.

Feinleib M, Rifkind B, Sempos C, Johnson C, Bachorik P, Lippel K, Carroll M, Ingster-Moore L, Murphy R. 1993. Methodological issues in the measurement of cardiovascular risk factors: Within-person variability in selected serum lipid measures—Results from the Third National Health and Nutrition Survey (NHANES III). *Can J Cardiol* 9:87D–88D.

Hay WW. 1994. Placental transport of nutrients to the fetus. *Horm Res* 42:215–222.

Health Canada. 1990. *Nutrition Recommendations. The Report of the Scientific Review Committee 1990*. Ottawa: Canadian Government Publishing Centre.

Heinig MJ, Nommsen LA, Peerson JM, Lonnerdal B, Dewey KG. 1993. Energy and protein intakes of breast-fed and formula-fed infants during the first year of life and their association with growth velocity: The DARLING Study. *Am J Clin Nutr* 58:152–161.

Heitmann BL, Lissner L. 1995. Dietary underreporting by obese individuals—Is it specific or non-specific? *Br Med J* 311:986–989.

Hill AB. 1971. *Principles of Medical Statistics*, 9th ed. New York: Oxford University Press.

Hofvander Y, Hagman U, Hillervik C, Sjolin S. 1982. The amount of milk consumed by 1–3 months old breast- or bottle-fed infants. *Acta Paediatr Scand* 71:953–958.

IOM (Institute of Medicine). 1990. *Nutrition During Pregnancy*. Washington, DC: National Academy Press.

IOM. 1991. *Nutrition During Lactation*. Washington, DC: National Academy Press.

IOM. 1997. *Dietary Reference Intakes for Calcium, Phosphorus, Magnesium, Vitamin D, and Fluoride*. Washington, DC: National Academy Press.

IOM. 2000. *Dietary Reference Intakes: Applications in Dietary Assessment*. Washington, DC: National Academy Press.

IOM. 2001. *Dietary Reference Intakes for Vitamin A, Vitamin K, Arsenic, Boron, Chromium, Copper, Iodine, Iron, Manganese, Molybdenum, Nickel, Silicon, Vanadium, and Zinc*. Washington, DC: National Academy Press.

Kleiber M. 1947. Body size and metabolic rate. *Physiol Rev* 27:511–541.

Lichtman SW, Pisarska K, Berman ER, Pestone M, Dowling H, Offenbacher E, Weisel H, Heshka S, Matthews DE, Heymsfield SB. 1992. Discrepancy between self-reported and actual caloric intake and exercise in obese subjects. *N Engl J Med* 327:1893–1898.

McDowell MA, Briefel RR, Alaimo K, Bischof AM, Caughman CR, Carroll MD, Loria CM, Johnson CL. 1994. Energy and macronutrient intakes of persons ages 2 months and over in the United States: Third National Health and Nutrition Examination Survey, Phase 1, 1988–91. *Adv Data* 255:1–24.

Mertz W, Tsui JC, Judd JT, Reiser S, Hallfrisch J, Morris ER, Steele PD, Lashley E. 1991. What are people really eating? The relation between energy intake derived from estimated diet records and intake determined to maintain body weight. *Am J Clin Nutr* 54:291–295.

Michaelsen KF, Larsen PS, Thomsen BL, Samuelson G. 1994. The Copenhagen Cohort Study on Infant Nutrition and Growth: Breast-milk intake, human milk macronutrient content, and influencing factors. *Am J Clin Nutr* 59:600–611.

Neville MC, Keller R, Seacat J, Lutes V, Neifert M, Casey C, Allen J, Archer P. 1988. Studies in human lactation: Milk volumes in lactating women during the onset of lactation and full lactation. *Am J Clin Nutr* 48:1375–1386.

NRC (National Research Council). 1986. *Nutrient Adequacy: Assessment Using Food Consumption Surveys.* Washington, DC: National Academy Press.

Nusser SM, Carriquiry AL, Dodd KW, Fuller WA. 1996. A semiparametric transformation approach to estimating usual daily intake distributions. *J Am Stat Assoc* 91:1440–1449.

Perloff BP, Rizek RL, Haytowitz DB, Reid PR. 1990. Dietary intake methodology. II. USDA's Nutrient Data Base for Nationwide Dietary Intake Surveys. *J Nutr* 120:1530–1534.

Schoeller DA, Bandini LG, Dietz WH. 1990. Inaccuracies in self-reported intake identified by comparison with the doubly labelled water method. *Can J Physiol Pharmacol* 68:941–949.

Sempos CT, Liu K, Ernst ND. 1999. Food and nutrient exposures: What to consider when evaluating epidemiologic evidence. *Am J Clin Nutr* 69:1330S–1338S.

West GB, Brown JH, Enquist BJ. 1997. A general model for the origin of allometric scaling laws in biology. *Science* 276:122–126.

Willett WC, Sampson L, Stampfer MJ, Rosner B, Bain C, Witschi J, Hennekens CH, Speizer FE. 1985. Reproducibility and validity of a semiquantitative food frequency questionnaire. *Am J Epidemiol* 122:51–65.

3

Relationship of Macronutrients and Physical Activity to Chronic Disease

OVERVIEW

Over the last 40 years, a growing body of evidence has accumulated regarding the relationships among consumption of dietary fat, carbohydrate, protein, and energy and risk of chronic disease. The fact that diets are usually composed of a variety of foods that include varying amounts of carbohydrate, protein, and various fats imposes some limits on the type of research that can be conducted to ascertain causal relationships. The available data regarding the relationships among major chronic diseases that have been linked with consumption of dietary energy and macronutrients (fats, carbohydrates, fiber, and protein), as well as physical inactivity, are discussed below and are reviewed in greater detail in the specific nutrient chapters (Chapters 5 through 11) and the chapter on physical activity (Chapter 12).

CANCER

Diet has long been suspected as a cancer-causing agent. Early studies in animals showed that diet could influence carcinogenesis (Tannenbaum, 1942; Tannenbaum and Silverstone, 1957). Cross-cultural studies that compare incidence rates of specific cancers across populations have found great differences in cancer incidence, and dietary factors, at least in part, have been implicated as causes of these differences (Armstrong and Doll, 1975; Gray et al., 1979; Rose et al., 1986). In addition, observational studies have found strong correlations among dietary components and incidence and mortality rates of cancer (Armstrong and Doll, 1975).

Associations among dietary fat, carbohydrates, and protein and cancer have been hypothesized. Many of these associations, however, have not been supported by clinical and interventional studies in humans.

Increased intakes of energy, total fat, n-6 polyunsaturated fatty acids, cholesterol, sugars, protein, and some amino acids have been thought to increase the risk of various cancers, whereas intakes of n-3 fatty acids, dietary fiber, and physical activity are thought to be protective. The major findings and potential mechanisms for these relationships are discussed below.

Energy

Animal studies suggest that restriction of energy intake may inhibit cell proliferation (Zhu et al., 1999) and tumor growth (Wang et al., 2000). A risk of mortality from cancer has been associated with increased energy intakes during childhood (Frankel et al., 1998; Must and Lipman, 1999). Excess energy intake is a contributing factor to obesity, which is thought to increase the risk of certain cancers (Carroll, 1998). To support this concept, a number of studies have observed a positive association between energy intake during adulthood and risk of cancer (Andersson et al., 1996; Lissner et al., 1992; Lyon et al., 1987), whereas other studies did not find an association (Stemmermann et al., 1985).

Dietary Fat

High intakes of dietary fat have been implicated in the development of certain cancers. Early cross-cultural and case-control studies reported strong associations between total fat intake and breast cancer (Howe et al., 1991; Miller et al., 1978; van't Veer et al., 1990), yet a number of epidemiological studies, most in the last 15 years, have found little or no association (Hunter et al., 1996; Jones et al., 1987; Kushi et al., 1992; van den Brandt et al., 1993; Velie et al., 2000; Willett et al., 1987, 1992). Evidence from epidemiological studies on the relationship between fat intake and colon cancer has been mixed as well (De Stefani et al., 1997b; Giovannucci et al., 1994; Willett et al., 1990). Howe and colleagues (1997) reported no association between fat intake and risk of colorectal cancer from the combined analysis of 13 case-control studies. Epidemiological studies tend to suggest that dietary fat intake is not associated with prostate cancer (Ramon et al., 2000; Veierød et al., 1997b). Giovannucci and coworkers (1993), however, reported a positive association between total fat consumption, primarily animal fat, and risk of advanced prostate cancer. Findings on the association between fat intake and lung cancer have been mixed (De Stefani et al., 1997a; Goodman et al., 1988; Veierød et al., 1997a; Wu et al.,

1994). Numerous mechanisms for the carcinogenic effect of dietary fat have been proposed, including eiconasanoid metabolism, cellular proliferation, and alteration of gene expression (Birt et al., 1999).

Experimental evidence suggests several mechanisms in which n-3 fatty acids may protect against cancer. n-3 Fatty acids, particularly docosahexaenoic acid and eicosapentaenoic acid, have been shown to suppress neoplastic transformation (Takahashi et al., 1992), inhibit cell growth and proliferation (Anti et al., 1992; Calviello et al., 1998; Grammatikos et al., 1994), induce apoptosis (Calviello et al., 1998; Lai et al., 1996), and inhibit angiogenesis (Rose and Connolly, 2000), which may occur by suppressing n-6 fatty acid eicosanoid production. Epidemiological studies have shown an inverse relationship between fish consumption and the risk of breast and colorectal cancer (Caygill and Hill, 1995; Caygill et al., 1996; Kaizer et al., 1989; Sasaki et al., 1993; Willett et al., 1990).

Monounsaturated fatty acids have been reported as being protective against breast, colon, and possibly prostate cancer (Bartsch et al., 1999). However, there is also some epidemiological evidence for a positive association between these fatty acids and breast cancer risk in women with no history of benign breast disease (Velie et al., 2000) and prostate cancer in men (Schuurman et al., 1999). There may be protective effects associated with olive oil (Rose, 1997; Trichopoulou et al., 1995; Willett, 1997); however, these benefits may reflect constituents other than monounsaturated fatty acids.

Dietary Carbohydrate

While the data on sugar intake and cancer are limited and insufficient, several case-control studies have shown an increased risk of colorectal cancer among individuals with high intakes of sugar-rich foods (Benito et al., 1990; Macquart-Moulin et al., 1986, 1987; Tuyns et al., 1988). Additionally, high vegetable and fruit consumption and avoidance of foods containing highly refined sugars were shown to be negatively correlated to the risk of colon cancer (Giovannucci and Willett, 1994).

Dietary Fiber

There is some evidence based on observational and case-control studies that fiber-rich diets are protective against colorectal cancer (Lanza, 1990; Trock et al., 1990). There is also some epidemiological evidence of a protective effect of cereals and cereal fiber against colon carcinogenesis (Hill, 1997). Despite these and other positive findings, a number of important studies (Fuchs et al., 1999; Giovannucci and Willett, 1994) and three recent clinical intervention trials (Alberts et al., 2000; Bonithon-Kopp et al., 2000;

Schatzkin et al., 2000) do not support a protective effect of dietary fiber against colon cancer, and the issue remains to be resolved.

High-fiber diets may also be protective against the development of colonic adenomas (Giovannucci et al., 1992; Hoff et al., 1986; Little et al., 1993; Macquart-Moulin et al., 1987; Neugut et al., 1993). However, not all studies have found a significant association between the dietary intake of total, cereal, or vegetable fiber and colorectal adenomas, although a slight reduction in risk was observed with increasing intake of fruit fiber (Platz et al., 1997).

There are numerous hypotheses as to how fiber might protect against the development of colon cancer. These include the dilution of carcinogens, procarcinogens, and tumor promoters in a bulky stool; a more rapid rate of transit through the colon with high-fiber diets; a reduction in the ratio of secondary bile acids to primary bile acids by acidifying colonic contents; the production of butyrate from the fermentation of dietary fiber by the colonic microflora; and the reduction of ammonia, which is known to be toxic to cells (Harris and Ferguson, 1993; Jacobs, 1986; Klurfeld, 1992; Van Munster and Nagengast, 1993; Visek, 1978).

Fiber has been shown to lower serum estrogen concentrations (Rose et al., 1991), and therefore may have a protective effect against hormone-related cancers. Recent studies have shown a decreased risk of endometrial cancer (Barbone et al., 1993; Goodman et al., 1997), ovarian cancer (Risch et al., 1994; Tzonou et al., 1993), and prostate cancer (Andersson et al., 1996) with high fiber intakes. More research is needed before conclusions can be drawn on these relationships.

Although fiber has the ability to decrease blood estrogen concentrations by a variety of different mechanisms (Rose et al., 1991), it is not yet known whether this action is sufficient to decrease the risk of breast cancer. Half of the epidemiological studies attempting to link low dietary fiber intake to breast cancer have failed to show this relationship (Gerber, 1998). The data on cereal intake and breast cancer risk are considerably stronger than overall fiber intake (Rohan et al., 1993), suggesting that certain cereal foods are protective or that only certain types and stages of breast cancer respond to these interventions.

Physical Activity

Regular exercise, as recommended in this report, has been shown to be negatively correlated with the risk of colon cancer (Colbert et al., 2001; White et al., 1996). This is, in part, due to the reduction in obesity, which is positively related to cancer (Carroll, 1998). In men and women who are physically active, the risk of colon cancer is reduced by 30 to 40 percent compared with those who are sedentary. A plausible mechanism for the effect of physical activity on colon cancer is the shortening of intestinal transit time, thus reducing contact time between intestinal mucosa and carcinogens and mutagens in the diet that are carried in the fecal stream (Batty and Thune, 2000).

Examination of more than 30 epidemiological studies concluded that regular physical activity decreased the risk of breast cancer by 20 to 40 percent (IARC, 2002). However, relatively few studies found a consistent association between physical activity and decreased incidence of endometrial cancer. For prostate cancer, results of about 20 studies were less consistent, with only moderately strong relationships. As endogenous sex steroids have been implicated in the development of breast, endometrial, and prostrate cancers, a plausible explanation for the inverse relationship among physical activity and reproductive organ cancers may involve the effect of exercise on the binding and turnover of sex steroids and glucoregulatory hormones, as well as the overall effect of exercise on body fat (IARC, 2002; Vainio and Bianchini, 2001).

With regard to the possible effect of exercise on other forms of cancer, such as pancreatic cancer (Michaud et al., 2001), exercise may also play a beneficial role by compensating for effects of excess energy intake; by modifying the effects of carcinogens, cocarcinogens, and cancer promoters; or by decreasing body fat and lessening the accumulation of cancer-causing substances in body tissues (Shephard, 1990, 1996). Regular activity may also bolster the immune system (Bruunsgaard et al., 1999; Mazzeo et al., 1998).

HEART DISEASE

The known risk factors for coronary heart disease (CHD) include high serum low density lipoprotein (LDL) cholesterol concentration, low serum high density lipoprotein (HDL) cholesterol concentration, a family history of CHD, hypertension, diabetes mellitus, cigarette smoking, advancing age, and obesity (Castelli, 1996; Hennekens, 1998; Parmley, 1997). There is a positive linear relationship between serum total cholesterol and LDL cholesterol concentrations and risk of CHD or mortality from CHD (Jousilahti et al., 1998; Neaton and Wentworth, 1992; Sorkin et al., 1992; Stamler et al., 1986). A low concentration of HDL cholesterol is positively correlated with risk of CHD, independent of other risk factors (Austin et al., 2000).

High concentrations of serum triacylglycerol may also contribute to CHD (Austin, 1989), but the evidence is less clear. Most studies show a positive relationship between serum triacylglycerol and CHD (Bainton et al., 1992; Carlson and Böttiger, 1972; Gordon et al., 1977; Hulley et al., 1980; Stampfer et al., 1996); however, Gordon and coworkers (1977) found that the statistical significance of this relationship disappears after controlling for total cholesterol, LDL cholesterol, or HDL cholesterol.

The role of diet in the promotion or prevention of heart disease is the subject of considerable research. New studies investigating dietary energy sources and physical activity for their potential to alter some of the risk factors for heart disease are underway (i.e., plasma cholesterol, hypertension, obesity, and diabetes).

Dietary Fat

Increasing the intake of saturated fat can increase serum total cholesterol and LDL cholesterol concentrations (Clarke et al., 1997; Hegsted et al., 1993; Kasim et al., 1993; Krauss and Dreon, 1995; Mensink and Katan, 1992). Furthermore, a meta-analysis of 37 intervention studies showed that a reduction in plasma total cholesterol and LDL cholesterol concentrations was correlated with reductions in percentages of total dietary fat that also included a decrease in saturated fats (Yu-Poth et al., 1999). The correlation between total fat and serum cholesterol concentration is due, in part, to the strong positive association between total fat and saturated fat intake and the weak association between total fat and polyunsaturated fat intake (Masironi, 1970; Stamler, 1979). Furthermore, the impact of saturated fats in increasing LDL cholesterol concentration is twofold greater than the impact of polyunsaturated fats in reducing LDL cholesterol (Hegsted et al., 1993; Mensink and Katan, 1992). This effect, however, is not seen with all saturated fatty acids. While lauric, myristic, and palmitic acids increase cholesterol concentration (Mensink et al., 1994), stearic acid has been shown to have a neutral effect (Bonanome and Grundy, 1988; Denke, 1994; Yu et al., 1995).

Similar to saturated fat, increasing intakes of *trans* fatty acids and cholesterol increase serum total cholesterol and LDL cholesterol concentrations (Ascherio et al., 1999; Clarke et al., 1997; Hegsted, 1986; Howell et al., 1997). Epidemiological studies have generally demonstrated a positive association between *trans* fatty acid intake and increased risk of heart disease (Ascherio et al., 1994, 1996b; Hu et al., 1997; Pietinen et al., 1997; Willett et al., 1993); however, the risk with cholesterol intake has been mixed (Ascherio et al., 1996b; Hu et al., 1997, 1999b; Kushi et al., 1985; Mann et al., 1997; Pietinen et al., 1997). There is wide interindividual variation in serum cholesterol response to dietary cholesterol (Hopkins, 1992), which may be due to genetic factors.

Monounsaturated and polyunsaturated fatty acids decrease serum total cholesterol and LDL cholesterol concentrations (Gardner and Kraemer, 1995). The epidemiological data indicate that monounsaturated fats are either not associated or are positively associated with risk of CHD (Hu et al., 1997; Kromhout and de Lezenne Coulander, 1984; Pietinen et al., 1997). High intakes of n-6 polyunsaturated fats have been associated with the reduced total cholesterol and LDL cholesterol concentrations that are associated with low risk of CHD (Arntzenius et al., 1985; Becker et al., 1983; Sonnenberg et al., 1996). In general, epidemiological studies have demonstrated an inverse association between n-6 polyunsaturated fatty acid intake and risk of CHD (Arntzenius et al., 1985; Gartside and Glueck, 1993).

n-3 Polyunsaturated fatty acids (eicosapentaenoic acid [EPA] and docosahexaenoic acid [DHA]) have been shown to reduce the risk of CHD and stroke by a multitude of mechanisms: by preventing arrhythmias (Billman et al., 1999; Kang and Leaf, 1996; McLennan, 1993), reducing atherosclerosis (von Schacky et al., 1999), decreasing platelet aggregation (Harker et al., 1993), lowering plasma triacylglycerol concentrations (Harris, 1989), decreasing proinflammatory eicosanoids (James et al., 2000), modulating endothelial function (De Caterina et al., 2000), and decreasing blood pressure in hypertensive individuals (Morris et al., 1993). Many epidemiological studies have used fish or fish oil intake as a surrogate for n-3 fatty acid intake because of the high content of EPA and DHA found in fish. A number of these studies have concluded that fish consumption reduced the risk of CHD mortality (Daviglus et al., 1997; Dolecek, 1992; Kromhout et al., 1985, 1995), while others found no association (Albert et al., 1998; Ascherio et al., 1995).

Dietary Carbohydrate

High carbohydrate (low fat) intakes tend to increase plasma triacylglycerol and decrease plasma HDL cholesterol concentrations (Borkman et al., 1991; Brussaard et al., 1982; Marckmann et al., 2000; West et al., 1990; Yost et al., 1998). This effect has been observed especially for increased sugar intake (Mann et al., 1973; Rath et al., 1974; Reiser et al., 1979; Yudkin et al., 1986). Fructose is a better substrate for de novo lipogenesis than glucose or starches (Cohen and Schall, 1988; Reiser and Hallfrisch, 1987), and Parks and Hellerstein (2000) concluded that hypertriacylglycerolemia is more extreme if the carbohydrate content of the diet consists primarily of monosaccharides, particularly fructose.

Dietary Fiber

Evidence supports a protective effect of dietary fiber for CHD, particularly viscous fibers that occur naturally in foods, which reduce total cholesterol and LDL cholesterol concentrations (see Chapter 7). Reduced rates of CHD were observed in individuals consuming high fiber diets (Jacobs et al., 1998; Kushi et al., 1985; Pietinen et al., 1996). These studies used fiber-containing foods; fiber supplements may not have the same effects. The type of fiber is important; oat bran (viscous fiber) significantly reduces total cholesterol, but wheat bran (primarily nonviscous fiber) may not (Behall, 1990). Viscous fibers are thought to lower serum cholesterol concentrations by interfering with absorption and recirculation of bile acids and cholesterol in the intestine and thus decreasing the concentration of circulating cholesterol. These fibers may also work by delaying absorption of fat and carbohydrate, which could result in increased insulin sensitivity (Hallfrisch et al., 1995) and lower triacylglycerol concentrations (Rivellese et al., 1980). Dietary fiber intake has also been shown to be negatively associated with hypertension in men (Ascherio et al., 1992), but not women (Ascherio et al., 1996a). Fiber intake was shown to have an inverse relationship with systolic and diastolic pressures (Ashcerio et al., 1996a).

Dietary Protein

An inverse relationship between protein intake and risk of CHD has been observed (Hu et al., 1999a). High protein intake has been shown to lower blood pressure (Obarzanek et al., 1996), and substitution of carbohydrate with protein resulted in lower LDL cholesterol and triacylglycerol concentrations (Wolfe and Piché, 1999). These results may, however, be confounded by the fact that dietary animal protein and dietary fat tend to be highly correlated. Independent effects of protein on CHD mortality have not been shown (Gordon et al., 1981; Keys et al., 1986). Soy-based protein may reduce serum cholesterol concentrations, but the evidence has been mixed (Anderson et al., 1995; Bakhit et al., 1994; Meinertz et al., 1989; van Raaij et al., 1982).

Physical Activity

Exercise improves and maintains vessel function. An inverse relationship between exercise and CHD mortality has been observed in numerous studies (Arraiz et al., 1992; Kannel et al., 1986; Lindsted et al., 1991; Paffenbarger et al., 1984). Regular exercise increases serum HDL cholesterol, decreases serum triacylglycerol, decreases blood pressure, enhances fibrinolysis, lessens platelet adherence, enhances glucose effectiveness and insulin sensitivity, and decreases risk of cardiac arrhythmias (Araújo-Vilar et al., 1997; Arroll and Beaglehole, 1992; El-Sayed, 1996; Hinkle et al., 1988; Huttunen et al., 1979).

The mechanisms by which exercise serves to mitigate progression of cardiovascular disease (CVD) and coronary artery disease (CAD) are numerous. For instance, patients with CAD who participated in exercise training showed improved endothelium-dependent vasodilatation in epicardial coronary vessels and in resistance vessels (Hambrecht et al., 2000). Thus, exercise serves to maintain conduit function in vessels impacted by CAD. An inverse dose–response relationship between physical activity and physical fitness and CVD mortality has been documented (Arraiz et al., 1992; Blair et al., 1993; Kannel and Sorlie, 1979; Kannel et al., 1986; Lindsted et al., 1991; Paffenbarger et al., 1984).

Activity may also influence CVD indirectly via an influence on lipoprotein metabolism. Vigorous physical activity increases plasma HDL cholesterol, HDL_2, and apolipoprotein A-I and decreases plasma triacylglycerol, very low density lipoprotein, and atherogenic small, dense LDL concentrations (Williams et al., 1986, 1990, 1992; Wood et al., 1988). Gradient gel electrophoresis shows that the protective HDL_{2b} subclass is increased while the HDL_{3b} subclass is decreased through exercise (Williams et al., 1992). The distribution of LDL is shifted toward larger and more buoyant particles of lower density that result in a decrease in the prevalence of the small, dense LDL phenotype among vigorously active men (Williams et al., 1990). Cross-sectional comparisons of high mileage and low mileage runners suggest that the benefits of vigorous exercise on the lipoprotein profile increase linearly with exercise dose through at least 40 mi (64 km)/wk for both HDL cholesterol and triacylglycerol (Williams, 1997). Physical activity prevents the rise in plasma triacylglycerols in individuals who consume high carbohydrate diets (Koutsari et al., 2001).

Many of the exercise-induced changes in lipoproteins may arise from the effects of lipolytic enzymes on lipoprotein size and composition, namely increases in lipoprotein lipase activity and decreases in hepatic lipase activity (Williams et al., 1986). Runners have significantly higher lipoprotein lipase activity in both muscle and adipose tissue (Nikkilä et al., 1978). Weight loss is known to both increase lipoprotein lipase and reduce hepatic lipase (Marniemi et al., 1990; Purnell et al., 2000). This may explain, in part, why increases in HDL cholesterol and HDL_2 mass in sedentary men who begin exercising vigorously are strongly associated with loss of body fat (Williams et al., 1983). Lipoprotein lipase activity may also explain why HDL cholesterol concentrations in sedentary men predict their success at running (Williams et al., 1994). Specifically, the enzyme's activity is positively correlated with HDL cholesterol concentrations and is higher in slow-twitch red muscle fibers. Thus, high HDL concentrations may be a marker for muscle fiber composition that facilitates endurance exercise.

DENTAL CARIES

Sugars play an important role in dental caries development (Walker and Cleaton-Jones, 1992). Sugars provide a favorable environment for bacteria in the mouth, and the presence of these sugars increases the rate and volume of plaque formation (Depaola et al., 1999). However, because development of caries involves other factors such as fluoride intake, oral hygiene, food composition, and frequency of meals and snacks, sugar intake alone is not the only cause of caries.

TYPE 2 DIABETES MELLITUS

Type 2 diabetes mellitus is characterized by a genetic predisposition to the disorder, decreased tissue sensitivity to insulin (insulin resistance), and impaired function of pancreatic β-cells, which control the timely release of insulin (Anderson, 1999). Obesity, physical inactivity, and advancing age are primary risk factors for insulin resistance and development of type 2 diabetes (Barrett-Connor, 1989; Colditz et al., 1990; Helmrich et al., 1991; Manson et al., 1991). Dietary factors have also been suggested as playing a major role in the development of insulin resistance and type 2 diabetes.

Dietary Fat

Intervention studies that have evaluated the effect of the level of fat intake on biochemical risk factors for diabetes have been mixed (Abbott et al., 1989; Borkman et al., 1991; Coulston et al., 1983; Fukagawa et al., 1990; Howard et al., 1991; Jeppesen et al., 1997; Leclerc et al., 1993; Straznicky et al., 1999; Swinburn et al., 1991; Thomsen et al., 1999; Yost et al., 1998). Some epidemiological studies have shown a correlation between higher fat intakes and insulin resistance (Marshall et al., 1991; Mayer-Davis et al., 1997; Parker et al., 1993). It is not clear, however, whether the correlation is due to fat in the diet or to obesity. Obesity, particularly abdominal obesity, is a risk factor for type 2 diabetes (Vessby, 2000). Decreased physical activity is also a significant predictor of higher postprandial insulin concentrations and may confound some studies (Feskens et al., 1994; Parker et al., 1993).

Findings from intervention studies tend to suggest a lack of adverse effect of saturated fat on risk indictors of diabetes in healthy individuals (Fasching et al., 1996; Roche et al., 1998; Thomsen et al., 1999). However, it was recently reported that the consumption of saturated fatty acids can significantly impair insulin sensitivity (Vessby et al., 2001).

Because of the favorable effects of n-3 fatty acids (eicosapentaenoic acid and docosahexaenoic acid) on risk indicators of coronary heart disease, they are often used in patients with lipid disorders. There has been concern about the use of these fatty acids for lipid disorders because many of these patients also have type 2 diabetes. A number of studies have suggested that n-3 polyunsaturated fatty acid intake may have adverse effects in individuals with type 2 diabetes (Glauber et al., 1988; Kasim et al., 1988), requiring increased doses of hypoglycemic agents (Friday et al., 1989; Stacpoole et al., 1989; Zambon et al., 1992).

Dietary Carbohydrate

There is little evidence that total dietary carbohydrate intake is associated with type 2 diabetes (Colditz et al., 1992; Lundgren et al., 1989). There may be an increased risk, however, when the glycemic index of a meal is considered instead of total carbohydrates (Salmerón et al., 1997a, 1997b). Some studies have found that reducing the glycemic index of a meal can result in short-term improved glucose tolerance and insulin sensitivity in healthy individuals (Frost et al., 1998; Jenkins et al., 1988; Liljeberg et al., 1999; Wolever et al., 1988). Additional long-term studies are needed to elucidate the true relationship between glycemic index and the development of type 2 diabetes and to determine its effect on glucose tolerance and insulin.

Dietary Fiber

Certain dietary fibers may attenuate the insulin response and thus be protective against type 2 diabetes. There is good epidemiological evidence for the protective effect of fiber against type 2 diabetes (Colditz et al., 1992; Meyer et al., 2000; Salmerón et al., 1997a, 1997b). Viscous soluble fibers, such as pectin and guar gum, have been found to produce a significant reduction in glycemic response in the majority of studies reviewed by Wolever and Jenkins (1993). It is believed that viscous soluble fibers reduce the glycemic response of food by delaying gastric emptying and therefore delaying the absorption of glucose (Jenkins et al., 1978; Wood et al., 1994).

Physical Activity

Increased levels of physical activity have been found to improve insulin sensitivity in individuals with type 2 diabetes (Horton, 1986; Mayer-Davis et al., 1998; Schneider et al., 1984). Physical inactivity was found to be associated with increased incidence of type 2 diabetes in cross-sectional (King et al., 1984; Taylor et al., 1983), cohort (Helmrich et al., 1991; Manson et al., 1991, 1992), and longitudinal training studies (Tuomilehto et al., 2001). Short- and long-term effects of physical activity on glucose tolerance, insulin action, and muscle glucose uptake show that contracting muscle has an "insulin-like" effect on promoting glucose uptake and metabolism (Bergman et al., 1999; Horton, 1991; Richter et al., 1981). This synergistic effect of contractions on insulin action is thought to increase insulin action and decrease circulating glucose and insulin concentrations. Further, by increasing muscle mass, decreasing total and abdominal obesity (Björntorp et al., 1979; Després et al., 1988), and diverting dietary carbohydrate to muscle for oxidation and glycogen repletion (Brooks et al., 2000), physical activity reduces the potential for energy intakes exceeding expenditures, leading to fat accumulation. Physical activity can reduce the risk of type 2 diabetes (Diabetes Prevention Program Research Group, 2002; Tuomilehto et al., 2001), and can also reduce total and abdominal obesity, both of which are risk factors for type 2 diabetes (Vessby, 2000).

OBESITY

Obesity results from an imbalance between energy intake and energy expenditure. The health risks associated with obesity include increased mortality, hypertension, cardiovascular disease, diabetes mellitus, gallbladder disease, some cancers, and changes in endocrine function and metabolism (NHLBI/NIDDK, 1998). The risk factors for becoming obese are not entirely understood but are thought to include genetics, food intake, physical inactivity, and some rare metabolic disorders (NHLBI/NIDDK, 1998).

Dietary Fat

The available data on whether diets high in total fat increase the risk for obesity are conflicting and are complicated by underreporting of food intake, notably fat intake (Bray and Popkin, 1998; Lissner and Heitmann, 1995; Lissner et al., 2000; Willett, 1998). Intervention studies have shown that high-fat diets, as compared with low-fat diets with equivalent energy intake, are not intrinsically fattening (Davy et al., 2001), whereas cross-cultural, animal, and some human studies have provided support for the theory that diets with a high percentage of fat increase the risk of obesity (Astrup et al., 1997; Lissner and Heitmann, 1995; West and York, 1998). Other studies have shown that as the proportion of fat in the diet increases, so does energy intake (Kendall et al., 1991; Lissner et al., 1987; Stubbs et al., 1995). Because energy density was not kept separate from fat content in these studies, recent investigators have questioned the conclusions of these studies and have found differing results. Further studies have shown that fat content does not affect energy intake (Saltzman et al., 1997; Stubbs et al., 1996; van Stratum et al., 1978), and that energy density has an effect on energy intake independent of the fat content of the diet (Bell et al., 1998).

Dietary Carbohydrate

A negative correlation between total sugars intake and body mass index has been reported in adults (Dreon et al., 1988; Dunnigan et al., 1970; Fehily et al., 1984; Gibson, 1993, 1996b; Miller et al., 1990). Increased added sugars intakes have been shown to result in increased energy intakes of children and adults (see Chapter 6) (Bowman, 1999; Gibson, 1996a, 1997; Lewis et al., 1992). In spite of this, a negative correlation between added sugars intake and body mass index has been observed in children (Bolton-Smith and Woodward, 1994; Gibson, 1996a; Lewis et al., 1992). Published reports disagree about whether a direct link exists between the trend toward higher intakes of sugars and increased rates of obesity. Any association between added sugars intake and body mass index is, in all likelihood, masked by the pervasive and serious problem of underreporting, which is more prevalent and severe among the obese population. In addition, foods and beverages high in added sugars are more likely to be underreported compared to other foods that may be perceived as "healthy" (Johnson, 2000).

Dietary Fiber

Consumption of soluble fibers, which are low in energy, delays gastric emptying (Roberfroid, 1993), which in turn can cause an extended feeling of fullness and therefore satiety (Bergmann et al., 1992). A number of intervention studies suggest that diets high in fiber may assist in weight loss (Birketvedt et al., 2000; Eliasson et al., 1992; Rigaud et al., 1990; Rössner et al., 1987; Ryttig et al., 1989), although other studies have not found this effect (Astrup et al., 1990; Baron et al., 1986). Thus, the evidence to support a role of fiber in the prevention of obesity is unclear at this time.

Physical Activity

Energy expenditure by physical activity (see Chapters 5 and 12) varies considerably between individuals, affecting the energy balance and the body composition by which energy balance and weight maintenance are achieved (Ballor and Keesey, 1991; Williamson et al., 1993). Indeed, physical inactivity is a major risk factor for development of obesity in children and adults (Astrup, 1999; Goran, 2001). In one study, increasing the level of physical activity in obese individuals appeared to have no effect on food intake, whereas in normal-weight individuals an increase in activity was coupled with an increase in food intake (Pi-Sunyer and Woo, 1985).

SKELETAL HEALTH

Physical activity has a beneficial effect on bone health in individuals of all ages (Anderson, 2000; French et al., 2000; Hurley and Roth, 2000; Khan et al., 2000; Layne and Nelson, 1999; Madsen et al., 1998). Physical activity increases bone mass in children and adolescents and maintains bone mass in adults (French et al., 2000; Khan et al., 2000). In elderly individuals, bone mineral density has been found to be higher in those who exercise than in those who do not (Hurley and Roth, 2000). The same is true for young athletes compared to nonathletes (Madsen et al., 1998). Physical activity results in muscle strength, coordination, and flexibility that may benefit elderly individuals by preventing falls and fractures.

SUMMARY

Many causal relationships among over- or underconsumption of macronutrients, physical inactivity, and chronic disease have been proposed. When the diet is modified for one energy-yielding nutrient, it invariably changes the intake of other nutrients, which makes it extremely difficult to have adequate substantiating evidence for providing clear and specific nutritional guidance. Acceptable Macronutrient Distribution Ranges can be estimated, however, by considering risk of chronic disease, as well as in the context of consuming adequate amounts of essential macronutrients and micronutrients. This information is provided in detail in Chapter 11.

REFERENCES

Abbott WGH, Boyce VL, Grundy SM, Howard BV. 1989. Effects of replacing saturated fat with complex carbohydrate in diets of subjects with NIDDM. *Diabetes Care* 12:102–107.

Albert CM, Hennekens CH, O'Donnell CJ, Ajani UA, Carey VJ, Willett WC, Ruskin JN, Manson JE. 1998. Fish consumption and risk of sudden cardiac death. *J Am Med Assoc* 279:23–28.

Alberts DS, Martínes ME, Roe DJ, Guillén-Rodríguez JM, Marshall JR, van Leeuwen JB, Reid ME, Ritenbaugh C, Vargas PA, Bhattacharyya AB, Earnest DL, Sampliner RE. 2000. Lack of effect of a high-fiber cereal supplement on the recurrence of colorectal adenomas. *N Engl J Med* 342:1156–1162.

Anderson JJB. 2000. The important role of physical activity in skeletal development: How exercise may counter low calcium intake. *Am J Clin Nutr* 71:1384–1386.

Anderson JW. 1999. Nutritional management of diabetes mellitus. In: Shils ME, Olson JA, Shike M, Ross AC, eds. *Modern Nutrition in Health and Disease,* 9th ed. Baltimore, MD: Williams and Wilkins. Pp. 1365–1394.

Anderson JW, Johnstone BM, Cook-Newell ME. 1995. Meta-analysis of the effects of soy protein intake on serum lipids. *N Engl J Med* 333:276–282.

Andersson S-O, Wolk A, Bergström R, Giovannucci E, Lindgren C, Baron J, Adami H-O. 1996. Energy, nutrient intake and prostate cancer risk: A population-based case-control study in Sweden. *Int J Cancer* 68:716–722.

Anti M, Marra G, Armelao F, Bartoli GM, Ficarelli R, Percesepe A, De Vitis I, Maria G, Sofo L, Rapaccini GL. 1992. Effect of omega-3 fatty acids on rectal mucosal cell proliferation in subjects at risk for colon cancer. *Gastroenterology* 103:883–891.

Araújo-Vilar D, Osifo E, Kirk M, García-Estévez DA, Cabezas-Cerrato J, Hockaday TDR. 1997. Influence of moderate physical exercise on insulin-mediated and non-insulin-mediated glucose uptake in healthy subjects. *Metabolism* 46:203–209.

Armstrong B, Doll R. 1975. Environmental factors and cancer incidence and mortality in different countries, with special reference to dietary practices. *Int J Cancer* 15:617–631.

Arntzenius AC, Kromhout D, Barth JD, Reiber JHC, Bruschke AVG, Buis B, van Gent CM, Kempen-Voogd N, Strikwerda S, van der Velde EA. 1985. Diet, lipoproteins, and the progression of coronary atherosclerosis. The Leiden Intervention Trial. *N Engl J Med* 312:805–811.

Arraiz GA, Wigle DT, Mao Y. 1992. Risk assessment of physical activity and physical fitness in the Canada Health Survey Mortality Follow-up Study. *J Clin Epidemiol* 45:419–428.

Arroll B, Beaglehole R. 1992. Does physical activity lower blood pressure? A review of the clinical trials. *J Clin Epidemiol* 45:439–447.

Ascherio A, Rimm EB, Giovannucci EL, Colditz GA, Rosner B, Willett WC, Sacks F, Stampfer MJ. 1992. A prospective study of nutritional factors and hypertension among US men. *Circulation* 86:1475–1484.

Ascherio A, Hennekens CH, Buring JE, Master C, Stampfer MJ, Willett WC. 1994. *Trans*-fatty acids intake and risk of myocardial infarction. *Circulation* 89:94–101.

Ascherio A, Rimm EB, Stampfer MJ, Giovannucci EL, Willett WC. 1995. Dietary intake of marine *n*-3 fatty acids, fish intake, and the risk of coronary disease among men. *N Engl J Med* 332:977–982.

Ascherio A, Hennekens C, Willett WC, Sacks F, Rosner B, Manson J, Witteman J, Stampfer MJ. 1996a. Prospective study of nutritional factors, blood pressure, and hypertension among US women. *Hypertension* 27:1065–1072.

Ascherio A, Rimm EB, Giovannucci EL, Spiegelman D, Stampfer M, Willett WC. 1996b. Dietary fat and risk of coronary heart disease in men: Cohort follow up study in the United States. *Br Med J* 313:84–90.

Ascherio A, Katan MB, Zock PL, Stampfer MJ, Willett WC. 1999. Trans fatty acids and coronary heart disease. *N Engl J Med* 340:1994–1998.

Astrup A. 1999. Macronutrient balances and obesity: The role of diet and physical activity. *Public Health Nutr* 2:341–347.

Astrup A, Vrist E, Quaade F. 1990. Dietary fibre added to very low calorie diet reduces hunger and alleviates constipation. *Int J Obes* 14:105–112.

Astrup A, Toubro S, Raben A, Skov AR. 1997. The role of low-fat diets and fat substitutes in body weight management: What have we learned from clinical studies? *J Am Diet Assoc* 97:S82–S87.

Austin MA. 1989. Plasma triglyceride as a risk factor for coronary heart disease. The epidemiologic evidence and beyond. *Am J Epidemiol* 129:249–259.

Austin MA, Rodriguez BL, McKnight B, McNeely MJ, Edwards KL, Curb DJ, Sharp DS. 2000. Low-density lipoprotein particle size, triglycerides, and high-density lipoprotein cholesterol as risk factors for coronary heart disease in older Japanese-American men. *Am J Cardiol* 86:412–416.

Bainton D, Miller NE, Bolton CH, Yarnell JWG, Sweetnam PM, Baker IA, Lewis B, Elwood PC. 1992. Plasma triglyceride and high density lipoprotein cholesterol as predictors of ischaemic heart disease in British men. The Caerphilly and Speedwell Collaborative Heart Disease Studies. *Br Heart J* 68:60–66.

Bakhit RM, Klein BP, Essex-Sorlie D, Ham JO, Erdman JW, Potter SM. 1994. Intake of 25 g of soybean protein with or without soybean fiber alters plasma lipids in men with elevated cholesterol concentrations. *J Nutr* 124:213–222.

Ballor DL, Keesey RE. 1991. A meta-analysis of the factors affecting exercise-induced changes in body mass, fat mass and fat-free mass in males and females. *Int J Obes* 15:717–726.

Barbone F, Austin H, Partridge EE. 1993. Diet and endometrial cancer: A case-control study. *Am J Epidemiol* 137:393–403.

Baron JA, Schori A, Crow B, Carter R, Mann JI. 1986. A randomized controlled trial of low carbohydrate and low fat/high fiber diets for weight loss. *Am J Public Health* 76:1293–1296.

Barrett-Connor E. 1989. Epidemiology, obesity, and non-insulin-dependent diabetes mellitus. *Epidemiol Rev* 11:172–181.

Bartsch H, Nair J, Owen RW. 1999. Dietary polyunsaturated fatty acids and cancers of the breast and colorectum: Emerging evidence for their role as risk modifiers. *Carcinogenesis* 20:2209–2218.

Batty D, Thune I. 2000. Does physical activity prevent cancer? Evidence suggests protection against colon cancer and probably breast cancer. *Br Med J* 321:1424–1425.

Becker N, Illingworth R, Alaupovic P, Connor WE, Sundberg EE. 1983. Effects of saturated, monounsaturated, and ω-6 polyunsaturated fatty acids on plasma lipids, lipoproteins, and apoproteins in humans. *Am J Clin Nutr* 37:355–360.

Behall KM. 1990. Effect of soluble fibers on plasma lipids, glucose tolerance and mineral balance. *Adv Exp Med Biol* 270:7–16.

Bell EA, Castellanos VH, Pelkman CL, Thorwart ML, Rolls BJ. 1998. Energy density of foods affects energy intake in normal-weight women. *Am J Clin Nutr* 67:412–420.

Benito R, Obrador A, Stiggelbout A, Bosch FX, Mulet M, Muñoz N, Kaldor J. 1990. A population-based case-control study of colorectal cancer in Majorca. I. Dietary factors. *Int J Cancer* 45:69–76.

Bergman BC, Butterfield GE, Wolfel EE, Lopaschuk GD, Casazza GA, Horning MA, Brooks GA. 1999. Muscle net glucose uptake and glucose kinetics after endurance training in men. *Am J Physiol* 277:E81–E92.

Bergmann JF, Chassany O, Petit A, Triki R, Caulin C, Segrestaa JM. 1992. Correlation between echographic gastric emptying and appetite: Influence of psyllium. *Gut* 33:1042–1043.

Billman GE, Kang JX, Leaf A. 1999. Prevention of sudden cardiac death by dietary pure ω-3 polyunsaturated fatty acids in dogs. *Circulation* 99:2452–2457.

Birketvedt GS, Aaseth J, Florholmen JR, Ryttig K. 2000. Long term effect of fibre supplement and reduced energy intake on body weight and blood lipids in overweight subjects. *Acta Medica (Hradec Králové)* 43:129–132.

Birt DF, Shull JD, Yaktine AL. 1999. Chemoprevention of cancer. In: Shils ME, Olson JA, Shike M, Ross AC, eds. *Modern Nutrition in Health and Disease*, 9th ed. Baltimore, MD: Williams and Wilkins. Pp. 1263–1295.

Björntorp P, Sjöström L, Sullivan L. 1979. The role of physical exercise in the management of obesity. In: Munro JF, ed. *The Treatment of Obesity*. Baltimore, MD: University Park Press. Pp. 123–138.

Blair SN, Kohl HW, Barlow CE. 1993. Physical activity, physical fitness, and all-cause mortality in women: Do women need to be active? *J Am Coll Nutr* 12:368–371.

Bolton-Smith C, Woodward M. 1994. Dietary composition and fat to sugar ratios in relation to obesity. *Int J Obes Relat Metab Disord* 18:820–828.

Bonanome A, Grundy SM. 1988. Effect of dietary stearic acid on plasma cholesterol and lipoprotein levels. *N Engl J Med* 318:1244–1248.

Bonithon-Kopp C, Kronborg O, Giacosa A, Räth U, Faivre J. 2000. Calcium and fibre supplementation in prevention of colorectal adenoma recurrence: A randomised intervention trial. *Lancet* 356:1300–1306.

Borkman M, Campbell LV, Chisholm DJ, Storlien LH. 1991. Comparison of the effects on insulin sensitivity of high carbohydrate and high fat diets in normal subjects. *J Clin Endocrinol Metab* 72:432–437.

Bowman SA. 1999. Diets of individuals based on energy intakes from added sugars. *Fam Econ Nutr Rev* 12:31–38.

Bray GA, Popkin BM. 1998. Dietary fat intake does affect obesity! *Am J Clin Nutr* 68:1157–1173.

Brooks GA, Fahey TD, White TP, Baldwin KM. 2000. *Exercise Physiology: Human Bioenergetics and its Applications*, 3rd ed. Mountain View, CA: Mayfield Publishing.

Brussaard JH, Katan MB, Groot PHE, Havekes LM, Hautvast JGAJ. 1982. Serum lipoproteins of healthy persons fed a low-fat diet or a polyunsaturated fat diet for three months. A comparison of two cholesterol-lowering diets. *Atherosclerosis* 42:205–219.

Bruunsgaard H, Jensen MS, Schjerling P, Halkjaer-Kristensen J, Ogawa K, Skinhøj P, Pedersen BK. 1999. Exercise induces recruitment of lymphocytes with an activated phenotype and short telomeres in young and elderly humans. *Life Sci* 65:2623–2633.

Calviello G, Palozza P, Piccioni E, Maggiano N, Frattucci A, Franceschelli P, Baroli GM. 1998. Dietary supplementation with eicosapentaenoic and docosahexaenoic acid inhibits growth of Morris hepatocarcinoma 3924A in rats: Effects on proliferation and apoptosis. *Int J Cancer* 75:699–705.

Carlson LA, Böttiger LE. 1972. Ischaemic heart-disease in relation to fasting values of plasma triglycerides and cholesterol. Stockholm Prospective Study. *Lancet* 1:865–868.

Carroll KK. 1998. Obesity as a risk factor for certain types of cancer. *Lipids* 33:1055–1059.

Castelli WP. 1996. Lipids, risk factors and ischaemic heart disease. *Atherosclerosis* 124:S1–S9.

Caygill CPJ, Hill MJ. 1995. Fish, *n*-3 fatty acids and human colorectal and breast cancer mortality. *Eur J Cancer Prev* 4:329–332.

Caygill CPJ, Charlett A, Hill MJ. 1996. Fat, fish, fish oil and cancer. *Br J Cancer* 74:159–164.

Clarke R, Frost C, Collins R, Appleby P, Peto R. 1997. Dietary lipids and blood cholesterol: Quantitative meta-analysis of metabolic ward studies. *Br Med J* 314:112–117.

Cohen JC, Schall R. 1988. Reassessing the effects of simple carbohydrates on the serum triglyceride responses to fat meals. *Am J Clin Nutr* 48:1031–1034.

Colbert LH, Hartman TJ, Malila N, Limburg PJ, Pietinen P, Virtamo J, Taylor PR, Albanes D. 2001. Physical activity in relation to cancer of the colon and rectum in a cohort of male smokers. *Cancer Epidemiol Biomarkers Prev* 10:265–268.

Colditz GA, Willett WC, Stampfer MJ, Manson JE, Hennekens CH, Arky RA, Speizer FE. 1990. Weight as a risk factor for clinical diabetes in women. *Am J Epidemiol* 132:501–513.

Colditz GA, Manson JE, Stampfer MJ, Rosner B, Willett WC, Speizer FE. 1992. Diet and risk of clinical diabetes in women. *Am J Clin Nutr* 55:1018–1023.

Coulston AM, Liu GC, Reaven GM. 1983. Plasma glucose, insulin and lipid responses to high-carbohydrate low-fat diets in normal humans. *Metabolism* 32:52–56.

Daviglus ML, Stamler J, Orencia AJ, Dyer AR, Liu K, Greenland P, Walsh MK, Morris D, Shekelle RB. 1997. Fish consumption and the 30-year risk of fatal myocardial infarction. *N Engl J Med* 336:1046–1053.

Davy KP, Horton T, Davy BM, Bessessen D, Hill JO. 2001. Regulation of macronutrient balance in healthy young and older men. *Int J Obes Relat Metab Disord* 25:1497–1502.

De Caterina R, Liao JK, Libby P. 2000. Fatty acid modulation of endothelial activation. *Am J Clin Nutr* 71:213–223.

Denke MA. 1994. Effects of cocoa butter on serum lipids in humans: Historical highlights. *Am J Clin Nutr* 60:1014S–1016S.

Depaola DP, Faine MP, Palmer CA. 1999. Nutrition in relation to dental medicine. In: Shils ME, Olson JA, Shike M, Ross AC, eds. *Modern Nutrition in Health and Disease*, 9th ed. Baltimore, MD: Williams and Wilkins. Pp. 1099–1124.

Després J-P, Tremblay A, Nadeau A, Bouchard C. 1988. Physical training and changes in regional adipose tissue distribution. *Acta Med Scand Suppl* 723:205–212.

De Stefani E, Deneo-Pellegrini H, Mendilaharsu M, Carzoglio JC, Ronco A. 1997a. Dietary fat and lung cancer: A case-control study in Uruguay. *Cancer Causes Control* 8:913–921.

De Stefani E, Mendilaharsu M, Deneo-Pellegrini H, Ronco A. 1997b. Influence of dietary levels of fat, cholesterol, and calcium on colorectal cancer. *Nutr Cancer* 29:83–89.

Diabetes Prevention Program Research Group. 2002. Reduction in the incidence of type 2 diabetes with lifestyle intervention or metformin. *N Engl J Med* 346:393–403.

Dolecek TA. 1992. Epidemiological evidence of relationships between dietary polyunsaturated fatty acids and mortality in the Multiple Risk Factor Intervention Trial. *Proc Soc Exp Med Biol* 200:177–182.

Dreon DM, Frey-Hewitt B, Ellsworth N, Williams PT, Terry RB, Wood PD. 1988. Dietary fat:carbohydrate ratio and obesity in middle-aged men. *Am J Clin Nutr* 47:995–1000.

Dunnigan MG, Fyfe T, McKiddie MT, Crosbie SM. 1970. The effects of isocaloric exchange of dietary starch and sucrose on glucose tolerance, plasma insulin and serum lipids in man. *Clin Sci* 38:1–9.

Eliasson K, Ryttig KR, Hylander B, Rossner S. 1992. A dietary fibre supplement in the treatment of mild hypertension. A randomized, double-blind, placebo-controlled trial. *J Hypertens* 10:195–199.

El-Sayed MS. 1996. Effects of exercise on blood coagulation, fibrinolysis and platelet aggregation. *Sports Med* 22:282–298.

Fasching P, Ratheiser K, Schneeweiss B, Rohac M, Nowotny P, Waldhausl W. 1996. No effect of short-term dietary supplementation of saturated and poly- and monounsaturated fatty acids on insulin secretion and sensitivity in healthy men. *Ann Nutr Metab* 40:116–122.

Fehily AM, Phillips KM, Yarnell JWG. 1984. Diet, smoking, social class, and body mass index in the Caerphilly Heart Disease Study. *Am J Clin Nutr* 40:827–833.

Feskens EJM, Loeber JG, Kromhout D. 1994. Diet and physical activity as determinants of hyperinsulinemia: The Zutphen Elderly Study. *Am J Epidemiol* 140: 350–360.

Frankel S, Gunnell DJ, Peters TJ, Maynard M, Smith GD. 1998. Childhood energy intake and adult mortality from cancer: The Boyd Orr Cohort Study. *Br Med J* 316:499–504.

French SA, Fulkerson JA, Story M. 2000. Increasing weight-bearing physical activity and calcium intake for bone mass growth in children and adolescents: A review of intervention trials. *Prev Med* 31:722–731.

Friday KE, Childs MT, Tsunehara CH, Fujimoto WY, Bierman EL, Ensinck JW. 1989. Elevated plasma glucose and lowered triglyceride levels from omega-3 fatty acid supplementation in type II diabetes. *Diabetes Care* 12:276–281.

Frost G, Leeds A, Trew G, Margara R, Dornhorst A. 1998. Insulin sensitivity in women at risk of coronary heart disease and the effect of a low glycemic diet. *Metabolism* 47:1245–1251.

Fuchs CS, Giovannucci EL, Colditz GA, Hunter DJ, Stampfer MJ, Rosner B, Speizer FE, Willett WC. 1999. Dietary fiber and the risk of colorectal cancer and adenoma in women. *N Engl J Med* 340:169–176.

Fukagawa NK, Anderson JW, Hageman G, Young VR, Minaker KL. 1990. High-carbohydrate, high-fiber diets increase peripheral insulin sensitivity in healthy young and old adults. *Am J Clin Nutr* 52:524–528.

Gardner CD, Kraemer HC. 1995. Monounsaturated versus polyunsaturated dietary fat and serum lipids. A meta-analysis. *Arterioscler Thromb Vasc Biol* 15:1917–1927.

Gartside PS, Glueck CJ. 1993. Relationship of dietary intake to hospital admission for coronary heart and vascular disease: The NHANES II National Probability Study. *J Am Coll Nutr* 6:676–684.

Gerber M. 1998. Fibre and breast cancer. *Eur J Cancer Prev* 7:S63–S67.

Gibson SA. 1993. Consumption and sources of sugars in the diets of British schoolchildren: Are high-sugar diets nutritionally inferior? *J Hum Nutr Diet* 6:355–371.

Gibson SA. 1996a. Are diets high in non-milk extrinsic sugars conducive to obesity? An analysis from the Dietary and Nutritional Survey of British Adults. *J Hum Nutr Diet* 9:283–292.

Gibson SA. 1996b. Are high-fat, high-sugar foods and diets conducive to obesity? *Int J Food Sci Nutr* 47:405–415.

Gibson SA. 1997. Non-milk extrinsic sugars in the diets of pre-school children: Association with intakes of micronutrients, energy, fat and NSP. *Br J Nutr* 78:367–378.

Giovannucci E, Willett WC. 1994. Dietary factors and risk of colon cancer. *Ann Med* 26:443–452.

Giovannucci E, Stampfer MJ, Colditz G, Rimm EB, Willett WC. 1992. Relationship of diet to risk of colorectal adenoma in men. *J Natl Cancer Inst* 84:91–98.

Giovannucci E, Rimm EB, Colditz GA, Stampfer MJ, Ascherio A, Chute CC, Willett WC. 1993. A prospective study of dietary fat and risk of prostate cancer. *J Natl Cancer Inst* 85:1571–1579.

Giovannucci E, Rimm EB, Stampfer MJ, Colditz GA, Ascherio A, Willett WC. 1994. Intake of fat, meat, and fiber in relation to risk of colon cancer in men. *Cancer Res* 54:2390–2397.

Glauber H, Wallace P, Griver K, Brechtel G. 1988. Adverse metabolic effect of omega-3 fatty acids in non-insulin-dependent diabetes mellitus. *Ann Intern Med* 108:663–668.

Goodman MT, Kolonel LN, Yoshizawa CN, Hankin JH. 1988. The effect of dietary cholesterol and fat on the risk of lung cancer in Hawaii. *Am J Epidemiol* 128:1241–1255.

Goodman MT, Wilkens LR, Hankin JH, Lyu L-C, Wu AH, Kolonel LN. 1997. Association of soy and fiber consumption with the risk of endometrial cancer. *Am J Epidemiol* 146:294–306.

Goran MI. 2001. Metabolic precursors and effects of obesity in children: A decade of progress, 1990–1999. *Am J Clin Nutr* 73:158–171.

Gordon T, Castelli WP, Hjortland MC, Kannel WB, Dawber TR. 1977. High density lipoprotein as a protective factor against coronary heart disease. The Framingham Study. *Am J Med* 62:707–714.

Gordon T, Kagan A, Garcia-Palmieri M, Kannel WB, Zukel WJ, Tillotson J, Sorlie P, Hjortland M. 1981. Diet and its relation to coronary heart disease and death in three populations. *Circulation* 63:500–515.

Grammatikos SI, Subbaiah PV, Victor TA, Miller WM. 1994. *n*-3 And *n*-6 fatty acid processing and growth effects in neoplastic and non-cancerous human mammary epithelial cell lines. *Br J Cancer* 70:219–227.

Gray GE, Pike MC, Henderson BE. 1979. Breast-cancer incidence and mortality rates in different countries in relation to known risk factors and dietary practices. *Br J Cancer* 39:1–7.

Hallfrisch J, Scholfield DJ, Behall KM. 1995. Diets containing soluble oat extracts improve glucose and insulin responses of moderately hypercholesterolemic men and women. *Am J Clin Nutr* 61:379–384.

Hambrecht R, Wolf A, Gielen S, Linke A, Hofer J, Erbs S, Schoene N, Schuler G. 2000. Effect of exercise on coronary endothelial function in patients with coronary artery disease. *N Eng J Med* 342:454–460.

Harker LA, Kelly AB, Hanson SR, Krupski W, Bass A, Osterud B, Fitzgerald GA, Goodnight SH, Connor WE. 1993. Interruption of vascular thrombus formation and vascular lesion formation by dietary *n*-3 fatty acids in fish oil in non-human primates. *Circulation* 87:1017–1029.

Harris PJ, Ferguson LR. 1993. Dietary fibre: Its composition and role in protection against colorectal cancer. *Mutat Res* 290:97–110.

Harris WS. 1989. Fish oils and plasma lipid and lipoprotein metabolism in humans: A critical review. *J Lipid Res* 30:785–807.

Hegsted DM. 1986. Serum-cholesterol response to dietary cholesterol: A re-evaluation. *Am J Clin Nutr* 44:299–305.

Hegsted DM, Ausman LM, Johnson JA, Dallal GE. 1993. Dietary fat and serum lipids: An evaluation of the experimental data. *Am J Clin Nutr* 57:875–883.

Helmrich SP, Ragland DR, Leung RW, Paffenbarger RS. 1991. Physical activity and reduced occurrence of non-insulin-dependent diabetes mellitus. *N Engl J Med* 325:147–152.

Hennekens CH. 1998. Risk factors for coronary heart disease in women. *Cardiol Clin* 16:1–8.

Hill MJ. 1997. Cereals, cereal fibre and colorectal cancer risk: A review of the epidemiological literature. *Eur J Cancer Prev* 6:219–225.

Hinkle LE, Thaler HT, Merke DP, Renier-Berg D, Morton NE. 1988. The risk factors for arrhythmic death in a sample of men followed for 20 years. *Am J Epidemiol* 127:500–515.

Hoff G, Moen IE, Trygg K, Frølich W, Sauar J, Vatn M, Gjone E, Larsen S. 1986. Epidemiology of polyps in the rectum and sigmoid colon. Evaluation of nutritional factors. *Scand J Gastroenterol* 21:199–204.

Hopkins PN. 1992. Effects of dietary cholesterol on serum cholesterol: A meta-analysis and review. *Am J Clin Nutr* 55:1060–1070.

Horton ES. 1986. Exercise and physical training: Effects on insulin sensitivity and glucose metabolism. *Diabetes Metab Rev* 2:1–17.

Horton ES. 1991. Exercise and decreased risk of NIDDM. *N Engl J Med* 325:196–197.

Howard BV, Abbott WGH, Swinburn BA. 1991. Evaluation of metabolic effects of substitution of complex carbohydrates for saturated fat in individuals with obesity and NIDDM. *Diabetes Care* 14:786–795.

Howe GR, Friedenreich CM, Jain M, Miller AB. 1991. A cohort study of fat intake and risk of breast cancer. *J Natl Cancer Inst* 83:336–340.

Howe GR, Aronson KJ, Benito E, Castelleto R, Cornée J, Duffy S, Gallagher RP, Iscovich JM, Deng-ao J, Kaaks R, Kune GA, Kune S, Lee HP, Lee M, Miller AB, Peters RK, Potter JD, Riboli E, Slattery ML, Trichopoulos D, Tuyns A, Tzonou A, Watson LF, Whittemore AS, Wu-Willimas AH, Shu Z. 1997. The relationship between dietary fat intake and risk of colorectal cancer: Evidence from the combined analysis of 13 case-control studies. *Cancer Causes Control* 8:215–228.

Howell WH, McNamara DJ, Tosca MA, Smith BT, Gaines JA. 1997. Plasma lipid and lipoprotein responses to dietary fat and cholesterol: A meta-analysis. *Am J Clin Nutr* 65:1747–1764.

Hu FB, Stampfer MJ, Manson JE, Rimm E, Colditz GA, Rosner BA, Hennekens CH, Willett WC. 1997. Dietary fat intake and the risk of coronary heart disease in women. *N Engl J Med* 337:1491–1499.

Hu FB, Stampfer MJ, Manson JE, Rimm E, Colditz GA, Speizer FE, Hennekens CH, Willett WC. 1999a. Dietary protein and risk of ischemic heart disease in women. *Am J Clin Nutr* 70:221–227.

Hu FB, Stampfer MJ, Rimm EB, Manson JE, Ascherio A, Colditz GA, Rosner BA, Spiegelman D, Speizer FE, Sacks FM, Hennekens CH, Willett WC. 1999b. A prospective study of egg consumption and risk of cardiovascular disease in men and women. *J Am Med Assoc* 281:1387–1394.

Hulley SB, Rosenman RH, Bawol RD, Brand RJ. 1980. Epidemiology as a guide to clinical decisions. The association between triglyceride and coronary heart disease. *N Engl J Med* 302:1383–1389.

Hunter DJ, Spiegelman D, Adami H-O, Beeson L, van den Brandt PA, Folsom AR, Fraser GE, Goldbohn A, Graham S, Howe GR, Kushi LH, Marshall JR, McDermott A, Miller AB, Speizer FE, Wolk A, Yaun S-S, Willett W. 1996. Cohort studies of fat intake and the risk of breast cancer—A pooled analysis. *N Engl J Med* 334:356–361.

Hurley BR, Roth SM. 2000. Strength training in the elderly. Effects on risk factors for age-related diseases. *Sports Med* 30:249–268.

Huttunen JK, Länsimies E, Voutilainen E, Ehnholm C, Hietanen E, Penttilä I, Siitonen O, Rauranaa R. 1979. Effect of moderate physical exercise on serum lipoproteins. A controlled clinical trial with special reference to serum high-density lipoproteins. *Circulation* 60:1220–1229.

IARC (International Agency for Research on Cancer). 2002. *IARC Handbooks of Cancer Prevention. Volume 6: Weight Control and Physical Activity.* Lyon, France: IARC Press.

Jacobs DR, Meyer KA, Kushi LH, Folsom AR. 1998. Whole-grain intake may reduce the risk of ischemic heart disease death in postmenopausal women: The Iowa Women's Health Study. *Am J Clin Nutr* 68:248–257.

Jacobs LR. 1986. Relationship between dietary fiber and cancer: Metabolic, physiologic, and cellular mechanisms. *Proc Soc Exp Biol Med* 183:299–310.

James MJ, Gibson RA, Cleland LG. 2000. Dietary polyunsaturated fatty acids and inflammatory mediator production. *Am J Clin Nutr* 71:343S–348S.

Jenkins DJA, Wolever TMS, Leeds AR, Gassull MA, Haisman P, Dilawari J, Goff DV, Metz GL, Alberti KGMM. 1978. Dietary fibres, fibre analogues, and glucose tolerance: Importance of viscosity. *Br Med J* 1:1392–1394.

Jenkins DJA, Wolever TMS, Buckley G, Lam KY, Giudici S, Kalmusky J, Jenkins AL, Patten RL, Bird J, Wong GS, Josse RG. 1988. Low-glycemic-index starchy food in the diabetic diet. *Am J Clin Nutr* 48:248–254.

Jeppesen J, Schaaf P, Jones C, Zhou M-Y, Chen Y-DI, Reaven GM. 1997. Effects of low-fat, high-carbohydrate diets on risk factors for ischemic heart disease in postmenopausal women. *Am J Clin Nutr* 65:1027–1033.

Johnson RK. 2000. What are people really eating and why does it matter? *Nutr Today* 35:40–45.

Jones DY, Schatzkin A, Green SB, Block G, Brinton LA, Ziegler RG, Hoover R, Taylor PR. 1987. Dietary fat and breast cancer in the National Health and Nutrition Examination Survey I. Epidemiologic follow-up study. *J Natl Cancer Inst* 79:465–471.

Jousilahti P, Vartiainen E, Pekkanen J, Tuomilehto J, Sundvall J, Puska P. 1998. Serum cholesterol distribution and coronary heart disease risk. Observations and predictions among middle-aged population in eastern Finland. *Circulation* 97:1087–1094.

Kaizer L, Boyd NF, Kriukov V, Tritchler D. 1989. Fish consumption and breast cancer risk: An ecologic study. *Nutr Cancer* 12:61–68.

Kang JX, Leaf A. 1996. Antiarrhythmic effects of polyunsaturated fatty acids: Recent studies. *Circulation* 94:1774–1780.

Kannel WB, Sorlie P. 1979. Some health benefits of physical activity. The Framingham Study. *Arch Intern Med* 139:857–861.

Kannel WB, Belanger A, D'Agostino R, Israel I. 1986. Physical activity and physical demand on the job and risk of cardiovascular disease and death: The Framingham Study. *Am Heart J* 112:820–825.

Kasim SE, Stern B, Khilnani S, McLin P, Baciorowski S, Jen K-LC. 1988. Effects of omega-3 fish oils on lipid metabolism, glycemic control, and blood pressure in type II diabetic patients. *J Clin Endocrinol Metab* 67:1–5.

Kasim SE, Martino S, Kim P-N, Khilnani S, Boomer A, Depper J, Reading BA, Heilbrun LK. 1993. Dietary and anthropometric determinants of plasma lipoproteins during a long-term low-fat diet in healthy women. *Am J Clin Nutr* 57:146–153.

Kendall A, Levitsky DA, Strupp BJ, Lissner L. 1991. Weight loss on a low-fat diet: Consequence of the imprecision of the control of food intake in humans. *Am J Clin Nutr* 53:1124–1129.

Keys A, Menotti A, Karvonen MJ, Aravanis C, Blackburn H, Buzina R, Djordjevic BS, Dontas AS, Fidanza F, Keys MH, Kromhout D, Nedeljkovic S, Punsar S, Seccareccia F, Toshima H. 1986. The diet and 15-year death rate in the seven countries study. *Am J Epidemiol* 124:903–915.

Khan K, McKay HA, Haapasalo H, Bennell KL, Forwood MR, Kannus P, Wark JD. 2000. Does childhood and adolescence provide a unique opportunity for exercise to strengthen the skeleton? *J Sci Med Sport* 3:150–164.

King H, Taylor R, Zimmet P, Pargeter K, Raper LR, Beriki T, Tekanene J. 1984. Non-insulin-dependent diabetes (NIDDM) in a newly independent Pacific nation: The Republic of Kiribati. *Diabetes Care* 7:409–415.

Klurfeld DM. 1992. Dietary fiber-mediated mechanisms in carcinogenesis. *Cancer Res* 52:2055S–2059S.

Koutsari C, Karpe F, Humphreys SM, Frayn KN, Hardman AE. 2001. Exercise prevents the accumulation of triglyceride-rich lipoproteins and their remnants seen when changing to a high-carbohydrate diet. *Arterioscler Thromb Vasc Biol* 21:1520–1525.

Krauss RM, Dreon DM. 1995. Low-density-lipoprotein subclasses and response to a low-fat diet in healthy men. *Am J Clin Nutr* 62:478S–487S.

Kromhout D, de Lezenne Coulander C. 1984. Diet, prevalence and 10-year mortality from coronary heart disease in 871 middle-aged men. *Am J Epidemiol* 119:733–741.

Kromhout D, Bosschieter EB, de Lezenne Coulander C. 1985. The inverse relation between fish consumption and 20-year mortality from coronary heart disease. *N Engl J Med* 312:1205–1209.

Kromhout D, Feskens EJM, Bowles CH. 1995. The protective effect of a small amount of fish on coronary heart disease mortality in an elderly population. *Int J Epidemiol* 24:340–345.

Kushi LH, Lew RA, Stare FJ, Ellison CR, el Lozy M, Bourke G, Daly L, Graham I, Hickey N, Mulcahy R, Kevaney J. 1985. Diet and 20-year mortality from coronary heart disease. The Ireland-Boston Diet-Heart Study. *N Engl J Med* 312:811–818.

Kushi LH, Sellers TA, Potter JD, Nelson CL, Munger RG, Kaye SA, Folsom AR. 1992. Dietary fat and postmenopausal breast cancer. *J Natl Cancer Inst* 84:1092–1099.

Lai PBS, Ross JA, Fearson KCH, Anderson JD, Carter DC. 1996. Cell cycle arrest and induction of apoptosis in pancreatic cancer cells exposed to eicosapentaenoic acid in vitro. *Br J Cancer* 74:1375–1383.

Lanza E. 1990. National Cancer Institute Satellite Symposium on Fiber and Colon Cancer. In: Kritchevsky D, Bonfield C, Anderson JW, eds. *Dietary Fiber: Chemistry, Physiology, and Health Effects*. New York: Plenum Press. Pp. 383–387.

Layne JE, Nelson ME. 1999. The effects of progressive resistance training on bone density: A review. *Med Sci Sports Exerc* 21:25–30.

Leclerc I, Davignon I, Lopez D, Garrel DR. 1993. No change in glucose tolerance and substrate oxidation after a high-carbohydrate, low-fat diet. *Metabolism* 42:365–370.

Lewis CJ, Park YK, Dexter PB, Yetley EA. 1992. Nutrient intakes and body weights of persons consuming high and moderate levels of added sugars. *J Am Diet Assoc* 92:708–713.

Liljeberg HGM, Åkerberg AKE, Björck IME. 1999. Effect of the glycemic index and content of indigestible carbohydrates of cereal-based breakfast meals on glucose tolerance at lunch in healthy subjects. *Am J Clin Nutr* 69:647–655.

Lindsted KD, Tonstad S, Kuzma JW. 1991. Self-report of physical activity and patterns of mortality in Seventh-day Adventist men. *J Clin Epidemiol* 44:355–364.

Lissner L, Heitmann BL. 1995. Dietary fat and obesity: Evidence from epidemiology. *Eur J Clin Nutr* 49:79–90.

Lissner L, Levitsky DA, Strupp BJ, Kalkwarf HJ, Roe DA. 1987. Dietary fat and the regulation of energy intake in human subjects. *Am J Clin Nutr* 46:886–892.

Lissner L, Helgesson Ö, Bengtsson C, Lapidus L, Hultén B, Branehög I, Holmberg E. 1992. Energy and macronutrient intake in relation to cancer incidence among Swedish women. *Eur J Clin Nutr* 46:501–507.

Lissner L, Heitmann BL, Bengtsson C. 2000. Population studies of diet and obesity. *Br J Nutr* 83:S21–S24.

Little J, Logan RFA, Hawtin PG, Hardcastle JD, Turner ID. 1993. Colorectal adenomas and diet: A case-control study of subjects participating in the Nottingham Faecal Occult Blood Screening Programme. *Br J Cancer* 67:177–84.

Lundgren H, Bengtsson C, Blohmé G, Isaksson B, Lapidus L, Lenner RA, Saaek A, Winther E. 1989. Dietary habits and incidence of noninsulin-dependent diabetes mellitus in a population study of women in Gothenburg, Sweden. *Am J Clin Nutr* 49:708–712.

Lyon JL, Mahoney AW, West DW, Gardner JW, Smith KR, Sorenson AW, Stanish W. 1987. Energy intake: Its relationship to colon cancer risk. *J Natl Cancer Inst* 78:853–861.

Macquart-Moulin G, Riboli E, Cornée J, Charnay B, Berthezène P, Day N. 1986. Case-control study on colorectal cancer and diet in Marseilles. *Int J Cancer* 38:183–191.

Macquart-Moulin G, Riboli E, Cornée J, Kaaks R, Berthezène P. 1987. Colorectal polyps and diet: A case-control study in Marseilles. *Int J Cancer* 40:179–188.

Madsen KL, Adams WC, Van Loan MD. 1998. Effects of physical activity, body weight and composition, and muscular strength on bone density in young women. *Med Sci Sports Exerc* 30:114–120.

Mann JI, Watermeyer GS, Manning EB, Randles J, Truswell AS. 1973. Effects on serum lipids of different dietary fats associated with a high sucrose diet. *Clin Sci* 44:601–604.

Mann JI, Appleby PN, Key TJ, Thorogood M. 1997. Dietary determinants of ischaemic heart disease in health conscious individuals. *Heart* 78:450–455.

Manson JE, Rimm EB, Stampfer MJ, Colditz GA, Willett WC, Krolewski AS, Rosner B, Hennekens CH, Speizer FE. 1991. Physical activity and incidence of non-insulin-dependent diabetes mellitus in women. *Lancet* 338:774–778.

Manson JE, Nathan DM, Krolewski AS, Stampfer MJ, Willett WC, Hennekens CH. 1992. A prospective study of exercise and incidence of diabetes among US male physicians. *J Am Med Assoc* 268:63–67.

Marckmann P, Raben A, Astrup A. 2000. Ad libitum intake of low-fat diets rich in either starchy foods or sucrose: Effects on blood lipids, factor VII coagulant activity, and fibrinogen. *Metabolism* 49:731–735.

Marniemi J, Seppänen A, Hakala P. 1990. Long-term effects on lipid metabolism of weight reduction on lactovegetarian and mixed diet. *Int J Obes* 14:113–125.

Marshall JA, Hamman RF, Baxter J. 1991. High-fat, low-carbohydrate diet and the etiology of non-insulin-dependent diabetes mellitus: The San Luis Valley Diabetes Study. *Am J Epidemiol* 134:590–603.

Masironi R. 1970. Dietary factors and coronary heart disease. *Bull World Health Organ* 42:103–114.

Mayer-Davis EJ, Monaco JH, Hoen HM, Carmichael S, Vitolins MZ, Rewers MJ, Haffner SM, Ayad MF, Bergman RN, Karter AJ. 1997. Dietary fat and insulin sensitivity in a triethnic population: The role of obesity. The Insulin Resistance Arteriosclerosis Study (IRAS). *Am J Clin Nutr* 65:79–87.

Mayer-Davis EJ, D'Agostino R, Karter AJ, Haffner SM, Rewers MJ, Saad M, Bergman RN. 1998. Intensity and amount of physical activity in relation to insulin sensitivity. The Insulin Resistance Atherosclerosis Study. *J Am Med Assoc* 279:669–674.

Mazzeo RS, Rajkumar C, Rolland J, Blaher B, Jennings G, Esler M. 1998. Immune response to a single bout of exercise in young and elderly subjects. *Mech Ageing Dev* 100:121–132.

McLennan PL. 1993. Relative effects of dietary saturated, monounsaturated, and polyunsaturated fatty acids on cardiac arrhythmias in rats. *Am J Clin Nutr* 57:207–212.

Meinertz H, Nilausen K, Faergeman O. 1989. Soy protein and casein in cholesterol-enriched diets: Effects on plasma lipoproteins in normolipidemic subjects. *Am J Clin Nutr* 50:786–793.

Mensink RP, Katan MB. 1992. Effect of dietary fatty acids on serum lipids and lipoproteins. A meta-analysis of 27 trials. *Arterioscler Thromb* 12:911–919.

Mensink RP, Temme EH, Hornstra G. 1994. Dietary saturated and trans fatty acids and lipoprotein metabolism. *Ann Med* 26:461–464.

Meyer KA, Kushi LH, Jacobs DR, Slavin J, Sellers TA, Folsom AR. 2000. Carbohydrates, dietary fiber, and incident type 2 diabetes in older women. *Am J Clin Nutr* 71:921–930.

Michaud DS, Giovannucci E, Willett WC, Colditz GA, Stampfer MJ, Fuchs CS. 2001. Physical activity, obesity, height, and the risk of pancreatic cancer. *J Am Med Assoc* 286:921–929.

Miller AB, Kelly A, Choi NW, Matthews V, Morgan RW, Munan L, Burch JD, Feather J, Howe GR, Jain M. 1978. A study of diet and breast cancer. *Am J Epidemiol* 107:499–509.

Miller WC, Lindeman AK, Wallace J, Niederpruem M. 1990. Diet composition, energy intake, and exercise in relation to body fat in men and women. *Am J Clin Nutr* 52:426–430.

Morris MC, Sacks F, Rosner B. 1993. Does fish oil lower blood pressure? A meta-analysis of controlled trials. *Circulation* 88:523–533.

Must A, Lipman RD. 1999. Childhood energy intake and cancer mortality in adulthood. *Nutr Rev* 57:21–24.

Neaton JD, Wentworth D. 1992. Serum cholesterol, blood pressure, cigarette smoking, and death from coronary heart disease. Overall findings and differences by age for 316,099 white men. *Arch Intern Med* 152:56–64.

Neugut AI, Garbowski GC, Lee WC, Murray T, Nieves JW, Forde KA, Treat MR, Waye JD, Fenoglio-Preiser C. 1993. Dietary risk factors for the incidence and recurrence of colorectal adenomatous polyps. A case-control study. *Ann Intern Med* 118:91–95.

NHLBI/NIDDK (National Heart, Lung, and Blood Institute/National Institute of Diabetes and Digestive and Kidney Diseases). 1998. *Clinical Guidelines on the Identification, Evaluation, and Treatment of Overweight and Obesity in Adults. The Evidence Report.* NIH Publication No. 98-4083. Bethesda, MD: National Institutes of Health.

Nikkilä EA, Taskinen M-R, Rehunen S, Härkönen M. 1978. Lipoprotein lipase activity in adipose tissue and skeletal muscle of runners: Relation to serum lipoproteins. *Metabolism* 27:1661–1671.

Obarzanek E, Velletri PA, Cutler JA. 1996. Dietary protein and blood pressure. *J Am Med Assoc* 275:1598–1603.

Paffenbarger RS, Hyde RT, Jung DL, Wing AL. 1984. Epidemiology of exercise and coronary heart disease. *Clin Sports Med* 3:297–318.

Parker DR, Weiss ST, Troisi R, Cassano PA, Vokonas PS, Landsberg L. 1993. Relationship of dietary saturated fatty acids and body habitus to serum insulin concentrations: The Normative Aging Study. *Am J Clin Nutr* 58:129–136.

Parks EJ, Hellerstein MK. 2000. Carbohydrate-induced hypertriacylglycerolemia: Historical perspective and review of biological mechanisms. *Am J Clin Nutr* 71:412–433.

Parmley WW. 1997. Nonlipoprotein risk factors for coronary heart disease: Evaluation and management. *Am J Med* 102:7–14.

Pietinen P, Rimm EB, Korhonen P, Hartman AM, Willett WC, Albanes D, Virtamo J. 1996. Intake of dietary fiber and risk of coronary heart disease in a cohort of Finnish men. The Alpha-Tocopherol, Beta-Carotene Cancer Prevention Study. *Circulation* 94:2720–2727.

Pietinen P, Ascherio A, Korhonen P, Hartman AM, Willett WC, Albanes D, Virtamo J. 1997. Intake of fatty acids and risk of coronary heart disease in a cohort of Finnish men. The Alpha-Tocopherol, Beta-Carotene Cancer Prevention Study. *Am J Epidemiol* 145:876–887.

Pi-Sunyer FX, Woo R. 1985. Effect of exercise on food intake in human subjects. *Am J Clin Nutr* 42:983–990.

Platz EA, Giovannucci E, Rimm EB, Rickett HRH, Stampfer MJ, Colditz GA, Willett WC. 1997. Dietary fiber and distal colorectal adenoma in men. *Cancer Epidemiol Biomarkers Prev* 6:661–670.

Purnell JQ, Kahn SE, Albers JJ, Nevin DN, Brunzell JD, Schwartz RS. 2000. Effect of weight loss with reduction of intra-abdominal fat on lipid metabolism in older men. *J Clin Endocrinol Metab* 85:977–982.

Ramon JM, Bou R, Romea S, Alkiza ME, Jacas M, Ribes J, Oromi J. 2000. Dietary fat intake and prostate cancer risk: A case-control study in Spain. *Cancer Causes Control* 11:679–685.

Rath R, Mas̆ek J, Kujalová V, Slabochová Z. 1974. Effect of a high sugar intake on some metabolic and regulatory indicators in young men. *Nahrung* 18:343–353.

Reiser S, Hallfrisch J. 1987. Lipogenesis and blood lipids. In: *Metabolic Effects of Dietary Fructose.* Boca Raton, FL: CRC Press. Pp. 83–111.

Reiser S, Hallfrisch J, Michaelis OE, Lazar FL, Martin RE, Prather ES. 1979. Isocaloric exchange of dietary starch and sucrose in humans. I. Effects on levels of fasting blood lipids. *Am J Clin Nutr* 32:1659–1669.

Richter EA, Ruderman NB, Schneider SH. 1981. Diabetes and exercise. *Am J Med* 70:201–209.

Rigaud D, Ryttig KR, Angel LA, Apfelbaum M. 1990. Overweight treated with energy restriction and a dietary fibre supplement: A 6-month randomized, double-blind, placebo-controlled trial. *Int J Obes* 14:763–769.

Risch HA, Jain M, Marrett LD, Howe GR. 1994. Dietary fat intake and risk of epithelial ovarian cancer. *J Natl Cancer Inst* 86:1409–1415.

Rivellese A, Riccardi G, Giacco A, Pacioni D, Genovese S, Mattioli PL, Mancini M. 1980. Effect of dietary fibre on glucose control and serum lipoproteins in diabetic patients. *Lancet* 2:447–450.

Roberfroid M. 1993. Dietary fiber, inulin, and oligofructose: A review comparing their physiological effects. *Crit Rev Food Sci Nutr* 33:103–148.

Roche HM, Zampelas A, Jackson KG, Williams CM, Gibney MJ. 1998. The effect of test meal monounsaturated fatty acid:saturated fatty acid ratio on postprandial lipid metabolism. *Br J Nutr* 79:419–424.

Rohan TE, Howe GR, Friedenreich CM, Jain M, Miller AB. 1993. Dietary fiber, vitamins A, C, and E, and risk of breast cancer: A cohort study. *Cancer Causes Control* 4:29–37.

Rose DP. 1997. Dietary fatty acids and cancer. *Am J Clin Nutr* 66:998S–1003S.

Rose DP, Connolly JM. 2000. Regulation of tumor angiogenesis by dietary fatty acids and eicosanoids. *Nutr Cancer* 37:119–127.

Rose DP, Boyar AP, Wynder EL. 1986. International comparisons of mortality rates for cancer of the breast, ovary, prostate, and colon, and per capita food consumption. *Cancer* 58:2363–2371.

Rose DP, Goldman M, Connolly JM, Strong LE. 1991. High-fiber diet reduces serum estrogen concentrations in premenopausal women. *Am J Clin Nutr* 54:520–525.

Rössner S, von Zweigbergk D, Öhlin A, Ryttig K. 1987. Weight reduction with dietary fibre supplements. Results of two double-blind randomized studies. *Acta Med Scand* 222:83–88.

Ryttig KR, Tellnes G, Haegh L, Boe E, Fagerthun H. 1989. A dietary fibre supplement and weight maintenance after weight reduction: A randomized, double-blind, placebo-controlled long-term trial. *Int J Obes* 13:165–171.

Salmerón J, Ascherio A, Rimm EB, Colditz GA, Spiegelman D, Jenkins DJ, Stampfer MJ, Wing AL, Willett WC. 1997a. Dietary fiber, glycemic load, and risk of NIDDM in men. *Diabetes Care* 20:545–550.

Salmerón J, Manson JE, Stampfer MJ, Colditz GA, Wing AL, Willett WC. 1997b. Dietary fiber, glycemic load, and risk of non-insulin-dependent diabetes mellitus in women. *J Am Med Assoc* 277:472–477.

Saltzman E, Dallal GE, Roberts SB. 1997. Effect of high-fat and low-fat diets on voluntary energy intake and substrate oxidation: Studies in identical twins consuming diets matched for energy density, fiber, and palatability. *Am J Clin Nutr* 66:1332–1339.

Sasaki S, Horacsek M, Kesteloot H. 1993. An ecological study of the relationship between dietary fat intake and breast cancer mortality. *Prev Med* 22:187–202.

Schatzkin A, Lanza E, Corle D, Lance P, Iber F, Caan B, Shike M, Weissfeld J, Burt R, Cooper MR, Kikendall JW, Cahill J. 2000. Lack of effect of a low-fat, high-fiber diet on the recurrence of colorectal adenomas. *N Engl J Med* 342:1149–1155.

Schneider SH, Amorosa LF, Khachadurian AK, Ruderman NB. 1984. Studies on the mechanism of improved glucose control during regular exercise in type 2 (non-insulin-dependent) diabetes. *Diabetologia* 26:355–360.

Schuurman AG, van den Brandt PA, Dorant E, Brants HAM, Goldbohm RA. 1999. Association of energy and fat intake with prostate carcinoma risk. Results from the Netherlands Cohort Study. *Cancer* 86:1019–1027.

Shephard RJ. 1990. Physical activity and cancer. *Int J Sports Med* 11:413–420.

Shephard RJ. 1996. Exercise and cancer: Linkages with obesity? *Crit Rev Food Sci Nutr* 36:321–339.

Sonnenberg LM, Quatromoni PA, Gagnon DR, Cupples LA, Franz MM, Ordovas JM, Wilson PWF, Schaefer EJ, Millen BE. 1996. Diet and plasma lipids in women. II. Macronutrients and plasma triglycerides, high-density lipoprotein, and the ratio of total to high-density lipoprotein cholesterol in women: The Framingham Nutrition Studies. *J Clin Epidemiol* 49:665–672.

Sorkin JD, Andres R, Muller DC, Baldwin HL, Fleg JL. 1992. Cholesterol as a risk factor for coronary heart disease in elderly men. The Baltimore Longitudinal Study of Aging. *Ann Epidemiol* 2:59–67.

Stacpoole PW, Alig J, Ammon L, Crockett SE. 1989. Dose–response effects of dietary marine oil on carbohydrate and lipid metabolism in normal subjects and patients with hypertriglyceridemia. *Metabolism* 38:946–956.

Stamler J. 1979. Population studies. In: Levy R, Rifkind B, Dennis B, Ernst N, eds. *Nutrition, Lipids, and Coronary Heart Disease.* New York: Raven Press. Pp. 25–88.

Stamler J, Wentworth D, Neaton JD. 1986. Is relationship between serum cholesterol and risk of premature death from coronary heart disease continuous and graded? Findings in 356,222 primary screenees of the Multiple Risk Factor Intervention Trial (MRFIT). *J Am Med Assoc* 256:2823–2828.

Stampfer MJ, Krauss RM, Ma J, Blanche PJ, Holl LG, Sacks FM, Hennekens CH. 1996. A prospective study of triglyceride level, low-density lipoprotein particle diameter, and risk of myocardial infarction. *J Am Med Assoc* 276:882–888.

Stemmermann GN, Nomura AM, Heilbrun LK. 1985. Cancer risk in relation to fat and energy intake among Hawaii Japanese: A prospective study. *Princess Takamatsu Symp* 16:265–274.

Straznicky NE, O'Callaghan CJ, Barrington VE, Louis WJ. 1999. Hypotensive effect of low-fat, high-carbohydrate diet can be independent of changes in plasma insulin concentrations. *Hypertension* 34:580–585.

Stubbs RJ, Ritz P, Coward WA, Prentice AM. 1995. Covert manipulation of the ratio of dietary fat to carbohydrate and energy density: Effect on food intake and energy balance in free-living men eating ad libitum. *Am J Clin Nutr* 62:330–337.

Stubbs RJ, Harbron CG, Prentice AM. 1996. Covert manipulation of the dietary fat to carbohydrate ratio of isoenergetically dense diets: Effect on food intake in feeding men ad libitum. *Int J Obes Relat Metab Disord* 20:651–660.

Swinburn BA, Boyce VL, Bergman RN, Howard BV, Bogardus C. 1991. Deterioration in carbohydrate metabolism and lipoprotein changes induced by modern, high fat diet in Pima Indians and Caucasians. *J Clin Endocrinol Metab* 73:156–165.

Takahashi M, Przetakiewicz M, Ong A, Borek C, Lowenstein JM. 1992. Effect of omega 3 and omega 6 fatty acids on transformation of cultured cells by irradiation and transfection. *Cancer Res* 52:154–162.

Tannenbaum A. 1942. The genesis and growth of tumors. II. Effects of caloric restriction per se. *Cancer Res* 2:460–467.

Tannenbaum A, Silverstone H. 1957. Nutrition and the genesis of tumours. In: Raven RW, ed. *Cancer,* Vol. 1. London: Butterworth. Pp. 306–334.

Taylor RJ, Bennett PH, LeGonidec G, Lacoste J, Combe D, Joffres M, Uili R, Charpin M, Zimmet PZ. 1983. The prevalence of diabetes mellitus in a traditional-living Polynesian population: The Wallis Island Survey. *Diabetes Care* 6:334–340.

Thomsen C, Rasmussen O, Christiansen C, Pedersen E, Vesterlund M, Storm H, Ingerslev J, Hermansen K. 1999. Comparison of the effects of a mono-unsaturated fat diet and a high carbohydrate diet on cardiovascular risk factors in first degree relatives to type-2 diabetic subjects. *Eur J Clin Nutr* 52:818–823.

Trichopoulou A, Katsouyanni K, Stuver S, Tzala L, Gnardellis C, Rimm E, Trichopoulos D. 1995. Consumption of olive oil and specific food groups in relation to breast cancer risk in Greece. *J Natl Cancer Inst* 87:110–116.

Trock B, Lanza E, Greenwald P. 1990. Dietary fiber, vegetables, and colon cancer: Critical review and meta-analyses of the epidemiologic evidence. *J Natl Cancer Inst* 82:650–661.

Tuomilehto J, Lindström J, Eriksson JG, Valle TT, Hämäläinen H, Ilanne-Parikka P, Keinänen-Kiukaanniemi S, Laakso M, Louheranta A, Rastas M, Salminen V, Uusitupa M. 2001. Prevention of type 2 diabetes mellitus by changes in lifestyle among subjects with impaired glucose tolerance. *N Engl J Med* 344:1343–1350.

Tuyns AJ, Kaaks R, Haelterman M. 1988. Colorectal cancer and the consumption of foods: A case-control study in Belgium. *Nutr Cancer* 11:189–204.

Tzonou A, Hsieh C-C, Polychronopoulou A, Kaprinis G, Toupadaki N, Trichopoulou A, Karakatsani A, Trichopoulos D. 1993. Diet and ovarian cancer: A case-control study in Greece. *Int J Cancer* 55:411–414.

Vainio H, Bianchini F. 2001. Physical activity and cancer prevention—Is 'no pain, no gain' passé? *Eur J Cancer Prev* 10:301–302.

van den Brandt PA, van't Veer P, Goldbohm RA, Dorant E, Volovics A, Hermus RJJ, Sturmans F. 1993. A prospective cohort study on dietary fat and the risk of postmenopausal breast cancer. *Cancer Res* 53:75–82.

Van Munster IP, Nagengast FM. 1993. The role of carbohydrate fermentation in colon cancer prevention. *Scand J Gastroenterol* 200:80–86.

van Raaij JMA, Katan MB, West CE, Hautvast JGAJ. 1982. Influence of diets con-taining casein, soy isolate, and soy concentrate on serum cholesterol and lipo-proteins in middle-aged volunteers. *Am J Clin Nutr* 35:925–934.

van Stratum P, Lussenburg RN, van Wezel LA, Vergroesen AJ, Cremer HD. 1978. The effect of dietary carbohydrate:fat ratio on energy intake by adult women. *Am J Clin Nutr* 31:206–212.

van't Veer P, Kok FJ, Brants HAM, Ockhuizen T, Sturmans F, Hermus RJJ. 1990. Dietary fat and the risk of breast cancer. *Int J Epidemiol* 19:12–18.

Veierød MB, Laake P, Thelle DS. 1997a. Dietary fat intake and risk of lung cancer: A prospective study of 51,452 Norwegian men and women. *Eur J Cancer Prev* 6:540–549.

Veierød MB, Laake P, Thelle DS. 1997b. Dietary fat intake and risk of prostate cancer: A prospective study of 25,708 Norwegian men. *Int J Cancer* 73:634–638.

Velie E, Kulldorff M, Schairer C, Block G, Albanes D, Schatzkin A. 2000. Dietary fat, fat subtypes, and breast cancer in postmenopausal women: A prospective cohort study. *J Natl Cancer Inst* 92:833–839.

Vessby B. 2000. Dietary fat and insulin action in humans. *Br J Nutr* 83:S91–S96.

Vessby B, Uusitupa M, Hermansen K, Riccardi G, Rivellese AA, Tapsell LC, Nälsén C, Berglund L, Louheranta A, Rasmussen BM, Calvert GD, Maffetone A, Pedersen E, Gustafsson I-B, Storlien LH. 2001. Substituting dietary saturated for monounsaturated fat impairs insulin sensitivity in healthy men and women: The KANWU study. *Diabetologia* 44:312–319.

Visek WJ. 1978. Diet and cell growth modulation by ammonia. *Am J Clin Nutr* 31:S216–S220.

von Schacky C, Angerer P, Kothny W, Theisen K, Mudra H. 1999. The effect of dietary ω-3 fatty acids on coronary atherosclerosis. A randomized, double-blind, placebo-controlled trial. *Ann Intern Med* 130:554–562.

Walker ARP, Cleaton-Jones PE. 1992. Sugar intake and dental caries. *Br Dent J* 172:7.

Wang G-S, Olsson JM, Eriksson LC, Stål P. 2000. Diet restriction increases ubiquinone contents and inhibits progression of hepatocellular carcinoma in the rat. *Scand J Gastroenterol* 35:83–89.

West CE, Sullivan DR, Katan MB, Halferkamps IL, van der Torre HW. 1990. Boys from populations with high-carbohydrate intake have higher fasting tri-glyceride levels than boys from populations with high-fat intake. *Am J Epidemiol* 131:271–282.

West DB, York B. 1998. Dietary fat, genetic predisposition, and obesity: Lessons from animal models. *Am J Clin Nutr* 67:505S–512S.

White E, Jacobs EJ, Daling JR. 1996. Physical activity in relation to colon cancer in middle-aged men and women. *Am J Epidemiol* 144:42–50.

Willett WC. 1997. Specific fatty acids and risks of breast and prostate cancer: Dietary intake. *Am J Clin Nutr* 66:1557S–1563S.

Willett WC. 1998. Is dietary fat a major determinant of body fat? *Am J Clin Nutr* 67:556S–562S.

Willett WC, Stampfer MJ, Colditz GA, Rosner BA, Hennekens CH, Speizer FE. 1987. Dietary fat and the risk of breast cancer. *N Engl J Med* 316:22–28.

Willett WC, Stampfer MJ, Colditz GA, Rosner BA, Speizer FE. 1990. Relation of meat, fat, and fiber intake to the risk of colon cancer in a prospective study among women. *N Engl J Med* 323:1664–1672.

Willett WC, Hunter DJ, Stampfer MJ, Colditz G, Manson JE, Spiegelman D, Rosner B, Hennekens CH, Speizer FE. 1992. Dietary fat and fiber in relation to risk of breast cancer. An 8-year follow-up. *J Am Med Assoc* 268:2037–2044.

Willett WC, Stampfer MJ, Mason JE, Colditz GA, Speizer FE, Rosner BA, Sampson LA, Hennekens CH. 1993. Intake of *trans* fatty acids and risk of coronary heart disease among women. *Lancet* 341:581–585.

Williams PT. 1997. Relationship of distance run per week to coronary heart disease risk factors in 8283 male runners. The National Runners' Health Study. *Arch Intern Med* 157:191–198.

Williams PT, Wood PD, Krauss RM, Haskell WL, Vranizan KM, Blair SN, Terry R, Farquhar JW. 1983. Does weight loss cause the exercise-induced increase in plasma high density lipoproteins? *Atherosclerosis* 47:173–185.

Williams PT, Krauss RM, Wood PD, Lindgren FT, Giotas C, Vranizan KM. 1986. Lipoprotein subfractions of runners and sedentary men. *Metabolism* 35:45–52.

Williams PT, Krauss RM, Vranizan KM, Wood PDS. 1990. Changes in lipoprotein subfractions during diet-induced and exercise-induced weight loss in moderately overweight men. *Circulation* 81:1293–1304.

Williams PT, Krauss RM, Vranizan KM, Albers JJ, Wood PDS. 1992. Effects of weight-loss by exercise and by diet on apolipoproteins A-I and A-II and the particle-size distribution of high-density lipoproteins in men. *Metabolism* 41:441–449.

Williams PT, Stefanick ML, Vranizan KM, Wood PD. 1994. The effects of weight loss by exercise or by dieting on plasma high-density lipoprotein (HDL) levels in men with low, intermediate, and normal-to-high HDL at baseline. *Metabolism* 43:917–924.

Williamson DF, Madans J, Anda RF, Kleinman JC, Kahn HS, Byers T. 1993. Recreational physical activity and ten-year weight change in a US national cohort. *Int J Obes Relat Metab Disord* 17:279–286.

Wolever TMS, Jenkins DJA. 1993. Effect of dietary fiber and foods on carbohydrate metabolism. In: Spiller G, ed. *CRC Handbook of Dietary Fiber in Human Nutrition.* Boca Raton, FL: CRC Press. Pp. 111–162.

Wolever TMS, Jenkins DJA, Ocana AM, Rao VA, Collier GR. 1988. Second-meal effect: Low-glycemic-index foods eaten at dinner improve subsequent breakfast glycemic response. *Am J Clin Nutr* 48:1041–1047.

Wolfe BMJ, Piché LA. 1999. Replacement of carbohydrate by protein in a conventional-fat diet reduces cholesterol and triglyceride concentrations in healthy normolipidemic subjects. *Clin Invest Med* 22:140–148.

Wood PD, Stefanick ML, Dreon DM, Frey-Hewitt B, Garay SC, Williams PT, Superko HR, Fortmann SP, Albers JJ, Vranizan KM, Ellsworth NM, Terry RB, Haskell WL. 1988. Changes in plasma lipids and lipoproteins in overweight men during weight loss through dieting as compared with exercise. *N Engl J Med* 319:1173–1179.

Wood PJ, Braaten JT, Scott FW, Riedel KD, Wolynetz MS, Collins MW. 1994. Effect of dose and modification of viscous properties of oat gum on plasma glucose and insulin following an oral glucose load. *Br J Nutr* 72:731–743.

Wu Y, Zheng W, Sellars TA, Kushi LH, Bostick RM, Potter JD. 1994. Dietary cholesterol, fat, and lung cancer incidence among older women: The Iowa Women's Health Study (United States). *Cancer Causes Control* 5:395–400.

Yost TJ, Jensen DR, Haugen BR, Eckel RH. 1998. Effect of dietary macronutrient composition on tissue-specific lipoprotein lipase activity and insulin action in normal-weight subjects. *Am J Clin Nutr* 68:296–302.

Yu S, Derr J, Etherton TD, Kris-Etherton PM. 1995. Plasma cholesterol-predictive equations demonstrate that stearic acid is neutral and monounsaturated fatty acids are hypocholesterolemic. *Am J Clin Nutr* 61:1129–1139.

Yudkin J, Eisa O, Kang SS, Meraji S, Bruckdorfer KR. 1986. Dietary sucrose affects plasma HDL cholesterol concentration in young men. *Ann Nutr Metab* 30: 261–266.

Yu-Poth S, Zhao G, Etherton T, Naglak M, Jonnalagadda S, Kris-Etherton PM. 1999. Effects of the National Cholesterol Education Program's Step I and Step II dietary intervention programs on cardiovascular disease risk factors: A meta-analysis. *Am J Clin Nutr* 69:632–646.

Zambon S, Friday KE, Childs MT, Fujimoto WY, Bierman EL, Ensinck JW. 1992. Effect of glyburide and ω3 fatty acid dietary supplements on glucose and lipid metabolism in patients with non-insulin-dependent diabetes mellitus. *Am J Clin Nutr* 56:447–454.

Zhu Z, Jiang W, Thompson HJ. 1999. Effect of energy restriction on tissue size regulation during chemically induced mammary carcinogenesis. *Carcinogenesis* 20:1721–1726.

4

A Model for the Development of Tolerable Upper Intake Levels

BACKGROUND

The *Tolerable Upper Intake Level* (UL) refers to the highest level of daily nutrient intake that is likely to pose no risk of adverse health effects for almost all individuals in the general population. As intake increases above the UL, the risk of adverse effects increases. The term *tolerable* is chosen because it connotes a level of intake that can, with high probability, be tolerated biologically by individuals; it does not imply acceptability of that level in any other sense. The setting of a UL does not indicate that nutrient intakes greater than the Recommended Dietary Allowance (RDA) or Adequate Intake (AI) are recommended as being beneficial to an individual. Many individuals are self-medicating with nutrients for curative or treatment purposes. It is beyond the scope of this report to address the possible therapeutic benefits of higher nutrient intakes that may offset the risk of adverse effects. The UL is not meant to apply to individuals who are treated with the nutrient under medical supervision or to individuals with predisposing conditions that modify their sensitivity to the nutrient. This chapter describes a model for developing ULs.

The term *adverse effect* is defined as any significant alteration in the structure or function of the human organism (Klaassen et al., 1986) or any impairment of a physiologically important function that could lead to a health effect that is adverse, in accordance with the definition set by the joint World Health Organization, Food and Agriculture Organization of the United Nations, and International Atomic Energy Agency Expert Consultation in Trace Elements in Human Nutrition and Health (WHO, 1996). In the case of nutrients, it is exceedingly important to consider the possi-

84

bility that the intake of one nutrient may alter, in detrimental ways, the health benefits conferred by another nutrient. Any such alteration (referred to as an adverse nutrient–nutrient interaction) is considered an adverse health effect. When evidence for such adverse interactions is available, it is considered in establishing a nutrient's UL.

ULs are useful because of the increased interest in, and availability of, fortified foods, the increased use of dietary supplements, and the growing recognition of the health consequences of excesses, as well as inadequacies of nutrient intakes. ULs are based on total intake of a nutrient from food, water, and supplements if adverse effects have been associated with total intake. However, if adverse effects have been associated with intake from supplements or food fortificants only, the UL is based on a nutrient intake from those sources only, not on total intake. The UL applies to chronic daily use.

For many nutrients, there are insufficient data on which to develop a UL. This does not mean that there is no potential for adverse effects resulting from high intake. When data about adverse effects are extremely limited, extra caution may be warranted.

Like all chemical agents, nutrients can produce adverse health effects if their intake from a combination of food, water, nutrient supplements, and pharmacological agents is excessive. Some lower level of nutrient intake will ordinarily pose no likelihood (or risk) of adverse health effects in normal individuals even if the level is above that associated with any benefit. It is not possible to identify a single risk-free intake level for a nutrient that can be applied with certainty to all members of a population. However, it is possible to develop intake levels that are unlikely to pose risk of adverse health effects for most members of the general population, including sensitive individuals. For some nutrients, these intake levels may pose a risk to subpopulations with extreme or distinct vulnerabilities.

Whether routine, long-term intake above the UL is safe is not well documented. Although members of the general population should not routinely exceed the UL, intake above the UL may be appropriate for investigation within well-controlled clinical trials. Clinical trials of doses above the UL should not be discouraged as long as subjects participating in these trials have signed informed consent documents regarding possible toxicity, and as long as these trials employ appropriate safety monitoring of trial subjects.

A MODEL FOR THE DERIVATION OF TOLERABLE UPPER INTAKE LEVELS

The possibility that the methodology used to derive Tolerable Upper Intake Levels (ULs) might be reduced to a mathematical model that could be generically applied to all nutrients was considered. Such a model might have several potential advantages, including ease of application and assurance of consistent treatment of all nutrients. It was concluded, however, that the current state of scientific understanding of toxic phenomena in general, and nutrient toxicity in particular, is insufficient to support the development of such a model. Scientific information about various adverse effects and their relationships to intake levels varies greatly among nutrients and depends on the nature, comprehensiveness, and quality of available data. The uncertainties associated with the unavoidable problem of extrapolating from the circumstances under which data are developed (e.g., in the laboratory or clinic) to other circumstances (e.g., to the healthy population) add to the complexity.

Given the current state of knowledge, any attempt to capture, in a mathematical model, all of the information and scientific judgments that must be made to reach conclusions about ULs would not be consistent with contemporary risk assessment practices. Instead, the model for the derivation of ULs consists of a set of scientific factors that always should be considered explicitly. The framework by which these factors are organized is called *risk assessment*. Risk assessment (NRC, 1983, 1994) is a systematic means of evaluating the probability of occurrence of adverse health effects in humans from excess exposure to an environmental agent (in this case, a nutrient) (FAO/WHO, 1995; Health Canada, 1993). The hallmark of risk assessment is the requirement to be explicit in all of the evaluations and judgments that must be made to document conclusions.

RISK ASSESSMENT AND FOOD SAFETY

Basic Concepts

Risk assessment is a scientific undertaking having as its objective a characterization of the nature and likelihood of harm resulting from human exposure to agents in the environment. The characterization of risk typically contains both qualitative and quantitative information and includes a discussion of the scientific uncertainties in that information. In the present context, the agents of interest are nutrients, and the environmental media are food, water, and nonfood sources such as nutrient supplements and pharmacological preparations.

Performing a risk assessment results in a characterization of the relationships between exposure to an agent and the likelihood that adverse health effects will occur in members of exposed populations. Scientific uncertainties are an inherent part of the risk assessment process and are discussed below. Deciding whether the magnitude of exposure is *acceptable* or *tolerable* in specific circumstances is not a component of risk assessment; this activity falls within the domain of *risk management*. Risk management decisions depend on the results of risk assessments, but may also involve the public health significance of the risk, the technical feasibility of achieving various degrees of risk control, and the economic and social costs of this control. Because there is no single, scientifically definable distinction between safe and unsafe exposures, risk management necessarily incorporates components of sound, practical decision making that are not addressed by the risk assessment process (NRC, 1983, 1994).

Risk assessment requires that information be organized in rather specific ways, but it does not require any specific scientific evaluation methods. Rather, risk assessors must evaluate scientific information using what they judge to be appropriate methods and must make explicit the basis for their judgments, the uncertainties in risk estimates, and, when appropriate, alternative scientifically plausible interpretations of the available data (NRC, 1994; OTA, 1993).

Risk assessment is subject to two types of scientific uncertainties: those related to data and those associated with inferences that are required when directly applicable data are not available (NRC, 1994). Data uncertainties arise during the evaluation of information obtained from the epidemiological and toxicological studies of nutrient intake levels that are the basis for risk assessments. Examples of inferences include the use of data from experimental animals to estimate responses in humans and the selection of uncertainty factors to estimate inter- and intraspecies variabilities in response to toxic substances. Uncertainties arise whenever estimates of adverse health effects in humans are based on extrapolations of data obtained under dissimilar conditions (e.g., from experimental animal studies). Options for dealing with uncertainties are discussed below and in detail in Appendix L.

Steps in the Risk Assessment Process

The organization of risk assessment is based on a model proposed by the National Research Council (NRC, 1983, 1994) that is widely used in public health and regulatory decision making. The steps of risk assessment as applied to nutrients follow (see also Figure 4-1).

• Step 1. Hazard identification involves the collection, organization, and evaluation of all information pertaining to the adverse effects of a given nutrient. It concludes with a summary of the evidence concerning the capacity of the nutrient to cause one or more types of toxicity in humans.
• Step 2. Dose–response assessment determines the relationship between nutrient intake (dose) and adverse effect (in terms of incidence

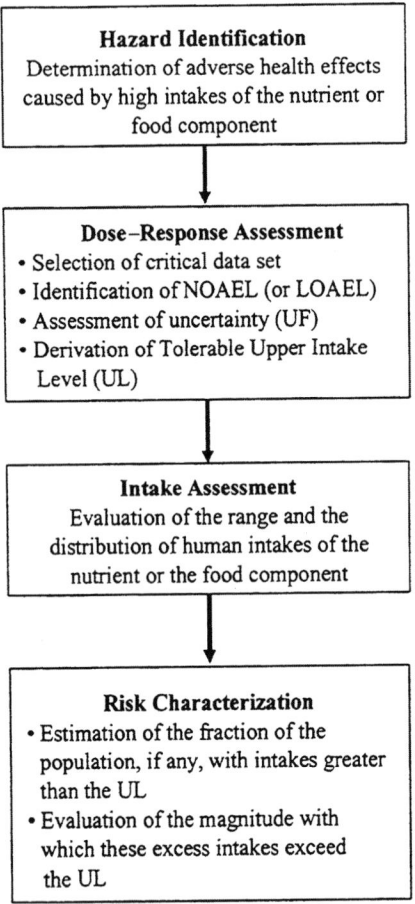

FIGURE 4-1 Risk assessment model for nutrient toxicity. NOAEL = no-observed-adverse-effect level; LOAEL = lowest-observed-adverse-effect level; UF = uncertainty factor.

and severity). This step concludes with an estimate of the Tolerable Upper Intake Level (UL)—it identifies the highest level of daily nutrient intake that is likely to pose no risk of adverse health effects for almost all individuals in the general population. Different ULs may be developed for various life stage groups.

• Step 3. Intake assessment evaluates the distribution of usual total daily nutrient intakes for members of the general population. In cases where the UL pertains only to supplement use and does not pertain to usual food intakes of the nutrient, the assessment is directed at supplement intakes only. It does not depend on Step 1 or 2.

• Step 4. Risk characterization summarizes the conclusions from Steps 1 and 2 with Step 3 to determine the risk. The risk is generally expressed as the fraction of the exposed population, if any, having nutrient intakes (Step 3) in excess of the estimated UL (Steps 1 and 2). If possible, characterization also covers the magnitude of any such excesses. Scientific uncertainties associated with both the UL and the intake estimates are described so that risk managers understand the degree of scientific confidence they can place in the risk assessment.

The risk assessment contains no discussion of recommendations for reducing risk; these are the focus of risk management.

Thresholds

A principal feature of the risk assessment process for noncarcinogens is the long-standing acceptance that no risk of adverse effects is expected unless a threshold dose (or intake) is exceeded. The adverse effects that may be caused by a nutrient almost certainly occur only when the threshold dose is exceeded (NRC, 1994; WHO, 1996). The critical issue concerns the methods used to identify the approximate threshold of toxicity for a large and diverse human population. Because most nutrients are not considered to be carcinogenic in humans, approaches used for carcinogenic risk assessment are not discussed here.

Thresholds vary among members of the general population (NRC, 1994). For any given adverse effect, if the distribution of thresholds in the population could be quantitatively identified, it would be possible to establish ULs by defining some point in the lower tail of the distribution of thresholds that would protect some specified fraction of the population. The method described here for identifying thresholds for a general population is designed to ensure that almost all members of the population will be protected, but it is not based on an analysis of the theoretical (but practically unattainable) distribution of thresholds. By using the model to derive the threshold, however, there is considerable confidence that the threshold, which becomes the UL for nutrients or food components, lies very near the low end of the theoretical distribution and is the end representing the most sensitive members of the population. For some nutrients there may be subpopulations that are not included in the general distribution because of extreme or distinct vulnerabilities to toxicity. Data relating to the effects observed in these groups are not used to derive ULs. Such distinct groups, whose conditions warrant medical supervision, may not be protected by the UL.

The Joint FAO/WHO Expert Committee on Food Additives and various national regulatory bodies have identified factors (called *uncertainty factors* [UFs]) that account for interspecies and intraspecies differences in response to the hazardous effects of substances and for other uncertainties (WHO, 1987). UFs are used to make inferences about the threshold dose of substances for members of a large and diverse human population from data on adverse effects obtained in epidemiological or experimental studies. These factors are applied consistently when data of specific types and quality are available. They are typically used to derive acceptable daily intakes for food additives and other substances for which data on adverse effects are considered sufficient to meet minimum standards of quality and completeness (FAO/WHO, 1982). These adopted or recognized UFs have sometimes been coupled with other factors to compensate for deficiencies in the available data and other uncertainties regarding data.

When possible, the UL is based on a no-observed-adverse-effect level (NOAEL), which is the highest intake (or experimental oral dose) of a nutrient at which no adverse effects have been observed in the individuals studied. This is identified for a specific circumstance in the hazard identification and dose–response assessment steps of the risk. If there are no adequate data demonstrating a NOAEL, then a lowest-observed-adverse-effect level (LOAEL) may be used. A LOAEL is the lowest intake (or experimental oral dose) at which an adverse effect has been identified. The derivation of a UL from a NOAEL (or LOAEL) involves a series of choices about which factors should be used to deal with uncertainties. Uncertainty factors are applied in an attempt to deal both with gaps in data and with incomplete knowledge about the inferences required (e.g., the expected variability in response within the human population). The problems of both data and inference uncertainties arise in all steps of the risk assessment. A discussion of options available for dealing with these uncertainties is presented below and in greater detail in Appendix L.

A UL is not, in itself, a description or estimate of human risk. It is derived by application of the hazard identification and dose–response evaluation steps (Steps 1 and 2) of the risk assessment model. To determine whether populations are at risk requires an intake or exposure assessment (Step 3, evaluation of intakes of the nutrient by the population) and a determination of the fractions of these populations, if any, whose intakes exceed the UL. In the intake assessment and risk characterization steps (Steps 3 and 4), the distribution of usual intakes for the population is used as a basis for determining whether, and to what extent, the population is at risk (Figure 4-1). A discussion of other aspects of the risk characterization that may be useful in judging the public health significance of the risk and in risk management decisions is provided in the final section of this chapter "Risk Characterization."

APPLICATION OF THE RISK ASSESSMENT MODEL TO NUTRIENTS

This section provides guidance for applying the risk assessment framework (the model) to the derivation of Tolerable Upper Intake Levels (ULs) for nutrients.

Special Problems Associated with Substances Required for Human Nutrition

Although the risk assessment model outlined above can be applied to nutrients to derive ULs, it must be recognized that nutrients possess some properties that distinguish them from the types of agents for which the risk assessment model was originally developed (NRC, 1983). In the application of accepted standards for risk assessment of environmental chemicals to risk assessment of nutrients, a fundamental difference between the two categories must be recognized: within a certain range of intakes, nutrients are essential for human well-being and usually for life itself. Nonetheless, they may share with other chemicals the production of adverse effects at excessive exposures. Because the consumption of balanced diets is consistent with the development and survival of humankind over many millennia, there is less need for the large uncertainty factors that have been used for the risk assessment of nonessential chemicals. In addition, if data on the adverse effects of nutrients are available primarily from studies in human populations, there will be less uncertainty than is associated with the types of data available on nonessential chemicals.

There is no evidence to suggest that nutrients consumed at the recommended intake (the Recommended Dietary Allowance or Adequate Intake) present a risk of adverse effects to the general population.[1] It is clear, however, that the addition of nutrients to a diet through the ingestion of large amounts of highly fortified food, nonfood sources such as supplements, or both, may (at some level) pose a risk of adverse health effects. The UL is the highest level of daily nutrient intake that is likely to pose no risk of adverse health effects for almost all individuals in the general population. As intake increases above the UL, the risk of adverse effects increases.

If adverse effects have been associated with total intake, ULs are based on total intake of a nutrient from food, water, and supplements. For cases in which adverse effects have been associated with intake only from supple-

---

[1]It is recognized that possible exceptions to this generalization relate to specific geochemical areas with excessive environmental exposures to certain trace elements (e.g., selenium) and to rare case reports of adverse effects associated with highly eccentric consumption of specific foods. Data from such findings are generally not useful for setting ULs for the general North American population.

ments and food fortificants, the UL is based on intake from these sources only, rather than on total intake. The effects of nutrients from fortified foods or supplements may differ from those of naturally occurring constituents of foods because of the chemical form of the nutrient, the timing of the intake and amount consumed in a single bolus dose, the matrix supplied by the food, and the relation of the nutrient to the other constituents of the diet. Nutrient requirements and food intake are related to the metabolizing body mass, which is also at least an indirect measure of the space in which the nutrients are distributed. This relation between food intake and space of distribution supports homeostasis, which maintains nutrient concentrations in that space within a range compatible with health. However, excessive intake of a single nutrient from supplements or fortificants may compromise this homeostatic mechanism. Such elevations alone may pose risks of adverse effects; imbalances among the nutrients may also be possible. These reasons and those discussed previously support the need to include the form and pattern of consumption in the assessment of risk from high nutrient or food component intake.

Consideration of Variability in Sensitivity

The risk assessment model outlined in this chapter is consistent with classical risk assessment approaches in that it must consider variability in the sensitivity of individuals to adverse effects of nutrients or food components. A discussion of how variability is dealt with in the context of nutritional risk assessment follows.

Physiological changes and common conditions associated with growth and maturation that occur during an individual's lifespan may influence sensitivity to nutrient toxicity. For example, sensitivity increases with declines in lean body mass and with the declines in renal and liver function that occur with aging; sensitivity changes in direct relation to intestinal absorption or intestinal synthesis of nutrients; sensitivity increases in the newborn infant because of rapid brain growth and limited ability to secrete or biotransform toxicants; and sensitivity increases with decreases in the rate of metabolism of nutrients. During pregnancy, the increase in total body water and glomerular filtration results in lower blood levels of water-soluble vitamins dose for dose, and therefore results in reduced susceptibility to potential adverse effects. However, in the unborn fetus this may be offset by active placental transfer, accumulation of certain nutrients in the amniotic fluid, and rapid development of the brain. Examples of life stage groups that may differ in terms of nutritional needs and toxicological sensitivity include infants and children, the elderly, and women during pregnancy and lactation.

Even within relatively homogeneous life stage groups, there is a range of sensitivities to toxic effects. The model described below accounts for the normal expected variability in sensitivity, but it excludes subpopulations with extreme and distinct vulnerabilities. Such subpopulations consist of individuals needing medical supervision; they are better served through the use of public health screening, product labeling, or other individualized health care strategies. Such populations may not be at *negligible risk* when their intakes reach the UL developed for the healthy population. The decision to treat identifiable vulnerable subgroups as distinct (not protected by the UL) is a matter of judgment and is discussed in the individual nutrient chapters, as applicable.

Bioavailability

In the context of toxicity, the bioavailability of an ingested nutrient can be defined as its accessibility to normal metabolic and physiological processes. Bioavailability influences a nutrient's beneficial effects at physiological levels of intake and also may affect the nature and severity of toxicity due to excessive intakes. The concentration and chemical form of the nutrient, the nutrition and health of the individual, and excretory losses all affect bioavailability. Bioavailability data for specific nutrients must be considered and incorporated into the risk assessment process.

Some nutrients may be less readily absorbed when part of a meal than when consumed separately. Supplemental forms of some nutrients may require special consideration if they have higher bioavailability since they may present a greater risk of producing adverse effects than equivalent amounts from the natural form found in food.

Nutrient–Nutrient Interactions

A diverse array of adverse health effects can occur as a result of the interaction of nutrients. The potential risks of adverse nutrient–nutrient interactions increase when there is an imbalance in the intake of two or more nutrients. Excessive intake of one nutrient may interfere with absorption, excretion, transport, storage, function, or metabolism of a second nutrient. Possible adverse nutrient–nutrient interactions are considered as a part of setting a UL. Nutrient–nutrient interactions may be considered either as a critical endpoint on which to base a UL, or as supportive evidence for a UL based on another endpoint.

Other Relevant Factors That Affect the Bioavailability of Nutrients

In addition to nutrient interactions, other considerations have the potential to influence nutrient bioavailability, such as the nutritional status of an individual and the form of intake. These issues are considered in the risk assessment. With regard to the form of intake, fat-soluble vitamins, such as vitamin A, are more readily absorbed when they are part of a meal that is high in fat. ULs must therefore be based on nutrients as part of the total diet, including the contribution from water. Nutrient supplements that are taken separately from food require special consideration because they are likely to have different bioavailabilities and therefore may represent a greater risk of producing adverse effects.

STEPS IN THE DEVELOPMENT OF THE TOLERABLE UPPER INTAKE LEVEL

Hazard Identification

Based on a thorough review of the scientific literature, the hazard identification step outlines the adverse health effects that have been demonstrated to be caused by the nutrient. The primary types of data used as background for identifying nutrient hazards in humans are:

- *Human studies.* Human data provide the most relevant kind of information for hazard identification and, when they are of sufficient quality and extent, are given the greatest weight. However, the number of controlled human toxicity studies conducted in a clinical setting is very limited because of ethical reasons. Such studies are generally most useful for identifying very mild (and ordinarily reversible) adverse effects. Observational studies that focus on well-defined populations with clear exposures to a range of nutrient intake levels are useful for establishing a relationship between exposure and effect. Observational data in the form of case reports or anecdotal evidence are used for developing hypotheses that can lead to knowledge of causal associations. Sometimes a series of case reports, if it shows a clear and distinct pattern of effects, may be reasonably convincing on the question of causality.
- *Animal data.* Most of the available data used in regulatory risk assessments come from controlled laboratory experiments in animals, usually mammalian species other than humans (e.g., rodents). Such data are used in part because human data on nonessential chemicals are generally very limited. Moreover, there is a long-standing history of the use of animal studies to identify the toxic properties of chemical substances, and there is no inherent reason why animal data should not be relevant to the evaluation of nutrient toxicity. Animal studies offer several advantages over human studies. They can, for example, be readily controlled so that causal relationships can be recognized. It is possible to identify the full range of toxic effects produced by a chemical, over a wide range of exposures, and

---

BOX 4-1
Development of Tolerable Upper Intake Levels (ULs)

COMPONENTS OF HAZARD IDENTIFICATION
- Evidence of adverse effects in humans
- Causality
- Relevance of experimental data
- Pharmacokinetic and metabolic data
- Mechanisms of toxic action
- Quality and completeness of the database
- Identification of distinct and highly sensitive subpopulations

COMPONENTS OF DOSE–RESPONSE ASSESSMENT
- Data selection and identification of critical endpoints
- Identification of no-observed-adverse-effect level (NOAEL) (or lowest-observed-adverse-effect level [LOAEL]) and critical endpoint
- Assessment of uncertainty and data on variability in response
- Derivation of a UL
- Characterization of the estimate and special considerations

---

to establish dose–response relationships. The effects of chronic exposures can be identified in far less time than they can with the use of epidemiological methods. All these advantages of animal data, however, may not always overcome the fact that species differences in response to chemical substances can sometimes be profound, and any extrapolation of animal data to predict human response needs to take this possibility into account.

Key issues that are addressed in the data evaluation of human and animal studies are described below (see Box 4-1).

Evidence of Adverse Effects in Humans

The hazard identification step involves the examination of human, animal, and in vitro published evidence that addresses the likelihood of a nutrient eliciting an adverse effect in humans. Decisions about which observed effects are adverse are based on scientific judgment. Although toxicologists generally regard any demonstrable structural or functional alteration as representing an adverse effect, some alterations may be considered to be of little or self-limiting biological importance. As noted earlier, adverse nutrient–nutrient interactions are considered in the definition of an adverse effect.

Causality

The identification of a hazard is strengthened by evidence of causality. As explained in Chapter 2, the criteria of Hill (1971) are considered in judging the causal significance of an exposure–effect association indicated by epidemiological studies.

Relevance of Experimental Data

Consideration of the following issues can be useful in assessing the relevance of experimental data.

Animal Data. Some animal data may be of limited utility in judging the toxicity of nutrients because of highly variable interspecies differences in nutrient requirements. Nevertheless, relevant animal data are considered in the hazard identification and dose–response assessment steps where applicable, and, in general, they are used for hazard identification unless there are data demonstrating they are not relevant to humans, or it is clear that the available human data are sufficient.

Route of Exposure.[2] Data derived from studies involving oral exposure (rather than parenteral, inhalation, or dermal exposure) are most useful for the evaluation of nutrients. Data derived from studies involving parenteral, inhalation, or dermal routes of exposure may be considered relevant if the adverse effects are systemic and data are available to permit interroute extrapolation.

Duration of Exposure. Because the magnitude, duration, and frequency of exposure can vary considerably in different situations, consideration needs to be given to the relevance of the exposure scenario (e.g., chronic daily dietary exposure versus short-term bolus doses) to dietary intakes by human populations.

Pharmacokinetic and Metabolic Data

When available, data regarding the rates of nutrient absorption, distribution, metabolism, and excretion may be important in derivation of Tolerable Upper Intake Levels (ULs). Such data may provide significant information regarding the interspecies differences and similarities in

---

[2]The terms *route of exposure* and *route of intake* refer to how a substance enters the body (e.g., by ingestion, injection, or dermal absorption). These terms should not be confused with *form of intake*, which refers to the medium or vehicle used (e.g., supplements, food, or drinking water).

nutrient behavior, and so may assist in identifying relevant animal data. They may also assist in identifying life stage differences in response to nutrient toxicity.

In some cases, there may be limited or even no significant data relating to nutrient toxicity. It is conceivable that in such cases pharmacokinetic and metabolic data may provide valuable insights into the magnitude of the UL. Thus, if there are significant pharmacokinetic and metabolic data over the range of intakes that meet nutrient requirements, and if it is shown that this pattern of pharmacokinetic and metabolic data does not change in the range of intakes greater than those required for nutrition, it may be possible to infer the absence of toxic risk in this range. In contrast, an alteration of pharmacokinetics or metabolism may suggest the potential for adverse effects. There has been no case encountered thus far in which sufficient pharmacokinetic and metabolic data are available for establishing ULs in this fashion, but it is possible such situations may arise in the future.

Mechanisms of Toxic Action

Knowledge of molecular and cellular events underlying the production of toxicity can assist in dealing with the problems of extrapolation between species and from high to low doses. It may also aid in understanding whether the mechanisms associated with toxicity are those associated with deficiency. In most cases, however, because knowledge of the biochemical sequence of events resulting from toxicity and deficiency is still incomplete, it is not yet possible to state with certainty whether these sequences share a common pathway.

Quality and Completeness of the Database

The scientific quality and quantity of the database are evaluated. Human or animal data are reviewed for suggestions that the nutrient has the potential to produce additional adverse health effects. If suggestions are found, additional studies may be recommended.

Identification of Distinct and Highly Sensitive Subpopulations

The ULs are based on protecting the most sensitive members of the general population from adverse effects of high nutrient intake. Some highly sensitive subpopulations have responses (in terms of incidence, severity, or both) to the agent of interest that are clearly distinct from the responses expected for the healthy population. The risk assessment process recognizes that there may be individuals within any life stage group who are more biologically sensitive than others, and thus their extreme sensitivities do not fall within the range of sensitivities expected for the general population. The UL for the general population may not be protective for these subgroups. As indicated earlier, the extent to which a distinct subpopulation will be included in the derivation of a UL for the general population is an area of judgment to be addressed on a case-by-case basis.

Dose–Response Assessment

The process for deriving the UL is described in this section and outlined in Box 4-1. It includes selection of the critical data set, identification of a critical endpoint with its no-observed-adverse-effect level (NOAEL) or lowest-observed-adverse-effect level (LOAEL), and assessment of uncertainty.

Data Selection and Identification of Critical Endpoints

The data evaluation process results in the selection of the most appropriate or critical data sets for deriving the UL. Selecting the critical data set includes the following considerations:

• Human data, when adequate to evaluate adverse effects, are preferable to animal data, although the latter may provide useful supportive information.
• In the absence of appropriate human data, information from an animal species with biological responses most like those of humans is most valuable. Pharmacokinetic, metabolic, and mechanistic data may be available to assist in the identification of relevant animal species.
• If it is not possible to identify such a species or to select such data, data from the most sensitive animal species, strain, and gender combination are given the greatest emphasis.
• The route of exposure that most resembles the route of expected human intake is preferable. This consideration includes the digestive state (e.g., fed or fasted) of the subjects or experimental animals. When this is not possible, the differences in route of exposure are noted as a source of uncertainty.
• The critical data set defines a dose–response relationship between intake and the extent of the toxic response known to be most relevant to humans. Data on bioavailability are considered and adjustments in expressions of dose–response are made to determine whether any apparent differences in response can be explained.
• The critical data set documents the route of exposure and the magnitude and duration of the intake. Furthermore, the critical data set documents the NOAEL (or LOAEL).

Identification of a NOAEL (or LOAEL)

A nutrient can produce more than one toxic effect (or endpoint), even within the same species or in studies using the same or different exposure durations. The NOAELs and LOAELs for these effects will ordinarily differ. The critical endpoint used to establish a UL is the adverse biological effect exhibiting the lowest NOAEL (e.g., the most sensitive indicator of a nutrient's toxicity). Because the selection of uncertainty factors (UFs) depends in part upon the seriousness of the adverse effect, it is possible that lower ULs may result from the use of the most *serious* (rather than most *sensitive*) endpoint. Thus, it is often necessary to evaluate several endpoints independently to determine which leads to the lowest UL.

For some nutrients, there may be inadequate data on which to develop a UL. The lack of reports of adverse effects following excess intake of a nutrient does not mean that adverse effects do not occur. As the intake of any nutrient increases, a point (see Figure 4-2) is reached at which intake begins to pose a risk. Above this point, increased intake increases the risk of adverse effects. For some nutrients and for various reasons, there are inadequate data to identify this point, or even to estimate its location.

Because adverse effects are almost certain to occur for any nutrient at some level of intake, it should be assumed that such effects may occur for nutrients for which a scientifically documentable UL cannot now be derived. Until a UL is set or an alternative approach to identifying protec-

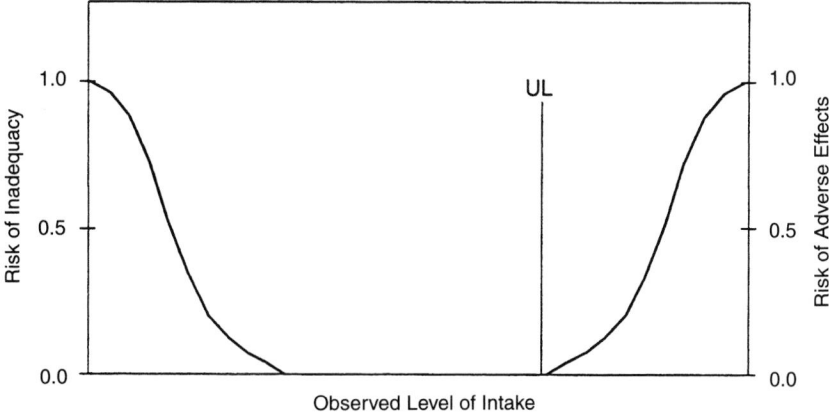

FIGURE 4-2 Theoretical description of health effects of a nutrient as a function of level of intake. The Tolerable Upper Intake Level (UL) is the highest level of daily nutrient intake that is likely to pose no risk of adverse health effects for almost all individuals in the general population. At intakes above the UL, the risk of adverse effects increases.

tive limits is developed, intakes greater than the Recommended Dietary Allowance (RDA) or Adequate Intake (AI) should be viewed with caution.

The absence of sufficient data to establish a UL points to the need for studies suitable for developing ULs.

Uncertainty Assessment

Several judgments must be made regarding the uncertainties and thus the uncertainty factor (UF) associated with extrapolating from the observed data to the general population (see Appendix L). Applying a UF to a NOAEL (or LOAEL) results in a value for the derived UL that is less than the experimentally derived NOAEL unless the UF is 1. The greater the uncertainty, the larger the UF and the smaller the resulting UL. This is consistent with the ultimate goal of the risk assessment: to provide an estimate of a level of intake that will protect the health of virtually all members of the healthy population (Mertz et al., 1994).

Although several reports describe the underlying basis for UFs (Dourson and Stara, 1983; Zielhuis and van der Kreek, 1979), the strength of the evidence supporting the use of a specific UF will vary. Because the imprecision of these UFs is a major limitation of risk assessment approaches, considerable leeway must be allowed for the application of scientific judgment in making the final determination. Because data are generally available regarding intakes of nutrients in human populations, the data on nutrient toxicity may not be subject to the same uncertainties as are data on nonessential chemical agents. The resulting UFs for nutrients and food components are typically less than the factors of 10 often applied to nonessential toxic substances. The UFs are lower with higher quality data and when the adverse effects are extremely mild and reversible.

In general, when determining a UF, the following potential sources of uncertainty are considered and combined in the final UF:

- *Interindividual variation in sensitivity.* Small UFs (close to 1) are used to represent this source of uncertainty if it is judged that little population variability is expected for the adverse effect, and larger factors (close to 10) are used if variability is expected to be great (NRC, 1994).
- *Extrapolation from experimental animals to humans.* A UF to account for the uncertainty in extrapolating animal data to humans is generally applied to the NOAEL when animal data are the primary data available. While a default UF of 10 is often used to extrapolate animal data to humans for nonessential chemicals, a lower UF may be used because of data showing some similarities between the animal and human responses (NRC, 1994).
- *LOAEL instead of NOAEL.* If a NOAEL is not available, a UF may be applied to account for the uncertainty in deriving a UL from the LOAEL.

The size of the UF involves scientific judgment based on the severity and incidence of the observed effect at the LOAEL and the steepness (slope) of the dose–response.

- *Subchronic NOAEL to predict chronic NOAEL.* When data are lacking on chronic exposures, scientific judgment is necessary to determine whether chronic exposures are likely to lead to adverse effects at lower intakes than those producing effects after subchronic exposures (exposures of shorter duration).

Derivation of a UL

The UL is derived by dividing the NOAEL (or LOAEL) by a single UF that incorporates all relevant uncertainties. ULs, expressed as amount per day, are derived for various life stage groups using relevant databases, NOAELs, LOAELs, and UFs. In cases where no data exist with regard to NOAELs or LOAELs for the group under consideration, extrapolations from data in other age groups or animal data are made on the basis of known differences in body size, physiology, metabolism, absorption, and excretion of the nutrient.

Generally, any age group adjustments are made based solely on differences in body weight, unless there are data demonstrating age-related differences in nutrient pharmacokinetics, metabolism, or mechanism of action.

The derivation of the UL involves the use of scientific judgment to select the appropriate NOAEL (or LOAEL) and UF. As shown in Figure 4-3, when using the same critical endpoint there is a greater level of uncertainty in setting the UL based on a LOAEL compared with a NOAEL. The risk assessment requires explicit consideration and discussion of all choices made regarding both the data used and the uncertainties accounted for. These considerations are discussed in the nutrient chapters.

Characterization of the Estimate and Special Considerations

If the data review reveals the existence of subpopulations having distinct and exceptional sensitivities to a nutrient's toxicity, these subpopulations are explicitly discussed and concerns related to adverse effects are noted; however, the use of the data is not included in the identification of the NOAEL or LOAEL, upon which the UL for the general population is based.

Circumstances in Which No UL Is Established

There are two general conditions under which ULs are not established. In some cases, the availability of insufficient evidence regarding a

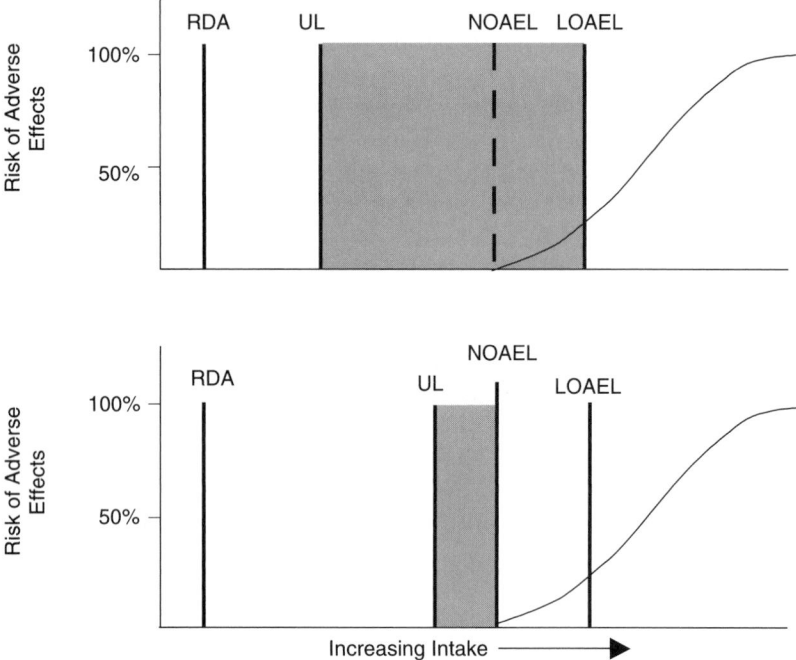

FIGURE 4-3 Effect of uncertainty assessment on the Tolerable Upper Intake Level (UL). Dashed line represents a hypothetical no-observed-adverse-effect level (NOAEL). Solid lines represent available data used to set the UL. Area containing diagonal lines represents theoretical range of uncertainty. LOAEL = lowest-observed-adverse-effect level; RDA = Recommended Dietary Allowance.

nutrient's capacity to cause adverse effects prohibits the application of the UL model. In other cases, the evidence is available, but meeting the UL derived from such evidence will necessarily result in the introduction of undesirable health effects because of the required adjustments in dietary patterns.

Insufficient Evidence of Adverse Effects

The scientific evidence relating to adverse effects of nutrient excess varies greatly among nutrients. The type of data and evidence of causation used to derive ULs have been described earlier in this chapter, but such data and evidence are simply unavailable for some nutrients. In some cases (e.g., the individual amino acids), some data relating to adverse effects may be available, but are of such uncertain relevance to human health that their use in deriving ULs is scientifically insupportable. In every instance in which ULs are not derived because of lack of adequate evidence, the specific limitations in the database are described.

Offsetting Benefits Reduction

In the case of macronutrients, particularly, problems arise because of the adjustments in dietary patterns that would be required to meet a derived UL. For saturated and *trans* fatty acids and dietary cholesterol, for example, there is evidence that any intake greater than zero will increase serum levels of low density lipoprotein cholesterol, an established risk for cardiovascular disease. In such cases, the UL model calls for the establishment of a UL of 0. But it is clear that, because saturated fat and cholesterol are both unavoidable in ordinary diets, achieving such a UL will require extraordinary changes in patterns of dietary intake. Such extraordinary adjustments may introduce other undesirable health effects (e.g., elimination of foods containing saturated fats may result in a large excess intake of carbohydrate and insufficient intake of micronutrients). In addition, unknown and unquantifiable health risks may also be introduced. For these reasons, no UL will be proposed in circumstances in which implementation of measures to achieve the UL may lead to undesirable dietary adjustments. In all such cases, the basis for failing to propose a UL will be described.

Lack of ULs for Macronutrients and Implications

ULs were not set for macronutrients because (1) there was insufficient evidence for identifying an adverse effect, and therefore a LOAEL, upon which to determine a UL (e.g., protein), (2) data relating to adverse effects were available (e.g., amino acids), but were of uncertain relevance to human health because their use in deriving ULs was not scientifically supportable, (3) macronutrients are interrelated in providing energy and therefore it is not known whether the adverse effect is due to a high intake of one macronutrient (e.g., fat), due to a low intake of another macronutrient (e.g., carbohydrate, which is usually low in a high fat diet), or both (high fat, low carbohydrate diet), and (4) adjustments of dietary patterns to prevent exceeding a UL of near 0 g/d (e.g., *trans* and saturated fatty acids and cholesterol), resulting in inadequate intakes of certain micronutrients (e.g., iron and zinc). In addition, the UL method is not applicable to energy since any intake above the requirement would be expected to result in weight gain and an increased risk of premature mortality.

The failure to establish a UL for any nutrient should not be interpreted as a lack of concern for adverse health effects (i.e., it is not equivalent to a recommendation that the nutrient can be consumed without limit). Lack of data regarding adverse effects is not evidence of safety. Indeed, in some cases (the previous example of saturated fat) there is clearly evidence of adverse health effects, but a UL is not established to avoid the need for drastic changes that may introduce undesirable health effects.

In every instance in which a UL is not established, it is necessary to offer specific advice regarding the need to avoid deficiency, or in some cases, to reduce intakes, consistent with the need to maintain healthy dietary patterns.

INTAKE ASSESSMENT

In order to assess the risk of adverse effects, information on the range of nutrient intakes in the general population is required. As noted earlier, in cases where the Tolerable Upper Intake Level (UL) pertains only to supplement use and not to usual food intakes of the nutrient, the assessment is directed at supplement intake only.

RISK CHARACTERIZATION

As described earlier, the question of whether nutrient intakes create a risk of toxicity requires a comparison of the range of nutrient intakes (from food, supplements, and other sources, or from supplements alone, depending upon the basis for the Tolerable Upper Intake Level [UL]) with the UL.

Figure 4-4 illustrates a distribution of chronic nutrient intakes in a population; the fraction of the population experiencing chronic intakes above the UL represents the potential at-risk group. A policy decision is needed to determine whether efforts should be made to reduce risk. No precedents are available for such policy decisions, although in the areas of food additives or pesticide regulations, federal regulatory agencies have generally sought to ensure that the 90th or 95th percentile of intake falls below the UL (or its approximate equivalent measure of risk). If this goal is achieved, the fraction of the population remaining above the UL is likely to experience intakes only slightly greater than the UL and is likely to be at little or no risk.

For risk management decisions, it is useful to evaluate the public health significance of the risk, and information contained in the risk characterization is critical for this purpose.

Thus, the significance of the risk to a population consuming a nutrient in excess of the UL is determined by the following:

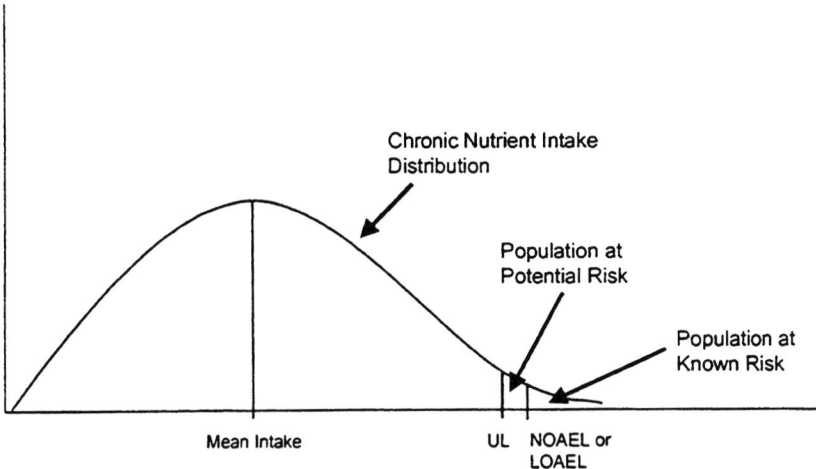

FIGURE 4-4 Illustration of the population at risk from excessive nutrient intakes. The fraction of the population consistently consuming a nutrient at intake levels in excess of the Tolerable Upper Intake Level (UL) is potentially at risk of adverse health effects. See text for a discussion of additional factors necessary to judge the significance of the risk. NOAEL = no-observed-adverse-effect level; LOAEL = lowest-observed-adverse-effect level.

1. the fraction of the population consistently consuming the nutrient at intake levels in excess of the UL,

2. the seriousness of the adverse effects associated with the nutrient,

3. the extent to which the effect is reversible when intakes are reduced to levels less than the UL, and

4. the fraction of the population with consistent intakes above the no-observed-adverse-effect level or even the lowest-observed-adverse-effect level.

Thus, the significance of the risk of excessive nutrient intake cannot be judged only by reference to Figure 4-4, but requires careful consideration of all of the above factors. Information on these factors is contained in sections of the nutrient chapters that describe the bases for each of the ULs.

REFERENCES

Dourson ML, Stara JF. 1983. Regulatory history and experimental support of uncertainty (safety) factors. *Regul Toxicol Pharmacol* 3:224–238.

FAO/WHO (Food and Agriculture Organization of the United Nations/World Health Organization). 1982. *Evaluation of Certain Food Additives and Contaminants.* Twenty-sixth report of the Joint FAO/WHO Expert Committee on Food Additives. WHO Technical Report Series No. 683. Geneva: WHO.

FAO/WHO. 1995. *The Application of Risk Analysis to Food Standard Issues.* Recommendations to the Codex Alimentarius Commission (ALINORM 95/9, Appendix 5). Geneva: WHO.

Health Canada. 1993. *Health Risk Determination—The Challenge of Health Protection.* Ottawa: Health Canada, Health Protection Branch.

Hill AB. 1971. *Principles of Medical Statistics,* 9th ed. New York: Oxford University Press.

Klaassen CD, Amdur MO, Doull J. 1986. *Casarett and Doull's Toxicology: The Basic Science of Poisons,* 3rd ed. New York: Macmillan.

Mertz W, Abernathy CO, Olin SS. 1994. *Risk Assessment of Essential Elements.* Washington, DC: ILSI Press.

NRC (National Research Council). 1983. *Risk Assessment in the Federal Government: Managing the Process.* Washington, DC: National Academy Press.

NRC. 1994. *Science and Judgment in Risk Assessment.* Washington, DC: National Academy Press.

OTA (Office of Technology Assessment). 1993. *Researching Health Risks.* Washington, DC: OTA.

WHO (World Health Organization). 1987. *Principles for the Safety Assessment of Food Additives and Contaminants in Food.* Environmental Health Criteria 70. Geneva: WHO.

WHO. 1996. *Trace Elements in Human Nutrition and Health.* Geneva: WHO.

Zielhuis RL, van der Kreek FW. 1979. The use of a safety factor in setting health-based permissible levels for occupational exposure. *Int Arch Occup Environ Health* 42:191–201.

5
Energy

SUMMARY

Energy is required to sustain the body's various functions, including respiration, circulation, physical work, and maintenance of core body temperature. The energy in foods is released in the body by oxidation, yielding the chemical energy needed to sustain metabolism, nerve transmission, respiration, circulation, and physical work. The heat produced during these processes is used to maintain body temperature. Energy balance in an individual depends on his or her dietary energy intake and energy expenditure. Imbalances between intake and expenditure result in gains or losses of body components, mainly in the form of fat, and these determine changes in body weight.

The Estimated Energy Requirement (EER) is defined as the average dietary energy intake that is predicted to maintain energy balance in a healthy, adult of a defined age, gender, weight, height, and level of physical activity consistent with good health. To calculate the EER, prediction equations for normal weight individuals were developed from data on total daily energy expenditure measured by the doubly labeled water technique. In children and pregnant or lactating women, the EER includes the needs associated with the deposition of tissues or the secretion of milk at rates consistent with good health. While the expected between-individual variability is calculated for the EER, there is no Recommended Dietary Allowance (RDA) for energy because energy intakes above the EER would be expected to result in weight gain. Similarly, the Tolerable Upper Intake Level (UL) concept does not apply to

107

energy, because any intake above an individual's energy requirement would lead to undesirable (and potentially hazardous) weight gain.

BACKGROUND INFORMATION

Humans and other mammals constantly need to expend energy to perform physical work; to maintain body temperature and concentration gradients; and to transport, synthesize, degrade, and replace small and large molecules that make up body tissue. This energy is generated by the oxidation of various organic substances, primarily carbohydrates, fats, and amino acids. In 1780, Lavoisier and LaPlace measured the heat production of mammals by calorimetry (Kleiber, 1975). They demonstrated that it was equal to the heat released when organic substances were burned, and that the same quantities of oxygen were consumed by animal metabolism as were used during the combustion of the same organic substrates (Holmes, 1985). Indeed, it has been verified by numerous experiments on animals and humans since then that the energy produced by oxidation of carbohydrates and fats in the body is the same as the heat of combustion of these substances (Kleiber, 1975). The crucial difference is that in organisms oxidation proceeds through many steps, allowing capture of some of the energy in an intermediate chemical form—the high energy pyrophosphate bond of adenosine triphosphate (ATP). Hydrolysis of these high-energy bonds can then be coupled to various chemical reactions, thereby driving them to completion, even if by themselves they would not proceed (Lipmann, 1941). Typically, the rates of energy expenditure in adults at rest are slightly less than 1 kcal/min in women (i.e., 0.8 to 1.0 kcal/min or 1,150 to 1,440 kcal/d), and slightly more than 1 kcal/min in men (i.e., 1.1 to 1.3 kcal/min or 1,580 to 1,870 kcal/d) (Owen et al., 1986, 1987). One kcal/min corresponds approximately to the heat released by a burning candle or by a 75-watt light bulb (i.e., 1 kcal/min corresponds to 70 J/sec or 70 W).

Energy Yields from Substrates

Carbohydrate, fat, protein, and alcohol provide all of the energy supplied by foods and are generally referred to as macronutrients (in contrast to vitamins and elements, usually referred to as micronutrients). The amount of energy released by the oxidation of carbohydrate, fat, protein, and alcohol (also known as Heat of Combustion, or ΔH) is shown in Table 5-1.

When alcohol (ethanol or ethyl alcohol) is consumed, it promptly appears in the circulation and is oxidized at a rate determined largely by its concentration and by the activity of liver alcohol dehydrogenase. Oxi-

TABLE 5-1 Heat of Combustion of Various Macronutrients

Macronutrient	Heat of Combustion[a] (kcal/g)	kcal[b]/L O_2	RQ[c] (CO_2/O_2)	Atwater Factor[d] (kcal/g)
Starch	4.18	5.05	1.0	4.0
Sucrose	3.94	5.01	1.0	4.0
Glucose	3.72	4.98	1.0	4.0
Fat	9.44	4.69	0.71	9.0
Protein by combustion[a]	5.6			
Protein through metabolism[a]	4.70	4.66	0.835	4.0
Alcohol[e]	7.09	4.86	0.67	—

[a] The energy derived by protein oxidation in living organisms is less than the heat of combustion of protein, because the nitrogen-containing end product of metabolism in mammals is urea (or uric acid in birds and reptiles), whereas nitrogen is converted into nitrous oxide when protein is combusted. The heat liberated by biological oxidation of proteins was long thought to be 4.3 kcal/g (Merrill and Watt, 1973), but a more recent demonstration showed that the actual value is 4.7 kcal/g (Livesey and Elia, 1988).

[b] One calorie is the amount of energy needed to increase the temperature of 1 g of water from 14.5° to 15.5°C. In the context of foods and nutrition, "large calorie" (i.e., Calories, with a capital C), which is more properly referred to as "kilocalorie" (kcal), has been traditionally used. In the International System of Units, the basic energy unit is the Joule (J). One J = 0.239 calories, so that 1 kcal = to 4.186 kJ. A daily energy expenditure of 2,400 kcal corresponds to the expenditure of 10,000 kJ, or 10 MJ (Mega Joules)/d.

[c] RQ = respiratory quotient, which is defined as the ratio of CO_2 produced divided by O_2 consumed (in terms of mols, or in terms of volumes of CO_2 and O_2).

[d] Atwater, a pioneer in the study and characterization of nutrients and metabolism, proposed to use the values of 4, 9, and 4 kcal/g of carbohydrate, fat, and protein, respectively (Merrill and Watt, 1973). This equivalent is now uniformly used in nutrient labeling and diet formulation. Nutrition Labeling of Food. 21 C.F.R. §101.9 (1991).

[e] Alcohol (ethanol) content of beverages is usually described in terms of percent by volume. The heat of combustion of alcohol is 5.6 kcal/mL. (One mL of alcohol weighs 0.789 g.)

dation of alcohol elicits a prompt reduction in the oxidation of other substrates used for ATP regeneration, demonstrating that ethanol oxidation proceeds in large part via conversion to acetate and oxidative phosphorylation. The phenomenon has been precisely measured by indirect calorimetry in human subjects, in whom ethanol consumption was found to primarily reduce fat oxidation (Suter et al., 1992). About 80 percent of the energy liberated by ethanol oxidation is used to drive ATP regeneration, so that the thermic effect of ethanol comes to about 20 percent (Siler et al., 1999). The thermic effect of food is the increase in energy expenditure as measured by heat produced upon ingestion of that food. The thermic effect of alcohol is about twice the thermic effect of carbohydrate, but less than the thermic effect of protein (see later section, "Thermic Effect of Food").

Reported food intake in individuals consuming alcohol is often similar to that of individuals who do not consume alcohol (de Castro and Orozco, 1990). As a result, it has sometimes been questioned whether alcohol contributes substantially to energy production. However, the biochemical and physiological evidence about the contribution made by ethanol to oxidative phosphorylation is so unambiguous that the apparent discrepancies between energy intake data and body weights must be attributed to inaccuracies in reported food intakes. In fact, in individuals consuming a healthy diet, the additional energy provided by alcoholic beverages can be a risk factor for weight gain (Suter et al., 1997), as opposed to alcoholics in whom the pharmacological impact of excessive amounts of ethanol tends to inhibit normal eating and may cause emaciation.

Energy Requirements Versus Nutrient Requirements

Recommendations for nutrient intakes are generally set to provide an ample supply of the various nutrients needed (i.e., enough to meet or exceed the requirements of almost all healthy individuals in a given life stage and gender group). For most nutrients, recommended intakes are thus set to correspond to the median amounts sufficient to meet a specific criterion of adequacy plus two standard deviations to meet the needs of nearly all healthy individuals (see Chapter 1). However, this is not the case with energy because excess energy cannot be eliminated, and is eventually deposited in the form of body fat. This reserve provides a means to maintain metabolism during periods of limited food intake, but it can also result in obesity.

The first alternate criterion that may be considered as the basis for a recommendation for energy is that energy intake should be commensurate with energy expenditure, so as to achieve energy balance. Although frequently applied in the past, this is not appropriate as a sole criterion, as described by the FAO/WHO/UNU publication, *Energy and Protein Requirements* (1985):

> The energy requirement of an individual is a level of energy intake from food that will balance energy expenditure when the individual has a body size and composition, and level of physical activity, consistent with long-term good health; and that would allow for the maintenance of economically necessary and socially desirable physical activity. In children and pregnant or lactating women the energy requirement includes the energy needs associated with

the deposition of tissues or the secretion of milk at rates consistent with good health (p. 12).

This definition indicates that desirable energy intakes for obese individuals are less than their current energy expenditure, as weight loss and establishment of a steady state at a lower body weight is desirable for them. In underweight individuals, on the other hand, desirable energy intakes are greater than their current energy expenditure to permit weight gain and maintenance of a higher body weight. Thus, it seems logical to base estimated values for energy intake on the amounts of energy that need to be consumed to maintain energy balance in adult men and women who are maintaining desirable body weights, taking into account the increments in energy expenditure elicited by their habitual level of activity.

There is another fundamental difference between the requirements for energy and those for other nutrients. Body weight provides each individual with a readily monitored indicator of the adequacy or inadequacy of habitual energy intake, whereas a comparably obvious and individualized indicator of inadequate or excessive intake of other nutrients is not usually evident.

Energy Balance

Because of the effectiveness in regulating the distribution and use of metabolic fuels, man and animals can survive on foods providing widely varying proportions of carbohydrates, fats, and proteins. The ability to shift from carbohydrate to fat as the main source of energy, coupled with the presence of substantial reserves of body fat, makes it possible to accommodate large variations in macronutrient intake, energy intake, and energy expenditure. The amount of fat stored in an adult of normal weight commonly ranges from 6 to 20 kg. Since one gram of fat provides 9.4 kcal, body fat energy reserves thus range typically from approximately 50,000 to 200,000 kcal, providing a large buffer capacity as well as the ability to provide energy to survive for extended periods (i.e., several months) of severe food deprivation. Large daily deviations from energy balance are thus readily tolerated, and accommodated primarily by gains or losses of body fat (Abbott et al., 1988; Stubbs et al., 1995). Coefficients of variation for intra-individual variability in daily energy intake average ± 23 percent (Bingham et al., 1994); variations in physical activity are not closely synchronized with adjustments in food intake (Edholm et al., 1970). Thus, substantial positive as well as negative energy balances of several hundred kcal/d occur as a matter of course under free-living conditions among normal and overweight subjects. Yet over the long term, energy balance is maintained with remarkable accuracy. Indeed, during long periods in the life of most individuals, gains or losses of adipose tissue are less than 1 to 2 kg over a year (McCargar et al., 1993), implying that the cumulative error in adjusting energy intake to expenditure amounts to less than 2 percent of energy expenditure.

Components of Energy Expenditure

Basal and Resting Metabolism

The basal metabolic rate (BMR) describes the rate of energy expenditure that occurs in the postabsorptive state, defined as the particular condition that prevails after an overnight fast, the subject having not consumed food for 12 to 14 hours and resting comfortably, supine, awake, and motionless in a thermoneutral environment. This standardized metabolic state corresponds to the situation in which food and physical activity have minimal influence on metabolism. The BMR thus reflects the energy needed to sustain the metabolic activities of cells and tissues, plus the energy needed to maintain blood circulation, respiration, and gastrointestinal and renal processing (i.e., the basal cost of living). BMR thus includes the energy expenditure associated with remaining awake (the cost of arousal), reflecting the fact that the sleeping metabolic rate (SMR) during the morning is some 5 to 10 percent lower than BMR during the morning hours (Garby et al., 1987).

BMR is commonly extrapolated to 24 hours to be more meaningful, and it is then referred to as basal energy expenditure (BEE), expressed as kcal/24 h. Resting metabolic rate (RMR), energy expenditure under resting conditions, tends to be somewhat higher (10 to 20 percent) than under basal conditions due to increases in energy expenditure caused by recent food intake (i.e., by the "thermic effect of food") or by the delayed effect of recently completed physical activity (see Chapter 12). Thus, it is important to distinguish between BMR and RMR and between BEE and resting energy expenditure (REE) (RMR extrapolated to 24 hours).

Basal, resting, and sleeping energy expenditures are related to body size, being most closely correlated with the size of the fat-free mass (FFM), which is the weight of the body less the weight of its fat mass. The size of the FFM generally explains about 70 to 80 percent of the variance in RMR (Nelson et al., 1992; Ravussin et al., 1986). However, RMR is also affected by age, gender, nutritional state, inherited variations, and by differences in the endocrine state, notably (but rarely) by hypo- or hyperthyroidism. The relationships among RMR, body weight, and FFM are illustrated in Figures 5-1 and 5-2 (Owen, 1988), which show that differences in RMR relative to body weight among diverse individuals such as men, women, and athletes mostly disappear when RMR is considered relative to FFM.

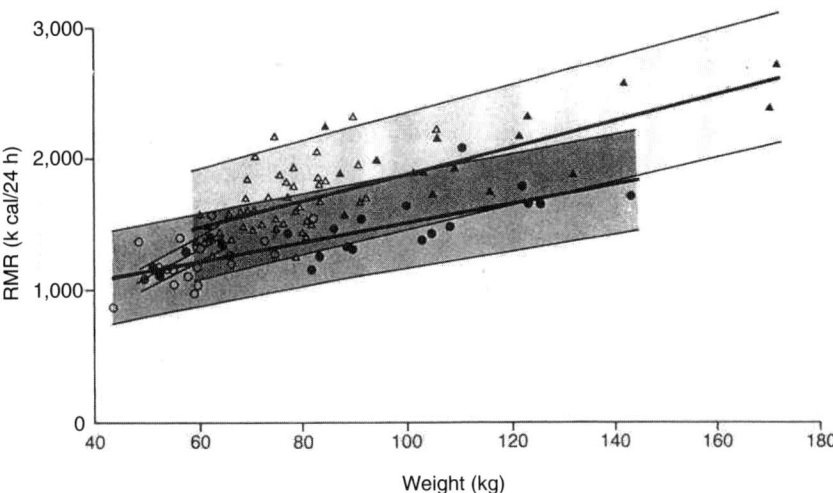

FIGURE 5-1 Resting metabolic rates (RMR) are contrasted against the weights of 44 lean (○) and obese (●) healthy women, 8 of whom were athletes (⊕), and 60 lean (△) and obese (▲) healthy men. Reprinted, with permission, from Owen (1988). Copyright 1988 by W.B. Saunders.

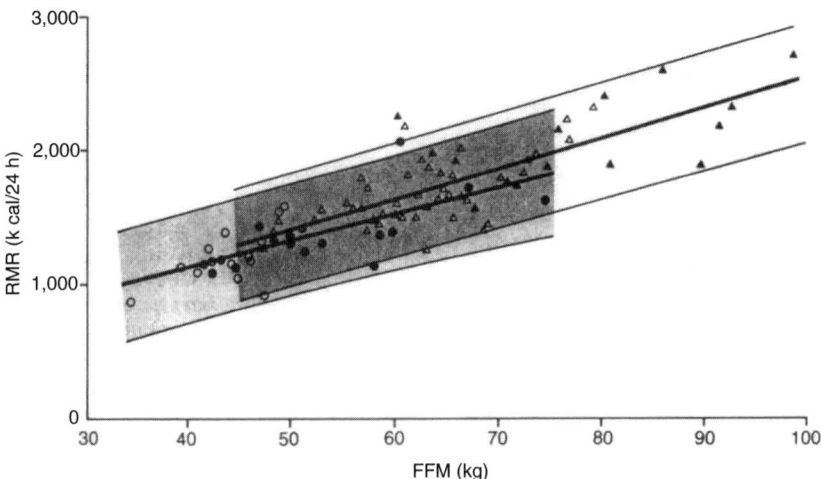

FIGURE 5-2 Resting metabolic rates (RMR) are contrasted against the fat-free masses (FFM) of 44 lean (○) and obese (●) healthy women, 8 of whom were athletes (⊕), and 60 lean (△) and obese (▲) healthy men. Reprinted, with permission, from Owen (1988). Copyright 1988 by W.B. Saunders.

BEE has been predicted from age, gender, and body size. Prediction equations were developed for each gender (WN Schofield, 1985) by pooling and analyzing reported measurements made in 7,393 individuals. A recent re-evaluation of all available data performed by Henry (2000) has led to a new set of predicting equations.

Thermic Effect of Food

It has long been known that food consumption elicits an increase in energy expenditure (Kleiber, 1975). Originally referred to as the Specific Dynamic Action (SDA) of food, this phenomenon is now more commonly referred to as the thermic effect of food (TEF). The intensity and duration of meal-induced TEF is determined primarily by the amount and composition of the foods consumed, mainly due to the metabolic costs incurred in handling and storing ingested nutrients (Flatt, 1978). Activation of the sympathetic nervous system elicited by dietary carbohydrate and by sensory stimulation causes an additional, but modest, increase in energy expenditure (Acheson et al., 1983). The increments in energy expenditure during digestion above baseline rates, divided by the energy content of the food consumed, vary from 5 to 10 percent for carbohydrate, 0 to 5 percent for fat, and 20 to 30 percent for protein. The high TEF for protein reflects the relatively high metabolic cost involved in processing the amino acids yielded by absorption of dietary protein, for protein synthesis, or for the synthesis of urea and glucose (Flatt, 1978; Nair et al., 1983). Consumption of the usual mixture of nutrients is generally considered to elicit increases in energy expenditure equivalent to 10 percent of the food's energy content (Kleiber, 1975). Since TEF occurs during a limited part of the day only, it can result in noticeable increases in REE if energy expenditure is measured during the hours following meals.

Thermoregulation

Birds and mammals, including humans, regulate their body temperature within narrow limits. This process, termed *thermoregulation*, can elicit increases in energy expenditure that are greater when ambient temperatures are below the zone of thermoneutrality. The environmental temperature at which oxygen consumption and metabolic rate are lowest is described as the critical temperature or thermoneutral zone (Hill, 1964). Because most people adjust their clothing and environment to maintain comfort, and thus thermoneutrality, the additional energy cost of thermoregulation rarely affects total energy expenditure to an appreciable extent. However, there does appear to be a small influence of ambient temperature on energy expenditure as described in more detail below.

Physical Activity

The energy expended for physical activity varies greatly among individuals as well as from day to day. In sedentary individuals, about two-thirds of total energy expenditure goes to sustain basal metabolism over 24 hours (the BEE), while one-third is used for physical activity. In very active individuals, 24-hour total energy expenditure can rise to twice as much as basal energy expenditure (Grund et al., 2001), while even higher total expenditures occur among heavy laborers and some athletes.

The efficiency with which energy from food is converted into physical work is remarkably constant when measured under conditions where body weight and athletic skill are not a factor, such as on bicycle ergometers (Kleiber, 1975; Nickleberry and Brooks, 1996; Pahud et al., 1980). For weight-bearing physical activities, the cost is roughly proportional to body weight. In the life of most persons, walking represents the most significant form of physical activity, and many studies have been performed to determine the energy expenditures induced by walking or running at various speeds (Margaria et al., 1963; Pandolf et al., 1977; Passmore and Durnin, 1955). Walking at a speed of 2 mph is considered to correspond to a mild degree of exertion, walking speeds of 3 to 4 mph correspond to moderate degrees of exertion, and a walking speed of 5 mph to vigorous exertion (Table 12-1, Fletcher et al., 2001). Over this range of speeds, the increment in energy expenditure amounts to some 60 kcal/mi walked for a 70-kg individual, or 50 kcal/mi walked for a 57-kg individual (see Chapter 12, Figure 12-4). The exertion caused by walking/jogging increases progressively at speeds of 4.5 mph and beyond, reaching 130 kcal/mi at 5 mph for a 70-kg individual.

The increase in daily energy expenditure is somewhat greater, however, because exercise induces an additional small increase in expenditure for some time after the exertion itself has been completed. This excess post-exercise oxygen consumption (EPOC) depends on exercise intensity and duration and has been estimated at some 15 percent of the increment in expenditure that occurs during exertions of the type described above (Bahr et al., 1987). This raises the cost of walking at 3 mph to 69 kcal/mi (60 kcal/mi × 1.15) for a 70-kg individual and to 58 kcal/mi (50 kcal/mi × 1.15) for a 57-kg individual. Taking into account the dissipation of 10 percent of the energy consumed on account of the thermic effect of food to cover the expenditure associated with walking, then walking 1 mile raises daily energy expenditure to 76 kcal/mi (69 kcal/mi × 1.1) in individuals weighing 70 kg, or 64 kcal/mi (58 kcal/mi × 1.1) for individuals weighing 57 kg. Since the cost of walking is proportional to body weight, it is convenient to consider that the overall cost of walking at moderate speeds is approximately 1.1 kcal/mi/kg body weight (75 kcal/mi/70 kg or 64 kcal/mi/57 kg). The effects of variations in body weights and the impact of various physical activities on energy expenditure are considered in more detail in Chapter 12.

Physical Activity Level

The level of physical activity is commonly described as the ratio of total to basal daily energy expenditure (TEE/BEE). This ratio is known as the Physical Activity Level (PAL), or the Physical Activity Index. Describing physical activity habits in terms of PAL is not entirely satisfactory because the increments above basal needs in energy expenditure, brought about by most physical activities where body weight is supported against gravity (e.g., walking, but not cycling on a stationary cycle ergometer), are directly proportional to body weight, whereas BEE is more nearly proportional to body weight$^{0.75}$. However, PAL is a convenient comparison and is used in this report to describe and account for physical activity habits. The effect of variations in activities on PAL is described in Chapter 12.

Total Energy Expenditure

Total Energy Expenditure (TEE) is the sum of BEE (which includes a small component associated with arousal, as compared to sleeping), TEF, physical activity, thermoregulation, and the energy expended in depositing new tissues and in producing milk. With the emergence of information on TEE by the doubly labeled water (DLW) method (Schoeller, 1995), it has become possible to determine energy expenditure of infants, children, and adults under free-living conditions. TEE from doubly labeled water does not include the energy content of the tissue constituents laid down during normal growth and pregnancy or the milk produced during lactation, as it refers to energy expended during oxidation of energy-yielding nutrients to water and carbon dioxide.

It should be noted that direct measurements of TEE represent a distinct advantage over previous TEE evaluations, which had to rely on the factorial approach and on food intake data, which have limited accuracy due to the inability to reliably determine average physical activity cost and nutrient intakes.

Estimated Energy Requirement

Information on energy expenditure obtained by DLW studies conducted by a number of research units (see Appendix I) are used in this report to estimate energy requirements, taking into account estimates of the energy content of new body constituents during growth and pregnancy and of the milk produced during lactation. Energy expenditure depends on age and varies primarily as a function of body size and physical activity, both of which vary greatly among individuals. Recommendations about energy intake vary accordingly, and are also subject to the criterion that an individual adult's body weight should remain stable and within the healthy range.

SELECTION OF INDICATORS FOR ESTIMATING THE REQUIREMENT FOR ENERGY

Reported Energy Intake

The reported energy intakes of weight-stable subjects (i.e., those in energy balance) could, in principle, be used to predict energy requirements for weight maintenance. However, it is now widely recognized that reported energy intakes in dietary surveys underestimate usual energy intake (Black et al., 1993).

The most compelling evidence about underreporting has come from measurements of total energy expenditure (TEE) by the doubly labeled water (DLW) method (Schoeller, 1995). The use of a measure or estimate of TEE to validate instruments that measure food intake is dependent on the principle of energy balance. That is, in weight-stable adults, energy intake must equal TEE. By comparing reported energy intake to TEE, the accuracy of food intake reporting can be assessed (Goldberg et al., 1991a).

A large body of literature documents the underreporting of food intake, which can range from 10 to 45 percent depending on the age, gender, and body composition of individuals in the sample population (Johnson, 2000). Underreporting tends to increase as children grow older (Livingstone et al., 1992b), is worse among women than in men (Johnson et al., 1994), and is more pronounced among overweight and obese than among lean individuals (Bandini et al., 1990a; Lichtman et al., 1992; Prentice et al., 1986). Low socioeconomic status, characterized by low income, low educational attainment, and low literacy levels increase the tendency to underreport energy intakes (Briefel et al., 1997; Johnson et al., 1998; Price et al., 1997; Pryer et al., 1997). Ethnic differences affecting sensitivities and psychological perceptions relating to eating and body weight can also affect the accuracy of reported food intakes (Tomoyasu et al., 2000). Finally, individuals with infrequent symptoms of hunger underreport to a greater degree than those who experience frequent hunger (Bathalon et al., 2000).

There is some evidence suggesting that underreporters often fail to report foods perceived to be bad or sinful, such as cakes/pies, savory snacks, cheese, fried potatoes, meat mixtures, soft drinks, spreads, condiments, and generally foods known to be high in fat (Bingham and Day, 1997; Krebs-Smith et al., 2000). Reported intakes of added sugars are also significantly lower than that consumed, due in part to the frequent omission of snack foods from 24-hour food recording (Poppitt et al., 1998).

Finally, there is no objective evidence for the existence of "small eaters," individuals who can survive long term on the low energy intakes that they report in dietary surveys (Black, 1999; Lichtman et al., 1992; Prentice et al., 1986). Clearly, it is no longer tenable to base energy requirements on self-reported food consumption data.

Factorial Approach

Previous Recommended Dietary Allowances for energy (NRC, 1989) used the factorial method to estimate TEE. This method calculates TEE using information on the amount of time devoted to different activities and the energy costs of each activity throughout a theoretical 24-hour period. The factorial method allowed theoretical estimation of TEE for a defined activity pattern (using measured average costs of standard activities and theoretical activity duration). Thus, mean expected energy requirements for different levels of physical activity were defined.

However, there are recognized problems with the factorial method and doubts about the validity of energy requirement predictions based on it (Roberts et al., 1991). The first problem is that there are a wide range of activities and physical efforts performed during normal life, and it is not feasible to measure the energy cost of each. Another concern with the factorial method is that the measurement of the energy costs of specific activities imposes constraints (due to mechanical impediments associated with performing an activity while wearing unfamiliar equipment) that may alter the measured energy costs of different activities. Although generalizations are essential in trying to account for the energy costs of daily activities, substantial errors may be introduced. In addition, energy expenditure during sleep, once considered to be equivalent to basal metabolic rate (BMR), is generally somewhat lower (–5 to –10 percent) than BMR (Garby et al., 1987).

Also, and perhaps most importantly, the factorial method only takes into account activities that can be specifically accounted for (e.g., sleeping, walking, household work, occupational activity, and so on). However, 24-hour room calorimeter studies have shown that a significant amount of energy is expended in spontaneous physical activities, some of which are part of a sedentary lifestyle (Ravussin et al., 1986; Zurlo et al., 1992). In addition, some individuals manifest a substantial amount of fidgeting. Together these were reported to average about 350 kcal/d, ranging from

140 to 700 kcal/d (Ravussin et al., 1986). Thus, the factorial method is bound to underestimate usual energy needs (Durnin, 1990; Roberts et al., 1991).

Most comparisons of the factorial approach with DLW determinations of TEE have shown significantly higher measured values for TEE than predicted by the factorial method (Haggarty et al., 1994; Jones et al., 1997; Roberts et al., 1991; Sawaya et al., 1995). In two direct comparisons of factorial energy requirement estimates with DLW, one confirmed that the factorial method underestimated energy needs (Leonard et al., 1997), while the other found no difference between the methods in an elderly population with a mean age of 70 years (Morio et al., 1997).

Measurement of Energy Expenditure by Doubly Labeled Water

The DLW method is a relatively new technique that measures TEE in free-living individuals. It was originally proposed and developed by Lifson for use in small animals (Lifson and McClintock, 1966; Lifson et al., 1955), but has been adapted for human studies and extensively used (Schoeller et al., 1986). Two stable isotopic forms of water ($H_2{}^{18}O$ and ^2H_2O) are administered, and their disappearance rates from a body fluid (i.e., urine or blood) are monitored for a period of time, optimally equivalent to 1 to 3 half lives for these isotopes (7 to 21 days in most human subjects). The disappearance rate of ^2H_2O relates to water flux, while that of $H_2{}^{18}O$ reflects water flux plus carbon dioxide (CO_2) production rate, because of the rapid equilibration of the body water and bicarbonate pools by carbonic anhydrase (Lifson et al., 1949). The difference between the two disappearance rates can therefore be used to calculate the CO_2 production rate, and with knowledge of the composition of the diet, TEE can be calculated.

To predict TEE from a measurement of CO_2 production, it is necessary to have an estimate of the average respiratory quotient (RQ = ratio of CO_2 produced to the O_2 consumed) of the subject during the period of measurement. This is because the energy released per liter of CO_2 varies with the RQ and hence with the substrate mix oxidized by the body (Elia, 1991). The ratio of the CO_2 produced to the O_2 consumed by the biological oxidation of a representative sample of the diet is commonly referred to as the food quotient, or FQ (Flatt, 1978).

Short-term measurements of RQ by indirect calorimetry are not useful for the DLW technique because RQ varies markedly during the day, particularly after meals. It is therefore more accurate to estimate the average RQ from information on the subjects' dietary intake. When energy balance prevails, the average RQ is equal to the FQ. If substantial gains or losses of body constituents are known to occur during the period of measurement, appropriate adjustments can be made in estimating the average RQ. Although food reports are inaccurate for measuring total energy intake, FQ calculations from food records can be used because FQ has a relatively small effect on DLW measurements of TEE.

Several validations of the DLW study have been conducted in which DLW-derived estimates of TEE were compared with measurements of TEE in whole-body calorimeters (Table 5-2). Although studies in whole-body calorimeters do not mimic normal life conditions, they do allow for an exact comparison of the DLW method with classic calorimetry, which is considered the most reliable measurement of energy expenditure. As shown in Table 5-2, there is a close agreement between means for the CO_2 production rate determined by the two methods in all the validation studies. The precision of DLW measurements, as assessed by the variability of individual DLW measurements from the calorimetry assessments, ranged from −2.5 to 5.9 percent in the different studies. These validation studies show that the DLW method can provide an accurate assessment of the CO_2 production rate and hence TEE in a wide range of human subjects.

One particular advantage of the DLW method is that it provides an index of TEE over a period of several days. Because 1 to 3 half-lives of isotope disappearance are needed for changes in isotopic abundance to be measured accurately by mass spectrometry, optimal time periods for DLW measurements of TEE range from 1 to 3 weeks in most groups of individuals (Schoeller, 1983). Thus, in contrast to other techniques, DLW can provide TEE estimates over biologically meaningful periods of time that can reduce the impact of spontaneous daily variations in physical activity. Moreover, because DLW is noninvasive (requiring only that the subject drink the stable isotopes and provide at least three urine samples over the study period), measurements can be made in subjects leading their normal daily lives. A critical mass of DLW data has now accumulated on a wide range of age groups and body sizes, so that the estimated energy requirements provided in this report could be based on DLW measurements of TEE.

The available DLW data (Appendix I) are not from randomly selected individuals, except in the recent study of Bratteby and coworkers (1997), and they do not constitute a sample representative of the population of the United States and Canada. However, the measurements were obtained in men, women, and children whose ages, body weights, heights, and physical activities varied over wide ranges. At the present time, a few age groups are underrepresented and interpolations had to be performed in these cases. Thus, while the available DLW data do not yet provide an entirely satisfactory set of data, they nevertheless offer the best currently available information.

A second potential criticism of using DLW-derived estimates of TEE as a basis for estimating energy requirements is that the approach assumes that TEE is relatively unaffected by fluctuations in energy balance. Although there is some capacity for TEE to increase or decrease spontaneously when energy intakes increase or decrease, these changes are small and attenuate the effect of energy imbalances only modestly (Levine et al., 1999; Roberts et al., 1990). Indeed, overfeeding studies show that overeating is inevitably accompanied by substantial weight gain, and that reduced energy intake induces weight loss (Saltzman and Roberts, 1995). Thus, although there may be some adaptive capacity to alter TEE in response to changes in dietary energy intake, the DLW-based evaluation of TEE at approximate weight maintenance provides an appropriate estimate of energy expenditure from which energy requirements for maintaining energy balance can be derived.

Body Mass Index

Adults

A growing literature supports the use of the body mass index (BMI, defined as weight in kilograms divided by the square of height in meters) as a predictor of the impact of body weight on morbidity and mortality risks (Seidell et al., 1996; Troiano et al., 1996). As an index of healthy weight and as a predictor of morbidity and mortality risk, it has supplanted weight-for-height tables, which were derived primarily from white populations and relied on questionable estimates of frame size (NHLBI/NIDDK, 1998). BMI, although only an indirect indicator of body composition, is now used to classify underweight and overweight individuals.

While sophisticated techniques are available to precisely measure fat-free mass (FFM) and fat mass (FM) of individuals, these techniques are used mainly in research protocols. For most clinical and epidemiological applications, body size is judged on the basis of the BMI, which is easy to determine, accurate, and reproducible. The main disadvantages of relying on BMI are that (1) it does not reliably reflect body fat content, which is an independent predictor of health risk, and (2) very muscular individuals may be misclassified as overweight (Willett et al., 1999).

The National Institutes of Health (NIH) clinical guidelines on the identification, evaluation, and treatment of normal, overweight and obese adults and the World Health Organization have defined BMI cutoffs for adults over 19 years of age, regardless of age or gender (NHLBI/NIDDK, 1998; WHO, 1998). Underweight is defined as a BMI of less than 18.5 kg/m^2, overweight as a BMI from 25 up to 30 kg/m^2, and obese as a BMI of 30 kg/m^2 or higher. A healthy or desirable BMI is considered to be from 18.5 up to

TABLE 5-2 Comparison of Carbon Dioxide Production Rates Measured by the Doubly Labeled Water Method and Indirect Calorimetry in Humans

Reference	Subjects	n	Time (d)
Coward et al., 1984	Adults, in energy balance[d]	4	12
Klein et al., 1984	Adults, in energy balance	1	5
Schoeller and Webb, 1984	Adults, in energy balance	5	5
Roberts et al., 1986	Preterm infants, growing	4	5
Schoeller et al., 1986	Adults, in energy balance		
	"Low" dose	6	4
	"High" dose	3	4
Jones et al., 1987	Infants, after surgery	9	5–6
Westerterp et al., 1988	Adults, in energy balance		
	Sedentary	5	6
	Active	4	3.5
Riumallo et al., 1989	Adults	6	7
Seale et al., 1990	Adults, in energy balance	4	13
Ravussin et al., 1991	Obese adults, in energy balance	12	7
Schulz et al., 1992	Adults, in energy balance	9	7
Seale and Rumpler, 1997	Adults, in energy balance	19	10

[a] Calculations for pool: I = 2-pool model using measured pool sizes as proposed by Coward et al. (1984) and detailed by Roberts et al. (1986), S = single-pool model as described by Lifson et al. (1955) and Lifson and McClintock (1966), F = 2-pool model with fixed ratio of 1.03 between pool sizes as described by Schoeller et al. (1986).
[b] Calculations for fractionated water loss: 50 = assumed to be 50 percent of total water output, 25 = assumed to be 25 percent of total water output, M = measured or calcu-

| $T_{1/2}$ (d) | Calculations | | | CO_2 % Error |
	Pool[a]	Fractionated[b]	Growth[c]	
	I	50	L	1.9
10.1	S	25	L	1.8
6.3–9.5	S	50	L	5.9 ± 7.6
2.5–3.6	I	M	E	−1.4 ± 4.8
6.7–9.8	F	P	L	5.0 ± 9.5
8.6–9.9	F	P	L	1.7 ± 4.5
2.9–4.5	F	P	L	−0.9 ± 6.2
5.7–9.0	F	P	L	1.4 ± 3.9
4.0–4.9	F	P	L	−1.0 ± 7.0
	F	P	L	
	F	P	L	−1.04 ± 0.63
	I	P	L	−2.5 ± 5.8
	I	P	L	
	F	P	L	

lated from data on water balance, P = assumed to be proportional to carbon dioxide output (Jones et al., 1987; Schoeller et al., 1986).

[c] Growth correction: L = no change or linear change in pool sizes, E = exponential change in pool sizes.

[d] Energy balance indicates that induction of positive or negative energy balance was not part of study protocol.

25 kg/m^2, a view adopted in this report. Although the healthy BMI range is the result of a consensus, there are reasons to suggest that slightly different mortality-based BMI ranges may be appropriate for different populations (NHLBI/NIDDK, 1998).

In establishing the 2000 Dietary Guidelines, the U.S. Departments of Agriculture and of Health and Human Services set the "healthy weight" upper limit at a BMI of 24.99 kg/m^2 for adult men and women because mortality increases significantly beyond this point (USDA/HHS, 2000). Although the incidence of diabetes, hypertension, and coronary heart disease begins to increase even below this cutoff, a BMI of 24.99 kg/m^2 is considered a reasonable upper limit of healthy weight. The lower BMI limit of 18.5 kg/m^2 is not as well substantiated. The point at which low BMI poses a health risk is poorly defined. The ability to identify persons with low BMIs who are at increased risk for morbidity and mortality is highly nonspecific.

Reference Weights. Weights corresponding to BMIs from 18.5 up to 25 kg/m^2 are tabulated for adult men and women with heights ranging from 1.47 to 1.98 m in Table 5-3 (men) and Table 5-4 (women). Reference weights used in this report correspond to a BMI of 22.5 kg/m^2 for men and a BMI of 21.5 kg/m^2 for women, which match the 50th percentile among 19-year-old individuals (Kuczmarski et al., 2000).

Relationship Between BMI and Body Fat Content. The Third National Health and Nutrition Examination Survey (NHANES III) data that provide the major anthropometric parameters, including waist circumference, skin-fold measurements, and bioimpedance data for some 15,000 women and men were examined to evaluate the body fat content typical for all BMI values (Appendix Table H-1) and among the 5,700 women and men whose BMIs were from 18.5 up to 25 kg/m^2 (Appendix Table H-2). Bioimpedance data were used to calculate percent body fat using equations developed by Sun and coworkers (2003).

The regressions of percent body fat versus BMI (Appendix Table H-3) were used to define the percent body fat ranges given in Table 5-5. The multiple regressions of percent body fat versus BMI and waist circumference (Appendix Table H-4) and of percent body fat versus BMI and triceps skinfold (Appendix Table H-5) were used to construct Figures 5-3 and 5-4.

One of the most commonly cited problems encountered in using BMI as a criterion for assessing the presence of excess body fat is that muscular subjects may have a BMI greater than 25 kg/m^2 without carrying excess body fat. In such cases, it is helpful to consider waist circumference in addition to BMI. As shown in Figure 5-3, a man with a BMI of 30 kg/m^2

TABLE 5-3 Reference Heights and Weights for Men Based on a Body Mass Index (BMI) Range from 18.5 up to 25 kg/m^2

Height (m[in])	Weight at BMI of 18.5 kg/m^2 (kg [lb])	Weight at BMI of 22.5 kg/m^{2a} (kg [lb])	Weight at BMI of 25 kg/m^2 (kg [lb])
1.47 (58)	40 (88)	49 (108)	54 (119)
1.50 (59)	42 (93)	51 (112)	56 (123)
1.52 (60)	43 (95)	52 (115)	58 (128)
1.55 (61)	44 (97)	54 (119)	60 (132)
1.57 (62)	46 (101)	55 (121)	62 (137)
1.60 (63)	47 (104)	58 (128)	64 (141)
1.63 (64)	49 (108)	60 (132)	66 (146)
1.65 (65)	50 (110)	61 (134)	68 (150)
1.68 (66)	52 (115)	64 (141)	70 (154)
1.70 (67)	53 (117)	65 (143)	72 (159)
1.73 (68)	55 (121)	67 (148)	75 (165)
1.75 (69)	57 (126)	69 (152)	76 (168)
1.77 (70)	58 (128)	70 (154)	78 (172)
1.78 (70)	59 (130)	71 (156)	79 (174)
1.80 (71)	60 (132)	73 (161)	81 (178)
1.83 (72)	62 (137)	75 (165)	84 (185)
1.85 (73)	63 (139)	77 (170)	86 (190)
1.88 (74)	65 (143)	80 (176)	88 (194)
1.91 (75)	67 (148)	82 (181)	91 (201)
1.93 (76)	69 (152)	84 (185)	93 (205)
1.96 (77)	71 (156)	86 (190)	96 (212)
1.98 (78)	72 (159)	88 (194)	98 (216)

[a] Weights for men at a BMI of 22.5 kg/m^2, equivalent to the 50th percentile for BMI at 19 years of age (Kuczmarski et al., 2000).

and a waist circumference of 85 cm (33.5 in) would still be expected to have less than 21 percent body fat. In women ($R^2 = 0.77$), BMI is a better predictor of differences in percentage of body fat than in men ($R^2 = 0.55$, Appendix Table H-3), and in women, triceps skinfold data ($R^2 = 0.82$, Appendix Table H-5) provide a better parameter than waist circumference ($R^2 = 0.79$, Appendix Table H-4) in complementing the indication of body fat percentage provided by BMI. In contrast, in men, waist circumference ($R^2 = 0.61$, Appendix Table H-4) provides a better parameter than triceps skinfold data ($R^2 = 0.58$, Appendix Table H-5) in complementing the indication of body fat percentage provided by BMI.

Relationship Between Height and Body Fat Content. The NHANES III data allowed examination of the impact of height on FFM, and hence on FM and on adiposity (as estimated by percent body fat). The impact of height

TABLE 5-4 Reference Heights and Weights for Women Based on a Body Mass Index (BMI) Range from 18.5 up to 25 kg/m^2

Height (m[in])	Weight at BMI of 18.5 kg/m^2 (kg [lb])	Weight at BMI of 21.5 kg/m^{2a} (kg [lb])	Weight at BMI of 25 kg/m^2 (kg [lb])
1.47 (58)	40 (88)	46 (101)	54 (119)
1.50 (59)	42 (93)	48 (106)	56 (123)
1.52 (60)	43 (95)	50 (110)	58 (128)
1.55 (61)	44 (97)	52 (115)	60 (132)
1.57 (62)	46 (101)	53 (117)	62 (137)
1.60 (63)	47 (104)	55 (121)	64 (141)
1.63 (64)	49 (108)	57 (126)	66 (146)
1.65 (65)	50 (110)	59 (130)	68 (150)
1.68 (66)	52 (115)	61 (134)	70 (154)
1.70 (67)	53 (117)	62 (137)	72 (159)
1.73 (68)	55 (121)	64 (141)	75 (165)
1.75 (69)	57 (126)	66 (146)	76 (168)
1.77 (70)	58 (128)	67 (148)	78 (172)
1.78 (70)	59 (130)	68 (150)	79 (174)
1.80 (71)	60 (132)	70 (154)	81 (178)
1.83 (72)	62 (137)	72 (159)	84 (185)
1.85 (73)	63 (139)	74 (163)	86 (190)
1.88 (74)	65 (143)	76 (168)	88 (194)
1.91 (75)	67 (148)	78 (172)	91 (201)
1.93 (76)	69 (152)	80 (176)	93 (205)
1.96 (77)	71 (156)	82 (181)	96 (212)
1.98 (78)	72 (159)	84 (185)	98 (216)

[a] Weights for women at a BMI of 21.5 kg/m^2, equivalent to the 50th percentile for BMI at 19 years of age (Kuczmarski et al., 2000).

TABLE 5-5 Body Weight Classification by Body Mass Index (BMI) and Body Fat Content[a]

BMI Range (kg/m^2)	Classification	Body Fat (%)[b]	
		Men	Women
From 18.5 up to 25	Normal	13–21	23–31
From 25 up to 30	Overweight	21–25	31–37
From 30 up to 35	Obese	25–31	37–42
35 or higher	Clinically obese	> 31	> 42

[a] Developed from regression of percent body fat versus BMI (kg/m^2) (Appendix H) using equations by Sun et al. (2003).
[b] Estimated from equations derived from bioimpedence data (Sun et al., 2003).

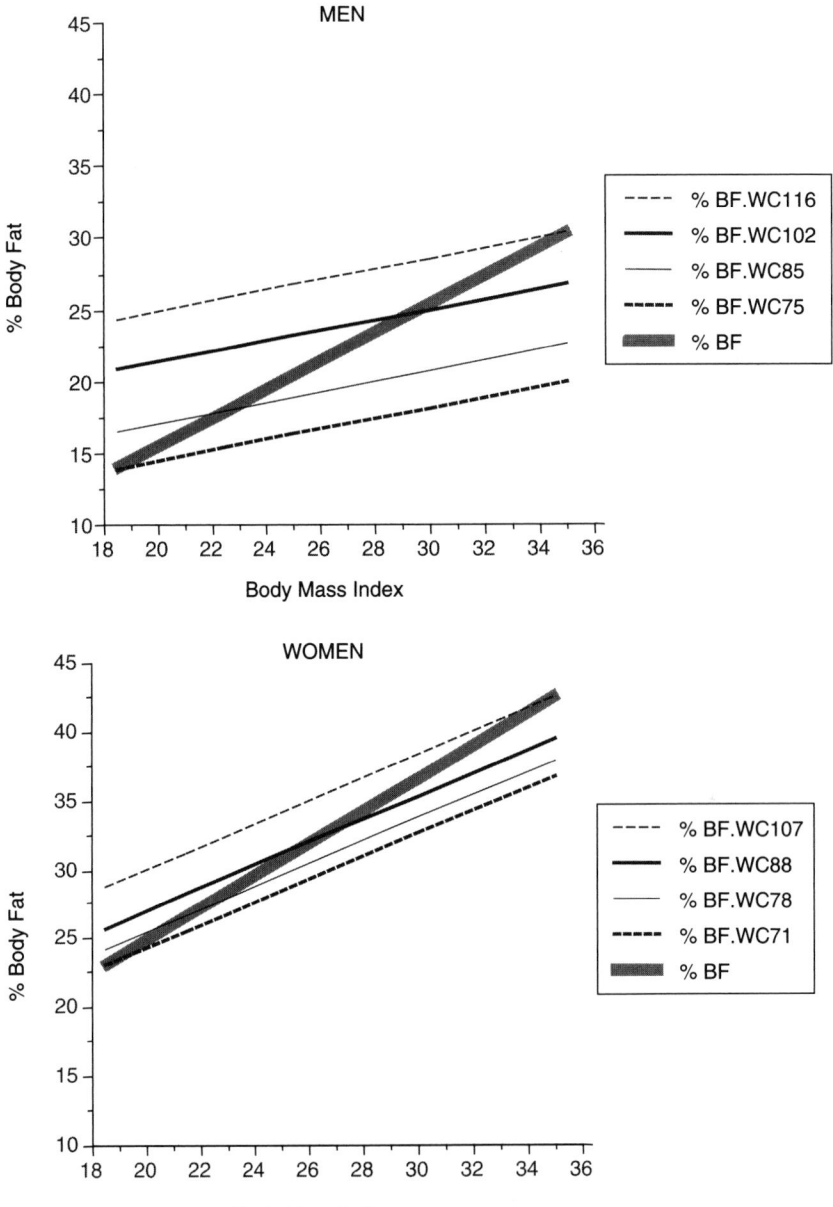

FIGURE 5-3 Regressions of percent body fat (% BF) vs. body mass index (BMI) (heavy lines), and vs. BMI relationships (thin lines) for adult men and women with BMI of 18.5 kg/m² and higher and with a specified waist circumference (WC) in men (WC = 116, 102, 85, or 75 cm) and women (WC = 107, 88, 78, or 71 cm).

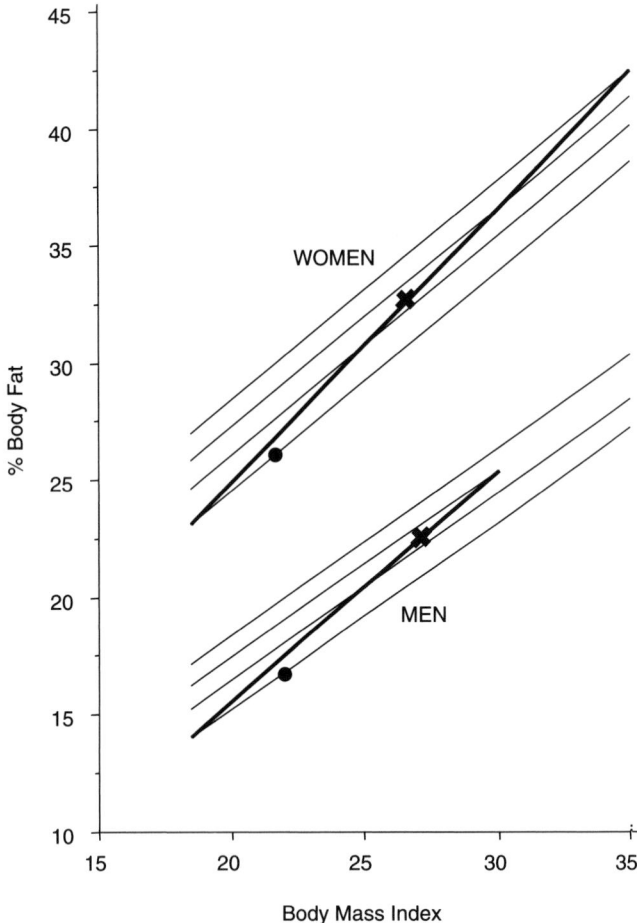

FIGURE 5-4 Regressions of percent body fat (% BF) versus body mass index (BMI) (heavy lines) and the % BF versus BMI relationships (thin lines) for adult men and women 19 years and older with BMI 18.5 kg/m^2 and higher and with specified triceps skinfold (TSF) thickness in men (TSF = 19.6, 15.8, 11.9, and 6.9 mm) and women (TSF = 30.7, 26.4, 22.2, and 16.7 mm). The • indicates the mean BMI and % BF for men and women with BMIs from 18.5 up to 25 kg/m^2 and the × indicates the mean BMI and % BF values for all men and women estimated in Appendix Table H-4.

on FFM for various BMI values is shown in Figure 5-5. BEE and REE are correlated with FFM. Yet no correlation can be detected between height and percent body fat in men, whereas in women a negative correlation exists, but with a very small R^2 value (0.0026) (Appendix Table H-6). Thus

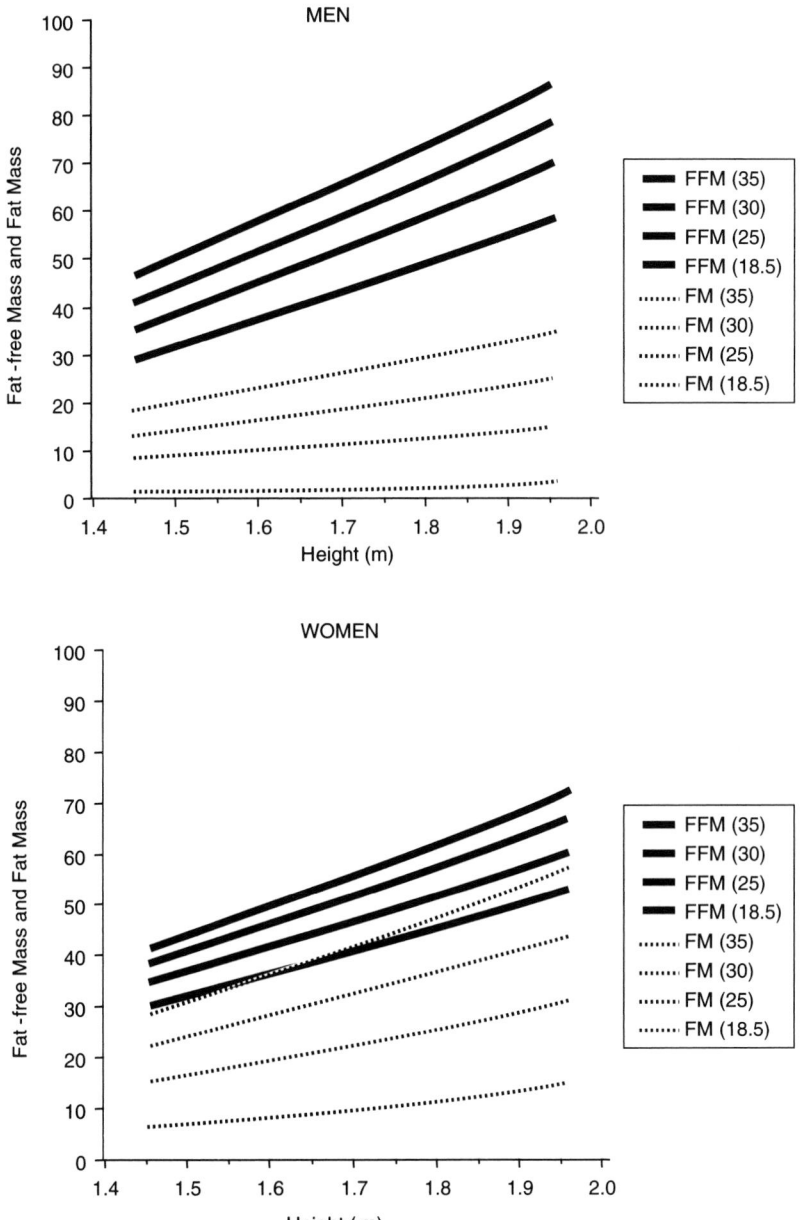

FIGURE 5-5 Regression of fat-free mass (FFM) and fat mass (FM) as a function of height in adult men and women with body mass indexes of 18.5, 25, 30, and 35 kg/m^2 (from Appendix H).

in women, as in men, differences in height have very little, if any, impact on adiposity.

Children

As children grow and develop, linear and ponderal growth do not occur at exactly commensurate rates; consequently, BMI is not constant throughout childhood. In U.S. children, BMI declines and reaches a minimum around 4 to 6 years, and then gradually increases through adolescence (Kuczmarski et al., 2000). Therefore, cutoff points to define underweight and overweight must be age- and gender-specific. The revised growth charts for the United States were derived from five national health examination surveys collected from 1963 to 1994 (Kuczmarski et al., 2000). Smoothed curves were developed for infants from birth to 36 months and for children 2 to 20 years, and BMI charts were developed for boys and girls greater than 2 years of age. Based on these data, the Centers for Disease Control and Prevention (CDC) defined underweight in children as a BMI of less than the 5th percentile. Children are considered to be at risk of overweight when their BMI is greater than the 85th percentile, and overweight when their BMI is greater than the 95th percentile (Kuczmarski et al., 2000).

Data from NHANES III on children 6 years of age and older were not used in the CDC analysis because of the recent rise in obesity among American youth. The most recent data from the NHANES III survey (1988–1994) (Troiano et al., 1995) show that substantially more than 22 percent of children in the United States now fall into the at-risk-for-overweight category (from the 85th BMI percentile) and more than 10 percent are in the overweight category (from the 95th BMI percentile). Childhood overweight is associated with several risk factors for later heart disease and other chronic diseases including hyperlipidemia, hyperinsulinemia, hypertension, and early arteriosclerosis (Must and Strauss, 1999).

Generally, an abnormal anthropometric measure is statistically defined as a value below –2 standard deviations (SD) or Z-scores (less than the 2.3 percentile) or above +2 SD or Z-scores (greater than the 97.7 percentile) relative to the reference mean (WHO Working Group, 1986). Undernutrition is defined as below the 3rd percentile for weight-for-length. Similarly, overweight has been defined as above the 97th percentile for weight-for-length. For lengths between the 3rd and 97th percentiles, the median and range of weights defined by the 3rd and 97th weight-for-length percentiles for children 0 to 3 years of age are presented in Tables 5-6 (boys) and 5-7 (girls) (Kuczmarski et al., 2000).

Reference heights and weights for boys and girls 3 to 18 years of age are given in Tables 5-8 (boys) and 5-9 (girls). Median and range of weights corresponding to the 5th and 85th BMI percentiles are designated for the 3rd and 97th height percentiles.

FACTORS AFFECTING ENERGY EXPENDITURE AND REQUIREMENTS

Body Composition and Body Size

While body size and body weight exert marked effects on energy expenditure, it is still disputed whether differences in body composition quantitatively affect energy expenditure. In adult men and women with moderate levels of body fat (20 to 35 percent), it has been suggested that the relative proportions of fat-free mass (FFM) and of fat mass are unlikely to influence energy metabolism at rest or while physically active in ways other than through their impact on body weight (Durnin, 1996). It is unlikely that body composition to any important extent affects energy expenditure at rest or the energy costs of physical activities among adults with body mass indexes from 18.5 up to 25 kg/m^2 (Heymsfield et al., 2002). In adults with higher percentages of body fat composition, mechanical hindrances can increase the energy expenditure associated with certain types of activity.

Effects on Basal and Resting Metabolic Rate

FFM includes the metabolically active compartments of the body, and the size of the FFM is the major parameter in determining the rate of energy expenditure under fasting basal metabolic rate (BMR) and resting metabolic rate (RMR) conditions. The contribution of FFM and FM to the variability in RMR was examined in a meta-analysis of seven published studies (Nelson et al., 1992). FFM was the single best predictor of RMR, accounting for 73 percent of the variability; FM accounted for only an additional 2 percent. Adjusted for FFM, RMR did not differ between genders, but it did between lean and obese individuals. In another compilation of studies, the relationship of RMR to FFM was found to be nonlinear across a wide range of individuals, from infants to adults (Weinsier et al., 1992). RMR/kg of weight or RMR/kg of FFM falls as mass increases because the relative contributions made by the most metabolically active tissues (brain, liver, and heart) decline as body size increases. The decline in BMR with increasing age is to some extent also the consequence of changes in the relative size of organs and tissues (Henry, 2000).

TABLE 5-6 Reference Lengths and Weights for Boys
1 Through 35 Months of Age Based on Median Length
and Median Weight for Age

Age (mo)	Median Length (cm [in])	Length Range 3rd–97th Percentile (cm [in])
1	54.7 (21.5)	50.2–59.6 (19.8–23.5)
2	58.1 (22.9)	53.8–63.1 (21.2–24.8)
3	60.8 (23.9)	56.6–65.9 (22.3–25.9)
4	63.1 (24.8)	58.8–68.3 (23.1–26.9)
5	65.2 (25.7)	60.8–70.4 (23.9–27.7)
6	67.0 (26.4)	62.5–72.3 (24.6–28.5)
7	68.7 (27.0)	64.1–74.1 (25.2–29.2)
8	70.2 (27.6)	65.6–75.7 (25.8–29.8)
9	71.6 (28.2)	66.9–77.2 (26.3–30.4)
10	73.0 (28.7)	68.1–78.7 (26.8–31.0)
11	74.3 (29.3)	69.3–80.0 (27.3–31.5)
12	75.5 (29.7)	70.4–81.3 (27.7–32.0)
15	78.9 (31.1)	73.4–84.9 (28.9–33.4)
18	81.9 (32.2)	76.1–88.1 (30.0–34.7)
21	84.7 (33.3)	78.5–91.1 (30.9–35.9)
24	87.2 (34.3)	80.7–93.8 (31.8–36.9)
27	89.6 (35.3)	82.9–96.5 (32.6–38.0)
30	91.8 (36.1)	85.0–99.0 (33.5–39.0)
33	93.8 (36.9)	87.0–101.3 (34.3–39.9)
35	95.1 (37.4)	88.2–102.7 (34.7–40.4)

SOURCE: Kuczmarski et al. (2000).

Effects on Total Energy Expenditure

Factors affecting total energy expenditure (TEE) were examined in a meta-analysis of 13 adult studies ($n = 162$) (Carpenter et al., 1995). The relationships between weight and TEE were highly variable across studies ($z = 0.68$; $r = 0.18$–1.0). Differences in RMR accounted for less than 50 percent of the variance in TEE ($z = 0.66$; $r = 0.42$–0.89). Adjusted for RMR, TEE was not affected by FM and was lower in women than men. In a separate study, Roberts and Dallal (1998) reported a negative relationship between FM and TEE consistent with the general perception that low physical activity and fat accumulation are correlated.

Obesity

Another question relevant to the effect of body composition on energy requirements is whether obese individuals taken as a group have altered energy requirements, either prior to the development of obesity (in

Median Weight (kg [lb])	Weight Range 3rd–97th Percentile (kg [lb])
4.4 (9.7)	3.2–5.6 (7.0–12.3)
5.3 (11.7)	4.0–6.6 (8.8–14.5)
6.0 (13.2)	4.7–7.6 (10.4–16.7)
6.7 (14.8)	5.3–8.4 (11.7–18.5)
7.3 (16.1)	5.8–9.2 (12.8–20.3)
7.9 (17.4)	6.3–9.8 (13.9–21.6)
8.4 (18.5)	6.8–10.5 (15.0–23.1)
8.9 (19.6)	7.2–11.0 (15.9–24.2)
9.3 (20.5)	7.5–11.5 (16.5–25.3)
9.7 (21.4)	7.8–12.0 (17.2–26.4)
10.0 (22.0)	8.1–12.4 (17.8–27.3)
10.3 (22.7)	8.4–12.7 (18.5–28.0)
11.1 (24.4)	9.1–13.7 (20.0–30.2)
11.7 (25.8)	9.6–14.4 (21.1–31.7)
12.2 (26.9)	10.0–15.0 (22.0–33.0)
12.7 (28.0)	10.4–15.6 (22.9–34.4)
13.1 (28.9)	10.7–16.1 (23.6–35.5)
13.5 (29.7)	11.1–16.7 (24.4–36.8)
13.9 (30.6)	11.4–17.3 (25.1–38.1)
14.2 (31.3)	11.6–17.7 (25.6–39.0)

which case they could potentially contribute to weight gain) or following weight stabilization at a high level. The information relating to the former issue is conflicting, as cross-sectional studies consistently show that overweight and obese individuals have higher absolute values for TEE than nonobese adults, as the effect of high RMR values associated with increased body size generally outweighs the influence of low energy expenditure of physical activity (EEPA) (Platte et al., 1995; Prentice et al., 1996a; Schoeller and Fjeld, 1991). In extremely obese adults, TEE can be as high as 4,500 kcal/d even when the physical activity level is low (where TEE is only 1.5 × BEE) (Prentice et al., 1996a).

Cross-sectionally, Goran and coworkers (1995a) and Griffiths and Payne (1976) reported significantly lower resting energy expenditure in children born to one or both overweight parents when the children were not themselves overweight. However, others (Davies et al., 1995; Goran et al., 1994b; Treuth et al., 2000), but not all (Roberts et al., 1988), reported no mean difference in energy expenditure between children of lean and overweight parents. While the thermic effect of food (TEF) has not been

TABLE 5-7 Reference Lengths and Weights for Girls
1 Through 35 Months of Age Based on Median Length
and Median Weight for Age

Age (mo)	Median Length (cm [in])	Length Range 3rd–97th Percentile (cm [in])
1	53.5 (21.1)	49.3–58.2 (19.4–22.9)
2	56.7 (22.3)	52.4–61.3 (20.6–24.1)
3	59.3 (23.3)	54.8–63.9 (21.6–25.2)
4	61.5 (24.2)	56.9–66.1 (22.4–26.0)
5	63.5 (25.0)	58.7–68.1 (23.1–26.8)
6	65.3 (25.7)	60.4–70.0 (23.8–27.6)
7	66.9 (26.3)	61.9–71.7 (24.4–28.2)
8	68.4 (26.9)	63.4–73.4 (25.0–28.9)
9	69.9 (27.5)	64.7–74.9 (25.5–29.5)
10	71.3 (28.1)	65.9–76.4 (25.9–30.1)
11	72.6 (28.6)	67.1–77.8 (26.4–30.6)
12	73.8 (29.1)	68.3–79.1 (26.9–31.1)
15	77.2 (30.4)	71.4–82.8 (28.1–32.6)
18	80.3 (31.6)	74.3–86.2 (29.3–33.9)
21	83.1 (32.7)	76.8–89.3 (30.2–35.2)
24	85.8 (33.8)	79.2–92.3 (31.2–36.3)
27	88.4 (34.8)	81.6–95.2 (32.1–37.5)
30	90.8 (35.7)	83.7–97.9 (33.0–38.5)
33	92.9 (36.6)	85.7–100.2 (33.7–39.4)
35	94.1 (37.0)	86.9–101.6 (34.2–40.0)

SOURCE: Kuczmarski et al. (2000).

widely studied in obese children, Tounian and colleagues (1993) reported no difference in TEF values among obese or overweight and normal-weight prepubertal children in contrast to the widespread finding of low TEF in obese adults (Segal et al., 1987, 1990a, 1990b, 1992).

In longitudinal studies of preobese adults and children, low RMR in apparently susceptible populations (Pima Indians and those infants of overweight mothers who themselves gained weight), 24-hour sedentary energy expenditure or TEE predicted excess weight gain over time in some studies (Ravussin et al., 1988; Roberts et al., 1988), but not in one other (Goran et al., 1998c).

There are also some studies that investigated apparently susceptible children (i.e., born to overweight parents) in whom weight gain was normal (Davies et al., 1995; Stunkard et al., 1999). In those studies, there was no relationship between TEE and growth rate, further suggesting that TEE is within the normal range in individuals who are apparently susceptible to excess weight gain but maintain a normal weight. The combina-

Median Weight (kg [lb])	Weight Range 3rd–97th Percentile (kg [lb])
4.2 (9.3)	3.1–5.2 (6.8–11.5)
4.9 (10.8)	3.7–6.1 (8.1–13.4)
5.5 (12.1)	4.3–6.9 (9.5–15.2)
6.1 (13.4)	4.8–7.6 (10.6–16.7)
6.7 (14.8)	5.3–8.3 (11.7–18.3)
7.2 (15.9)	5.7–8.9 (12.6–19.6)
7.7 (17.0)	6.2–9.5 (13.7–20.9)
8.1 (17.8)	6.5–10.0 (14.3–22.0)
8.5 (18.7)	6.9–10.4 (15.2–22.9)
8.9 (19.6)	7.2–10.9 (15.9–24.0)
9.2 (20.3)	7.5–11.3 (16.5–24.9)
9.5 (20.9)	7.8–11.7 (17.2–25.8)
10.3 (22.7)	8.5–12.7 (18.7–28.0)
11.0 (24.2)	9.1–13.5 (20.0–29.7)
11.6 (25.6)	9.6–14.3 (21.1–31.5)
12.1 (26.7)	10.0–15.0 (22.0–33.0)
12.5 (27.5)	10.3–15.5 (22.7–34.1)
13.0 (28.6)	10.7–16.4 (23.6–36.1)
13.4 (29.5)	11.0–17.1 (24.2–37.7)
13.7 (30.2)	11.2–17.6 (24.7–38.8)

tion of these findings from different studies suggests that low energy expenditure is a risk factor for weight gain in a subgroup of individuals susceptible to excess weight gain, but not in all susceptible individuals and not in individuals with a normal level of risk. As such, these data are consistent with the general view that obesity is a multifactor problem.

The question of whether obese individuals may have decreased energy requirements after weight loss, a factor that would help explain the common phenomenon of weight regain following weight loss, has also been investigated. As reviewed by Saltzman and Roberts (1995), RMR is consistently depressed during active weight loss out of proportion to the loss of FFM, but controversy exists over whether RMR remains depressed after weight has stabilized at a lower level. Most of the cross-sectional studies comparing post-obese with never-obese individuals have reported no difference between groups, suggesting no long-term effect of weight loss or susceptibility to depressed RMR in individuals who have been obese (Larson et al., 1995; Saltzman and Roberts, 1995; Weinsier et al., 2000). In

TABLE 5-8 Reference Heights and Weights for Boys 3 Through 18 Years of Age Based on Median Height and Median Weight for Age

Age (y)	Median Height (m [in])	Height Range 3rd–97th Percentile (m [in])
3	0.95 (37.4)	0.88–1.03 (34.6–40.6)
4	1.02 (40.2)	0.94–1.10 (37.0–43.3)
5	1.09 (42.9)	1.00–1.18 (39.4–46.5)
6	1.15 (45.3)	1.06–1.25 (41.7–49.2)
7	1.22 (48.0)	1.12–1.32 (44.1–52.0)
8	1.28 (50.4)	1.17–1.39 (46.1–54.7)
9	1.34 (52.8)	1.22–1.45 (48.0–57.1)
10	1.39 (54.7)	1.26–1.51 (49.6–59.4)
11	1.44 (56.7)	1.31–1.57 (51.6–61.8)
12	1.49 (58.7)	1.35–1.63 (53.1–64.2)
13	1.56 (61.4)	1.41–1.71 (55.5–67.3)
14	1.64 (64.6)	1.48–1.79 (58.3–70.5)
15	1.70 (66.9)	1.54–1.84 (60.6–72.4)
16	1.74 (68.5)	1.59–1.87 (62.6–73.6)
17	1.75 (68.9)	1.61–1.89 (63.4–74.4)
18	1.76 (69.3)	1.62–1.89 (63.8–74.4)

SOURCE: Kuczmarski et al. (2000).

TABLE 5-9 Reference Heights and Weights for Girls 3 Through 18 Years of Age Based on Median Height and Median Weight for Age

Age (y)	Median Height (m [in])	Height Range 3rd–97th Percentile (m [in])
3	0.94 (37.0)	0.87–1.01 (34.3–39.8)
4	1.01 (39.8)	0.93–1.09 (36.6–42.9)
5	1.08 (42.5)	0.99–1.17 (39.0–46.1)
6	1.15 (45.3)	1.06–1.25 (41.7–49.2)
7	1.21 (47.6)	1.12–1.32 (44.1–52.0)
8	1.28 (50.4)	1.17–1.39 (46.1–54.7)
9	1.33 (52.4)	1.22–1.45 (48.0–57.1)
10	1.38 (54.3)	1.26–1.51 (49.6–59.4)
11	1.44 (56.7)	1.30–1.58 (51.2–62.2)
12	1.51 (59.4)	1.37–1.65 (53.9–65.0)
13	1.57 (61.8)	1.44–1.70 (56.7–66.9)
14	1.60 (63.0)	1.48–1.73 (58.3–68.1)
15	1.62 (63.8)	1.50–1.74 (59.1–68.5)
16	1.63 (64.2)	1.50–1.75 (59.1–68.9)
17	1.63 (64.2)	1.51–1.75 (59.4–68.9)
18	1.63 (64.2)	1.51–1.75 (59.4–68.9)

SOURCE: Kuczmarski et al. (2000).

Median Weight (kg [lb])	Weight Range 3rd–97th Percentile (kg [lb])
14.3 (31.5)	11.8–17.9 (26.0–39.4)
16.2 (35.7)	13.2–20.9 (29.1–46.0)
18.4 (40.5)	14.8–24.3 (32.6–53.5)
20.7 (45.6)	16.4–28.1 (36.1–61.9)
23.1 (50.9)	18.2–32.3 (37.9–67.2)
25.6 (56.4)	20.0–37.2 (44.1–81.9)
28.6 (63.0)	22.0–42.8 (48.5–94.3)
31.9 (70.3)	24.1–49.1 (53.1–108.1)
35.9 (79.1)	26.5–56.0 (58.4–123.3)
40.5 (89.2)	29.3–63.0 (64.5–138.8)
45.6 (100.4)	32.8–70.0 (72.2–154.2)
51.0 (112.3)	36.9–76.7 (81.3–168.9)
56.3 (124.0)	41.3–83.0 (91.0–182.8)
60.9 (134.1)	45.6–88.7 (100.4–195.4)
64.6 (142.3)	49.2–93.6 (108.4–206.2)
67.2 (148.0)	51.6–97.1 (113.7–213.9)

Median Weight (kg [lb])	Weight Range 3rd–97th Percentile (kg [lb])
13.9 (30.6)	11.3–17.9 (24.9–39.4)
15.8 (34.8)	12.7–21.1 (28.0–46.5)
17.9 (39.4)	14.3–24.8 (31.5–54.6)
20.2 (44.5)	15.9–28.7 (35.0–63.2)
22.8 (50.2)	17.7–33.2 (39.0–73.1)
25.6 (56.4)	19.5–38.3 (43.0–84.4)
29.0 (63.9)	21.5–44.3 (47.4–97.6)
32.9 (72.5)	23.9–51.1 (52.6–112.6)
37.2 (81.9)	26.7–58.4 (58.8–128.6)
41.6 (91.6)	29.9–65.6 (65.9–144.5)
45.8 (100.9)	33.3–72.1 (73.3–158.8)
49.4 (108.8)	36.6–77.5 (80.6–170.7)
52.0 (114.5)	39.5–81.5 (87.0–179.5)
53.9 (118.7)	41.7–84.3 (91.9–185.7)
55.1 (121.4)	43.3–86.1 (95.4–189.6)
56.2 (123.8)	44.2–87.4 (97.4–192.5)

contrast, most longitudinal studies following individuals over the course of weight loss and subsequent weight stabilization have observed low RMR after adjusting for body composition change (Saltzman and Roberts, 1995). Notable exceptions to the latter conclusion are from studies of Amatruda and colleagues (1993) and Weinsier and colleagues (2000), which compared individuals longitudinally over the course of weight loss with a cross-sectional, never-obese control group. In these studies, there was no significant difference in TEE among the groups after adjusting for body composition. The combination of these data from different types of studies does not permit any general conclusion at the current time, and further studies in this area are needed.

Physical Activity

The impact of physical activity on energy expenditure is discussed briefly here and in more detail in Chapter 12. EEPA is the most variable component of TEE (Schoeller, 2001). Given that the basal oxygen (O_2) consumption rate of adults is approximately 250 mL/min, and that athletes such as elite marathon runners can sustain O_2 consumption rates of 5,000 mL/min, the scale of metabolic responses to exercise varies over a 20-fold range. The increase in energy expenditure elicited while physical activities take place accounts for the largest part of the effect of physical activity on overall energy expenditure, which is the product of the cost of particular activities and their duration (see Table 12-1 for examples of the energy cost of typical activities).

Recent studies have focused on using doubly labeled water to quantify the effects of physical activity on TEE. In cross-sectional studies, there is a substantial difference in physical activity level (PAL) between long-term exercising women and sedentary women. For example, Withers and co-workers (1998) observed a mean PAL value of 2.48 in long-term active women reporting a mean of 8.6 h/wk of aerobic exercise compared with a mean PAL value of 1.87 in nonexercisers. Intensive exercise programs such as those undertaken by subjects training to run a half-marathon and requiring 8 to 10 h/wk of strenuous exercise can also effect a substantial 15 to 50 percent increase in TEE in both adults and children (Eliakim et al., 1996; Goran et al., 1994a; Westerterp et al., 1992). However, more moderate exercise programs are reported to have a much smaller effect, with two studies (one in children and one in elderly individuals) reporting no significant increase in TEE (Goran and Poehlman, 1992; Treuth et al., 1998b). This lack of effect of a moderate increase in planned physical activity on TEE emphasizes the fact that intentional and spontaneous energy expenditures are interrelated. In some circumstances an increase in one component may be balanced by a decrease in another, so that TEE remains relatively unaffected.

Effect of Exercise on Postexercise Energy Expenditure

In addition to the immediate energy cost of individual activities, physical activity also affects energy expenditure in the post-exercise period. Excess postexercise O_2 consumption depends on exercise intensity and duration as well as other factors, such as environmental temperatures, state of hydration, and degree of trauma, demonstrable sometimes up to 24 hours after exercise (Bahr et al., 1987; Benedict and Cathcart, 1913; Bielinski et al., 1985; Gaesser and Brooks, 1984). In one study, residual effects of exercise could be seen following 15 hours of exercise, but not after 30 hours (Herring et al., 1992). However, a significant decrease in RMR over 3 days following cessation of training in athletes has been observed (Tremblay et al., 1988).

There may also be chronic changes in energy expenditure associated with regular physical activity as a result of changes in body composition and alterations in the metabolic rate of muscle tissue, neuroendocrine status, and changes in spontaneous physical activity associated with altered levels of fitness (van Baak, 1999; Webber and Macdonald, 2000). However, the magnitude and direction of change in energy expenditure associated with these factors remain controversial due to the variable effects of exercise on the coupling of oxidative phosphorylation in mitochondria, on ion shifts, on substrates, and on other factors (Gaesser and Brooks, 1984).

Since FFM is the major predictor of BMR and RMR, increases in FFM due to increased physical activity would be expected to increase BMR or RMR. However, three studies reported no measurable increase in BMR or RMR with increased physical activity (Bingham et al., 1989; Tremblay et al., 1990; Treuth et al., 1998b). This may be explained by the fact that energy expenditure in resting muscle is relatively low, accounting for only 20 to 25 percent of RMR even though muscle constitutes some 75 percent of the body cell mass (Moore, 1963).

Spontaneous Nonexercise Activity

Spontaneous nonexercise activity has been reported to be quantitatively important, accounting for 100 to 700 kcal/d, even in subjects residing in a whole-body calorimeter chamber (Ravussin et al., 1986). Sitting without or with fidgeting raises energy expenditure by 4 or 54 percent respectively, compared to lying supine (Levine et al., 2000), whereas standing motionless or while fidgeting raised energy expenditure by 13 or 94 percent, respectively. The impact of fidgeting was positively correlated with body weight while standing, but not while sitting. (For comparison, walking at speeds of 2 or 3 mph increases energy expenditure by 150 or 230 percent, respectively.) It is not known to what extent spontaneous nonexercise activity is affected by intentional physical activity and by its intensity.

Shah and coworkers (1988) reported a 5 percent mean increase in 24-hour TEE with a program of moderate exercise (walking) compared with a 3 percent increase with an equivalent amount of strenuous aerobic training. This suggests that the subjects had lower levels of spontaneous movement after strenuous exercise because they were more tired. In contrast, Schulz and coworkers (1991) reported no difference in sedentary 24-hour TEE between aerobically fit and sedentary individuals, and Pacy and coworkers (1996) showed no differential effect of moderate versus strenuous activity on 24-hour TEE after accounting for the energy costs of the exercise itself. On the other hand, Van Etten and colleagues (1997) showed no significant increase in 24-hour TEE with a standardized exercise program beyond that immediately associated with the exercise program. Similarly, Blaak and coworkers (1992) reported no measurable change in spontaneous physical activity in obese boys enrolled in an exercise-training program.

The combination of these different results indicates that the effects of planned physical activity on activity at other times are highly variable (ranging from overall positive to negative effects on overall energy expenditure). This most likely depends on a number of factors, including the nature of the exercise (strenuous versus moderate), the initial fitness of the subjects, body composition, and gender.

Gender

There are substantial data on the effects of gender on energy expenditure throughout the lifespan. In adult premenopausal women, the majority of studies show that RMR, BMR, or sleeping metabolic rate (SMR) is slightly increased in the luteal phase of the menstrual cycle compared to the follicular phase (Bisdee et al., 1989; Hessemer and Bruck, 1985; Meijer et al., 1992; Melanson et al., 1996; Solomon et al., 1982), but two studies reported no increase in the luteal phase compared to the follicular phase (Howe et al., 1993; Piers et al., 1995a). However, Howe and colleagues (1993) reported that both sleeping metabolic rate and sedentary 24-hour TEE were significantly increased. Twenty-four hour sedentary TEE (measured in a whole-body calorimeter) was increased in the luteal phase compared to the follicular phase in two studies (Ferraro et al., 1992; Howe et al., 1993), whereas Bisdee and colleagues (1989) found no significant change.

Because of the weight of evidence indicating cyclical changes in BMR and perhaps also sedentary 24-hour TEE in premenopausal adult women, studies of 24-hour TEE have necessarily adjusted or averaged for stage of the menstrual cycle when comparing men and women. In such adjusted studies, two studies reported lower 24-hour sedentary TEE in women compared to men after adjusting for FFM and FM (Dionne et al., 1999; Ferraro et al., 1992), while one study reported no significant gender effect in adjusted data (Klausen et al., 1997).

DLW data show a 16 percent lower TEE in women than men after controlling for FFM (Carpenter et al., 1998). This was partly accounted for by lower RMR and partly by other factors (presumably lower EEPA). Finally, menopause has also been associated with decreased RMR and EEPA and increased FM in women receiving no hormone replacement therapy (Poehlman et al., 1995).

Thus, the question of whether the hormonal differences between premenopausal women and men are responsible for the observed differences in TEE, or whether they are a secondary consequence of differences in body composition remain uncertain. Although most of the above studies adjusted data for gender differences in FFM and FM, it was not possible to adjust for differences in the *make-up* of FFM (the contribution made by different tissues and organs). It is recognized that different body tissues have different metabolic rates, with brain and organ tissues having the highest values and muscle and adipose tissues having the lowest values (FAO/WHO/UNU, 1985). Therefore, it is possible that the lower RMR in women compared to men is due to a different balance of organ and brain tissue and skeletal muscle, rather than lower energy expenditure per unit of individual tissues. Further studies are needed to address this issue.

Two of three studies investigating differences in prepubertal children reported that girls have lower values for REE than boys when adjusted for differences in body composition (Goran et al., 1994b, 1995b). The one study that reported no gender effect on REE in prepubertal children (Grund et al., 2000) used imprecise methods for assessing body composition. A separate longitudinal study (Goran et al., 1998a) reported a fall-off in TEE prior to puberty in girls but not boys.

Because commonly used BMR equations are based on body weight (Henry, 2000; WN Schofield, 1985), differences in BMR between genders are due both to the greater level of body fatness in women and to differences in the RMR–FFM relationship. These differences are ultimately reflected by lower numerical coefficients for height and weight in women compared with men in various equations to predict basal energy expenditure (BEE), or for weight and height when both variables are considered to predict BEE and TEE.

Growth

In infants and children, the energy requirement includes the energy associated with the deposition of tissues at rates consistent with good health. Although the energy requirement for growth relative to maintenance is low, except for the first months of life, satisfactory growth is a sensitive indicator of whether energy needs are being met. The energy cost of growth as a percentage of total energy requirements decreases from around 35 percent at 1 month to 3 percent at 12 months of age, and remains low until the pubertal growth spurt, at which time it increases to about 4 percent (Butte, 2000).

Growth is most impressive during infancy. Infants double their birth weight by 6 months of age, and triple it by 12 months (Butte et al., 2000a). At birth, the newborn is about 11 percent body fat. Progressive fat deposition in the early months results in a peak in the percentage body weight that is fat at 3 to 6 months (about 31 percent) and body fatness subsequently declines to an average of 27 percent at 12 months (Butte et al., 2000a). During infancy and childhood, girls grow slightly slower than boys, and girls have slightly more body fat (Butte et al., 2000a). During adolescence the gender differences in body composition are accentuated (Ellis, 1997; Ellis et al., 1997; Forbes, 1987; Tanner, 1955). Adolescence in boys is characterized by rapid acquisition of FFM and a modest increase in FM in early puberty, followed by a decline. FFM accretion coincides with the rapid spurt in height, though height gain may also continue until 20 to 25 years of age. Adolescence in girls is characterized by a modest increase in FFM and a continual accumulation of FM. The pubertal increase in FFM ceases at about 18 years, following the decrease in the rate of height gain after menarche (Forbes, 1987; Tanner, 1955).

Growth velocity is a sensitive indicator of energy status and use of growth velocity charts will detect growth faltering earlier than detected using attained growth charts. There is a wide range of variation in the growth rate of infants and children. Growth occurs in spurts, even in healthy children. Problems with measurement precision and high variability in individual growth rates over short time periods complicate the interpretation of growth velocity data. The timing of the adolescent growth spurt, which typically lasts 2 to 3 years, is also very variable, with the onset typically between 10 and 13 years of age in the majority of children (Forbes, 1987; Tanner, 1955). In general, weight velocity reflects acute episodes of dietary intake, whereas length velocity is affected by chronic factors.

Older Age

All three major components of energy expenditure decrease with aging: RMR, TEF, and EEPA. There is an average decline in BMR of 1 to 2 percent per decade in men who maintain constant weight (Keys et al., 1973). The suggested breakpoint for a more rapid decline apparently occurs around 40 years of age in men and 50 years of age in women (Poehlman, 1992, 1993). For women, this may be due to an accelerated loss of FFM during menopause (Svendsen et al., 1995).

In addition to the loss of FFM being a cause of age-associated decline in RMR, several (Fukagawa et al., 1990; Klausen et al., 1997; Pannemans and Westerterp, 1995; Poehlman et al., 1991; Roberts et al., 1995; Vaughan et al., 1991; Visser et al., 1995), though not all (Tzankoff and Norris, 1977), studies suggest that RMR adjusted for the change in FFM is decreased by about 5 percent in older adults compared to younger adults. However, in individuals who gain significant amounts of weight as they get older, RMR may actually increase due to gains of FM and FFM.

There is evidence suggesting that the RMR response to changes in energy balance may be attenuated in old versus young adults (Roberts and Dallal, 1998). The primary connection between RMR changes with age and FFM is also emphasized by research showing that endurance training (which increases FFM) increases RMR in elders (Poehlman and Danforth, 1991).

Concerning TEF, some studies report a decrease with aging (Golay et al., 1982; Morgan and York, 1983; Schutz et al., 1984; Schwartz et al., 1990; Thorne and Wahren, 1990), while other studies report no change or a nonsignificant increase (Bloesch et al., 1988; Fukagawa et al., 1991; Melanson et al., 1998; Poehlman et al., 1991; Tuttle et al., 1953; Visser et al., 1995). Although this controversy cannot currently be resolved, a suggested explanation is that TEF does not decline with aging per se, but that some studies may have included subjects with factors that decrease TEF independent of aging, such as obesity and digestive problems that limit nutrient absorption (Melanson et al., 1998).

PAL has been shown to decrease progressively with age and is lower in elderly adults compared to young adults (Roberts et al., 1992). Twenty-four-hour sedentary TEE measured in a whole-body calorimeter is also lower in elderly subjects compared with young adults (Vaughan et al., 1991). However, in whole body calorimeter protocols in which sedentary activity protocols were standardized, TEE did not differ between young and old adults (Pannemans et al., 1995).

The apparent decline in EEPA is consistent with the reported decreased frequency of strenuous physical activities in elderly men (Roberts, 1996). In addition, the decrease in TEE with age closely parallels the increase in

FM (Roberts and Dallal, 1998). However, the extent to which the increase in FM with age is a consequence or a cause of the age-related decrease in EEPA is not known. In relation to this observation, it should be noted that some elderly individuals clearly are able to maintain very high levels of TEE; Withers and coworkers (1998) report PAL values of 2.48 among older women with routine exercise habits compared to 1.87 in nonexercising women. However, mean maximal oxygen consumption declines 0.70 to 1 percent/y after age 35 in both sedentary adults and active adults (Suominen et al., 1977). Further studies are needed to determine the extent to which EEPA can be maintained in older adults in the general population.

Genetics

Energy requirements vary substantially between individuals due to combinations of differences in body size and composition, differences in RMR independent of body composition, differences in TEF, and differences in physical activity and in EEPA. All of these determinants of energy requirements are potentially influenced by genetic inheritance, with transmissible and nontransmissible cultural factors contributing to variability as well. Currently there is insufficient research data to predict differences in energy requirements among specific genetic groups, but as data accumulate this may become possible.

The effects of genetic inheritance on body composition are well known, with most studies reporting that 25 to 50 percent of interindividual variability in body composition can be attributed to genetic factors (Bouchard and Perusse, 1993). Because FFM and FM are major determinants of both RMR and TEE (Roberts and Dallal, 1998), these genetic influences on FFM and FM must be expected to influence energy requirements.

In addition to genetic influences on energy requirements mediated by genetic influences on body composition, there also appear to be genetic influences on TEE independent of body composition. Bogardus and coworkers (1986) reported a significant familial (intra-family) influence on RMR independent of FFM, age, and gender. Although the origin of this familial association is not currently known, it may potentially be due to differences in the relative sizes of FFM components (e.g., muscle, brain, organs) because recent work has suggested that organ size determined by magnetic resonance imaging strongly predicts RMR (Illner et al., 2000). In addition, Bouchard and coworkers (1989) reported that about 40 percent or more of the variances in RMR, TEF, and the energy costs of low-to-moderate intensity exercise are explained by inherited characteristics. The same group also reported that there is a genetic component to the weight-gain response to 1,000 kcal/d of overfeeding (Bouchard et al., 1990).

The question of which specific genes underlie genetic differences in TEE components is starting to be addressed, but few data are yet available. Valve and coworkers (1998) reported that polymorphisms within the UCP1 gene had no effect on BMR, but a combination of polymorphisms in the UCP1 and β_3-adrenergic receptor genes were associated with a significant 79 kcal/d decrease in BEE. Klannemark and coworkers (1998) reported no association between polymorphisms in the UCP2 gene and BMR, while Astrup and coworkers (1999) reported significant associations of these polymorphisms with TEE determined in a whole-body calorimeter and adjusted for FFM.

The study of Astrup and coworkers (1999) suggesting an association of specific gene polymorphisms with sedentary TEE is also consistent with the work of Heitmann and coworkers (1997) suggesting genetic influences on voluntary physical activity. Since EEPA is the major variable component of TEE, it is likely that genetic influences on EEPA may contribute substantially to intra-individual variability in TEE. Further work in this area is needed.

Ethnicity

African Americans and Caucasians

Most (Albu et al., 1997; Carpenter et al., 1998; Forman et al., 1998; Foster et al., 1997, 1999; Jakicic and Wing, 1998; Weyer et al., 1999a), but not all (Kushner et al., 1995; Nicklas et al., 1997), studies comparing RMR, BMR, or SMR between African-American and Caucasian adults have reported that RMR or SMR, adjusted for differences in body composition, are significantly lower in African Americans by about 10 percent. Foster and colleagues (1999) reported that the decrease in RMR with weight loss (adjusted for body composition change) is greater in African-American women than in Caucasian women, with weight loss of the African-American women in that study less than that of the Caucasian women. Similarly, the majority of studies reported lower RMR or BMR adjusted for body composition in African-American children than in Caucasian children (Kaplan et al., 1996; Morrison et al., 1996; Treuth et al., 2000; Wong et al., 1999; Yanovski et al., 1997); only one study found no difference between groups (Sun et al., 1998).

In addition, free-living EEPA, measured using the DLW method, appears to be lower in African-American compared to Caucasian individuals by about 10 to 20 percent (Carpenter et al., 1998; Kushner et al., 1995). These studies are consistent with the reports of lower levels of reported physical activity in African-American versus Caucasian adults (Washburn et al., 1992) and also lower maximal oxygen consumption (Vo_2max)

(Hunter et al., 2000). However, 24-hour sedentary TEE measured by whole-body calorimetry was not significantly different between African-American and Caucasian groups (Weyer et al., 1999a).

In children, EEPA adjusted for body composition was reported to be lower in African Americans than Caucasians (Wong et al., 1999). This finding is consistent with another study (Trowbridge et al., 1997) showing a 15 percent lower Vo_2max in African-American compared with Caucasian children. However, another DLW study observed no significant difference in TEE or EEPA between African-American and Caucasian children (Sun et al., 1998). Further studies in this area are needed.

The combination of data from these studies in adults and children indicate that BMR is usually lower in African Americans compared to Caucasians. Currently, insufficient data exist to create prediction equations for BMRs in African-American adults that would be accurate for both males and females throughout the life stages. In this report, therefore, the general prediction equations are used for all races, recognizing their potential to overestimate BMR in some groups such as African Americans.

Other Ethnic Groups

In addition to African Americans and Caucasians, other ethnic groups have been investigated for potential differences in energy requirements. In Pima Indians, an ethnic group widely considered to have a form of genetic obesity, RMR or SMR is not different from RMR or SMR in Caucasians after adjustment for body composition (Fontvieille et al., 1992; Weyer et al., 1999b). Similarly, physical activity levels were not different between Pima Indian and Caucasian children (Salbe et al., 1997), although the same group observed that spontaneous physical activity is a familial trait (Zurlo et al., 1992). Mohawk Indian children were reported to have higher values for TEE than Caucasian children, due to high levels of EEPA (Goran et al., 1995b). Thus, there are currently insufficient data to define specific differences in energy requirements between different racial groups and more research is needed in this area.

Environment

Climate

In the United States and Canada, indoor temperatures are typically controlled to remain within the 20°C to 25°C (68°F to 77°F) range during winter, and are frequently maintained to within a similar range in summer (EPA, 1991). In addition, most individuals intentionally create a relatively consistent temperature microenvironment for themselves by using more insulating clothing in cold weather and cooler clothes in hot weather. The question of whether normal variations in ambient temperature influence energy requirements is therefore complex.

Potential effects of ambient temperature on energy requirements include the postprandial and postabsorptive metabolic rate (which would also include energy expenditure for shivering and nonshivering thermogenesis), the amount and types of voluntary and required physical activity, and EEPA. Ambient temperature effects are probably only significant when there is prolonged exposure to substantial cold or heat. The energy cost of work was judged to be 5 percent greater in a cold environment as compared to a warm environment (Consolazio et al., 1963). There can also be an additional energy cost (2 to 5 percent) of both the increased weight of clothing worn and the hobbling effect of that clothing in cold weather compared with clothing worn in warm weather (Consolazio et al., 1963). In addition, temperatures low enough to induce shivering or increased muscular activity will increase energy needs because of the increase in mechanical work (Timmons et al., 1985). More recent work also suggests that the recognized increase in energy expenditure in markedly cold climates may be greater in physically active individuals than in sedentary ones (Armstrong, 1998).

High ambient temperatures may also increase energy requirements. There is an increase in the energy expenditure of standard tasks when ambient temperatures are very high (Consolazio et al., 1963). However, this increase in energy expenditure may be attenuated by continued exposure. Garby and colleagues (1990) reported that the extra energy expenditure for 2 hours of light activity at 34°C fell progressively a total of 3 to 8 percent with acclimatization over 8 days of the study compared with activity at 20°C to 24°C.

Relative to high-normal ambient temperatures (26°C to 28°C), low-normal ambient temperatures (20°C to 22°C) were associated with increased sedentary TEE values in lean female subjects (Blaza and Garrow, 1983; Dauncey, 1981). More recent studies have reported a significant effect of variations in ambient temperature within the usual range on energy requirements. Lean and colleagues (1988) reported a 4 percent increase in the sleeping metabolic rate of women at an ambient temperature of 22°C compared with 28°C. Warwick and Busby (1990) reported a 5 percent increase in sedentary TEE at 20°C in men and women wearing clothing of their own choice and performing a standardized pattern of physical activity compared with similar activity at 28°C. Buemann and co-workers (1992) reported a significant 2 percent increase in TEE at 16°C compared with 24°C (with no difference in response seen between post-obese and normal women). Men showed a significant increase in sedentary TEE at the lowest (20°C) and highest (30°C) temperatures studied compared to temperatures in the middle range (23°C and 26°C) (Valencia et al., 1992). This study also confirmed earlier findings (Nielsen, 1987) that humidity did not significantly affect RMR. These data consistently suggest that low-normal temperatures (20°C to 22°C) and high-normal temperatures (28°C to 30°C) are associated with an increase in sedentary TEE of 2 to 5 percent compared to temperatures of 24°C to 27°C. This conclusion is also consistent with the report of Lanzola and colleagues (1990) that skin temperature closely predicts BMR in normal individuals.

A summary of changes in BMR among individuals migrating between the tropic and temperate climates has demonstrated that changes in ambient temperature do not produce a long-term change in metabolic rate (Hayter and Henry, 1993). Instead, the effect of ambient temperature appears to be confined to the period of time during which the ambient temperature is altered. Nevertheless, the energy expenditure response to cold temperatures may be enhanced with previous acclimatization by prolonged exposure to a cool environment (Kashiwazaki et al., 1990).

The question of whether there are gender differences in the apparent increase in sedentary TEE at low-normal ambient temperatures compared to high-normal temperatures remains uncertain. In a re-analysis of the data of Warwick and Busby (1990), Murgatroyd and coworkers (1990) reported that the increase in sedentary TEE was only statistically significant in women, raising the question of whether women may be more responsive to low-normal ambient temperatures than men. Since most of the recent data has been collected in women, further research in this area is needed.

In addition to the effects of normal variations in ambient temperature on sedentary TEE, there may also be season-related influences on the amount of voluntary physical activity and EEPA, but these potential effects are less well defined. Burstein and coworkers (1996) reported a nonsignificant increase in TEE in soldiers participating in an intense exercise regimen in winter compared to summer. There was also no significant difference in season-related values for physical activity in free-living adult Dutch women, but in contrast to the values reported above for soldiers, the values tended to be higher in summer than in winter (van Staveren et al., 1986). However, unlike these nonsignificant effects of season and temperature on TEE in adults, children were reported to have significantly greater TEE in the spring than in the fall (Bitar et al., 1999; Goran et al. 1998b).

The combination of these results indicates that there is a modest 2 to 5 percent increase in sedentary TEE at low-normal ambient temperatures compared to high-normal ambient temperatures. However, it is not possible to generalize these results to seasonal effects on TEE because of the potentially important and variable impact of seasonal changes in physical activity that are likely dependent on local temperature fluctuations and cultural factors. For this reason, no specific allowance is made for ambient temperature in the requirements for energy. It should also be noted that the TEE values used to predict the energy requirements of different groups were made throughout the year, and can be considered values averaged for the ambient temperatures of the different seasons.

Altitude

Hypoxia increases glucose utilization whether measurements are made on isolated muscle tissue (Cartee et al., 1991), tissues in situ (Zinker et al., 1995), or intact functioning individuals (Brooks et al., 1991, 1992). The hypobaric hypoxia of high altitude increases BMR and TEE but it is unclear at which heights the effect becomes prominent. A study on men at 4,300 m (14,100 ft) found an increase in BMR of about 200 to 500 kcal/d when energy intakes were maintained (Butterfield et al., 1992). However, in a subsequent study on women, the effect of altitude on raising BMR and TEE was less prominent (Mawson et al., 2000).

Adaptation and Accommodation

There are two key differences between nutritional adaptation and accommodation (Waterlow, 1999). First, while adaptation implies maintenance of essentially unchanged functional capacity in spite of some alteration in steady-state conditions, accommodation allows maintenance of adequate functional capacity under altered steady-state conditions. Second, whereas accommodation involves relatively short-term adjustments, such as the responses needed to maintain homeostasis, adaptation involves changes in body composition that occur over a more extended period of time.

Adaptation

The term adaptation describes the normal physiological responses of humans to different environmental conditions. A good example of adaptation is the increase in hemoglobin concentration that occurs when individuals live at high altitudes (Leon-Velarde et al., 2000).

Energy balance is regulated by a complex set of feedback mechanisms. Changes in energy intake or in energy expenditure trigger metabolic and behavioral responses aimed at restoring energy balance in adults. These responses involve the endocrine system, the central nervous system, and the body energy stores. When effective, these regulatory mechanisms result in the maintenance of a stable body weight (Jequier and Tappy, 1999).

The estimation of energy requirements from energy expenditure implicitly assumes that the efficiency of energy utilization is more or less uniform across all individuals. Otherwise, individuals with higher efficiency would require less energy for equal energy expenditure than persons with lower efficiency. The experimental data supports the notion that differences in efficiency of energy utilization among healthy individuals living under similar conditions fluctuate within a narrow range (James et al., 1990; Waterlow et al., 1989).

Body weight can be remarkably stable in many healthy adults, demonstrating the human potential for maintaining energy balance and stable body composition in spite of conditions that have promoted the recent secular trends in increasing body weights. Maintenance of stable body weight and composition are affected by genetic factors, energy intake, and diet composition, as well as by other environmental factors (Hill and Peters, 1998). Environmental conditions favoring high energy consumption and low physical activity can overwhelm these mechanisms and lead to positive energy balance, resulting in body fat accumulation and weight gain until another state of weight maintenance becomes established. Thus, weight gain and obesity can be seen as a form of adaptation that brings about a new steady state (Astrup et al., 1994).

Adaptation has been defined as "a process by which a new or different steady state is reached in response to a change or difference in the intake of food and nutrients" (FAO/WHO/UNU, 1985). A more practical definition, applied to the study of energy requirements, would be the ability to compensate for changes in energy (energy intake, expenditure, or balance) without any discernible detriment to health.

Although the concept applies both to increases and decreases in energy intake or energy expenditure, a focus of controversy has been its application to the definition of energy needs in poor areas of the world. In studies that specifically attempted to assess whether some adaptive mechanism may permit those populations to subsist with lower than predicted energy intakes, no reduction in weight-adjusted basal metabolic rates could be detected (Soares et al., 1991).

Studies by numerous investigators (Minghelli et al., 1990; Ravussin et al., 1988; Weinsier et al., 1998; Weyer et al., 1999a, 1999b) tend to confirm the limited capacity of homeostasis to prevent or attenuate the impact of changes in energy intake on weight gain or weight loss without discernible impact on activity. Thus, a reduction in BEE or REE is generally associated with reduced body weight (Minghelli et al., 1990). Reports on the ethnic and gender differences in energy efficiency have yielded conflicting results, but the overall contributions such differences can make toward the maintenance of energy balance appears to be small (Soares et al., 1998; Weyer et al., 1999a, 1999b). The TEF component of the energy balance equation accounts for only a small fraction of TEE and does not appear to vary adaptively in relationship to changes in energy balance. Thus, maintenance of energy balance is largely dependent on adjustments in food intake and physical activity.

Some studies suggest a capacity for TEE to increase or decrease spontaneously when energy intake increases or decreases (Levine et al., 1999; Roberts et al., 1990). However, most overfeeding studies show that overeating is accompanied by substantial weight gain, and likewise reduced energy intake induces weight loss (Saltzman and Roberts, 1995). Thus, although there is some adaptive capacity of TEE to adjust to changes in dietary energy intake, the extent of this adjustment (other than what can be attributed to change in body size) is much too small to offset the impact observed by changes in energy intake. Body weight is a direct indicator of the relationship between food intake or availability and TEE.

Accommodation

The term accommodation was proposed to characterize an adaptive response that allows survival but results in some more or less serious consequences on health or physiological function. The most common example is a decrease in growth velocity in children. By reducing growth rate, children are able to save energy and may subsist for prolonged periods of time on marginal energy intakes, though at the cost of eventually becoming stunted. Another common example of accommodation is a reduction in physical activity. This can result in reduced productivity of physical work or in decreased leisure physical activity, which in children is important for behavioral and mental development (Twisk, 2001).

APPROACH USED TO DETERMINE TOTAL ENERGY EXPENDITURE

Based on the preceding review of possible approaches to estimating energy requirements, direct measurement of total energy expenditure (TEE) by the doubly labeled water (DLW) method represents a distinct advantage over previous TEE evaluations that had to rely on the factorial approach and/or on food intake data, both of which have limited reliability.

Description of the Doubly Labeled Water Database

Total energy expenditure data obtained by the DLW method were solicited for this report from investigators identified in the literature. Over 20 investigators responded and submitted individual TEE and ancillary data including age, gender, height, weight, basal energy expenditure (BEE) (observed or estimated), and descriptors for each individual in the data set (see Appendix I; also available at www.iom.edu/fnb). A normative

DLW database was created based on the inclusion/exclusion criteria described below.

Since the DLW data were not obtained in randomly selected individuals (except in the recent study of Bratteby and coworkers [1997]), they do not therefore constitute a representative sample of the populations of the United States and Canada. However, the measurements were obtained from men, women, and children whose ages, body weight, height, and physical activities varied over wide ranges, so they provide an appropriate base to estimate energy expenditures and requirements at different life stages in relation to gender, body weight, height, age, and for different activity estimations. A few age groups are underrepresented in the data set and interpolations had to be performed in these cases. Thus, while the available DLW data set used is not entirely satisfactory, it nevertheless offers the best currently available information. This data set, used to estimate the current energy recommendations, can be used to refine other existing communicated recommendations or guidelines developed by other organizations and agencies.

Inclusion/Exclusion Criteria

Normative Database. To arrive at estimates of TEE, the normative DLW database, as summarized in Table 5-10, included infants and very young children (0 through 2 years of age) within the 3rd to 97th percentile for weight-for-height (Kuczmarski et al., 2000) (Appendix Table I-1), children (3 through 18 years of age) within the 5th to 85th percentile for body mass index (BMI) (Kuczmarski et al., 2000) (Appendix Table I-2), and adults (19 years of age and older) with BMI from 18.5 up to 25 kg/m^2 (Appendix Table I-3). Subjects were required to be healthy, free-living, maintaining their body weight, and with measured heights and weights. Exclusion criteria included undernutrition, acute and chronic diseases, underfeeding and overfeeding protocols, and lifestyles involving uncommonly high levels of physical activity (e.g., elite athletes, astronauts, military trainees, and those with a physical activity level [PAL] greater than 2.5). A subset of DLW data was formulated for pregnant (Appendix Table I-4) and lactating (Appendix Table I-5) women meeting the inclusion/exclusion criteria prior to pregnancy.

There are 407 adults in the normative database (Appendix Table I-3), 169 men and 238 women. Among the men whose ethnicity was reported, there are 33 Caucasians, 7 African Americans, and 2 Asians, and among the women there are 94 Caucasians, 13 African Americans, 3 Asians, and 3 Hispanics. The majority of the adult data come from studies that were conducted in the United States or the Netherlands, with the remainder from studies done in the United Kingdom, Australia, and Sweden. For the 100 adults for whom data were provided on occupation, the most commonly reported types of occupations were offices workers, followed by teachers and students, scientists, medical workers, active occupations (e.g., aerobics instructor, police officer, physical therapist, dog trainer), homemakers, artists, and the unemployed.

The database for normal-weight children (n = 525) (Appendix Table I-2) includes 167 boys (73 Caucasians, 13 African Americans, 4 Hispanics, and 62 American Indians) and 358 girls (197 Caucasians 58 African Americans, 20 Hispanics, 10 Asians, and 60 American Indians); ethnicity was not provided for 15 boys and 13 girls. All data on children were collected in the United States.

Overweight and Obese Database. DLW databases of overweight and obese children and adults were also developed and are summarized in Table 5-11. Children (3 through 18 years of age) above the 85th percentile for BMI (Kuczmarski et al., 2000) (Appendix Table I-6) and adults (19 years of age and older) with BMIs from 25 kg/m^2 and higher (Appendix Table I-7) were included in the database. Subjects were required to be free-living. Diet and exercise intervention studies were excluded. There were insufficient data to address pregnancy and lactation in overweight and obese women.

The database for overweight and obese adults contains information on 360 individuals—165 men and 195 women (Appendix Table I-7). Among the men whose ethnicity was reported, there are 22 Caucasians and 21 African Americans; among the women there are 51 Caucasians, 34 African Americans, and 5 Hispanics. The majority of the data come from studies conducted in the United States and the Netherlands; the rest are from studies conducted in the United Kingdom, Sweden, and Australia. Occupations were not provided for 326 individuals. For those 34 individuals for whom an occupation was given, the most common types were office workers, followed by medical personnel, homemakers, active occupations (e.g., firefighter, fitness instructors), teachers and students, researchers, and artists.

The database for overweight and obese children (n = 319) (Appendix Table I-6) includes 127 boys (33 Caucasian, 20 African-American, 2 Hispanic, and 71 American Indian) and 192 girls (63 Caucasian, 48 African-American, 6 Hispanic, 68 American Indian, and 1 Asian; ethnicity was not provided for 1 boy and 6 girls. All data were collected in the United States.

TABLE 5-10 Doubly Labeled Water Databases for All Individuals with a Body Mass Index (BMI) in the Range from 18.5 up to 25 kg/m^{2a}

Age (y)	n	Mean Weight (kg [lb])	Mean Height (m [in])
0–0.5	116	6.9 (15)	0.64 (25)
0.6–1.0	72	9.0 (20)	0.72 (28)
1–2	132	11.0 (24)	0.82 (32)
Males			
3–8	129	20.4 (45)	1.15 (45)
9–13	28	35.8 (79)	1.44 (57)
14–18	10	58.8 (130)	1.70 (67)
19–30	48	71.0 (156)	1.80 (71)
31–50	59	71.4 (157)	1.78 (70)
51–70	24	70.0 (154)	1.74 (69)
71+	38	68.9 (152)	1.74 (69)
Females			
3–8	227	22.9 (50)	1.20 (47)
9–13	89	36.4 (80)	1.44 (57)
14–18	42	54.1 (119)	1.63 (64)
19–30	82	59.3 (131)	1.66 (65)
31–50	61	58.6 (129)	1.64 (65)
51–70	71	59.1 (130)	1.63 (63)
71+	24	54.8 (121)	1.58 (62)

a Summary of data in Appendix Tables I-1 through I-5.
b For adults (19 years of age and over), the observed BEE was used to calculate the mean BEE. BEE and physical activity level were not used for infants. For children, BEE

Data Analysis and Assumptions Made for the Total Energy Expenditure Equations

For the normative DLW database, prediction equations of TEE from age, gender, height, and weight were developed. The validity of these equations to predict TEE rest on three general assumptions: that the database represents the phenomena of interest, that the model describes the physiological phenomena of the data, and that the fitted equations accurately describe the data. As in any realistic statistical modeling activity, the balance is between fitting the data and fitting the phenomena, while making optimal use of the available data.

The available data were reviewed and analyzed and it is assumed that they are representative of the phenomena of interest—the energy metabo-

Mean Body Mass Index (kg/m^2)	Mean Basal Energy Expenditure (BEE) (kcal/d)[b]	Mean Total Energy Expenditure (TEE) (kcal/d)	Mean Physical Activity Level (TEE/BEE)
16.9	—	501	—
17.2	—	713	—
16.2	—	869	—
15.4	1,035	1,441	1.39
17.2	1,320	2,079	1.56
20.4	1,729	3,116	1.80
22.0	1,769	3,081	1.74
22.6	1,675	3,021	1.81
23.0	1,524	2,469	1.63
22.8	1,480	2,238	1.52
15.6	1,004	1,487	1.48
17.4	1,186	1,907	1.60
20.4	1,361	2,302	1.69
21.4	1,361	2,436	1.80
21.6	1,322	2,404	1.83
22.2	1,226	2,066	1.70
21.8	1,183	1,564	1.33

was predicted based on the following equations (see "TEE Equations for Normal-Weight Children"):

Boys: BEE (kcal/d) = 68 – 43.3 × age (y) + 712 × height (m) + 19.2 × weight (kg).
Girls: BEE (kcal/d) = 189 – 17.6 × age (y) + 625 × height (m) + 7.9 × weight (kg).

lism of healthy individuals over the normal range of age, height, weight, and energy expenditure. The analyses were restricted to include individuals within the specific ranges of body sizes and excluded individuals who were identified as being full-time in physical training.

An additive model was chosen as the default, with the relative contributions of height and weight kept constant for each gender. Because of the difficulty of estimating physical activity in the field, a four-level ordinal variable was generated, estimated from PAL data and used in the model to modify the total height and weight contribution to TEE. Various transformations of the data and the inclusion of multiplicative terms were explored, but none significantly improved how well the model described the data.

TABLE 5-11 Doubly Labeled Water Database for Overweight and Obese Males and Females[a]

Age (y)	n	Mean Weight (kg [lb])	Mean Height (m [in])
Males			
3–8	91	28.6 (63)	1.19 (46)
9–13	36	54.7 (120)	1.46 (57)
14–18	—	—	—
19–30	11	98.5 (217)	1.82 (72)
31–50	68	98.3 (217)	1.78 (70)
51–70	54	90.4 (199)	1.75 (69)
71+	32	82.3 (181)	1.72 (68)
Females			
3–8	123	30.5 (67)	1.22 (48)
9–13	56	55.8 (123)	1.50 (59)
14–18	13	73.9 (163)	1.64 (65)
19–30	37	82.3 (181)	1.66 (65)
31–50	51	88.3 (194)	1.66 (65)
51–70	79	79.7 (176)	1.62 (64)
71+	28	69.0 (152)	1.58 (62)

[a] Summary of data in Appendix Tables I-6 and I-7.
[b] For adults (ages 19 and over), the observed BEE was used to calculate the mean BEE. For children, BEE was predicted based on the following equations (see "Estimation of Energy Expenditure in Overweight Children Ages 3 through 18 Years"):

Finally, although the equations are essentially linear (within each PAL), a nonlinear regression procedure was used, with a least squares loss function. During the exploratory phase, evaluations of alternative models were based on the magnitude of residual error and examination of residual plots. These residual plots showed that while errors are not constant over the whole range of the variables, there is no simple pattern. As noted above, various transformations of the dependent variable (TEE) were explored, and in light of these results it was decided that assuming a least squares loss function did not lead to serious bias in the fitted models, and that the effect on error estimates was not important given the large amount of unexplained variability in the data. Since nonlinear regression is an iterative approach, the influence of varying the starting point was investigated and was found not to be a problem. The standard errors of the coefficients were estimated asymptotically; for a sample of the fits estimates were determined by jackknife techniques; these were found not to change the conclusions.

Mean Body Mass Index (kg/m^2)	Mean Basal Energy Expenditure (BEE) (kcal/d)[b]	Mean Total Energy Expenditure (TEE) (kcal/d)	Mean Physical Activity Level (TEE/BEE)
19.8	1,210	1,728	1.42
25.4	1,612	2,451	1.52
—	—	—	—
29.6	1,970	3,599	1.85
30.8	1,955	3,598	1.85
29.6	1,722	2,946	1.72
27.8	1,667	2,510	1.52
20.3	1,149	1,669	1.45
24.7	1,443	2,346	1.63
27.6	1,596	2,798	1.75
29.8	1,524	2,677	1.77
31.9	1,629	2,895	1.79
30.4	1,380	2,176	1.59
27.6	1,258	1,763	1.40

Boys: BEE (kcal/d) = 419.9 − 33.5 × age (y) + 418.9 × height (m) + 16.7 × weight (kg).
Girls: BEE (kcal/d) = 515.8 − 26.8 × age (y) + 347 × height (m) + 12.4 × weight (kg).

Examination of the normative DLW database showed an initial increase of TEE with age until a plateau from age 20 to 45 in women, followed by a decline (Figure 5-6). Men peaked around 35 years of age, and then declined (Figure 5-6). Increased TEE is related to greater heights (Figure 5-7) and weights (Figure 5-8). For adults, TEE was independent of BMI when the analysis was adjusted for height. Analyses indicated that the best predictions for TEE were obtained by fitting all the data separately for adults (ages 19 years and older), children and adolescents (ages 3 through 18 years), and young children (ages 0 through 2 years).

Gender-specific equations were found to be unnecessary in children less than 3 years of age. All data were entered into and analyzed with SPSS, version 10.0.

Physical Activity Level Categories

The PAL categories were defined as sedentary (PAL ≥ 1.0 < 1.4), low active (PAL ≥ 1.4 < 1.6), active (PAL ≥ 1.6 < 1.9), and very active (PAL ≥

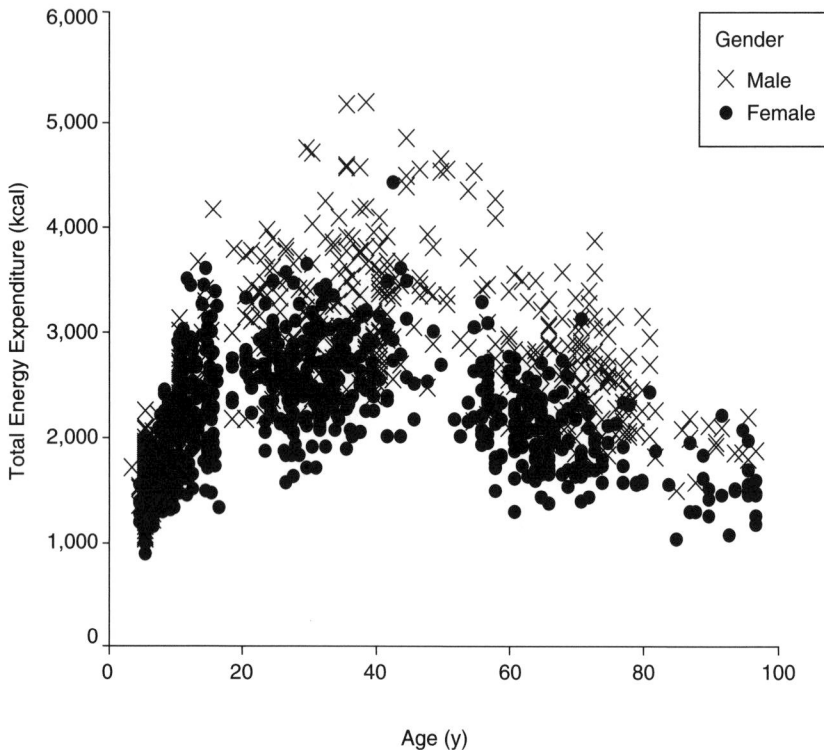

FIGURE 5-6 Total energy expenditure and age in all individuals (excluding infants and pregnant or lactating women) in the doubly labeled water database (Appendix I).

1.9 < 2.5) (Table 5-12). The mean PALs for the four categories are shown in Table 5-13. The energy expenditure in sedentary individuals is set to reflect their BEE, the thermic effect of food, and the physical activities that are required for independent living. A low-active lifestyle (PAL = 1.5) for an adult weighing 70 kg is set to include an exertion *equivalent to* walking 2.2 mi/d at a rate of 3 to 4 mph or the equivalent energy expenditure in other activities, in addition to the activities that are part of independent living (Table 5-12). The active lifestyle was set at a PAL of 1.6 to 1.89. The physical activities performed by active, mid-weight individuals with a PAL of 1.75 (midpoint in this PAL category) would on average to be equivalent to walking 7 mi/d at the rate of 3 to 4 mph, while walking ~17 mi/d would be equivalent to the sum of the activities above independent living carried out by a very active, mid-weight individual with a PAL of 2.2 (Table 5-12). The PAL range set for a "very active" lifestyle is 1.9 to 2.49. As shown in

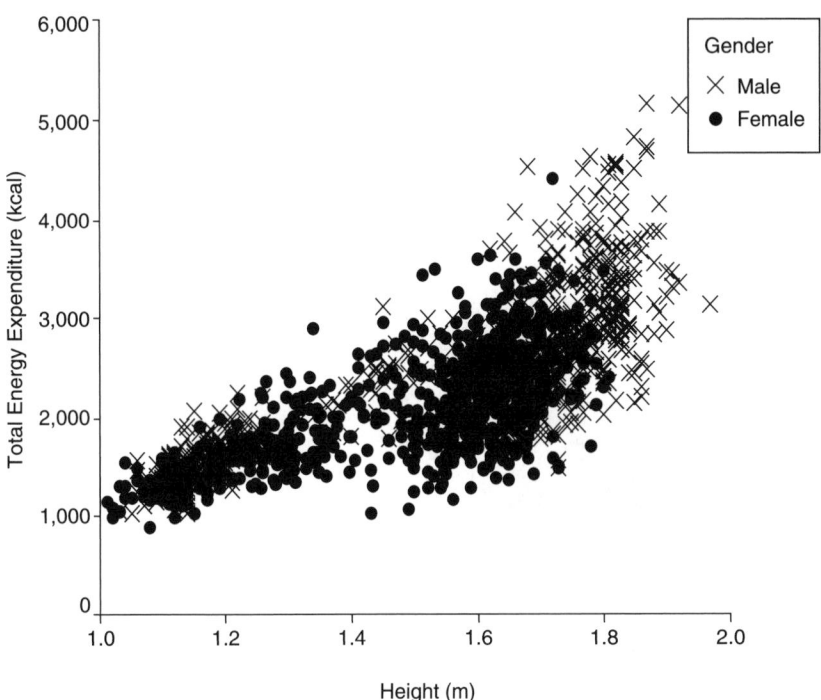

FIGURE 5-7 Total energy expenditure and height in all individuals (excluding infants and pregnant and lactating women) in the doubly labeled water database (Appendix I).

Table 5-12, these distances vary with the actual PAL value as well as with body weights. Tables are included in Chapter 12 that indicate how an individual can estimate his or her PAL on a daily (Table 12-2) or weekly (Table 12-3) basis.

Regression of Total Energy Expenditure on Age, Height, Weight, and Physical Activity Level Category

While stepwise multiple linear regressions were used to identify gender, age, height, and weight as the important variables for predicting TEE, physiological considerations determined that the form of the best predictive equation was nonlinear:

$$TEE = A + B \times age + PA \times (D \times weight + E \times height)$$

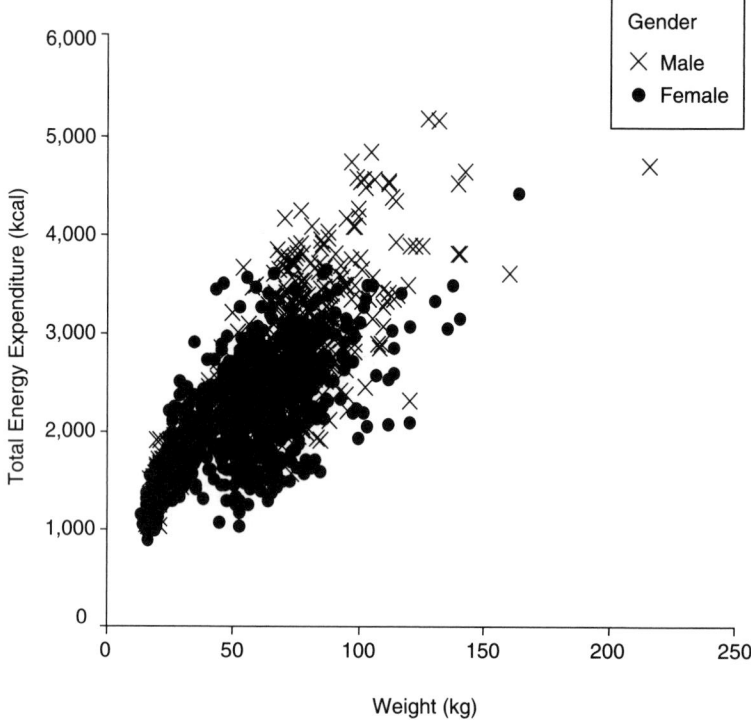

FIGURE 5-8 Total energy expenditure and weight in all individuals (excluding infants and pregnant and lactating women in the doubly labeled water database (Appendix I).

where TEE is in kcal/d, age is in years, weight is in kilograms, and height is in meters. In this equation, A is the constant term; B is the age coefficient; PA is the physical activity coefficient, which depends on whether the individual is estimated to be in the sedentary, low-active, active, or very active PAL categories; D is the weight coefficient; and E is the height coefficient. It should be noted that this approach is equivalent to fitting the individuals in each PAL category separately but keeping their equations parallel.

In the above equation the relative importance of height and weight is constant for different activity levels but the magnitude of their combined contribution changes for different PAL levels. Because of the mathematical interdependencies between the physical activity coefficients and the height and weight coefficients, the physical activity coefficient for the sedentary PAL category is set to 1.0.

The standard error of fit (the standard deviation of the residuals) represents how variable the measurements of the energy requirements of

TABLE 5-12 Physical Activity Level (PAL) Categories and Walking Equivalence

| PAL Category | PAL Range | PAL | Walking Equivalence (mi/d at 3–4 mph)[a] | | |
			Light-Weight Individual (44 kg)	Middle-Weight Individual (70 kg)	Heavy-Weight Individual (120 kg)
Sedentary	1.0-1.39	1.25	~ 0	~ 0	~ 0
Low active	1.4-1.59				
Mean		1.5	2.9	2.2	1.5
Active	1.6-1.89				
Minimum		1.6	5.8	4.4	3.0
Mean		1.75	9.9	7.3	5.3
Very active	1.9-2.49				
Minimum		1.9	14.0	10.3	17.5
Mean		2.2	22.5	16.7	12.3
Maximum		2.5	31.0	23.0	17.0

[a] In addition to energy spent for the generally unscheduled activities that are part of a normal daily life.
SOURCE: Chapter 12.

individuals with similar characteristics might be. In order to estimate the true between-individual variability, it was necessary to partition this observed variability into biological and experimental; in the light of limited data, and following the suggestion of the 1981 FAO/WHO/UNU Expert Consultation, it is assumed that the biological and the experimental variance are equal. Therefore, values for individual standard deviations are recommended as 70 percent of the observed standard error of fit (Table 5-14).

The data were fitted to this equation using nonlinear regression and the Levenberg-Marquardt method for searching for convergence based on minimizing the sum of residuals squared. For each fit an R-squared was calculated as the ratio of the explained sum of squared error to the total sum of squared error, and asymptotic standard errors of the coefficients were calculated.

TEE Equations for Normal-Weight Children

Separate TEE predictive equations were developed for normal-weight boys and girls from age, height, weight, and PAL category using the same definitions as that for adults (see Table 5-12) using nonlinear regression techniques. In order to utilize all the TEE data, PAL categorization was determined using predicted rather than observed BEE, since only 71 percent (256/358) of the girls and 66 percent (111/167) of the boys had

TABLE 5-13 Sample Size, Mean Total Energy Expenditure (TEE), Body Mass Index (BMI), and Physical Activity Level (PAL) for each of the PAL Categories in Adults Included in the DLW Database[a]

BMI (kg/m²)	Gender	PAL Category	n
18.5 to 25	Women	Sedentary	35
		Low active	45
		Active	87
		Very active	71
		Total	238
	Men	Sedentary	22
		Low active	36
		Active	76
		Very active	35
		Total	169
25 and higher	Women	Sedentary	39
		Low active	43
		Active	78
		Very active	35
		Total	195
	Men	Sedentary	20
		Low active	35
		Active	58
		Very active	52
		Total	165

[a] From Appendix I.
[b] Mean ± standard deviation.

observed BEE (Appendix Table I-2). The following predictive equations for BEE were derived from the observed BEE provided in the DLW database.

For boys:
BEE (kcal/d) = 68 − (43.3 × age [y]) + 712 × height (m) + 19.2 × weight (kg) [standard error = 88; R^2 = 0.89]

For girls:
BEE (kcal/d) = 189 − (17.6 × age [y]) + 625 × height (m) + 7.9 × weight (kg) [standard error = 95; R^2 = 0.75]

TEE Measured (kcal/d)[b]	BMI Measured (kg/m^2)[b]	PAL Measured[b]
1,567 ± 261	22.1 ± 1.7	1.23 ± 0.11
2,036 ± 252	22.1 ± 1.8	1.52 ± 0.05
2,303 ± 288	21.8 ± 1.7	1.74 ± 0.09
2,588 ± 348	21.2 ± 1.6	2.09 ± 0.16
2,229 ± 447	21.7 ± 1.7	1.73 ± 0.31
1,992 ± 263	23.0 ± 1.5	1.29 ± 0.10
2,500 ± 381	22.4 ± 1.5	1.51 ± 0.05
2,892 ± 402	22.5 ± 1.5	1.74 ± 0.08
3,338 ± 419	22.4 ± 1.6	2.06 ± 0.01
2,784 ± 561	22.5 ± 1.5	1.70 ± 0.25
1,788 ± 373	30.3 ± 5.0	1.25 ± 0.10
2,205 ± 344	30.2 ± 4.3	1.52 ± 0.06
2,594 ± 452	31.0 ± 6.6	1.74 ± 0.08
2,888 ± 347	28.9 ± 3.3	2.04 ± 0.11
2,400 ± 545	30.3 ± 5.3	1.65 ± 0.27
2,378 ± 546	30.3 ± 6.3	1.27 ± 0.09
2,719 ± 544	29.7 ± 6.5	1.50 ± 0.06
3,142 ± 425	29.4 ± 4.1	1.73 ± 0.09
3,821 ± 608	29.9 ± 4.2	2.10 ± 0.14
3,174 ± 727	29.7 ± 5.0	1.74 ± 0.30

Prediction equations of TEE for normal-weight boys and girls ages 3 through 18 years were then developed using age, height, weight, and PAL category as predicted from the above BEE equations. Data were not used in the derivation of the TEE equations if the PAL value was less than 1.0 or greater than 2.5.

Plots of the residuals (predicted versus observed TEE) for each PAL category did not differ from zero and showed no evidence of nonlinear patterns of bias. Standard deviation (SD) of the residuals ranged from 56 to 167, with the highest SD for the very active PAL category. The residuals were not correlated with weight, height, BMI, or age.

TABLE 5-14 Estimated Standard Deviation of Estimated Energy Requirements (kcal/d) Derived from Regression Equations for Individuals of a Specific Age, Height, Weight, and Physical Activity Level Category[a]

Age (y)	Body Mass Index	Males	Females
3–18	≥ 3rd < 85th percentile	58	68
3–18	≥ 85th percentile	69	75
3–18	≥ 3rd percentile	67	70
≥ 19	≥ 18.5 < 25 kg/m²	199	162
≥ 19	≥ 25 kg/m²	208	160
≥ 19	≥ 18.5 kg/m²	202	160

[a] Observed variance = biological variance + experimental variance, for the square root of biological variance = biological standard deviation, assuming biological variance = experimental variance.

The coefficients and standard error for the prediction of TEE in boys and girls ages 3 through 18 years of age in the normative database are described in Appendix Table I-8.

FINDINGS BY LIFE STAGE AND GENDER GROUP

Infants and Children Ages 0 Through 2 Years

Evidence Considered in Determining the Estimated Energy Requirement

Energy Expenditure and Energy Deposition. The energy requirements of infants and young children should balance energy expenditure at a level of physical activity consistent with normal development and allow for deposition of tissues at a rate consistent with health. This approach requires knowledge of what constitutes developmentally appropriate levels of physical activity, normal growth, and body composition. Although the energy requirement for growth relative to maintenance is small, except during the first months of life, satisfactory growth is a sensitive indicator of whether energy needs are being met. To determine the energy cost of growth, the energy content of the newly synthesized tissues must be estimated, preferably from the separate costs of protein and fat deposition.

Basal Metabolism. The brain, liver, heart, and kidney account for most of the basal metabolism of infants. Holliday (1971) analyzed basal metabolic rate (BMR) in relation to body and organ weight, and noted that oxygen (O_2) consumption increased at a rate greater than that of organ or body weight during the intrauterine and postnatal periods. There is also an increase in O_2 consumption during the transition to extrauterine life. After birth, the O_2 consumption of these vital organs increases in proportion to increases in organ weight. The contribution of the brain to BMR is exceptionally high in the newborn period (70 percent) and throughout the first years of life (60 to 65 percent).

Basal metabolism of term infants has been investigated extensively. Karlberg (1952) and Benedict and Talbot (1921) reported BMR ranges from 43 to 60 kcal/kg/d. The high variability is attributable to biological differences in body composition and technical differences in experimental conditions and methods. (In most studies of infants, BMR is measured while they are either asleep or sedated, which may lead to an underestimate of BEE.) Nevertheless, it should be appreciated that energy expenditure per kg is approximately two times greater in infants than in adults (Denne and Kalhan, 1987).

The basal metabolism of infants is dependent on gender, age, and feeding mode. Significant differences between breast-fed and formula-fed infants have been reported at 3 and 6 months (Butte, 1990; Butte et al., 2000b; Wells and Davies, 1995). BMR predicted from Schofield equations (WN Schofield, 1985) was equal to 0.88 measured BMR at 3–12 months (Butte et al., 2000b). Schofield compiled approximately 300 measurements from Benedict and Talbot (1914, 1921), Clagett and Hathaway (1941), Harris and Benedict (1919), and Karlberg (1952) to develop predictive models based on weight and length (C Schofield, 1985). Experimental conditions varied across studies in which indirect calorimetry was used to measure SMR or resting metabolic rate (RMR) rather than BMR. In the older studies, the influence of neonatal age, sedation, or experimental techniques in some of the older studies may explain the lower values predicted by the Schofield equation compared to measured BMR.

Thermic Effect of Feeding. Since infants normally are fed frequently and not subjected to prolonged fasting, the thermic effect of food (TEF) will exert a continual, albeit variable, influence on energy expenditure. The TEF in preterm infants (Reichman et al., 1982) and in infants recovering from malnutrition (Ashworth, 1969) has been shown to be proportional to the rate of weight gain. These observations support the view that some of the observed energy expenditure is due to the metabolic costs of tissue synthesis.

Thermoregulation. In the first 24 hours after birth, thermoneu-trality is reported to be at 34°C to 36°C for the naked infant and falls to 30°C to

32°C by 7 to 10 days of age (Sinclair, 1978). The amount of energy required to maintain normal body temperature is greater at lower than at higher temperatures (Sinclair, 1978). Basal oxygen consumption rates increase from 4.8 ml O_2/kg/min at 0 to 6 hours postpartum to 7.0 ml O_2/kg/min at 6 to 10 days of life and remain fairly constant thereafter throughout the first year of life (Widdowson, 1974). The neonate responds to mild cold exposure with an increase in nonshivering thermogenesis, which increases metabolic rate and may be mediated by increased sympathetic tone (Penn and Schmidt-Sommerfeld, 1989). Increased oxidation of fatty acids in brown adipose tissue located between the scapulae and around major vessels and organs of the mediastinum and abdomen is thought to make the most important contribution to nonshivering thermogenesis in infants (Penn and Schmidt-Sommerfeld, 1989). Shivering thermogenesis occurs at lower ambient temperatures when nonshivering thermogenesis is insufficient to maintain body temperature.

Physical Activity. Physical activity represents an increasingly larger component of the total energy expenditure (TEE) as the young child grows and develops. In a longitudinal study of 76 developmentally normal infants, PAL (TEE/BEE) increased significantly from 1.2 at 3 months of age to 1.4 at 24 months of age (Butte et al., 2000b).

Total Energy Expenditure (TEE). While application of the doubly labeled water (DLW) method is subject to errors in infants and small children, the method has been validated in term and preterm infants (Jensen et al., 1992; Jones et al., 1987; Roberts et al., 1986; Westerterp et al., 1991). Mean discrepancies between the DLW method and respiration calorimetry were 0.3 ± 2.6 percent (Roberts et al., 1986), –0.9 ± 6.2 percent (Jones et al., 1987), –4.5 ± 6.0 percent (Westerterp et al., 1991), and –0.4 ± 11.5 percent (Jensen et al., 1992).

TEE is influenced by age, gender, and feeding mode (Butte et al., 2000b). In a longitudinal study of children from 3 to 24 months of age, absolute TEE differed by age (older greater than younger), gender (boys greater than girls), and feeding mode (human milk-fed less than formula-fed infants). Adjusted for body weight, TEE still differed by age and feeding mode, but not by gender. Adjusted for fat-free mass (FFM) and fat mass (FM), TEE differed by feeding mode, but not by age or gender (Butte et al., 2000b). TEE has been shown to be lower in breast-fed than formula-fed infants in a number of other studies (Butte et al., 1990; Davies et al., 1990; Jiang et al., 1998).

Growth. Body composition data may be used to compute the energy cost of growth. The energy content of the newly synthesized tissues is theoretically more accurate when the separate costs of protein and fat deposition are taken into account since the composition of weight gain varies with age. Much understanding of the energy cost of growth has been derived from preterm infants or children recovering from malnutrition (Butte et al., 1989; Roberts and Young, 1988). Typically, the energy cost of growth in these studies ranges from 2.4 to 6.0 kcal/g (10 to 25 kJ/g). In practicality, the energy cost of growth is an issue only during the first half of infancy when energy deposition contributes significantly to energy requirements.

In this report, the energy content of tissue deposition was computed from rates of protein and fat deposition observed in a longitudinal study of infants from 0.5 to 24 months of age (Butte et al., 2000b). The energy content of tissue deposition (kcal/g) derived from the above study was applied to the 50th percentile of weight gain published by Guo and colleagues (1991) as shown in Table 5-15 for infants and children 0 through 24 months of age. The estimated energy cost of tissue deposition averaged approximately 175 kcal/d for the age interval 0 to 3 months, 60 kcal/d for

TABLE 5-15 Weight Gain and Energy Deposition of Boys and Girls 0 Through 2 Years of Age

Age Interval (mo)	Protein Gain (g/d)[a]	Fat Mass Gain (g/d)[a]	Energy Cost of Tissue Deposition (kcal/g)	Weight Gain (g/d)[b]	Energy Deposition (kcal/d)
Boys					
0–3	2.6	19.6	6.0	31	186
4–6	2.3	3.9	2.8	18	50
7–9	2.3	0.5	1.5	12	18
10–12	1.6	1.7	2.7	10	27
13–15	1.3	1.0	2.2	9	20
16–18	1.3	1.0	2.2	8	17
19–24	1.1	2.1	4.7	7	33
Girls					
0–3	2.2	19.7	6.3	26	163
4–6	1.9	5.8	3.7	17	63
7–9	2.0	0.8	1.8	12	21
10–12	1.8	1.1	2.3	10	23
13–15	1.3	1.4	2.5	9	23
16–18	1.3	1.4	2.5	8	20
19–24	1.0	0.8	2.2	7	15

[a] Body composition (Butte et al., 2000a).
[b] Increments in weight at the 50th percentile (Guo et al., 1991).

4 to 6 months, 22 kcal/d for 7 to 12 months, and 20 kcal for 13 to 35 months.

Estimated Energy Requirements (EER). Total energy requirements of infants and young children have thus been shown to vary by age, gender, and feeding mode. Total energy requirements increase as children grow and are higher in boys than girls. Weight or FFM and FM accounted for the differences in energy requirements between ages and genders. The effect of feeding mode on energy requirements was apparent throughout the first year, primarily due to the higher TEE in formula-fed than human milk-fed infants (Butte et al., 2000b). Energy requirements (kcal/kg/d) were 7, 8, 9, and 3 percent higher in formula-fed than human milk-fed infants at 3, 6, 9, 12 months, respectively. The differences in energy requirements between feeding groups appeared to diminish beyond the first year of life.

Based upon analysis of the DLW data for infants and very young children (Appendix Table I-1), a single equation to predict total energy expenditure involving only weight was found to fit all of the individuals (n = 320 measurements) regardless of gender. Because the data included repeated measurements of individuals, dummy variables were used to link those individual data. While age, height, and weight were all independently correlated with TEE, weight was the best predictor. TEE values, adjusted for weight, were not correlated with age or height. Gender was not a statistically significant predictor of TEE, once body weight was accounted for. Because of the small sample size and limited range of estimated physical activity, the physical activity level (PAL) category was not included in the TEE equation. Examination of the residuals revealed no bias and including the squares of age, height, and weight added nothing to the prediction of TEE. Additionally, the inclusion of mean published data (Butte et al., 1990; Davies et al., 1989, 1991, 1997; de Bruin et al., 1998; Lucas et al., 1987; Stunkard et al., 1999; Wells et al., 1996), weighted for sample size, did not change the predictive equations.

Because of the lack of gender differences, it was decided to use a single equation for individuals 0 through 2 years of age:

$$\text{TEE (kcal/d)} = 89 \ (\pm 3 \ [\text{standard error}]) \times \text{weight of the child (kg)} \\ - 100 \ (\pm 56 \ [\text{standard error}])$$

EER Summary, Ages 0 Through 2 Years

Since infants and very young children are growing, an allowance for energy deposition (estimated in Table 5-15) must be added to the TEE to derive the EER. This energy deposition allowance is the average of energy deposition for boys and girls of similar ages. The EER is equal to the sum of TEE from the equation above plus energy deposition. Specific EERs are given in Tables 5-16 (boys) and 5-17 (girls) and are summarized for each age group below. The estimated energy deposition is the average of boys and girls taken from Table 5-15.

EER for Ages 0 Through 36 Months

EER = TEE + energy deposition

0–3 months	**($89 \times$ weight [kg] – 100) + 175 kcal**
4–6 months	**($89 \times$ weight [kg] – 100) + 56 kcal**
7–12 months	**($89 \times$ weight [kg] – 100) + 22 kcal**
13–36 months	**($89 \times$ weight [kg] – 100) + 20 kcal**

TABLE 5-16 Estimated Energy Requirement (EER) for Boys 0 Through 2 Years of Age

Age (mo)	Reference Weight (kg [lb])[a]	Total Energy Expenditure[b] (TEE) (kcal/d)	Energy Deposition[c] (ED) (kcal/d)	EER (kcal/d) (TEE + ED)
1	4.4 (9.7)	292	180	472
2	5.3 (11.7)	372	195	567
3	6.0 (13.2)	434	138	572
4	6.7 (14.8)	496	52	548
5	7.3 (16.1)	550	46	596
6	7.9 (17.4)	603	42	645
7	8.4 (18.5)	648	20	668
8	8.9 (19.6)	692	18	710
9	9.3 (20.5)	728	18	746
10	9.7 (21.4)	763	30	793
11	10.0 (22.0)	790	27	817
12	10.3 (22.7)	817	27	844
15	11.1 (24.4)	888	20	908
18	11.7 (25.8)	941	20	961
21	12.2 (26.9)	986	20	1,006
24	12.7 (28.0)	1,030	20	1,050
27	13.1 (28.9)	1,066	20	1,086
30	13.5 (29.7)	1,101	20	1,121
33	13.9 (30.6)	1,137	20	1,157
35	14.2 (31.3)	1,164	20	1,184

[a] From Table 5-6.
[b] Estimated from TEE = $89 \times$ weight (kg) – 100 derived from DLW data (Appendix I).
[c] From Table 5-15.

TABLE 5-17 Estimated Energy Requirement (EER) for Girls
0 Through 2 Years of Age

Age (mo)	Reference Weight (kg [lb])[a]	Total Energy Expenditure[b] (TEE) (kcal/d)	Energy Deposition[c] (ED) (kcal/d)	EER (kcal/d) (TEE + ED)
1	4.2 (9.3)	274	164	438
2	4.9 (10.8)	336	164	500
3	5.5 (12.1)	389	132	521
4	6.1 (13.4)	443	65	508
5	6.7 (14.8)	496	57	553
6	7.2 (15.9)	541	52	593
7	7.7 (17.0)	585	23	608
8	8.1 (17.8)	621	22	643
9	8.5 (18.7)	656	22	678
10	8.9 (19.6)	692	25	717
11	9.2 (20.3)	719	23	742
12	9.5 (20.9)	745	23	768
15	10.3 (22.7)	817	20	837
18	11.0 (24.2)	879	20	899
21	11.6 (25.6)	932	20	952
24	12.1 (26.7)	977	20	997
27	12.5 (27.5)	1,013	20	1,033
30	13.0 (28.6)	1,057	20	1,077
33	13.4 (29.5)	1,093	20	1,113
35	13.7 (30.2)	1,119	20	1,139

[a] From Table 5-6.
[b] Estimated from TEE = 89 × weight (kg) − 100 derived from DLW data (Appendix I).
[c] From Table 5-15.

EERs for energy calculated by these equations are slightly lower than those estimated by Prentice and colleagues (1988). Their estimates were 95, 85, 83, and 83 kcal/kg/d at 3, 6, 9, and 12 months, respectively. These estimates of total energy expenditures are approximately 80 percent of the 1985 FAO/WHO/UNU recommendations for energy intake of infants and toddlers (FAO/WHO/UNU, 1985), which were based upon observed energy intakes of infants compiled by Whitehead and colleagues (1981) from the literature predating 1940 and up to 1980.

More recent intake data are 2 to 15 percent lower than those on which the 1985 FAO/WHO/UNU recommendations were based (Davies et al., 1997; Prentice et al., 1988). In addition, an extra 5 percent allowance was factored into the FAO/WHO/UNU recommendations to correct for a presumed underestimation of energy intake (FAO/WHO/UNU, 1985).

Human Milk

Human milk is recognized as the optimal milk source for infants throughout at least the first year of life and is recommended as the sole nutritional milk source for infants through the first 4 to 6 months of life (IOM, 1991). Infants receiving human milk for this period would have an energy intake of some 500 kcal/d based on an average volume of milk intake of 0.78 L/d (Heinig et al., 1993; Neville et al., 1988) and an average caloric density of human milk of 650 kcal/L (Anderson et al., 1983; Butte and Calloway, 1981; Butte et al., 1984a; Dewey et al., 1984; Nommsen et al., 1991) (Table 5-18). The EERs derived in this report are thus more consistent with energy intakes of human milk-fed infants than the recommendations in the 1985 FAO/WHO/UNU report; it should be noted that the EERs based on the equations given *do* exceed the calculated 500 kcal/d from human milk for some infant boys and girls (Tables 5-16 and 5-17), which is in agreement with studies that have shown that infants fed human milk as a sole source of nutrients have lower TEE values than formula-fed infants.

Children Ages 3 Through 8 Years

Evidence Considered in Determining the Estimated Energy Requirement

Basal Metabolism. BMR may be measured by indirect calorimetry or estimated from weight using the Schofield equations (WN Schofield, 1985). Validation of the Schofield equations has been undertaken by comparing predicted values with measured values (Torun et al., 1996) in British 7- to 10-year-old children (Livingstone et al., 1992a) and Dutch 8- to 10-year-old children (Saris et al., 1989). Mean differences between the measured and calculated BMR ranged from 7.6 to 9.9 percent, suggesting that the Schoefield equations are adequate for use in this population.

In this report, predictive equations for basal energy expenditure (BEE) (BMR extrapolated to 24 hours) were derived from observed BEE measured in the children in the DLW database and are described in the earlier section "TEE Equations for Normal-Weight Children."

Thermic Effect of Food. The TEF was studied in prepubertal children for 3 hours after ingestion of a mixed meal in liquid form (Maffeis et al., 1993). In normal-weight children, the rise in energy expenditure was equivalent to 14 percent RMR or to 5.9 percent of the energy ingested.

Physical Activity. Energy needs per unit body weight for maintenance and growth decrease in relation to the increased energy needed for physi-

TABLE 5-18 Human Milk Intake and Composition

Study	Country	n	Stage of Lactation	Energy Intake from Milk (As Reported in Study)[a]
Anderson et al., 1981	Canada	10 women	3–5 d 8–11 d 15–18 d 26–29 d	Not reported
Anderson et al., 1983	United States	9 women	3 d 7 d 14 d	Not reported
Butte and Calloway, 1981	United States	23	1 mo	Not reported
Butte et al., 1984a, 1984b	United States	37 infants 40 infants 37 infants 41 infants	1 mo 2 mo 3 mo 4 mo	520 ± 131 kcal/d 468 ± 115 kcal/d 458 ± 124 kcal/d 477 ± 111 kcal/d
Dewey et al., 1984	United States	12 women	7–20 mo	610 kcal/d at 7 mo 735 kcal/d at 11–16 mo
Ferris et al., 1998	United States	12 women	2 wk 6 wk 12 wk 16 wk	Not reported
Lammi-Keefe et al., 1990	United States	6 women	8 wk	Not reported
Nommsen et al., 1991	United States	58 infants 45 infants 28 infants 21 infants	3 mo 6 mo 9 mo 12 mo	Not reported
Heinig et al., 1993	United States	38 F, 33 M 30 F, 26 M 22 F, 24 M 21 F, 19 M	3 mo 6 mo 9 mo 12 mo	535.37 ± 81.26 kcal/d 518.64 ± 114.72 kcal/d 439.77 ± 143.40 kcal/d 303.54 ± 172.08 kcal/d

[a] Mean ± SD, unless otherwise noted.

Energy Content of Milk[a]	Maternal Intake[a]	Comments
50 kcal/dL 60 kcal/dL 60 kcal/dL 60 kcal/dL	Not reported	Full-term infants Milk energy content was approximated from study figure
51 ± 9 kcal/dL 63 ± 9 kcal/dL 67 ± 10 kcal/dL	Not reported	Full-term pregnancies
66 ± 12 kcal/dL	Not reported	Navajo women
0.68 ± 0.08 kcal/g 0.64 ± 0.08 kcal/g 0.62 ± 0.09 kcal/g 0.64 ± 0.10 kcal/g	2,334 ± 536 kcal/d 2,125 ± 582 kcal/d 2,170 ± 629 kcal/d 2,092 ± 498 kcal/d	Healthy term infants, exclusively breast-fed
65 kcal/dL	Not reported	Breast-feeding mothers
78.1 ± 12.5 kcal/dL 75.3 ± 7.7 kcal/dL 79.2 ± 9.3 kcal/dL 82.9 ± 12.2 kcal/dL	2,315 ± 658 kcal/d 2,439 ± 806 kcal/d 2,384 ± 845 kcal/d 2,337 ± 724 kcal/d	Full-term pregnancies, healthy nonsmokers, exclusively breast- feeding Energy content measured by bomb calorimetry
66.5 kcal/dL ± 7.74 (range 51.9–81.2 kcal/dL)	2,531 ± 442 kcal/d	Exclusively breast- feeding Full-term pregnancies
69.7 ± 6.7 kcal/dL 70.7 ± 9.2 kcal/dL 70.9 ± 7.4 kcal/dL 70.6 ± 11.0 kcal/dL	2,340 kcal/d (range: 1,477– 3,201 kcal/d)	Healthy, exclusively breast-feeding mothers
66.9 kcal/dL 69.3 kcal/dL 71.7 kcal/dL 71.7 kcal/dL	Not reported	Healthy, full-term, exclusively breast-fed No additional solid foods consumed before 4 mo of age

cal activity in healthy, active children. An index of physical activity, PAL, defined as the ratio of TEE:BEE, reflects differences in lifestyle, geographic habitat, and socioeconomic conditions. Torun and coworkers (1996) reviewed PALs estimated by DLW, heart rate monitoring, and time-motion/ activity diary techniques in children. Mean PALs were between 1.4 and 1.5 for children less than 5 years of age and between 1.5 and 1.8 for children 6 to 18 years of age living in urban settings in industrialized countries.

Total Energy Expenditure. TEE has been measured by the DLW method in a number of studies of children. Black and coworkers (1996) compiled DLW studies on 2- to 6-year-old children from around the world. In their analysis of cross sectional data on 196 children they found the mean TEE per kg of body weight was significantly higher in boys ($p < 0.05$) than in girls, but not for BMR or PAL.

Growth. The energy cost of growth for children (Table 5-19) was computed based on rates of weight gain of children enrolled in the FELS Longitudinal Study (Baumgartner et al., 1986) and estimated rates of protein and fat deposition for children (Fomon et al., 1982). It is recognized that the energy content of newly synthesized tissues varies in childhood, particularly during the childhood adiposity rebound (Rolland-Cachera, 2001; Rolland-Cachera et al., 1984), but these variations are assumed to minimally impact total energy requirements of children, as only from 8 to 32 kcal/d are estimated to be required for tissue deposition.

EER Summary, Ages 3 Through 8 Years

Marked variability exists for boys and girls in the EER because of variations in growth rate and physical activity (Zlotkin, 1996). To derive total energy requirements, the DLW data (Appendix Table I-2) were utilized to develop equations to predict TEE based on a child's gender, age, height, weight and PAL category (Appendix Table I-8 gives the constants and standard errors of the predictive equations). The calculated TEE is increased by an average of 20 kcal/d for estimated energy deposition (Table 5-19) to get the EER. EER predictions for children with reference weights for ages 3 through 8 years are given below and values are summarized at yearly intervals for reference-weight children in Tables 5-20 (boys) and 5-21 (girls).

EER for Boys 3 Through 8 years
  EER = TEE + energy deposition
  EER = 88.5 − (61.9 × age [y]) + PA × (26.7 × weight [kg] + 903
       × height [m]) + 20 kcal

TABLE 5-19 Weight Gain and Energy Deposition of Boys and Girls 3 Through 18 Years of Age

Age at End of Interval (y)	Weight Gain (kg/6 mo)[a]	Weight Gain (g/d)[a]	Energy Deposition (kcal/g)[b]	Energy Deposition (kcal/d)[b]
Boys				
3.5	1.0	5	1.5	8.1
4.5	1.1	6	1.5	8.7
5.5	1.2	6	1.5	9.5
6.5	1.2	6	1.7	10.8
7.5	1.4	8	2.4	18.2
8.5	1.4	8	2.4	18.8
9.5	1.5	8	2.6	22.0
10.5	1.6	9	2.9	25.6
11.5	1.9	10	3.1	32.6
12.5	2.5	13	1.8	24.1
13.5	3.1	17	1.3	22.1
14.5	3.7	20	1.5	29.3
15.5	2.6	14	1.7	24.3
16.5	1.7	9	1.9	18.0
17.5	1.1	6	2.0	12.2
Girls				
3.5	1.0	5	1.7	9.3
4.5	0.9	5	2.0	10.3
5.5	1.0	5	2.2	11.7
6.5	1.2	7	2.6	17.0
7.5	1.3	7	2.9	21.0
8.5	1.5	8	3.1	25.2
9.5	1.5	8	3.3	27.7
10.5	2.0	11	2.8	30.1
11.5	2.5	14	2.3	31.8
12.5	2.8	15	1.9	28.3
13.5	2.3	13	3.0	37.9
14.5	1.5	8	4.1	33.7
15.5	0.9	5	5.1	25.7
16.5	0.8	4	4.9	20.3
17.5	0.4	2	4.0	8.8

[a] Increments in weight at the 50th percentile (Baumgartner et al., 1986).
[b] Rates of protein and fat deposition (Fomon et al., 1982; Haschke, 1989).

Where PA is the physical activity coefficient:
    PA = 1.00 if PAL is estimated to be ≥ 1.0 < 1.4 (sedentary)
    PA = 1.13 if PAL is estimated to be ≥ 1.4 < 1.6 (low active)
    PA = 1.26 if PAL is estimated to be ≥ 1.6 < 1.9 (active)
    PA = 1.42 if PAL is estimated to be ≥ 1.9 < 2.5 (very active)

TABLE 5-20 Estimated Energy Requirement (EER) for Boys 3 Through 18 Years of Age

Age (y)	Reference Weight (kg [lb])[a]	Reference Height (m [in])	Total Energy Expenditure[b] (TEE) (kcal/d)			
			Sedentary PAL	Low Active PAL	Active PAL	Very Active PAL
3	14.3 (31.5)	0.95 (37.4)	1,142	1,304	1,465	1,663
4	16.2 (35.7)	1.02 (40.2)	1,195	1,370	1,546	1,763
5	18.4 (40.5)	1.09 (42.9)	1,255	1,446	1,638	1,874
6	20.7 (45.6)	1.15 (45.3)	1,308	1,515	1,722	1,977
7	23.1 (50.9)	1.22 (48.0)	1,373	1,597	1,820	2,095
8	25.6 (56.4)	1.28 (50.4)	1,433	1,672	1,911	2,205
9	28.6 (63.0)	1.34 (52.8)	1,505	1,762	2,018	2,334
10	31.9 (70.3)	1.39 (54.7)	1,576	1,850	2,124	2,461
11	35.9 (79.1)	1.44 (56.7)	1,666	1,960	2,254	2,615
12	40.5 (89.2)	1.49 (58.7)	1,773	2,088	2,403	2,792
13	45.6 (100.4)	1.56 (61.4)	1,910	2,251	2,593	3,013
14	51.0 (112.3)	1.64 (64.6)	2,065	2,434	2,804	3,258
15	56.3 (124.0)	1.70 (66.9)	2,198	2,593	2,988	3,474
16	60.9 (134.1)	1.74 (68.5)	2,295	2,711	3,127	3,638
17	64.6 (142.3)	1.75 (68.9)	2,341	2,771	3,201	3,729
18	67.2 (148.0)	1.76 (69.3)	2,358	2,798	3,238	3,779

[a] From Table 5-8.
[b] Based on equations given in Appendix Table I-8. PAL = physical activity level.
[c] EER = TEE + 20 kcal/d − estimate of energy deposition during childhood.

EER for Girls 3 Through 8 Years
 EER = TEE + energy deposition
 EER = 135.3 − (30.8 × age [y]) + PA × (10.0 × weight [kg] + 934 × height [m]) + 20 kcal

Where PA is the physical activity coefficient:
 PA = 1.00 if PAL is estimated to be ≥ 1.0 < 1.4 (sedentary)
 PA = 1.16 if PAL is estimated to be ≥ 1.4 < 1.6 (low active)
 PA = 1.31 if PAL is estimated to be ≥ 1.6 < 1.9 (active)
 PA = 1.56 if PAL is estimated to be ≥ 1.9 < 2.5 (very active)

EER^c (kcal/d)

Sedentary PAL	Low Active PAL	Active PAL	Very Active PAL
1,162	1,324	1,485	1,683
1,215	1,390	1,566	1,783
1,275	1,466	1,658	1,894
1,328	1,535	1,742	1,997
1,393	1,617	1,840	2,115
1,453	1,692	1,931	2,225
1,530	1,787	2,043	2,359
1,601	1,875	2,149	2,486
1,691	1,985	2,279	2,640
1,798	2,113	2,428	2,817
1,935	2,276	2,618	3,038
2,090	2,459	2,829	3,283
2,223	2,618	3,013	3,499
2,320	2,736	3,152	3,663
2,366	2,796	3,226	3,754
2,383	2,823	3,263	3,804

Children Ages 9 Through 18 Years

Evidence Considered in Determining the Estimated Energy Requirement

Energy requirements of adolescents are defined to maintain health, promote optimal growth and maturation, and support a desirable level of physical activity. Growth refers to increases in height and weight and changes in physique, body composition, and organ systems. Maturation refers to the rate and timing of progress toward the mature biological state. Developmental changes occur in the reproductive organs, and lead to the development of secondary gender characteristics and to changes in the cardiorespiratory and muscular systems leading to an increases in strength and endurance. As a result of these changes, energy requirements of adolescents increase. In adolescents, changes in occupational and recreational activities further alter energy requirements.

TABLE 5-21 Estimated Energy Requirement (EER) for Girls
3 Through 18 Years of Age

Age (y)	Reference Weight (kg [lb])[a]	Reference Height (m [in])	Total Energy Expenditure[b] (TEE) (kcal/d)			
			Sedentary PAL[b]	Low Active PAL	Active PAL	Very Active PAL
3	13.9 (30.6)	0.94 (37.0)	1,060	1,223	1,375	1,629
4	15.8 (34.8)	1.01 (39.8)	1,113	1,290	1,455	1,730
5	17.9 (39.4)	1.08 (42.5)	1,169	1,359	1,537	1,834
6	20.2 (44.5)	1.15 (45.3)	1,227	1,431	1,622	1,941
7	22.8 (50.2)	1.21 (47.6)	1,278	1,495	1,699	2,038
8	25.6 (56.4)	1.28 (50.4)	1,340	1,573	1,790	2,153
9	29.0 (63.9)	1.33 (52.4)	1,390	1,635	1,865	2,248
10	32.9 (72.5)	1.38 (54.3)	1,445	1,704	1,947	2,351
11	37.2 (81.9)	1.44 (56.7)	1,513	1,788	2,046	2,475
12	41.6 (91.6)	1.51 (59.4)	1,592	1,884	2,158	2,615
13	45.8 (100.9)	1.57 (61.8)	1,659	1,967	2,256	2,737
14	49.4 (108.8)	1.60 (63.0)	1,693	2,011	2,309	2,806
15	52.0 (114.5)	1.62 (63.8)	1,706	2,032	2,337	2,845
16	53.9 (118.7)	1.63 (64.2)	1,704	2,034	2,343	2,858
17	55.1 (121.4)	1.63 (64.2)	1,685	2,017	2,328	2,846
18	56.2 (123.8)	1.63 (64.2)	1,665	1,999	2,311	2,833

[a] From Table 5-9.
[b] Based on equations given in Appendix Table I-8. PAL = physical activity level.
[c] EER = TEE + 20 kcal/d – estimate of energy deposition during childhood.

Basal Metabolism. The effect of age on basal metabolism is a function of changes in body composition through adolescence. FFM comprises the bulk of the active metabolic tissue, and energy expenditure is strongly correlated with FFM (Webb, 1981). Marked gender differences in intensity and duration of the adolescent growth spurt in FFM dictates higher energy and nutrient needs in boys than girls (Butte, 2000).

The accuracy of the Schofield equations (WN Schofield, 1985) for the prediction of BEE has been evaluated by comparing predicted BEE values with measured BEE values from several studies of adolescents (Torun et al., 1996). Predicted BEE values were within –4.9, and –0.2 percent of measured values in American adolescents (Bandini et al., 1990b) and were within –4.8, –2.9, –7.2, and +16.8 percent of measured values in British adolescents (Livingstone et al., 1992a); however, the sample size was small in some of the age and gender categories.

In a large-scale study of 5- to 16-year-old children, predicted BEE agreed within ± 8 percent of measured values (Firouzbakhsh et al., 1993),

EER^c (kcal/d)

Sedentary PAL	Low Active PAL	Active PAL	Very Active PAL
1,080	1,243	1,395	1,649
1,133	1,310	1,475	1,750
1,189	1,379	1,557	1,854
1,247	1,451	1,642	1,961
1,298	1,515	1,719	2,058
1,360	1,593	1,810	2,173
1,415	1,660	1,890	2,273
1,470	1,729	1,972	2,376
1,538	1,813	2,071	2,500
1,617	1,909	2,183	2,640
1,684	1,992	2,281	2,762
1,718	2,036	2,334	2,831
1,731	2,057	2,362	2,870
1,729	2,059	2,368	2,883
1,710	2,042	2,353	2,871
1,690	2,024	2,336	2,858

while in another study, the Schofield equations overestimated the BEE of African-American girls in the United States by 8 percent compared to measured values (Wong et al., 1999). The tendency for the equations to overestimate BEE of some adolescents will require further research to determine if universal equations or specific equations for different ethnic groups are warranted.

In this report, predictive equations for BEE were derived from the observed BEE provided in the DLW database as described in the earlier section "TEE Equations for Normal-Weight Children."

Thermic Effect of Food. No publications describing TEF in this age group were available.

Physical Activity. Physical activity reflects the energy expended in activities beyond basal processes for survival and for the attainment of physical, intellectual, and social well-being. Physical fitness entails muscular, motor, and cardiorespiratory fitness. Dietary energy recommendations include recommendations for physical activity compatible with health, prevention of obesity, and appropriate social and psychological development.

The assessment of habitual physical activity and its impact on the energy needs of adolescents is difficult because of the wide variability in lifestyles. PALs of 1.60 to 1.73 at 11 to 14 years of age and 1.50 to 1.65 at 15 to 18 years of age were designated as typical for adolescent boys and girls, respectively, in the 1985 FAO/WHO/UNU report. A detailed categorization of adolescent lifestyles was also provided that allowed for individualization of energy requirements (FAO/WHO/UNU, 1985).

Physical activity in adolescents has been estimated by the DLW method, heart rate monitoring, and activity–time allocation studies. Although heart rate monitors, calibrated against indirect calorimetry, can be used to predict TEE of individuals (Treuth et al., 1998a), the DLW method shows closer agreement when validated against calorimetry than heart rate monitoring or activity–time allocation studies. Torun and co-workers (1996) extensively reviewed PALs as estimated by DLW, heart rate monitoring, and activity–time allocation studies conducted in urban and rural areas of industrialized and developing countries. Mean PALs were between 1.45 and 2.05 for children 6 to 18 years of age engaged in light, moderate, or heavy levels of physical activity.

Physical activity is generally viewed as having a favorable influence on the growth and physical fitness of youth, but longitudinal data addressing these relationships are limited. Regular physical activity has no apparent effect on statural growth and biological maturation (i.e., skeletal age, age at peak height velocity, and age at menarche) (Malina, 1994; Geithner et al. 1998; Beunen et al., 1992). Data suggesting later menarche in female athletes are associational and retrospective, and do not control for other factors that influence the age at menarche (e.g., genotype, physique, and dietary practices). Regular physical activity is often associated with decreased body fat in both genders and, sometimes, increased FFM, at least in males (Parizkova, 1974; Sunnegardh et al., 1986; Deheeger et al., 1997). It is also associated with greater skeletal mineralization, bone density, and bone mass (Bailey and McCulloch, 1990). However, excessive training associated with, or causing, sustained weight loss and maintenance of excessively low body weights may contribute to bone loss and increased susceptibility to stress fractures (Dhuper et al., 1990; Warren et al., 1986).

Information is scant on the relationship between children's physical activity and fitness and present and future health status (Malina, 1994; Twisk, 2001). Most evidence is limited to cross-sectional comparisons of active and nonactive children. Active children tend to have lower skinfold thickness than inactive children (Raitakari et al., 1994; Moore et al., 1995). Short-term training does not seem to alter high blood pressure, low HDL cholesterol, and triacylglycerols in otherwise healthy children (Gilliam and Freedson, 1980; Hunt and White, 1980; Linder et al., 1983; Savage et al., 1986). Exercise training has been shown to slightly reduce the percentage body fat and improve lipoprotein profile in obese children (Gutin et al., 2002; Owens et al., 1999; Sasaki et al., 1987). The tracking of body fatness, blood pressure, and lipoprotein profile appears to be moderate from adolescence into adulthood (Clarke et al., 1978; Webber et al., 1983; Newman et al., 1986).

Total Energy Expenditure. A number of investigators have measured the TEE of adolescents using the DLW method (Davies et al., 1991; Livingstone et al., 1992a; Wong, 1994). While absolute energy expenditure increases with age, energy expenditure per unit body weight decreases across adolescence, primarily due to the decrease in BEE.

Growth. The energy cost of growth comprises the energy deposited in newly accrued tissues and the energy expended for tissue synthesis. It is recognized that the energy deposited in newly synthesized tissues varies in childhood, particularly around the adolescent growth spurt, but these variations minimally impact total energy requirements. Longitudinal data on the body composition of normally growing adolescents are not available. However, Haschke (1989) estimated the typical body composition of male and female adolescents from literature values of total body water, potassium, and calcium. FFM increased dramatically from approximately 28 kg at 10.5 years of age to 61 kg at 18.5 years of age in boys of median height and weight, with peak deposition coinciding with peak rates of height gains. The FFM:height ratio was higher in boys than girls, while FM deposition was greater in girls, increasing from 8 kg at 10.5 years of age to 14 kg at 18.5 years of age. As a percentage of body weight, FM increased during this period from 23.5 to 25 percent in girls, and actually declined in boys from 16 to 13 percent by 18.5 years.

In this report, the energy cost of growth was computed based on rates of weight gain of children enrolled in the FELS Longitudinal Study (Baumgartner et al., 1986) and rates of protein and fat deposition for children (Fomon et al., 1982) and adolescents (Haschke, 1989) (Table 5-19). The energy cost of tissue deposition was approximately 20 kcal/d, increasing to 30 kcal/d at peak growth velocity.

EER Summary, Ages 9 Through 18 Years

EERs for adolescents have been based on estimates of energy expenditure and requirements for growth based on tissue deposition. Energy requirements of adolescents must take into account habitual physical activity level and lifestyle consistent with the maintenance of health, optimal growth and maturation, and social and economic demands.

Marked variability exists in the energy requirements of adolescents due to varying rates of growth and physical activity levels (Zlotkin, 1996). In adolescents, growth is relatively slow except around the adolescent growth spurt, which varies considerably in timing and magnitude between individuals. Occupational and recreational activities also variably affect energy requirements.

To derive the EER for children, the DLW data (Appendix Table I-2) were utilized to develop equations (Appendix Table I-8) to predict TEE based on a child's gender, age, height, weight, and PAL category and added to 25 kcal/d as an estimate of energy deposition (Table 5-19). The TEE equations allow for four levels of activity as shown in Table 5-12. EERs for children with reference heights and weights (Tables 5-8 and 5-9) for ages 9 through 18 are given below and values are summarized in yearly intervals for children with reference weights in Tables 5-20 (boys) and 5-21 (girls). The equations below are the same as those used for children ages 3 to 8 years, but the additional amount added to cover energy deposition resulting from growth is somewhat larger (25 kcal/d compared with 20 kcal/d).

EER for Boys 9 Through 18 Years
    EER = TEE + energy deposition
    EER = 88.5 – (61.9 × age [y]) + PA × (26.7 × weight [kg] + 903
        × height [m]) + 25 kcal

Where PA is the physical activity coefficient:
    PA = 1.00 if PAL is estimated to be ≥ 1.0 < 1.4 (sedentary)
    PA = 1.13 if PAL is estimated to be ≥ 1.4 < 1.6 (low active)
    PA = 1.26 if PAL is estimated to be ≥ 1.6 < 1.9 (active)
    PA = 1.42 if PAL is estimated to be ≥ 1.9 < 2.5 (very active)

EER for Girls 9 Through 18 Years
    EER = TEE + energy deposition
    EER = 135.3 – (30.8 × age [y]) + PA × (10.0 × weight [kg] + 934
        × height [m]) + 25 kcal

Where PA is the physical activity coefficient:
    PA = 1.00 if PAL is estimated to be ≥ 1.0 < 1.4 (sedentary)
    PA = 1.16 if PAL is estimated to be ≥ 1.4 < 1.6 (low active)
    PA = 1.31 if PAL is estimated to be ≥ 1.6 < 1.9 (active)
    PA = 1.56 if PAL is estimated to be ≥ 1.9 < 2.5 (very active)

Adults Ages 19 Years and Older

Evidence Considered in Determining the Estimated Energy Requirement

Weight and Height. In adults, BEE predictions are not generally or significantly improved by considering weight and height, as compared to weight alone (WN Schofield, 1985). In the present approach for evaluating TEE in adults with body weights in the desirable range, however, height becomes a significant factor because desirable body weights (i.e., those corresponding to BMIs in the range from 18.5 up to 25 kg/m^2) depend on an individual's height. The impact of height and weight on TEE are shown quantitatively in Figures 5-7 and 5-8.

Age. Age comes out as a significant parameter in the multiple regression analysis performed on the DLW database for subjects with BMIs from 18.5 up to 25 kg/m^2 (Appendix Table I-3). The age-related decline in TEE was found to amount to approximately 10 and 7 kcal/y for adult men and women, respectively.

Physical Activity. The physical activities carried out by free-living individuals vary greatly in intensity as well as duration, and assessment of physical activity-induced increments in TEE in individuals is fraught with considerable uncertainties. For this reason, individuals in the DLW database are classified as sedentary, low active, active, or very active (Table 5-12). Currently available reliable data on PAL can be obtained only by the DLW technique. The 407 individuals studied in this manner have been included in the DLW database shown in Appendix Table I-3. Other techniques involving heart rate monitors and accelerometers have also been used to estimate TEE, but their accuracy depends on careful individual calibration of these instruments for each subject studied.

In spite of concerns about obtaining accurate estimates, it is important to be able to evaluate PAL and TEE in individuals for whom such data are not available or for whom these approaches are not practical. One way to do this is to evaluate physical efforts by estimating how many miles an individual would have to walk in one day to induce a comparable level of exertion (in terms of kcal expended). For example, individuals who have 30 minutes of moderately intense activity (equivalent to walking 2 miles in 30 minutes or an equivalent amount of physical exertion in addition to the activities involved in maintaining a sedentary lifestyle) have a PAL of about 1.5 (see Table 12-2), and they are classified as "low active" in this report. To raise a PAL from 1.5 to 1.75, in addition to activity equivalent to walking 2 miles in 30 minutes, each day one would to need increase activity to the equivalent of walking an additional 1 hour at 4.5 mph (an equivalent activity would be to bicycle for 1 hour at 10 to 12 mph, use a stair-treadmill for 1 hour, or run for 30 minutes at 6 mph while maintaining the habitual daily routine of other activities).

The change in PAL induced by various types of physical activities can be estimated with the help of Table 12-1, which contains a list of the physical activities typically performed and the impact on PAL when they are performed for 10 minutes or 1 hour. Unlike food intake, which is generally underreported, physical activities tend to be overestimated, and activities of one kind may cause a reduction in activities of another. Thus, subjective determination of PAL has errors similar to using dietary intake to obtain EERs.

Body Weight and PAL. PAL describes the ratio of TEE divided by BEE extrapolated to one day. Whereas the energy cost of weight-bearing physical activities is approximately proportional to body weight, BEE is not proportional to body weight, as the contribution of FFM to basal metabolism is much greater than FM (resulting in a substantial intercept in the equations relating BEE to body weight). The relationship between miles walked per day (or between other weight bearing activities) and PAL is thus not linear, and it will take fewer miles at a given walking speed to raise PAL in a heavy compared to a light-weight individual (see Table 5-12).

EER Summary, Ages 19 Years and Older

Separate TEE predictive equations for EER were developed for adult men and women from age, height, weight, and PAL category, which were determined using the observed BEE for individuals in the DLW database (Appendix Table I-3). Individual data were not used in the derivation of the TEE equations if the PAL value was less than 1.0 or greater than 2.5.

Plots of the residuals showed no evidence of nonlinear patterns of bias (although there was a general increased magnitude of residuals with increasing values of each variable). The additional predictive value of BMI and the squares of age, height, and weight were explored for the linear predictions and none of these significantly reduced the standard error of the fit. The coefficients and standard error for the prediction of TEE of adults, ages 19 years and older, are described in Appendix Table I-9 and are summarized below. EERs for 30-year-old adult women and men of various heights with BMIs from 18.5 up to 25 kg/m^2 are shown in Table 5-22.

EER for Men Ages 19 Years and Older
    EER = 662 – (9.53 × age [y]) + PA × (15.91 × weight [kg]
         + 539.6 × height [m])

Where PA is the physical activity coefficient:
    PA = 1.00 if PAL is estimated to be ≥ 1.0 < 1.4 (sedentary)
    PA = 1.11 if PAL is estimated to be ≥ 1.4 < 1.6 (low active)
    PA = 1.25 if PAL is estimated to be ≥ 1.6 < 1.9 (active)
    PA = 1.48 if PAL is estimated to be ≥ 1.9 < 2.5 (very active)

EER for Women Ages 19 Years and Older
    EER = 354 – (6.91 × age [y]) + PA × (9.36 × weight [kg]
         + 726 × height [m])

Where PA is the physical activity coefficient:
    PA = 1.00 if PAL is estimated to be ≥ 1.0 < 1.4 (sedentary)
    PA = 1.12 if PAL is estimated to be ≥ 1.4 < 1.6 (low active)
    PA = 1.27 if PAL is estimated to be ≥ 1.6 < 1.9 (active)
    PA = 1.45 if PAL is estimated to be ≥ 1.9 < 2.5 (very active)

Pregnancy

Evidence Considered to Determine the Estimated Energy Requirement

Basal Metabolism. Basal metabolism increases during pregnancy due to the metabolic contribution of the uterus and fetus and increased work of the heart and lungs. The increase in basal metabolism is one of the major components of the increased energy requirements during pregnancy (Hytten, 1991a). Variation in energy expenditure between individuals is largely due to differences in FFM, which in pregnancy is comprised of low energy-requiring expanded blood volume, high energy-requiring fetal and uterine tissues, and moderate energy-requiring skeletal muscle mass (Hytten, 1991a). In late pregnancy, approximately one-half the increment in energy expenditure can be attributed to the fetus (Hytten, 1991a). The fetus uses about 8 ml O_2/kg body weight/min or 56 kcal/kg body weight/d; for a 3-kg fetus, this would be equivalent to 168 kcal/d (Sparks et al., 1980). FM, a low energy-requiring tissue, contributes to the variation in energy expenditure, but to a much lesser extent than FFM, which has been found to be the strongest predictor of BEE (Butte et al., 1999).

The basal metabolism of pregnant women has been estimated longitudinally in a number of studies using a Douglas bag, ventilated hood, or whole-body respiration calorimeter (Durnin et al., 1987; Forsum et al.,

TABLE 5-22 Estimated Energy Requirements (EER) for Men and Women 30 Years of Age[a]

Height (m [in])	PAL[b]	Weight for BMI of 18.5 kg/m^2 (kg [lb])	Weight for BMI of 24.99 kg/m^2 (kg [lb])
1.45 (57)	Sedentary Low active Active Very active	38.9 (86)	52.5 (116)
1.50 (59)	Sedentary Low active Active Very active	41.6 (92)	56.2 (124)
1.55 (61)	Sedentary Low active Active Very active	44.4 (98)	60.0 (132)
1.60 (63)	Sedentary Low active Active Very active	47.4 (104)	64.0 (141)
1.65 (65)	Sedentary Low active Active Very active	50.4 (111)	68.0 (150)
1.70 (67)	Sedentary Low active Active Very active	53.5 (118)	72.2 (159)
1.75 (69)	Sedentary Low active Active Very active	56.7 (125)	76.5 (168)
1.80 (71)	Sedentary Low active Active Very active	59.9 (132)	81.0 (178)
1.85 (73)	Sedentary Low active Active Very active	63.3 (139)	85.5 (188)

EER, Men (kcal/d)[c]		EER, Women (kcal/d)[d]	
BMI of 18.5 kg/m²	BMI of 24.99 kg/m²	BMI of 18.5 kg/m²	BMI of 24.99 kg/m²
1,777	1,994	1,563	1,691
1,931	2,172	1,733	1,877
2,128	2,399	1,946	2,108
2,450	2,771	2,201	2,386
1,848	2,080	1,625	1,762
2,010	2,268	1,803	1,956
2,216	2,506	2,025	2,198
2,554	2,898	2,291	2,489
1,919	2,168	1,688	1,834
2,089	2,365	1,873	2,036
2,305	2,616	2,104	2,290
2,661	3,028	2,382	2,593
1,993	2,257	1,752	1,907
2,171	2,464	1,944	2,118
2,397	2,728	2,185	2,383
2,769	3,160	2,474	2,699
2,068	2,349	1,816	1,981
2,254	2,566	2,016	2,202
2,490	2,842	2,267	2,477
2,880	3,296	2,567	2,807
2,144	2,442	1,881	2,057
2,339	2,670	2,090	2,286
2,586	2,959	2,350	2,573
2,993	3,434	2,662	2,916
2,222	2,538	1,948	2,134
2,425	2,776	2,164	2,372
2,683	3,078	2,434	2,670
3,108	3,576	2,758	3,028
2,301	2,636	2,015	2,211
2,513	2,884	2,239	2,459
2,782	3,200	2,519	2,769
3,225	3,720	2,855	3,140
2,382	2,735	2,082	2,290
2,602	2,995	2,315	2,548
2,883	3,325	2,605	2,869
3,344	3,867	2,954	3,255

continued

TABLE 5-22 Continued

Height (m [in])	PAL[b]	Weight for BMI of 18.5 kg/m^2 (kg [lb])	Weight for BMI of 24.99 kg/m^2 (kg [lb])
1.90 (75)	Sedentary Low active Active Very active	66.8 (147)	90.2 (198)
1.95 (77)	Sedentary Low active Active Very active	70.3 (155)	95.0 (209)

[a] For each year below 30, add 7 kcal/d for women and 10 kcal/d for men. For each year above 30, subtract 7 kcal/d for women and 10 kcal/d for men.
[b] PAL = physical activity level.
[c] EER for men calculated as: EER = 662 − (9.53 × age [y]) + PA × (15.91 × weight [kg] + 539.6 × height [m]), where PA is the physical activity coefficient of 1.00 for sedentary

1988; Goldberg et al., 1993; van Raaij et al., 1990). Cumulative changes in BEE throughout pregnancy ranged from 29,636 to 50,300 kcal or 106 to 180 kcal/d (Table 5-23). Marked variation in the basal metabolic response to pregnancy was seen in 12 British women measured before and throughout pregnancy (Goldberg et al., 1993; Prentice et al., 1989). By 36 weeks of gestation, the increment in absolute BEE ranged from 8.6 to 35.4 percent, or −9.2 to 18.6 percent/kg FFM. Energy-sparing or energy-profligate responses to pregnancy were dependent on prepregnancy body fatness. In 12 Dutch women, the late-pregnancy increment in absolute TEE varied from 9.5 to 26 percent (de Groot et al., 1994). Mean increments in BEE over prepregnancy values were 48, 96, and 263 kcal/d, or 4, 7, and 19 percent in the first, second, and third trimesters in healthy women with positive pregnancy outcomes (Prentice et al., 1996b). The cumulative increase in BEE was positively correlated with weight gain and body fatness.

Prediction equations for the BEE of pregnant women have not been published. Nonpregnant prediction equations based on weight are not accurate during pregnancy since metabolic rate increases disproportionately to the increase in total body weight. Prentice and colleagues (1996b) suggested that BEE could be predicted from weight using the Schofield equations, plus an additional 48, 96, and 263 kcal/d during the first, second, and third trimesters.

EER, Men (kcal/d)[c]		EER, Women (kcal/d)[d]	
BMI of 18.5 kg/m^2	BMI of 24.99 kg/m^2	BMI of 18.5 kg/m^2	BMI of 24.99 kg/m^2
2,464	2,837	2,151	2,371
2,694	3,107	2,392	2,637
2,986	3,452	2,692	2,971
3,466	4,018	3,053	3,371
2,548	2,940	2,221	2,452
2,786	3,222	2,470	2,728
3,090	3,581	2,781	3,074
3,590	4,171	3,154	3,489

PAL ($\geq 1.0 < 1.4$), 1.11 for low active PAL ($\geq 1.4 < 1.6$), 1.25 for active PAL ($\geq 1.6 < 1.9$), and 1.48 for very active PAL ($\geq 1.9 < 2.5$).

[d] EER for women calculated as: EER = 354 − (6.91 × age [y]) + PA × (9.36 × weight [kg] + 726 × height [m]), where PA is the physical activity coefficient of 1.00 for sedentary PAL, 1.12 for low active PAL, 1.27 for active PAL, and 1.45 for very active PAL.

In late gestation, the anti-insulinogenic and lipolytic effects of human chorionic somatomammotropin, prolactin, cortisol, and glucagon contribute to glucose intolerance, insulin resistance, decreased hepatic glycogen, and mobilization of adipose tissue (Kalkhoff et al., 1978). Although levels of serum prolactin, cortisol, glucagon, and fatty acids were elevated and serum glucose levels were lower in one study, a greater utilization of fatty acids was not observed during late pregnancy (Butte et al., 1999). On the contrary, higher mean respiratory quotients (RQs) were observed for BEE and TEE compared with the postpartum period. Higher basal RQs have been observed in pregnancy by several (Bronstein et al., 1995; Denne et al., 1991; Knuttgen and Emerson, 1974; van Raaij et al., 1989), but not all (Spaaij et al., 1994b) investigators. These observations are consistent with persistent glucose production in fasted pregnant women, despite lower fasting plasma glucose concentrations. After fasting, the total rates of glucose production and total gluconeogenesis were increased, even though the fraction of glucose oxidized and the fractional contribution of gluconeogenesis to glucose production remained unchanged (Assel et al., 1993; Kalhan et al., 1997). In pregnant women, the sustained energy expenditure and higher RQ may reflect the obligatory oxygen consumption of the fetus and the contribution of glucose as the primary oxidative substrate of the fetus. In late gestation, the fetus is estimated to use 17 to 26 g/d of

TABLE 5-23 Cumulative Changes in Basal Energy Expenditure (BEE) Throughout Pregnancy

Reference	n	Pregravid Weight (kg [lb])	Gestation Interval
Durnin et al., 1987	88	57.3±7.5 (126.1±16.5)	Prepregnancy to 40 wk
van Raaij et al., 1987	57	62.5±8.1 (137.5±17.8)	3 wk to term
Forsum et al., 1988	22	61.0± 9.9 (134.2±21.8)	Prepregnancy to 40 wk
Goldberg et al., 1993	12	61.7±8.8 (135.7±19.3)	Prepregnancy to 40 wk
Kopp-Hoolihan et al., 1999	10	NA	Prepregnancy to 35 wk

[a] The Douglas bag technique of indirect calorimetry was used to estimate BEE.

glucose (Hay, 1994), well within the increment of carbohydrate oxidation observed in pregnancy.

Thermic Effect of Food. In studies of pregnant women, TEF has been shown to be unchanged (Bronstein et al., 1995; Nagy and King, 1984; Spaaij et al., 1994b) or lower (Schutz et al., 1988) than values of nonpregnant women.

Physical Activity. Until late gestation, the gross energy cost of standardized nonweight-bearing activity does not significantly change. In the last month of pregnancy, the energy expended while cycling was increased on the order of 10 percent. However, when corrected for increased BMR the increased energy expenditure due to the activity of cycling was 6 percent (Prentice et al., 1996b). The energy cost of standardized weight-bearing activities such as treadmill walking was unchanged until 25 weeks of gestation, after which it increased by 19 percent (Prentice et al., 1996b). Standardized protocols, however, do not allow for behavioral changes in pace and intensity of physical activity, which may occur and conserve energy during pregnancy.

Growth of Maternal and Fetal Tissues. Gestational weight gain includes the products of conception (fetus, placenta, and amniotic fluid) and accretion of maternal tissues (uterus, breasts, blood, extracellular fluid, and adipose). The energy cost of deposition can be calculated from the amount of protein and fat deposited. Hytten (1991b) made theoretical

Cumulative Increase in BEE (kcal)	Cumulative Increase in BEE (kcal/d)	Method Used to Estimate BEE
30,114	108	Indirect calorimetry[a]
34,416	133	Indirect calorimetry[a]
50,300	180	DLW
29,636	106	DLW
36,089	147	DLW

calculations based on a weight gain of 12.5 kg and birth weight of 3.4 kg. The energy equivalents for protein and fat deposition were assumed to be 5.6 kcal/g and 9.5 kcal/g, respectively. The energy cost of tissue deposition was equivalent to 3.32 kcal/g gained (Table 5-24).

Current recommendations for weight gain during pregnancy are specified for a woman's prepregnancy BMI (IOM, 1990). Total weight gain during pregnancy varies widely among women. For normal-weight women, the mean rate of weight gain is 1.6 kg in the first trimester and 0.44 kg/wk in the second and third trimesters (IOM, 1990). For underweight women, the mean rate of weight gain is 2.3 kg in the first trimester and 0.49 kg/wk in the second and third trimesters. For overweight women, the mean rate of weight gain is 0.9 kg in the first trimester and 0.30 kg/wk in the second and third trimesters.

Fat gains associated with gestational weight gains within the IOM recommended ranges were measured in 200 women with varying prepregnancy BMIs using a four-component body composition model (Lederman et al., 1997). The total energy deposition between 14 and 37+ weeks of gestation was calculated based on an assumed protein deposition of 925 g of protein, and energy equivalences of 5.65 kcal/g of protein and 9.25 kcal/g of fat (Table 5-25).

Empirical data on the longitudinal changes in the body composition of well-nourished, normal weight (prepregnancy BMI from 18.5 up to 25 kg/m^2) pregnant women were used to estimate the energy deposition during pregnancy. Studies in which a prepregnancy baseline or first trimester value was available and methodology was appropriately corrected

TABLE 5-24 Theoretical Energy Cost of Tissue Deposition During Pregnancy

	Protein Gain (g)	Fat Gain (g)	Protein Gain (kcal)	Fat Gain (kcal)	Total Energy Deposition[a] (kcal)
Fetus	440	440	2,464	4,180	6,644
Placenta	100	4	560	38	598
Amniotic fluid	3	0	17	0	17
Uterus	166	4	930	38	968
Breasts	81	12	454	114	568
Blood	135	20	756	190	946
Maternal stores		3,345		31,778	31,778
Total	925	3,825	5,180	36,338	41,518

[a] Based on 5.6 kcal/g for protein gained and 9.5 kcal/g for fat gained.
SOURCE: Adapted from Hytten (1991b).

TABLE 5-25 Estimated Energy Deposition During Pregnancy

Prepregnancy Body Mass Index (BMI) (kg/m²)	Recommended Gestational Weight Gain[a] (GWG) (kg [lb])	Actual GWG (kg [lb])	Fat Gain (kg)	Estimated Energy Deposition[b] (kcal)
Low (BMI < 19.8)	12.5–18.0 (28–40)	12.6±2.4 (28±5.3)	6.0±2.6	60,726
Normal (BMI = 19.8–26.0)	11.5–16.0 (25–35)	12.1±3.4 (27±7.5)	3.8±3.5	40,376
High (BMI > 26.0–29.0)	7.0–11.5 (15–25)	9.1±3.1 (20±6.8)	2.8±4.1	31,126
Obese (BMI > 29.0)	At least 6.8 (15)[c]	6.9±4.4 (15±9.7)	−0.6±4.6	−324

[a] As recommended by IOM (1990).
[b] Calculated based on assumed 5.65 kcal/g of protein gained and 9.25 kcal/g of fat gained.
[c] Lederman et al. (1997), used 7–9.2 kg (15–20 lb).
SOURCE: Adapted from Lederman et al. (1997).

for pregnancy-induced changes in the hydration or density of FFM were used (Table 5-26). Total energy deposition during pregnancy was estimated from the mean fat gain of 3.7 kg from these studies, plus an assumed deposition of 925 g of protein, applying energy equivalencies of 5.65 kcal/g of protein and 9.25 kcal/g of fat. Mean total energy deposition was equal to 39,862 kcal or 180 kcal/d (Table 5-26).

Total Energy Expenditure. The DLW method has been employed in four studies of well-nourished, pregnant women to measure free-living TEE (Forsum et al., 1992; Goldberg et al., 1991b, 1993; Kopp-Hoolihan et al., 1999) (Table 5-27). There appeared to be a steady decrease in PAL as pregnancy advanced, primarily due to the increase in the denominator, BEE. In the British (Goldberg et al., 1993) and Swedish women (Forsum et al., 1992) studied, the energy expenditure for activity (TEE – BEE) decreased in the 36th week of gestation; this decrease was not observed in the American women (Kopp-Hoolihan et al., 1999).

EER Summary, Pregnancy

The DLW database on pregnant women with prepregnancy BMIs from 18.5 up to 25 kg/m^2 (Appendix Table I-4) consists of longitudinal measurements of TEE throughout pregnancy, and in most cases includes a TEE measurement prior to pregnancy. Therefore, the average TEE change/gestational week was computed for each woman, and the median value of these data were assumed to represent the general trend. The median change in TEE was 8 kcal per week of gestation with a range of –57 to 107 kcal/wk. There was great variability in the average TEE change/ week between women and studies; however, few predictive factors were identified. The change in TEE was not related to maternal age, prepregnancy weight, prepregnancy BMI, or weight gain or loss during pregnancy. The change in TEE, however, is negatively correlated to the baseline PAL.

The EER for energy during pregnancy is derived from the sum of the TEE of the woman in the nonpregnant state plus a median change in TEE of 8 kcal/wk plus the energy deposition during pregnancy of 180 kcal/d (Table 5-26). Since TEE changes little and weight gain is minor during the first trimester, no increase in energy intake during the first trimester is recommended.

EER for Pregnancy
   14–18 years
    EER$_{pregnant}$ = adolescent EER$_{nonpregnant}$ + additional
        energy expended during pregnancy + energy deposition
    1st trimester = adolescent EER + 0 + 0
    2nd trimester = adolescent EER + 160 kcal (8 kcal/wk × 20 wk)
        + 180 kcal
    3rd trimester = adolescent EER + 272 kcal (8 kcal/wk × 24 wk)
        + 180 kcal

TABLE 5-26 Energy Deposition During Pregnancy

Reference	n	Gestation Interval (wk)	Observed Gestational Weight Gain (kg [lb])	Body Composition Method[a]
Pipe et al., 1979	27	12–37	10.40 (23)	TBW TBK
Forsum et al., 1988	22	0–36	13.60 (30)	TBW TBK
van Raaij et al., 1988	42	11–35	9.15 (20) 11.60 (26)	UWW
Goldberg et al., 1993	12	0–36	11.91 (26)	TBW
de Groot et al., 1994	12	0–34	11.70 (26)	UWW
Lederman et al., 1997	46	14–37	12.10 (27)	TBW UWW BMC
Lindsay et al., 1997	27	0–33/36	12.61 (28)	UWW
Sohlstrom and Forsum, 1997	16	0–5/10 d postpartum	15.80 (35)	MRI
Kopp-Hoolihan et al., 1999	10	0–34	11.60 (26)	TBW UWW BMC
Mean				

[a] TBW = total body water, TBK = total body potassium, UWW = underwater weighing, BMC = bone mineral content, MRI = magnetic resonance imaging.

19–50 years

$EER_{pregnant} = EER_{nonpregnant}$ + additional energy expended during pregnancy + energy deposition

1st trimester = adult EER + 0 + 0

2nd trimester = adult EER + 160 kcal (8 kcal/wk × 20 wk) + 180 kcal

3rd trimester = adult EER + 272 kcal (8 kcal/wk × 34 wk) + 180 kcal

Theoretical Protein Gain[b] (kg)	Measured Fat Gain (kg)	Energy Deposition (kcal)	Energy Deposition[c] (kcal/d)	Energy Deposition (kcal/g)
0.925	2.40	27,426	157	2.64
0.925	5.8	58,876	234	4.33
0.925	1.9	22,801	136	2.49
0.925	2.8	31,126	124	2.61
0.925	3.4	36,676	154	3.13
0.925	3.8	40,376	251	3.34
0.925	5.9	59,801	247	4.74
0.925	3.6	38,526	138	2.44
0.925	4.5	43,151	176	3.85
	3.7	38,862	180	

[b] From Hytten (1991b) (see Table 5-24).
[c] Based on 5.65 kcak/g of protein gained and 9.25 kcal/g of fat gained.

Lactation

Evidence Considered in Determining the Estimated Energy Requirement

Basal Metabolism. Increased RMRs and SMRs have been observed in lactating women on the order of 4 to 5 percent (Butte et al., 1999; Forsum et al., 1992; Sadurskis et al., 1988; Spaaij et al., 1994a). The increased energy expenditure is consistent with the additional energy cost of milk synthesis. Others have reported lower (Guillermo-Tuazon et al., 1992) or

TABLE 5-27 Doubly Labeled Water Pregnancy Studies

Reference	n	Gestation Week	Pregravid Weight (kg)	Gestational Weight Gain (kg)
Goldberg et al., 1991b	10	36	—	—
Forsum et al., 1992	22	0	60.8	13.5
	22	16–18		
	22	30		
	19	36		
Goldberg et al., 1993	12	0	61.7	11.91
		6		
		12		
		18		
		24		
		30		
		36		
Kopp-Hoolihan et al., 1999	10	0	—	11.6
		8–10		
		24–26		
		34–36		

a Physical activity level = total energy expenditure/basal energy expenditure.

similar BEE or RMR in lactating women compared to the nonlactating state (Frigerio et al., 1991; Goldberg et al., 1991b; Illingworth et al., 1986; Motil et al., 1990; Piers et al., 1995b; van Raaij et al., 1991). Interpretation of these studies is difficult because BEE or RMR was not always adjusted for differences in body weight or body composition between comparison groups. In general, it would appear that BEE or RMR is unchanged or slightly elevated during lactation; there is little evidence of energy conservation.

Higher RQs and rates of carbohydrate utilization have been reported in lactating compared with nonlactating women, consistent with the preferential use of glucose by the mammary gland (Butte et al., 1999). Conflicting results of lower fasting RQ (0.82 versus 0.85) (Spaaij et al., 1994a), as well as no significant differences in RQ during lactation, have been reported (Frigerio et al., 1991; Piers et al., 1995b; van Raaij et al., 1991).

Thermic Effect of Food. TEF was reported to be 30 percent lower during than after lactation in one study (Illingworth et al., 1986), but unchanged

Total Energy Expenditure (kcal/d)	Physical Activity Level[a]	Activity Energy Expenditure (kcal/d)
2,470	1.42	731
2,484	1.87	1,147
2,293	1.65	860
2,986	1.82	1,338
2,914	1.66	1,171
2,274	1.58	835
2,322	1.54	818
2,426	1.64	939
2,456	1.65	964
2,621	1.66	1,042
2,675	1.62	1,026
2,688	1.50	885
2,205	1.68	892
2,047	1.57	743
2,410	1.56	867
2,728	1.61	1,038

in another (Spaaij et al., 1994a). Although results are conflicting, it is unlikely that TEF contributes significantly to the energetic economy of lactating women.

Physical Activity. Theoretically, the energy cost of lactation could be met by a reduction in the time spent in physical activity or an increase in the efficiency of performing routine tasks. The energetic cost of nonweight-bearing and weight-bearing activities has been measured in lactating women (Spaaij et al., 1994a; van Raaij et al., 1990). Adaptations in the level of physical activity are not always seen in lactating women. Reductions in physical activity have been reported in early lactation (4 to 5 weeks postpartum) in the Netherlands (van Raaij et al., 1991), the United States (Butte et al., 2001), and Great Britain (Goldberg et al., 1991b). Physical activity increased in the lactating Dutch women from 5 to 27 weeks postpartum (van Raaij et al., 1991). By 3 months postpartum, the American women (Butte et al., 2001) had resumed their prepregnancy occupational and recreational lifestyles in addition to their child-rearing responsibilities

TABLE 5-28 Doubly Labeled Water Lactation Studies

Reference	n	Stage of Lactation (mo)	Total Energy Expenditure (kcal/d)	Total Energy Expenditure (kcal/kg/d)	Basal Estimation (kcal/d)
Goldberg et al.,	10	1	2,109	35.8	1,406
1991b		2	2,171	36.9	1,397
		3	2,138	36.5	1,345
Forsum et al., 1992	23	2	2,532	39.3	1,409
		6	2,580	41.0	1,433
Lovelady et al., 1993	9[e]	3–6	2,413	37.2	1,376
Kopp-Hoolihan et al., 1999	10	1	2,146	—	1,328
Butte et al., 2001[f]	24	3	2,391	38.1	1,331

[a] Unless otherwise noted AEE includes TEF.

[b] Estimated to be 0.67 kcal/g (Butte et al., 1984a, 1984b; Neville, 1995).

[c] Observed change in body composition during lactation.

and their physical activity had returned to prepregnancy levels. While a decrease in moderate and discretionary activities appears to occur in most lactating women in the early postpartum period, activity patterns beyond this period are highly variable.

Total Energy Expenditure. TEEs of lactating women have been measured by the DLW method in five studies (Butte et al., 2001; Forsum et al., 1992; Goldberg et al., 1991b; Kopp-Hoolihan et al., 1999; Lovelady et al., 1993) as shown in Table 5-28. There are several potential sources of error in using the DLW method in lactation studies. These sources of error may be attributed to isotope exchange and sequestration that occurs during the de novo synthesis of milk fat and lactose, and to increased water flux into milk (Butte et al., 2001). Underestimation of carbon dioxide by 1.0 to 1.3 percent may theoretically occur due to the export of exchangeable hydrogen bound to solids in milk (IDECG, 1990). This underestimation may increase to 1.5 to 3.4 percent due to ^{2}H sequestration.

As shown in Table 5-28, mean TEE values of 2,391 kcal/d (PAL = 1.79) (Butte et al., 2001) and 2,413 kcal/d (PAL = 1.76) (Lovelady et al., 1993) in American women were higher than average values reported for British women (2,139 kcal/d; PAL = 1.55) (Goldberg et al., 1991b), and lower than average values in Swedish women (2,556 kcal/d, PAL = 1.80) (Forsum et al., 1992) during lactation. The energy expended in activity (TEE –

Activity Energy Expenditure[a] (kcal/d)	Physical Activity Level	Milk Energy Output[b] (kcal/d)	Energy Mobilization[c] (kcal/d)	Energy Requirement[d] (kcal/d)
703	1.50	536	Gained fat	2,645
774	1.55	532	mass	2,703
793	1.59	530		2,668
1,123	1.82	502	72	2,962
1,123	1.79			
1,037	1.75	538	287	2,664
816	1.62	—	—	—
1,061	1.79	483	155	2,719

[d] Energy requirement = measured TEE_{DLW} + energy of milk output − energy mobilized from tissues.
[e] All subjects breast-fed, except one.
[f] TEF only for Butte et al. (2001). TEF was 239.

BEE) ranged from 700 to 1,100 kcal/d in American, British, and Swedish lactating women.

Milk Energy Output. Milk energy output is computed from milk production and the energy density of human milk. Milk production rates increase during the first 6 months of full lactation. Beyond 6 months postpartum, typical milk production rates are variable and depend on weaning practices. Mean milk production rates of American women were 0.78 L/d in term infants from birth through 6 months of age (Allen et al., 1991; Heinig et al., 1993), and 0.6 L/d in term infants from 7 through 12 months of age (Dewey et al., 1984).

The energy density of human milk has been measured by bomb calorimetry or proximate macronutrient analysis of representative 24-hour pooled milk samples. The mean energy density of human milk ranged from 0.64 to 0.74 kcal/g (Butte et al., 1984a, 1984b; Neville, 1995). The value of 0.67 kcal/g is used in this report.

Energy Mobilization. The changes in weight and therefore energy mobilization from tissues occur in some, but not all, lactating women (Butte and Hopkinson, 1998; Butte et al., 2001; IOM, 1991). In general, during the first 6 months postpartum, well-nourished lactating women experience a mild, gradual weight loss, averaging −0.8 kg/mo (Butte et al.,

2001). In some women, the energy costs of lactation may be met by an increase in energy intake or a decrease in physical activity, with no change or even an increase in weight or FM.

After monitoring FM in 23 Swedish women, Sadurskis and colleagues (1988) found that FM decreased from 34.3 to 32.4 percent from 2 to 6 months postpartum by ^{18}O dilution and total body potassium counting. Consistent with a minor weight loss and sedentary lifestyle, British women ($n = 10$) displayed a nonsignificant increase in percent of FM (30.3 to 31.4 percent between 1 to 3 months postpartum) estimated by ^2H and ^{18}O dilution (Goldberg et al., 1991b). In American women, FM decreased from 28.0 percent at 1 month to 26.3 percent at 4 months postpartum, measured by underwater weighing (Butte et al., 1984b). Changes in adipose tissue volume in 15 Swedish women were measured by magnetic resonance imaging (Sohlstrom and Forsum, 1995). In the first 6 months postpartum, the subcutaneous region accounted for the entire reduction in adipose tissue volume, which decreased from 23.2 L to 20.0 L; nonsubcutaneous adipose tissue volume actually increased. Mobilization of tissue reserves is a general, but not obligatory, feature of lactation.

Total Energy Requirements. The energy requirements of lactating women were estimated from measurements of TEE, milk energy output, and energy mobilization from tissue stores in the following studies in which DLW was used (Butte et al., 2001; Forsum et al., 1992; Goldberg et al., 1991b; Lovelady et al., 1993) (Table 5-28). In the 10 lactating British women, the total energy requirements (and net energy requirements, since there was no fat mobilization) were 2,646, 2,702, and 2,667 kcal/d (11.1, 11.3, and 11.2 MJ/d) at 1, 2, and 3 months postpartum, respectively. Milk energy output averaged 533 kcal/d (2.2 MJ/d) (Goldberg et al., 1991b). In 23 lactating Swedish women, the total energy requirement at 2 months postpartum was 3,034 kcal/d (12.7 MJ/d), offset by 72 kcal/d (0.3 MJ/d) from tissue stores to yield a net requirement of 2,962 kcal/d (12.4 MJ/d) (Forsum et al., 1992). In nine lactating American women, the total energy requirement was 2,413 kcal/d (10.1 MJ/d), with 538 kcal/d (2.3 MJ/d) exported into milk and 287 kcal/d (1.2 MJ/d) mobilized from tissues, yielding a net requirement of 2,663 kcal/d (11.1 MJ/d) (Lovelady et al., 1993). Data from other lactating American women (Butte et al., 2001) give similar results. The women in the above studies were fully breastfeeding their infants, who were less than 6 months of age. In these studies, mean milk energy outputs during full lactation were similar (483 to 538 kcal/d or 2.0 to 2.3 MJ/d). The energetic inefficiency of milk synthesis is encompassed in the measurement of TEE.

The stage and extent of breastfeeding affect the incremental energy requirements for lactation. During the first 6 months of lactation, milk production rates are increased (Butte et al., 2001). Customary milk production rates beyond 6 months postpartum typically vary and depend on weaning practices (Butte et al., 2001).

EER Summary, Lactation

The DLW database provided TEE values for lactating women with prepregnancy BMIs from 18.5 up to 25 kg/m^2 at 1, 2, 3, 4, and 6 months postpartum (Appendix Table I-5). Analysis of the DLW database showed a small but significant change in TEE over these postpartum time periods (ANOVA, $P = 0.05$). A comparison was made between observed TEE of lactating women and TEE calculated from age, height, weight, and PAL using the prediction equation for adult women (see earlier section, "Adults Ages 19 Years and Older"). At 1 month postpartum, observed TEE was about 200 kcal less than predicted, while no differences were apparent at later months. For derivation of the EER for lactation, the TEE is based on the EER for normal-weight adult women using current age, weight, and PAL.

The EERs to be used during lactation are estimated from TEE, milk energy output, and energy mobilization from tissue stores. Because adaptations in basal metabolism and physical activity are not evident in well-nourished women, energy requirements of lactating women are met partially by mobilization of tissue stores, but primarily from the diet. In the first 6 months postpartum, well-nourished lactating women experience an average weight loss of 0.8 kg/mo, which is equivalent to 170 kcal/d (6,500 kcal/kg) (Butte and Hopkinson, 1998). Weight stability is assumed after 6 months postpartum. Milk production rates average 0.78 L/d from birth through 6 months of age and 0.6 L/d from 7 through 12 months of age. At 0.67 kcal/g of milk (Table 5-18), the milk energy output would be 523 kcal/d, which is rounded to 500 kcal/d, in the first 6 months and 402 kcal/d, which is rounded to 400 kcal/d, in the second 6 months of lactation.

EER for Lactation
   14–18 Years
   EER$_{lactation}$ = adolescent EER$_{prepregnancy}$ + milk energy output
                     – weight loss
      1st 6 mo   adolescent EER + 500 – 170
      2nd 6 mo   adolescent EER + 400 – 0

19–50 Years

$EER_{lactation}$ = adult $EER_{prepregnancy}$ + milk energy output
  – weight loss
  1st 6 mo   adult EER + 500 – 170
  2nd 6 mo   adult EER + 400 – 0

Special Considerations

Method Used to Estimate Weight Maintenance in Overweight and Obese Adults

Since Dietary Reference Intakes are designed to apply to apparently health individuals, the EERs are defined as values appropriate for maintenance of long-term good health. Overweight and obese individuals have greater weight than is consistent with long-term good health, thus EER values given in previous sections are not intended for overweight or obese individuals or for those who desire to lose weight. Instead, weight maintenance TEE values are discussed, along with information on the relationship between reduction in energy intake and change in body composition.

Equations to predict TEE for all adults from age, height, weight, gender, and activity level were generated from the combined DLW database of normal, overweight, and obese individuals (Appendix Tables I-3 and I-7). In addition, the DLW database of overweight and obese individuals (Appendix Table I-7) was used to generate equations to predict TEE in overweight and obese adult men and women (BMI 25 kg/m² and higher) from age, height, weight, and physical activity category using nonlinear regression. PAL categorization was determined using the adults' observed BEE. Data were not used in the derivation of the TEE equations if the PAL value was less than 1.0 or greater than 2.5.

The coefficients and standard error derived for only overweight and obese men and women are provided in Appendix Table I-10. For the overweight and obese equations, the standard deviations of the residuals ranged from 190 to 331, with the highest value in the very active PAL category. The equations are shown below (see Table I-10 for coefficients used).

Overweight and Obese Men Ages 19 Years and Older
  TEE = 1086 – (10.1 × age [y]) + PA × (13.7 × weight [kg]
    + 416 × height [m])

Where PA is the physical activity coefficient:
  PA = 1.00 if PAL is estimated to be ≥ 1.0 < 1.4 (sedentary)
  PA = 1.12 if PAL is estimated to be ≥ 1.4 < 1.6 (low active)

PA = 1.29 if PAL is estimated to be ≥ 1.6 < 1.9 (active)
PA = 1.59 if PAL is estimated to be ≥ 1.9 < 2.5 (very active)

Overweight and Obese Women Ages 19 Years and Older
TEE = 448 – (7.95 × age [y]) + PA × (11.4 × weight [kg] + 619 × height [m])

Where PA is the physical activity coefficient:
PA = 1.00 if PAL is estimated to be ≥ 1.0 < 1.4 (sedentary)
PA = 1.16 if PAL is estimated to be ≥ 1.4 < 1.6 (low active)
PA = 1.27 if PAL is estimated to be ≥ 1.6 < 1.9 (active)
PA = 1.44 if PAL is estimated to be ≥ 1.9 < 2.5 (very active)

Method Used to Estimate Weight Maintenance in Normal-weight, Overweight, and Obese Adults

TEE predictive equations were also developed combining normal-weight, overweight, and obese adults (BMI 18.5 kg/m^2 and higher) as mentioned earlier; the coefficients and standard errors are shown in Appendix Table I-11. Mean of the residuals did not differ from zero. For the combined data sets, the standard deviations of the residuals ranged from 182 to 321.

The adult predictive equations for TEE were subjected to statistical testing of their estimated coefficients and asymptotic standard deviations using a chi-square distribution (Hotelling T-squared test). The specific equations for the overweight and obese men and women (BMI from 25 kg/m^2 and higher) given above were not statistically different from the equations derived solely from normal-weight individuals given in the previous section (BMI from 18.5 up to 25 kg/m^2; $P > 0.99$) or normal plus overweight and obese individuals shown below (BMI from 18.5 kg/m^2 and higher; $P = 0.96–0.99$).

In addition, the equations generated to predict TEE from the combined data set of normal plus overweight and obese individuals had a larger sample size, thus reducing the standard error of the coefficients, and improved the continuity of predicted TEEs at the BMI junction between normal-weight and overweight individuals. For these reasons, the combined data from normal-weight and overweight and obese individuals were used to develop equations to predict TEE in overweight and obese adults. The resulting equations, described in the following sections, are accurate for use in both normal-weight and overweight and obese adults, and are thus suitable for prediction of energy requirements both in overweight and obese groups and in mixed groups containing normal-weight and overweight adults. The equations are shown below (see Table I-11 for coefficients used).

Normal-weight, Overweight, and Obese Men Ages 19 Years and Older
$$TEE = 864 - (9.72 \times age~[y]) + PA \times (14.2 \times weight~[kg]$$
$$+ 503 \times height~[m])$$

Where PA is the physical activity coefficient:
PA = 1.00 if PAL is estimated to be ≥ 1.0 < 1.4 (sedentary)
PA = 1.12 if PAL is estimated to be ≥ 1.4 < 1.6 (low active)
PA = 1.27 if PAL is estimated to be ≥ 1.6 < 1.9 (active)
PA = 1.54 if PAL is estimated to be ≥ 1.9 < 2.5 (very active)

Normal-weight, Overweight, and Obese Women Ages 19 Years and Older
$$TEE = 387 - (7.31 \times age~[y]) + PA \times (10.9 \times weight~[kg]$$
$$+ 660.7 \times height~[m])$$

Where PA is the physical activity coefficient:
PA = 1.00 if PAL is estimated to be ≥ 1.0 < 1.4 (sedentary)
PA = 1.14 if PAL is estimated to be ≥ 1.4 < 1.6 (low active)
PA = 1.27 if PAL is estimated to be ≥ 1.6 < 1.9 (active)
PA = 1.45 if PAL is estimated to be ≥ 1.9 < 2.5 (very active)

Current consensus guidelines for the management of obesity in adults (BMI 30 kg/m^2 and higher) recommend weight loss of around 10 percent of initial weight over a 6-month period (NIH, 2000). For overweight individuals (BMI from 25 up to 30 kg/m^2) who have no other risk factors, a motivation and desire to lose weight is an important consideration for recommending weight loss. Persons who do not wish to lose weight should receive advice and monitoring aimed at weight maintenance and risk reduction. Nevertheless, there is consensus that BMIs of 25 kg/m^2 and higher increase risk of premature morbidity and mortality (Chan et al., 1994; Colditz GA et al., 1995; Rimm et al., 1995; Stevens et al., 1998; Willett et al., 1999), and that relatively modest weight loss can improve blood pressure (Huang Z et al., 1998; Kannel et al., 1967; Reisin et al., 1978; Schotte and Stunkard, 1990), serum lipid (Grundy et al., 1979; Kesaniemi and Grundy, 1983; Osterman et al., 1992; Wood et al., 1988, 1991), and glucose tolerance (Amatruda et al., 1988; Doar et al., 1975; Hadden et al., 1975; Wing et al., 1991).

Rationale for Recommending Use of Equations Based on Combined Database for Overweight and Obese Individuals

Tables 5-29 and 5-30 show 24-h BEE and TEE values for 30-year-old men and women of different BMIs. The tables illustrate that obese men and women have consistently higher TEE than normal-weight men and women of comparable height and PAL, which implies that, on average, overweight and obese individuals need to consume more dietary energy to maintain weight than individuals within the healthy weight range to maintain their larger body weights.

The following predictive equations for BEE were derived from the observed BEE values in the DLW database (Appendix Tables I-3 and I-7):

For normal-weight men:
$$\text{BEE (kcal/d)} = 204 - (4 \times \text{age [y]}) + 450.5 \times \text{height (m)}$$
$$+ 11.69 \times \text{weight (kg)}$$
$$\text{residual} = 0 \pm 149, R^2 = 0.46.$$

For normal-weight, overweight, and obese men:
$$\text{BEE (kcal/d)} = 293 - (3.8 \times \text{age [y]}) + 456.4 \times \text{height (m)}$$
$$+ 10.12 \times \text{weight (kg)}$$
$$\text{residual} = 0 \pm 156, R^2 = 0.64.$$

For normal-weight women:
$$\text{BEE (kcal/d)} = 255 - 2.35 \times \text{age (y)} + 361.6 \times \text{height (m)}$$
$$+ 9.39 \times \text{weight (kg)}$$
$$\text{residual} = \pm 125, R^2 = 0.39.$$

For normal-weight, overweight, and obese women:
$$\text{BEE (kcal/d)} = 247 - (2.67 \times \text{age [y]}) + 401.5 \times \text{height (m)}$$
$$+ 8.60 \times \text{weight (kg)}$$
$$\text{residual} = \pm 156, R^2 = 0.62.$$

The residuals (differences between the observed and predicted BEE) can be compared with the differences between the BEE values calculated for the adults in the DLW database using the BEE predictive equations by Henry (2000) and WN Schofield (1985) based on body weight, and the predictive BEE equation of WN Schofield (1985) based on body weight and height and the observed BEE in the DLW database. These differences (averages ± standard deviation [SD]) are: –35 ± 168, –9 ± 169, and –34 ± 184 in men, and –33 ± 134, 8 ± 137, and 16 ± 135 in women, respectively.

For the normal-weight adults with BMIs from 18.5 up to 25 kg/m^2 in Tables 5-29 and 5-30, BEE was calculated using the above BEE prediction

TABLE 5-29 Basal and Total Daily Energy Expenditure in Men 30 Years of Age as Calculated from Total Energy Expenditure (TEE) Equations for Normal-weight, Overweight, and Obese Men[a]

Height (m [in])	PAL[b]	Weight (kg [lb]) for a Body Mass Index (kg/m²) of:						
		18.5	22.5	24.99	25	30	35	40
1.45	BEE	38.9	47.3	52.5	52.6	63.1	73.6	84.1
(57)	Sedentary	(86)	(104)	(116)	(116)	(139)	(162)	(185)
	Low active							
	Active							
	Very active							
1.50	BEE	41.6	50.6	56.2	56.3	67.5	78.8	90.0
(59)	Sedentary	(92)	(111)	(124)	(124)	(149)	(173)	(198)
	Low active							
	Active							
	Very active							
1.55	BEE	44.4	54.1	60.0	60.1	72.1	84.1	96.1
(61)	Sedentary	(98)	(119)	(132)	(132)	(159)	(185)	(211)
	Low active							
	Active							
	Very active							
1.60	BEE	47.4	57.6	64.0	64.0	76.8	89.6	102.4
(63)	Sedentary	(104)	(127)	(141)	(141)	(169)	(197)	(225)
	Low active							
	Active							
	Very active							
1.65	BEE	50.4	61.3	68.0	68.1	81.7	95.3	108.9
(65)	Sedentary	(111)	(135)	(150)	(150)	(180)	(210)	(240)
	Low active							
	Active							
	Very active							
1.70	BEE	53.5	65.0	72.2	72.3	86.7	101.2	115.6
(67)	Sedentary	(118)	(143)	(159)	(159)	(191)	(223)	(254)
	Low active							
	Active							
	Very active							
1.75	BEE	56.7	68.9	76.5	76.6	91.9	107.2	122.5
(69)	Sedentary	(125)	(152)	(168)	(168)	(202)	(236)	(270)
	Low active							
	Active							
	Very active							

TEE[c] (kcal/d) for a Body Mass Index (kg/m^2) of:

18.5	22.5	24.99	25	30	35	40
1,192	1,290	1,351	1,373	1,479	1,585	1,692
1,777	1,911	1,994	2,048	2,197	2,347	2,496
1,931	2,080	2,172	2,225	2,393	2,560	2,727
2,128	2,295	2,399	2,447	2,636	2,826	3,015
2,450	2,648	2,771	2,845	3,075	3,305	3,535
1,246	1,352	1,417	1,433	1,547	1,661	1,774
1,848	1,991	2,080	2,126	2,285	2,445	2,605
2,010	2,169	2,268	2,312	2,491	2,670	2,849
2,216	2,395	2,506	2,545	2,748	2,951	3,154
2,554	2,766	2,898	2,964	3,210	3,456	3,702
1,302	1,414	1,484	1,494	1,616	1,737	1,859
1,920	2,073	2,168	2,205	2,376	2,546	2,717
2,089	2,259	2,365	2,401	2,592	2,783	2,974
2,305	2,497	2,616	2,646	2,862	3,079	3,296
2,661	2,887	3,028	3,087	3,349	3,612	3,875
1,358	1,478	1,553	1,557	1,686	1,816	1,946
1,993	2,156	2,257	2,286	2,468	2,650	2,831
2,171	2,352	2,464	2,492	2,695	2,899	3,102
2,397	2,601	2,728	2,749	2,980	3,210	3,441
2,769	3,010	3,160	3,211	3,491	3,771	4,051
1,416	1,543	1,623	1,621	1,759	1,896	2,034
2,068	2,241	2,349	2,369	2,562	2,755	2,949
2,254	2,446	2,566	2,584	2,801	3,017	3,234
2,491	2,707	2,842	2,854	3,099	3,345	3,590
2,880	3,136	3,296	3,339	3,637	3,934	4,232
1,475	1,610	1,694	1,686	1,832	1,979	2,125
2,144	2,328	2,442	2,453	2,659	2,864	3,069
2,339	2,542	2,670	2,679	2,909	3,139	3,369
2,586	2,816	2,959	2,961	3,222	3,483	3,743
2,993	3,265	3,434	3,469	3,785	4,101	4,417
1,535	1,678	1,767	1,753	1,907	2,062	2,217
2,222	2,417	2,538	2,540	2,757	2,975	3,192
2,425	2,641	2,776	2,776	3,019	3,263	3,507
2,683	2,927	3,079	3,071	3,347	3,623	3,899
3,108	3,396	3,576	3,602	3,937	4,272	4,607

continued

TABLE 5-29 Continued

Height (m [in])	PAL[b]	Weight (kg [lb]) for a Body Mass Index (kg/m²) of:						
		18.5	22.5	24.99	25	30	35	40
1.80	BEE	59.9	72.9	81.0	81.0	97.2	113.4	129.6
(71)	Sedentary	(132)	(160)	(178)	(178)	(214)	(249)	(285)
	Low active							
	Active							
	Very active							
1.85	BEE	63.3	77.0	85.5	85.6	102.7	119.8	136.9
(73)	Sedentary	(139)	(169)	(188)	(188)	(226)	(264)	(301)
	Low active							
	Active							
	Very active							
1.90	BEE	66.8	81.2	90.2	90.3	108.3	126.4	144.4
(75)	Sedentary	(147)	(179)	(198)	(199)	(239)	(278)	(318)
	Low active							
	Active							
	Very active							
1.95	BEE	70.3	85.6	95.0	95.1	114.1	133.1	152.1
(77)	Sedentary	(155)	(188)	(209)	(209)	(251)	(293)	(335)
	Low active							
	Active							
	Very active							

[a] For each year below 30, add 4 kcal/d to BEE and 10 kcal/d to TEE. For each year above 30, subtract 4 kcal/d from BEE and 10 kcal/d from TEE. Equations determined from combined DLW databases (Appendix Table I-11).

equations for normal-weight men and women, and TEE was calculated utilizing the EER equations in the section "Adults Ages 19 Years and Older." For overweight and obese adults with BMIs from 25 up to 40 kg/m², the above BEE prediction equations for normal, overweight, and obese men and women were utilized to calculate BEE, and the above TEE equations for normal, overweight, and obese individuals were used to predict the TEE. The differences between the predictions made for BMI of 24.99 kg/m² and BMI of 25 kg/m² in Tables 5-29 and 5-30 show that the discrepancies at the junction of the two prediction ranges are essentially negligible as average differences (± SD) are 0.4 ± 2.1 percent in men, and 0.9 ± 1.1 percent in women, respectively.

TEE^c (kcal/d) for a Body Mass Index (kg/m^2) of:						
18.5	22.5	24.99	25	30	35	40
1,596	1,747	1,841	1,820	1,984	2,148	2,312
2,301	2,507	2,635	2,628	2,858	3,088	3,318
2,513	2,742	2,884	2,875	3,132	3,390	3,648
2,782	3,040	3,200	3,183	3,475	3,767	4,059
3,225	3,530	3,720	3,738	4,092	4,447	4,801
1,658	1,818	1,917	1,889	2,062	2,236	2,409
2,382	2,600	2,735	2,718	2,961	3,204	3,447
2,602	2,844	2,995	2,975	3,248	3,520	3,792
2,883	3,155	3,325	3,297	3,606	3,915	4,223
3,344	3,667	3,867	3,877	4,251	4,625	4,999
1,721	1,889	1,995	1,959	2,142	2,325	2,507
2,464	2,694	2,837	2,810	3,066	3,322	3,579
2,694	2,949	3,107	3,078	3,365	3,652	3,939
2,986	3,273	3,452	3,414	3,739	4,065	4,390
3,466	3,806	4,018	4,018	4,412	4,807	5,202
1,785	1,963	2,073	2,031	2,223	2,416	2,608
2,548	2,790	2,940	2,903	3,173	3,443	3,713
2,786	3,055	3,222	3,183	3,485	3,788	4,090
3,090	3,393	3,581	3,532	3,875	4,218	4,561
3,590	3,948	4,171	4,162	4,578	4,993	5,409

^{b} PAL = physical activity level, BEE = basal energy expenditure.

Weight Reduction in Overweight and Obese Adults

When obese individuals need to lose weight, the necessary negative energy balance can theoretically be achieved by either a reduction in energy intake or an increase in energy expenditure of physical activity (EEPA). Most usually, a combination of both is desirable (NIH, 2000) because it is hard to achieve the high levels of negative energy balance necessary for 1 to 2 lb/wk weight loss with exercise alone. In support of this contention, meta-analyses show very low levels of weight loss in structured exercise programs (Ballor and Keesey, 1991), but at the same time several studies suggest that the combination of dietary change and increased physical activity appears effective for promoting weight loss and successful weight maintenance after weight loss, perhaps by promoting

TABLE 5-30 Basal and Total Daily Energy Expenditure in Women 30 Years of Age as Calculated from Total Energy Expenditure (TEE) Equations for Normal-weight, Overweight, and Obese Women[a]

Height (m [in])	PAL[b]	Weight (kg [lb]) for a Body Mass Index (kg/m²) of:						
		18.5	22.5	24.99	25	30	35	40
1.45	BEE	38.9	45.2	52.5	52.6	63.1	73.6	84.1
(57)	Sedentary	(86)	(100)	(116)	(116)	(139)	(162)	(185)
	Low active							
	Active							
	Very active							
1.50	BEE	41.6	48.4	56.2	56.3	67.5	78.8	90.0
(59)	Sedentary	(92)	(107)	(124)	(124)	(149)	(174)	(198)
	Low active							
	Active							
	Very active							
1.55	BEE	44.4	51.7	60.0	60.1	72.1	84.1	96.1
(61)	Sedentary	(98)	(114)	(132)	(132)	(159)	(185)	(212)
	Low active							
	Active							
	Very active							
1.60	BEE	47.4	55.0	64.0	64.0	76.8	89.6	102.4
(63)	Sedentary	(104)	(121)	(141)	(141)	(169)	(197)	(226)
	Low active							
	Active							
	Very active							
1.65	BEE	50.4	58.5	68.0	68.1	81.7	95.3	108.9
(65)	Sedentary	(111)	(129)	(150)	(150)	(180)	(210)	(240)
	Low active							
	Active							
	Very active							
1.70	BEE	53.5	62.1	72.2	72.3	86.7	101.2	115.6
(67)	Sedentary	(118)	(137)	(159)	(159)	(191)	(223)	(255)
	Low active							
	Active							
	Very active							
1.75	BEE	56.7	65.8	76.5	76.6	91.9	107.2	122.5
(69)	Sedentary	(125)	(145)	(169)	(169)	(202)	(236)	(270)
	Low active							
	Active							
	Very active							

TEE (kcal/d) for a Body Mass Index (kg/m^2) of:

18.5	22.5	24.99	25	30	35	40
1,074	1,133	1,202	1,201	1,291	1,382	1,472
1,564	1,623	1,691	1,698	1,813	1,927	2,042
1,734	1,800	1,877	1,912	2,043	2,174	2,304
1,946	2,021	2,108	2,112	2,257	2,403	2,548
2,201	2,287	2,386	2,387	2,553	2,719	2,886
1,118	1,181	1,255	1,253	1,349	1,446	1,543
1,625	1,689	1,762	1,771	1,894	2,017	2,139
1,803	1,874	1,956	1,996	2,136	2,276	2,415
2,025	2,105	2,198	2,205	2,360	2,516	2,672
2,291	2,382	2,489	2,493	2,671	2,849	3,027
1,163	1,230	1,309	1,306	1,409	1,512	1,615
1,688	1,756	1,834	1,846	1,977	2,108	2,239
1,873	1,949	2,037	2,081	2,230	2,380	2,529
2,104	2,190	2,290	2,299	2,466	2,632	2,798
2,382	2,480	2,593	2,601	2,791	2,981	3,171
1,208	1,280	1,364	1,360	1,470	1,580	1,690
1,752	1,824	1,907	1,922	2,061	2,201	2,340
1,944	2,025	2,118	2,168	2,327	2,486	2,645
2,185	2,276	2,383	2,396	2,573	2,750	2,927
2,474	2,578	2,699	2,712	2,914	3,116	3,318
1,254	1,331	1,420	1,415	1,532	1,649	1,766
1,816	1,893	1,982	1,999	2,148	2,296	2,444
2,016	2,102	2,202	2,256	2,425	2,594	2,763
2,267	2,364	2,477	2,494	2,682	2,871	3,059
2,567	2,678	2,807	2,824	3,039	3,254	3,469
1,301	1,383	1,478	1,471	1,595	1,719	1,843
1,881	1,963	2,057	2,078	2,235	2,393	2,550
2,090	2,180	2,286	2,345	2,525	2,705	2,884
2,350	2,453	2,573	2,594	2,794	2,994	3,194
2,662	2,780	2,917	2,938	3,166	3,395	3,623
1,350	1,436	1,536	1,528	1,659	1,791	1,923
1,948	2,034	2,134	2,158	2,325	2,492	2,659
2,164	2,260	2,372	2,437	2,627	2,817	3,007
2,434	2,543	2,670	2,695	2,907	3,119	3,331
2,758	2,883	3,028	3,054	3,296	3,538	3,780

continued

TABLE 5-30 Continued

Height (m [in])	PAL[b]	Weight (kg [lb]) for a Body Mass Index (kg/m^2) of:						
		18.5	22.5	24.99	25	30	35	40
1.80	BEE	59.9	69.7	81.0	81.0	97.2	113.4	129.6
(71)	Sedentary	(132)	(154)	(178)	(178)	(214)	(250)	(285)
	Low active							
	Active							
	Very active							
1.85	BEE	63.3	73.6	85.5	85.6	102.7	119.8	136.9
(73)	Sedentary	(139)	(162)	(188)	(189)	(226)	(264)	(302)
	Low active							
	Active							
	Very active							
1.90	BEE	66.8	77.6	90.2	90.3	108.3	126.4	144.4
(75)	Sedentary	(147)	(171)	(198)	(199)	(239)	(278)	(318)
	Low active							
	Active							
	Very active							
1.95	BEE	70.3	81.8	95.0	95.1	114.1	133.1	152.1
(77)	Sedentary	(155)	(180)	(209)	(209)	(251)	(293)	(335)
	Low active							
	Active							
	Very active							

[a] For each year below 30, add 2.5 kcal/d to BEE and 7 kcal/d to TEE. For each year above 30, subtract 2.5 kcal/d from BEE and 7 kcal/d from TEE. Equations determined from combined DLW databases (Appendix Table I-11).

favorable metabolic changes or improved dietary compliance (DePue et al., 1995; Dunn et al., 1999; Hartman et al., 1993; Holden et al., 1992; Miller et al., 1997).

Several studies indicate that energy expenditure decreases when energy intake is less than TEE, with the result that weight loss is less than anticipated based on the reduction in energy intake. As shown in Figure 5-9, a summary of studies on changes in resting energy expenditure (REE) with negative energy balance in adults have shown that the decline in REE with weight loss is greater than predicted from the loss of FFM that occurs concomitantly during negative energy balance. This suggests that there is a decrease in REE per unit of FFM during active weight loss (underfeeding).

TEE (kcal/d) for a Body Mass Index (kg/m^2) of:						
18.5	22.5	24.99	25	30	35	40
1,398	1,490	1,596	1,586	1,725	1,865	2,004
2,015	2,106	2,211	2,239	2,416	2,593	2,769
2,239	2,341	2,459	2,529	2,731	2,932	3,133
2,519	2,634	2,769	2,799	3,023	3,247	3,472
2,855	2,987	3,141	3,172	3,428	3,684	3,940
1,448	1,545	1,657	1,645	1,792	1,940	2,087
2,083	2,179	2,290	2,322	2,509	2,695	2,882
2,315	2,422	2,548	2,624	2,836	3,049	3,262
2,605	2,727	2,869	2,904	3,141	3,378	3,615
2,954	3,093	3,255	3,292	3,562	3,833	4,103
1,499	1,601	1,719	1,706	1,861	2,016	2,171
2,151	2,253	2,371	2,406	2,603	2,800	2,996
2,392	2,505	2,637	2,720	2,944	3,168	3,393
2,693	2,821	2,971	3,011	3,261	3,511	3,760
3,053	3,200	3,371	3,414	3,699	3,984	4,270
1,550	1,657	1,782	1,767	1,931	2,094	2,258
2,221	2,328	2,452	2,492	2,699	2,906	3,113
2,470	2,589	2,729	2,817	3,053	3,290	3,526
2,781	2,917	3,074	3,119	3,383	3,646	3,909
3,154	3,309	3,489	3,538	3,838	4,139	4,439

[b] PAL = Physical activity level, BEE = basal energy expenditure.

Role of Decreased Food Intake with or Without Increased Physical Activity

There are also four underfeeding studies that have examined changes in TEE with negative energy balance achieved by a reduction in energy intake. As shown in Table 5-31, the reduction in energy intake in these studies ranged from 758 to 1,620 kcal/d and was associated with a reduction in TEE that averaged 36 percent of the reduction in energy intake. It should be noted that there was a period of 3 to 52 weeks of underfeeding between the measurements of TEE made during weight maintenance and negative energy balance. Thus, some of the reduction in TEE was due to reduced energy requirements associated with reduced body weight.

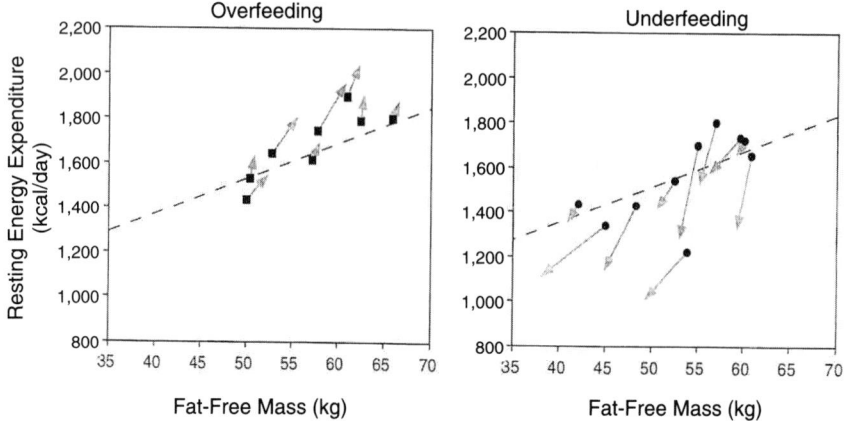

FIGURE 5-9 Relationship between changes in fat-free mass and resting energy expenditure during overfeeding and underfeeding. Reprinted, with permission, from Saltzman and Roberts (1995). Copyright 1995 by International Life Sciences Institute.

    In multiple regression analyses using the DLW data of the studies in Table 5-31, weight, age, and gender significantly predicted TEE, and the b-coefficient for the weight term was 16.6 kcal/d. This implies that for weight-stable individuals, differences in body weight of 1 kg are associated with differences in TEE of 16.6 kcal/d. By correcting the changes in TEE that can be attributed to the decrease in body size in the four underfeeding studies described in Table 5-31, 8.4 percent of the reduction in TEE was unaccounted for by weight loss and appears therefore to be associated with a state of negative energy balance. This could be due to a reduction in energy expenditure per kg body weight or to a decrease in physical activity.

    These values can be used to estimate the anticipated reduction in metabolizable energy intake necessary to achieve a given level of weight loss, if weight loss is achieved solely by a reduction in energy intake and there is no change in energy expenditure for physical activity. For example, a weight loss of 1 to 2 lb/wk (65 to 130 g/d) is equivalent to a body energy loss of 468 to 936 kcal/d, because the energy content of weight loss averages 7.2 kcal/g (i.e., 75 percent fat containing 9.25 kcal/g and 25 percent FFM containing 1 kcal/g) (Saltzman and Roberts, 1995). Taking into account the decrease in TEE due to weight loss (16.6 kcal/kg) and due to negative energy balance (8.4 percent of initial TEE), the total expected reduction in TEE after 10 weeks of dieting is predicted to be 376 to

TABLE 5-31 Changes (Δ) in Total Energy Expenditure (TEE) During Underfeeding Studies[a]

Reference	ΔTEE (kcal/d)	ΔBE[b] (kcal/d)	ΔEI[c] (kcal/d)	ΔTEE/ΔEI	CoorΔTEE/ΔEI[d]
Heyman et al., 1992	−297	−461	−758	0.392	0.076
Kempen et al., 1995	−359	−765	−1,124	0.319	0.087
Racette et al., 1995	−349	−695	−1,044	0.334	0.079
van Gemert et al., 2000	−645	−975	−1,620	0.398	0.093
Means				0.361	0.084

[a] Where all values are in kcal/d, Δ describes changes in value between weight maintenance and underfeeding.
[b] BE = body energy.
[c] EI = energy intake (calculated as ΔBE + ΔTEE).
[d] CorrΔTEE is change in total energy expenditure after subtracting the estimated change in TEE due to weight loss in the underfeeding period prior to measurement of TEE. This value indicates the change in TEE is due to negative energy balance rather than weight loss. It was estimated as weight loss prior to the underfeeding TEE × 16.6, where 16.6 is the weight coefficient in the relationship, TEE = constant + weight + age + gender in the doubly labeled water data from these studies.

542 kcal/d for an individual with an initial weight maintenance TEE of 2,500 kcal/d. Therefore, to maintain a rate of weight loss of 1 to 2 lb/wk, the reduction in energy intake would need to be 844 (468 + 376) to 1,478 kcal/d (936 + 542) after 10 weeks of weight loss.

This calculation serves both to emphasize the importance of exercise in helping prevent reduced TEE during weight loss, and to illustrate the relatively high level of reduction in energy intake needed when weight loss is to be achieved by dieting alone. It should be noted that the above calculations were based on TEE data derived from studies in adults in which reduction in energy intake was in the range of 758 to 1,620 kcal/d. The impact on energy expenditure of weight loss regimens involving lesser or greater reductions in energy intake need to be assessed before rates of weight reduction can be more precisely predicted. However, it must be appreciated that reduction in resting rates of energy expenditure per kilogram of body weight have a small impact on the prediction of energy deficits imposed by food restriction, and the greatest cause of deviation from projected rates of weight loss lies in the degree of compliance. The coefficient of 16.6 kcal/kg of weight loss calculated from the data in Table 5-31 could be utilized to anticipate the reduction in energy intake required for maintaining lower body weights. Further studies in this area are needed.

Estimation of Energy Expenditure for Weight Maintenance in Overweight Children Ages 3 Through 18 Years

While the Centers for Disease Control and Prevention (CDC) currently defines childhood "risk of overweight" as greater than the 85th percentile for BMI and "overweight" as greater than the 95th percentile of BMI, it gives no definition for obesity in childhood. Several organizations, however, define childhood obesity as a BMI above the 95th age-adjusted percentile (Barlow and Dietz, 1998; Bellizzi and Dietz, 1999). An international standardized approach was also recently proposed, based on identifying the childhood BMI at different ages that would be equivalent to a BMI of 25 kg/m^2 (for overweight) or 30 kg/m^2 (for obese) at age 18 years (Cole et al., 2000). Using this approach, the cutoff for obesity would fall near the 97th percentile of the current CDC growth charts (Figure 5-10). For this report, the CDC definitions of risk of overweight and overweight are accepted for children, namely BMI above the 95th percentile for overweight and above the 85th percentile for risk of overweight.

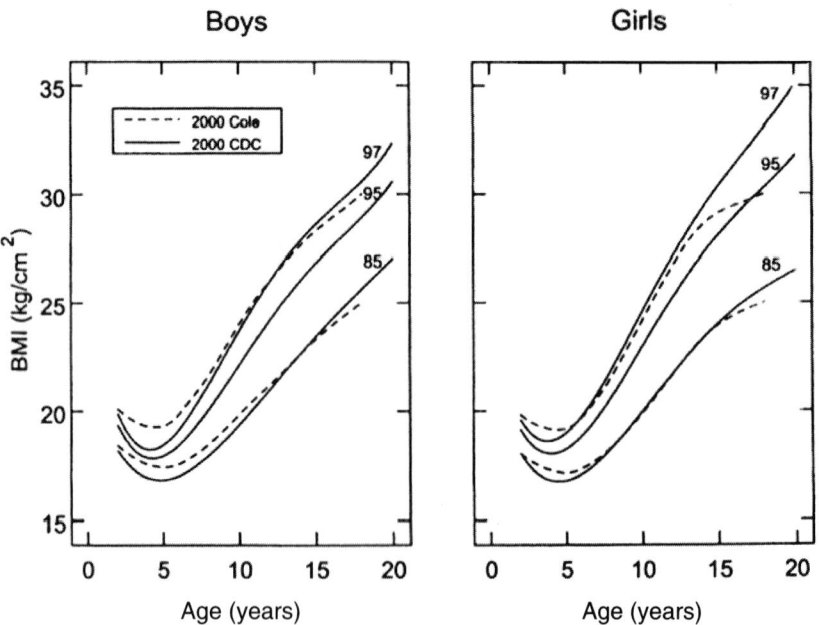

FIGURE 5-10 Comparison of body mass index (BMI) definitions of overweight and obesity during childhood with percentiles for BMI (85th, 95th, 97th). Reprinted, with permission, from Roberts and Dallal (2001). Copyright 2001 by International Life Sciences Institute.

Rapid weight loss is undesirable in children due to the risks of stunting and micronutrient deficiencies. In addition, children under 2 years of age should not be placed on energy-restricted diets out of concern that brain development may inadvertently be compromised by inadequate dietary intake of fatty acids and micronutrients. A recent expert pediatric committee recommended that weight maintenance be the goal for most children over 2 years of age in the 85th to 95th percentiles for BMI (Barlow and Dietz, 1998). In addition, the committee recommended that weight loss be at a rate of 1 lb/mo for children over 7 years of age at or greater than the 95th percentile BMI and for children between the 85th and 95th percentiles who have comorbidities that would be anticipated to be improved by weight loss.

Separate TEE predictive equations were developed from the DLW data for 3- through 18-year-old overweight and obese boys and girls (Appendix Table I-6) from age, height, weight, and PAL categories using nonlinear regression techniques. In order to utilize all the TEE data, PAL categorization was determined using predicted BEE rather than observed BEE, since only 67 percent (85/127) of the boys and 64 percent (123/192) of the girls and had observed BEEs. The following predictive equations for BEE were derived from the observed BEEs provided in the DLW database (Appendix Table I-6).

For overweight and obese boys:
$$\text{BEE (kcal/d)} = 420 - 33.5 \text{ age (y)} + 418.9 \times \text{height (m)} + 16.7 \text{ weight (kg)}$$
$$\text{SE} = 89.9, R^2 = 0.88.$$

For overweight and obese girls:
$$\text{BEE (kcal/d)} = 516 - (26.8 \times \text{age [y]}) + 347 \text{ height (m)} + 12.4 \text{ weight (kg)}$$
$$\text{SE} = 113.4, R^2 = 0.79.$$

For normal-weight, overweight, and obese boys:
$$\text{BEE (kcal/d)} = 79 - 934.2 \times \text{age [y]}) + 730 \times \text{height (m)} + 15.3 \text{ weight (kg)}$$
$$\text{SE} = 90.6, R^2 = 0.89.$$

For normal-weight, overweight, and obese girls:
$$\text{BEE (kcal/d)} = 322 - 926.0 \times \text{age [y]}) + 504 \times \text{height (m)} + 11.6 \text{ weight (kg)}$$
$$\text{SE} = 102.1, R^2 = 0.80.$$

Prediction equations of TEE for overweight and obese girls and boys were developed using age, height, weight, and PAL category as predicted from the above BEE equations. Data were not used in the derivation of the TEE equations if the PAL value was less than 1.0 or greater than 2.5. In addition, TEE predictive equations were developed combining normal-weight, overweight, and obese children. The coefficients and SE for boys and girls in the overweight and obese database (Appendix Table I-6) are provided in Appendix Table I-12. Mean of the residuals did not differ from zero, and the standard deviation of the residuals ranged from 74 to 213. The coefficients and SE for boys and girls in the combined normal-weight, overweight, and obese database are described in Appendix Table I-13. The mean of the residuals did not differ from zero and the standard deviation of the residuals ranged from 73 to 208.

The children's predictive equations for TEE were subjected to statistical testing of their estimated coefficients and asymptotic standard deviations using a chi-square distribution (Hotelling T-squared test). The specific equation for the overweight and obese boys was statistically different from the equation derived solely from normal-weight boys ($P > 0.032$), and tended to differ from the combined equation derived from normal, overweight, and obese boys ($P = 0.086$). The specific equation for the overweight and obese girls was statistically different from the equation derived solely from normal-weight girls ($P > 0.001$), but not from the combined equation derived from normal, overweight, and obese girls ($P = 0.99$). The equations for the normal-weight boys and girls differed from the combined equation ($P = 0.001$).

Despite the suggestion of differences in the predictive equations for the TEE of boys, and because of the larger sample size, reduced SEs of the coefficients and increased stability, and consistency between the genders, *the prediction equations for TEE based on the combined database are recommended for use in overweight and obese children for weight maintenance—they do not include growth.* (See Table I-13 for coefficients used in the equations.)

Weight Maintenance TEE in Overweight Boys Ages 3 Through 18 Years
TEE = 114 – (50.9 × age [y]) + PA × (19.5 × weight [kg]
+ 1161.4 × height [m])

Where PA is the physical activity coefficient:
PA = 1.00 if PAL is estimated to be ≥ 1.0 < 1.4 (sedentary)
PA = 1.12 if PAL is estimated to be ≥ 1.4 < 1.6 (low active)
PA = 1.24 if PAL is estimated to be ≥ 1.6 < 1.9 (active)
PA = 1.45 if PAL is estimated to be ≥ 1.9 < 2.5 (very active)

Weight Maintenance TEE in Overweight Girls Ages 3 Through 18 Years
    TEE = 389 − (41.2 × age [y]) + PA × (15.0 × weight [kg]
            + 701.6 × height [m])

Where PA is the physical activity coefficient:
    PA = 1.00 if PAL is estimated to be ≥ 1.0 < 1.4 (sedentary)
    PA = 1.18 if PAL is estimated to be ≥ 1.4 < 1.6 (low active)
    PA = 1.35 if PAL is estimated to be ≥ 1.6 < 1.9 (active)
    PA = 1.60 if PAL is estimated to be ≥ 1.9 < 2.5 (very active)

As in adults, these TEE equations do not form the basis of EER values since the weight of the group is considered high (when BMI is greater than the 95th percentile) or at risk of being high (when BMI is greater than the 85th percentile). Nevertheless, TEE values are equivalent to EER values when weight maintenance is the goal. It should be noted that EER values for energy in children of healthy weight also include an amount that will provide sufficient energy for normal rates of growth. When weight maintenance is the goal, as in most children between the 85th and 95th BMI percentiles, it is assumed that linear growth and lean tissue growth can occur at a normal rate when body weight gain is prevented, because over time body fat content gradually decreases in parallel with the increase in FFM.

Weight Reduction in Overweight Children Ages 3 Through 18 Years

Weight reduction at a rate of 1 lb/m (15 g/d) is equivalent to a body energy loss of 108 kcal/d (assuming the energy content of weight loss averages 7.2 kcal/g [Saltzman and Roberts, 1995]), an amount that is small enough to be achievable by either an increase in EEPA, a reduction in energy intake, or a combination of both. There is currently no information on changes in TEE with negative energy balance in children, and no information even from adults on changes in TEE at low levels of negative energy balance. Thus, the extent to which TEE falls when energy intake is reduced with the intention of producing very slow weight loss in children is not known. This lack of data makes it impossible to describe the relationship between change in energy intake and change in body energy for children in whom weight loss is indicated. However, if the negative energy balance is achieved by a reduction in energy intake alone, at least a 108 kcal/d decrease in energy intake (i.e., equivalent to the indicated loss of body energy) would be necessary to result in a slow weight loss, and perhaps more if a reduction in TEE occurs. Small reductions in energy intake of the magnitude required to resolve childhood overweight gradually over time are within the potential for ad libitum changes induced by improvements in dietary composition.

Undernutrition

Undernutrition is still a frequent condition in many parts of the world, particularly in children. When energy intake is unable to match energy needs (due to insufficient dietary intake, excessive intestinal losses, or a combination thereof) several mechanisms of adaptation come into play (see earlier section, "Adaptation and Accommodation"). Reduction in voluntary physical activity is a rapid means of reducing energy needs to match limited energy input. In children, reduction in growth rates is another important mechanism of accommodation to energy deficit. Under conditions of persistent energy deficit, the low growth rate will result in short stature and low weight-for-age, a condition termed *stunting*.

A chronic energy deficit elicits mobilization of energy reserves, progressively depleting its main source: adipose tissue. Thus, an energy deficit of certain duration is associated with changes in body weight and body composition. As body weights decrease, so do energy requirements, although energy turnover may be higher when expressed per kg of body weight due to a predominant loss of fat tissue relative to lean tissue. In healthy, normal-weight individuals who face a sustained energy deficit, several hormonal mechanisms come into play, including a reduction in insulin release by the pancreas, a reduction in the active thyroid hormone T_3, and a decrease in adrenergic tone. These steps are aimed at reducing cellular energy demands by reducing the rates of key energy-consuming metabolic processes. However, there is less evidence that similar mechanisms are available to individuals who already have a chronic energy deficit when they are faced with further reductions in energy input (Shetty et al., 1994).

The effects of chronic undernutrition in children include decreased school performance, delayed bone age, and increased susceptibility to infections. In adults, an abnormally low BMI is associated with decreased work capacity and limited voluntary physical activity.

Additional Energy Requirements to Restore Normal Weight

In an adult with a low BMI (less than 18.5 kg/m²), the additional energy intake required to normalize body weight will depend on the initial deficit and the desired rate of recovery. Although estimates of energy needs can be made based on the initial deficit, body weight gain will include not only energy stored as fat tissue, but also some amount in the form of skeletal muscle and even visceral tissues. Thus, as recovery of body weight proceeds, the energy requirement will vary not only as a function of body weight but in response to changes in body composition.

Catch-up Growth in Children. The energy needs for catch-up growth for children can be estimated from the energy cost of tissue deposition. The average energy cost of tissue synthesis and deposition was estimated at 5 kcal/g of tissue deposited (FAO/WHO/UNU, 1985). Based on experimental data from DLW studies in infants, Butte and colleagues (1989) estimated this cost as 4.8 kcal/g. Median weight for height has been used in the past as a target for recovery. Using BMI, the 50th BMI percentile for age may be considered as a target. However, in practical terms, the target for recovery depends on the initial deficit and the conditions of nutritional treatment: clinical unit or community. Under the controlled conditions of a clinical setting, undernourished children can exhibit rates of growth of 10 to 15 g/kg body weight/d (Fjeld et al., 1989), which are tenfold higher than normal rates of weight gain at 1 year of age. Under less controlled conditions (e.g., community-dwelling children), the rates of growth are likely to be much lower. The 1985 FAO/WHO/UNU report estimated these rates as twice the normal rate (FAO/WHO/UNU, 1985). Undoubtedly, this figure would be highly dependent on the magnitude and effectiveness of the nutritional intervention.

Dewey and coworkers (1996) estimated the energy needs for recovery growth for children with moderate or severe wasting, assuming that the latter would require a higher proportion of energy relative to protein. These estimates are presented in Table 5-32.

Catch-up Grown Following Stunting. The above estimates apply to children with a weight deficit relative to height. If a child is stunted, however, weight may be adequate for height, and unless an increased energy intake elicits both gains in height and in weight, the child may become overweight without correcting his or her height. In fact, this phenomenon is increasingly documented in urban settings of developing countries. It is a matter of debate whether significant catch-up gains in longitudinal growth are possible beyond about 3 years of age. Clearly, height gain is far more regulated than weight, which is primarily influenced by substrate availability and energy balance. Furthermore, longitudinal growth may also be dependent on the availability of other dietary constituents, such as zinc (Gibson et al., 1989; Walravens et al., 1983).

Athletes

With minor exceptions, dietary recommendations for athletes are not distinguished from the general population. As described in Chapter 12, the amount of dietary energy from the recommended nutrient mix should be adjusted to achieve or maintain optimal body weight for competitive athletes and others engaged in similarly demanding physical activities. As

TABLE 5-32 Energy Needs for Catch-up Growth at Different Rates of Weight Gain

Rate of Gain[a] (g/kg/d)	Normal Composition of Weight Gain[b]		High Rate of Fat Deposition[c]	
	EE[d] = 80 Energy[e] (kcal/kg/d)	EE = 90 Energy[e] (kcal/kg/d)	EE = 80 Energy[e] (kcal/kg/d)	EE = 90 Energy[e] (kcal/kg/d)
1	83	93	86	96
2	87	97	92	102
5	97	107	110	120
10	113	123	140	150
20	146	156	200	210

[a] In normal children, average rates of weight gain are about 1.3 g/kg/d at 6–12 months, 0.8 g/kg/d at 12–18 months, and 0.5 g/kg/d at 18–24 months.

[b] 17 percent protein, 9 percent fat; assume energy cost of growth = 3.3 kcal/g (based on 5.65 kcal/g protein and 9.25 kcal/g fat, with efficiencies of synthesis of 42 percent and 85 percent, respectively [Roberts and Young, 1988: 0.17 g protein × 5.65 kcal/g/0.42 = 2.3 kcal; 0.09 g fat × 9.25 kcal/g/0.85 = 1.0 kcal]); protein needs for growth = protein need/efficiency = 0.17/0.7 = 0.24 g/kg/d.

[c] 10 percent protein, 43 percent fat; assume energy cost of growth = 6.0 kcal/g (based on 5.65 kcal/g protein and 9.25 kcal/g fat, with efficiencies of synthesis of 42 percent and 85 percent, respectively [Roberts and Young, 1988: 0.10 g protein × 5.65 kcal/g/0.42 = 1.3 kcal; 0.43 g fat × 9.25 kcal/g/0.85 = 4.7 kcal]); protein needs for growth = protein need/efficiency = 0.10/0.7 = 0.14 g/kg/d.

[d] EE = energy expenditure for maintenance and activity expressed as kcal/kg/d. As described by Dewey and colleagues (1996), the lower value is similar to average energy expenditure of preschool children and to energy expenditure for maintenance and activity of recovering malnourished children in Peru. The higher value is typical of normal infants at 9–12 months of age, but may be higher than would be expected of malnourished children if they are less active.

[e] Metabolizable energy intake.

SOURCE: Adapted from Dewey et al. (1996).

in the general population, the need to balance energy intake and expenditure over a wide range of body sizes, body compositions, and forms of exercise means that athletes will, in fact, require vastly different meal sizes and frequencies (e.g., female gymnasts compared to male American football linemen). While some athletes may be able to sustain extremely high power outputs over days or even weeks (such as in the Tour de France bicycle race), such endeavors are episodic and cannot be sustained indefinitely. Further, the recommendation for athletes to select foods in accordance with the same dietary guidelines as the general population is intended to teach sound dietary practices to men and women whose lifestyles will become more typical when their athletic careers diminish.

Despite the difference in scope of energy flux associated with participation in sports and extremely demanding physical activities such as marathon running and military operations, several advantages are associated with different forms of exercise. For example, resistance exercise promotes muscle hypertrophy and changes in body composition by increasing the ratio of muscle to total body mass (Brooks et al., 2000). Hence, the height-weight values given in Tables 5-4 and 5-5 are of little relevance to lean, but highly muscular individuals such as speed/power athletes who, because of muscle hypertrophy, will have BMIs in excess of 25 kg/m^2. Athletes needing to increase strength will necessarily employ resistance exercises while ensuring that dietary energy is sufficient to increase muscle mass. Total body mass may increase, remain the same, or decrease depending on energy balance. Athletes needing to decrease body mass to obtain biomechanical advantages will necessarily increase total exercise energy output, reduce energy input, or use a combination of the two approaches. As distinct from weight loss by diet alone, having a major exercise component will serve to preserve lean body mass even in the face of negative energy balance.

ADVERSE EFFECTS OF OVERCONSUMPTION OF ENERGY

Hazard Identification

Adverse Effects

Adaptation to High Levels of Energy Intake. The ability of healthy individuals to compensate for increases in energy intake by increasing energy expenditure (either for physical activity or resting metabolism) depends on physiological and behavioral factors. When individuals are given a diet providing a fixed (but limited) amount of energy in excess of the requirements to maintain body weight, they will initially gain weight. However, over a period of several weeks, their energy expenditure will increase, mostly (Durnin, 1990; Ravussin et al., 1991), but perhaps not entirely (Leibel et al., 1995), on account of their increased body size, so that body weight eventually will stabilize at a higher level. A reduction of energy intake will produce the opposite effect. Some reports indicate that the magnitude of the reduction in energy expenditure when energy intake is reduced is greater than the corresponding increase in energy expenditure when energy intake is increased (Saltzman and Roberts, 1995). Nevertheless, weight changes invariably occur under conditions of increased and decreased energy intake. It is likely that for most individuals the principal mechanism for maintaining body weight is by controlling food intake rather than physical activity (Jequier and Tappy, 1999).

Body Weight Gain and Chronic Disease. Weight gain that causes body mass index (BMI) to reach and exceed 25 kg/m^2 is associated with an increased risk of premature mortality (NHLBI/NIDDK, 1998). As shown in Tables 5-33 through 5-38, cohort studies have shown that morbidity risk for type 2 diabetes, hypertension, coronary heart disease, stroke, gallbladder disease, osteoarthritis, and some types of cancer also increases with increasing BMI of 25 kg/m^2 and higher.

Some data from large cohort studies suggest that disease risk begins to increase at BMI levels lower than those associated with increased risk of mortality (Manson et al., 1990). Thus, some investigators have recommended that individuals should aim at having a BMI of 22 kg/m^2 at the end of adolescence (NHLBI/NIDDK, 1998). This level would also provide some margin for weight gain in mid-life without surpassing the 25 kg/m^2 threshold.

For these reasons, energy intakes associated with adverse risk are defined as those that cause weight gain for individuals with a body weight within the healthy range (BMI from 18.5 up to 25 kg/m^2) and overweight individuals (BMI from 25 up to 30 kg/m^2). In the case of obese individuals who need to lose weight to improve their health, energy intakes that cause adverse risk are those that are higher than those needed to lose weight without causing negative health consequences.

Summary

Because of the direct impact of deviations from energy balance on body weight and of changes in body weight, body-weight data represent critical indicators of the adequacy of energy intake. Energy requirements are defined as the amounts of energy that need to be consumed by individuals to sustain stable body weights in the range desired for good health (BMI from 18.5 up to 25 kg/m^2) while maintaining lifestyles that include adequate levels of physical activity to maintain social, cultural, and economic activity. Since any energy intake above the Estimated Energy Requirement (EER) would be expected to result in weight gain and a likely increased risk of morbidity, the Tolerable Upper Intake Levels are not applicable to energy. If weight gain was identified as the hazard, the lowest-observed-adverse-effect level (LOAEL) would be any intake above the EER for adults. The uncertainty factor would be one as there is no uncertainty in the fact that overconsumption of energy leads to weight gain.

Intake Assessment

Based on distribution data from the 1994–1996, 1998 Continuing Survey of Food Intakes by Individuals, the highest mean intake of energy from diet for any gender and life stage group was estimated to be about 2,840 kcal/d (Appendix Table E-1), the intake of boys ages 14 through 18 years. Men 19 through 30 years of age had the highest reported energy intake with the 99th percentile of intake at 5,378 kcal/d.

RESEARCH RECOMMENDATIONS

- The number of available doubly labeled water studies for the determination of total energy expenditure (TEE) in certain age and gender categories is limited and should be expanded. This is particularly true for young children 3 to 5 years of age, adolescent boys, and adult men and women 40 through 60 years of age.
- Development of reliable methods to track dietary energy intakes in population groups is needed.
- Identification of biological markers of risk of excess weight gain in children and young adults is needed.
- Methods suitable for free-living population-based studies or applications should be developed to measure physical activity levels in order to classify children and adults into sedentary, low active, active, and very active levels of physical activity.
- More studies are necessary to determine whether and which dietary composition patterns facilitate permanent weight loss in adults and children.
- Development of practical, accurate means to assess body composition in populations is needed.
- Physical activity patterns consistent with normal health and development of children should be described that are applicable across age, gender, and ethnic backgrounds.
- Factors affecting the energy intake required to satisfy nutrient requirements should be explored, including diet digestibility, viscosity, and energy and nutrient density.
- Factors affecting the changes in TEE during pregnancy, as well as equations to predict the basal metabolic rate throughout pregnancy, are needed to better predict the energy requirements of nonobese, overweight, and obese pregnant women.
- More information is needed on the energy requirements of overweight and obese adults and children. It would be desirable for this additional TEE information to be collected in studies that also document physical activity patterns, so that the relationship between activity and TEE can be further evaluated.

TABLE 5-33 Body Mass Index (BMI) and Risk of
Noninsulin-Dependent Diabetes Mellitus

Reference	Country	Study Population	Length of Follow-Up
Westlund and Nicolaysen, 1972	Sweden	3,751 men, 40–49 y	10 y
Medalie et al., 1974	Israel	10,059 men, 40+ y	5 y
Ohlson et al., 1985	Sweden	792 men, 54 y	13.5 y
Despres et al., 1989	Canada	52 premenopausal obese women	Not applicable
Lundgren et al., 1989	Sweden	1,462 women, 38–60 y	12 y
Colditz et al., 1990	United States	113,861 women, 30–55 y	8 y
Haffner et al., 1991	United States	254 men and 366 women	8 y

Obesity Index	Outcome[a]
Weight-height relationship	Incidence of diabetes (%)
Normal ± 10%	0.6
10–15% overweight	1.8
15–25% overweight	2.5
25–35% overweight	3.7
35–45% overweight	7.1
> 45% overweight	12.6
Weight/height index (kg/cm)	Incidence rate of diabetes
0.24–0.39	26/1,000
0.40–0.45	39/1,000
0.46–0.69	57/1,000
BMI, waist-to-hip ratio	Risk of development of diabetes was significantly associated with BMI ($p = 0.0003$) and waist-to-hip ratio ($p < 0.0001$)
BMI, body fat mass	BMI and body fat mass were significantly associated with plasma glucose and insulin
BMI	Significant correlation between initial BMI and incidence of diabetes during follow-up ($p < 0.001$)
BMI (kg/m^2)	Proportional hazards RR for diabetes (95% CI)
< 22	1.0
22–22.9	2.1 (1.4–3.3)
23–23.9	3.5 (2.3–5.1)
24–24.9	2.9 (1.9–4.5)
25–26.9	5.2 (3.7–7.5)
27–28.9	9.6 (6.8–13.6)
29–30.9	19.0 (13.6–26.4)
31–32.9	28.0 (19.9–39.4)
33–34.9	38.5 (27.0–54.9)
≥ 35	58.2 (42.4–79.9)

	OR for diabetes (95% CI)	
BMI (kg/m^2)	Men	Women
< 24.6	1.00	1.00
24.6–28.2	1.33 (0.25–7.27)	1.38 (0.32–6.08)
> 28.2	2.51 (0.49–12.6)	3.70 (1.03–13.3)

continued

TABLE 5-33 Continued

Reference	Country	Study Population	Length of Follow-Up
Chan et al., 1994	United States	27,983 men, 40–75 y	5 y
Ford et al., 1997	United States	8,545 adults	10 y

a RR = relative risk, CI = confidence interval, OR = odds ratio, CVD = cardiovascular disease.

Obesity Index	Outcome[a]
BMI (kg/m^2)	RR for diabetes (95% CI)
< 23	1.0
23–23.9	1.0 (0.5–2.0)
24–24.9	1.5 (0.8–2.9)
25–26.9	2.2 (1.3–3.8)
27–28.9	4.4 (2.6–7.7)
29–30.9	6.7 (3.8–12.0)
31–32.9	11.6 (6.3–21.5)
33–34.9	21.3 (11.4–41.2)
≥ 35	42.1 (22.0–80.6)
Weight gain since age 21	RR for diabetes (95% CI)
0–2 kg	1.0
3–5 kg	0.9 (0.5–1.8)
6–7 kg	1.9 (1.0–3.7)
8–9 kg	3.5 (2.0–6.3)
10–14 kg	3.4 (2.0–5.8)
15+ kg	8.9 (5.5–14.7)
BMI at baseline (kg/m^2)	Hazard ratio for diabetes (95% CI)
< 22	1.00
22–22.9	1.16 (0.48–2.82)
23–23.9	2.39 (1.30–4.40)
24–24.9	2.82 (1.45–5.50)
25–26.9	2.75 (1.55–4.91)
27–28.9	4.63 (2.69–7.96)
29–30.9	4.88 (2.77–8.59)
31–32.9	6.96 (3.79–12.81)
33–34.9	9.28 (4.60–18.72)
≥ 35	11.24 (6.66–18.96)
Weight gain since baseline	Hazard ratio for diabetes (95% CI)
< 5 kg	1.00
5 to < 8 kg	2.11 (1.40–3.18)
8 to < 11 kg	1.19 (0.75–1.89)
11 to < 20 kg	2.66 (1.84–3.85)
≥ 20 kg	3.84 (2.04–7.22)

NOTE: BMI = kg/m^2 unless noted otherwise. Multivariate-adjusted relative risk/hazard risk/odds ratio estimates were used in this table whenever possible.

TABLE 5-34 Body Mass Index (BMI) and Risk of Hypertension and Stroke

Reference	Country	Study Population	Length of Follow-Up
Hypertension			
Ballantyne et al., 1978	UK	637 men and 835 women, mean 45–49 y	Not applicable
Brennan et al., 1980	Australia	600 men and 400 women, 20–49 y	Not applicable
Criqui et al., 1982	United States	2,482 men and 2,298 women, 20+ y	Not applicable
MacMahon et al., 1984	Australia	5,550 men and women, 25–64 y	Not applicable
Brown et al., 2000	United States	16,681 adults, 20+ y	Not applicable
Stroke			
Walker et al., 1996	United States	28,643 men, 40–75 y	5 y
Rexrode et al., 1997	United States	116,759 women, 30–55 y	16 y

[a] RR = relative risk, OR = odds ratio.

Obesity Index	Outcome[a]
Ponderal Index (height/weight$^{1/3}$)	Ponderal index was significantly associated with blood pressure only in hypertensive, male nonsmokers
BMI	Significant correlation between BMI and hypertension in men ($p < 0.05$) and women ($p < 0.01$)
BMI	BMI was significantly associated with diastolic and systolic blood pressure in both men and women

BMI in men (kg/m^2)	RR for hypertension (95% CI)
19.5–25.4	1.00
25.5–30.4	1.72 (1.44–2.05)
≥ 30.5	2.47 (1.83–3.34)

BMI in women (kg/m^2)	RR for hypertension (95% CI)
18.5–24.4	1.00
24.5–30.4	2.09 (1.72–2.55)
≥ 30.5	2.96 (2.14–4.10)

	OR for high blood pressure	
BMI (kg/m^2)	Men	Women
< 25	1.0	1.0
25 to <27	2.4	1.7
27 to <30	3.1	2.3
≥ 30	8.7	9.7

BMI (kg/m^2)	RR for stroke (95% CI)
< 23	1.00
23.1–24.4	0.61 (0.32–1.16)
24.5–25.8	1.00 (0.57–1.75)
25.9–27.6	1.16 (0.67–2.02)
≥ 27.7	1.25 (0.72–2.19)

BMI (kg/m^2)	RR for ischemic stroke (95% CI)
< 21	1.00
21 to <23	1.01 (0.70–1.45)
23 to <25	1.20 (0.83–1.71)
25 to <27	1.15 (0.78–1.70)
27 to <29	1.75 (1.17–2.59)
29 to <32	1.90 (1.28–2.82)
≥ 32	2.37 (1.60–3.50)

NOTE: BMI = kg/m^2 unless noted otherwise. Multivariate-adjusted relative risk/ hazard risk/odds ratio estimates were used in this table whenever possible.

TABLE 5-35 Body Mass Index (BMI) and Risk of Coronary Heart Disease

Reference	Country	Study Population	Length of Follow-Up
Hubert et al., 1983	United States	2,252 men and 2,818 women, 28–62 y	26 y
Willett et al., 1995	United States	115,818 women, 30–55 y	14 y
Rexrode et al., 2001	United States	16,164 men, 40–84 y	9 y

a RR = relative risk, CI = confidence interval.
NOTE: BMI = kg/m^2 unless noted otherwise. Multivariate-adjusted relative risk/hazard risk/odds ratio estimates were used in this table whenever possible.

Obesity Index	Outcome[a]
Metropolitan relative weight (MRW) at baseline (% of desirable weight)	MRW predicted incidence of coronary disease, coronary death, and congestive heart failure in men In women, MRW was positively associated with coronary disease, stroke, congestive failure, and coronary and cardiovascular disease death
BMI at baseline (kg/m^2)	RR for coronary heart disease (95% CI)
< 21	1.00
21–22.9	1.19 (0.98–1.44)
23–24.9	1.46 (1.20–1.77)
25–28.9	2.06 (1.72–2.48)
≥ 29	3.56 (2.96–4.29)
Weight Gain from age 18	RR for coronary heart disease (95% CI)
< 5 kg	1.00
5–7.9 kg	1.25 (1.01–1.55)
8–10.9 kg	1.65 (1.33–2.05)
11–19 kg	1.92 (1.61–2.29)
≥ 20 kg	2.65 (2.17–3.22)
BMI (kg/m^2)	RR for coronary heart disease (95% CI)
< 22.8	1.00
22.8 to < 24.3	1.33 (0.99–1.79)
24.3 to < 25.7	1.28 (0.95–1.73)
25.7 to < 27.6	1.74 (1.31–2.30)
≥ 27.6	1.89 (1.43–2.51)

TABLE 5-36 Body Mass Index (BMI) and Risk of Gallbladder Disease

Reference	Country	Study Population	Length of Follow-Up
Kato et al., 1992	United States	7,831 men, 45+ y	22 y
Stampfer et al., 1992	United States	90,302 women, 34–59 y	8 y
Sahi et al., 1998	United States	16,785 men, 15–24 y	61 y

[a] RR = relative risk, CI = confidence interval.

Obesity Index	Outcome[a]
BMI (kg/m^2)	RR for gallbladder disease (95% CI)
< 21.65	1.0
21.65–23.79	1.1 (0.9–1.5)
23.80–25.80	1.4 (1.1–1.9)
> 25.80	1.8 (1.4–2.3)
	RR for cholecystectomy or unremoved
BMI (kg/m^2)	gallstones (95% CI)
< 24	1.00
24 to <25	1.36 (1.16–1.60)
25 to <26	1.60 (1.36–1.88)
26 to <27	1.92 (1.60–2.30)
27 to <29	2.32 (2.02–2.66)
29 to <30	2.63 (2.16–3.19)
30 to <35	3.52 (3.11–3.98)
35 to <40	4.64 (3.86–5.57)
40 to <45	5.42 (4.01–7.34)
45+	6.99 (4.48–10.90)
BMI at baseline (kg/m^2)	Rate ratio for gallbladder disease
< 20.0	1.00
20.0–21.9	1.05
22.0–23.9	1.12
≥ 24.0	1.43
BMI change from baseline (kg/m^2)	Rate ratio for gallbladder disease
≤ 0.9	1.00
1.0–2.9	1.01
3.0–5.9	1.74
≥ 6.0	2.16

NOTE: BMI = kg/m^2 unless noted otherwise. Multivariate-adjusted relative risk/hazard risk/odds ratio estimates were used in this table whenever possible.

TABLE 5-37 Body Mass Index (BMI) and Risk of Osteoarthritis

Reference	Country	Study Population	Length of Follow-Up
Felson et al., 1988	United States	1,420 adults, 63–94 at follow-up	~ 36 y
Hart and Spector, 1993	United Kingdom	985 women, 45–64 y	Not applicable
Carman et al., 1994	United States	588 men and 688 women, 50–74 y at follow-up	23 y
Hochberg et al., 1995	United States	465 men and 275 women, 40+ y	Not applicable
Cicuttini et al., 1996	United Kingdom	658 women, twins, 48–69 y	Not applicable

a OR = odds ratio.

Obesity Index	Outcome[a]
Metropolitan relative weight at baseline	Cumulative incidence rate of knee osteoarthritis (n/n [%])

Men	Women	Men	Women
< 105	< 100	34/110 (30.9)	28/155 (18.1)
105–112	100–108	26/113 (23.0)	42/173 (24.3)
113–120	109–116	38/128 (29.7)	58/170 (34.1)
121–128	117–127	31/112 (27.7)	60/157 (38.2)
≥ 129	≥ 128	53/126 (42.1)	98/176 (55.7)

BMI (kg/m^2)	OR for osteoarthritis of the knee (95% CI)
< 23.4	1.00
23.4–26.4	2.86 (1.44–5.68)
> 26.4	6.17 (3.26–11.71)

Relative weight index at baseline (% of ideal weight)	Incidence rate for osteoarthritis of the hand and wrist
< 100	70.0/100
100–109	74.1/100
110–119	80.7/100
120–129	83.7/100
≥ 130	88.9/100

	OR for osteoarthritis of the knee (95% CI)	
BMI	Men	Women
Tertile 1	1.00	1.00
Tertile 2	0.94 (0.52–1.70)	2.03 (0.89–4.66)
Tertile 3	2.40 (1.32–4.35)	4.34 (1.89–9.98)

BMI	OR for developing a radiological feature of osteoarthritis per unit of BMI ranged from 1.07 (0.91–1.25) to 1.63 (1.09–2.44) for all twins

NOTE: BMI = kg/m^2 unless noted otherwise. Multivariate-adjusted relative risk/hazard risk/odds ratio estimates were used in this table whenever possible.

TABLE 5-38 Body Mass Index (BMI) and Risk of Cancer

Reference	Country	Study Population	Length of Follow-Up
Helmrich et al., 1983	United States, Canada, Israel	1,185 women breast cancer cases, median 52 y 3,227 women controls, median 47 y	~ 3 y
Rosenberg et al., 1990	Canada	607 women breast cancer cases, < 70 y 1,214 women controls	4 yr
Chu et al., 1991	United States	4,323 cases and 4,358 controls, women, 20–54 y	Not applicable
Giovannucci et al., 1995	United States	47,723 men, 40–75 y	6 y
Giovannucci et al., 1996	United States	13,057 women, 40–65 y	6 y
Huang et al., 1997	United States	95,256 women, 30–55 y	16 y

[a] RR = relative risk, CI = confidence interval.

Obesity Index	Outcome[a]	
	RR for breast cancer in postmenopausal women	
BMI (kg/m^2)	(95% CI)	
< 21	1.0	
21–24	1.5 (1.1–1.9)	
25–27	1.6 (1.2–2.1)	
≥ 28	1.3 (1.0–1.8)	
	RR for breast cancer (95% CI)	
BMI (kg/m^2)	Premenopausal	Postmenopausal
< 21	1.0	1.0
21–25	0.9 (0.7–1.3)	0.8 (0.5–1.1)
≥ 26	0.8 (0.5–1.2)	1.2 (0.8–1.7)
	RR for breast cancer in menopausal	
BMI (kg/m^2)	women (95% CI)	
< 20.0	1.0	
20.0–21.99	1.1 (0.7–1.5)	
22.0–24.89	1.5 (1.0–2.2)	
24.9–27.29	2.2 (1.4–3.5)	
27.3–32.29	1.8 (1.1–2.8)	
≥ 32.3	2.7 (1.5–5.4)	
BMI (kg/m^2)	RR for colon cancer (95% CI)	
< 22	1.0	
22–24.9	0.87 (0.54–1.39)	
25–26.9	1.31 (0.85–2.02)	
27–28.9	1.48 (0.89–2.56)	
≥ 29	1.48 (0.89–2.46)	
BMI (kg/m^2)	RR for distal colon adenomas (95% CI)	
< 21	1.00	
21–22	0.82 (0.59–1.15)	
23–24	1.18 (0.85–1.63)	
25–28	1.03 (0.72–1.47)	
≥ 29	1.50 (1.02–2.21)	
	RR for breast cancer in postmenopausal women	
Weight gain from age 18	(95% CI)	
≤ 2.0 kg	1.00	
2.1–5.0 kg	1.20 (0.96–1.51)	
5.1–10.0 kg	1.18 (0.96–1.45)	
10.1–20.0 kg	1.20 (0.98–1.47)	
20.1–25.0 kg	1.40 (1.10–1.78)	
> 25.0 kg	1.41 (1.12–1.78)	

NOTE: BMI = kg/m^2 unless noted otherwise. Multivariate-adjusted relative risk/hazard risk/odds ratio estimates were used in this table whenever possible.

- Additional research is needed on the extent to which energy expenditure changes when a hypocaloric diet is consumed, and whether dietary composition affects the extent of change in energy expenditure.
- Independent of energy, identification of dietary components, if any, that could favorably affect body composition is needed.

REFERENCES

Abbott WG, Howard BV, Christin L, Freymond D, Lillioja S, Boyce VL, Anderson TE, Bogardus C, Ravussin E. 1988. Short-term energy balance: Relationship with protein, carbohydrate, and fat balances. *Am J Physiol* 255:E332–E337.

Acheson K, Jéquier E, Wahren J. 1983. Influence of beta-adrenergic blockade on glucose-induced thermogenesis in man. *J Clin Invest* 72:981–986.

Albu J, Shur M, Curi M, Murphy L, Heymsfield SB, Pi-Sunyer FX. 1997. Resting metabolic rate in obese, premenopausal black women. *Am J Clin Nutr* 66:531–538.

Allen JC, Keller RP, Archer P, Neville MC. 1991. Studies in human lactation: Milk composition and daily secretion rates of macronutrients in the first year of lactation. *Am J Clin Nutr* 54:69–80.

Amatruda JM, Richeson F, Welle SL, Brodows RG, Lockwood DH. 1988. The safety and efficacy of a controlled low-energy ('very-low-calorie') diet in the treatment of non-insulin-dependent diabetes and obesity. *Arch Intern Med* 148:873–877.

Amatruda JM, Statt MC, Welle SL. 1993. Total and resting energy expenditure in obese women reduced to ideal body weight. *J Clin Invest* 92:1236–1242.

Anderson DM, Williams FH, Merkatz RB, Schulman PK, Kerr DS, Pittard WB. 1983. Length of gestation and nutritional composition of human milk. *Am J Clin Nutr* 37:810–814.

Anderson GH, Atkinson SA, Bryan MH. 1981. Energy and macronutrient content of human milk during early lactation from mothers giving birth prematurely and at term. *Am J Clin Nutr* 34:258–265.

Armstrong DW. 1998. Metabolic and endocrine responses to cold air in women differing in aerobic capacity. *Med Sci Sport Exerc* 30:880–884.

Ashworth A. 1969. Metabolic rates during recovery from protein–calorie malnutrition: The need for a new concept of specific dynamic action. *Nature* 223:407–409.

Assel B, Rossi K, Kalhan S. 1993. Glucose metabolism during fasting through human pregnancy: Comparison of tracer method with respiratory calorimetry. *Am J Physiol* 265:E351–E356.

Astrup A, Buemann B, Western P, Toubro S, Raben A, Christensen NJ. 1994. Obesity as an adaptation to a high-fat diet: Evidence from a cross-sectional study. *Am J Clin Nutr* 59:350–355.

Astrup A, Toubro S, Dalgaard LT, Urhammer SA, Sorensen TI, Pedersen O. 1999. Impact of the v/v 55 polymorphism of the uncoupling protein 2 gene on 24-h energy expenditure and substrate oxidation. *Int J Obes Relat Metab Disord* 23:1030–1034.

Bahr R, Ingnes I, Vaage O, Sejersted OM, Newsholme EA. 1987. Effect of duration of exercise on excess postexercise O_2 consumption. *J Appl Physiol* 62:485–490.

Bailey DA, McCulloch RG. 1990. Bone tissue and physical activity. *Can J Sport Sci* 15:229–239.

Ballantyne D, Devine BL, Fife R. 1978. Interrelation of age, obesity, cigarette smoking, and blood pressure in hypertensive patients. *Br Med J* 1:880–881.

Ballor DL, Keesey RE. 1991. A meta-analysis of the factors affecting exercise-induced changes in body mass, fat mass and fat-free mass in males and females. *Int J Obes* 15:717–726.

Bandini LG, Schoeller DA, Cyr HN, Dietz WH. 1990a. Validity of reported energy intake in obese and nonobese adolescents. *Am J Clin Nutr* 52:421–451.

Bandini LG, Schoeller DA, Dietz WH. 1990b. Energy expenditure in obese and nonobese adolescents. *Pediatr Res* 27:198–203.

Barlow SE, Dietz WH. 1998. Obesity evaluation and treatment: Expert Committee recommendations. *Pediatrics* 102:E29.

Bathalon GP, Tucker KL, Hays NP, Vinken AG, Greenberg AS, McCrory MA, Roberts SB. 2000. Psychological measures of eating behavior and the accuracy of 3 common dietary assessment methods in healthy postmenopausal women. *Am J Clin Nutr* 71:739–745.

Baumgartner RN, Roche AF, Himes JH. 1986. Incremental growth tables: Supplementary to previously published charts. *Am J Clin Nutr* 43:711–722.

Bellizzi MC, Dietz WH. 1999. Workshop on childhood obesity: Summary of the discussion. *Am J Clin Nutr* 70:173S–175S.

Benedict FG, Cathcart EP. 1913. *Muscular Work. A Metabolic Study with Special Reference to the Efficiency of the Human Body as a Machine.* Washington, DC: Carnegie Institution. Pp. 163–176.

Benedict FG, Talbot FB. 1914. *The Gaseous Metabolism of Infants, with Special Reference to its Relation of Pulse-Rate and Muscular Activity.* Washington, DC: Carnegie Institution.

Benedict FG, Talbot FB. 1921. *Metabolism and Growth from Birth to Puberty.* Washington, DC: Carnegie Institution.

Bielinski R, Schutz Y, Jequier E. 1985. Energy metabolism during the postexercise recovery in man. *Am J Clin Nutr* 42:69–82.

Bingham SA, Day NE. 1997. Using biochemical markers to assess the validity of prospective dietary assessment methods and the effect of energy adjustment. *Am J Clin Nutr* 65:1130S–1137S.

Bingham SA, Goldberg GR, Coward WA, Prentice AM, Cummings JH. 1989. The effect of exercise and improved physical fitness on basal metabolic rate. *Br J Nutr* 61:155–173.

Bingham SA, Gill C, Welch A, Day K, Cassidy A, Khaw KT, Sneyd MJ, Key TJ, Roe L, Day NE. 1994. Comparison of dietary assessment methods in nutritional epidemiology: Weighed records v. 24 h recalls, food-frequency questionnaires and estimated-diet records. *Br J Nutr* 72:619–643.

Bisdee JT, James WP, Shaw MA. 1989. Changes in energy expenditure during the menstrual cycle. *Br J Nutr* 61:187–199.

Bitar A, Fellmann N, Vernet J, Coudert J, Vermorel M. 1999. Variations and determinants of energy expenditure as measured by whole-body indirect calorimetry during puberty and adolescence. *Am J Clin Nutr* 69:1209–1216.

Blaak EE, Westerterp KR, Bar-Or O, Wouters LJ, Saris WH. 1992. Total energy expenditure and spontaneous activity in relation to training in obese boys. *Am J Clin Nutr* 55:777–782.

Black AE. 1999. Small eaters or under-reporters? In: Guy-Grand B, Ailhaud G, eds. *Progress in Obesity Research 8.* London: John Libbey. Pp. 223–228.

Black AE, Prentice AM, Goldberg GR, Jebb SA, Bingham SA, Livingstone MB, Coward WA. 1993. Measurements of total energy expenditure provide insights into the validity of dietary measurements of energy intake. *J Am Diet Assoc* 93:572–579.

Black AE, Coward WA, Prentice AM. 1996. Human energy expenditure in affluent societies: An analysis of 574 doubly-labelled water measurements. *Eur J Clin Nutr* 50:72–92.

Blaza S, Garrow JS. 1983. Thermogenic response to temperature, exercise and food stimuli in lean and obese women, studied by 24 h direct calorimetry. *Br J Nutr* 49:171–180.

Bloesch D, Schutz Y, Breitenstein E, Jequier E, Felber JP. 1988. Thermogenic response to an oral glucose load in man: Comparison between young and elderly subjects. *J Am Coll Nutr* 7:471–483.

Bogardus C, Lillioja S, Ravussin E, Abbott W, Zawadzki JK, Young A, Knowler WC, Jacobowitz R, Moll PP. 1986. Familial dependence of the resting metabolic rate. *N Engl J Med* 315:96–100.

Bouchard C, Perusse L. 1993. Genetics of obesity. *Annu Rev Nutr* 13:337–354.

Bouchard C, Tremblay A, Nadeau A, Despres JP, Theriault G, Boulay MR, Lortie G, Leblanc C, Fournier G. 1989. Genetic effect in resting and exercise metabolic rates. *Metabolism* 38:364–370.

Bouchard C, Tremblay A, Despres JP, Nadeau A, Lupien PJ, Theriault G, Dussault J, Moorjani S, Pinault S, Fournier G. 1990. The response to long-term overfeeding in identical twins. *N Engl J Med* 322:1477–1482.

Bratteby LE, Sandhagen B, Lotborn M, Samuelson G. 1997. Daily energy expenditure and physical activity assessed by an activity diary in 374 randomly selected 15-year-old adolescents. *Eur J Clin Nutr* 51:592–600.

Brennan PJ, Simpson JM, Blacket RB, McGilchrist CA. 1980. The effects of body weight on serum cholesterol, serum triglycerides, serum urate and systolic blood pressure. *Aust N Z J Med* 10:15–20.

Briefel RR, Sempos CT, McDowell MA, Chien S, Alaimo K. 1997. Dietary methods research in the Third National Health and Nutrition Examination Survey: Underreporting of energy intake. *Am J Clin Nutr* 65:1203S–1209S.

Bronstein MN, Mak RP, King JC. 1995. The thermic effect of food in normalweight and overweight pregnant women. *Br J Nutr* 74:261–275.

Brooks GA, Butterfield GE, Wolfe RR, Groves BM, Mazzeo RS, Sutton JR, Wolfel EE, Reeves JT. 1991. Increased dependence on blood glucose after acclimatization to 4,300 m. *J Appl Physiol* 70:919–927.

Brooks GA, Wolfel EE, Groves BM, Bender PR, Butterfield GE, Cymerman A, Mazzeo RS, Sutton JR, Wolfe RR, Reeves JT. 1992. Muscle accounts for glucose disposal but not lactate appearance during exercise after acclimatization to 4,300 m. *J Appl Physiol* 72:2435–2445.

Brooks GA, Fahey TD, White TP, Baldwin KM. 2000. *Exercise Physiology: Human Bioenergetics and Its Applications*, 3rd ed. Mountain View, CA: Mayfield Publishing.

Brown CD, Higgins M, Donato KA, Rohde FC, Garrison R, Obarzanek E, Ernst ND, Horan M. 2000. Body mass index and the prevalence of hypertension and dyslipidemia. *Obes Res* 8:605–619.

Buemann B, Astrup A, Christensen NJ, Madsen J. 1992. Effect of moderate cold exposure on 24-h energy expenditure: Similar response in postobese and nonobese women. *Am J Physiol* 263:E1040–1045.

Buenen GP, Malina RM, Renson R, Simons J, Ostyn M, Lefevre J. 1992. Physical activity and growth, maturation and performance: A longitudinal study. *Med Sci Sports Exerc* 24(5):576–585.

Burstein R, Coward AW, Askew WE, Carmel K, Irving C, Shpilberg O, Moran D, Pikarsky A, Ginot G, Sawyer M, Golan R, Epstein Y. 1996. Energy expenditure variations in soldiers performing military activities under cold and hot climate conditions. *Mil Med* 161:750–754.

Butte NF. 1990. Basal metabolism of infants. In: Schürch B, Scrimshaw NS, eds. *Activity, Energy Expenditure and Energy Requirements of Infants and Children.* Switzerland: Nestlé Foundation. Pp. 117–137.

Butte NF. 2000. Fat intake of children in relation to energy requirements. *Am J Clin Nutr* 72:1246S–1252S.

Butte NF, Calloway DH. 1981. Evaluation of lactational performance in Navajo women. *Am J Clin Nutr* 34:2210–2215.

Butte NF, Hopkinson JM. 1998. Body composition changes during lactation are highly variable among women. *J Nutr* 128:381S–385S.

Butte NF, Garza C, O'Brian Smith E, Nichols BL. 1984a. Human milk intake and growth in exclusively breast-fed infants. *J Pediatr* 104:187–195.

Butte NF, Garza C, Stuff JE, Smith EO, Nichols BL. 1984b. Effect of maternal diet and body composition on lactational performance. *Am J Clin Nutr* 39:296–306.

Butte NF, Wong WW, Garza C. 1989. Energy cost of growth during infancy. *Proc Nutr Soc* 48:303–312.

Butte NF, Wong WW, Ferlic L, Smith EO, Klein PD, Garza C. 1990. Energy expenditure and deposition of breast-fed and formula-fed infants during early infancy. *Pediatr Res* 28:631–640.

Butte NF, Hopkinson JM, Mehta N, Moon JK, Smith EO. 1999. Adjustments in energy expenditure and substrate utilization during late pregnancy and lactation. *Am J Clin Nutr* 69:299–307.

Butte NF, Hopkinson JM, Wong WW, Smith EO, Ellis KJ. 2000a. Body composition during the first two years of life: An updated reference. *Pediatr Res* 47:578–585.

Butte NF, Wong WW, Hopkinson JM, Heinz CJ, Mehta NR, Smith EO. 2000b. Energy requirements derived from total energy expenditure and energy deposition during the first 2 y of life. *Am J Clin Nutr* 72:1558–1569.

Butte NF, Wong WW, Hopkinson JM. 2001. Energy requirements of lactating women derived from doubly labeled water and milk energy output. *J Nutr* 131:53–58.

Butterfield GE, Gates J, Fleming S, Brooks GA, Sutton JR, Reeves JT. 1992. Increased energy intake minimizes weight loss in men at high altitude. *J Appl Physiol* 72:1741–1748.

Carman WJ, Sowers M, Hawthorne VM, Weissfeld LA. 1994. Obesity as a risk factor for osteoarthritis of the hand and wrist: A prospective study. *Am J Epidemiol* 139:119–129.

Carpenter WH, Poehlman ET, O'Connell M, Goran MI. 1995. Influence of body composition and resting metabolic rate on variation in total energy expenditure: A meta-analysis. *Am J Clin Nutr* 61:4–10.

Carpenter WH, Fonong T, Toth MJ, Ades PA, Calles-Escandon J, Walston JD, Poehlman ET. 1998. Total daily energy expenditure in free-living older African-Americans and Caucasians. *Am J Physiol* 274:E96–E101.

Cartee GD, Douen AG, Ramlal T, Klip A, Holloszy JO. 1991. Stimulation of glucose transport in skeletal muscle by hypoxia. *J Appl Physiol* 70:1593–1600.

Chan JM, Rimm EB, Colditz GA, Stampfer MJ, Willett WC. 1994. Obesity, fat distribution, and weight gain as risk factors for clinical diabetes in men. *Diabetes Care* 17:961–969.

Chu SY, Lee NC, Wingo PA, Senie RT, Greenberg RS, Peterson HB. 1991. The relationship between body mass and breast cancer among women enrolled in the Cancer and Steroid Hormone Study. *J Clin Epidemiol* 44:1197–1206.

Cicuttini FM, Baker JR, Spector TD. 1996. The association of obesity with osteo-arthritis of the hand and knee in women: A twin study. *J Rheumatol* 23:1221–1226.

Clagett DD, Hathaway ML. 1941. Basal metabolism of normal infants from three to fifteen months of age. *Am J Dis Child* 62:967–980.

Clarke WR, Schrott HG, Leaverton PE, Connor WE, Lauer RM. 1978. Tracking of blood lipids and blood pressures in school age children: the Muscatine study. *Circulation* 58:626–634.

Colditz GA, Willett SC, Stampfer MJ, Manson JE, Hennekens CH, Arky RA, Speizer FE. 1990. Weight as a risk factor for clinical diabetes in women. *Am J Epidemiol* 132:501–513.

Colditz GA, Willett WC, Rotnitzky A, Manson JE. 1995. Weight gain as a risk factor for clinical diabetes mellitus in women. *Ann Intern Med* 122:481–486.

Cole TJ, Bellizzi MC, Flegal KM, Dietz WH. 2000. Establishing a standard defini-tion for child overweight and obesity worldwide: International survey. *Br Med J* 320:1–6.

Consolazio CF, Johnson RE, Pecora LJ. 1963. *Physiological Measurements of Metabolic Functions in Man.* New York: McGraw-Hill. Pp. 414–436.

Coward WA, Prentice AM, Murgatroyd PR, Davies HL, Cole TJ, Sawyer M, Goldberg GR, Halliday D, MacNamara JP. 1984. Measurement of CO_2 and water produc-tion rates in man using ^2H, ^{18}O-labelled H_2O: Comparisons between calorimeter and isotope values. In: Van Es AJ, ed. *Human Energy Metabolism: Physical Activity and Energy Expenditure Measurements in Epidemiological Research Based upon Direct and Indirect Calorimetry.* Den Haag: CIP-gegevens Koninklijke Bibliotheek. Pp. 126–128.

Criqui MH, Mebane I, Wallace RB, Heiss G, Holdbrook MJ. 1982. Multivariate correlates of adult blood pressures in nine North American populations: The Lipid Research Clinics Prevalence Study. *Prev Med* 11:391–402.

Dauncey MJ. 1981. Influence of mild cold on 24 h energy expenditure, resting metabolism and diet-induced thermogenesis. *Br J Nutr* 45:257–267.

Davies PS, Ewing G, Lucas A. 1989. Energy expenditure in early infancy. *Br J Nutr* 62:621–629.

Davies PS, Ewing G, Coward WA, Lucas A. 1990. Energy metabolism in breast and formula fed infants. In: Atkinson SA, Hanson LA, Chandra RK, eds. *Breast-Feeding, Nutrition, Infection and Infant Growth in Developed and Emerging Countries.* St. John's, Newfoundland: Arts Biomedical. P. 521.

Davies PS, Day JM, Lucas A. 1991. Energy expenditure in early infancy and later body fatness. *Int J Obes* 15:727–731.

Davies PS, Wells JC, Fieldhouse CA, Day JM, Lucas A. 1995. Parental body composi-tion and infant energy expenditure. *Am J Clin Nutr* 61:1026–1029.

Davies PS, Wells JC, Hinds A, Day JM, Laidlaw A. 1997. Total energy expenditure in 9 month and 12 month infants. *Eur J Clin Nutr* 51:249–252.

de Bruin NC, Degenhart HJ, Gal S, Westerterp KR, Stijnen T, Visser HK. 1998. Energy utilization and growth in breast-fed and formula-fed infants measured prospectively during the first year of life. *Am J Clin Nutr* 67:885–896.

de Castro JM, Orozco S. 1990. Moderate alcohol intake and spontaneous eating patterns of humans: Evidence of unregulated supplementation. *Am J Clin Nutr* 52:246–253.

de Groot LC, Boekholt HA, Spaaij CJ, van Raaij JM, Drijvers JJ, van der Heijden LJ, van der Heide D, Hautvast JG. 1994. Energy balances of healthy Dutch women before and during pregnancy: Limited scope for metabolic adaptations in pregnancy. *Am J Clin Nutr* 59:827–832.

Deheeger M, Rolland-Cachera MF, Fontvieille AM. 1997. Physical activity and body composition in 10 year old French children: linkages with nutritional intake? *Int J Obes Relat Metab Disord* 21:372-379.

Denne SC, Kalhan SC. 1987. Leucine metabolism in human newborns. *Am J Physiol* 253:E608–E615.

Denne SC, Patel D, Kalhan SC. 1991. Leucine kinetics and fuel utilization during a brief fast in human pregnancy. *Metabolism* 40:1249–1256.

DePue JD, Clark MM, Ruggiero L, Medeiros ML, Pera V. 1995. Maintenance of weight loss: A needs assessment. *Obes Res* 3:241–248.

Despres J-P, Nadeau A, Tremblay A, Ferland M, Moorjani S, Lupien PJ, Thériault G, Pinault S, Bouchard C. 1989. Role of deep abdominal fat in the association between regional adipose tissue distribution and glucose tolerance in obese women. *Diabetes* 38:304–309.

Dewey KG, Finley DA, Lonnerdal B. 1984. Breast milk volume and composition during late lactation (7–20 months). *J Pediatr Gastroenterol Nutr* 3:713–720.

Dewey KG, Beaton G, Fjeld C, Lonnerdal B, Reeds P. 1996. Protein requirements of infants and children. *Eur J Clin Nutr* 50:S119–S150.

Dhuper S, Warren MP, Brooks-Gunn J, Fox R. 1990. Effects of hormonal status on bone density in adolescent girls. *J Clin Endocrinol Metab* 71:1083–1088.

Dionne I, Despres JP, Bouchard C, Tremblay A. 1999. Gender difference in the effect of body composition on energy metabolism. *Int J Obes Relat Metab Disord* 23:312–319.

Doar JWH, Wilde, Thompson ME, Stewell PFJ. 1975. Influence of treatment with diet alone on oral glucose-tolerance test and plasma sugar and insulin levels in patients with maturity-onset diabetes mellitus. *Lancet* 1:1263–1266.

Dunn AL, Marcus BH, Kampert JB, Garcia ME, Kohl HW, Blair SN. 1999. Comparison of lifestyle and structured interventions to increase physical activity and cardiorespiratory fitness: A randomized trial. *J Am Med Assoc* 281:327–334.

Durnin JV. 1990. Low energy expenditures in free-living populations. *Eur J Clin Nutr* 44:95–102.

Durnin JV. 1996. Energy requirements: General principles. *Eur J Clin Nutr* 50: S2–S10.

Durnin JV, McKillop FM, Grant S, Fitzgerald G. 1987. Energy requirements of pregnancy in Scotland. *Lancet* 2:897–900.

Edholm OG, Adam JM, Healey MJ, Wolff HS, Goldsmith R, Best TW. 1970. Food intake and energy expenditure of army recruits. *Br J Nutr* 24:1091–1107.

Elia M. 1991. Energy equivalents of CO_2 and their importance in assessing energy expenditure when using tracer techniques. *Am J Physiol* 260:E75–E88.

Eliakim A, Barstow TJ, Brasel JA, Ajie H, Lee WN, Renslo R, Berman N, Cooper DM. 1996. Effect of exercise training on energy expenditure, muscle volume, and maximal oxygen uptake in female adolescents. *J Pediatr* 129:537–543.

Ellis KJ. 1997. Body composition of a young, multiethnic, male population. *Am J Clin Nutr* 66:1323–1331.

Ellis KJ, Abrams SA, Wong WW. 1997. Body composition of a young, multiethnic female population. *Am J Clin Nutr* 65:724–731.

EPA (Environmental Protection Agency). 1991. *Building Air Quality: A Guide for Building Owners and Facility Managers*. Washington, DC: U.S. Government Printing Office.

FAO/WHO/UNU (Food and Agriculture Organization/World Health Organization/United Nations University). 1985. *Energy and Protein Requirements.* Report of a Joint FAO/WHO/UNU Expert Consultation. Technical Report Series No. 724. Geneva: WHO.

Felson DT, Anderson JJ, Naimark A, Walker AM, Meenan RF. 1988. Obesity and knee osteoarthritis. The Framingham Study. *Ann Intern Med* 109:18–24.

Ferraro R, Lillioja S, Fontvieille AM, Rising R, Bogardus C, Ravussin E. 1992. Lower sedentary metabolic rate in women compared with men. *J Clin Invest* 90:780–784.

Ferris AM, Dotts MA, Clark RM, Ezrin M, Jensen RG. 1988. Macronutrients in human milk at 2, 12, and 16 weeks postpartum. *J Am Diet Assoc* 88:694–697.

Firouzbakhsh S, Mathis RK, Dorchester WL, Oseas RS, Groncy PK, Grant KE, Finklestein JZ. 1993. Measured resting energy expenditure in children. *J Pediatr Gastroenterol Nutr* 16:136–142.

Fjeld CR, Schoeller DA, Brown KH. 1989. Body composition of children recovering from severe protein-energy malnutrition at two rates of catch-up growth. *Am J Clin Nutr* 50:1266–1275.

Flatt JP. 1978. The biochemistry of energy expenditure. In: Bray GA, ed. *Recent Advances in Obesity Research II.* London: Newman Publishing. Pp. 211–228.

Fletcher GF, Balady GJ, Amsterdam EA, Chaitman B, Eckel R, Fleg J, Froelicher VF, Leon AS, Piña IL, Rodney R, Simons-Morton DG, Williams MA, Bazzarre T. 2001. Exercise standards for testing and training: A statement for healthcare professionals from the American Heart Association. *Circulation* 104:1694–1740.

Fomon SJ, Haschke F, Ziegler EE, Nelson SE. 1982. Body composition of reference children from birth to age 10 years. *Am J Clin Nutr* 35:1169–1175.

Fontvieille AM, Dwyer J, Ravussin E. 1992. Resting metabolic rate and body composition of Pima Indian and Caucasian children. *Int J Obes Relat Metab Disord* 16:535–542.

Forbes GB. 1987. *Human Body Composition. Growth, Aging, Nutrition, and Activity.* New York: Springer-Verlag.

Ford ES, Williamson DF, Liu S. 1997. Weight change and diabetes incidence: Findings from a national cohort of US adults. *Am J Epidemiol* 146:214–222.

Forman JN, Miller WC, Szymanski LM, Fernhall B. 1998. Differences in resting metabolic rates of inactive obese African-American and Caucasian women. *Int J Obes Relat Metab Disord* 22:215–221.

Forsum E, Sadurskis A, Wager J. 1988. Resting metabolic rate and body composition of healthy Swedish women during pregnancy. *Am J Clin Nutr* 47:942–947.

Forsum E, Kabir N, Sadurskis A, Westerterp K. 1992. Total energy expenditure of healthy Swedish women during pregnancy and lactation. *Am J Clin Nutr* 56:334–342.

Foster GD, Wadden TA, Vogt RA. 1997. Resting energy expenditure in obese African American and Caucasian women. *Obes Res* 5:1–8.

Foster GD, Wadden TA, Swain RM, Anderson DA, Vogt RA. 1999. Changes in resting energy expenditure after weight loss in obese African American and white women. *Am J Clin Nutr* 69:13–17.

Frigerio C, Schutz Y, Whitehead R, Jequier E. 1991. A new procedure to assess the energy requirements of lactation in Gambian women. *Am J Clin Nutr* 54:526–533.

Fukagawa NK, Bandini LG, Young JB. 1990. Effect of age on body composition and resting metabolic rate. *Am J Physiol* 259:E233–E238.

Fukagawa NK, Bandini LG, Lim PH, Roingeard F, Lee MA, Young JB. 1991. Protein-induced changes in energy expenditure in young and old individuals. *Am J Physiol* 260:E345–E352.

Gaesser GA, Brooks GA. 1984. Metabolic bases of excess post-exercise oxygen consumption: A review. *Med Sci Sports Exerc* 16:29–43.

Garby L, Kurzer MS, Lammert O, Nielsen E. 1987. Energy expenditure during sleep in men and women: Evaporative and sensible heat losses. *Hum Nutr Clin Nutr* 41:225–233.

Garby L, Lammert O, Nielsen E. 1990. Changes in energy expenditure of light physical activity during a 10 day period at 34°C environmental temperature. *Eur J Clin Nutr* 44:241–244.

Geithner CA, Woynarowska B, Malina RM. 1998. The adolescent spurt and sexual maturation in girls active and nonactive in sport. *Ann Hum Biol* 25(5):415–423.

Gibson RS, Vanderkooy PD, MacDonald AC, Goldman A, Ryan BA, Berry M. 1989. A growth-limiting, mild zinc-deficiency syndrome in some Southern Ontario boys with low height percentiles. *Am J Clin Nutr* 49:1266–1276.

Gilliam TB, Freedson. 1980. Effects of a 12-week school physical fitness program on peak VO2, body composition and blood lipids in 7 to 9 year old children. *Int J Sports Med* 1:73–78.

Giovannucci E, Ascherio A, Rimm EB, Colditz GA, Stampfer MJ, Willett WC. 1995. Physical activity, obesity, and risk for colon cancer and adenoma in men. *Ann Intern Med* 122:327–334.

Giovannucci E, Colditz GA, Stampfer MJ, Willett WC. 1996. Physical activity, obesity, and risk of colorectal adenoma in women (United States). *Cancer Causes Control* 7:253–263.

Golay A, Schutz Y, Meyer HU, Thiebaud D, Curchod B, Maeder E, Felber JP, Jequier E. 1982. Glucose-induced thermogenesis in nondiabetic and diabetic obese subjects. *Diabetes* 31:1023–1028.

Goldberg GR, Black AE, Jebb SA, Cole TJ, Murgatroyd PR, Coward WA, Prentice AM. 1991a. Critical evaluation of energy intake data using fundamental principles of energy physiology: 1. Derivation of cut-off limits to identify under-recording. *Eur J Clin Nutr* 45:569–581.

Goldberg GR, Prentice AM, Coward WA, Davies HL, Murgatroyd PR, Sawyer MB, Ashford J, Black AE. 1991b. Longitudinal assessment of the components of energy balance in well-nourished lactating women. *Am J Clin Nutr* 54:788–798.

Goldberg GR, Prentice AM, Coward WA, Davies HL, Murgatroyd PR, Wensing C, Black AE, Harding M, Sawyer M. 1993. Longitudinal assessment of energy expenditure in pregnancy by the doubly labeled water method. *Am J Clin Nutr* 57:494–505.

Goran MI, Poehlman ET. 1992. Endurance training does not enhance total energy expenditure in healthy elderly persons. *Am J Physiol* 263:E950–E957.

Goran MI, Calles-Escandon J, Poehlman ET, O'Connell M, Danforth E. 1994a. Effects of increased energy intake and/or physical activity on energy expenditure in young healthy men. *J Appl Physiol* 77:366–372.

Goran MI, Kaskoun M, Johnson R. 1994b. Determinants of resting energy expenditure in young children. *J Pediatr* 125:362–367.

Goran MI, Carpenter WH, McGloin A, Johnson R, Hardin JM, Weinsier RL. 1995a. Energy expenditure in children of lean and obese parents. *Am J Physiol* 268:E917–E924.

Goran MI, Kaskoun M, Johnson R, Martinez C, Kelly B, Hood V. 1995b. Energy expenditure and body fat distribution in Mohawk children. *Pediatrics* 95:89–95.

Goran MI, Gower BA, Nagy TR, Johnson RK. 1998a. Developmental changes in energy expenditure and physical activity in children: Evidence for a decline in physical activity in girls before puberty. *Pediatrics* 101:887–891.

Goran MI, Nagy TR, Gower BA, Mazariegos M, Solomons N, Hood V, Johnson R. 1998b. Influence of sex, seasonality, ethnicity, and geographic location on the components of total energy expenditure in young children: Implications for energy requirements. *Am J Clin Nutr* 68:675–682.

Goran MI, Shewchuk R, Gower BA, Nagy TR, Carpenter WH, Johnson RK. 1998c. Longitudinal changes in fatness in white children: No effect of childhood energy expenditure. *Am J Clin Nutr* 67:309–316.

Griffiths M, Payne PR. 1976. Energy expenditure in small children of obese and non-obese parents. *Nature* 260:698–700.

Grund A, Vollbrecht H, Frandsen W, Krause H, Siewers M, Rieckert H, Muller MJ. 2000. No effect of gender on different components of daily energy expenditure in free living prepubertal children. *Int J Obes Relat Metab Disord* 24:299–305.

Grund A, Krause H, Kraus M, Siewers M, Rieckert H, Müller MJ. 2001. Association between different attributes of physical activity and fat mass in untrained, endurance- and resistance-trained men. *Eur J Appl Physiol* 84:310–320.

Grundy SM, Mok HYI, Zech L, Steinberg D, Berman M. 1979. Transport of very low density lipoprotein triglycerides in varying degrees of obesity and hypertriglyceridemia. *J Clin Invest* 63:1274–1283.

Guillermo-Tuazon MA, Barba CV, van Raaij JM, Hautvast JG. 1992. Energy intake, energy expenditure, and body composition of poor rural Philippine women throughout the first 6 mo of lactation. *Am J Clin Nutr* 56:874–880.

Gutin B, Barbeau P, Owens S, Lemmon CR, Bauman M, Allison J, Kang HS, Litaker MS. 2002. Effects of exercise intensity on cardiovascular fitness, total body composition, and visceral adiposity of obese adolescents. *Am J Clin Nutr* 75:818–826.

Guo S, Roche AF, Fomon SJ, Nelson SE, Chumlea WC, Rogers RR, Baumgartner RN, Ziegler EE, Siervogel RM. 1991. Reference data on gains in weight and length during the first two years of life. *J Pediatr* 119:355–362.

Hadden DR, Montgomery DAD, Skelly RJ, Trimble ER, Weaver JA, Wilson EA, Buchanan KD. 1975. Maturity onset diabetes mellitus: response to intensive dietary management. *Br Med J* 2:276–278.

Haffner SM, Mitchell BD, Hazuda HP, Stern MP. 1991. Greater influence of central distribution of adipose tissue on incidence of non-insulin-dependent diabetes in women than men. *Am J Clin Nutr* 53:1312–1317.

Haggarty P, McNeill G, Abu Manneh MK, Davidson L, Milne E, Duncan G, Ashton J. 1994. The influence of exercise on the energy requirements of adult males in the UK. *Br J Nutr* 72:799–813.

Harris JA, Benedict FG. 1919. *A Biometric Study of Basal Metabolism in Man.* Washington, DC: Carnegie Institution.

Hart DJ, Spector TD. 1993. The relationship of obesity, fat distribution and osteoarthritis in women in the general population: The Chingford Study. *J Rheumatol* 20:331–335.

Hartman WM, Stroud M, Sweet DM, Saxton J. 1993. Long-term maintenance of weight loss following supplemented fasting. *Int J Eat Disord* 14:87–93.

Haschke F. 1989. Body composition during adolescence. In: *Body Composition Measurements in Infants and Children: Report of the 98th Ross Conference on Pediatric Research.* Columbus, OH: Ross Laboratories. Pp. 76–83.

Hay WW. 1994. Placental supply of energy and protein substrates to the fetus. *Acta Paediatr Suppl* 405:13–19.

Hayter JE, Henry CJ. 1993. Basal metabolic rate in human subjects migrating between tropical and temperate regions: A longitudinal study and review of previous work. *Eur J Clin Nutr* 47:724–734.

Heinig MJ, Nommsen LA, Peerson JM, Lonnerdal B, Dewey KG. 1993. Energy and protein intakes of breast-fed and formula-fed infants during the first year of life and their association with growth velocity: The DARLING Study. *Am J Clin Nutr* 58:152–161.

Heitmann BL, Kaprio J, Harris JR, Rissanen A, Korkeila M, Koskenvuo M. 1997. Are genetic determinants of weight gain modified by leisure-time physical activity? A prospective study of Finnish twins. *Am J Clin Nutr* 66:672–678.

Helmrich SP, Shapiro S, Rosenberg L, Kaufman DW, Slone D, Bain C, Miettinen OS, Stolley PD, Rosenshein NB, Knapp RC, Leavitt T, Schottenfeld D, Engle RL, Levy M. 1983. Risk factors for breast cancer. *Am J Epidemiol* 117:35–45.

Henry CJ. 2000. Mechanisms of changes in basal metabolism during ageing. *Eur J Clin Nutr* 54:S77–S91.

Herring JL, Mole PA, Meredith CN, Stern JS. 1992. Effect of suspending exercise training on resting metabolic rate in women. *Med Sci Sports Exerc* 24:59–65.

Hessemer V, Bruck K. 1985. Influence of menstrual cycle on thermoregulatory, metabolic, and heart rate responses to exercise at night. *J Appl Physiol* 59:1911–1917.

Heyman MB, Young VR, Fuss P, Tsay R, Joseph L, Roberts SB. 1992. Underfeeding and body weight regulation in normal-weight young men. *Am J Physiol* 263:R250–R257.

Heymsfield SB, Gallagher D, Kotler DP, Wang Z, Allison DB, Heshka S. 2002. Body-size dependence of resting energy expenditure can be attributed to nonenergetic homogeneity of fat-free mass. *Am J Physiol* 282:E132–E138.

Hill JO, Peters JC. 1998. Environmental contributions to the obesity epidemic. *Science* 280:1371–1374.

Hill JR. 1964. The development of thermal stability in the newborn baby. In: Jonxis JH, Visser HK, Troelstra JA, eds. *The Adaptation of the Newborn Infant to Extra-Uterine Life.* Springfield, IL: Charles Thomas. Pp. 223–228.

Hochberg MC, Lethbridge-Cejku M, Scott WW, Reichle R, Plato CC, Tobin JD. 1995. The association of body weight, body fatness and body fat distribution with osteoarthritis of the knee: Data from the Baltimore Longitudinal Study of Aging. *J Rheumatol* 22:488–493.

Holden JH, Darga LL, Olson SM, Stettner DC, Ardito EA, Lucas CP. 1992. Long-term follow-up of patients attending a combination very-low calorie diet and behaviour therapy weight loss programme. *Int J Obes Relat Metab Disord* 16:605–613.

Holliday MA. 1971. Metabolic rate and organ size during growth from infancy to maturity and during late gestation and early infancy. *Pediatrics* 47:169–179.

Holmes FL. 1985. *Lavoisier and the Chemistry of Life.* Madison, WI: University of Wisconsin Press.

Howe JC, Rumpler WV, Seale JL. 1993. Energy expenditure by indirect calorimetry in premenopausal women: Variation within one menstrual cycle. *J Nutr Biochem* 4:268–273.

Huang Z, Hankinson SE, Colditz GA, Stampfer MJ, Hunter DJ, Manson JE, Hennekens CH, Rosner B, Speizer FE, Willett WC. 1997. Dual effects of weight and weight gain on breast cancer risk. *J Am Med Assoc* 278:1407–1411.

Huang Z, Willett WC, Manson JE, Rosner B, Stampfer MJ, Speizer FE, Colditz GA. 1998. Body weight, weight change, and risk for hypertension in women. *Ann Intern Med* 128:81–88.

Hubert HB, Feinleib M, McNamara PM, Castelli WP. 1983. Obesity as an independent risk factor for cardiovascular disease: A 26-year follow-up of participants in the Framingham Heart Study. *Circulation* 67:968–977.

Hunt JF, White JR. 1980. Effect of ten weeks of vigorous daily exercise on serum lipids and lipoproteins in teenage males. *Med Sci Sports Exerc* 12:93.

Hunter GR, Weinsier RL, Darnell BE, Zuckerman PA, Goran MI. 2000. Racial differences in energy expenditure and aerobic fitness in premenopausal women. *Am J Clin Nutr* 71:500–506.

Hytten FE. 1991a. Nutrition. In: Hytten FE, Chamberlain G, eds. *Clinical Physiology in Obstetrics*. Oxford: Blackwell Scientific. Pp. 150–172.

Hytten FE. 1991b. Weight gain in pregnancy. In: Hytten FE, Chamberlain G, eds. *Clinical Physiology in Obstetrics*. Oxford: Blackwell Scientific. Pp. 173–203.

IDECG (International Dietary Energy Consulting Group). 1990. *The Doubly-Labelled Water Method for Measuring Energy Expenditure: A Consensus Report by the IDECG Working Group. Technical Recommendations for Use in Humans*. Vienna, Austria: NAHRES-4, International Atomic Energy Agency.

Illingworth PJ, Jung RT, Howie PW, Leslie P, Isles TE. 1986. Diminution in energy expenditure during lactation. *Br Med J* 292:437–441.

Illner K, Brinkmann G, Heller M, Bosy-Westphal A, Muller MJ. 2000. Metabolically active components of fat free mass and resting energy expenditure in non-obese adults. *Am J Physiol* 278:E308–E315.

IOM (Institute of Medicine). 1990. *Nutrition During Pregnancy*. Washington, DC: National Academy Press.

IOM. 1991. *Nutrition During Lactation*. Washington, DC: National Academy Press.

Jakicic JM, Wing RR. 1998. Differences in resting energy expenditure in African-American vs. Caucasian overweight females. *Int J Obes Relat Metab Disord* 22:236–242.

James WPT, McNeill G, Ralph A. 1990. Metabolism and nutritional adaptation to altered intakes of energy substrates. *Am J Clin Nutr* 51:264–269.

Jensen CL, Butte NF, Wong WW, Moon JK. 1992. Determining energy expenditure in preterm infants: Comparison of $^2H_2{}^{18}O$ method and indirect calorimetry. *Am J Physiol* 263:R685–R692.

Jequier E, Tappy L. 1999. Regulation of body weight in humans. *Physiol Rev* 79:451–480.

Jiang Z, Yan Q, Su Y, Acheson KJ, Thelin A, Piguet-Welsch C, Ritz P, Ho Z. 1998. Energy expenditure of Chinese infants in Guangdong Province, south China, determined with use of the doubly labeled water method. *Am J Clin Nutr* 67:1256–1264.

Johnson RK. 2000. What are people really eating and why does it matter? *Nutr Today* 35:40–45.

Johnson RK, Goran MI, Poehlman ET. 1994. Correlates of over- and under-reporting of energy intake in healthy older men and women. *Am J Clin Nutr* 59:1286–1290.

Johnson RK, Soultanakis RP, Matthews DE. 1998. Literacy and body fatness are associated with underreporting of energy intake in U.S. low-income women using the multiple-pass 24-hour recall: A doubly labeled water study. *J Am Diet Assoc* 98:1136–1140.

Jones PJ, Winthrop AL, Schoeller DA, Swyer PR, Smith J, Filler RM, Heim T. 1987. Validation of doubly labeled water for assessing energy expenditure in infants. *Pediatr Res* 21:242–246.

Jones PJ, Martin LJ, Su W, Boyd NF. 1997. Canadian Recommended Nutrient Intakes underestimate true energy requirements in middle-aged women. *Can J Public Health* 88:314–319.

Kalhan S, Rossi K, Gruca L, Burkett E, O'Brien A. 1997. Glucose turnover and gluconeogenesis in human pregnancy. *J Clin Invest* 100:1775–1781.

Kalkhoff RK, Kissebah AH, Kim H-J. 1978. Carbohydrate and lipid metabolism during normal pregnancy: Relationship to gestational hormone action. *Semin Perinatol* 2:291–307.

Kannel WB, Brand N, Skinner JJ, Dawber TR, McNamara PM. 1967. The relation of adiposity to blood pressure and development of hypertension. *Ann Intern Med* 67:48–59.

Kaplan AS, Zemel BS, Stallings VA. 1996. Differences in resting energy expenditure in prepubertal black children and white children. *J Pediatr* 129:643–647.

Karlberg P. 1952. Determinations of standard energy metabolism (basal metabolism) in normal infants. *Acta Paediatr Scand* 41:11–151.

Kashiwazaki H, Dejima Y, Suzuki T. 1990. Influence of upper and lower thermoneutral room temperatures (20°C and 25°C) on fasting and post-prandial resting metabolism under different outdoor temperatures. *Eur J Clin Nutr* 44:405–413.

Kato I, Nomura A, Stemmermann GN, Chyou P-H. 1992. Prospective study of clinical gallbladder disease and its association with obesity, physical activity, and other factors. *Dig Dis Sci* 37:784–790.

Kempen KP, Saris WH, Westerterp KR. 1995. Energy balance during an 8-wk energy-restricted diet with and without exercise in obese women. *Am J Clin Nutr* 62:722–729.

Kesaniemi YA, Grundy SM. 1983. Increased low density lipoprotein production associated with obesity. *Arteriosclerosis* 3:170–177.

Keys A, Taylor H, Grande F. 1973. Basal metabolism and age of adult man. *Metabolism* 22:579–587.

Klannemark M, Orho M, Groop L. 1998. No relationship between identified variants in the uncoupling protein 2 gene and energy expenditure. *Eur J Endocrinol* 139:217–223.

Klausen B, Toubro S, Astrup A. 1997. Age and sex effects on energy expenditure. *Am J Clin Nutr* 65:895–907.

Kleiber M. 1975. *The Fire of Life. An Introduction to Animal Energetics.* New York: Robert E. Krieger Publishing.

Klein PD, James WP, Wong WW, Irving CS, Murgatroyd PR, Cabrera M, Dallosso HM, Klein ER, Nichols BL. 1984. Calorimetric validation of the doubly-labelled water method for determination of energy expenditure in man. *Hum Nutr Clin Nutr* 38C:95–106.

Knuttgen HG, Emerson K. 1974. Physiological response to pregnancy at rest and during exercise. *J Appl Physiol* 36:549–553.

Kopp-Hoolihan LE, Van Loan MD, Wong WW, King JC. 1999. Longitudinal assessment of energy balance in well-nourished, pregnant women. *Am J Clin Nutr* 69:697–704.

Krebs-Smith SM, Graubard B, Kahle L, Subar A, Cleveland L, Ballard-Barbash R. 2000. Low energy reporters vs. others: A comparison of reported food intakes. *Eur J Clin Nutr* 54:281–287.

Kuczmarski RJ, Ogden CL, Grummer-Strawn LM, Flegal KM, Guo SS, Wei R, Mei Z, Curtin LR, Roche AF, Johnson CL. 2000. CDC growth charts: United States. *Adv Data* 314:1–28.

Kushner RF, Racette SB, Neil K, Schoeller DA. 1995. Measurement of physical activity among black and white obese women. *Obes Res* 3:261S–265S.

Lammi-Keefe CJ, Ferris AM, Jensen RG. 1990. Changes in human milk at 0600, 1000, 1400, 1800, and 2200 h. *J Pediatr Gastroenterol Nutr* 11:83–88.

Lanzola E, Tagliabue A, Cena H. 1990. Skin temperature and energy expenditure. *Ann Nutr Metab* 34:311–316.

Larson DE, Ferraro RT, Robertson DS, Ravussin E. 1995. Energy metabolism in weight-stable postobese individuals. *Am J Clin Nutr* 62:735–739.

Lean ME, Murgatroyd PR, Rothnie I, Reid IW, Harvey R. 1988. Metabolic and thyroidal responses to mild cold are abnormal in obese diabetic women. *Clin Endocrinol* 28:665–673.

Lederman SA, Paxton A, Heymsfield SB, Wang J, Thornton J, Pierson RN. 1997. Body fat and water changes during pregnancy in women with different body weight and weight gain. *Obstet Gynecol* 90:483–488.

Leibel RL, Rosenbaum M, Hirsch J. 1995. Changes in energy expenditure resulting from altered body weight. *N Engl J Med* 332:621–628.

Leonard WR, Galloway VA, Ivakine E. 1997. Underestimation of daily energy expenditure with the factorial method: Implications for anthropological research. *Am J Phys Anthropol* 103:443–454.

Leon-Velarde F, Gamboa A, Chuquiza JA, Esteba WA, Rivera-Chira M, Monge CC. 2000. Hematological parameters in high altitude residents living at 4,355, 4,660, and 5,500 meters above sea level. *High Alt Med Biol* 1:97–104.

Levine JA, Eberhardt NL, Jensen MD. 1999. Role of nonexercise activity thermogenesis in resistance to fat gain in humans. *Science* 283:212–214.

Levine JA, Schleusner SJ, Jensen MD. 2000. Energy expenditure of nonexercise activity. *Am J Clin Nutr* 72:1451–1454.

Lichtman SW, Pisarska K, Berman ER, Pestone M, Dowling H, Offenbacher E, Weisel H, Heshka S, Matthews DE, Heymsfield SB. 1992. Discrepancy between self-reported and actual caloric intake and exercise in obese subjects. *N Engl J Med* 327:1893–1898.

Lifson N, McClintock R. 1966. Theory of use of the turnover rates of body water for measuring energy and material balance. *J Theoret Biol* 12:46–74.

Lifson N, Gordon GB, Visscher MB, Nier AO. 1949. The fate of utilized molecular oxygen and the source of the oxygen of respiratory carbon dioxide, studied with the aid of heavy oxygen. *J Biol Chem* 180:803–811.

Lifson N, Gordon GB, McClintock R. 1955. Measurement of total carbon dioxide production by means of D_2O^{18}. *J Appl Physiol* 7:704–710.

Linder CW, Durant RH, Mahoney OM. 1983. The effect of physical conditioning on serum lipids and lipoproteins in white male adolescents. *Med Sci Sports Exerc* 15:232–236.

Lindsay CA, Huston L, Amini SB, Catalano PM. 1997. Longitudinal changes in the relationship between body mass index and percent body fat in pregnancy. *Obstet Gynecol* 89:377–382.

Lipmann F. 1941. Metabolic generation and utilization of phosphate bond energy. *Adv Enzymol* 1:99–162.

Livesey G, Elia M. 1988. Estimation of energy expenditure, net carbohydrate utilization, and net fat oxidation and synthesis by indirect calorimetry: Evaluation of errors with special reference to the detailed composition of fuels. *Am J Clin Nutr* 47:608–628.

Livingstone MB, Coward WA, Prentice AM, Davies PS, Strain JJ, McKenna PG, Mahoney CA, White JA, Stewart CM, Kerr MJ. 1992a. Daily energy expenditure in free-living children: Comparison of heart-rate monitoring with the doubly labeled water ($^2H_2$$^{18}O$) method. *Am J Clin Nutr* 56:343–352.

Livingstone MB, Prentice AM, Coward WA, Strain JJ, Black AE, Davies PS, Stewart CM, McKenna PG, Whitehead RG. 1992b. Validation of estimates of energy intake by weighed dietary record and diet history in children and adolescents. *Am J Clin Nutr* 56:29–35.

Lovelady CA, Meredith CN, McCrory MA, Nommsen LA, Joseph LJ, Dewey KG. 1993. Energy expenditure in lactating women: A comparison of doubly labeled water and heart-rate-monitoring methods. *Am J Clin Nutr* 57:512–518.

Lucas A, Ewing G, Roberts SB, Coward WA. 1987. How much energy does the breast fed infant consume and expend? *Br Med J* 295:75–77.

Lundgren H, Bengtsson C, Blohme G, Lapidus L, Sjöström L. 1989. Adiposity and adipose tissue distribution in relation to incidence of diabetes in women: Results from a prospective population study in Gothenburg, Sweden. *Int J Obes* 13:413–423.

MacMahon SW, Blacket RB, Macdonald GJ, Hall W. 1984. Obesity, alcohol consumption and blood pressure in Australian men and women. The National Heart Foundation of Australia Risk Factor Prevalence Study. *J Hypertens* 2:85–91.

Maffeis C, Schutz Y, Zoccante L, Micciolo R, Pinelli L. 1993. Meal-induced thermogenesis in lean and obese prepubertal children. *Am J Clin Nutr* 57:481–485.

Malina RM. 1994. Physical activity: Relationship to growth, maturation, and physical fitness. In: Bouchard C, Shephard RJ, Stephens T, eds. *Physical Activity, Fitness, and Health. International Proceedings and Consensus Statement.* Champaign, IL: Human Kinetics. Pp. 918–930.

Manson JE, Colditz GA, Stampfer MJ, Willett WC, Rosner B, Monson RR, Speizer FE, Hennekens CH. 1990. A prospective study of obesity and risk of coronary heart disease in women. *N Engl J Med* 322:882–889.

Margaria R, Cerretelli P, Aghemo P, Sassi G. 1963. Energy cost of running *J Appl Physiol* 18:367–370.

Mawson JT, Braun B, Rock PB, Moore LG, Mazzeo R, Butterfield GE. 2000. Women at altitude: Energy requirement at 4,300 m. *J Appl Physiol* 88:272–281.

McCargar L, Taunton J, Birmingham CL, Paré S, Simmons D. 1993. Metabolic and anthropometric changes in female weight cyclers and controls over a 1-year period. *J Am Diet Assoc* 93:1025–1030.

Medalie JH, Papier C, Herman JB, Goldbourt U, Tamir S, Neufeld HN, Riss E. 1974. Diabetes mellitus among 10,000 adult men. I. Five-year incidence and associated variables. *Isr J Med Sci* 10:681–697.

Meijer GA, Westerterp KR, Saris WH, ten Hoor F. 1992. Sleeping metabolic rate in relation to body composition and the menstrual cycle. *Am J Clin Nutr* 55:637–640.

Melanson KJ, Saltzman E, Russell R, Roberts SB. 1996. Postabsorptive and postprandial energy expenditure and substrate oxidation do not change during the menstrual cycle in young women. *J Nutr* 126:2531–2538.

Melanson KJ, Saltzman E, Vinken AG, Russell R, Roberts SB. 1998. The effects of age on postprandial thermogenesis at four graded energetic challenges: Findings in young and older women. *J Gerontol A Biol Sci Med Sci* 53:B409–B414.

Merrill AL, Watt BK. 1973. *Energy Value of Foods, Basis and Derivation*. Agricultural Handbook No.74. Human Nutrition Research Branch, Agricultural Research Service, United States Department of Agriculture. U.S. Government Printing Office, Washington, D.C.

Miller WC, Koceja DM, Hamilton EJ. 1997. A meta-analysis of the past 25 years of weight loss research using diet, exercise or diet plus exercise intervention. *Int J Obes Relat Metab Disord* 21:941–947.

Minghelli G, Schutz Y, Charbonnier A, Whitehead R, Jequier E. 1990. Twenty-four-hour energy expenditure and basal metabolic rate measured in a whole-body indirect calorimeter in Gambian men. *Am J Clin Nutr* 51:563–570.

Moore FS. 1963. *The Body Cell Mass and Its Supporting Environment: Body Composition in Health and Disease*. Philadelphia, PA: Saunders.

Moore LL, Nguyen USDT, Rothman KJ, Cupples LA, Ellison RC. 1995. Preschool physical activity level and change in body fatness in young children. *Am J Epidemiol* 142:982–988.

Morgan JB, York DA. 1983. Thermic effect of feeding in relation to energy balance in elderly men. *Ann Nutr Metab* 27:71–77.

Morio B, Ritz P, Verdier E, Montaurier C, Beaufrere B, Vermorel M. 1997. Critical evaluation of the factorial and heart-rate recording methods for the determination of energy expenditure of free-living elderly people. *Br J Nutr* 78:709–722.

Morrison JA, Alfaro MP, Khoury P, Thornton BB, Daniels SR. 1996. Determinants of resting energy expenditure in young black girls and young white girls. *J Pediatr* 129:637–642.

Motil KJ, Montandon CM, Garza C. 1990. Basal and postprandial metabolic rates in lactating and nonlactating women. *Am J Clin Nutr* 52:610–615.

Murgatroyd PR, Goldberg GR, Diaz E, Prentice AM. 1990. The influence of mild cold on human energy expenditure: Is there a sex difference in the response? *Br J Nutr* 64:777.

Must A, Strauss RS. 1999. Risks and consequences of childhood and adolescent obesity. *Int J Obes Relat Metab Disord* 23:S2–S11.

Nagy LE, King JC. 1984. Postprandial energy expenditure and respiratory quotient during early and late pregnancy. *Am J Clin Nutr* 40:1258–1263.

Nair KS, Halliday D, Garrow JS. 1983. Thermic response to isoenergetic protein, carbohydrate or fat meals in lean and obese subjects. *Clin Sci* 65:307–312.

Nelson KM, Weinsier RL, Long CL, Schutz Y. 1992. Prediction of resting energy expenditure from fat-free mass and fat mass. *Am J Clin Nutr* 56:848–856.

Neville MC. 1995. Determinants of milk volume and composition. In: Jensen RG, ed. *Handbook of Milk Composition*. San Diego, CA: Academic Press. Pp. 87–113.

Neville MC, Keller R, Seacat J, Lutes V, Neifert M, Casey C, Allen J, Archer P. 1988. Studies in human lactation: Milk volumes in lactating women during the onset of lactation and full lactation. *Am J Clin Nutr* 48:1375–1386.

Newman WP 3rd, Freedman DS, Voors AW, Gard PD, Srinivasan SR, Cresanta JL, Williamson GD, Webber LS, Berenson GS. 1986. Relation of serum lipoprotein levels and systolic blood pressure to early artherosclerosis. The Bolgalusa heart study. *N Engl J Med* 314:138–144.

NHLBI/NIDDK (National Heart, Lung, and Blood Institute/National Institute of Diabetes and Digestive and Kidney Diseases). 1998. *Clinical Guidelines on the Identification, Evaluation, and Treatment of Overweight and Obesity in Adults. The Evidence Report.* NIH Publication No. 98-4083. Bethesda, MD: National Institutes of Health.

Nicklas BJ, Toth MJ, Goldberg AP, Poehlman ET. 1997. Racial differences in plasma leptin concentrations in obese postmenopausal women. *J Clin Endocrinol Metab* 82:315–317.

Nickleberry BL, Brooks GA. 1996. No effect of cycling experience on leg cycle ergometer efficiency. *Med Sci Sports Exerc* 28:1396–1401.

Nielsen E. 1987. Acute modest changes in relative humidity do not affect energy expenditure at rest in human subjects. *Hum Nutr Clin Nutr* 41:485–488.

NIH (National Institutes of Health). 2000. *The Practical Guide. Identification, Evaluation, and Treatment of Overweight and Obesity in Adults.* NIH Publication No. 00-4084. Bethesda, MD: National Institutes of Health.

Nommsen LA, Lovelady CA, Heinig MJ, Lonnerdal B, Dewey KG. 1991. Determinants of energy, protein, lipid, and lactose concentrations in human milk during the first 12 mo of lactation: The DARLING Study. *Am J Clin Nutr* 53:457–465.

NRC (National Research Council). 1989. *Recommended Dietary Allowances,* 10th ed. Washington, DC: National Academy Press.

Ohlson L-O, Larsson B, Svärdsudd K, Welin L, Eriksson H, Wilhelmsen L, Björntorp P, Tibblin G. 1985. The influence of body fat distribution on the incidence of diabetes mellitus. 13.5 years of follow-up of the participants in the study of men born in 1913. *Diabetes* 34:1055–1058.

Osterman J, Lin Tu, Nankin HR, Brown KA, Hornung CA. 1992. Serum cholesterol profiles during treatment of obese outpatients with a very low calorie diet. Effect of initial cholesterol levels. *Int J Obes Relat Metab Disord* 16:49–58.

Owen OE. 1988. Regulation of energy and metabolism. In: MJ Kinney, Jeejeebhoy KN, Hill GH, Owen OE, eds. *Nutrition and Metabolism in Patient Care.* Philadelphia: W.B. Saunders. Pp. 35–59.

Owen OE, Kavle E, Owen RS, Polansky M, Caprio S, Mozzoli MA, Kendrick ZV, Bushman MC, Boden G. 1986. A reappraisal of caloric requirements in healthy women. *Am J Clin Nutr* 44:1–19.

Owen OE, Holup JL, D'Alessio DA, Craig ES, Polansky M, Smalley KJ, Kavle EC, Bushman MC, Owen LR, Mozzoli MA, Kendrick ZV, Boden GH. 1987. A reappraisal of the caloric requirements of men. *Am J Clin Nutr* 46:875–885.

Owens S, Gutin B, Allison J, Riggs S, Ferguson M, Litaker M, Thompson W. 1999. Effect of physical training on total and visceral fat in obese children. *Med Sci Sports Exerc* 31:143–148.

Pacy PJ, Cox M, Khalouha M, Elkins S, Robinson AC, Garrow JS. 1996. Does moderate aerobic activity have a stimulatory effect on 24 h resting energy expenditure: A direct calorimeter study. *Int J Food Sci Nutr* 47:299–305.

Pahud P, Ravussin E, Jequier E. 1980. Energy expended during oxygen deficit period of submaximal exercise in man. *J Appl Physiol* 48:770–775.

Pandolf KB, Givoni B, Goldman RF. 1977. Predicting energy expenditure with loads while standing or walking very slowly. *J Appl Physiol* 43:577–581.

Pannemans DL, Westerterp KR. 1995. Energy expenditure, physical activity and basal metabolic rate of elderly subjects. *Br J Nutr* 73:571–581.

Pannemans DL, Bouten CV, Westerterp KR. 1995. 24 h Energy expenditure during a standardized activity protocol in young and elderly men. *Eur J Clin Nutr* 49:49–56.

Parizkova J. 1974. Particularities of lean body mass and fat development in growing boys as related to their motor activity. *Acta Paediatrica Belgica* 28:233S–243S.

Passmore R, Durnin JV. 1955. Human energy expenditure. *Physiol Rev* 35:801–840.

Penn D, Schmidt-Sommerfeld E. 1989. Lipids as an energy source for the fetus and newborn infant. In: Lebenthal E, ed. *Textbook of Gastroenterology and Nutrition in Infancy*. New York: Raven Press. Pp. 293–310.

Piers LS, Diggavi SN, Rijskamp J, van Raaij JM, Shetty PS, Hautvast JG. 1995a. Resting metabolic rate and thermic effect of a meal in the follicular and luteal phases of the menstrual cycle in well-nourished Indian women. *Am J Clin Nutr* 61:296–302.

Piers LS, Diggavi SN, Thangam S, van Raaij JM, Shetty PS, Hautvast JG. 1995b. Changes in energy expenditure, anthropometry, and energy intake during the course of pregnancy and lactation in well-nourished Indian women. *Am J Clin Nutr* 61:501–513.

Pipe NG, Smith T, Halliday D, Edmonds CJ, Williams C, Coltart TM. 1979. Changes in fat, fat-free mass and body water in human normal pregnancy. *Br J Obstet Gynaecol* 86:929–940.

Platte P, Pirke KM, Wade SE, Trimborn P, Fichter MM. 1995. Physical activity, total energy expenditure, and food intake in grossly obese and normal weight women. *Int J Eating Disord* 17:51–57.

Poehlman ET. 1992. Energy expenditure and requirements in aging humans. *J Nutr* 122:2057–2065.

Poehlman ET. 1993. Regulation of energy expenditure in aging humans. *J Am Geriatr Soc* 41:552–559.

Poehlman ET, Danforth E. 1991. Endurance training increases metabolic rate and norepinephrine appearance rate in older individuals. *Am J Physiol* 261:E233–E239.

Poehlman ET, Melby CL, Badylak SF. 1991. Relation of age and physical exercise status on metabolic rate in younger and older healthy men. *J Gerontol* 46:B54–B58.

Poehlman ET, Toth MJ, Gardner AW. 1995. Changes in energy balance and body composition at menopause: A controlled longitudinal study. *Ann Intern Med* 123:673–675.

Poppitt SD, Swann D, Black AE, Prentice AM. 1998. Assessment of selective under-reporting of food intake by both obese and non-obese women in a metabolic facility. *Int J Obesity Relat Metab Disord* 22:303–311.

Prentice AM, Black AE, Coward WA, Davies HL, Goldberg GR, Murgatroyd PR, Ashford J, Sawyer M, Whitehead RG. 1986. High levels of energy expenditure in obese women. *Br Med J* 292:983–987.

Prentice AM, Lucas A, Vasquez-Velasquez L, Davies PS, Whitehead RG. 1988. Are current dietary guidelines for young children a prescription for overfeeding? *Lancet* 2:1066–1069.

Prentice AM, Goldberg GR, Davies HL, Murgatroyd PR, Scott W. 1989. Energy-sparing adaptations in human pregnancy assessed by whole-body calorimetry. *Br J Nutr* 62:5–22.

Prentice AM, Black AE, Coward WA, Cole TJ. 1996a. Energy expenditure in over-weight and obese adults in affluent societies: An analysis of 319 doubly-labelled water measurements. *Eur J Clin Nutr* 50:93–97.

Prentice AM, Spaaij CJ, Goldberg GR, Poppitt SD, van Raaij JM, Totton M, Swann D, Black AE. 1996b. Energy requirements of pregnant and lactating women. *Eur J Clin Nutr* 50:S82–S111.

Price GM, Paul AA, Cole TJ, Wadsworth ME. 1997. Characteristics of the low-energy reporters in a longitudinal national dietary survey. *Br J Nutr* 77:833–851.

Pryer JA, Vrijheid M, Nichols R, Kiggins M, Elliot P. 1997. Who are the 'low energy reporters' in the dietary and nutritional survey of British adults? *Int J Epidemiol* 26:146–154.

Racette SB, Schoeller DA, Kushner RF, Neil KM, Herling-Iaffaldano K. 1995. Effects of aerobic exercise and dietary carbohydrate on energy expenditure and body composition during weight reduction in obese women. *Am J Clin Nutr* 61:486–494.

Raitakari OT, Porkka KVK, Taimela S, Telama R, Rasanen L, Viikari JSA. 1994. Effects of persistent physical activity and inactivity on coronary risk factors in children and young adults. *Am J Epidemiol* 140:195–205.

Ravussin E, Lillioja S, Anderson TE, Christin L, Bogardus C. 1986. Determinants of 24-hour energy expenditure in man: Methods and results using a respiratory chamber. *J Clin Invest* 78:1568–1578.

Ravussin E, Lillioja S, Knowler WC, Christin L, Freymond D, Abbott WG, Boyce V, Howard BV, Bogardus C. 1988. Reduced rate of energy expenditure as a risk factor for body-weight gain. *N Engl J Med* 318:467–472.

Ravussin E, Harper IT, Rising R, Bogardus C. 1991. Energy expenditure by doubly labeled water: Validation in lean and obese subjects. *Am J Physiol* 261:E402–E409.

Reichman BL, Chessex P, Putet G, Verellen GJ, Smith JM, Heim T, Swyer PR. 1982. Partition of energy metabolism and energy cost of growth in the very low-birth-weight infant. *Pediatrics* 69:446–451.

Reisin E, Abel R, Modan M, Silverberg DS, Eliahou HE, Modan B. 1978. Effect of weight loss without salt restriction on the reduction of blood pressure in over-weight hypertensive patients. *N Engl J Med* 298:1–6.

Rexrode KM, Hennekens CH, Willett WC, Colditz GA, Stampfer MJ, Rich-Edwards JW, Speizer FE, Manson JE. 1997. A prospective study of body mass index, weight change, and risk of stroke in women. *J Am Med Assoc* 277:1539–1545.

Rexrode KM, Buring JE, Manson JE. 2001. Abdominal and total adiposity and risk of coronary heart disease in men. *Int J Obes Relat Metab Disord* 25:1047–1056.

Rimm EB, Stampfer MJ, Giovannucci F, Ascherio A, Spiegelman D, Colditz GA, Willett WC. 1995. Body size and fat distribution as predictors of coronary heart disease among middle-aged and older US women. *Am J Epidemiol* 15:1117–1127.

Riumallo JA, Schoeller D, Barrera G, Gattas V, Uauy R. 1989. Energy expenditure in underweight free-living adults: Impact of energy supplementation as deter-mined by doubly labeled water and indirect calorimetry. *Am J Clin Nutr* 49:239–246.

Roberts SB. 1996. Energy requirements of older individuals. *Eur J Clin Nutr* 50:S112–S118.

Roberts SB, Dallal GE. 1998. Effects of age on energy balance. *Am J Clin Nutr* 68:975S–979S.

Roberts SB, Dallal GE. 2001. The new childhood growth charts. *Nutr Rev* 59:31–36.

Roberts SB, Young VR. 1988. Energy costs of fat and protein deposition in the human infant. *Am J Clin Nutr* 48:951–955.

Roberts SB, Coward WA, Schlingenseipen K-H, Nohria V, Lucas A. 1986. Comparison of the doubly labeled water ($^2H_2{}^{18}O$) method with indirect calorimetry and a nutrient-balance study for simultaneous determination of energy expenditure, water intake, and metabolizable energy intake in preterm infants. *Am J Clin Nutr* 44:315–322.

Roberts SB, Savage J, Coward WA, Chew B, Lucas A. 1988. Energy expenditure and intake in infants born to lean and overweight mothers. *N Engl J Med* 318:461–466.

Roberts SB, Young VR, Fuss P, Fiatarone MA, Richard B, Rasmussen H, Wagner D, Joseph L, Holehouse E, Evans WJ. 1990. Energy expenditure and subsequent nutrient intakes in overfed young men. *Am J Physiol* 259:R461–R469.

Roberts SB, Heyman MB, Evans WJ, Fuss P, Tsay R, Young VR. 1991. Dietary energy requirements of young adult men, determined by using the doubly labeled water method. *Am J Clin Nutr* 54:499–505.

Roberts SB, Young VR, Fuss P, Heyman MB, Fiatarone M, Dallal GE, Cortiella J, Evans WJ. 1992. What are the dietary energy needs of elderly adults? *Int J Obes Relat Metab Disord* 16:969–976.

Roberts SB, Fuss P, Heyman MB, Young VR. 1995. Influence of age on energy requirements. *Am J Clin Nutr* 62:1053S–1058S.

Rolland-Cachera MF, Deheeger M, Bellisle F, Sempe M, Guilloud-Bataille M, Patois E. 1984. Adiposity rebound in children: a simple indicator for predicting obesity. *Am J Clin Nutr* 39:129–135.

Rolland-Cachera MF. 2001. Early adiposity rebound is not associated with energy or fat intake in infancy. *Pediatrics* 108:218–219.

Rosenberg L, Palmer JR, Miller DR, Clarke EA, Shapiro S. 1990. A case-control study of alcoholic beverage consumption and breast cancer. *Am J Epidemiol* 131:6–14.

Sadurskis A, Kabir N, Wager J, Forsum E. 1988. Energy metabolism, body composition, and milk production in healthy Swedish women during lactation. *Am J Clin Nutr* 48:44–49.

Sahi T, Paffenbarger RS, Hsieh C-C, Lee I-M. 1998. Body mass index, cigarette smoking, and other characteristics as predictors of self-reported, physician-diagnosed gallbladder disease in male college alumni. *Am J Epidemiol* 147:644–651.

Salbe AD, Fontvieille AM, Harper IT, Ravussin E. 1997. Low levels of physical activity in 5-year-old children. *J Pediatr* 131:423–429.

Saltzman E, Roberts SB. 1995. The role of energy expenditure in energy regulation: Findings from a decade of research. *Nutr Rev* 53:209–220.

Saris WHM, Emons HJG, Groenenboom DC, Westerterp KR. 1989. Discrepancy between FAO/WHO energy requirements and actual energy expenditure in healthy 7-11 year old children. In: Beunen G, Ghesquiere J, Reybrouck T, Claessens AL, eds. *Children and Exercise: 14th International Seminar on Pediatric Work Physiology.* Stuttgart, Germany: Ferdinand Enke Verlag Press.

Sasaki J, Shindo M, Tanaka M, Ando M, Arakawa K. 1987. A long-term aerobic exercise program decreases the obesity index and increases high density lipoprotein cholesterol concentration in obese children. *Int J Obes* 11:339–345.

Savage MP, Petratis MM, Thomson WH, Berg K, Smith JL, Sady SP. 1986. Exercise training effects on serum lipids of prepubescent boys and adult men. *Med Sci Sports Exerc* 18:197–204.

Sawaya AL, Saltzman E, Fuss P, Young VR, Roberts SB. 1995. Dietary energy requirements of young and older women determined by using the doubly labeled water method. *Am J Clin Nutr* 62:338–344.

Schoeller DA. 1983. Energy expenditure from doubly labeled water: Some fundamental considerations in humans. *Am J Clin Nutr* 38:999–1005.

Schoeller DA. 1995. Limitations in the assessment of dietary energy intake by self-report. *Metabolism* 44:18–22.

Schoeller DA. 2001. The importance of clinical research: The role of thermogenesis in human obesity. *Am J Clin Nutr* 73:511–516.

Schoeller DA, Fjeld CR. 1991. Human energy metabolism: What we have learned from the doubly labeled water method? *Annu Rev Nutr* 11:355–373.

Schoeller DA, Webb P. 1984. Five-day comparison of the doubly labeled water method with respiratory gas exchange. *Am J Clin Nutr* 40:153–158.

Schoeller DA, Ravussin E, Schutz Y, Acheson KJ, Baertschi P, Jequier E. 1986. Energy expenditure by doubly labeled water: Validation in humans and proposed calculation. *Am J Physiol* 250:R823–R830.

Schofield C. 1985. An annotated bibliography of source material for basal metabolic rate data. *Hum Nutr Clin Nutr* 39C:42–91.

Schofield WN. 1985. Predicting basal metabolic rate, new standards and review of previous work. *Hum Nutr Clin Nutr* 39C:5–41.

Schotte DE, Stunkard AJ. 1990. The effects of weight reduction on blood pressure in 301 obese patients. *Ann Intern Med* 150:1701–1704.

Schulz LO, Nyomba BL, Alger S, Anderson TE, Ravussin E. 1991. Effect of endurance training on sedentary energy expenditure measured in a respiratory chamber. *Am J Physiol* 260:E257–E261.

Schulz LO, Alger S, Harper I, Wilmore JH, Ravussin E. 1992. Energy expenditure of elite female runners measured by respiratory chamber and doubly labeled water. *J Appl Physiol* 72:23–28.

Schutz Y, Golay A, Felber JP, Jéquier E. 1984. Decreased glucose-induced thermogenesis after weight loss in obese subjects: A predisposing factor for relapse obesity? *Am J Clin Nutr* 39:380–387.

Schutz Y, Golay A, Jéquier E. 1988. 24 h Energy expenditure (24-EE) in pregnant women with a standardized activity level. *Experentia* 44:A31.

Schwartz RS, Jaeger LF, Veith RC. 1990. The thermic effect of feeding in older men: The importance of the sympathetic nervous system. *Metabolism* 39:733–737.

Seale JL, Rumpler WV. 1997. Comparison of energy expenditure measurements by diet records, energy intake balance, doubly labeled water and room calorimetry. *Eur J Clin Nutr* 51:856–863.

Seale JL, Rumpler WV, Conway JM, Miles CW. 1990. Comparison of doubly labeled water, intake-balance, and direct- and indirect-calorimetry methods for measuring energy expenditure in adult men. *Am J Clin Nutr* 52:66–71.

Segal KR, Gutin B, Albu J, Pi-Sunyer FX. 1987. Thermic effects of food and exercise in lean and obese men of similar lean body mass. *Am J Physiol* 252:E110–E117.

Segal KR, Edano A, Blando L, Pi-Sunyer FX. 1990a. Comparison of thermic effects of constant and relative caloric loads in lean and obese men. *Am J Clin Nutr* 51:14–21.

Segal KR, Edano A, Tomas MB. 1990b. Thermic effect of a meal over 3 and 6 hours in lean and obese men. *Metabolism* 39:985–992.

Segal KR, Chun A, Coronel P, Cruz-Noori A, Santos R. 1992. Reliability of the measurement of postprandial thermogenesis in men of three levels of body fatness. *Metabolism* 41:754–762.

Seidell JC, Verschuren WM, Van Leer EM, Kromhout D. 1996. Overweight, under-weight, and mortality: A prospective study of 48,287 men and women. *Arch Intern Med* 156:958–963.

Shah M, Geissler CA, Miller DS. 1988. Metabolic rate during and after aerobic exercise in post-obese and lean women. *Eur J Clin Nutr* 42:455–464.

Shetty PS, Soares MJ, James WPT. 1994. Body mass index: Its relationship to basal metabolic rates and energy requirements. *Eur J Clin Nutr* 48:S28–S38.

Siler SQ, Neese RA, Hellerstein MK. 1999. De novo lipogenesis, lipid kinetics, and whole-body lipid balances in humans after acute alcohol consumption. *Am J Clin Nutr* 70:928–936.

Sinclair JC. 1978. *Temperature Regulation and Energy Metabolism in the Newborn.* New York: Grune and Stratton.

Soares MJ, Piers LS, Shetty PS, Robinson S, Jackson AA, Waterlow CJ. 1991. Basal metabolic rate, body composition and whole-body protein turnover in Indian men with differing nutritional status. *Clin Sci* 81:419–425.

Soares MJ, Piers LS, O'Dea K, Shetty PS. 1998. No evidence for an ethnic influence on basal metabolism: An examination of data from India and Australia. *Br J Nutr* 79:333–341.

Sohlstrom A, Forsum E. 1995. Changes in adipose tissue volume and distribution during reproduction in Swedish women as assessed by magnetic resonance imaging. *Am J Clin Nutr* 61:287–295.

Sohlstrom A, Forsum E. 1997. Changes in total body fat during the human repro-ductive cycle as assessed by magnetic resonance imaging, body water dilution, and skinfold thickness: A comparison of methods. *Am J Clin Nutr* 66:1315–1322.

Solomon SJ, Kurzer MS, Calloway DH. 1982. Menstrual cycle and basal metabolic rate in women. *Am J Clin Nutr* 36:611–616.

Spaaij CJK, van Raaij JMA, de Groot LC, van der Heijden LJ, Boekholt HA, Hautvast JG. 1994a. Effect of lactation on resting metabolic rate and on diet- and work-induced thermogenesis. *Am J Clin Nutr* 59:42–47.

Spaaij CJK, van Raaij JMA, van der Heijden LJ, Schouten FJM, Drijvers JJ, de Groot LC, Boekholt HA, Hautvast JG. 1994b. No substantial reduction of the thermic effect of a meal during pregnancy in well-nourished Dutch women. *Br J Nutr* 71:335–344.

Sparks JW, Girard JR, Battaglia FC. 1980. An estimate of the caloric requirements of the human fetus. *Biol Neonate* 38:113–119.

Stampfer MJ, Maclure KM, Colditz GA, Manson JE, Willett WC. 1992. Risk of symp-tomatic gallstones in women with severe obesity. *Am J Clin Nutr* 55:652–658.

Stevens J, Cai J, Pamuk ER, Williamson DF, Thun MJ, Wood JL. 1998. The effect of age on the association between body-mass index and mortality. *N Engl J Med* 338:1–7.

Stubbs RJ, Harbron CG, Murgatroyd PR, Prentice AM. 1995. Covert manipulation of dietary fat and energy density: Effect on substrate flux and food intake in men eating ad libitum. *Am J Clin Nutr* 62:316–329.

Stunkard AJ, Berkowitz RI, Stallings VA, Schoeller DA. 1999. Energy intake, not energy output, is a determinant of body size in infants. *Am J Clin Nutr* 69:524–530.

Sun M, Gower BA, Nagy TR, Trowbridge CA, Dezenberg C, Goran MI. 1998. Total, resting, and activity-related energy expenditures are similar in Caucasian and African-American children. *Am J Physiol* 274:E232–E237.

Sun SS, Chumlea WC, Heymsfield SB, Lukaski HC, Schoeller D, Friedl K, Kuczmarski RJ, Flegal KM, Johnson CL, Hubbard VS. 2003. Development of bioelectrical impedance analysis prediction equations for body composition with the use of a multicomponent model for use in epidemiologic surveys. *Am J Clin Nutr* 77: 331–340.

Sunnegardh J, Bratteby LE, Hagman U, Samuelson G, Sjolin S. 1986. Physical activity in relation to energy intake and body fat in 8- and 13-year-old children in Sweden. *Acta Paediatr Scand* 75:955–963.

Suominen H, Heikkinen E, Parkatti T, Frosberg S, Kiiskinen A. 1977. Effects of 'lifelong' physical training on functional aging in men. *Scand J Soc Med* 14:225–240.

Suter PM, Schutz Y, Jequier E. 1992. The effect of ethanol on fat storage in healthy subjects. *N Engl J Med* 326:983–987.

Suter PM, Hasler E, Vetter W. 1997. Effects of alcohol on energy metabolism and body weight regulation: Is alcohol a risk factor for obesity? *Nutr Rev* 55:157–171.

Svendsen OL, Hassager C, Christiansen C. 1995. Age- and menopause-associated variations in body composition and fat distribution in healthy women as measured by dual-energy x-ray absorptiometry. *Metabolism* 44:369–373.

Tanner JM. 1955. *Growth at Adolescence*. Springfield, IL: Charles C. Thomas.

Thorne A, Wahren J. 1990. Diminished meal-induced thermogenesis in elderly man. *Clin Physiol* 10:427–437.

Timmons BA, Araujo J, Thomas TR. 1985. Fat utilization enhanced by exercise in a cold environment. *Med Sci Sports Exerc* 17:673–678.

Tomoyasu NJ, Toth MJ, Poehlman ET. 2000. Misreporting of total energy intake in older African Americans. *Int J Obes Relat Metab Disord* 24:20–26.

Torun B, Davies PSW, Livingstone MBE, Paolisso M, Sackett R, Spurr GB. 1996. Energy requirements and dietary energy recommendations for children and adolescents 1 to 18 years old. *Eur J Clin Nutr* 50:S37–S81.

Tounian P, Girardet J, Carlier L, Frelut ML, Veinberg F, Fontaine JL. 1993. Resting energy expenditure and food-induced thermogenesis in obese children. *J Pediatr Gastroenterol Nutr* 16:451–457.

Tremblay A, Nadeau A, Fournier G, Bouchard C. 1988. Effect of a three-day interruption of exercise-training on resting metabolic rate and glucose-induced thermogenesis in training individuals. *Int J Obes* 12:163–168.

Tremblay A, Nadeau A, Despres JP, St-Jean L, Theriault G, Bouchard C. 1990. Long-term exercise training with constant energy intake. 2: Effect on glucose metabolism and resting energy expenditure. *Int J Obes* 14:75–84.

Treuth MS, Adolph AL, Butte NF. 1998a. Energy expenditure in children predicted from heart rate and activity calibrated against respiration calorimetry. *Am J Physiol* 275:E12–E18.

Treuth MS, Hunter GR, Pichon C, Figueroa-Colon R, Goran MI. 1998b. Fitness and energy expenditure after strength training in obese prepubertal girls. *Med Sci Sports Exerc* 30:1130–1136.

Treuth MS, Butte NF, Wong W. 2000. Effects of familial predisposition to obesity on energy expenditure in multiethnic prepubertal girls. *Am J Clin Nutr* 71:893–900.

Troiano RP, Flegal KM, Kuczmarski RJ, Campbell SM, Johnson CL. 1995. Overweight prevalence and trends for children and adolescents. The National Health and Nutrition Examination Surveys, 1963 to 1991. *Arch Pediatr Adolesc Med* 149:1085–1091.

Troiano RP, Frongillo EA, Sobal J, Levitsky DA. 1996. The relationship between body weight and mortality: A quantitative analysis of combined information from existing studies. *Int J Obes Relat Metab Disord* 20:63–75.

Trowbridge CA, Gower BA, Nagy TR, Hunter GR, Treuth MS, Goran MI. 1997. Maximal aerobic capacity in African-American and Caucasian prepubertal children. *Am J Physiol* 273:E809–E814.

Tuttle WW, Horvath SM, Presson LF, Daum K. 1953. Specific dynamic action of protein in men past 60 years of age. *J Appl Physiol* 5:631–634.

Twisk JWR. 2001. Physical activity guidelines for children and adolescents. A critical review. *Sports Med* 31:617–627.

Tzankoff SP, Norris AH. 1977. Effect of muscle mass decrease on age-related BMR changes. *J Appl Physiol* 43:1001–1006.

USDA/HHS (U.S. Department of Agriculture/U.S. Department of Health and Human Services). 2000. *Nutrition and Your Health: Dietary Guidelines for Americans.* Home and Garden Bulletin No. 232. Washington, DC: U.S. Government Printing Office.

Valencia ME, McNeill G, Brockway JM, Smith JS. 1992. The effect of environmental temperature and humidity on 24 h energy expenditure in men. *Br J Nutr* 68:319–327.

Valve R, Heikkinen S, Rissanen A, Laakso M, Uusitupa M. 1998. Synergistic effect of polymorphisms in uncoupling protein 1 and β_3-adrenergic receptor genes on basal metabolic rate in obese Finns. *Diabetologia* 41:357–361.

van Baak MA. 1999. Physical activity and energy balance. *Public Health Nutr* 2:335–339.

Van Etten LM, Westerterp KR, Verstappen FT, Boon BJ, Saris WH. 1997. Effect of an 18-wk weight-training program on energy expenditure and physical activity. *J Appl Physiol* 82:298–304.

van Gemert WG, Westerterp KR, van Acker BA, Wagenmakers AJ, Halliday D, Greve JM, Soeters PB. 2000. Energy, substrate and protein metabolism in morbid obesity before, during and after massive weight loss. *Int J Obes Relat Metab Disord* 24:711–718.

van Raaij JMA, Vermaat-Miedema SH, Schonk CM, Peek ME, Hautvast JG. 1987. Energy requirements of pregnancy in the Netherlands. *Lancet* 2:953–955.

van Raaij JMA, Peek ME, Vermaat-Miedema SH, Schonk CM, Hautvast JG. 1988. New equations for estimating body fat mass in pregnancy from body density or total body water. *Am J Clin Nutr* 48:24–29.

van Raaij JMA, Schonk CM, Vermaat-Miedema SH, Peek ME, Hautvast JG. 1989. Body fat mass and basal metabolic rate in Dutch women before, during, and after pregnancy: A reappraisal of energy cost of pregnancy. *Am J Clin Nutr* 49:765–772.

van Raaij JMA, Schonk CM, Vermaat-Miedema SH, Peek ME, Hautvast JG. 1990. Energy cost of physical activity throughout pregnancy and the first year postpartum in Dutch women with sedentary lifestyles. *Am J Clin Nutr* 52:234–239.

van Raaij JMA, Schonk CM, Vermaat-Miedema SH, Peek ME, Hautvast JG. 1991. Energy cost of lactation, and energy balances of well-nourished Dutch lactating women: Reappraisal of the extra energy requirements of lactation. *Am J Clin Nutr* 53:612–619.

van Staveren WA, Deurenberg P, Burema J, de Groot LC, Hautvast JG. 1986. Seasonal variation in food intake, pattern of physical activity and change in body weight in a group of young adult Dutch women consuming self-selected diets. *Int J Obes* 10:133–145.

Vaughan L, Zurlo F, Ravussin E. 1991. Aging and energy expenditure. *Am J Clin Nutr* 53:821–825.

Visser M, Deurenberg P, van Staveren WA, Hautvast JG. 1995. Resting metabolic rate and diet-induced thermogenesis in young and elderly subjects: Relationship with body composition, fat distribution, and physical activity level. *Am J Clin Nutr* 61:772–778.

Walker SP, Rimm EB, Ascherio A, Kawachi I, Stampfer MJ, Willett WC. 1996. Body size and fat distribution as predictors of stroke among US men. *Am J Epidemiol* 144:1143–1150.

Walravens PA, Krebs NF, Hambidge KM. 1983. Linear growth of low income preschool children receiving a zinc supplement. *Am J Clin Nutr* 38:195–201.

Warren MP, Brooks-Gunn J, Hamilton LH, Warren LF, Hamilton WG. 1986. Scoliosis and fractures in young ballet dancers. Relation to delayed menarche and secondary amenorrhea. *N Engl J Med* 314:1348–1353.

Warwick PM, Busby R. 1990. Influence of mild cold on 24 h energy expenditure in "normally" clothed adults. *Br J Nutr* 63:481–488.

Washburn RA, Kline G, Lackland DT, Wheeler FC. 1992. Leisure time physical activity: Are there black/white differences? *Prev Med* 21:127–135.

Waterlow JC. 1999. The nature and significance of nutritional adaptation. *Eur J Clin Nutr* 53:S2–S5.

Waterlow JC, James WPT, Healy MJR. 1989. Nutritional adaptation and variability. *Eur J Clin Nutr* 43:203–210.

Webb P. 1981. Energy expenditure and fat-free mass in men and women. *Am J Clin Nutr* 34:1816–1826.

Webber J, Macdonald IA. 2000. Signalling in body-weight homeostasis: Neuroendocrine efferent signals. *Proc Nutr Soc* 59:397–404.

Webber LS, Cresanta JL, Voors AW, Berenson GS. 1983. Tracking of cardiovascular disease risk factor variables in school-age children. *J Chron Dis* 36:647–660.

Weinsier RL, Schutz Y, Bracco D. 1992. Reexamination of the relationship of resting metabolic rate to fat-free mass and to the metabolically active components of fat-free mass in humans. *Am J Clin Nutr* 55:790–794.

Weinsier RL, Hunter GR, Heini AF, Goran MI, Sell SM. 1998. The etiology of obesity: Relative contribution of metabolic factors, diet, and physical activity. *Am J Med* 105:145–150.

Weinsier RL, Nagy TR, Hunter GR, Darnell BE, Hensrud DD, Weiss HL. 2000. Do adaptive changes in metabolic rate favor weight regain in weight-reduced individuals? An examination of the set-point theory. *Am J Clin Nutr* 72:1088–1094.

Wells JC, Davies PS. 1995. The effect of diet and sex on sleeping metabolic rate in 12-week old infants. *Eur J Clin Nutr* 49:329–335.

Wells JC, Cole TJ, Davies PS. 1996. Total energy expenditure and body composition in early infancy. *Arch Dis Child* 75:423–426.

Westerterp KR, Brouns F, Saris WHM, ten Hoor F. 1988. Comparison of doubly labeled water with respirometry at low and high activity levels. *J Appl Physiol* 65:53–56.

Westerterp KR, Lafeber HN, Sulkers EJ, Sauer PJ. 1991. Comparison of short term indirect calorimetry and doubly labeled water method for the assessment of energy expenditure in preterm infants. *Biol Neonate* 60:75–82.

Westerterp KR, Meijer GA, Janssen EM, Saris WH, ten Hoor F. 1992. Long-term effect of physical activity on energy balance and body composition. *Br J Nutr* 68:21–30.

Westlund K, Nicolaysen R. 1972. Ten-year mortality and morbidity related to se-rum cholesterol. A follow-up of 3,751 men aged 40–49. *Scand J Clin Lab Invest* 30:1–24.

Weyer C, Snitker S, Bogardus C, Ravussin E. 1999a. Energy metabolism in African Americans: Potential risk factors for obesity. *Am J Clin Nutr* 70:13–20.

Weyer C, Snitker S, Rising R, Bogardus C, Ravussin E. 1999b. Determinants of energy expenditure and fuel utilization in man: Effects of body composition, age, sex, ethnicity and glucose tolerance in 916 subjects. *Int J Obes Relat Metab Disord* 23:715–722.

Whitehead RG, Paul AA, Cole TJ. 1981. A critical analysis of measured food energy intakes during infancy and early childhood in comparison with current inter-national recommendations. *J Hum Nutr* 35:339–348.

WHO (World Health Organization). 1998. *Obesity: Preventing and Managing the Global Epidemic. Report of a World Health Organization Consultation on Obesity.* Geneva: WHO.

WHO Working Group. 1986. Use and interpretation of anthropometric indicators of nutritional status. *Bull World Health Organ* 64:929–941.

Widdowson EM. 1974. Nutrition. In: Davis JA, Dobbing J, eds. *Scientific Foundations of Paediatrics.* London: William Heinemann Medical Books. Pp. 44–55.

Willett WC, Manson JE, Stampfer MJ, Colditz GA, Rosner B, Speizer FE, Hennekens CH. 1995. Weight, weight change, and coronary heart disease in women. Risk within the 'normal' weight range. *J Am Med Assoc* 273:461–465.

Willett WC, Dietz WH, Colditz GA. 1999. Guidelines for healthy weight. *N Engl J Med* 341:427–434.

Wing RR, Marcus MD, Salata R, Epstein LH, Miaskiewicz S, Blair EH. 1991. Effects of a very-low-calorie diet on long-term glycemic control in obese Type 2 dia-betic subjects. *Arch Intern Med* 151:1334–1340.

Withers RT, Smith DA, Tucker RC, Brinkman M, Clark DG. 1998. Energy metabolism in sedentary and active 49- to 70-yr-old women. *J Appl Physiol* 84:1333–1340.

Wong WW. 1994. Energy expenditure of female adolescents. *J Am Coll Nutr* 13:332–337.

Wong WW, Butte NF, Ellis KJ, Hergenroeder AC, Hill RB, Stuff JE, Smith E. 1999. Pubertal African-American girls expend less energy at rest and during physical activity than Caucasian girls. *J Clin Endocrinol Metab* 84:906–911.

Wood PD, Stefanick ML, Dreon DM, Frey-Hewitt B, Garay SC, William PT, Superko HR, Fortmann SP, Albers JJ, Vranizan KM, et al. 1988. Changes in plasma lipids and lipoproteins in overweight men during weight loss through dieting as compared with exercise. *N Engl J Med* 319(18):1173-1179.

Wood PD, Stefanick ML, Williams PT, Haskell WL. 1991. The effects on plasma lipoproteins of a prudent weight-reducing diet, with or without exercise, in overweight men and women. *N Engl J Med* 325:461–466.

Yanovski SZ, Reynolds JC, Boyle AJ, Yanovski JA. 1997. Resting metabolic rate in African-American and Caucasian girls. *Obes Res* 5:321–325.

Zinker BA, Wilson RD, Wasserman DH. 1995. Interaction of decreased arterial PO_2 and exercise on carbohydrate metabolism in the dog. *Am J Physiol* 269:E409–E417.

Zlotkin SH. 1996. A review of the Canadian "Nutrition Recommendations Update: Dietary Fat and Children." *J Nutr* 126:1022S–1027S.

Zurlo F, Ferraro RT, Fontvieille AM, Rising R, Bogardus C, Ravussin E. 1992. Spon-taneous physical activity and obesity: Cross-sectional and longitudinal studies in Pima Indians. *Am J Physiol* 263:E296–E300.

6

Dietary Carbohydrates: Sugars and Starches

SUMMARY

The primary role of carbohydrates (sugars and starches) is to provide energy to cells in the body, particularly the brain, which is the only carbohydrate-dependent organ in the body. The Recommended Dietary Allowance (RDA) for carbohydrate is set at 130 g/d for adults and children based on the average minimum amount of glucose utilized by the brain. This level of intake, however, is typically exceeded to meet energy needs while consuming acceptable intake levels of fat and protein (see Chapter 11). The median intake of carbohydrates is approximately 220 to 330 g/d for men and 180 to 230 g/d for women. Due to a lack of sufficient evidence on the prevention of chronic diseases in generally healthy individuals, no recommendations based on glycemic index are made.

BACKGROUND INFORMATION

Classification of Dietary Carbohydrates

Carbohydrates can be subdivided into several categories based on the number of sugar units present. A *monosaccharide* consists of one sugar unit such as glucose or fructose. A *disaccharide* (e.g., sucrose, lactose, and maltose) consists of two sugar units. *Oligosaccharides,* containing 3 to 10 sugar units, are often breakdown products of *polysaccharides,* which contain more than 10 sugar units. Oligosaccharides such as raffinose and stachyose are found in small amounts in legumes. Examples of polysaccharides include starch and glycogen, which are the storage forms of carbohydrates in plants and animals, respectively. Finally, *sugar alcohols*, such as sorbitol and mannitol, are alcohol forms of glucose and fructose, respectively.

Definition of Sugars

The term "sugars" is traditionally used to describe mono- and disaccharides (FAO/WHO, 1998). Sugars are used as sweeteners to improve the palatability of foods and beverages and for food preservation (FAO/WHO, 1998). In addition, sugars are used to confer certain functional attributes to foods such as viscosity, texture, body, and browning capacity. The monosaccharides include glucose, galactose, and fructose, while the disaccharides include sucrose, lactose, maltose, and trehalose. Some commonly used sweeteners contain trisaccharides and higher saccharides. Corn syrups contain large amounts of these saccharides; for example, only 33 percent or less of the carbohydrates in some corn syrups are mono- and disaccharides; the remaining 67 percent or more are trisaccharides and higher saccharides (Glinsmann et al., 1986). This may lead to an underestimation of the intake of sugars if the trisaccharides and higher saccharides are not included in an analysis.

Extrinsic and Intrinsic Sugars

The terms extrinsic and intrinsic sugars originate from the United Kingdom Department of Health. Intrinsic sugars are defined as sugars that are present within the cell walls of plants (i.e., naturally occurring), while extrinsic sugars are those that are typically added to foods. An additional phrase, "non-milk extrinsic sugars," was developed due to the lactose in milk also being an extrinsic sugar (FAO/WHO, 1998). The terms were developed to help consumers differentiate sugars inherent to foods from sugars that are not naturally occurring in foods.

Added Sugars

The U.S. Department of Agriculture (USDA) has defined "added sugars" for the purpose of analyzing the nutrient intake of Americans using nationwide surveys, as well as for use in the Food Guide Pyramid. The Food Guide Pyramid, which is the food guide for the United States, translates recommendations on nutrient intakes into recommendations for food intakes (Welsh et al., 1992). Added sugars are defined as sugars and syrups that are added to foods during processing or preparation. Major sources of added sugars include soft drinks, cakes, cookies, pies, fruitades, fruit punch, dairy desserts, and candy (USDA/HHS, 2000). Specifically, added sugars include white sugar, brown sugar, raw sugar, corn syrup, corn-syrup solids, high-fructose corn syrup, malt syrup, maple syrup, pancake syrup, fructose sweetener, liquid fructose, honey, molasses, anhydrous dextrose, and crystal dextrose. Added sugars do not include naturally occurring sugars such as lactose in milk or fructose in fruits.

The Food Guide Pyramid places added sugars at the tip of the pyramid and advises consumers to use them sparingly (USDA, 1996). Table 6-1 shows the amounts of added sugars that could be included in diets that meet the Food Guide Pyramid for three different calorie levels.

Since USDA developed the added sugars definition, the added sugars term has been used in the scientific literature (Bowman, 1999; Britten et al., 2000; Forshee and Storey, 2001; Guthrie and Morton, 2000). The 2000 *Dietary Guidelines for Americans* used the term to aid consumers in identifying beverages and foods that are high in added sugars (USDA/HHS, 2000). Although added sugars are not chemically different from naturally occurring sugars, many foods and beverages that are major sources of added sugars have lower micronutrient densities compared with foods and beverages that are major sources of naturally occurring sugars (Guthrie and Morton, 2000). Currently, U.S. food labels contain information on total sugars per serving, but do not distinguish between sugars naturally present in foods and added sugars.

Definition of Starch

Starch consists of less than 1,000 to many thousands of α-linked glucose units. Amylose is the linear form of starch that consists of α-(1,4) linkages of glucose polymers. Amylopectin consists of the linear

TABLE 6-1 Amount of Sugars That Can Be Added for Three Different Energy Intakes That Meet the Food Guide Pyramid

Food Guide Pyramid Patterns at Three Calorie Levels	Pattern A	Pattern B	Pattern C
Kilocalories (approximate)	1,600	2,200	2,800
Bread/grain group (servings)	6	9	11
Vegetable group (servings)	3	4	5
Fruit group (servings)	2	3	4
Milk group (servings)	2–3	2–3	2–3
Meat group (oz)	5	6	7
Total fat (g)	53	73	93
Total added sugars (tsp)[a]	6	12	18

[a] 1 tsp added sugars = 4 g added sugars.
SOURCE: USDA (1996).

α-(1,4) glucose polymers, as well as branched 1-6 glucose polymers. The amylose starches are compact, have low solubility, and are less rapidly digested. They are prone to retrogradation (hydrogen bonding between amylose units) to form resistant starches (RS_3). The amylopectin starches are digested more rapidly, presumably because of the more effective enzymatic attack of the more open-branched structure.

Definition of Glycemic Response, Glycemic Index, and Glycemic Load

Foods containing carbohydrate have a wide range of effects on blood glucose concentration during the time course of digestion (glycemic response), with some resulting in a rapid rise followed by a rapid fall in blood glucose concentration, and others resulting in a slow extended rise and a slow extended fall. Prolonging the time over which glucose is available for absorption in healthy individuals greatly reduces the postprandial glucose response (Jenkins et al., 1990). Holt and coworkers (1997), however, reported that the insulin response to consumption of carbohydrate foods is influenced by the level of the glucose response, but varies among individuals and with the amount of carbohydrate consumed. Adults with type 1 or type 2 diabetes have been shown to have similar glycemic responses to specific foods (Wolever et al., 1987), whereas glycemic responses were shown to vary with severity of diabetes (Gannon and Nuttall, 1987). Individuals with lactose maldigestion have reduced glycemic responses to lactose-containing items (Maxwell et al., 1970).

The glycemic index (GI) is a classification proposed to quantify the relative blood glucose response to foods containing carbohydrate (Jenkins et al., 1981). It is defined as the area under the curve for the increase in blood glucose after the ingestion of a set amount of carbohydrate in an individual food (e.g., 50 g) in the 2-hour postingestion period as compared with ingestion of the same amount of carbohydrate from a reference food (white bread or glucose) tested in the same individual, under the same conditions, using the initial blood glucose concentration as a baseline. The average daily dietary GI of a meal is calculated by summing the products of the carbohydrate content per serving for each food, times the average number of servings of that food per day, multiplied by the GI, and all divided by the total amount of carbohydrate (Wolever and Jenkins, 1986). Individual foods have characteristic values for GI (Foster-Powell and Brand Miller, 1995), although within-subject and between-subject variability is relatively large (Wolever et al., 1991). Because GI has been determined by using 50-g carbohydrate portions of food, it is possible that there is a nonlinear response between the amount of food ingested, as is the case for fructose (Nuttall et al., 1992) and the glycemic response.

The average glycemic load is derived the same way as the GI, but without dividing by the total amount of carbohydrate consumed. Thus, glycemic load is an indicator of glucose response or insulin demand that is induced by total carbohydrate intake.

GI is referred to throughout this chapter because many studies have used this classification system. This does not imply that it is the best or only system for classifying glycemic responses or other statistical associations. The GI approach does not consider different metabolic responses to the ingestion of sugars versus starches, even though they may have the same GI values (Jenkins et al., 1988b).

Utilization of the Glycemic Index

Several food characteristics that influence GI are summarized in Table 6-2. Broadly speaking, the two main factors that influence GI are carbohydrate type and physical determinants of the rate of digestion, such as whether grains are intact or ground into flour, food firmness resulting from cooking, ripeness, and soluble fiber content (Wolever, 1990). Intrinsic factors such as amylose:amylopectin ratio, particle size and degree of gelatinization, as well as extrinsic factors such as enzyme inhibitors and food preparation and processing, affect GI in their ability to interact with digestive enzymes and the consequent production of monosaccharides. With progressive ripeness of foods, there is a decrease in starch and an increase in free sugar content. The ingestion of fat and protein has been shown to decrease the GI of foods by increasing plasma glucose disposal through the increased secretion of insulin and possibly other hormones (Gannon et al., 1993; Nuttall et al., 1984). Significantly high correlations between GI and protein, fat, and total caloric content were observed and

TABLE 6-2 Factors That Reduce the Rate of Starch Digestibility and the Glycemic Index

Intrinsic	Extrinsic
High amylose:amylopectin ratio	Protective insoluble fiber seed coat as in whole intact grains
Intact grain/large particle size	Viscous fibers
Intact starch granules	Enzyme inhibitors
Raw, ungelatinized or unhydrated starch	Raw foods (vs. cooked foods)
Physical interaction with fat or protein	Minimal food processing
	Reduced ripeness in fruit
	Minimal (compared to extended) storage

explained 87 percent of the variation in glycemic response among foods (Hollenbeck et al., 1986). In addition to these factors, the GI of a meal can affect the glycemic response of the subsequent meal (Ercan et al., 1994; Wolever et al., 1988). Examples of published values for the GI of pure carbohydrates and other food items are shown in Table 6-3.

A number of research groups have reported a significant relationship between mixed-meal GI predicted from individual food items and either the GI measured directly (Chew et al., 1988; Collier et al., 1986; Gulliford et al., 1989; Indar-Brown et al., 1992; Järvi et al., 1995; Wolever and Jenkins, 1986; Wolever et al., 1985, 1990) or metabolic parameters such as high

TABLE 6-3 Glycemic Index (GI) of Common Foods

Food Item	GI (White Bread = 100)
Rice, white, low-amylose	126
Baked potato	121
Corn flakes	119
Rice cakes	117
Jelly beans	114
Cheerios	106
Carrots	101
White bread	101
Wheat bread	99
Soft drink	97
Angel food cake	95
Sucrose	92
Cheese pizza	86
Spaghetti (boiled)	83
Popcorn	79
Sweet corn	78
Banana	76
Orange juice	74
Rice, Uncle Ben's converted long-grain	72
Green peas	68
Oat bran bread	68
Orange	62
All-Bran cereal	60
Apple juice	58
Pumpernickel bread	58
Apple	52
Chickpeas	47
Skim milk	46
Kidney beans	42
Fructose	32

SOURCE: Foster-Powell and Brand Miller (1995).

density lipoprotein cholesterol concentration that are known to be influenced by GI (Liu et al., 2001). Although the glycemic response of diabetics is distinctly higher than that of healthy individuals, the relative response to different types of mixed meals is similar (Indar-Brown et al., 1992; Wolever et al., 1985). The prediction of GI in mixed meals by Wolever and Jenkins (1986) is shown in Figure 6-1. In contrast, some studies reported no such relationship between the calculated and measured GI of mixed meals (Coulston et al., 1984; Hollenbeck et al., 1986; Laine et al., 1987).

There are a number of reasons why different groups have reported different findings on the calculation of GI in mixed meals. As previously discussed, there are a number of intrinsic (e.g., particle size) and extrinsic (e.g., ingestion of fat and protein, degree of food preparation) factors that can affect the glycemic response of a meal (Table 6-2), some of which are known to also affect the absorption of other nutrients such as vitamins and minerals. For instance, coingestion of dietary fat and protein can sometimes have a significant influence on the glucose response of a carbohydrate-containing food, with a reduction in the glucose response generally seen with increases in fat or protein content (Gulliford et al., 1989; Holt et al.,

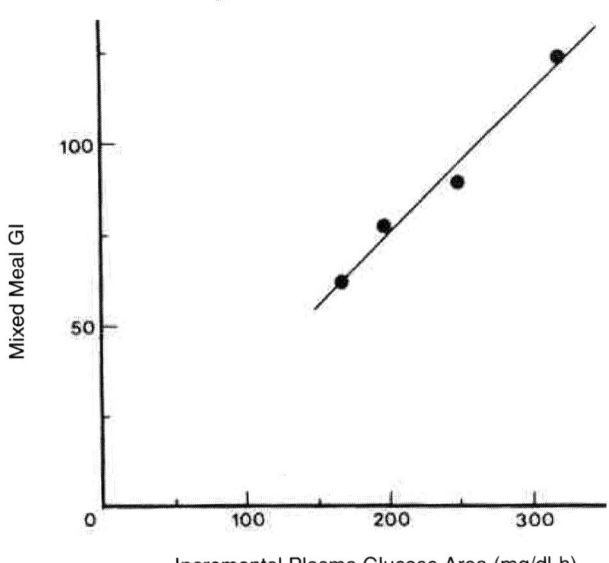

Incremental Plasma Glucose Area (mg/dl-h)

FIGURE 6-1 Correlation between calculated glycemic index (GI) of four test meals (•) and incremental blood glucose response areas. Based on data from Coulston et al. (1984). Reproduced, with permission, from Wolever and Jenkins (1986). Copyright 1986 by the American Society for Clinical Nutrition.

1997). Palatability can have an influence on GI, independent of food type and composition (Sawaya et al., 2001). Furthermore, there are expected inherent biological variations in glucose control and carbohydrate tolerance that are unrelated to the GI of a meal. Finally, varied experimental design and methods for calculating the area under the blood glucose curve can result in a different glycemic response to meals of a similar predicted GI (Coulston et al., 1984; Wolever and Jenkins, 1986). For instance, it is important that the incremental area, rather than the absolute area, under the blood glucose curve be measured (Wolever and Jenkins, 1986). Taken together, the results from these different studies indicate that the GI of mixed meals can usually be predicted from the GI of individual food components.

Physiology of Digestion, Absorption, and Metabolism

Digestion

Starch. The breakdown of starch begins in the mouth where salivary amylase acts on the interior α-(1,4) linkages of amylose and amylopectin. The digestion of these linkages continues in the intestine where pancreatic amylase is released. Amylase digestion produces large oligosaccharides (α-limit dextrins) that contain approximately eight glucose units of one or more α-(1,6) linkages. The α-(1,6) linkages are cleaved more easily than the α-(1,4) linkages.

Oligosaccharides and Sugars. The microvilli of the small intestine extend into an unstirred water layer phase of the intestinal lumen. When a limit dextrin, trisaccharide, or disaccharide enters the unstirred water layer, it is rapidly hydrolyzed by enzymes bound to the brush border membrane. These limit dextrins, produced from starch digestion, are degraded by glucoamylase, which removes glucose units from the nonreducing end to yield maltose and isomaltose. Maltose and isomaltose are degraded by intestinal brush border disaccharidases (e.g., maltase and sucrase). Maltase, sucrase, and lactase digest sucrose and lactose to monosaccharides prior to absorption.

Intestinal Absorption

Monosaccharides first diffuse across to the enterocyte surface, followed by movement across the brush border membrane by one of two mechanisms: active transport or facilitated diffusion.

Active Transport. The intestine is one of two organs that vectorially transports hexoses across the cell into the bloodstream. The mature enterocytes capture the hexoses directly ingested from food or produced from the digestion of di- and polysaccharides. Active transport of sugars involves sodium dependent glucose transporters (SGLTs) in the brush border membrane (Díez-Sampedro et al., 2001). Sodium is pumped from the cell to create a gradient between the interior of the cell and the lumen of the intestine, requiring the hydrolysis of adenosine triphosphate (ATP). The resultant gradient results in the cotransport of one molecule each of sodium and glucose. Glucose is then transported across the basolateral membrane of the small intestine by glucose transporter (GLUT) 2. Similar to glucose, galactose utilizes SGLT cotransporters and basolateral GLUT 2. Fructose is not transported by SGLT cotransporters.

Facilitated Diffusion. There are also transporters of glucose that require neither sodium nor ATP. The driving force for glucose transport is the glucose gradient and the energy change that occurs when the unstirred water layer is replaced with glucose. In this type of transport, called facilitated diffusion, glucose is transported down its concentration gradient (from high to low). Fructose is also transported by facilitated diffusion. One facilitated glucose transporter, GLUT 5, has been identified in the small intestine (Levin, 1999). GLUT 5 appears to transport glucose poorly and is the main transporter of fructose.

Metabolism

Cellular Uptake. Absorbed sugars are transported throughout the body to cells as a source of energy. The concentration of glucose in the blood is highly regulated by the release of insulin. Uptake of glucose by the adipocyte and muscle cell is dependent upon the binding of insulin to a membrane-bound insulin receptor that increases the translocation of intracellular glucose transporters (GLUT 4) to the cell membrane surface for uptake of glucose. GLUT 1 is the transporter of the red blood cell; however, it is also present in the plasma membrane of many other tissues (Levin, 1999). Besides its involvement in the small intestine, GLUT 2 is expressed in the liver and can also transport galactose, mannose, and fructose (Levin, 1999). GLUT 3 is important in the transport of glucose into the brain (Levin, 1999).

Intracellular Utilization of Galactose. Absorbed galactose is primarily the result of lactose digestion. The majority of galactose is taken up by the liver where it is metabolized to galactose-1-phosphate, which is then converted to glucose-1-phosphate. Most of the glucose-1-phosphate derived from galactose metabolism is converted to glycogen for storage.

Intracellular Utilization of Fructose. Absorbed fructose, from either direct ingestion of fructose or digestion of sucrose, is transported to the liver and phosphorylated to fructose-1-phosphate, an intermediate of the glycolytic pathway, which is further cleaved to glyceraldehyde and dihydroxyacetone phosphate (DHAP). DHAP is an intermediary metabolite in both the glycolytic and gluconeogenic pathways. The glyceraldehyde can be converted to glycolytic intermediary metabolites that serve as precursors for glycogen synthesis. Glyceraldehyde can also be used for triacylglycerol synthesis, provided that sufficient amounts of malonyl coenzyme A (CoA) (a precursor for fatty acid synthesis) are available.

Intracellular Utilization of Glucose. Glucose is a major fuel used by most cells in the body. In muscle, glucose is metabolized anaerobically to lactate via the glycolytic pathway. Pyruvate is decarboxylated to acetyl CoA, which enters the tricarboxylic acid (TCA) cycle. Reduced coenyzmes generated in the TCA cycle pass off their electrons to the electron transport system, where it is completely oxidized to carbon dioxide and water. This results in the production of the high-energy ATP that is needed for many other metabolic reactions. After the consumption of carbohydrates, fat oxidation is markedly curtailed, allowing glucose oxidation to provide most of the body's energy needs. In this manner, the body's glucose and glycogen content can be reduced toward more normal concentrations.

Gluconeogenesis. Glucose can be synthesized via gluconeogenesis, a metabolic pathway that requires energy. Gluconeogenesis in the liver and renal cortex is inhibited via insulin following the consumption of carbohydrates and is activated during fasting, allowing the liver to continue to release glucose to maintain adequate blood glucose concentrations.

Glycogen Synthesis and Utilization. Glucose can also be converted to glycogen (glycogenesis), which contains α-(1-4) and α-(1-6) linkages of glucose units. Glycogen is present in the muscle for storage and utilization and in the liver for storage, export, and maintenance of blood glucose concentrations. Glycogenesis is activated in skeletal muscle by a rise in insulin concentration following the consumption of carbohydrate. In the liver, glycogenesis is activated directly by an increase in circulating glucose, fructose, galactose, or insulin concentration. Muscle glycogen is mainly used in the muscle. Following glycogenolysis, glucose can be exported from the liver for maintenance of normal blood glucose concentrations and for use by other tissues.

Formation of Amino Acids and Fatty Acids from Carbohydrates. Pyruvate and intermediates of the TCA cycle are precursors of certain nonessential amino acids. A limited amount of carbohydrate is converted to fat because de novo lipogenesis is generally quite minimal (Hellerstein, 1999; Parks and Hellerstein, 2000). This finding is true for those who are obese, indicating that the vast majority of deposited fat is not derived from dietary carbohydrate when consumed at moderate levels.

Insulin. Based on the metabolic functions of insulin discussed above, the ingestion of carbohydrate produces an immediate increase in plasma insulin concentrations. This immediate rise in plasma insulin concentration minimizes the extent of hyperglycemia after a meal. The effects of insulin deficiency (elevated blood glucose concentration) are exemplified by type 1 diabetes. Individuals who have type 2 diabetes may or may not produce insulin and insulin-dependent muscle and adipose tissue cells may or may not respond to increased insulin concentrations (insulin resistant); therefore, circulating glucose is not effectively taken up by these tissues and metabolized.

Clinical Effects of Inadequate Intake

The lower limit of dietary carbohydrate compatible with life apparently is zero, provided that adequate amounts of protein and fat are consumed. However, the amount of dietary carbohydrate that provides for optimal health in humans is unknown. There are traditional populations that ingested a high fat, high protein diet containing only a minimal amount of carbohydrate for extended periods of time (Masai), and in some cases for a lifetime after infancy (Alaska and Greenland Natives, Inuits, and Pampas indigenous people) (Du Bois, 1928; Heinbecker, 1928). There was no apparent effect on health or longevity. Caucasians eating an essentially carbohydrate-free diet, resembling that of Greenland natives, for a year tolerated the diet quite well (Du Bois, 1928). However, a detailed modern comparison with populations ingesting the majority of food energy as carbohydrate has never been done.

It has been shown that rats and chickens grow and mature successfully on a carbohydrate-free diet (Brito et al., 1992; Renner and Elcombe, 1964), but only if adequate protein and glycerol from triacylglycerols are provided in the diet as substrates for gluconeogenesis. It has also been shown that rats grow and thrive on a 70 percent protein, carbohydrate-free diet (Gannon et al., 1985). Azar and Bloom (1963) also reported that nitrogen balance in adults ingesting a carbohydrate-free diet required the ingestion of 100 to 150 g of protein daily. This, plus the glycerol obtained from triacylglycerol in the diet, presumably supplied adequate substrate for gluconeogenesis and thus provided at least a minimal amount of completely oxidizable glucose.

The ability of humans to starve for weeks after endogenous glycogen supplies are essentially exhausted is also indicative of the ability of humans to survive without an exogenous supply of glucose or monosaccharides convertible to glucose in the liver (fructose and galactose). However, adaptation to a fat and protein fuel requires considerable metabolic adjustments.

The only cells that have an absolute requirement for glucose as an oxidizable fuel are those in the central nervous system (i.e., brain) and those cells that depend upon anaerobic glycolysis (i.e., the partial oxidation of glucose to produce lactate and alanine as a source of energy), such as red blood cells, white blood cells, and medulla of the kidney. The central nervous system can adapt to a dietary fat-derived fuel, at least in part (Cahill, 1970; Sokoloff, 1973). Also, the glycolyzing cells can obtain their complete energy needs from the indirect oxidation of fatty acids through the lactate and alanine-glucose cycles.

In the absence of dietary carbohydrate, de novo synthesis of glucose requires amino acids derived from the hydrolysis of endogenous or dietary protein or glycerol derived from fat. Therefore, the marginal amount of carbohydrate required in the diet in an energy-balanced state is conditional and dependent upon the remaining composition of the diet. Nevertheless, there may be subtle and unrecognized, untoward effects of a very low carbohydrate diet that may only be apparent when populations not genetically or traditionally adapted to this diet adopt it. This remains to be determined but is a reasonable expectation.

Of particular concern in a Western, urbanized society is the long-term consequences of a diet sufficiently low in carbohydrate such that it creates a chronically increased production of β-hydroxybutyric and acetoacetic acids (i.e., keto acids). The concern is that such a diet, deficient in water-soluble vitamins and some minerals, may result in bone mineral loss, may cause hypercholesterolemia, may increase the risk of urolithiasis (Vining, 1999), and may affect the development and function of the central nervous system. It also may adversely affect an individual's general sense of well being (Bloom and Azar, 1963), although in men starved for an extended period of time, encephalographic tracings remained unchanged and psychometric testing showed no deficits (Owen et al., 1967). It also may not provide for adequate stores of glycogen. The latter is required for hypoglycemic emergencies and for maximal short-term power production by muscles (Hultman et al., 1999).

EVIDENCE CONSIDERED FOR ESTIMATING THE AVERAGE REQUIREMENT FOR CARBOHYDRATE

The endogenous glucose production rate, and thus the utilization rate, depends on the duration of starvation. Glucose production has been determined in a number of laboratories using isotopically labeled glucose (Amiel et al., 1991; Arslanian and Kalhan, 1992; Bier et al., 1977; Denne and Kalhan, 1986; Kalhan et al., 1986; King et al., 1982; Patel and Kalhan, 1992). In overnight fasted adults (i.e., postabsorptive state), glucose production is approximately 2 to 2.5 mg/kg/min, or approximately 2.8 to 3.6 g/kg/d. In a 70-kg man, this represents approximately 210 to 270 g/d. In the postabsorptive state, approximately 50 percent of glucose production comes from glycogenolysis in liver and 50 percent from gluconeogenesis in the liver (Chandramouli et al., 1997; Landau et al., 1996).

The minimal amount of carbohydrate required, either from endogenous or exogenous sources, is determined by the brain's requirement for glucose. The brain is the only true carbohydrate-dependent organ in that it oxidizes glucose completely to carbon dioxide and water. Normally, the brain uses glucose almost exclusively for its energy needs. The endogenous glucose production rate in a postabsorptive state correlates very well with the estimated size of the brain from birth to adult life. However, not all of the glucose produced is utilized by the brain (Bier et al., 1977; Felig, 1973). The requirement for glucose has been reported to be approximately 110 to 140 g/d in adults (Cahill et al., 1968). Nevertheless, even the brain can adapt to a carbohydrate-free, energy-sufficient diet, or to starvation, by utilizing ketoacids for part of its fuel requirements. When glucose production or availability decreases below that required for the complete energy requirements for the brain, there is a rise in ketoacid production in the liver in order to provide the brain with an alternative fuel. This has been referred to as "ketosis." Generally, this occurs in a starving person only after glycogen stores in the liver are reduced to a low concentration and the contribution of hepatic glycogenolysis is greatly reduced or absent (Cahill et al., 1968). It is associated with approximately a 20 to 50 percent decrease in circulating glucose and insulin concentration (Carlson et al., 1994; Owen et al., 1998; Streja et al., 1977). These are signals for adipose cells to increase lipolysis and release nonesterified fatty acids and glycerol into the circulation. The signal also is reinforced by an increase in circulating epinephrine, norepinephrine, glucagon, and growth hormone concentration (Carlson et al., 1994). The nonesterified fatty acids are removed by the liver and converted into ketoacids, which then diffuse out of the liver into the circulation. The increase in nonesterified fatty acids results in a concentration-dependent exponential increase in ketoacids (Hanson et al., 1965); glucagon facilitates this process (Mackrell and Sokal, 1969).

In an overnight fasted person, the circulating ketoacid concentration is very low, but with prolonged starvation the concentration increases dramatically and may exceed the molar concentration of glucose (Cahill, 1970; Streja et al., 1977). In individuals fully adapted to starvation, ketoacid oxidation can account for approximately 80 percent of the brain's energy requirements (Cahill et al., 1973). Thus, only 22 to 28 g/d of glucose are required to fuel the brain. This is similar to the total glucose oxidation rate integrated over 24 hours determined by isotope-dilution studies in these starving individuals (Carlson et al., 1994; Owen et al., 1998).

Overall, the key to the metabolic adaptation to extended starvation is the rise in circulating nonesterified fatty acid concentrations and the large increase in ketoacid production. The glycerol released from the hydrolysis of triacylglycerols stored in fat cells becomes a significant source of substrate for gluconeogenesis, but the conversion of amino acids derived from protein catabolism into glucose is also an important source. Interestingly, in people who consumed a protein-free diet, total nitrogen excretion was reported to be in the range of 2.5 to 3.5 g/d (35 to 50 mg/kg), or the equivalent of 16 to 22 g of catabolized protein in a 70-kg man (Raguso et al., 1999). Thus, it is similar to that in starving individuals (3.7 g/d) (Owen et al., 1998). Overall, this represents the minimal amount of protein oxidized through gluconeogenic pathways (Du Bois, 1928). This amount of protein is considerably less than the Recommended Dietary Allowance (RDA) of 0.8 g/kg/d for adults with a normal body mass index (Chapter 10). For a 70-kg lean male, this equals 56 g/d of protein, which is greater than the estimated obligate daily loss in body protein from the shedding of cells, secretions, and other miscellaneous functions (approximately 6 to 8 g/d for a 70-kg man; see Chapter 10) and has been assumed to be due to inefficient utilization of amino acids for synthesis of replacement proteins and other amino acid-derived products (Gannon and Nuttall, 1999). In part, it also may represent the technical difficulty in determining a minimal daily protein requirement (see Chapter 10).

If 56 g/d of dietary protein is required for protein homeostasis, but the actual daily loss of protein is only approximately 7 g, then presumably the remaining difference (49 g) is metabolized and may be utilized for new glucose production. It has been determined that for ingested animal protein, approximately 0.56 g of glucose can be derived from every 1 g of protein ingested (Janney, 1915). Thus, from the 49 g of protein not directly utilized to replace loss of endogenous protein or not used for other synthetic processes, approximately 27 g (0.56 × 49) of glucose may be produced. In people on a protein-free diet or who are starving, the 16 to 22 g of catabolized protein could provide 10 to 14 g of glucose.

If the starving individual's energy requirement is 1,800 kcal/d and 95 percent is supplied by fat oxidation either directly or indirectly through oxidation of ketoacids (Cahill et al., 1973), then fat oxidation represents 1,710 kcal/d, or 190 g based upon approximately 9 kcal/g fat. The glycerol content of a typical triacylglycerol is 10 percent by weight, or in this case 19 g of glycerol, which is equivalent to approximately 19 g of glucose. This, plus the amount of glucose potentially derived from protein, gives a total of approximately 30 to 34 g ([10 to 14] + 19). Thus, a combination of protein and fat utilization is required to supply the small amount of glucose still required by the brain in a person fully adapted to starvation. Presumably this also would be the obligatory glucose requirement in people adapted to a carbohydrate-free diet. Thus, the normal metabolic adaptation to a lack of dietary protein, as occurs in a starving person in whom the protein metabolized is in excess of that lost daily, is to provide the glucose required by the brain. Nevertheless, utilization of this amount of glucose by the brain is vitally important. Without it, function deteriorates dramatically, at least in the brain of rats (Sokoloff, 1973).

The required amount of glucose could be derived easily from ingested protein alone if the individual was ingesting a carbohydrate-free, but energy-adequate diet containing protein sufficient for nitrogen balance. However, ingested amounts of protein greater than 30 to 34 g/d would likely stimulate insulin secretion unless ingested in small amounts throughout a 24-hour period. For example, ingestion of 25 to 50 g of protein at a single time stimulates insulin secretion (Krezowski et al., 1986; Westphal et al., 1990), despite a lack of carbohydrate intake. This rise in insulin would result in a diminution in the release of fatty acids from adipose cells and as a consequence, reduce ketoacid formation and fatty acid oxidation. The ultimate effect would be to increase the requirement for glucose of the brain and other organs. Thus, the minimal amount of glucose irreversibly oxidized to carbon dioxide and water requires utilization of a finely balanced ratio of dietary fat and protein.

Azar and Bloom (1963) reported that 100 to 150 g/d of protein was necessary for maintenance of nitrogen balance. This amount of protein could typically provide amino acid substrate sufficient for the production of 56 to 84 g of glucose daily. However, daily infusion of 90 g of an amino acid mixture over 6 days to both postoperative and nonsurgical starving adults has been reported to reduce urinary nitrogen loss without a significant change in glucose or insulin concentration, but with a dramatic increase in ketoacids (Hoover et al., 1975). Thus, the issue becomes complex in nonstarving people.

Glucose utilization by the brain has been determined either by measuring arteriovenous gradients of glucose, oxygen, lactate, and ketones across the brain and the respiratory quotient (Kety, 1957; Sokoloff, 1973), or with estimates of brain blood flow determined by different methods (e.g., NO_2 diffusion). A major problem with studies based on arteriovenous differences is the limited accuracy of the blood flow methods used (Settergren et al., 1976, 1980). Using ^{18}F-2-fluoro-2-deoxyglucose and positron emission tomography, the rate of glucose accumulation in the brain also has been determined (Chugani, 1993; Chugani and Phelps, 1986; Chugani et al., 1987; Hatazawa et al., 1987). This is an indirect method for measuring glucose utilization, and also has limitations (Hatazawa et al., 1987). Brain O_2 consumption in association with the brain respiratory quotient also has been used as an indirect estimate of glucose utilization (Kalhan and Kiliç, 1999).

Only data determined by direct measurement of glucose arteriovenous difference across the brain in association with determination of brain blood flow can be considered for setting an Estimated Average Requirement (EAR), although the other, indirect methods yield similar results. The glucose consumption by the brain can be used along with information from Dobbing and Sands (1973) and Dekaban and Sadowsky (1978), which correlated weight of the brain with body weight to calculate glucose utilization.

FINDINGS BY LIFE STAGE AND GENDER GROUP

Infants Ages 0 Through 12 Months

Methods Considered to Set the AI

Carbohydrate Utilization by the Brain. In infants, the brain size relative to body size is greater than that in adults. The brain utilizes approximately 60 percent of the infant's total energy intake (Gibbons, 1998). Therefore, the turnover of glucose per kilogram of body weight can be up to fourfold greater in the infant compared to the adult (Kalhan and Kiliç, 1999).

The infant brain is fully capable of using ketoacids as fuel. In species in which the mothers' milk is very high in fat, such as in rats, the circulating ketoacid concentration is very high in the suckling pups, and the ketoacids are an important source of fuel for the developing brain (Edmond et al., 1985; Sokoloff, 1973). In addition, the gluconeogenic pathway is well developed even in premature human infants (Sunehag et al., 1999). Indeed, provided that adequate lipid and protein substrates are supplied, gluconeogenesis can account for the majority of glucose turnover. Whether gluconeogenesis can account for the entire glucose requirement in infants has not been tested.

Growth. Studies have been performed using artificial formula feedings and varying the fat and carbohydrate content while keeping the protein content constant (9 percent) (Fomon et al., 1976). Fomon and coworkers (1976) provided infants with formulas containing either 34 or 62 percent of energy from carbohydrate for 104 days. There were no significant differences in the length or weight of the infants fed the two formulas. Interestingly, it also did not affect the total food energy consumed over the 6 or 12 months of life. From the limited data available, the lowest intake that has been documented to be adequate is 30 percent of total food energy. However, it is likely that infants also may grow and develop normally on a very low or nearly carbohydrate-free diet since their brains' enzymatic machinery for oxidizing ketoacids is more efficient than it is in adults (Sokoloff, 1973).

Human Milk. The lower limit of dietary carbohydrate compatible with life or for optimal health in infants is unknown. Human milk is recognized as the optimal milk source for infants throughout at least the first year of life and is recommended as the sole nutritional milk source for infants during the first 4 to 6 months of life (IOM, 1991). Carbohydrate in human milk is almost exclusively lactose (Table 6-4). The only source of lactose in the animal kingdom is from the mammary gland and therefore is found only in mammals. Lactose is readily hydrolyzed in the infant intestine. The resulting glucose and galactose also readily pass into the portal venous system. They are carried to the liver where the galactose is converted to glucose and either stored as glycogen or released into the general circulation and oxidized. The net result is the provision of two glucose molecules for each lactose molecule ingested. The reason why lactose developed as the carbohydrate fuel produced by the mammary gland is not understood. One reason may be that the provision of a disaccharide compared to a monosaccharide reduces the osmolality of milk. Lactose has also been reported to facilitate calcium absorption from the gut, which otherwise is not readily absorbed from the immature infant intestine (Condon et al., 1970; Ziegler and Fomon, 1983). However, isotopic tracer data have not confirmed this (Kalhan and Kiliç, 1999).

The lactose content of human milk is approximately 74 g/L and changes little over the total nursing period (Dewey and Lönnerdal, 1983; Dewey et al., 1984; Lammi-Keefe et al., 1990; Nommsen et al., 1991) (Table 6-4). However, the volume of milk consumed by the infant decreases gradually over the first 12 months of life as other foods are gradually introduced into the feeding regimen. Over the first 6 months of life, the volume consumed is about 0.78 L/d (see Chapter 2); therefore approximately 60 g of carbohydrate represents about 37 percent of total food energy (see Chapter 5) (Nommsen et al., 1991). This amount of carbohydrate and the ratio of carbohydrate to fat in human milk can be assumed to be optimal for infant growth and development over the first 6 months of life.

TABLE 6-4 Total Carbohydrate Content of Human Milk

Reference	Stage of Lactation	Total Carbohydrate Content (g/L)	Total Lactose Content (g/L)	Total Glucose Content (g/L)
Anderson et al., 1981	3–5 d		51.4 ± 2.2	
	8–11 d		59.8 ± 2.3	
	26–29 d		65.1 ± 2.3	
Anderson et al., 1983	3 d	62 ± 9		
	7 d	67 ± 5		
	14 d	67 ± 6		
Dewey and Lönnerdal, 1983	1 mo		70.5 ± 5.6	
	2 mo		72.1 ± 6.2	
	3 mo		71.3 ± 7.9	
	4 mo		76.1 ± 4.0	
	5 mo		76.2 ± 3.3	
	6 mo		77.5 ± 2.7	
Dewey et al., 1984	4–6 mo		77.1 ± 3.0	
	7–11 mo		75.7 ± 3.6	
	12–20 mo		72.3 ± 4.3	
Neville et al., 1984	33–210 d Median 115 d		Mid-feed: 72.1 Pooled pumped: 71.8	Mid-feed: 0.27 Pooled pumped: 0.27
Ferris et al., 1988	2 wk		62.5 ± 6.5	
	6 wk		67.8 ± 6.4	
	12 wk		68.5 ± 7.3	
	16 wk		70.0 ± 6.5	
Lammi-Keefe et al., 1990	8 wk		76.2 ± 3.2	0.26 ± 0.05
			73.6 ± 3.8	0.31 ± 0.05
			77.4 ± 6.7	0.33 ± 0.06
			74.2 ± 4.7	0.33 ± 0.08
			80.1 ± 4.6	0.33 ± 0.06
Allen et al., 1991	21 d		63.4 ± 0.7	0.27 ± 0.01
	45 d		65.6 ± 0.4	0.27 ± 0.01
	90 d		67.7 ± 0.7	0.31 ± 0.01
	180 d		68.8 ± 1.4	0.32 ± 0.02
Nommsen et al., 1991	3 mo		74.4 ± 1.5	
	6 mo		74.4 ± 1.9	
	9 mo		73.5 ± 2.9	
	12 mo		74.0 ± 2.7	

continued

TABLE 6-4 Continued

Reference	Stage of Lactation	Total Carbohydrate Content (g/L)	Total Lactose Content (g/L)	Total Glucose Content (g/L)
Coppa et al., 1993	4 d	78.1 ± 8.08	56.0 ± 6.06	
	10 d	83.8 ± 6.45	62.5 ± 5.74	
	30 d	80.6 ± 6.90	64.1 ± 6.45	
	60 d	79.8 ± 7.01	66.2 ± 6.88	
	90 d	79.3 ± 7.03	66.3 ± 7.08	
	120 d	82.2 ± 10.31	68.9 ± 8.16	

The method used to set the Adequate Intake (AI) for older infants is carbohydrate intake from human milk and complementary foods (see Chapter 2). According to the Third National Health and Nutrition Examination Survey, the median carbohydrate intake from weaning food for ages 7 through 12 months was 50.7 ± 5 g/d (standard error of the mean). Based on an average volume of 0.6 L/d of human milk that is secreted (Chapter 2), the carbohydrate intake from human milk is 44 g/d (0.6 L/d × 74 g/L). Therefore, the total intake of carbohydrate from human milk and complementary foods is 95 g/d (44 + 51).

Carbohydrate AI Summary, Ages 0 Through 12 Months

The AI is based on the average intake of carbohydrate consumed from human milk and complementary foods.

AI for Infants
    0–6 months   **60 g/d of carbohydrate**
    7–12 months   **95 g/d of carbohydrate**

Special Considerations

The carbohydrate content of milk protein-based formulas for term infants is similar to that of human milk (70 to 74 g/L). Whole cow milk contains lower concentrations of carbohydrate than human milk (48 g/L) (Newburg and Neubauer, 1995). In addition to lactose, conventional infant formulas can also contain sucrose or glucose polymers.

Children and Adolescents Ages 1 Through 18 Years

Evidence Considered in Estimating the Average Requirement

In the newborn, the brain weight is approximately 380 g; by age 1 year this has increased to approximately 1,000 g in boys and approximately 980 g in girls (Dekaban and Sadowsky, 1978; Dobbing and Sands, 1973), with a corresponding increase in energy requirement. After 1 year of age, there is a further increase in brain weight up to 5 years of age (approximately 1,300 g in boys and 1,150 g in girls). Subsequently, the brain size increases only modestly. The consumption of glucose by the brain after age 1 year also remains rather constant or increases modestly and is in the range reported for adults (approximately 31 µmol/100 g of brain/min) (Kennedy and Sokoloff, 1957; Sokoloff et al., 1977). Therefore, the Estimated Average Requirement (EAR) for carbohydrate is set based on information used for adults (see "Adults Ages 19 Years and Older"). As for adults, the EAR is the same for both genders since differences in brain glucose utilization are small.

The amount of glucose produced from obligatory endogenous protein catabolism in children is not known. Therefore, this information was not considered in the derivation of the EAR for children. Children ages 2 to 9 years have requirements for carbohydrate that are similar to adults. This is based on population data in which animal-derived foods are ingested exclusively (e.g., Alaska and Greenland natives), as well as in children with epilepsy who have been treated with ketogenic diets for extended periods of time (Swink et al., 1997; Vining, 1999). In these children, the ketoacid concentration was in the range of 2 to 3 mmol/L (i.e., similar to that in a starving adult) (Nordli et al., 1992).

Carbohydrate EAR and RDA Summary, Ages 1 Through 18 Years

EAR for Children
1–3 years	100 g/d of carbohydrate
4–8 years	100 g/d of carbohydrate

EAR for Boys
9–13 years	100 g/d of carbohydrate
14–18 years	100 g/d of carbohydrate

EAR for Girls
9–13 years	100 g/d of carbohydrate
14–18 years	100 g/d of carbohydrate

The Recommended Dietary Allowance (RDA) for carbohydrate is set by using a coefficient of variation (CV) of 15 percent based on the variation in brain glucose utilization. The RDA is defined as equal to the EAR plus twice the CV to cover the needs of 97 to 98 percent of the individuals in the group (therefore, for carbohydrate the RDA is 130 percent of the EAR).

RDA for Children
| 1–3 years | 130 g/d of carbohydrate |
| 4–8 years | 130 g/d of carbohydrate |

RDA for Boys
| 9–13 years | 130 g/d of carbohydrate |
| 14–18 years | 130 g/d of carbohydrate |

RDA for Girls
| 9–13 years | 130 g/d of carbohydrate |
| 14–18 years | 130 g/d of carbohydrate |

Adults Ages 19 Years and Older

Evidence Considered in Estimating the Average Requirement

Glucose Utilization by the Brain. Long-term data in Westernized populations, which could determine the minimal amount of carbohydrate compatible with metabolic requirements and for optimization of health, are not available. Therefore, it is provisionally suggested that an EAR for carbohydrate ingestion in the context of overall food energy sufficiency be based on an amount of digestible carbohydrate that would provide the brain (i.e., central nervous system) with an adequate supply of glucose fuel without the requirement for additional glucose production from ingested protein or triacylglycerols. This amount of glucose should be sufficient to supply the brain with fuel in the absence of a rise in circulating acetoacetate and β-hydroxybutyrate concentrations greater than that observed in an individual after an overnight fast (see "Evidence Considered for Estimating the Average Requirement for Carbohydrate"). This assumes the consumption of an energy-sufficient diet containing an Acceptable Macronutrient Distribution Range of carbohydrate intake (approximately 45 to 65 percent of energy) (see Chapter 11).

Brain glucose utilization based on O_2 consumption is summarized in Table 6-5. Only data determined by direct measurement of glucose arteriovenous difference across the brain in association with determination of

TABLE 6-5 Indirect Estimates of Glucose Utilization by Measuring Brain Oxygen (O_2) Consumption

Reference	Study Population	O_2 Consumption (mL/100 g/min)	O_2 Consumption (L/100 g/d)
Kennedy and Sokoloff, 1957	2 children, 3 y	6.2	8.93
		5.6	8.06
Kennedy and Sokoloff, 1957	5 children, 4–7 y	5.3	7.63
		4.3	6.19
		4.4	6.34
		5.7	8.21
		4.4	6.34
Kennedy and Sokoloff, 1957	2 children, 10 and 11 y	5.7	8.21
		4.9	7.06
Kennedy and Sokoloff, 1957	12 adults	4.18	6.02

[a] For males, based on Dekaban and Sadowsy (1978) and Dobbing and Sands (1973).
[b] O_2 = 4.8 kcal/L = 1.2 g of glucose/L.

brain blood flow (Table 6-6) were considered for setting an EAR, although both methods yielded similar results. Data on glucose consumption by the brain for various age groups using information from Dobbing and Sands (1973) and Dekaban and Sadowsky (1978) were also used, which correlated weight of the brain with body weight. The average rate of brain glucose utilization in the postabsorptive state of adults based on several studies is approximately 33 µmol/100 g of brain/min (5.5 mg/100 g of brain/min or 8.64 g/100 g of brain/d) (Table 6-6). Based on these data, the brain's requirement for carbohydrate is in the range of approximately 117 to 142 g/d (Gottstein and Held, 1979; Reinmuth et al., 1965; Scheinberg and Stead, 1949; Sokoloff et al., 1977). Regardless of age and the associated change in brain mass, the glucose utilization rate/100 g of brain tissue remains rather constant, at least up to age 73 years (Reinmuth et al., 1965). In 351 men (aged 21 to 39 years), the average brain weight at autopsy was reported to be 1.45 kg, with a standard deviation of only 0.02 kg. In 201 women of the same age range, the average brain weight was 1.29 kg with a standard deviation of 0.03 kg. There was excellent correlation between body weight and height and brain weight in adults of all ages.

The glucose produced from the obligatory turnover of protein plus the glucose produced from glycerol is approximately 30 g/d (see "Evi-

Estimated Brain Weight (g)[a]	O₂ Consumption (L/d)	Glucose Consumption (g/d)[b]
1,200	107.1	129
1,200	96.8	116
1,260	96.2	115
1,260	78.0	94
1,300	82.4	99
1,300	109.2	131
1,300	84.3	101
1,360	111.6	134
1,360	96.0	115
1,450	84.3	101

dence Considered for Estimating the Average Requirement for Carbohydrate"). Therefore, the overall dietary carbohydrate requirement in the presence of an energy-adequate diet would be approximately 87 (117 − 30) to 112 (142 − 30) g/d. This amount of carbohydrate is similar to that reported to be required for the prevention of ketosis (50 to 100 g) (Bell et al., 1969; Calloway, 1971; Gamble, 1946; Sapir et al., 1972) and to that reported to have a maximal protein sparing effect when glucose was ingested daily (Gamble, 1946). The carbohydrate requirement is modestly greater than the potential glucose that can be derived from an amount of ingested protein required for nitrogen balance in people ingesting a carbohydrate-free diet (Azar and Bloom, 1963).

This amount of carbohydrate will not provide sufficient fuel for those cells that are dependent on anaerobic glycolysis for their energy supply (e.g., red and white blood cells). For glycolyzing cells, approximately 36 g/d are necessary (Cahill, 1970). Glycolyzing cells can obtain energy through the functioning of the Cori cycle (i.e., lactate to glucose to lactate) and the alanine-glucose cycle. That is, the cyclic interconversion of glucose with lactate or alanine occurs without a net loss of carbon.

In the absence of carbohydrate in the diet, and in the absence of a rise in ketoacids above the overnight fasting reference range, ingested protein

TABLE 6-6 Direct Estimates of Glucose Utilization by Measuring Brain Glucose Consumption

Reference	Study Population	Glucose Consumption (μmol/100 g of brain/min)	Estimated Brain Weight (g)[a]	Glucose Consumption	
				(mg/min)	(g/d)
Settergren et al., 1976	12 infants, average 5 mo	27	400	19.4	28
Mehta et al., 1977	10 infants, average 11 mo	66	1,000	118	170
Settergren et al., 1980	42 infants and children, 3 wk–14 y	25	400–1,450	18–65	26–94
Scheinberg and Stead, 1949	18 adults, 18–36 y	34	1,450	88	127
Reinmuth et al., 1965	13 adults, 21–29 y	38	1,450	99	142
Sokoloff et al., 1977	Adults	31	1,450	81	117
Gottstein and Held, 1979	24 adults, 21–43 y	31	1,450	81	117

[a] Based on Dekaban and Sadowsy (1978) and Dobbing and Sands (1973).

sufficient to provide the brain with glucose fuel is theoretically possible, but is not likely to be acceptable. The amount of dietary protein required approaches the theoretical maximal rate of gluconeogenesis from amino acids in the liver (135 g of glucose/24 h) (Brosnan, 1999).

In summary, the EAR for total carbohydrate is set at 100 g/d. This amount should be sufficient to fuel central nervous system cells without having to rely on a partial replacement of glucose by ketoacids. Although the latter are used by the brain in a concentration-dependent fashion (Sokoloff, 1973), their utilization only becomes quantitatively significant when the supply of glucose is considerably reduced and their circulating concentration has increased several-fold over that present after an overnight fast.

Diets contain a combination of carbohydrate, fat, and protein, and therefore available glucose is not limiting to the brain unless carbohydrate energy intake is insufficient to meet the glucose needs of the brain. Nevertheless, it should be recognized that the brain can still receive enough glucose from the metabolism of the glycerol component of fat and from the gluconeogenic amino acids in protein when a very low carbohydrate diet is consumed.

Aging. It is well known that the overall rate of energy metabolism decreases with aging (Roberts, 2000a). Also, the total body glucose oxidation rate is decreased, but only modestly. In adults 70 years of age or older, the glucose oxidation rate was only about 10 percent less than in young adults between 19 and 29 years of age (Robert et al., 1982).

The actual brain mass slowly decreases after age 45 to 55 years. In 76- to 80-year-old men, the average brain mass was 1.33 kg, and for women in the same age range it was 1.19 kg (i.e., a loss of 8 to 9 percent of mass) (Dekaban and Sadawosky, 1978). This decrease is similar to that reported from autopsy data in Japan (mean 1,422 to 1,336 g) (Yamaura et al., 1980). Whether glucose oxidation changes out of proportion to brain mass remains a controversial issue (Gottstein and Held, 1979; Leenders et al., 1990). In any case, the decrease in brain glucose oxidation rate is not likely to be substantially less. Therefore, the EAR is the same for all adults. There is no evidence to indicate that a certain amount of carbohydrate should be provided as starch or sugars. However, most individuals do not choose to eat a diet in which sugars exceed approximately 30 percent of energy (Nuttall and Gannon, 1981).

Carbohydrate EAR and RDA Summary, Ages 19 Years and Older

EAR for Men

19–30 years	100 g/d of carbohydrate
31–50 years	100 g/d of carbohydrate
51–70 years	100 g/d of carbohydrate
> 70 years	100 g/d of carbohydrate

EAR for Women

19–30 years	100 g/d of carbohydrate
31–50 years	100 g/d of carbohydrate
51–70 years	100 g/d of carbohydrate
> 70 years	100 g/d of carbohydrate

The RDA for carbohydrate is set by using a CV of 15 percent based on the variation in brain glucose utilization. The RDA is defined as equal to the

EAR plus twice the CV to cover the needs of 97 to 98 percent of the individuals in the group (therefore, for carbohydrate the RDA is 130 percent of the EAR).

RDA for Men
19–30 years	130 g/d of carbohydrate
31–50 years	130 g/d of carbohydrate
51–70 years	130 g/d of carbohydrate
> 70 years	130 g/d of carbohydrate

RDA for Women
19–30 years	130 g/d of carbohydrate
31–50 years	130 g/d of carbohydrate
51–70 years	130 g/d of carbohydrate
> 70 years	130 g/d of carbohydrate

Pregnancy

Evidence Considered in Estimating the Average Requirement

Pregnancy results in an increased metabolic rate and thus an increased fuel requirement. This increased fuel requirement is due to the establishment of the placental–fetal unit and an increased energy supply for growth and development of the fetus. It is also necessary for the maternal adaptation to the pregnant state and for moving about the increased mass of the pregnant woman. This increased need for metabolic fuel often includes an increased maternal storage of fat early in pregnancy, as well as sufficient energy to sustain the growth of the fetus during the last trimester of pregnancy (Knopp et al., 1973).

In spite of the recognized need for increased energy-yielding substrates imposed by pregnancy, the magnitude of need, as well as how much of the increased requirement needs to be met from exogenous sources, remains incompletely understood and is highly variable (Tables 5-23 through 5-27). There is general agreement that the additional food energy requirement is relatively small. Several doubly labeled water studies indicate a progressive increase in total energy expenditure over the 36 weeks of pregnancy (Forsum et al., 1992; Goldberg et al., 1993; Kopp-Hoolihan et al., 1999) (Table 5-27). The mean difference in energy expenditure between week 0 and 36 in the studies was approximately 460 kcal/d and is proportional to body weight.

The developing fetus utilizes glucose as an energy-yielding substrate. However, there is some evidence that the fetus can utilize maternally provided ketoacids. The fetus does not utilize significant amounts of free fatty acids (Rudolf and Sherwin, 1983).

As part of the adaptation to pregnancy, there is a decrease in maternal blood glucose concentration, a development of insulin resistance, and a tendency to develop ketosis (Burt and Davidson, 1974; Cousins et al., 1980; Phelps et al., 1981; Rudolf and Sherwin, 1983; Ryan et al., 1985).

A higher mean respiratory quotient for both the basal metabolic rate and total 24-hour energy expenditure has also been reported in pregnant women when compared to the postpartum period. This indicates an increased utilization of glucose by the maternal–fetal unit. The increased glucose utilization rate persists after fasting, indicating an increased endogenous production rate as well (Assel et al., 1993; Kalhan et al., 1997) (see Chapter 5). Thus, irrespective of whether there is an increase in total energy expenditure, these data indicate an increase in glucose utilization. Earlier, it was reported that the glucose turnover in the overnight fasted state based on maternal weight gain remains unchanged from that in the nonpregnant state (Cowett et al., 1983; Kalhan et al., 1979).

The fetus reportedly uses approximately 8 ml O_2/kg/min or 56 kcal/ kg/d (Sparks et al., 1980). For a 3-kg term fetus, this is equivalent to 168 kcal/d. The transfer of glucose from the mother to the fetus has been estimated to be 17 to 26 g/d in late gestation (Hay, 1994). If this is the case, then glucose can only account for approximately 51 percent of the total oxidizable substrate transferred to the fetus at this stage of gestation.

The mean newborn infant brain weight is reported to be approximately 380 g (Dekaban and Sadowsky, 1978). Assuming the glucose consumption rate is the same for infants and adults (approximately 33 µmol/100 g of brain/min or 8.64 g/100 g of brain/d) (see "Adults Ages 19 Years and Older"), and that ketoacids do not supply a significant amount of oxidizable substrate for the fetal brain in utero, the glucose requirement at the end of pregnancy would be approximately 32.5 g/d. This is greater than the total amount of glucose transferred daily from the mother to the fetus.

Data obtained in newborns indicate that glucose oxidation can only account for approximately 70 percent of the brain's estimated fuel requirement (Denne and Kalhan, 1986). Whether this is the case in the late-term fetus is not known. However, the fetal brain can clearly utilize ketoacids (Patel et al., 1975). In addition, an increase in circulating ketoacids is common in pregnant women (Homko et al., 1999). Taken together, these data suggest that ketoacids may be utilized by the fetal brain in utero. If nonglucose sources (largely ketoacids) supply 30 percent of the fuel requirement of the fetal brain, then the brain glucose utilization rate would be 23 g/d (32.5 g × 0.70). This is essentially the same as the average maternal–fetal glucose transfer rate (mean 22 g, range 17 to 26 g) (Hay,

1994). These data also indicate that the fetal brain utilizes essentially all of the glucose derived from the mother.

In order to assure provision of glucose to the fetal brain (approximately 33 g/d) as a fuel in the absence of utilization of a lipid-derived fuel, as well as to supply the glucose fuel requirement for the mother's brain independent of utilization of ketoacids (or other substrates), the EAR for metabolically available dietary carbohydrate is the EAR for nonpregnant women (100 g/d) plus the additional amount required during the last trimester of pregnancy (35 g/d), or 135 g/d. There is no evidence to indicate that a certain portion of the carbohydrate must be consumed as starch or sugars.

EAR and RDA Summary, Pregnancy

EAR for Pregnancy
14–18 years	135 g/d of carbohydrate
19–30 years	135 g/d of carbohydrate
31–50 years	135 g/d of carbohydrate

The RDA for carbohydrate is set by using a CV of 15 percent based on the variation in brain glucose utilization. The RDA is defined as equal to the EAR plus twice the CV to cover the needs of 97 to 98 percent of the individuals in the group (therefore, for carbohydrate the RDA is 130 percent of the EAR). The calculated values for the RDAs have been rounded.

RDA for Pregnancy
14–18 years	175 g/d of carbohydrate
19–30 years	175 g/d of carbohydrate
31–50 years	175 g/d of carbohydrate

Lactation

Evidence Considered in Estimating the Average Requirement

The requirement for carbohydrate is increased during lactation. The lactose content of human milk is approximately 74 g/L; this concentration changes very little during the nursing period. Therefore, the amount of precursors necessary for lactose synthesis must increase. Lactose is synthesized from glucose and as a consequence, an increased supply of glucose must be obtained from ingested carbohydrate or from an increased supply of amino acids in order to prevent utilization of the lactating woman's endogenous proteins. Glycerol derived from endogenous or exogenous fat may contribute to the increased production of glucose through gluco-neogenesis. However, the amount of fat that can be oxidized daily greatly limits the contribution of glycerol to glucose production and thus lactose formation.

The EAR during lactation is the sum of the carbohydrate intake neces-sary to replace the carbohydrate secreted in human milk (60 g/d) and the EAR for adolescent girls and women (100 g/d). The EAR for carbohydrate during lactation is set at 160 g/d.

EAR and RDA Summary, Lactation

EAR for Lactation
14–18 years	**160 g/d of carbohydrate**
19–30 years	**160 g/d of carbohydrate**
31–50 years	**160 g/d of carbohydrate**

The RDA for carbohydrate is set by using a CV of 15 percent based on the variation in brain glucose utilization. The RDA is defined as equal to the EAR plus twice the CV to cover the needs of 97 to 98 percent of the individuals in the group (therefore, for carbohydrate the RDA is 130 per-cent of the EAR). The calculated values for the RDAs have been rounded.

RDA for Lactation
14–18 years	**210 g/d of carbohydrate**
19–30 years	**210 g/d of carbohydrate**
31–50 years	**210 g/d of carbohydrate**

Special Considerations

Individuals adapted to a very low carbohydrate diet can perform ade-quately for extended periods of time at power outputs represented by exercise at less than 65 percent O_2 max (Miller and Wolfe, 1999). For extended periods of power output exceeding this level, the dependence on carbohydrate as a fuel increases rapidly to near total dependence (Miller and Wolfe, 1999). Therefore, for such individuals there must be a corre-sponding increase in carbohydrate derived directly from carbohydrate-containing foods. Additional consumption of dietary protein may assist in meeting the need through gluconeogenesis, but it is unlikely to be con-sumed in amounts necessary to meet the individual's need. A requirement for such individuals cannot be determined since the requirement for carbohydrate will depend on the particular energy expenditure for some defined period of time (Brooks and Mercier, 1994).

INTAKE OF CARBOHYDRATES

Food Sources

White, brown, and raw sugars represent different forms and purification of sucrose. Corn syrups are the hydrolytic products of starch digestion. They are composed of various proportions of glucose (dextrose), maltose, trisaccharides, and higher molecular-weight products including some starch itself. Another source of carbohydrate, high fructose corn syrup, is often misunderstood. These syrups are also derived from cornstarch through the conversion of a portion of the glucose present in starch into fructose. The fructose content present in corn syrup is 42, 55, or 90 percent. The great majority of the remaining content is glucose. Other sources of sugars include malt syrup, comprised largely of sucrose; honey, which resembles sucrose in its composition but is composed of individual glucose and fructose molecules; and molasses, a by-product of table sugar production.

With the introduction of high fructose corn sweeteners in 1967, the amount of "free" fructose in the diet of Americans has increased considerably (Hallfrisch, 1990). Nonalcoholic beverages (e.g., soft drinks and fruit-flavored drinks) are the major dietary sources of added fructose; fruits and fruit products are the major dietary sources of naturally occurring fructose (Park and Yetley, 1993).

Using 1994–1996 U.S. Department of Agriculture food consumption survey data, nondiet soft drinks were the leading source of added sugars in Americans' diets, accounting for one-third of added sugars intake (Guthrie and Morton, 2000). This was followed by sugars and sweets (16 percent), sweetened grains (13 percent), fruit ades/drinks (10 percent), sweetened dairy (9 percent), and breakfast cereals and other grains (10 percent). Together, these foods and beverages accounted for 90 percent of Americans' added sugars intake. Gibney and colleagues (1995) reported that dairy foods contributed 31 percent of the total sugar intakes in children, and fruits contributed 17 percent of the sugars for all ages.

Grains and certain vegetables are the major contributors of starch. The majority of carbohydrate occurs as starch in corn, tapioca, flour, cereals, popcorn, pasta, rice, potatoes, and crackers. Fruits and darkly colored vegetables contain little or no starch.

Dietary Intake

Data from the 1994–1996, 1998 Continuing Food Survey of Intakes by Individuals (CSFII) indicates that the median intake of carbohydrate was approximately 220 to 330 g/d for men and 180 to 230 g/d for women in the United States (Appendix Table E-2). This represents 49 to 50 percent of energy intake (Appendix Table E-3). Between 10 and 25 percent of adults consumed less than 45 percent of energy from carbohydrate. Less than 5 percent of adults consumed more than 65 percent of energy from carbohydrate (Appendix Table E-3).

Median carbohydrate intakes of Canadian men and women during 1990 to 1997 ranged from approximately 47 to 50 percent of energy intake (Appendix Table F-2). More than 25 percent of men consumed less than 45 percent of energy from carbohydrate, whereas between 10 and 25 percent of women consumed below this level. Less than 5 percent of Canadian men and women consumed more than 65 percent of energy from carbohydrate.

Data from the Third National Health and Nutrition Examination Survey shows that the median intake of added sugars widely ranged from 10 to 30 tsp/d for adults, which is equivalent to 40 to 120 g/d of sugars (1 tsp = 4 g of sugar) (Appendix Table D-1). Based on data from CFSII, the mean intake of added sugars in the U.S. population aged 2 and older was 82 g, accounting for 15.8 percent of the total energy intake (Guthrie and Morton, 2000).

ADVERSE EFFECTS OF OVERCONSUMPTION

Hazard Identification

Sugars such as sucrose (e.g., white sugar), fructose (e.g., high-fructose corn syrup), and dextrose that are present in foods have been associated with various adverse effects. These sugars may be either naturally occurring or added to foods. Potential adverse effects from consuming a high carbohydrate diet, including sugars and starches, are discussed in detail in Chapter 11.

Behavior

The concept that sugars might adversely affect behavior was first reported by Shannon (1922). The notion that intake of sugars is related to hyperactivity, especially in children, is based on two physiological theories: (1) an allergic reaction to refined sugars (Egger et al., 1985; Speer, 1954) and (2) a hypoglycemic response (Cott, 1977). A number of studies have been conducted to find a correlation between intake of sugars and adverse behavior; some have been reviewed by White and Wolraich (1995). Most of the intervention studies looked at the behavior effects of sugars within a few hours after ingestion, and therefore the long-term effects are unclear. The cross-sectional studies are not capable of determining if the sugars caused adverse behavior or adverse behavior resulted in increased sugar consumption. A meta-analysis of 23 studies conducted over a 12-year period concluded that sugar intake does not affect either behavior or cognitive performance in children (Wolraich et al., 1995) (Figure 6-2). Therefore, altered behavior cannot be used as an adverse effect for setting a Tolerable Upper Intake Level (UL) for sugars.

Dental Caries

Sugars play a significant role in the development of dental caries (Walker and Cleaton-Jones, 1992), but much less information is known about the role of starch in the development of dental caries (Lingstrom et al., 2000). Early childhood dental caries, also known as baby-bottle tooth decay or nursing caries, affects about 3 to 6 percent of children (Fitzsimons et al., 1998). This is associated with frequent, prolonged use of baby bottles containing fermentable sugars (e.g., cow's milk, infant formula, fruit juice, soft drinks, and other sweetened drinks), at-will breast-feeding, and continual use of a sweetened pacifier (Fitzsimons et al., 1998). Increased consumption of sugar-containing foods has been associated with a deterioration of dental health in 5-year-old children (Holbrook et al., 1995). Children 5 or 8 years of age who consumed sweet snacks between meals more than five times a day had significantly higher mean decayed and missing teeth and filled scores than children with a lower consumption (Kalsbeek and Verrips, 1994). Root caries in middle-aged and elderly adults was significantly associated with sucrose consumption (Papas et al., 1995).

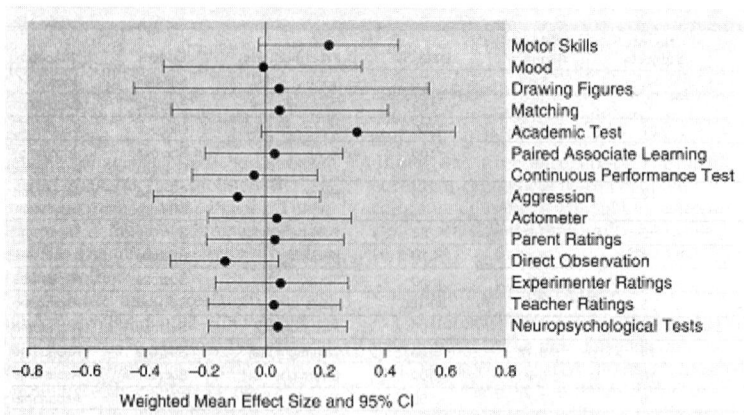

FIGURE 6-2 Weighted mean effect sizes and 95 percent confidence intervals (CI) by measurement construct following meta-analysis of 23 studies on the effect of sugar intake on behavior and cognition. Reprinted, with permission, from Wolraich et al. (1995). Copyright 1995 by the American Medical Association.

Dental caries is a disorder of multifactorial causation. Hence, it is difficult to rationalize the relationship of sugars and dental caries as simply "cause-and-effect" (Walker and Cleaton-Jones, 1992). Caries occurrence is influenced by frequency of meals and snacks, oral hygiene (tooth-brushing frequency), water fluoridation, fluoride supplementation, and fluoride toothpaste (Holbrook et al., 1995; Mascarenhas, 1998; McDonagh et al., 2000; Shaw, 1987). Fluoride alters the sugars–caries dose–response curve. Caries has declined in many industrialized countries and in areas with water fluoridation (McDonagh et al., 2000). Because of the various factors that can contribute to dental caries, it is not possible to determine an intake level of sugars at which increased risk of dental caries can occur.

Triacylglycerol, LDL, and HDL Cholesterol Concentration

Sugars. Fructose is more lipogenic than glucose or starches (Cohen and Schall, 1988; Reiser and Hallfrisch, 1987); however, the precise biochemical basis for this mechanism has not been elucidated (Roche, 1999). There is some evidence that increased intake of sugars is positively associated with plasma triacylglycerol and low density lipoprotein (LDL) cholesterol concentrations (Table 6-7). The data on triacylglycerol concentration is mixed with a number of studies showing an increase in concentration with increased sucrose, glucose, or fructose concentration (Albrink and Ullrich, 1986; Hayford et al., 1979; Kaufmann et al., 1966; Mann et al., 1973, Rath et al., 1974; Reiser et al., 1979a, 1989; Yudkin et al., 1986), whereas other studies have shown no effect (Bossetti et al., 1984; Crapo and Kolterman, 1984; Dunnigan et al., 1970; Hallfrisch et al., 1983; Mann and Truswell, 1972; Surwit et al., 1997; Swanson et al., 1992).

Smith and colleagues (1996) demonstrated that hypertriacylglycerolemia could be reduced in some people with the reduction (73 percent) of extrinsic sucrose in the diet. The investigators reported reduced plasma triacylglycerol concentrations in 32 hypertriacylglycerolemic individuals by greater than 20 percent, and the reduction remained significant with the control of weight loss. Parks and Hellerstein (2000) published an exhaustive review of carbohydrate-induced hypertriacylglycerolemia and concluded that it is more extreme if the carbohydrate content of a high carbohydrate diet consists primarily of monosaccharides, particularly fructose, rather than oligo- and polysaccharides. Purified diets, whether based on starch or monosaccharides, induce hypertriacylglycerolemia more readily than diets higher in fiber in which most of the carbohydrate is derived from unprocessed whole foods, and possibly result in a lower glycemic index and reduced postprandial insulin response (Jenkins et al., 1987b).

TABLE 6-7 Dietary Sugars and Blood Lipid Concentrations in Healthy Subjects

Reference	Study Population/ Dietary Intervention	Triacylglycerol Concentration (mmol/L)			
Kaufmann et al., 1966	3 men and 1 woman, 10–35 d/diet 30% starch 30% sucrose 30% fructose	2 males: no difference between diets 1 male (ad lib to sucrose to fructose): 0.98–1.98 to 2.76 to 4.50 1 female (starch to fructose): 1.32–1.78 to 2.30–2.58			
Dunnigan et al., 1970	9 men and women, 4-wk crossover 31% sucrose sucrose-free	1.05[a] 1.04[a]			
Mann and Truswell, 1972	9 men, 2-wk crossover 23% sucrose 23% starch	1.10[a] 1.11[a]			
Mann et al., 1973	9 men, 2-wk crossover 17% sucrose 34% sucrose 34% sucrose + polyunsaturated fatty acids	1.66[a] 1.84[b] 1.50[a]			
Rath et al., 1974	6 men, 2- to 5-wk crossover 17% sucrose 52% sucrose	Significant increase with 52% sucrose			
Hayford et al., 1979	8 men, 10-d crossover 45% sucrose 65% sucrose 45% glucose 65% glucose	0.87[a] 1.31[b] 0.80[a] 1.33[b]			
Reiser et al., 1979a	19 men and women, 6-wk crossover 30% starch 30% sucrose	Men Baseline 1.28[a] 1.54[a]	6 wk 1.42[a] 1.86[b]	Women Baseline 1.06[a] 1.06[a]	6 wk 0.98[a] 1.23[b]
Hallfrisch et al., 1983	12 men, 5-wk crossover 0% fructose, 15% starch 7.5% fructose, 7.5% starch 15% fructose, 0% starch	0.97[a] 1.07[a] 1.04[a]			
Bossetti et al., 1984	8 men and women, 140-d crossover 11–16% sucrose 11–16% fructose	Baseline 0.60[a] 0.80[a]	14 d 0.63[a] 0.56[a]		

Low Density Lipoprotein Cholesterol Concentration (mmol/L)		High Density Lipoprotein Cholesterol Concentration (mmol/L)	
3.52^a		1.01^a	
3.76^b		1.05^a	
3.70^b		1.07^a	
Baseline	14 d	Baseline	14 d
2.38^a	2.35^a	1.42^a	1.37^a
2.59^a	2.48^a	1.42^a	1.40^a

continued

TABLE 6-7 Continued

Reference	Study Population/ Dietary Intervention	Triacylglycerol Concentration (mmol/L)	
Crapo and Kolterman, 1984	11 men and women, 14-d crossover 24% sucrose 24% fructose	No significant difference	
Albrink and Ullrich, 1986	6 men per group, 11 d 0% sucrose 18% sucrose 36% sucrose 52% sucrose	Significant increase when fed 36% or 52% sucrose and a diet containing less than 14 g of fiber	
Yudkin et al., 1986	14 men, 14-d crossover 18% sucrose 37% sucrose 19% sucrose	1.02^a 1.11^a 1.09^a	
	26 men, 14-d crossover 23% sucrose 9% sucrose 24% sucrose	1.33^a 1.05^b 1.23^a	
Reiser et al., 1989	11 men, 5-wk crossover 20% fructose 20% starch	0.84^a 0.70^b	
Swanson et al., 1992	14 men and women, 4-wk crossover 19% fructose, 25% starch < 3% fructose, 39% starch	Baseline 1.16^a 1.02^a	4 wk 0.96^a 0.94^a
Surwit et al., 1997	42 women, 6-wk intervention 4% sucrose 43% sucrose	1.05^a 1.08^a	
Marckmann et al., 2000	20 women, 2-wk crossover 2.5% sucrose, 59% carbohydrate 23.2% sucrose, 59% carbohydrate	0.81^a 0.96^b	
Saris et al., 2000	390 adults, 6-mo parallel 18.8% sugar, 52% carbohydrate 29.5% sugar, 56% carbohydrate	1.29^a 1.46^a	

^{a,b} Different lettered superscripts within each study indicate that values were significantly different.

Low Density Lipoprotein Cholesterol Concentration (mmol/L)		High Density Lipoprotein Cholesterol Concentration (mmol/L)	
		Significant reduction in high density lipoprotein concentration with fructose	
Significant decline observed for 0% and 18% sucrose diets		Significantly lower for 18%, 36%, and 52% sucrose diets	
		1.27[a]	
		1.07[b]	
		1.42[a]	
		1.30[a]	
		1.27[a]	
		1.26[a]	
3.06[a]		1.16[a]	
2.73[b]		1.11[a]	
Baseline	4 wk	Baseline	4 wk
2.62[a]	2.73[a]	1.28[a]	1.30[a]
2.65[a]	2.46[b]	1.32[a]	1.22[a]
2.38[a]		1.03[a]	
2.60[b]		1.06[a]	
2.43[a]		1.34[a]	
2.72[b]		1.38[a]	
3.68[a]		1.20[a]	
3.61[a]		1.15[a]	

Increases in LDL cholesterol concentration have been observed more consistently with increases in sugar intake (Table 6-7). Increases in LDL cholesterol concentration were reported when 7.5 and 15 percent fructose replaced an equal amount of starch (Hallfrisch et al., 1983), 36 and 52 percent sucrose were fed compared with 0 and 18 percent sucrose (Albrink and Ullrich, 1986), 20 percent fructose replaced an equal amount of starch (Reiser et al., 1989), and 19 percent fructose was fed compared with less than 3 percent fructose (Swanson et al., 1992).

In general, most epidemiological studies have shown an inverse relationship between sugar intake and high density lipoprotein (HDL) cholesterol concentration (Archer et al., 1998; Bolton-Smith et al., 1991; Ernst et al., 1980; Tillotson et al., 1997). Of the nine intervention studies reviewed, five showed no difference in HDL cholesterol concentration with varying intakes of sugars (Bossetti et al., 1984; Hallfrisch et al., 1983; Reiser et al., 1989; Swanson et al., 1992; Surwit et al., 1997). A significant decrease in HDL cholesterol concentration was observed when 24 percent fructose replaced the same amount of sucrose (Crapo and Kolterman, 1984); 37 percent sucrose was fed compared with 18 or 19 percent sucrose (Yudkin et al., 1986); and 18, 36, and 52 percent sucrose was fed compared with 0 percent sucrose (Albrink and Ullrich, 1986).

Kant (2000) used the Third National Health and Nutrition Examination Survey (NHANES III) survey to examine the association between the consumption of energy-dense, nutrient-poor (EDNP) foods on lipid profiles. EDNP foods such as visible fats, nutritive sweeteners and sweetened beverages, desserts, and snacks have high fat and/or high carbohydrate and poor micronutrient content. HDL cholesterol concentration was inversely related and serum homocysteine concentration was positively related to EDNP food intake. Both serum homocysteine and HDL cholesterol concentrations are independent risk factors for cardiovascular disease (Aronow and Ahn, 1998; Boushey et al., 1995).

GI. In controlled studies, the consumption of high glycemic index (GI) diets has generally resulted in modest increases in circulating concentrations of hemoglobin A_{1c}, total serum cholesterol, and triacylglycerols, as well as decreased circulating HDL cholesterol and urinary C-peptide concentrations in diabetic and hyperlipidemic individuals (Table 6-8). Furthermore, studies on dyslipidemic individuals show that a low GI diet can reduce cholesterol and triacylglycerol concentrations (Jenkins et al., 1985, 1987b). Data are limited for healthy individuals as only one study has measured the effect of predicted GI on blood lipid concentrations (Jenkins et al., 1987a). This study showed a 15 and 13 percent reduction in total cholesterol and LDL cholesterol concentration, respectively, when the GI was reduced by 41 (Jenkins et al., 1987a).

A significant negative relationship between GI and HDL cholesterol concentration was reported in two epidemiological studies (Ford and Liu, 2001; Frost et al., 1999) (Table 6-9 and Figure 6-3). Only the negative relationship to glycemic load was significant for postmenopausal women (Liu et al., 2001). HDL cholesterol concentrations were more responsive to changes in GI in women than in men (Figure 6-3). In contrast, Ford and Liu (2001) reported a more pronounced response in men than in women. Thus, although there is evidence for an association between high GI and risk factors for cardiovascular disease (Haffner et al., 1988a; Morris and Zemel, 1999), further controlled studies are needed.

CHD. Four epidemiological studies have shown no risk of coronary heart disease (CHD) from consuming naturally occurring or added sugars (Bolton-Smith and Woodward, 1994a; Kushi et al., 1985; Liu et al., 1982, 2000; McGee et al., 1984) (see Table 11-7). Two epidemiological studies have been conducted to relate the risk of CHD with GI (Liu et al., 2000; van Dam et al., 2000) (Table 6-9). One study showed increased risk of CHD with increasing GI, but for only those with a body mass index greater than 23 (Liu et al., 2000). van Dam and coworkers (2000) observed no association between GI and risk of CHD in elderly men. Thus, there are insufficient data for setting a UL based on increased risk for CHD.

Insulin Sensitivity and Type 2 Diabetes

Sugars. Insulin has three major effects on glucose metabolism: it decreases hepatic glucose output, it increases glucose utilization in muscle and adipose tissue, and it enhances glycogen production in the liver and muscle. Insulin sensitivity measures the ability to do these effectively. Individuals vary genetically in their insulin sensitivity, some being much more efficient than others (Reaven, 1999). Obesity is related to decreased insulin sensitivity (Kahn et al., 2001), which can also be influenced by fat intake (see Chapter 11) and exercise.

Two prospective cohort studies showed no risk of diabetes from consuming increased amounts of sugars (Colditz et al., 1992; Meyer et al., 2000). Furthermore, a negative association was observed between increased sucrose intake and risk of diabetes (Meyer et al., 2000). Intervention studies that have evaluated the effect of sugar intakes on insulin concentration and insulin resistance portray mixed results. Dunnigan and coworkers (1970) reported no difference in glucose tolerance and plasma insulin concentration after 0 or 31 percent sucrose was consumed for 4 weeks. Reiser and colleagues (1979b) reported that when 30 percent starch was replaced with 30 percent sucrose, insulin concentration was significantly elevated; however, serum glucose concentration did not differ.

TABLE 6-8 Controlled Studies of Low Glycemic Index (GI) Diets on Carbohydrate and Lipid Metabolism in Healthy, Diabetic, and Hyperlipidemic Subjects

Reference	Study Design	Change in Diet GI	Type of Glycated Proteins
Healthy subjects			
Jenkins et al., 1987a	6 men, 2 wk	−41	Fructosamine
Kiens and Richter, 1996	7 young men, 30 d	−24	Not reported
Frost et al., 1998	25 women, 3 wk	−18	Not reported
Diabetic subjects			
Collier et al., 1988	7 type I children, 6 wk	−12	Albumin
Fontvieille et al., 1988	8 type I men and women, 3 wk	−14	Fructosamine
Jenkins et al., 1988a	8 type II men and women, 2 wk	−23	HbA_{1c} Fructosamine
Brand et al., 1991	16 type II men and women, 12 wk	−14	HbA_{1c}
Fontvieille et al., 1992	18 type I and II men and women, 5 wk	−26	Fructosamine
Wolever et al., 1992a	15 type II men and women, 2 wk	−27	Fructosamine
Wolever et al., 1992b	6 type II overweight men and women, 6 wk	−28	Fructosamine

Change in Glycated Proteins (%)	Change in Blood Lipids[a] (%)	Comments[b]
−7[c,d]	−15[c,d] TC −13[c,d] LDL-C	−32%[c,e] urinary C-peptide excretion −10%[c,e] creatinine clearance during the day
Not reported	Not reported	Euglycemic hyperinsulinemic clamp showed no difference in glucose uptake between high and low GI diets at low plasma insulin, but glucose uptake was reduced at high plasma insulin with low GI diet
Not reported	Not reported	Using short insulin tolerance test, in vivo insulin sensitivity improved after low GI diet
−19[c,d]	−14[c,d] TC	Reduced postprandial glucose response to standard test meal with low GI diet
−18.1[c,d]	−5.8[c,d] TAG	−8.9%[c,d] plasma phospholipids −6.1%[c,d] daily insulin needs
−6.6[c,d] −6.6[c,d]	−5.8[c,d] TC	−30%[c,d] fasting blood glucose
−11[c,e]	Not significant	−11%[c,e] plasma glucose response to standard meal
−12.1[c,e]	−21.1[c,e] TAG	−11%[c,e] fasting blood glucose −13.3%[c,e] mean daily blood glucose
−3.4[c,e]	−7[c,e] TC	−30%[c,e] urinary C-peptide excretion −29%[c,e] postbreakfast blood glucose TAG rose on high GI diet ($p = 0.027$) and fell on low GI diet, but the difference between the two diets was not significant
−8[c,e]	−6.8[c,e] TC	−22.4%[c,e] TAG for the 5 subjects with TAG > 2.2 mmol/L

continued

TABLE 6-8 Continued

Reference	Study Design	Change in Diet GI	Type of Glycated Proteins
Frost et al., 1994	25 type II men and women, 12 wk	−5	Fructosamine
Järvi et al., 1999	20 type II men and women, 2 d	−26	HbA$_{1c}$ Fructosamine
Luscombe et al., 1999	21 type II men and women, 4 wk	−20	Fructosamine
Hyperlipidemic subjects			
Jenkins et al., 1987b	30 men and women, 4 wk	−17	Fructosamine

[a] TC = total cholesterol, LDL-C = low density lipoprotein cholesterol, TAG = triacylglycerols, HDL-C = high density lipoprotein cholesterol.
[b] PAI-1 = plasminogen activator inhibitor-1.

GI. There are well-recognized, short-term effects of high versus low GI carbohydrates on several key hormones and metabolites. In particular, compared to regular consumption of low GI carbohydrates, regular consumption of high GI carbohydrates results in high concentrations of circulating glucose and insulin (Table 6-8). In healthy individuals, there also appears to be an amplification of glucose and insulin responses to consumption of high GI foods with repeated consumption (Liljeberg et al., 1999). Based on associations between these metabolic parameters and risk of disease (DeFronzo et al., 1992; Groop and Eriksson, 1992; Haffner et al., 1988b, 1990; Martin et al., 1992; Rossetti et al., 1990; Warram et al., 1990), further controlled studies on GI and risk factors for diabetes are needed. Furthermore, studies are needed on the extent to which consumption of high GI diets might influence the development of diabetes compared to other putative dietary variables that also influence insulin secretion (e.g., dietary fiber).

In prospective epidemiological studies, three of the four published studies support an association between GI and the development of type 2 diabetes (Table 6-9). Data from the Nurses' Health Study illustrated a significant association between the dietary glycemic index and risk of type 2 diabetes that was significant both with and without an adjustment for

Change in Glycated Proteins (%)	Change in Blood Lipids[a] (%)	Comments[b]
−15.8[c,d]	−11.3[c,d] TC −26.3[c,d] TAG	−21.3%[c,d] fasting blood glucose
−5.9[c,d] −2.5[c,e]	−5.2[c,e] TC −8.3[c,e] LDL-C	−31%[c,e] 9-h blood glucose profile −53%[c,d] PAI-1 activity
Not significant	+5.7[c,e] HDL-C	Fasting plasma glucose did not significantly differ between the diets
Not significant	When TAG > 2 mmol/L −8.8[c,e] TC −9.1[c,e] LDL-C −19.3[c,e] TAG	24-h urinary C-peptide was not significantly different Changes in weight loss and fat intake did not explain the lipid effects

[c] Significant effect ($p < 0.05$).
[d] Treatment difference (across treatment).
[e] Endpoint difference (between treatment).

cereal fiber intake (Salmerón et al., 1997b). In contrast, the Iowa Women's Health Study showed no significant relationship between GI and the development of type 2 diabetes after adjusting for total dietary fiber, although the association was positive in the GI range of 59 to 71 and then declined with GI values greater than 71 (Meyer et al., 2000). The reasons for the discrepancy between studies are not known, but may be related to the accuracy of dietary intake records, the imprecision in calculating GI from reported diets, and the age of individuals entering the investigations. There are currently no intervention trials in which dietary GI is manipulated and development of chronic diseases monitored; such studies are needed.

Obesity

Sugars. Several studies have been conducted to determine the relationship between total (intrinsic plus added) and added sugars intake and energy intake (Table 6-10). The Department of Health Survey of British School Children showed that as total sugar intake increased from less than 20.7 percent of energy to up to 25.2 percent of energy, intake increased by approximately 100 kcal/d (Gibson, 1993). In contrast, the Bogalusa Heart

TABLE 6-9 Cross-Sectional and Cohort Studies on the Relation of Glycemic Index (GI) to the Risk of Diabetes, Coronary Heart Disease (CHD), and Cancer and Its Association with High Density Lipoprotein Cholesterol (HDL-C) Concentration and Glucated Hemoglobin (HbA$_{1c}$) in Diabetes

References	Study Design	GI
Diabetes		
Salmerón et al., 1997a	42,759 healthy, male health professionals Cohort, 6-y follow-up	Quintile mean 65 70 73 75 79
Salmerón et al., 1997b	65,173 healthy, female nurses Cohort, 6-y follow-up	Quintile mean 64 68 71 73 77
Meyer et al., 2000	35,988 postmenopausal women Cohort, 6-y follow-up	< 58 59–65 66–71 72–80 > 80
Buyken et al., 2001	2,810 type I diabetic men and women Cross-sectional study	58.2–77.7 79.8–81.5 81.5–85.5 85.5–111.5
Hu et al., 2001	84,941 healthy, female nurses Cohort, 16-y follow-up	
CHD and related parameters		
Frost et al., 1999	1,420 British adults Cross-sectional study	Mean: 86

Main Effect[a]	Comments[b]
RR of diabetes	p for trend = 0.03 after adjustment for
1.00	cereal fiber intake
1.16	For high GL plus low cereal fiber intake, the
1.19	RR of diabetes was 2.17 (1.04–4.54)
1.20	
1.37	
RR of diabetes	p for trend = 0.005 after adjustment for
1.00	cereal fiber intake
1.21	Significant association between glycemic
1.37	load and risk of diabetes (RR = 1.47
1.37	for 5th quintile)
1.37	
RR of diabetes	GI and GL were not associated with risk
1.00	of diabetes
1.19	
1.26	
0.96	
0.89	
HbA_{1c} (%)	Using bivariate model, serum HDL-C
6.05	was inversely associated with GI
6.27	(p for trend = 0.0001), and TAG
6.59	was positively associated with GI
6.55	(p for trend = 0.01)
	Significant association between GL and
	risk of diabetes (p trend < 0.001); this
	is an updated analysis from Salmerón et al.
	(1997b) that includes 3,300 new cases of
	type 2 diabetes
Negative	
relationship	
between GI	
and HDL-C	
(p < 0.0001)	

continued

TABLE 6-9 Continued

References	Study Design	GI
Liu et al., 2000	75,521 female nurses Cohort, 10-y follow-up	GI quintile mean by GL score 72 75 77 78 80
van Dam et al., 2000	646 elderly Dutch men Prospective analysis	Tertile median 77 82 85
Ford and Liu, 2001	13,907 men and women Cross-sectional study	< 76 76–79 80–83 84–87 > 87
Liu et al., 2001	280 postmenopausal women Prospective analysis	Quintile mean 68 73 75 77 81
Cancer Franceschi et al., 2001	Italian men and women with colon cancer 1,953 cases 4,154 controls	< 70.8 70.8–73.8 73.9–76.5 76.6–79.6 > 79.6

[a] RR = relative risk, OR = odds ratio.
[b] GL = glycemic load, TAG = triacylglycerol, BMI = body mass index.

Study reported a significant decrease in energy intake with increased total sugar intake (Nicklas et al., 1996). A negative correlation between total sugar intake and body mass index (BMI) has been consistently reported for children and adults (Bolton-Smith and Woodward, 1994b; Dreon et al., 1988; Dunnigan et al., 1970; Fehily et al., 1984; Gibson, 1993, 1996b; Miller

Main Effect[a]		Comments[b]
RR of CHD		RR of CHD associated with high glycemic load only for those with BMI > 23
1.00		
1.01		
1.25		
1.51		
1.98		
RR of CHD		No association between GI and risk of CHD (p for trend = 0.7)
1.00		
1.12		
1.11		
Serum HDL-C (mmol/L)		p for trend < 0.001
1.36		The decrease in HDL-C was similar for subjects with BMI < 25 and those with BMI ≥ 25
1.31		
1.30		
1.27		
1.28		
Plasma HDL-C (mmol/L)	Plasma TAG (mmol/L)	Nonsignificant negative association between GI and HDL-C concentration
1.45	1.16	(p for trend = 0.1)
1.42	1.20	Nonsignificant positive association between GI and TAG concentration
1.42	1.14	(p for trend = 0.03)
1.40	1.27	
1.29	1.37	
OR of colon and rectum cancer		p for trend < 0.001
1.0		Similar findings for glycemic load
1.3		
1.6		
1.5		
1.7		

et al., 1990) (Table 6-11). A study of 42 women compared the effects of a high sucrose (43 percent of total energy) and low sucrose (4 percent of total energy), low fat (11 percent total energy) hypoenergetic diet (Surwit et al., 1997). There were no significant differences between groups in total body weight lost during the intervention. On the other hand, a study using

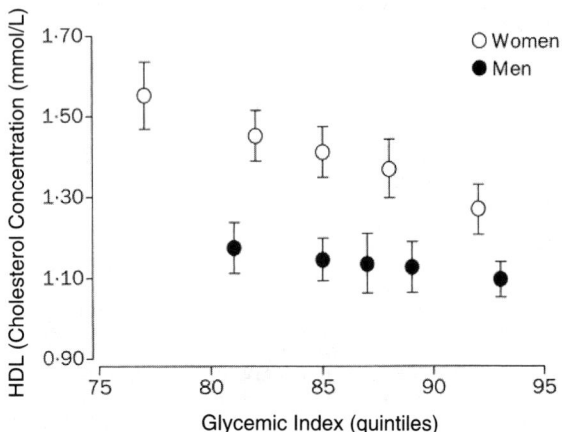

FIGURE 6-3 Relation between high density lipoprotein (HDL) cholesterol concentration and five quintiles of glycemic index in men and women. Reprinted, with permission, from Frost et al. (1999). Copyright 1999 by Elsevier Science (*The Lancet*).

23 lean men, 23 obese men, 17 lean women, and 15 obese women found that lean and obese individuals of the same gender had similar total sugar intake (Miller et al., 1994). However, the obese individuals derived a greater percentage (38.0 to 47.9 percent) of their sugar intake from added sugars compared with lean individuals (25.2 to 31.4 percent).

Increased added sugars intakes have been shown to result in increased energy intakes for children and adults (Bowman, 1999; Gibson 1996a, 1997; Lewis et al., 1992). Despite these observations, a negative correlation between added sugars intake and BMI has been observed (Bolton-Smith and Woodward, 1994b; Gibson, 1996a; Lewis et al., 1992). For adolescents, nonconsumers of soft drinks consumed 1,984 kcal/d in contrast to 2,604 kcal/d for those teens who consumed 26 or more oz of soft drinks per day (Harnack et al., 1999). Using NHANES III data, Troiano and colleagues (2000) found that soft drinks contributed a higher proportion of daily energy intake for overweight than for nonoverweight children and adolescents. Kant (2000) demonstrated a positive association between energy-dense, micronutrient-poor food and beverage consumption (visible fats, nutritive sweeteners, sweetened beverages, desserts, and snacks) and energy intake.

Ludwig and colleagues (2001) examined the relationship between consumption of drinks sweetened with sugars and childhood obesity. They concluded that for each additional serving of the drinks consumed, the odds of becoming obese increased by 60 percent. Drinks sweetened with sugars, such as soft drinks, have been suggested to promote obesity because compensation at subsequent meals for energy consumed in the form of a liquid could be less complete than for energy consumed as solid food (Mattes, 1996).

Published reports disagree about whether a direct link exists between the trend toward increased intakes of sugars and increased rates of obesity. The lack of association in some studies may be partially due to the pervasive problem of underreporting food intake, which is known to occur with dietary surveys (Johnson, 2000). Underreporting is more prevalent and severe by obese adolescents and adults than by their lean counterparts (Johnson, 2000). In addition, foods high in added sugars are selectively underreported (Krebs-Smith et al., 2000). Thus, it can be difficult to make conclusions about associations between sugars intake and BMI by using self-reported data.

Based on the above data, it appears that the effects of increased intakes of total sugars on energy intake are mixed, and the increased intake of added sugars are most often associated with increased energy intake. There is no clear and consistent association between increased intake of added sugars and BMI. Therefore, the above data cannot be used to set a UL for either added or total sugars.

GI. Although there have been several short-term studies on the relationship between dietary GI and hunger, satiety, and energy intake at single meals, many of the studies are confounded by differences between test diets in variables other than GI (Roberts, 2000b). Among relatively controlled studies (Guss et al., 1994; Holt and Brand Miller, 1995; Ludwig et al., 1999; Rodin, 1991; Spitzer and Rodin, 1987), voluntary energy intake was 29 percent higher following consumption of high GI test meals or preloads compared to those of low GI, as summarized in Figure 6-4 (Roberts, 2000b). These data strongly suggest an effect of GI on short-term energy intake, but there are currently little data on the effect of GI on energy intake from longer-term clinical trials. Such data are necessary before the effects of the GI of carbohydrate-containing foods on energy regulation can be appropriately evaluated because the effects of GI on energy intake might become smaller over time. Obtaining data from clinical trials is especially important because although one nonblinded study reported greater weight loss success in obese patients treated with a low GI diet compared with a conventional low fat diet (Spieth et al., 2000), the two epidemiological studies reporting BMI in their evaluations of the relationship between GI and development of chronic diseases observed no significant association between GI and BMI (Liu et al., 2000; Salmerón et al., 1997a, 1997b).

TABLE 6-10 Sugar and Energy Intake

Reference	Design and Study	Sugar Intake (% of Energy)
Total sugar		
Gibson, 1993	2,705 boys and girls Department of Health Survey of British School Children	< 20.7 20.7–25.2 > 25.2
Nicklas et al., 1996	568 boys and girls, 10 y Bogalusa Heart Study	18.0 22.0 26.4 31.2
Farris et al., 1998	568 boys and girls, 10 y Bogalusa Heart Study	16.1 23.5 28.2 35.6
Added sugar		
Lewis et al., 1992	Nationwide Food Consumption Survey (1977–1978)	
Gibson, 1996a	1,087 men and 1,110 women Dietary and Nutritional Survey of British Adults	< 10 10–13 14–16 17–20 > 20
Gibson, 1997	1,675 boys and girls, 1.5–4.5 y U.K. National Diet and Nutrition Survey of Children	< 12 12–16 16–20 20–25 > 25
Bowman, 1999	Continuing Survey of Food Intakes by Individuals (1994–1996)	< 10 10–18 > 18

[a,b,c] Different lettered superscripts within each study indicate that values were significantly different.

Energy Intake (kcal)

Boys		Girls	
10–11 y	14–15 y	10–11 y	14–15 y
1,954[a]	2,401[a]	1,753[a]	1,819[a]
2,095[b]	2,526[b]	1,838[b]	1,961[b]
2,066[b]	2,549[b]	1,871[b]	1,901[a,b]

2,291
2,245
2,274
2,016

2,249
2,286
2,144
2,061

High consumers of added sugars had greater
energy intakes than consumers of moderate
and low added sugars

Men	Women
2,219[a]	1,438[a]
2,430[b]	1,681[b]
2,455[b,c]	1,738[b]
2,549[b,c]	1,773[b]
2,596[c]	1,774[b]

Boys	Girls
1,129[a]	1,097[a]
1,168[a,b]	1,102[a]
1,187[a,b]	1,139[a]
1,188[a,b]	1,115[a]
1,217[b]	1,116[a]

1,860[a]
2,040[b]
2,049[b]

TABLE 6-11 Interventional and Epidemiological Data on Sugar Intake and Body Mass Index (BMI)

Reference	Study Design	Sugar Intake (% of energy)
Total sugars		
Dunnigan et al., 1970	9 men and women, 4-wk crossover	31% sucrose sucrose-free
Fehily et al., 1984	493 men, 45–59 y 7-d weighed dietary record	
Dreon et al., 1988	155 obese men, 30–59 y 7-d dietary record	13.7 ± 8.4 g/1,000 kcal
Miller et al., 1990	107 men and 109 women, 18–71 y 24-h recall and 2-d dietary questionnaire	
Gibson, 1993	2,705 boys and girls Department of Health Survey of British School Children	< 20.7 20.7–25.2 < 25.2
Bolton-Smith and Woodward, 1994b	11,626 men and women, 25–64 y Scottish Heart Health and MONICA studies	Quintile 1 2 3 4 5
Gibson, 1996b	1,087 men and 1,110 women, 16–64 y Dietary and Nutritional Survey of British Adults	Quintile 1 2 3 4 5

BMI (kg)

62.4
63.8

Significant negative association between sucrose intake and BMI

Significant negative correlation between sucrose intake and BMI

Significant negative correlation between sugar intake and
    percentage of body fat for women; no association for men

Boys		Girls	
10–11 y	14–15 y	10–11 y	14–15 y
18.6^a	20.2^a	18.2^a	21.2^a
$17.9^{a,b}$	$20.0^{a,b}$	18.1^a	20.2^b
17.5^b	19.2^b	17.9^a	19.8^b

Men	Women
27.0	26.5
26.4	26.0
26.0	25.5
25.5	25.1
24.7	24.4

Significant negative correlation between sugar intake and BMI

Men	Women
24.9	25.4
25.3	24.7
25.2	24.5
24.8	23.8
24.4	24.4

Weak negative association between sugar intake and BMI

continued

TABLE 6-11 Continued

Reference	Study Design	Sugar Intake (% of energy)
Added sugars		
Lewis et al., 1992	Nationwide Food Consumption Survey (1977–1978)	
Bolton-Smith and Woodward, 1994b	11,626 men and women, 25–64 y Scottish Heart Health and MONICA studies	Quintile 1 2 3 4 5
Gibson, 1996a	1,087 men and 1,110 women, 16–64 y Dietary and Nutritional Survey of British Adults	< 10 10–13 14–16 17–20 > 20
Ludwig et al., 2001	Planet Health intervention and evaluation project	

a,b,c,d Different lettered superscripts within each study indicate that values were significantly different.

Physical Activity

Although consumption of high GI test foods increases glucose oxidation and suppresses the availability of free fatty acids (Ritz et al., 1991), for factors that would be predicted to have an adverse effect on the capacity for endurance exercise there are conflicting reports on whether consumption of high GI diets prior to exercise results in measurably adverse exercise performance. Some studies report a negative effect of consumption of high GI carbohydrates prior to exercise compared with consumption of low GI carbohydrates (DeMarco et al., 1999; Gleeson et al., 1986; Okano et al., 1988; Thomas et al., 1991), while other studies report no effect on exercise performance (Chryssanthopoulos et al., 1994; Décombaz et al., 1985; Febbraio et al., 2000; Hargreaves et al., 1987; Sparks et al., 1998). It is possible that the level and duration of exercise and amount of test food have critical influences on the results obtained in such studies. Since the

BMI (kg)

High consumers of added sugars tended to weigh less than
  moderate consumers

Men	Women
27.2	26.5
26.4	25.8
26.1	25.6
25.4	25.4
24.5	24.1

Significant negative correlation between added sugar intake and BMI

Men	Women
25.9^a	26.0^a
$25.5^{a,b}$	$24.9^{a,b}$
$24.8^{b,c}$	24.2^b
$24.4^{c,d}$	24.1^b
$24.1^{c,d}$	23.8^b

Significant negative correlation between added sugar intake and BMI

For each additional serving of sugar-sweetened drink consumed,
  BMI and frequency of obesity increased; baseline consumption
  of sugar-sweetened drinks was independently associated with
  change in BMI

available studies are in considerable conflict, the potential for GI to impact exercise performance at submaximal levels of exercise seems limited.

Lung Cancer

One case-control study in Uruguay (463 cases and 465 controls) suggested that foods rich in sugars, total sucrose intake, sucrose-to-dietary fiber ratio, and GI were associated with increased risk of lung cancer (De Stefani et al., 1998).

Breast Cancer

The data examining sugars intake and breast cancer have been inconsistent (World Cancer Research Fund/American Institute for Cancer

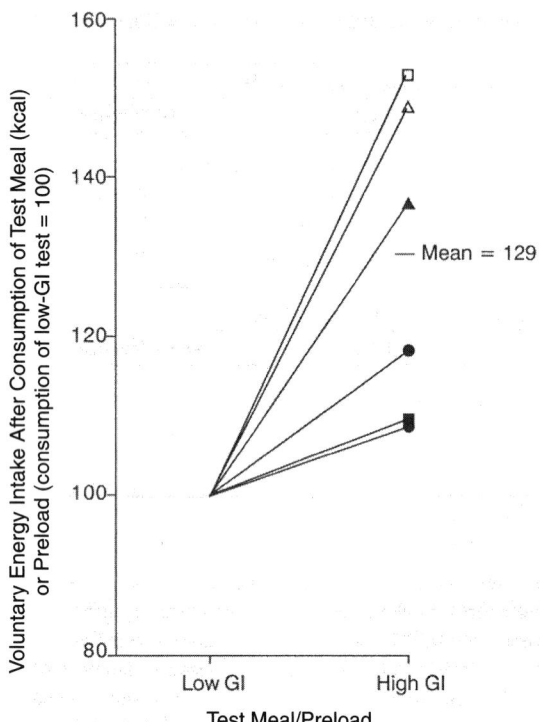

FIGURE 6-4 Summary of data from crossover studies examining the effects of the glycemic index (GI) of test meals or preloads on subsequent energy intake. Δ from Spitzer and Rodin (1987), ▲ from Rodin (1991), ■ from Guss et al. (1994), • from Holt and Brand Miller (1995), □ from Ludwig et al. (1999). All published studies that used pairs of diets differing in GI that contained physiologic amounts of energy, were isocaloric, and were approximately matched for all factors are summarized (i.e., data from 10% sugar solutions in Guss et al. [1994] and the high and medium GI meals only in Ludwig et al. [1999]). Where energy intake was assessed at more than one time point, data from the longest period were used. Reprinted, with permission, from Roberts (2000b). Copyright 2000 by the International Life Sciences Institute.

Research, 1997) and therefore are insufficient to determine a role of sugars in breast cancer (Burley, 1998). There are indications that insulin resistance and insulin-like growth factors may play a role in the development of breast cancer (Bruning et al., 1992; Kazer, 1995).

Prostate Cancer

The Health Professionals Follow-Up Study (n = 47,781 men) demonstrated a reduced risk of advanced prostate cancer associated with increased fructose intakes. Both fruit intake and nonfruit sources of fructose predicted reduced risk of advanced prostate cancer (Giovannucci et al., 1998), but evidence to suggest a role of sugars in prostate cancer is lacking (Burley, 1998).

Colorectal Cancer

The World Cancer Research Fund and American Institute for Cancer Research (1997) reviewed the literature linking foods, nutrients, and dietary patterns with the risk of human cancers worldwide. Data from five case-control studies showed an increase in colorectal polyps and colorectal cancer risk across intakes of sugars and foods rich in sugars (Benito et al., 1990; Macquart-Moulin et al., 1986, 1987; Miller et al., 1983; Tuyns et al., 1988). The subgroups studied showed an elevated risk for those consuming 30 g or more per day compared with those eating less than 10 g/d. Others have concluded that high consumption of fruits and vegetables, as well as the avoidance of foods containing highly refined sugars, are likely to reduce the risk of colon cancer (Giovannucci and Willett, 1994). In many of the studies, sugars increased the risk of colorectal cancer while fiber and starch had the opposite effect. One investigator suggested that the positive association between high sugars consumption and colorectal cancer reflects a global dietary habit that is generally associated with an increased risk of colorectal cancer and may not indicate a biological effect of sugars on colon carcinogenesis (Macquart-Moulin et al., 1987). Burley (1997) concluded from a review of the available literature that there was insufficient evidence to conclude whether sugars had a role in colon cancer.

Concerning a possible relationship between GI and colon cancer, two groups recently reported a case-control study suggesting increased risk of colon cancer among individuals consuming a high versus a low GI diet (Franceschi et al., 2001; Slattery et al., 1997). However, data from other types of investigations are currently unavailable.

Summary

GI

There is a significant body of data suggesting that more slowly absorbed starchy foods that are less processed, or have been processed in traditional ways, may have health advantages over those that are rapidly digested and absorbed. These foods have been classified as having a low GI and reduce the glycemic load of the diet. Not all studies of low GI or low glycemic load diets have resulted in beneficial effects. However, none have shown negative effects. At a time when populations are increasingly obese, inactive, and prone to insulin resistance, there are theoretical reasons that dietary interventions that reduce insulin demand may have advantages. In this section of the population, it is likely that more slowly absorbed carbohydrate foods and low glycemic load diets will have the greatest advantage.

Dietary GI and glycemic load have relatively predicable effects on circulating glucose, hemoglobin A_{1c}, insulin, triacylglycerol, HDL cholesterol, and urinary C-peptide concentrations, particularly in individuals with diabetes and hyperlipidemia. Although the data are lacking in healthy individuals, on theoretical grounds, these effects would be expected to result in reduced risks of type 2 diabetes and cardiovascular disease in individuals consuming low GI versus high GI carbohydrates. However, the results of epidemiological studies are not always consistent, perhaps because of the difficulty of predicting dietary GI precisely from the relatively simple dietary assessment tools used in some studies. Thus, although there may be beneficial metabolic and disease prevention effects of consuming a greater proportion of carbohydrate from low GI sources, further studies are needed before general recommendations on this issue can be made for the general healthy population.

Further research is especially needed because recommendations to reduce the GI of carbohydrate consumed by the general healthy population would have a significant impact on recommended food sources. Currently, recommended healthy carbohydrate sources with a high GI include whole wheat breads, some breakfast cereals, and potatoes. A recommendation to replace bread and potatoes in the U.S. diet with foods of lower GI would involve major changes in current dietary patterns, and thus substantial evidence of significant beneficial effects of GI is needed. Another important practical issue in considering recommendations on GI is that dietary fiber somewhat decreases GI and may have a beneficial role in several chronic diseases, including the prevention of cardiovascular disease (see Chapter 7). Currently, the median intake of *Dietary Fiber* is only about half the Adequate Intake (AI) for *Total Fiber* (see Appendix Table E-4 and Chapter 7), and the question of whether lowering the GI has measurable beneficial effects on chronic diseases among individuals consuming recommended fiber intakes has received little attention (Luscombe et al., 1999).

Concerning obesity, there is limited evidence suggesting an effect of GI on short-term energy intake. Data from long-term clinical trials on the effects on energy intake are lacking and further studies are needed in this area.

In summary, a UL based on GI is not made at the present time because, although several lines of evidence suggest adverse effects of high GI carbohydrates, it is difficult to eliminate other contributing factors, and the critical mass of evidence necessary for recommending substantial dietary change is not available. Furthermore, it should be noted that sugars have a lower GI than starch yet are rapidly absorbed. However, the principle of slowing carbohydrate absorption, which may underpin the positive findings made in relation to GI, is a potentially important principal with respect to the beneficial health effects of carbohydrate. Further research in this area is needed.

Sugars

Based on the data available on dental caries, behavior, cancer, risk of obesity, and risk of hyperlipidemia, there is insufficient evidence to set a UL for total or added sugars. Although a UL is not set for sugars, a maximal intake level of 25 percent or less of energy from added sugars is suggested based on the decreased intake of some micronutrients of American subpopulations exceeding this level (see Chapter 11 and Appendix J). Because not all micronutrients and other nutrients such as fiber were not examined, the association between added sugars and these nutrients it is not known. While it is recognized that hypertriglyceridemia can occur with increasing intakes of total (intrinsic plus added) sugars, total sugars intake can be limited by minimizing the intake of added sugars and consuming naturally occurring sugars present in nutrient-rich milk, dairy products, and fruits.

Intake Assessment

Median intakes of added sugars were highest in young adults, particularly adolescent males (35.7 tsp or 143 g), and progressively declined with age (Appendix Table D-1). At the 95th percentile of intake, added sugars intakes were as high as 52 tsp (208 g or 832 kcal) for men aged 19 to 50 years.

RESEARCH RECOMMENDATIONS

• There is a need for more research to elucidate the metabolic and long-term health differences resulting from the ingestion of high versus low glycemic index carbohydrates using larger, diverse sample sizes and whole-food diets.

• There is a need for research to determine if the energy density approach to weight reduction is effective in the long-term.

- Experimental studies are needed to determine whether there is a metabolic effect of sugars in enhancing energy expenditure or in suppressing fat intake at a fixed level of energy.
- Research is needed to determine the effect of low glycemic index foods and low glycemic-load diets on serum lipids and other risk factors for chronic disease and complications, especially in high-risk groups.

REFERENCES

Albrink MJ, Ullrich IH. 1986. Interaction of dietary sucrose and fiber on serum lipids in healthy young men fed high carbohydrate diets. *Am J Clin Nutr* 43:419–428.

Allen JC, Keller RP, Archer P, Neville MC. 1991. Studies in human lactation: Milk composition and daily secretion rates of macronutrients in the first year of lactation. *Am J Clin Nutr* 54:69–80.

Amiel SA, Caprio S, Sherwin RS, Plewe G, Haymond MW, Tamborlane WV. 1991. Insulin resistance of puberty: A defect restricted to peripheral glucose metabolism. *J Clin Endocrinol Metab* 72:277–282.

Anderson DM, Williams FH, Merkatz RB, Schulman PK, Kerr DS, Pittard WB. 1983. Length of gestation and nutritional composition of human milk. *Am J Clin Nutr* 37:810–814.

Anderson GH, Atkinson SA, Bryan MH. 1981. Energy and macronutrient content of human milk during early lactation from mothers giving birth prematurely and at term. *Am J Clin Nutr* 34:258–265.

Archer SL, Liu K, Dyer AR, Ruth KJ, Jacobs DR, Van Horn L, Hilner JE, Savage PJ. 1998. Relationship between changes in dietary sucrose and high density lipoprotein cholesterol: The CARDIA Study. *Ann Epidemiol* 8:433–438.

Aronow WS, Ahn C. 1998. Risk factors for new coronary events in older African-American men and women. *Am J Cardiol* 82:902–904.

Arslanian S, Kalhan S. 1992. Effects of growth hormone releasing hormone on insulin action and insulin secretion in a hypopituitary patient evaluated by the clamp technique. *Acta Endocrinol* 127:93–96.

Assel B, Rossi K, Kalhan S. 1993. Glucose metabolism during fasting through human pregnancy: Comparison of tracer method with respiratory calorimetry. *Am J Physiol* 265:E351–E356.

Azar GJ, Bloom WL. 1963. Similarities of carbohydrate deficiency and fasting. II. Ketones, nonesterified fatty acids, and nitrogen excretion. *Arch Intern Med* 112:338–343.

Bell JD, Margen S, Calloway DH. 1969. Ketosis, weight loss, uric acid, and nitrogen balance in obese women fed single nutrients at low caloric levels. *Metabolism* 18:193–208.

Benito R, Obrador A, Stiggelbout A, Bosch FX, Mulet M, Muñoz N, Kaldor J. 1990. A population-based case-control study of colorectal cancer in Majorca. I. Dietary factors. *Int J Cancer* 45:69–76.

Bier DM, Leake RD, Haymond MW, Arnold KJ, Gruenke LD, Sperling MA, Kipnis DM. 1977. Measurement of "true" glucose production rates in infancy and childhood with 6,6-dideuteroglucose. *Diabetes* 26:1016–1023.

Bloom WL, Azar GJ. 1963. Similarities of carbohydrate deficiency and fasting. I. Weight loss, electrolyte excretion, and fatigue. *Arch Intern Med* 112:333–337.

Bolton-Smith C, Woodward M. 1994a. Coronary heart disease: Prevalence and dietary sugars in Scotland. *J Epidemiol Community Health* 48:119–122.

Bolton-Smith C, Woodward M. 1994b. Dietary composition and fat to sugar ratios in relation to obesity. *Int J Obes Relat Metab Disord* 18:820–828.

Bolton-Smith C, Woodward M, Smith WCS, Tunstall-Pedoe H. 1991. Dietary and non-dietary predictors of serum total and HDL-cholesterol in men and women: Results from the Scottish Heart Health Study. *Int J Epidemiol* 20:95–104.

Bossetti BM, Kocher LM, Moranz JF, Falko JM. 1984. The effects of physiologic amounts of simple sugars on lipoprotein, glucose, and insulin levels in normal subjects. *Diabetes Care* 7:309–312.

Boushey CJ, Beresford SA, Omenn GS, Motulsky AG. 1995. A quantitative assessment of plasma homocysteine as a risk factor for vascular disease: Probable benefits of increasing folic acid intakes. *J Am Med Assoc* 274:1049–1057.

Bowman SA. 1999. Diets of individuals based on energy intakes from added sugars. *Fam Econ Nutr Rev* 12:31–38.

Brand JC, Colagiuri S, Crossman S, Allen A, Roberts DCK, Truswell AS. 1991. Low-glycemic index foods improve long-term glycemic control in NIDDM. *Diabetes Care* 14:95–101.

Brito MN, Brito NA, Migliorini RH. 1992. Thermogenic capacity of brown adipose tissue is reduced in rats fed a high protein, carbohydrate-free diet. *J Nutr* 122:2081–2086.

Britten P, Basiotis PP, Davis CA, Anand R. 2000. Is intake of added sugars associated with diet quality? Online. *Nutrition Insights* No 21. USDA Center for Nutrition Policy and Promotion. Available at http://www.usda.gov/cnpp/insights.htm. Accessed June 8, 2001.

Brooks GA, Mercier J. 1994. Balance of carbohydrate and lipid utilization during exercise: The "crossover" concept. *J Appl Physiol* 76:2253–2261.

Brosnan JT. 1999. Comments on metabolic needs for glucose and the role of gluconeogenesis. *Eur J Clin Nutr* 53:S107–S111.

Bruning PF, Bonfrèr JMG, van Noord PAH, Hart AAM, de Jong-Bakker M, Nooijen WJ. 1992. Insulin resistance and breast-cancer risk. *Int J Cancer* 52:511–516.

Burley VJ. 1997. Sugar consumption and cancers of the digestive tract. *Eur J Cancer Prev* 6:422–434.

Burley VJ. 1998. Sugar consumption and human cancer in sites other than the digestive tract. *Eur J Cancer Prev* 7:253–277.

Burt RL, Davidson IWF. 1974. Insulin half-life and utilization in normal pregnancy. *Obstet Gynecol* 43:161–170.

Buyken AE, Toeller M, Heitkamp G, Karamanos B, Rottiers R, Muggeo M, Fuller JH. 2001. Glycemic index in the diet of European outpatients with type 1 diabetes: Relations to glycated hemoglobin and serum lipids. *Am J Clin Nutr* 73:574–581.

Cahill GF. 1970. Starvation in man. *N Engl J Med* 282:668–675.

Cahill GF, Owen OE, Morgan AP. 1968. The consumption of fuels during prolonged starvation. *Adv Enzyme Reg* 6:143–150.

Cahill GF, Aoki TT, Ruderman NB. 1973. Ketosis. *Trans Am Clin Climatol Assoc* 84:184–202.

Calloway DH. 1971. Dietary components that yield energy. *Environ Biol Med* 1:175–186.

Carlson MG, Snead WL, Campbell PJ. 1994. Fuel and energy metabolism in fasting humans. *Am J Clin Nutr* 60:29–36.

Chandramouli V, Ekberg K, Schumann WC, Kalhan SC, Wahren J, Landau BR. 1997. Quantifying gluconeogenesis during fasting. *Am J Physiol* 273:E1209–E1215.

Chew I, Brand JC, Thornburn AW, Truswell AS. 1988. Application of glycemic index to mixed meals. *Am J Clin Nutr* 47:53–56.

Chryssanthopoulos C, Hennessy LCM, Williams C. 1994. The influence of pre-exercise glucose ingestion on endurance running capacity. *Br J Sports Med* 28:105–109.

Chugani HT. 1993. Positron emission tomography scanning: Applications in newborns. *Clin Perinatol* 20:395–409.

Chugani HT, Phelps ME. 1986. Maturational changes in cerebral function in infants determined by [18]FDG positron emission tomography. *Science* 231:840–843.

Chugani HT, Phelps ME, Mazziotta JC. 1987. Positron emission tomography study of human brain functional development. *Ann Neurol* 22:487–497.

Cohen JC, Schall R. 1988. Reassessing the effects of simple carbohydrates on the serum triglyceride responses to fat meals. *Am J Clin Nutr* 48:1031–1034.

Colditz GA, Manson JE, Stampfer MJ, Rosner B, Willett WC, Speizer FE. 1992. Diet and risk of clinical diabetes in women. *Am J Clin Nutr* 55:1018–1023.

Collier GR, Wolever TMS, Wong GS, Josse RG. 1986. Prediction of glycemic response to mixed meals in noninsulin-dependent diabetic subjects. *Am J Clin Nutr* 44:349–352.

Collier GR, Giudici S, Kalmusky J, Wolever TMS, Helman G, Wesson V, Ehrlich RM, Jenkins DJA. 1988. Low glycaemic index starchy foods improve glucose control and lower serum cholesterol in diabetic children. *Diabetes Nutr Metab* 1:11–19.

Condon JR, Nassim JR, Millard FJC, Hilbe A, Stainthorpe EM. 1970. Calcium and phosphorus metabolism in relation to lactose tolerance. *Lancet* 1:1027–1029.

Coppa GV, Gabrielli O, Pierani P, Catassi C, Carlucci A, Giorgi PL. 1993. Changes in carbohydrate composition in human milk over 4 months of lactation. *Pediatrics* 91:637–641.

Cott A. 1977. Treatment of learning disabilities. In: Williams RJ, Kalita DK, eds. *A Physician's Handbook on Orthomolecular Medicine.* New York: Pergamon Press. Pp. 90–94.

Coulston AM, Hollenbeck CB, Liu GC, Williams RA, Starich GH, Mazzaferri EL, Reaven GM. 1984. Effect of source of dietary carbohydrate on plasma glucose, insulin, and gastric inhibitory polypeptide responses to test meals in subjects with noninsulin-dependent diabetes mellitus. *Am J Clin Nutr* 40:965–970.

Cousins L, Rigg L, Hollingsworth D, Brink G, Aurand J, Yen SSC. 1980. The 24-hour excursion and diurnal rhythm of glucose, insulin, and C-peptide in normal pregnancy. *Am J Obstet Gynecol* 136:483–488.

Cowett RM, Susa JB, Kahn CB, Giletti B, Oh W, Schwartz R. 1983. Glucose kinetics in nondiabetic and diabetic women during the third trimester of pregnancy. *Am J Obstet Gynecol* 146:773–780.

Crapo PA, Kolterman OG. 1984. The metabolic effects of 2-week fructose feeding in normal subjects. *Am J Clin Nutr* 39:525–534.

Décombaz J, Sartori D, Arnaud M-J, Thélin A-L, Schürch P, Howald H. 1985. Oxidation and metabolic effects of fructose or glucose ingested before exercise. *Int J Sports Med* 6:282–286.

DeFronzo RA, Bonadonna RC, Ferrannini E. 1992. Pathogenesis of NIDDM. A balanced overview. *Diabetes Care* 15:318–368.

Dekaban AS, Sadowsky D. 1978. Changes in brain weights during the span of human life: Relation of brain weights to body heights and body weights. *Ann Neurol* 4:345–356.

DeMarco HM, Sucher KP, Cisar CJ, Butterfield GE. 1999. Pre-exercise carbohydrate meals: Application of glycemic index. *Med Sci Sports Exerc* 31:164–170.

Denne SC, Kalhan SC. 1986. Glucose carbon recycling and oxidation in human newborns. *Am J Physiol* 251:E71–E77.

De Stefani E, Deneo-Pellegrini H, Mendilaharsu M, Ronco A, Carzoglio JC. 1998. Dietary sugar and lung cancer: A case-control study in Uruguay. *Nutr Cancer* 31:132–137.

Dewey KG, Lönnerdal B. 1983. Milk and nutrient intake of breast-fed infants from 1 to 6 months: Relation to growth and fatness. *J Pediatr Gastroenterol Nutr* 2:497–506.

Dewey KG, Finley DA, Lönnerdal B. 1984. Breast milk volume and composition during late lactation (7–20 months). *J Pediatr Gastroenterol Nutr* 3:713–720.

Díez-Sampedro A, Eskandari S, Wright EM, Hirayama BA. 2001. Na+-to-sugar stoichiometry of SGLT3. *Am J Physiol Renal Physiol* 280:F278–F282.

Dobbing J, Sands J. 1973. Quantitative growth and development of human brain. *Arch Dis Child* 48:757–767.

Dreon DM, Frey-Hewitt B, Ellsworth N, Williams PT, Terry RB, Wood PD. 1988. Dietary fat:carbohydrate ratio and obesity in middle-aged men. *Am J Clin Nutr* 47:995–1000.

Du Bois EF. 1928. The control of protein in the diet. *J Am Diet Assoc* 4:53–76.

Dunnigan MG, Fyfe T, McKiddie MT, Crosbie SM. 1970. The effects of isocaloric exchange of dietary starch and sucrose on glucose tolerance, plasma insulin and serum lipids in man. *Clin Sci* 38:1–9.

Edmond J, Austad N, Robbins RA, Bergstrom JD. 1985. Ketone body metabolism in the neonate: Development and effect of diet. *Fed Proc* 44:2359–2364.

Egger J, Carter CM, Graham PJ, Gumley D, Soothill JF. 1985. Controlled trial of oligoantigenic treatment in the hyperkinetic syndrome. *Lancet* 1:540–545.

Ercan N, Gannon MC, Nuttall FQ. 1994. Effect of added fat on the plasma glucose and insulin response to ingested potato given in various combinations as two meals in normal individuals. *Diabetes Care* 17:1453–1459.

Ernst N, Fisher M, Smith W, Gordon T, Rifkind BM, Little JA, Mishkel MA, Williams OD. 1980. The association of plasma high-density lipoprotein cholesterol with dietary intake and alcohol consumption. The Lipid Research Clinics Program Prevalence Study. *Circulation* 62:IV41–IV52.

FAO/WHO (Food and Agriculture Organization/World Health Organization). 1998. *Carbohydrates in Human Nutrition*. Rome: FAO.

Farris RP, Nicklas TA, Myers L, Berenson GS. 1998. Nutrient intake and food group consumption of 10-year-olds by sugar intake level: The Bogalusa Heart Study. *J Am Coll Nutr* 17:579–585.

Febbraio MA, Keenan J, Angus DJ, Campbell SE, Garnham AP. 2000. Preexercise carbohydrate ingestion, glucose kinetics, and muscle glycogen use: Effect of the glycemic index. *J Appl Physiol* 89:1845–1851.

Fehily AM, Phillips KM, Yarnell JWG. 1984. Diet, smoking, social class, and body mass index in the Caerphilly Heart Disease Study. *Am J Clin Nutr* 40:827–833.

Felig P. 1973. The glucose-alanine cycle. *Metabolism* 22:179–207.

Ferris AM, Dotts MA, Clark RM, Ezrin M, Jensen RG. 1988. Macronutrients in human milk at 2, 12, and 16 weeks postpartum. *J Am Diet Assoc* 88:694–697.

Fitzsimons D, Dwyer JT, Palmer C, Boyd LD. 1998. Nutrition and oral health guidelines for pregnant women, infants, and children. *J Am Diet Assoc* 98:182–189.

Fomon SJ, Thomas LN, Filer LJ, Anderson TA, Nelson SE. 1976. Influence of fat and carbohydrate content of diet on food intake and growth of male infants. *Acta Paediatr Scand* 65:136–144.

Fontvieille AM, Acosta M, Rizkalla SW, Bornet F, David P, Letanoux M, Tchobroutsky G, Slama G. 1988. A moderate switch from high to low glycaemic-index foods for 3 weeks improves the metabolic control of type I (IDDM) diabetic subjects. *Diabetes Nutr Metab* 1:139–143.

Fontvieille AM, Rizkalla SW, Penfornis A, Acosta M, Bornet FRJ, Slama G. 1992. The use of low glycaemic index foods improves metabolic control of diabetic patients over five weeks. *Diabet Med* 9:444–450.

Ford ES, Liu S. 2001. Glycemic index and serum high-density lipoprotein cholesterol concentration among US adults. *Arch Intern Med* 161:572–576.

Forshee RA, Storey ML. 2001. The role of added sugars in the diet quality of children and adolescents. *J Am Coll Nutr* 20:32–43.

Forsum E, Kabir N, Sadurskis A, Westerterp K. 1992. Total energy expenditure of healthy Swedish women during pregnancy and lactation. *Am J Clin Nutr* 56:334–342.

Foster-Powell K, Brand Miller J. 1995. International tables of glycemic index. *Am J Clin Nutr* 62:871S–890S.

Franceschi S, Dal Maso L, Augustin L, Negri E, Parpinel M, Boyle P, Jenkins DJA, La Vecchia C. 2001. Dietary glycemic load and colorectal cancer risk. *Ann Oncol* 12:173–178.

Frost G, Wilding J, Beecham J. 1994. Dietary advice based on the glycaemic index improves dietary profile and metabolic control in type 2 diabetic patients. *Diabet Med* 11:397–401.

Frost G, Leeds A, Trew G, Margara R, Dornhorst A. 1998. Insulin sensitivity in women at risk of coronary heart disease and the effect of a low glycaemic diet. *Metabolism* 47:1245–1251.

Frost G, Leeds AA, Doré CJ, Madeiros S, Brading S, Dornhorst A. 1999. Glycaemic index as a determinant of serum HDL-cholesterol concentration. *Lancet* 353:1045–1048.

Gamble JL. 1946. Physiological information gained from studies on the life raft ration. *Harvey Lect* 42:247–273.

Gannon MC, Nuttall FQ. 1987. Factors affecting interpretation of postprandial glucose and insulin areas. *Diabetes Care* 10:759–763.

Gannon MC, Nuttall FQ. 1999. Protein and diabetes. In: Franz MJ, Bantle JP, eds. *American Diabetes Association Guide to Medical Nutrition Therapy for Diabetes.* Alexandria, VA: American Diabetes Association. Pp. 107–125.

Gannon MC, Niewoehner CB, Nuttall FQ. 1985. Effect of insulin administration on cardiac glycogen synthase and synthase phosphatase activity in rats fed diets high in protein, fat or carbohydrate. *J Nutr* 115:243–251.

Gannon MC, Nuttall FQ, Westphal SA, Seaquist ER. 1993. The effect of fat and carbohydrate on plasma glucose, insulin, C-peptide, and triglycerides in normal male subjects. *J Am Coll Nutr* 12:36–41.

Gibbons A. 1998. Solving the brain's energy crisis. *Science* 280:1345–1347.

Gibney M, Sigman-Grant M, Stanton JL, Keast DR. 1995. Consumption of sugars. *Am J Clin Nutr* 62:178S–194S.

Gibson SA. 1993. Consumption and sources of sugars in the diets of British schoolchildren: Are high-sugar diets nutritionally inferior? *J Hum Nutr Diet* 6:355–371.

Gibson SA. 1996a. Are diets high in non-milk extrinsic sugars conducive to obesity? An analysis from the Dietary and Nutritional Survey of British Adults. *J Hum Nutr Diet* 9:283–292.

Gibson SA. 1996b. Are high-fat, high-sugar foods and diets conducive to obesity? *Int J Food Sci Nutr* 47:405–415.

Gibson SA. 1997. Non-milk extrinsic sugars in the diets of pre-school children: Association with intakes of micronutrients, energy, fat and NSP. *Br J Nutr* 78:367–378.

Giovannucci E, Willett WC. 1994. Dietary factors and risk of colon cancer. *Ann Med* 26:443–452.

Giovannucci E, Rimm EB, Wolk A, Ascherio A, Stampfer MJ, Colditz GA, Willett WC. 1998. Calcium and fructose intake in relation to risk of prostate cancer. *Cancer Res* 58:442–447.

Gleeson M, Maughan RJ, Greenhaff PL. 1986. Comparison of the effects of pre-exercise feeding of glucose, glycerol and placebo on endurance and fuel homeostasis in man. *Eur J Appl Physiol* 55:645–653.

Glinsmann WH, Irausquin H, Park YK. 1986. Evaluation of health aspects of sugars contained in carbohydrate sweeteners. Report of Sugars Task Force. *J Nutr* 116:S1–S216.

Goldberg GR, Prentice AM, Coward WA, Davies HL, Murgatroyd PR, Wensing C, Black AE, Harding M, Sawyer M. 1993. Longitudinal assessment of energy expenditure in pregnancy by the doubly labeled water method. *Am J Clin Nutr* 57:494–505.

Gottstein U, Held K. 1979. Effects of aging on cerebral circulation and metabolism in man. *Acta Neurologica Scand* 60:54–55.

Groop LC, Eriksson JG. 1992. The etiology and pathogenesis of non-insulin-dependent diabetes. *Ann Med* 24:483–489.

Gulliford MC, Bicknell EJ, Scarpello JH. 1989. Differential effect of protein and fat ingestion on blood glucose responses to high- and low-glycemic-index carbohydrates in noninsulin-dependent diabetic subjects. *Am J Clin Nutr* 50:773–777.

Guss JL, Kissileff HR, Pi-Sunyer FX. 1994. Effects of glucose and fructose solutions on food intake and gastric emptying in nonobese women. *Am J Physiol* 267:R1537–R1544.

Guthrie JF, Morton JF. 2000. Food sources of added sweeteners in the diets of Americans. *J Am Diet Assoc* 100:43–48, 51.

Haffner SM, Fong D, Hazuda HP, Pugh JA, Patterson JK. 1988a. Hyperinsulinemia, upper body adiposity, and cardiovascular risk factors in non-diabetics. *Metabolism* 37:338–345.

Haffner SM, Stern MP, Hazuda HP, Mitchell BD, Patterson JK. 1988b. Increased insulin concentrations in nondiabetic offspring of diabetic parents. *N Engl J Med* 319:1297–1301.

Haffner SM, Stern MP, Mitchell BD, Hazuda HP, Patterson JK. 1990. Incidence of type II diabetes in Mexican Americans predicted by fasting insulin and glucose levels, obesity, and body-fat distribution. *Diabetes* 39:283–288.

Hallfrisch J. 1990. Metabolic effects of dietary fructose. *FASEB J* 4:2652–2660.

Hallfrisch J, Reiser S, Prather ES. 1983. Blood lipid distribution of hyperinsulinemic men consuming three levels of fructose. *Am J Clin Nutr* 37:740–748.

Hanson PG, Johnson RE, Zaharko DS. 1965. Correlation between ketone body and free fatty acid concentrations in the plasma during early starvation in man. *Metabolism* 14:1037–1040.

Hargreaves M, Costill DL, Fink WJ, King DS, Fielding RA. 1987. Effect of pre-exercise carbohydrate feedings on endurance cycling performance. *Med Sci Sports Exerc* 19:33–36.

Harnack L, Stang J, Story M. 1999. Soft drink consumption among US children and adolescents: Nutritional consequences. *J Am Diet Assoc* 99:436–441.

Hatazawa J, Brooks RA, Di Chiro G, Bacharach SL. 1987. Glucose utilization rate versus brain size in humans. *Neurology* 37:583–588.

Hay WW. 1994. Placental supply of energy and protein substrates to the fetus. *Acta Paediatr Suppl* 405:13–19.

Hayford JT, Danney MM, Wiebe D, Roberts S, Thompson RG. 1979. Triglyceride integrated concentrations: Effect of variation of source and amount of dietary carbohydrate. *Am J Clin Nutr* 32:1670–1678.

Heinbecker P. 1928. Studies on the metabolism of Eskimos. *J Biol Chem* 80:461–475.

Hellerstein MK. 1999. De novo lipogenesis in humans: Metabolic and regulatory aspects. *Eur J Clin Nutr* 53:S53–S65.

Holbrook WP, Árnadóttir IB, Takazoe E, Birkhed D, Frostell G. 1995. Longitudinal study of caries, cariogenic bacteria and diet in children just before and after starting school. *Eur J Oral Sci* 103:42–45.

Hollenbeck CB, Coulston AM, Reaven GM. 1986. Glycemic effects of carbohydrates: A different perspective. *Diabetes Care* 9:641–647.

Holt SH, Brand Miller J. 1995. Increased insulin responses to ingested foods are associated with lessened satiety. *Appetite* 24:43–54.

Holt SHA, Brand Miller JC, Petocz P. 1997. An insulin index of foods: The insulin demand generated by 1000-kJ portions of common foods. *Am J Clin Nutr* 66:1264–1276.

Homko CJ, Sivan E, Reece EA, Boden G. 1999. Fuel metabolism during pregnancy. *Semin Reprod Endocrinol* 17:119–125.

Hoover HC, Grant JP, Gorschboth C, Ketcham AS. 1975. Nitrogen-sparing intravenous fluids in postoperative patients. *N Engl J Med* 293:172–175.

Hu FB, Manson JE, Stampfer MJ, Colditz G, Liu S, Solomon CG, Willett WC. 2001. Diet, lifestyle, and the risk of type 2 diabetes mellitus in women. *N Engl J Med* 345:790–797.

Hultman E, Harris RC, Spriet LL. 1999. Diet in work and exercise performance. In: Shils ME, Olson JA, Shike M, Ross AC, eds. *Modern Nutrition in Health and Disease*, 9th ed. Baltimore, MD: Williams and Wilkins. Pp. 761–782.

Indar-Brown K, Norenberg C, Madar Z. 1992. Glycemic and insulinemic responses after ingestion of ethnic foods by NIDDM and healthy subjects. *Am J Clin Nutr* 55:89–95.

IOM (Institute of Medicine). 1991. *Nutrition During Lactation*. Washington, DC: National Academy Press.

Janney NW. 1915. The metabolic relationship of the proteins to glucose. *J Biol Chem* 20:321–350.

Järvi AE, Karlström BE, Granfeldt YE, Björk IME, Vessby BOH, Asp N-GL. 1995. The influence of food structure on postprandial metabolism in patients with non-insulin-dependent diabetes mellitus. *Am J Clin Nutr* 61:837–842.

Järvi AE, Karlström BE, Granfeldt YE, Björck IE, Asp N-GL, Vessby BOH. 1999. Improved glycemic control and lipid profile and normalized fibrinolytic activity on a low-glycemic index diet in type 2 diabetic patients. *Diabetes Care* 22:10–18.

Jenkins DJA, Wolever TMS, Taylor RH, Barker H, Fielden H, Baldwin JM, Bowling AC, Newman HC, Jenkins AL, Goff DV. 1981. Glycemic index of foods: A physiological basis for carbohydrate exchange. *Am J Clin Nutr* 34:362–366.

Jenkins DJA, Wolever TMS, Kalmusky J, Giudici S, Giordano C, Wong GS, Bird JN, Patten R, Hall M, Buckley G, Little JA. 1985. Low glycemic index carbohydrate foods in the management of hyperlipidemia. *Am J Clin Nutr* 42:604–617.

Jenkins DJA, Wolever TMS, Collier GR, Ocana A, Rao AV, Buckley G, Lam Y, Mayer A, Thompson LU. 1987a. Metabolic effects of a low-glycemic-index diet. *Am J Clin Nutr* 46:968–975.

Jenkins DJA, Wolever TMS, Kalmusky J, Guidici S, Girodano C, Patten R, Wong GS, Bird J, Hall M, Buckley G, Csima A, Little JA. 1987b. Low-glycemic index diet in hyperlipidemia: Use of traditional starchy foods. *Am J Clin Nutr* 46:66–71.

Jenkins DJA, Wolever TMS, Buckley G, Lam KY, Giudici S, Kalmusky J, Jenkins AL, Patten RL, Bird J, Wong GS, Josse RG. 1988a. Low-glycemic-index starchy food in the diabetic diet. *Am J Clin Nutr* 48:248–254.

Jenkins DJA, Wolever TMS, Jenkins AL. 1988b. Starchy foods and glycemic index. *Diabetes Care* 11:149–159.

Jenkins DJA, Jenkins AL, Wolever TM, Vuksan V, Brighenti F, Testolin G. 1990. Fiber and physiological and potentially therapeutic effects of slowing carbohydrate absorption. *Adv Exp Med Biol* 270:129–134.

Johnson RK. 2000. What are people really eating and why does it matter? *Nutr Today* 35:40–46.

Kahn SE, Prigeon RL, Schwartz RS, Fujimoto WY, Knopp RH, Brunzell JD, Porte D. 2001. Obesity, body fat distribution, insulin sensitivity and islet β-cell function as explanations for metabolic diversity. *J Nutr* 131:354S–360S.

Kalhan SC, Kiliç İ. 1999. Carbohydrate as nutrient in the infant and child: Range of acceptable intake. *Eur J Clin Nutr* 53:S94–S100.

Kalhan SC, D'Angelo LJ, Savin SM, Adam PAJ. 1979. Glucose production in pregnant women at term gestation. Sources of glucose for human fetus. *J Clin Invest* 63:388–394.

Kalhan SC, Oliven A, King KC, Lucero C. 1986. Role of glucose in the regulation of endogenous glucose production in the human newborn. *Pediatr Res* 20:49–52.

Kalhan S, Rossi K, Gruca L, Burkett E, O'Brien A. 1997. Glucose turnover and gluconeogenesis in human pregnancy. *J Clin Invest* 100:1775–1781.

Kalsbeek H, Verrips GH. 1994. Consumption of sweet snacks and caries experience of primary school children. *Caries Res* 28:477–483.

Kant AK. 2000. Consumption of energy-dense, nutrient-poor foods by adult Americans: Nutritional and health implications. The Third National Health and Nutrition Examination Survey, 1988–1994. *Am J Clin Nutr* 72:929–936.

Kaufmann NA, Poznanski R, Blondheim SH, Stein Y. 1966. Effect of fructose, glucose, sucrose and starch on serum lipids in carbohydrate induced hypertriglyceridemia and in normal subjects. *Israel J Med Sci* 2:715–726.

Kazer RR. 1995. Insulin resistance, insulin-like growth factor I and breast cancer: A hypothesis. *Int J Cancer* 62:403–406.

Kennedy C, Sokoloff L. 1957. An adaptation of the nitrous oxide method to the study of the cerebral circulation in children: Normal values for cerebral blood flow and cerebral metabolic rate in childhood. *J Clin Invest* 36:1130–1137.

Kety SS. 1957. The general metabolism of the brain in vivo. In: Richter D, ed. *Metabolism of the Nervous System.* London: Pergamon Press. Pp. 221–237.

Kiens B, Richter EA. 1996. Types of carbohydrate in an ordinary diet affect insulin action and muscle substrates in humans. *Am J Clin Nutr* 63:47–53.

King KC, Tserng K-Y, Kalhan SC. 1982. Regulation of glucose production in newborn infants of diabetic mothers. *Pediatr Res* 16:608–612.

Knopp RH, Saudek CD, Arky RA, O'Sullivan JB. 1973. Two phases of adipose tissue metabolism in pregnancy: Maternal adaptations for fetal growth. *Endocrinology* 92:984–988.

Kopp-Hoolihan LE, van Loan MD, Wong WW, King JC. 1999. Longitudinal assessment of energy balance in well-nourished, pregnant women. *Am J Clin Nutr* 69:697–704.

Krebs-Smith SM, Graubard BI, Kahle LL, Subar AF, Cleveland LE, Ballard-Barbash R. 2000. Low energy reporters vs. others: A comparison of reported food intakes. *Eur J Clin Nutr* 54:281–287.

Krezowski PA, Nuttall FQ, Gannon MC, Bartosh NH. 1986. The effect of protein ingestion on the metabolic response to oral glucose in normal individuals. *Am J Clin Nutr* 44:847–856.

Kushi LK, Lew RA, Stare FJ, Ellison CR, el Lozy M, Bourke G, Daly L, Graham I, Hickey N, Mulcahy R, Kevaney J. 1985. Diet and 20-year mortality from coronary heart disease. The Ireland–Boston Diet–Heart Study. *N Engl J Med* 312:811–888.

Laine DC, Thomas W, Levitt MD, Bantle JP. 1987. Comparison of predictive capabilities of diabetic exchange lists and glycemic index of foods. *Diabetes Care* 10:387–394.

Lammi-Keefe CJ, Ferris AM, Jensen RG. 1990. Changes in human milk at 0600, 1000, 1400, 1800, and 2200 h. *J Pediatr Gastroenterol Nutr* 11:83–88.

Landau BR, Wahren J, Chandramouli V, Schumann WC, Ekberg K, Kalhan SC. 1996. Contributions of gluconeogenesis to glucose production in the fasted state. *J Clin Invest* 98:378–385.

Leenders KL, Perani D, Lammertsma AA, Heather JD, Buckingham P, Healy MJR, Gibbs JM, Wise RJS, Hatazawa J, Herold S, Beaney RP, Brooks DJ, Spinks T, Rhodes C, Frackowiak RSJ, Jones T. 1990. Cerebral blood flow, blood volume and oxygen utilization. Normal values and effect of age. *Brain* 113:27–47.

Levin RJ. 1999. Carbohydrates. In: Shils ME, Olson JA, Shike M, Ross AC, eds. *Modern Nutrition in Health and Disease*, 9th ed. Baltimore, MD: Williams and Wilkins. Pp. 49–65.

Lewis CJ, Park YK, Dexter PB, Yetley EA. 1992. Nutrient intakes and body weights of persons consuming high and moderate levels of added sugars. *J Am Diet Assoc* 92:708–713.

Liljeberg HGM, Åkerberg AKE, Björck IME. 1999. Effect of the glycemic index and content of indigestible carbohydrates of cereal-based breakfast meals on glucose tolerance at lunch in healthy subjects. *Am J Clin Nutr* 69:647–655.

Lingstrom P, van Houte J, Kashket S. 2000. Food starches and dental caries. *Crit Rev Oral Biol Med* 11:366–380.

Liu K, Stamler J, Trevisan M, Moss D. 1982. Dietary lipids, sugar, fiber, and mortality from coronary heart disease. Bivariate analysis of international data. *Arteriosclerosis* 2:221–227.

Liu S, Willett WC, Stampfer MJ, Hu FB, Franz M, Sampson L, Hennekens CH, Manson JE. 2000. A prospective study of dietary glycemic load, carbohydrate intake, and risk of coronary heart disease in US women. *Am J Clin Nutr* 71:1455–1461.

Liu S, Manson JE, Stampfer MJ, Holmes MD, Hu FB, Hankinson SE, Willett WC. 2001. Dietary glycemic load assessed by food-frequency questionnaire in relation to plasma high-density-lipoprotein cholesterol and fasting plasma triacylglycerols in postmenopausal women. *Am J Clin Nutr* 73:560–566.

Ludwig DS, Majzoub JA, Al-Zahrani A, Dallal GE, Blanco I, Roberts SB. 1999. High glycemic index foods, overeating, and obesity. *Pediatrics* 103:E26.

Ludwig DS, Peterson KE, Gortmaker SL. 2001. Relation between consumption of sugar-sweetened drinks and childhood obesity: A prospective, observational analysis. *Lancet* 357:505–508.

Luscombe ND, Noakes M, Clifton PM. 1999. Diets high and low in glycemic index versus high monounsaturated fat diets: Effects on glucose and lipid metabolism in NIDDM. *Eur J Clin Nutr* 53:473–478.

Mackrell DJ, Sokal JE. 1969. Antagonism between the effects of insulin and glucagon on the isolated liver. *Diabetes* 18:724–732.

Macquart-Moulin G, Riboli E, Cornée J, Charnay B, Berthezène P, Day N. 1986. Case-control study on colorectal cancer and diet in Marseilles. *Int J Cancer* 38:183–191.

Macquart-Moulin G, Riboli E, Cornée J, Kaaks R, Berthezène P. 1987. Colorectal polyps and diet: A case-control study in Marseilles. *Int J Cancer* 40:179–188.

Mann JI, Truswell AS. 1972. Effects of isocaloric exchange of dietary sucrose and starch on fasting serum lipids, postprandial insulin secretion and alimentary lipaemia in human subjects. *Br J Nutr* 27:395–405.

Mann JI, Watermeyer GS, Manning EB, Randles J, Truswell AS. 1973. Effects on serum lipids of different dietary fats associated with a high sucrose diet. *Clin Sci* 44:601–604.

Marckmann P, Raben A, Astrup A. 2000. Ad libitum intake of low-fat diets rich in either starchy foods or sucrose: Effects on blood lipids, factor VII coagulant activity, and fibrinogen. *Metabolism* 49:731–735.

Martin BC, Warram JH, Krolewski AS, Bergman RN, Soeldner JS, Kahn CR. 1992. Role of glucose and insulin resistance in development of type 2 diabetes mellitus: Results of a 25-year follow-up study. *Lancet* 340:925–929.

Mascarenhas AK. 1998. Oral hygiene as a risk indicator of enamel and dentin caries. *Community Dent Oral Epidemiol* 26:331–339.

Mattes RD. 1996. Dietary compensation by humans for supplemental energy provided as ethanol or carbohydrate in fluids. *Physiol Behav* 59:179–187.

Maxwell JD, McKiddie MT, Ferguson A, Buchanan KD. 1970. Plasma insulin response to oral carbohydrate in patients with glucose and lactose malabsorption. *Gut* 11:962–965.

McDonagh MS, Whiting PF, Wilson PM, Sutton AJ, Chestnutt I, Cooper J, Misso K, Bradley M, Treasure E, Kleijnen J. 2000. Systemic review of water fluoridation. *Br Med J* 321:855–859.

McGee DL, Reed DM, Yano K, Kagan A, Tillotson J. 1984. Ten-year incidence of coronary heart disease in the Honolulu Heart Program. Relationship to nutrient intake. *Am J Epidemiol* 119:667–676.

Mehta S, Kalsi HK, Nain CK, Menkes JH. 1977. Energy metabolism of brain in human protein-calorie malnutrition. *Pediatr Res* 11:290–293.

Meyer KA, Kushi LH, Jacobs DR, Slavin J, Sellers TA, Folsom AR. 2000. Carbohydrates, dietary fiber, and incident of type 2 diabetes in older women. *Am J Clin Nutr* 71:921–930.

Miller AB, Howe GR, Jain M, Craib KJP, Harrison L. 1983. Food items and food groups as risk factors in a case-control study of diet and colorectal cancer. *Int J Cancer* 32:155–161.

Miller SL, Wolfe RR. 1999. Physical exercise as a modulator of adaptation to low and high carbohydrate and low and high fat intakes. *Eur J Clin Nutr* 53:S112–S119.

Miller WC, Lindeman AK, Wallace J, Niederpruem M. 1990. Diet composition, energy intake, and exercise in relation to body fat in men and women. *Am J Clin Nutr* 52:426–430.

Miller WC, Niederpruem MG, Wallace JP, Lindman AK. 1994. Dietary fat, sugar, and fiber predict body fat content. *J Am Diet Assoc* 94:612–615.

Morris KL, Zemel MB. 1999. Glycemic index, cardiovascular disease, and obesity. *Nutr Rev* 57:273–276.

Neville MC, Keller RP, Seacat J, Casey CE, Allen JC, Archer P. 1984. Studies on human lactation. I. Within-feed and between-breast variation in selected components of human milk. *Am J Clin Nutr* 40:635–646.

Newburg DS, Neubauer SH. 1995. Carbohydrates in milks: Analysis, quantities, and significance. In: Jensen RG, ed. *Handbook of Milk Composition*. New York: Academic Press. Pp. 273–349.

Nicklas TA, Myers L, Farris RP, Srinivasan SR, Berenson GS. 1996. Nutritional quality of a high carbohydrate diet as consumed by children: The Bogalusa Heart Study. *J Nutr* 126:1382–1388.

Nommsen LA, Lovelady CA, Heinig MJ, Lönnerdal B, Dewey KG. 1991. Determinants of energy, protein, lipid, and lactose concentrations in human milk during the first 12 mo of lactation: The DARLING Study. *Am J Clin Nutr* 53:457–465.

Nordli DR, Koenigsberger D, Schroeder J, deVivo DC. 1992. Ketogenic diets. In: Resor SR, Kutt H, eds. *The Medical Treatment of Epilepsy*. New York: Marcel Dekker. Pp. 455–472.

Nuttall FQ, Gannon MC. 1981. Sucrose and disease. *Diabetes Care* 4:305–310.

Nuttall FQ, Mooradian AD, Gannon MC, Billington C, Krezowski P. 1984. Effect of protein ingestion on the glucose and insulin response to a standardized oral glucose load. *Diabetes Care* 7:465–470.

Nuttall FQ, Gannon MC, Burmeister LA, Lane JT, Pyzdrowski KL. 1992. The metabolic response to various doses of fructose in type II diabetic subjects. *Metabolism* 41:510–517.

Okano G, Takeda H, Morita I, Katoh M, Mu Z, Miyake S. 1988. Effect of pre-exercise fructose ingestion on endurance performance in fed men. *Med Sci Sports Exerc* 20:105–109.

Owen OE, Morgan AP, Kemp HG, Sullivan JM, Herrera MG, Cahill GF. 1967. Brain metabolism during fasting. *J Clin Invest* 46:1589–1595.

Owen OE, Smalley KJ, D'Alessio DA, Mozzoli MA, Dawson EK. 1998. Protein, fat, and carbohydrate requirements during starvation: Anaplerosis and cataplerosis. *Am J Clin Nutr* 68:12–34.

Papas AS, Joshi A, Palmer CA, Giunta JL, Dwyer JT. 1995. Relationship of diet to root caries. *Am J Clin Nutr* 61:423S–429S.

Park YK, Yetley EA. 1993. Intakes and food sources of fructose in the United States. *Am J Clin Nutr* 58:737S–747S.

Parks EJ, Hellerstein MK. 2000. Carbohydrate-induced hypertriacylglycerolemia: Historical perspective and review of biological mechanisms. *Am J Clin Nutr* 71:412–433.

Patel D, Kalhan S. 1992. Glycerol metabolism and triglyceride-fatty acid cycling in the human newborn: Effect of maternal diabetes and intrauterine growth retardation. *Pediatr Res* 31:52–58.

Patel MS, Johnson CA, Rajan R, Owen OE. 1975. The metabolism of ketone bodies in developing human brain: Development of ketone-body-utilizing enzymes and ketone bodies as precursors for lipid synthesis. *J Neurochem* 25:905–908.

Phelps RL, Metzger BE, Freinkel N. 1981. Carbohydrate metabolism in pregnancy. XVII. Diurnal profiles of plasma glucose, insulin, free fatty acids, triglycerides, cholesterol, and individual amino acids in late normal pregnancy. *Am J Obstet Gynecol* 140:730–736.

Raguso CA, Pereira P, Young VR. 1999. A tracer investigation of obligatory oxidative amino acid losses in healthy, young adults. *Am J Clin Nutr* 70:474–483.

Rath R, Mas˘ek J, Kujalová V, Slabochová Z. 1974. Effect of a high sugar intake on some metabolic and regulatory indicators in young men. *Nahrung* 18:343–353.

Reaven GM. 1999. Insulin resistance: A chicken that has come to roost. *Ann N Y Acad Sci* 892:45–57.

Reinmuth OM, Scheinberg P, Bourne B. 1965. Total cerebral blood flow and metabolism. *Arch Neurol* 12:49–66.

Reiser S, Hallfrisch J. 1987. *Metabolic Effects of Dietary Fructose.* Boca Raton, FL: CRC Press.

Reiser S, Hallfrisch J, Michaelis OE, Lazar FL, Martin RE, Prather ES. 1979a. Isocaloric exchange of dietary starch and sucrose in humans. I. Effects on levels of fasting blood lipids. *Am J Clin Nutr* 32:1659–1669.

Reiser S, Handler HB, Gardner LB, Hallfrisch JG, Michaelis OE, Prather ES. 1979b. Isocaloric exchange of dietary starch and sucrose in humans. II. Effect on fasting blood insulin, glucose, and glucagon and on insulin and glucose response to a sucrose load. *Am J Clin Nutr* 32:2206–2216.

Reiser S, Powell AS, Scholfield DJ, Panda P, Ellwood KC, Canary JJ. 1989. Blood lipids, lipoproteins, apoproteins, and uric acid in men fed diets containing fructose or high-amylose cornstarch. *Am J Clin Nutr* 49:832–839.

Renner R, Elcombe AM. 1964. Factors affecting the utilization of "carbohydrate-free" diets by the chick. II. Level of glycerol. *J Nutr* 84:327–330.

Ritz P, Krempf M, Cloarec D, Champ M, Charbonnel B. 1991. Comparative continuous-indirect-calorimetry study of two carbohydrates with different glycemic indices. *Am J Clin Nutr* 54:855–859.

Robert J-J, Cummins JC, Wolfe RR, Durkot M, Matthews DE, Zhao XH, Bier DM, Young VR. 1982. Quantitative aspects of glucose production and metabolism in healthy elderly subjects. *Diabetes* 31:203–211.

Roberts SB. 2000a. A review of age-related changes in energy regulation and suggested mechanisms. *Mech Ageing Dev* 116:157–167.

Roberts SB. 2000b. High-glycemic index foods, hunger, and obesity: Is there a connection? *Nutr Rev* 58:163–169.

Roche HM. 1999. Dietary carbohydrates and triacylglycerol metabolism. *Proc Nutr Soc* 58:201–207.

Rodin J. 1991. Effects of pure sugar vs. mixed starch fructose loads on food intake. *Appetite* 17:213–219.

Rossetti L, Giaccari A, DeFronzo RA. 1990. Glucose toxicity. *Diabetes Care* 13:610–630.

Rudolf MCJ, Sherwin RS. 1983. Maternal ketosis and its effects on the fetus. *Clin Endocrinol Metab* 12:413–428.

Ryan EA, O'Sullivan MJ, Skyler JS. 1985. Insulin action during pregnancy. Studies with the euglycemic clamp technique. *Diabetes* 34:380–389.

Salmerón J, Ascherio A, Rimm EB, Colditz GA, Spiegelman D, Jenkins DJ, Stampfer MJ, Wing AL, Willett WC. 1997a. Dietary fiber, glycemic load, and risk of NIDDM in men. *Diabetes Care* 20:545–550.

Salmerón J, Manson JE, Stampfer MJ, Colditz GA, Wing AL, Willett WC. 1997b. Dietary fiber, glycemic load, and risk of non-insulin-dependent diabetes mellitus in women. *J Am Med Assoc* 277:472–477.

Sapir DG, Owen OE, Cheng JT, Ginsberg R, Boden G, Walker WG. 1972. The effect of carbohydrates on ammonium and ketoacid excretion during starvation. *J Clin Invest* 51:2093–2102.

Saris WH, Astrup A, Prentice AM, Zunft HJ, Formiguera X, Verboeket-van de Venne WP, Raben A, Poppitt SD, Seppelt B, Johnston S, Vasilaras TH, Keogh GF. 2000. Randomized controlled trial of changes in dietary carbohydrate/fat ratio and simple vs. complex carbohydrates on body weight and blood lipids: The CARMEN study. *Int J Obes Relat Metab Disord* 24:1310–1318.

Sawaya AL, Fuss PJ, Dallal GE, Tsay R, McCrory MA, Young V, Roberts SB. 2001. Meal palatability, substrate oxidation and blood glucose in young and older men. *Physiol Behav* 72:5–12.

Scheinberg P, Stead EA. 1949. The cerebral blood flow in male subjects as measured by the nitrous oxide technique. Normal values for blood flow, oxygen utilization, glucose utilization, and peripheral resistance, with observations on the effect of tiliting and anxiety. *J Clin Invest* 28:1163–1171.

Settergren G, Lindblad BS, Persson B. 1976. Cerebral blood flow and exchange of oxygen, glucose, ketone bodies, lactate, pyruvate and amino acids in infants. *Acta Paediatr Scand* 65:343–353.

Settergren G, Lindblad BS, Persson B. 1980. Cerebral blood flow and exchange of oxygen, glucose, ketone bodies, lactate, pyruvate and amino acids in anesthetized children. *Acta Paediatr Scand* 69:457–465.

Shannon WR. 1922. Neuropathologic manifestations in infants and children as a result of anaphylactic reaction to foods contained in their diet. *Am J Dis Child* 24:89–94.

Shaw JH. 1987. Causes and control of dental caries. *N Engl J Med* 317:996–1004.

Slattery ML, Benson J, Berry TD, Duncan D, Edwards SL, Caan BJ, Potter JD. 1997. Dietary sugar and colon cancer. *Cancer Epidemiol Biomarkers Prev* 6:677–685.

Smith JB, Niven BE, Mann JI. 1996. The effect of reduced extrinsic sucrose intake on plasma triglyceride levels. *Eur J Clin Nutr* 50:498–504.

Sokoloff L. 1973. Metabolism of ketone bodies by the brain. *Annu Rev Med* 24:271–280.

Sokoloff L, Fitzgerald GG, Kaufman EE. 1977. Cerebral nutrition and energy metabolism. In: Wurtman RJ, Wurtman JJ, eds. *Nutrition and the Brain.* New York: Raven Press. Pp. 87–139.

Sparks JW, Girard JR, Battaglia FC. 1980. An estimate of the caloric requirements of the human fetus. *Biol Neonate* 38:113–119.

Sparks MJ, Selig SS, Febbraio MA. 1998. Pre-exercise carbohydrate ingestion: Effect of the glycemic index on endurance exercise performance. *Med Sci Sports Exerc* 30:844–849.

Speer F. 1954. The allergenic tension-fatigue syndrome. *Pediatr Clin North Am* 1:1029–1037.

Spieth LE, Harnish JD, Lenders CM, Raezer LB, Pereira MA, Hangen SJ, Ludwig DS. 2000. A low-glycemic index diet in the treatment of pediatric obesity. *Arch Pediatr Adolesc Med* 154:947–951.

Spitzer L, Rodin J. 1987. Effects of fructose and glucose preloads on subsequent food intake. *Appetite* 8:135–145.

Streja DA, Steiner G, Marliss EB, Vranic M. 1977. Turnover and recycling of glucose in man during prolonged fasting. *Metabolism* 26:1089–1098.

Sunehag AL, Haymond MW, Schanler RJ, Reeds PJ, Bier DM. 1999. Gluconeogenesis in very low birth weight infants receiving total parenteral nutrition. *Diabetes* 48:791–800.

Surwit RS, Feinglos MN, McCaskill CC, Clay SL, Babyak MA, Brownlow BS, Plaisted CS, Lin P-H. 1997. Metabolic and behavioral effects of a high-sucrose diet during weight loss. *Am J Clin Nutr* 65:908–915.

Swanson JE, Laine DC, Thomas W, Bantle JP. 1992. Metabolic effects of dietary fructose in healthy subjects. *Am J Clin Nutr* 55:851–856.

Swink TD, Vining EPG, Freeman JM. 1997. The ketogenic diet: 1997. *Adv Pediatr* 44:297–329.

Thomas DE, Brotherhood JR, Brand JC. 1991. Carbohydrate feeding before exercise: Effect of glycemic index. *Int J Sports Med* 12:180–186.

Tillotson JL, Grandits GA, Bartsch GE, Stamler J. 1997. Relation of dietary carbohydrates to blood lipids in the special intervention and usual care groups in the Multiple Risk Factor Intervention Trial. *Am J Clin Nutr* 65:314S–326S.

Troiano RP, Briefel RR, Carroll MD, Bialostosky K. 2000. Energy and fat intakes of children and adolescents in the United States: Data from the National Health and Nutrition Examination Surveys. *Am J Clin Nutr* 72:1343S–1353S.

Tuyns AJ, Kaaks R, Haelterman M. 1988. Colorectal cancer and the consumption of foods: A case-control study in Belgium. *Nutr Cancer* 11:189–204.

USDA (U.S. Department of Agriculture). 1996. *The Food Guide Pyramid.* Home and Garden Bulletin No. 252. Washington, DC: U.S. Government Printing Office.

USDA/HHS (U.S. Department of Agriculture/U.S. Department of Health and Human Services). 2000. *Nutrition and Your Health: Dietary Guidelines for Americans.* Home and Garden Bulletin No. 232. Washington, DC: U.S. Government Printing Office.

van Dam RM, Visscher AWJ, Feskens EJM, Verhoef P, Kromhout D. 2000. Dietary glycemic index in relation to metabolic risk factors and incidence of coronary heart disease: The Zutphen Elderly Study. *Eur J Clin Nutr* 54:726–731.

Vining EPG. 1999. Clinical efficacy of the ketogenic diet. *Epilepsy Res* 37:181–190.

Walker ARP, Cleaton-Jones PE. 1992. Sugar intake and dental caries. *Br Dent J* 172:7.

Warram JH, Martin BC, Krolewski AS, Soeldner JS, Kahn CR. 1990. Slow glucose removal rate and hyperinsulinemia precede the development of type II diabetes in the offspring of diabetic parents. *Ann Intern Med* 113:909–915.

Welsh S, Davis C, Shaw A. 1992. Development of the Food Guide Pyramid. *Nutr Today* 27:12–23.

Westphal SA, Gannon MC, Nuttall FQ. 1990. Metabolic response to glucose ingested with various amounts of protein. *Am J Clin Nutr* 52:267–272.

White JW, Wolraich M. 1995. Effect of sugar on behavior and mental performance. *Am J Clin Nutr* 62:242S–249S.

Wolever TMS. 1990. Relationship between dietary fiber content and composition in foods and the glycemic index. *Am J Clin Nutr* 51:72–75.

Wolever TMS, Jenkins DJA. 1986. The use of the glycemic index in predicting the blood glucose response to mixed meals. *Am J Clin Nutr* 43:167–172.

Wolever TMS, Nuttal FQ, Lee R, Wong GS, Josse RG, Csima A, Jenkins DJA. 1985. Prediction of the relative blood glucose response of mixed meals using the white bread glycemic index. *Diabetes Care* 8:418–428.

Wolever TMS, Jenkins DJA, Josse RG, Wong GS, Lee R. 1987. The glycemic index: Similarity of values derived in insulin-dependent and non-insulin-dependent diabetic patients. *J Am Coll Nutr* 6:295–305.

Wolever TMS, Jenkins DJA, Ocana AM, Rao VA, Collier GR. 1988. Second-meal effect: Low-glycemic-index foods eaten at dinner improve subsequent breakfast glycemic response. *Am J Clin Nutr* 48:1041–1047.

Wolever TMS, Jenkins DJA, Vuksan V, Josse RG, Wong GS, Jenkins AL. 1990. Glycemic index of foods in individual subjects. *Diabetes Care* 13:126–132.

Wolever TMS, Jenkins DJA, Jenkins AL, Josse RG. 1991. The glycemic index: Methodology and clinical implications. *Am J Clin Nutr* 54:846–854.

Wolever TMS, Jenkins DJA, Vuksan V, Jenkins AL, Buckley GC, Wong GS, Josse RG. 1992a. Beneficial effect of a low glycaemic index diet in type 2 diabetes. *Diabet Med* 9:451–458.

Wolever TMS, Jenkins DJA, Vuksan V, Jenkins AL, Wong GS, Josse RG. 1992b. Beneficial effect of low-glycemic index diet in overweight NIDDM subjects. *Diabetes Care* 15:562–564.

Wolraich ML, Wilson DB, White JW. 1995. The effect of sugar on behavior or cognition in children. A meta-analysis. *J Am Med Assoc* 274:1617–1621.

World Cancer Research Fund/American Institute for Cancer Research. 1997. *Food, Nutrition and the Prevention of Cancer: A Global Perspective*. Washington, DC: American Institute for Cancer Research.

Yamaura H, Ito M, Kubota K, Matsuzawa T. 1980. Brain atrophy during aging: A quantitative study with computed tomography. *J Gerontol* 35:492–498.

Yudkin J, Eisa O, Kang SS, Meraji S, Bruckdorfer KR. 1986. Dietary sucrose affects plasma HDL cholesterol concentration in young men. *Ann Nutr Metab* 30:261–266.

Ziegler EE, Fomon SJ. 1983. Lactose enhances mineral absorption in infancy. *J Pediatr Gastroenterol Nutr* 2:288–294.

7

Dietary, Functional, and Total Fiber

SUMMARY

Dietary Fiber consists of nondigestible carbohydrates and lignin that are intrinsic and intact in plants. *Functional Fiber* consists of isolated, nondigestible carbohydrates that have beneficial physiological effects in humans. *Total Fiber* is the sum of *Dietary Fiber* and *Functional Fiber*. Fibers have different properties that result in different physiological effects. For example, viscous fibers may delay the gastric emptying of ingested foods into the small intestine, resulting in a sensation of fullness, which may contribute to weight control. Delayed gastric emptying may also reduce postprandial blood glucose concentrations and potentially have a beneficial effect on insulin sensitivity. Viscous fibers can interfere with the absorption of dietary fat and cholesterol, as well as with the enterohepatic recirculation of cholesterol and bile acids, which may result in reduced blood cholesterol concentrations. Consumption of *Dietary* and certain *Functional Fibers*, particularly those that are poorly fermented, is known to improve fecal bulk and laxation and ameliorate constipation. The relationship of fiber intake to colon cancer is the subject of ongoing investigation and is currently unresolved. An Adequate Intake (AI) for *Total Fiber* in foods is set at 38 and 25 g/d for young men and women, respectively, based on the intake level observed to protect against coronary heart disease. Median intakes of *Dietary Fiber* ranged from 16.5 to 17.9 g/d for men and 12.1 to 13.8 g/d for women (Appendix Table E-4). There was insufficient evidence to set a Tolerable Upper Intake Level (UL) for *Dietary Fiber* or *Functional Fiber*.

BACKGROUND INFORMATION
Overview

Definitions of Fiber

A variety of definitions of fiber exist worldwide (IOM, 2001). Some are based solely on one or more analytical methods for isolating fiber, while others are physiologically based. For instance, in the United States fiber is defined by a number of analytical methods that are accepted by the Association of Official Analytical Chemists International (AOAC); these methods isolate nondigestible animal and plant carbohydrates. In Canada, however, a formal definition has been in place that recognizes nondigestible food of plant origin—but not of animal origin—as fiber. As nutrition labeling becomes uniform throughout the world, it is recognized that a single definition of fiber may be needed. Furthermore, new products are being developed or isolated that behave like fiber, yet do not meet the traditional definitions of fiber, either analytically or physiologically.

Without an accurate definition of fiber, compounds can be designed or isolated and concentrated using available methods without necessarily providing beneficial health effects, which most people consider to be an important attribute of fiber. Other compounds can be developed that are nondigestible and provide beneficial health effects, yet do not meet the current U.S. definition based on analytical methods. For these reasons, the Food and Nutrition Board, under the oversight of the Standing Committee on the Scientific Evaluation of Dietary Reference Intakes, assembled a Panel on the Definition of Dietary Fiber to develop a proposed definition of fiber (IOM, 2001). Based on the panel's deliberations, consideration of public comments, and subsequent modifications, the following definitions have been developed:

Dietary Fiber consists of nondigestible carbohydrates and lignin that are intrinsic and intact in plants.
Functional Fiber consists of isolated, nondigestible carbohydrates that have beneficial physiological effects in humans.
Total Fiber is the sum of *Dietary Fiber* and *Functional Fiber*.

This two-pronged approach to define edible, nondigestible carbohydrates recognizes the diversity of carbohydrates in the human food supply that are not digested: plant cell wall and storage carbohydrates that predominate in foods, carbohydrates contributed by animal foods, and isolated and low molecular weight carbohydrates that occur naturally or have been synthesized or otherwise manufactured. These definitions recognize a continuum of carbohydrates and allow for flexibility to incorporate new fiber sources developed in the future (after demonstration of beneficial physiological effects in humans). While it is not anticipated that the new definitions will significantly impact recommended levels of intake, information on both *Dietary Fiber* and *Functional Fiber* will more clearly delineate the source of fiber and the potential health benefits. Although sugars and sugar alcohols could potentially be categorized as *Functional Fibers*, for labeling purposes they are not considered to be *Functional Fibers* because they fall under "sugars" and "sugar alcohols" on the food label.

Distinguishing Features of Dietary Fiber Compared with Functional Fiber

Dietary Fiber consists of nondigestible food plant carbohydrates and lignin in which the plant matrix is largely intact. Specific examples are provided in Table 7-1. Nondigestible means that the material is not digested and absorbed in the human small intestine. Nondigestible plant carbohydrates in foods are usually a mixture of polysaccharides that are integral components of the plant cell wall or intercellular structure. This definition recognizes that the three-dimensional plant matrix is responsible for some of the physicochemical properties attributed to *Dietary Fiber*. Fractions of plant foods are considered *Dietary Fiber* if the plant cells and their three-dimensional interrelationships remain largely intact. Thus, mechanical treatment would still result in intact fiber. Another distinguishing feature of *Dietary Fiber* sources is that they contain other macronutrients (e.g., digestible carbohydrate and protein) normally found in foods. For example, cereal brans, which are obtained by grinding, are anatomical layers of the grain consisting of intact cells and substantial amounts of starch and protein; they would be categorized as *Dietary Fiber* sources.

TABLE 7-1 Characteristics of *Dietary Fiber*

Characteristic	*Dietary Fiber*
Nondigestible animal carbohydrate	No
Carbohydrates not recovered by alcohol precipitation[a]	Yes
Nondigestible mono- and disaccharides and polyols	No
Lignin	Yes
Resistant starch	Some
Intact, naturally occurring food source only	Yes
Resistant to human enzymes	Yes
Specifies physiological effect	No

[a] Includes inulin, oligosaccharides (3–10 degrees of polymerization), fructans, polydextrose, methylcellulose, resistant maltodextrins, and other related compounds.

Resistant starch that is naturally occurring and inherent in a food or created during normal processing of a food, as is the case for flaked corn cereal, would be categorized as *Dietary Fiber*. Examples of oligosaccharides that fall under the category of *Dietary Fiber* are those that are normally constituents of a *Dietary Fiber* source, such as raffinose, stachyose, and verbacose in legumes, and the low molecular weight fructans in foods, such as Jerusalem artichoke and onions.

Functional Fiber consists of isolated or extracted nondigestible carbohydrates that have beneficial physiological effects in humans. *Functional Fibers* may be isolated or extracted using chemical, enzymatic, or aqueous steps. Synthetically manufactured or naturally occurring isolated oligosaccharides and manufactured resistant starch are included in this definition. Also included are those naturally occurring polysaccharides or oligosaccharides usually extracted from their plant source that have been modified (e.g., to a shorter polymer length or to a different molecular arrangement). Although they have been inadequately studied, animal-derived carbohydrates such as connective tissue are generally regarded as nondigestible. The fact that animal-derived carbohydrates are not of plant origin forms the basis for including animal-derived, nondigestible carbohydrates in the *Functional Fiber* category. Isolated, manufactured, or synthetic oligosaccharides of three or more degrees of polymerization are considered to be *Functional Fiber*. Nondigestible monosaccharides, disaccharides, and sugar alcohols are not considered to be *Functional Fibers* because they fall under "sugars" or "sugar alcohols" on the food label. Also, rapidly changing lumenal fluid balance resulting from large amounts of nondigestible mono- and disaccharides or low molecular weight oligosaccharides, such as that which occurs when sugar alcohols are consumed, is not considered a mechanism of laxation for *Functional Fibers*.

Rationale for Definitions

Nondigestible carbohydrates are frequently isolated to concentrate a desirable attribute of the mixture from which it was extracted. Distinguishing a category of *Functional Fiber* allows for the desirable characteristics of such components to be highlighted. In the relatively near future, plant and animal synthetic enzymes may be produced as recombinant proteins, which in turn may be used in the manufacture of fiber-like materials. The definition will allow for the inclusion of these materials and will provide a viable avenue to synthesize specific oligosaccharides and polysaccharides that are part of plant and animal tissues.

In summary, one definition has been proposed for *Dietary Fiber* because many other substances in high fiber foods, including a variety of vitamins and minerals, often have made it difficult to demonstrate a significant health benefit specifically attributable to the fiber in foods. Thus, it is difficult to separate out the effect of fiber per se from the high fiber food. Attempts have been made to do this, particularly in epidemiological studies, by controlling for other substances in those foods, but these attempts were not always successful. The advantage, then, of adding isolated nondigestible carbohydrates as a fiber source to a food is that one may be able to draw conclusions about *Functional Fiber* itself with regard to its physiological role rather than that of the vehicle in which it is found. The proposed definitions do not preclude research directed towards the health benefits of *Dietary Fiber* in foods, but it is not necessary to demonstrate a physiological effect in order for a food fiber to be listed as *Dietary Fiber*.

An important aspect of the recommended definitions is that a substance is required to demonstrate a beneficial physiological effect to be classified as *Functional Fiber*. Research has shown that extraction or isolation of a polysaccharide, usually through chemical, enzymatic, or aqueous means, can either enhance its health benefit (usually because it is a more concentrated source) or diminish the beneficial effect. These recommendations should be helpful in evaluating diet and disease relationship studies as it will be possible to classify fiber-like components as *Functional Fibers* due to their documented health benefits. Although databases are not currently constructed to delineate potential beneficial effects of specific fibers, there is no reason that this could not be accomplished in the future.

Examples of Dietary and Functional Fibers

As described in the report, *Dietary Reference Intakes: Proposed Definition of Dietary Fiber* (IOM, 2001), *Dietary Fiber* includes plant nonstarch polysaccharides (e.g., cellulose, pectin, gums, hemicellulose, β-glucans, and fibers contained in oat and wheat bran), plant carbohydrates that are not recovered by alcohol precipitation (e.g., inulin, oligosaccharides, and fructans), lignin, and some resistant starch. Potential *Functional Fibers* for food labeling include isolated, nondigestible plant (e.g., resistant starch, pectin, and gums), animal (e.g., chitin and chitosan), or commercially produced (e.g., resistant starch, polydextrose, inulin, and indigestible dextrins) carbohydrates.

How the Definitions Affect the Interpretation of This Report

The reason that a definition of fiber is so important is that what *is* or *is not* considered to be dietary fiber in, for example, a major epidemiological study on fiber and heart disease or fiber and colon cancer, could determine the results and interpretation of that study. In turn, that would affect recommendations regarding fiber intake. Clearly, the definitions described above were developed after the studies cited in this report, which form the basis for fiber intake recommendations. However, that should not detract from the relevance of the recommendations, as the database used to measure fiber for these studies will be noted.

For example, most epidemiological studies use the U.S. Department of Agriculture (USDA) database for fiber, along with other databases and data added by the investigators for missing values (Hallfrisch et al., 1988; Heilbrun et al., 1989; Miller et al., 1983; Platz et al., 1997). Such a database represents *Dietary Fiber*, since *Functional Fibers* that serve as food ingredients contribute a minor amount to the *Total Fiber* content of foods. In 1987, the U.S. Food and Drug Administration (FDA) adopted AOAC method 985.29 for regulatory purposes to identify fiber as a mixture of nonstarch polysaccharides, lignin, and some resistant starch (FDA, 1987). Related methods that isolated the same components as AOAC method 985.29 were developed independently and accepted by AOAC and FDA in subsequent years. These methods exclude all oligosaccharides (3 to 9 degrees of polymerization) from the definition and include all polysaccharides, lignin, and some of the resistant starch that is resistant to the enzymes (protease, amylase, and amyloglucosidase) used in the AOAC methods. It is these methods that are used to measure the fiber content of foods that is entered into the USDA database.

Other epidemiological studies have assessed intake of specific high fiber foods, such as legumes, breakfast cereals, fruits, and vegetables (Hill, 1997; Thun et al., 1992). Intervention studies often use specific fiber supplements such as pectin, psyllium, and guar gum, which would, by the above definition, be considered *Functional Fibers* if their role in human health is documented. For the above reasons, the type of fiber (*Dietary, Functional,* or *Total Fiber*) used in the studies discussed later in this chapter is identified.

Description of the Common Dietary and Functional Fibers

Below is a description of the *Dietary Fibers* that are most abundant in foods and the *Functional Fibers* that are commonly added to foods or provided as supplements. To be classified as a *Functional Fiber* for food labeling purposes, a certain level of information on the beneficial physiological effects in humans will be needed. For some of the known beneficial effects of *Dietary* and potential *Functional Fibers*, see "Physiological Effects of Isolated and Synthetic Fibers" and "Evidence Considered for Estimating the Requirement for *Dietary Fiber* and *Functional Fiber*."

Cellulose. Cellulose, a polysaccharide consisting of linear β-(1,4)–linked glucopyranoside units, is the main structural component of plant cell walls.

Humans lack digestive enzymes to cleave β-(1,4) linkages and thus cannot absorb glucose from cellulose. Powdered cellulose is a purified, mechanically disintegrated cellulose obtained as a pulp from wood or cotton and is added to food as an anticaking, thickening, and texturizing agent. Dietary cellulose can be classified as *Dietary Fiber* or *Functional Fiber*, depending on whether it is naturally occurring in food (*Dietary Fiber*) or added to foods (*Functional Fiber*).

Chitin and Chitosan. Chitin is an amino-polysaccharide containing β-(1,4) linkages as is present in cellulose. Chitosan is the deacetylated product of chitin. Both chitin and chitosan are found in the exoskeletons of arthropods (e.g., crabs and lobsters) and in the cell walls of most fungi. Neither chitin nor chitosan is digested by mammalian digestive enzymes. Chitin and chitosan are primarily consumed as a supplement and potentially can be classified as *Functional Fibers* if sufficient data on physiological benefits in humans are documented.

β-Glucans. β-glucans are homopolysaccharides of branched glucose resides. These β-linked D-glucopyranose polymers are constituents of fungi, algae, and higher plants (e.g., barley and oats). Naturally occurring β-glucans can be classified as *Dietary Fibers*, whereas added or isolated β-glucans are potential *Functional Fibers*.

Gums. Gums consist of a diverse group of polysaccharides usually isolated from seeds and have a viscous feature. Guar gum is produced by the milling of the endosperm of the guar seed. The major polysaccharide in guar gum is galactomannan. Galactomannans are highly viscous and are therefore used as food ingredients for their thickening, gelling, and stabilizing properties. Gums in the diet can be classified as *Dietary* or *Functional Fibers*.

Hemicelluloses. Hemicelluloses are a group of polysaccharides found in plant cell walls that surround cellulose. These polymers can be linear or branched and consist of glucose, arabinose, mannose, xylose, and galacturonic acid. Dietary hemicelluoses are classified as *Dietary Fibers*.

Inulin, Oligofructose, and Fructooligosaccharides. Inulin and oligofructose are naturally occurring in a variety of plants. Most of the commercially available inulin and oligofructose is either synthesized from sucrose or extracted and purified from chicory roots. Oligofructose is also formed by partial hydrolysis of inulin. Inulin is a polydisperse β-(2,1)-linked fructan with a glucose molecule at the end of each fructose chain. The chain length is usually 2 to 60 units, with an average degree of polymerization of ten. The β-(2,1) linkage is resistant to enzymatic digestion. Synthetic oligofructose contains β-(2,1) fructose chains with and without terminal glucose units. The chain ranges from two to eight monosaccharide residues. Synthetic fructooligosaccharides have the same chemical and structural composition as oligofructose, except that the degree of polymerization ranges from two to four. Because many current definitions of dietary fiber are based on methods involving ethanol precipitation, oligosaccharides and fructans that are endogenous in foods, but soluble in ethanol, are not analyzed as dietary fiber. Thus, the USDA database does not currently include these fiber sources. With respect to the definitions outlined in this chapter, the naturally occurring fructans that are found in plants, such as chicory, onions, and Jerusalem artichoke, would be classified as *Dietary Fibers*; the synthesized or extracted fructans could be classified as *Functional Fibers* when there are sufficient data to show positive physiological effects in humans.

Lignin. Lignin is a highly branched polymer comprised of phenyl-propanoid units and is found within "woody" plant cell walls, covalently bound to fibrous polysaccharides (*Dietary Fibers*). Although not a carbohydrate, because of its association with *Dietary Fiber*, and because it affects the physiological effects of *Dietary Fiber*, lignin is classified as a *Dietary Fiber* if it is relatively intact in the plant. Lignin isolated and added to foods could be classified as *Functional Fiber* given sufficient data on positive physiological effects in humans.

Pectins. Pectins, which are found in the cell wall and intracellular tissues of many fruits and berries, consist of galacturonic acid units with rhamnose interspersed in a linear chain. Pectins frequently have side chains of neutral sugars, and the galactose units may be esterified with a methyl group, a feature that allows for its viscosity. While fruits and vegetables contain 5 to 10 percent naturally occurring pectin, pectins are industrially extracted from citrus peels and apple pomace. Isolated, high methoxylated pectins are mainly added to jams due to their gelling properties with high amounts of sugar. Low methoxylated pectins are added to low-calorie gelled products, such as sugar-free jams and yogurts. Thus, pectins in the diet are classified as *Dietary* and/or *Functional Fiber*.

Polydextrose. Polydextrose is a polysaccharide that is synthesized by random polymerization of glucose and sorbitol. Polydextrose serves as a bulking agent in foods and sometimes as a sugar substitute. Polydextrose is not digested or absorbed in the small intestine and is partially fermented in the large intestine, with the remaining excreted in the feces. Polydextrose can potentially be classified as a *Functional Fiber* when sufficient data on physiological benefits in humans are documented.

Psyllium. Psyllium refers to the husk of psyllium seeds and is a very viscous mucilage in aqueous solution. The psyllium seed, also known as plantago or flea seed, is small, dark, reddish-brown, odorless, and nearly tasteless. *P. ovata*, known as blond or Indian plantago seed, is the species from which husk is usually derived. *P. ramosa* is known as Spanish or French psyllium seed. Psyllium, also known as ispaghula husk, may be classified as a *Functional Fiber.*

Resistant Dextrins. Indigestible components of starch hydrolysates, as a result of heat and enzymatic treatment, yield indigestible dextrins that are also called resistant maltodextrins. Unlike gums, which have a high viscosity that can lead to problems in food processing and unpleasant organoleptic properties, resistant maltodextrins are easily added to foods and have a good mouth feel. Resistant maltodextrins are produced by heat/acid treatment of cornstarch, followed by enzymatic (amylase) treatment. The average molecular weight of resistant maltodextrins is 2,000 daltons and consists of polymers of glucose containing α-(1-4) and α-(1-6) glucosidic bonds, as well as 1-2 and 1-3 linkages. Resistant dextrins can potentially be classified as *Functional Fibers* when sufficient data on physiological benefits in humans are documented.

Resistant Starch. Resistant starch is naturally occurring, but can also be produced by the modification of starch during the processing of foods. Starch that is included in a plant cell wall and thus physically inaccessible to α-amylase is called RS_1. Native starch that can be made accessible to the enzyme by gelatinization is called RS_2. Resistant starch that is formed during processing is called RS_3 or RS_4 and is considered to be fiber that is isolated rather than intact and naturally occurring. RS_3 (retrograded starch) is formed from the cooking and cooling or extrusion of starchy foods (e.g., potato chips and cereals). RS_4 (chemically modified starch) includes starch esters, starch ethers, and cross-bonded starches that have been produced by the chemical modification of starch. RS_3 and RS_4 are not digested by mammalian intestinal enzymes and are partly fermented in the colon (Cummings et al., 1996; Englyst et al., 1992). Resistant starch is estimated to be approximately 10 percent (2 to 20 percent) of the amount of starch consumed in the Western diet (Stephen et al., 1983). Thus, RS_1 and RS_2 are classified as *Dietary Fibers*, and RS_3 and RS_4 may be classified as *Functional Fibers.*

Physiology of Absorption, Metabolism, and Excretion

By definition, *Dietary Fiber* and *Functional Fiber* are not digested by mammalian enzymes. Therefore, they pass into the large intestine relatively intact. Along the gastrointestinal tract, properties of fiber result in different physiological effects.

Effect on Gastric Emptying and Satiety

Consumption of viscous fibers delays gastric emptying (Low, 1990; Roberfroid, 1993) and expands the effective unstirred layer, thus slowing the process of absorption once in the small intestine (Blackburn et al., 1984). This in turn can cause an extended feeling of fullness (Bergmann et al., 1992). A slower emptying rate means delayed digestion and absorption of nutrients (Jenkins et al., 1978; Ritz et al., 1991; Roberfroid, 1993; Truswell, 1992), resulting in decreased absorption of energy (Heaton, 1973). For example, Stevens and coworkers (1987) showed an 11 percent reduction in energy intake with psyllium gum intake. Postprandial glucose concentration in the blood is thus lower after the consumption of viscous fiber than after consumption of digestible carbohydrate alone (Benini et al., 1995; Holt et al., 1992; Leathwood and Pollet, 1988). The extended presence of nutrients in the upper small intestine may promote satiety (Sepple and Read, 1989).

Fermentation

Fibers may be fermented by the colonic microflora to carbon dioxide, methane, hydrogen, and short-chain fatty acids (primarily acetate, propionate, and butyrate). Foods rich in hemicelluloses and pectins, such as fruits and vegetables, contain *Dietary Fiber* that is more completely fermentable than foods rich in celluloses, such as cereals (Cummings, 1984; Cummings and Englyst, 1987; McBurney and Thompson, 1990). There appears to be no relationship between the level of *Dietary Fiber* intake and fermentability up to very high levels (Livesey, 1990). Resistant starch is highly fermentable (van Munster et al., 1994). Butyrate, a four-carbon, short-chain fatty acid, is the preferred energy source for colon cells (Roediger, 1982), and lack of butyrate production, absorption, or metabolism is thought by some to contribute to ulcerative colitis (Roediger, 1980; Roediger et al., 1993). Others have suggested that butyrate may be protective against colon cancer (see *"Dietary Fiber* and the Prevention of Colon Cancer"). However, the relationship between butyrate and colon cancer is controversial and the subject of ongoing investigation (Lupton, 1995).

Contribution of Fiber to Energy

When a metabolizable carbohydrate is absorbed in the small intestine, its energy value is 16.7 kJ/g (4 kcal/g); when fiber is anaerobically fermented by colonic microflora in the large intestine, short-chain fatty acids (e.g., butyrate, acetate, and propionate) are produced and absorbed as an energy source. Once absorbed into the colon cells, butyrate can be used as an energy source by colonocytes (Roediger, 1982); acetate and propionate travel through the portal vein to the liver, where propionate is then utilized by the liver. Acetate can be metabolized peripherally. A small proportion of energy from fermented fiber is used for bacterial growth and maintenance, and bacteria are excreted in feces, which also contain short-chain fatty acids (Cummings and Branch, 1986). Differences in food composition, patterns of food consumption, the administered dose of fiber, the metabolic status of the individual (e.g., obese, lean, malnourished), and the digestive capability of the individual influence the digestible energy consumed and the metabolizable energy available from various dietary fibers. Because the process of fermentation is anaerobic, less energy is recovered from fiber than the 4 kcal/g that is recovered from carbohydrate. While it is still unclear as to the energy yield of fibers in humans, current data indicate that the yield is in the range of 1.5 to 2.5 kcal/g (Livesey, 1990; Smith et al., 1998).

Physiological Effects of Isolated and Synthetic Fibers

This section summarizes the fibers for which there is a sufficient database that documents their beneficial physiological human effects, which is the rationale for categorizing them as *Functional Fibers*. It is important to note that discussions on the potential benefits of what might eventually be classified as *Functional Fibers* should not be construed as endorsements of those fibers. While plant-based foods are a good source of *Dietary Fiber*, isolated or synthetic fibers have been developed for their use as food ingredients and because of their beneficial role in human health. In 1988 Health Canada published guidelines for what they considered to be "novel fiber sources" and food products containing them that could be labeled as a source of fiber in addition to those included in their 1985 definition (Health Canada, 1988). The rationale for these guidelines was that there were safety issues unique to novel sources of fiber, and if a product was represented as containing fiber, it should have the beneficial physiological effects associated with dietary fiber that the public expects. The guidelines indicated that both safety and efficacy of the fiber source had to be established in order for the product to be identified as a source of dietary fiber in Canada, and this had to be done through experiments using humans.

Three measures of efficacy were identified: (1) laxation, (2) normalization of blood lipid concentrations, and (3) attenuation of blood glucose responses. Detailed guidelines were later produced for the clinical studies required to assess laxation effects, as this was the physiological function most often used by industry when seeking approval for a novel fiber source (Health Canada, 1997). For each of the fiber sources discussed below, studies will be summarized that relate to one of the three measures of efficacy identified by Health Canada, as these are the three most commonly accepted beneficial effects of fibers. A more complete discussion of these three measures of efficacy may be found later in this chapter. In addition, other potentially efficacious effects will be noted where studies are available.

As interest has increased in fiber, manufacturers have isolated various types of fiber from a wide range of carbohydrate sources added to foods. Many of these isolated materials are used as food additives based on functional properties such as thickening or fat reduction. As enzymatic and other technologies evolve, many types of polysaccharides will continue to be designed and manufactured using plant and animal synthetic enzymes. Examples in this category include modified cellulose, in which the hydroxyl groups on the glucose residues have been substituted to varying degrees with alkyl groups such as methyl and propyl; fructooligosaccharides manufactured from sucrose; and polydextrose synthesized from glucose. In some instances, fibers isolated from plants or manufactured chemically or synthetically have demonstrated more powerful beneficial physiological effects than a food source of the fiber polysaccharide.

Cellulose

Laxation. From a meta-analysis of about 100 studies of changes in stool weight with various fiber sources, investigators have calculated the increase in fecal weight due to fiber ingestion (Cummings, 1993). As noted later in this chapter, an increase in fecal weight does not necessarily equate with enhanced laxation, so this needs to be considered in interpreting the results of fecal bulking studies. Cellulose was shown to increase fecal bulk by 3 g/g of cellulose fed. This is lower than that achieved by bran (5.7 g/g of bran), but higher than that of isolated, fermentable fibers such as pectin (1.3 g/g of pectin) (Cummings, 1993). In a randomized, crossover study designed to compare the effects of supplemental pectin (12 g/d), cellulose (15 g/d), and lignin (12 g/d) on stool characteristics of healthy volunteers, cellulose was the only fiber that significantly decreased (–27 percent) mean stool transit time and increased mean wet stool weight (+57 percent) (Hillman et al., 1983).

Normalization of Blood Lipid Concentrations. Cellulose is often used as the placebo in studies designed to test the efficacy of fibers on decreasing serum cholesterol concentrations. Cellulose is either neutral with respect to blood cholesterol concentrations (Hillman et al., 1985; Niemi et al., 1988) or, in some studies, it actually shows a slight increase (Anderson et al., 1999).

Attenuation of Blood Glucose Responses. Similar to the relationship between cellulose and serum cholesterol concentrations, cellulose is also often used as a placebo in studies that evaluate the effect of fiber on blood glucose and insulin concentrations. Cellulose is ineffective in decreasing the postprandial glucose response (Librenti et al., 1992; Niemi et al., 1988).

Chitin and Chitosan

Laxation. There is no evidence that chitin or chitosan function as laxatives in humans.

Normalization of Blood Lipid Concentrations. There are a number of animal studies that have suggested that chitin and chitosan may decrease lipid absorption and thus the amount of fat entering the blood (Gallaher et al., 2000; Razdan and Pettersson, 1994; Sugano et al., 1980; Zacour et al., 1992). Therefore, blood cholesterol and triacylglycerol concentrations have been shown to be reduced with chitosan intake in animals (Chiang et al., 2000; Jennings et al., 1988; Razdan and Pettersson, 1994, 1996; Razdan et al., 1997).

These results, however, have not always been observed in controlled intervention trials with humans. When adult volunteers were given 2.7 g of chitosan for 7 days, there was no effect on fecal fat excretion (Guerciolini et al., 2001). When 2.4 g of chitosan was consumed daily by women, a significant reduction in low density lipoprotein (LDL) cholesterol concentration was observed (Wuolijoki et al., 1999). More intervention studies are needed to further understand the role of chitin and chitosan in the attenuation of blood lipid concentration in humans.

Attenuation of Blood Glucose Responses. There are no known reports in humans on chitin or chitosan intake and the attenuation of blood glucose responses.

Other Potential Physiological Effects. Because chitosan has been shown in some animal studies to reduce fat absorption, it has been proposed that chitosan intake can aid in weight reduction. When rats were fed up to

5 percent of their diet as chitosan, there was no effect on weight gain (Jennings et al., 1988; Sugano et al., 1980). Significantly reduced body weights were observed when chickens were fed 30 g/kg of chitosan (Razdan et al., 1997). There was no change in body weight in women consuming 2.4 g/d of chitosan for 8 weeks (Wuolijoki et al., 1999). Furthermore, no change in body weight was observed in women who consumed 2 g/d of chitosan for 28 days (Pittler et al., 1999). Similarly, in a study of 88 obese Asians, Ho and colleagues (2001) found no effect of chitosan supplementation (3 g/d) on weight, body mass index, or lean body mass compared to placebo.

Guar Gum

Laxation. As a viscous, highly fermentable fiber, guar gum has little effect on fecal bulk or laxation (Slavin, 1987).

Normalization of Blood Lipid Concentrations. Jenkins and coworkers (1975) reported the hypocholesterolemic effect of guar gum, which is often added to foods. Since 1975 there have been a number of studies with guar gum supplementation and findings of an 11 to 16 percent reduction in serum cholesterol concentration (Anderson and Tietyen-Clark, 1986; Penagini et al., 1986). For example, when type 2 diabetics were provided guar gum (21 g/d) for 3 months, the mean serum total and LDL cholesterol concentrations were significantly lower than controls (Aro et al., 1981). Furthermore, hypercholesterolemic men who received 15 g/d of guar gum had significantly lower serum total cholesterol and LDL cholesterol concentrations compared to the placebo controls after 6 weeks (Aro et al., 1984). Blake and coworkers (1997) evaluated the effect of depolymerized guar galactomannan on fasting plasma lipid concentrations in volunteers with moderately raised plasma cholesterol. There were significant reductions in plasma total cholesterol (9.7 percent) and LDL cholesterol (11 percent) concentrations after the guar treatment ($p < 0.001$). In addition to decreasing blood cholesterol concentrations, guar gum has also been shown to decrease concentrations of triacylglycerols (Bosello et al., 1984), as well as systolic and diastolic blood pressure (Krotkiewski, 1987).

Attenuation of Blood Glucose Responses. Viscous fibers, such as pectin and guar gum and those present in oat products and beans, produced significant reductions in glycemic response in 33 of 50 studies (66 percent) as reviewed in Wolever and Jenkins (1993). This is in contrast to only 3 of 14 studies conducted with insoluble fiber (21 percent). For example, when individuals with type 2 diabetes were given 21 g/d of guar gum, there was a significant reduction in both basal and postprandial hyper-glycemia compared to the placebo controls (Aro et al., 1981). In addition, the provision of 30 g/d of guar gum decreased fasting blood glucose concentration and increased insulin sensitivity (Landin et al., 1992).

In a dose–response study to determine the amount of guar gum needed to decrease postprandial glycemia and insulinemia, guar gum was supplied at 0, 2.9, 6.0, and 9.1 g/d in the form of biscuits to eight nondiabetics (Ellis et al., 1988). A reduction of 209 mU/min/L in the integrated insulin curve was estimated for every 1 g of guar gum incorporated into the biscuit. The addition of 10 g/d of guar gum to a test meal generated an overall decrease in blood glucose concentrations in both normal ($n = 5$) and diabetic ($n = 6$) individuals (Goulder et al., 1978).

Guar gum has also been shown to be effective when sprinkled on food. In a study with 18 type 2-diabetic patients, 5 g of guar gum granules or 5 g of wheat bran were sprinkled over food at each main meal for 4 weeks (Fuessl et al., 1987). There was a 50 percent reduction in the incremental area under the postprandial glycemic curve with the guar gum. Mean fasting plasma glucose and glycosylated hemoglobin concentrations were lower after treatment with guar gum compared with the wheat bran control.

Not all studies, however, have found a glycemic benefit from guar administration. In one study with type 2 diabetics with near-normal fasting plasma glucose concentrations, 15 g/d of guar gum did not reduce the excessive postprandial glycemic response (Holman et al., 1987). Although the mechanism for improved glycemic response seen with guar gum in most studies is not entirely clear, guar gum has been shown to increase C-peptide response over time, thus suggesting enhanced insulin secretion by guar gum (Groop et al., 1993). When the standard glucose test was performed after ingestion of 15 g/d of guar gum, improved glucose tolerance was observed in all but one pregnant women. In addition, guar gum generated significant reductions in mean serum glucose concentrations at 1, 2, and 3 hours after feeding (Gabbe et al., 1982).

Inulin, Oligofructose, and Fructooligosaccharides

Laxation. A few studies have demonstrated an increase in fecal bulk and increased stool frequency upon the ingestion of inulin or oligofructose. Fecal weight was increased after consuming 15 g/d of inulin or oligofructose (Gibson et al., 1995), and inulin (20 to 40 g/d) was shown to reduce constipation (Kleessen et al., 1997). A multicenter trial was conducted to test whether fructooligosaccharides worsen gastrointestinal symptoms in people with irritable bowel syndrome (Olesen and Gudmand-

Høyer, 2000). After 2 to 6 weeks of treatment with 20 g/d of fructo-oligosaccharides or placebo, symptoms of irritable bowel syndrome improved more in the placebo group than in the fructooligosaccharide group; however, there was no difference between the groups after continuous treatment for 12 weeks.

Normalization of Blood Lipid Concentrations. Studies on the effect of inulin or oligofructose ingestion on plasma lipid concentrations have provided mixed results. Significant reductions in plasma triacylglycerol concentrations occurred with the intake of 10 g/d of inulin, particularly in those individuals with a baseline triacylglycerol concentration greater than 1.5 mmol/L (Jackson et al., 1999). The ingestion of 9 g/d of inulin significantly reduced plasma total cholesterol and triacylglycerol concentrations in young men (Brighenti et al., 1999). Nonsignificant changes in plasma total or high density lipoprotein (HDL) cholesterol and triacylglycerol concentrations were reported for individuals consuming 14 g/d of inulin (Pedersen et al., 1997) or 20 g/d of fructooligosaccharide (Luo et al., 1996). In young, healthy males, 15 g/d of nondigestible oligosaccharides (inulin or fructooligosaccharides) did not decrease blood lipids or affect glucose absorption compared to controls (van Dokkum et al., 1999).

Attenuation of Blood Glucose Responses. A placebo-controlled parallel study showed that a daily intake of 10 g of inulin significantly reduced fasting insulin concentrations (Jackson et al., 1999). Fasting blood glucose concentrations were significantly reduced by 15 mg/dL in type 2 diabetics who were fed 8 g/d of fructooligosaccharides (Yamashita et al., 1984). Daily intake of 20 g of fructooligosaccharides significantly decreased basal hepatic glucose production (Luo et al., 1996). No difference, however, was observed in the incremental area under the curve for glucose when individuals were fed 50 g of a rice-based cereal containing 0 or 9 g of inulin (Brighenti et al., 1999).

Other Potential Physiological Effects. An important effect of inulin intake is considered to be the production of *Bifidobacteria*. *Bifidobacteria* contain high amounts of β-fructosidase, which are specific for the β-(1,2) bond present in inulin and oligofructose. A number of studies in humans have shown that the ingestion of fructooligosaccharides leads to an increase in fecal *Bifidobacteria* (Bouhnik et al., 1996, 1999; Buddington et al., 1996; Tuohy et al., 2001; Williams et al., 1994). *Bifidobacteria* have been shown to promote beneficial health effects in animals (Grizard and Barthomeuf, 1999); however, potential beneficial effects in humans are not well understood.

Oat Products and β-Glucans

Laxation. Extracted β-glucans are highly fermentable and therefore their contribution to fecal bulk is minimal (McBurney, 1991). This may contribute, in part, to the lack of an effect in preventing constipation. Oat bran increases stool weight by supplying rapidly fermented viscous fiber to the proximal colon for bacterial growth (Chen et al., 1998).

Normalization of Blood Lipid Concentrations. In one study, oat gum supplementation (9 g/d of β-glucan) did not significantly decrease serum total cholesterol concentration compared to the placebo, leading the authors to conclude that the cholesterol-lowering capacity of oat gum in healthy young men is weak (Beer et al., 1995). In contrast, when hypercholesterolemic individuals were fed oat gum providing 5.8 g/d of β-glucan or a maltodextrin placebo for 4 weeks, mean total and LDL cholesterol concentrations decreased throughout the oat gum phase, and both concentrations were reduced 9 percent relative to initial values (Braaten et al., 1994b). In a larger study, adults with multiple risk factors and LDL cholesterol concentrations above 4.14 mmol/L or between 3.37 and 4.14 mmol/L were randomized to one of seven groups to receive either oatmeal or oat bran at various levels or a placebo control (Davidson et al., 1991). There was a dose-dependent reduction in LDL cholesterol concentrations with the oat cereals. However, when a modest level of β-glucan (3 g/d) was provided to 62 healthy adults with mild to moderate hyperlipidemia, there was no significant reduction in plasma total or LDL cholesterol concentrations (Lovegrove et al., 2000).

Oat bran concentrate has been incorporated into bread products. The long-term effects of such products were tested in men with type 2 diabetes (Pick et al., 1996). Total plasma and LDL cholesterol concentrations were lower in the oat bran concentrate period (9 g/d of viscous fiber) than in the white bread period.

Attenuation of Blood Glucose Responses. In one study, individuals with type 2 diabetes were fed meals containing wheat farina, wheat farina with oat gum, or oat bran (Braaten et al., 1994a). Both the oat bran and wheat farina with oat gum meals reduced the postprandial rise in plasma glucose and insulin concentrations compared to the wheat farina meal without the oat gum. This is an example of the extracted form of oat bran (*Functional Fiber*) having a similar effect to the native form (*Dietary Fiber*). Oat gum has also been compared to guar gum with respect to glucose and insulin responses after an oral glucose load in healthy, fasting individuals (Braaten et al., 1991). In this study, the glucose and insulin responses to the oat and guar gum meals were nearly identical. In addition, both gum meals resulted in increases in plasma glucose and insulin concentrations that were lower than glucose alone ($p < 0.01$). Hallfrisch and colleagues (1995) studied glucose responses in 16 women and 7 men with moderately high cholesterol concentrations who supplemented their normal diets with oat extracts in which either 1 or 10 percent viscous β-glucans were added. Glucose responses were reduced at both the 1 and 10 percent β-glucan supplementation level.

Pectin

Laxation. In a meta-analysis of approximately 100 studies on stool weight changes with various fiber sources, investigators were able to calculate the increase in fecal weight due to fiber ingestion (Cummings, 1993). This meta-analysis concluded that pectin ingestion leads to an increase of about 1.3 g of stool/g of pectin as compared to 5.4 g/g produced from wheat bran, suggesting that pectin is not an important fecal bulking agent (Cummings, 1993). In a randomized crossover study designed to compare the effects of pectin (12 g/d), cellulose (15 g/d), and lignin (12 g/d) on stool characteristics in healthy volunteers, pectin did not alter transit time or increase 24-hour stool wet weight, whereas cellulose decreased mean stool transit time and increased mean wet stool weight (Hillman et al., 1983).

Normalization of Blood Lipid Concentrations. Pectin has been tested in a number of studies for its hypocholesterolemic effect. For example, in a 16-week, double-blind crossover study, grapefruit pectin supplementation decreased plasma cholesterol concentration by 7.6 percent and LDL cholesterol concentration by 10.8 percent in individuals at moderate to high risk of coronary heart disease (Cerda et al., 1988). When 12 g/d of pectin was taken with meals for 3 weeks, there was a mean decrease in total serum cholesterol concentration of 0.48 ± 0.18 mmol/L (Durrington et al., 1976). This decrease was mainly due to a reduction in LDL cholesterol concentration. When 15 g/d of citrus pectin was provided in metabolically controlled diets for 3 weeks, plasma cholesterol concentrations were reduced by 13 percent and fecal fat excretion increased by 44 percent; however, plasma triacylglycerol concentrations did not change (Kay and Truswell, 1977). Gold and coworkers (1980) did not observe reductions in serum cholesterol concentrations following the consumption of 10 g of pectin with 100 g of glucose. The consumption of 7.2 g/d of psyllium that had been added to foods did not result in a significant decrease in LDL cholesterol concentration. However, total cholesterol and triacylglycerol concentrations were significantly decreased (Jenkins et al., 2002).

There is some documentation that the hypocholesterolemic effects of pectin are due to increased excretion of bile acids and cholesterol. Supplementation with 15 g of pectin increased bile acid excretion by 35 percent and net cholesterol excretion by 14 percent in ileostomy patients, whereas 16 g of wheat bran produced no significant changes (Bosaeus et al., 1986).

Attenuation of Blood Glucose Responses. Viscous fibers such as pectin have been found to produce a significant reduction in glycemic response in 33 of 50 studies (66 percent) (Wolever and Jenkins, 1993). This is in contrast to only 3 of 14 studies with insoluble fiber (21 percent).

Polydextrose

Laxation. Polydextrose has been shown to increase fecal mass and sometimes stool frequency. Tomlin and Read (1988) showed that 30 g/d of polydextrose increased fecal mass without affecting transit time and stool frequency. Achour and coworkers (1994) observed no significant changes in fecal weight or transit time when seven men consumed 30 g/d of polydextrose. When 4, 8, or 12 g/d of polydextrose was provided, fecal weight increased and ease and frequency of defecation improved in a dose–response manner (Jie et al., 2000).

Findings on the effect of polydextrose intake on fecal bacterial production are mixed. Achour and colleagues (1994) reported no changes in bacterial mass in the feces of individuals who consumed 30 g/d of polydextrose. This lack of difference may be explained, in part, by the findings of Jie and coworkers (2000). Following the ingestion of 4, 8, or 12 g/d of polydextrose (*n* = 30 treatment), there was a dose-dependent decrease in *Bacteriodes*, whereas the beneficial *Lactobacillus* and *Bifidobacteria* species increased.

Normalization of Blood Lipid Concentrations. Sixty-one healthy volunteers received 15 g/d of polydextrose for 2 months. Serum concentrations of total cholesterol, triacylglycerols, and LDL cholesterol did not change during this period; however, concentrations of HDL cholesterol decreased (Saku et al., 1991).

Psyllium

Laxation. Psyllium is the active ingredient in laxatives, and thus from an over-the-counter drug viewpoint, there is extensive literature on its efficacy in this regard. After 8 weeks of psyllium treatment to patients with idiopathic constipation, both stool frequency and stool weight increased significantly, stool consistency improved, and pain on defecation was reduced (Ashraf et al., 1995). The authors concluded that the beneficial effects of psyllium with regard to constipation are largely related to a facilitation of the defecatory process (Ashraf et al., 1995). Similarly, psyllium was tested in a multisite study of 170 individuals with chronic idiopathic constipation for 2 weeks (McRorie et al., 1998). Psyllium increased stool water content, stool water weight, total stool output, bowel movement frequency, and a score combining objective measures of constipation. Four months of psyllium treatment significantly improved bowel function and fecal output in 12 elderly patients (Burton and Manninen, 1982). In a multicenter trial with 394 individuals, psyllium improved bowel function better than other laxatives (mainly lactulose), with superior stool consistency and decreased incidence of adverse events (Dettmar and Sykes, 1998). Prior and Whorwell (1987) tested psyllium (ispaghula husk) in 80 patients with irritable bowel syndrome and found that constipation was significantly improved and transit time decreased in patients taking psyllium.

Normalization of Blood Lipid Concentrations. A number of studies have been conducted to ascertain the beneficial effects of psyllium on blood lipid concentrations. Several of these studies provided 10.2 g/d of psyllium for up to 26 weeks and all showed marked reductions in serum total and LDL cholesterol concentrations compared to cellulose (Anderson et al., 1988, 1999, 2000b; Levin et al., 1990). The dose–response effect of psyllium at 0, 3.4, 6.8, or 10.2 g/d was tested in a double-blind controlled study in 286 adults with LDL cholesterol concentrations between 3.36 and 5.68 mmol/L (Davidson et al., 1998). The effects of 10.2 g/d of psyllium seed husk on serum LDL cholesterol concentrations were modest, with levels 5.3 percent below that of the control group at week 24 ($p < 0.05$).

In a 3-week intervention with 21 g/d of psyllium ($n = 7$), plasma total, LDL, and HDL cholesterol concentrations were significantly reduced (Abraham and Mehta, 1988). Psyllium decreased plasma concentrations of total cholesterol by 5.6 percent and LDL cholesterol by 8.6 percent; concentrations were unchanged in the cellulose group. Serum cholesterol concentration was reduced by 20 percent in 12 elderly patients receiving psyllium supplementation (Burton and Manninen, 1982). In a large, multicenter trial conducted in the United Kingdom, 7 or 10.5 g/d of psyllium was provided to 340 patients with mild to moderate hypercholesterolemia over 12 weeks (MacMahon and Carless, 1998). After 12 weeks, LDL cholesterol concentrations decreased by 8.7 percent for the 7-g/d group and 9.7 percent for the 10.5-g/d group. After a 6-month follow-up period, psyllium combined with diet modification was shown to reduce LDL cholesterol concentrations by 10.6 to 13.2 percent and total cholesterol concentrations by 7.7 to 8.9 percent (MacMahon and Carless, 1998). Danielsson and coworkers (1979) treated 13 patients with essential hyperlipoproteinemia over 2 to 29 months with psyllium hydrophilic colloid. Serum cholesterol and triacylglycerol concentrations were reduced an average of 16.9 and 52.0 percent, respectively. If blood lipid concentrations were normal at baseline, no reductions were observed when individuals consumed psyllium colloid (Danielsson et al., 1979).

Studies also have been conducted using a ready-to-eat cereal enriched with psyllium. Hypercholesterolemic individuals consuming 114 g/d of a psyllium-flake cereal for 6 weeks showed significantly lower serum total and LDL cholesterol concentrations than those consuming the same amount of wheat-bran flake cereal (Anderson et al., 1992b). Similarly, Bell and coworkers (1990) tested the cholesterol-lowering effects of viscous fiber (psyllium or pectin) cereals as part of a diet in 58 men with mild to moderate hypercholesterolemia. During the cereal-plus-diet phase of the study, total and LDL cholesterol concentrations in the psyllium-enriched cereal group decreased by 5.9 and 5.7 percent, respectively.

A meta-analysis was conducted to determine the effect of consumption of psyllium-enriched cereal products on blood lipid concentrations in 404 adults with mild to moderate hypercholesterolemia consuming a low fat diet (Olson et al., 1997). Compared to the control cereals, individuals who consumed psyllium cereals had lower total and LDL cholesterol concentrations, whereas HDL cholesterol concentrations were not affected. Anderson and coworkers (2000a) conducted a meta-analysis of eight controlled trials to define the hypolipidemic effects of psyllium when used in combination with a low fat diet in hypercholesterolemic men and women. There were a total of 384 individuals receiving psyllium in the eight studies covered by the meta-analysis and these individuals were compared to those consuming cellulose ($n = 272$). Consumption of 10.2 g/d of psyllium ($n = 384$) lowered serum total cholesterol by 4 percent and serum LDL cholesterol by 7 percent, relative to the cellulose control ($n = 272$).

Everson and colleagues (1992) evaluated the mechanisms of the hypocholesterolemic effect of psyllium by measuring intestinal cholesterol absorption, cholesterol synthesis in isolated peripheral blood mononuclear cells, bile acid kinetics, gallbladder motility, and intestinal transit. The researchers concluded that psyllium decreases LDL cholesterol concentrations mainly by the stimulation of bile acid production.

Attenuation of Blood Glucose Responses. In an 8-week intervention study in 34 men with type 2 diabetes and hypercholesterolemia consuming either 10.2 g/d of psyllium or cellulose, daily and postlunch postprandial glucose concentration were 11.0 and 19.2 percent lower, respectively, in the psyllium group (Anderson et al., 1999). Also, psyllium has been shown to reduce the glycemic index of foods when added to a meal (Frati-Munari et al., 1998). The effect of psyllium or placebo on postprandial serum glucose and insulin concentrations was tested in 18 type 2 diabetic patients in a crossover design (Pastors et al., 1991). Compared to placebo, postprandial glucose elevation was reduced by 14 percent at breakfast and 20 percent at dinner, and postprandial serum insulin concentration was reduced by 12 percent after breakfast. However, this depression of the normal postprandial increase in serum glucose and insulin concentrations seen with psyllium does not appear to be due to a delay in gastric emptying (Rigaud et al., 1998).

Resistant Dextrins

Laxation. There are no human studies to support a laxative benefit from ingestion of indigestible dextrins.

Normalization of Blood Lipid Concentrations. The intake of 60 g/d of resistant maltodextrin was shown to reduce serum total cholesterol and triacylglycerol concentrations in type 2 diabetics as compared with type 2 diabetics or healthy adults who consumed 30 g/d of resistant maltodextrin (Ohkuma and Wakabayashi, 2001). No difference was observed in the concentration of HDL cholesterol.

Attenuation of Blood Glucose Responses. Reduced blood glucose concentrations and insulin secretion were observed when rats were given resistant maltodextrins after sucrose or maltose loading (Wakabayashi et al., 1993, 1995). Furthermore, an intake of 5 g of resistant maltodextrin reduced the postprandial blood glucose concentrations in healthy men and women (Tokunaga and Matsuoka, 1999). The ingestion of 60 g/d, but not 30 g/d, of resistant maltodextrin resulted in a significant reduction of fasting blood glucose concentrations in type 2 diabetics (Ohkuma and Wakabayashi, 2001).

Resistant Starch

Laxation. Increased fecal bulk due to increased starch intake has been reported (Shetty and Kurpad, 1986). The impact of resistant starch (RS_3) from a corn-based cereal on colonic function was measured in eight male volunteers (Tomlin and Read, 1990). After consuming 10.33 g/d of RS_3 for 1 week, there was no significant difference in fecal output, stool frequency, ease of defecation, whole-gut transit time, or degree of flatulence compared to an intake of 0.86 g/d of RS_3 from a rice-based cereal. A significant increase in stool weight, however, was observed when men consumed 32 g/d RS_3 for 4 weeks (Heijnen et al., 1998). Jenkins and coworkers (1998) determined the effects of low fiber (control), wheat bran supplements providing an additional 30 g of fiber (high fiber control), or the equivalent amount of resistant starch as RS_2 or RS_3. Compared to the low fiber control, the wheat bran supplement increased fecal bulk by 96 ± 14 g/d ($p < 0.001$) and the mean for both resistant starches was 22 ± 8 g/d greater than controls ($p = 0.013$). This is consistent with the small increase in fecal bulk seen with resistant starch intake in other studies (Behall and Howe, 1996; Cummings et al., 1996; Heijnen et al., 1998; Hylla et al., 1998; Phillips et al., 1995).

Because resistant starch is partly fermented in the colon, intake may lead to increased production of short-chain fatty acids. When 39 g/d of a mixture of naturally occurring and processed resistant starch was consumed, there was a significant increase in fecal butyrate and acetate concentrations, and therefore a significant reduction in fecal pH (Phillips et al., 1995). However, when glucose or 32 g/d of RS_3 was consumed for 4 weeks, there was no difference in fecal pH, fecal short-chain fatty acid concentrations, or fecal secondary bile acid concentrations (Heijnen et al., 1998).

Normalization of Blood Lipid Concentrations. Several animal studies have demonstrated a lowering of blood cholesterol and triacylglycerol concentrations with resistant starch intake (de Deckere et al., 1993; Ranhotra et al., 1997; Younes et al., 1995). When healthy, normolipidemic individuals were given glucose or 30 g/d of RS_3 supplements for 3 weeks, there were no significant differences in fasting serum total, LDL, and HDL cholesterol concentrations or triacylglycerol concentrations (Heijnen et al., 1996). Resistant starch does not appear to provide the cholesterol-lowering effects of viscous fiber, but rather acts more like nonviscous fiber (Jenkins et al., 1998). Neither Jenkins and coworkers (1998) nor Heijnen and coworkers (1996) showed a lowering effect of resistant starch on serum lipids.

Attenuation of Blood Glucose Responses. Adding resistant starch to bread at various levels (0, 5, 10, and 20 percent) was shown to reduce the glycemic index in a dose-dependent manner (100, 96, 74, and 53) (Brown et al., 1995). The consumption of 30 g/d of RS_3 was shown to significantly reduce the urinary excretion of C-peptide, indicating reduced insulin secretion (de Roos et al., 1995).

Clinical Effects of Inadequate Intake

Dietary and *Functional Fibers* are not essential nutrients, so inadequate intakes do not result in biochemical or clinical symptoms of a deficiency. A lack of these fibers in the diet, however, can result in inadequate fecal bulk and may detract from optimal health in a variety of different ways depending on other factors, such as the rest of the diet and the stage of the life cycle.

EVIDENCE CONSIDERED FOR ESTIMATING THE REQUIREMENT FOR *DIETARY FIBER* AND *FUNCTIONAL FIBER*

There is no biochemical assay that reflects *Dietary Fiber* or *Functional Fiber* nutritional status. Clearly one cannot measure blood fiber concentration since, by definition, fiber is not absorbed. Instead, the potential health benefits of fiber consumption, which may be compromised by a lack of fiber in the diet, have been reviewed. Throughout each section and the discussion of each indicator, a delineation is made between *Dietary Fiber* and *Functional Fiber*. It should be kept in mind that although high *Dietary Fiber* intake is associated with decreased risk or improvements in several chronic diseases, a report of the National Academy of Sciences states "there is no conclusive evidence that it is dietary fiber rather than the other components of vegetables, fruits, and cereal products that reduces the risk of those diseases" (NRC, 1989). The definition of *Dietary Fiber* in this report states that it must be "intrinsic and intact in plants." Thus, the reported benefits are due to the fiber *source*, not necessarily to the fiber per se. In contrast, *Functional Fiber* (which consists of isolated, nondigestible carbohydrates that have beneficial physiological effects in humans), by definition, must show that the beneficial physiological effect in humans is due to the isolated or synthesized fiber itself.

A number of epidemiological studies have been conducted to evaluate the relationship between fiber intake and risk of chronic disease. While *Functional Fibers*, such as pectins and gums, are added to foods as ingredients, these levels are minimal and therefore fiber intakes that are estimated from food composition tables generally represent *Dietary Fiber*.

Dietary Fiber, Functional Fiber, *and the Prevention of Hyperlipidemia, Hypertension, and Coronary Heart Disease*

Epidemiological Studies

There are no epidemiological studies that have evaluated the relationship between *Functional Fiber* and the risk of coronary heart disease (CHD). A number of epidemiological studies, however, have found reduced CHD rates in individuals consuming high amounts of *Dietary Fiber* and fiber-rich foods (Bolton-Smith et al., 1992; Fraser et al., 1992; Humble et al., 1993; Jacobs et al., 1998; Khaw and Barrett-Connor, 1987; Kushi et al., 1985;

Morris et al., 1977; Pietinen et al., 1996; Rimm et al., 1996; Todd et al., 1999; Wolk et al., 1999). For example, Fraser and colleagues (1992) reported that in a cohort of 31,208 California Seventh-day Adventists, there was a 44 percent reduced risk of nonfatal CHD and an 11 percent reduced risk of fatal CHD for those who ate whole wheat bread compared with those who ate white bread. In the Iowa Women's Health Study, Jacobs and coworkers (1998) found that the risk of CHD death was reduced by approximately one-third for women consuming one or more servings of a whole grain product each day compared with those rarely eating any whole grain products. Similarly, Morris and coworkers (1977) followed 337 men in London, England for 10 to 20 years and found that men with a high intake of cereal fiber had a lower rate of CHD than men with a low cereal fiber intake.

In the Health Professionals Follow-up Study, the relative risk for fatal coronary disease and total myocardial infarction were 0.45 and 0.59, respectively, for men in the highest quintile of *Dietary Fiber* intake (28.9 g/d) compared with the lowest quintile (12.4 g/d) (Rimm et al., 1996) (Table 7-2). Cereal fiber was more strongly associated with the reduced risk of CHD than were fiber from fruits and vegetables. Wolk and coworkers (1999) examined the relationship between intake of *Dietary Fiber* and risk of CHD in the Nurses' Health Study and found a significant inverse association, which was confined to *Dietary Fiber* from cereal sources (Table 7-2). Compared with the lowest quintile of cereal fiber intake (2.2 g/d), women in the highest quintile (7.7 g/d) had a 34 percent lower risk of total CHD. In a large cohort of 21,930 Finnish men, there was a significant inverse association between *Dietary Fiber* intake and CHD, with a multivariate relative risk of 0.84 for men in the highest quintile of intake (34.8 g/d) compared with the lowest quintile of intake (16.1 g/d) (Pietinen et al., 1996) (Table 7-2).

In summary, the large-scale, adequately powered, prospective studies all show a substantial protective effect of *Dietary Fiber* for CHD. Specifically, these three studies—which used multivariate models to control for energy, saturated fat, alcohol, body mass index, and various vitamins—showed a strong relationship between cereal fibers and a weak or no relationship between vegetable and fruit fibers. In terms of setting intake recommendations and actual numbers as a primary determinant of fiber requirements, these studies are most useful as they are adequately powered, divide *Dietary Fiber* into quintiles of intake, and provide data on energy intake (Pietinen et al., 1996; Rimm et al., 1996; Wolk et al., 1999). Using these studies, it is also possible to relate the number of grams of *Dietary Fiber* per day to the decrease in CHD incidence.

Although not reporting quintiles of intake, a fourth study by Khaw and Barrett-Connor (1987) can be considered because it showed that an

TABLE 7-2 Prospective Cohort Studies on *Dietary Fiber* Intake and Risk of Coronary Heart Disease (CHD)

Reference	Study Design	Quintile	Relative Risk for CHD
Pietinen et al., 1996	21,930 Finnish men, 50–69 y 6-y follow-up	1 2 3 4 5	1.00 0.91 0.88 0.86 0.84 *p* for trend = 0.03
Rimm et al., 1996	43,757 U.S. men, 40–75 y 6-y follow-up	1 2 3 4 5	1.00 0.97 0.91 0.87 0.59 *p* for trend < 0.001
Wolk et al., 1999	68,782 U.S. women, 37–64 y 10-y follow-up	1 2 3 4 5	1.00 0.98 0.92 0.87 0.77 *p* for trend = 0.07

a Dietary Fiber intake is energy-adjusted to 2,000 kcals.
b Dietary Fiber intake is energy-adjusted to 1,600 kcals.

increased intake of 6 g/d of *Dietary Fiber* was associated with a 33 percent risk reduction for CHD in women and 24 percent in men, and the reduction in CHD mortality was independent of other dietary variables. The Health Professionals Follow-up Study reported a 19 percent decrease in risk for total myocardial infarction per 10-g/d increase of *Dietary Fiber* and a 29 percent decrease per 10-g/d increase of cereal fiber (Rimm et al., 1996). A similar result for women was reported by Wolk and coworkers (1999) with a 19 percent decrease in risk for total CHD events per 10-g/d increase of *Dietary Fiber*, but a stronger relationship was reported for cereal fiber (37 percent decrease per 5-g/d increase).

Dietary Fiber Intake (g/d)	Energy Intake (kcal/d)	Grams of Dietary Fiber/ 1,000 kcal
16.1	2,722	5.9
20.7	2,787	7.4
24.3	2,781	8.7
28.3	2,754	10.3
34.8	2,705	12.9
12.4	2,000[a]	6.2
16.6	2,000	8.3
19.6	2,000	9.8
23.0	2,000	11.5
28.9	2,000	14.45
11.5	1,600[b]	7.2
14.3	1,600	8.9
16.4	1,600	10.25
18.8	1,600	11.75
22.9	1,600	14.31

Intervention Trials

There have been a large number of intervention trials to ascertain whether fiber supplementation can alter blood lipid concentrations and therefore alter the risk of CHD. These trials are briefly summarized below. All but one are small trials; often these interventions are performed in people with high initial serum cholesterol concentrations. The strongest data are for oat products and beans (Dietary Fiber). In addition, viscous Functional Fibers such as guar, pectin, and psyllium, have been tested in intervention trials and found to decrease serum total and low density lipoprotein (LDL) cholesterol concentration in most studies. For example,

Anderson and coworkers (1984b) compared the effects of oat bran or bean supplementation on 20 hypercholesterolemic adult males, providing approximately 47 g/d of plant *Dietary Fiber* and 17 g/d of viscous *Dietary Fiber*. Both the oat bran and bean diets significantly decreased serum total cholesterol concentrations by 19 percent. In a similar metabolic ward study of 10 hypercholesterolemic men, oat bran and bean diets decreased both serum total and LDL cholesterol concentrations by 23 percent after 3 weeks on the test diets (Anderson et al., 1984a). A review of the oat bran and bean fiber intervention trials where *Dietary Fiber* supplementation was combined with a low fat diet shows that reductions in serum total cholesterol concentrations ranged from 8 to 26 percent (Anderson and Gustafson, 1988; Anderson et al., 1984a, 1984b; Judd and Truswell, 1981; Kirby et al., 1981). Smaller portions of oat bran or oat meal (60 g, dry measure) have been shown to decrease serum total cholesterol concentrations by approximately 8 to 11 percent (Bartram et al., 1992; Van Horn et al., 1986).

Other viscous fibers, in addition to those from oats and beans, have also been shown to decrease serum cholesterol concentrations. For example, Jenkins and coworkers (1975) reported the hypocholesterolemic effect of guar gum (*Functional Fiber*), which is often added to foods. Since that time, there have been a number of studies with guar gum supplementation that resulted in a reduction in serum cholesterol concentrations of between 11 and 15 percent (Anderson and Tietyen-Clark, 1986). In a 3-week intervention that provided 21 g/d of psyllium, total, LDL, and high density lipoprotein cholesterol concentrations were all significantly reduced (Abraham and Mehta, 1988). A meta-analysis testing the effects of pectin, oat bran, guar gum, and psyllium on blood lipid concentrations showed that 2 to 10 g/d of viscous fiber were associated with small but significant decreases in total and LDL cholesterol concentrations (Brown et al., 1999). The different viscous fibers reduced serum total and LDL cholesterol concentrations by similar amounts. Resistant starch does not appear to provide the cholesterol-lowering effects of viscous fibers, but rather acts more like nonviscous fibers (Jenkins et al., 1998). Neither Heijnen and coworkers (1996) nor Jenkins and coworkers (1998) showed a lipid-lowering effect of resistant starch on serum lipid concentrations.

It should also be noted that the effect of fiber on decreasing serum cholesterol concentration is not due to its replacement of fat in the diet. In a prospective, randomized, controlled trial with a low fat and a low fat plus high *Dietary Fiber* groups, the group consuming high *Dietary Fiber* exhibited a greater average reduction (13 percent) in serum total cholesterol concentration than the low fat (9 percent) and the usual diet (7 percent) groups (Anderson et al., 1992a). Mathur and coworkers (1968) conducted a study in 20 men supplemented with Bengal gram. Serum total cholesterol concentrations averaged 23 percent lower on the high fat, Bengal gram diet than on the high fat diet alone.

Not all fibers decrease serum cholesterol concentration. For example, Anderson and coworkers (1991) randomly allocated 20 hypercholesterolemic men to either a wheat bran or oat bran diet. After 21 days, oat bran significantly decreased serum total cholesterol concentration by 12.8 percent; however, there was no effect with wheat bran. Behall (1990) compared a low fiber diet with a diet containing an average of 19.5 g/d of added cellulose (a nonviscous fiber) or the viscous fibers carboxymethylcellulose gum, karaya gum, or locust bean gum. The diets containing the viscous fibers led to significantly lower plasma cholesterol concentrations. Although these relatively small-scale intervention trials using viscous *Functional Fibers* have reported substantial cholesterol-lowering effects and therefore should be protective against CHD, no protective effect against CHD was seen in a large-scale clinical trial with individuals who had a previous myocardial infarction (Burr et al., 1989). These individuals were encouraged to increase grain fiber intake by increasing consumption of whole meal bread, high fiber breakfast cereals, and wheat bran, which resulted in an increased grain fiber intake from 9 to 17 g/d in the intervention group. Wheat bran and other poorly fermented fibers (e.g., cellulose) have also failed to decrease serum lipids in animal studies. Increasing the intake of *Dietary Fiber* by increasing the consumption of fruits and vegetables can attenuate plasma triacylglycerol concentrations. Obarzanek and coworkers (2001) showed that increasing *Dietary Fiber* intake from 11 to 30 g/d as a result of increased consumption of fruits, vegetables, and whole grains prevented a rise in plasma triacylglycerol concentrations in those fed a low fat diet, especially in those individuals with initially high concentrations. Plasma triacylglycerol concentrations were significantly reduced (Chandalia et al., 2000) or unchanged (Lichtenstein et al., 2002) by increasing *Dietary Fiber* intake when consuming a low fat diet. These studies suggest that *Dietary Fiber* prevents the rise in plasma triacylglycerol concentrations that occurs when consuming a low fat, high carbohydrate diet (see Chapter 11).

Summary of the Intervention Trials

Viscous *Functional Fibers* and foods sources of viscous *Dietary Fiber* reduce both total and LDL cholesterol concentrations, and may also reduce serum triglycerides. The amount of cholesterol reduction appears to be related to the amount of fiber consumed, although only a few studies report dose–response data. A meta-analysis of 20 trials that used high doses of oat bran, which is rich in viscous *Dietary Fiber*, showed that the reductions in serum cholesterol concentrations ranged from 0.1 to 2.5 percent/g of intake (Ripsin et al., 1992). If one accepts the proposed 2 percent risk reduction for CHD for every 1 percent reduction in serum cholesterol (Lipid Research Clinics Program, 1984), these results suggest substantial benefits from consumption of high amounts of viscous *Dietary* and *Functional Fibers* and support the epidemiological findings regarding fiber and CHD. It is of interest to compare the hypothetical risk reduction for CHD per gram of oat bran consumed (in the clinical intervention trials) to that for total dietary fiber intake in the epidemiological studies. For example, in the oat bran meta-analysis, using a 1.2 percent reduction in serum cholesterol per gram of oat bran (the midpoint of the range of 0.1 to 2.5 percent) and multiplying by 2 (proposed 2 percent reduction for risk of CHD for every 1 percent reduction in serum cholesterol) would suggest a reduced risk of CHD of 2.4 percent/g of oat bran consumed. This can then be compared with the data on total fiber consumption and risk for CHD in the three primary epidemiological studies shown in Table 7-2.

In the Health Professionals Follow-Up Study (Rimm et al., 1996), there is a difference of 16.5 g of fiber intake between the highest and lowest intake groups (28.9–12.4), and a reported relative risk of 0.45 for fatal coronary disease and 0.59 for total myocardial infarction for men in the highest compared to the lowest quintile for fiber intake. This equates to a risk reduction of 3.3 percent/g of fiber for fatal coronary disease and 2.5 percent/g of fiber for total myocardial infarction. In the Nurses' Health Study (Wolk et al., 1999) there is a difference of 11.4 g of fiber between the highest and lowest intake groups (22.9–11.5) and a relative risk of 0.77 for total CHD. This equates to a risk reduction of 2.02 percent/g of fiber. Finally, in a study of Finnish men (Pietinen et al., 1996), there is a difference of 18.7 g of fiber between the highest and lowest intake groups (34.8–16.1) and a relative risk of 0.68 for coronary death. This equates to a risk reduction of 1.71 percent/g of fiber.

Although the calculations above are hypothetical and are based on a number of assumptions, (including the linearity of response of fiber consumption to risk reduction), the finding that the degree of risk reductions per gram of fiber consumed are within a reasonable range of each other are suggestive that the results of the clinical trials for viscous fibers are supportive of the epidemiological finding. It is also clear that the effect of viscous fibers on decreasing blood cholesterol concentrations cannot explain the multitude of studies cited above that generally show *Dietary Fiber* to be protective against CHD, even though a mixed fiber diet is only approximately one-third viscous fiber. This suggests that mechanisms in addition to cholesterol-lowering may be involved.

Mechanisms by Which Dietary Fibers May Protect Against CHD

While not explicit, several hypotheses exist to explain the mechanisms by which *Dietary Fiber* may protect against CHD. The lowering of serum cholesterol concentration by viscous *Dietary* or *Functional Fibers* is thought to involve changes in cholesterol or bile acid absorption, hepatic production of lipoproteins, or peripheral clearance of lipoproteins (Chen and Anderson, 1986). Viscous fibers may interfere with the absorption and enterohepatic recirculation of bile acids and cholesterol in the intestine, forcing the liver to synthesize more cholesterol to meet the need for bile acid synthesis, and thus decreasing circulating cholesterol. This cannot be the sole explanation, however, since not all viscous fibers increase fecal bile acid excretion, and the magnitude of the increase, when present, is often small. In addition to delaying or interfering with the absorption of cholesterol and bile acids, viscous fibers may delay the absorption of macronutrients, including fat and carbohydrate. Delayed carbohydrate absorption, in turn, could lead to increased insulin sensitivity (Hallfrisch et al., 1995) and decreased triacylglycerol concentrations (Rivellese et al., 1980), also considered risk factors for CHD. Ascherio and coworkers (1992) have shown a strong inverse association between *Dietary Fiber* intake and risk of hypertension in men, with hypertension being an important risk factor for CHD.

Diets high in *Dietary Fiber* also may favorably affect plasminogen activator inhibitor type 1 and factor VII activity (Djoussé et al., 1998; Mennen et al., 1997; Sundell and Ranby, 1993). In addition, a large number of studies (described above) show whole-grain cereal products as being protective against CHD. Whole grain cereals are also sources of phytochemicals, such as phytate and phytoestrogens, which may independently impact CHD.

Summary

On the basis of the evidence provided on fiber intake and CHD, certain sources of *Dietary Fiber* (cereal foods) and certain *Functional Fibers* (viscous) are associated with reduced risk of CHD. In prospective population studies, there is a strong relationship between *Total Fiber* intake from foods and CHD. Therefore, a recommended intake level can be set for *Total Fiber* based on prevention of CHD and recognizing that the greatest benefit comes from the ingestion of cereal fibers and viscous *Functional Fibers*, including gums and pectins. Further discussion is provided in the later section, "Findings by Life Stage and Gender Group."

Fiber Intake and Gastrointestinal Health

Fiber Intake and Duodenal Ulcer

In a prospective cohort of 47,806 men with 138 newly diagnosed cases of duodenal ulcer, *Dietary Fibers*, and particularly the viscous fibers, were strongly associated with a decreased risk of duodenal ulcer (relative risk of 0.40 for the highest quintile of viscous fiber intake) (Aldoori et al., 1997). In this study, fiber from fruit, vegetable, and leguminous sources, but not cereal fiber, was associated with a reduced risk of duodenal ulcer. Although the mechanism behind this proposed positive effect of viscous fibers on duodenal ulcer is not known, one hypothesis is that the delay in gastric emptying, known to result from the ingestion of viscous fibers, may play a role.

Dietary Fiber, Functional Fiber, and Colon Health

Constipation, Laxation, and the Contribution of Fiber to Fecal Weight. Consumption of certain *Dietary* and *Functional Fibers* is known to improve laxation and ameliorate constipation (Burkitt et al., 1972; Cummings et al., 1978; Kelsay et al., 1978; Lupton et al., 1993). In most reports there is a strong positive correlation between intake of *Dietary Fiber* and daily fecal weight (Birkett et al., 1997). Also, *Dietary Fiber* intake is usually negatively correlated with transit time (Birkett et al., 1997). Although what constitutes "constipation" is variously defined, diets that increase the number of bowel movements per day, improve the ease with which a stool is passed, or increase fecal bulk are considered to be of benefit. For example, in a weight-loss study, obese individuals were put on a very low energy diet with or without 30 g/d of isolated plant fiber (Astrup et al., 1990). Those receiving the fiber supplement had a higher number of bowel movements per day (1.0) compared to those not receiving the fiber supplement (0.7/d). Not all reports, however, support the concept that fiber serves as a laxative (Cameron et al., 1996; Kochen et al., 1985). Because water is also important for laxation, some have suggested that increasing fiber intake alone is not sufficient, and that more water should be consumed as well (Anti et al., 1998). Determining a stool weight that might promote laxation and ameliorate constipation is very difficult. In one study, although fecal weight ranged from 41 to 340 g and transit time ranged from 22 to 123 hours, no subject reported suffering either constipation or diarrhea (Birkett et al., 1997). At the same time, a number of studies have shown that low fiber intake is associated with constipation. For example, Morais and coworkers (1999) reported that children with chronic constipation had lower *Dietary*

Fiber intake than the control group. The authors concluded that a low intake of fiber is a risk factor for chronic constipation in children.

In a meta-analysis of about 100 studies of stool-weight changes with various fiber sources, investigators were able to calculate the increase in fecal weight due to *Dietary* or *Functional Fiber* ingestion (Cummings, 1993). Such calculations yielded the following increases in fecal weight: 5.4 g of stool/g of wheat-bran fiber, 4.9 g/g of fruits and vegetables, 3 g/g of isolated cellulose, and 1.3 g/g of isolated pectin (Cummings, 1993). The contribution of resistant starch to fecal bulk has also been assessed. For example, Jenkins and colleagues (1998) determined the bulking effects of wheat bran supplements (30 g) or the equivalent amount as resistant starch (RS_2 or RS_3). Compared to the low fiber control, the wheat bran supplement increased fecal bulk by 96 ± 14 g/d ($p < 0.001$) and the mean for both resistant starches was 22 ± 8 g/d greater ($p = 0.013$). This is consistent with the small increase in fecal bulk seen with resistant starch intake in other studies (Behall and Howe, 1996; Cummings et al., 1996; Heijnen et al., 1998; Hylla et al., 1998; Phillips et al., 1995). Additional discussion of the effects of *Functional Fibers*, such as psyllium, is included in the earlier section, "Physiological Effects of Isolated and Synthetic Fibers."

Fiber Fermentation Products as an Energy Source for the Colon. Butyrate is the primary energy source for the colonocyte (Roediger, 1982). One study showed high acetate and low butyrate ratios of short-chain fatty acids in patients with adenomatous polyps and colon cancer (Weaver et al., 1988). Increased fecal butyrate outputs have been demonstrated using both whole food and commercial sources of resistant starch in some studies (Jenkins et al., 1998; Macfarlane and Englyst, 1986; Phillips et al., 1995; Silvester et al., 1995), but not in others (Heijnen et al., 1998; Hylla et al., 1998). It has been proposed that colonic diseases, including ulcerative colitis, are disorders of energy utilization (Roediger, 1980), although this remains an unresolved issue.

Fiber and the Prevention of Diverticular Disease. Diverticular disease is characterized by saccular herniations of the colonic wall and is highly prevalent in elderly populations in Western societies (Watters and Smith, 1990). Although usually asymptomatic, when diverticula become inflamed, the condition is known as diverticulitis. Current estimates for the North American population indicate that one-third of those older than 45 years and two-thirds of those older than 85 years have diverticular disease (Roberts and Veidenheimer, 1990).

Several types of studies have shown a relationship between fiber intake and diverticular disease. In the prospective Health Professionals Follow-Up Study, there was a strong negative association between *Dietary Fiber* intake and the incidence of symptomatic diverticular disease (Aldoori et al., 1994, 1995), which persisted after adjustment for several other risk factors. The data showed that the inverse relationship was particularly strong for the nonviscous *Dietary Fiber*, particularly cellulose (Aldoori et al., 1998). Case-control studies have consistently found that patients with diverticula consumed less *Dietary Fiber* than did nonpatients. For example, Gear and coworkers (1979) reported on the prevalence of symptomless diverticular disease in vegetarians and nonvegetarians in England. Twelve percent of the vegetarians had diverticular disease compared with 33 percent of the nonvegetarians. In addition, the vegetarians had a mean daily *Dietary Fiber* intake of 41.5 g/d in comparison to 21.4 g/d for the non-vegetarians. Similarly, Manousos and coworkers (1985) reported a lower prevalence of diverticular disease in rural Greece compared with that found in urban areas. In addition, those individuals with diverticular disease consumed fewer vegetables, brown bread, potatoes, and fruit. In an intervention trial, Findlay and coworkers (1974) showed a protective effect of unprocessed bran. In another study, Brodribb (1977) treated 18 patients with diverticular disease by providing either a high fiber, bran-containing bread (6.7 g) or ordinary wheat bread (0.6 g). Relief of symptoms was significantly greater in the high fiber group compared with the low fiber control group.

Although the mechanism by which fiber may be protective against diverticular disease is unknown, several hypotheses have been proposed. For example, some scientists report that it is due to decreased transit time, increased stool weight, and decreased intracolonic pressure with fiber supplementation (Cummings, 2000).

Summary and Conclusions. The majority of the studies cited above show a relationship between *Dietary Fiber* and gastrointestinal health. There are data that show the benefits of certain *Dietary* and *Functional Fibers* on gastrointestinal health, including the effect of fiber on duodenal ulcers, constipation, laxation, fecal weight, energy source for the colon, and prevention of diverticular disease. For duodenal ulcer and diverticular disease, the data are promising for a protective effect, but insufficient data exist at this time upon which to base a recommended intake level. It is clear that fiber fermentation products provide energy for colonocytes and other cells of the body, but again this is not sufficient to use as a basis for a recommendation for fiber intake. With regard to the known fecal bulking and laxative effects of certain fibers, these are very well documented in numerous studies. A recommended intake level for *Total Fiber* based on prevention of CHD should be sufficient to reduce constipation in most normal people given adequacy of hydration of the large bowel.

Dietary Fiber *and the Prevention of Colon Cancer*

Marked international differences in rates of colon cancer (Boyle et al., 1985), coupled with findings from migratory studies showing that individuals take on the cancer demographics of the population to which they move (Haenszel and Kurihara, 1968), have suggested a strong role for environmental factors in colon cancer incidence.

Epidemiological Studies

Thun and coworkers (1992) found a significant inverse relation between the intake of citrus fruits, vegetables, and high fiber grains and colon cancer, although *Dietary Fiber* intake was not specifically analyzed. Fuchs and colleagues (1999) prospectively examined the relationship between *Dietary Fiber* intake and the risk of colon cancer in a large cohort of women. The same study group found a minimal nonsignificant inverse association in an earlier report that was based on 150 cases of colon cancer reported during 6 years of follow-up (Willett et al., 1990). In addition, the follow-up study revealed no relationship (Fuchs et al., 1999). Likewise, in six large, prospective studies, inverse associations between *Dietary Fiber* intake and the risk of colon cancer were weak or nonexistent (Giovannucci et al., 1994; Heilbrun et al., 1989; Kato et al., 1997; Key et al., 1996; Pietinen et al., 1999; Steinmetz et al., 1994).

Inverse relationships have been reported between *Dietary Fiber* intake and risk of colon cancer in some case-control studies (Bidoli et al., 1992; Dales et al., 1979; Freudenheim et al., 1990; Gerhardsson de Verdier et al., 1990; Iscovich et al., 1992; Lyon et al., 1987; Modan et al., 1975; Tuyns et al., 1987; West et al., 1989), but not all (Berta et al., 1985; Jain et al., 1980; Macquart-Moulin et al., 1986). A critical review of 37 observational epidemiological studies and a meta-analysis of 23 case-control studies showed that the majority suggest that *Dietary Fiber* is protective against colon cancer, with an odds ratio of 0.57 for the highest fiber group compared with the lowest (Trock et al., 1990). Furthermore, a meta-analysis of case-control studies demonstrated a combined relative risk of 0.53 for colon cancer in the highest as compared with the lowest quintile of fiber intake (Howe et al., 1992).

Lanza (1990) reviewed 48 epidemiological studies on the relationship between diets containing *Total Fiber* and colon cancer and found that 38 reported an inverse relationship, 7 reported no association, and 3 reported a direct association. In the Netherlands, *Dietary Fiber* intake was reported to be inversely related to total cancer deaths, as the 10-year cancer death rate was approximately threefold higher in individuals with low fiber intake compared with high fiber intake (Kromhout et al., 1982). Despite these and other positive findings, a number of important studies (Fuchs et al., 1999; Giovannucci and Willett, 1994) and three recent clinical intervention trials (Alberts et al., 2000; Bonithon-Kopp et al., 2000; Schatzkin et al., 2000) do not support a protective effect of *Dietary Fiber* intake against colon cancer. This issue remains to be resolved.

Intervention Studies

There have been a number of small clinical interventions addressing various surrogate markers for colon cancer, primarily changes in rectal cell proliferation and polyp recurrence. Generally, the small intervention trials have shown either no effect of fiber on the marker of choice or a very small effect. For example, Alberts and coworkers (1990) supplemented individuals with 13.5 g/d of wheat-bran fiber (*Dietary Fiber*) for 8 weeks and analyzed rectal mucosa cell biopsies for changes in cell proliferation. There was no overall decrease in rectal cell proliferation as a result of fiber supplementation unless the groups were divided into those with initially high and those with initially normal labeling indices. With this statistical division, there was a significant decrease in cell proliferation as a result of the fiber supplementation in six of the eight patients with initially high labeling indices and three of the eight patients with initially low indices, which suggests that wheat-bran fiber is protective against colon cancer. In a separate trial from the same group, supplemental dietary wheat-bran fiber (2.0 or 13.5 g/d) was provided to participants with a history of colon adenoma resection (Alberts et al., 1997). Wheat-bran fiber did not reduce the labeling index at either 3 or 9 months. Additionally, two randomized, placebo-controlled trials found no significant reduction in the incidence of colon tumor indicators among subjects who supplemented their diet with wheat bran or consumed high fiber diets (MacLennan et al., 1995; McKeown-Eyssen et al., 1994).

Recently, findings from three major trials on fiber and colonic polyp recurrence were reported (Alberts et al., 2000; Bonithon-Kopp et al., 2000; Schatzkin et al., 2000). All were well-designed, well-executed trials in individuals who previously had polyps removed. The Polyp Prevention Trial, which incorporated eight clinical centers, included an intervention that consisted of a diet that was low in fat, high in fiber, and high in fruits and vegetables (*Dietary Fiber*) (Schatzkin et al., 2000). There was no difference in polyp recurrence between the intervention and control groups. The Arizona Wheat-bran Fiber Trial provided 13.5 g/d versus 2 g/d of wheat-bran fiber (*Dietary Fiber*) (Alberts et al., 2000). Again, there was no difference between the control group and the intervention group in terms of polyp recurrence. The third trial used 3.5 g/d of psyllium (ispaghula husk) as the intervention (a potential *Functional Fiber*) (Bonithon-Kopp et al.,

2000). The adjusted odds ratio for the psyllium fiber intervention on polyp recurrence was 1.67 ($p = 0.042$).

Potential Mechanisms

Many hypotheses have been proposed as to how fiber might protect against colon cancer development; these hypotheses have been tested primarily in animal models. The hypotheses include the dilution of carcinogens, procarcinogens, and tumor promoters in a bulky stool; a more rapid rate of transit through the colon with high fiber diets; a reduction in the ratio of secondary bile acids to primary bile acids by acidifying colonic contents; the production of butyrate from the fermentation of dietary fiber by the colonic microflora; and the reduction of ammonia, which is known to be toxic to cells (Harris and Ferguson, 1993; Jacobs, 1986; Klurfeld, 1992; Van Munster and Nagengast, 1993; Visek, 1978). Unfortunately, most of the epidemiological and even the clinical intervention trials did not measure functional aspects of potential mechanisms by which fiber may be protective, and they did not attempt to relate aspects of colon physiology such as fecal weight or transit time to a protective effect against tumor development. Cummings and colleagues (1992) suggest that a daily fecal weight greater than 150 g is protective against colon cancer. In a study by Birkett and coworkers (1997), it was necessary to achieve a stool weight of 150 g to improve fecal markers for colon cancer, including fecal bulk, primary to secondary bile acid ratios, fecal pH, ammonia, and transit time. *Dietary Fiber* intake was 18 ± 8 g in the less than 150-g fecal-weight group and 28 ± 9 g in the greater than 150-g group ($p < 0.01$).

Dietary Fiber Intake and Colonic Adenomas

People with colonic adenomas are at elevated risk of developing colon cancer (Lev, 1990). Several epidemiological studies have reported that high *Dietary Fiber* and low fat intakes are associated with a lower incidence of colonic adenomas (Giovannucci et al., 1992; Hoff et al., 1986; Little et al., 1993; Macquart-Moulin et al., 1987; Neugut et al., 1993). For example, Giovannucci and coworkers (1992) studied a population of 7,284 men from the Health Professionals Follow-up Study and found a significant negative relationship between *Dietary Fiber* intake and colonic adenomas. The inverse relationship with *Dietary Fiber* persisted when they adjusted for other nutrients commonly found in fruits and vegetables. The overall median dietary intake of *Dietary Fiber* in this population was 21 g/d, with a median intake of 13 g/d for the lowest quintile and 34 g/d for the highest quintile. A reanalysis of 16,448 men from the Health Professionals Follow-Up Study that controlled for folate intake did not find a significant association between intake of *Dietary Fiber* and colon adenomas, although a slight reduction in risk was observed with increasing intake of fruit fiber (Platz et al., 1997).

Possible Reasons for the Lack of a Protective Effect of Dietary Fiber in Some Trials

There is considerable debate and speculation as to why clinical intervention trials on the relationship between fiber intake and colon cancer have not shown the expected beneficial effect of fiber. Some of the possible reasons for these results are discussed below.

Timing of the Intervention. Some of the recent prospective studies, such as the Nurses' Health Study (Fuchs et al., 1999) and the Health Professionals Follow-Up Study (Giovannucci et al., 1994), have failed to show a protective effect of *Dietary Fiber* intake against colon cancer when early indications from these same cohorts suggested that they would. As noted above, the Health Professionals Follow-up Study showed a protective effect of *Dietary Fiber* from the diet against colonic adenomas (Giovannucci et al., 1992). However, when the same cohort was later investigated for the relationship between intake of *Dietary Fiber* and colon carcinoma, no relationship was found (Giovannucci et al., 1994). A partial explanation for the difference is due to differences in ways that the data were analyzed based on information that was known at the time of analysis.

A similar situation was found in the Nurses' Health Study cohort, which initially found that the combination of high *Dietary Fiber* and low saturated or animal fat intake was associated with a reduced risk of adenomas (Willett et al., 1990), whereas a low intake of fiber alone did not contribute to the risk of colon cancer. Again, at follow-up in the same cohort, no relationship was found between *Dietary Fiber* intake and colon cancer incidence (Fuchs et al., 1999). This may also account for the lack of a protective effect of *Dietary Fiber* in the three recently reported clinical intervention trials (Alberts et al., 2000; Bonithon-Kopp et al., 2000; Schatzkin et al., 2000) since the participants already had colonic adenomas. Perhaps, as Giovannucci and colleagues (1992) suggest, intake of *Dietary Fiber* may influence the early stages of carcinogenesis, whereas dietary fat may have a greater influence on the progression of initiated cells into cancer.

The Confounding Role of Other Dietary Factors. Another possible explanation for the lack of a positive effect of fiber on colon cancer involves the potential confounding role of starch. As discussed in Chapter 6, starch may be divided into glycemic and nonglycemic starch, with nonglycemic starch being resistant to digestion by mammalian enzymes and thus reaching the colon. Resistant starch intake has been associated with increased concentrations of fecal ammonia (Birkett et al., 1997). This association was reversed when nonstarch polysaccharides were added. Ammonia is toxic to normal colonic cells and stimulates the growth of malignant cells (Visek, 1978). Thus, diets that are high in resistant starch, but low in fiber, may have adverse effects (Birkett et al., 1997).

Individuals May Not Consume Sufficient Amounts of Fiber or the Right Type of Fiber. Neither the prospective studies nor the three large intervention trials reported aspects of colonic function (Alberts et al., 2000; Bonithon-Kopp et al., 2000; Schatzkin et al., 2000). It is possible that bulkier stools or faster transit through the colon reduce the risk of bowel cancer (Cummings et al., 1992), but that the amounts or types of *Dietary Fibers* consumed did not result in these physiological effects. In addition, positive benefits of fiber with respect to colon cancer may not occur until *Dietary Fiber* intake is sufficiently high; for example, greater than the median 32 g/d for the highest quintile in The Health Professionals Follow-Up Study of men (Giovannucci et al., 1994; Platz et al., 1997) and 25 g/d in the Nurses' Health Study (Fuchs et al., 1999).

Summary

All but one of the studies (Bonithon-Kopp et al., 2000) cited in this section examined the relationship of *Dietary Fiber* to colon cancer. Information is lacking on the role of *Functional Fibers* in the incidence of colon cancer because of the lack of intake data on specific *Functional Fibers* collected in epidemiological studies. Most animal studies on fiber and colon cancer, however, have used what could be termed *Functional Fibers* (Jacobs, 1986). Because evidence available is either too conflicting or inadequately understood, a recommended intake level based on the prevention of colon cancer cannot be set.

Dietary Fiber *and Protection Against Breast Cancer*

A growing number of studies have reported on the relationship of *Dietary Fiber* intake and breast cancer incidence, and the strongest case can be made for cereal consumption rather than consumption of *Dietary Fiber* per se (for an excellent review see Gerber [1998]). Between-country studies, such as England versus Wales (Ingram, 1981), southern Italy versus northern Italy versus the United States (Taioli et al., 1991), and China versus the United States (Yu et al., 1991), and one study within Spain (Morales and Llopis, 1992), all showed an inverse correlation between bread and cereal consumption and breast cancer risk. The findings of

Caygill and coworkers (1998) showed an inverse correlation between breast cancer incidence and both the current diet ($p < 0.001$) and the diet 20 years previously ($p < 0.001$). However, starchy root, vegetable, and fruit intakes were not related to breast cancer risk for either diet.

Prospective Studies

There have been at least two prospective studies relating *Dietary Fiber* intake to breast cancer incidence in the United States and both found no significant association (Graham et al., 1992; Willett et al., 1992). A Canadian study showed a significant protective trend for the intake of cereals, with borderline significance for *Dietary Fiber* (Rohan et al., 1993). Verhoeven and coworkers (1997) investigated the relationship between *Dietary Fiber* intake and breast cancer risk in The Netherlands Cohort Study. This prospective cohort study showed no evidence that a high intake of *Dietary Fiber* decreased the risk of breast cancer.

Case-Control Studies

Eight of eleven reported case-control studies showed a protective effect of *Dietary Fiber* against breast cancer (Baghurst and Rohan, 1994; De Stefani et al., 1997; Franceschi et al., 1996; Freudenheim et al., 1996; Graham et al., 1991; Lubin et al., 1986; Rohan et al., 1988; Ronco et al., 1999; van't Veer et al., 1990; Witte et al., 1997; Yuan et al., 1995). For studies that showed this protection, the range of the odds ratio or relative risk was 0.40 to 0.74.

Intervention Studies

Most intervention studies on fiber and breast cancer have examined fiber intake and plasma or urinary indicators of estrogen (e.g., estrone, estradiol). Since certain breast cancers are hormone dependent, the concept is that fiber may be protective by decreasing estrogen concentrations. Rose and coworkers (1991) provided three groups of premenopausal women with a minimum of 30 g/d of *Dietary Fiber* from wheat, oats, or corn. After 2 months, wheat bran was shown to decrease plasma estrone and estradiol concentrations, but oats and corn were not effective. Bagga and coworkers (1995) provided 12 premenopausal women a very low fat diet (10 percent of energy) that provided 25 to 35 g/d of *Dietary Fiber*. After 2 months there were significant decreases in serum estradiol and estrone concentrations, with no effects on ovulation. Woods and colleagues (1989) found that a low fat (25 percent of energy), high fiber (40 g of *Dietary Fiber*) diet significantly reduced serum estrone sulfate concentrations in healthy premenopausal women compared with consumption of a typical Western diet (40 percent of energy from fat, 12 g of *Dietary Fiber*). In a separate study, the same researchers again provided a low fat (20 percent of energy), high fiber (40 g of *Dietary Fiber*) diet to premenopausal African-American women and observed reduced concentrations of serum estradiol and estrone sulfate when compared with a typical Western diet (Woods et al., 1996).

Mechanisms

A variety of different mechanisms have been proposed as to how fiber might protect against breast cancer, but the primary hypothesis is through decreasing serum estrogen concentrations. Fiber can reduce the entero-hepatic circulation of estrogen by binding unconjugated estrogens in the gastrointestinal tract (Shultz and Howie, 1986), making them unavailable for absorption (Gorbach and Goldin, 1987). Goldin and coworkers (1982) reported decreased plasma concentrations of estrone and increased fecal excretion of estrogens with increasing fecal weight. Alternatively, certain fibers can modify the colonic microflora to produce bacteria with low deconjugating activity (Rose, 1990), and deconjugated estrogens are reabsorbed. With less reabsorption of estrogens, plasma concentrations decrease. Another related hypothesis is that fiber speeds up transit through the colon, thus allowing less time for bacterial deconjugation. In fact, Petrakis and King (1981) noted abnormal cells in the mammary fluid of severely constipated women. Also, fiber sources contain phytoestrogens, which may compete with endogenous estrogens and act as antagonists (Lee et al., 1991; Rose, 1992). Finally, one report showed that *Dietary Fiber* intake was negatively correlated with total body fat mass, intra-abdominal adipose tissue, and subcutaneous abdominal adipose tissue in 135 men and 214 women (Larson et al., 1996). Since estrogen synthesis can occur in lipid stores, a decreased lipid mass should result in decreased synthesis. In addition to decreasing serum estrogen concentrations, fiber may be protective by adsorbing carcinogens or speeding their transit through the colon and providing less opportunity for their absorption. Carcinogens known to be related to breast cancer that may be affected include hetero-cyclic amines (Ito et al., 1991; Knekt et al., 1994), which have been shown to adsorb to fiber (Harris et al., 1996).

Summary

There are no reports on the role of *Functional Fibers* in the risk of breast cancer. Clearly, fiber has the potential capacity to decrease blood estrogen concentrations by a variety of different mechanisms, but whether or not this is sufficient to decrease the risk of breast cancer has not been thoroughly investigated. Because of the lack of evidence to support a role of *Dietary Fiber* in preventing breast cancer, this clinical endpoint cannot be used to set a recommended intake level.

Dietary Fiber *and Other Cancers*

Although the preponderance of the literature on fiber intake and cancer involves colon cancer and breast cancer, several studies have shown decreased risk for other types of cancer. Because *Dietary Fiber* has been shown to decrease serum estrogen concentrations, some researchers have hypothesized a protective effect against hormone-related cancers such as endometrial, ovarian, and prostate. Studies on *Dietary Fiber* intake and endometrial cancer have shown both significant and nonsignificant decreases in risk (Barbone et al., 1993; Goodman et al., 1997; McCann et al., 2000). In addition, studies have shown a decreased risk in ovarian cancer with a high intake of *Dietary Fiber* (McCann et al., 2001; Risch et al., 1994; Tzonou et al., 1993). However, no significant associations have been observed between *Dietary Fiber* intake and risk of prostate cancer (Andersson et al., 1996; Ohno et al., 1988; Rohan et al., 1995). Although interesting to note, this literature is in its infancy and cannot be used to set a recommended intake level for *Dietary Fiber.*

Dietary Fiber *and* Functional Fiber *and Glucose Tolerance, Insulin Response, and Amelioration of Diabetes*

Epidemiological Studies

Epidemiological evidence suggests that intake of certain fibers may delay glucose uptake and attenuate the insulin response, thus providing a protective effect against diabetes. Evidence for the protective effect of *Dietary Fiber* intake against type 2 diabetes comes from several prospective studies that have reported on the relationship between food intake and type 2 diabetes (Colditz et al., 1992; Meyer et al., 2000; Salmerón et al., 1997a, 1977b). One study examined the relationship between specific dietary patterns and risk of type 2 diabetes in a cohort of 42,759 men, while controlling for major known risk factors (Salmerón et al., 1997a). The results suggest that diets with a high glycemic load and low cereal fiber content are positively associated with risk of type 2 diabetes, independent of other currently known risk factors (Figure 7-1). In a second study, diet and risk of type 2 diabetes in a cohort of 65,173 women were evaluated (Salmerón et al., 1997b). Again, diets with a high glycemic load and

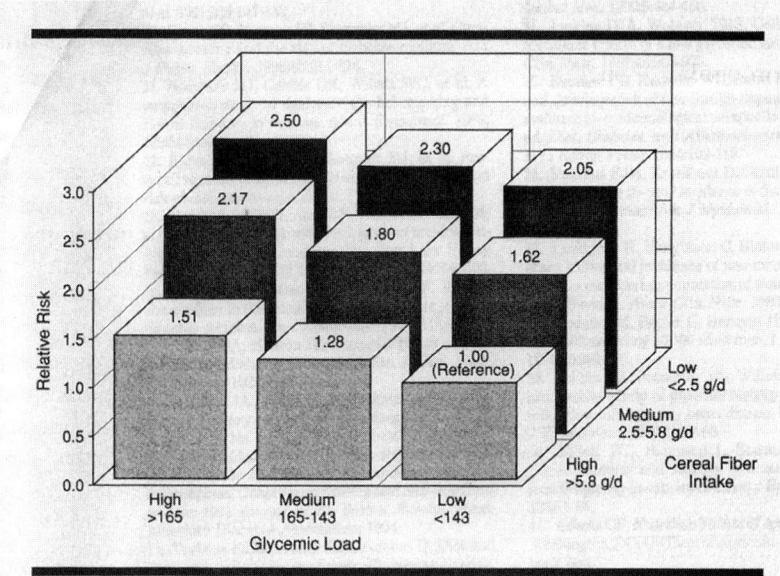

FIGURE 7-1 Relative risk of type 2 diabetes by different levels of cereal fiber intake and glycemic load. Reprinted, with permission, from Salmerón et al. (1997b). Copyright 1997 by the American Medical Association.

low cereal fiber content were positively associated with risk of type 2 diabetes, independent of other dietary factors and currently known risk factors. Of particular importance is that this combination resulted in a relative risk of 2.17 for men (Salmerón et al., 1997a) and 2.5 for women (Salmerón et al., 1997b), which is more than twofold greater relative to consumption of a diet high in cereal fiber and low in glycemic load (Figure 7-1).

In theory, the hypothesis as to how *Dietary Fiber* may be protective against type 2 diabetes is that it attenuates the glucose response and decreases insulin concentrations. This theory is supported by results from the Zutphen Elderly Study, where a negative relationship was observed between *Dietary Fiber* intake and insulin concentrations (Feskens et al., 1994).

Intervention Studies

In some clinical intervention trials ranging from 2 to 17 weeks, consumption of *Dietary Fiber* was shown to decrease insulin requirements in type 2 diabetics (Anderson et al., 1987; Rivellese et al., 1980; HCR Simpson et al., 1981). However, Behall (1990) compared the addition of 19.5 g of one of four different *Functional Fibers* (cellulose, carboxymethycellulose gum, karaya gum, and locust bean gum) to a low fiber diet with respect to glucose and insulin response curves from a standard glucose tolerance test and found no significant differences between the diets after 4 weeks. In addition, resistant starch has not been shown to have an effect on glycemic index. This is in contrast to the differences in "slow release" versus "fast release" starches, which have differential effects on postprandial glycemic and insulinemic profiles (Golay et al., 1992; Jenkins et al., 1987).

Viscous *Dietary* and *Functional Fibers*, such as are found in oat products, beans, isolated pectin, and isolated guar gum, have been found to produce significant reductions in glycemic response in 33 of 50 studies (66 percent) reviewed by Wolever and Jenkins (1993), which is in contrast to only 3 of 14 studies with nonviscous fiber (21 percent). Mechanistic data and hypotheses support this effect of viscous fibers as they delay gastric emptying and delay the absorption of glucose and other nutrients (Jenkins et al., 1978; Wood et al., 1994). However, a seeming anomaly is that the blood glucose response of foods is more closely related to their nonviscous fiber content than to their viscous fiber content (Wolever, 1995). It is not clear as to how significant the viscosity of fiber is to its contribution to the reduction in glycemic response in the overall observation of a lower incidence of type 2 diabetes with high fiber diets. Therefore, viscosity should not be considered the most important attribute of fiber with respect to this endpoint.

Summary

There is evidence that *Total Fiber* reduces the risk of diabetes; this can be used as a secondary endpoint to support a recommended intake level for *Total Fiber* that is primarily based on prevention of CHD. Further discussion is provided in the later section, "Findings by Life Stage and Gender Group."

Fiber Intake, Satiety, and Weight Maintenance

Epidemiological Studies

Since foods rich in fiber tend to be low in energy, researchers have hypothesized that fiber consumption may help with weight maintenance. This is an important consideration since obesity is such a prevalent problem and contributes to the risk of many diseases. Support for the concept that fiber consumption helps with weight maintenance is provided by studies showing that daily *Dietary Fiber* intake is lower for obese men (20.9 ± 1.8 g) and women (15.7 ± 1.1 g) than for lean men (26.9 ± 1.8 g) and women (22.7 ± 2.1 g) (Miller et al., 1994). Furthermore, in a study of 1,914 men and 3,378 women, mean body mass index (BMI) was significantly lower in the high *Dietary Fiber* group for both men and women (Appleby et al., 1998).

Intervention Studies

Several intervention studies suggest that diets high in fiber may assist in weight loss (Birketvedt et al., 2000; Eliasson et al., 1992; Rigaud et al., 1990; Rössner et al., 1987; Ryttig et al., 1989), although other studies have not found this effect (Astrup et al., 1990; Baron et al., 1986). For example, Birketvedt and coworkers (2000) conducted a study in which 53 moderately overweight females consumed a reduced energy diet (1,200 kcal/d) with or without a fiber supplement, which was 6 g/d for 8 weeks and then 4 g/d thereafter. The women on the fiber-supplemented diets lost 8.0 kg versus 5.8 kg for the placebo group ($p < 0.05$). High fiber diets are characterized by a very low energy density compared to diets high in fat, and a greater volume must be consumed in order to reach a certain energy level (Duncan et al., 1983; Tremblay et al., 1991), which again could result in cessation of eating. The issue of whether fiber has implications in the modulation of appetite has been reviewed (Blundell and Burley, 1987; Levine and Billington, 1994). Consumption of viscous fibers delays gastric emptying (Roberfroid, 1993), which in turn can cause an extended feeling of fullness (Bergmann et al., 1992) and delayed absorption of glucose and other nutrients (Jenkins et al., 1978; Ritz et al., 1991; Roberfroid, 1993; Truswell, 1992). Some investigators suggest that the delayed absorption of nutrients is associated with an extended feeling of satiety and delayed return of appetite (Grossman, 1986; Holt et al., 1992; Leathwood and Pollet, 1988), but not all investigators have found this effect (de Roos et al., 1995; Krishnamachar and Mickelsen, 1987; Sepple and Read, 1989).

A number of studies investigated the effect of consumption of a high fiber meal and food intake at a later eating occasion. For example, eating a breakfast supplemented with 29 g of sugar beet fiber resulted in 14 percent less energy consumption at the subsequent lunch (Burley et al., 1993). In contrast, other investigators have failed to demonstrate any postingestive effect of fiber on food intake (Delargy et al., 1995; Levine and Billington, 1994). One study found that there was no difference between a high fiber and a low fiber diet on later food intake if the energy content of the initial diets was similar (Delargy et al., 1995). These authors used 20 g of *Dietary Fiber* for their test breakfast meal, which is much lower than the 29 g used by Burley and coworkers (1993). The authors concluded that for *Dietary Fiber* to have an effect, there has to be greater than 20 g in the test meal

(Delargy et al., 1995). Similar findings of no effect of a test meal on appetite throughout the day have been found for substituting resistant starch for digestible starch (Raben et al., 1994). In addition, much of the data on chitin and chitosan in promoting weight loss have been negative (see earlier section, "Physiological Effects of Isolated and Synthetic Fibers").

Summary

The strongest data supporting a relationship between fiber and weight maintenance come from the few epidemiological studies showing that *Dietary Fiber* intake is lower for obese men and women than for lean men and women and that BMI is lower with higher fiber consumption for both men and women. Efforts to show that eating specific fibers increases satiety and thus results in a decreased food intake have been inconclusive. In terms of the attribute of fiber that may result in decreased food intake, some have suggested that viscosity is important as it delays gastric emptying and may lead to feeling more full for a longer period of time. However, this hypothesis has not been validated in clinical trials.

Although the finding that the overall data on *Dietary Fiber* intake are negatively correlated with BMI is suggestive of a role for fiber in weight control, the studies designed to determine how fiber intake might impact overall energy intake have not shown a major effect. In fact, it appears that very high amounts of fiber (e.g., 30 g/meal) are required to diminish subsequent energy intake after that meal. For humans, there is no overwhelming evidence that *Dietary Fiber* has an effect on satiety or weight maintenance, therefore this endpoint is not used to set a recommended intake level.

FINDINGS BY LIFE STAGE AND GENDER GROUP

Expression of the Total Fiber Requirement

Total Fiber requirements (the sum of *Dietary Fiber* and *Functional Fiber*) may be expressed in a variety of different ways, including age plus number of grams per day (Williams et al., 1995), grams per kilogram of body weight (AAP, 1993), grams per day (Health and Welfare Canada, 1985; LSRO, 1987), and grams per 1,000 kcal (LSRO, 1987). Each of these methods has its advantages and disadvantages. Because the available evidence suggests that the beneficial effects of fiber in humans are most likely related to the amount of food consumed—not to the individual's age or body weight—the best approach is to set an Adequate Intake (AI) based on grams per 1,000 kcal. However, since many people do not know how many kilocalories they consume in a day, the AI is based on the usual daily intake of energy (Appendix Table E-1) for each age group and is expressed in grams per day. Those with energy intakes significantly above or below the reference intakes for their age and gender may want to consider adjusting their total fiber intake accordingly.

Infants Ages 0 Through 12 Months

There are no functional criteria for fiber status that reflect response to dietary intake in infants. Since human milk is recognized as the optimal source of nourishment for infants throughout at least the first year of life and as a sole nutritional source for infants during the first 4 to 6 months of life (IOM, 1991), and because human milk contains no *Dietary Fiber*, there is no AI for infants 0 through 6 months of age. During the 7- through 12-month age period, the intake of solid foods becomes more significant, and *Dietary Fiber* intake may increase. However, there are no data on *Dietary Fiber* intake in this age group and no theoretical reason to establish an AI for infants 7 through 12 months of age.

Children and Adolescents Ages 1 Through 18 Years

Method Used to Set the AI

Although guidelines have been endorsed for recommended dietary intakes of total fat and fatty acids, protein, carbohydrate, and cholesterol in children 2 years of age and older by a variety of different organizations (AHA, 1983; Dwyer, 1980; USDA/HHS, 2000), none of these guidelines recommend a specific level of fiber intake during childhood. Data suggest that North American children, like adults, consume inadequate amounts of fiber for optimal health, and that consumption of fiber should be increased to promote normal laxation, to help prevent diet-related cancer, to help reduce serum cholesterol concentrations and therefore the risk of coronary heart disease (CHD), and to help prevent obesity and the risk of adult-onset diabetes (AHA, 1983; AMA Council on Scientific Affairs, 1989; Wynder and Berenson, 1984). National pediatric dietary goals are targeted for children older than 2 years of age, with a suggestion that age 2 to 3 years be a transition year (National Cholesterol Education Program, 1991).

Constipation is a common problem during childhood, as it is in adults, and accounts for 25 percent of visits to pediatric gastroenterology clinics (Loening-Baucke, 1993). As discussed in the earlier section, "*Dietary Fiber, Functional Fiber*, and Colon Health," there are strong data showing the contribution of high fiber diets, along with adequate fluid intake, to laxation in adults. However, fiber intake and constipation data in children are limited. Studies correlate low *Dietary Fiber* intake with constipation

(Hunt et al., 1993; Roma et al., 1999). Two studies by the same research group addressed fiber intake in American children and found that children with constipation consumed, on average, about half as much fiber as the healthy control group (McClung et al., 1993, 1995). Morais and coworkers (1999) reported that children with chronic constipation ingested less *Dietary Fiber* than age-matched controls.

The AI for *Total Fiber* for children and adolescents is based on the data cited for adults, which showed that 14 g/1,000 kcal reduced the risk of CHD (see "Adults Ages 19 Years and Older"). The AI (14 g/1,000 kcal × median energy intake [kcal/1,000 kcal/d]) is then set for each age and gender group. The median energy intake for 1- to 3-year-old children is 1,372 kcal/d (Appendix Table E-1). Thus, 19 g/d (14 × 1.37) of total fiber would be recommended for this age group. It should be kept in mind that recommendations for fiber intake are based on a certain amount of total fiber as a function of energy intake. This means that those who consume less than the median energy intake of a particular category need less fiber than the recommendation (which is based on the mean energy intake). For example, the median energy intake for 1- to 3-year-old children is 1,372 kcal/d and the recommendation for total fiber is 19 g/d. However, 1-year-old children not meeting this energy consumption level will not require 19 g/d and their intake should be scaled back accordingly.

The median energy intake for 4- to 8-year-old children is 1,759 kcal/d (Appendix Table E-1). Thus, 25 g/d (14 × 1.76) of *Total Fiber* would be recommended for these children. The AIs for *Total Fiber* for boys and girls 9 to 18 years of age have been calculated in a similar manner using the energy intake values in Appendix Table E-1.

Total Fiber *AI Summary, Ages 1 Through 18 Years*

AI for Children
1–3 years	19 g/d of *Total Fiber*
4–8 years	25 g/d of *Total Fiber*

AI for Boys
9–13 years	31 g/d of *Total Fiber*
14–18 years	38 g/d of *Total Fiber*

AI for Girls
9–13 years	26 g/d of *Total Fiber*
14–18 years	26 g/d of *Total Fiber*

Adults Ages 19 Years and Older

Methods Used to Set the AI

Fiber Intake and Risk of CHD. Although the preponderance of the data shows a protective effect of consumption of high fiber and high fiber-containing foods against CHD (see earlier section, "*Dietary Fiber, Functional Fiber*, and the Prevention of Hyperlipidemia, Hypertension, and Coronary Heart Disease"), there are exceptions to these findings. A more important consideration for establishing a requirement for fiber is the fact that the dietary intake data from epidemiological studies are on fiber-containing foods, which are considered *Dietary Fiber*. Certain investigators specifically analyzed diets for *Dietary Fiber* (Burr and Sweetnam, 1982; Hallfrisch et al., 1988; Khaw and Barrett-Connor, 1987; Kromhout et al., 1982; Kushi et al., 1985; Morris et al., 1977; Pietinen et al., 1996; Rimm et al., 1996), but others used indicators of *Dietary Fiber* intake such as cereals, vegetables, fruits, whole grains, or legumes. There are many constituents of whole grains, in addition to *Dietary Fiber*, that may reduce the risk of CHD (Slavin et al., 1997; Thompson, 1994). Despite these cautions, the data on the relationship between *Dietary Fiber* intake and risk of CHD based on epidemiological, clinical, and mechanistic data are strong enough to warrant using this relationship as a basis for setting a recommended level of intake. Both men and women appear to benefit from increasing their intake of foods rich in fibers, particularly cereal fibers, with women appearing to benefit more from increasing fiber consumption than men.

Because the prospective studies of Pietinen and coworkers (1996), Rimm and coworkers (1996), and Wolk and coworkers (1999) are adequately powered, divide fiber intake into quintiles, and provide data on energy intake (Table 7-2), it is possible to set a recommended intake level. Data from 21,930 Finnish men showed that at the highest quintile of *Dietary Fiber* intake (34.8 g/d), median energy intake was 2,705 kcal/d, which equates to 12.9 g of *Dietary Fiber*/1,000 kcal (Pietinen et al., 1996). The Health Professionals Follow-up Study of men reported a *Dietary Fiber* intake of 28.9 g/d in the highest quintile, with a normalized energy intake of 2,000 kcal/d, which equates to 14.45 g of *Dietary Fiber*/1,000 kcal (Rimm et al., 1996). In the Nurses' Health Study of women, the median *Dietary Fiber* intake at the highest quintile was 22.9 g/d, with a normalized energy intake of 1,600 kcal/d (Wolk et al., 1999), which equates to 14.3 g of *Dietary Fiber*/1,000 kcal. In these three studies, there was a significant negative trend in *Dietary Fiber* intake and risk of CHD. Specifically, there was a strong negative correlation between cereal fiber intake and risk of CHD, whereas the correlation was weak or nonexistent for fruit and vegetable fibers. Taken collectively and averaging to the nearest gram, these data suggest an intake of 14 g of *Dietary Fiber*/1,000 kcal, particularly from cereals, to promote heart health. Data from the intervention trials are in line with these recommendations, as are data from epidemiological studies.

Fiber Intake and Risk of Type 2 Diabetes. The literature on *Dietary Fiber* intake and glucose tolerance, insulin response, and amelioration of diabetes alone is insufficient at this time to use as a basis for a recommendation (see "Evidence Considered for Estimating the Requirement for *Dietary Fiber* and *Functional Fiber*"). However, it should be noted that the positive effects seen in two large prospective studies (Salmerón et al., 1997a, 1997b) were achieved with the same levels of fiber that have previously been reported as being protective against CHD (Pietinen et al., 1996; Rimm et al., 1996; Wolk et al., 1999). Therefore, the recommendations made using the effect of *Dietary Fiber* intake on CHD are supported by the data on *Dietary Fiber* intake and type 2 diabetes.

Summary. Prospective studies have shown that the impact of *Dietary Fiber* on the advent of CHD occurs continuously across a range of intakes. Therefore, an Estimated Average Requirement (EAR) cannot be set.

Based on the average intake of *Dietary Fiber* and its effect on CHD, as well as the beneficial role of *Functional Fibers* (such as gums, pectin and psyllium), an AI for *Total Fiber* is set for each age and gender group by multiplying 14 g/1,000 kcal × median energy intake (kcal/1,000 kcal/d). The highest median intake level for each gender-specific age group (from Appendix Table E-1) was used in the equation to set the AI for young adults (19 to 50 years of age) and older adults (51 years of age and older). There is no information to indicate that fiber intake as a function of energy intake differs during the life cycle.

By definition, the AI is expected to meet or exceed the EAR or the average amount needed to maintain a defined nutritional state or criterion of adequacy in essentially all members of a specific healthy population. Thus, where data are insufficient to be used as the basis of an AI, *Total Fiber* at the recommended levels may also help to ameliorate constipation and diverticular disease, provide fuel for colonic cells, attenuate blood glucose and lipid concentrations, and provide a source of nutrient-rich, low energy-dense foods that could contribute to satiety.

Total Fiber AI Summary, Ages 19 Years and Older

AI for Men
19–30 years	38 g/d of *Total Fiber*
31–50 years	38 g/d of *Total Fiber*
51–70 years	30 g/d of *Total Fiber*
> 70 years	30 g/d of *Total Fiber*

AI for Women
19–30 years	25 g/d of *Total Fiber*
31–50 years	25 g/d of *Total Fiber*
51–70 years	21 g/d of *Total Fiber*
> 70 years	21 g/d of *Total Fiber*

Pregnancy

Method Used to Set the AI

There is no evidence to suggest the beneficial effects of fiber in reducing the risk of CHD for pregnant adolescent girls and women is different from nonpregnant adolescent girls and women. Therefore, the AI for *Total Fiber* is 28 g/d (14 g/1,000 kcal × 1,978 kcal/1,000 kcal/d).

Total Fiber *AI Summary, Pregnancy*

AI for Pregnant Women
14–18 years	28 g/d of *Total Fiber*
19–30 years	28 g/d of *Total Fiber*
31–50 years	28 g/d of *Total Fiber*

Lactation

Method Used to Set the AI

There is no evidence to suggest the beneficial effects of fiber in reducing the risk of CHD for lactating adolescent girls and women are different from nonpregnant adolescent girls and women. Therefore, the AI for *Total Fiber* is 29 g/d (14 g/1,000 kcal × 2,066 kcal/1,000 kcal/d).

Total Fiber *AI Summary, Lactation*

AI for Lactating Women
    14–18 years   29 g/d of *Total Fiber*
    19–30 years   29 g/d of *Total Fiber*
    31–50 years   29 g/d of *Total Fiber*

INTAKE OF *DIETARY FIBER*

Food Sources

Marlett (1992) reported on the *Dietary Fiber* content of 117 frequently consumed foods. *Dietary Fiber* was present in the majority of fruits, vegetables, refined grains, and miscellaneous foods such as ketchup, olives, and soups, at concentrations of 1 to 3 percent, or 1 to 3 g/100 g of fresh weight. Nuts, legumes, and high fiber grains typically contained more than 3 percent *Dietary Fiber.* About one-third of the fiber in legumes, nuts, fruits, and vegetables was present as hemicelluloses. Approximately one-fourth of the fiber in grains and fruit and one-third in nuts and vegetables consisted of cellulose. Although fruits contained the greatest amount of pectin, 15 to 20 percent of the fiber content in legumes, nuts, and vegetables was pectin.

The major sources of naturally occurring inulin and oligofructose are wheat and onions, which provide about 70 and 25 percent of these components, respectively (Moshfegh et al., 1999). Isolated inulin provides a creamy texture and is added to replace fat in table spreads, dairy products, frozen desserts, baked goods, fillings, and dressings. Oligofructose is most commonly added to cereals, fruit preparations for yogurt, cookies, dairy products, and frozen desserts.

Depending on one's chosen diet, naturally occurring and manufactured resistant starch, as well as that produced during normal processing of foods for human consumption, could make a significant contribution to daily *Total Fiber* intake. Legumes are the largest source of naturally occurring resistant starch (Marlett and Longacre, 1996). In addition, green bananas (Englyst and Cummings, 1986) and cooled, cooked potatoes (Englyst and Cummings, 1987) can provide a significant amount of resistant starch. Resistant starch resulting from normal processing of a foodstuff is a more modest contributor to a typical daily intake. Starches specifically manufactured to be resistant to endogenous human digestion are a rapidly growing segment of commercially available resistant starches.

Dietary Intake

National nutrition surveys use the U.S. Department of Agriculture (USDA) food composition database to estimate the intake of various nutrients. This database primarily measures *Dietary Fiber* intake because isolated *Functional Fibers*, such as pectins and gums, that are used as ingredients represent a very minor amount of the fiber present in foods. For instance, the fiber content of fat-free ice creams and yogurts, which contain *Functional Fibers* as additives, is much less than 1 g/serving and therefore is often labeled as having 0 g of fiber. Based on intake data from the Continuing Survey of Food Intakes by Individuals (CSFII) (1994–1996, 1998), median *Dietary Fiber* intakes ranged from 16.5 to 17.9 g/d for men and 12.1 to 13.8 g/d for women (Appendix Table E-4). Based on the Adequate Intakes (AI) set for the various age and gender groups, 10 percent or less of a particular group consumed greater than the AI.

Based on additional intake data from CSFII, American diets provided on average 2.6 g/d of inulin and 2.5 g/d of oligofructose (Moshfegh et al., 1999). Since inulin and oligofructose have not been analyzed as fiber previously, they would not be in the USDA database. This would mean that people are actually consuming approximately 5.1 g/d more fiber than reported in the CSFII database (Appendix Table E-4). Although there is a seemingly large gap between current fiber intake and the recommended intake, it is not difficult to consume recommended levels of *Total Fiber* by choosing foods recommended by the Food Guide Pyramid. Two sample menus are provided that meet the Estimated Energy Requirement (EER) and AI for *Total Fiber* for men (Table 7-3) and women (Table 7-4).

These menus show that a 19-year-old active male and a 19-year-old active female can meet their AI for *Total Fiber* without exceeding their EER. These diets also meet the Recommended Dietary Allowances and AIs for all of the micronutrients.

ADVERSE EFFECTS OF OVERCONSUMPTION

Adverse Effects of Dietary Fiber

Mineral Bioavailability

Within the last 20 years, several animal and human studies have shown that foods or diets rich in fibers may alter mineral metabolism, especially when phytate is present (Sandstead, 1992). Fibers may reduce the bioavailability of minerals such as iron, calcium, and zinc (AAP, 1981; Williams and Bollella, 1995). However, levels of 10 to 12 g of *Dietary Fiber*/1,000 kcal have been suggested as safe even for Japanese adolescents, who tradition-

TABLE 7-3 Fiber Intake from an Omnivorous Diet Adequate in Essential Micronutrients to Meet the Estimated Energy Requirement for a Male 19 Years of Age (3,078 kcal/d)

Meal	Foods Eaten	Energy (kcal)	Total Fiber (g)
Breakfast	Grapefruit, pink or red ($^1/_2$ medium)	38	1.4
	Banana (1 medium)	109	2.8
	Cereal, ready-to-eat shredded oats (1 cup)	112	3.0
	English muffin (white, 1 whole)	134	1.5
	Margarine (2 tsp)	68	0
	Milk, 1% (1 cup)	102	0
	Total for meal	563	8.7
Snack	Crackers, whole wheat (6 each)	109	0.9
	Cheddar cheese (1.5 oz)	171	0
	Juice ($^3/_4$ cup)	78	0.4
	Total for snack	358	1.3
Lunch	Tossed salad (1 cup)	16	1.5
	Salad dressing (1 tbs)	66	0
	Chili with beans and beef (1 cup)	273	6.5
	Cornbread (1 piece)	173	1.3
	Margarine (1 tsp)	34	0
	Grapes ($^1/_2$ cup)	57	0.8
	Fig bar cookies (2)	111	1.5
	Milk, 1% (1 cup)	102	0
	Total for meal	832	11.6
Dinner	Salmon in soy sauce (3.5 oz)	169	0.2
	Rice with vegetables ($^3/_4$ cup)	167	1.4
	Broccoli (1-$^1/_2$ cup)	40	4.4
	Roll, whole wheat (2 medium)	177	5.0
	Margarine (2 tsp)	68	0
	Ice cream ($^1/_2$ cup)	98	0.3
	Total for meal	719	11.3
Snack	Carrots, raw (12 medium baby)	51	3.6
	Spinach dip (2 tbs)	58	0.4
	Turkey sandwich	344	1.2
	Cola (1 can)	153	0
	Total for snack	606	5.2
Daily total		3,078	38.1

NOTE: Source of food composition data: NDS-R Food and Nutrient Data Base, Version 4.04_32, 2001, Nutrition Coordinating Center, University of Minnesota.

TABLE 7-4 Fiber Intake from an Omnivorous Diet Adequate in Essential Micronutrients to Meet the Estimated Energy Requirement for a Female 19 Years of Age (2,393 kcal/d)

Meal	Foods Eaten	Energy (kcal)	Total Fiber (g)
Breakfast	Banana ($^1/_2$ medium)	54	1.4
	Cereal, ready-to-eat shredded oats ($^3/_4$ cup)	84	2.3
	English muffin (white, 1 whole)	134	1.5
	Margarine (2 tsp)	68	0
	Milk, skim (1 cup)	86	0
	Total for meal	426	5.2
Snack	Crackers, whole wheat (5 each)	90	0.7
	Cheddar cheese (1.5 oz)	171	0
	Juice ($^3/_4$ cup)	78	0.4
	Total for snack	339	1.1
Lunch	Tossed salad ($^3/_4$ cup)	12	1.1
	Salad dressing (1 tbs)	66	0
	Chili with beans and beef ($^3/_4$ cup)	205	4.9
	Cornbread (1 piece)	173	1.3
	Margarine (1 tsp)	34	0
	Grapes ($^1/_2$ cup)	57	0.8
	Milk, skim (1 cup)	86	0
	Total for meal	633	8.1
Dinner	Salmon in soy sauce (3.5 oz)	169	0.2
	Rice with vegetables ($^1/_2$ cup)	111	1.0
	Broccoli ($^1/_2$ cup)	14	1.5
	Roll, whole wheat (1 medium)	89	2.5
	Margarine (1 tsp)	34	0
	Ice cream ($^1/_2$ cup)	98	0.3
	Total for meal	515	5.5
Snack	Apple (1 medium)	81	3.7
	Pretzels (1 oz)	108	0.9
	Peanut butter sandwich	138	1.3
	Cola (1 can)	153	0
	Total for snack	480	5.9
Daily total		2,393	25.8

NOTE: Source of food composition data: NDS-R Food and Nutrient Data Base, Version 4.04_32, 2001, Nutrition Coordinating Center, University of Minnesota.

ally have low levels of calcium intake (Nishimune et al., 1993). Most studies that assess the effect of fiber intake on mineral status have looked at calcium, magnesium, iron, or zinc.

Calcium. Most studies investigating the effects of cereal, vegetable, and fruit fibers on the absorption of calcium in animals and humans have reported no effect on calcium absorption or balance (Spencer et al., 1991; Wisker et al., 1991). However, some studies described a decrease in calcium absorption with ingestion of *Dietary Fiber* under certain conditions (Knox et al., 1991; O'Brien et al., 1993). Slavin and Marlett (1980) found that supplementing the diet with 16 g/d of cellulose resulted in significantly greater fecal excretion of calcium resulting in an average loss of approximately 200 mg/d. There was no effect on the apparent absorption of calcium after the provision of 15 g/d of citrus pectin (Sandberg et al., 1983).

Magnesium. Studies report no differences in magnesium balance with intake of certain *Dietary Fibers* (Behall et al., 1987; Hallfrisch et al., 1987; Spencer et al., 1991). Astrup and coworkers (1990) showed no effect of the addition of 30 g/d of plant fiber to a very low energy diet on plasma concentrations of magnesium. There was no effect on the apparent absorption of magnesium after the provision of 15 g/d of citrus pectin (Sandberg et al., 1983). Magnesium balance was not significantly altered with the consumption of 16 g/d of cellulose (Slavin and Marlett, 1980).

Iron and Zinc. A number of studies have looked at the impact of fiber-containing foods, such as cereal fibers, on iron and zinc absorption. These cereals typically contain levels of phytate that are known to impair iron and zinc absorption. Coudray and colleagues (1997) showed no effect of isolated viscous inulin or partly viscous sugar beet fibers on either iron or zinc absorption when compared to a control diet. Metabolic balance studies conducted in adult males who consumed four oat bran muffins daily showed no changes in zinc balance due to the supplementation (Spencer et al., 1991). Brune and coworkers (1992) have suggested that the inhibitory effect of bran on iron absorption is due to its phytate content rather than its *Dietary Fiber* content. However, the addition of 12 g/d of bran to a meal decreased iron absorption by 51 to 74 percent, and the inhibition was not explained by the presence of phytate (KM Simpson et al., 1981).

Gastrointestinal Distress. There are limited studies to suggest that chronic high intakes of *Dietary Fibers* can cause gastrointestinal distress. The consumption of wheat bran at levels up to 40 g/d did not result in significant increases in gastrointestinal distress compared to a placebo (McRorie et al., 2000). However, flatulence did increase with increased intake of *Dietary*

Fiber (Bolin and Stanton, 1998; Tomlin et al., 1991). Adverse effects have been observed under certain special circumstances. For instance, 75 to 80 g/d of *Dietary Fiber* has been associated with sensations of excessive abdominal fullness and increased flatulence in individuals with pancreatic disease (Dutta and Hlasko, 1985). Furthermore, the consumption of 160 to 200 g/d of unprocessed bran resulted in intestinal obstruction in a woman who was taking an antidepressant (Kang and Doe, 1979).

Summary

Dietary Fiber can have variable compositions and therefore it is difficult to link a specific fiber with a particular adverse effect, especially when phytate is also often present. It is concluded that as part of an overall healthy diet, a high intake of *Dietary Fiber* will not produce significant deleterious effects in healthy people. Therefore, a Tolerable Upper Intake Level (UL) is not set for *Dietary Fiber*.

Special Considerations

Dietary Fiber is a cause of gastrointestinal distress in people with irritable bowel syndrome. Those who suffer from excess gas production can consume a low gas-producing diet, which is low in dietary fiber (Cummings, 2000).

Hazard Identification for Isolated and Synthetic Fibers

Unlike *Dietary Fiber*, it may be possible to concentrate large amounts of *Functional Fiber* in foods, beverages, and supplements. Since the potential adverse health effects of *Functional Fiber* are not completely known, they should be evaluated on a case-by-case basis. In addition, projections regarding the potential contribution of *Functional Fiber* to daily *Total Fiber* intake at anticipated patterns of food consumption would be informative. *Functional Fiber*, like *Dietary Fiber*, is not digested by mammalian enzymes and passes into the colon. Thus, like *Dietary Fiber*, most potentially deleterious effects of *Functional Fiber* ingestion will be on the interaction with other nutrients in the gastrointestinal tract. Data from human studies on adverse effects of consuming what may be considered as *Functional Fibers* (if sufficient data exist to show a potential health benefit) are summarized below under the particular fiber.

Chitin and Chitosan

Studies on the adverse effects of chitin and chitosan are limited. A study in rats fed up to 5 percent chitin for 13 weeks showed no adverse effects based on clinical signs, hematology, serum biochemistry, and histopathology analysis (Niho et al., 1999).

Gums

Gastrointestinal Distress. While the adverse gastrointestinal effects of gums are limited, incidences of moderate to severe degrees of flatulence were reported from a trial in which 4 to 12 g/d of a hydrolyzed guar gum were provided to 16 elderly patients (Patrick et al., 1998).

Allergic Reactions. Gums such as the exudate gums, gum arabic, and gum tragacanth have been shown to elicit an immune response in mice (Strobel et al., 1982). Occupational asthma caused by guar gum has been reported (Lagier et al., 1990).

Inulin, Oligofructose, and Fructooligosaccharide

Cancer. When F-344 rats, known to have a high incidence of neoplastic lesions, were given 0, 8,000, 20,000, or 50,000 ppm doses of fructooligosaccharide, the incidence of pituitary adenomas was 20, 26, 38, and 44 percent, respectively (Haseman et al., 1990). The incidence was significantly higher for intakes at 20,000 and 50,000 ppm. Clevenger and coworkers (1988) reported no difference in the onset of cancer in F-344 rats fed 0, 8,000 (341 to 419 mg/kg/d), 20,000 (854 to 1,045 mg/kg/d), or 50,000 ppm (2,170 to 2,664 mg/kg/d) doses of fructooligosaccharide compared with the controls.

Development and Reproduction. Henquin (1988) observed a lack of developmental toxicity when female rats were fed a diet containing 20 percent fructooligosaccharide during gestation. When pregnant rats were fed diets containing 5, 10, or 20 percent fructooligosaccharide during gestation, no adverse developmental effects were observed (Sleet and Brightwell, 1990).

Genotoxicity. Fructooligosaccharide has been tested for genotoxicity using a wide range of test doses (0 to 50,000 ppm); the results indicated no genotoxic potential from use of fructooligosaccharide (Clevenger et al., 1988).

Gastrointestinal Distress. A number of studies have observed gastrointestinal distress (e.g., diarrhea, flatulence, bloating, and cramping) with inulin, oligofructose, or fructooligosaccharide intake. Cramping, bloating, flatulence, and diarrhea was observed at intakes ranging from 14 to 18 g/d of inulin (Davidson and Maki, 1999; Pedersen et al., 1997). Consumption of 5 or 15 g/d of fructooligosaccharide produced a gaseous response in healthy men (Alles et al., 1996). Briet and coworkers (1995) reported increased flatulence as a result of consuming more than 30 g/d of fructo-oligosaccharide, increased bloating at greater than 40 g/d, and cramps and diarrhea at 50 g/d. Increased flatulence and bloating were observed when 10 g/d of fructooligosaccharide was consumed (Stone-Dorshow and Levitt, 1987).

The role carbohydrate malabsorption plays in the onset of diarrhea most likely depends upon the balance between the osmotic force of the carbohydrate and the capacity of the colon to remove the carbohydrate via bacterial fermentation. In order to evaluate the significance of osmolarity, Clausen and coworkers (1998) compared the severity of diarrhea after consumption of fructooligosaccharide and lactulose, both of which are nonabsorbable carbohydrates. Although both carbohydrates are fermented by colonic microflora, they differ in osmolarity. The osmotic force is twice as high for lactulose as for frutooligosaccharide. In a crossover design, 12 individuals were given fructooligosaccharide or lactulose in increasing doses of 0, 20, 40, 80, and 160 g/d. The increase in fecal volume measured as a function of the dose administered was twice as high for lactulose as for fructooligosaccharide; however, there was substantial interindividual variation in the response. The researchers concluded that fecal volume in carbohydrate-induced diarrhea is proportional to the osmotic force of the malabsorbed saccharide, even though most is degraded by colonic bacteria (Clausen et al., 1998).

Allergic Reactions. Data on the allergenicity of inulin and oligofructose is very limited. Anaphylaxis was observed following the intravenous administration of inulin for determining the glomerular filtration rate (Chandra and Barron, 2002). Separate episodes of anaphylaxis were observed following the ingestion of artichoke leaves, a margarine containing inulin extracted from chicory (Raftiline HP), and a candy containing inulin (Raftiline HP) or oligofructose (Raftilose P95) (Gay-Crosier et al., 2000). A skin-pricking test revealed hypersensitivity to each of the above foods or ingredients (Gay-Crosier et al., 2000).

Pectin

Pectin has been shown to have a negligible effect on zinc retention in humans (Lei et al., 1980). Also, Behall and coworkers (1987) found that refined fibers had no effect on mineral balance as long as people were consuming recommended dietary allowance levels of iron and zinc when fed as part of their control diet.

Polydextrose

Polydextrose has showed no reproductive toxicity, teratology, mutagenicity, genotoxicity, or carcinogenesis in experimental animals (Burdock and Flamm, 1999). In humans, no reports of abdominal cramping or diarrhea were reported in men and women who were given up to 12 g/d of polydextrose (Jie et al., 2000). Furthermore, there were no complaints of abdominal distress with the consumption of 30 g/d of polydextrose (Achour et al., 1994). However, flatulence and gas-related problems were reported following the intake of 30 g/d of polydextrose (Tomlin and Read, 1988). Diarrhea was reported with the consumption of 15 g/d of polydextrose; however, this symptom ceased after 1 month of intake (Saku et al., 1991).

Psyllium

Gastrointestinal Distress. In a meta-analysis of eight studies regarding psyllium intake, the authors found that psyllium was well tolerated and safe (Anderson et al., 2000a). There have been certain situations in which adverse effects have been observed. Esophageal obstruction was noted in an elderly man who regularly took a "heaping" teaspoon with some water (Noble and Grannis, 1984). Furthermore, an elderly woman who was given 2 tbs of a psyllium-based laxative three times daily suffered from small-bowel obstruction (Berman and Schultz, 1980). It was determined that her water intake was insufficient for this dose. Thus, psyllium generally does not cause gastrointestinal distress provided adequate amounts of water are consumed.

Cancer. In the European Center Prevention Organization Study, psyllium (*Functional Fiber*) was provided at a level of 3.5 g/d (Bonithon-Kopp et al., 2000). Patients ($n = 655$) with a history of colon adenomas were randomly assigned to one of three treatment groups: 2 g/d of calcium, 3.5 g/d of psyllium, or placebo. Participants in the study also had a colonoscopy after 3 years of follow-up. The adjusted odds ratio for colon adenoma recurrence for the psyllium fiber intervention was 1.67 ($p = 0.042$). The authors concluded that supplementation with psyllium may have adverse effects on colon adenoma recurrence.

Allergic Reactions. Several reports of anaphylaxis have been reported following the ingestion of psyllium-containing cereals (Drake et al., 1991; James et al., 1991; Lantner et al., 1990). Subsequent IgE antibodies to psyllium were confirmed in these reports. Symptoms of asthma have also been reported in individuals exposed to psyllium powder (Busse and Schoenwetter, 1975).

Resistant Starch

Ninety-one percent of individuals who consumed 32 g/d of RS_3 (retrograded starch; formed from the cooking and cooling or extrusion of starchy foods) experienced flatulence and 41 percent reported bloated feelings (Heijnen et al., 1998). Other gastrointestinal discomforts were reported by 14 percent of those consuming 32 g/d of RS_3, whereas only 5 percent of individuals consuming an equal amount of glucose reported such discomforts.

Summary

While occasional adverse gastrointestinal symptoms are observed when consuming some of the isolated or synthetic fibers, serious chronic adverse effects have not been observed. Furthermore, due to the bulky nature of fibers, excess consumption is likely to be self-limiting. Therefore, a UL was not set for these individual fibers.

RESEARCH RECOMMENDATIONS

The relationship of fiber to health is of great importance, particularly since novel fiber sources are appearing on the market, and these fiber sources may or may not produce the same physiological effects as fiber from traditional foods. Research that provides human data and does the following is assigned the highest priority:

- Evaluate the protective effect of fiber against colon cancer in subsets of the population by applying genotyping and phenotyping to those participating in fiber and colon cancer trials. There also needs to be increased validation of intermediate markers, such as polyp recurrence, and assessment of functional markers (e.g., fecal bulk) and its relationship to these endpoints.
- Conduct a dose–response study to determine the amount of fiber that needs to be ingested to promote optimum laxation so that this could form the basis for a recommendation for fiber intake and provide a basis for determining functional fibers.

- Attempt to relate changes in the colonic microflora due to fiber ingestion to functional endpoints (e.g., decreased irritable bowel syndrome, increased laxation).

- Conduct longer-term studies on low energy-dense food sources (high in dietary fiber) and satiety and weight control to see if a higher fiber diet will help with weight maintenance or promote adherence to reduced calorie diets for weight reduction.

- Examine the relation between *Dietary Fiber* intake, energy intake, and long-term body weight in existing prospective epidemiological studies in addition to intervention studies.

- Conduct long-term studies on the effects of both viscous and whole-grain cereal fibers on coronary heart disease and diabetes risk factors.

REFERENCES

AAP (American Academy of Pediatrics). 1981. Plant fiber intake in the pediatric diet. *Pediatrics* 67:572–575.

AAP. 1993. Carbohydrate and dietary fiber. In: Barness LA, ed. *Pediatric Nutrition Handbook*, 3rd ed. Elk Grove Village, IL: AAP. Pp. 100–106.

Abraham ZD, Mehta T. 1988. Three-week psyllium-husk supplementation: Effect on plasma cholesterol concentrations, fecal steroid excretion, and carbohydrate absorption in men. *Am J Clin Nutr* 47:67–74.

Achour L, Flourié B, Briet F, Pellier P, Marteau P, Rambaud J-C. 1994. Gastrointestinal effects and energy value of polydextrose in healthy nonobese men. *Am J Clin Nutr* 59:1362–1368.

AHA (American Heart Association). 1983. AHA committee report. Diet in the healthy child. Task Force Committee of the Nutrition Committee and the Cardiovascular Disease in the Young Council of the American Heart Association. *Circulation* 67:1411A–1414A.

Alberts DS, Einspahr J, Rees-McGee S, Ramanujam P, Buller MK, Clark L, Ritenbaugh C, Atwood J, Pethigal P, Earnest D, Villar H, Phelps J, Lipkin M, Wargovich M, Meyskens FL. 1990. Effects of dietary wheat-bran fiber on rectal epithelial cell proliferation in patients with resection for colorectal cancers. *J Natl Cancer Inst* 82:1280–1285.

Alberts DS, Einspahr J, Ritenbaugh C, Aickin M, Rees-McGee S, Atwood J, Emerson S, Mason-Liddil N, Bettinger L, Patel J, Bellapravalu S, Ramanujam PS, Phelps J, Clark L. 1997. The effect of wheat-bran fiber and calcium supplementation on rectal mucosal proliferation rates in patients with resected adenomatous colorectal polyps. *Cancer Epidemiol Biomarkers Prev* 6:161–169.

Alberts DS, Martínez ME, Roe DJ, Guillén-Rodríguez JM, Marshall JR, van Leeuwen JB, Reid ME, Ritenbaugh C, Vargas PA, Bhatacharyya AB, Earnest DL, Sampliner RE. 2000. Lack of effect of a high-fiber cereal supplement on the recurrence of colorectal adenomas. *N Engl J Med* 342:1156–1162.

Aldoori WH, Giovannucci EL, Rimm EB, Wing AL, Trichopoulos DV, Willett WC. 1994. A prospective study of diet and the risk of symptomatic diverticular disease in men. *Am J Clin Nutr* 60:757–764.

Aldoori WH, Giovannucci EL, Rimm EB, Ascherio A, Stampfer MJ, Colditz GA, Wing AL, Trichopoulos DV, Willett WC. 1995. Prospective study of physical activity and the risk of symptomatic diverticular disease in men. *Gut* 36:276–282.

Aldoori WH, Giovannucci EL, Stampfer MJ, Rimm EB, Wing AL, Willett WC. 1997. Prospective study of diet and the risk of duodenal ulcer in men. *Am J Epidemiol* 145:42–50.

Aldoori WH, Giovannucci EL, Rockett HRH, Sampson L, Rimm EB, Willett WC. 1998. A prospective study of dietary fiber types and symptomatic diverticular disease in men. *J Nutr* 128:714–719.

Alles MS, Hautvast JG, Nagengast FM, Hartemink R, Van Laere KM, Jansen JB. 1996. Fate of fructo-oligosaccharides in the human intestine. *Br J Nutr* 76:211–221.

AMA (American Medical Association) Council on Scientific Affairs. 1989. Dietary fiber and health. *J Am Med Assoc* 262:542–546.

Anderson JW, Gustafson NJ. 1988. Hypocholesterolemic effects of oat and bean products. *Am J Clin Nutr* 48:749–753.

Anderson JW, Tietyen-Clark J. 1986. Dietary fiber: Hyperlipidemia, hypertension, and coronary heart disease. *Am J Gastroenterol* 81:907–919.

Anderson JW, Story L, Sieling B, Chen W-JL. 1984a. Hypocholesterolemic effects of high-fibre diets rich in water-soluble plant fibres. *J Can Diet Assoc* 45:140–148.

Anderson JW, Story L, Sieling B, Chen W-JL, Petro MS, Story J. 1984b. Hypocholesterolemic effects of oat-bran or bean intake for hypercholesterolemic men. *Am J Clin Nutr* 40:1146–1155.

Anderson JW, Gustafson NJ, Bryant CA, Tietyen-Clark J. 1987. Dietary fiber and diabetes: A comprehensive review and practical application. *J Am Diet Assoc* 87:1189–1197.

Anderson JW, Zettwoch N, Feldman T, Tietyen-Clark J, Oeltgen P, Bishop CW. 1988. Cholesterol-lowering effects of psyllium hydrophilic mucilloid for hypercholesterolemic men. *Arch Intern Med* 148:292–296.

Anderson JW, Gilinsky NH, Deakins DA, Smith SF, O'Neal DS, Dillon DW, Oeltgen PR. 1991. Lipid responses of hypercholesterolemic men to oat-bran and wheat-bran intake. *Am J Clin Nutr* 54:678–683.

Anderson JW, Garrity TF, Wood CL, Whitis SE, Smith BM, Oeltgen PR. 1992a. Prospective, randomized, controlled comparison of the effects of low-fat and low-fat plus high-fiber diets on serum lipid concentrations. *Am J Clin Nutr* 56:887–894.

Anderson JW, Riddell-Mason S, Gustafson NJ, Smith SF, Mackey M. 1992b. Cholesterol-lowering effects of psyllium-enriched cereal as an adjunct to a prudent diet in the treatment of mild to moderate hypercholesterolemia. *Am J Clin Nutr* 56:93–98.

Anderson JW, Allgood LD, Turner J, Oeltgen PR, Daggy BP. 1999. Effects of psyllium on glucose and serum lipid responses in men with type 2 diabetes and hypercholesterolemia. *Am J Clin Nutr* 70:466–473.

Anderson JW, Allgood LD, Lawrence A, Altringer LA, Jerdack GR, Hengehold DA, Morel JG. 2000a. Cholesterol-lowering effects of psyllium intake adjunctive to diet therapy in men and women with hypercholesterolemia: Meta-analysis of 8 controlled trials. *Am J Clin Nutr* 71:472–479.

Anderson JW, Davidson MH, Blonde L, Brown WV, Howard JW, Ginsberg H, Allgood LD, Weingand KW. 2000b. Long-term cholesterol-lowering effects of psyllium as an adjunct to diet therapy in the treatment of hypercholesterolemia. *Am J Clin Nutr* 71:1433–1438.

Andersson S-O, Wolk A, Bergström R, Giovannucci E, Lindgren C, Baron J, Adami H-O. 1996. Energy, nutrient intake and prostate cancer risk: A population-based case-control study in Sweden. *Int J Cancer* 68:716–722.

Anti M, Pignataro G, Armuzzi A, Valenti A, Iascone E, Marmo R, Lamazza A, Pretaroli AR, Pace V, Leo P, Castelli A, Gasbarrini G. 1998. Water supplementation enhances the effect of high-fiber diet on stool frequency and laxative consumption in adult patients with functional constipation. *Hepatogastroenterology* 45:727–732.

Appleby PN, Thorogood M, Mann JI, Key TJ. 1998. Low body mass index in non-meat eaters: The possible roles of animal fat, dietary fibre and alcohol. *Int J Obes Relat Metab Disord* 22:454–460.

Aro A, Uusitupa M, Voutilainen E, Hersio K, Korhonen T, Siitonen O. 1981. Improved diabetic control and hypocholesterolaemic effect induced by long-term dietary supplementation with guar gum in type-2 (insulin-independent) diabetes. *Diabetologia* 21:29–33.

Aro A, Uusitupa M, Voutilainen E, Korhonen T. 1984. Effects of guar gum in male subjects with hypercholesterolemia. *Am J Clin Nutr* 39:911–916.

Ascherio A, Rimm EB, Giovannucci EL, Colditz GA, Rosner B, Willett WC, Sacks F, Stampfer MJ. 1992. A prospective study of nutritional factors and hypertension among US men. *Circulation* 86:1475–1484.

Ashraf W, Park F, Lof J, Quigley EM. 1995. Effects of psyllium therapy on stool characteristics, colon transit and anorectal function in chronic idiopathic constipation. *Aliment Pharmacol Ther* 9:639–647.

Astrup A, Vrist E, Quaade F. 1990. Dietary fibre added to very low calorie diet reduces hunger and alleviates constipation. *Int J Obes* 14:105–112.

Bagga D, Ashley JM, Geffrey SP, Wang HJ, Barnard RJ, Korenman S, Heber D. 1995. Effects of a very low fat, high fiber diet on serum hormones and menstrual function. Implications for breast cancer prevention. *Cancer* 76:2491–2496.

Baghurst PA, Rohan TE. 1994. High-fiber diets and reduced risk of breast cancer. *Int J Cancer* 56:173–176.

Barbone F, Austin H, Partridge EE. 1993. Diet and endometrial cancer: A case-control study. *Am J Epidemiol* 137:393–403.

Baron JA, Schori A, Crow B, Carter R, Mann JI. 1986. A randomized controlled trial of low carbohydrate and low fat/high fiber diets for weight loss. *Am J Public Health* 76:1293–1296.

Bartram P, Gerlach S, Scheppach W, Keller F, Kasper H. 1992. Effect of a single oat bran cereal breakfast on serum cholesterol, lipoproteins, and apolipoproteins in patients with hyperlipoproteinemia type IIa. *J Parenter Enteral Nutr* 16:533–537.

Beer MU, Arrigoni E, Amado R. 1995. Effects of oat gum on blood cholesterol levels in healthy young men. *Eur J Clin Nutr* 49:517–522.

Behall KM. 1990. Effect of soluble fibers on plasma lipids, glucose tolerance and mineral balance. *Adv Exp Med Biol* 270:7–16.

Behall KM, Howe JC. 1996. Resistant starch as energy. *J Am Coll Nutr* 15:248–254.

Behall KM, Scholfield DJ, Lee K, Powell AS, Moser PB. 1987. Mineral balance in adult men: Effect of four refined fibers. *Am J Clin Nutr* 46:307–314.

Bell LP, Hectorn KJ, Reynolds H, Hunninghake DB. 1990. Cholesterol-lowering effects of soluble-fiber cereals as part of a prudent diet for patients with mild to moderate hypercholesterolemia. *Am J Clin Nutr* 52:1020–1026.

Benini L, Castellani G, Brighenti F, Heaton KW, Brentegani MT, Casiraghi MC, Sembenini C, Pellegrini N, Fioretta A, Minniti G. 1995. Gastric emptying of a solid meal is accelerated by the removal of dietary fibre naturally present in food. *Gut* 36:825–830.

Bergmann JF, Chassany O, Petit A, Triki R, Caulin C, Segrestaa JM. 1992. Correlation between echographic gastric emptying and appetite: Influence of psyllium. *Gut* 33:1042–1043.

Berman JI, Schultz MJ. 1980. Bulk laxative ileus. *J Am Geriatr Soc* 28:224–226.

Berta JL, Coste T, Rautureau J, Guilloud-Bataille M, Pequignot G. 1985. Diet and rectocolonic cancers. Results of a case-control study. *Gastroenterol Clin Biol* 9:348–353.

Bidoli E, Franceschi S, Talamini R, Barra S, La Vecchia C. 1992. Food consumption and cancer of the colon and rectum in north-eastern Italy. *Int J Cancer* 50:223–229.

Birkett AM, Jones GP, de Silva AM, Young GP, Muir JG. 1997. Dietary intake and faecal excretion of carbohydrate by Australians: Importance of achieving stool weights greater than 150 g to improve faecal markers relevant to colon cancer risk. *Eur J Clin Nutr* 51:625–632.

Birketvedt GS, Aaseth J, Florholmen JR, Ryttig K. 2000. Long term effect of fibre supplement and reduced energy intake on body weight and blood lipids in overweight subjects. *Acta Medica (Hradec Králové)* 43:129–132.

Blackburn NA, Holgate AM, Read NW. 1984. Does guar gum improve post-prandial hyperglycaemia in humans by reducing small intestinal contact area? *Br J Nutr* 52:197–204.

Blake DE, Hamblett CJ, Frost PG, Judd PA, Ellis PR. 1997. Wheat bread supplemented with depolymerized guar gum reduces the plasma cholesterol concentration in hypercholesterolemic human subjects. *Am J Clin Nutr* 65:107–113.

Blundell JE, Burley VJ. 1987. Satiation, satiety and the action of fibre on food intake. *Int J Obesity* 11:9–25.

Bolin TD, Stanton RA. 1998. Flatus emission patterns and fibre intake. *Eur J Surg* 582:115–118.

Bolton-Smith C, Woodward M, Tunstall-Pedoe H. 1992. The Scottish Heart Health Study. Dietary intake by food frequency questionnaire and odds ratios for coronary heart disease risk. II. The antioxidant vitamins and fibre. *Eur J Clin Nutr* 46:85–93.

Bonithon-Kopp C, Kronborg O, Giacosa A, Räth U, Faivre J. 2000. Calcium and fibre supplementation in prevention of colorectal adenoma recurrance: A randomised intervention trial. *Lancet* 356:1300–1306.

Bosaeus I, Carlsson NG, Sandberg AS, Andersson H. 1986. Effect of wheat bran and pectin on bile acid and cholesterol excretion in ileostomy patients. *Hum Nutr Clin Nutr* 40:429–440.

Bosello O, Cominacini L, Zocca I, Garbin U, Ferrari F, Davoli A. 1984. Effects of guar gum on plasma lipoproteins and apolipoproteins C-II and C-III in patients affected with familial combined hyperlipoproteinemia. *Am J Clin Nutr* 40:1165–1174.

Bouhnik Y, Flourié B, Riottot M, Bisetti N, Gailing M-F, Guibert A, Bornet F, Rambaud J-C. 1996. Effects of fructo-oligosaccharides ingestion on fecal bifidobacteria and selected metabolic indexes of colon carcinogenesis in healthy humans. *Nutr Cancer* 26:21–29.

Bouhnik Y, Vahedi K, Achour L, Attar A, Salfati J, Pochart P, Marteau P, Flourié B, Bornet F, Rambaud J-C. 1999. Short-chain fructo-oligosaccharide administration dose-dependently increases fecal bifidobacteria in healthy humans. *J Nutr* 129:113–116.

Boyle P, Zaridze DG, Smans M. 1985. Descriptive epidemiology of colorectal cancer. *Int J Cancer* 36:9–18.

Braaten JT, Wood PJ, Scott FW, Riedel KD, Poste LM, Collins MW. 1991. Oat gum lowers glucose and insulin after an oral glucose load. *Am J Clin Nutr* 53:1425–1430.

Braaten JT, Scott FW, Wood PJ, Riedel KD, Wolynetz MS, Brulé D, Collins MW. 1994a. High β-glucan oat bran and oat gum reduce postprandial blood glucose and insulin in subjects with and without type 2 diabetes. *Diabetic Med* 11:312–318.

Braaten JT, Wood PJ, Scott FW, Wolynetz MS, Lowe MK, Bradley-White P, Collins MW. 1994b. Oat beta-glucan reduces blood cholesterol concentration in hypercholesterolemic subjects. *Eur J Clin Nutr* 48:465–474.

Briet F, Achour L, Flourié B, Beaugerie L, Pellier P, Franchisseur C, Bornet F, Rambaud JC. 1995. Symptomatic response to varying levels of fructo-oligosaccharides consumed occasionally or regularly. *Eur J Clin Nutr* 49:501–507.

Brighenti F, Casiraghi MC, Canzi E, Ferrari A. 1999. Effect of consumption of a ready-to-eat breakfast cereal containing inulin on the intestinal milieu and blood lipids in healthy male volunteers. *Eur J Clin Nutr* 53:726–733.

Brodribb AJM. 1977. Treatment of symptomatic diverticular disease with a high-fibre diet. *Lancet* 1:664–666.

Brown IL, McNaught KJ, Moloney E. 1995. Hi-maize: New directions in starch technology and nutrition. *Food Aust* 47:273–279.

Brown L, Rosner B, Willett W, Sacks FM. 1999. Cholesterol-lowering effects of dietary fiber: A meta-analysis. *Am J Clin Nutr* 69:30–42.

Brune M, Rossander-Hulten L, Hallberg L, Gleerup A, Sandberg AS. 1992. Iron absorption from bread in humans: Inhibiting effects of cereal fiber, phytate and inositol phosphates with different numbers of phosphate groups. *J Nutr* 122:442–449.

Buddington RK, Williams CH, Chen S-C, Witherly SA. 1996. Dietary supplementation of neosugar alters the fecal flora and decreases activities of some reductive enzymes in human subjects. *Am J Clin Nutr* 63:709–716.

Burdock GA, Flamm WG. 1999. A review of the studies of the safety of polydextrose in food. *Food Chem Toxicol* 37:233–264.

Burkitt DP, Walker ARP, Painter NS. 1972. Effect of dietary fibre on stools and transit-times, and its role in the causation of disease. *Lancet* 2:1408–1412.

Burley VJ, Paul AW, Blundell JE. 1993. Sustained post-ingestive action of dietary fibre: Effects of a sugar-beet-fibre-supplemented breakfast on satiety. *J Hum Nutr Diet* 6:43–50.

Burr ML, Sweetnam PM. 1982. Vegetarianism, dietary fiber, and mortality. *Am J Clin Nutr* 36:873–877.

Burr ML, Fehily AM, Gilbert JF, Rogers S, Holliday RM, Sweetnam PM, Elwood PC, Deadman NM. 1989. Effects of changes in fat, fish, and fibre intakes on death and myocardial reinfarction: Diet and Reinfarction Trial (DART). *Lancet* 2:757–761.

Burton R, Manninen V. 1982. Influence of psyllium-based fibre preparation on faecal and serum parameters. *Acta Med Scand Suppl* 668:91–94.

Busse WW, Schoenwetter WF. 1975. Asthma from psyllium in laxative manufacture. *Ann Intern Med* 83:361–362.

Cameron KJ, Nyulasi IB, Collier GR, Brown DJ. 1996. Assessment of the effect of increased dietary fibre intake on bowel function in patients with spinal cord injury. *Spinal Cord* 34:277–283.

Caygill CPJ, Charlett A, Hill MJ. 1998. Relationship between the intake of high-fibre foods and energy and the risk of cancer of the large bowel and breast. *Eur J Cancer Prev* 7:S11–S17.

Cerda JJ, Robbins FL, Burgin CW, Baumgartner TG, Rice RW. 1988. The effects of grapefruit pectin on patients at risk for coronary heart disease without altering diet or lifestyle. *Clin Cardiol* 11:589–594.

Chandalia M, Garg A, Lutjohann D, von Bergmann K, Grundy SM, Brinkley LJ. 2000. Beneficial effects of high dietary fiber intake in patients with type 2 diabetes mellitus. *N Engl J Med* 342:1392–1398.

Chandra R, Barron JL. 2002. Anaphylactic reaction to intravenous sinistrin (Inutest). *Ann Clin Biochem* 39:76.

Chen H-L, Haack VS, Janecky CW, Vollendorf NW, Marlett JA. 1998. Mechanisms by which wheat bran and oat bran increase stool weight in humans. *Am J Clin Nutr* 68:711–719.

Chen WJL, Anderson JW. 1986. Hypocholesterolemic effects of soluble fibers. In: Vahouny GV, Kritchevsky D, eds. *Dietary Fiber: Basic and Clinical Aspects.* New York: Plenum Press. Pp. 275–286.

Chiang MT, Yao HT, Chen HC. 2000. Effect of dietary chitosans with different viscosity on plasma lipids and lipid peroxidation in rats fed on a diet enriched with cholesterol. *Biosci Biotechnol Biochem* 64:965–971.

Clausen MR, Jorgensen J, Mortensen PB. 1998. Comparison of diarrhea induced by ingestion of fructooligosaccharide Idolax and disaccharide lactulose (role of osmolarity versus fermentation of malabsorbed carbohydrate). *Dig Dis Sci* 43:2696–2707.

Clevenger MA, Turnbill D, Inoue H, Enomoto M, Allen JA, Henderson LM, Jones E. 1988. Toxicological evaluation of neosugar: Genotoxicity, carcinogenicity, and chronic toxicity. *J Am Coll Toxicol* 7:643–662.

Colditz GA, Manson JE, Stampfer MJ, Rosner B, Willett WC, Speizer FE. 1992. Diet and risk of clinical diabetes in women. *Am J Clin Nutr* 55:1018–1023.

Coudray C, Bellanger J, Castiglia-Delavaud C, Remesy C, Vermorel M, Rayssignuier Y. 1997. Effect of soluble or partly soluble dietary fibres supplementation on absorption and balance of calcium, magnesium, iron and zinc in healthy young men. *Eur J Clin Nutr* 51:375–380.

Cummings JH. 1984. Microbial digestion of complex carbohydrates in man. *Proc Nutr Soc* 43:35–44.

Cummings JH. 1993. The effect of dietary fiber on fecal weight and composition. In: Spiller GA, ed. *CRC Handbook of Dietary Fiber in Human Nutrition,* 2nd ed. Boca Raton, FL: CRC Press. Pp. 263–349.

Cummings JH. 2000. Nutritional management of diseases of the gut. In: Garrow JS, James WPT, Ralph A, eds. *Human Nutrition and Dietetics,* 10th ed. Edinburgh: Churchill Livingston. Pp. 547–573.

Cummings JH, Branch WJ. 1986. Fermentation and the production of short-chain fatty acids in the human large intestine. In: Vahouny GV, Kritchevsky D, eds. *Dietary Fiber: Basic and Clinical Aspects.* New York: Plenum Press. Pp. 131–149.

Cummings JH, Englyst HN. 1987. Fermentation in the human large intestine and the available substrates. *Am J Clin Nutr* 45:1243–1255.

Cummings JH, Southgate DAT, Branch W, Houston H, Jenkins DJA, James WPT. 1978. Colonic responses to dietary fibre from carrot, cabbage, apple, bran, and guar gum. *Lancet* 1:5–9.

Cummings JH, Bingham SA, Heaton KW, Eastwood MA. 1992. Fecal weight, colon cancer risk, and dietary intake of nonstarch polysaccharides (dietary fiber). *Gastroenterology* 103:1783–1789.

Cummings JH, Beatty ER, Kingman SM, Bingham SA, Englyst HN. 1996. Digestion and physiological properties of resistant starch in the human large bowel. *Br J Nutr* 75:733–747.

Dales LG, Friedman GD, Ury HK, Grossman S, Williams SR. 1979. A case-control study of relationships of diet and other traits to colorectal cancer in American blacks. *Am J Epidemiol* 109:132–144.

Danielsson A, Ek B, Nyhlin H, Steen L. 1979. Effect of long term treatment with hydrophilic colloid on serum lipids. *Acta Hepatogastroenterol (Stuttg)* 26:148–153.

Davidson MH, Maki KC. 1999. Effects of dietary inulin on serum lipids. *J Nutr* 129:1474S–1477S.

Davidson MH, Dugan LD, Burns JH, Bova J, Story K, Drennan KB. 1991. The hypocholesterolemic effects of β-glucan in oatmeal and oat bran. A dose-controlled study. *J Am Med Assoc* 265:1833–1839.

Davidson MH, Maki KC, Kong JC, Dugan LD, Torri SA, Hall HA, Drennan KB, Anderson SM, Fulgoni VL, Saldanha LG, Olson BH. 1998. Long-term effects of consuming foods containing psyllium seed husk on serum lipids in subjects with hypercholesterolemia. *Am J Clin Nutr* 67:367–376.

de Deckere EA, Kloots WJ, van Amelsvoort JM. 1993. Resistant starch decreases serum total cholesterol and triacylglycerol concentrations in rats. *J Nutr* 123:2142–2151.

Delargy HJ, Burley VJ, O'Sullivan KR, Fletcher RJ, Blundell JE. 1995. Effects of different soluble:insoluble fibre ratios at breakfast on 24-h pattern of dietary intake and satiety. *Eur J Clin Nutr* 49:754–766.

de Roos N, Heijnen M-L, de Graaf C, Woestenenk G, Hobbel E. 1995. Resistant starch has little effect on appetite, food intake and insulin secretion of healthy young men. *Eur J Clin Nutr* 49:532–541.

De Stefani E, Correa P, Ronco A, Mendilaharsu M, Guidobono M, Deneo-Pellegrini H. 1997. Dietary fiber and risk of breast cancer: A case-control study in Uruguay. *Nutr Cancer* 28:14–19.

Dettmar PW, Sykes J. 1998. A multi-centre, general practice comparison of ispaghula husk with lactulose and other laxatives in the treatment of simple constipation. *Curr Med Res Opin* 14:227–233.

Djoussé L, Ellison RC, Zhang Y, Arnett DK, Sholinsky P, Borecki I. 1998. Relation between dietary fiber consumption and fibrinogen and plasminogen activator inhibitor type 1: The National Heart, Lung, and Blood Institute Family Heart Study. *Am J Clin Nutr* 68:568–575.

Drake CL, Moses ES, Tandberg D. 1991. Systemic anaphylaxis after ingestion of a psyllium-containing breakfast cereal. *Am J Emerg Med* 9:449–451.

Duncan KH, Bacon JA, Weinsier RL. 1983. The effects of high and low energy density diets on satiety, energy intake, and eating time of obese and nonobese subjects. *Am J Clin Nutr* 37:763–767.

Durrington PN, Manning AP, Bolton CH, Hartog M. 1976. Effect of pectin on serum lipids and lipoproteins, whole-gut transit-time, and stool weight. *Lancet* 2:394–396.

Dutta SK, Hlasko J. 1985. Dietary fiber in pancreatic disease: Effect of high fiber diet on fat malabsorption in pancreatic insufficiency and in vitro study of the interaction of dietary fiber with pancreatic enzymes. *Am J Clin Nutr* 41:517–525.

Dwyer J. 1980. Diets for children and adolescents that meet the dietary goals. *Am J Dis Child* 134:1073–1080.

Eliasson K, Ryttig KR, Hylander B, Rossner S. 1992. A dietary fibre supplement in the treatment of mild hypertension. A randomized, double-blind, placebo-controlled trial. *J Hypertens* 10:195–199.

Ellis PR, Kamalanathan T, Dawoud FM, Strange RN, Coultate TP. 1988. Evaluation of guar biscuits for use in the management of diabetes: Tests of physiological effects and palatability in non-diabetic volunteers. *Eur J Clin Nutr* 42:425–435.

Englyst HN, Cummings JH. 1986. Digestion of the carbohydrates of banana (*Musa paradisiaca sapientum*) in the human small intestine. *Am J Clin Nutr* 44:42–50.

Englyst HN, Cummings JH. 1987. Digestion of polysaccharides of potato in the small intestine of man. *Am J Clin Nutr* 45:423–431.

Englyst HN, Kingman SM, Cummings JH. 1992. Classification and measurement of nutritionally important starch fractions. *Eur J Clin Nutr* 46:S33–S50.

Everson GT, Daggy BP, McKinley C, Story JA. 1992. Effects of psyllium hydrophilic muccilloid on LDL-cholesterol and bile acid synthesis in hypercholesterolemic men. *J Lipid Res* 33:1183–1192.

FDA (U.S. Food and Drug Administration). 1987. Nutrition labeling of food; calorie content. *Fed Regis* 52:28590–28691.

Feskens EJM, Loeber JG, Kromhout D. 1994. Diet and physical activity as determinants of hyperinsulinemia: The Zutphen Elderly Study. *Am J Epidemiol* 140:350–360.

Findlay JM, Smith AN, Mitchell WD, Anderson AJB, Eastwood MA. 1974. Effects of unprocessed bran on colon function in normal subjects and in diverticular disease. *Lancet* 1:146–149.

Franceschi S, Favero A, Decarli A, Negri E, La Vecchia C, Ferraroni M, Russo A, Salvini S, Amadori D, Conti E, Montella M, Giacosa A. 1996. Intake of macronutrients and risk of breast cancer. *Lancet* 347:1351–1356.

Fraser GE, Sabaté J, Beeson WL, Strahan TM. 1992. A possible protective effect of nut consumption on risk of coronary heart disease. The Adventist Health Study. *Arch Intern Med* 152:1416–1424.

Frati-Munari AC, Benitez-Pinto W, Raul Ariza-Andraca C, Casarrubias M. 1998. Lowering glycemic index of food by acarbose and Plantago psyllium mucilage. *Arch Med Res* 29:137–141.

Freudenheim JL, Graham S, Horvath PJ, Marshall JR, Haughey BP, Wilkinson G. 1990. Risks associated with source of fiber and fiber components in cancer of the colon and rectum. *Cancer Res* 50:3295–3300.

Freudenheim JL, Marshall JR, Vena JE, Laughlin R, Brasure JR, Swanson MK, Nemoto T, Graham S. 1996. Premenopausal breast cancer risk and intake of vegetables, fruits, and related nutrients. *J Natl Cancer Inst* 88:340–348.

Fuchs CS, Giovannucci EL, Colditz GA, Hunter DJ, Stampfer MJ, Rosner B, Speizer FE, Willett WC. 1999. Dietary fiber and the risk of colorectal cancer and adenoma in women. *N Engl J Med* 340:169–176.

Fuessl HS, Williams G, Adrian TE, Bloom SR. 1987. Guar sprinkled on food: Effect on glycaemic control, plasma lipids and gut hormones in non-insulin dependent diabetic patients. *Diabetic Med* 4:463–468.

Gabbe SG, Cohen AW, Herman GO, Schwartz S. 1982. Effect of dietary fiber on the oral glucose tolerance test in pregnancy. *Am J Obstet Gynecol* 143:514–517.

Gallaher CM, Munion J, Hesslink R, Wise J, Gallaher DD. 2000. Cholesterol reduction by glucomannan and chitosan is mediated by changes in cholesterol absorption and bile acid and fat excretion in rats. *J Nutr* 130:2753–2759.

Gay-Crosier F, Schreiber G, Hauser C. 2000. Anaphylaxis from inulin in vegetables and processed food. *N Engl J Med* 342:1372.

Gear JSS, Ware A, Fursdon P, Mann JI, Nolan DJ, Brodribb AJM, Vessey MP. 1979. Symptomless diverticular disease and intake of dietary fibre. *Lancet* 1:511–514.

Gerber M. 1998. Fibre and breast cancer. *Eur J Cancer Prev* 7:S63–S67.

Gerhardsson de Verdier M, Hagman U, Steineck G, Rieger Å, Norell SE. 1990. Diet, body mass and colorectal cancer: A case-referent study in Stockholm. *Int J Cancer* 46:832–838.

Gibson GR, Beatty ER, Wang X, Cummings JH. 1995. Selective stimulation of bifidobacteria in the human colon by oligofructose and inulin. *Gastroenterology* 108:975–982.

Giovannucci E, Willett WC. 1994. Dietary factors and risk of colon cancer. *Ann Med* 26:443–452.

Giovannucci E, Stampfer MJ, Colditz G, Rimm EB, Willett WC. 1992. Relationship of diet to risk of colorectal adenoma in men. *J Natl Cancer Inst* 84:91–98.

Giovannucci E, Rimm EB, Stampfer MJ, Colditz GA, Ascherio A, Willett WC. 1994. Intake of fat, meat, and fiber in relation to risk of colon cancer in men. *Cancer Res* 54:2390–2397.

Golay A, Koellreutter B, Bloise D, Assal JP, Wursch P. 1992. The effect of muesli or cornflakes at breakfast on carbohydrate metabolism in type 2 diabetic patients. *Diabetes Res Clin Pract* 15:135–141.

Gold LA, McCourt JP, Merimee TJ. 1980. Pectin: An examination in normal subjects. *Diabetes Care* 3:50–52.

Goldin BR, Adlercreutz H, Gorbach SL, Warram JH, Dwyer JT, Swenson L, Woods MN. 1982. Estrogen excretion patterns and plasma levels in vegetarian and omnivorous women. *N Engl J Med* 307:1542–1547.

Goodman MT, Wilkens LR, Hankin JH, Lyu L-C, Wu AH, Kolonel LN. 1997. Association of soy and fiber consumption with the risk of endometrial cancer. *Am J Epidemiol* 146:294–306.

Gorbach SL, Goldin BR. 1987. Diet and the excretion and enterohepatic cycling of estrogens. *Prev Med* 16:525–529.

Goulder TJ, Alberti KGMM, Jenkins DA. 1978. Effect of added fiber on the glucose and metabolic response to a mixed meal in normal and diabetic subjects. *Diabetes Care* 1:351–355.

Graham S, Hellmann R, Marshall J, Freudenheim J, Vena J, Swanson M, Zielezny M, Nemoto T, Stubbe N, Raimondo T. 1991. Nutritional epidemiology of postmenopausal breast cancer in western New York. *Am J Epidemiol* 134:552–566.

Graham S, Zielezny M, Marshall J, Priore R, Freudenheim J, Brasure J, Haughey B, Nasca P, Zdeb M. 1992. Diet in the epidemiology of postmenopausal breast cancer in the New York State Cohort. *Am J Epidemiol* 136:1327–1337.

Grizard D, Barthomeuf C. 1999. Non-digestible oligosaccharides used as prebiotic agents: Mode of production and beneficial effects on animal and human health. *Reprod Nutr Dev* 39:563–588.

Groop P-H, Aro A, Stenman S, Groop L. 1993. Long-term effects of guar gum in subjects with non-insulin-dependent diabetes mellitus. *Am J Clin Nutr* 58:513–518.

Grossman SP. 1986. The role of glucose, insulin and glucagon in the regulation of food intake and body weight. *Neurosci Biobehav Rev* 10:295–315.

Guerciolini R, Radu-Radulescu L, Boldrin M, Dallas J, Moore R. 2001. Comparative evaluation of fecal fat excretion induced by orlistat and chitosan. *Obes Res* 9:364–367.

Haenszel W, Kurihara M. 1968. Studies of Japanese migrants. I. Mortality from cancer and other diseases among Japanese in the United States. *J Natl Cancer Inst* 40:43–68.

Hallfrisch J, Powell A, Carafelli C, Reiser S, Prather ES. 1987. Mineral balances of men and women consuming high fiber diets with complex or simple carbohydrate. *J Nutr* 117:48–55.

Hallfrisch J, Tobin JD, Muller DC, Andres R. 1988. Fiber intake, age, and other coronary risk factors in men of the Baltimore Longitudinal Study (1959–1975). *J Gerontol Med Sci* 43:M64–M68.

Hallfrisch J, Scholfield DJ, Behall KM. 1995. Diets containing soluble oat extracts improve glucose and insulin responses of moderately hypercholesterolemic men and women. *Am J Clin Nutr* 61:379–384.

Harris PJ, Ferguson LR. 1993. Dietary fibre: Its composition and role in protection against colorectal cancer. *Mutat Res* 290:97–110.

Harris PJ, Triggs CM, Roberton AM, Watson ME, Ferguson LR. 1996. The adsorption of heterocyclic aromatic amines by model dietary fibres with contrasting compositions. *Chem Biol Interact* 100:13–25.

Haseman JK, Arnold J, Eustis SL. 1990. Tumor incidences in Fischer 344 rats: NTP historical data. In: GA Boorman, ed. *Pathology of the Fischer Rat*. San Diego, CA: Academic Press. Pp. 557–564.

Health and Welfare Canada. 1985. *Report of the Expert Advisory Committee on Dietary Fibre*. Ottawa: Supply and Services Canada.

Health Canada. 1988. *Guideline Concerning the Safety and Physiological Effects of Novel Fibre Sources and Food Products Containing Them*. Ottawa: Food Directorate, Health Protection Branch, Health Canada.

Health Canada. 1997. Appendix 2. Guideline for planning and statistical review of clinical laxation studies for dietary fibre. In: *Guideline Concerning the Safety and Physiological Effects of Novel Fibre Sources and Food Products Containing Them*. Ottawa: Food Directorate, Health Protection Branch, Health Canada.

Heaton KW. 1973. Food fibre as an obstacle to energy intake. *Lancet* 2:1418–1421.

Heijnen M-LA, van Amelsvoort JMM, Deurenberg P, Beynen AC. 1996. Neither raw nor retrograded resistant starch lowers fasting serum cholesterol concentrations in healthy normolipidemic subjects. *Am J Clin Nutr* 64:312–318.

Heijnen M-LA, van Amelsvoort JMM, Deurenberg P, Beynen AC. 1998. Limited effect of consumption of uncooked (RS_2) or retrograded (RS_3) resistant starch on putative risk factors for colon cancer in healthy men. *Am J Clin Nutr* 67:322–331.

Heilbrun LK, Nomura A, Hankin JH, Stemmermann GN. 1989. Diet and colorectal cancer with special reference to fiber intake. *Int J Cancer* 44:1–6.

Henquin JC. 1988. *Reproduction Toxicity: Study on the Influence of Fructooligosaccharides on the Development of Foetal and Postnatal Rat*. Raffinerie Tirlemontoise Internal Report. Photocopy.

Hill MJ. 1997. Cereals, cereal fibre and colorectal cancer risk: A review of the epidemiological literature. *Eur J Cancer Prev* 6:219–225.

Hillman LC, Peters SG, Fisher CA, Pomare EW. 1983. Differing effects of pectin, cellulose and lignin on stool pH, transit time and weight. *Br J Nutr* 50:189–195.

Hillman LC, Peters SG, Fisher CA, Pomare EW. 1985. The effects of the fiber components pectin, cellulose and lignin on serum cholesterol levels. *Am J Clin Nutr* 42:207–213.

Ho SC, Tai ES, Eng PHK, Tan CE, Fok ACK. 2001. In the absence of dietary surveillance, chitosan does not reduce plasma lipids or obesity in hyper-cholesterolaemic obese Asian subjects. *Singapore Med J* 42:6–10.

Hoff G, Moen IE, Trygg K, Frølich W, Sauar J, Vatn M, Gjone E, Larsen S. 1986. Epidemiology of polyps in the rectum and sigmoid colon. Evaluation of nutritional factors. *Scand J Gastroenterol* 21:199–204.

Holman RR, Steemson J, Darling P, Turner RC. 1987. No glycemic benefit from guar administration in NIDDM. *Diabetes Care* 10:68–71.

Holt S, Brand J, Soveny C, Hansky J. 1992. Relationship of satiety to postprandial glycaemic, insulin and cholecystokinin responses. *Appetite* 18:129–141.

Howe GR, Benito E, Castelleto R, Cornée J, Estéve J, Gallagher RP, Iscovich JM, Deng-ao J, Kaaks R, Kune GA, Kune S, L'Abbé KA, Lee HP, Lee M, Miller AB, Peters RK, Potter JD, Riboli E, Slattery ML, Trichopoulos D, Tuyns A, Tzonou A, Whittemore AS, Wu-Williams AH, Shu Z. 1992. Dietary intake of fiber and decreased risk of cancers of the colon and rectum: Evidence from the combined analysis of 13 case-control studies. *J Natl Cancer Inst* 84:1887–1896.

Humble CG, Malarcher AM, Tyroler HA. 1993. Dietary fiber and coronary heart disease in middle-aged hypercholesterolemic men. *Am J Prev Med* 9:197–202.

Hunt R, Fedorak R, Frohlich J, McLennan C, Pavilanis A. 1993. Therapeutic role of dietary fibre. *Can Fam Physician* 39:897–910.

Hylla S, Gostner A, Dusel G, Anger H, Bartram H-P, Christl SU, Kasper H, Scheppach W. 1998. Effects of resistant starch on the colon in healthy volunteers: Possible implications for cancer prevention. *Am J Clin Nutr* 67:136–142.

Ingram DM. 1981. Trends in diet and breast cancer mortality in England and Wales 1928–1977. *Nutr Cancer* 3:75–80.

IOM (Institute of Medicine). 1991. *Nutrition During Lactation.* Washington, DC: National Academy Press.

IOM. 2001. *Dietary Reference Intakes: Proposed Definition of Dietary Fiber.* Washington, DC: National Academy Press.

Iscovich JM, L'Abbé KA, Castelleto R, Calzona A, Bernedo A, Chopita NA, Jmelnitzsky AC, Kaldor J, Howe GR. 1992. Colon cancer in Argentina. II: Risk from fibre, fat and nutrients. *Int J Cancer* 51:858–861.

Ito N, Hasegawa R, Sano M, Tamano S, Esumi H, Takayama S, Sugimura T. 1991. A new colon and mammary carcinogen in cooked food, 2-amino-1-methyl-6-phenylimidazo[4,5-b]pyridine (PhIP). *Carcinogenesis* 12:1503–1506.

Jackson KG, Taylor GRJ, Clohessy AM, Williams CM. 1999. The effect of the daily intake of inulin fasting lipid, insulin and glucose concentrations in middle-aged men and women. *Br J Nutr* 82:23–30.

Jacobs DR, Meyer KA, Kushi LH, Folsom AR. 1998. Whole-grain intake may reduce the risk of ischemic heart disease death in postmenopausal women: The Iowa Women's Health Study. *Am J Clin Nutr* 68:248–257.

Jacobs LR. 1986. Relationship between dietary fiber and cancer: Metabolic, physiologic, and cellular mechanisms. *Proc Soc Exp Biol Med* 183:299–310.

Jain M, Cook GM, Davis FG, Grace MG, Howe GR, Miller AB. 1980. A case-control study of diet and colo-rectal cancer. *Int J Cancer* 26:757–768.

James JM, Cooke SK, Barnett A, Sampson HA. 1991. Anaphylactic reactions to a psyllium-containing cereal. *J Allergy Clin Immunol* 88:402–408.

Jenkins DJA, Newton C, Leeds AR, Cummings JH. 1975. Effect of pectin, guar gum, and wheat fibre on serum cholesterol. *Lancet* 1:1116–1117.

Jenkins DJA, Wolever TMS, Leeds AR, Gassull MA, Haisman P, Dilawari J, Goff DV, Metz GL, Alberti KGMM. 1978. Dietary fibres, fibre analogues, and glucose tolerance: Importance of viscosity. *Br Med J* 1:1392–1394.

Jenkins DJA, Wolever TMS, Collier GR, Ocana A, Rao AV, Buckley G, Lam Y, Mayer A, Thompson LU. 1987. Metabolic effects of a low-glycemic-index diet. *Am J Clin Nutr* 46:968–975.

Jenkins DJA, Vuksan V, Kendall CWC, Würsch P, Jeffcoat R, Waring S, Mehling CC, Vidgen E, Augustin LSA, Wong E. 1998. Physiological effects of resistant starches on fecal bulk, short chain fatty acids, blood lipids and glycemic index. *J Am Coll Nutr* 17:609–616.

Jenkins DJA, Kendall CWC, Vuksan V, Vidgen E, Parler T, Faulkner D, Mehling CC, Garsetti M, Testolin G, Cunnane SC, Ryan MA, Corey PN. 2002. Soluble fiber intake at a dose approved by the US Food and Drug Administration for a health claim of health benefits: Serum lipid risk factors for cardiovascular disease assessed in a randomized controlled crossover trial. *Am J Clin Nutr* 75:834–839.

Jennings CD, Boleyn K, Bridges SR, Wood PJ, Anderson JW. 1988. A comparison of the lipid-lowering and intestinal morphological effects of cholestyramine, chitosan, and oat gum in rats. *Proc Soc Exp Biol Med* 189:13–20.

Jie Z, Bang-Yao L, Ming-Jie X, Hai-Wei L, Zu-Kang Z, Ting-Song W, Craig SAS. 2000. Studies on the effects of polydextrose intake on physiologic function in Chinese people. *Am J Clin Nutr* 72:1503–1509.

Judd PA, Truswell AS. 1981. The effect of rolled oats on blood lipids and fecal steroid excretion in man. *Am J Clin Nutr* 34:2061–2067.

Kang JY, Doe WF. 1979. Unprocessed bran causing intestinal obstruction. *Br Med J* 1:1249–1250.

Kato I, Akhmedkhanov A, Koenig K, Toniolo PG, Shore RE, Riboli E. 1997. Prospective study of diet and female colorectal cancer: The New York University Women's Health Study. *Nutr Cancer* 28:276–281.

Kay RM, Truswell AS. 1977. Effect of citrus pectin on blood lipids and fecal steroid excretion in man. *Am J Clin Nutr* 30:171–175.

Kelsay JL, Behall KM, Prather ES. 1978. Effect of fiber from fruits and vegetables on metabolic responses of human subjects. I. Bowel transit time, number of defecations, fecal weight, urinary excretions of energy and nitrogen and apparent digestibilities of energy, nitrogen, and fat. *Am J Clin Nutr* 31:1149–1153.

Key TJA, Thorogood M, Appleby PN, Burr ML. 1996. Dietary habits and mortality in 11,000 vegetarians and health conscious people: Results of a 17 year follow up. *Br Med J* 313:775–779.

Khaw K, Barrett-Connor E. 1987. Dietary fiber and reduced ischemic heart disease mortality rates in men and women: A 12-year prospective study. *Am J Epidemiol* 126:1093–1102.

Kirby RW, Anderson JW, Sieling B, Rees ED, Chen W-JL, Miller RE, Kay RM. 1981. Oat-bran intake selectively lowers serum low-density lipoprotein cholesterol concentrations of hypercholesterolemic men. *Am J Clin Nutr* 34:824–829.

Kleessen B, Sykura B, Zunft HJ, Blaut M. 1997. Effects of inulin and lactose on fecal microflora, microbial activity, and bowel habit in elderly constipated persons. *Am J Clin Nutr* 65:1397–1402.

Klurfeld DM. 1992. Dietary fiber-mediated mechanisms in carcinogenesis. *Cancer Res* 52:2055S–2059S.

Knekt P, Steineck G, Järvinen R, Hakulinen T, Aromaa A. 1994. Intake of fried meat and risk of cancer: A follow-up study in Finland. *Int J Cancer* 59:756–760.

Knox TA, Kassarjian Z, Dawson-Hughes B, Golner BB, Dallal GE, Arora S, Russell RM. 1991. Calcium absorption in elderly subjects on high- and low-fiber diets: Effect of gastric acidity. *Am J Clin Nutr* 53:1480–1486.

Kochen MM, Wegscheider K, Abholz HH. 1985. Prophylaxis of constipation by wheat bran: A randomized study in hospitalized patients. *Digestion* 31:220–224.

Krishnamachar S, Mickelsen O. 1987. The influence of different carbohydrate sources on blood glucose levels and satiety: Effect of physical activity on blood glucose response. *Hum Nutr Food Sci Nutr* 41F:29–39.

Kromhout D, Bosschieter EB, de Lezenne Coulander C. 1982. Dietary fibre and 10-year mortality from coronary heart disease, cancer, and all causes. The Zutphen Study. *Lancet* 2:518–522.

Krotkiewski M. 1987. Effect of guar gum on the arterial blood pressure. *Acta Med Scand* 222:43–49.

Kushi LH, Lew RA, Stare FJ, Ellison CR, el Lozy M, Bourke G, Daly L, Graham I, Hickey N, Mulcahy R, Kevaney J. 1985. Diet and 20-year mortality from coronary heart disease. The Ireland-Boston Diet-Heart Study. *N Engl J Med* 312:811–818.

Lagier F, Cartier A, Somer J, Dolovich J, Malo JL. 1990. Occupational asthma caused by guar gum. *J Allergy Clin Immunol* 85:785–790.

Landin K, Holm G, Tengborn L, Smith U. 1992. Guar gum improves insulin sensitivity, blood lipids, blood pressure, and fibrinolysis in healthy men. *Am J Clin Nutr* 56:1061–1065.

Lantner RR, Espiritu BR, Zumerchik P, Tobin MC. 1990. Anaphylaxis following ingestion of a psyllium-containing cereal. *J Am Med Assoc* 264:2534–2536.

Lanza E. 1990. National Cancer Institute Satellite Symposium on Fiber and Colon Cancer. In: Kritchevsky D, Bonfield C, Anderson JW, eds. *Dietary Fiber: Chemistry, Physiology, and Health Effects.* New York: Plenum Press. Pp. 383–387.

Larson DE, Hunter GR, Williams MJ, Kekes-Szabo T, Nyikos I, Goran MI. 1996. Dietary fat in relation to body fat and intraabdominal adipose tissue: A cross-sectional analysis. *Am J Clin Nutr* 64:677–684.

Leathwood P, Pollet P. 1988. Effects of slow release carbohydrates in the form of bean flakes on the evolution of hunger and satiety in man. *Appetite* 10:1–11.

Lee HP, Gourley L, Duffy SW, Estève J, Lee J, Day NE. 1991. Dietary effects on breast-cancer risk in Singapore. *Lancet* 337:1197–1200.

Lei KY, Davis MW, Fang MM, Young LC. 1980. Effect of pectin on zinc, copper and iron balances in humans. *Nutr Rep Int* 22:459–466.

Lev R. 1990. Malignant potential of adenomatous polyps. In: *Adenomatous Polyps of the Colon: Pathobiological and Clinical Features.* New York: Springer-Verlag. Pp. 53–89.

Levin EG, Miller VT, Muesing RA, Stoy DB, Balm TK, LaRosa JC. 1990. Comparison of psyllium hydrophilic mucilloid and cellulose as adjuncts to a prudent diet in the treatment of mild to moderate hypercholesterolemia. *Arch Intern Med* 150:1822–1827.

Levine AS, Billington CJ. 1994. Dietary fiber: Does it affect food intake and body weight? In: Fernstrom JD, Miller GD, eds. *Appetite and Body Weight Regulation: Sugar, Fat, and Macronutrient Substitutes.* Boca Raton, FL: CRC Press. Pp. 191–200.

Librenti MC, Cocchi M, Orsi E, Pozza G, Micossi P. 1992. Effect of soya and cellulose fibers on postprandial glycemic response in type II diabetic patients. *Diabetes Care* 15:111–113.

Lichtenstein AH, Ausman LM, Jalbert SM, Vilella-Bach M, Jauhiainen M, McGladdery S, Erkkila AT, Ehnholm C, Frohlich J, Schaefer EJ. 2002. Efficacy of a Therapeutic Lifestyle Change/Step 2 diet in moderately hypercholesterolemic middle-aged and elderly female and male subjects. *J Lipid Res* 43:264–273.

Lipid Research Clinics Program. 1984. The Lipid Research Clinics Coronary Primary Prevention Trial results. II. The relationship of reduction in incidence of coronary heart disease to cholesterol lowering. *J Am Med Assoc* 251:365–374.

Little J, Logan RFA, Hawtin PG, Hardcastle JD, Turner ID. 1993. Colorectal adenomas and diet: A case-control study of subjects participating in the Nottingham Faecal Occult Blood Screening Programme. *Br J Cancer* 67:177–184.

Livesey G. 1990. Energy values of unavailable carbohydrate and diets: An inquiry and analysis. *Am J Clin Nutr* 51:617–637.

Loening-Baucke V. 1993. Chronic constipation in children. *Gastroenterology* 105:1557–1564.

Lovegrove JA, Clohessy A, Milon H, Williams CM. 2000. Modest doses of β-glucan do not reduce concentrations of potentially atherogenic lipoproteins. *Am J Clin Nutr* 72:49–55.

Low AG. 1990. Nutritional regulation of gastric secretion, digestion and emptying. *Nutr Res Rev* 3:229–252.

LSRO (Life Sciences Research Office). 1987. *Physiological Effects and Health Consequences of Dietary Fiber.* Bethesda, MD: LSRO.

Lubin F, Wax Y, Modan B. 1986. Role of fat, animal protein, and dietary fiber in breast cancer etiology: A case-control study. *J Natl Cancer Inst* 77:605–612.

Luo J, Rizkalla SW, Alamowitch C, Boussairi A, Blayo A, Barry J-L, Laffitte A, Guyon F, Bornet FRJ, Slama G. 1996. Chronic consumption of short-chain fructo-oligosaccharides by healthy subjects decreased basal hepatic glucose production but had no effect on insulin-stimulated glucose metabolism. *Am J Clin Nutr* 63:939–945.

Lupton JR. 1995. Butyrate and colonic cytokinetics: Differences between in vitro and in vivo studies. *Eur J Cancer Prev* 4:373–378.

Lupton JR, Morin JL, Robinson MC. 1993. Barley bran flour accelerates gastrointestinal transit time. *J Am Diet Assoc* 93:881–885.

Lyon JL, Mahoney AW, West DW, Gardner JW, Smith KR, Sorenson AW, Stanish W. 1987. Energy intake: Its relationship to colon cancer risk. *J Natl Cancer Inst* 78:853–861.

Macfarlane GT, Englyst HN. 1986. Starch utilization by the human large intestinal microflora. *J Appl Bacteriol* 60:195–201.

MacLennan R, Macrae F, Bain C, Battistutta D, Chapuis P, Gratten H, Lambert J, Newland RC, Ngu M, Russell A, Ward M, Wahlqvist ML. 1995. Randomized trial of intake of fat, fiber, and beta carotene to prevent colorectal adenomas. *J Natl Cancer Inst* 87:1760–1766.

MacMahon M, Carless J. 1998. Ispaghula husk in the treatment of hypercholesterolemia: A double-blind controlled study. *J Cardiovasc Risk* 5:167–172.

Macquart-Moulin G, Riboli E, Cornée J, Charnay B, Berthezène P, Day N. 1986. Case-control study on colorectal cancer and diet in Marseilles. *Int J Cancer* 38:183–191.

Macquart-Moulin G, Riboli E, Cornée J, Kaaks R, Berthezène P. 1987. Colorectal polyps and diet: A case-control study in Marseilles. *Int J Cancer* 40:179–188.

Manousos O, Day NE, Tzonou A, Papadimitriou C, Kapetanakis A, Polychronopoulou-Trichopoulou A, Trichopoulos D. 1985. Diet and other factors in the aetiology of diverticulosis: An epidemiological study in Greece. *Gut* 26:544–549.

Marlett JA. 1992. Content and composition of dietary fiber in 117 frequently consumed foods. *J Am Diet Assoc* 92:175–186.

Marlett JA, Longacre MJ. 1996. Comparison of in vitro and in vivo measures of resistant starch in selected grain products. *Cereal Chem* 73:63–68.

Mathur KS, Khan MA, Sharma RD. 1968. Hypocholesterolaemic effect of Bengal gram: A long-term study in man. *Br Med J* 1:30–31.

McBurney MI. 1991. Potential water-holding capacity and short-chain fatty acid production from purified fiber sources in a fecal incubation system. *Nutrition* 7:421–424.

McBurney MI, Thompson LU. 1990. Fermentative characteristics of cereal brans and vegetable fibers. *Nutr Cancer* 13:271–280.

McCann SE, Freudenheim JL, Marshall JR, Brasure JR, Swanson MK, Graham S. 2000. Diet in the epidemiology of endometrial cancer in western New York (United States). *Cancer Causes Control* 11:965–974.

McCann SE, Moysich KB, Mettlin C. 2001. Intakes of selected nutrients and food groups and risk of ovarian cancer. *Nutr Cancer* 39:19–28.

McClung HJ, Boyne LJ, Linsheid T, Heitlinger LA, Murray RD, Fyda J, Li BUK. 1993. Is combination therapy for encopresis nutritionally safe? *Pediatrics* 91:591–594.

McClung HJ, Boyne L, Heitlinger L. 1995. Constipation and dietary fiber intake in children. *Pediatrics* 96:999–1001.

McKeown-Eyssen GE, Bright-See E, Bruce WR, Jazmaji V. 1994. A randomized trial of a low fat high fibre diet in the recurrence of colorectal polyps. *J Clin Epidemiol* 47:525–536.

McRorie JW, Daggy BP, Morel JG, Diersing PS, Miner PB, Robinson M. 1998. Psyllium is superior to docusate sodium for treatment of chronic constipation. *Aliment Pharmacol Ther* 12:491–497.

McRorie J, Kesler J, Bishop L, Filloon T, Allgood G, Sutton M, Hunt T, Laurent A, Rudolph C. 2000. Effects of wheat bran and Olestra on objective measures of stool and subjective reports of GI symptoms. *Am J Gastroenterol* 95:1244–1252.

Mennen LI, Witteman JCM, den Breeijen JH, Schouten EG, de Jong PTVM, Hofman A, Grobbee DE. 1997. The association of dietary fat and fiber with coagulation factor VII in the elderly: The Rotterdam Study. *Am J Clin Nutr* 65:732–736.

Meyer KA, Kushi LH, Jacobs DR, Slavin J, Sellers TA, Folsom AR. 2000. Carbohydrates, dietary fiber, and incident type 2 diabetes in older women. *Am J Clin Nutr* 71:921–930.

Miller AB, Howe GR, Jain M, Craib KJP, Harrison L. 1983. Food items and food groups as risk factors in a case-control study of diet and colo-rectal cancer. *Int J Cancer* 32:155–161.

Miller WC, Niederpruem MG, Wallace JP, Lindeman AK. 1994. Dietary fat, sugar, and fiber predict body fat content. *J Am Diet Assoc* 94:612–615.

Modan B, Barell V, Lubin F, Modan M, Greenberg RA, Graham S. 1975. Low-fiber intake as an etiologic factor in cancer of the colon. *J Natl Cancer Inst* 55:15–18.

Morais MB, Vítolo MR, Aguirre ANC, Fagundes-Neto U. 1999. Measurement of low dietary fiber intake as a risk factor for chronic constipation in children. *J Pediatr Gastroenterol Nutr* 29:132–135.

Morales M, Llopis A. 1992. Breast cancer and diet in Spain. *J Environ Pathol Toxicol Oncol* 11:157–167.

Morris JN, Marr JW, Clayton DG. 1977. Diet and heart: A postscript. *Br Med J* 2:1307–1314.

Moshfegh AJ, Friday JE, Goldman JP, Ahuja JKC. 1999. Presence of inulin and oligofructose in the diets of Americans. *J Nutr* 129:1407S–1411S.

National Cholesterol Education Program. 1991. *Report of the Expert Panel on Blood Cholesterol Levels in Children and Adolescents*. NIH Publication No. 91-2732. Bethesda, MD: National Heart, Lung, and Blood Institute.

Neugut AI, Garbowski GC, Lee WC, Murray T, Nieves JW, Forde KA, Treat MR, Waye JD, Fenoglio-Preiser C. 1993. Dietary risk factors for the incidence and recurrence of colorectal adenomatous polyps. A case-control study. *Ann Intern Med* 11:91–95.

Niemi MK, Keinänen-Kiukaanniemi SM, Salmela PI. 1988. Long-term effects of guar gum and microcrystalline cellulose on glycaemic control and serum lipids in type 2 diabetes. *Eur J Clin Pharmacol* 34:427–429.

Niho N, Tamura T, Toyoda K, Uneyama C, Shibutani M, Hirose M. 1999. A 13-week subchronic toxicity study of chitin in F344 rats. *Kokuritsu Iyakuhin Shokuhin Eisei Kenkyusho Hokoku* 117:129–134.

Nishimune T, Sumimoto T, Konishi Y, Yakushiji T, Komachi Y, Mitsuhashi Y, Nakayama I, Okazaki K, Tsuda T, Ichihashi A, Adachi T, Imanaka M, Kirigaya T, Ushio H, Kasuga Y, Saeki K, Yamamoto Y, Ichikawa T, Nakahara S, Oda S. 1993. Dietary fiber intake of Japanese younger generations and the recommended daily allowance. *J Nutr Sci Vitaminol (Tokyo)* 39:263–278.

Noble JA, Grannis FW. 1984. Acute esophageal obstruction by a psyllium-based bulk laxative. *Chest* 86:800.

NRC (National Research Council). 1989. *Diet and Health: Implications for Reducing Chronic Disease Risk*. Washington, DC: National Academy Press.

Obarzanek E, Sacks FM, Vollmer WM, Bray GA, Miller ER, Lin P-H, Karanja NM, Most-Windhauser MM, Moore TJ, Swain JF, Bales CW, Proschan MA. 2001. Effects on blood lipids of a blood pressure-lowering diet: The Dietary Approaches to Stop Hypertension (DASH) Trial. *Am J Clin Nutr* 74:80–89.

O'Brien KO, Allen LH, Quatromoni P, Siu-Caldera M-L, Vieira NE, Perez A, Holick MF, Yergey AL. 1993. High fiber diets slow bone turnover in young men but have no effect on efficiency of intestinal calcium absorption. *J Nutr* 123:2122–2128.

Ohkuma K, Wakabayashi S. 2001. Fibersol-2: A soluble, non-digestible, starch-derived dietary fibre. In: McCleary BV, Prosky L, eds. *Advanced Dietary Fibre Technology*. Oxford: Blackwell Science. Pp. 510–523.

Ohno Y, Yoshida O, Oishi K, Okada K, Yamabe H, Schroeder FH. 1988. Dietary β-carotene and cancer of the prostate: A case-control study in Kyoto, Japan. *Cancer Res* 48:1331–1336.

Olesen M, Gudmand-Høyer E. 2000. Efficacy, safety, and tolerability of fructo-oligosaccharides in the treatment of irritable bowel syndrome. *Am J Clin Nutr* 72:1570–1575.

Olson BH, Anderson SM, Becker MP, Anderson JW, Hunninghake DB, Jenkins DJA, LaRose JC, Rippe JM, Roberts DCK, Stoy DB, Summerbell CD, Truswell AS, Wolever TMS, Morris DH, Fulgoni VL. 1997. Psyllium-enriched cereals lower blood total cholesterol and LDL cholesterol, but not HDL cholesterol, in hypercholesterolemic adults: Results of a meta-analysis. *J Nutr* 127:1973–1980.

Pastors JG, Blaisdell PW, Balm TK, Asplin CM, Pohl SL. 1991. Psyllium fiber reduces rise in postprandial glucose and insulin concentrations in patients with non-insulin-diabetes mellitus. *Am J Clin Nutr* 53:1431–1435.

Patrick PG, Gohman SM, Marx SC, DeLegge MH, Greenberg NA. 1998. Effect of supplements of partially hydrolyzed guar gum on the occurrence of constipation and use of laxative agents. *J Am Diet Assoc* 98:912–914.

Pedersen A, Sandstrom B, Van Amelsvoort JM. 1997. The effect of ingestion of inulin on blood lipids and gastrointestinal symptoms in healthy females. *Br J Nutr* 78:215–222.

Penagini R, Velio P, Vigorelli R, Bozzani A, Castagnone D, Ranzi T, Bianchi PA. 1986. The effect of dietary guar on serum cholesterol, intestinal transit, and fecal output in man. *Am J Gastroenterol* 81:123–125.

Petrakis NL, King EB. 1981. Cytological abnormalities in nipple aspirates of breast fluid from women with severe constipation. *Lancet* 2:1203–1204.

Phillips J, Muir JG, Birkett A, Lu ZX, Jones GP, O'Dea K, Young GP. 1995. Effect of resistant starch on fecal bulk and fermentation-dependent events in humans. *Am J Clin Nutr* 62:121–130.

Pick ME, Hawrysh ZJ, Gee MI, Toth E, Garg ML, Hardin RT. 1996. Oat bran concentrate bread products improve long-term control of diabetes: A pilot study. *J Am Diet Assoc* 96:1254–1261.

Pietinen P, Rimm EB, Korhonen P, Hartman AM, Willett WC, Albanes D, Virtamo J. 1996. Intake of dietary fiber and risk of coronary heart disease in a cohort of Finnish men. The Alpha-Tocopherol, Beta-Carotene Cancer Prevention Study. *Circulation* 94:2720–2727.

Pietinen P, Malila N, Virtanen M, Hartman TJ, Tangrea JA, Albanes D, Virtamo J. 1999. Diet and risk of colorectal cancer in a cohort of Finnish men. *Cancer Causes Control* 10:387–396.

Pittler MH, Abbot NC, Harkness EF, Ernst E. 1999. Randomized, double-blind trial of chitosan for body weight reduction. *Eur J Clin Nutr* 53:379–381.

Platz EA, Giovannucci E, Rimm EB, Rockett HRH, Stampfer MJ, Colditz GA, Willett WC. 1997. Dietary fiber and distal colorectal adenoma in men. *Cancer Epidemiol Biomarkers Prev* 6:661–670.

Prior A, Whorwell PJ. 1987. Double blind study of ispagula in irritable bowel syndrome. *Gut* 28:1510–1513.

Raben A, Tagliabue A, Christensen NJ, Madsen J, Holst JJ, Astrup A. 1994. Resistant starch: The effect on postprandial glycemia, hormonal response, and satiety. *Am J Clin Nutr* 60:544–551.

Ranhotra GS, Gelroth JA, Leinen SD. 1997. Hypolipidemic effect of resistant starch in hamsters is not dose dependent. *Nutr Res* 17:317–323.

Razdan A, Pettersson D. 1994. Effect of chitin and chitosan on nutrient digestibility and plasma lipid concentrations in broiler chickens. *Br J Nutr* 72:277–288.

Razdan A, Pettersson D. 1996. Hypolipidaemic, gastrointestinal and related responses of broiler chickens to chitosans of different viscosity. *Br J Nutr* 76:387–397.

Razdan A, Pettersson D, Pettersson J. 1997. Broiler chicken body weights, feed intakes, plasma lipid and small-intestinal bile acid concentrations in response to feeding of chitosan and pectin. *Br J Nutr* 78:283–291.

Rigaud D, Ryttig KR, Angel LA, Apfelbaum M. 1990. Overweight treated with energy restriction and a dietary fibre supplement: A 6-month randomized, double-blind, placebo-controlled trial. *Int J Obes* 14:763–769.

Rigaud D, Paycha F, Meulemans A, Merrouche M, Mignon M. 1998. Effect of psyllium on gastric emptying, hunger feeling and food intake in normal volunteers: A double blind study. *Eur J Clin Nutr* 52:239–245.

Rimm EB, Ascherio A, Giovannucci E, Spiegelman D, Stampfer MJ, Willett WC. 1996. Vegetable, fruit, and cereal fiber intake and risk of coronary heart disease among men. *J Am Med Assoc* 275:447–451.

Ripsin CM, Keenan JM, Jacobs DR, Elmer PJ, Welch RR, Van Horn L, Liu K, Turnbull WH, Thye FW, Kestin M, Hegsted M, Davidson DM, Davidson MH, Dugan LD, Demark-Wahnefried W, Beling S. 1992. Oat products and lipid lowering. A meta-analysis. *J Am Med Assoc* 267:3317–3325.

Risch HA, Jain M, Marrett LD, Howe GR. 1994. Dietary fat intake and risk of epithelial ovarian cancer. *J Natl Cancer Inst* 86:1409–1415.

Ritz P, Krempf M, Cloarec D, Champ M, Charbonnel B. 1991. Comparative continuous-indirect-calorimetry study of two carbohydrates with different glycemic indices. *Am J Clin Nutr* 54:855–859.

Rivellese A, Riccardi G, Giacco A, Pacioni D, Genovese S, Mattioli PL, Mancini M. 1980. Effect of dietary fibre on glucose control and serum lipoproteins in diabetic patients. *Lancet* 2:447–450.

Roberfroid M. 1993. Dietary fiber, inulin, and oligofructose: A review comparing their physiological effects. *Crit Rev Food Sci Nutr* 33:103–148.

Roberts PL, Veidenheimer MC. 1990. Diverticular disease of the colon. In: Bayless TM, ed. *Current Therapy in Gastroenterology and Liver Disease—3*. Toronto: Decker Mosby. Pp. 416–419.

Roediger WEW. 1980. The colonic epithelium in ulcerative colitis: An energy-deficiency disease? *Lancet* 2:712–715.

Roediger WEW. 1982. Utilization of nutrients by isolated epithelial cells of the rat colon. *Gastroenterology* 83:424–429.

Roediger WE, Duncan A, Kapaniris O, Millard S. 1993. Reducing sulfur compounds of the colon impair colonocyte nutrition: Implications for ulcerative colitis. *Gastroenterology* 104:802–809.

Rohan TE, McMichael AJ, Baghurst PA. 1988. A population-based case-control study of diet and breast cancer in Australia. *Am J Epidemiol* 128:478–489.

Rohan TE, Howe GR, Friedenreich CM, Jain M, Miller AB. 1993. Dietary fiber, vitamins A, C, and E, and risk of breast cancer: A cohort study. *Cancer Causes Control* 4:29–37.

Rohan TE, Howe GR, Burch JD, Jain M. 1995. Dietary factors and risk of prostate cancer: A case-control study in Ontario, Canada. *Cancer Causes Control* 6:145–154.

Roma E, Adamidis D, Nikolara R, Constantopoulos A, Messaritakis J. 1999. Diet and chronic constipation in children: The role of fiber. *J Pediatr Gastroenterol Nutr* 28:169–174.

Ronco A, De Stefani E, Boffetta P, Deneo-Pellegrini H, Mendilaharsu M, Leborgne F. 1999. Vegetables, fruits, and related nutrients and risk of breast cancer: A case-control study in Uruguay. *Nutr Cancer* 35:111–119.

Rose DP. 1990. Dietary fiber and breast cancer. *Nutr Cancer* 13:1–8.

Rose DP. 1992. Dietary fiber, phytoestrogens, and breast cancer. *Nutrition* 8:47–51.

Rose DP, Goldman M, Connoly JM, Strong LE. 1991. High-fiber diet reduces serum estrogen concentrations in premenopausal women. *Am J Clin Nutr* 54:520–525.

Rössner S, von Zweigbergk D, Öhlin A, Ryttig K. 1987. Weight reduction with dietary fibre supplements. Results of two double-blind randomized studies. *Acta Med Scand* 222:83–88.

Ryttig KR, Tellnes G, Haegh L, Boe E, Fagerthun H. 1989. A dietary fibre supplement and weight maintenance after weight reduction: A randomized, double-blind, placebo-controlled long-term trial. *Int J Obes* 13:165–171.

Saku K, Yoshinaga K, Okura Y, Ying H, Harada R, Arakawa K. 1991. Effects of polydextrose on serum lipids, lipoproteins, and apolipoproteins in healthy subjects. *Clin Ther* 13:254–258.

Salmerón J, Ascherio A, Rimm EB, Colditz GA, Spiegelman D, Jenkins DJ, Stampfer MJ, Wing AL, Willett WC. 1997a. Dietary fiber, glycemic load, and risk of NIDDM in men. *Diabetes Care* 20:545–550.

Salmerón J, Manson JE, Stampfer MJ, Colditz GA, Wing AL, Willett WC. 1997b. Dietary fiber, glycemic load, and risk of non-insulin-dependent diabetes mellitus in women. *J Am Med Assoc* 277:472–477.

Sandberg AS, Ahderinne R, Andersson H, Hallgren B, Hulten L. 1983. The effect of citrus pectin on the absorption of nutrients in the small intestine. *Hum Nutr Clin Nutr* 37:171–183.

Sandstead HH. 1992. Fiber, phytates, and mineral nutrition. *Nutr Rev* 50:30–31.

Schatzkin A, Lanza E, Corle D, Lance P, Iber F, Caan B, Shike M, Weissfeld J, Burt R, Cooper MR, Kikendall JW, Cahill J. 2000. Lack of effect of a low-fat, high-fiber diet on the recurrence of colorectal adenomas. *N Engl J Med* 342:1149–1155.

Sepple CP, Read NW. 1989. Gastrointestinal correlates of the development of hunger in man. *Appetite* 13:183–191.

Shetty PS, Kurpad AV. 1986. Increasing starch intake in the human diet increases fecal bulking. *Am J Clin Nutr* 43:210–212.

Shultz TD, Howie BJ. 1986. In vitro binding of steroid hormones by natural and purified fibers. *Nutr Cancer* 8:141–147.

Silvester KR, Englyst HN, Cummings JH. 1995. Ileal recovery of starch from whole diets containing resistant starch measured in vitro and fermentation of ileal effluent. *Am J Clin Nutr* 62:403–411.

Simpson HCR, Simpson RW, Lousley S, Carter RD, Geekie M, Hockaday TDR, Mann JI. 1981. A high carbohydrate leguminous fibre diet improves all aspects of diabetic control. *Lancet* 1:1–15.

Simpson KM, Morris ER, Cook JD. 1981. The inhibitory effect of bran on iron absorption in man. *Am J Clin Nutr* 34:1469–1478.

Slavin JL. 1987. Dietary fiber: Classification, chemical analyses, and food sources. *J Am Diet Assoc* 87:1164–1171.

Slavin JL, Marlett JA. 1980. Influence of refined cellulose on human bowel function and calcium and magnesium retention. *Am J Clin Nutr* 33:1932–1939.

Slavin J, Jacobs D, Marquart L. 1997. Whole-grain consumption and chronic disease: Protective mechanisms. *Nutr Cancer* 27:14–21.

Sleet R, Brightwell J. 1990. *FS-Teratology Study in Rats*. Raffinerie Tirlemontoise Internal Report. Photocopy.

Smith T, Brown JC, Livesey G. 1998. Energy balance and thermogenesis in rats consuming nonstarch polysaccharides of various fermentabilities. *Am J Clin Nutr* 68:802–819.

Spencer H, Norris C, Derler J, Osis D. 1991. Effect of oat bran muffins on calcium absorption and calcium, phosphorus, magnesium and zinc balance in men. *J Nutr* 121:1976–1983.

Steinmetz KA, Kushi LH, Bostick RM, Folsom AR, Potter JD. 1994. Vegetables, fruit, and colon cancer in the Iowa Women's Health Study. *Am J Epidemiol* 139:1–15.

Stephen AM, Haddad AC, Phillips SF. 1983. Passage of carbohydrate into the colon. Direct measurements in humans. *Gastroenterology* 85:589–595.

Stevens J, Levitsky DA, VanSoest PJ, Robertson JB, Kalkwarf HJ, Roe DA. 1987. Effect of psyllium gum and wheat bran on spontaneous energy intake. *Am J Clin Nutr* 46:812–817.

Stone-Dorshow T, Levitt MD. 1987. Gaseous response to ingestion of a poorly absorbed fructo-oligosaccharide sweetener. *Am J Clin Nutr* 46:61–65.

Strobel S, Ferguson A, Anderson DM. 1982. Immunogenicity of foods and food additives—In vivo testing of gums arabic, karaya, and tragacanth. *Toxicol Lett* 14:247–252.

Sugano M, Fujikawa T, Hiratsuji Y, Nakashima K, Fukuda N, Hasegawa Y. 1980. A novel use of chitosan as a hypocholesterolemic agent in rats. *Am J Clin Nutr* 33:787–793.

Sundell IB, Ranby M. 1993. Oat husk fiber decreases plasminogen activator inhibitor type 1 activity. *Haemostasis* 23:45–50.

Taioli E, Nicolosi A, Wynder EL. 1991. Dietary habits and breast cancer: A comparative study of United States and Italian data. *Nutr Cancer* 16:259–265.

Thompson LU. 1994. Antioxidants and hormone-mediated health benefits of whole grains. *Crit Rev Food Sci Nutr* 34:473–497.

Thun MJ, Calle EE, Namboodiri MM, Flanders WD, Coates RJ, Byers T, Boffetta P, Garfinkel L, Heath CW. 1992. Risk factors for fatal colon cancer in a large prospective study. *J Natl Cancer Inst* 84:1491–1500.

Todd S, Woodward M, Tunstall-Pedoe H, Bolton-Smith C. 1999. Dietary antioxidant vitamins and fiber in the etiology of cardiovascular disease and all-causes mortality: Results from the Scottish Heart Health Study. *Am J Epidemiol* 150:1073–1080.

Tokunaga K, Matsuoka A. 1999. Effects of a Food for Specified Health Use (FOSHU) which contains indigestible dextrin as an effective ingredient on glucose and lipid metabolism. *J Jpn Diabetes Soc* 42:61–65.

Tomlin J, Read NW. 1988. A comparative study of the effects on colon function caused by feeding ispaghula husk and polydextrose. *Aliment Pharmacol Ther* 2:513–519.

Tomlin J, Read NW. 1990. The effect of resistant starch on colon function in humans. *Br J Nutr* 64:589–595.

Tomlin J, Lowis C, Read NW. 1991. Investigation of normal flatus production in healthy volunteers. *Gut* 32:665–669.

Tremblay A, Lavallée N, Alméras N, Allard L, Després J-P, Bouchard C. 1991. Nutritional determinants of the increase in energy intake associated with a high-fat diet. *Am J Clin Nutr* 53:1134–1137.

Trock B, Lanza E, Greenwald P. 1990. Dietary fiber, vegetables, and colon cancer: Critical review and meta-analyses of the epidemiologic evidence. *J Natl Cancer Inst* 82:650–661.

Truswell AS. 1992. Glycaemic index of foods. *Eur J Clin Nutr* 46:S91–S101.

Tuohy KM, Kolida S, Lustenberger AM, Gibson GR. 2001. The prebiotic effects of biscuits containing partially hydrolysed guar gum and fructo-oligosaccharides—A human volunteer study. *Br J Nutr* 86:341–348.

Tuyns AJ, Haelterman M, Kaaks R. 1987. Colorectal cancer and the intake of nutrients: Oligosaccharides are a risk factor, fats are not. A case-control study in Belgium. *Nutr Cancer* 10:181–196.

Tzonou A, Hsieh C-C, Polychronopoulou A, Kaprinis G, Toupadaki N, Trichopoulou A, Karakatsani A, Trichopoulos D. 1993. Diet and ovarian cancer: A case-control study in Greece. *Int J Cancer* 55:411–414.

USDA/HHS (U.S. Department of Agriculture/U.S. Department of Health and Human Services). 2000. *Nutrition and Your Health: Dietary Guidelines for Americans.* Home and Garden Bulletin No. 232. Washington, DC: U.S. Government Printing Office.

van Dokkum W, Wezendonk B, Srikumar TS, van den Heuvel EGHM. 1999. Effect of nondigestible oligosaccharides on large-bowel functions, blood lipid concentrations and glucose absorption in young healthy male subjects. *Eur J Clin Nutr* 53:1–7.

Van Horn LV, Liu K, Parker D, Emidy L, Liao Y, Pan WH, Giumetti D, Hewitt J, Stamler J. 1986. Serum lipid response to oat product intake with a fat-modified diet. *J Am Diet Assoc* 86:759–764.

van Munster IP, Nagengast FM. 1993. The role of carbohydrate fermentation in colon cancer prevention. *Scand J Gastroenterol* 200:80–86.

van Munster IP, de Boer HM, Jansen MC, de Haan AF, Katan MB, van Amelsvoort JM, Nagengast FM. 1994. Effect of resistant starch on breath-hydrogen and methane excretion in healthy volunteers. *Am J Clin Nutr* 59:626–630.

van't Veer P, Kolb CM, Verhoef P, Kok FJ, Schouten EG, Hermus RJ, Sturmans F. 1990. Dietary fiber, beta-carotene and breast cancer: Results from a case-control study. *Int J Cancer* 45:825–828.

Verhoeven DTH, Assen N, Goldbohm RA, Dorant E, van't Veer P, Sturmans F, Hermus RJJ, van den Brandt PA. 1997. Vitamins C and E, retinol, beta-carotene and dietary fibre in relation to breast cancer risk: A prospective cohort study. *Br J Cancer* 75:149–155.

Visek WJ. 1978. Diet and cell growth modulation by ammonia. *Am J Clin Nutr* 31:S216–S220.

Wakabayashi S, Ueda Y, Matsuoka A. 1993. Effects of indigestible dextrin on blood glucose and insulin levels after various sugar loads in rats. *J Jpn Soc Nutr Food Sci* 46:131–137.

Wakabayashi S, Kishimoto Y, Matsuoka A. 1995. Effects of indigestible dextrin on glucose tolerance in rats. *J Endocrinol* 144:533–538.

Watters DAK, Smith AN. 1990. Strength of the colon wall in diverticular disease. *Br J Surg* 77:257–259.

Weaver GA, Krause JA, Miller TL, Wolin MJ. 1988. Short chain fatty acid distributions of enema samples from a sigmoidoscopy population: An association of high acetate and low butyrate ratios with adenomatous polyps and colon cancer. *Gut* 29:1539–1543.

West DW, Slattery ML, Robison LM, Schuman KL, Ford MH, Mahoney AW, Lyon JL, Sorensen AW. 1989. Dietary intake and colon cancer: Sex- and anatomic site-specific associations. *Am J Epidemiol* 130:883–894.

Willett WC, Stampfer MJ, Colditz GA, Rosner BA, Speizer FE. 1990. Relation of meat, fat, and fiber intake to the risk of colon cancer in a prospective study among women. *N Engl J Med* 323:1664–1672.

Willett WC, Hunter DJ, Stampfer MJ, Colditz G, Manson JE, Spiegelman D, Rosner B, Hennekens CH, Speizer FE. 1992. Dietary fat and fiber in relation to risk of breast cancer. An 8-year follow-up. *J Am Med Assoc* 268:2037–2044.

Williams CH, Witherly SA, Buddington RK. 1994. Influence of dietary neosugar on selected bacterial groups of the human faecal microbiota. *Microb Ecol Health Dis* 7:91–97.

Williams CL, Bollella M. 1995. Is a high-fiber diet safe for children? *Pediatrics* 96:1014–1019.

Williams CL, Bollella M, Wynder EL. 1995. A new recommendation for dietary fiber in childhood. *Pediatrics* 96:985–988.

Wisker E, Nagel R, Tanudjaja TK, Feldheim W. 1991. Calcium, magnesium, zinc, and iron balances in young women: Effects of a low-phytate barley-fiber concentrate. *Am J Clin Nutr* 54:553–559.

Witte JS, Ursin G, Siemiatycki J, Thompson WD, Paganini-Hill A, Haile RW. 1997. Diet and premenopausal bilateral breast cancer: A case-control study. *Breast Cancer Res Treat* 42:243–251.

Wolever TMS. 1995. In vitro and in vivo models for predicting the effect of dietary fiber and starchy foods on carbohydrate metabolism. In: Kritchevsky D, Bonfield C, eds. *Dietary Fiber in Health and Disease.* St. Paul, MN: Eagan Press. Pp. 360–377.

Wolever TMS, Jenkins DJA. 1993. Effect of dietary fiber and foods on carbohydrate metabolism. In: Spiller G, ed. *CRC Handbook of Dietary Fiber in Human Nutrition.* Boca Raton, FL: CRC Press. Pp. 111–162.

Wolk A, Manson JE, Stampfer MJ, Colditz GA, Hu FB, Speizer FE, Hennekens CH, Willett WC. 1999. Long-term intake of dietary fiber and decreased risk of coronary heart disease among women. *J Am Med Assoc* 281:1998–2004.

Wood PJ, Braaten JT, Scott FW, Riedel KD, Wolynetz MS, Collins MW. 1994. Effect of dose and modification of viscous properties of oat gum on plasma glucose and insulin following an oral glucose load. *Br J Nutr* 72:731–743.

Woods MN, Gorbach SL, Longcope C, Goldin BR, Dwyer JT, Morrill-LaBrode A. 1989. Low-fat, high-fiber diet and serum estrone sulfate in premenopausal women. *Am J Clin Nutr* 49:1179–1183.

Woods MN, Barnett JB, Spiegelman D, Trail N, Hertzmark E, Longcope C, Gorbach SL. 1996. Hormone levels during dietary changes in premenopausal African-American women. *J Natl Cancer Inst* 88:1369–1374.

Wuolijoki E, Hirvelä T, Ylitalo P. 1999. Decrease in serum LDL cholesterol with microcrystalline chitosan. *Methods Find Exp Clin Pharmacol* 21:357–361.

Wynder EL, Berenson GS. 1984. Preventive strategies for reducing hyperlipidemia in childhood. *Prev Med* 13:327–329.

Yamashita K, Kawai K, Itakura M. 1984. Effects of fructo-oligosaccharides on blood glucose and serum lipids in diabetic subjects. *Nutr Res* 4:961–966.

Younes H, Levrat MA, Demigne C, Remesy C. 1995. Resistant starch is more effective than cholestyramine as a lipid-lowering agent in the rat. *Lipids* 30:847–853.

Yu H, Harris RE, Gao Y-T, Gao R, Wynder RL. 1991. Comparative epidemiology of cancers of the colon, rectum, prostate and breast in Shanghai, China versus the United States. *Int J Epidemiol* 20:76–81.

Yuan J-M, Wang Q-S, Ross RK, Henderson BE, Yu MC. 1995. Diet and breast cancer in Shanghai and Tianjin, China. *Br J Cancer* 71:1353–1358.

Zacour AC, Silva ME, Cecon PR, Bambirra EA, Vieira EC. 1992. Effect of dietary chitin on cholesterol absorption and metabolism in rats. *J Nutr Sci Vitaminol (Tokyo)* 38:609–613.

8

Dietary Fats: Total Fat and Fatty Acids

SUMMARY

Fat is a major source of fuel energy for the body and aids in the absorption of fat-soluble vitamins and carotenoids. Neither an Adequate Intake (AI) nor Recommended Dietary Allowance (RDA) is set for total fat because there are insufficient data to determine a defined level of fat intake at which risk of inadequacy or prevention of chronic disease occurs. An Acceptable Macronutrient Distribution Range (AMDR), however, has been estimated for total fat—it is 20 to 35 percent of energy (see Chapter 11). A Tolerable Upper Intake Level (UL) is not set for total fat because there is no defined intake level of fat at which an adverse effect occurs.

Saturated fatty acids are synthesized by the body to provide an adequate level needed for their physiological and structural functions; they have no known role in preventing chronic diseases. Therefore, neither an AI nor RDA is set for saturated fatty acids. There is a positive linear trend between total saturated fatty acid intake and total and low density lipoprotein (LDL) cholesterol concentration and increased risk of coronary heart disease (CHD). A UL is not set for saturated fatty acids because any incremental increase in saturated fatty acid intake increases CHD risk. It is neither possible nor advisable to achieve 0 percent of energy from saturated fatty acids in typical whole-food diets. This is because all fat and oil sources are mixtures of fatty acids, and consuming 0 percent of energy would require extraordinary changes in patterns of dietary intake. Such extraordinary adjustments may introduce undesirable effects (e.g., inadequate intakes of protein and certain micronutrients) and unknown and unquantifiable health risks. The AMDR for total fat is set at 20 to 35 percent of energy. It is possible to have a diet low in saturated fatty acids by following the dietary guidance provided in Chapter 11.

n-9 *cis* Monounsaturated fatty acids are synthesized by the body and have no known independent beneficial role in human health and are not required in the diet. Therefore, neither an AI nor an RDA is set. There is insufficient evidence to set a UL for n-9 *cis* monounsaturated fatty acids.

Linoleic acid is the only n-6 polyunsaturated fatty acid that is an essential fatty acid; it serves as a precursor to eicosanoids. A lack of dietary n-6 polyunsaturated fatty acids is characterized by rough and scaly skin, dermatitis, and an elevated eicosatrienoic acid:arachidonic acid (triene:tetraene) ratio. The AI for linoleic acid is based on the median intake in the United States where an n-6 fatty acid deficiency is nonexistent in healthy individuals. The AI is 17 g/d for young men and 12 g/d for young women. While intake levels much lower than the AI occur in the United States without the presence of a deficiency, the AI can provide the beneficial health effects associated with the consumption of linoleic acid (see Chapter 11). There is insufficient evidence to set a UL for n-6 polyunsaturated fatty acids.

n-3 Polyunsaturated fatty acids play an important role as structural membrane lipids, particularly in nerve tissue and the retina, and are precursors to eicosanoids. A lack of α-linolenic acid in the diet can result in clinical symptoms of a deficiency (e.g., scaly dermatitis). An AI is set for α-linolenic acid based on median intakes in the United States where an n-3 fatty acid deficiency is nonexistent in healthy individuals. The AI is 1.6 and 1.1 g/d for men and women, respectively. While intake levels much lower than the AI occur in the United States without the presence of a deficiency, the AI can provide the beneficial health effects associated with the consumption of n-3 fatty acids (see Chapter 11). There is insufficient evidence to set a UL for n-3 fatty acids.

Trans fatty acids are not essential and provide no known benefit to human health. Therefore, no AI or RDA is set. As with saturated fatty acids, there is a positive linear trend between *trans* fatty acid intake and LDL cholesterol concentration, and therefore increased risk of CHD. A UL is not set for *trans* fatty acids because any incremental increase in *trans* fatty acid intake increases CHD risk. Because *trans* fatty acids are unavoidable in ordinary, nonvegan diets, consuming 0 percent of energy would require significant changes in patterns of dietary intake. As with saturated fatty acids, such adjustments may introduce undesirable effects (e.g., elimination of commercially prepared foods, dairy products, and meats that contain *trans* fatty acids may result in inadequate intakes of protein and certain micronutrients) and unknown and unquantifiable health risks. Nevertheless, it is recommended that *trans* fatty acid consumption be as low as possible while consuming a nutritionally adequate diet. Dietary guidance in minimizing *trans* fatty acid intake is provided in Chapter 11.

BACKGROUND INFORMATION

Total Fat

Fat is a major source of fuel energy for the body. It also aids in the absorption of the fat-soluble vitamins A, D, E, and K and carotenoids. Dietary fat consists primarily (98 percent) of triacylglycerol, which is composed of one glycerol molecule esterified with three fatty acid molecules, and smaller amounts of phospholipids and sterols. Fatty acids are hydrocarbon chains that contain a methyl (CH_3-) and a carboxyl (-COOH) end. The fatty acids vary in carbon chain length and degree of unsaturation (number of double bonds in the carbon chain). The fatty acids can be classified into the following categories:

- Saturated fatty acids
- *Cis* monounsaturated fatty acids
- *Cis* polyunsaturated fatty acids
  — *n*-6 fatty acids
  — *n*-3 fatty acids
- *Trans* fatty acids

Dietary fat derives from both animal and plant products. In general, animal fats have higher melting points and are solid at room temperature, which is a reflection of their high content of saturated fatty acids. Plant fats (oils) tend to have lower melting points and are liquid at room temperature (oils); this is explained by their high content of unsaturated fatty acids. Exceptions to this rule are the seed oils (e.g., coconut oil and palm kernel oil), which are high in saturated fat and solid at room temperature. *Trans* fatty acids have physical properties generally resembling saturated fatty acids and their presence tends to harden fats. In the discussion below, total fat intake refers to the intake of all forms of triacylglycerol, regardless of fatty acid composition, in terms of percentage of total energy intake.

In addition to the functions of fat and fatty acids described above, fatty acids also function in cell signaling and alter expression of specific genes involved in lipid and carbohydrate metabolism (Jump and Clarke, 1999; Sessler and Ntambi, 1998). Fatty acids may themselves be ligands for, or serve as precursors for, the synthesis of unknown endogenous ligands for nuclear peroxisome proliferator activating receptors (Kliewer et al., 1997; Latruffe and Vamecq, 1997). These receptors are important regulators of adipogenesis, inflammation, insulin action, and neurological function.

Phospholipids

Phospholipids are a form of fat that contains one glycerol molecule that is esterified with two fatty acids and either inositol, choline, serine, or ethanolamine. Phospholipids are primarily located in the membranes of cells in the body and the globule membranes in milk. A very small amount of dietary fat occurs as phospholipid. The metabolism of phospholipids is described below for total fat. The various fatty acids that are contained in phospholipids are the same as those present in triglycerides.

Saturated Fatty Acids

The majority of dietary saturated fatty acids come from animal products such as meat and dairy products (USDA, 1996). The remaining comes from plant sources. These sources provide a series of saturated fatty acids for which the major dietary fatty acids range in chain length from 8 to 18 carbon atoms. These are:

- 8:0   Caprylic acid
- 10:0   Caproic acid
- 12:0   Lauric acid
- 14:0   Myristic acid
- 16:0   Palmitic acid
- 18:0   Stearic acid

The saturated fatty acids are not only a source of body fuel, but are also structural components of cell membranes. Various saturated fatty acids are also associated with proteins and are necessary for their normal function. Saturated fatty acids can be synthesized by the body.

Fats in general, including saturated fatty acids, play a role in providing desirable texture and palatability to foods used in the diet. Palmitic acid is particularly useful for enhancing the organoleptic properties of fats used in commercial products. Stearic acid, in contrast, has physical properties that limit the amount that can be incorporated into dietary fat.

Cis *Monounsaturated Fatty Acids*

Cis monounsaturated fatty acids are characterized by having one double bond with the hydrogen atoms present on the same side of the double bond. Typically, plant sources rich in *cis* monounsaturated fatty acids (e.g., canola oil, olive oil, and the high oleic safflower and sunflower oils) are liquid at room temperature. Monounsaturated fatty acids are present in foods with a double bond located at 7 (*n*-7) or 9 (*n*-9) carbon atoms from the methyl end. Monounsaturated fatty acids that are present in the diet include:

- 18:1*n*-9　Oleic acid
- 14:1*n*-7　Myristoleic acid
- 16:1*n*-7　Palmitoleic acid
- 18:1*n*-7　Vaccenic acid
- 20:1*n*-9　Eicosenoic acid
- 22:1*n*-9　Erucic acid

Oleic acid accounts for about 92 percent of dietary monounsaturated fatty acids. Monounsaturated fatty acids, including oleic acid and nervonic acid (24:1*n*-9), are important in membrane structural lipids, particularly nervous tissue myelin. Other monounsaturated fatty acids, such as palmitoleic acid, are present in minor amounts in the diet.

n-6 *Polyunsaturated Fatty Acids*

The primary *n*-6 polyunsaturated fatty acids are:

- 18:2　　Linoleic acid
- 18:3　　γ-Linolenic acid
- 20:3　　Dihomo-γ-linolenic acid
- 20:4　　Arachidonic acid
- 22:4　　Adrenic acid
- 22:5　　Docosapentaenoic acid

Linoleic acid cannot be synthesized by humans and a lack of it results in adverse clinical symptoms, including a scaly rash and reduced growth. Therefore, linoleic acid is essential in the diet. Linoleic acid is the precursor to arachidonic acid, which is the substrate for eicosanoid production in tissues, is a component of membrane structural lipids, and is also important in cell signaling pathways. Dihomo-γ-linolenic acid, also formed from linoleic acid, is also an eicosanoid precursor. *n*-6 Polyunsaturated fatty acids also play critical roles in normal epithelial cell function (Jones and

Kubow, 1999). Arachidonic acid and other unsaturated fatty acids are involved with regulation of gene expression resulting in decreased expression of proteins that regulate the enzymes involved with fatty acid synthesis (Ou et al., 2001). This may partly explain the ability of unsaturated fatty acids to influence the hepatic synthesis of fatty acids.

n-3 Polyunsaturated Fatty Acids

n-3 Polyunsaturated fatty acids tend to be highly unsaturated with one of the double bonds located at 3 carbon atoms from the methyl end. This group includes:

- 18:3   α-Linolenic acid
- 20:5   Eicosapentaenoic acid
- 22:5   Docosapentaenoic acid
- 22:6   Docosahexaenoic acid

α-Linolenic acid is not synthesized by humans and a lack of it results in adverse clinical symptoms, including neurological abnormalities and poor growth. Therefore, α-linolenic acid is essential in the diet. It is the precursor for synthesis of eicosapentaenoic acid (EPA) and docosahexaenoic acid (DHA), which are formed in varying amounts in animal tissues, especially fatty fish, but not in plant cells. EPA is the precursor of n-3 eicosanoids, which have been shown to have beneficial effects in preventing coronary heart disease, arrhythmias, and thrombosis (Kinsella et al., 1990).

Trans Fatty Acids

Trans fatty acids are unsaturated fatty acids that contain at least one double bond in the trans configuration. The trans double-bond configuration results in a larger bond angle than the cis configuration, which in turn results in a more extended fatty acid carbon chain more similar to that of saturated fatty acids rather than that of cis unsaturated, double-bond–containing fatty acids. The conformation of the double bond impacts on the physical properties of the fatty acid. Those fatty acids containing a trans double bond have the potential for closer packing or aligning of acyl chains, resulting in decreased mobility; hence fluidity is reduced when compared to fatty acids containing a cis double bond. Partial hydrogenation of polyunsaturated oils causes isomerization of some of the remaining double bonds and migration of others, resulting in an increase in the trans fatty acid content and the hardening of fat. Hydrogenation of oils, such as corn oil, can result in both cis and trans double bonds anywhere between carbon 4 and carbon 16. A major trans fatty acid is elaidic acid (9-trans 18:1).

During hydrogenation of polyunsaturated fatty acids, small amounts of several other *trans* fatty acids (9-*trans*,12-*cis* 18:2; 9-*cis*,12-*trans* 18:2) are produced. In addition to these isomers, dairy fat and meats contain 9-*trans* 16:1 and conjugated dienes (9-*cis*,11-*trans* 18:2). The *trans* fatty acid content in foods tends to be higher in foods containing hydrogenated oils (Emken, 1995).

Conjugated Linoleic Acid

Conjugated linoleic acid (CLA) is a collective term for a group of geometric and positional isomers of linoleic acid in which the *trans*/*cis* double bonds are conjugated; that is, the double bonds occur without an intervening carbon atom not part of a double bond. At least nine different isomers of CLA have been reported as minor constituents of food (Ha et al., 1989), but only two of the isomers, *cis*-9,*trans*-11 and *trans*-10,*cis*-12, possess biological activity (Pariza et al., 2001). There is limited evidence to suggest that the *trans*-10,*cis*-12 isomer reduces the uptake of lipids by the adipocyte, and that the *cis*-9,*trans*-11 isomer is active in inhibiting carcinogenesis. Similarly, there are limited data to show that *cis*-9,*trans*-11 and *trans*-10,*cis*-12 isomers inhibit atherogenesis (Kritchevsky et al., 2000).

CLA is naturally present in dairy products and ruminant meats as a consequence of biohydrogenation in the rumen. *Butyrivibrio fibrisolvens*, a ruminant microorganism, is responsible for the production of the *cis*-9,*trans*-11 CLA isomer that is synthesized as a result of the biohydrogenation of linoleic acid (Noble et al., 1974). The *cis*-9,*trans*-11 CLA isomer may be directly absorbed or further metabolized to *trans*-11 octadecenoic acid (vaccenic acid) (Pariza et al., 2001). After absorption, vaccenic acid can then be converted back to *cis*-9,*trans*-11 CLA within mammalian cells by Δ9 desaturase (Adlof et al., 2000; Chin et al., 1994; Griinari et al., 2000; Santora et al., 2000). Additionally, the biohydrogenation of several other polyunsaturated fatty acids has been shown to produce vaccenic acid as an intermediate (Griinari and Bauman, 1999), thus providing additional substrate for the endogenous production of *cis*-9,*trans*-11 CLA. Griinari and coworkers (2000) estimate that approximately 64 percent of the CLA in cow's milk is of endogenous origin.

Verhulst and coworkers (1987) isolated a microorganism, *Propionibacterium acnes*, that appears to have the ability to convert linoleic acid to *trans*-10,*cis*-12 CLA, an isomer of CLA that is found in rumen digesta (Fellner et al., 1999). *Trans*-10 octadecenoic acid is formed in the rumen via biohydrogenation of *trans*-10,*cis*-12 CLA, and both have been reported to be found in cow's milk (Griinari and Bauman, 1999). However, endogenous production of *trans*-10,*cis*-12 CLA from *trans*-10 octadecenoic acid does not occur because mammalian cells do not possess the Δ12 desaturase enzyme (Adlof et al., 2000; Pariza et al., 2001). Therefore, any *trans*-10,*cis*-12 CLA isomer that is reported in mammalian tissue or sera would likely originate from gastrointestinal absorption.

Physiology of Absorption, Metabolism, and Excretion

Total Fat

Absorption. Dietary fat undergoes lipolysis by lipases in the gastrointestinal tract prior to absorption. Although there are lipases in the saliva and gastric secretion, most lipolysis occurs in the small intestine. The hydrolysis of triacylglycerol is achieved through the action of pancreatic lipase, which requires colipase, also secreted by the pancreas, for activity. In the intestine, fat is emulsified with bile salts and phospholipids secreted into the intestine in bile, hydrolyzed by pancreatic enzymes, and almost completely absorbed. Pancreatic lipase has high specificity for the *sn*-1 and *sn*-3 positions of dietary triacylglycerols, resulting in the release of free fatty acids from the *sn*-1 and *sn*-3 positions and 2-monoacylglycerol. These products of digestion are absorbed into the enterocyte, and the triacylglycerols are reassembled, largely via the 2-monoacylglycerol pathway. This pathway conserves the fatty acid at the *sn*-2 position. The triacylglycerols are then assembled together with cholesterol, phospholipid, and apoproteins into chylomicrons. Following absorption, fatty acids of carbon chain length 12 or less may be transported as unesterified fatty acids bound to albumin directly to the liver via the portal vein, rather than acylated into triacylglycerols.

Dietary phospholipids are hydrolyzed by pancreatic phospholipase A_2 and cholesterol esters by pancreatic cholesterol ester hydrolase. The lysophospholipids are re-esterified and packaged together with cholesterol and triacylglycerols in intestinal lipoproteins or transported as lysophospholipid via the portal system to the liver.

Chylomicrons enter the circulation through the thoracic duct. These particles enter the circulation and within the capillaries of muscle and adipose tissue. Chylomicrons come into contact with the enzyme lipoprotein lipase, which is located on the surface of capillaries. Activation of lipoprotein lipase apolipoprotein CII, an apoprotein present on chylomicrons, results in the hydrolysis of the chylomicron triacylglycerol fatty acids. Most of the fatty acids released in this process are taken up by adipose tissue and re-esterified into triacylglycerol for storage. Triacylglycerol fatty acids also are taken up by muscle and oxidized for energy or are released into the systemic circulation and returned to the liver.

Metabolism. Most newly absorbed fatty acids enter adipose tissue for storage as triacylglycerol. However, in the postabsorptive state or during exercise when fat is needed for fuel, adipose tissue triacylglycerol undergoes lipolysis and free fatty acids are released into the circulation. Hydrolysis occurs via the action of the adipose tissue enzyme hormone-sensitive lipase. The activity of this lipase is suppressed by insulin. When plasma insulin concentrations fall in the postabsorptive state, hormone-sensitive lipase is activated to release more free fatty acids into the circulation. Thus, in the postabsorptive state, free fatty acid concentrations in plasma are high; conversely, in the postprandial state, hormone-sensitive lipase activity is suppressed and free fatty acid concentrations in plasma are low.

Free fatty acids circulate in the blood bound to albumin. The major site of fatty acid oxidation is skeletal muscle. When free fatty acid concentrations are relatively high, muscle uptake of fatty acids is also high. As in liver, fatty acids in the muscle are transported via a carnitine-dependent pathway into mitochondria where they undergo β-oxidation, which involves removal of two carbon fragments. These two carbon units enter the citric acid cycle as acetyl coenzyme A (CoA), through which they are completely oxidized to carbon dioxide with the generation of large quantities of high-energy phosphate bonds, or they condense to form ketone bodies. Muscle can oxidize both fatty acids and glucose for energy. However, the uptake of fatty acids in excess of the needs for oxidation for energy by muscle does result in temporary storage as triacylglycerol (Bessesen et al., 1995). High uptake of fatty acids by skeletal muscle also reduces glucose uptake by muscle and glucose oxidation (Pan et al., 1997; Roden et al., 1996).

Fatty acids released from adipose tissue or to a lesser extent during hydrolysis of chylomicron and very low density lipoprotein (VLDL) triacylglycerols are also taken up and oxidized by the liver. Oxidation of fatty acids containing up to 18 carbon atoms occurs mainly in the mitochondria. Oxidation of excess fatty acids in the liver, which occurs in prolonged fasting and with high intakes of medium-chain fatty acids, results in formation of large amounts of acetyl CoA that exceed the capacity for entry to the citric acid cycle. These 2-carbon acetyl CoA units condense to form ketone bodies (e.g., acetoacetate and β-hydroxybutyrate) that are released into the circulation. During starvation or prolonged low carbohydrate intake, ketone bodies can become an important alternate energy substrate to glucose for the brain and muscle. High dietary intakes of medium-chain fatty acids also result in the generation of ketone bodies. This is explained by the carnitine-independent influx of medium-chain fatty acids into the mitochondria, thus by-passing this regulatory step of fatty acid entry into β-oxidation. Fatty acids of greater than 18 carbon atoms require chain shortening in peroxisomes prior to mitochondrial β-oxidation.

Fatty acids that do not enter into oxidative pathways can be re-esterified into triacylglycerols or other lipids. The major pathway for triacylglycerol synthesis in liver is the 3-glycerophosphate pathway, which shows a high degree of specificity for saturated fatty acids at the *sn*-1(3) position and for unsaturated fatty acids at the *sn*-2 position. In the liver, triacylglycerols can either be stored temporarily or incorporated into triacylglycerol-rich VLDL and released into the plasma. The triacylglycerol fatty acids of VLDL have the same fate as chylomicron triacylglycerol fatty acids. When VLDL triacylglycerols undergo lipolysis, the remaining triacylglycerol-depleted particle is called a VLDL remnant. These remnants are either removed directly by the liver or they are further metabolized in the vascular compartment to form low density lipoproteins (LDL).

Excretion. Fatty acids are generally catabolized entirely by oxidative processes from which the only excretion products are carbon dioxide and water. Small amounts of ketone bodies produced by fatty acid oxidation are excreted in urine. Fatty acids are present in the cells of the skin and intestine, thus small quantities are lost when these cells are sloughed.

Saturated Fatty Acids

Absorption. When saturated fatty acids are ingested along with fats containing appreciable amounts of unsaturated fatty acids, they are absorbed almost completely by the small intestine. In general, the longer the chain length of the fatty acid, the lower will be the efficiency of absorption. However, unsaturated fatty acids are well absorbed regardless of chain length. Studies with human infants have shown the absorption to be 75, 62, 92, and 94 percent of palmitic acid, stearic acid, oleic acid, and linoleic acid, respectively, from vegetable oils (Jensen et al., 1986). The absorption of palmitic acid and stearic acid from human milk is higher than from cow milk and vegetable oils (which are commonly used in infant formulas) because of the specific positioning of these long-chain saturated fatty acids at the *sn*-2 position of milk triacylglycerols (Carnielli et al., 1996a; Jensen, 1999). The intestinal absorption of palmitic acid and stearic acid from vegetable oils was 75 to 78 percent compared with 91 to 97 percent from fats with these fatty acids in the *sn*-2 position (Carnielli et al., 1996a). Still, absorption of stearic acid was over 90 percent complete in healthy adults when contained in triacylglycerols of mixed fatty acids (Bonanome and Grundy, 1989). Long-chain saturated fatty acids released into the lumen through the action of pancreatic lipase are less readily solubilized into mixed micelles than are unsaturated fatty acids; in the alkaline pH of the intestine they can form insoluble soaps with calcium and other divalent cations and can be excreted (Carnielli et al., 1996a; Lucas et al., 1997; Tomarelli et al., 1968). Following absorption, long-chain saturated fatty acids are re-esterified along with other fatty acids into triacylglycerols and released in chylomicrons. Medium-chain saturated fatty acids (C8:0 and C10:0) are absorbed and transported bound to albumin as free fatty acids in the portal circulation and cleared by the liver. About two-thirds of lauric acid (C12:0) is transported with chylomicron triacylglycerols, whereas the remaining one-third enters the portal circulation as free fatty acids.

Metabolism. Pathways of oxidation of saturated fatty acids are similar to those for other types of fatty acids (see earlier section, "Total Fat"). Unoxidized stearic acid (9 to 14 percent) is rapidly desaturated and converted to the monounsaturated fatty acid, oleic acid (Emken, 1994; Rhee et al., 1997). For this reason, dietary stearic acid has metabolic effects that are closer to those of oleic acid rather than those of other long-chain saturated fatty acids. The saturated fatty acids, in contrast to *cis* mono- or polyunsaturated fatty acids, have a unique property in that they suppress the expression of LDL receptors (Spady et al., 1993). Through this action, dietary saturated fatty acids raise serum LDL cholesterol concentrations (Mustad et al., 1997).

Excretion. Saturated fatty acids, like other fatty acids, are generally completely oxidized to carbon dioxide and water.

cis-*Monounsaturated Fatty Acids*

Absorption. The absorption of *cis*-monounsaturated fatty acids (based on oleic acid data) is in excess of 90 percent in adults and infants (Jensen et al., 1986; Jones et al., 1985). The pathways of *cis*-monounsaturated fat digestion and absorption are similar to those of other fatty acids (see earlier section, "Total Fat").

Metabolism. Oleic acid, the major monounsaturated fatty acid in the body, is derived mainly from the diet. Small amounts also come from desaturation of stearic acid. Stable isotope tracer methods have shown that approximately 9 to 14 percent of dietary stearic acid is converted to oleic acid in vivo (Emken, 1994; Rhee et al., 1997). Based on the amount of stearic acid in the average diet (approximately 3 percent of energy), desaturation of dietary stearic acid is not a main source of oleic acid in the body. Oleic acid is oxidized, as are all other fatty acids, by β-oxidation. However, there is some evidence that oxidation of chylomicron-derived oleic acid is significantly greater than for palmitic acid (Schmidt et al.,

1999). The metabolic implications of the differential rates of oxidation of saturated, monounsaturated, and *cis* n-6 and n-3 fatty acids are not clear.

Excretion. Because oleic acid is highly absorbed, little is excreted. As for other fatty acids, the oxidation of monounsaturated fatty acids results in production of carbon dioxide and water.

n-6 *Polyunsaturated Fatty Acids*

Absorption. The digestion and absorption of *n*-6 fatty acids is efficient and occurs via the same pathways as that of other long-chain fatty acids (see earlier section, "Total Fat").

Metabolism. Both saturated and *n*-9 monounsaturated fatty acids can be synthesized from the carbon moieties of carbohydrate and protein. Mammalian cells do not have the enzymatic ability to insert a *cis* double bond at the *n*-6 position of a fatty acid chain, thus *n*-6 fatty acids are essential nutrients. The parent fatty acid of the *n*-6 series is linoleic acid. Studies using isotopically labeled linoleic acid have shown that adults and newborn infants can desaturate and elongate linoleic acid to form arachidonic acid (Emken et al., 1998, 1999; Salem et al., 1996; Sauerwald et al., 1997). The elongation of linoleic acid involves the sequential addition of two carbon units and desaturation involves insertion of a methylene-interrupted double bond towards the carboxyl terminus, thus preserving the position of the first *n*-6 double bond. These longer-chain, more polyunsaturated *n*-6 fatty acids are found primarily in membrane phospholipids, and since they can be formed only in animal cells, arachidonic acid is present in the diet only in animal tissue lipids.

Recent studies using stable isotopically labeled fatty acids to investigate the effect of gestational age and intrauterine growth on essential fatty acid desaturation and elongation have shown that the conversion of linoleic to arachidonic acid occurs as early as 26 weeks of gestation, and is in fact more active at earlier gestational ages (Uauy et al., 2000a). In addition to its role as a precursor to dihomo-γ-linolenic acid and arachidonic acid, linoleic acid has a specific role in acylceramides, which are important in maintaining the epidermal water barrier (Hansen and Jensen, 1985).

The 18 and 20 carbon *n*-9, *n*-6, and *n*-3 fatty acids compete for a common Δ6 and Δ5 desaturase. In vitro studies have shown the Δ6 desaturase enzymes preference occurs in the order 18:3*n*-3 > 18:2*n*-6 > 18:1*n*-9 (Brenner, 1974; Castuma et al., 1977). The formation of arachidonic acid and *n*-3 fatty acid metabolites also appears to be inhibited by the products of the reaction and by high amounts of substrate. Thus, high intakes of *n*-3 fatty acids or arachidonic and linoleic acids will reduce the efficiency of conversion of linoleic acid to arachidonic acid and α-linolenic acid to its products (Emken et al., 1994, 1998, 1999). For example, Emken and coworkers (1994) reported that an intake of 30 g/d of linoleic acid resulted in a 40 to 54 percent lower conversion of stable isotopically labeled linoleic and α-linolenic acid to their metabolites compared to an intake of 15 g/d in healthy men. High dietary intakes of n-3 fatty acids result in reduced tissue arachidonic acid concentrations and synthesis of arachidonic acid-derived eicosanoids, with consequent effects on the balance of n-6 and n-3 fatty acid-derived eicosanoids that are produced. The reduction in arachidonic acid-derived eicosanoids due to high n-3 fatty acid intake involves effects on pathways of eicosanoid formation, in addition to reducing concentrations of precursor arachidonic acid availability.

Both the rate of oxidation to carbon dioxide and water and the acylation into different lipids differ among fatty acids of different chain length and unsaturation. Arachidonic acid is primarily found in tissue phospholipids, rather than in triacylglycerols or cholesterol esters. Retroconversion of adrenic acid to arachidonic acid occurs through cleavage of a 2-carbon unit from the carboxyl end of the fatty acid and may be important in maintaining adequate tissue concentrations of arachidonic acid. Besides being elongated to longer-chain fatty acids, arachidonic acid is the precursor to a number of eicosanoids (prostaglandins, thromboxanes, and leukotienes) that are involved in platelet aggregation, hemodynamics, and coronary vascular tone, which can have an effect on the onset of atherogenesis and coronary infarction (Kinsella et al., 1990).

Excretion. n-6 Fatty acids are almost completely absorbed and are either incorporated into tissue lipids, utilized in eicosanoid synthesis, or oxidized to carbon dioxide and water. Small amounts are lost during sloughing of cells from skin and other epithelial membranes.

n-3 Polyunsaturated Fatty Acids

Absorption. The digestion and absorption of n-3 fatty acids is similar to that of other long-chain fatty acids.

Metabolism. Humans are unable to insert a double bond at the n-3 position (*cis* 15) of a fatty acid of 18 carbons in length, and thus require a dietary source of n-3 fatty acids. The n-3 fatty acids cannot be formed from saturated, n-9 monounsaturated, or n-6 polyunsaturated fatty acids. The parent fatty acid of the n-3 series is α-linolenic acid, which can be further metabolized by elongation and desaturation to longer-chain, more highly unsaturated metabolites using the same pathway and enzymes as those used for the n-6 fatty acids. α-Linolenic acid is desaturated by Δ6 desaturase, elongated, and then desaturated by Δ5 desaturase to form EPA, which is the precursor for series 3 eicosanoids and series 5 leukotrienes. The pathway leading from EPA to more highly unsaturated fatty acids involves the addition of two 2-carbon units, then a second Δ6 desaturation, after which the 24-carbon-chain fatty acid is transported to the peroxisomes and converted to DHA through one step of β-oxidation (Sprecher et al., 1995; Voss et al., 1991). DHA is a component of membrane structural lipids that are enriched in certain phospholipids, such as the ethanolamine phosphoglycerides and phosphatidylserine in nervous tissue, retina, and spermatozoa. α-Linolenic acid is not known to have any specific functions other than to serve as a precursor for synthesis of EPA and DHA.

High dietary intakes of EPA and DHA result in decreased tissue concentrations of arachidonic acid and increased concentrations of EPA and DHA, respectively. This results in changes in the balance of eicosanoids synthesized from the n-6 and n-3 fatty acids. The ability to convert α-linolenic acid to EPA and DHA differs among mammalian species. Studies using isotopically labeled α-linolenic acid, however, have shown that adults and newborn infants can desaturate and elongate α-linolenic acid to form DHA (Carnielli et al., 1996b; Salem et al., 1996; Sauerwald et al., 1996, 1997; Uauy et al., 2000a; Vermunt et al., 2000). Recent studies with infants have shown that the rates of conversion of α-linolenic acid to DHA appear to be higher in preterm infants and decrease with increasing gestational age (Uauy et al., 2000a). These types of studies have also shown that high intakes of α-linolenic acid result in reduced conversion to DHA (Vermunt et al., 2000).

Whereas the retroconversion of adrenic acid to maintain tissue arachidonic acid requires the removal of only a single 2-carbon unit, the retroconversion of DHA to EPA is more complex and involves the removal of the double bond at the Δ4 position, in addition to a 2-carbon unit. Supplementation with DHA is accompanied by an increase in EPA, which could be explained by retroconversion of DHA to EPA or by inhibition of further metabolism of EPA formed from α-linolenic acid (Brossard et al., 1996; Conquer and Holub, 1996; Nelson et al., 1997; Vidgren et al., 1997).

Excretion. n-3 Fatty acids are almost completely absorbed and either oxidized to carbon dioxide and water, incorporated into tissue lipids, or utilized in eicosanoid synthesis. Small amounts of n-3 fatty acids are lost during sloughing of skin and other epithelial cells.

Trans *Fatty Acids*

Absorption. As with other fatty acids, the coefficient of absorption of elaidic acid (18:1*t*) is about 95 percent (Emken, 1979). Studies in humans using pure triacylglycerols containing deuterated *cis* and *trans* octadecenoic acid isomers varying in melting point and double bond position suggest that the presence of *trans* double bonds in the fatty acyl chain has no measurable effect on efficiency of absorption (Emken, 1979, 1984).

Transport. *Trans* fatty acids are transported similarly to other dietary fatty acids and are distributed within the cholesteryl ester, triacylglycerol, and phospholipid fractions of lipoproteins (Vidgren et al., 1998). Platelet lipids also contain *trans* fatty acids and their composition reflects *trans* fatty acid intake, as do other tissues (except the brain) (Mensink and Hornstra, 1995).

Metabolism. The *trans* isomers of oleic acid and linoleic acid that are formed during partial hydrogenation of unsaturated vegetable oils have been suggested to have potential adverse effects on fetal and infant growth and development through inhibition of the desaturation of linoleic acid and α-linolenic acid to arachidonic acid and DHA, respectively (Koletzko, 1992; van Houwelingen and Hornstra, 1994). Many animal and in vitro studies, however, have involved much higher amounts of *trans* than all-*cis* polyunsaturated fatty acids (Hwang et al., 1982; Shimp et al., 1982). Other animal studies have suggested that the deleterious effects seen with high intakes of *trans* fatty acid do not occur with amounts comparable to those consumed in a normal human diet containing sufficient amounts of linoleic acid (Bruckner et al., 1982; Zevenbergen et al., 1988).

Available animal and human data indicate that adipose tissue *trans* fatty acid content reflects the content of the diet and that selective accumulation does not occur (Emken, 1984). More recent attention has been focused on validating the use of adipose *trans* fatty acid content as a measure of long-term dietary intake. In a study of Canadian individuals, Chen and colleagues (1995b) reported that adipose tissue *trans* fatty acid patterns, particularly those isomers found in partially hydrogenated vegetable fat, reflected dietary sources. Garland and coworkers (1998) also reported that adipose tissue *trans* fatty acid patterns correlated with intake and noted a stronger relationship with the isomers found in vegetable fat rather than animal fat. The authors cautioned that the later conclusion may have been due to the smaller between-person variability with animal versus vegetable *trans* fatty acid intake. In a letter to the editor regarding this study, Aro and Salminen (1998) suggested that the stronger correlation between adipose tissue *trans* fatty acid isomers found in hydrogenated vegetable fat rather than animal fat may be attributable to different rates of metabolism of the *trans* isomers. Two groups have used adipose tissue *trans* fatty acid to corroborate dietary *trans* fatty acid intake derived from food frequency questionnaires and found a strong relationship (Lemaitre et al., 1998; London et al., 1991). Despite these observations, it should be noted that adipose tissue *trans* fatty acid profiles can be confounded by the retention of intermediate products of β-oxidation (Emken, 1995).

Excretion. *Trans* fatty acids are completely catabolized to carbon dioxide and water.

Clinical Effects of Inadequate Intakes

Total Fat

Impaired Growth. Dietary fat is a major source of body fuel. If intakes of fat, along with carbohydrate and protein, are inadequate to meet energy needs, the individual will be in negative energy balance. Depending on the severity and duration, this may lead to malnutrition or starvation. In an energy-sufficient diet, carbohydrate can replace fat as a source of energy. In some populations, fat intakes are very low and body weight and health are maintained by high intakes of carbohydrate (Bunker et al., 1996; Falase et al., 1973; Shintani et al., 2001). Clearly, humans have the ability to adapt metabolically to a wide spectrum of fat-to-carbohydrate intake ratios. In the short term, an isocaloric diet can be either very high or very low in fat with no obvious differences in health. The critical question therefore is, Are there optimal fat-to-carbohydrate ratios for long-term health, and if so, what are they? One potential concern over fat restriction is the potential for reduction in total energy intake, which is of particular relevance for infants and children, as well as during pregnancy when there is a relatively high energy requirement for both energy expenditure and for fetal development. Chapter 11 provides a detailed discussion on fat intake and growth.

Increased Risk of Chronic Diseases. Compared to higher fat intakes, low fat, high carbohydrate diets may modify the metabolic profile in ways that are considered to be unfavorable with respect to chronic diseases such as coronary heart disease (CHD) and diabetes (see Chapters 6 and 11). These changes include a reduction in high density lipoprotein cholesterol concentration, an increase in serum triacylglycerol concentration, and higher responses in postprandial glucose and insulin concentrations. This metabolic pattern has been associated with increased risk for CHD and type 2 diabetes in intervention and prospective studies (see Chapter 11). Although changes in the metabolic profile do occur, strong evidence that low fat diets actually predispose to either CHD or diabetes does not exist. In fact, some populations that consume low fat diets and in which habitual energy intake is relatively high have a low prevalence of these chronic diseases (Falase et al., 1973; Shintani et al., 2001). Similarly, populations with high fat diets (i.e., $\geq$ 40 percent of energy) and a low prevalence of chronic diseases often include people who engage in heavy physical labor, are lean, and have a low family history of chronic diseases. Conversely, in sedentary populations, such as that of the United States where overweight and obesity are common, high carbohydrate, low fat diets induce changes in lipoprotein and glucose/insulin metabolism in ways that could raise risk for chronic diseases (see Chapter 11). Available prospective studies have not concluded whether low fat, high carbohydrate diets provide a health risk in the North American population.

Chronic nonspecific diarrhea in children has been suggested as a potential adverse effect of low fat diets. It is considered a disorder of intestinal motility that may improve with an increase in dietary fat intake in order to slow gastric emptying and alter intestinal motility (Cohen et al., 1979). Detailed discussion on fat intake and risk of chronic disease is provided in Chapter 11.

n-6 Polyunsaturated Fatty Acids

Certain polyunsaturated fatty acids were first identified as being essential in rats fed diets almost completely devoid of fat (Burr and Burr, 1929). Subsequently, studies in infants and children fed skimmed cow milk (Hansen et al., 1958, 1963) and patients receiving parenteral nutrition without an adequate source of essential fatty acids (Collins et al., 1971; Holman et al., 1982; Paulsrud et al., 1972) demonstrated clinical symptoms of a deficiency in humans. Because adipose tissue lipids in free-living, healthy adults contain about 10 percent of total fatty acids as linoleic acid, biochemical and clinical signs of essential fatty acid deficiency do not appear during dietary fat restriction or malabsorption when they are accompanied by an energy deficit. In this situation, release of linoleic acid and small amounts of arachidonic acid from adipose tissue reserves may prevent development of essential fatty acid deficiency. However, during parenteral nutrition with dextrose solutions, insulin concentrations are high and mobilization of adipose tissue is prevented, resulting in development of the characteristic signs of essential fatty acid deficiency. Studies on patients given fat-free parenteral feeding have provided great insight into defining levels at which essential fatty acid deficiency may occur. Without intervention, these patients develop clinical signs of a deficiency in 2 to 4 weeks (Fleming et al., 1976; Goodgame et al., 1978; Jeppesen et al., 1998; Riella et al., 1975). In rapidly growing infants, feeding with milk containing very low amounts of n-6 fatty acids results in characteristic signs of an essential fatty acid deficiency and elevated plasma triene:tetraene ratios (see "n-6:n-3 Polyunsaturated Fatty Acid Ratio").

When dietary essential fatty acid intake is inadequate or absorption is impaired, tissue concentrations of arachidonic acid decrease, inhibition of the desaturation of oleic acid is reduced, and synthesis of eicosatrienoic acid from oleic acid increases. The characteristic signs of deficiency attributed to the n-6 fatty acids are scaly skin rash, increased transepidermal water loss, reduced growth, and elevation of the plasma ratio of eicosatrienoic acid:arachidonic acid ($20:3n$-$9:20:4n$-6) to values greater than 0.4 (Goodgame et al., 1978; Holman, 1960; Jeppesen et al., 2000; Mascioli et al., 1996; O'Neill et al., 1977). Other studies have utilized a ratio of 0.2 as indicative of an essential fatty acid deficiency (Holman et al., 1991; Jeppesen et al., 1998). In addition to the clinical signs mentioned above, essential fatty acid deficiency in special populations has been linked to hematologic disturbances and diminished immune response (Bistrian et al., 1981; Boissonneault and Johnston, 1983). Further discussion on this topic is included in "Findings by Life Stage and Gender Group—n-6 Polyunsaturated Fatty Acids."

n-3 Polyunsaturated Fatty Acids

Tissue levels of arachidonic acid, as well as the amounts of arachidonic acid and EPA- derived eicosanoids that are formed, have important effects on many physiological processes (e.g., platelet aggregation, vessel wall constriction, and immune cell function) via the biosynthesis of eicosanoids. Thus, the amount of n-3 fatty acids and their effects on arachidonic acid metabolism are relevant to many chronic diseases. EPA also appears to have specific effects on fatty acid metabolism, resulting in inhibition of hepatic triacylglycerol synthesis and VLDL secretion (Berge et al., 1999; Wong and Nestel, 1987). DHA, on the other hand, is highly enriched in specific phospholipids of the retina and nonmyelin membranes of the nervous system.

Studies in rodents and nonhuman primates have consistently demonstrated that prolonged feeding with diets containing very low amounts of α-linolenic acid result in reductions of visual acuity thresholds and electroretinogram A and B wave recordings, which were prevented when α-linolenic acid was included in the diet (Anderson et al., 1974; Benolken et al., 1973; Bourre et al., 1989; Neuringer et al., 1984, 1986; Wheeler et al., 1975). A variety of changes in learning behaviors in animals fed α-linolenic acid-deficient diets have also been reported (Innis, 1991). These studies have involved feeding oils such as safflower oil, which contains less than 0.1 percent α-linolenic acid and is high in linoleic acid, as the sole source of fat for prolonged periods. The reduction in visual function is accompanied by decreased brain and retina DHA with an increase in docosapentaenoic acid (DPA, 22:5n-6). The compensatory increase in 22 carbon chain n-6 fatty acids results in maintenance of the total amount of n-6 and n-3 polyunsaturated fatty acids in neural tissue. DPA is formed from linoleic acid by similar desaturation and elongation steps used in the synthesis of DHA from α-linolenic acid. However, α-linolenic acid is clearly handled differently from linoleic acid. For example, rates of β-oxidation of α-linolenic acid are much higher than for linoleic acid (Clouet et al., 1989). This may suggest that immaturity or reduced enzyme activity is unlikely to explain lower DHA in the brain of young animals fed diets with low amounts of α-linolenic acid, and that DHA has specific metabolic functions that cannot be accomplished by DPA despite its structural similarity. Stable isotope studies have shown that infants can convert linoleic acid to arachidonic acid and α-linolenic acid to DHA (Carnielli et al., 1996b; Salem et al., 1996; Sauerwald et al., 1996, 1997; Uauy et al., 2000a), with the rate of conversion apparently higher in infants of younger gestational ages (Uauy et al., 2000a).

Unlike essential fatty acid deficiency (n-6 and n-3 fatty acids), plasma eicosatrienoic acid (20:3n-9) remains within normal ranges and skin atrophy and scaly dermatitis are absent when the diet is deficient in only n-3 fatty acids. Tissue concentrations of 22-carbon chain n-6 fatty acids increase, and DHA concentration decreases with a prolonged dietary deficiency of n-3 fatty acids accompanied by adequate n-6 fatty acids. Currently, there are no accepted plasma n-3 fatty acid or n-3 fatty acid-derived eicosanoid concentrations for indicating impaired neural function or impaired health endpoints. Further discussion on this topic is included in the next section.

EVIDENCE CONSIDERED FOR ESTIMATING THE REQUIREMENTS FOR TOTAL FAT AND FATTY ACIDS

Total Fat

Clinical endpoints of fat intake are trends, rather than defined endpoints, and therefore cannot be used to set an Estimated Average Requirement (EAR). The endpoints that strongly predict the relation of total fat intake to the development of chronic disease have been identified and are discussed in Chapter 11 for estimating Acceptable Macronutrient Distribution Ranges (AMDRs).

Growth

Because the amount of fat in the diet can have an impact on energy intake, a number of studies have been conducted to determine if diets containing less than 30 percent of energy from fat can impair growth of children (Boulton and Magarey, 1995; Foman et al., 1976; Lagström et al., 1999; Lapinleimu et al., 1995; Niinikoski et al., 1997a, 1997b; Obarzanek et al., 1997; Shea et al., 1993; Uauy et al., 2000b; Vobecky et al., 1995). These studies showed no effect of the level of dietary fat on growth when energy intake is adequate. Chapter 11 provides further discussion on this topic.

Fat Balance (Maintenance of Body Weight)

Because fat is an important source of energy, studies have been conducted to ascertain whether dietary fat influences energy expenditure and the amount of fat needed in the diet to achieve fat balance and therefore maintain body weight. These studies demonstrated that the amount of fat in the diet does not affect energy expenditure and thus the amount of energy required to maintain body weight (Hill et al., 1991; Leibel et al., 1992). Chapter 11 provides further discussion on this topic.

Saturated Fatty Acids

Saturated fatty acids are a potential fuel source for the body. In addition, they are important structural fatty acids for cell membranes and other functions and therefore are essential for body functions. These fatty acids, however, can be synthesized as needed for these functions from other fuel sources and have not been associated with any beneficial role in preventing chronic disease. Consequently, saturated fatty acids are not essential in the diet.

cis-Monounsaturated Fatty Acids

Monounsaturated fatty acids are a potential fuel source for the body and are a critical structural fatty acid for cell membranes and other functions. Monounsaturated fatty acids undoubtedly are required for many body functions. Nevertheless, monounsaturated fatty acids can be biosynthesized from other fuel sources and therefore are not essential in the diet.

n-6 *Polyunsaturated Fatty Acids*

Clinical signs of essential fatty acid deficiency are generally only found in patients with chronic fat malabsorption on parenteral nutrition and without an enteral or parenteral source of polyunsaturated fat. Early signs of essential fatty acid deficiency include rough and scaly skin, which if left untreated, develops into dermatitis (Jeppesen et al., 1998). In studies of patients with dermatitis who were receiving parenteral nutrition, the ratio of eicosatrienoic acid:arachidonic acid ($20:3n-9:20:4n-6$) in plasma was elevated. As described earlier, when present in adequate amounts, linoleic acid is converted to arachidonic acid through a multi-step process involving $\Delta 6$ and $\Delta 5$ desaturases (see Figure 8-1); however, in the absence of linoleic acid, $\Delta 6$ and $\Delta 5$ desaturases convert oleic acid to eicosatrienoic acid. The increase in eicosatrienoic acid concentration, which occurs in the absence of $n-6$ fatty acids or the combined absence of $n-6$ and $n-3$ fatty acids, led Holman (1960) to define a plasma triene:tetraene ratio of greater than 0.4 as evidence of essential fatty acid deficiency. More recently, a lower threshold of greater than 0.2 has been suggested (Holman et al., 1979; Jeppesen et al., 1998; Mascioli et al., 1996) because the average ratio was found to be 0.1 ± 0.08 (standard deviation) in populations of normal $n-6$ fatty acid status. Optimal plasma or tissue lipid concentrations of linoleic acid, arachidonic acid, and other $n-6$ fatty acids or the ratios of certain $n-6:n-3$ fatty acids have not been established.

Because the $n-6$ fatty acid intake is generally well above the levels needed to maintain a triene:tetraene ratio below 0.2 (even for very low fat diets), data on $n-6$ fatty acid requirements from traditional metabolic feeding studies are not available. Instead, studies with patients on total parenteral nutrition (TPN) solutions that contained very low amounts or were completely devoid of $n-6$ fatty acids have been used. In these studies, after developing an essential fatty acid deficiency, patients were treated with linoleic acid. Several case reports, small studies of two or three patients in which varying feeding designs were employed, or larger studies of patients with $n-6$ fatty acid deficiency caused by TPN have been documented (Barr et al., 1981; Collins et al., 1971; Goodgame et al., 1978; Jeppesen et al., 1998; Mascioli et al., 1979; Meng, 1983; Richardson and Sgoutas, 1975; Riella et al., 1975; Siguel et al., 1986; Wene et al., 1975; Wong and Deitel, 1981). These studies observed symptoms such as rash, scaly skin, and ectopic dermatitis; reduced serum tetraene concentrations; increased serum triene concentration; and a triene:tetraene ratio greater than 0.4 after 2 to 4 weeks of TPN. Because of the lack of data on the $n-6$ fatty acid requirement in healthy individuals, an EAR cannot be set based on correction of a deficiency.

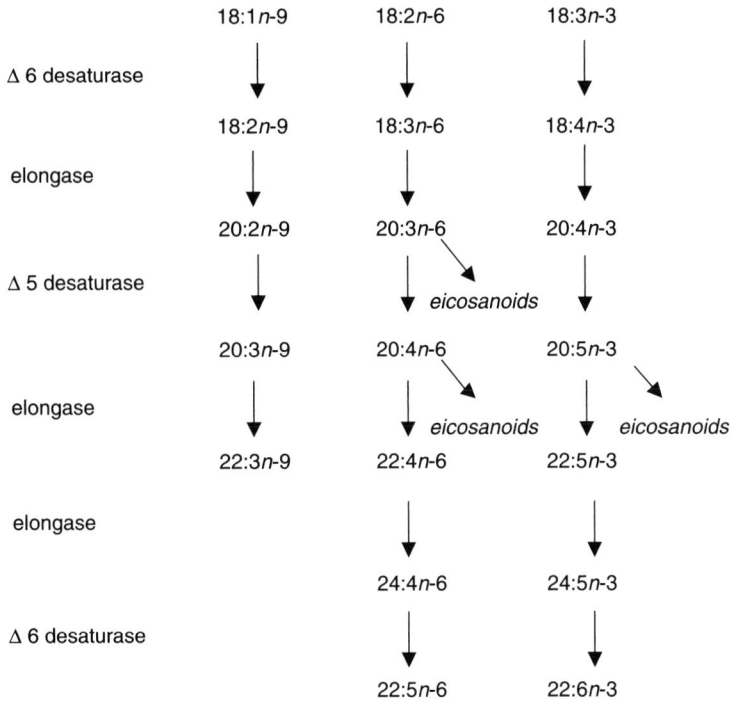

FIGURE 8-1 Biosynthesis of long-chain fatty acids.

n-3 Polyunsaturated Fatty Acids

n-3 Polyunsaturated Fatty Acid Deficiency

Some evidence for the essentiality of *n*-3 fatty acids in humans can be drawn from case reports of patients receiving parenteral nutrition with intravenous lipids containing an emulsion of safflower oil, which is very low in α-linolenic acid and high in linoleic acid. Biochemical changes of *n*-3 fatty acid deficiency include a decrease in plasma and tissue docosahexaenoic acid (DHA) concentrations. There is no accepted cut-off concentration of plasma or tissue DHA concentrations below which functions ascribed to *n*-3 fatty acids, such as visual or neural function, are impaired. Similarly, there are no accepted normal ranges for eicosapentaenoic acid (EPA) with respect to synthesis of EPA-derived eicosanoids or regulation of arachidonic acid metabolism and its eicosanoid metabolites, nor are there accepted clinical functional endpoints such as immune response.

Dietary or intravenous supplementation with oils containing α-linolenic acid, such as soybean oil, has been shown to increase red blood cell and plasma phospholipid DHA concentration in hospitalized patients with a long history of dietary n-3 fatty acid restriction (Bjerve et al., 1987a, 1987b; Holman et al., 1982). Sensory neuropathy and visual problems in a young girl given parenteral nutrition with an intravenous lipid emulsion containing only a small amount of α-linolenic acid were corrected when the emulsion was changed to one containing generous amounts of α-linolenic acid (Holman et al., 1982). Nine patients with an n-3 fatty acid deficiency had scaly and hemorrhagic dermatitis, hemorrhagic folliculitis of the scalp, impaired wound healing, and growth retardation (Bjerve, 1989). The possibility of other nutrient deficiencies, such as vitamin E and selenium, has been raised (Anderson and Connor, 1989; Meng, 1983). A series of papers have described low tissue n-3 fatty acid concentrations in nursing home patients fed by gastric tube for several years with a powdered diet formulation that provided about 0.5 to 0.6 percent of energy (0.65 to 0.86 g) as linoleic acid, and 0.02 percent of energy (30 to 50 mg) as α-linolenic acid (Bjerve et al., 1987a, 1987b). Skin lesions were resolved following supplementation with cod liver oil and soybean oil or ethyl linolenate (Bjerve et al., 1987a, 1987b). Concurrent deficiency of both n-6 and n-3 fatty acids in these patients, as in studies of patients supported by lipid-free parenteral nutrition, limits interpretation of the specific problems caused by inadequate intakes of n-3 fatty acids. Supplementation with cod liver oil and soybean oil, or feeding with a formula providing linoleic acid and α-linolenic acid or ethyl α-linolenic acid for 14 days, increased red blood cell arachidonic acid and DHA concentrations and gave some resolution of skin signs (Bjerve et al., 1987a, 1987b). Because of the lack of data on the n-3 fatty acid requirement in healthy individuals, an EAR cannot be set based on correction of a deficiency.

Growth and Neural Development

The membrane lipids of brain gray matter and the retina contain very high concentrations of DHA, particularly in the amino phospholipids phosphatidylethanolamine and phosphatidylserine. In these tissues, the concentration of DHA can exceed 50 percent of the fatty acids resulting in the presence of di-DHA phospholipid species. During n-3 fatty acid deficiency, DHA is tenaciously retained, thus most animal studies investigating the importance of n-3 fatty acids have used rats deprived of n-3 fatty acids for two or more generations. Small amounts of DHA are also present in cell membranes throughout the body. In these tissues, the phospholipid sn-1 chain is usually a saturated fatty acid (e.g., 16:0) and DHA is found on the sn-2 position. The developing brain accumulates large amounts of DHA during pre- and postnatal development and this accumulation continues throughout the first two years after birth (Martinez, 1992). Evidence from autopsy analysis indicates that accumulation of DHA in the retina is complete by term birth (Martinez et al., 1988). Due to the accumulation of DHA during brain growth, the developing brain is more susceptible to n-3 fatty acid deficiency than the mature brain. However, the presence of DHA within the membrane hydrophobic interior can influence membrane order (fluidity), thickness, domain size, hydration, and permeability and activity of associated proteins and ion channels. Unesterified DHA also regulates the expression of a variety of genes and influences cell signaling mechanisms (Salem et al., 2001; Sinclair et al., 2000). Animal studies have shown that feeding a diet very low in α-linolenic acid results in reduced brain and retina DHA concentration, which is accompanied by reduced visual function and behavior in learning tasks (Benolken et al., 1973; Bourre et al., 1989; Neuringer et al., 1984; Wheeler et al., 1975). The decrease in DHA concentration in the brain and retina is compensated for by an increase in the n-6 fatty acid docosapentaenoic acid, and this leads to maintenance of the total polyunsaturated fatty acid content of the membrane. Reduced growth or changes in food intake have not been noted in the extensive number of studies in animals, including nonhuman primates fed for extended periods on otherwise adequate diets lacking n-3 fatty acids.

The essential role of α-linolenic acid appears to be its role as precursor for synthesis of EPA and DHA. Thus, the dietary n-3 fatty acid requirement involves the activity of the desaturase enzymes and factors that influence the desaturation of α-linolenic acid in addition to the amount of the n-3 fatty acid. The questions of whether term gestation infants can form DHA, or if DHA is required in the infant diet, has been studied extensively. Activity of $\Delta 6$ and $\Delta 5$ desaturases has been demonstrated in human fetal tissue from as early as 17 to 18 weeks of gestation (Chambaz et al., 1985; Rodriguez et al., 1998), and stable isotope studies have confirmed that preterm and term infants are able to convert α-linolenic acid to DHA (Carnielli et al., 1996b; Salem et al., 1996; Sauerwald et al., 1996, 1997; Uauy et al., 2000a). Furthermore, the ability to convert α-linolenic acid appears to be greater in premature infants than in older term infants (Uauy et al., 2000a), although variability among infants is large. Current information from stable isotope tracer studies does not provide quantitative whole body or organ data on the conversion of α-linolenic acid to DHA, whether the rate of conversion can meet the needs of the developing brain for DHA, or the effect of varying linoleic and α-linolenic acid intakes and ratios on conversion. Experimental studies suggest that the eye and certain brain cells, such as astrocytes, are able to synthesize DHA from α-linolenic acid (Moore et al., 1991; Wetzel et al., 1991). The contribution of synthesis of DHA in the brain and retina to the accumulation of

DHA in these organs is not known. In vivo studies, however, have shown that the brain does take up DHA from plasma (de la Presa Owens and Innis, 1999; Greiner et al., 1997).

A large number of clinical trials have been completed comparing growth, as well as measures of visual, motor, and mental development, in term infants fed formula with no DHA or with addition of DHA to approximate the amount in human milk. Some have included arachidonic acid or γ-linolenic acid (18:3n-6), the Δ6 desaturase product of linoleic acid. The results of these trials are summarized in Table 8-1. Several aspects of design are important in evaluating these studies. These include a prospective, double-blind design with a sufficient number of infants randomized to control for the multiple genetic, environmental, and dietary factors that influence infant development and to detect meaningful treatment effects (Gore, 1999; Morley, 1998); the amount and balance of linoleic and α-linolenic acid; the duration of supplementation; the age at testing and tests used; and the physiological significance of any statistical differences found. None of the studies in Table 8-1 reported differences in growth among infants fed formulas with DHA added.

Recent large, randomized trials did not find differences in visual evoked potential, visual acuity, or tests of mental and psychomotor development through at least the first 18 months in term infants fed formulas supplemented with DHA or DHA plus arachidonic acid (Auestad et al., 1997, 2001; Lucas et al., 1999; Scott et al., 1998). These studies used formulas with at least 1.1 percent α-linolenic acid and had linoleic:α-linolenic acid ratios close to 10:1. In the study by Scott and coworkers (1998), indices of early vocabulary development were lower in infants fed formula with DHA, but not in those fed formulas lacking DHA and arachidonic acid or containing both DHA and arachidonic acid. Birch and coworkers (1998, 2000) reported better visual evoked potential, but not visual acuity, and higher Bayley mental developmental indices scores in infants fed formulas with DHA or DHA plus arachidonic acid than in infants fed standard formula. Carlson and coworkers (1996a) on the other hand, found higher visual acuity at 2 months, but not at 4, 6, 9, or 12 months, in infants fed formula with DHA and arachidonic acid. Early studies by Makrides and colleagues (1995) reported better visual evoked potential acuity in infants fed formula with 0.36 percent DHA than infants given no dietary DHA. However, this group did not confirm this finding in subsequent studies with formulas containing 0.34 or 0.35 percent DHA (Makrides et al., 2000b). In addition, greater problem-solving ability has been reported among infants fed formula with DHA and arachidonic acid than in infants fed standard formula (Willatts et al., 1998).

The effect of low n-6:n-3 ratios (high n-3 fatty acids) on arachidonic acid metabolism is also of concern in growing infants. Several studies in premature infants have reported an association between feeding *n*-3 long-chain fatty acids in the absence of arachidonic acid and reduced growth (Carlson et al., 1992, 1993, 1996b; Ryan et al., 1999). Scott and coworkers (1998) reported lower indices of language development in term infants fed formula with DHA, although not in infants fed formula with both DHA and arachidonic acid or with no DHA and arachidonic acid. Human milk from women in the United States and Canada following usual diets contains both arachidonic acid and DHA, usually in the range of 1:1 to 2:1. No evidence of reduced growth or outcome on developmental tests have been reported for infants fed formulas with both arachidonic acid and DHA in amounts similar to that contained in human milk. Infants fed formula with a ratio of linoleic:α-linolenic acid of 4.8:1 and no arachidonic acid had lower growth, as well as lower plasma arachidonic acid status, than infants fed a formula with a ratio of 44:1 (Jensen et al., 1997), and no differences in growth were found between infants fed formulas containing linoleic:α-linolenic acid ratios of 9.7:1 and 18.2:1. Additionally, no differences in growth were found among infants fed formulas with 1.7 or 3.3 percent α-linolenic acid with linoleic:α-linolenic acid ratios of 10:1 or 5:1, respectively (Makrides et al., 2000a).

In conclusion, randomized clinical studies on growth or neural development with term infants fed formulas currently yield conflicting results on the requirements for *n*-3 fatty acids in young infants, but do raise concern over supplementation with long-chain *n*-3 fatty acids without arachidonic acid. For these reasons, growth and neural development could not be used to set an EAR.

Trans *Fatty Acids and Conjugated Linoleic Acid*

Small amounts of *trans* fatty acids and conjugated linoleic acid are present in all diets. They can serve as a source of fuel energy for the body. However, there are no known requirements for *trans* fatty acids and conjugated linoleic acid for specific body functions.

FACTORS AFFECTING THE REQUIREMENTS

Fat Absorption and Aging

Aging in humans has been associated with a decrease in liver size and hepatic blood flow, slightly decreased serum albumin concentrations, and normal routine liver chemistries (Russell, 1992). Pancreatic secretion after initial stimulation with either secretin or pancreozymin is not diminished with age (Bartoš and Groh, 1969). Similarly, 72-hour fecal fat excretion in response to a dietary fat challenge in young (19 to 44 years of age) and old

TABLE 8-1 Randomized Studies of *n*-3 Fatty Acids and Neural and Visual Development in Full-Term, Formula-Fed Infants

Reference	Study Population[a]	Test/Age[b]	Fatty Acid[c]
Agostoni et al., 1995	*n* = 29 formula *n* = 29 formula + LC-PUFA	Brunet-Lézine psychomotor development test 4 mo	18:2*n*-6 18:3*n*-3 18:3*n*-6 (GLA) 20:4*n*-6 (AA) 22:6*n*-3 (DHA)
Makrides et al., 1995	*n* = 14 formula *n* = 12 formula + LC-PUFA	VEP acuity 16, 30 wk	18:2*n*-6 18:3*n*-3 18:3*n*-6 (GLA) 20:4*n*-6 (AA) 22:6*n*-3 (DHA)
Carlson et al., 1996a	*n* = 20 formula *n* = 19 formula + DHA + AA	Visual acuity 2, 4, 6, 9, 12 mo	18:2*n*-6 18:3*n*-3 20:4*n*-6 (AA) 22:6*n*-3 (DHA)
Agostoni et al., 1997	*n* = 30 formula *n* = 26 formula + LC-PUFA	DQ 24 mo	18:2*n*-6 18:3*n*-3 18:3*n*-6 (GLA) 20:4*n*-6 (AA) 22:6*n*-3 (DHA)
Auestad et al., 1997	*n* = 45 formula *n* = 43 formula + DHA *n* = 46 formula + DHA + AA	Sweep VEP 2, 4, 6, 9, 12 mo Visual acuity 2, 4, 6, 9, 12 mo	18:2*n*-6 18:3*n*-3 20:4*n*-6 (AA) 22:6*n*-3 (DHA)
Jensen et al., 1997	*n* = 20 each group	VER 4 mo	18:2*n*-6 18:3*n*-3 18:2*n*-6:18:3*n*-3 ratio
Birch et al., 1998	*n* = 21 formula *n* = 20 formula + DHA *n* = 19 formula + DHA + AA	Sweep VEP acuity 6, 17, 26, 52 wk Visual acuity 6, 17, 26, 52 wk	18:2*n*-6 18:3*n*-3 20:4*n*-6 (AA) 22:6*n*-3 (DHA)

Fatty Acid Content (% of fatty acids)				Results
Formula	Formula + LC-PUFA			Infants consuming formula
11.1	10.8			supplemented with LC-PUFA
0.70	0.73			scored significantly higher than
—	0.30			standard formula group
—	0.44			
—	0.30			
Formula	Formula + LC-PUFA			VEP acuity better in infants fed
16.79	17.44			supplemented formula than in
1.58	1.52			infants fed standard formula
0.05	0.27			
—	0.01			
	0.36			
Formula	Formula + DHA + AA			Infants fed formula supplemented
21.9	21.8			with DHA + AA had higher
2.2	2.0			visual acuity than infants fed
—	0.43			standard formula at 2 mo, but
—	0.10			not at 4, 6, 9, or 12 mo
Formula	Formula + LC-PUFA			No differences in DQ values
11.1	10.8			
0.70	0.73			
—	0.30			
—	0.44			
—	0.30			
Formula	Formula + DHA	Formula + DHA + AA		No differences in VEP or visual acuity
21.9	20.7	21.7		
2.2	1.9	1.9		
—	—	0.43		
—	0.23	0.12		
Formula #1	#2	#3	#4	No differences in VER
17.6	17.3	16.5	15.6	Infants fed formula with a ratio of
0.4	0.95	1.7	3.2	4.8 weighed less than infants fed
44.0	18.2	9.7	4.8	formula with a ratio of 44
Formula	Formula + DHA	Formula + DHA + AA		Sweep VEP acuity better in infants
14.6	15.1	14.9		fed supplemented formulas than
1.49	1.54	1.53		in infants fed standard formula at
—	0.02	0.72		6, 17, and 52 wk, but not 26 wk
—	0.35	0.36		Visual acuity not different between groups

continued

TABLE 8-1 Continued

Reference	Study Population[a]	Test/Age[b]	Fatty Acid[c]
Jørgensen et al., 1998	n = 11 formula n = 12 formula + DHA n = 14 formula + DHA + GLA	Sweep VEP acuity 4 mo	18:2n-6 18:3n-3 18:3n-6 (GLA) 20:4n-6 (AA) 22:6n-3 (DHA)
Scott et al., 1998	n = 42–45 formula n = 33–43 formula + DHA n = 38–46 formula + DHA + AA	Bayley scales of infant development 12 mo MacArthur communicative development 14 mo	18:2n-6 18:3n-3 20:4n-6 (AA) 22:6n-3 (DHA)
Lucas et al., 1999	n = 125 formula n = 125 formula + LC-PUFA	Bayley scales of infant development 18 mo	18:2n-6 18:3n-3 20:4n-6 (AA) 22:6n-3 (DHA)
Makrides et al., 2000a	n = 30 10:1 formula n = 28 5:1 formula	VEP acuity 16, 34 wk	18:2n-6 18:3n-3
Makrides et al., 2000b	n = 21 formula n = 23 formula + DHA n = 24 formula + DHA + AA	VEP acuity 16, 34 wk Bayley scales of infant development 12, 24 mo	18:2n-6 18:3n-3 20:4n-6 (AA) 22:6n-3 (DHA)

[a] LC-PUFA = long chain polyunsaturated fatty acids.
[b] VEP = visual evoked potential, DQ = developmental quotient, VER = visual evoked response.

(70 to 91 years of age) individuals suggests little change in the capacity to absorb fat (Arora et al., 1989). The ratio of mean surface area to volume of jejunal mucosa has been reported not to differ between young and old individuals (Corazza et al., 1986). Total gastrointestinal transit time appears to be similar between young and elderly individuals (Brauer et al.,

Fatty Acid Content (% of fatty acids)			Results
Formula	Formula + DHA	Formula + DHA + GLA	No differences in VEP acuity
12.01	11.95	12.67	
1.20	1.20	1.17	
—	—	0.54	
—	0.06	0.06	
—	0.32	0.32	
Formula	Formula + DHA	Formula + DHA + AA	No differences in mental and psychomotor development
21.9	20.7	21.7	Vocabulary production and comprehension lower in the formula + DHA group
2.2	1.9	1.9	
—	—	0.43	
—	0.23	0.12	
Formula	Formula + LC-PUFA		No differences in mental and psychomotor development
12.4	15.9		
1.1	1.4		
—	0.30		
—	0.32		
10:1 Formula	5:1 Formula		No differences in VEP acuity
16.9	16.6		
1.7	3.3		
Formula	Formula + DHA	Formula + DHA + AA	No differences in VEP acuity or Bayley scales of mental and psychomotor development
16.8	16.8	16.6	
1.5	1.2	1.0	
—	—	0.34	
—	0.35	0.34	

c GLA = γ-linolenic acid, AA = arachidonic acid, DHA = docosahexaenoic acid.

1981). Documented changes with age may be confounded by the inclusion of a subgroup with clinical disorders (e.g., atrophic gastritis). The presence of bile salt-splitting bacteria normally present in the small intestine of humans is of potential significance to fat absorption. No evidence of bacterial overgrowth has been reported in older individuals (Arora et al., 1989). In addition, increases in fat malabsorption have not been demonstrated in normal elderly compared to younger individuals (Russell, 1992).

Exercise

Imposed physical activity decreased the magnitude of weight gain in nonobese volunteers given access to high fat diets (60 percent of energy) (Murgatroyd et al., 1999). In the exercise group, energy and fat balances (fat intake + fat synthesis – fat utilization) were not different from zero. Thus, high fat diets may cause positive fat balance, and therefore weight gain, only under sedentary conditions. These results are consistent with epidemiological evidence that show interactions between dietary fat, physical activity, and weight gain (Sherwood et al., 2000). Higher total fat diets can probably be consumed safely by active individuals while maintaining body weight. Although in longitudinal studies of weight gain, where dietary fat predicts weight gain independent of physical activity, it is important to note that physical activity may account for a greater percentage of the variance in weight gain than does dietary fat (Hill et al., 1989). Another endpoint that merits consideration is physical performance. High fat diets (69 percent of energy) do not appear to compromise endurance in trained athletes (Goedecke et al., 1999); however, athletes may not be able to train as effectively on short-term (less than 6 days) intakes of a high fat diet as on a high carbohydrate diet (Helge, 2000). This effect on training was not observed following long-term adaptation of high fat diets.

Genetic Factors

Studies of the general population may underestimate the importance of dietary fat in the development of obesity in subsets of individuals. Some data indicate that genetic predisposition may modify the relationship between diet and obesity (Heitmann et al., 1995). Additionally, some individuals with relatively high metabolic rates appear to be able to consume high fat diets (44 percent of energy) without obesity (Cooling and Blundell, 1998). Intervention studies have shown that those individuals susceptible to weight gain and obesity appear to have an impaired ability to increase fat oxidation when challenged with high fat meals and diets (Astrup et al., 1994; Raben et al., 1994). Animal studies show that there are important gene and dietary fat interactions that influence the tendency to gain excessive weight on a high fat diet (West and York, 1998). Once these genes are identified, further studies in humans will be feasible.

Alcohol

Alcohol is metabolized to acetylcoenzyme A in the liver and can enter all normal pathways for acetate metabolism, including the synthesis of fatty acids. The formation of nicotinamide adenine dinucleotide, resulting from ethanol oxidation, serves as a cofactor for fatty acid biosynthesis (Eisenstein, 1982). Similar to carbohydrate, alcohol consumption creates a shift in postprandial substrate utilization to reduce the oxidation of fatty acids (Schutz, 2000). Significant intake of alcohol (23 percent of energy) can depress fatty acid oxidation to a level equivalent to storing as much as 74 percent as fat (Murgatroyd et al., 1996). If the energy derived from alcohol is not utilized, the excess is stored as fat (Suter et al., 1992).

Interaction of n-6 and n-3 Fatty Acid Metabolism

The n-6 and n-3 unsaturated fatty acids are believed to be desaturated and elongated using the same series of desaturase and elongase enzymes (see Figure 8-1). The rate-limiting steps are the desaturases, rather than the elongase, enzymes. In vitro, the Δ6 desaturase shows clear substrate preference in the following order: α-linolenic acid > linoleic acid > oleic acid (Brenner, 1974). In addition, the formation of docosahexaenoic acid (DHA) from tetracosapentenoic acid (24:5n-3) involves a Δ6 desaturation to 24:6n-3 and then β-oxidation to yield 22:6n-3 (DHA) (Sprecher, 1992). It is not known if these are the Δ6 desaturases that are responsible for metabolism of linoleic acid and α-linolenic acid or a different enzyme (Cho et al., 1999). Many studies, primarily in laboratory animals, have provided evidence that the balance of linoleic and α-linolenic acid is important in determining the amounts of arachidonic acid, eicosapentaenoic acid (EPA), and DHA in tissue lipids. An inappropriate ratio may involve too high an intake of either linoleic acid or α-linolenic acid, too little of one fatty acid, or a combination leading to an imbalance between the two series. The provision of preformed carbon chain n-6 and n-3 fatty acids results in rapid incorporation into tissue lipids. Thus, the linoleic:α-linolenic acid ratio is likely to be of most importance for diets that are very low in or devoid of arachidonic acid, EPA, and DHA. The importance of the dietary linoleic:α-linolenic acid ratio for diets rich in arachidonic acid, EPA, and DHA is not known. Arachidonic acid is important for normal growth in rats (Mohrhauer and Holman, 1963). Later in life, risk of certain diseases may be altered by arachidonic acid and arachidonic acid-derived eicosanoids. Consequently, the desirable range of n-6:n-3 fatty acids may differ with life stage.

The regulation of n-6 and n-3 fatty acid metabolism is complex as the conversion of linoleic acid to arachidonic acid is inhibited by EPA and

DHA in humans, as well as arachidonic acid, α-linolenic acid, and linoleic acid itself (Chen and Nilsson, 1993; Emken et al., 1994, 1998, 1999; Sauerwald et al., 1996). Similarly, stable isotope studies have shown that increased intakes of α-linolenic acid result in decreased conversion of linoleic acid to its metabolites, and the amounts metabolized to longer-chain metabolites is inversely related to the amount oxidized (Vermunt et al., 2000). Unfortunately, very few studies are available on the rates of formation of arachidonic acid and DHA from their precursors in humans fed diets differing in linoleic acid and α-linolenic acid content, and with or without controlled amounts of arachidonic acid, EPA, and DHA.

Arachidonic acid is a precursor to a number of eicsanoids (e.g., thromboxane A_2, prostacylcin, and leukotriene B_4). These eicosanoids have been shown to have beneficial and adverse effects in the onset of platelet aggregation, hemodynamics, and coronary vascular tone. EPA has been shown to compete with the biosynthesis of n-6 eicosanoids and is the precursor of several n-3 eicosanoids (e.g., thromboxane A_3, prostaglandin I_3, and leukotriene B_5), resulting in a less thrombotic and atherogenic state (Kinsella et al., 1990).

n-6:n-3 Polyunsaturated Fatty Acid Ratio

Jensen and coworkers (1997) reported that infants fed formulas containing a linoleic acid:α-linolenic acid ratio of 4.8:1 had lower arachidonic acid concentrations and impaired growth compared to infants fed formulas containing ratios of 9.7:1 or higher. More recent, large clinical trials with infants fed formulas providing linoleic acid:α-linolenic acid ratios of 5:1 to 10:1 found no evidence of reduced growth or other problems that could be attributed to decreased arachidonic acid concentrations (Auestad et al., 1997, 2001; Makrides et al., 2000a). Clark and coworkers (1992) concluded that intake ratios less than 4:1 were likely to result in fatty acid profiles markedly different from those from infants fed human milk. Based on the limited studies, the linoleic acid:α-linolenic acid or total n-3:n-6 fatty acids ratios of 5:1 to 10:1, 5:1 to 15:1, and 6:1 to 16:1 have been recommended for infant formulas (Aggett et al., 1991; ISSFAL, 1994; LSRO, 1998).

In adult rats it has been determined that a linoleic acid:α-linolenic acid ratio of 8:1 was optimal in maintaining normal-tissue fatty acid concentrations (Bourre et al., 1996). Increasing the intake of linoleic acid from 15 to 30 g/d, with an increase in the linoleic:α-linolenic acid ratio from 8:1 to 30:1, resulted in a 40 to 54 percent decreased conversion of linoleic acid and α-linolenic acid to their metabolites in healthy men (Emken et al., 1994). Clinical studies with patients supported by total parenteral nutrition found resolution of signs of deficiency when a parenteral lipid containing a linoleic acid:α-linolenic acid ratio of 6:1 was provided (Holman et al., 1982).

Clinical and epidemiological studies have addressed the *n*-6:*n*-3 fatty acid ratio, focusing on beneficial effects on risk of certain diseases associated with higher intakes of the *n*-3 fatty acids EPA and DHA, as reviewed in Chapter 11. The specific importance of the ratio in these studies cannot be assessed because the decreased ratio is secondary to an increased intake of fish or EPA and DHA from supplements. For example, low rates of heart disease in Japan, compared with the United States, have been attributed in part to a total *n*-6:*n*-3 fatty acid ratio of 4:1 (Lands et al., 1990), with about 5 percent energy as linoleic acid, 0.6 percent energy from α-linolenic acid, and 2 percent energy from EPA+DHA in Japan, compared with intakes of 6 percent energy from linoleic acid, 0.7 percent energy from α-linolenic acid, and less than 0.1 percent energy from EPA+DHA in the United States (Lands et al., 1992). Similarly, an inverse association between the dietary total *n*-6:*n*-3 fatty acid ratio and cardiovascular disease, cancer, and all-cause mortality (Dolecek and Grandits, 1991), as well as between fish intake and coronary heart disease mortality (Kromhout et al., 1985; Shekelle et al., 1985), have been reported. In other studies, however, no differences were found in coronary heart disease risk factors when a diet containing a total *n*-6:*n*-3 ratio of 4:1 compared to 1:1 was consumed (Ezaki et al., 1999), or in thrombotic conditions with a diet containing a total *n*-6:*n*-3 ratio of 3.3:1 compared with 10:1 (Nelson et al., 1991). Hu and coworkers (1999b) observed a weak relationship between the *n*-6:*n*-3 ratio and fatal ischemic heart disease since both α-linolenic acid and linoleic acid were inversely related to risk. Based on the limited studies in animals, children, and adults, a reasonable linoleic:α-linolenic acid ratio of 5:1 to 10:1 has been recommended for adults (FAO/WHO, 1994).

Impact of Trans Fatty Acids on n-6 and n-3 Metabolism

The *trans* isomers of oleic acid and linoleic acid, which are present in hydrogenated vegetable oils and meats, have been suggested to have adverse effects on growth and development through inhibition of the desaturation of linoleic acid and α-linolenic acid to arachidonic acid and DHA, respectively (Sugano and Ikeda, 1996). Desaturation and elongation of *trans* linoleic and α-linolenic acid isomers containing a double bond at the *cis*-12 and *cis*-15 position, respectively, with formation of 20 and 22 carbon chain metabolites that could be incorporated into mem-brane lipids, have also been suggested. In vitro studies and studies with animals fed diets high in *trans* fatty acids have found evidence of reduced essential *n*-6 and *n*-3 fatty acid desaturation (Cook, 1981; Rosenthal and Doloresco, 1984). An inverse association between total *trans* fatty acids and arachidonic acid and DHA concentrations in plasma cholesteryl esters, and between plasma cholesteryl esters, elaidic acid (18:1 *trans*), and birth weight of premature infants has been reported (Koletzko, 1992). Studies in term infants found no relation between *trans* fatty acids and length of gestation, birth weight, or birth length (Elias and Innis, 2001). Similarly, an inverse association between plasma phospholipid *trans* fatty acids and arachidonic acid has been found for children aged 1 to 15 years (Decsi and Koletzko, 1995). The industrial hydrogenation of vegetable oils results in destruction of *cis* essential *n*-6 and *n*-3 fatty acids and the formation of *trans* fatty acids (Valenzuela and Morgado, 1999). It is not clear if differences in dietary intakes of *n*-6 and *n*-3 fatty acids, rather than inhibition of linoleic acid and α-linolenic acid desaturation by *trans* fatty acids, explains the statistical inverse associations between *trans* and *n*-6 and *n*-3 fatty acids reported in some studies (Craig-Schmidt, 2001). Based on the much greater affinity of the Δ6 desaturase for *cis* *n*-6 and *n*-3 fatty acids than monounsaturated fatty acids (Brenner, 1974; Castuma et al., 1977), and on experimental work that shows that inhibition of the Δ6 desaturation of linoleic acid is not of concern with linoleic acid intakes above about 2 percent of energy (Zevenbergen et al., 1988), it seems unlikely that inhibition of essential fatty acid metabolism by *trans* fatty acids is of concern for practical human diets.

FINDINGS BY LIFE STAGE AND GENDER GROUP

Total Fat
Infants Ages 0 Through 12 Months

Method Used to Set the Adequate Intake

No functional criteria of fat have been demonstrated that reflects a response to dietary intake in infants. Thus, the recommended intakes of total fat are based on an Adequate Intake (AI) that reflects the observed mean fat intake of infants principally fed human milk.

Ages 0 Through 6 Months. Fat is the major single source of energy in the diet of infants exclusively fed human milk. The high intake of fat and the energy density that it provides to the diet are important in providing the energy needed for rapid growth during early infancy. Thus, the recommended intake of total fat for infants 0 through 6 months of age is based on an AI that reflects the observed mean fat intake of infants fed human milk. Table 8-2 shows the concentration and proportion of energy from fat provided by mature human milk from women delivering at term gestation. Assuming an intake of 0.78 L/d of human milk by infants exclusively fed human milk (Chapter 1) and a mean milk fat content of 40 g/L, the AI for fat is 31 g/d. This AI assumes that the energy requirements of the young infant are being met. The mean energy content of mature human milk is 650 kcal/L (Chapter 5), thus dietary fat represents 55 percent of total energy intake for infants 0 through 6 months of age. Fomon and coworkers (1976) reported that the length and weight of infants were not different when fed formula and strained food providing 29 or 57 percent of energy from fat. Thus, an intake of 55 percent energy most likely exceeds the minimum percent needed for optimal growth of healthy infants.

Ages 7 Through 12 Months. The proportion of energy from dietary fat decreases during the second 6 months of age when complementary foods, specifically infant cereals, vegetables, and fruits, are added to the diet of the infant. The average concentration of fat in milk is approximately 40 g/L during the second 6 months of lactation (Table 8-2). The infant consumes about 0.6 L/d of human milk during the second 6 months (Chapter 1), with additional energy and nutrients provided by complementary foods, thus achieving total energy and essential nutrient needs of the infant 7 through 12 months of age.

The AI for the older infants is set based on the average intake of fat ingested from human milk and complementary foods (Chapter 1). Data from the Continuing Survey of Food Intakes by Individuals (CFSII) indicate that the average intake of fat from complementary foods by older infants is approximately 5.7 g/d. Therefore, the average fat intake from human milk and complementary foods would be 30 g/d ([0.6 L/d × 40 g/L] + 5.7) after rounding. The average energy intake from human milk is 390 kcal/d (0.6 L/d × 650 kcal/L) and from complementary foods is 281 kcal/d (CFSII), or a total energy intake of 671 kcal/d. Therefore, for infants 7 though 12 months of age, 40 percent of energy from fat is consumed from human milk and complementary foods.

Total Fat AI Summary, Ages 0 Through 12 Months

AI for Infants
    0–6 months   **31 g/d of fat**
    7–12 months   **30 g/d of fat**

Special Considerations

Conventional milk-based infant formulas contain approximately 48 percent of energy intake as fat (LSRO, 1998). The most common sources of fat in infant formulas are soybean oil, safflower oil, sunflower oil, coconut oil, and palm oil.

TABLE 8-2 Total Fat Content in Term Human Milk of Women in the United States and Canada

Reference	Study Population/ Stage of Lactation[a]	Total Fat Content (g/L)	Total Fat Content (% of total energy)	Total Energy[b] (kcal/L)
Anderson et al., 1983	9 women			
	3 d pp	18 ± 6	31.3	510 ± 90
	7 d pp	31 ± 10	43.6	630 ± 98
	14 d pp	37 ± 10	49.0	670 ± 100
Bitman et al., 1983	8–41 women			
	3 d pp	20.4 ± 3.2		
	7 d pp	28.9 ± 3.1		
	21 d pp	34.5 ± 3.7		
	42 d pp	31.9 ± 4.3		
	84 d pp	48.7 ± 6.2		
Dewey and Lönnerdal, 1983	13–18 women			
	1 mo pp	49.2 ± 10.5	55.9	781 ± 100
	2 mo pp	45.8 ± 9.7	54.0	753 ± 92
	3 mo pp	45.8 ± 16.5	55.2	736 ± 148
	4 mo pp	46.2 ± 18.6	52.1	787 ± 173
	5 mo pp	43.6 ± 16.7	51.8	747 ± 148
	6 mo pp	43.0 ± 19.6	51.0	748 ± 183
Butte et al., 1984	45 women			
	1 mo pp		47.8	
	2 mo pp		47.8	
	3 mo pp		45.7	
	4 mo pp		47.6	
Dewey et al., 1984	119 samples			
	4–6 mo pp	44.1 ± 18.5	60.2[c]	
	7–11 mo pp	34.5 ± 15.3	47.1[c]	
	12–20 mo pp	48.4 ± 1.19	66.0[c]	
Ferris et al., 1988	12 women			
	2 wk pp	39.8 ± 9.9	45.2	781 ± 125
	6 wk pp	44.1 ± 11.7	51.9	753 ± 77
	12 wk pp	48.7 ± 11.9	54.5	792 ± 93
	16 wk pp	55.0 ± 10.9	58.8	829 ± 122
Innis and Kuhnlein, 1988	12 Vancouver women	31 ± 3		

TABLE 8-2 Continued

Reference	Study Population/ Stage of Lactation[a]	Total Fat Content (g/L)	Total Fat Content (% of total energy)	Total Energy[b] (kcal/L)
Nommsen et al., 1991	46–70 women			
	3 mo pp	36.2 ± 7.0	46.1	697 ± 67
	6 mo pp	37.7 ± 9.6	47.3	707 ± 92
	9 mo pp	38.1 ± 8.0	47.7	709 ± 74
	12 mo pp	37.0 ± 11.3	46.7	706 ± 110
Chen et al., 1995a	198 samples 3–4 wk pp	31.58 ± 9.37		

[a] pp = postpartum.
[b] Calculated using 8.87 kcal/g of fat.
[c] Percent of energy determined from mean energy content of all milk samples during 7–20 mo pp (650 kcal/L).

Children and Adolescents Ages 1 Through 18 Years

A number of studies have been conducted to ascertain whether a certain amount of fat is needed in the diet to provide normal growth in children. These data generally conclude that there is no effect of fat intake on growth when consumed at levels as low as 21 percent of energy and provided that the energy intake is adequate (Boulton and Magarey, 1995; Fomon et al., 1976; Lagström et al., 1999; Lapinleimu et al., 1995; Niinikoski et al., 1997a, 1997b; Obarzanek et al., 1997; Shea et al., 1993) (see Chapter 11). There is insufficient evidence to identify a defined intake level of fat to prevent obesity or chronic diseases. Based on this lack of evidence and the lack of an effect of fat intake on growth, neither an AI nor an Estimated Average Requirement (EAR) and Recommended Dietary Allowance (RDA) are set for children and adolescents.

Adults Ages 19 Years and Older

The amount of total energy as fat in the diet can vary from 10 to 50 percent without differing effects on short-term health (Jéquier, 1999). When men and women were fed isocaloric diets containing 20, 40, or 60 percent fat, there was no difference in total daily energy expenditure (Hill et al., 1991). Similar observations were reported for individuals who consumed diets containing 10, 40, or 70 percent fat (Leibel et al., 1992) and men fed 9 to 79 percent fat (Shetty et al., 1994). In addition, a number of studies have reported on the impact of or the relationship between low and high fat diets and the indicators for and risk of chronic diseases (e.g., coronary heart disease, diabetes, and obesity) (see Chapter 11). There are insufficient data, however, to identify a defined intake level for fat based on maintaining fat balance or on the prevention of chronic diseases. Therefore, neither an AI nor an EAR and RDA are set.

Saturated Fatty Acids

There is no evidence to indicate that saturated fatty acids are essential in the diet or have a beneficial role in the prevention of chronic diseases. Therefore, neither an AI nor an EAR and RDA are set.

cis n-9 Monounsaturated Fatty Acids

There is no evidence to indicate that monounsaturated fatty acids are essential in the diet, and monounsaturated fatty acids have no known independent role in preventing chronic diseases. Therefore, neither an AI nor an EAR and RDA are set.

n-6 Polyunsaturated Fatty Acids
Infants Ages 0 Through 12 Months

Method Used to Set the AI

A series of papers reported skin lesions and poor growth in infants fed skimmed cow milk, which is very low in n-6 fatty acids (Hansen et al., 1958, 1963). Cuthbertson (1976) concluded that less than 50 mg/100 kcal of linoleic acid (0.45 percent energy) can provide normal health and well-being during infancy. Studies on the essential fatty acid status of older individuals have established that about 2 percent energy from n-6 poly-unsaturated fatty acids (linoleic acid) will prevent abnormal elevation of the triene:tetraene ratio ($20:3n-9:20:4n-6$) and clinical signs of essential fatty acid deficiency during parenteral nutrition (Barr et al., 1981). Inter-pretation, however, is complicated because linoleic acid in the soybean oil emulsion used to provide n-6 fatty acids can also be expected to inhibit synthesis of eicosatrienoic acid ($20:3n-9$) (Brenner, 1974), and thus reduce the triene:tetraene ratio. Furthermore, children are expected to require higher amounts of n-6 fatty acids than adults in order to support deposi-tion of n-6 fatty acids in cell membranes of growing tissues. This suggests that a margin of safety is prudent.

Ages 0 Through 6 Months. An AI can be set based on the average amount of *n*-6 polyunsaturated fatty acids provided by human milk. Table 8-2 provides the fat and energy content of human milk. Human milk contains 5.6 g/L (14 percent *n*-6 fatty acid in milk × 40 g/L) of *n*-6 polyunsaturated fatty acids (Table 8-3).

Based on an average intake of 0.78 L/d of human milk (Chapter 1), the AI is 4.4 g/d (0.78 L/d × 5.6 g/L). The energy content of human milk is approximately 650 kcal/L (Chapter 5) and therefore provides 507 kcal/d (650 kcal/L × 0.78 L/d). Thus, *n*-6 polyunsaturated fatty acids contribute approximately 8 percent of daily energy intake. The various *n*-6 fatty acids that are naturally present in human milk can contribute to this AI.

Ages 7 Through 12 Months. The period from 7 through 12 months of age is a time of major transition in the diet, from infants exclusively fed human milk or infant formulas that provide large amounts of dietary fat to a diet containing a variety of foods in addition to milk or formula. The infant consumes about 0.6 L/d of human milk during the second 6 months of life (Chapter 1), with additional energy and nutrients provided by complementary foods, thus achieving total energy and essential nutrient needs. The AI for older infants is set based on the average intake of *n*-6 polyunsaturated fatty acids ingested from human milk and complementary foods (Chapter 1). Data from CFSII indicates that the average intake of *n*-6 polyunsaturated fatty acids from complementary foods by older infants is approximately 1.2 g/d. Therefore, the AI for *n*-6 polyunsaturated fatty acids is 4.6 g/d ([0.6 L/d × 5.6 g/L] + 1.2) after rounding. The average fat energy coming from human milk is 390 kcal/d (0.6 L/d × 650 kcal/L), and from complementary foods is 281 kcal/d (CFSII), for a total energy intake of 671 kcal/d. Therefore, 6 percent of energy from *n*-6 polyunsaturated fat is consumed via human milk and complementary foods.

n-6 Polyunsaturated Fatty Acids AI Summary, Ages 0 Through 12 Months

AI for Infants
    0–6 months   **4.4 g/d of *n*-6 polyunsaturated fatty acids**
    7–12 months   **4.6 g/d of *n*-6 polyunsaturated fatty acids**

Special Considerations

The polyunsaturated vegetables oils (e.g., safflower oil and soybean oil) used in the manufacture of infant formulas contain abundant amounts (45 to 70 percent of total fatty acids) of linoleic acid. The minimum permissible amount of linoleic acid found in infant formulas is 2.7 percent of

TABLE 8-3 *n*-6 Polyunsaturated Fatty Acid Content in Term Human Milk of Women in the United States and Canada

Reference	*n*	*n*-6 Fatty Acid	Content in Human Milk	
			% of Total Fatty Acids	% of Total Energy[a]
Putnam et al., 1982	9	18:2	15.8 ± 0.61	8.62
		20:2	0.4 ± 0.03	0.22
		20:3	0.4 ± 0.03	0.22
		20:4	0.6 ± 0.03	0.33
		22:4	0.2 ± 0.02	0.11
		22:5	0.1 ± 0.02	0.05
		Total	17.50	9.55
Bitman et al., 1983	6	18:2	15.58 ± 1.99	8.50
		20:2	0.18 ± 0.20	0.10
		20:3	0.53 ± 0.15	0.29
		20:4	0.60 ± 0.29	0.33
		22:4	0.07 ± 0.16	0.04
		22:5	0.03 ± 0.08	0.02
		Total	16.99	9.28
Harris et al., 1984	8	18:2	15.3 ± 3.3	8.35
		20:3	0.3 ± 0.1	0.16
		20:4	0.4 ± 0.1	0.22
		Total	16.0	8.73
Finley et al., 1985	172	18:2	16.49 ± 4.80	9.00
		20:2	0.38 ± 0.15	0.21
		20:3	0.28 ± 0.09	0.15
		20:4	0.29 ± 0.08	0.16
		Total	17.44	9.52
Innis and Kuhnlein, 1988	12	18:2	12.7 ± 1.8	6.93
		20:2	0.4 ± 0.1	0.22
		20:4	0.7 ± 0.0	0.38
		22:5	0.2 ± 0.1	0.11
		Total	14.0	7.64
Chen et al., 1995a	198	18:2	10.47 ± 2.62	5.72
		18:3	0.08 ± 0.06	0.04
		20:2	0.17 ± 0.37	0.09
		20:3	0.26 ± 0.09	0.14
		20:4	0.35 ± 0.11	0.19
		22:4	0.04 ± 0.05	0.02
		22:5	0.01 ± 0.02	0.01
		Total	11.38	6.21

TABLE 8-3 Continued

| Reference | n | n-6 Fatty Acid | Content in Human Milk | |
			% of Total Fatty Acids	% of Total Energy[a]
Innis and	103	18:2	12.1 ± 0.35	6.60
King, 1999		18:3	0.1 ± 0.00	0.05
		20:2	0.3 ± 0.01	0.16
		20:3	0.3 ± 0.01	0.16
		20:4	0.4 ± 0.01	0.22
		22:4	0.1 ± 0.00	0.05
		Total	13.3	7.24

[a] Calculated using the following values: 40 g of fat/L of milk, 8.87 kcal/g of fat, 650 kcal/L of milk.

energy (Infant Formula. Nutrient Specifications. 21 C.F.R. §107.100, 1985); however, formulas provide higher amounts than this level.

Children and Adolescents Ages 1 Through 18 Years

Method Used to Set the AI

No specific information is available on the amount of linoleic acid required to correct the symptoms of an n-6 polyunsaturated fatty acid deficiency. In the absence of this information, an AI is set based on the median intake of linoleic acid consumed in the United States where the presence of an n-6 fatty acid deficiency is basically nonexistent in the free-living population (Appendix Table E-9), and rounding.

Linoleic Acid AI Summary, Ages 1 Through 18 Years

AI for Children
1–3 years	**7 g/d of linoleic acid**
4–8 years	**10 g/d of linoleic acid**

AI for Boys
9–13 years	**12 g/d of linoleic acid**
14–18 years	**16 g/d of linoleic acid**

AI for Girls
   9–13 years   10 g/d of linoleic acid
  14–18 years   11 g/d of linoleic acid

Adults Ages 19 Years and Older

Method Used to Set the AI

Various studies on adult patients receiving total parenteral nutrition have shown that linoleic acid intakes of as little as 7.4 to 8 g/d reverses the symptoms of deficiency (Barr et al., 1981; Collins et al., 1971; Goodgame et al., 1978; Jeppesen et al., 1998; Wong and Deitel, 1981). There is inadequate information, however, to set an EAR for healthy individuals. In the absence of this information, an AI is set based on the median intake of linoleic acid in the United States where the presence of an n-6 fatty acid deficiency is basically nonexistent in the free-living population (Appendix Table E-9). The highest median intakes have been used, each for men and women 19 to 50 years of age. Energy expenditure increases fat oxidation (Calles-Escandon et al., 1996) and linoleic acid is readily used for energy (Cunnane et al., 2001). Therefore, the AI for older men and women (greater than 50 years of age), whose energy expenditure is less than younger adults, is based on the highest median intake within this age range and rounding.

Linoleic Acid AI Summary, Ages 19 Years and Older

AI for Men
  19–30 years   17 g/d of linoleic acid
  31–50 years   17 g/d of linoleic acid
  51–70 years   14 g/d of linoleic acid
  > 70 years   14 g/d of linoleic acid

AI for Women
  19–30 years   12 g/d of linoleic acid
  31–50 years   12 g/d of linoleic acid
  51–70 years   11 g/d of linoleic acid
  > 70 years   11 g/d of linoleic acid

Pregnancy

Method Used to Set the AI

The demand for *n*-6 fatty acids for incorporation into placental tissue and the developing fetus during gestation must be met by *n*-6 fatty acids from maternal tissues or through dietary intake. Longitudinal studies have reported a decrease in plasma arachidonic acid concentration in pregnant women (Ghebremeskel et al., 2000; Sanjurjo et al., 1993). Lower arachidonic acid concentrations have also been reported for red blood cell phospholipids of pregnant women compared with nonpregnant women (Ghebremeskel et al., 2000). It is not clear that this reflects an increased need for *n*-6 fatty acids that was not met in the women in these studies, or whether changes in maternal *n*-6 fatty acid concentrations are normal physiological responses explained by the changes in endocrine status, lipoprotein and lipid metabolism, or nutrient transfer to the fetus. There is no evidence that maternal dietary intervention with *n*-6 fatty acids has any effect on fetal or infant growth and development in women meeting the requirements for *n*-6 fatty acids.

Because of a lack of evidence for determining the requirement during pregnancy, the AI is set based on the median linoleic acid intake of pregnant women in the United States where a deficiency is basically nonexistent in noninstitutionalized populations (Appendix Table E-9), and rounding.

Linoleic Acid AI Summary, Pregnancy

AI for Pregnant Women
14–18 years	**13 g/d of linoleic acid**
19–30 years	**13 g/d of linoleic acid**
31–50 years	**13 g/d of linoleic acid**

Lactation

Method Used to Set the AI

As stated above, there is no evidence that maternal dietary intervention with *n*-6 fatty acids has any effect on infant growth and development in women meeting the requirements for *n*-6 fatty acids. Because of a lack of evidence for determining the requirement during lactation, the AI is set based on the median linoleic acid intake of lactating women in the United States where a deficiency is basically nonexistent in noninstitutionalized populations (Appendix Table E-9), and rounding.

Linoleic Acid AI Summary, Lactation

AI for Lactation
    14–18 years   13 g/d of linoleic acid
    19–30 years   13 g/d of linoleic acid
    31–50 years   13 g/d of linoleic acid

n-3 Polyunsaturated Fatty Acids
Infants Ages 0 Through 12 Months

Method Used to Set the AI

Human milk contains α-linolenic acid (18:3), eicosapentaenoic acid (EPA, 20:5), and docosahexaenoic acid (DHA, 22:6) (Table 8-4), but the amounts present are highly variable and depend on the amounts present in the mother's diet. Concentrations of about 0.7 to 1.4 percent DHA have been reported for women who eat large amounts of fish and other marine foods (Innis and Kuhnlein, 1988; Kneebone et al., 1985). Blood concentrations of DHA appear to show little metabolic regulation and increase with increasing DHA intake in breast-fed infants (Gibson et al., 1997; Innis and King, 1999; Sanders and Reddy, 1992) or formula-fed infants (Auestad et al., 1997; Carlson et al., 1996a; Innis et al., 1996; Makrides et al., 1995), as they do in adults. Numerous studies have shown that infants fed formulas with no DHA have lower plasma and red blood cell DHA concentrations than infants fed human milk or formulas with DHA (Auestad et al., 1997; Carlson et al., 1986, 1996a; Innis et al., 1996; Makrides et al., 1995; Ponder et al., 1992; Putnam et al., 1982). Similarly, the plasma and red blood cell DHA concentrations are lower in infants breast-fed by mothers with vegetarian rather than omnivorous diets (Sanders and Reddy, 1992). Evidence of DHA depletion based on functional endpoints has not been reported for populations or subgroups that have diets containing no DHA but with adequate α-linolenic acid.

Several autopsy studies have reported lower DHA concentrations in the brains of infants fed formulas that contain no DHA compared with infants fed human milk (Byard et al., 1995; Farquharson, 1994; Farquharson et al., 1992, 1995; Jamieson et al., 1994, 1999; Makrides et al., 1994). In addition, brain DHA accumulation continues in both breast-fed and formula-fed infants for at least 40 weeks of life, but the accumulation is at a greatly reduced rate in formula-fed infants (Makrides et al., 1996). Although many infant formulas contain similar amounts of α-linolenic acid as human milk, the dietary supply of only α-linolenic acid and no DHA in formulas may be inadequate to supply the infant brain with DHA (Farquharson,

TABLE 8-4 *n*-3 Polyunsaturated Fatty Acid Content in Term Human Milk of Women in the United States and Canada

Reference	*n*	*n*-3 Fatty Acid	Content in Human Milk	
			% of Total Fatty Acids	% of Total Energy[a]
Putnam et al., 1982	9	18:3	0.8 ± 0.09	0.44
		20:5	0.1 ± 0.03	0.05
		22:5	0.1 ± 0.01	0.05
		22:6	0.1 ± 0.01	0.05
		Total	1.1	0.59
Bitman et al., 1983	6	18:3	1.03 ± 0.21	0.56
		20:5	trace	trace
		22:5	0.11 ± 0.15	0.06
		22:6	0.23 ± 0.14	0.13
		Total	1.37	0.75
Harris et al., 1984	8	18:3	0.8 ± 0.5	0.44
		20:5	trace	trace
		22:5	trace	trace
		22:6	0.1 ± 0.1	0.05
		Total	0.9	0.49
Finley et al., 1985	172	18:3	1.56 ± 0.43	0.85
		22:6	0.06 ± 0.004	0.03
		Total	1.62	0.88
Innis and Kuhnlein, 1988	12	18:3	0.6 ± 0.2	0.33
		20:5	0.2 ± 0.2	0.11
		22:5	0.4 ± 0.1	0.22
		22:6	0.4 ± 0.1	0.22
		Total	1.6	0.88
Chen et al., 1995a	198	18:3	1.16 ± 0.37	0.63
		20:4	0.06 ± 0.06	0.03
		20:5	0.05 ± 0.05	0.03
		22:5	0.08 ± 0.06	0.04
		22:6	0.14 ± 0.10	0.08
		Total	1.49	0.81
Innis and King, 1999	103	18:3	1.4 ± 0.07	0.76
		20:5	0.1 ± 0.01	0.05
		22:5	0.2 ± 0.02	0.11
		22:6	0.2 ± 0.03	0.11
		Total	1.9	1.03

[a] Calculated using the following values: 40 g of fat/L of milk, 8.87 kcal/g of fat, 650 kcal/L of milk.

1994). Animal studies have shown that dietary DHA is incorporated into brain tissue to a greater extent than is DHA that is biosynthesized from α-linolenic acid (Abedin et al., 1999; Sinclair, 1975). Furthermore, administration of dietary α-linolenic acid was not effective in restoring brain DHA concentrations in chicks deficient in n-3 fatty acids (Anderson et al., 1990). Therefore, the DHA content of the brain may depend more heavily upon the dietary supply of DHA rather than its precursor, α-linolenic acid. Randomized clinical studies on growth or neural development with term infants fed formulas currently yield conflicting results on the requirement for n-3 fatty acids in young infants (see "Evidence Considered for Estimating the Requirement for Total Fat and Fatty Acids").

Ages 0 Through 6 Months. n-3 Polyunsaturated fatty acids provide DHA that is important for the developing brain and retina. Human milk is assumed to meet the n-3 fatty acid requirements of the infants fed human milk. Therefore, an AI for n-3 fatty acids is based on the amount of n-3 fatty acids, total fat, and energy provided by human milk. Table 8-2 shows the fat and energy content of human milk. Human milk contains approximately 0.63 g/L (1.58 percent n-3 fatty acids × 40 g/L total fat) of n-3 polyunsaturated fatty acids (Table 8-4). The AI is based on the average amount of milk consumed by the infant (0.78 L/d) and the n-3 fatty acid concentration in human milk. Therefore, the AI is set at 0.5 g/d (0.78 L/d × 0.63 g/L), after rounding, which provides approximately 4.5 kcal/d. Because human milk provides 650 kcal/L (Chapter 5) or 507 kcal/d (650 kcal/L × 0.78 L/d), an AI of 0.5 g/d of n-3 polyunsaturated fatty acids represents approximately 1 percent (4.5 ÷ 507) energy intake, after rounding. The various n-3 fatty acids that are naturally present in human milk can contribute to this AI.

Ages 7 Through 12 Months. While the energy requirement relative to body weight decreases in the second 6 months of life (see Chapter 5), autopsy analyses suggest that brain DHA accretion continues at a similar rate from 0 through 24 months of age (Martinez, 1992). The AI for older infants is set based on the average intake of n-3 fatty acids ingested from human milk and complementary foods (Chapter 1). Data from CFSII indicate that the average intake of n-3 fatty acids from complementary foods by older infants is approximately 0.11 g/d. Therefore, the AI is 0.5 g/d [0.6 L/d × 0.63 g/L] + 0.11), after rounding, which represents approximately 4.5 kcal/d. The average energy intake from human milk is 390 kcal/d (0.6 L/d × 650 kcal/L), and from complementary foods is 281 kcal/d (CFSII), for a total energy intake of 671 kcal/d. Therefore, approximately 0.67 percent (4.5 kcal/d ÷ 671 kcal/d) of energy is consumed as n-3 polyunsaturated fatty acids from human milk and complementary foods.

n-3 Polyunsaturated Fatty Acid AI Summary, Ages 0 Through 12 Months

AI for Infants
  0–6 months   0.50 g/d of n-3 polyunsaturated fatty acids
  7–12 months   0.50 g/d of n-3 polyunsaturated fatty acids

Special Considerations

Vegetable oils that provide α-linolenic acid are used in the manufacture of infant formulas. The U.S. Code of Federal Regulations does not currently specify minimum or maximum levels of α-linolenic acid for infant formulas. At the present time, DHA is not directly added to infant formulas. Information from clinical trials with term infants fed formulas with DHA are inconsistent, and associations between lower growth and delays on some developmental tests have been noted in preterm and term infants fed formulas containing DHA, but not arachidonic acid. Definitive evidence that this is due to the absence of arachidonic acid or explained by antagonism between DHA and n-6 fatty acids is not available. DHA is added to infant formula ingredients in the form of oils from fish oils, egg total lipids, egg phospholipids, and oil from single cell microorganisms.

Children and Adolescents Ages 1 Through 18 Years

Method Used to Set the AI

One case study of a 6-year-old girl on total parenteral nutrition (TPN) reported that the TPN solution, which was low in α-linolenic acid and provided approximately 0.08 g/d, resulted in episodes of numbness, weakness, blurred vision, and the inability to walk (Holman et al., 1982). Analysis of the girl's plasma fatty acids confirmed a low n-3 fatty acid concentration. It was determined that 1.625 g/d of α-linolenic acid reversed the abnormal neurological symptoms. Bjerve and coworkers (1988) reported low plasma n-3 fatty acid concentrations and poor growth in a child fed approximately 0.54 g/d of α-linolenic acid via a gastric tube. Growth was somewhat improved by the addition of 0.56 g/d of α-linolenic acid.

Because of a lack of evidence for determining the requirement for n-3 fatty acids during childhood, an AI is set based on the median intake of α-linolenic acid in the United States where a deficiency is basically nonexistent in noninstitutionalized populations (Appendix Table E-11), and rounding. Small amounts of EPA and DHA can contribute toward reversing an n-3 fatty acid deficiency (Bjerve, 1989; Bjerve et al., 1987a, 1987b, 1989) and can therefore contribute toward the AI for α-linolenic acid.

EPA and DHA contribute approximately 10 percent of the total n-3 fatty acid intake and therefore this percent contributes toward the AI for α-linolenic acid (Appendix Tables E-10, E-12, and E-14).

α-Linolenic Acid AI Summary, Ages 1 Through 18 Years

AI for Children
1–3 years	0.7 g/d of α-linolenic acid
4–8 years	0.9 g/d of α-linolenic acid

AI for Boys
9–13 years	1.2 g/d of α-linolenic acid
14–18 years	1.6 g/d of α-linolenic acid

AI for Girls
9–13 years	1.0 g/d of α-linolenic acid
14–18 years	1.1 g/d of α-linolenic acid

Adults Ages 19 Years and Older

Method Used to Set the AI

Several studies involving adult patients who were fed by gastric tube showed that an n-3 fatty acid (α-linolenic acid) deficiency could occur with intakes ranging from 0.015 to 0.095 g/d of α-linolenic acid (Bjerve, 1989; Bjerve et al., 1987a, 1987b, 1989), whereas intakes of as low as 0.3 g/d prevented the symptoms of a deficiency (Bjerve et al., 1987a). There were insufficient data, however, to set an EAR for free-living healthy adults.

Because of a lack of evidence for determining the requirement for n-3 fatty acids, an AI is set based on the highest median intake of α-linolenic acid by adults in the United States where a deficiency is basically non-existent in noninstitutionalized populations (Appendix Table E-11), and rounding. Small amounts of EPA and DHA can contribute toward reversing an n-3 fatty acid deficiency (Bjerve, 1989; Bjerve et al., 1987a, 1987b, 1989). EPA and DHA contribute approximately 10 percent of the total n-3 fatty acid intake and therefore this percent contributes toward the AI for α-linolenic acid (Appendix Tables E-10, E-12, and E-14).

α-Linolenic Acid AI Summary, Ages 19 Years and Older

AI for Men
19–30 years	1.6 g/d of α-linolenic acid
31–50 years	1.6 g/d of α-linolenic acid
51–70 years	1.6 g/d of α-linolenic acid
> 70 years	1.6 g/d of α-linolenic acid

AI for Women
19–30 years	1.1 g/d of α-linolenic acid
31–50 years	1.1 g/d of α-linolenic acid
51–70 years	1.1 g/d of α-linolenic acid
> 70 years	1.1 g/d of α-linolenic acid

Pregnancy and Lactation

Method Used to Set the AI

The demand for n-3 polyunsaturated fatty acids for incorporation into placental tissue and for the developing fetus during gestation, as well as for secretion of n-3 polyunsaturated fatty acids in milk during lactation, must be met by n-3 fatty acids from maternal tissues or through dietary intake. Several studies have reported lower plasma and red blood cell lipid DHA concentrations in pregnant and lactating women compared with nonpregnant, nonlactating women (Ghebremeskel et al., 2000; Holman et al., 1991). It is not clear that this reflects declining DHA status due to inadequate n-3 fatty acid intakes in the women in these studies. An alternative explanation is that changes in maternal DHA concentrations are normal physiological responses to the changes in endocrine status, lipoprotein and lipid metabolism, or nutrient transfer that accompany pregnancy and lactation. However, supplementation with fish oil during pregnancy does increase DHA in both the mother and the newborn infant, and supplementation with fish oil during lactation increases the concentration of DHA in the mother's milk and in the infant's blood (Connor et al., 1996; Henderson et al., 1992; van Houwelingen et al., 1995). Dietary fatty acids are almost completely absorbed, and an increase in blood DHA concentration following the increase in intake with fish oil supplementation is to be expected. Evidence is not available to show that increasing intakes of DHA in pregnant and lactating women consuming diets that meet requirements for n-6 and n-3 fatty acids have any physiologically significant benefit to the infant. Population comparative studies have found higher birthweights and longer gestation for women in the Faroe Islands than in Denmark (Olsen et al., 1989). This has been attributed to a higher intake of EPA from fish and other marine foods, leading to n-3 fatty acid-induced inhibition of the n-6 fatty acid-derived eicosanoids that are important in cervical ripening and initiation of parturition. Subsequent intervention studies indicate that 10.8 g of supplemental n-3 fatty acids from fish oil is associated with an increase in gestation of about 4 days (Olsen et al., 1992).

Because of a lack of evidence for determining the requirement for n-3 fatty acids during pregnancy and lactation, an AI is set based on the median intake of α-linolenic acid in the United States where a deficiency is basically nonexistent in noninstitutionalized populations (Appendix Table E-11), and rounding. Small amounts of EPA and DHA can contribute toward reversing an n-3 fatty acid deficiency (Bjerve, 1989; Bjerve et al., 1987a, 1987b, 1989), and can therefore contribute toward the AI for α-linolenic acid.

α-Linolenic Acid AI Summary, Pregnancy and Lactation

AI for Pregnancy

14–18 years	**1.4 g/d of α-linolenic acid**
19–30 years	**1.4 g/d of α-linolenic acid**
31–50 years	**1.4 g/d of α-linolenic acid**

AI for Lactation

14–18 years	**1.3 g/d of α-linolenic acid**
19–30 years	**1.3 g/d of α-linolenic acid**
31–50 years	**1.3 g/d of α-linolenic acid**

Special Considerations

The ratio of linoleic acid:α-linolenic acid in the diet is important because linoleic acid and α-linolenic acid compete for the same desaturase enzymes. Thus, a high ratio of linoleic acid:α-linolenic acid can inhibit the conversion of α-linolenic acid to DHA, while a low ratio will inhibit the desaturation of linoleic acid to arachidonic acid. The linoleic acid:α-linolenic acid ratio, however, is likely to be of greatest importance in diets that are very low or devoid of arachidonic acid, EPA, and DHA.

The available data, although limited, suggest that linoleic:α-linolenic acid ratios below 5:1 may be associated with impaired growth in infants (Jensen et al., 1997). Although a ratio of 30:1 has been shown to reduce further metabolism of α-linolenic acid, sufficient dose–response data are not available to set an upper range for this ratio with confidence. Assuming an intake of n-6 fatty acids of 5 percent energy, with this being mostly linoleic acid, the α-linolenic acid intake at a 5:1 ratio would be 1 percent of energy.

Trans *Fatty Acids*

There are no data available to indicate a health benefit from consuming *trans* fatty acids. Therefore, neither an AI nor an EAR and RDA are established for *trans* fatty acids.

INTAKES OF TOTAL FAT AND FATTY ACIDS

Total Fat

Food Sources

Both animal- and plant-derived food products contain fat. The principal foods that contribute to fat intake are butter, margarine, vegetable oils, visible fat on meat and poultry products, whole milk, egg yolks, nuts, and baked goods (e.g., cookies, doughnuts, and cakes). Over 95 percent of total fat intake is in the form of triacylglycerols. As discussed below, the type of fat present in these food products varies.

Dietary Intake

Intake data from the Continuing Survey of Food Intakes of Individuals (CFSII) (1994–1996, 1998) showed that the median total fat intake ranged from 65 to 100 g/d for men and 48 to 63 g/d for women (Appendix Table E-5). These intake ranges represent approximately 32 to 34 percent of total energy (Appendix Table E-6). During 1990 to 1997, median intakes of fat ranged from 32 to 34 percent and 30 to 33 percent of energy in Canadian men and women, respectively (Appendix Table F-3).

A longitudinal study in the United States found that dietary fat represented 48, 41, 35, and 30 percent of total energy intakes at 3, 6, 12, and 24 months of age, respectively (Butte, 2000). The Third National Health and Nutrition Examination Survey (NHANES) estimated that children 2 to 19 years of age consumed an average of 34 percent of total energy as fat, with little difference across the individual age groups (Troiano et al., 2000). Comparison of data collected across the three NHANES studies conducted since the early 1970s shows that children and adolescents across all race, gender, and age groups have decreased their total fat intake. Mean age-adjusted fat intakes have declined from 36 to 37 percent to 33 to 34 percent of total energy (Troiano et al., 2000). About 23 percent of children 2 to 5 years old, 16 percent of children 6 to 11 years old, and 15 percent of adolescents 12 to 19 years old had dietary fat intakes equal to or less than 30 percent of total energy intakes.

Saturated Fatty Acids

Food Sources

Sources of saturated fatty acids tend to be foods of animal sources, including whole milk, cream, butter, cheese, and fatty meats such as pork and beef (USDA/HHS, 2000). Certain oils, however, such as coconut, palm, and palm kernel oil, also contain relatively high amounts of saturated fatty acids. Saturated fatty acids provide approximately 20 to 25 percent of energy in human milk (Table 8-5).

Dietary Intake

Based on intake data from CFSII (1994–1996, 1998), median saturated fatty acid intake ranged from approximately 21 to 34 g/d for men and 15 to 21 g/d for women (Appendix Table E-7). Data from NHANES III indicated that saturated fatty acids provided 11 to 12 percent of energy in adult diets and ranged from 12.2 to 13.9 percent of energy for children and adolescents (CDC, 1994). NHANES III reported that 9 percent of children 2 to 11 years old and 7 percent of those 12 to 19 years old had saturated fatty acid intakes of less than 10 percent of total energy (Troiano et al., 2000). During 1990 to 1997, median intakes of saturated fatty acids ranged from approximately 10 to 12 percent of energy for Canadian men and women (Appendix Table F-4).

Cis-Monounsaturated Fatty Acids

Food Sources

About 50 percent of monounsaturated fatty acids are provided by animal products, primarily meat fat (Jonnalagadda et al., 1995). Oils that contain monounsaturated fatty acids include canola and olive oils. Monounsaturated fatty acids provide approximately 20 percent of energy in human milk (Table 8-6).

Dietary Intake

Based on intake data from CFSII (1994–1996, 1998), median monounsaturated fatty acid intake ranged from approximately 25 to 39 g/d for men and 18 to 24 g/d for women (Appendix Table E-8). Data from the 1987–1988 Nationwide Food Consumption Survey indicated that mean intakes of monounsaturated fatty acids were 13.6 to 14.3 percent of energy (Ganji and Betts, 1995).

TABLE 8-5 Saturated Fatty Acid Content in Term Human Milk of Women in the United States and Canada

Reference	n	Saturated Fatty Acid	Content in Human Milk	
			% of Total Fatty Acids	% of Total Energy[a]
Putnam et al., 1982	9	8:0	0.3	0.16
		10:0	1.4	0.76
		12:0	6.2	3.38
		14:0	7.6	4.15
		16:0	20.5 ± 0.70	11.19
		18:0	9.0 ± 0.46	4.91
		20:0	0.3 ± 0.02	0.16
		21:0	0.1 ± 0.02	0.05
		24:0	0.5 ± 0.01	0.27
		Total	45.9	25.03
Bitman et al., 1983	6	10:0	0.97 ± 0.28	0.53
		12:0	4.46 ± 1.17	2.43
		14:0	5.68 ± 1.36	3.10
		15:0	0.31 ± 0.07	0.17
		16:0	22.20 ± 2.28	12.12
		17:0	0.49 ± 0.36	0.27
		18:0	7.68 ± 1.85	4.19
		20:0	0.32 ± 0.11	0.17
		21:0	0.17 ± 0.12	0.09
		Total	42.28	23.07
Harris et al., 1984	8	10:0	trace	trace
		12:0	4.2 ± 1.3	2.29
		14:0	5.9 ± 0.7	3.22
		16:0	22.8 ± 1.6	12.45
		18:0	8.2 ± 1.2	4.48
		Total	41.1	22.44
Finley et al., 1985	172	8:0	0.16 ± 0.11	0.09
		10:0	1.10 ± 0.30	0.60
		12:0	5.56 ± 1.68	3.03
		14:0	8.01 ± 2.46	4.37
		16:0	23.28 ± 3.35	12.71
		18:0	8.06 ± 1.58	4.40
		Total	46.17	25.20
Innis and Kuhnlein, 1988	12	10:0	1.2 ± 0.2	0.66
		12:0	5.2 ± 0.7	2.84
		14:0	6.7 ± 0.5	3.66
		16:0	22.1 ± 2.7	12.06
		18:0	8.2 ± 0.8	4.48
		Total	43.4	23.70

continued

TABLE 8-5 Continued

Reference	n	Saturated Fatty Acid	Content in Human Milk	
			% of Total Fatty Acids	% of Total Energy[a]
Chen et al., 1995a	198	10:0	1.39 ± 0.59	0.76
		12:0	5.68 ± 2.01	3.10
		14:0	6.10 ± 1.73	3.33
		15:0	0.37 ± 0.12	0.20
		16:0	18.30 ± 2.25	9.99
		17:0	0.32 ± 0.08	0.17
		18:0	6.15 ± 0.97	3.36
		20:0	0.15 ± 0.09	0.08
		Total	38.46	20.99
Innis and King, 1999	103	10:0	0.6 ± 0.03	0.33
		12:0	4.1 ± 0.15	2.24
		14:0	6.1 ± 0.21	3.33
		16:0	19.4 ± 0.28	10.59
		18:0	7.2 ± 0.15	3.93
		20:0	0.2 ± 0.00	0.11
		22:0	0.1 ± 0.00	0.05
		24:0	0.1 ± 0.00	0.05
		Total	37.8	20.63

[a] Calculated using the following values: 40 g of fat/L of milk, 8.87 kcal/g of fat, 650 kcal/L of milk.

n-6 Polyunsaturated Fatty Acids

Food Sources

Sources of n-6 polyunsaturated fatty acids include nuts, seeds, certain vegetables, and vegetable oils such as soybean oil, safflower oil, and corn oil. Certain oils, such as blackcurrant seed oil and evening primrose oil, are high in γ-linolenic acid (18:3n-6), which is an intermediate in the conversion of linoleic acid to arachidonic acid. Arachidonic acid is formed from linoleic acid in animal cells, but not plant cells, and is present in the diet in small amounts in meat, poultry, and eggs. Arachidonic acid is not present in plant-derived fats and oils.

TABLE 8-6 Monounsaturated Fatty Acid Content in Term Human Milk of Women in the United States and Canada

Reference	n	Monounsaturated Fatty Acid	Content in Human Milk % of Total Fatty Acids	% of Total Energy[a]
Putnam et al., 1982	9	18:1	37.6 ± 0.75	20.52
		20:1	0.9 ± 0.07	0.49
		22:1	0.1 ± 0.02	0.05
		Total	38.6	21.06
Bitman et al., 1983	6	16:1	3.83 ± 0.39	2.09
		18:1	35.51 ± 2.73	19.38
		Total	39.34	21.47
Harris et al., 1984	8	16:1	2.5 ± 0.6	1.36
		18:1	32.6 ± 3.3	17.79
		20:1	0.5 ± 0.1	0.27
		Total	35.6	19.42
Finley et al., 1985	172	16:1	3.02 ± 0.77	1.65
		18:1	31.72 ± 3.81	17.31
		Total	34.74	18.96
Innis and Kuhnlein, 1988	12	16:1	3.3 ± 0.6	1.80
		18:1	36.3 ± 2.7	19.81
		20:1	0.7 ± 0.3	0.38
		22:1	0.2 ± 0.1	0.11
		Total	40.5	22.10
Chen et al., 1995a	198	14:1	0.28 ± 0.08	0.15
		16:1	2.68 ± 0.69	1.46
		17:1	0.21 ± 0.06	0.11
		18:1	36.09 ± 3.51	19.70
		20:1	0.53 ± 0.22	0.29
		22:1	0.02 ± 0.03	0.01
		Total	39.81	21.72
Innis and King, 1999	103	14:1	0.2 ± 0.01	0.11
		16:1	2.5 ± 0.08	1.36
		18:1	35.7 ± 0.41	19.49
		20:1	0.6 ± 0.05	0.33
		22:1	0.2 ± 0.02	0.11
		24:1	0.1 ± 0.01	0.05
		Total	39.3	21.45

[a] Calculated using the following values: 40 g of fat/L of milk, 8.87 kcal/g of fat, 650 kcal/L of milk.

Dietary Intake

Based on intake data from CFSII (1994–1996, 1998), median *n*-6 poly-unsaturated fatty acid (linoleic acid) intake ranged from approximately 12 to 17 g/d for men and 9 to 11 g/d for women (Appendix Table E-9).

Polyunsaturated fatty acids have been reported to contribute approximately 5 to 7 percent of total energy intake in diets of adults (Allison et al., 1999; Fischer et al., 1985). Most (approximately 85 to 90 percent) *n*-6 polyunsaturated fatty acids are consumed in the form of linoleic acid. Other *n*-6 polyunsaturated fatty acids, such as arachidonic acid and γ-linolenic acid, are present in small amounts in the diet.

n-3 Polyunsaturated Fatty Acids

Food Sources

The major sources of *n*-3 fatty acids include certain vegetable oils and fish (Kris-Etherton et al., 2000). Vegetable oils such as soybean and flax-seed oils contain high amounts of α-linolenic acid. Fish oils provide a mixture of eicosapentaenoic acid (EPA) and docosahexaenoic acid (DHA), and fatty fish are the major dietary sources of EPA and DHA. Smaller amounts are also present in meat and eggs.

Dietary Intake

Based on intake data from CFSII (1994–1996, 1998), the total *n*-3 fatty intake for men and women ranged from approximately 1.3 to 1.8 g/d and 1.0 to 1.2 g/d, respectively (Appendix Table E-10). These findings are similar to that reported by Kris-Etherton and coworkers (2000), who also reported that the average intake of *n*-3 polyunsaturated fatty acids was approximately 0.7 percent of energy. The median intake of α-linolenic acid ranged from approximately 1.2 to 1.6 g/d for men and 0.9 to 1.1 g/d for women (Appendix Table E-11). For all adults, the median intakes of EPA and DHA ranged from 0.004 to 0.007 and 0.052 to 0.093 g/d, respectively (Appendix Tables E-12 and E-14). The median intake of DHA ranged from 0.066 to 0.093 g/d for men and 0.052 to 0.069 g/d for women (Appendix Table E-14). Docosapentaenoic acid provided only 0.001 to 0.005 g/d (Appendix Table E-13).

Trans *Fatty Acids*

Food Sources

Reports listing the *trans* fatty acid level in selected food items are available from the United States (Enig et al., 1990; Litin and Sacks, 1993; Michels and Sacks, 1995), Canada (Ratnayake et al., 1993), and Europe (Aro et al., 1998a, 1998b, 1998c; Michels and Sacks, 1995; van Erp-baart et al., 1998; van Poppel et al., 1998). More recently, a comprehensive U.S. database was compiled by the U.S. Department of Agriculture (ARS, 2001) that included a description of the methodology used to formulate the nutrient values (Schakel et al., 1997). *Trans* fatty acids are present in foods containing traditional stick margarine (3.04 g *trans* fatty acids/serving) and vegetable shortenings (2.54 g/serving) that have been subjected to hydrogenation, as well as in milk (0.22 g/serving), butter (0.40 g/serving) and meats (0.01 to 0.21 g/serving) (Emken, 1995). Therefore, foods that are contributors of *trans* fatty acids include pastries, fried foods (e.g., doughnuts and french fries), dairy products, and meats. Human milk contains approximately 1 to 5 percent of total energy as *trans* fatty acids (Table 8-7) and similarly, infant formulas contain approximately 1 to 3 percent (Ratnayake et al., 1997).

Dietary Intake

Estimating the amount of *trans* fatty acids in the food supply has been hampered by the lack of an accurate and comprehensive database from which to derive the data and the trend towards the reformulation of products over the past decade to reduce levels. This latter issue complicates analysis of historical food intake data. Additionally, the variability in the *trans* fatty acid content of foods within a food category is extensive and can introduce substantial error when the calculations are based on food frequency questionnaires that heavily rely on the grouping of similar foods (Innis et al., 1999). *trans* Fatty acid intake is not currently collected in U.S. national surveys.

Early reports suggested a wide range of *trans* fatty acid intakes, from 2.6 to 12.8 g/d (Emken, 1995). The lower estimated intakes tended to be derived from food frequency data, whereas the higher estimated intakes tended to be derived from food availability data. More recent data from food frequency questionnaires collected in the United States suggest average *trans* fatty acid intakes of 1.5 to 2.2 percent of energy (Ascherio et al., 1994; Hu et al., 1997), or 5.2 percent of total dietary fat (Lemaitre et al., 1998). Intakes of about 1 to 2 percent of energy have been reported for women in Canada, although the range of intakes was wide (Elias and Innis,

TABLE 8-7 *Trans* Fatty Acid Content in Term Human Milk of Women in the United States and Canada

Reference	Study Population/Stage of Lactation[a]	*Trans* Fatty Acid	Content in Human Milk % of Total Fatty Acids	% of Total Energy[b]
Gibson and Kneebone, 1981	120 women, 40–45 d pp	16:1 18:1	trace ~ 10	trace ~ 5.46
Chappell et al., 1985	7 women, 1–37 d pp	18:1(9) 18:1(7) 18:1(5) 18:2(6) c,t+t,c[c] Total	2.6 ± 0.4 0.1 ± 0.03 0.1 ± 0.04 0.1 ± 0.4 2.9	1.42 0.05 0.05 0.05 1.57
Chen et al., 1995a	198 samples, 3–4 wk pp	Total *trans*	7.19 ± 3.03	3.92
Innis and King, 1999	103 women, 2 mo pp	Total *trans*	7.1 ± 0.32	3.88

[a] pp = postpartum.
[b] Calculated using the following values: 40 g of fat/L of milk, 8.87 kcal/g of fat, 650 kcal/L of milk.
[c] c,t+t,c = *cis, trans* and *trans, cis.*

2001, 2002). Most recently, *trans* fatty acid intake was estimated from existing CFSII data (Allison et al., 1999). The mean *trans* fatty acid intake for the U.S. population aged 3 years and older was 2.6 percent of total energy intake.

Conjugated Linoleic Acid

Food Sources

The average concentration of conjugated linoleic acid (CLA) in dairy products and ruminant meats is approximately 5 mg of CLA/g of fat (Chin et al., 1992). Although numerous CLA isomers have been reported to be found in meat, milk, and dairy products (Ha et al., 1989), the *cis*-9,*trans*-11 isomer is the predominant form of CLA present in these foods (Ma et al., 1999). The conjugated linoleic acid content of milk can vary depending on a number of factors, such as animal feed diet, pasture grazing, supplement use, and number of lactations (MacDonald, 2000). Ma and coworkers (1999) reported values of 1.8 mg of CLA/g of fat for skim milk, 3.4 mg/g for whole milk, 4.3 mg/g for 1 percent milk, 5.0 mg/g for 2 percent milk, and 5.5 mg/g for half-and-half cream. In addition, values ranged from 2.7 to 6.2 mg of CLA/g of fat for various cheeses and 1.2 to 3.2 mg of CLA/g of fat for different types of raw and cooked beef products.

Dietary Intake

Recent analysis of duplicate food portions indicates CLA intake in the United States is in the range of 151 to 212 mg/d (Ritzenthaler et al., 2001). The average intake of cis-9,trans-11 octadecadienoic acid in a small group of Canadians was recently estimated to be about 95 mg/d (Ens et al., 2001). Based on the CLA content in the Health Canada National Nutritious Food Basket 1998 for purchased quantities, cis-9,trans-11 CLA intake for men and women was 332 and 295 mg/d, respectively. These values assume that all food purchased is actually eaten. From food records it is clear that the pattern of CLA intake is highly variable among individuals and from day-to-day for individuals themselves. Estimates from information on foods purchased, however, are higher than estimates from reported food intake data; therefore, the two data sets are not comparable.

ADVERSE EFFECTS OF OVERCONSUMPTION

Total Fat

A Tolerable Upper Intake Level (UL) was not set for total fat because of the lack of a defined intake level at which an adverse effect, such as obesity, can occur (see Chapter 11). An Acceptable Macronutrient Distribution Range (AMDR) for fat intake, however, has been estimated based on adverse effects from consuming low fat and high fat diets (Chapter 11).

Saturated Fatty Acids

Hazard Identification

Elevated LDL Cholesterol Concentration and Risk of CHD. Several hundred studies have been conducted to assess the effect of saturated fatty acids on serum cholesterol concentration. In general, the higher the intake of saturated fatty acids, the higher the serum total (Figure 8-2) and low density lipoprotein (LDL) cholesterol concentrations (Figure 8-3). Regression analyses of such studies have suggested that for each 1 percent increase

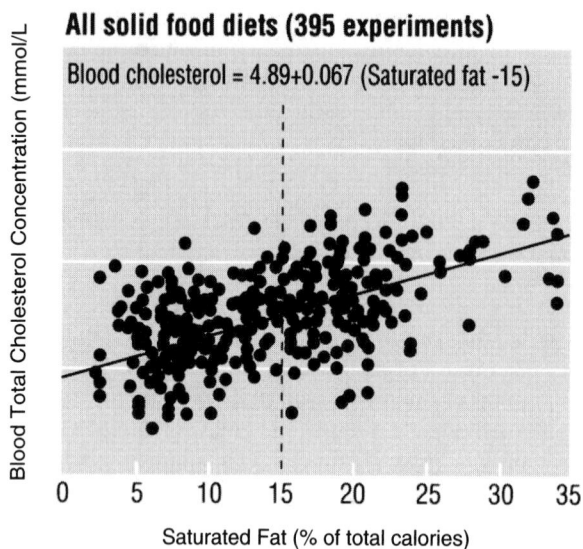

FIGURE 8-2 Relationship between blood total cholesterol concentrations and saturated fatty acid intake. Reprinted, with permission, from Clarke et al. (1997). Copyright 1997 by the *British Medical Journal.*

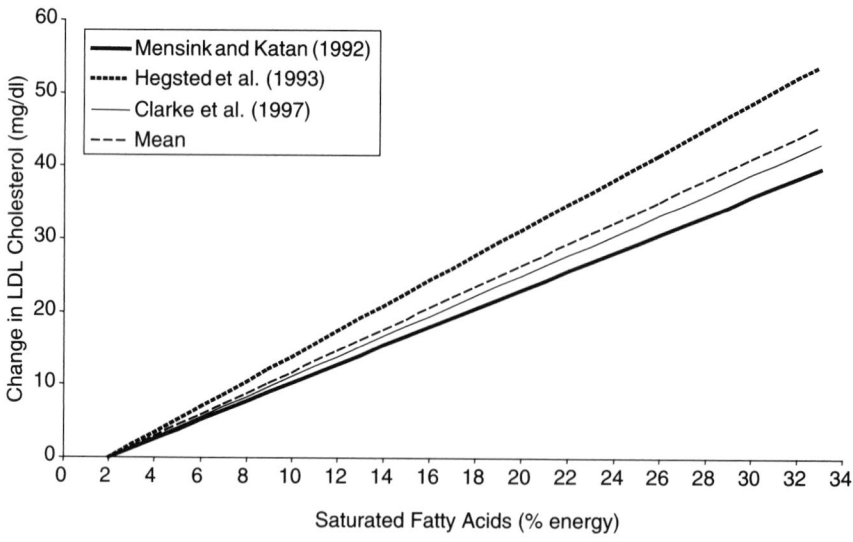

FIGURE 8-3 Calculated changes in serum low density lipoprotein cholesterol concentration in response to percent change in dietary saturated fatty acids. Three regression equations were used to establish the response curves. The range in saturated fatty acid intake was 2.2 to 33 percent of energy.

in energy from saturated fatty acids, serum LDL cholesterol concentration increases by 0.033 mmol/L (Mensink and Katan, 1992), 0.036 mmol/L (Clarke et al., 1997), or 0.045 mmol/L (Hegsted et al., 1993). Although all fats will increase serum high density lipoprotein (HDL) cholesterol concentration relative to carbohydrate, the increase attributable to saturated fats is greater than that observed for monounsaturated and polyunsaturated fatty acids. Serum HDL cholesterol concentration increases by 0.011 to 0.013 mmol/L for each 1 percent increase in saturated fat (Clarke et al., 1997; Hegsted et al., 1993; Mensink and Katan, 1992).

Similar to that observed for saturated fatty acid intake and LDL cholesterol concentration, there is a positive linear relationship between serum total and LDL cholesterol concentrations and risk of coronary heart disease (CHD) or mortality from CHD (Jousilahti et al., 1998; Neaton and Wentworth, 1992; Sorkin et al., 1992; Stamler et al., 1986; Weijenberg et al., 1996). Results from the Zutphen Elderly Study estimated that the relative risk of CHD mortality was 1.4 with a corresponding increase of 1 mmol/L of total serum cholesterol concentration (Weijenberg et al., 1996). It has been estimated that a 10 percent reduction in serum cholesterol concentration would reduce CHD mortality by 20 percent (Jousilahti et al., 1998).

A number of epidemiological studies have reported an association between saturated fatty acid intake and risk of CHD. The majority of these studies have reported a positive relationship between saturated fatty acid intake and risk of CHD and CHD mortality (Goldbourt et al., 1993; Hu et al., 1997, 1999a, 1999c; Keys et al., 1980; McGee et al., 1984). Ascherio and coworkers (1996) concluded that the association between saturated fatty acid intake and risk of CHD was not strong; however, saturated fat and the predicted effects on blood cholesterol concentrations did affect risk. No association between saturated fatty acid intake and coronary deaths was observed in the Zutphen Study or the Alpha-Tocopherol, Beta-Carotene Cancer Prevention Study (Kromhout and de Lezenne Coulander, 1984; Pietinen et al., 1997).

Although all saturated fatty acids were originally considered to be associated with increased adverse health outcomes, including increased blood cholesterol concentrations, it later became apparent that saturated fatty acids differ in their metabolic effects (e.g., potency in raising blood cholesterol concentrations). In general, stearic acid has been shown to have a neutral effect on total and LDL cholesterol concentrations (Bonanome and Grundy, 1988; Denke, 1994; Hegsted et al., 1965; Keys et al., 1965; Yu et al., 1995; Zock and Katan, 1992). While palmitic, lauric, and myristic acids increase cholesterol concentrations (Mensink et al., 1994), stearic acid is more similar to oleic acid in its neutral effect (Kris-Etherton et al., 1993). Furthermore, a stearic acid-rich diet has been shown to improve thrombogenic and atherogenic risk factor profiles (Kelly et al., 2001). However, it is impractical at the current time to make recommendations for saturated fatty acids on the basis of individual fatty acids.

Mortality. A number of studies have demonstrated a positive association between serum cholesterol concentration and the incidence of mortality (Conti et al., 1983; Corti et al., 1997; Haheim et al., 1993; Klag et al., 1993; Martin et al., 1986). Some studies, however, have reported an increased risk of non-CHD mortality, especially cancer, with low serum cholesterol concentration, suggesting a "U" or "J" shaped curve (Agner and Hansen, 1983; Frank et al., 1992; Kagan et al., 1981). The Poland and United States Collaborative Study on Cardiovascular Epidemiology showed an increased risk for cancer with low serum cholesterol concentrations in Poland, but not in the United States (Rywik et al., 1999). It was concluded that various nutritional and non-nutritional factors (obesity, smoking, alcohol use) were confounding factors, resulting in the differences observed between the two countries. As a specific example, body fat was shown to have a "U" shaped relation to mortality (Yao et al., 1991).

Obesity. A number of studies have attempted to ascertain the relationship between saturated fatty acid intake and body mass index, and these results are mixed. Saturated fatty acid intake was shown to be positively associated with body mass index or percent of body fat (Doucet et al., 1998; Gazzaniga and Burns, 1993; Larson et al., 1996; Ward et al., 1994). In contrast, no relationship was observed for saturated fatty acid intake and body weight (González et al., 2000; Ludwig et al., 1999; Miller et al., 1994).

Impaired Glucose Tolerance and Risk of Diabetes. Epidemiological studies have been conducted to ascertain the association between the intake of saturated fatty acids and the risk of diabetes. A number of these studies found no relationship (Colditz et al., 1992; Costa et al., 2000; Salmerón et al., 2001; Sevak et al., 1994; Virtanen et al., 2000). Several large epidemiological studies, however, showed increased risk of diabetes with increased intake of saturated fatty acids (Feskens et al., 1995; Hu et al., 2001; Marshall et al., 1997; Parker et al., 1993). The Normative Aging Study found that a diet high in saturated fatty acids was an independent predictor for both fasting and postprandial insulin concentration (Parker et al., 1993). A reduction in saturated fatty acid intake from 13.9 to 7.8 percent of energy was associated with an 18 percent decrease in fasting insulin and a 25 percent decrease in postprandial insulin concentrations.

Findings from short-term intervention studies tend to suggest a lack of adverse effect of saturated fatty acids on risk indicators for diabetes in healthy individuals. Postprandial glucose and insulin concentrations were not significantly different in men who ingested three different levels of saturated fatty acids (Roche et al., 1998). Fasching and coworkers (1996) reported no difference in insulin secretion or sensitivity in men who consumed a 33 percent saturated, monounsaturated, or polyunsaturated fatty acid diet. There was no difference in postprandial glucose or insulin concentration when healthy adults were fed butter or olive oil (Thomsen et al., 1999). Louheranta and colleagues (1998) found no difference in glucose tolerance and insulin sensitivity in healthy women fed either a high oleic or stearic acid diet. In contrast, results of the KANWU study indicate that consumption of high levels (18 percent of energy) of saturated fats can significantly impair insulin sensitivity (Vessby et al., 2001).

Summary

Intakes above an identified UL indicate a potential risk of an adverse health effects. There is a positive linear trend between total saturated fatty acid intake and total and LDL cholesterol concentration and increased risk of CHD. A UL is not set for saturated fatty acids because any incremental increase in saturated fatty acid intake increases CHD risk. It is neither possible nor advisable to achieve 0 percent of energy from saturated fatty acids in typical whole-food diets. This is because all fat and oil sources are mixtures of fatty acids, and consuming 0 percent of energy would require extraordinary changes in patterns of dietary intake, such as the inclusion of fats and oils devoid of saturated fatty acids, which are presently unavailable. Such extraordinary adjustments may introduce undesirable effects (e.g., inadequate intakes of protein and certain micronutrients) and unknown and unquantifiable health risks. It is possible to consume a diet low in saturated fatty acids by following the dietary guidance provided in Chapter 11.

Cis-Monounsaturated Fatty Acids

Hazard Identification

Cardiovascular Disease. Within the range of usual intake, there are no clearly established adverse effects of n-9 monounsaturated fatty acids in humans. There is some preliminary evidence that a meal providing 50 g of fat from olive oil reduced brachial artery flow-mediated vasodilation by 31 percent in 10 healthy, normolipidemic individuals versus canola oil or salmon (Vogel et al., 2000). In addition, there is evidence from nonhuman primates that a diet rich in n-9 monounsaturated fatty acids promotes atherosclerosis just as much as a diet containing isocaloric amounts of saturated or polyunsaturated fatty acids (Rudel et al., 1997). Dietary monounsaturated fatty acids induce atherogenesis due to greater hepatic lipid concentrations (i.e., triacylglycerol, free cholesterol, and cholesteryl ester), as well as the high degree of cholesteryl oleate enrichment in plasma cholesteryl esters. Overconsumption of energy related to a high n-9 monounsaturated fatty acid and high fat diet is another potential risk associated with excess consumption of monounsaturated fatty acids. n-9 Monounsaturated fatty acid intake may result in an increase in energy intake from saturated fatty acids due to the simultaneous occurrence of saturated and n-9 monounsaturated fatty acids in animal fats.

The n-7 monounsaturated fatty acid, palmitoleic acid, behaves like saturated fatty acids in raising LDL cholesterol concentration (Nestel et al., 1994). Watts and coworkers (1996) reported a positive correlation between palmitoleic acid and progression of CHD.

Cancer. While most epidemiological studies indicate that monounsaturated fatty acid intake is not associated with increased risk of most cancers (Holmes et al., 1999; Hursting et al., 1990; van Dam et al., 2000; van den Brandt et al., 1993), a few studies have observed a positive association. There is some epidemiological evidence for a positive association between oleic acid intake and breast cancer risk in women with no history of benign breast disease (Velie et al., 2000). In addition, one study reported that women with a family history of colorectal cancer who consumed a diet high in mono- and polyunsaturated fatty acids were at greater risk of colon cancer than women without a family history (Slattery et al., 1997). Giovannucci and coworkers (1993) reported a positive association between monounsaturated fatty acid intake and risk of advanced prostate cancer, while two studies observed increased risk of lung cancer (De Stefani et al., 1997; Veierød et al., 1997).

Summary

Based on the lack of adequate data on adverse effects of monounsaturated fatty acids, a UL is not set.

n-6 Polyunsaturated Fatty Acids

A UL is not set for n-6 polyunsaturated fatty acids because of the lack of a defined intake level at which an adverse effect can occur (see Chapter 11). An AMDR for n-6 polyunsaturated fatty acids, however, is estimated based on adverse effects from consuming a diet low or high in n-6 polyunsaturated fatty acids (Chapter 11).

n-3 Polyunsaturated Fatty Acids

Because the longer-chain *n*-3 fatty acids, eicosapentaenoic acid (EPA) and docosahexaenoic acid (DHA), are biologically more potent than their precursor, α-linolenic acid, much of the work on the adverse effects of this group of fatty acids has been on DHA and EPA.

Hazard Identification

Immune Function. Numerous studies have shown suppression of various aspects of human immune function in vitro or ex vivo in peripheral blood mononuclear cells, or in isolated neutrophils or monocytes in individuals provided *n*-3 polyunsaturated fatty acids as a supplement or as an experimental diet compared with baseline values before the intervention (Table 8-8). The minimum dose observed for such an effect was 0.9 g/d of EPA and 0.6 g/d of DHA given as fish oil for 6 to 8 weeks to healthy adults (Cooper et al., 1993). The level of EPA that caused some type of immuno-suppression ranged from 0.9 to 9.4 g/d when fed for 3 to 24 weeks. The level of DHA that caused immunosuppression ranged from 0.6 to 6.0 g/d (Table 8-8).

The data in single treatment studies comparing baseline versus post-supplementation immune function indicate that *n*-3 polyunsaturated fatty acids, especially EPA and DHA at levels 7 to 15 times greater than typical current U.S. intakes, diminish the potential of the immune system to attack pathogens (Kelley et al., 1998, 1999; Lee et al., 1985; Schmidt et al., 1989). This diminished ability, however, is also associated with suppression of inflammatory responses, suggesting benefits for individuals suffering from autoimmune diseases such as rheumatoid arthritis. It seems that the same doses of *n*-3 fatty acids that may be beneficial in chronic disease prevention are doses that are also immunosuppressive.

Several studies using a design of comparison across treatment groups (Blok et al., 1997; Kelley et al., 1998; Mølvig et al., 1991; Yaqoob et al., 2000), rather than comparison within individuals with a baseline, have shown a lack of several potential adverse effects of EPA and DHA supplementation on human immune cell functions. In one key study, 58 healthy men were given daily supplements of 0, 3, 6, or 9 g/d of a fish-oil supplement (EPA intake of 0, 0.81, 1.62, or 2.43 g/d and DHA intake of 0, 0.16, 0.33, or 0.49 g/d) for 1 year (Blok et al., 1997). Ex vivo endotoxin-stimulated production of interleukin (IL)-1β, tumor necrosis factor (TNF)-α, or IL-1Ra (IL-1 receptor antagonist) did not differ among treatments up to 6 months after the fish-oil supplementation was stopped. These data support a lack of long-term adverse effect of fish-oil supplementation on cytokine activity.

TABLE 8-8 Effects of *n*-3 Fatty Acid Intake on Immune Function

Reference	Study Design	*n*-3 Fatty Acid Dose (Daily)[a]
Lee et al., 1985	7 men 6 wk	MaxEPA (3.2 g EPA, 2.2 g DHA)
Endres et al., 1989	9 men 6 wk	MaxEPA (2.75 g EPA, 1.85 g DHA)
Schmidt et al., 1989	12 men 6 wk	Cod liver oil (2.5 g EPA)
Kelley et al., 1991	10 men 56-d crossover	Basal diet Flaxseed oil-supplemented diet (20 g 18:3*n*-3)
Meydani et al., 1991	6 young women, 6 older women 12 wk	ProMega (1.68 g EPA, 0.72 g DHA)
Mølvig et al., 1991	8 men 9 men 8 men 7 wk	Placebo oil Fish oil (1 g EPA, 0.5 g DHA) Fish oil (2 g EPA, 1 g DHA)
Thompson et al., 1991	6 men, 6 women 4-wk crossover	MaxEPA (2.16 g EPA) 12 g olive oil
Virella et al., 1991	4 men fed fish oil, 2 men fed olive oil 6 wk	Fish oil (2.4 g EPA)
Yamashita et al., 1991	3 adults 1 d	3 g EPA, infused
Cooper et al., 1993	8 men and women 6–8 wk	Fish oil (0.9 g EPA, 0.6 g DHA)
Endres et al., 1993	9 men 6 wk	MaxEPA (2.75 g EPA, 1.85 g DHA)
Meydani et al., 1993	7 women, 3 men 24 wk after 6 wk on typical U.S. diet (baseline)	Low fat, high fish diet (1.23 g EPA + DHA)
Sperling et al., 1993	5 women and 3 men with rheumatoid arthritis 10 wk	SuperEPA (9.4 g EPA, 5.0 g DHA)

Results[b]

Depressed neutrophil LTB_4, 6-*trans*-LTB_4, 5-HETE, and endothelial adherence, monocyte LTB_4 and 5-HETE, neutrophil chemotaxis

Depressed PBMC IL-1β, IL-1α, TNF, PGE_2, and neutrophil chemotaxis

Depressed neutrophil migration, monocyte cell density (marker of monocyte migration)

Depressed PBMC proliferation in response to T-cell mitogen but not to B-cell mitogen with flaxseed oil-supplemented diet

Depressed PBMC IL-1β and IL-6 (greater in older women), TNF and IL-2 (older women only)

Depressed PBMC proliferation, IL-1β in PBMCs and monocytes with *n*-3 fatty acids
PBMC secretion of IL-1β, TNF-α, PGE_2 or LTB_4 not affected by *n*-3 fatty acids

Depressed neutrophil chemiluminescence (marker of neutrophil function) with MaxEPA diet

Depressed PBMC IL-2

Depressed NK cell activity of PBMCs

Typhoid vaccine injection site less inflamed, postvaccination tachycardia inhibited, depressed blood IL-1 and IL-6 concentrations

Depressed PBMC IL-2 and proliferation

Depressed PBMC IL-1β, TNF, IL-6, PGE_2, CD_{4+} lymphocytes, and lymphocyte proliferation, delayed-type hypersensitivity

Depressed neutrophil chemotaxis, inositol tris-phosphate formation, and LTB_4, monocyte LTB_4

continued

TABLE 8-8 Continued

Reference	Study Design	n-3 Fatty Acid Dose (Daily)[a]
Gallai et al., 1995	20 patients with relapsing/remitting multiple sclerosis and 15 controls 6 mo	Fish oil (3.06 g EPA, 1.86 g DHA)
Caughey et al., 1996	30 men 4-wk diet + 4-wk diet with fish oil	Flaxseed oil-enriched diet and fish oil (EPA 1.62 g, DHA 1.08 g) Sunflower oil diet and fish oil (EPA 1.62 g, DHA 1.08 g)
Hughes et al., 1996	3 men, 3 women 3 wk	EPA Forte (0.93 g EPA, 0.63 g DHA)
Blok et al., 1997	58 men 1 y	0, 3, 6, or 9 g fish oil (0, 0.81, 1.62, or 2.43 g EPA; 0, 0.16, 0.33, or 0.49 g DHA)
Kelley et al., 1998	4 men 7 men 120 d	Basal diet DHA-enriched oil (6 g DHA)
Kelley et al., 1999	4 men 7 men 120 d	Basal diet DHA-enriched oil (6 g DHA)
Yaqoob et al., 2000	5 men, 3 women 7 men, 1 woman 3 other groups of 8 fed other oils, but all comparable to placebo 12-wk parallel	Placebo oil (3:1 coconut and soybean oils) Fish oil (2.1 g EPA, 1.1 g DHA)

[a] EPA = eicosapentaenoic acid, DHA = docosahexaenoic acid.
[b] LTB$_4$ = leukotriene B$_4$, 5-HETE = 5-hydroxyeicosatetraenoic acid, PBMC = peripheral blood mononuclear cell, IL = interleukin, TNF = tumor necrosis factor, PGE$_2$ = prosta-

In studies using multitreatment parallel designs, potential adverse effects of n-3 fatty acids on immune function that were observed include decreased expression of monocyte major histocompatibility complex antigens and cell surface adhesion proteins (Hughes et al., 1996), decreased peripheral blood mononuclear cell (PBMC) proliferation and IL-1β in

Results[b]

Depressed PBMC IL-1β, TNF-α, IL-2 and IFN-γ, PGE_2, and LTB_4, serum-soluble IL-2 receptors

Depressed PBMC TNF-α, IL-1β, TxB_2, and PGE_2 with flaxseed oil-enriched diet
Greater decreases in PBMC TNF-α, IL-1β, and TxB_2 in both groups after fish-oil supplementation

Depressed monocyte surface proteins: HLA-DR, HLA-DP, HLA-DQ, ICAM-1, LFA-1

No effect on whole blood IL-1β, TNF-α, or IL-1 receptor antagonist

Decreased white blood cells
PBMC proliferation and delayed-type hypersensitivity not different between groups

Depressed PBMC IL-1β and TNF-α production, in vitro PBMC PGE_2 and LTB_4 secretion

No effect of fish oil on PBMC NK cell activity, proliferation, types of blood lymphocytes, IL-1α, IL-1β, TNF-α, IL-2, IL-10, and IFN-γ

glandin E_2, NK cell = natural killer cell, IFN-γ = interferon-γ, TxB_2 = thromboxane B_2, HLA = human leukocytes antigen, ICAM = intercellular adhesion molecule, LFA = leukocyte function-associated antigen.

PBMCs and monocytes (Mølvig et al., 1991), decreased PBMC IL-2 (Virella et al., 1991), decreased but still clinically normal neutrophils (Kelley et al., 1998), and decreased tachycardia and inflammation after typhoid vaccine (Cooper et al., 1993).

All of the single treatment studies comparing individuals fed n-3 polyunsaturated fatty acids before and after supplementation showed immunosuppressive effects. Differences in study design (single treatment versus multitreatment parallel designs) seem to be quite significant in determining whether n-3 fatty acid supplementation exerts immunosuppression or not. There is no clear basis to prefer one type of study design to the other. For example, the difference in results between Caughey and colleagues (1996) (a baseline comparison study) and Blok and colleagues (1997) (a group comparison study) is not accounted for by greater variability in measurements by the latter group. The standard deviation for whole blood TNF-α was no more than 5 percent of the mean in the study by Blok and coworkers (1997), and the standard deviation for mononuclear cell TNF-α was 25 to 45 percent of the mean in the study by Caughey and coworkers (1996). In another study using intertreatment comparisons of control versus men given fish oil for 7 weeks, secretions of IL-1β and TNF-α were not suppressed by fish-oil feeding, but lysates of peripheral blood mononuclear cells from people given fish oil contained less IL-1β and TNF-α than did cells from controls (Mølvig et al., 1991). Therefore, the study by Mølvig and colleagues (1991) showed some concurrence with that of Blok and colleagues (1997) and Caughey and colleagues (1996).

Another alternative is to extrapolate from animal studies using model species that are known to have similar immune system components and responsiveness compared to humans. Detailed characterization of appropriateness of animal models for extrapolation to humans with respect to immunosuppression has not been done. A few animal studies have shown the effects of dietary n-3 fatty acids on response to infection (Chang et al., 1992; Fritsche et al., 1997). At this time, there are not sufficient data to support establishing an UL for EPA and DHA based on infection responsiveness.

Bleeding and Increased Risk of Hemorrhagic Stroke. One of a number of factors that has been suggested to link n-3 polyunsaturated fatty acid intake with reduced risk of CHD is reduced platelet aggregation, and therefore prolonged bleeding time. The platelet count can decline by as much as 35 percent; however, the count does not usually fall below the lower limit of normal (Goodnight et al., 1981). Although prolonged bleeding times have been shown to be beneficial in preventing heart disease, bleeding times can become prolonged enough to result in excessive bleeding and bruising. Intervention studies that have examined the effects of n-3 fatty acids on bleeding time are mixed. A number of short-term studies (4 to 11 weeks) have shown significant increased bleeding time with taking EPA/DHA supplements ranging from 2 to 15 g/d (Cobiac et al., 1991; De

Caterina et al., 1990; Levinson et al., 1990; Lorenz et al., 1983; Mortensen et al., 1983; Sanders et al., 1981; Schmidt et al., 1990, 1992; Smith et al., 1989; Thorngren and Gustafson, 1981; Wojenski et al., 1991; Zucker et al., 1988), whereas other studies using similar intake levels resulted in no difference (Blonk et al., 1990; Freese and Mutanen, 1997; Rogers et al., 1987). Analysis of these studies collectively indicated no dose–response for EPA and DHA intake and the percent increase in bleeding time. Schmidt and coworkers (1992) reported increased bleeding times when 3.1 g/d of EPA and DHA were given for 6 weeks and 9 months. None of the above studies reported excessive bleeding times, bleeding episodes, or bruising.

Dietary feeding studies that provided approximately 2 percent of energy as EPA and DHA from salmon did not result in increased bleeding time compared to a stabilization diet that contained only 0.3 percent of energy as EPA and DHA (Nelson et al., 1991). Excessive cutaneous bleeding time and reduced in vitro platelet aggregability have been reported in Greenland Eskimos (Dyerberg and Bang, 1979; Dyerberg et al., 1978) who ingest on average 6.5 g/d (3.8 percent of energy) of EPA and DHA derived mainly from seal (Bang et al., 1980). A tendency to bleed from the nose and urinary tract was observed among the Greenland Eskimos (Bang and Dyerberg, 1980). One study comparing perirenal adipose tissue fatty acid profiles with incidence of hemorrhagic stroke in human autopsy cases from Greenland showed that the amounts of EPA and DHA in the adipose tissue of 4 hemorrhagic stroke victims was greater than in 26 control cases with no cerebral pathology (Pedersen et al., 1999). Furthermore, ecological studies have suggested an increased risk of hemorrhagic stroke among Greenland Eskimos (Kristensen, 1983; Kromann and Green, 1980). A recent prospective study in the United States showed no association between intake of n-3 fatty acids and risk of hemorrhagic stroke (Iso et al., 2001). The median intake levels for the quintiles of n-3 polyunsaturated fat intake, however, ranged from only 0.077 to 0.481 g/d, which reflects the relatively low intake level of n-3 fatty acids in the Unites States.

Oxidative Damage. Long-chain polyunsaturated fatty acids, particularly DHA and EPA, are vulnerable to lipid peroxidation, resulting in oxidative damage of various tissues. Numerous feeding studies using laboratory animals have demonstrated increased lipid peroxidation and oxidative damage of erythrocytes, liver, and kidney membranes and bone marrow DNA with consumption of DHA (Ando et al., 1998; Song and Miyazawa, 2001; Umegaki et al., 2001; Yasuda et al., 1999). The oxidative damage was shown to be reduced or prevented with the coconsumption of vitamin E (Ando et al., 1998; Leibovitz et al., 1990; Yasuda et al., 1999).

Summary

While there is evidence to suggest that high intakes of *n*-3 polyunsaturated fatty acids, particularly EPA and DHA, may impair immune response and result in excessively prolonged bleeding times, it is not possible to establish a UL. Studies on immune function were done in vitro and it is difficult, if not impossible, to know how well these artificial conditions simulate human immune cell response in vivo. Data on EPA and DHA intakes and bleeding times are mixed and a dose–response effect was not observed. Although excessively prolonged bleeding times and increased incidence of bleeding have been observed in Eskimos, whose diets are rich in EPA and DHA, information is lacking to conclude that EPA and DHA were the sole basis for these observations. At the 99th percentile of intake, the highest intakes of dietary EPA and DHA were 0.662 and 0.651 g/d, respectively, in men 71 years of age and older (Appendix Tables E-12 and E-14). This EPA + DHA intake (1.31 g/d) is much lower than that for Greenland Eskimos (6.5 g/d). EPA and DHA are available as dietary supplements, and until more information is available on the adverse effects of EPA and DHA, these supplements should be taken with caution.

Special Considerations

A few special populations have been reported to exhibit adverse effects from consuming *n*-3 polyunsaturated fatty acids. Despite the favorable effects of *n*-3 fatty acids on glucose homeostasis, caution has been suggested for the use of n-3 fatty acids in those individuals who already exhibit glucose intolerance or diabetic conditions (Glauber et al., 1988; Kasim et al., 1988) that require increased doses of hypoglycemic agents (Friday et al., 1989; Stacpoole et al., 1989; Zambon et al., 1992). Increased episodes of nose bleeds have been observed in individuals with familial hypercholesterolemia during fish-oil supplementation (Clarke et al., 1990). Anticoagulants, such as aspirin, warfarin, and coumadin, will prolong bleeding times and the simultaneous ingestion of n-3 fatty acids by individuals may excessively prolong bleeding times (Thorngren and Gustafson, 1981). Therefore, the subpopulations described above should take supplements containing EPA and DHA with caution.

Trans *Fatty Acids*

Hazard Identification

Total and LDL Cholesterol Concentrations. Prior to 1980 there was generally little concern about the trend toward increased consumption of hydrogenated fat in the U.S. diet, especially when the hydrogenated fats displaced fats relatively high in saturated fatty acids (Denke, 1995). During the early 1980s studies showed a hypercholesterolemic effect of *trans* fatty acids in rabbits (Kritchevsky, 1982; Ruttenberg et al., 1983). Renewed interest in the topic of hydrogenated fat in human diets, or more precisely *trans* fatty acid intake, started in the early 1990s. The availability of a methodology to distinguish the responses of individual lipoprotein classes to dietary modification expanded the depth to which the topic could be readdressed.

A report from the Netherlands suggested that a diet enriched with elaidic acid (a subfraction of 18:1 *trans*) compared to one enriched with oleic acid (18:1 *cis*) increased total and LDL cholesterol concentrations and decreased HDL cholesterol concentrations, hence resulting in a less favorable total cholesterol:HDL cholesterol ratio (Mensink and Katan, 1990). Consumption of a diet enriched with saturated fatty acids resulted in LDL cholesterol concentrations similar to those observed after individuals consumed the diet high in elaidic acid, but HDL cholesterol concentrations were similar to those observed after individuals consumed the diet high in oleic acid. A number of similar studies have been published since then and have reported that hydrogenated fat/*trans* fatty acid consumption increases LDL cholesterol concentrations (Aro et al., 1997; Judd et al., 1994, 1998; Louheranta et al., 1999; Müller et al., 1998; Sundram et al., 1997) (Tables 8-9, 8-10, and 8-11). Recent data have demonstrated a dose-dependent relationship between *trans* fatty acid intake and the LDL:HDL ratio and when combining a number of studies, the magnitude of this effect is greater for *trans* fatty acids compared with saturated fatty acids (Figure 8-4) (Ascherio et al., 1999).

Similar to the metabolic clinical trial data, studies in free-living individuals asked to substitute hydrogenated fat for other fat in their habitual diet resulted in higher concentrations of total and LDL cholesterol (Table 8-11) (Nestel et al., 1992b; Noakes and Clifton, 1998; Seppänen-Laakso et al., 1993).

No studies have been conducted to evaluate the effect of *trans* fatty acids that are present in meats and dairy products on LDL concentrations. The relative effect of *trans* fatty acids in meat and dairy products on LDL cholesterol concentration would be small compared to hydrogenated oils because of the lower levels that are present, and because any rise in concentration would most likely be due to the abundance of saturated fatty acids.

HDL Cholesterol Concentrations. The data related to the impact of hydrogenated fat/*trans* fatty acids compared with unhydrogenated oil/*cis* fatty acids on HDL cholesterol concentrations are less consistent than for LDL cholesterol concentrations (Tables 8-9, 8-10, and 8-11). As reported

TABLE 8-9 Dietary *Trans* Fatty Acids (TFA) and Blood Lipid Concentration: Controlled Feeding Trials

Reference	Study Population	Diet[a]
Mensink and Katan, 1990; Mensink et al., 1992	79 men and women, avg 25–26 y	3-wk crossover, 40% fat 10% 18:1 10% SF 10% TFA
Zock and Katan, 1992	56 healthy men and women	3 wk crossover, 41% fat 18:2 18:0 TFA
Judd et al., 1994	58 men and women	6-wk crossover, 40% fat 18:1 SFA moderate TFA high TFA
Aro et al., 1997	80 healthy men and women, 20–52 y	5-wk intervention, 33% fat 18:0 TFA
Sundram et al., 1997	27 men and women, 19–39 y	4-wk crossover, 31% fat 18:1 16:0 12:0 + 14:0 TFA
Louheranta et al., 1999	14 healthy women, avg 23 y	4-wk crossover, 37% fat 18:1 TFA
Judd et al., 2002	50 men	5-wk crossover, 39% fat 18:1 18:0 TFA/18:0 TFA

[a] SF = saturated fat, SFA = saturated fatty acids.
[b] LDL-C = low density lipoprotein cholesterol, HDL-C = high density lipoprotein cholesterol, Lp(a) = lipoprotein(a).

TFA (% of energy)	Blood Lipid Concentrations[b]		
	LDL-C (mmol/L)	HDL-C (mmol/L)	Lp(a) (mg/L)
0	2.67^c	1.42^c	32^c
1.8	3.14^d	1.42^c	26^d
10.9	3.04^e	1.25^d	45^e
0.1	2.83^c	1.47^c	
0.3	3.00^d	1.41^d	
7.7	3.07^d	1.37^d	
0.7	3.34^c	1.42^c	
0.7	3.64^d	$1.40^{c,d}$	
3.8	3.54^e	1.47^e	
6.6	$3.60^{d,e}$	1.38^d	
0.4	2.89^c	1.42^c	270^c
8.7	3.13^d	1.22^d	308^d
0	3.17	1.25	128.3
0	3.15	1.26	122.0
0	3.57	1.18	134.3
6.9	3.81	1.05	153.3
0	2.53	1.37	225 (units/L)
5.1	2.64	1.31	220 (units/L)
0	2.95^c		
0	3.10^d		
4	3.32^e		
8	3.36^e		

[c,d,e] Within each study, LDL-C, HDL-C, or Lp(a) concentrations that are significantly different between treatment groups have a different superscript.

TABLE 8-10 Hydrogenated Fat Intake and Blood Lipid Concentrations: Controlled Feeding Trials

Reference	Study Population	Diet[a]
Lichtenstein et al., 1993	14 men and women, 44–78 y	32-d crossover, 30% fat Baseline Corn oil Corn oil margarine
Almendingen et al., 1995	31 men, 21–46 y	3-wk crossover, 33–36% fat Butter PHFO PHSO
Judd et al., 1998b	46 men and women, 28–65 y	5-wk crossover, 34% fat PUFA-M Butter TFA-M
Müller et al., 1998	16 healthy females, 19–30 y	14-d crossover, 31–32% fat Vegetable oil PHFO
Lichtenstein et al., 1999	36 men and women, > 50 y	35-d crossover, 30% fat Soybean oil Semiliquid margarine Butter Soft margarine Shortening Stick margarine

[a] PHFO = partially hydrogenated fish oil, PHSO = partially hydrogenated soybean oil, PUFA-M = margarine containing polyunsaturated fatty acids, TFA-M = margarine containing *trans* fatty acids.
[b] TFA = *trans* fatty acids.

for LDL cholesterol concentrations, the effect of hydrogenated fat/*trans* fatty acids on HDL cholesterol concentrations, if present, is likely to be dose-dependent (Judd et al., 1994). The preponderance of the data suggests that hydrogenated fat/*trans* fatty acids, relative to saturated fatty acids, result in lower HDL cholesterol concentrations (Ascherio et al., 1999; Zock and Mensink, 1996; Zock et al., 1995). Because of the potentially

| TFA[b] | Blood Lipid Concentrations[c] | | |
(% of energy)	LDL-C (mmol/L)	HDL-C (mmol/L)	Lp(a) (mg/L)
0.77	3.96[d]	1.24[d]	140[d]
0.44	3.23[e]	1.14[e]	160[d]
4.16	3.49[e]	1.11[e]	130[d]
0.9	3.81[d]	1.05[d]	194[d]
8.0	3.94[d,f]	0.98[e]	234[e]
8.5	3.58[e]	1.05[d]	238[e]
2.4	3.21[d]	1.24[d]	197[d]
2.7	3.44[e]	1.27[d]	186[e]
3.9	3.27[f]	1.24[d]	202[d]
1.1	2.63[d]	1.32[d]	212[d]
1.7	2.87[e]	1.28[d]	225[d]
0.55	3.98[d]	1.11[d,e]	230
0.91	4.01[d,e]	1.11[d,e]	230
1.25	4.58[f]	1.16[e]	220
3.30	4.11[d,e]	1.11[d,e]	240
4.15	4.24[e]	1.11[d,e]	240
6.72	4.34[e]	1.01[d]	240

[c] LDL-C = low density lipoprotein cholesterol, HDL-C = high density lipoprotein cholesterol, Lp(a) = lipoprotein(a).
[d,e,f] Within each study, LDL-C, HDL-C, or Lp(a) concentrations that are significantly different between treatment groups have a different superscript.

differential effects of hydrogenated fat/*trans* fatty acids on LDL and HDL cholesterol concentrations, concern has been raised regarding their effect on the total cholesterol or LDL cholesterol:HDL cholesterol ratio (Ascherio et al., 1999). However, with respect to dietary fat recommendations, the strategy to improve the total cholesterol or LDL cholesterol:HDL

TABLE 8-11 Dietary *Trans* Fatty Acids (TFA), Hydrogenated Fat, and Blood Lipid Concentrations: Free-Living Trials

Reference	Study Population	Diet[a]
Nestel et al., 1992a	26 mildly hypercholesterolemic men, 27–57 y	4-wk crossover, 42% fat Control 1 Control 2 Blend 1 Blend 2
Nestel et al., 1992b	27 mildly hypercholesterolemic men, 30–63 y	3-wk crossover, 36–37% fat Control 18:1 TFA 16:0
Seppänen-Laakso et al., 1993	57 men and women, middle-aged	12-wk crossover to 1 of 2 diets, 39–43% fat Margarine Rapeseed Olive oil
Wood et al., 1993a	38 healthy men, 30–60 y	6-wk crossover, 38% fat Butter Butter-sunflower Butter-olive Hard margarine Soft margarine
Wood et al., 1993b	29 healthy men, 30–60 y	6-wk crossover, 37% fat Butter Crude palm Margarine Refined palm Refined palm+sunflower Sunflower oil
Chisholm et al., 1996	49 hypercholesterolemic men and women, avg 47 y	6-wk crossover, 26–27% fat Butter Margarine

TFA (% of energy)	Blood Lipid Concentrations[c]		
	LDL-C (mmol/L)	HDL-C (mmol/L)	Lp(a) (units/L)
3.8	4.13[c]	1.11[c]	
3.7	4.03[c,d]	1.15[c]	
6.7	3.92[d,e]	1.10[c]	
6.6	3.83[e]	1.11[c]	
< 1	4.22[c]	0.98[c]	235[c]
1.4	3.90[d]	0.98[c]	236[c]
5.7	4.27[c]	0.98[c]	296[d]
< 1	4.16[c]	1.09[d]	249[e]
	Change from baseline	Change from baseline	
2.9	−0.20	+0.05	
0	−0.30	−0.01	
0	−0.32	0.00	
2.1	3.78[c]	1.22[c]	
1.0	3.49[d]	1.19[c]	
1.0	3.59[d]	1.22[c]	
11.1	3.47[d]	1.16[c]	
0	3.26[e]	1.16[c]	
0.2	3.52[c]	1.03[c]	
0	3.36[c]	1.03[c]	
3.0	3.36[c]	1.00[c]	
0	3.41[c]	1.06[d]	
0	3.41[c]	1.03[c]	
0	3.23[d]	1.00[c]	
1.4	4.21[c]	1.26[c]	223[c]
3.6	3.82[d]	1.24[c]	249[c]

continued

TABLE 8-11 Continued

Reference	Study Population	Diet[a]
Noakes and Clifton, 1998	38 mildly hyperlipidemic men and women	3-wk crossover, 2 groups, 31–35% fat Canola + TFA TFA-free canola Butter PUFA + TFA TFA-free PUFA Butter

[a] PUFA = polyunsaturated fatty acids.
[b] LDL-C = low density lipoprotein cholesterol, HDL-C = high density lipoprotein cholesterol, Lp(a) = lipoprotein(a).

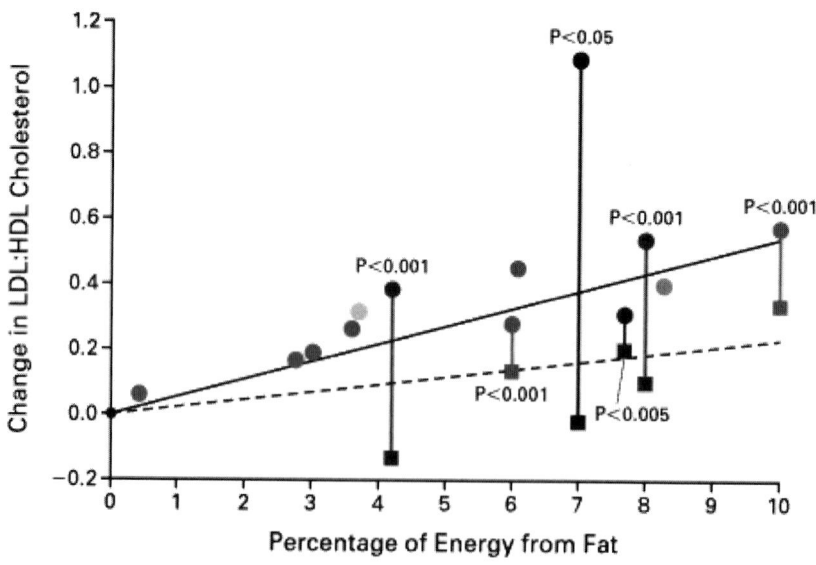

FIGURE 8-4 Change in the low density lipoprotein (LDL):high density lipoprotein (HDL) cholesterol concentration with increasing energy intake from saturated and *trans* fatty acids. Solid line represents the best-fit regression for *trans* fatty acids. Dotted line represents the best-fit regression for saturated fatty acids. Reprinted, with permission, from Ascherio et al. (1999). Copyright 1999 by the Massachusetts Medical Society.

TFA (% of energy)	Blood Lipid Concentrations[c]		
	LDL-C (mmol/L)	HDL-C (mmol/L)	Lp(a) (units/L)
3.3	3.64[c]	1.19[c]	
0	3.61[c]	1.28[c]	
1.1	4.14[d]	1.20[c]	
3.6	4.23[c]	1.17[c]	
0	3.98[d]	1.23[c]	
1.2	4.70[e]	1.27[c]	

thin each study, LDL-C, HDL-C, or Lp(a) concentrations that are significantly
it between treatment groups have a different superscript.

cholesterol ratio would not be different from that to decrease LDL cholesterol concentrations.

Lp(a) Concentrations. Lipoprotein(a) (Lp(a)) concentrations in plasma
have been associated with increased risk for developing cardiovascular and
cerebrovascular disease, possibly via inhibition of plasminogen activity
(Lippi and Guidi, 1999; Nielsen, 1999; Wild et al., 1997). Lp(a) is a lipoprotein particle similar to LDL with respect to its cholesterol and apolipoprotein
B100 content, but it also contains an additional apolipoprotein termed
apo(a) (Lippi and Guidi, 1999; Nielsen, 1999). Lp(a) concentrations have
been reported by some investigators to be increased after the consumption
of diets enriched in hydrogenated fat/*trans* fatty acids (Tables 8-9, 8-10,
and 8-11) (Almendingen et al., 1995; Aro et al., 1997; Lichtenstein et al.,
1999; Mensink et al., 1992; Nestel et al., 1992b; Sundram et al., 1997), but
not by all (Chisholm et al., 1996; Judd et al., 1998; Lichtenstein et al.,
1993; Louheranta et al., 1999; Müller et al., 1998). The magnitude of the
mean increases in Lp(a) concentrations reported to date that is associated
with *trans* fatty acid intake for the most part would not be predicted to
have a physiologically significant effect on cardiovascular disease risk. However, an unresolved issue at this time is the potential effect of relatively
high levels of *trans* fatty acids in individuals with initially high concentrations of Lp(a).

Hemostatic Factors. The effect of *trans* fatty acids on hemostatic factors has been assessed by a number of investigators (Almendingen et al., 1996; Mutanen and Aro, 1997; Sanders et al., 2000; Turpeinen et al., 1998; Wood et al., 1993b) (Table 8-12). In general, these researchers have concluded that hydrogenated fat/*trans* fatty acids had little effect on a variety of hemostatic variables. Similarly, Müller and colleagues (1998) reported that hemostatic variables were unaffected by the substitution of a vegetable oil-based margarine relatively high in saturated fatty acids when compared with a hydrogenated fish oil-based margarine.

Susceptibility of LDL to Oxidation. Hydrogenated fat/*trans* fatty acids have consistently been reported to have little effect on the susceptibility of LDL to oxidation (Cuchel et al., 1996; Halvorsen et al., 1996; Nestel et al., 1992b; Sørensen et al., 1998) (Table 8-12).

Blood Pressure. A few reports addressed the issue of *trans* fatty acid intake and blood pressure (Mensink et al., 1991; Zock et al., 1993) (Table 8-12). The authors concluded that consumption of diets high in saturated, mono-unsaturated, or *trans* fatty acids resulted in similar diastolic and systolic blood pressures.

CHD. Similar to saturated fatty acids, there is a positive linear trend between *trans* fatty acid intake and LDL cholesterol concentrations (Judd et al., 1994; Lichtenstein et al., 1999; Zock and Katan, 1992). Some evidence also suggests that *trans* fatty acids result in lower HDL cholesterol concentrations (Table 8-13). Hence, the net result is a higher total cholesterol or LDL cholesterol:HDL cholesterol ratio (Judd et al., 1994; Lichtenstein et al., 1999; Zock and Katan, 1992). This finding, combined with data from prospective cohort studies (Ascherio et al., 1996; Gillman et al., 1997; Hu et al., 1997; Pietinen et al., 1997; Willett et al., 1993) (Table 8-13), has lead to the concern that dietary *trans* fatty acids are more deleterious with respect to CHD than saturated fatty acids (Ascherio et al., 1999).

Summary

Similar to saturated fatty acids, there is a positive linear trend between *trans* fatty acid intake and LDL cholesterol concentration, and therefore increased risk of CHD. A UL is not set for *trans* fatty acids because any incremental increase in *trans* fatty acid intake increases CHD risk. Because *trans* fatty acids are unavoidable in ordinary, nonvegan diets, consuming 0 percent of energy would require significant changes in patterns of dietary intake. Such adjustments may introduce undesirable effects (e.g., elimination of commercially prepared foods and dairy products and meats that contain *trans* fatty acids may result in inadequate intakes of protein and certain micronutrients) and unknown and unquantifiable health risks. It is possible to consume a diet low in *trans* fatty acids by following the dietary guidance provided in Chapter 11.

RESEARCH RECOMMENDATIONS

Total Fat

- Studies are needed that examine the effects of alterations in the level of total fat in the context of a low saturated fatty acid diet on blood lipid concentrations and glucose-insulin homeostasis in individuals with defined metabolic syndromes, such as type 1 and type 2 diabetes.
- Randomized and blinded long-term (greater than 1 year) studies are needed on the effect of dietary fat versus carbohydrate on body fatness.

Saturated Fatty Acids

- Further examination of intakes at which significant risk of chronic diseases can occur is needed.
- Data that examine the indicators for and risk of chronic disease at low levels of saturated fatty acid intake are necessary.

Cis-*Monounsaturated Fatty Acids*

- Information is needed to assess energy balance in free-living individuals who have implemented a diet high in monounsaturated fatty acids versus a diet lower in monounsaturated fatty acids (and higher in carbohydrate).
- Additional information is needed on the effects of alterations in the level of monounsaturated fatty acid in the context of a low saturated fatty acid diet on blood lipid concentrations and glucose–insulin homeostasis in individuals with defined metabolic syndromes, such as type 1 and type 2 diabetes.
- Studies are needed to evaluate cardiovascular disease risk status and risk of other chronic diseases in individuals consuming a high monounsaturated fatty acid diet versus a diet lower in monounsaturated fatty acids (and higher in carbohydrate).
- An evaluation of the nutritional adequacy and nutrient profile of free-living individuals following a self-selected high monounsaturated fatty acid diet is necessary.
- Studies that assess the effects of a high monounsaturated fatty acid diet on endothelial function and atherogenesis are needed.

TABLE 8-12 *Trans* Fatty Acid (TFA) Intake and Blood Clotting, Low Density Lipoprotein (LDL) Oxidation, and Blood Pressure

Reference	Study Population	Diet[a]	TFA (% of energy)
Clotting			
Wood et al., 1993b	29 men, 30–60 y	6-wk crossover, 37% fat	
		Butter	0.2
		Crude palm oil	0
		Margarine	3.0
		Refined palm oil	0
		Refined palm+sunflower	0
		Sunflower oil	0
Almendingen et al., 1996	31 men, avg 27 y	3-wk crossover, 33–36% fat	
		PHSO	8.5
		PHFO	8.0
		Butter	0.9
Mutanen and Aro, 1997	80 men and women, 20–52 y	5-wk crossover to 1 of 2 diets, 33–34% fat	
		High 18:0	0.4
		High TFA	8.7
Turpeinen et al., 1998	80 men and women, 20–52 y	5-wk crossover to 1 of 2 diets, 32–34% fat	
		18:0	0.4
		TFA	8.7
Sanders et al., 2000	16 men and women, 18–32 y	1 test-meal crossover, 7% or 65% fat	
		18:1	0.1
		18:1 trans	24.7
		18:0	0
		16:0	0.2
		MCT	0
		Low fat	0
Oxidation			
Cuchel et al., 1996	14 men and women, 44–78 y	32-d crossover, 30% fat	
		Corn oil	0.44
		Corn oil+margarine	4.16

Results[b]		Comments
TxB$_2$ (pg/mL)	6-keto-PGF$_{1\alpha}$ (pg/mL)	
35	89	
41	94	
40	86	
40	87	
36	100	
62	95	
Fibrinogen (g/L)	PAI-1 activity (units/mL)	For PHSO, greater PAI-1 activity than PHFO or butter
3.0	13.5	Increased fibrinogen with butter diet
2.9	10.7	No significant difference in factor VII,
3.1	8.8	fibrinogen peptide A, β-thromboglobulin, or tissue plasminogen activator
		No marked difference in factor VII coagulation activity, tissue type plasminogen activity, or PAI-1 activity
Fibrinogen (g/L)		
3.62		
3.61		
		No difference in TxB$_2$ production or ADP-induced platelet aggregation in vitro Significant increase in collagen-induced aggregation with 18:0 diet
FVII$_c$ (% standard)	FVII$_a$ (ng/mL)	No significant differences in factor VII coagulation activity; factor VII-activated
124	2.7	concentrations were significantly higher
122	1.9	with 18:1, 18:1 trans, 18:0, and 16:0 diets
114	1.9	
112	2.1	
112	1.5	
99	1.4	
		No difference in susceptibility to LDL oxidation

continued

TABLE 8-12 Continued

Reference	Study Population	Diet[a]	TFA (% of energy)
Halvorsen et al., 1996	29 men, 21–46 y	19-d crossover, 33–36% fat	
		Butter	0.9
		PHSO	8.5
		PHFO	8.0
Sørensen et al., 1998	47 men, 29–60 y	4 wk, consumed 30 g/d of 1 of 2 margarines	mol % of fat
		Sunflower oil	0.79
		Fish oil, enriched	0.98
Blood pressure			
Mensink et al., 1991	59 men and women, 19–57 y, normo-tensive	3-wk crossover, 39–40% fat	
		18:1	0
		TFA	10.9
		SFA	1.8
Zock et al., 1993	55 men and women, 19–49 y	3-wk crossover, 40–43% fat	
		18:2	0.1
		18:0	0.3
		TFA	7.7

[a] PHSO = partially hydrogenated soybean oil, PHFO = partially hydrogenated fish oil, MCT = medium-chain triacylglycerol, SFA = saturated fatty acid.

n-6 Polyunsaturated Fatty Acids

- In metabolic and large observational studies, comparison should be made of the benefits of α-linolenic acid, eicosapentaenoic acid (EPA), and docosahexaenoic acid (DHA) across a range of *n*-6 polyunsaturated fatty acid intakes.

- Using good biomarkers for low density lipoprotein oxidation and cancer susceptibility, assessments are needed of the potential adverse effects of diets at levels of *n*-6 polyunsaturated fatty acids greater than 10 percent of energy.

- Studies that assess the effects of a high *n*-6 polyunsaturated fatty acid diet on markers of endothelial function and inflammation are needed.

Results[b]		Comments
Dienes (nmol/mg LDL)	Formation rate (nmol/mg LDL × min)	No significant differences in conjugated dienes, lipid peroxides, uptake by macrophages, or electrophoretic mobility of LDL
1,020	10	
1,034	10	TFA does not alter susceptibility to LDL oxidation
1,107	10	
	Oxidation rate (nmol/mg × min)	Fish oil consumption compared with sunflower oil margarine had no effect on LDL size and led to minor changes in LDL oxidation resistance
Dienes (nmol/g)		
445	10.4	
468	10.2	
		No effect of TFA intake on blood pressure
SBP (mmHg)	DBP (mmHg)	
113	66	
112	67	
112	67	
		No effect of TFA intake on blood pressure
SBP (mmHg)	SBP (mmHg)	
114	68	
113	70	
113	69	

[b] TxB_2 = thromboxane B_2, 6-keto-$PGF_{1\alpha}$ = 6-keto-prostaglandin $F_{1\alpha}$, PAI-1 = plasminogen activator inhibitor type 1, $FVII_c$ = factor VII coagulant activity, $FVII_a$ = factor VII activated, SBP = systolic blood pressure, DBP = diastolic blood pressure.

- Further research is needed to address the potentially important relationships between the amount of n-3 and n-6 fatty acids and glucose tolerance suggested by studies of fatty acid composition in affected individuals.

n-3 Polyunsaturated Fatty Acids

- Randomized clinical trials are needed of EPA+DHA, EPA, and DHA to evaluate their impact on cancer (i.e., colon, breast, prostate). The use of biomarkers for cancer susceptibility may expedite such studies.

TABLE 8-13 Dietary *Trans* Fatty Acids (TFA): Epidemiological Studies

Reference	Study Design[a]	Dietary and Other Information
Lipoprotein concentration		
Siguel and Lerman, 1993	47 CAD cases 56 controls Case-control	No dietary intake information
Coronary heart disease (CHD)		
Hudgins et al., 1991	76 men, 23–78 y Cross-sectional	No dietary intake information
Troisi et al., 1992	748 men, 43–85 y Cross-sectional	Food frequency questionnaire, multivariate analysis
Willett et al., 1993	Women, 431 CHD cases Cohort, 8-y follow-up	Food frequency questionnaire, multivariate analysis
Ascherio et al., 1994	239 MI cases 282 controls Case-control	Food frequency questionnaire, multivariate analysis
Kromhout et al., 1995	12,763 men, 40–59 y Cohort, 25-y follow-up	Weighed food record
Ascherio et al., 1996	43,757 men, 40–75 y Cohort, 6-y follow-up	Food frequency questionnaire, multivariate analysis

Results[b]			Comments[c]
Plasma	Case	Control	TFA negatively associated with HDL
TFA (%)	1.38	1.11	TFA positively associated with LDL and
HDL (mmol/L)	0.88	1.34	TAG
LDL (mmol/L)	3.78	2.97	
TAG (mmol/L)	1.78	0.97	

Total TFA in adipose tissue was 4.4% of total fatty acids

Total TFA content in adipose tissue was not significantly related to risk factors of CHD (e.g., age, BMI, LDL, cholesterol, blood pressure)

TFA intake was directly related to total ($r = 0.07$, $P = 0.04$) and LDL ($r = 0.09$, $P = 0.01$) cholesterol

An increased TFA intake from 2.1 to 4.9 g/d increased the risk of MI by 27%

TFA intake (% energy)	RR of CHD	Positive association with TFA intake and risk of CHD
1.3	1.0	
1.8	1.4	
2.2	1.25	
2.6	1.55	
3.2	1.8	

TFA intake (g/d)	RR of MI	Positive association of TFA intake and risk of myocardial infarction
1.69	1.0	
2.48	0.73	
3.35	1.24	
4.52	1.63	
6.51	2.28	

Correlation between 18:1 *trans* intake and CHD mortality is 0.78 (p < 0.001)

TFA intake (g/d)	RR of MI	TFA intake directly associated with risk of MI
1.5	1.0	
2.2	1.20	
2.7	1.24	
3.3	1.27	
4.3	1.40	

continued

TABLE 8-13 Continued

Reference	Study Design[a]	Dietary and Other Information
Gillman et al., 1997	Men, 45–64 y 267 CHD cases Cohort, 21-y follow-up	24-h recall, multivariate analysis
Hu et al., 1997	Women, 34–59 y 939 MI cases Cohort, 14-y follow-up	Food frequency questionnaire, multivariate analysis
Pietinen et al., 1997	Smoking men, 50–69 y 1,399 coronary events 635 coronary deaths Cohort, 6.1-y follow-up	Food frequency questionnaire, multivariate analysis
Tavani et al., 1997	Women, 18–74 y 429 MI cases 866 controls Case-control	Questionnaire on selected indicator foods, multivariate analysis
Cancer Kohlmeier et al., 1997	Women, 50–74 y 291 breast cancer cases 407 controls Case-control	No diet information

Results[b]			Comments[c]
	No. of events		RR for CHD for each increment of 1 tsp/d was
Margarine	(/1,000)		0.99 for follow-up period 1 and 1.12 for
intake (tsp/d)	Period 1	Period 2	period 2
0	77	65	Modest risk of CHD with increasing
1–4	42	35	margarine intake
≥ 5	18	30	
TFA intake			RR for 2% increment in energy from TFA
(% energy)	RR of MI		intake was 1.93
1.3	1.0		
1.7	1.07		
2.0	1.10		
2.4	1.13		
2.9	1.27		
	RR of major		Positive association between TFA intake and
TFA intake (g)	coronary event		risk of coronary death
1.0	1.00		
1.7	1.10		
2.0	0.97		
2.7	1.07		
6.2	1.14		
	RR of coronary		
TFA intake (g)	death		
1.0	1.00		
1.7	1.05		
2.0	1.12		
2.7	0.90		
6.2	1.39		
Margarine			The association with margarine could
intakes	RR of MI		explain about 6% of MI in this population
No or low	1.0		
Medium or high	1.5		
Adipose TFA	OR of breast		Risk for breast cancer is based on
concentration	cancer		the relative concentration of TFA and PUFA
TFA	1.46		
TFA within	3.65		
lowest PUFA			
tertile			
TFA within			
highest			
PUFA tertile	0.97		

continued

TABLE 8-13 Continued

Reference	Study Design[a]	Dietary and Other Information
Tuyns et al., 1988	35–75 y 453 colon cancer cases 365 rectal cancer cases 2,851 controls Case-control	Dietary history

[a] CAD = coronary artery disease, CHD = coronary heart disease, MI = myocardial infarction.
[b] HDL = high density lipoprotein cholesterol, LDL = low density lipoprotein cholesterol, TAG = triacylglycerol, RR = relative risk, OR = odds ratio, PUFA = polyunsaturated fatty acid.

- Randomized clinical trials on the use of EPA+DHA, EPA, and DHA in treatment of inflammatory disorders (e.g., Crohn's disease, arthritis, psoriasis, asthma) and infections are needed.
- Studies of EPA+DHA, EPA, and DHA supplementation in the elderly to prevent degenerative diseases of the central nervous system and retina, such as dementia, age-related macular degeneration, and night blindness are needed.

Trans *Fatty Acids*

- A comprehensive database needs to be developed for the *trans* fatty acid content of the United States food supply; this database could then be used to determine the *trans* fatty acid intakes in different age and socio-economic groups.
- An assessment of major sources of *trans* fatty acids currently in the marketplace is needed, along with development of alternatives similar to that done for foods high in saturated fatty acids.
- Studies that distinguish *trans* fatty acid isomers from plants and animals with respect to the relative impact on blood lipid and lipoprotein concentrations are needed.
- In light of the wide variability of *trans* fatty acid intakes within food categories, the development of a biochemical marker for *trans* fatty acid intake, independent of self-reported intake data, is needed.

Results[b]	Comments[c]
	There was no increased risk of either cancers with increased consumption of margarine

[c] BMI = body mass index.

REFERENCES

Abedin L, Lien EL, Vingrys AJ, Sinclair AJ. 1999. The effects of dietary α-linolenic acid compared with docosahexaenoic acid on brain, retina, liver, and heart in the guinea pig. *Lipids* 34:475–482.

Adlof RO, Duval S, Emken EA.! Ç00. Biosynthesis of conjugated linoleic acid in humans. *Lipids* 35:131–135.

Aggett PJ, Haschke F, Heine W, Hernell O, Koletzko B, Launiala K, Rey J, Rubino A, Schöch G, Senterre J, Tormo R. 1991. Comment on the content and composition of lipids in infant formulas. *Acta Paediatr Scand* 80:887–896.

Agner E, Hansen PF. 1983. Fasting serum cholesterol and triglycerides in a ten-year prospective study in old age. *Acta Med Scand* 214:33–41.

Agostoni C, Trojan S, Bellù R, Riva E, Giovannini M. 1995. Neurodevelopment quotient of healthy term infants at 4 months and feeding practice: The role of long-chain polyunsaturated fatty acids. *Pediatr Res* 38:262–266.

Agostoni C, Trojan S, Bellù R, Riva E, Bruzzese MG, Giovannini M. 1997. Developmental quotient at 24 months and fatty acid composition of diet in early infancy: A follow up study. *Arch Dis Child* 76:421–424.

Allison DB, Egan SK, Barraj LM, Caughman C, Infante M, Heimbach JT. 1999. Estimated intakes of *trans* fatty and other fatty acids in the US population. *J Am Diet Assoc* 99:166–174.

Almendingen K, Jordal O, Kierulf P, Sandstad B, Pedersen JI. 1995. Effects of partially hydrogenated fish oil, partially hydrogenated soybean oil, and butter on serum lipoproteins and Lp[a] in men. *J Lipid Res* 36:1370–1384.

Almendingen K, Seljeflot I, Sandstad B, Pedersen JI. 1996. Effects of partially hydrogenated fish oil, partially hydrogenated soybean oil, and butter on hemostatic variables in men. *Arterioscler Thromb Vasc Biol* 16:375–380.

Anderson DM, Williams FH, Merkatz RB, Schulman PK, Kerr DS, Pittard WB. 1983. Length of gestation and nutritional composition of human milk. *Am J Clin Nutr* 37:810–814.

Anderson GJ, Connor WE. 1989. On the demonstration of ω-3 essential-fatty-acid deficiency in humans. *Am J Clin Nutr* 49:585–587.

Anderson GJ, Connor WE, Corliss JD. 1990. Docosahexaenoic acid is the preferred dietary *n*-3 fatty acid for the development of the brain and retina. *Pediatr Res* 27:89–97.

Anderson RE, Benolken RM, Dudley PA, Landis DJ, Wheeler TG. 1974. Polyunsaturated fatty acids of photoreceptor membranes. *Exp Eye Res* 18:205–213.

Ando K, Nagata K, Beppu M, Kikugawa T, Kawabata T, Hasegawa K, Suzuki M. 1998. Effect of *n*-3 fatty acid supplementation on lipid peroxidation and protein aggregation in rat erythrocyte membranes. *Lipids* 33:505–512.

Aro A, Salminen I. 1998. Difference between animal and vegetable *trans* fatty acids. *Am J Clin Nutr* 68:918–919.

Aro A, Jauhiainen M, Partanen R, Salminen I, Mutanen M. 1997. Stearic acid, *trans* fatty acids, and dairy fat: Effects on serum and lipoprotein lipids, apolipoproteins, lipoprotein(a), and lipid transfer proteins in healthy subjects. *Am J Clin Nutr* 65:1419–1426.

Aro A, Amaral E, Kesteloot H, Rimestad A, Thamm M, van Poppel G. 1998a. *Trans* fatty acids in French fries, soups, and snacks from 14 European countries: The TRANSFAIR Study. *J Food Comp Anal* 11:170–177.

Aro A, Antoine JM, Pizzoferrato L, Reykdal O, van Poppel G. 1998b. *Trans* fatty acids in dairy and meat products from 14 European countries: The TRANSFAIR Study. *J Food Comp Anal* 11:150–160.

Aro A, Van Amelsvoort J, Becker W, van Erp-Baart M-A, Kafatos A, Leth T, van Poppel G. 1998c. *Trans* fatty acids in dietary fats and oils from 14 European countries: The TRANSFAIR Study. *J Food Comp Anal* 11:137–149.

Arora S, Kassarjian Z, Krasinski SD, Croffey B, Kaplan MM, Russell RM. 1989. Effect of age on tests of intestinal and hepatic function in healthy humans. *Gastroenterology* 96:1560–1565.

ARS (Agricultural Research Service). 2001. *USDA Nutrient Database for Standard Reference, Release 14.* Online. U.S. Department of Agriculture. Available at http:// www.nal.usda.gov/fnic/foodcomp/Data/SR14/sr14.html. Accessed November 13, 2001.

Ascherio A, Hennekens CH, Buring JE, Master C, Stampfer MJ, Willett WC. 1994. *Trans*-fatty acids intake and risk of myocardial infarction. *Circulation* 89:94–101.

Ascherio A, Rimm EB, Giovannucci EL, Spiegelman D, Stampfer M, Willett WC. 1996. Dietary fat and risk of coronary heart disease in men: Cohort follow up study in the United States. *Br Med J* 313:84–90.

Ascherio A, Katan MB, Zock PL, Stampfer MJ, Willett WC. 1999. Trans fatty acids and coronary heart disease. *N Engl J Med* 340:1994–1998.

Astrup A, Buemann B, Christensen NJ, Toubro S. 1994. Failure to increase lipid oxidation in response to increasing dietary fat content in formerly obese women. *Am J Physiol* 266:E592–E599.

Auestad N, Montalto MB, Hall RT, Fitzgerald KM, Wheeler RE, Connor WE, Neuringer M, Connor SL, Taylor JA, Hartmann EE. 1997. Visual acuity, erythrocyte fatty acid composition, and growth in term infants fed formulas with long chain polyunsaturated fatty acids for one year. *Pediatr Res* 41:1–10.

Auestad N, Halter R, Hall RT, Blatter M, Bogle ML, Burks W, Erickson JR, Fitzgerald KM, Dobson V, Innis SM, Singer LT, Montalto MB, Jacobs JR, Qiu W, Bornstein MH. 2001. Growth and development in term infants fed long-chain polyunsaturated fatty acids: A double-masked, randomized, parallel, prospective, multivariate study. *Pediatrics* 108:372–381.

Bang HO, Dyerberg J. 1980. The bleeding tendency in Greenland Eskimos. *Dan Med Bull* 27:202–205.

Bang HO, Dyerberg J, Sinclair HM. 1980. The composition of the Eskimo food in north western Greenland. *Am J Clin Nutr* 33:2657–2661.

Barr LH, Dunn GD, Brennan MF. 1981. Essential fatty acid deficiency during total parenteral nutrition. *Ann Surg* 193:304–311.

Bartoš V, Groh J. 1969. The effect of repeated stimulation of the pancreas on the pancreatic secretion in young and aged men. *Gerontol Clin* 11:56–62.

Benolken RM, Anderson RE, Wheeler TG. 1973. Membrane fatty acids associated with the electrical response in visual excitation. *Science* 182:1253–1254.

Berge RK, Madsen L, Vaagenes H, Tronstad KJ, Göttlicher M, Rustan AC. 1999. In contrast with docosahexaenoic acid, eicosapentaenoic acid and hypolipidaemic derivatives decrease hepatic synthesis and secretion of triacylglycerol by decreased diacylglycerol acyltransferase activity and stimulation of fatty acid oxidation. *Biochem J* 343:191–197.

Bessesen DH, Rupp CL, Eckel RH. 1995. Trafficking of dietary fat in lean rats. *Obes Res* 3:191–203.

Birch EE, Hoffman DR, Uauy R, Birch DG, Prestidge C. 1998. Visual acuity and the essentiality of docosahexaenoic acid and arachidonic acid in the diet of term infants. *Pediatr Res* 44:201–209.

Birch EE, Garfield S, Hoffman DR, Uauy R, Birch DG. 2000. A randomized controlled trial of early dietary supply of long-chain polyunsaturated fatty acids and mental development in term infants. *Dev Med Child Neurol* 42:174–181.

Bistrian BR, Bothe A, Blackburn GL, DeFriez AI. 1981. Low plasma cortisol and hematologic abnormalities associated with essential fatty acid deficiency in man. *J Parenter Enteral Nutr* 5:141–144.

Bitman J, Wood DL, Hamosh M, Hamosh P, Mehta NR. 1983. Comparison of the lipid composition of breast milk from mothers of term and preterm infants. *Am J Clin Nutr* 38:300–312.

Bjerve KS. 1989. *n*-3 Fatty acid deficiency in man. *J Intern Med* 225:171–175.

Bjerve KS, Mostad IL, Thoresen L. 1987a. Alpha-linolenic acid deficiency in patients on long-term gastric-tube feeding: Estimation of linolenic acid and long-chain unsaturated *n*-3 fatty acid requirement in man. *Am J Clin Nutr* 45:66–77.

Bjerve KS, Thoresen L, Mostad IL, Alme K. 1987b. Alpha-linolenic acid deficiency in man: Effect of essential fatty acids on fatty acid composition. *Adv Prostaglandin Thromboxane Leukot Res* 17:862–865.

Bjerve KS, Thoresen L, Børsting S. 1988. Linseed and cod liver oil induce rapid growth in a 7-year-old girl with *n*-3 fatty acid deficiency. *J Parenter Enteral Nutr* 12:521–525.

Bjerve KS, Fischer S, Wammer F, Egeland T. 1989. α-Linolenic acid and long-chain ω-3 fatty acid supplementation in three patients with ω-3 fatty acid deficiency: Effect on lymphocyte function, plasma and red cell lipids, and prostanoid formation. *Am J Clin Nutr* 49:290–300.

Blok WL, Deslypere J-P, Demacker PNM, van der Ven-Jongekrijg J, Hectors MPC, van der Meer JWM, Katan MB. 1997. Pro- and anti-inflammatory cytokines in healthy volunteers fed various doses of fish oil for 1 year. *Eur J Clin Invest* 27:1003–1008.

Blonk MC, Bilo HJG, Nauta JJP, Popp-Snijders C, Mulder C, Donker AJM. 1990. Dose-response effects of fish-oil supplementation in healthy volunteers. *Am J Clin Nutr* 52:120–127.

Boissonneault GA, Johnston PV. 1983. Essential fatty acid deficiency, prostaglandin synthesis and humoral immunity in Lewis rats. *J Nutr* 113:1187–1194.

Bonanome A, Grundy SM. 1988. Effect of dietary stearic acid on plasma cholesterol and lipoprotein levels. *N Engl J Med* 318:1244–1248.

Bonanome A, Grundy SM. 1989. Intestinal absorption of stearic acid after consumption of high fat meals in humans. *J Nutr* 119:1556–1560.

Boulton TJC, Magarey AM. 1995. Effects of differences in dietary fat on growth, energy and nutrient intake from infancy to eight years of age. *Acta Paediatr* 84:146–150.

Bourre J-M, Francois M, Youyou A, Dumont O, Piciotti M, Pascal G, Durand G. 1989. The effects of dietary α-linolenic acid on the composition of nerve membranes, enzymatic activity, amplitude of electrophysiological parameters, resistance to poisons and performance of learning tasks in rats. *J Nutr* 119:1880–1892.

Bourre J-M, Dumont O, Durand G. 1996. Does an increase in dietary linoleic acid modify tissue concentrations of cervonic acid and consequently alter alpha-linolenic requirements? Minimal requirement of linoleic acid in adult rats. *Biochem Mol Biol Int* 39:607–619.

Brauer PM, Slavin JL, Marlett JA. 1981. Apparent digestibility of neutral detergent fiber in elderly and young adults. *Am J Clin Nutr* 34:1061–1070.

Brenner RR. 1974. The oxidative desaturation of unsaturated fatty acids in animals. *Mol Cell Biochem* 3:41–52.

Brossard N, Croset M, Pachiaudi C, Riou JP, Tayot JL, Lagarde M. 1996. Retroconversion and metabolism of [^{13}C]22:6n-3 in humans and rats after intake of a single dose of [^{13}C]22:6n-3-triacylglycerols. *Am J Clin Nutr* 64:577–586.

Bruckner G, Shimp J, Goswami S, Mai J, Kinsella JE. 1982. Dietary trilinoelaidate: Effects on metabolic parameters related to EFA metabolism in rats. *J Nutr* 112:126–135.

Bunker CH, Ukoli FA, Okoro FI, Olomu AB, Kriska AM, Huston SL, Markovic N, Kuller LH. 1996. Correlates of serum lipids in a lean black population. *Atherosclerosis* 123:215–225.

Burr GO, Burr MM. 1929. A new deficiency disease produced by the rigid exclusion of fat from the diet. *J Biol Chem* 82:345–367.

Butte NF. 2000. Fat intake of children in relation to energy requirements. *Am J Clin Nutr* 72:1246S–1252S.

Butte NF, Garza C, Smith EO, Nichols BL. 1984. Human milk intake and growth in exclusively breast-fed infants. *J Pediatr* 104:187–195.

Byard RW, Makrides M, Need M, Neumann MA, Gibson RA. 1995. Sudden infant death syndrome: Effect of breast and formula feeding on frontal cortex and brainstem lipid composition. *J Paediatr Child Health* 31:14–16.

Calles-Escandon J, Goran MI, O'Connell M, Nair KS, Danforth E. 1996. Exercise increases fat oxidation at rest unrelated to changes in energy balance or lipolysis. *Am J Physiol* 270:E1009–E1014.

Carlson SE, Rhodes PG, Ferguson MG. 1986. Docosahexaenoic acid status of preterm infants at birth and following feeding with human milk or formula. *Am J Clin Nutr* 44:798–804.

Carlson SE, Cooke RJ, Werkman SH, Tolley EA. 1992. First year growth of preterm infants fed standard compared to marine oil n-3 supplemented formula. *Lipids* 27:901–907.

Carlson SE, Werkman SH, Peeples JM, Cooke RJ, Tolley EA. 1993. Arachidonic acid status correlates with first year growth in preterm infants. *Proc Natl Acad Sci USA* 90:1073–1077.

Carlson SE, Ford AJ, Werkman SH, Peeples JM, Koo WWK. 1996a. Visual acuity and fatty acid status of term infants fed human milk and formulas with and without docosahexaenoate and arachidonate from egg yolk lecithin. *Pediatr Res* 39:882–888.

Carlson SE, Werkman SH, Tolley EA. 1996b. Effect of long-chain *n*-3 fatty acid supplementation on visual acuity and growth of preterm infants with and without bronchopulmonary dysplasia. *Am J Clin Nutr* 63:687–697.

Carnielli VP, Luijendijk IHT, Van Goudoever JB, Sulkers EJ, Boerlage AA, Degenhart HJ, Sauer PJJ. 1996a. Structural position and amount of palmitic acid in infant formulas: Effects on fat, fatty acid, and mineral balance. *J Pediatr Gastroenterol Nutr* 23:553–560.

Carnielli VP, Wattimena DJL, Luijendijk IHT, Boerlage A, Degenhart HJ, Sauer PJJ. 1996b. The very low birth weight premature infant is capable of synthesizing arachidonic and docosahexaenoic acids from linoleic and linolenic acids. *Pediatr Res* 40:169–174.

Castuma JC, Brenner RR, Kunau W. 1977. Specificity of Δ6 desaturase—Effect of chain length and number of double bonds. *Adv Exp Med Biol* 83:127–134.

Caughey GE, Mantzioris E, Gibson RA, Cleland LG, James MJ. 1996. The effect on human tumor necrosis factor α and interleukin 1β production of diets enriched in *n*-3 fatty acids from vegetable oil or fish oil. *Am J Clin Nutr* 63:116–122.

CDC (Centers for Disease Control and Prevention). 1994. Daily dietary fat and total food-energy intakes—Third National Health and Nutrition Examination Survey, Phase 1, 1988–91. *Morb Mortal Wkly Rep* 43:116–117, 123–125.

Chambaz J, Ravel D, Manier M-C, Pepin D, Mulliez N, Bereziat G. 1985. Essential fatty acids interconversion in the human fetal liver. *Biol Neonate* 47:136–140.

Chang HR, Dulloo AG, Vladoianu IR, Piguet PF, Arsenijevic D, Girardier L, Pechère JC. 1992. Fish oil decreases natural resistance of mice to infection with *Salmonella typhimurium*. *Metabolism* 41:1–2.

Chappell JE, Clandinin MT, Kearney-Volpe C. 1985. Trans fatty acids in human milk lipids: Influence of maternal diet and weight loss. *Am J Clin Nutr* 42:49–56.

Chen Q, Nilsson Å. 1993. Desaturation and chain elongation of *n*-3 and *n*-6 polyunsaturated fatty acids in the human CaCo-2 cell line. *Biochim Biophys Acta* 1166:193–201.

Chen ZY, Pelletier G, Hollywood R, Ratnayake WMN. 1995a. *Trans* fatty acid isomers in Canadian human milk. *Lipids* 30:15–21.

Chen ZY, Ratnayake WMN, Fortier L, Ross R, Cunnane SC. 1995b. Similar distribution of *trans* fatty acid isomers in partially hydrogenated vegetable oils and adipose tissue of Canadians. *Can J Physiol Pharmacol* 73:718–723.

Chin SF, Liu W, Storkson JM, Ha YL, Pariza MW. 1992. Dietary sources of conjugated dienoic isomers of linoleic acid, a newly recognized class of anticarcinogens. *J Food Comp Anal* 5:185–197.

Chin SF, Storkson JM, Liu W, Albright KJ, Pariza MW. 1994. Conjugated linoleic acid (9,11- and 10,12-octadecadienoic acid) is produced in conventional but not germ-free rats fed linoleic acid. *J Nutr* 124:694–701.

Chisholm A, Mann J, Sutherland W, Duncan A, Skeaff M, Frampton C. 1996. Effect on lipoprotein profile of replacing butter with margarine in a low fat diet: Randomised crossover study with hypercholesterolaemic subjects. *Br Med J* 312:931–934.

Cho HP, Nakamura MT, Clarke SD. 1999. Cloning, expression, and nutritional requirements of the mammalian Δ-6 desaturase. *J Biol Chem* 274:471–477.

Clark KJ, Makrides M, Neumann MA, Gibson RA. 1992. Determination of the optimal ratio of linoleic acid to α-linolenic acid in infant formulas. *J Pediatr* 120:S151–S158.

Clarke JTR, Cullen-Dean G, Regelink E, Chan L, Rose V. 1990. Increased incidence of epistaxis in adolescents with familial hypercholesterolemia treated with fish oil. *J Pediatr* 116:139–141.

Clarke R, Frost C, Collins R, Appleby P, Peto R. 1997. Dietary lipids and blood cholesterol: Quantitative meta-analysis of metabolic ward studies. *Br Med J* 314:112–117.

Clouet P, Niot I, Bézard J. 1989. Pathway of α-linolenic acid through the mitochondrial outer membrane in the rat liver and influence on the rate of oxidation. Comparison with linoleic and oleic acids. *Biochem J* 263:867–873.

Cobiac L, Clifton PM, Abbey M, Belling GB, Nestel PJ. 1991. Lipid, lipoprotein, and hemostatic effects of fish vs. fish-oil *n-3* fatty acids in mildly hyperlipidemic males. *Am J Clin Nutr* 53:1210–1216.

Cohen SA, Hendricks KM, Eastham EJ, Mathis RK, Walker WA. 1979. Chronic nonspecific diarrhea. A complication of dietary fat restriction. *Am J Dis Child* 133:490–492.

Colditz GA, Manson JE, Stampfer MJ, Rosner B, Willett WC, Speizer FE. 1992. Diet and risk of clinical diabetes in women. *Am J Clin Nutr* 55:1018–1023.

Collins FD, Sinclair AJ, Royle JP, Coats DA, Maynard AT, Leonard RF. 1971. Plasma lipids in human linoleic acid deficiency. *Nutr Metab* 13:150–167.

Connor WE, Lowensohn R, Hatcher L. 1996. Increased docosahexaenoic acid levels in human newborn infants by administration of sardines and fish oil during pregnancy. *Lipids* 31:S183–S187.

Conquer JA, Holub BJ. 1996. Supplementation with an algae source of docosahexaenoic acid increases (*n-3*) fatty acid status and alters selected risk factors for heart disease in vegetarian subjects. *J Nutr* 126:3032–3039.

Conti S, Farchi G, Menotti A. 1983. Coronary risk factors and excess mortality from all causes and specific causes. *Int J Epidemiol* 12:301–307.

Cook HW. 1981. The influence of *trans*-acids on desaturation and elongation of fatty acids in developing brain. *Lipids* 16:920–926.

Cooling J, Blundell J. 1998. Differences in energy expenditure and substrate oxidation between habitual high fat and low fat consumers (phenotypes). *Int J Obes Relat Metab* 22:612–618.

Cooper AL, Gibbons L, Horan MA, Little RA, Rothwell NJ. 1993. Effect of dietary fish oil supplementation on fever and cytokine production in human volunteers. *Clin Nutr* 12:321–328.

Corazza GR, Frazzoni M, Gatto MR, Gasbarrini G. 1986. Ageing and small-bowel mucosa: A morphometric study. *Gerontology* 32:60–65.

Corti MC, Guralnik JM, Salive ME, Harris T, Ferrucci L, Glynn RJ, Havlik RJ. 1997. Clarifying the direct relation between total cholesterol levels and death from coronary heart disease in older persons. *Ann Intern Med* 126:753–760.

Costa MB, Ferreira SRG, Franco LJ, Gimeno SGA, Iunes M, Japanese-Brazilian Diabetes Study Group. 2000. Dietary patterns in a high-risk population for glucose intolerance. *J Epidemiol* 10:111–117.

Craig-Schmidt MC. 2001. Isomeric fatty acids: Evaluating status and implications for maternal and child health. *Lipids* 36:997–1006.

Cuchel M, Schwab US, Jones PJH, Vogel S, Lammi-Keefe C, Li Z, Ordovas J, McNamara JR, Schaefer EJ, Lichtenstein AH. 1996. Impact of hydrogenated fat consumption on endogenous cholesterol synthesis and susceptibility of low-density lipoprotein to oxidation in moderately hypercholesterolemic individuals. *Metabolism* 45:241–247.

Cunnane SC, Ross R, Bannister JL, Jenkins DJA. 2001. β-Oxidation of linoleate in obese men undergoing weight loss. *Am J Clin Nutr* 73:709–714.

Cuthbertson WFJ. 1976. Essential fatty acid requirements in infancy. *Am J Clin Nutr* 29:559–568.

De Caterina R, Giannessi D, Mazzone A, Berini W, Lazzerini G, Maffei S, Cerri M, Salvatore L, Weksler B. 1990. Vascular prostacyclin is increased in patients ingesting ω-3 polyunsaturated fatty acids before coronary artery bypass graft surgery. *Circulation* 82:428–438.

Decsi T, Koletzko B. 1995. Do trans fatty acids impair linoleic acid metabolism in children? *Ann Nutr Metab* 39:36–41.

de la Presa Owens S, Innis SM. 1999. Docosahexaenoic and arachidonic acid prevent a decrease in dopaminergic and serotoninergic neurotransmitters in frontal cortex caused by a linoleic and α-linolenic acid deficient diet in formula-fed piglets. *J Nutr* 129:2088–2093.

Denke MA. 1994. Effects of cocoa butter on serum lipids in humans: Historical highlights. *Am J Clin Nutr* 60:1014S–1016S.

Denke MA. 1995. Serum lipid concentrations in humans. *Am J Clin Nutr* 62:693S–700S.

De Stefani E, Deneo-Pellegrini H, Mendilaharsu M, Carzoglio JC, Ronco A. 1997. Dietary fat and lung cancer: A case-control study in Uruguay. *Cancer Causes Control* 8:913–921.

Dewey KG, Lönnerdal B. 1983. Milk and nutrient intake of breast-fed infants from 1 to 6 months: Relation to growth and fatness. *J Pediatr Gastroenterol Nutr* 2:497–506.

Dewey KG, Finley DA, Lönnerdal B. 1984. Breast milk volume and composition during late lactation. *J Pediatr Gastroenterol Nutr* 3:713–720.

Dolecek TA, Grandits G. 1991. Dietary polyunsaturated fatty acids and mortality in the Multiple Risk Factor Intervention Trial (MRFIT). *World Rev Nutr Diet* 66:205–216.

Doucet E, Alméras N, White MD, Després J-P, Bouchard C, Tremblay A. 1998. Dietary fat composition and human adiposity. *Eur J Clin Nutr* 52:2–6.

Dyerberg J, Bang HO. 1979. Haemostatic function and platelet polyunsaturated fatty acids in Eskimos. *Lancet* 2:433–435.

Dyerberg J, Bang HO, Stoffersen E, Moncada S, Vane JR. 1978. Eicosapentaenoic acid and prevention of thrombosis and atherosclerosis? *Lancet* 2:117–119.

Eisenstein AB. 1982. Nutritional and metabolic effects of alcohol. *J Am Diet Assoc* 81:247–251.

Elias SL, Innis SM. 2001. Infant plasma *trans*, n-6, and n-3 fatty acids and conjugated linoleic acids are related to maternal plasma fatty acids, length of gestation, and birth weight and length. *Am J Clin Nutr* 73:807–814.

Elias SL, Innis SM. 2002. Bakery foods are the major dietary source of *trans*-fatty acids among pregnant women with diets providing 30 percent energy from fat. *J Am Diet Assoc* 102:46–51.

Emken EA. 1979. Utilization and effects of isomeric fatty acids in humans. In: Emken EA, Dutton HJ, eds. *Geometrical and Positional Fatty Acid Isomers*. Champaign, IL: American Oil Chemists' Society. Pp. 99–129.

Emken EA. 1984. Nutrition and biochemistry of *trans* and positional fatty acid isomers in hydrogenated oils. *Annu Rev Nutr* 4:339–376.

Emken EA. 1994. Metabolism of dietary stearic acid relative to other fatty acids in human subjects. *Am J Clin Nutr* 60:1023S–1028S.

Emken EA. 1995. Physiochemical properties, intake, and metabolism. *Am J Clin Nutr* 62:659S–669S.

Emken EA, Adlof RO, Gulley RM. 1994. Dietary linoleic acid influences desaturation and acylation of deuterium-labeled linoleic and linolenic acids in young adult males. *Biochim Biophys Acta* 1213:277–288.

Emken EA, Adlof RO, Duval SM, Nelson GJ. 1998. Effect of dietary arachidonic acid on metabolism of deuterated linoleic acid by adult male subjects. *Lipids* 33:471–480.

Emken EA, Adlof RO, Duval SM, Nelson GJ. 1999. Effect of dietary docosahexaenoic acid on desaturation and uptake *in vivo* of isotope-labeled oleic, linoleic, and linolenic acids by male subjects. *Lipids* 34:785–791.

Endres S, Ghorbani R, Kelley VE, Georgilis K, Lonnemann G, van der Meer JWM, Cannon JG, Rogers TS, Klempner MS, Weber PC, Schaefer EJ, Wolff SM, Dinarello CA. 1989. The effect of dietary supplementation with *n*-3 polyunsaturated fatty acids on the synthesis of interleukin-1 and tumor necrosis factor by mononuclear cells. *N Engl J Med* 320:265–271.

Endres S, Meydani SN, Ghorbani R, Schindler R, Dinarello CA. 1993. Dietary supplementation with *n*-3 fatty acids suppresses interleukin-2 production and mononuclear cell proliferation. *J Leukoc Biol* 54:599–603.

Enig MG, Atal S, Keeney M, Sampugna J. 1990. Isomeric *trans* fatty acids in the U.S. diet. *J Am Coll Nutr* 5:471–486.

Ens JG, Ma DW, Cole KS, Field CJ, Clandinin MT. 2001. An assessment of *c*9,*t*11 linoleic acid intake in a small group of young Canadians. *Nutr Res* 21:955–960.

Ezaki O, Takahashi M, Shigematsu T, Shimamura K, Kimura J, Ezaki H, Gotoh T. 1999. Long-term effects of dietary α-linolenic acid from perilla oil on serum fatty acids composition and on the risk factors of coronary heart disease in Japanese elderly subjects. *J Nutr Sci Vitaminol* 45:759–772.

Falase AO, Cole TO, Osuntokun BO. 1973. Myocardial infarction in Nigerians. *Trop Geogr Med* 25:147–150.

FAO/WHO (Food and Agricultural Organization/World Health Organization). 1994. General conclusions and recommendations of the consultation. In: *Fats and Oils in Human Nutrition*. Rome: FAO. Pp. 3–7.

Farquharson J. 1994. Infant cerebral cortex and dietary fatty acids. *Eur J Clin Nutr* 48:S24–S26.

Farquharson J, Cockburn F, Patrick WA, Jamieson EC, Logan RW. 1992. Infant cerebral cortex phospholipid fatty-acid composition and diet. *Lancet* 340:810–813.

Farquharson J, Jamieson EC, Abbasi KA, Patrick WJA, Logan RW, Cockburn F. 1995. Effect of diet on the fatty acid composition of the major phospholipids of infant cerebral cortex. *Arch Dis Child* 72:198–203.

Fasching P, Ratheiser K, Schneeweiss B, Rohac M, Nowotny P, Waldhausl W. 1996. No effect of short-term dietary supplementation of saturated and poly- and monounsaturated fatty acids on insulin secretion and sensitivity in healthy men. *Ann Nutr Metab* 40:116–122.

Fellner V, Sauer FD, Kramer JKG. 1999. Effect of ionophores on conjugated linoleic acid in ruminal cultures and in the milk of dairy cows. In: Yurawecz MP, Mossoba MM, Kramer JKG, Pariza MW, Nelson GJ, eds. *Advances in Conjugated Linoleic Acid Research*, Vol. 1. Champaign, IL: AOCS Press. Pp. 209–214.

Ferris AM, Dotts MA, Clark RM, Ezrin M, Jensen RG. 1988. Macronutrients in human milk at 2, 12, and 16 weeks postpartum. *J Am Diet Assoc* 88:694–697.

Feskens EJM, Virtanen SM, Räsänen L, Tuomilehto J, Stengard J, Pekkanen J, Nissinen A, Kromhout D. 1995. Dietary factors determining diabetes and impaired glucose tolerance: A 20-year follow-up of the Finnish and Dutch cohorts of the Seven Countries Study. *Diabetes Care* 18:1104–1112.

Finley DA, Lönnerdal B, Dewey KG, Grivetti LE. 1985. Breast milk composition: Fat content and fatty acid composition in vegetarians and non-vegetarians. *Am J Clin Nutr* 41:787–800.

Fischer DR, Morgan KJ, Zabik ME. 1985. Cholesterol, saturated fatty acids, polyunsaturated fatty acids, sodium, and potassium intakes of the United States population. *J Am Coll Nutr* 4:207–224.

Fleming CR, Smith LM, Hodges RE. 1976. Essential fatty acid deficiency in adults receiving total parenteral nutrition. *Am J Clin Nutr* 29:976–983.

Fomon SJ, Thomas LN, Filer LJ, Anderson TA, Nelson SE. 1976. Influence of fat and carbohydrate content of diet on food intake and growth of male infants. *Acta Paediatr Scand* 65:136–144.

Frank JW, Reed DM, Grove JS, Benfante R. 1992. Will lowering population levels of serum cholesterol affect total mortality? Expectations from the Honolulu Heart Program. *J Clin Epidemiol* 45:333–346.

Freese R, Mutanen M. 1997. α-Linolenic acid and marine long-chain *n*-3 fatty acids differ only slightly in their effects on hemostatic factors in healthy subjects. *Am J Clin Nutr* 66:591–598.

Friday KE, Childs MT, Tsunehara CH, Fujimoto WY, Bierman EL, Ensinck JW. 1989. Elevated plasma glucose and lowered triglyceride levels from omega-3 fatty acid supplementation in type II diabetes. *Diabetes Care* 12:276–281.

Fritsche KL, Shahbazian LM, Feng C, Berg JN. 1997. Dietary fish oil reduces survival and impairs bacterial clearance in C3H/Hen mice challenged with *Listeria monocytogenes*. *Clin Sci* 92:95–101.

Gallai V, Sarchielli P, Trequattrini A, Franceschini M, Floridi A, Firenze C, Alberti A, Di Benedetto D, Stragliotto E. 1995. Cytokine secretion and eicosanoid production in the peripheral blood mononuclear cells of MS patients undergoing dietary supplementation with *n*-3 polyunsaturated fatty acids. *J Neuroimmunol* 56:143–153.

Ganji V, Betts N. 1995. Fat, cholesterol, fiber and sodium intakes of US population: Evaluation of diets reported in 1987–88 Nationwide Food Consumption Survey. *Eur J Clin Nutr* 49:915–920.

Garland M, Sacks FM, Colditz GA, Rimm EB, Sampson LA, Willett WC, Hunter DJ. 1998. The relation between dietary intake and adipose tissue composition of selected fatty acids in US women. *Am J Clin Nutr* 67:25–30.

Gazzaniga JM, Burns TL. 1993. Relationship between diet composition and body fatness, with adjustment for resting energy expenditure and physical activity, in preadolescent children. *Am J Clin Nutr* 58:21–28.

Ghebremeskel K, Min Y, Crawford MA, Nam J-H, Kim A, Koo J-N, Suzuki H. 2000. Blood fatty acid composition of pregnant and nonpregnant Korean women: Red cells may act as a reservoir of arachidonic acid and docosahexaenoic acid for utilization by the developing fetus. *Lipids* 35:567–574.

Gibson RA, Kneebone GM. 1981. Fatty acid composition of human colostrum and mature breast milk. *Am J Clin Nutr* 34:252–257.

Gibson RA, Neumann MA, Makrides M. 1997. Effect of increasing breast milk docosahexaenoic acid on plasma and erythrocyte phospholipid fatty acids and neural indices of exclusively breast fed infants. *Eur J Clin Nutr* 51:578–584.

Gillman MW, Cupples LA, Gagnon D, Millen BE, Ellison RC, Castelli WP. 1997. Margarine intake and subsequent coronary heart disease in men. *Epidemiology* 8:144–149.

Giovannucci E, Rimm EB, Colditz GA, Stampfer MJ, Ascherio A, Chute CC, Willett WC. 1993. A prospective study of dietary fat and risk of prostate cancer. *J Natl Cancer Inst* 85:1571–1579.

Glauber H, Wallace P, Griver K, Brechtel G. 1988. Adverse metabolic effect of omega-3 fatty acids in non-insulin-dependent diabetes mellitus. *Ann Intern Med* 108:663–668.

Goedecke JH, Christie C, Wilson G, Dennis SC, Noakes TD, Hopkins WG, Lambert EV. 1999. Metabolic adaptations to a high-fat diet in endurance cyclists. *Metabolism* 48:1509–1517.

Goldbourt U, Yaari S, Medalie JH. 1993. Factors predictive of long-term coronary heart disease mortality among 10,059 male Israeli civil servants and municipal employees. A 23-year mortality follow-up in the Israeli Ischemic Heart Disease Study. *Cardiology* 82:100–121.

González CA, Pera G, Quirós JR, Lasheras C, Tormo MJ, Rodriguez M, Navarro C, Martinez C, Dorronsoro M, Chirlaque MD, Beguiristain JM, Barricarte A, Amiano P, Agudo A. 2000. Types of fat intake and body mass index in a Mediterranean country. *Public Health Nutr* 3:329–336.

Goodgame JT, Lowry SF, Brennan MF. 1978. Essential fatty acid deficiency in total parenteral nutrition: Time course of development and suggestions for therapy. *Surgery* 84:271–277.

Goodnight SH, Harris WS, Connor WE. 1981. The effects of dietary ω3 fatty acids on platelet composition and function in man: A prospective, controlled study. *Blood* 58:880–885.

Gore SM. 1999. Statistical considerations in infant nutrition trials. *Lipids* 34:185–197.

Greiner RCS, Winter J, Nathanielsz PW, Brenna JT. 1997. Brain docosahexaenoate accretion in fetal baboons: Bioequivalence of dietary α-linolenic and docosahexaenoic acids. *Pediatr Res* 42:826–834.

Griinari JM, Bauman DE. 1999. Biosynthesis of conjugated linoleic acid and its incorporation into meat and milk ruminants. In: Yurawecz MP, Mossoba MM, Kramer JKG, Pariza MW, Nelson GJ, eds. *Advances in Conjugated Linoleic Acid Research*, Vol. 1. Champaign, IL: AOCS Press. Pp. 180–200.

Griinari JM, Corl BA, Lacy SH, Chouinard PY, Nurmela KVV, Bauman DE. 2000. Conjugated linoleic acid is synthesized endogenously in lactating cows by Δ^9-desaturase. *J Nutr* 130:2285–2291.

Ha YL, Grimm NK, Pariza MW. 1989. Newly recognized anticarcinogenic fatty acids: Identification and quantification in natural and processed cheeses. *J Agric Food Chem* 37:75–81.

Haheim LL, Holme I, Hjermann I, Leren P. 1993. The predictability of risk factors with respect to incidence and mortality of myocardial infarction and total mortality. A 12-year follow-up of the Oslo Study, Norway. *J Intern Med* 234:17–24.

Halvorsen B, Almendingen K, Nenseter MS, Pedersen JI, Christiansen EN. 1996. Effects of partially hydrogenated fish oil, partially hydrogenated soybean oil and butter on the susceptibility of low density lipoprotein to oxidative modification in men. *Eur J Clin Nutr* 50:364–370.

Hansen AE, Haggard ME, Boelsche AN, Adam DJD, Wiese HF. 1958. Essential fatty acids in infant nutrition. III. Clinical manifestations of linoleic acid deficiency. *J Nutr* 66:565–576.

Hansen AE, Wiese HF, Boelsche AN, Haggard ME, Adam DJD, Davis H. 1963. Role of linoleic acid in infant nutrition. Clinical and chemical study of 428 infants fed on milk mixtures varying in kind and amount of fat. *Pediatrics* 31:171–192.

Hansen HS, Jensen B. 1985. Essential function of linoleic acid esterified in acylglucosylceramide and acylceramide in maintaining the epidermal water permeability barrier. Evidence from feeding studies with oleate, linoleate, arachidonate, columbinate and α-linolenate. *Biochim Biophys Acta* 834:357–363.

Harris WS, Connor WE, Lindsey S. 1984. Will dietary ω-3 fatty acids change the composition of human milk? *Am J Clin Nutr* 40:780–785.

Hegsted DM, McGandy RB, Myers ML, Stare FJ. 1965. Quantitative effects of dietary fat on serum cholesterol in man. *Am J Clin Nutr* 17:281–295.

Hegsted DM, Ausman LM, Johnson JA, Dallal GE. 1993. Dietary fat and serum lipids: An evaluation of the experimental data. *Am J Clin Nutr* 57:875–883.

Heitmann BL, Lissner L, Sørensen TIA, Bengtsson C. 1995. Dietary fat intake and weight gain in women genetically predisposed for obesity. *Am J Clin Nutr* 61:1213–1217.

Helge JW. 2000. Adaptation to a fat-rich diet. Effects on endurance performance in humans. *Sports Med* 30:347–357.

Henderson RA, Jensen RG, Lammi-Keefe CJ, Ferris AM, Dardick KR. 1992. Effect of fish oil on the fatty acid composition of human milk and maternal and infant erythrocytes. *Lipids* 27:863–869.

Hill JO, Schlundt DG, Sbrocco T, Sharp T, Pope-Cordle J, Stetson B, Kaler M, Heim C. 1989. Evaluation of an alternating-calorie diet with and without exercise in the treatment of obesity. *Am J Clin Nutr* 50:248–254.

Hill JO, Peters JC, Reed GW, Schlundt DG, Sharp T, Greene HL. 1991. Nutrient balance in humans: Effects of diet composition. *Am J Clin Nutr* 54:10–17.

Holman RT. 1960. The ratio of trienoic:tetraenoic acids in tissue lipids as a measure of essential fatty acid requirement. *J Nutr* 70:405–410.

Holman RT, Smythe L, Johnson S. 1979. Effect of sex and age on fatty acid composition of human serum lipids. *Am J Clin Nutr* 32:2390–2399.

Holman RT, Johnson SB, Hatch TF. 1982. A case of human linolenic acid deficiency involving neurological abnormalities. *Am J Clin Nutr* 35:617–623.

Holman RT, Johnson SB, Ogburn PL. 1991. Deficiency of essential fatty acids and membrane fluidity during pregnancy and lactation. *Proc Natl Acad Sci USA* 88:4835–4839.

Holmes MD, Hunter DJ, Colditz GA, Stampfer MJ, Hankinson SE, Speizer FE, Rosner B, Willett WC. 1999. Association of dietary intake of fat and fatty acids with risk of breast cancer. *J Am Med Assoc* 281:914–920.

Hu FB, Stampfer MJ, Manson JE, Rimm E, Colditz GA, Rosner BA, Hennekens CH, Willett WC. 1997. Dietary fat intake and the risk of coronary heart disease in women. *N Engl J Med* 337:1491–1499.

Hu FB, Stampfer MJ, Manson JE, Ascherio A, Colditz GA, Speizer FE, Hennekens CH, Willett WC. 1999a. Dietary saturated fats and their food sources in relation to the risk of coronary heart disease in women. *Am J Clin Nutr* 70:1001–1008.

Hu FB, Stampfer MJ, Manson JE, Rimm EB, Wolk A, Colditz GA, Hennekens CH, Willett WC. 1999b. Dietary intake of α-linolenic acid and risk of fatal ischemic heart disease among women. *Am J Clin Nutr* 69:890–897.

Hu FB, Stampfer MJ, Rimm E, Ascherio A, Rosner BA, Spiegelman D, Willett WC. 1999c. Dietary fat and coronary heart disease: A comparison of approaches for adjusting for total energy intake and modeling repeated dietary measurements. *Am J Epidemiol* 149:531–540.

Hu FB, van Dam RM, Liu S. 2001. Diet and risk of type II diabetes: The role of types of fat and carbohydrate. *Diabetologia* 44:805–817.

Hudgins LC, Hirsch J, Emken EA. 1991. Correlation of isomeric fatty acids in human adipose tissue with clinical risk factors for cardiovascular disease. *Am J Clin Nutr* 53:474–482.

Hughes DA, Pinder AC, Piper Z, Johnson IT, Lund EK. 1996. Fish oil supplementation inhibits the expression of major histocompatibility complex class II molecules and adhesion molecules on human monocytes. *Am J Clin Nutr* 63:267–272.

Hursting SD, Thornquist M, Henderson MM. 1990. Types of dietary fat and the incidence of cancer at five sites. *Prev Med* 19:242–253.

Hwang DH, Chanmugam P, Anding R. 1982. Effects of dietary 9-*trans*,12-*trans* linoleate on arachidonic acid metabolism in rat platelets. *Lipids* 17:307–313.

Innis SM. 1991. Essential fatty acids in growth and development. *Prog Lipid Res* 30:39–103.

Innis SM, King DJ. 1999. *Trans* fatty acids in human milk are inversely associated with concentrations of essential *all-cis* n-6 and n-3 fatty acids and determine *trans*, but not n-6 and n-3, fatty acids in plasma lipids of breast-fed infants. *Am J Clin Nutr* 70:383–390.

Innis SM, Kuhnlein HV. 1988. Long-chain n-3 fatty acids in breast milk of Inuit women consuming traditional foods. *Early Hum Dev* 18:185–189.

Innis SM, Auestad N, Siegman JS. 1996. Blood lipid docosahexaenoic and arachidonic acid in term gestation infants fed formulas with high docosahexaenoic acid, low eicosapentaenoic acid fish oil. *Lipids* 31:617–625.

Innis SM, Green TJ, Halsey TK. 1999. Variability in the *trans* fatty acid content of foods within a food category: Implications for estimation of dietary trans fatty acid intakes. *J Am Coll Nutr* 18:255–260.

Iso H, Rexrode KM, Stampfer MJ, Manson JE, Colditz GA, Speizer FE, Hennekens CH, Willett WC. 2001. Intake of fish and omega-3 fatty acids and risk of stroke in women. *J Am Med Assoc* 285:304–312.

ISSFAL (International Society for the Study of Fatty Acids and Lipids). 1994. *Recommendations for the Essential Fatty Acid Requirement for Infant Formulas.* Online. Available at http://www.issfal.org.uk/infantnutr.htm. Accessed July 2, 2001.

Jamieson EC, Abbasi KA, Cockburn F, Farquharson J, Logan RW, Patrick WA. 1994. Effect of diet on term infant cerebral cortex fatty acid composition. *World Rev Nutr Diet* 75:139–141.

Jamieson EC, Farquharson J, Logan RW, Howatson AG, Patrick WJA, Weaver LT, Cockburn F. 1999. Infant cerebral gray and white matter fatty acids in relation to age and diet. *Lipids* 34:1065–1071.

Jensen C, Buist NRM, Wilson T. 1986. Absorption of individual fatty acids from long chain or medium chain triglycerides in very small infants. *Am J Clin Nutr* 43:745–751.

Jensen CL, Prager TC, Fraley JK, Chen H, Anderson RE, Heird WC. 1997. Effect of dietary linoleic/alpha-linolenic acid ratio on growth and visual function of term infants. *J Pediatr* 131:200–209.

Jensen RG. 1999. Lipids in human milk. *Lipids* 34:1243–1271.

Jeppesen PB, Høy C-E, Mortensen PB. 1998. Essential fatty acid deficiency in patients receiving home parenteral nutrition. *Am J Clin Nutr* 68:126–133.

Jeppesen PB, Hoy CE, Mortensen PB. 2000. Deficiencies of essential fatty acids, vitamin A and E and changes in plasma lipoproteins in patients with reduced fat absorption or intestinal failure. *Eur J Clin Nutr* 54:632–642.

Jéquier E. 1999. Response to and range of acceptable fat intake in adults. *Eur J Clin Nutr* 53:S84–S93.

Jones PJH, Kubow S. 1999. Lipids, sterols, and their metabolites. In: Shils ME, Olson JA, Shike M, Ross AC, eds. *Modern Nutrition in Health and Disease,* 9th ed. Baltimore, MD: Williams and Wilkins. Pp. 67–94.

Jones PJH, Pencharz PB, Clandinin MT. 1985. Whole body oxidation of dietary fatty acids: Implications for energy utilization. *Am J Clin Nutr* 42:769–777.

Jonnalagadda SS, Egan SK, Heimbach JT, Harris SS, Kris-Etherton PM. 1995. Fatty acid consumption pattern of Americans: 1987–1988 USDA Nationwide Food Consumption Survey. *Nutr Res* 15:1767–1781.

Jørgensen MG, Hølmer G, Lund P, Hernell O, Michaelsen KM. 1998. Effect of formula supplemented with docosahexaenoic acid and γ-linolenic acid on fatty acid status and visual acuity in term infants. *J Pediatr Gastroenterol Nutr* 26:412–421.

Jousilahti P, Vartiainen E, Pekkanen J, Tuomilehto J, Sundvall J, Puska P. 1998. Serum cholesterol distribution and coronary heart disease risk. Observations and predictions among middle-aged population in eastern Finland. *Circulation* 97:1087–1094.

Judd JT, Clevidence BA, Muesing RA, Wittes J, Sunkin ME, Podczasy JJ. 1994. Dietary *trans* fatty acids: Effects on plasma lipids and lipoproteins of healthy men and women. *Am J Clin Nutr* 59:861–868.

Judd JT, Baer DJ, Clevidence BA, Muesing RA, Chen SC, Weststrate JA, Meijer GW, Wittes J, Lichtenstein AH, Vilella-Bach M, Schaefer EJ. 1998. Effects of margarine compared with those of butter on blood lipid profiles related to cardiovascular disease risk factors in normolipemic adults fed controlled diets. *Am J Clin Nutr* 68:768–777.

Judd JT, Baer DJ, Clevidence BA, Kris-Etherton P, Muesing RA, Iwane M. 2002. Dietary *cis* and *trans* monounsaturated and saturated FA and plasma lipids and lipoproteins in men. *Lipids* 37:123–131.

Jump DB, Clarke SD. 1999. Regulation of gene expression by dietary fat. *Annu Rev Nutr* 19:63–90.

Kagan A, McGee DL, Yano K, Rhoads GG, Nomura A. 1981. Serum cholesterol and mortality in a Japanese-American population: The Honolulu Heart Program. *Am J Epidemiol* 114:11–20.

Kasim SE, Stern B, Khilnani S, McLin P, Baciorowski S, Jen K-LC. 1988. Effects of omega-3 fish oils on lipid metabolism, glycemic control, and blood pressure in type II diabetic patients. *J Clin Endocrinol Metab* 67:1–5.

Kelley DS, Branch LB, Love JE, Taylor PC, Rivera YM, Iacono JM. 1991. Dietary αlinolenic acid and immunocompetence in humans. *Am J Clin Nutr* 53:40–46.

Kelley DS, Taylor PC, Nelson GJ, Mackey BE. 1998. Dietary docosahexaenoic acid and immunocompetence in young healthy men. *Lipids* 33:559–566.

Kelley DS, Taylor PC, Nelson GJ, Schmidt PC, Ferretti A, Erickson KL, Yu R, Chandra RK, Mackey BE. 1999. Docosahexaenoic acid ingestion inhibits natural killer cell activity and production of inflammatory mediators in young healthy men. *Lipids* 34:317–324.

Kelly FD, Sinclair AJ, Mann NJ, Turner AH, Abedin L, Li D. 2001. A stearic acid-rich diet improves thrombogenic and atherogenic risk factor profiles in healthy males. *Eur J Clin Nutr* 55:88–96.

Keys A, Anderson JT, Grande F. 1965. Serum cholesterol response to changes in the diet. IV. Particular saturated fatty acids in the diet. *Metabolism* 14:776–787.

Keys A, Aravanis C, Blackburn H, Buzina R, Djordevic´ BS, Dontas AS, Fidanza F, Karvonen MJ, Kimura N, Menotti A, Mohac˘ek I, Nedeljkovic´ S, Puddu V, Punsar S, Taylor HL, van Buchem FSP. 1980. *Seven Countries. A Multivariate Analysis of Death and Coronary Heart Disease.* Cambridge, MA: Harvard University Press.

Kinsella JE, Lokesh B, Stone RA. 1990. Dietary *n*-3 polyunsaturated fatty acids and amelioration of cardiovascular disease: Possible mechanisms. *Am J Clin Nutr* 52:1–28.

Klag MJ, Ford DE, Mead LA, He J, Whelton PK, Liang KY, Levine DM. 1993. Serum cholesterol in young men and subsequent cardiovascular disease. *N Engl J Med* 328:313–318.

Kliewer SA, Sundseth SS, Jones SA, Brown PJ, Wisely GB, Koble CS, Devchand P, Wahli W, Willson TM, Lenhard JM, Lehmann JM. 1997. Fatty acids and eicosanoids regulate gene expression through direct interactions with peroxisome proliferator-activated receptors α and γ. *Proc Natl Acad USA* 94:4318–4323.

Kneebone GM, Kneebone R, Gibson R. 1985. Fatty acid composition of breast milk from three racial groups from Penang, Malaysia. *Am J Clin Nutr* 41:765–769.

Kohlmeier L, Simonsen N, van't Veer P, Strain JJ, Martin-Moreno JM, Margolin B, Huttunen JK, Fernández-Crehuet Navajas J, Martin BC, Thamm M, Kardinaal AFM, Kok FJ. 1997. Adipose tissue *trans* fatty acids and breast cancer in the European Community Multicenter Study on Antioxidants, Myocardial Infarction, and Breast Cancer. *Cancer Epidemiol Biomarkers Prev* 6:705–710.

Koletzko B. 1992. *Trans* fatty acids may impair biosynthesis of long-chain polyunsaturates and growth in man. *Acta Paediatr* 81:302–306.

Kris-Etherton PM, Derr J, Mitchell DC, Mustad VA, Russell ME, McDonnell ET, Salabsky D, Pearson TA. 1993. The role of fatty acid saturation on plasma lipids, lipoproteins, and apolipoproteins: I. Effects of whole food diets high in cocoa butter, olive oil, soybean oil, dairy butter, and milk chocolate on the plasma lipids of young men. *Metabolism* 42:121–129.

Kris-Etherton PM, Taylor DS, Yu-Poth S, Huth P, Moriarty K, Fishell V, Hargrove RL, Zhao G, Etherton TD. 2000. Polyunsaturated fatty acids in the food chain in the United States. *Am J Clin Nutr* 71:179S–188S.

Kristensen MØ. 1983. Increased incidence of bleeding intracranial aneurysms in Greenlandic Eskimos. *Acta Neurochir* 67:37–43.

Kritchevsky D. 1982. Trans fatty acid effects in experimental atherosclerosis. *Fed Proc* 41:2813–2817.

Kritchevsky D, Tepper SA, Wright S, Tso P, Czarnecki SK. 2000. Influence of conjugated linoleic acid (CLA) on establishment and progression of atherosclerosis in rabbits. *J Am Coll Nutr* 19:472S–477S.

Kromann N, Green A. 1980. Epidemiological studies in the Upernavik district, Greenland. Incidence of some chronic diseases 1950–1974. *Acta Med Scand* 208:401–406.

Kromhout D, de Lezenne Coulander C. 1984. Diet, prevalence and 10-year mortality from coronary heart disease in 871 middle-aged men. *Am J Epidemiol* 119:733–741.

Kromhout D, Bosschieter EB, de Lezenne Coulander C. 1985. The inverse relation between fish consumption and 20-year mortality from coronary heart disease. *N Engl J Med* 312:1205–1209.

Kromhout D, Menotti A, Bloemberg B, Aravanis C, Blackburn H, Buzina R, Dontas AS, Fidanza F, Giampaoli S, Jansen A, Karvonen M, Katan M, Nissinen A, Nedeljkovic S, Pekkanen J, Pekkarinen M, Punsar S, Räsänen L, Simic B, Toshima H. 1995. Dietary saturated and *trans* fatty acids and cholesterol and 25-year mortality from coronary heart disease: The Seven Countries Study. *Prev Med* 24:308–315.

Lagström H, Seppänen R, Jokinen E, Niinikoski H, Rönnemaa T, Viikari J, Simell O. 1999. Influence of dietary fat on the nutrient intake and growth of children from 1 to 5 y of age: The Special Turku Coronary Risk Factor Intervention Project. *Am J Clin Nutr* 69:516–523.

Lands WEM, Hamazaki T, Yamazaki K, Okuyama H, Sakai K, Goto Y, Hubbard VS. 1990. Changing dietary patterns. *Am J Clin Nutr* 51:991–993.

Lands WEM, Libelt B, Morris A, Kramer NC, Prewitt TE, Bowen P, Schmeisser D, Davidson MH, Burns JH. 1992. Maintenance of lower proportions of (*n*-6) eicosanoid precursors in phospholipids of human plasma in response to added dietary (*n*-3) fatty acids. *Biochim Biophys Acta* 1180:147–162.

Lapinleimu H, Viikari J, Jokinen E, Salo P, Routi T, Leino A, Rönnemaa R, Seppänen R, Välimäki I, Simell O. 1995. Prospective randomised trial in 1062 infants of diet low in saturated fat and cholesterol. *Lancet* 345:471–476.

Larson DE, Hunter GR, Williams MJ, Kekes-Szabo T, Nyikos I, Goran MI. 1996. Dietary fat in relation to body fat and intraabdominal adipose tissue: A cross-sectional analysis. *Am J Clin Nutr* 64:677–684.

Latruffe N, Vamecq J. 1997. Peroxisome proliferators and peroxisome proliferator activated receptors (PPARs) as regulators of lipid metabolism. *Biochimie* 79:81–94.

Lee TH, Hoover RL, Williams JD, Sperling RI, Ravalese JD, Spur BW, Robinson DR, Corey EJ, Lewis RA, Austen KF. 1985. Effect of dietary enrichment with eicosapentaenoic and docosahexaenoic acids on in vitro neutrophil and monocyte leukotriene generation and neutrophil function. *N Engl J Med* 312:1217–1224.

Leibel RL, Hirsch J, Appel BE, Checani GC. 1992. Energy intake required to maintain body weight is not affected by wide variation in diet composition. *Am J Clin Nutr* 55:350–355.

Leibovitz BE, Hu ML, Tappel AL. 1990. Lipid peroxidation in rat tissue slices: Effect of dietary vitamin E, corn oil-lard and mehaden oil. *Lipids* 25:125–129.

Lemaitre RN, King IB, Patterson RE, Psaty BM, Kestin M, Heckbert SR. 1998. Assessment of *trans*-fatty acid intake with a food frequency questionnaire and validation with adipose tissue levels of *trans*-fatty acids. *Am J Epidemiol* 148:1085–1093.

Levinson PD, Iosiphidis AH, Saritelli AL, Herbert PN, Steiner M. 1990. Effects of *n*-3 fatty acids in essential hypertension. *Am J Hypertens* 3:754–760.

Lichtenstein AH, Ausman LM, Carrasco W, Jenner JL, Ordovas JM, Schaefer EJ. 1993. Hydrogenation impairs the hypolipidemic effect of corn oil in humans. Hydrogenation, *trans* fatty acids, and plasma lipids. *Arterioscler Thromb* 13:154–161.

Lichtenstein AH, Ausman LM, Jalbert SM, Schaefer EJ. 1999. Effects of different forms of dietary hydrogenated fats on serum lipoprotein cholesterol levels. *N Engl J Med* 340:1933–1940.

Lippi G, Guidi G. 1999. Biochemical risk factors and patient's outcome: The case of lipoprotein(a). *Clin Chim Acta* 280:59–71.

Litin L, Sacks F. 1993. *Trans*-fatty-acid content of common foods. *N Engl J Med* 329:1969–1970.

London SJ, Sacks FM, Caesar J, Stampfer MJ, Siguel E, Willett WC. 1991. Fatty acid composition of subcutaneous adipose tissue and diet in postmenopausal US women. *Am J Clin Nutr* 54:340–345.

Lorenz R, Spengler U, Fischer S, Duhm J, Weber PC. 1983. Platelet function, thromboxane formation and blood pressure control during supplementation of the Western diet with cod liver oil. *Circulation* 67:504–511.

Louheranta AM, Turpeinen AK, Schwab US, Vidgren HM, Parviainen MT, Uusitupa MIJ. 1998. A high-steric acid diet does not impair glucose tolerance and insulin sensitivity in healthy women. *Metabolism* 47:529–534.

Louheranta AM, Turpeinen AK, Vidgren HM, Schwab US, Uusitupa MIJ. 1999. A high-*trans* fatty acid diet and insulin sensitivity in young healthy women. *Metabolism* 48:870–875.

LSRO (Life Sciences Research Office). 1998. Fat. In: Raiten DJ, Talbot JM, Waters JH, eds. *Assessment of Nutrient Requirements for Infant Formulas*. Bethesda, MD: LSRO. Pp. 19–46.

Lucas A, Quinlan P, Abrams S, Ryan S, Meah S, Lucas PJ. 1997. Randomised controlled trial of a synthetic triglyceride milk formula for preterm infants. *Arch Dis Child* 77:F178–F184.

Lucas A, Stafford M, Morley R, Abbott R, Stephenson T, MacFadyen U, Elias-Jones A, Clements H. 1999. Efficacy and safety of long-chain polyunsaturated fatty acid supplementation of infant-formula milk: A randomised trial. *Lancet* 354:1948–1954.

Ludwig DS, Pereira MA, Kroenke CH, Hilner JE, Van Horn L, Slattery ML, Jacobs DR. 1999. Dietary fiber, weight gain, and cardiovascular disease risk factors in young adults. *J Am Med Assoc* 282:1539–1546.

Ma DWL, Wierzbicki AA, Field CJ, Clandinin MT. 1999. Conjugated linoleic acid in Canadian dairy and beef products. *J Agric Food Chem* 47:1956–1960.

MacDonald HB. 2000. Conjugated linoleic acid and disease prevention: A review of current knowledge. *J Am Coll Nutr* 19:111S–118S.

Makrides M, Neumann MA, Byard RW, Simmer K, Gibson RA. 1994. Fatty acid composition of brain, retina, and erythrocytes in breast- and formula-fed infants. *Am J Clin Nutr* 60:189–194.

Makrides M, Neumann M, Simmer K, Pater J, Gibson R. 1995. Are long-chain polyunsaturated fatty acids essential nutrients in infancy? *Lancet* 345:1463–1468.

Makrides M, Neumann MA, Gibson RA. 1996. Is dietary docosahexaenoic acid essential for term infants? *Lipids* 31:115–119.

Makrides M, Neumann MA, Jeffrey B, Lien EL, Gibson RA. 2000a. A randomized trial of different ratios of linoleic to α-linolenic acid in the diet of term infants: Effects on visual function and growth. *Am J Clin Nutr* 71:120–129.

Makrides M, Neumann MA, Simmer K, Gibson RA. 2000b. A critical appraisal of the role of dietary long-chain polyunsaturated fatty acids on neural indices of term infants: A randomized controlled trial. *Pediatrics* 105:32–38.

Marshall JA, Bessesen DH, Hamman RF. 1997. High saturated fat and low starch and fibre are associated with hyperinsulinemia in a non-diabetic population: The San Luis Valley Diabetes Study. *Diabetologia* 40:430–438.

Martin MJ, Hulley SB, Browner WS, Kuller LH, Wentworth D. 1986. Serum cholesterol, blood pressure, and mortality: Implications from a cohort of 361,662 men. *Lancet* 2:933–936.

Martinez M. 1992. Tissue levels of polyunsaturated fatty acids during early human development. *J Pediatr* 120:S129–S138.

Martinez M, Ballabriga A, Gil-Gibernau JJ. 1988. Lipids of the developing human retina: I. Total fatty acids, plasmalogens, and fatty acid composition of ethanolamine and choline phosphoglycerides. *J Neurosci Res* 20:484–490.

Mascioli EA, Smith MF, Trerice MS, Meng HC, Blackburn GL. 1979. Effect of total parenteral nutrition with cycling on essential fatty acid deficiency. *J Parenter Enteral Nutr* 3:171–173.

Mascioli EA, Lopes SM, Champagne C, Driscoll DF. 1996. Essential fatty acid deficiency and home total parenteral nutrition patients. *Nutrition* 12:245–249.

McGee DL, Reed DM, Yano K, Kagan A, Tillotson J. 1984. Ten-year incidence of coronary heart disease in the Honolulu Heart Program. Relationship to nutrient intake. *Am J Epidemiol* 119:667–676.

Meng HC. 1983. A case of human linolenic acid deficiency involving neurological abnormalities. *Am J Clin Nutr* 37:157–159.

Mensink RP, Hornstra G. 1995. The proportion of *trans* monounsaturated fatty acids in serum triacylglycerols or platelet phospholipids as an objective indicator of their short-term intake in healthy men. *Br J Nutr* 73:605–612.

Mensink RP, Katan MB. 1990. Effect of dietary *trans* fatty acids on high-density and low-density lipoprotein cholesterol levels in healthy subjects. *N Engl J Med* 323:439–445.

Mensink RP, Katan MB. 1992. Effect of dietary fatty acids on serum lipids and lipoproteins. A meta-analysis of 27 trials. *Arterioscler Thromb* 12:911–919.

Mensink RP, de Louw MHJ, Katan MB. 1991. Effects of dietary *trans* fatty acids on blood pressure in normotensive subjects. *Eur J Clin Nutr* 45:375–382.

Mensink RP, Zock PL, Katan MB, Hornstra G. 1992. Effect of dietary *cis* and *trans* fatty acids on serum lipoprotein[a] levels in humans. *J Lipid Res* 33:1493–1501.

Mensink RP, Temme EH, Hornstra G. 1994. Dietary saturated and *trans* fatty acids and lipoprotein metabolism. *Ann Med* 26:461–464.

Meydani SN, Endres S, Woods MM, Goldin BR, Soo C, Morrill-Labrode A, Dinarello CA, Gorbach SL. 1991. Oral (*n*-3) fatty acid supplementation suppresses cytokine production and lymphocyte proliferation: Comparison between young and older women. *J Nutr* 121:547–555.

Meydani SN, Lichtenstein AH, Cornwall S, Meydani M, Goldin BR, Rasmussen H, Dinarello CA, Schaefer EJ. 1993. Immunologic effects of National Cholesterol Education Panel Step-2 Diets with and without fish-derived *n*-3 fatty acid enrichment. *J Clin Invest* 92:105–113.

Michels K, Sacks F. 1995. Trans fatty acids in European margarines. *N Engl J Med* 332:541–542.

Miller WC, Niederpruem MG, Wallace JP, Lindeman AK. 1994. Dietary fat, sugar, and fiber predict body fat content. *J Am Diet Assoc* 94:612–615.

Mohrhauer H, Holman RT. 1963. The effect of dose level of essential fatty acids upon fatty acid composition of the rat liver. *J Lipid Res* 4:151–159.

Mølvig J, Pociot F, Worsaae H, Wogensen LD, Baek L, Christensen P, Mandrup-Poulsen T, Andersen K, Madsen P, Dyerberg J, Nerup J. 1991. Dietary supplementation with ω-3-polyunsaturated fatty acids decreases mononuclear cell proliferation and interleukin-1β content but not monokine secretion in healthy and insulin-dependent diabetic individuals. *Scand J Immunol* 34:399–410.

Moore SA, Yoder E, Murphy S, Dutton GR, Spector AA. 1991. Astrocytes, not neurons, produce docosahexaenoic acid (22:6ω-3) and arachidonic acid (20:4ω-6). *J Neurochem* 56:518–524.

Morley R. 1998. Nutrition and cognitive development. *Nutrition* 14:752–754.

Mortensen JZ, Schmidt EB, Nielsen AH, Dyerberg J. 1983. The effect of *n*-6 and *n*-3 fatty acids on hemostasis, blood lipids and blood pressure. *Thromb Haemostas* 50:543–546.

Müller H, Jordal O, Seljeflot I, Kierulf P, Kirkhus B, Ledsaak O, Pedersen JI. 1998. Effect on plasma lipids and lipoproteins of replacing partially hydrogenated fish oil with vegetable fat in margarine. *Br J Nutr* 80:243–251.

Murgatroyd PR, Van De Ven MLHM, Goldberg GR, Prentice AM. 1996. Alcohol and the regulation of energy balance: Overnight effects on diet-induced thermogenesis and fuel storage. *Br J Nutr* 75:33–45.

Murgatroyd PR, Goldberg GR, Leahy FE, Gilsenan MB, Prentice AM. 1999. Effects of inactivity and diet composition on human energy balance. *Int J Obes Relat Metab Disord* 23:1269–1275.

Mustad VA, Etherton TD, Cooper AD, Mastro AM, Pearson TA, Jonnalagadda SS, Kris-Etherton PM. 1997. Reducing saturated fat intake is associated with increased levels of LDL receptors on mononuclear cells in healthy men and women. *J Lipid Res* 38:459–468.

Mutanen M, Aro A. 1997. Coagulation and fibrinolysis factors in healthy subjects consuming high stearic or *trans* fatty acid diets. *Thromb Haemost* 77:99–104.

Neaton JD, Wentworth D. 1992. Serum cholesterol, blood pressure, cigarette smoking, and death from coronary heart disease. Overall findings and differences by age for 316,099 white men. *Arch Intern Med* 152:56–64.

Nelson GJ, Schmidt PC, Corash L. 1991. The effect of a salmon diet on blood clotting, platelet aggregation and fatty acids in normal adult men. *Lipids* 26:87–96.

Nelson GJ, Schmidt PC, Bartolini GL, Kelley DS, Kyle D. 1997. The effect of dietary docosahexaenoic acid on plasma lipoproteins and tissue fatty acid composition in humans. *Lipids* 32:1137–1146.

Nestel PJ, Noakes M, Belling GB, McArthur R, Clifton PM, Abbey M. 1992a. Plasma cholesterol-lowering potential of edible-oil blends suitable for commercial use. *Am J Clin Nutr* 55:46–50.

Nestel PJ, Noakes M, Belling B, McArthur R, Clifton P, Janus E, Abbey M. 1992b. Plasma lipoprotein lipid and Lp[a] changes with substitution of elaidic acid for oleic acid in the diet. *J Lipid Res* 33:1029–1036.

Nestel P, Clifton P, Noakes M. 1994. Effects of increasing dietary palmitoleic acid compared with palmitic and oleic acids on plasma lipids of hypercholesterolemic men. *J Lipid Res* 35:656–662.

Neuringer M, Connor WE, Van Petten C, Barstad L. 1984. Dietary omega-3 fatty acid deficiency and visual loss in infant rhesus monkeys. *J Clin Invest* 73:272–276.

Neuringer M, Connor WE, Lin DS, Barstad L, Luck S. 1986. Biochemical and functional effects of prenatal and postnatal ω3 fatty acid deficiency on retina and brain in rhesus monkeys. *Proc Natl Acad Sci USA* 83:4021–4025.

Nielsen LB. 1999. Atherogenecity of lipoprotein(a) and oxidized low density lipoprotein: Insight from in vivo studies of arterial wall influx, degradation and efflux. *Atherosclerosis* 143:229–243.

Niinikoski H, Lapinleimu H, Viikari J, Rönnemaa T, Jokinen E, Seppänen R, Terho P, Tuominen J, Välimäki I, Simell O. 1997a. Growth until 3 years of age in a prospective, randomized trial of a diet with reduced saturated fat and cholesterol. *Pediatrics* 99:687–694.

Niinikoski H, Viikari J, Rönnemaa T, Helenius H, Jokinen E, Lapinleimu H, Routi T, Lagström H, Seppänen R, Välimäki I, Simell O. 1997b. Regulation of growth of 7- to 36-month-old children by energy and fat intake in the prospective, randomized STRIP baby trial. *Pediatrics* 100:810–816.

Noakes M, Clifton PM. 1998. Oil blends containing partially hydrogenated or interesterified fats: Differential effects on plasma lipids. *Am J Clin Nutr* 68:242–247.

Noble RC, Moore JH, Harfoot CG. 1974. Observations on the pattern of biohydrogenation of esterified and unesterified linoleic acid in the rumen. *Br J Nutr* 31:99–108.

Nommsen LA, Lovelady CA, Heinig MJ, Lönnerdal B, Dewey KG. 1991. Determinants of energy, protein, lipid, and lactose concentrations in human milk during the first 12 mo of lactation: The DARLING Study. *Am J Clin Nutr* 53:457–465.

Obarzanek E, Hunsberger SA, Van Horn L, Hartmuller VV, Barton BA, Stevens VJ, Kwiterovich PO, Franklin FA, Kimm SYS, Lasser NL, Simons-Morton DG, Lauer RM. 1997. Safety of a fat-reduced diet: The Dietary Intervention Study in Children (DISC). *Pediatrics* 100:51–59.

Olsen SF, Hansen HS, Jensen B, Sørensen TIA. 1989. Pregnancy duration and the ratio of long-chain *n*-3 fatty acids to arachidonic acid in erythrocytes from Faroese women. *J Intern Med* 225:185–189.

Olsen SF, Sørensen JD, Secher NJ, Hedegaard M, Henriksen TB, Hansen HS, Grant A. 1992. Randomised controlled trial of effect of fish-oil supplementation on pregnancy duration. *Lancet* 339:1003–1007.

O'Neill JA, Caldwell MD, Meng HC. 1977. Essential fatty acid deficiency in surgical patients. *Ann Surg* 185:535–542.

Ou J, Tu H, Luk A, DeBose-Boyd RA, Bashmakov Y, Goldstein JL, Brown MS. 2001. Unsaturated fatty acids inhibit transcription of the sterol regulatory element-binding protein-1c (SREBP-1c) gene by antagonizing ligand-dependent activation of the LXR. *Proc Natl Acad Sci USA* 98:6027–6032.

Pan DA, Lillioja S, Kriketos AD, Milner MR, Baur LA, Bogardus C, Jenkins AB, Storlien LH. 1997. Skeletal muscle triglyceride levels are inversely related to insulin action. *Diabetes* 46:983–988.

Pariza MW, Park Y, Cook ME. 2001. The biologically active isomers of conjugated linoleic acid. *Prog Lipid Res* 40:283–298.

Parker DR, Weiss ST, Troisi R, Cassano PA, Vokonas PS, Landsberg L. 1993. Relationship of dietary saturated fatty acids and body habitus to serum insulin concentrations: The Normative Aging Study. *Am J Clin Nutr* 58:129–136.

Paulsrud JR, Pensler L, Whitten CF, Stewart S, Holman RT. 1972. Essential fatty acid deficiency in infants induced by fat-free intravenous feeding. *Am J Clin Nutr* 25:897–904.

Pedersen HS, Mulvad G, Seidelin KN, Malcom GT, Boudreau DA. 1999. *n*-3 Fatty acids as a risk factor for haemorrhagic stroke. *Lancet* 353:812–813.

Pietinen P, Ascherio A, Korhonen P, Hartman AM, Willett WC, Albanes D, Virtamo J. 1997. Intake of fatty acids and risk of coronary heart disease in a cohort of Finnish men. The Alpha-Tocopherol, Beta-Carotene Cancer Prevention Study. *Am J Epidemiol* 145:876–887.

Ponder DL, Innis SM, Benson JD, Siegman JS. 1992. Docosahexaenoic acid status of term infants fed breast milk or infant formula containing soy oil or corn oil. *Pediatr Res* 32:683–688.

Putnam JC, Carlson SE, DeVoe PW, Barness LA. 1982. The effect of variations in dietary fatty acids on the fatty acid composition of erythrocyte phosphatidyl-choline and phosphatidylethanolamine in human infants. *Am J Clin Nutr* 36:106–114.

Raben A, Andersen HB, Christensen NJ, Madsen J, Holst JJ, Astrup A. 1994. Evidence for an abnormal postprandial response to a high-fat meal in women predisposed to obesity. *Am J Physiol* 267:E549–E559.

Ratnayake WMN, Hollywood R, O'Grady E, Pelletier G. 1993. Fatty acids in some common food items in Canada. *J Am Coll Nutr* 12:651–660.

Ratnayake WM, Chardigny JM, Wolff RL, Bayard CC, Sebedio JL, Martine L. 1997. Essential fatty acids and their *trans* geometrical isomers in powdered and liquid infant formulas sold in Canada. *J Pediatr Gastroenterol* 25:400–407.

Rhee SK, Kayani AJ, Ciszek A, Brenna JT. 1997. Desaturation and interconversion of dietary stearic and palmitic acids in human plasma and lipoproteins. *Am J Clin Nutr* 65:451–458.

Richardson TJ, Sgoutas D. 1975. Essential fatty acid deficiency in four adult patients during total parenteral nutrition. *Am J Clin Nutr* 28:258–263.

Riella MC, Broviac JW, Wells M, Scribner BH. 1975. Essential fatty acid deficiency in human adults during total parenteral nutrition. *Ann Intern Med* 83:786–789.

Ritzenthaler KL, McGuire MK, Falen R, Shultz TD, Dasgupta N, McGuire MA. 2001. Estimation of conjugated linoleic acid intake by written dietary assessment methodologies underestimates actual intake evaluated by food duplicate methodology. *J Nutr* 131:1548–1554.

Roche HM, Zampelas A, Jackson KG, Williams CM, Gibney MJ. 1998. The effect of test meal monounsaturated fatty acid:saturated fatty acid ratio on postprandial lipid metabolism. *Br J Nutr* 79:419–424.

Roden M, Price TB, Perseghin G, Petersen KF, Rothman DL, Cline GW, Shulman GI. 1996. Mechanism of free fatty acid-induced insulin resistance in humans. *J Clin Invest* 97:2859–2865.

Rodriguez A, Sarda P, Nessmann C, Boulot P, Poisson J-P, Leger CL, Descomps B. 1998. Fatty acid desaturase activities and polyunsaturated fatty acid composition in human fetal liver between the seventeenth and thirty-sixth gestational weeks. *Am J Obstet Gynecol* 179:1063–1070.

Rogers S, James KS, Butland BK, Etherington MD, O'Brien JR, Jones JG. 1987. Effects of a fish oil supplement on serum lipids, blood pressure, bleeding time, haemostatic and rheological variables. A double blind randomised controlled trial in healthy volunteers. *Atherosclerosis* 63:137–143.

Rosenthal MD, Doloresco MA. 1984. The effects of *trans* fatty acids on fatty acyl Δ5 desaturation by human skin fibroblasts. *Lipids* 19:869–874.

Rudel LL, Haines J, Sawyer JK, Shah R, Wilson MS, Carr TP. 1997. Hepatic origin of cholesteryl oleate in coronary artery atherosclerosis in African green monkeys. *J Clin Invest* 100:74–83.

Russell RM. 1992. Changes in gastrointestinal function attributed to aging. *Am J Clin Nutr* 55:1203S–1207S.

Ruttenberg H, Davidson LM, Little NA, Klurfeld DM, Kritchevsky D. 1983. Influence of *trans* unsaturated fats on experimental atherosclerosis in rabbits. *J Nutr* 113:835–844.

Ryan AS, Montalto MB, Groh-Wargo S, Mimouni F, Sentipal-Walerius J, Doyle J, Siegman JS, Thomas AJ. 1999. Effect of DHA-containing formula on growth of preterm infants to 59 weeks postmenstrual age. *Am J Hum Biol* 11:457–467.

Rywik SL, Manolio TA, Pajak A, Piotrowski W, Davids CE, Broda GB, Kawalec E. 1999. Association of lipids and lipoprotein level with total mortality and mortality caused by cardiovascular and cancer diseases (Poland and United States collaborative study on cardiovascular epidemiology). *Am J Cardiol* 84:540–548.

Salem N, Wegher B, Mena P, Uauy R. 1996. Arachidonic and docosahexaenoic acids are biosynthesized from their 18-carbon precursors in human infants. *Proc Natl Acad Sci USA* 93:49–54.

Salem N, Litman B, Kim H-Y, Gawrisch K. 2001. Mechanisms of action of docosahexaenoic acid in the nervous system. *Lipids* 36:945–959.

Salmerón J, Hu FB, Manson JE, Stampfer MJ, Colditz GA, Rimm EB, Willett WC. 2001. Dietary fat intake and risk of type 2 diabetes in women. *Am J Clin Nutr* 73:1019–1026.

Sanders TAB, Reddy S. 1992. The influence of a vegetarian diet on the fatty acid composition of human milk and the essential fatty acid status of the infant. *J Pediatr* 120:S71–S77.

Sanders TAB, Vickers M, Haines AP. 1981. Effect of blood lipids and haemostasis of a supplement of cod-liver oil, rich in eicosapentaenoic and docosahexaenoic acids, in healthy young men. *Clin Sci* 61:317–324.

Sanders TAB, de Grassi T, Miller GJ, Morrissey JH. 2000. Influence of fatty acid chain length and *cis/trans* isomerization on postprandial lipemia and factor VII in healthy subjects (postprandial lipids and factor VII). *Atherosclerosis* 149:413–420.

Sanjurjo P, Matorras R, Ingunza N, Alonso M, Rodriguez-Alarcón J, Perteagudo L. 1993. Cross-sectional study of percentual changes in total plasmatic fatty acids during pregnancy. *Horm Metab Res* 25:590–592.

Santora JE, Palmquist DL, Roehrig KL. 2000. *Trans*-vaccenic acid is desaturated to conjugated linoleic acid in mice. *J Nutr* 130:208–215.

Sauerwald TU, Hachey DL, Jensen CL, Chen H, Anderson RE, Heird WC. 1996. Effect of dietary α-linolenic acid intake on incorporation of docosahexaenoic and arachidonic acids into plasma phospholipids of term infants. *Lipids* 31:S131–S135.

Sauerwald TU, Hachey DL, Jensen CL, Chen H, Anderson RE, Heird WC. 1997. Intermediates in endogenous synthesis of C22:6ω3 and C20:4ω6 by term and preterm infants. *Pediatr Res* 41:183–187.

Schakel SF, Buzzard IM, Gebhardt SE. 1997. Procedures for estimating nutrient values for food composition databases. *J Food Comp Anal* 10:102–114.

Schmidt DE, Allred JB, Kien CL. 1999. Fractional oxidation of chylomicron-derived oleate is greater than that of palmitate in healthy adults fed frequent small meals. *J Lipid Res* 40:2322–2332.

Schmidt EB, Pedersen JO, Ekelund S, Grunnet N, Jersild C, Dyerberg J. 1989. Cod liver oil inhibits neutrophil and monocyte chemotaxis in healthy males. *Atherosclerosis* 77:53–57.

Schmidt EB, Varming K, Ernst E, Madsen P, Dyerberg J. 1990. Dose–response studies on the effect of *n*-3 polyunsaturated fatty acids on lipids and haemostasis. *Thromb Haemost* 63:1–5.

Schmidt EB, Lervang H-H, Varming K, Madsen P, Dyerberg J. 1992. Long-term supplementation with *n*-3 fatty acids. I: Effect on blood lipids, haemostasis and blood pressure. *Scand J Clin Lab Invest* 52:221–228.

Schutz Y. 2000. Role of substrate utilization and thermogenesis on body-weight control with particular reference to alcohol. *Proc Nutr Soc* 59:511–517.

Scott DT, Janowsky JS, Carroll RE, Taylor JA, Auestad N, Montalto MB. 1998. Formula supplementation with long-chain polyunsaturated fatty acids: Are there developmental benefits? *Pediatrics* 102:E59.

Seppänen-Laakso T, Vanhanen H, Laakso I, Kohtamäki H, Viikari J. 1993. Replacement of margarine on bread by rapeseed and olive oils: Effects on plasma fatty acid composition and serum cholesterol. *Ann Nutr Metab* 37:161–174.

Sessler AM, Ntambi JM. 1998. Polyunsaturated fatty acid regulation of gene expression. *J Nutr* 128:923–926.

Sevak L, McKeigue PM, Marmot MG. 1994. Relationship of hyperinsulinemia to dietary intake in South Asian and European men. *Am J Clin Nutr* 59:1069–1074.

Shea S, Basch CE, Stein AD, Contento IR, Irigoyen M, Zybert P. 1993. Is there a relationship between dietary fat and stature or growth in children three to five years of age? *Pediatrics* 92:579–586.

Shekelle RB, Missell L, Paul O, Shyrock AM, Stamler J. 1985. Fish consumption and mortality from coronary heart disease. *N Engl J Med* 313:820.

Sherwood NE, Jeffery RW, French SA, Hannan PJ, Murray DM. 2000. Predictors of weight gain in the Pound of Prevention Study. *Int J Obes Relat Metab Disord* 24:395–403.

Shetty PS, Prentice AM, Goldberg GR, Murgatroyd PR, McKenna APM, Stubbs RJ, Volschenk PA. 1994. Alterations in fuel selection and voluntary food intake in response to isoenergetic manipulation of glycogen stores in humans. *Am J Clin Nutr* 60:534–543.

Shimp JL, Bruckner G, Kinsella JE. 1982. The effects of dietary trilinoelaidin on fatty acid and acyl desaturases in rat liver. *J Nutr* 112:722–735.

Shintani TT, Beckham S, Brown AC, O'Connor HK. 2001. The Hawaii Diet: Ad libitum high carbohydrate, low fat multi-cultural diet for the reduction of chronic disease risk factors: Obesity, hypertension, hypercholesterolemia, and hyperglycemia. *Hawaii Med J* 60:69–73.

Siguel EN, Lerman RH. 1993. *Trans*-fatty acid patterns in patients with angiographically documented coronary artery disease. *Am J Cardiol* 71:916–920.

Siguel EN, Blumberg JB, Caesar J. 1986. Monitoring the optimal infusion of intravenous lipids. *Arch Pathol Lab Med* 110:792–797.

Sinclair AJ. 1975. Incorporation of radioactive polyunsaturated fatty acids into liver and brain of developing rat. *Lipids* 10:175–184.

Sinclair AJ, Murphy KJ, Li D. 2000. Marine lipids: Overview "news insights and lipid composition of Lyprinol™" *Allerg Immunol (Paris)* 32:261–271.

Slattery ML, Potter JD, Duncan DM, Berry TD. 1997. Dietary fats and colon cancer: Assessment of risk associated with specific fatty acids. *Int J Cancer* 73:670–677.

Smith P, Arnesen H, Opstad T, Dahl KH, Eritsland J. 1989. Influence of highly concentrated n-3 fatty acids on serum lipids and hemostatic variables in survivors of myocardial infarction receiving either oral anticoagulants or matching placebo. *Thromb Res* 53:467–474.

Song JH, Miyazawa T. 2001. Enhanced level of n-3 fatty acid in membrane phospholipids induces lipid peroxidation in rats fed dietary docosahexaenoic acid oil. *Atherosclerosis* 155:9–18.

Sørensen NS, Marckmann P, Høy C-E, van Duyvenvoorde W, Princen HMG. 1998. Effect of fish-oil-enriched margarine on plasma lipids, low-density-lipoprotein particle composition, size, and susceptibility to oxidation. *Am J Clin Nutr* 68:235–241.

Sorkin JD, Andres R, Muller DC, Baldwin HL, Fleg JL. 1992. Cholesterol as a risk factor for coronary heart disease in elderly men. The Baltimore Longitudinal Study of Aging. *Ann Epidemiol* 2:59–67.

Spady DK, Woolett LA, Dietschy JM. 1993. Regulation of plasma LDL-cholesterol levels by dietary cholesterol and fatty acids. *Annu Rev Nutr* 13:355–361.

Sperling RI, Benincaso AI, Knoell CT, Larkin JK, Austen KF, Robinson DR. 1993. Dietary ω-3 polyunsaturated fatty acids inhibit phosphoinositide formation and chemotaxis in neutrophils. *J Clin Invest* 91:651–660.

Sprecher H. 1992. Interconversions between 20- and 22-carbon *n*-3 and *n*-6 fatty acids via 4-desaturase independent pathways. In: Sinclair AJ, Gibson R, eds. *Essential Fatty Acids and Eicosanoids: Invited Papers from the Third International Congress.* Champaign, IL: American Oil Chemists' Society. Pp. 18–22.

Sprecher H, Luthria DL, Mohammed BS, Baykousheva SP. 1995. Reevaluation of the pathways for the biosynthesis of polyunsaturated fatty acids. *J Lipid Res* 36:2471–2477.

Stacpoole PW, Alig J, Ammon L, Crockett SE. 1989. Dose–response effects of dietary marine oil on carbohydrate and lipid metabolism in normal subjects and patients with hypertriglyceridemia. *Metabolism* 38:946–956.

Stamler J, Wentworth D, Neaton JD. 1986. Is relationship between serum cholesterol and risk of premature death from coronary heart disease continuous and graded? Findings in 356,222 primary screenees of the Multiple Risk Factor Intervention Trial (MRFIT). *J Am Med Assoc* 256:2823–2828.

Sugano M, Ikeda I. 1996. Metabolic interactions between essential and *trans*-fatty acids. *Curr Opin Lipidol* 7:38–42.

Sundram K, Ismail A, Hayes KC, Jeyamalar R, Pathmanathan R. 1997. *Trans* (elaidic) fatty acids adversely affect the lipoprotein profile relative to specific saturated fatty acids in humans. *J Nutr* 127:514S–520S.

Suter PM, Schutz Y, Jequier E. 1992. The effect of ethanol on fat storage in healthy subjects. *N Engl J Med* 326:983–987.

Tavani A, Negri E, D'Avanzo B, La Vecchia C. 1997. Margarine intake and risk of nonfatal acute myocardial infarction in Italian women. *Eur J Clin Nutr* 51:30–32.

Thompson PJ, Misso NLA, Passarelli M, Phillips MJ. 1991. The effect of eicosapentaenoic acid consumption on human neutrophil chemiluminescence. *Lipids* 26:1223–1226.

Thomsen C, Rasmussen O, Lousen T, Holst JJ, Fenselau S, Schrezenmeir J, Hermansen K. 1999. Differential effects of saturated and monounsaturated fatty acids on postprandial lipemia and incretin responses in healthy subjects. *Am J Clin Nutr* 69:1135–1143.

Thorngren M, Gustafson A. 1981. Effects of 11-week increase in dietary eicosapentaenoic acid on bleeding time, lipids, and platelet aggregation. *Lancet* 2:1190–1193.

Tomarelli RM, Meyer BJ, Weaber JR, Bernhart FW. 1968. Effect of positional distribution on the absorption of the fatty acids of human milk and infant formulas. *J Nutr* 95:583–590.

Troiano RP, Briefel RR, Carroll MD, Bialostosky K. 2000. Energy and fat intakes of children and adolescents in the United States: Data from the National Health and Nutrition Examination Surveys. *Am J Clin Nutr* 72:1343S–1353S.

Troisi R, Willett WC, Weiss ST. 1992. *Trans*-fatty acid intake in relation to serum lipid concentrations in adult men. *Am J Clin Nutr* 56:1019–1024.

Turpeinen AM, Wübert J, Aro A, Lorenz R, Mutanen M. 1998. Similar effects of diets rich in stearic acid or *trans*-fatty acids on platelet function and endothelial prostacyclin production in humans. *Arterioscler Thromb Vasc Biol* 18:316–322.

Tuyns AJ, Kaaks R, Haelterman M. 1988. Colorectal cancer and the consumption of foods: A case-control study in Belgium. *Nutr Cancer* 11:189–204.

Uauy R, Mena P, Wegher B, Nieto S, Salem N. 2000a. Long chain polyunsaturated fatty acid formation in neonates: Effect of gestational age and intrauterine growth. *Pediatr Res* 47:127–135.

Uauy R, Mize CE, Castillo-Duran C. 2000b. Fat intake during childhood: Metabolic responses and effects on growth. *Am J Clin Nutr* 72:1354S–1360S.

Umegaki K, Hashimoto M, Yamasaki H, Fujii Y, Yoshimura M, Sugisawa A, Shinozuka K. 2001. Docosahexaenoic acid supplementation-increased oxidative damage in bone marrow DNA in aged rats and its relation to antioxidant vitamins. *Free Radic Res* 34:427–435.

USDA (U.S. Department of Agriculture). 1996. *The Food Guide Pyramid*. Home and Garden Bulletin No. 252. Washington, DC: U.S. Government Printing Office.

USDA/HHS (U.S. Department of Health and Human Services). 2000. *Nutrition and Your Health: Dietary Guidelines for Americans*, 5th ed. Home and Garden Bulletin No. 232. Washington, DC: U.S. Government Printing Office.

Valenzuela A, Morgado N. 1999. *Trans* fatty acid isomers in human health and in the food industry. *Biol Res* 32:273–287.

van Dam RM, Huang Z, Giovannucci E, Rimm EB, Hunter DJ, Colditz GA, Stampfer MJ, Willett WC. 2000. Diet and basal cell carcinoma of the skin in a prospective cohort of men. *Am J Clin Nutr* 71:135–141.

van den Brandt PA, van't Veer P, Goldbohm RA, Dorant E, Volovics A, Hermus RJJ, Sturmans F. 1993. A prospective cohort study on dietary fat and the risk of postmenopausal breast cancer. *Cancer Res* 53:75–82.

van Erp-baart M-A, Couet C, Cuadrado C, Kafatos A, Stanley J, van Poppel G. 1998. *Trans* fatty acids in bakery products from 14 European countries: The TRANSFAIR Study. *J Food Comp Anal* 11:161–169.

van Houwelingen AC, Hornstra G. 1994. *Trans* fatty acids in early human development. *World Rev Nutr Diet* 75:175–178.

van Houwelingen AC, Sørensen JD, Hornstra G, Simonis MMG, Boris J, Olsen SF, Secher NJ. 1995. Essential fatty acid status in neonates after fish-oil supplementation during late pregnancy. *Br J Nutr* 74:723–731.

van Poppel G, van Erp-baart M-A, Leth T, Gevers E, Van Amelsvoort J, Lanzmann-Petithory D, Kafatos A, Aro A. 1998. *Trans* fatty acids in foods in Europe: The TRANSFAIR Study. *J Food Comp Anal* 11:112–136.

Veierød MB, Laake P, Thelle DS. 1997. Dietary fat intake and risk of lung cancer: A prospective study of 51,452 Norwegian men and women. *Eur J Cancer Prev* 6:540–549.

Velie E, Kulldorff M, Schairer C, Block G, Albanes D, Schatzkin A. 2000. Dietary fat, fat subtypes, and breast cancer in postmenopausal women: A prospective cohort study. *J Natl Cancer Inst* 92:833–839.

Verhulst A, Janssen G, Parmentier G, Eyssen H. 1987. Isomerization of polyunsaturated long chain fatty acids by propionibacteria. *Syst Appl Microbiol* 9:12–15.

Vermunt SHF, Mensink RP, Simonis MMG, Hornstra G. 2000. Effects of dietary α-linolenic acid on the conversion and oxidation of ^{13}C-α-linolenic acid. *Lipids* 35:137–142.

Vessby B, Uusitupa M, Hermansen K, Riccardi G, Rivellese AA, Tapsell LC, Nälsén C, Berglund L, Louheranta A, Rasmussen BM, Calvert GD, Maffetone A, Pedersen E, Gustafsson I-B, Storlien LH. 2001. Substituting dietary saturated for monounsaturated fat impairs insulin sensitivity in healthy men and women: The KANWU study. *Diabetologia* 44:312–319.

Vidgren HM, Ågren JJ, Schwab U, Rissanen T, Hänninen O, Uusitupa MIJ. 1997. Incorporation of *n*-3 fatty acids into plasma lipid fractions, and erythrocyte membranes and platelets during dietary supplementation with fish, fish oil, and docosahexaenoic acid-rich oil among healthy young men. *Lipids* 32:697–705.

Vidgren HM, Louheranta AM, Ågren JJ, Schwab US, Uusitupa MIJ. 1998. Divergent incorporation of dietary *trans* fatty acids in different serum lipid fractions. *Lipids* 33:955–962.

Virella G, Fourspring K, Hyman B, Haskill-Stroud R, Long L, Virella I, La Via M, Gross AJ, Lopes-Virella M. 1991. Immunosuppressive effects of fish oil in normal human volunteers: Correlation with the in vitro effects of eicosapentanoic acid on human lymphocytes. *Clin Immunol Immunopathol* 61:161–176.

Virtanen SM, Feskens EJM, Räsänen L, Fidanza F, Tuomilehto J, Giampaoli S, Nissinen A, Kromhout D. 2000. Comparison of diets of diabetic and non-diabetic elderly men in Finland, The Netherlands and Italy. *Eur J Clin Nutr* 54:181–186.

Vobecky JS, Vobecky J, Normand L. 1995. Risk and benefit of low fat intake in childhood. *Ann Nutr Metab* 39:124–133.

Vogel RA, Corretti MC, Plotnick GD. 2000. The postprandial effect of components of the Mediterranean diet on endothelial function. *J Am Coll Cardiol* 36:1455–1460.

Voss A, Reinhart M, Sankarappa S, Sprecher H. 1991. The metabolism of 7,10,13,16,19-docosapentaenoic acid to 4,7,10,13,16,19-docosahexaenoic acid in rat liver is independent of a 4-desaturase. *J Biol Chem* 266:19995–20000.

Ward KD, Sparrow D, Vokonas PS, Willett WC, Landsberg L, Weiss ST. 1994. The relationships of abdominal obesity, hyperinsulinemia and saturated fat intake to serum lipid levels: The Normative Aging Study. *Int J Obes Relat Metab Disord* 18:137–144.

Watts GF, Jackson P, Burke V, Lewis B. 1996. Dietary fatty acids and progression of coronary artery disease in men. *Am J Clin Nutr* 64:202–209.

Weijenberg MP, Feskens EJM, Kromhout D. 1996. Total and high density lipo-protein cholesterol as risk factors for coronary heart disease in elderly men during 5 years of follow-up. The Zutphen Elderly Study. *Am J Epidemiol* 143:151–158.

Wene JD, Connor WE, DenBesten L. 1975. The development of essential fatty acid deficiency in healthy men fed fat-free diets intravenously and orally. *J Clin Invest* 56:127–134.

West DB, York B. 1998. Dietary fat, genetic predisposition, and obesity: Lessons from animal models. *Am J Clin Nutr* 67:505S–512S.

Wetzel MG, Li J, Alvarez RA, Anderson RE, O'Brien PJ. 1991. Metabolism of linolenic acid and docosahexaenoic acid in rat retinas and rod outer segments. *Exp Eye Res* 53:437–446.

Wheeler TG, Benolken RM, Anderson RE. 1975. Visual membranes: Specificity of fatty acid precursors for the electrical response to illumination. *Science* 188:1312–1314.

Wild SH, Fortmann SP, Marcovina SM. 1997. A prospective case-control study of lipoprotein(a) levels and apo(a) size and risk of coronary heart disease in Stanford Five-City Project participants. *Arterioscler Thromb Vasc Biol* 17:239–245.

Willatts P, Forsyth JS, DiModugno MK, Varma S, Colvin M. 1998. Effect of long-chain polyunsaturated fatty acids in infant formula on problem solving at 10 months of age. *Lancet* 352:688–691.

Willett WC, Stampfer MJ, Mason JE, Colditz GA, Speizer FE, Rosner BA, Sampson LA, Hennekens CH. 1993. Intake of *trans* fatty acids and risk of coronary heart disease among women. *Lancet* 341:581–585.

Wojenski CM, Silver MJ, Walker J. 1991. Eicosapentaenoic acid ethyl ester as an antithrombotic agent: Comparison to an extract of fish oil. *Biochim Biophys Acta* 1081:33–38.

Wong KH, Deitel M. 1981. Studies with a safflower oil emulsion in total parenteral nutrition. *Can Med Assoc J* 125:1328–1334.

Wong S, Nestel PJ. 1987. Eicosapentaenoic acid inhibits the secretion of triacylglycerol and of apoprotein B and the binding of LDL in Hep G2 cells. *Atherosclerosis* 64:139–146.

Wood R, Kubena K, O'Brien B, Tseng S, Martin G. 1993a. Effect of butter, mono- and polyunsaturated fatty acid-enriched butter, *trans* fatty acid margarine, and zero *trans* fatty acid margarine on serum lipids and lipoproteins in healthy men. *J Lipid Res* 34:1–11.

Wood R, Kubena K, Tseng S, Martin G, Crook R. 1993b. Effect of palm oil, margarine, butter, and sunflower oil on the serum lipids and lipoproteins of normocholesterolemic middle-aged men. *J Nutr Biochem* 4:286–297.

Yamashita N, Maruyama M, Yamazaki K, Hamazaki T, Yano S. 1991. Effect of eicosapentaenoic and docosahexaenoic acid on natural killer cell activity in human peripheral blood lymphocytes. *Clin Immunol Immunopathol* 59:335–345.

Yao CH, Slattery ML, Jacobs DR, Folsom AR, Nelson ET. 1991. Anthropometric predictors of coronary heart disease and total mortality: Findings from the US Railroad Study. *Am J Epidemiol* 134:1278–1289.

Yaqoob P, Pala HS, Cortina-Borja M, Newsholme EA, Calder PC. 2000. Encapsulated fish oil enriched in α-tocopherol alters plasma phospholipid and mononuclear cell fatty acid compositions but not mononuclear cell functions. *Eur J Clin Invest* 30:260–274.

Yasuda S, Watanabe S, Kobayashi T, Hata N, Misawa Y, Utsumi H, Okuyama H. 1999. Dietary docosahexaenoic acid enhances ferric nitrilotriacetate-induced oxidative damage in mice but not when additional alpha-tocopherol is supplemented. *Free Radic Res* 30:199–205.

Yu S, Derr J, Etherton TD, Kris-Etherton PM. 1995. Plasma cholesterol-predictive equations demonstrate that stearic acid is neutral and monounsaturated fatty acids are hypocholesterolemic. *Am J Clin Nutr* 61:1129–1139.

Zambon S, Friday KE, Childs MT, Fujimoto WY, Bierman EL, Ensinck JW. 1992. Effect of glyburide and ω3 fatty acid dietary supplements on glucose and lipid metabolism in patients with non-insulin-dependent diabetes mellitus. *Am J Clin Nutr* 56:447–454.

Zevenbergen JL, Houtsmuller UMT, Gottenbos JJ. 1988. Linoleic acid requirement of rats fed *trans* fatty acids. *Lipids* 23:178–186.

Zock PL, Katan MB. 1992. Hydrogenation alternatives: Effects of *trans* fatty acids and stearic acid versus linoleic acid on serum lipids and lipoproteins in humans. *J Lipid Res* 33:399–410.

Zock PL, Mensink RP. 1996. Dietary *trans*-fatty acids and serum lipoproteins in humans. *Curr Opin Lipidol* 7:34–37.

Zock PL, Blijlevens RAMT, de Vries JHM, Katan MB. 1993. Effects of stearic acid and *trans* fatty acids versus linoleic acid on blood pressure in normotensive women and men. *Eur J Clin Nutr* 47:437–444.

Zock PL, Katan MB, Mensink RP. 1995. Dietary *trans* fatty acids and lipoprotein cholesterol. *Am J Clin Nutr* 61:617.

Zucker ML, Bilyeu DS, Helmkamp GM, Harris WS, Dujovne CA. 1988. Effects of dietary fish oil on platelet function and plasma lipids in hyperlipoproteinemic and normal subjects. *Atherosclerosis* 73:13–22.

9

Cholesterol

SUMMARY

Cholesterol plays an important role in steroid hormone and bile acid biosynthesis and serves as an integral component of cell membranes. Given the capability of all tissues to synthesize sufficient amounts of cholesterol for their metabolic and structural needs, there is no evidence for a biological requirement for dietary cholesterol. Therefore, neither an Adequate Intake nor a Recommended Dietary Allowance is set for cholesterol.

There is much evidence to indicate a positive linear trend between cholesterol intake and low density lipoprotein cholesterol concentration, and therefore increased risk of coronary heart disease (CHD). A Tolerable Upper Intake Level is not set for cholesterol because any incremental increase in cholesterol intake increases CHD risk. Because cholesterol is unavoidable in ordinary diets, eliminating cholesterol in the diet would require significant changes in patterns of dietary intake. Such significant adjustments may introduce undesirable effects (e.g., inadequate intakes of protein and certain micronutrients) and unknown and unquantifiable health risks. Nonetheless, it is possible to have a diet low in cholesterol while consuming a nutritionally adequate diet. Dietary guidance for minimizing cholesterol intake is provided in Chapter 11.

BACKGROUND INFORMATION

Function

Cholesterol is a sterol that is present in all animal tissues. Tissue cholesterol occurs primarily as free (unesterified) cholesterol, but is also bound covalently to fatty acids as cholesteryl esters and to certain proteins. Free cholesterol is an integral component of cell membranes and serves as a precursor for steroid hormones such as estrogen, testosterone, and aldosterone, as well as bile acids.

Physiology of Absorption and Metabolism

Absorption

After emulsification and bile acid micellar solubilization, dietary cholesterol, as well as cholesterol derived from hepatic secretion and sloughed intestinal epithelium, is absorbed in the proximal jejunum. Cholesteryl esters, comprising 10 to 15 percent of total dietary cholesterol, are hydrolyzed by a specific pancreatic esterase. Cholesterol absorption by enterocytes is believed to occur primarily by passive diffusion across a concentration gradient established by the solubilization of cholesterol in bile acid micelles. However, recent evidence has shown that scavenger receptor class B type I is present in the small intestine brush-border membrane where it facilitates the uptake of micellar cholesterol (Hauser et al., 1998). In addition, as described further below, two recently identified adenosine triphosphate binding-cassette (ABC) proteins (ABCG5 and ABCG8) have been found to form heterodimers that export plant sterols and cholesterol from enterocytes into the gut lumen, thereby decreasing net sterol absorption (Berge et al., 2000). ABC1, a transporter involved in high density lipoprotein–(HDL) mediated cellular cholesterol efflux, may also participate in this process (Repa et al., 2000).

Esterification of cholesterol and subsequent secretion of both esterified and unesterified cholesterol into lymph and plasma in intestinally synthesized chylomicron and HDL particles may also affect net cholesterol uptake by enterocytes. Key components of this process include cholesterol esterification by acylCoA:cholesterol acyltransferase; lipoprotein assembly with the structural protein apoB48 (chylomicrons) and apoAI (HDL), as well as with triacylglycerols and phospholipids; and lipoprotein secretion into lymphatics facilitated by microsomal triacylglycerol transfer protein.

Cholesterol balance studies in humans have indicated a wide variation in efficiency of intestinal cholesterol absorption (from 20 to 80 percent), with most individuals absorbing between 40 and 60 percent of ingested cholesterol (Ros, 2000). As discussed below, such variability, which is likely due in part to genetic factors, may contribute to interindividual differences in plasma cholesterol response to dietary cholesterol. In addition, cholesterol absorption may be reduced by the cholesterol content of a meal and by decreased intestinal transit time (Ros, 2000). Although fatty acids are required for intestinal micelle formation, there is no strong evidence that fat content (or other dietary constituents such as fiber) has a significant effect on cholesterol absorption.

An average of 250 mg/d of plant sterols (e.g., sitosterol, stigmasterol, and campesterol) are consumed in the diet, but the absorption of such sterols (approximately 5 percent) is considerably lower than that for cholesterol (Ling and Jones, 1995; Salen et al., 1970). They are not known to have important biological effects in humans at the levels consumed in the diet. An exception is sitosterolemia, a rare genetic disorder that is characterized by markedly increased absorption and tissue accumulation of plant sterols and elevated plasma cholesterol levels (Lütjohann et al., 1996; Salen et al., 1992). Recently, patients with this disorder have been shown to have mutations in genes encoding ABCG5 and ABCG8, indicating the importance of these transporters in regulating sterol absorption presumably by promoting the export of nearly all plant sterols, and a portion of cholesterol, from intestinal cells (Berge et al., 2000). Moreover, increased expression of these genes induced by cholesterol feeding may be of importance in limiting cholesterol absorption (Berge et al., 2000). The ability of very high intakes of plant sterols to lower plasma cholesterol concentrations by reducing cholesterol absorption may also involve regulation of this transport process (Miettinen and Gylling, 1999).

Metabolism

Intestinally derived cholesterol is transported in the circulation to other tissues via chylomicrons, and to a lesser extent HDL, mainly in the form of cholesteryl ester. The hydrolysis of chylomicron triacylglycerols in peripheral tissues by lipoprotein lipase and subsequent remodeling by lipid transfer proteins yields a "remnant" particle that is internalized by receptors, primarily in the liver, that recognize apoprotein E and perhaps other constituents. Cholesterol released by intracellular cholesteryl esterase activity can be stored in hepatocytes; re-esterified and secreted into plasma in lipoproteins, primarily very low density lipoproteins (VLDL); oxidized and excreted as bile acids; or directly secreted into the bile. Free and esterified cholesterol circulate in the blood in humans principally in low density lipoproteins (LDL).

Cholesterol homeostasis in hepatocytes is of critical importance for the regulation of plasma LDL cholesterol concentrations (Dietschy et al.,

1993). Increased cellular cholesterol content leads to suppression of synthesis of LDL receptors via a series of steps resulting in interaction of sterol regulatory element-binding protein (SREBP) 1 and 2 transcription factors with a sterol response element in the LDL receptor gene (Brown and Goldstein, 1999). Increased plasma LDL concentrations can result from reduced hepatic LDL uptake, as well as reduced uptake of VLDL and intermediate density lipoproteins, leading to increased metabolic conversion of these particles to LDL (Kita et al., 1982). Metabolic studies in humans have indicated that a high cholesterol diet induces both increased LDL synthesis and reduced receptor-dependent fractional removal rate of LDL particles (Packard et al., 1983).

There are a number of other genes involved in cholesterol and lipoprotein metabolism in which hepatic regulation can be affected by cholesterol availability either directly via SREBPs or indirectly by the action of other transcription factors, such as liver X receptors (Repa and Mangelsdorf, 2000). These genes play a role in cholesterol regulatory pathways, including those involved in cholesterol synthesis that are suppressed by cholesterol (e.g., 3-hydroxy-3-methylglutaryl coenzyme A [HMG CoA] reductase) and others involved in bile acid production from cholesterol that are activated by cholesterol (e.g., 7 α-hydroxylase). Thus, increased hepatic cholesterol delivery from diet and other sources results in a complex admixture of metabolic effects that are generally directed at maintaining tissue and plasma cholesterol homeostasis. However, as described below, empirical observations in humans have indicated that increased dietary cholesterol does result in a net increase in plasma LDL cholesterol concentrations, probably as a consequence of reduced hepatic LDL receptor activity.

All cells are capable of synthesizing cholesterol in sufficient amounts for their structural and metabolic needs. However, certain tissues (e.g., adrenal glands and gonads) derive a significant proportion of cholesterol by uptake from plasma lipoproteins. Cholesterol synthesis via a series of intermediates from acetyl CoA is highly regulated. The enzyme HMG CoA reductase catalyzes the rate-limiting step in cholesterol synthesis—the formation of mevalonic acid from HMG CoA. The genes for this enzyme and a number of other proteins involved in cholesterol metabolism, such as the LDL receptor, are regulated by intracellular sterols and other signaling molecules to maintain tissue cholesterol homeostasis, as described above. Endogenous cholesterol synthesis in humans is approximately 12 to 13 mg/kg/d (840 to 910 mg/d for a 70-kg individual) (Di Buono et al., 2000).

Another group of diet-derived sterols with potential biological effects are oxysterols (Vine et al., 1998), which are cholesterol oxidation products that can be found in cholesterol-rich processed foods such as dried egg yolk, although typical levels of oxysterols in the diet are generally low (van de Bovenkamp et al., 1988). These cholesterol oxidation products can have major effects on cholesterol metabolism and have been shown to be highly atherogenic in animal models (Staprans et al., 2000; Vine et al., 1998). Their role in human nutrition remains to be established.

Overall, body cholesterol homeostasis is highly regulated by balancing intestinal absorption and endogenous synthesis with hepatic excretion of cholesterol and bile acids derived from hepatic cholesterol oxidation.

FINDINGS BY LIFE STAGE AND GENDER GROUP

Given the capability of all tissues to synthesize sufficient cholesterol for their metabolic and structural needs, there is no evidence for a biological requirement for dietary cholesterol. As an example, many Tarahumara Indians of Mexico consume very low amounts of dietary cholesterol and have no reported developmental or health problems that could be attributed to this aspect of their diet (McMurry et al., 1982). Therefore, neither an Adequate Intake (AI) nor an Estimated Average Requirement (EAR) and Recommended Dietary Allowance (RDA) are set for cholesterol.

The question of whether cholesterol in the infant diet plays some essential role on lipid and lipoprotein metabolism that is relevant to growth and development or to the atherosclerotic process in adults has been difficult to resolve. The idea that the early diet might have relevance to later lipid metabolism was first raised by Hahn and Koldovský (1966) in prematurely weaned rat pups and later supported by observations that normal weaning to a high intake of cholesterol resulted in greater resistance to dietary cholesterol in later adulthood (Reiser and Sidelman, 1972; Reiser et al., 1979). This led to the hypothesis that cholesterol in human milk may play some important role in establishing regulation of cholesterol homeostasis. Since human milk typically provides about 100 to 200 mg/L (Table 9-1), whereas infant formulas contain very little cholesterol (10 to 30 mg/L) (Huisman et al., 1996; Wong et al., 1993), it is not surprising that plasma cholesterol concentrations are higher in infants fed human milk than in formula-fed infants. Formula-fed infants also have a higher rate of cholesterol synthesis (Bayley et al., 1998; Cruz et al., 1994; Wong et al., 1993). However, the available evidence suggests that this effect is transient. Differences in cholesterol synthesis and plasma cholesterol concentration are not sustained once complementary feeding is introduced (Darmady et al., 1972; Friedman and Goldberg, 1975; Mize et al., 1995). Also, no clinically significant effects on growth and development due to these differences in plasma cholesterol concentration have been noted between breast-fed and formula-fed infants under 1 year of age. One explanation may be that the developing brain synthesizes the cholesterol required for myelination in situ and does not take up cholesterol from

TABLE 9-1 Cholesterol Content in Term Human Milk of Women in the United States

Reference	n	Stage of Lactation	Cholesterol Content (mg/L)
Picciano et al., 1978	18	6–12 wk postpartum (pp)	
		Early morning	157
		Midday	151
		Evening	178
Mellies et al., 1979	33	1 mo pp	201
		2 mo pp	195
		3 mo pp	97
		4 mo pp	220
		5 mo pp	156
		6 mo pp	283
		7 mo pp	289
		8 mo pp	220
		9 mo pp	260
		10 mo pp	210
		11 mo pp	135
		12–13 mo pp	151
Clark et al., 1982	10	2 wk pp	110
		6 wk pp	97
		12 wk pp	103
		16 wk pp	104
Bitman et al., 1983	6	3 wk pp	122
		6 wk pp	112
		12 wk pp	103
Lammi-Keefe et al., 1990	6	8 wk pp	
		0600 h	88
		1000 h	107
		1400 h	111
		1800 h	110
		2200 h	112
Jensen et al., 1995	10	12 wk pp	
		0600–1000 h	140
		1000–1400 h	162
		1400–1800 h	217
		1800–2200 h	220
		2200–0600 h	129
Bayley et al., 1998	14	4 mo pp	120

plasma (Edmond et al., 1991; Haave and Innis, 2001; Jurevics and Morell, 1994).

The effects of early cholesterol intake and weaning on cholesterol metabolism later in life have been studied in a number of different animal species (Hamosh, 1988; Kris-Etherton et al., 1979; Mott et al., 1990) and in short-term studies with infants and children. Studies in baboons fed breast milk or formulas with or without cholesterol and with varying fat compositions found that early cholesterol intake had little effect on serum cholesterol concentrations in young adults up to about 8 years of age (Mott et al., 1990). However, adult baboons that had been breast fed had lower high density lipoprotein (HDL) cholesterol concentrations, higher very low density lipoprotein + low density lipoprotein (LDL):HDL ratios, and more extensive atherosclerotic lesions than those that had been formula fed (Lewis et al., 1988; Mott et al., 1990, 1995). These differences were not explained by variations in the saturated and unsaturated fat content of the formulas and milk. The major metabolic difference associated with the differences in plasma lipoproteins was lower rates of bile acid synthesis and excretion among the baboons that had been breast fed.

The possible relations of early breast and bottle feeding with later cholesterol concentrations and other coronary heart disease risk factors were explored in several short-term studies and larger retrospective epidemiological studies, but these observations are inconsistent (Fall et al., 1992; Kolaček et al., 1993; Leeson et al., 2001; Ravelli et al., 2000).

The relationship between early dietary cholesterol intake from milk or formula and serum cholesterol concentration in infancy and that observed in children and young adults following their usual diets was either absent (Andersen et al., 1979; Friedman and Goldberg, 1975; Glueck et al., 1972; Huttunen et al., 1983), in favor of formula feeding compared to breast feeding during infancy in 7- to 12-year-old children (Hodgson et al., 1976), or in favor of feeding human milk compared to formula feeding in men and women. The disparate findings may be due to confounding factors such as duration of breast feeding, since human-milk feeding for less than 3 months was associated with higher serum cholesterol concentrations in men at 18 to 23 years of age, or the type of formula fed since formula composition, especially quality of fat, which has changed dramatically in the last century (Kolaček et al., 1993). A follow-up study of nearly 6,000 elderly men for whom early feeding methods had been recorded found higher total and LDL cholesterol concentrations and increased risk of coronary heart disease (CHD) mortality in men who had been exclusively fed human milk than in those who had been fed human milk and bottle fed or fed human milk and weaned at 1 year of age. Men who had been exclusively bottle-fed during infancy also had higher total and LDL cholesterol concentrations and CHD mortality than men who had previously been fed human milk (Fall et al., 1992).

The available data do not warrant a recommendation with respect to dietary cholesterol intake for infants who are not fed human milk. However, further research to identify possible mechanisms whereby early nutritional experiences affect the atherosclerotic process in adults, as well as the sensitive periods in development when this may occur, would be valuable.

INTAKE OF CHOLESTEROL

Food Sources

Cholesterol is present in foods of animal origin. High amounts of cholesterol are present in liver (375 mg/3 oz slice) and egg yolk (250 mg/ yolk). Although generally low in total fat, some seafood, including shrimp, lobster, and certain fish, contain moderately high amounts of cholesterol (60 to 100 g/half-cup serving). One cup of whole milk contains approximately 30 mg of cholesterol, whereas the cholesterol contained in 2 percent and skim milk is 15 and 7 mg/cup, respectively. Therefore, products that contain milk (e.g., cheese, ice cream, and cottage cheese) are moderate sources of cholesterol. One tablespoon of butter contains approximately 12 mg of cholesterol, whereas margarine does not contain cholesterol. The majority of cholesterol is consumed from eggs and meat (FASEB, 1995).

Dietary Intake

Based on intake data from the Continuing Survey of Food Intakes by Individuals (1994–1996, 1998), the median cholesterol intake ranged from approximately 250 to 325 mg/d for men and 180 to 205 mg/d for women (Appendix Table E-15).

ADVERSE EFFECTS OF OVERCONSUMPTION

Hazard Identification

Plasma Total, HDL, and LDL Cholesterol Concentrations

Numerous studies in humans have examined the effects of dietary cholesterol on plasma total and lipoprotein cholesterol concentrations (Tables 9-2 and 9-3, Figures 9-1 and 9-2), and empirical formulas have been derived to describe these relationships. Although most studies have

TABLE 9-2 Effects of Adding Dietary Cholesterol to Defined Diets with Strict Control of Dietary Intake on Serum Cholesterol Concentration

Reference	n	Baseline Dietary Cholesterol (mg/d)	Added Dietary Cholesterol (mg/d)
Beveridge et al.,	6	13	81
1960	9	13	140
	9	13	280
	9	13	621
	6	13	1,282
	10	13	2,481
	9	13	4,490
Connor et al.,	2	0	475
1961a	2	0	950
	2	0	1,425
Connor et al.,	3	0	2,400
1961b	1	0	1,650
	1	0	1,900
	1	0	4,800
Steiner et al., 1962	6	0	3,000
Wells and Bronte-	3	0	17
Stewart, 1963	3	0	42
	3	0	67
	3	0	88
	3	0	142
	3	0	267
	3	0	517
	3	0	1,017
	3	0	1,517
	3	0	3,017
Connor et al., 1964	6	0	729
	5	0	725
Erickson et al.,	6	0	742
1964	6	0	742
Hegsted et al., 1965	10	116	570
	10	306	380
	10	116	570

Change in Serum Total Cholesterol (mmol/L)	Percent of Calories from Fat	P:S Ratio
0.06	30	0.08
0.10	30	0.08
1.17	30	0.08
0.43	30	0.08
0.59	30	0.08
1.20	30	0.08
0.87	30	0.08
1.71	40	0.76
1.64	40	0.76
1.99	40	0.76
1.47	40	0.88
2.43	40	0.88
2.97	40	0.88
2.53	40	0.88
1.30	40	0.68
0.44	15	
0.56	15	
0.66	15	
0.80	15	
0.96	15	
1.03	15	
1.18	15	
1.09	15	
1.29	15	
1.23	15	
1.03	40	0.25
0.74	40	1.7
0.61	41	1.6
0.69	41	1.6
0.75	39	5.4
0.29	39	0.05
0.70	39	0.68

continued

TABLE 9-2 Continued

Reference	n	Baseline Dietary Cholesterol (mg/d)	Added Dietary Cholesterol (mg/d)
Keys et al., 1965	22	50	470
	22	50	1,410
	22	50	33
	22	50	1,400
	22	50	1,410
National Diet-Heart	81	126	495
Study Research	81	126	495
Group,1968	57	401	495
	57	154	495
Quintão et al., 1971	4	43	2,441
	1	43	499
	1	44	197
	2	53.5	4,002
Mattson et al., 1972	14	0	297
	14	0	594
	14	0	888
Anderson et al.,	12	3	291
1976	12	3	291
Nestel and Poyser,	4	210	500
1976	2	257	500
	2	334	532
	1	103	439
Quintão et al., 1977	6	0	3,250
Bronsgeest-Schoute	21	98	567
et al., 1979a,	21	98	567
1979b	9	124	607
	9	124	607
Lin and Connor, 1980	2	45	1,081
McMurry et al., 1981	12	0	600

Change in Serum Total Cholesterol (mmol/L)	Percent of Calories from Fat	P:S Ratio
0.36	40	
0.70	40	
0.41	40	
0.80	40	1.3
0.75	40	0.08
0.12	30	2.31
0.27	39	0.5
0.32	40	0.08
0.18	40	0.96
0.96	40	0.93
0.88	40	0.93
−0.80	40	0.93
0.13	40	0.93
0.34	39	0.31
0.61	39	0.31
1.05	39	0.31
0.23	35	0.26
0.21	35	4.7
1.56	40	1.9
0.25	40	1.9
0.76	40	1.9
0.67	40	1.9
0.74		
0.32	44	2
0.25	44	2
0.70	34	0.2
0.66	34	0.2
2.45	40	0.8
0.93	40	0.8

continued

TABLE 9-2 Continued

Reference	n	Baseline Dietary Cholesterol (mg/d)	Added Dietary Cholesterol (mg/d)
McMurry et al., 1982	8	0	905
Nestel et al., 1982	6	200	1,500
Schonfeld et al., 1982	11	300	750
	9	300	1,500
	6	300	750
	6	300	1,500
	6	300	750
	6	300	1,500
Maranhão and Quintdo, 1983	13	40	1,350
Applebaum-Bowden et al., 1984	9	137	897
Beynen and Katan, 1985b	6	114	526
Katan et al., 1986	94	110	500
Zanni et al., 1987	9	130	745
	9	130	745
Johnson and Greenland, 1990	10	200	400
Ginsberg et al., 1994	20	128	155
	20	128	340
	20	128	730
Sundram et al., 1994	17	192	7
	17	192	13
Fielding et al., 1995	20	200	403
	22	200	435
Ginsberg et al., 1995	13	108	169
	13	108	559

Change in Serum Total Cholesterol (mmol/L)	Percent of Calories from Fat	P:S Ratio
0.88	20	0.7
0.42	31	1
0.47	40	0.32
0.72	40	0.32
0.13	40	0.8
0.70	40	0.8
0.05	40	2.5
0.26	40	2.5
1.19	40	0.93
0.28	40	0.82
0.25	42	0.46
0.5	42	0.16
0.58	31	2.1
0.39	31	0.64
0.26	30	1.5
0.14	27	0.89
0.16	27	0.93
0.29	28	0.87
0.06	31	0.21
−0.35	31	0.25
0.50	39	0.81
0.76	36	0.28
0.16	28	0.89
0.41	28	0.86

TABLE 9-3 Effects of Adding Dietary Cholesterol to Self-Selected Diets with Strict Control of Dietary Intake on Serum Cholesterol Concentration

Reference	n	Baseline Dietary Cholesterol (mg/d)	Added Dietary Cholesterol (mg/d)
Slater et al., 1976	25	314	482
Kummerow et al., 1977	21	250	470
Porter et al., 1977	55	301	235
	59	301	235
Flynn et al., 1979	56	260	540
	60	260	540
Mistry et al., 1981	37	522	1,500
	14	480	750
Roberts et al., 1981	16	196	532
Packard et al., 1983	7	180	1,290
Beynen and Katan, 1985a	6	207	1,596
	6	207	1,596
Oh and Miller, 1985	21	474	654
Edington et al., 1987	33	120	188
	135	120	188
McNamara et al., 1987	39	192	628
	36	288	575
Kestin et al., 1989	10	180	686
	15	204	735
Clifton et al., 1990	Normal: 11	185	681
	Hypercholesterolemic diet-insensitive: 22	185	681
	Hypercholesterolemic diet-sensitive: 23	185	681

Change in Serum Total Cholesterol (mmol/L)	Percent of Calories from Fat	P:S Ratio
−0.09		
0.05	40	
0.16	38	
0.03	38	
0.49	38	
0.00	38	
0.75	41	
0.62	41	
0.40	40	
1.47	38	0.17
0.48	46	0.5
0.61	46	0.5
0.27	35	0.62
0.13	26	0.8
0.12	35	0.6
0.16	35	1.45
0.13	35	0.27
−0.02	41	0.37
0.04	36	0.85
0.06	29	0.6
0.19	29	0.6
0.36	29	0.6

continued

TABLE 9-3 Continued

Reference	n	Baseline Dietary Cholesterol (mg/d)	Added Dietary Cholesterol (mg/d)
Kern, 1994	8	585	2,393
	8	548	2,462
McCombs et al., 1994	12	213	938
	11	197	888
Clifton et al., 1995	67	151	691
	53	208	939
Sutherland et al., 1997	12	349	250
	14	349	250
Romano et al., 1998	10	200	800
	11	200	800

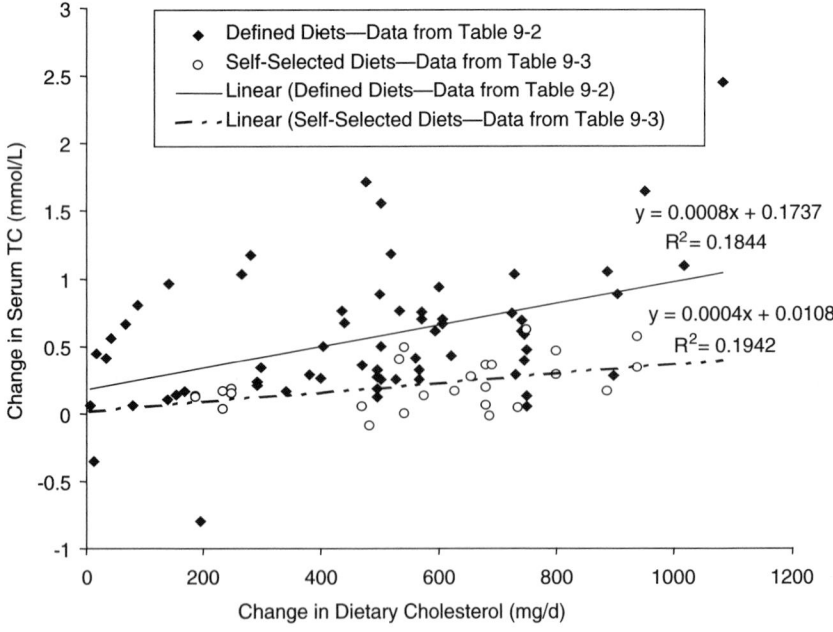

FIGURE 9-1 Relationship between change in dietary cholesterol (0 to 1,000 mg/d) and change in serum total cholesterol (TC) concentration.

Change in Serum Total Cholesterol (mmol/L)	Percent of Calories from Fat	P:S Ratio
0.14	44	0.59
−0.22	44	0.65
0.57	35	0.49
0.16	34	0.54
0.36	35	0.31
0.34	35	0.30
0.18	34	
0.15	34	
0.29	30	
0.46	30	

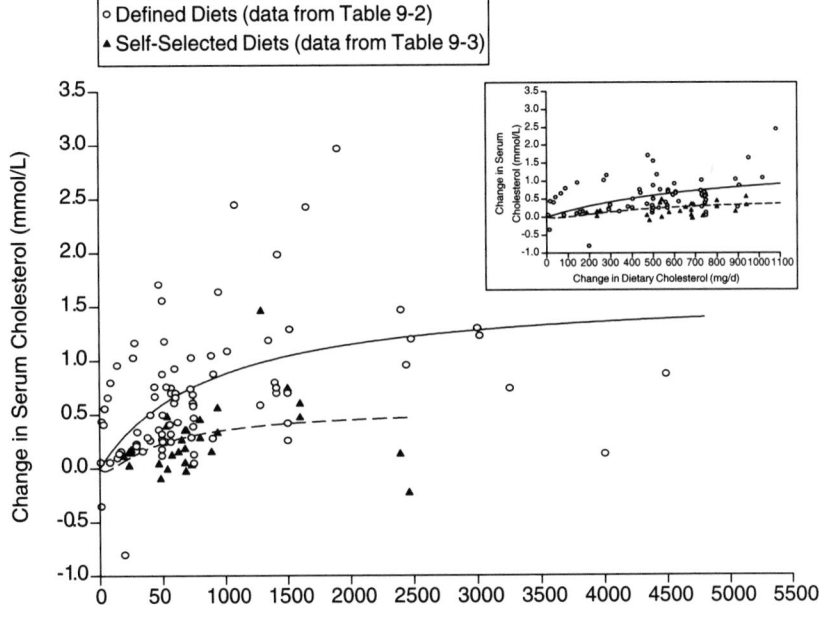

FIGURE 9-2 Relationship between change in dietary cholesterol (0 to 4,500 mg/d) and change in serum cholesterol (TC) concentration.

reported a linear relationship between changes in dietary cholesterol and total serum cholesterol concentration, other studies, including a meta-analysis of 27 controlled metabolic feeding studies of added dietary cholesterol (Hopkins, 1992), have indicated a curvilinear univariate relationship that is quasilinear in the range from 0 to 300 to 400 mg/d of added dietary cholesterol. The range of added dietary cholesterol in the studies was 17 to 4,800 mg/d. The meta-analysis also identified a diminishing increment of serum cholesterol with increasing baseline dietary cholesterol intake. With a baseline cholesterol intake of 0, the estimated increases in serum total cholesterol concentration for intakes from 100 to 400 mg/d of added dietary cholesterol were 0.16 to 0.51 mmol/L, whereas for a baseline cholesterol intake of 300 mg/d, the estimated increases in serum total cholesterol were 0.05 to 0.16 mmol/L (Hopkins, 1992). Another meta-analysis showed that dietary cholesterol raises the ratio of total cholesterol to high density lipoprotein (HDL) cholesterol, therefore adversely affecting the cholesterol profile (Weggemans et al., 2001).

Other predictive formulas for the effect of 100 mg/d of added dietary cholesterol, which did not consider baseline cholesterol intake and are based on compilations of studies with a variety of experimental conditions, have yielded estimates of 0.1 mmol/L (Hegsted, 1986), 0.057 mmol/L (Howell et al., 1997), and 0.065 mmol/L (Clarke et al., 1997), the latter two involving meta-analyses with adjustment for other dietary variables. Furthermore, pooled analyses of the effects of 100 mg/d of added dietary cholesterol on plasma lipoprotein cholesterol concentrations (Clarke et al., 1997) indicated an estimated increase of 0.05 mmol/L in low density lipoprotein (LDL) and 0.01 mmol/L in HDL (ratio of 5 LDL:1 HDL). There is evidence that the increase in HDL is largely accounted for by higher levels of apoE-containing HDL particles (Mahley et al., 1978), but the significance in atherosclerosis protection is not established. Hegsted and coworkers (1993) reported that the majority of the increase in serum total cholesterol concentration with increased cholesterol intake was due to an increase in LDL cholesterol concentration.

The incremental serum cholesterol response to a given amount of dietary cholesterol appears to diminish as baseline serum cholesterol intake increases (Hopkins, 1992). There is also evidence from a number of studies that increases in serum cholesterol concentration due to dietary cholesterol are blunted by diets low in saturated fat, high in polyunsaturated fat, or both (Fielding et al., 1995; National Diet-Heart Study Research Group, 1968; Schonfeld et al., 1982), although this effect has not been observed by others (Kestin et al., 1989; McNamara et al., 1987).

There is considerable evidence for interindividual variation in serum cholesterol response to dietary cholesterol, ranging from 0 to greater than 100 percent (Hopkins, 1992). It has been reported that such responsiveness is relatively stable within individuals (Beynen and Katan, 1985b) and appears to be correlated with serum cholesterol response to saturated fatty acids (Katan et al., 1988). Intrinsic differences in intestinal cholesterol absorption (Sehayek et al., 1998), suppression of hepatic cholesterol synthesis by dietary cholesterol (Dietschy et al., 1993; McNamara et al., 1987; Nestel and Poyser, 1976; Quintão et al., 1971), and LDL catabolism (Dietschy et al., 1993; Mistry et al., 1981) may all contribute to the observed variation in dietary cholesterol response.

There is increasing evidence that genetic factors underlie a substantial portion of interindividual variation in response to dietary cholesterol. An instructive case is that of the Tarahumara Indians, who in addition to consuming a diet low in cholesterol, have both low intestinal cholesterol absorption and increased transformation of cholesterol to bile acids (McMurry et al., 1985). However, with an increase in dietary cholesterol from 0 to 905 mg/d, their average plasma cholesterol concentration increased 0.88 mmol/L (from 2.92 to 3.8 mmol/L), the same value predicted by the formula of Hopkins (1992), indicating the likelihood of above-average responsiveness of other aspects of cholesterol or lipoprotein metabolism.

Variations in several genes have been associated with altered responsiveness to dietary cholesterol. The common E4 polymorphism of the apoE gene has been associated with increased cholesterol absorption (Kesäniemi et al., 1987) and with increased plasma LDL cholesterol response to dietary saturated fat and cholesterol in some, but not all studies (Dreon and Krauss, 1997). The recent finding that apoE is of importance in regulating cholesterol absorption and bile acid formation in apoE knockout mice (Sehayek et al., 2000) lends support to a possible role for this gene in modulating dietary cholesterol responsiveness in humans. The A-IV-2 variant allele of the apo A-IV gene has been found to attenuate the plasma cholesterol response to dietary cholesterol (McCombs et al., 1994). Recently, the A-IV-2 allele has been associated with reduced intestinal cholesterol absorption in diets high in polyunsaturated fat but not in diets high in saturated fat (Weinberg et al., 2000). However, this has not been confirmed in other studies (Weggemans et al., 2000). Finally, the recent discovery that defects in the ABCG5 and ABCG8 genes can lead to markedly increased intestinal absorption of both cholesterol and plant sterols (Berge et al., 2000) points to the possibility that more common variants of these genes may contribute to variation in cholesterol absorption and dietary cholesterol response in the general population.

There are numerous other candidate genes that could modulate plasma lipid and lipoprotein response to dietary cholesterol by affecting cholesterol absorption, cellular cholesterol homeostasis, and plasma lipoprotein metabolism. Among the most likely candidates are those regulated by lipid-responsive nuclear transcription factors, including sterol regulatory element-binding proteins, peroxisome proliferator-activated receptors, and orphan nuclear receptors. Studies in animal models have generated data in support of the possibility that variations among these genes may be of importance in influencing dietary cholesterol response in humans, but to date such human data are lacking. Nevertheless, the existence of marked interindividual variability in dietary cholesterol response among and within various animal models points to the likelihood that some of the mechanisms underlying this variability will also apply to humans.

Cardiovascular Disease and CHD

An association of dietary cholesterol with cardiovascular disease is based on several lines of evidence, including studies in animal models, epidemiological data in humans, and the effects of dietary cholesterol on plasma lipoproteins (Table 9-4). There is compelling evidence that dietary cholesterol can induce atherosclerosis in several animal species, including rabbits, pigs, nonhuman primates, and transgenic mice (Bocan, 1998; McNamara, 2000; Rudel, 1997). However, given the existence of marked inter- and intraspecies differences in cholesterol metabolism and atherogenic mechanisms, it is not possible to extrapolate these data directly to humans.

A number of prospective epidemiological studies have investigated the relationship of dietary cholesterol and other nutrients to the development of coronary heart disease (CHD) (reviewed in Kritchevsky and Kritchevsky, 2000; McNamara, 2000). Significant univariate relationships of cholesterol intake to risk for CHD have been observed in the Seven Countries Study (Kromhout et al., 1995) and the Honolulu Heart Program (McGee et al., 1984). A significant relative risk was also observed in the Western Electric Study, which remained significant after adjustment for a number of covariates, including dietary fat and serum cholesterol concentration (Stamler and Shekelle, 1988). More recently, in a study of 10,802 health-conscious men and women in the United Kingdom, a univariate relationship of cholesterol intake to ischemic heart disease mortality was observed (Mann et al., 1997).

However, a number of other epidemiological studies have not demonstrated a significant independent relationship of dietary cholesterol intake and CHD (Esrey et al., 1996; Kromhout and de Lezenne Coulander, 1984; Pietinen et al., 1997; Posner et al., 1991). In a cohort of 43,757 male health professionals, dietary cholesterol intake was significantly related to age-adjusted risk for myocardial infarction and fatal CHD ($p < 0.003$ and 0.002, respectively) across cholesterol quintiles ranging from median intakes of 189 to 422 mg/d (Ascherio et al., 1996). However, the risk was attenuated with multivariate analyses ($p < 0.07$ and 0.03), which included other risk factors such as body mass index, smoking habits, alcohol consumption, physical activity, history of hypertension or high blood cholesterol, family history of myocardial infarction, and profession. The risk became insignificant after adjustment for fiber intake, which was reported to be significantly inversely related to CHD risk in this cohort. A similar cohort analysis in a group of 80,082 female nurses showed a positive but nonsignificant relationship between dietary cholesterol and CHD in quintiles of median intakes ranging from 132 to 273 mg/1,000 kcal/d (Hu et al., 1997). In both the male Health Professionals Follow-up Study and the female Nurses' Health Study cohorts, there was no relationship of egg intake to CHD risk with intakes of up to 1 egg/d (Hu et al., 1999). There was, however, a significant increase of CHD risk associated with higher ranges of egg consumption in patients with diabetes. This finding was corroborated in a European study, but after multivariate analysis adjusting for fiber intake, the association was no longer significant (Toeller et al., 1999).

Measures of atherosclerosis using imaging techniques have also been assessed in relation to diet. Angiographically assessed coronary artery disease progression over 39 months in 50 men was weakly related to cholesterol intake in univariate, but not multivariate, analysis (Watts et al., 1994). In 13,148 male and female participants in the Atherosclerosis Risk in Communities Study, carotid artery wall thickness, an index of early atherosclerosis, was significantly related to dietary cholesterol intake by univariate analyses; multivariate analysis was not performed (Tell et al., 1994).

The lack of consistency in observations relating dietary cholesterol intake to clinical cardiovascular disease and CHD endpoints may be due to many factors, including the limited ability to detect such effects (e.g., due to relatively small increases in LDL cholesterol concentration and inaccuracies in dietary intake data) and to the limited ability to distinguish the effects of dietary cholesterol independent of energy intake and other dietary variables that may be positively (e.g., saturated fat intake) or negatively (e.g., fiber intake) associated with dietary cholesterol and heart disease risk. Another uncertainty relates to interpreting the effects of dietary cholesterol on blood cholesterol concentrations. Evidence indicates that increased dietary cholesterol results, on average, in increased blood concentrations of both LDL and HDL cholesterol, and it is possible that the net impact on cardiovascular disease risk depends on the relative changes in these lipoproteins, as well as on other unmeasured mediators of atherogenesis. Finally, the considerable interindividual variation in lipid response to dietary cholesterol may result in differing outcomes in different populations or population subgroups.

TABLE 9-4 Dietary Cholesterol and Coronary Heart Disease (CHD)

Reference	Study Design	Diet Information
Kromhout and de Lezenne Coulander, 1984	Men, 40–59 y 14 cases 857 controls Cohort, 10-y follow-up	Dietary history
McGee et al., 1984	456 cases 6,632 controls Cohort, 10-y follow-up	24-h recall Adjusted for age
Kushi et al., 1985	Men 110 cases 891 controls Cohort, 20-y follow-up	Dietary history Adjusted for age and cohort
McGee et al., 1985	8,006 men Cohort, 10-y follow-up	24-h recall Adjusted for age
Posner et al., 1991	Men 45–55 y Cohort, 16-y follow-up	24-h recall Multivariate analysis
Tzonou et al., 1993	Men and women 329 cases 570 controls Case-control	Dietary history
Tell et al., 1994	Men and women, 45–64 y Cohort	Food frequency questionnaire
Watts et al., 1994	50 men 26 lipid-lowering diet 24 usual care Intervention	Dietary history

Results[a]		Comments
Mean cholesterol intake (mg/1,000 kcal)		No association between cholesterol intake and CHD
Cases	145	
Controls	143	
Mean cholesterol intake (mg/1,000 kcal)		Significant positive association between cholesterol intake and incidence of CHD
Cases	256	
Controls	241	
Mean cholesterol intake (mg/1,000 kcal)		Significantly greater cholesterol intake in CHD deaths
Cases	266	
Controls	248	

Cholesterol intake (mg/1,000 kcal)	Rate of CHD death (per 1,000)	Cholesterol intake as mg/1,000 kcal positively associated with CHD death, but not when intake measured as mg/d
< 125	≈ 8	
125–175	≈ 16	
175–225	≈ 14	
225–275	≈ 12	
275–325	≈ 13	
> 325	≈ 20	

Cholesterol intake (mg/d)	RR of CHD	No association between cholesterol intake and risk of CHD
300	1.0	
529	0.99	

Mean cholesterol intake (mg/d)			No association between cholesterol intake and CHD
	Men	Women	
Cases	345	322	
Controls	350	292	

Cholesterol intake was positively associated with carotid artery wall thickness

Mean cholesterol intake (mg/d)		Cholesterol was positively associated with progression of coronary artery disease
Diet	215	
Usual	341	

continued

TABLE 9-4 Continued

Reference	Study Design	Diet Information
Ascherio et al., 1996	Men 40–75 y 734 cases Cohort, 6-y follow-up	Food frequency questionnaire Multivariate analysis (including fiber intake)
Esrey et al., 1996	52 cases, 30–59 y 3,873 controls 40 cases, 60–79 y 581 controls Cohort, 12-y follow-up	24-h recall Multivariate analysis
Hu et al., 1997	80,082 women, 34–59 y Cohort, 14-y follow-up	Food frequency questionnaire Multivariate analysis
Mann et al., 1997	Men and women, 16–79 y Prospective observation	Food frequency questionnaire Adjusted for age, sex, smoking, and social class
Pietinen et al., 1997	Smoking men, 50–69 y Cohort, 6.1-y follow-up	Food frequency questionnaire Multivariate analysis

Results[a]		Comments
Mean cholesterol intake (mg/d)	RR for MI or fatal CHD	No significant association between cholesterol intake and risk for MI or fatal CHD after adjustment for fiber intake
189	1.00	
246	0.86	
290	0.98	
338	0.94	
422	1.03	

Mean cholesterol intake (mg/d)			Cholesterol intake was not significantly associated with CHD mortality
Age (y)	30–59	60–79	
Cases	427	423	
Controls	416	355	

Quintile of cholesterol intake	RR of CHD	A positive but nonsignificant association between cholesterol intake and risk of CHD
1	1.00	
2	1.19	
3	1.14	
4	1.32	
5	1.25	

Tertile of cholesterol intake	IHD death rate ratio	Increased IHD mortality with increased cholesterol intake
1st	100	
2nd	181	
3rd	353	

Median cholesterol intake (mg/d)	RR of coronary death	No association between cholesterol intake and risk of coronary death
390	1.00	
477	0.90	
543	0.81	
621	0.86	
768	0.92	

continued

TABLE 9-4 Continued

Reference	Study Design	Diet Information
Hu et al., 1999	37,851 men, 40–75 y 866 cases Cohort, 8-y follow-up 80,082 women, 34–59 y 939 cases Cohort, 14-y follow-up	Food frequency questionnaire Multivariate analysis
Toeller et al., 1999	Diabetic men and women, 14–61 y Cross-sectional	3-d dietary records Multivariate analysis (including fiber intake)

a RR = relative risk, MI = myocardial infarction, IHD = ischemic heart disease, OR = odds ratio, CVD = cardiovascular disease.

Cancer

As shown in Tables 9-5 through 9-8, no consistent significant associations have been established between dietary cholesterol intake and cancer, including lung, breast, colon, and prostate. Several case-control studies have suggested that a high consumption of cholesterol may be associated with an increased risk of lung cancer (Alavanja et al., 1993; Byers et al., 1987; Goodman et al., 1988; Hinds et al., 1983; Jain et al., 1990). This positive association was shown in one cohort study (Shekelle et al., 1991), but not in three others (Heilbrun et al., 1984; Knekt et al., 1991; Wu et al., 1994).

Dose–Response Assessment

The main adverse effect of dietary cholesterol is increased serum LDL cholesterol concentration, which would be predicted to result in increased risk for CHD. Serum HDL concentration also increases, although to a

Results[a]			Comments
Egg intake (eggs/wk) Men	Mean cholesterol intake (mg/d)	RR of CHD	No significant association between egg consumption (up to 1 egg/d) and risk of CHD
< 1	237	1.00	
1	266	1.06	
2–4	330	1.12	
5–6	404	0.90	
≥ 7	536	1.08	
Women			
< 1	228	1.00	
1	258	0.82	
2–4	342	0.99	
5–6	436	0.95	
≥ 7	557	0.82	
Cholesterol intake (mg/d)	OR for CVD		No significant association between cholesterol intake and CVD risk after adjusting for fiber intake
15–236	1.00		
236–335	0.80		
335–461	0.86		
462–2,165	0.96		

lesser extent, but the impact of such a diet-induced change in CHD risk is uncertain.

As reviewed above, on average, an increase of 100 mg/d of dietary cholesterol is predicted to result in a 0.05 to 0.1 mmol/L increase in total serum cholesterol, of which approximately 80 percent is in the LDL fraction. This effect of added cholesterol is highly variable among individuals and is considerably attenuated at higher baseline cholesterol intakes. The LDL cholesterol concentration increase would predict approximately a 1 to 2 percent increase in CHD, with possibly offsetting effects of increased HDL cholesterol concentration. Epidemiological studies have limited power to detect effects of such magnitude and thus do not provide a meaningful basis for establishing adverse effects of dietary cholesterol. Therefore, it would seem reasonable to define the lowest-observed-adverse-effect level for dietary cholesterol as the lowest level shown to increase total or LDL cholesterol concentration. However, no studies have examined the effects of very small increments of dietary cholesterol in numbers of subjects sufficiently large enough to permit statistical treatment of the data. An increase

TABLE 9-5 Dietary Cholesterol and Risk of Lung Cancer

Reference	Study Design	Dietary and Other Information
Hinds et al., 1983	Men 188 cases 294 controls Case-control	Dietary history Adjusted for smoking, age, ethnicity, and occupational exposure
Heilbrun et al., 1984	Men 109 cases 7,420 controls Cohort, 15-y follow-up	24-h recall Adjusted for age and smoking
Byers et al., 1987	Men and women 450 cases 902 controls Case-control	Food frequency questionnaire Adjusted for age and smoking
Goodman et al., 1988	Men and women 336 cases 865 controls Case-control	Dietary history Adjusted for age, ethnicity, and pack-years of smoking
Jain et al., 1990	Men and women 839 cases 772 controls Case-control	Dietary history Adjusted for cumulative cigarette smoking
Knekt et al., 1991	Men 117 cases 4,421 controls Cohort, 20-y follow-up	Dietary history Adjusted for age, smoking, and energy intake

Results[a]			Comments
Cholesterol intake (mg/d)	RR of lung cancer		Increased lung cancer risk was positively associated with cholesterol intake
0–143	1.00		
144–285	1.65		
286–500	2.28		
≥ 501	3.50		
Cholesterol intake (mg/d)	RR of lung cancer		No significant association between lung cancer risk and cholesterol intake
0–299	1.00		
300–499	0.71		
500–749	0.99		
≥ 750	0.98		
Quartile of cholesterol intake	RR of lung cancer		Weak but nonsignificant association between cholesterol intake and lung cancer risk in men, but not in women
	Men	Women	
1 (low)	0.7	1.1	
2	0.9	1.7	
3	1.2	1.2	
4 (high)	1.0	1.0	
Mean cholesterol intake (mg/d)			Significant positive association between lung cancer risk and cholesterol intake in men, but not in women
	Men	Women	
Cases	385	249	
Controls	332	245	
Quartile of cholesterol intake	OR for lung cancer		
	Men	Women	
1 (low)	1.0	1.0	
2	2.3	0.6	
3	1.8	1.5	
4 (high)	2.2	0.9	
Cholesterol intake (mg/d)	OR for lung cancer		Significant increase in risk of lung cancer in highest quartile with cholesterol intake > 468 mg/d
< 235	1.00		
235–342	0.87		
343–468	0.99		
> 468	1.58		
Cholesterol intake (mg/d)	RR of lung cancer		Cholesterol intake was not associated with risk of lung cancer
< 441	1.00		
441–609	0.80		
> 609	1.03		

continued

TABLE 9-5 Continued

Reference	Study Design	Dietary and Other Information
Shekelle et al., 1991	Men 57 cases 1,821 controls Cohort, 24-y follow-up	Dietary history Adjusted for age, smoking, β-carotene intake, and percent of calories from fat
Alavanja et al., 1993	Women 429 cases 1,021 controls All nonsmokers Case-control	Food frequency questionnaire, Multivariate analysis
Wu et al., 1994	Women 212 cases Cohort, 6-y follow-up	Food frequency questionnaire Adjusted for age, smoking, occupation, physical activity, and total energy intake
Swanson et al., 1997	Women 587 cases 624 controls Case-control	Food frequency questionnaire Multivariate analysis

[a] RR = relative risk, M = men, W = women, OR = odds ratio.

in serum cholesterol concentration was observed with as little as 17 mg/d of cholesterol added to a cholesterol-free diet, but only three subjects were studied (Wells and Bronte-Stewart, 1963).

Serum cholesterol concentrations increase with increased dietary cholesterol (Figures 9-1 and 9-2), and the relationship of serum cholesterol concentration to CHD risk or mortality increases progressively (Neaton and Wentworth, 1992; Sorkin et al., 1992; Stamler et al., 1986; Weijenberg et al., 1996). Therefore, it is not appropriate to set a Tolerable Upper Intake Level (UL) for dietary cholesterol because increased risk may occur at a very low intake level and at a level that is exceeded by usual diets.

Results[a]		Comments
Cholesterol intake (mg/d)	RR of lung cancer	Cholesterol intake (specific to
198–604	1.00	consumption of eggs) was
605–794	1.30	positively associated with
795–1,909	1.94	risk of lung cancer
Cholesterol intake (mg/d)	OR for lung cancer	No significant association
< 120	1.00	between cholesterol intake
120–162	0.63	and risk of lung cancer
163–214	0.71	
215–302	1.14	
> 302	1.09	
Quartile of		Cholesterol intake was not
cholesterol intake	RR of lung cancer	associated with risk of
1 (low)	1.0	lung cancer
2	0.6	
3	0.9	
4 (high)	0.9	
Cholesterol intake		Cholesterol intake was not
(mg/1,000 kcal)	RR of lung cancer	associated with risk of
< 102	1.00	lung cancer
102–126	1.21	
127–148	0.88	
149–176	1.04	
> 176	1.22	

RISK CHARACTERIZATION

Intakes above an identified Tolerable Upper Intake Level (UL) indicate a potential risk of an adverse health effect. There is much evidence to indicate a positive linear trend between cholesterol intake and low density lipoprotein cholesterol concentration, and therefore increased risk of coronary heart disease (CHD). A UL is not set for cholesterol because any incremental increase in cholesterol intake increases CHD risk. Because cholesterol is unavoidable in ordinary, nonvegan diets, eliminating cholesterol in the diet would require significant changes in patterns of dietary intake. Such significant adjustments may introduce undesirable effects (e.g., inadequate intakes of protein and certain micronutrients) and unknown and unquantifiable health risks. Nonetheless, it is possible to

TABLE 9-6 Dietary Cholesterol and Risk of Breast Cancer

Reference	Study Design	Dietary and Other Information
Hirohata et al., 1987	Caucasian women 161 cases 161 hospital controls 161 neighborhood controls Case-control	Dietary history
Jones et al., 1987	Women 99 cases 5,386 controls Cohort, mean 10-y follow-up	24-h recall Multivariate analysis
Willett et al., 1987	Women 601 cases Cohort, 6-y follow-up	Food frequency questionnaire Multivariate analysis
van den Brandt et al., 1993	Women 55–69 y Cohort, 3.3-y follow-up	Food frequency questionnaire Multivariate analysis
Franceschi et al., 1996	Women 2,569 cases 2,588 controls Case-control	Food frequency questionnaire Multivariate analysis

[a] RR = relative risk, OR = odds ratio.

have a diet low in cholesterol while consuming a nutritionally adequate diet. Dietary guidance for minimizing cholesterol intake is provided in Chapter 11.

RESEARCH RECOMMENDATIONS

• Studies are needed to identify possible mechanisms whereby early nutritional experiences, such as dietary cholesterol, affect the atherosclerotic

Results[a]		Comments
Mean cholesterol intake (mg/d) Cases 286 Controls 267–289		No significant differences in cholesterol intake between breast cancer cases and controls
Cholesterol intake (mg/d) < 130 130–233 233–415 > 415	RR of breast cancer 1.00 1.33 0.79 0.70	No association between cholesterol intake and risk of breast cancer
Mean cholesterol intake (mg/d) 204 262 325 345 436	RR of breast cancer 1.00 1.06 1.02 1.07 0.91	No association between cholesterol intake and breast cancer
Quintile of cholesterol intake 1 2 3 4 5	RR of breast cancer 1.00 0.84 0.85 0.85 1.09	No association between cholesterol intake and risk of breast cancer
Cholesterol intake (mg/d) < 224 225–281 282–335 336–414 > 414	OR for breast cancer 1.00 0.93 0.90 0.97 0.91	No association between cholesterol intake and risk of breast cancer

process in adults and the sensitive periods in development when this may occur.

• The molecular mechanisms that regulate absorption of dietary cholesterol need to be determined.

• Specific genetic variants that contribute to wide interindividual variation in low density lipoprotein (LDL) cholesterol response to dietary cholesterol need to be delineated.

TABLE 9-7 Dietary Cholesterol and Risk of Colon Cancer

Reference	Study Design	Dietary and Other Information
Willett et al., 1990	Women Cohort, 6-y follow-up	Food frequency questionnaire Adjusted for age and total energy intake
Sandler et al., 1993	Men and women 236 cases 409 controls Case-control	Food frequency questionnaire Adjusted for age, alcohol intake, body mass index, and calories
Giovannucci et al., 1994	Men 205 cases Cohort, 6-y follow-up	Food frequency questionnaire Adjusted for age and total energy intake
Le Marchand et al., 1997	698 male case-control pairs 494 female case-control pairs Case-control	Food frequency questionnaire Multivariate analysis
Pietinen et al., 1999	Male smokers Cohort, 8-y follow-up	Food frequency questionnaire Multivariate analysis

[a] RR = relative risk, OR = odds ratio.

Results[a]			Comments
Cholesterol intake (mg/d)	RR of colon cancer		Increased risk of colon
< 247	1.00		cancer associated with
247–299	1.09		cholesterol intake
300–344	0.75		> 406 mg/d
345–406	1.07		
> 406	1.39		
	OR for colorectal		No association between
Cholesterol intake (mg/d)	adenomas		cholesterol intake and
< 156	1.0		risk of colorectal
156–189	0.78		adenomas
190–227	0.73		
228–289	0.89		
> 289	0.99		
Quintile/median			No association between
cholesterol intake (mg/d)	RR of colon cancer		cholesterol intake and
1/198	1.0		risk of colon cancer
2/262	1.27		
3/313	0.99		
4/369	1.07		
5/467	1.07		
Quartile of cholesterol	OR for colorectal cancer		Cholesterol intake
intake from eggs	Men	Women	(limited to cholesterol
1 (low)	1.0	1.0	from eggs) was
2	1.8	1.3	positively associated
3	1.8	1.5	with risk of colorectal
4 (high)	2.0	2.0	cancer
Quartile/median			No association between
cholesterol intake (mg/d)	RR of colorectal cancer		cholesterol intake and
1/378	1.0		risk of colorectal
2/501	1.2		cancer
3/594	1.1		
4/759	1.0		

TABLE 9-8 Dietary Cholesterol and Risk of Prostate Cancer

Reference	Study Design	Dietary and Other Information
Kolonel et al., 1988	452 cases 899 controls Case-control	Dietary history Adjusted for age and ethnicity

Andersson et al., 1996	522 cases
	536 controls
	Case-control
		Food frequency
		  questionnaire
		Adjusted for age
		  and energy

Key et al., 1997	328 cases 328 controls Case-control	Food frequency questionnaire
Vlajinac et al., 1997	101 cases 202 controls Case-control	Dietary history Adjusted for energy and significant nutrients

[a] OR = odds ratio.

- Other factors (dietary and constitutional) that contribute to the wide interindividual variation in LDL cholesterol response to dietary cholesterol also need to be delineated.
- Studies are needed to better define the relation between dietary cholesterol intakes and LDL cholesterol concentrations over a broad range of cholesterol intakes, from very low to high.
- The relationship between dietary cholesterol intakes and body pools of cholesterol needs to be determined.

REFERENCES

Alavanja MCR, Brown CC, Swanson C, Brownson RC. 1993. Saturated fat intake and lung cancer risk among nonsmoking women in Missouri. *J Natl Cancer Inst* 85:1906–1916.

Andersen GE, Lifschitz C, Friis-Hansen B. 1979. Dietary habits and serum lipids during first 4 years of life. A study of 95 Danish children. *Acta Paediatr Scand* 68:165–170.

Results[a]			Comments
Quartile of cholesterol intake	Age and OR for prostate cancer		Significant positive association between cholesterol intake and risk of prostate cancer, but no clear gradient effect
	≤ 70	≥ 70	
1 (low)	1.0	1.0	
2	1.2	1.6	
3	1.2	1.7	
4 (high)	1.3	1.6	
Cholesterol intake (mg/d)	OR for prostate cancer		No association between cholesterol intake and risk of prostate cancer
< 241	1.00		
241–301	0.71		
302–390	0.85		
> 390	0.96		
Mean cholesterol intake (mg/d)			No significant difference in cholesterol intake between prostate cancer cases andcontrols
Cases 341			
Controls 351			
Tertile of cholesterol intake	OR for prostate cancer		No significant association between cholesterol intake and risk of prostate cancer
1	1.00		
2	0.97		
3	0.60		

Anderson JT, Grande F, Keys A. 1976. Independence of the effects of cholesterol and degree of saturation of the fat in the diet on serum cholesterol in man. *Am J Clin Nutr* 29:1184–1189.

Andersson S-O, Wolk A, Bergström R, Giovannucci E, Lindgren C, Baron J, Adami H-O. 1996. Energy, nutrient intake and prostate cancer risk: A population-based case-control study in Sweden. *Int J Cancer* 68:716–722.

Applebaum-Bowden D, Haffner SM, Hartsook E, Luk KH, Albers JJ, Hazzard WR. 1984. Down-regulation of the low-density lipoprotein receptor by dietary cholesterol. *Am J Clin Nutr* 39:360–367.

Ascherio A, Rimm EB, Giovannucci EL, Spiegelman D, Stampfer M, Willett WC. 1996. Dietary fat and risk of coronary heart disease in men: Cohort follow up study in the United States. *Br Med J* 313:84–90.

Bayley TM, Alasmi M, Thorkelson T, Krug-Wispe S, Jones PJH, Bulani JL, Tsang RC. 1998. Influence of formula versus breast milk on cholesterol synthesis rates in four-month-old infants. *Pediatr Res* 44:60–67.

Berge KE, Tian H, Graf GA, Yu L, Grishin NV, Schultz J, Kwiterovich P, Shan B, Barnes R, Hobbs HH. 2000. Accumulation of dietary cholesterol in sitosterolemia caused by mutations in adjacent ABC transporters. *Science* 290:1771–1775.

Beveridge JMR, Connell WF, Mayer GA, Haust HL. 1960. The response of man to dietary cholesterol. *J Nutr* 71:61–65.

Beynen AC, Katan MB. 1985a. Effect of egg yolk feeding on the concentration and composition of serum lipoproteins in man. *Atherosclerosis* 54:157–166.

Beynen AC, Katan MB. 1985b. Reproducibility of the variations between humans in the response of serum cholesterol to cessation of egg consumption. *Atherosclerosis* 57:19–31.

Bitman J, Wood L, Hamosh M, Hamosh P, Mehta NR. 1983. Comparison of the lipid composition of breast milk from mothers of term and preterm infants. *Am J Clin Nutr* 38:300–312.

Bocan TMA. 1998. Animal models of atherosclerosis and interpretation of drug intervention studies. *Curr Pharm Des* 4:37–52.

Bronsgeest-Schoute DC, Hautvast JGAJ, Hermus RJJ. 1979a. Dependence of the effects of dietary cholesterol and experimental conditions on serum lipids in man. I. Effects of dietary cholesterol in a linoleic acid-rich diet. *Am J Clin Nutr* 33:2183–2187.

Bronsgeest-Schoute DC, Hermus RJJ, Dallinga-Thie GM, Hautvast JGAJ. 1979b. Dependence of the effects of dietary cholesterol and experimental conditions on serum lipids in man. II. Effects of dietary cholesterol in a linoleic acid-poor diet. *Am J Clin Nutr* 33:2188–2192.

Brown MS, Goldstein JL. 1999. A proteolytic pathway that controls the cholesterol content of membranes, cells, and blood. *Proc Natl Acad Sci USA* 96:11041–11048.

Byers TE, Graham S, Haughey BP, Marshall JR, Swanson MK. 1987. Diet and lung cancer risk: Findings from the Western New York Diet Study. *Am J Epidemiol* 125:351–363.

Clark RM, Ferris AM, Fey M, Brown PB, Hundrieser KE, Jensen RG. 1982. Changes in the lipids of human milk from 2 to 16 weeks postpartum. *J Pediatr Gastroenterol Nutr* 1:311–315.

Clarke R, Frost C, Collins R, Appleby P, Peto R. 1997. Dietary lipids and blood cholesterol: Quantitative meta-analysis of metabolic ward studies. *Br Med J* 314:112–117.

Clifton PM, Kestin M, Abbey M, Drysdale M, Nestel PJ. 1990. Relationship between sensitivity to dietary fat and dietary cholesterol. *Arteriosclerosis* 10:394–401.

Clifton PM, Abbey M, Noakes M, Beltrame S, Rumbelow N, Nestel PJ. 1995. Body fat distribution is a determinant of the high-density lipoprotein response to dietary fat and cholesterol in women. *Arterioscler Thromb Vasc Biol* 15:1070–1078.

Connor WE, Hodges RE, Bleiler RE. 1961a. Effect of dietary cholesterol upon serum lipids in man. *J Lab Clin Med* 57:331–342.

Connor WE, Hodges RE, Bleiler RE. 1961b. The serum lipids in men receiving high cholesterol and cholesterol-free diets. *J Clin Invest* 40:894–901.

Connor WE, Stone DB, Hodges RE. 1964. The interrelated effects of dietary cholesterol and fat upon human serum lipid levels. *J Clin Invest* 43:1691–1696.

Cruz MLA, Wong WW, Mimouni F, Hachey DL, Setchell KDR, Klein PD, Tsang RC. 1994. Effects of infant nutrition on cholesterol synthesis rates. *Pediatr Res* 35:135–140.

Darmady JM, Fosbrooke AS, Lloyd JK. 1972. Prospective study of serum cholesterol levels during first year of life. *Br Med J* 2:685–688.

Di Buono M, Jones PJH, Beaumier L, Wykes LJ. 2000. Comparison of deuterium incorporation and mass isotopomer distribution analysis for measurement of human cholesterol biosynthesis. *J Lipid Res* 41:1516–1523.

Dietschy JM, Turley SD, Spady DK. 1993. Role of liver in the maintenance of cholesterol and low density lipoprotein homeostasis in different animal species, including humans. *J Lipid Res* 34:1637–1659.

Dreon DM, Krauss RM. 1997. Diet-gene interactions in human lipoprotein metabolism. *J Am Coll Nutr* 16:313–324.

Edington J, Geekie M, Carter R, Benfield L, Fisher K, Ball M, Mann J. 1987. Effect of dietary cholesterol on plasma cholesterol concentration in subjects following reduced fat, high fibre diet. *Br Med J* 294:333–336.

Edmond J, Korsak RA, Morrow JW, Torok-Both G, Catlin DH. 1991. Dietary cholesterol and the origin of cholesterol in the brain of developing rats. *J Nutr* 121:1323–1330.

Erickson BA, Coots RH, Mattson FH, Kligman AM. 1964. The effect of partial hydrogenation of dietary fats, of the ratio of polyunsaturated to saturated fatty acids, and of dietary cholesterol upon plasma lipids in man. *J Clin Invest* 43:2017–2025.

Esrey KL, Joseph L, Grover SA. 1996. Relationship between dietary intake and coronary heart disease mortality: Lipid research clinics prevalence follow-up study. *J Clin Epidemiol* 49:211–216.

Fall CHD, Barker DJP, Osmond C, Winter PD, Clark PMS, Hales CN. 1992. Relation of infant feeding to adult serum cholesterol concentration and death from ischaemic heart disease. *Br Med J* 304:801–805.

FASEB (Federation of American Societies for Experimental Biology). 1995. *Third Report on Nutrition Monitoring in the United States.* Washington, DC: U.S. Government Printing Office.

Fielding CJ, Havel RJ, Todd KM, Yeo KE, Schloetter MC, Weinberg V, Frost PH. 1995. Effects of dietary cholesterol and fat saturation on plasma lipoproteins in an ethnically diverse population of healthy young men. *J Clin Invest* 95:611–618.

Flynn MA, Nolph GB, Flynn TC, Kahrs R, Krause G. 1979. Effect of dietary egg on human serum cholesterol and triglycerides. *Am J Clin Nutr* 32:1051–1057.

Franceschi S, Favero A, Decarli A, Negri E, La Vecchia C, Ferraroni M, Russo A, Salvini S, Amadori D, Conti E, Montella M, Giacosa A. 1996. Intake of macronutrients and risk of breast cancer. *Lancet* 347:1351–1356.

Friedman G, Goldberg SJ. 1975. Concurrent and subsequent serum cholesterols of breast- and formula-fed infants. *Am J Clin Nutr* 28:42–45.

Ginsberg HN, Karmally W, Siddiqui M, Holleran S, Tall AR, Rumsey SC, Deckelbaum RJ, Blaner WS, Ramakrishnan R. 1994. A dose-response study of the effects of dietary cholesterol on fasting and postprandial lipid and lipoprotein metabolism in healthy young men. *Arterioscler Thromb* 14:576–586.

Ginsberg HN, Karmally W, Siddiqui M, Holleran S, Tall AR, Blaner WS, Ramakrishnan R. 1995. Increases in dietary cholesterol are associated with modest increases in both LDL and HDL cholesterol in healthy young women. *Arterioscler Thromb Vasc Biol* 15:169–178.

Giovannucci E, Rimm EB, Stampfer MJ, Colditz GA, Ascherio A, Willett WC. 1994. Intake of fat, meat, and fiber in relation to risk of colon cancer in men. *Cancer Res* 54:2390–2397.

Glueck CJ, Tsang R, Balistreri W, Fallat R. 1972. Plasma and dietary cholesterol in infancy: Effects of early low or moderate dietary cholesterol intake on subsequent response to increased dietary cholesterol. *Metabolism* 21:1181–1192.

Goodman MT, Kolonel LN, Yoshizawa CN, Hankin JH. 1988. The effect of dietary cholesterol and fat on the risk of lung cancer in Hawaii. *Am J Epidemiol* 128:1241–1255.

Haave NC, Innis SM. 2001. Cholesterol synthesis and accretion within various tissues of the fetal and neonatal rat. *Metabolism* 50:12–18.

Hahn P, Koldovský O. 1966. *Utilization of Nutrients During Postnatal Development.* New York: Pergamon Press.

Hamosh M. 1988. Does infant nutrition affect adiposity and cholesterol levels in the adult? *J Pediatr Gastroenterol Nutr* 7:10–16.

Hauser H, Dyer JH, Nandy A, Vega MA, Werder M, Bieliauskaite E, Weber FE, Compassi S, Gemperli A, Boffelli D, Wehrli E, Schulthess G, Phillips MC. 1998. Identification of a receptor mediating absorption of dietary cholesterol in the intestine. *Biochemistry* 37:17843–17850.

Hegsted DM. 1986. Serum-cholesterol response to dietary cholesterol: A re-evaluation. *Am J Clin Nutr* 44:299–305.

Hegsted DM, McGandy RB, Myers ML, Stare FJ. 1965. Quantitative effects of dietary fat on serum cholesterol in man. *Am J Clin Nutr* 17:281–295.

Hegsted DM, Ausman LM, Johnson JA, Dallal GE. 1993. Dietary fat and serum lipids: An evaluation of the experimental data. *Am J Clin Nutr* 57:875–883.

Heilbrun LK, Nomura AMY, Stemmermann GN. 1984. Dietary cholesterol and lung cancer risk among Japanese men in Hawaii. *Am J Clin Nutr* 39:375–379.

Hinds MW, Kolonel LN, Lee J, Hankin JH. 1983. Dietary cholesterol and lung cancer risk among men in Hawaii. *Am J Clin Nutr* 37:192–193.

Hirohata T, Nomura AMY, Hankin JH, Kolonel LN, Lee J. 1987. An epidemiological study on the association between diet and breast cancer. *J Natl Cancer Inst* 78:595–600.

Hodgson PA, Ellefson RD, Elveback LR, Harris LE, Nelson RA, Weidman WH. 1976. Comparison of serum cholesterol in children fed high, moderate, or low cholesterol milk diets during neonatal period. *Metabolism* 25:739–746.

Hopkins PN. 1992. Effects of dietary cholesterol on serum cholesterol: A meta-analysis and review. *Am J Clin Nutr* 55:1060–1070.

Howell WH, McNamara DJ, Tosca MA, Smith BT, Gaines JA. 1997. Plasma lipid and lipoprotein responses to dietary fat and cholesterol: A meta-analysis. *Am J Clin Nutr* 65:1747–1764.

Hu FB, Stampfer MJ, Manson JE, Rimm E, Colditz GA, Rosner BA, Hennekens CH, Willett WC. 1997. Dietary fat intake and the risk of coronary heart disease in women. *N Engl J Med* 337:1491–1499.

Hu FB, Stampfer MJ, Rimm EB, Manson JE, Ascherio A, Colditz GA, Rosner BA, Spiegelman D, Speizer FE, Sacks FM, Hennekens CH, Willett WC. 1999. A prospective study of egg consumption and risk of cardiovascular disease in men and women. *J Am Med Assoc* 281:1387–1394.

Huisman M, van Beusekom CM, Lanting CI, Nijeboer HJ, Muskiet FAJ, Boersma ER. 1996. Triglycerides, fatty acids, sterols, mono- and disaccharides and sugar alcohols in human milk and current types of infant formula milk. *Eur J Clin Nutr* 50:255–260.

Huttunen JK, Saarinen UM, Kostiainen E, Siimes MA. 1983. Fat composition of the infant diet does not influence subsequent serum lipid levels in man. *Atherosclerosis* 46:87–94.

Jain M, Burch JD, Howe GR, Risch HA, Miller AB. 1990. Dietary factors and risk of lung cancer: Results from a case-control study, Toronto, 1981–1985. *Int J Cancer* 45:287–293.

Jensen RG, Lammi-Keefe CJ, Ferris AM, Jackson MB, Couch SC, Capacchione CM, Ahn HS, Murtaugh M. 1995. Human milk total lipid and cholesterol are dependent on interval of sampling during 24 hours. *J Pediatr Gastroenterol Nutr* 20:91–94.

Johnson C, Greenland P. 1990. Effects of exercise, dietary cholesterol, and dietary fat on blood lipids. *Arch Intern Med* 150:137–141.

Jones DY, Schatzkin A, Green SB, Block G, Brinton LA, Ziegler RG, Hoover R, Taylor PR. 1987. Dietary fat and breast cancer in the National Health and Nutrition Examination Survey. I. Epidemiologic follow-up study. *J Natl Cancer Inst* 79:465–471.

Jurevics HA, Morell P. 1994. Sources of cholesterol for kidney and nerve during development. *J Lipid Res* 35:112–120.

Katan MB, Beynen AC, De Vries JHM, Nobels A. 1986. Existence of consistent hypo- and hyperresponders to dietary cholesterol in man. *Am J Epidemiol* 123:221–234.

Katan MB, Berns MAM, Glatz JFC, Knuiman JT, Nobels A, de Vries JHM. 1988. Congruence of individual responsiveness to dietary cholesterol and to saturated fat in humans. *J Lipid Res* 29:883–892.

Kern F. 1994. Effects of dietary cholesterol on cholesterol and bile acid homeostasis in patients with cholesterol gallstones. *J Clin Invest* 93:1186–1194.

Kesäniemi YA, Ehnholm C, Miettinen TA. 1987. Intestinal cholesterol absorption efficiency in man is related to apoprotein E phenotype. *J Clin Invest* 80:578–581.

Kestin M, Clifton PM, Rouse IL, Nestel PJ. 1989. Effect of dietary cholesterol in normolipidemic subjects is not modified by nature and amount of dietary fat. *Am J Clin Nutr* 50:528–532.

Key TJA, Silcocks PB, Davey GK, Appleby PN, Bishop DT. 1997. A case-control study of diet and prostate cancer. *Br J Cancer* 76:678–687.

Keys A, Anderson JT, Grande F. 1965. Serum cholesterol response to changes in the diet. II. The effect of cholesterol in the diet. *Metabolism* 14:759–765.

Kita T, Brown MS, Bilheimer DW, Goldstein JL. 1982. Delayed clearance of very low density and intermediate density lipoproteins with enhanced conversion to low density lipoprotein in WHHL rabbits. *Proc Natl Acad Sci USA* 79:5693–5697.

Kolaček S, Kapetanović T, Zimolo A, Lužar V. 1993. Early determinants of cardiovascular risk factors in adults. A. Plasma lipids. *Acta Paediatr* 82:699–704.

Kolonel LN, Yoshizawa CN, Hankin JH. 1988. Diet and prostatic cancer: A casecontrol study in Hawaii. *Am J Epidemiol* 127:999–1012.

Knekt P, Seppänen R, Järvinen R, Virtamo J, Hyvönen L, Pukkala E, Teppo L. 1991. Dietary cholesterol, fatty acids, and the risk of lung cancer among men. *Nutr Cancer* 16:267–275.

Kris-Etherton PM, Layman DK, York PV, Frantz ID. 1979. The influence of early nutrition on the serum cholesterol of the adult rat. *J Nutr* 109:1244–1257.

Kritchevsky SB, Kritchevsky D. 2000. Egg consumption and coronary heart disease: An epidemiologic overview. *J Am Coll Nutr* 19:549S–555S.

Kromhout D, de Lezenne Coulander C. 1984. Diet, prevalence and 10-year mortality from coronary heart disease in 871 middle-aged men. The Zutphen Study. *Am J Epidemiol* 119:733–741.

Kromhout D, Menotti A, Bloemberg B, Aravanis C, Blackburn H, Buzina R, Dontas AS, Fidanza F, Giampaoli S, Jansen A, Karvonen M, Katan M, Nissinen A, Nedeljkovic S, Pekkanen J, Pekkarinen M, Punsar S, Räsänen L, Simic B, Toshima H. 1995. Dietary saturated and *trans* fatty acids and cholesterol and 25-year mortality from coronary heart disease: The Seven Countries Study. *Prev Med* 24:308–315.

Kummerow FA, Kim Y, Hull J, Pollard J, Ilinov P, Dorossiev DL, Valek J. 1977. The influence of egg consumption on the serum cholesterol level in human subjects. *Am J Clin Nutr* 30:664–673.

Kushi LH, Lew RA, Stare FJ, Ellison CR, el Lozy M, Bourke G, Daly L, Graham I, Hickey N, Mulcahy R, Kevaney J. 1985. Diet and 20-year mortality from coronary heart disease. The Ireland-Boston Diet-Heart Study. *N Engl J Med* 312:811–818.

Lammi-Keefe CJ, Ferris AM, Jensen RG. 1990. Changes in human milk at 0600, 1000, 1400, 1800, and 2200 h. *J Pediatr Gastroenterol Nutr* 11:83–88.

Leeson CPM, Kattenhorn M, Deanfield JE, Lucas A. 2001. Duration of breast feeding and arterial distensibility in early adult life: Population based study. *Br Med J* 322:643–647.

Le Marchand L, Wilkens LR, Hankin JH, Kolonel LN, Lyu L-C. 1997. A case-control study of diet and colorectal cancer in a multiethnic population in Hawaii (United States): Lipids and foods of animal origin. *Cancer Causes Control* 8:637–648.

Lewis DS, Mott GE, McMahan CA, Masoro EJ, Carey KD, McGill HC. 1988. Deferred effects of preweaning diet on atherosclerosis in adolescent baboons. *Arteriosclerosis* 8:274–280.

Lin DS, Connor WE. 1980. The long term effects of dietary cholesterol upon the plasma lipids, lipoproteins, cholesterol adsorption, and the sterol balance in man: The demonstration of feedback inhibition of cholesterol biosynthesis and increased bile acid excretion. *J Lipid Res* 21:1042–1052.

Ling WH, Jones PJH. 1995. Dietary phytosterols: A review of metabolism, benefits, and side effects. *Life Sci* 57:195–206.

Lütjohann D, Björkhem I, Ose L. 1996. Phytosterolaemia in a Norwegian family: Diagnosis and characterization of the first Scandinavian case. *Scand J Clin Lab Invest* 56:229–240.

Mahley RW, Innerarity TL, Bersot TP, Lipson A, Margolis S. 1978. Alterations in human high-density lipoproteins, with or without increased plasma-cholesterol, induced by diets high in cholesterol. *Lancet* 2:807–809.

Mann JI, Appleby PN, Key TJ, Thorogood M. 1997. Dietary determinants of ischaemic heart disease in health conscious individuals. *Heart* 78:450–455.

Maranhão RC, Quintão ECR. 1983. Long term steroid metabolism balance studies in subjects on cholesterol-free and cholesterol-rich diets: Comparison between normal and hypercholesterolemic individuals. *J Lipid Res* 24:167–173.

Mattson FH, Erickson BA, Kligman AM. 1972. Effect of dietary cholesterol on serum cholesterol in man. *Am J Clin Nutr* 25:589–594.

McCombs RJ, Marcadis DE, Ellis J, Weinberg RB. 1994. Attenuated hypercholesterolemic response to a high-cholesterol diet in subjects heterozygous for the apolipoprotein A-IV-2 allele. *N Engl J Med* 331:706–710.

McGee DL, Reed DM, Yano K, Kagan A, Tillotson J. 1984. Ten-year incidence of coronary heart disease in the Honolulu Heart Program. Relationship to nutrient intake. *Am J Epidemiol* 119:667–676.

McGee D, Reed D, Stemmerman G, Rhoads G, Yano K, Feinleib M. 1985. The relationship of dietary fat and cholesterol to mortality in 10 years: The Honolulu Heart Program. *Int J Epidemiol* 14:97–105.

McMurry MP, Connor WE, Goplerud CP. 1981. The effects of dietary cholesterol upon the hypercholesterolemia of pregnancy. *Metabolism* 30:869–879.

McMurry MP, Connor WE, Cerqueira MT. 1982. Dietary cholesterol and the plasma lipids and lipoproteins in the Tarahumara Indians: A people habituated to a low cholesterol diet after weaning. *Am J Clin Nutr* 35:741–744.

McMurry MP, Connor WE, Lin DS, Cerqueira MT, Connor SL. 1985. The absorption of cholesterol and the sterol balance in the Tarahumara Indians of Mexico fed cholesterol-free and high cholesterol diets. *Am J Clin Nutr* 41:1289–1298.

McNamara DJ. 2000. Dietary cholesterol and atherosclerosis. *Biochim Biophys Acta* 1529:310–320.

McNamara DJ, Kolb R, Parker TS, Batwin H, Samuel P, Brown CD, Ahrens EH. 1987. Heterogeneity of cholesterol homeostasis in man. Response to changes in dietary fat quality and cholesterol quantity. *J Clin Invest* 79:1729–1739.

Mellies MJ, Burton K, Larsen R, Fixler D, Glueck CJ. 1979. Cholesterol, phytosterols, and polyunsaturated/saturated fatty acid ratios during the first 12 months of lactation. *Am J Clin Nutr* 32:2383–2389.

Miettinen TA, Gylling H. 1999. Regulation of cholesterol metabolism by dietary plant sterols. *Curr Opin Lipidol* 10:9–14.

Mistry P, Miller NE, Laker M, Hazzard WR, Lewis B. 1981. Individual variation in the effects of dietary cholesterol on plasma lipoproteins and cellular cholesterol homeostasis in man. Studies of low density lipoprotein receptor activity and 3-hydroxy-3-methylglutaryl coenzyme A reductase activity in blood mononuclear cells. *J Clin Invest* 67:493–502.

Mize CE, Uauy R, Kramer R, Benser M, Allen S, Grundy SM. 1995. Lipoprotein-cholesterol responses in healthy infants fed defined diets from ages 1 to 12 months: Comparison of diets predominant in oleic acid versus linoleic acid, with parallel observations in infants fed a human milk-based diet. *J Lipid Res* 36:1178–1187.

Mott GE, Jackson EM, McMahan CA, McGill HC. 1990. Cholesterol metabolism in adult baboons is influenced by infant diet. *J Nutr* 120:243–251.

Mott GE, Jackson EM, DeLallo L, Lewis DS, McMahan CA. 1995. Differences in cholesterol metabolism in juvenile baboons are programmed by breast-versus formula-feeding. *J Lipid Res* 36:299–307.

National Diet-Heart Study Research Group. 1968. Faribault second study. National Diet-Heart Study final report. *Circulation* 37:I260–I274.

Neaton JD, Wentworth D. 1992. Serum cholesterol, blood pressure, cigarette smoking, and death from coronary heart disease. Overall findings and differences by age for 316,099 white men. Multiple Risk Factor Intervention Trial Research Group. *Arch Intern Med* 152:56–64.

Nestel PJ, Poyser A. 1976. Changes in cholesterol synthesis and excretion when cholesterol intake is increased. *Metabolism* 25:1591–1599.

Nestel P, Tada N, Billington T, Huff M, Fidge N. 1982. Changes in very low density lipoproteins with cholesterol loading in man. *Metabolism* 31:398–405.

Oh SY, Miller LT. 1985. Effect of dietary egg on variability of plasma cholesterol levels and lipoprotein cholesterol. *Am J Clin Nutr* 42:421–431.

Packard CJ, McKinney L, Carr K, Shepherd J. 1983. Cholesterol feeding increases low density lipoprotein synthesis. *J Clin Invest* 72:45–51.

Picciano MF, Guthrie HA, Sheehe DM. 1978. The cholesterol content of human milk. A variable constituent among women and within the same women. *Clin Pediatr* 17:359–362.

Pietinen P, Ascherio A, Korhonen P, Hartman AM, Willett WC, Albanes D, Virtamo J. 1997. Intake of fatty acids and risk of coronary heart disease in a cohort of Finnish men. The Alpha-Tocopherol, Beta-Carotene Cancer Prevention Study. *Am J Epidemiol* 145:876–887.

Pietinen P, Malila N, Virtanen M, Hartman TJ, Tangrea JA, Albanes D, Virtamo J. 1999. Diet and risk of colorectal cancer in a cohort of Finnish men. *Cancer Causes Control* 10:387–396.

Porter MW, Yamanaka W, Carlson SD, Flynn MA. 1977. Effect of dietary egg on serum cholesterol and triglyceride of human males. *Am J Clin Nutr* 30:490–495.

Posner BM, Cobb JL, Belanger AJ, Cupples LA, D'Agostino RB, Stokes J. 1991. Dietary lipid predictors of coronary heart disease in men. The Framingham Study. *Arch Intern Med* 151:1181–1187.

Quintão E, Grundy SM, Ahrens EH. 1971. Effects of dietary cholesterol on the regulation of total body cholesterol in man. *J Lipid Res* 12:233–247.

Quintão ECR, Brumer S, Stechhahn K. 1977. Tissue storage and control of cholesterol metabolism in man on high cholesterol diets. *Atherosclerosis* 26:297–310.

Ravelli ACJ, van der Meulen JHP, Osmond C, Barker DJP, Bleker OP. 2000. Infant feeding and adult glucose tolerance, lipid profile, blood pressure, and obesity. *Arch Dis Child* 82:248–252.

Reiser R, Sidelman Z. 1972. Control of serum cholesterol homeostasis by cholesterol in the milk of the suckling rat. *J Nutr* 102:1009–1016.

Reiser R, O'Brien BC, Henderson GR, Moore RW. 1979. Studies on a possible function for cholesterol in milk. *Nutr Rept Int* 19:835–849.

Repa JJ, Mangelsdorf DJ. 2000. The role of orphan nuclear receptors in the regulation of cholesterol homeostasis. *Annu Rev Cell Dev Biol* 16:459–481.

Repa JJ, Turley SD, Lobaccaro J-MA, Medina J, Li L, Lustig K, Shan B, Heyman RA, Dietschy JM, Mangelsdorf DJ. 2000. Regulation of absorption and ABC1-mediated efflux of cholesterol by RXR heterodimers. *Science* 289:1524–1529.

Roberts SL, McMurry MP, Connor WE. 1981. Does egg feeding (i.e., dietary cholesterol) affect plasma cholesterol levels in humans? The results of a double-blind study. *Am J Clin Nutr* 34:2092–2099.

Romano G, Tilly-Kiesi MK, Patti L, Taskinen M-R, Pacioni D, Cassader M, Riccardi G, Rivellese AA. 1998. Effects of dietary cholesterol on plasma lipoproteins and their subclasses in IDDM patients. *Diabetologia* 41:193–200.

Ros E. 2000. Intestinal absorption of triglyceride and cholesterol. Dietary and pharmacological inhibition to reduce cardiovascular risk. *Atherosclerosis* 151:357–379.

Rudel LL. 1997. Genetic factors influence the atherogenic response of lipoproteins to dietary fat and cholesterol in nonhuman primates. *J Am Coll Nutr* 16:306–312.

Salen G, Ahrens EH, Grundy SM. 1970. Metabolism of β-sitosterol in man. *J Clin Invest* 49:952–967.

Salen G, Shefer S, Nguyen L, Ness GC, Tint GS, Shore V. 1992. Sitosterolemia. *J Lipid Res* 33:945–955

Sandler RS, Lyles CM, Peipins LA, McAuliffe CA, Woosley JT, Kupper LL. 1993. Diet and risk of colorectal adenomas: Macronutrients, cholesterol, and fiber. *J Natl Cancer Inst* 85:884–891.

Schonfeld G, Patsch W, Rudel LL, Nelson C, Epstein M, Olson RE. 1982. Effects of dietary cholesterol and fatty acids on plasma lipoproteins. *J Clin Invest* 69:1072–1080.

Sehayek E, Nath C, Heinemann T, McGee M, Seidman CE, Samuel P, Breslow JL. 1998. U-shape relationship between change in dietary cholesterol absorption and plasma lipoprotein responsiveness and evidence for extreme inter-individual variation in dietary cholesterol absorption in humans. *J Lipid Res* 39:2415–2422.

Sehayek E, Shefer S, Nguyen LB, Ono JG, Merkel M, Breslow JL. 2000. Apolipoprotein E regulates dietary cholesterol absorption and biliary cholesterol excretion: Studies in C57BL/6 apolipoprotein E knockout mice. *Proc Natl Acad Sci USA* 97:3433–3437.

Shekelle RB, Rossof AH, Stamler J. 1991. Dietary cholesterol and incidence of lung cancer: The Western Electric Study. *Am J Epidemiol* 134:480–484.

Slater G, Mead J, Dhopeshwarkar G, Robinson S, Alfin-Slater RB. 1976. Plasma cholesterol and triglycerides in men with added eggs in the diet. *Nutr Rep Int* 14:249–260.

Sorkin JD, Andres R, Muller DC, Baldwin HL, Fleg JL. 1992. Cholesterol as a risk factor for coronary heart disease in elderly men. The Baltimore Longitudinal Study of Aging. *Ann Epidemiol* 2:59–67.

Stamler J, Shekelle R. 1988. Dietary cholesterol and human coronary heart disease. The epidemiologic evidence. *Arch Pathol Lab Med* 112:1032–1040.

Stamler J, Wentworth D, Neaton JD. 1986. Is relationship between serum cholesterol and risk of premature death from coronary heart disease continuous and graded? Findings in 356,222 primary screenees of the Multiple Risk Factor Intervention Trial (MRFIT). *J Am Med Assoc* 256:2823–2828.

Staprans I, Pan X-M, Rapp JH, Grunfeld C, Feingold KR. 2000. Oxidized cholesterol in the diet accelerates the development of atherosclerosis in LDL receptor- and apolipoprotein E-deficient mice. *Arterioscler Thromb Vasc Biol* 20:708–714.

Steiner A, Howard EJ, Akgun S. 1962. Importance of dietary cholesterol in man. *J Am Med Assoc* 181:186–190.

Sundram K, Hayes KC, Siru OH. 1994. Dietary palmitic acid results in lower serum cholesterol than does a lauric-myristic acid combination in normolipemic humans. *Am J Clin Nutr* 59:841–846.

Sutherland WHF, Ball MJ, Walker H. 1997. The effect of increased egg consumption on plasma cholesteryl ester transfer activity in healthy subjects. *Eur J Clin Nutr* 51:172–176.

Swanson CA, Brown CC, Sinha R, Kulldorff M, Brownson RC, Alavanja MCR. 1997. Dietary fats and lung cancer risk among women: The Missouri Women's Health Study (United States). *Cancer Causes Control* 8:883–893.

Tell GS, Evans GW, Folsom AR, Shimakawa T, Carpenter MA, Heiss G. 1994. Dietary fat intake and carotid artery wall thickness: The Atherosclerosis Risk in Communities (ARIC) Study. *Am J Epidemiol* 139:979–989.

Toeller M, Buyken AE, Heitkamp G, Scherbaum WA, Krans HMJ, Fuller JH. 1999. Associations of fat and cholesterol intake with serum lipid levels and cardiovascular disease: The EURODIAB IDDM Complications Study. *Exp Clin Endocrinol Diabetes* 107:512–521.

Tzonou A, Kalandidi A, Trichopoulou A, Hsieh C-C, Toupadaki N, Willett W, Trichopoulos D. 1993. Diet and coronary heart disease: A case-control study in Athens, Greece. *Epidemiology* 4:511–516.

van de Bovenkamp P, Kosmeijer-Schuil TG, Katan MB. 1988. Quantification of oxysterols in Dutch foods: Egg products and mixed diets. *Lipids* 23:1079–1085.

van den Brandt PA, van't Veer P, Goldbohm RA, Dorant E, Volovics A, Hermus RJJ, Sturmans F. 1993. A prospective cohort study on dietary fat and the risk of postmenopausal breast cancer. *Cancer Res* 53:75–82.

Vine DF, Mamo JCL, Beilin LJ, Mori TA, Croft KD. 1998. Dietary oxysterols are incorporated in plasma triglyceride-rich lipoproteins, increase their susceptibility to oxidation and increase aortic cholesterol concentration of rabbits. *J Lipid Res* 39:1995–2004.

Vlajinac HD, Marinkovic´ JM, Ilic´ MD, Kocev NI. 1997. Diet and prostate cancer: A case-control study. *Eur J Cancer* 33:101–107.

Watts GF, Jackson P, Mandalia S, Brunt JNH, Lewis ES, Coltart DJ, Lewis B. 1994. Nutrient intake and progression of coronary artery disease. *Am J Cardiol* 73:328–332.

Weggemans RM, Zock PL, Meyboom S, Funke H, Katan MB. 2000. Apolipoprotein A4-1/2 polymorphism and response of serum lipids to dietary cholesterol in humans. *J Lipid Res* 41:1623–1628.

Weggemans RM, Zock PL, Katan MB. 2001. Dietary cholesterol from eggs increases the ratio of total cholesterol to high-density lipoprotein cholesterol in humans: A meta-analysis. *Am J Clin Nutr* 73:885–891.

Weijenberg MP, Feskens EJM, Kromhout D. 1996. Total and high density lipoprotein cholesterol as risk factors for coronary heart disease in elderly men during 5 years of follow-up. The Zutphen Elderly Study. *Am J Epidemiol* 143:151–158.

Weinberg RB, Geissinger BW, Kasala K, Hockey KJ, Terry JG, Easter L, Crouse JR. 2000. Effect of apolipoprotein A-IV genotype and dietary fat on cholesterol absorption in humans. *J Lipid Res* 41:2035–2041.

Wells VM, Bronte-Stewart B. 1963. Egg yolk and serum-cholesterol levels: Importance of dietary cholesterol intake. *Br Med J* 1:577–581.

Willett WC, Stampfer MJ, Colditz GA, Rosner BA, Hennekens CH, Speizer FE. 1987. Dietary fat and the risk of breast cancer. *N Engl J Med* 316:22–28.

Willett WC, Stampfer MJ, Colditz GA, Rosner BA, Speizer FE. 1990. Relation of meat, fat, and fiber intake to the risk of colon cancer in a prospective study among women. *N Engl J Med* 323:1664–1672.

Wong WW, Hachey DL, Insull W, Opekun AR, Klein PD. 1993. Effect of dietary cholesterol on cholesterol synthesis in breast-fed and formula-fed infants. *J Lipid Res* 34:1403–1411.

Wu Y, Zheng W, Sellers TA, Kushi LH, Bostick RM, Potter JD. 1994. Dietary cholesterol, fat, and lung cancer incidence among older women: The Iowa Women's Health Study (United States). *Cancer Causes Control* 5:395–400.

Zanni EE, Zannis VI, Blum CB, Herbert PN, Breslow JL. 1987. Effect of egg cholesterol and dietary fats on plasma lipids, lipoproteins, and apoproteins of normal women consuming natural diets. *J Lipid Res* 28:518–527.

10

Protein and Amino Acids

SUMMARY

Protein is the major structural component of all cells in the body. Proteins also function as enzymes, in membranes, as transport carriers, and as hormones; and their component amino acids serve as precursors for nucleic acids, hormones, vitamins, and other important molecules. The Recommended Dietary Allowance (RDA) for both men and women is 0.80 g of good quality protein/kg body weight/d and is based on careful analyses of available nitrogen balance studies. For amino acids, isotopic tracer methods and linear regression analysis were used whenever possible to determine the requirements. The estimated average requirements for amino acids were used to develop amino acid scoring patterns for various age groups based on the recommended intake of dietary protein. The recommended protein digestibility corrected amino acid scoring pattern (PDCAAS) for proteins for children 1 year of age and older and all other age groups is as follows (in mg/g of protein): isoleucine, 25; leucine, 55; lysine, 51, methionine + cysteine (SAA), 25; phenylalanine + tyrosine, 47; threonine, 27; tryptophan, 7; valine, 32; and histidine, 18. While an upper range for total protein in the diet as a percent of total energy intake was set at no more than 35 percent to decrease risk of chronic disease (see Chapter 11), there were insufficient data to provide dose–response relationships to establish a Tolerable Upper Intake Level (UL) for total protein or for any of the amino acids. However, the absence of a UL means that caution is warranted in using any single amino acid at levels significantly above that normally found in food.

BACKGROUND INFORMATION

Chemistry of Proteins and Amino Acids

Protein

Protein is the major functional and structural component of all the cells of the body; for example, all enzymes, membrane carriers, blood transport molecules, the intracellular matrices, hair, fingernails, serum albumin, keratin, and collagen are proteins, as are many hormones and a large part of membranes. Moreover, the constituent amino acids of protein act as precursors of many coenzymes, hormones, nucleic acids, and other molecules essential for life. Thus an adequate supply of dietary protein is essential to maintain cellular integrity and function, and for health and reproduction.

Proteins in both the diet and body are more complex and variable than the other energy sources, carbohydrates and fats. The defining characteristic of protein is its requisite amino (or imino) nitrogen group. The average content of nitrogen in dietary protein is about 16 percent by weight, so nitrogen metabolism is often considered to be synonymous with protein metabolism. Carbon, oxygen, and hydrogen are also abundant elements in proteins, and there is a smaller proportion of sulfur.

Proteins are macromolecules consisting of long chains of amino acid subunits. The structures for the common L-amino acids found in typical dietary proteins are shown in Figure 10-1. In the protein molecule, the amino acids are joined together by peptide bonds, which result from the elimination of water between the carboxyl group of one amino acid and the α-amino (or imino in the case of proline) group of the next in line. In biological systems, the chains formed might be anything from a few amino acid units (di, tri, or oligopeptide) to thousands of units long (polypeptide), corresponding to molecular weights ranging from hundreds to hundreds of thousands of Daltons. The sequence of amino acids in the chain is known as the primary structure.

A critical feature of proteins is the complexity of their physical structures. Polypeptide chains do not exist as long straight chains, nor do they curl up into random shapes, but instead fold into a definite three-dimensional structure. The chains of amino acids tend to coil into helices (secondary structure) due to hydrogen bonding between side chain residues, and sections of the helices may fold on each other due to hydrophobic interactions between nonpolar side chains and, in some proteins, to disulfide bonds so that the overall molecule might be globular or rod-like (tertiary structure). Their exact shape depends on their function and for some proteins, their interaction with other molecules (quaternary structure).

Name	Abbreviation	Form
Aliphatic side chains		
Glycine	Gly	H–CH–COOH, NH$_2$
Alanine	Ala	CH$_3$–CH–COOH, NH$_2$
Valine[a]	Val	CH$_3$–CH–CH–COOH (CH$_3$, NH$_2$)
Leucine[a]	Leu	CH$_3$–CH–CH$_2$–CH–COOH (CH$_3$, NH$_2$)
Isoleucine[a]	Ile	CH$_3$–CH$_2$–CH–CH–COOH (CH$_3$, NH$_2$)
Aromatic side chains		
Phenylalanine	Phe	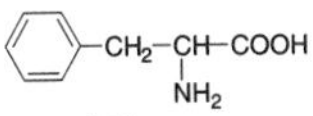 ⬡–CH$_2$–CH–COOH, NH$_2$
Tyrosine	Tyr	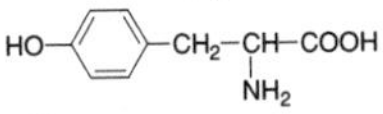 HO–⬡–CH$_2$–CH–COOH, NH$_2$
Tryptophan	Trp	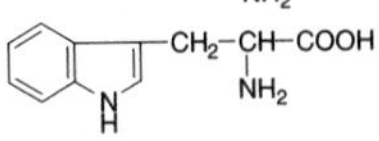 (indole)–CH$_2$–CH–COOH, NH$_2$
Hydroxyl groups in side chains		
Serine	Ser	CH$_2$–CH–COOH (OH, NH$_2$)
Threonine	Thr	CH$_2$–CH–CH–COOH (OH, NH$_2$)
Sulfur-containing side chains		
Cysteine[b]	Cys	HS–CH$_2$–CH–COOH, NH$_2$
Methionine	Met	CH$_3$–S–CH$_2$–CH$_2$–CH–COOH, NH$_2$
Imino Acids		
Proline[c]	Pro	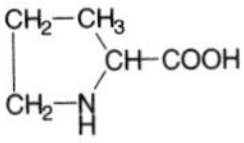 CH$_2$–CH$_2$ / CH–COOH / CH$_2$–N (H)
Acidic side chains and their amides		
Glutam	Glu	HOOC–CH$_2$–CH$_2$–CH–COOH, NH$_2$
Glutamine	Gln	H$_2$N–C(=O)–CH$_2$–CH$_2$–CH–COOH, NH$_2$
Aspartic acid	Asp	HOOC–CH$_2$–CH–COOH, NH$_2$
Asparagione	Asn	H$_2$N–C(=O)–CH$_2$–CH–COOH, NH$_2$
Basic side chains		
Lysine	Lys	H$_2$N–CH$_2$–CH$_2$–CH$_2$–CH$_2$–CH–COOH, NH$_2$
Arginine	Arg	H$_2$N–C(=NH)–N(H)–CH$_2$–CH$_2$–CH$_2$–CH–COOH, NH$_2$
Histidine	His	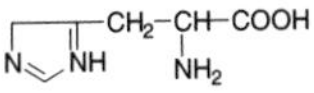 (imidazole)–CH$_2$–CH–COOH, NH$_2$

Amino acids in italics are classed as nutritionally indispensable to humans.
[a] Leucine, valine, and isoleucine are known as the branched-chain amino acids.
[b] Cysteine is often found as a dimer (cysteine), linked through sulfur atoms (-S-S-) by oxidation.
[c] Proline is, strictly speaking, an imino acid rather than an amino acid.

FIGURE 10-1 L-amino acids of nutritional significance.

Many proteins are composed of several separate peptide chains held together by ionic or covalent links, an example being hemoglobin, in which each active unit consists of two pairs of dissimilar subunits (the α and β chains).

The most important aspect of a protein from a nutritional point of view is its amino acid composition, but the protein's structure may also influence its digestibility. Some proteins, such as keratin, are highly insoluble in water and hence are resistant to digestion, while highly glycosylated proteins, such as the intestinal mucins, are resistant to attack by the proteolytic enzymes of the intestine.

Amino Acids

The amino acids that are incorporated into mammalian protein are α-amino acids, with the exception of proline, which is an α-imino acid. This means that they have a carboxyl group, an amino nitrogen group, and a side chain attached to a central α-carbon (Figure 10-1). Functional differences among the amino acids lie in the structure of their side chains. In addition to differences in size, these side groups carry different charges at physiological pH (e.g., nonpolar, uncharged but polar, negatively charged, positively charged); some groups are hydrophobic (e.g., branched chain and aromatic amino acids) and some hydrophilic (most others).

These side chains have an important bearing on the ways in which the higher orders of protein structure are stabilized and are intimate parts of many other aspects of protein function. Attractions between positive and negative charges pull different parts of the molecule together. Hydrophobic groups tend to cluster together in the center of globular proteins, while hydrophilic groups remain in contact with water on the periphery. The ease with which the sulfhydryl group in cysteine forms a disulfide bond with the sulfhydryl group of another cysteine in a polypeptide chain is an important factor in the stabilization of folded structures within the polypeptide and is a crucial element in the formation of inter-polypeptide bonds. The hydroxyl and amide groups of amino acids provide the sites for the attachment of the complex oligosaccharide side chains that are a feature of many mammalian proteins such as lactase, sucrase, and the mucins. Histidine and amino acids with the carboxyl side chains (glutamic acid and aspartic acid) are critical features in ion-binding proteins, such as the calcium-binding proteins (e.g., troponin C), critical for muscular contraction, and the iron-binding proteins (e.g., hemoglobin) responsible for oxygen transport.

Some amino acids in protein only achieve their final structure after their precursors have been incorporated into the polypeptide. Notable examples of such post-translational modifications are the hydroxyproline and hydroxylysine residues found in collagen (proline and lysine are converted to these after they have been incorporated into procollagen) and 3-methylhistidine present in actin and myosin. The former hydroxylated amino acids are critical parts of the cross-linking of collagen chains that lead to rigid and stable structures. The role of methylated histidine in contractile protein function is unknown.

Nutritional and Metabolic Classification of Amino Acids

Older views of the nutritional classification of amino acids categorized them into two groups: indispensable (essential) and dispensable (nonessential). The nine indispensable amino acids (Table 10-1) are those that have carbon skeletons that cannot be synthesized to meet body needs from simpler molecules in animals, and therefore must be provided in the diet. Although the classification of the indispensable amino acids and their assignment into a single category has been maintained in this report, the definition of dispensable amino acids has become blurred as more information on the intermediary metabolism and nutritional characteristics of these compounds has accumulated. Laidlaw and Kopple (1987) divided dispensable amino acids into two classes: truly dispensable and conditionally indispensable. Five of the amino acids in Table 10-1 are termed dispensable as they can be synthesized in the body from either other amino

TABLE 10-1 Indispensable, Dispensable, and Conditionally Indispensable Amino Acids in the Human Diet

Indispensable	Dispensable	Conditionally Indispensable[a]	Precursors of Conditionally Indispensable
Histidine[b]	Alanine	Arginine	Glutamine/glutamate, asparate
Isoleucine	Aspartic acid	Cysteine	Methionine, serine
Leucine	Asparagine	Glutamine	Gl utamic acid/ammonia
Lysine	Glutamic acid	Glycine	Serine, choline
Methionine	Serine	Proline	Glutamate
Phenylalanine		Tyrosine	Phenylalanine
Threonine			
Tryptophan			
Valine			

[a] Conditionally indispensable is defined as requiring a dietary source when endogenous synthesis cannot meet metabolic need.
[b] Although histidine is considered indispensable, unlike the other eight indispensable amino acids, it does not fulfill the criteria used in this report of reducing protein deposition and inducing negative nitrogen balance promptly upon removal from the diet.
SOURCE: Laidlaw and Kopple (1987).

acids or other complex nitrogenous metabolites. In addition, six other amino acids, including cysteine and tyrosine, are conditionally indispensable as they are synthesized from other amino acids or their synthesis is limited under special pathophysiological conditions (Chipponi et al., 1982; Harper, 1983; Laidlaw and Kopple, 1987). This is even more of an issue in the neonate where it has been suggested that only alanine, aspartate, glutamate, serine, and probably asparagine are truly dietarily dispensable (Pencharz et al., 1996).

The term conditionally indispensable recognizes the fact that under most normal conditions the body can synthesize these amino acids to meet metabolic needs. However, there may be certain physiological circumstances: prematurity in the young infant where there is an inadequate rate at which cysteine can be produced from methionine; the newborn, where enzymes that are involved in quite complex synthetic pathways may be present in inadequate amounts as in the case of arginine (Brunton et al., 1999), which results in a dietary requirement for this amino acid; or pathological states, such as severe catabolic stress in an adult, where the limited tissue capacity to produce glutamine to meet increased needs and to balance increased catabolic rates makes a dietary source of these amino acids required to achieve body nitrogen homeostasis. The cells of the small intestine become important sites of conditionally indispensable amino acid, synthesis, with some amino acids (e.g., glutamine and arginine) becoming nutritionally indispensable under circumstances of intestinal metabolic dysfunction (Stechmiller et al., 1997). However, the quantitative requirement levels for conditionally indispensable amino acids have not been determined and these, presumably, vary greatly according to the specific condition.

There now appears to be a requirement for preformed α-amino nitrogen in the form of glutamate, alanine, or aspartate, for example (Katagiri and Nakamura, 2002). It was previously thought that, in addition to the indispensable amino acids, simple sources of nitrogen such as urea and diammonium citrate together with carbon sources would be sufficient to maintain nitrogen homeostasis (FAO/WHO, 1965). However, there are now good theoretical reasons to conclude that this is not likely in the human (Katagiri and Nakamura, 2002). The mixture of dispensable and conditionally indispensable amino acids as supplied by food proteins at adequate intakes of total nitrogen will assure that both the nitrogen and specific amino acid needs are met.

Protein and Amino Acid Homeostasis

Maintenance of Body Protein

Body Protein Reserve. The body of a 70-kg man contains about 11 kg of protein. Nearly half of this protein (about 43 percent) is present as skeletal muscle, while other structural tissues such as skin and blood each contain approximately 15 percent of the total protein (Lentner, 1981). The metabolically active visceral tissues (e.g., liver and kidney) contain comparatively small amounts of protein (together about 10 percent of the total). Other organs such as the brain, lung, heart, and bone contribute the remainder. The distribution among the organs varies with developmental age, as the newborn infant has proportionately less muscle and much more brain and visceral tissue than the adult. It is also notable that, despite the very wide variety of enzymes and proteins within a single organism, almost one half of the total protein content of the human is present in just four proteins (myosin, actin, collagen, and hemoglobin). Collagen in particular may comprise 25 percent of the total. Moreover, in induced malnutrition, this proportion can rise to 50 percent because of the substantial loss of noncollagen proteins, whereas collagen itself is retained (Picou et al., 1966).

Even in the adult, when the protein mass of the body has reached a plateau, it can be influenced by a variety of nutritional and pathological factors. Thus, when diets high or low in protein are given, there is a gain or loss of body protein over the first few days, before re-equilibration of protein intake with the rates of oxidation and excretion (Swick and Benevenga, 1977). This phenomenon has led to the concept of a "labile protein reserve," which can be gained or lost from the body as a short-term store for use in emergencies or to take account of day-to-day variations in dietary intake. Studies in animals have suggested that this immediate labile protein store is contained in the liver and visceral tissues, as their protein content decreases very rapidly during starvation or protein depletion (by as much as 40 percent), while skeletal muscle protein drops much more slowly (Swick and Benevenga, 1977). During this situation, protein breakdown becomes a source of indispensable amino acid needs for synthesis of proteins critical to maintaining essential body function (Reeds et al., 1994).

This labile protein reserve in humans is unlikely to account for more than about 1 percent of total body protein (Waterlow, 1969; Young et al., 1968). Thus, the immediately accessible stores of protein (which serve as the source of indispensable amino acids and amino nitrogen) cannot be considered in the same light as the huge energy stores in the form of body fat; the labile protein reserve is similar in weight to the glycogen store. However, it should be recognized that this protein reserve is unlike the fat and glycogen stores, whose primary roles are for energy use. The protein lost during fasting is functional body protein and thus there is no evidence for a protein reserve that serves only as a store to meet future needs.

There is a wide range of variation in daily dietary protein intake, from the protein requirement and beyond, to which the body is able to adapt over a period of days, after which no further change in body protein content occurs. However, pathological conditions, such as severe disease states, can cause substantial rates of protein loss due to the increased demand for either amino acids or carbon skeletons to meet local energy demands. If these conditions go unchecked for more than a few days, there may be a serious depletion of the body's protein mass, which might eventually become life threatening. Although the evidence from short-term changes in diet suggests that the main loss of protein is from the viscera (de Blaauw et al., 1996), in chronic illness skeletal muscle, which comprises over 40 percent of the protein mass of a healthy individual, becomes the largest single contributor to protein loss (Hansen et al., 2000).

Free Amino Acids. Although the free amino acids dissolved in the body fluids are only a very small proportion of the body's total mass of amino acids, they are very important for the nutritional and metabolic control of the body's proteins.

The content of free and protein-bound amino acids in rat muscle is shown in Table 10-2. It can be seen that their ranges are considerable and that their concentrations in the free pool are in no way related to their concentrations in body proteins. In the human, free phenylalanine comprises less than 2 percent of its total body pool, and corresponds to only about 1.5 hour worth of protein synthesis, or 25 percent of the day's intake of protein (Waterlow et al., 1978). Free glutamate and alanine comprise a larger proportion of their respective body pools, but they could not be considered as reserves for more than a very short time. In human muscle, glutamine has an exceptionally large free pool, containing about 10 to 15 g of nitrogen. After trauma, this pool can become depleted by more than 50 percent (Labow and Souba, 2000); its loss may then make a significant contribution to the total loss of nitrogen.

Although the plasma compartment is most easily sampled, the concentration of most amino acids is higher in tissue intracellular pools. Typically, large neutral amino acids, such as leucine and phenylalanine, are essentially in equilibrium with the plasma. Others, notably glutamine, glutamic acid, and glycine, are 10- to 50-fold more concentrated in the intracellular pool. Dietary variations or pathological conditions can result in substantial changes in the concentrations of the individual free amino acids in both the plasma and tissue pools (Furst, 1989; Waterlow et al., 1978).

TABLE 10-2 Comparison of the Pool Sizes of Free and Protein-Bound Amino Acids in Rat Muscle

	μmol/g Wet Weight		
	Protein	Free	Protein: Free Ratio
Indispensable amino acids			
Histidine	26	0.39	67
Isoleucine	50	0.16	306
Leucine	109	0.20	556
Lysine	58	1.86	31
Methionine	36	0.16	225
Phenylalanine	45	0.07	646
Threonine	60	1.94	31
Valine	83	0.31	272
Dispensable and some conditionally indispensable amino acids			
Alanine	111	2.77	40
Arginine	67	0.25	269
Aspartic acid (+ amide)	110	1.13	97
Glutamic acid (+ amide)	148	9.91	15
Glycine	117	1.94	60
Serine	74	1.96	38
Tyrosine	36	0.14	266

SOURCE: Data of E.B. Fern, quoted by Waterlow et al. (1978).

Pathways of Amino Acid Metabolism

The exchange between body protein and the free amino acid pool is illustrated by the highly simplified scheme shown in Figure 10-2. Here, all the proteins in the tissues and circulation are grouped into one pool. Similarly, there is a second pool, consisting of the free amino acids dissolved in body fluids. The arrows into and out of the protein pool show the continual degradation and resynthesis of these macromolecules (i.e., protein turnover). The other major pathways that involve the free amino acid pool are the supply of amino acids by the gut from the absorbed amino acids derived from dietary proteins, the de novo synthesis in cells (including those of the gut, which are a source of dispensable amino acids), and the loss of amino acids by oxidation, excretion, or conversion to other metabolites. Although this scheme represents protein metabolism in the human as a whole, with minor modifications it can also be used to repre-

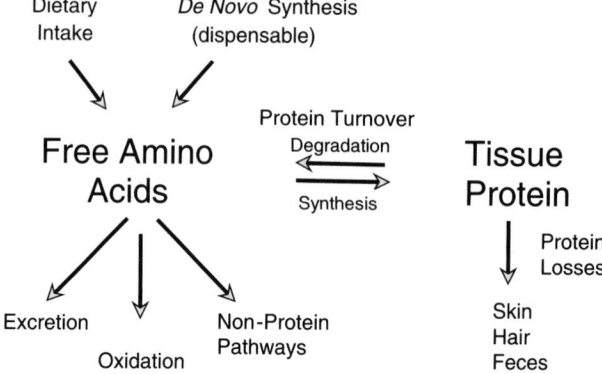

FIGURE 10-2 Exchange between body protein and free amino acid pools.

sent protein metabolism in individual organs, or indeed the metabolism of a single protein.

Amino Acid Utilization for Growth

Dietary protein is not only needed for maintaining protein turnover and the synthesis of physiologically important products of amino acid metabolism but is, of course, laid down as new tissue. Studies in animals show that the composition of amino acids needed for growth is very similar to the composition of body protein (Dewey et al., 1996). It is important to note, however, that the amino acid composition of human milk is not the same as that of body protein (Dewey et al., 1996), and although the present recommendations for the dietary amino acids for infants provided in this report continue to be based on human milk as the standard, recent authors (Dewey et al., 1996) have cautioned that the composition of human milk proteins is not necessarily a definition of the biological amino acid requirements of the growing neonate.

Maintenance Protein Needs

Even when mammals consume no protein, nitrogen continues to be lost. Provided that the energy intake is adequate, these "basal" losses are closely related to body weight and basal metabolic rate (Castaneda et al., 1995b; Scrimshaw et al., 1972). In man, normal growth is very slow and the dietary requirement to support growth is small in relation to maintenance needs except at very young ages. Moreover, the human being is a long-lived species. It follows that maintenance needs are of particular importance to humans and account for a very large majority of lifetime needs for dietary protein.

It has been known for decades (Said and Hegsted, 1970) that the body's capacity to conserve individual amino acids at low intakes varies, so the pattern of amino acids needed in the diet to match their individual catabolic rates does not correspond precisely with the composition of body protein. For example, the indispensable amino acid requirements for adults may provide a quarter of their minimum total need for amino nitrogen, compared with the need for noncollagen body protein in which approximately half of the amino acids are indispensable (FAO/WHO/UNU, 1985). This implies that there is very effective recycling of indispensable amino acids released continuously from protein degradation back into protein synthesis. Under conditions where the diet is devoid of protein, the efficiency of amino acid recycling is over 90 percent for both indispensable and dispensable amino acids (Neale and Waterlow, 1974). While highly efficient, some amino acids are recycled at different rates than others.

Physiology of Absorption, Metabolism, and Excretion

Protein Digestion and Absorption

After ingestion, proteins are denatured by the acid in the stomach, where they are also cleaved into smaller peptides by the enzyme pepsin, which is activated by the increase in stomach acidity that occurs on feeding. The proteins and peptides then pass into the small intestine, where the peptide bonds are hydrolyzed by a variety of enzymes. These bond-specific enzymes originate in the pancreas and include trypsin, chymotrypsins, elastase, and carboxypeptidases. The resultant mixture of free amino acids and small peptides is then transported into the mucosal cells by a number of carrier systems for specific amino acids and for di- and tri-peptides, each specific for a limited range of peptide substrates. After intracellular hydrolysis of the absorbed peptides, the free amino acids are then secreted into the portal blood by other specific carrier systems in the mucosal cell or are further metabolized within the cell itself. Absorbed amino acids pass into the liver, where a portion of the amino acids are taken up and used; the remainder pass through into the systemic circulation and are utilized by the peripheral tissues.

Although there are good reasons to suppose that dietary protein digestion is incomplete and variable among different diets, recent studies using proteins intrinsically labeled with ^{15}N added to a diet suggest that many common dietary proteins, including proteins from casein, mixed whey, wheat, and legumes, are digested with an efficiency of greater than 90 percent when fed as isolates, concentrates, or flours (Bergner et al., 1990; Gausserès et al., 1997). Thus, a significant portion (at least 50 percent) of fecal nitrogen losses represents the fixation by the colonic and cecal bacteria of nitrogenous substances (urea, ammonia, and protein secretions) that have been secreted into the intestinal lumen.

Some authors have argued that the host-colon nitrogen cycle, by which nitrogenous compounds that diffuse into the gut are converted to ammonia by the microflora and are reabsorbed, is a regulated function and serves as a mechanism of nitrogen conservation (Jackson, 1989). The theoretical basis of this proposition has been partly confirmed by the recent demonstration of the availability to the host of indispensable amino acids synthesized by intestinal microbes (Metges et al., 1999a, 1999b). However, not all investigators have obtained results indicative of regulated nitrogen cycling (Raguso et al., 1999; Young et al., 2000).

Although it seems clear that the efficiency of dietary protein digestion (in the sense of removal of amino acids from the small intestinal lumen) is high, there is now good evidence to show that nutritionally significant quantities of indispensable amino acids are metabolized by the tissues of the splanchnic bed, including the mucosal cells of the intestine (Fuller and Reeds, 1998). Thus, less than 100 percent of the amino acids removed from the intestinal lumen appear in the peripheral circulation, and the quantities that are metabolized by the splanchnic bed vary among the amino acids, with intestinal threonine metabolism being particularly high (Stoll et al., 1998). Currently, there is a lack of systematic information about the relationship between dietary amino acid intake and splanchnic metabolism, although there are indications that there is a nonlinear relationship between amino acid intake and appearance in the peripheral blood (van der Schoor et al., 2001).

Intestinal Protein Losses

Protein secretion into the intestine continues even under conditions of protein-free feeding, and fecal nitrogen losses (i.e., nitrogen lost as bacteria in the feces) may account for 25 percent of the obligatory loss of nitrogen (Fuller and Reeds, 1998). Under this dietary circumstance, the amino acids secreted into the intestine as components of proteolytic enzymes and from sloughed mucosal cells are the only sources of amino acids for the maintenance of the intestinal bacterial biomass. In those studies in which highly digestible protein-containing diets have been given to individuals previously ingesting protein-free diets, fecal nitrogen excretion increased by only a small amount. For highly digestible proteins, it also is likely that when humans consume diets that do not provide an excessive quantity of protein, a high proportion of the fecal nitrogen losses originate from a combination of gastrointestinal secretions and the partial capture of the significant quantities of secreted urea that are hydrolyzed and subsequently used by the microflora in the large intestine (Jackson, 1989).

The following points support the view that the intestinal route of protein (amino acid) loss is of quantitative significance to maintenance protein needs. First, continued mucosal cell turnover and enzyme and mucin secretion are necessary for maintaining the integrity of the gastrointestinal tract and its normal digestive physiology. Second, animal studies show that the amino acid composition of the proteins leaving the ileum for bacterial fermentation in the colon is quite different from that of body protein (Taverner et al., 1981). In particular, the secretions are relatively rich in dispensable amino acids as well as threonine and cysteine (Dekker et al., 1991; Khatri et al., 1998; Taverner et al., 1981), probably because mucin secretions make a substantial contribution to the endogenous outflow. These two amino acids are of significance in meeting amino acid needs when intake is close to the requirement (Laidlaw and Kopple, 1987).

Other routes of loss of intact amino acids are via the urine and through skin and hair loss. These losses are small by comparison with those described above, but nonetheless may have a significant impact on estimates of requirements, especially in disease states (Matthews, 1999).

Protein Synthesis

Amino acids are selected for protein synthesis by binding with transfer RNA (tRNA) in the cell cytoplasm. The information on the amino acid sequence of each individual protein is contained in the sequence of nucleotides in the messenger RNA (mRNA) molecules, which are synthesized in the nucleus from regions of DNA by the process of transcription. The mRNA molecules then interact with various tRNA molecules attached to specific amino acids in the cytoplasm to synthesize the specific protein by linking together individual amino acids; this process, known as translation, is regulated by amino acids (e.g., leucine) (Jefferson and Kimball, 2001), and hormones. Which specific proteins are expressed in any particular cell and the relative rates at which the different cellular proteins are synthesized, are determined by the relative abundances of the different mRNAs and the availability of specific tRNA-amino acid combinations, and hence by the rate of transcription and the stability of the messages.

From a nutritional and metabolic point of view, it is important to recognize that protein synthesis is a continuing process that takes place in most cells of the body. In a steady state, when neither net growth nor protein loss is occurring, protein synthesis is balanced by an equal amount of protein degradation. The major consequence of inadequate protein intakes, or diets low or lacking in specific indispensable amino acids relative to other amino acids (often termed limiting amino acids), is a shift in this balance so that rates of synthesis of some body proteins decrease while protein degradation continues, thus providing an endogenous source of those amino acids most in need.

Protein Degradation

The mechanism of intracellular protein degradation, by which protein is hydrolyzed to free amino acids, is more complex and is not as well characterized at the mechanistic level as that of synthesis (Kirschner, 1999). A wide variety of different enzymes that are capable of splitting peptide bonds are present in cells. However, the bulk of cellular proteolysis seems to be shared between two multienzyme systems: the lysosomal and proteasomal systems. The lysosome is a membrane-enclosed vesicle inside the cell that contains a variety of proteolytic enzymes and operates mostly at acid pH. Volumes of the cytoplasm are engulfed (autophagy) and are then subjected to the action of the protease enzymes at high concentration. This system is thought to be relatively unselective in most cases, although it can also degrade specific intracellular proteins (Cuervo and Dice, 1998). The system is highly regulated by hormones such as insulin and glucocorticoids, and by amino acids (Inubushi et al., 1996).

The second system is the ATP-dependent ubiquitin-proteasome system, which is present in the cytoplasm. The first step is to join molecules of ubiquitin, a basic 76-amino acid peptide, to lysine residues in the target protein. Several enzymes are involved in this process, which selectively targets proteins for degradation by a second component, the proteasome. This is a very large complex of proteins, possessing a range of different proteolytic activities. The ubiquitin-proteasome system is highly selective, so can account for the wide range of degradation rates (half-lives ranging from minutes to days) observed for different proteins. It is thought to be particularly responsible for degrading abnormal or damaged proteins, along with regulatory proteins that typically are synthesized and degraded very rapidly (Ciechanover et al., 1991; Goldberg and Rock, 1992; Hershko and Ciechanover, 1998).

Protein Turnover

The process by which all body proteins are being continuously broken down and resynthesized is known as protein turnover. In the adult human body, upward of 250 g/d of protein is synthesized and degraded (Waterlow, 1984). This compares with a median daily adult intake of about 55 to 100 g/d (Appendix Table E-16). The daily amount of protein turned over is greater in infants and less in the elderly, when compared with young adults on a body-weight basis (Table 10-3). Some tissues are more active in protein turnover than others. Thus the liver and intestine, despite their rather small contribution to the total protein content of the body, are together believed to contribute as much as 50 percent of whole body protein turnover (McNurlan and Garlick, 1980; Waterlow, 1984). Conversely, skeletal muscle is the largest single component of body protein mass (43 percent), but contributes only about 25 percent to total body protein turnover (Reeds and Garlick, 1984; Waterlow, 1984).

At the tissue level, proteins are continually being synthesized and degraded as a sensitive means of regulating the amount of each separate enzyme or structural component. Other proteins may be secreted from the cell after synthesis and subsequently degraded at a distant site. Examples of such proteins are serum albumin synthesized in the liver, antibodies in the B-lymphocytes, digestive enzymes in the pancreas, and peptide hormones formed in the endocrine glands.

Amino Acid Catabolism

Nitrogen Metabolism

About 11 to 15 g of nitrogen are excreted each day in the urine of a healthy adult consuming 70 to 100 g of protein, mostly in the form of urea, with smaller contributions from ammonia, uric acid, creatinine, and some free amino acids (Table 10-4). These are the end products of protein metabolism, with urea and ammonia arising from the partial oxidation of amino acids. Uric acid and creatinine are indirectly derived from amino acids as well.

The removal of nitrogen from the individual amino acids and its conversion to a form that can be excreted by the kidney can be considered as a two-part process. The first step usually takes place by one of two types of

TABLE 10-3 Whole-Body Protein Synthesis in Humans at Different Life Stages

Life Stage	Protein Synthesis (g/kg/d)
Newborn (preterm)	17.4
Infant	6.9
Adult	3.0
Elderly	1.9

SOURCE: Young et al. (1975b).

TABLE 10-4 Approximate Distribution of Nitrogen in Urinary Constituents in Humans Consuming 100 g of Protein per Day (~16 g of Nitrogen)

Compound	Nitrogen (g/d)
Urea	12.8
Ammonia	0.7
Amino acids	0.7
Creatine/Creatinine	0.7
Uric acid	0.3
Hippuric acid	0.1
Total	15.3

SOURCE: Diem (1962).

enzymatic reactions: transamination or deamination. Transamination is a reversible reaction that uses ketoacid intermediates of glucose metabolism (e.g., pyruvate, oxaloacetate, and α-ketoglutarate) as recipients of the amino nitrogen. Most amino acids can take part in these reactions, with the result that their amino nitrogen is transferred to just three amino acids: alanine from pyruvate, aspartate from oxaloacetate, and glutamate from α-ketoglutarate.

Unlike many amino acids, branched-chain amino acid transamination occurs throughout the body, particularly in skeletal muscle. Here the main recipients of amino nitrogen are alanine and glutamine (from pyruvate and glutamate, respectively), which then pass into the circulation. These serve as important carriers of nitrogen from the periphery (skeletal muscle) to the intestine and liver. In the small intestine, glutamine is extracted and metabolized to ammonia, alanine, and citrulline, which are then conveyed to the liver via the portal circulation (Harper et al., 1984).

Nitrogen is also removed from amino acids by deamination reactions, which result in the formation of ammonia. A number of amino acids can be deaminated, either directly (histidine), by dehydration (serine, threonine), by way of the purine nucleotide cycle (aspartate), or by oxidative deamination (glutamate). These latter two processes are important because glutamate and aspartate are recipients of nitrogen by transamination from other amino acids, including alanine. Glutamate is also formed in the specific degradation pathways of arginine and lysine. Thus, nitrogen from any amino acid can be funneled into the two precursors of urea synthesis, ammonia and aspartate.

Urea synthesis takes place in the liver by the cyclic pathway known as the Krebs-Henseleit cycle. Among the essential reactions in this process is the hydrolysis of the amino acid arginine by the enzyme arginase to yield urea and another amino acid, ornithine, which is not incorporated into body protein. The remaining part of the cycle involves the resynthesis of arginine using nitrogen from ammonia and aspartate. Thus, although arginine is the direct precursor of urea, it is not consumed in the process, as the nitrogen excreted as urea is all derived from ammonia and aspartate.

After synthesis, the urea is carried by the circulation from the liver to the kidney, where it is excreted into the urine. Although the excretion of urea dominates nitrogen excretion as a whole, significant quantities of ammonium ions are also excreted. There are some metabolic pathways, notably the purine nucleotide cycle, whereby purine nitrogen is converted to ammonium ions. It is generally believed that much of the ammonia produced by this cycle in skeletal muscle is transported in the blood as glutamine. Some of this glutamine is metabolized in the kidneys, where the enzyme glutaminase leads to the release of ammonium ions and glutamate. This glutamate, after losing its amino group, is then utilized in the synthesis of glucose in the kidney. The generation of ammonium ions from glutamine has a specific role in acid–base homeostasis, as ammonium ion excretion serves as the main vehicle for the excretion of excess hydrogen ions to prevent acidosis.

Carbon Metabolism

For most amino acids, removal of the amino nitrogen group generates their ketoacid analogues. Many of these are already in a form for entry into the pathways of oxidative metabolism (Figure 10-3). For example, both α-ketoglutarate (from glutamate) and pyruvate (from alanine) are intermediates of the glycolysis-tricarboxylic acid (TCA) pathway of glucose oxidation. All the others have specific degradation systems that give rise to intermediates that can be metabolized in these oxidative pathways. Thus, protein can make a significant contribution to the body's energy supply. This is particularly true in non-growing adults, who on average consume, and therefore oxidize, about 10 to 15 percent of their dietary energy as protein (Appendix Table E-17).

The contribution of protein to energy needs may be significant during periods of energy restriction or following the utilization of the body's limited endogenous carbohydrate stores. Protein oxidation also has been shown to rise considerably in highly traumatized or septic individuals, which results in large amounts of body protein loss; this loss can compromise recovery or even lead to death (see below) (Klein, 1990). It is much less in periods of chronic starvation because of various metabolic adaptations related to ketone utilization, or on protein-restricted diets.

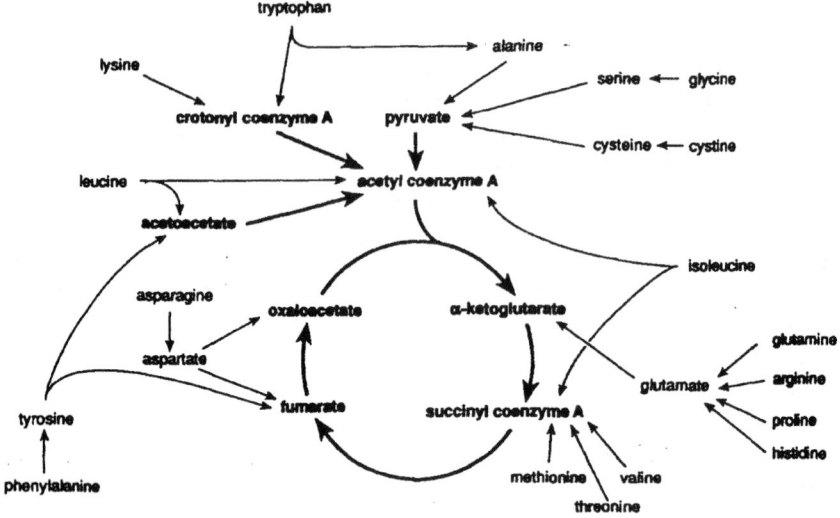

FIGURE 10-3 Metabolism of the carbon skeletons of the amino acid chains (light arrows) and their points of entry into the general pathways of metabolism of glucose and fat (bold arrows).
SOURCE: Garlick and Reeds (1993).

Once the amino acid deamination products enter the TCA cycle (also known as the citric acid cycle or Krebs cycle) or the glycolytic pathway, their carbon skeletons are also available for use in biosynthetic pathways, particularly for glucose and fat. Whether glucose or fat is formed from the carbon skeleton of an amino acid depends on its point of entry into these two pathways. If they enter as acetyl-CoA, then only fat or ketone bodies can be formed. The carbon skeletons of other amino acids can, however, enter the pathways in such a way that their carbons can be used for gluconeogenesis. This is the basis for the classical nutritional description of amino acids as either ketogenic or glucogenic (i.e., able to give rise to either ketones [or fat] or glucose).

Some amino acids produce both products upon degradation and so are considered both ketogenic and glucogenic (Figure 10-3). It has been argued that the majority of hepatic amino acid catabolism is directed in an obligatory fashion to glucose synthesis (Jungas et al., 1992). The synthesis of glucose in the liver from amino acids is dominated by alanine and glutamate, which derive much of their carbon from peripheral metabolism of glucose to lactate and TCA cycle intermediates. Thus, much of gluconeogenesis in metabolism is the result of a metabolic cycle of glucose carbon between the peripheral tissues (especially muscle) and the liver and kidney. This cycle also involves the peripheral synthesis of glutamine, an amino acid that is utilized in substantial quantities by the intestinal cells in which it is used for energy and for the synthesis of proline, citrulline, and nucleic acids.

A significant proportion of the glucose synthesized in the liver is due to recapture and recycling via the liver of 3-carbon units in the form of lactate derived from anaerobic glucose breakdown in muscle (the Cori cycle). Hepatic gluconeogenesis also occurs via the glucose–alanine cycle (a direct parallel of the Cori cycle) and the glucose–glutamine cycle. Since the nitrogen donors may be either glucogenic or ketogenic amino acids, these cycles function as mechanisms for transporting nitrogen from the periphery to the liver as well as for glucose production. The cycle involving glutamine transport from the periphery to the gastrointestinal tract is also vital to the synthesis of arginine and proline and is critical to the prevention of the build up of excessive ammonia in the circulation.

Nonprotein Pathways of Amino Acid Nitrogen Utilization

Although in general the utilization of dietary amino acids is dominated by their incorporation into protein and their role in energy metabolism, amino acids are also involved in the synthesis of other nitrogenous compounds important to physiological viability as shown in Table 10-5. Some pathways have the potential for exerting a substantial impact on the utilization of certain amino acids, and may be of potential significance for the requirements for these amino acids. This is particularly true for glycine, which is a precursor for six nitrogenous compounds, as shown in Table 10-5. Its utilization in the synthesis of creatine (muscle function), heme (oxygen transport and oxidative phosphorylation), and glutathione (protective reactions which are limited by the amount of available cysteine) is not only of physiological importance, but can also involve substantial quantities of the amino acid. For example, in the absence of a dietary source of creatine, adults require at least 1.1 g/d of glycine in order to sustain an adequate rate of creatine synthesis (calculated from a creatinine excretion of 1.8 g/d for a 70-kg man [Young et al., 1984] assuming 1 mole of glycine is used to synthesize 1 mole of creatine which gives rise to 1 mole of urinary creatinine). In premature infants, mainly fed human milk, there is evidence that the glycine supply may be a primary nutritional limitation to growth (Jackson, 1991). This so-called dispensable amino acid is then needed in the diet for optimum growth and may be termed "conditionally indispensable."

Similarly, the synthesis of carnitine (involved in intracellular fatty acid transport) could, under some circumstances, become of quantitative sig-

TABLE 10-5 Amino Acid Precursors of Nonprotein Products

Precursor Amino Acids	End Product
Tryptophan	Serotonin
Tryptophan	Nicotinic acid
Tyrosine	Catecholamines
Tyrosine	Thyroid hormones
Tyrosine	Melanin
Lysine	Carnitine
Cysteine	Taurine
Arginine	Nitric oxide
Glycine	Heme
Glycine, arginine, methionine	Creatine
Methionine, glycine, serine	"Methyl group metabolism"
Glycine, taurine	Bile acids
Glutamate, cysteine, glycine	Glutathione
Glutamate, aspartate, glycine	Nucleic acid bases

nificance to lysine requirements. These may be important nutritional considerations in individuals consuming marginal amounts of proteins of plant origin and undoubtedly have an impact on overall amino acid utilization when protein intake is very low.

Clinical Effects of Inadequate Protein Intake

As outlined above, protein is the fundamental component necessary for cellular and organ function. Not only must sufficient protein be provided, but also sufficient nonprotein energy (i.e., carbohydrates, fats) must be available so that the carbon skeletons of amino acids are not used to meet energy needs (Duffy et al., 1981). Similarly, unless amino acids are present in the diet in the right balance (see later section, "Protein Quality"), protein utilization will be affected (Duffy et al., 1981). In the world as a whole, protein-energy malnutrition (PEM) is fairly common in both children and adults (Stephenson et al., 2000), and is associated with the deaths of about 6 million children each year (FAO, 2000). In the industrialized world, PEM is seen predominantly in hospitals (Bistrian, 1990; Willard et al., 1980), is associated with disease (Wilson and Pencharz, 1997), and often found in the elderly (Allison, 1995). Hypoalbuminemic malnutrition has been described in hospitalized adults (Bistrian, 1990) and has also been called adult kwashiorkor (Hill, 1992).

Clearly, protein deficiency has adverse effects on all organs (Corish and Kennedy, 2000). In infants and young children, it has been shown to have harmful effects on the brain and may have longer-term effects on brain function (Pollitt, 2000). Furthermore, protein deficiency has been shown to have adverse effects on the immune system, resulting in a higher risk of infections (Bistrian, 1990). It also affects gut mucosal function and permeability, which, in turn, affects absorption and makes possible bacterial invasion from the gut, which can result in septicemia (Reynolds et al., 1996). Protein deficiency has also been shown to adversely affect kidney function, where it has adverse effects on both glomerular and tubular function (Benabe and Martinez-Moldonado, 1998).

Total starvation will result in death in initially normal-weight adults in 60 to 70 days (Allison, 1992). For comparison, protein and energy reserves are much smaller in premature infants, and survival of 1,000-g neonates is only about 5 days (Heird et al., 1972).

Clinical Assessment of Protein Nutritional Status

No single parameter is completely reliable to assess protein nutritional status. Borderline inadequate protein intakes in infants and children are reflected in failure to grow as estimated by length or height (Jelliffe, 1966; Pencharz, 1985). However, weight-height relationships can be distorted by edema and ascites (Corish and Kennedy, 2000). Mid-upper arm parameters such as arm muscle circumference have been used to measure protein status (Young et al., 1990). The triceps skinfold is reflective of energy nutritional status while the arm muscle circumference (or diameter) is reflective of protein nutritional status (unless a myopathy or neuropathy is present) (Patrick et al., 1994).

In addition, urinary creatinine excretion has been used as a reflection of muscle mass (Corish and Kennedy, 2000; Forbes, 1987; Young et al., 1990), but it is not very sensitive. The most commonly used methods to clinically evaluate protein status measure serum proteins; the strengths and weaknesses of these indicators are summarized in Table 10-6. In practical terms, acute protein depletion is not clinically important as it is rare, while chronic deficiency is important. Serum proteins as shown in Table 10-6 are useful, especially albumin and transferrin (an iron-binding protein). In a study from Nigeria, low transferrin levels were more predictive of risk of death in children with PEM than were albumin levels (Ramsey et al., 1992). Due to their very short half-lives, prealbumin and retinol binding protein (apart from their dependence on vitamin A status) may reflect more acute protein intake than risk of protein malnutrition (which is a process with an onset of period of 7 to 10 days (Ramsey et al., 1992). Hence, albumin and transferrin remain the best measures of protein malnutrition, but with all of the caveats listed in Table 10-6.

Physical examination related to protein malnutrition focuses attention on the skin and hair as they are rapidly growing protein-containing

TABLE 10-6 Use of Serum Proteins to Assess Protein Nutritional Status

	Half-Life	Clinical Use	Limitations
Albumin	18 d	Severe malnutrition	Affected by protein losing enteropathy, renal loss, burn, and by liver disease
Transferrin	8–9 d	Limited—chronic deficiency	Affected by iron deficiency and by infection
Pre-albumin	2 d	Acute depletion	Affected by vitamin A deficiency
Retinol-binding protein	12 h	Acute depletion	Affected by vitamin A deficiency

SOURCE: Adapted from Young et al. (1990).

tissues. In protein malnutrition, the skin becomes thinner and appears dull; the hair first does not grow, then it may fall out or show color changes (Pencharz, 1985). Over a longer period of time, assessment of changes in lean body mass reflects protein nutritional status. The clinical tools most available to assess lean mass are dual emission x-ray absorptiometry and bioelectrical impedance (Pencharz and Azcue, 1996).

SELECTION OF INDICATORS FOR ESTIMATING THE REQUIREMENT FOR PROTEIN (NITROGEN)

In the framework for Dietary Reference Intakes, as described in Chapter 1 and Appendix B, adequacy of requirements is defined as the lowest daily intake value for a nutrient that will meet the need, as defined by the specified indicator or criterion of adequacy, of apparently healthy individuals. This section reviews some of the possible indicators used or proposed for use in analyses estimating human protein requirements.

Factorial Method

The factorial method is based on estimating the nitrogen (obligatory) losses that occur when a person is fed a diet that meets energy needs but is essentially protein free and, when appropriate, also relies on estimates of the amount of nitrogen that is accreted during periods of growth or lost to mothers during lactation. The major losses of nitrogen under most conditions are in urine and feces, but also include sweat and miscellaneous losses, such as nasal secretions, menstrual losses, or seminal fluid. In this method, the protein requirement is estimated by interpolating or extrapolating the obligatory losses to the zero balance point in which protein needs (as nitrogen) are assumed to equal the obligatory protein lost as nitrogen (nitrogen equilibrium).

This is where the factorial method has its greatest weakness, since the relationship between protein intake and nitrogen retention is somewhat curvilinear; the efficiency of nitrogen retention becomes less as the zero balance point is approached (Rand and Young, 1999; Young et al., 1973). Additionally, in order to utilize the factorial approach when determining the protein requirement for infants and children, their needs for protein accreted as a result of growth must be added to their maintenance needs.

Nitrogen Balance Method

This classical method has been viewed by many as theoretically the most satisfactory way of determining the protein requirement. Nitrogen balance is the difference between nitrogen intake and the amount excreted in urine, feces, skin, and miscellaneous losses. As discussed below, nitrogen balance remains the only method that has generated sufficient data for the determination of the total protein (nitrogen) requirement. It is assumed that when needs are met or exceeded adults come into nitrogen balance; when intakes are inadequate, negative nitrogen balance results. In determining total protein (nitrogen) needs, high-quality proteins are utilized as test proteins to prevent negative nitrogen balance resulting from the inadequate intake of a limiting indispensable amino acid. A significant literature exists regarding the methods and procedures to use in determining nitrogen balance amount (Manatt and Garcia, 1992; Rand et al., 1981).

Limitations of the Method

The nitrogen balance method does have substantial practical limitations and problems. First, the rate of urea turnover in adults is slow, so several days of adaptation are required for each level of dietary protein tested to attain a new steady state of nitrogen excretion (Meakins and Jackson, 1996; Rand et al., 1976). Second, the execution of accurate nitrogen balance measurements requires very careful attention to all the details of the procedures involved. Since it is easy to overestimate intake and underestimate excretion, falsely positive nitrogen balances may be obtained (Hegsted, 1976). Indeed, an overestimate of nitrogen balance seems consistent throughout the literature because there are many observations of quite considerable apparent retention of nitrogen in adults (Oddoye and Margen, 1979). This observation is biologically implausible because (a) adults do not normally accrete body protein, and (b) the magnitude of the positive nitrogen balances is inconsistent with stability of body weight. A third limitation of the nitrogen balance method is that since the requirement is defined for the individual, and studies rarely provide exactly the amount of protein necessary to produce zero balance, individuals must be studied at several levels of protein intake in the region of the requirement so that estimates of individual requirements can be interpolated (Rand et al., 1976; Zello et al., 1990). Finally, dermal and miscellaneous losses of nitrogen must be included in the calculation. These are inordinately difficult to measure, and vary with the environmental conditions (e.g., ambient temperature). In fact, the literature indicates marked (at least twofold) differences between studies (Calloway et al., 1971). The inclusion of dermal and miscellaneous nitrogen losses can have a significant effect on estimates of amino acid requirements via nitrogen balance, especially in adults (Calloway et al., 1971; Millward, 1998; Rand and Young, 1999).

Statistical Analysis of Nitrogen Balance Data

In studies with healthy adults in presumably good nutritional status, it is generally assumed that the protein requirement is achieved when an individual is in zero nitrogen balance. To some extent, this assumption poses problems that may lead to underestimates of the true protein requirement. First, there are sufficient observations of paradoxically high positive nitrogen balances in the literature to imply that when individuals are in *measured* body nitrogen equilibrium, they are in fact in a small negative nitrogen balance (Kopple, 1987). The large majority of the studies have concentrated their measurements of protein adequacy at levels of intake below nitrogen balance and as a result, the intercept of protein intake at zero nitrogen balance is lower than the true intercept as the efficiency of protein utilization decreases as zero balance is reached (Young et al., 1973).

The empirical solution is to carry out measurements that span nitrogen equilibrium, ideally by using multiple levels of intake in the same individual and interpolating individual requirement levels. Three different interpolation schemes have been proposed, based on (1) a smooth nonlinear model (Hegsted, 1963; Rand and Young, 1999), (2) a two-phase linear model (also called bilinear or breakpoint) (Kurpad et al., 2001a; Zello et al., 1995), and (3) a linear model (Rand et al., 1976; Rand et al., 2003). Since the physiological response relationship between nitrogen intake and balance is theoretically expected not to be linear, the more complex models (1 and 2 above) would be appropriate bases for arriving at a requirement estimate. However, in order to set the Recommended Dietary Allowance (RDA), it is necessary to determine the variability of the requirement between individuals, free from the considerable within-individual variability, and both these models require more data points on each individual than are currently available in published studies.

Thus, while it is recognized that the first two models above are more realistic biologically, because of the lack of available data the method adopted for this report is to use linear interpolation to estimate the individual requirements (the intakes predicted to result in zero balance) that in turn are used to estimate the distribution of protein requirements. The bilinear model was used to estimate requirements for some of the amino acids; however, estimates of population variability (between individuals) were derived from the analysis of protein requirements.

SELECTION OF INDICATORS FOR ESTIMATING THE REQUIRMENT FOR INDIVIDUAL AMINO ACIDS

Irrespective of whether a design involving multiple studies in a limited number of individuals or single studies in a larger number of subjects has been used, the uniform approach to the determination of the requirement for an individual indispensable amino acid involves measuring the relationship between the intake of the amino acid (in an otherwise adequate diet) and some predetermined marker of nutritional adequacy. The marker can be one that follows the state of protein metabolism or balance (e.g., nitrogen balance or whole body protein turnover) or the status of the metabolism and utilization of the amino acid under investigation (e.g., its concentration). These approaches give somewhat different information about the requirement for the amino acid. Moreover, each method has peculiar theoretical and practical disadvantages, thus the level of consistency of estimates based on different approaches should be examined. The following approaches have been proposed.

Nitrogen Balance Method

This classical method is discussed earlier in more detail under "Selection of Indicators for Estimating the Requirement for Protein (Nitrogen)." It has been apparent for at least 15 years that the nitrogen balance–derived values for amino acid requirements in adults are lower than values derived by the other methods described below, which provide results similar to each other (Millward et al., 1990; Young, 1987; Young et al., 1989). Many explanations have been put forward for the lower results using nitrogen balance methodology, including the fact that excess nonprotein energy may have been used in many nitrogen balance studies (Garza et al., 1976, 1977a, 1977b, 1978).

Rand and Young (1999) analyzed the data of Jones and coworkers (1956) in which young women were fed up to five different intake levels of lysine. The design of that study allowed for the determination of between-individual variance by studying each individual at several levels of lysine intake. In fact, within the large nitrogen balance and amino acid requirement literature, only one other study (Reynolds et al., 1958) was found in which adults were studied at four or more different intakes of amino acids with constant levels of total nitrogen (Reynolds et al., 1958). These investigators studied four different levels of methionine and cysteine.

With these two data sets, nonlinear regression can be utilized. The reanalysis of the 1956 Jones study produced an estimate of nitrogen equilibrium for lysine of 30 mg/kg/d, which is comparable to the values derived by the other methods described below (Rand and Young, 1999). In addition, most of the classic amino acid work using nitrogen balance (Leverton et al., 1956a, 1956b, 1956c, 1956d; Rose, 1957; Rose et al., 1955a, 1955b, 1955c, 1955d, 1955e, 1955f) did not include dermal and miscellaneous losses, which result in further underestimation of indispensable amino acid requirements.

Unfortunately, for infants and children the only data available are those based on nitrogen balance, and considerable uncertainty about the accuracy of the estimates remains. However, recent factorial estimates are in reasonable agreement with the nitrogen balance estimates (Dewey et al., 1996).

Plasma Amino Acid Response Method

This method was the first that focused on the physiology of the individual amino acid (Longnecker and Hause, 1959; Munro, 1970). The reasoning behind this approach is that when the intake of the test amino acid is below its dietary requirement, then its circulating concentration is not only low, but also is relatively insensitive to changes in intake. As intakes of the target amino acid approach the requirement level by increasing the intake of the limiting amino acid, the plasma level of the amino acid starts to increase progressively (see Figure 10-4). The point at which the "constant" portion of the relationship between intake and plasma concentration intersects the linear portion is considered to be an estimate of the requirement.

A variation on this method involves the examination of the changes in the plasma concentration of the test amino acid as the adult moves from the post absorptive to the fed state post-consumption (Longnecker and Hause, 1961). At intakes below the requirement, the plasma concentration of the test amino acid is expected to fall in the fed state and rise only when the dietary supply of the amino acid is greater than the individual's

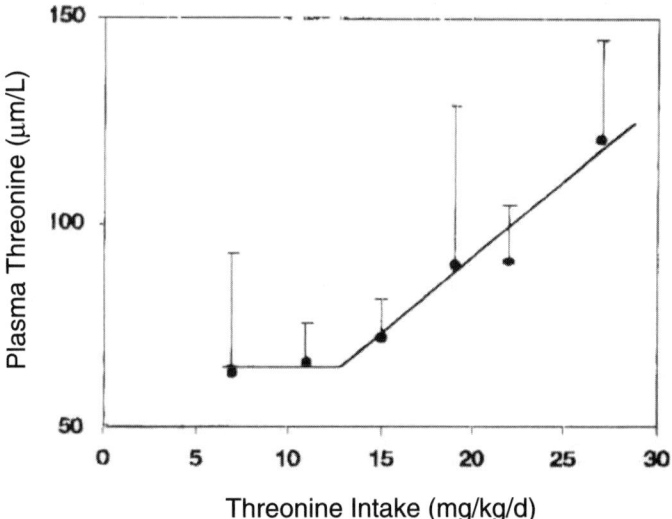

FIGURE 10-4 Plasma threonine levels in the fed state with increasing levels of threonine intake in well-nourished men. Two-phase regression revealed a breakpoint at about 13 mg/kg/d. Taken from Kurpad and Young (2001), with permission.

requirement. The theoretical basis of the approach is sound but the method has disadvantages. The main difficulty is that amino acid metabolism is so complex that factors other than the level of amino acid intake, such as gastric emptying time, can influence its concentration (Munro, 1970). Furthermore, the relationship between the intake of the amino acid and its circulating concentration is not necessarily bilinear, so it is difficult to determine a "breakpoint" (Young et al., 1972). Although in some regards this problem applies also to the oxidation methods discussed below, over the last 20 years these later methods have supplanted plasma amino acid concentration–based approaches.

Direct Amino Acid Oxidation (DAAO) Method

In the 1980s, Young and his coworkers introduced the use of measurements of the carbon oxidation of single indispensable amino acids as indicators of adequacy of the amino acids (Young et al., 1989). This marked a major theoretical advance over the nitrogen balance and plasma amino acid response methods. The theoretical basis of the direct amino acid oxidation (DAAO) method is that the nutritional indispensability of an amino acid is a function of its inability to synthesize its carbon skeleton.

Thus, when the test amino acid is labeled with ^{13}C, the production of breath $^{13}CO_2$ is assumed to be a good measure of the irreversible oxidative loss of the amino acid.

The method has been applied in a similar manner to the plasma amino acid response approach by designing experiments to determine a break-point in the relationship between the carbon catabolism of the amino acid (as measured as breath $^{13}CO_2$) and its intake. Thus by analogy to the concentration method, it is assumed that below the requirement the test amino acid is conserved and that there is a low constant oxidation rate, but once the requirement is reached, the oxidation of the test amino acid increases progressively.

Although the DAAO method was an important advance beyond nitrogen balance, it also presented limitations, which have been discussed in depth (Fuller and Garlick, 1994). The most salient problem arises from the reliance on the determination of a breakpoint in the oxidation of the test amino acid. This reliance requires studies at very low intakes of the test amino acid. However, at these low dietary intakes, the intake of the infused labeled amino acid becomes significant in relation to dietary intake. This can lead to errors in the estimation of amino acid oxidation based on the production of labeled CO_2. Thus, values of amino acid oxidation based on the production of $^{13}CO_2$ are likely to be overestimated. The second limitation is that the DAAO method can only be used with full accuracy for those amino acids whose carboxyl group is released directly to the body bicarbonate pools. This limits its use largely to the branched chain amino acids, phenylalanine, and lysine. Other amino acids, such as threonine and tryptophan, pose particular problems (Zhao et al., 1986).

A criticism of this method has been that measurements were only made during a short period during which food was given at regular hourly intervals. This period was therefore not representative of the day as a whole. A later modification of this approach was to infuse the labeled amino acid during a period of fasting followed by a period of hourly meals, thus acknowledging the discontinuous way in which food is normally taken (Young et al., 1987). However, although this was an advance on the earlier approach, assumptions still had to be made to extrapolate the results from the short periods to a full day.

Twenty-four Hour Amino Acid Balance Method

Over the last decade, the DAAO method has been adapted in such a way that it allows the carbon balance of the amino acid under investigation to be determined over a full 24-hour period (El-Khoury et al., 1994a, 1994b). In some respects, the development of the 24-hour amino acid balance method stemmed from the fact that the DAAO method had been criticized because measurements were made only in the fed state. Thus the 24-hour amino acid balance method was developed to determine the balance of the test amino acid over a 24-hour period that encompassed periods of fasting and feeding. This marked a significant advance in determining amino acid requirements because it moved investigations away from the simple study of nitrogen metabolism and allowed, in principle at least, direct measurements of the quantities of the amino acid lost under different nutritional circumstances.

There also are drawbacks to this method. The first limitation arises from the unresolved questions related to the method's theoretical basis. Although the end point of the method is the measurement of the body's balance of the test amino acid, the base measurement is the proportion of the dose of ^{13}C-amino acid that is excreted as $^{13}CO_2$. In order to convert the measured rate of production of labeled CO_2 to a rate of oxidation of the amino acid, it is necessary to know the isotopic enrichment of the amino acid at the intracellular site of oxidation. This is difficult because amino acid metabolism is compartmentalized and measurements of plasma amino acid labeling likely underestimate true turnover, and hence true oxidative loss, of the amino acid. Although for some amino acids this problem can be circumvented by administering a labeled metabolic product of the amino acid (e.g., α-keto isocaproic acid in studies of leucine metabolism).

The second drawback is practical—measuring the oxidation of the test amino acid over a complete 24-hour period makes the method labor intensive. This probably underlies the fact that to date this method has been applied to only three amino acids: leucine (El-Khoury et al., 1994a, 1994b; Kurpad et al., 2001b), lysine (El-Khoury et al., 2000; Kurpad et al., 2001a), and phenylalanine with and without tyrosine (Basile-Filho et al., 1998), and only a limited number of different levels of amino acid intake have been investigated.

Indicator Amino Acid Oxidation (IAAO) Method

The indicator amino acid oxidation (IAAO) method arose from work on the amino acid requirements of neonatal pigs (Kim et al., 1983). Although the IAAO method is based on measurements of amino acid oxidation, it uses measurements of the carbon catabolism of a nonlimiting amino acid (called the indicator amino acid) as a carbon analogue of nitrogen balance. The reasoning is that when a single indispensable amino acid is provided below its requirement, it acts as the single and primary limitation to the ability to retain other nonlimiting amino acids in body protein. These other amino acids, including the indicator amino acid, are then in nutritional excess and are oxidized (Zello et al., 1995). When the intake of the test amino acid is zero, then protein synthesis is minimal and oxidation of the indicator is maximal. As the intake of the test amino acid is increased, protein retention increases and the oxidation of the indicator amino acid falls until the requirement level of the test amino acid is reached, after which the oxidation of the indicator amino acid is lower and essentially constant. The data are then analyzed to obtain as estimate of the intersection of the constant and linear portions of the relationship (the breakpoint).

The IAAO method has some advantages over the direct oxidation and carbon balance methods and has been validated in growing piglets by comparing estimates based on growth and body composition (Kim et al., 1983). The first advantage is that the metabolic restrictions of carbon dioxide release apply only to the indicator amino acid. Thus amino acids such as threonine, whose peculiar metabolism makes them problematical in the DAAO method, can be studied. Second, the pool size of the indicator amino acid does not change radically as the intake of the test amino acid is varied. Thus to some extent, potential problems of compartmentation are minimized and, in principle, the method does not require estimates of the turnover of the indicator amino acid.

However, the IAAO method also has several limitations as it has been applied. First, like the DAAO approach, it has only been used in the fed state and the extent to which the fasting-state oxidation of the indicator amino acid is altered by the status of the limiting amino acid has not been determined. Second, the dependence of the result on the amount of total protein given during the isotope infusion has not been established. Third, the choice of the best indicator is still under study so that data obtained with the method are dependent on the assumption of the general applicability of the indicator amino acids (phenylalanine and lysine) that have been used most frequently.

Classical nitrogen balance studies in humans show that it takes 7 to 10 days for urinary nitrogen to equilibrate in adults put on a protein-free diet (Rand et al., 1976). On the other hand, it has been shown that most (about 90 percent) of the adaptation in leucine kinetics is complete in 24 hours (Motil et al., 1994). Zello and coworkers (1990) studied 2- to 8-day adaptation periods to either 4.2 or 14 mg/kg/d of phenylalanine on rates of phenylalanine oxidation at phenylalanine intakes of 5, 7, 10, 14, 21, 28, or 60 mg/kg/d. These investigators were unable to show any effect of prior adaptation to these two different phenylalanine intakes on the rates of phenylalanine oxidation at changing phenylalanine intakes, where the adaptation to the test level was about 4 hours. Clearly, from this study, adaptations in amino acid metabolism appear to take place much more quickly than do adaptations in urinary nitrogen excretion and are (at least for leucine [Motil et al., 1994]) virtually complete within 24 hours.

The most satisfactory statistical models for determining amino acid requirements use regression to define the population mean and variance. For the regression models to work, ranges of intake (particularly at the low end) have to be fed. In practical terms, this has greatly hampered studies in infants, children, and other vulnerable groups. On the other hand, if the individual only needs to be on a low or even zero intake of the test amino acid for a matter of 8 hours, then it becomes feasible to study indispensable amino acids in these and other vulnerable groups.

Such a minimally invasive indicator oxidation model has been developed (Bross et al., 1998) and applied to determine tyrosine requirements in children with phenylketonuria (Bross et al., 2000). In this model the oxidation study is conducted after only 6 hours of adaptation to the level of the test amino acid, which is administered every 30 minutes.

For amino acid oxidation measurements, two-phase linear crossover regression analysis was introduced during the validation of indicator amino acid oxidation in piglets (Kim et al., 1983). Later, this approach was transferred to humans in a direct oxidation study (Zello et al., 1990) and in indicator oxidation studies (Bross et al., 2000; Zello et al., 1993). This technique permits a precise determination of the breakpoint, which is used as the estimate of the requirement for the amino acid Estimated Average Requirement (EAR).

As pointed out above, the drawbacks of the indicator method are the short period of measurement in the fed state only, and the lack of a period of adaptation to the test diets. To avoid these drawbacks, a 24-hour indicator method has been developed (Kurpad et al., 2001a), which takes advantage of the strengths of the indicator approach, as well as the 24-hour period of measurements including feeding and fasting. On theoretical grounds, this method has advantages over other methods for estimating amino acid requirements, and is the chosen method for estimated amino acids requirements where data are available.

FINDINGS BY LIFE STAGE AND GENDER GROUP FOR TOTAL PROTEIN

Infants Ages 0 Through 6 Months

Method Used to Set the Adequate Intake

The recommended intakes of protein are based on an Adequate Intake (AI) that reflects the observed mean protein intake of infants fed principally with human milk.

Human Milk. Human milk is recognized as the optimal source of nutrients for infants throughout at least the first year of life and is recommended as the sole nutritional source for infants during the first 4 to 6 months of life (IOM, 1991). There are no reports of apparently healthy, full-term infants, exclusively fed human milk, who manifest any signs of protein deficiency (Heinig et al., 1993). Therefore, determination of the AI for protein for infants is based on data from infants fed human milk as the principal source of nutrients during the period 0 through 6 months of age. As is described in Chapter 2, the AI is set at the mean value calculated from studies in which the volume of human milk was measured by test weighing, and the average concentration of the protein content in human milk was determined using average values from several reported studies.

The protein content of human milk at various stages of lactation is shown in Table 10-7. In general, protein concentrations decline in the later stages of lactation. Nonprotein nitrogen contributes 20 to 27 percent of total milk nitrogen (Atkinson et al., 1980; Butte et al., 1984a, 1984b; Dewey et al., 1996). These nonprotein nitrogenous components include free amino acids, pyrimidine nucleotides, creatine, and glutathione, but the large majority is urea. Using data from 13 lactating mothers of term infants, Butte and coworkers (1984a) reported that the protein content of human milk was 1.29 g/dL at 2 weeks of lactation, 1.08 g/dL at 4 weeks, 1.01 g/dL at 6 weeks, 0.94 g/dL at 8 weeks, and 0.91 g/dL from 10 to 12 weeks. Similar results of 0.91 g/dL were reported by Lammi-Keefe and coworkers (1990) at 8 weeks of lactation in 6 mothers of term infants. Both of these studies analyzed nitrogen by the Kjeldahl method. However, higher human milk protein content has been reported by Nommsen and coworkers (1991): 1.21 g/dL at 3 months, 1.14 g/dL at 6 months, 1.16 g/dL at 9 months, and 1.24 g/dL at 12 months of lactation. Dewey and coworkers (1984) reported values of approximately 1.25 g/dL at 4 to 11 months of lactation. These latter investigators attribute the higher values to their utilization of the modified Lowry assay for total protein, which tends to result in slightly higher values (Nommsen et al., 1991).

Ages 0 Through 6 Months. The AI for infants 0 through 6 months is based on the estimated average volume of milk intake of 0.78 L/d (Allen et al., 1991; Heinig et al., 1993) for this age group, and an average protein content of human milk of 11.7 g/L. This is the average protein content of human milk during the first six months of lactation from studies (Butte et al., 1984a; Dewey and Lönnerdal, 1983; Dewey et al., 1984; Nommsen et al., 1991) in which the sample size was at least 10 and actual data were provided (see Table 10-7). This value is in the range of protein content reported in other studies (Table 10-7). Multiplying this amount by the estimated average volume of intake of human milk for infants 0 through

6 months, the AI would be 11.7 g/L × 0.78 L/d = 9.1 g/d or 1.52 g/kg/d based on the reference weight of 6 kg for the 2- through 6-month-old infant from Chapter 1 (Table 1-1).

Protein AI Summary, Ages 0 Through 6 Months

AI for Infants
  0–6 months   **1.52 g/kg/d**

Special Considerations

Although protein intakes have been reported to be 66 to 70 percent higher in infants fed formula compared with those fed human milk for up to 12 months of age, there is no evidence that the lower protein intakes in the breast-fed infants were associated with adverse outcomes (Heinig et al., 1993). In fact, despite their lower protein intakes, some studies have demonstrated that infants fed human milk have better immune function and behavioral development than formula-fed infants (IOM, 1991; Lucas et al., 1992; Rogan and Gladen, 1993). As expected, gains in weight and lean body mass are higher in the formula-fed than breast-fed infants, but when controlled for energy intake, protein intake is not associated with weight or length gain within the breast-fed infants (Heinig et al., 1993). Several studies have shown that infants fed formula with a true protein level ([total nitrogen – nonprotein nitrogen] multiplied by 6.25) of 15 g/L have higher urea nitrogen and plasma amino acid levels than those seen in breast-fed infants (Janas et al., 1985, 1987; Järvenpää et al., 1982a, 1982b; Räihä et al., 1986a, 1986b), a true protein intake of 13 g/L of infant formula based on cow milk has been shown to result in a similar plasma amino acid profile in formula-fed infants to that seen in breast-fed infants (Lönnerdal and Chen, 1990).

It is recognized that casein and whey in cow milk is not the same as human casein and whey and that the absorption and digestibility of amino acids from formula is different than that of human milk. The 1985 Joint FAO/WHO/UNU expert group (FAO/WHO/UNU, 1985) recommended a factor of 0.70 for protein in cow milk, finding that it is 70 percent as efficiently utilized as the protein in human milk based on studies in 1-year-old infants. Later Fomon (1991) recommended a conversion estimate of 90 percent for infants receiving infant formula as the only source of dietary protein and suggested that infant formula should contain a minimum of 1.6 g α-amino nitrogen/100 kcal. Thus in determining the level of protein to be included in infant formula based on various possible protein sources, it is important to evaluate the digestibility and comparative protein quality (see "Protein Quality") as indicated above.

TABLE 10-7 Protein Content of Human Milk in the United States and Canada

Reference	Country	n	Stage of Lactation	Protein Content in Milk (g/dL)[a]	Comments
Anderson et al., 1981	Canada	10	3–5 d 8–11 d 15–18 d 25–29 d	1.9 1.7 1.5 1.3	Milk protein content was approximated from study figure Nitrogen determined by Kjeldahl analysis
Lemons et al., 1982	United States	7	7 d 14 d 21 d 28 d	1.59 ± 0.08 1.23 ± 0.09 1.18 ± 0.04 1.10 ± 0.05	Nitrogen determined by Kjeldahl analysis Protein determined by multiplying milk protein nitrogen by 6.25
Anderson et al., 1983	United States	9	3 d 7 d 14 d	2.3 ± 0.6 1.7 ± 0.2 1.3 ± 0.4	Nitrogen determined by Kjeldahl analysis
Dewey and Lönnerdal, 1983	United States	13 16 18 16 14 15	1 mo 2 mo 3 mo 4 mo 5 mo 6 mo	**1.44 ± 0.20** **1.33 ± 0.16** **1.32 ± 0.16** **1.30 ± 0.24** **1.25 ± 0.17** **1.27 ± 0.36**	Protein analyzed by dye-binding assay
Neville et al., 1984	United States	10	33–210 d (median 115 d)	1.41 ± 0.06 (SEM)	Protein analyzed by the Biuret reaction Mid-feed sample

Reference	Country	Age	n	Protein (g/L)	Notes
Dewey et al., 1984	United States	4–6 mo 7–11 mo	40 27	**1.26 ± 0.27** *1.24 ± 0.22*	Protein analyzed by a modified Lowry assay
Butte et al., 1984a	United States	2 wk 4 wk 6 wk 8 wk 10 wk 12 wk	13	1.29 ± 0.18 **1.08 ± 0.16** **1.01 ± 0.10** **0.94 ± 0.15** **0.91 ± 0.16** **0.91 ± 0.16**	Nitrogen determined by Kjeldahl analysis. Protein determined by multiplying milk protein nitrogen by 6.25
Lönnerdal et al., 1987	United States	1–3 d 7–20 d 32–166 d	3 4 7	2.70 ± 0.18 (SEM) 1.61 ± 0.10 1.02 ± 0.05	Nitrogen determined by Kjeldahl analysis. Protein determined by multiplying milk protein nitrogen by 6.25
Lammi-Keefe et al., 1990	United States	8 wk	6	0.91	Nitrogen determined by Kjeldahl analysis. Protein determined by multiplying milk protein nitrogen by 6.25
Nommsen et al., 1991	United States	3 mo 6 mo 9 mo 12 mo	58 45 28 21	**1.21 ± 0.15** **1.14 ± 0.15** *1.16 ± 0.18* *1.24 ± 0.15*	Protein analyzed by a modified Lowry assay

[a] Mean ± standard deviation, unless otherwise noted. Values in bold used to estimate average protein content of human milk as 11.7 g/L during months 1 through 6 of lactation. Values in italics used to estimate average protein content of human milk as 12.3 g/L during months 7 through 12 of lactation.

Infants Ages 7 Through 12 Months

Method Used to Estimate Average Intakes

During the second 6 months of life, solid foods become a more important part of the diet of infants and add a significant amount of protein to the diet. Although limited data are available for typical protein intakes from foods by infants fed human milk, mean protein intake from complementary foods for infants aged 7 through 12 months was estimated to be 7.1 g/d for human milk–fed infants based on data from the Third National Health and Nutrition Examination Survey. Heinig and coworkers (1993) reported slightly higher values for nonmilk protein intake during the second 6 months of life. Based on their data, the average volume of human milk consumed during the second 6 months of life would be about 0.6 L/d. Thus, protein intake from human milk with a protein content of about 12.1 g/L at 7 to 12 months of lactation from the data for this age group (Dewey et al., 1984; Nommsen et al., 1991) would be approximately 7.3 g/d (12.1 g/L × 0.6 L/d). It should be noted that this is greater than that derived from the studies of content of milk from earlier lactation periods, primarily due to the use of the Lowry methods by both of these reports and the small number of studies available from this lactation period.

Adding the intake from milk (7.3 g/d) and food (7.1 g/d), the total average protein intake is estimated to be 14.4 g/d or 1.6 g/kg/d based on the reference weight of 9 kg for the 7- through 12-month-old infant from Chapter 1 (Table 1-1).

Method Used to Estimate the Average Requirement

Published data on the relationship between protein (nitrogen) intake and nitrogen balance were utilized to estimate protein requirements by the factorial method for infants 7 through 12 months of age as well as for children and adolescents through 18 years of age. The factorial method includes: (1) estimates of the maintenance requirement, which is determined by regression analysis of the relationship between nitrogen intake and nitrogen balance, (2) measurement of the rates of protein deposition, which are derived from body composition analysis, and (3) estimates of the efficiency of protein utilization, which is derived from the slope of the line relating intake and balance from the available data on infants and children.

Several nitrogen balance studies that involved children in the age range of 9 months to about 14 years were identified and analyzed (Table 10-8). The studies fall into three groups: (1) studies designed to measure "basal" nitrogen loss at very low or zero protein intakes, (2) studies involving children receiving only one of a variety of protein levels, and (3) studies involving a limited number of individuals but with each individual receiving a range of protein intakes. Included in the analysis were studies in which the children consumed diets containing milk/egg, legume/cereal, and mixed vegetable/animal protein sources. The results, summarized in Table 10-8, were obtained in mostly boys and include a number of different ethnic groups including European, African, Central American, and Chinese.

Miscellaneous Losses. A critical aspect of the analysis is the inclusion of an estimate for integumental and unaccounted losses that were based on direct measurements in children, mostly boys, aged 7 months through 14 years. On the basis of five reports (Howat et al., 1975; Huang et al., 1980; Korslund et al., 1976; Uauy et al., 1981; Viteri and Martinez, 1981), the mean miscellaneous nitrogen losses are estimated to be 6.5 (± 2.3) mg/kg/d with a range of 5 to 9 mg/kg/d. In deriving the protein requirement, this estimate of miscellaneous losses was included as an adjustment to the reported nitrogen balances for the studies included in Table 10-8. The miscellaneous losses from both boys and girls are assumed to be the same since data from girls were limited.

Maintenance Requirement. Individual maintenance protein requirements were estimated by first regressing nitrogen balance on nitrogen intake for the individuals studied at several different intake levels, and then using these individual regression equations to interpolate the intakes that would be expected to produce zero nitrogen balance (adjusting for 6.5 mg/kg/d for miscellaneous losses). Table 10-8 contains seven studies that permit estimation of individual requirements and three studies that were used to estimate pooled requirements. As shown in the table, the average individual maintenance requirement was estimated as the median of the individual nitrogen requirements (108 mg/kg/d). For each study, an estimate was calculated as the median of the individual studies or the study pooled nitrogen requirement for those studies without individual data, and was 110 mg/kg/d . Since data for girls were sparse and could not be separated from that for boys, the protein maintenance requirement for both boys and girls is set at the same level. In addition, the maintenance protein requirement was not adjusted for age, as the requirement per kg of body weight for children 8 years of age and above appeared to be similar to that of younger children ranging in age from 9 months to 5 years (Table 10-8). Supporting this decision are the data of Widdowson and Dickerson (1964), which demonstrated that around 4 years of age, body protein concentration reaches the adult value of 18 to 19 percent of body weight.

TABLE 10-8 Maintenance Protein Requirement for Children Based on Nitrogen Balance Data[a]

Reference	Country	Diet	Age
Huang et al., 1980	China	Milk	9–17 mo
Huang et al., 1980	China	Egg	9–17 mo
Intengan et al., 1981	Philippines	Rice and fish	18–26 mo
Torun and Viteri, 1981	Guatemala	Milk	17–31 mo
Torun et al., 1981	Guatemala	Soy	17–31 mo
Egana et al., 1984	Chile	Milk	34–62 mo
Egana et al., 1984	Chile	Soy	34–62 mo
Intengan, 1984	Philippines	Rice and beans	22–29 mo
Gattas et al., 1990	Chile	Mixed	8–10 y
Gattas et al., 1992	Chile	Mixed	12–14 y
Median of all individual estimates (n = 7 studies)			
Median of all studies (n = 10)			

[a] Entries are medians (mean ± standard deviation).
[b] Multiple data on each individual not available.
[c] Regression estimate of study requirement.

Protein Deposition. Estimates of rates of protein deposition for infants from 9 months through 3 years of age (Butte et al., 2000) and total body protein content from 4 through 18 years of age (Ellis et al., 2000) were utilized to estimate rates of body protein deposition and are shown in Table 10-9. This table contains longitudinal (Butte et al., 2000) and cross-

n	Intercept at 6.5 mg N/kg/d	Slope	Maintenance Requirement Including 6.5 mg N/kg/d
32 points[b] (24 boys)	−77.5[c]	0.69[c]	112[c]
29 points[b] (10 boys)	−81.6[c]	0.71[c]	116[c]
7 boys	−53.6 (−47.4 ± 26.0)	0.52 (0.49 ± 0.10)	102 (91 ± 37)
10 boys	−52.0 (−51.1 ± 22.1)	0.70 (0.71 ± 0.12)	66 (71 ± 28)
10 boys	−55.5 (−52.2 ± 14.5)	0.55 (0.58 ± 0.09)	90 (89 ± 18)
6 boys and girls	−35.4 (−40.1 ± 16.2)	0.52 (0.51 ± 0.08)	76 (79 ± 27)
7 boys and girls	−58.2 (−59.4 ± 9.9)	0.51 (0.49 ± 0.10)	127 (124 ± 19)
5 boys	−98.1 (−121.1 ± 43.7)	0.68 (0.77 ± 0.24)	149 (156 ± 15)
8 boys	−67.3 (−55.4 ± 39.2)	0.54 (0.43 ± 0.29)	126 (126 ± 11)
8 boys (pooled)[b]	−61.4[c]	0.57[c]	107[c]
53	−57.5 (−57.9 ± 32.3)	0.56 (0.57 ± 0.19)	108 (101 ± 35)
	−57.4	0.58	110

sectional (Ellis et al., 2000) data based on a combination of water dilution, whole body potassium, and dual-energy x-ray absorptiometry (DXA) scanning methods used to estimate body composition. To obtain protein deposition rates since the data in young children were longitudinal (Butte et al., 2000), and the data in older children were cross-sectional (Ellis et

TABLE 10-9 Mean Daily Rates of Protein Deposition and Factorial Model Calculations of Mean Requirements for Protein

Age (y)	Girls		Boys	
	Protein Deposition[a] (mg/kg/d)	Mean Requirement[b] (g/kg/d)	Protein Deposition[a] (mg/kg/d)	Mean Requirement[b] (g/kg/d)
0.75	183	1.00	180	1.00
1	150	0.94	150	0.94
1.5	112	0.88	116	0.89
2	91	0.84	96	0.85
3	57	0.78	54	0.78
1–3	103	0.86	104	0.87
4	48	0.77	44	0.76
5	44	0.76	40	0.76
6	48	0.77	42	0.76
7	46	0.76	46	0.76
8	42	0.76	51	0.77
4–8	46	0.77	45	0.77
9	48	0.77	55	0.78
10	36	0.74	51	0.77
11	35	0.75	48	0.77
12	39	0.75	48	0.77
13	29	0.74	41	0.76
9–13	37	0.75	49	0.77
14	23	0.73	38	0.75
15	19	0.72	34	0.74
16	8	0.70	28	0.73
17	0	0.69	19	0.72
18	0	0.69	6	0.70
14–18	10	0.71	25	0.71

[a] Deposition was derived from the data for protein accumulation in children (Butte et al., 2000; Ellis et al., 2000), which were fitted to the following polynomial equations. The gradients at specific ages in the range 4 through 17 years were determined by differentiation of the regression equation. The growth rates given by Butte et al. (2000) were employed for ages 0.75 through 2 years.

Girls protein content = $-0.00027 \times$ age $(y)^4 + 0.00816 \times$ age $(y)^3 - 0.0665 \times$ age $(y)^2 + 0.51819 \times$ age $(y) + 0.60856$ ($R^2 = 0.9946$).

Boys protein content = $-0.00047 \times$ age $(y)^4 + 0.01663 \times$ age $(y)^3 - 0.16613 \times$ age $(y)^2 + 0.95166 \times$ age $(y) + 0.36037$ ($R^2 = 0.9966$).

notes continue

al., 2000), the data for body protein content from the two studies were pooled and regressed on age, giving a smooth curve and yielding the polynomial equations that are shown in footnote a in Table 10-9. Inclusion of data from the young children (Butte et al., 2000) improved the fit over the range of ages 4 through 18 years, but the fit at the younger ages, near the tail of the curve, was not satisfactory. Hence, the gradients at specific ages in the age range 4 through 18 years were determined by differentiation of the regression equation, whereas for ages 9 months through 2 years, the growth rates given by Butte and coworkers (2000) were employed.

Protein EAR Summary, Ages 7 Through 12 Months

The Estimated Average Requirement (EAR) is estimated by the factorial method by taking the median (110 mg nitrogen/kg/d equivalent to 688 mg protein/kg/d) of the nitrogen intake for nitrogen equilibrium (thus measuring maintenance requirement only) derived from Table 10-8, plus the product of 1.72 (the reciprocal of the slope [0.58] of those data, which estimates the efficiency of protein utilization for growth) and the mean protein deposition (Table 10-9) for boys and for girls. The resulting mean protein requirement is estimated to be 1.0 g/kg/d for boys and for girls.

EAR for Older Infants
7–12 months   1.0 g/kg/d

Protein RDA Summary, Ages 7 Through 12 Months

The Recommended Dietary Allowance (RDA) is defined as covering 97.5 percent of the age group. Thus, the EAR must be increased by an amount equal to two times its standard deviation to cover the needs of almost all of this age group. The variation in requirements is based on both the variation in maintenance needs and the variation in the rate of protein deposition (protein for growth).

---

b Mean requirement = maintenance requirement from Table 10-8 or 10-12 + dietary amount needed from protein deposition by life stage and gender group.

Median requirement for ages 0.75 through 13 years = 688 mg protein/kg/d (110 mg N/kg/d [Table 10-8] × 6.25 mg protein/kg N) + (1.72 [efficiency of protein utilization derived from reciprocal of slope in Table 10-8] × mean protein deposition for life stage and gender group).

Median requirement for ages 14 through 18 years = 656 mg protein/kg/d (105 mg N/kg/d [Table 10-12] × 6.25 mg protein/kg N) + (2.13 [the efficiency of protein utilization derived from reciprocal of slope in Table 10-12 = 0.47] × mean protein deposition).

Due to lack of adequate data on this age group, the variation in maintenance requirement for protein was assumed to be the same in children of all ages as in adults. Thus, the coefficient of variation (CV) for maintenance for this age group is 12 percent, the same as the CV of the protein requirement for adults developed by Rand and coworkers (2003) (see "Adults Ages 19 Through 30 Years"). A coefficient of variation for growth of 43 percent was determined in a study of whole body potassium-40 content in children (Butte et al., 2002). The total variation from both sources combined is calculated from the formula:

$$SD_T = (\sqrt{[CV_M \times \text{maintenance requirement}]^2 + [CV_G \times \text{growth requirement}]^2}),$$

where CV_M is 0.12, the maintenance requirement is 0.688 g protein/kg/d, CV_G is 0.43, and the growth requirement is the rate of protein deposition divided by the efficiency of dietary protein utilization. This yields the following formula:

$$SD_T = (\sqrt{[0.12 \times 0.688 \text{ g protein/kg/d}]^2 + [0.43 \times 1.72 \times Y \text{ g protein/kg/d}^2]}),$$

where $Y = 0.182$ g/kg/d (average of value for boys and girls from Table 10-9).

The RDA is then calculated as the RDA = EAR + 2 × SD_T, yielding the formula:

$$RDA = EAR + 2 \times (\sqrt{[0.12 \times 0.688 \text{ g protein/kg/d}]^2 + [0.43 \times 1.72 \times 0.182 \text{ g protein/kg/d}]^2})$$

The estimated amount by which to increase the EAR to cover 97.5 percent of older infants is thus the EAR + 2 (0.101 g protein/kg/d) = 1.0 + 0.2 g protein/kg/d for a total of 1.2 g/kg/d of protein. This value is slightly lower than the AI for protein based on mean protein content of human milk and the intake from complementary foods of 1.6 g/kg/d.

RDA for Older Infants
7–12 months   1.2 g/kg/d or 11.0 g/d of protein[1]

---

[1]Due to a calculation error in the prepublication copy, the value is changed from 1.5 g/kg/d to 1.2 g/kg/d and for the reference infant from 13.5 g/d to 11.0 g/d.

Children Ages 1 Through 13 Years

Protein EAR Summary, Ages 1 Through 13 Years

The Estimated Average Requirement (EAR) is estimated by the factorial method, which adds the amount needed for maintenance based on body weight to the amount estimated to be needed for protein deposition. The mean of the nitrogen intake for nitrogen equilibrium (thus measuring maintenance requirement only) is derived from all of the individual estimates for children and is 110 mg nitrogen/kg/d or 688 mg protein/kg/d (110 × 6.25) (Table 10-8). This is increased by the product of 1.72 (the reciprocal of the slope [0.58] of that data, which estimates the amount of protein utilization) and the efficiency of utilization as estimated by Rand and coworkers (2003) for adults (see "Adults Ages 19 Years and Older"). This is multiplied by the mean protein deposition (Table 10-9) for boys and for girls for each age group. Given the assumptions in this method and the few girls in the studies included in Tables 10-8 and 10-9, the EAR is set at the average for boys and girls in each age group.

EAR for Boys and Girls
1–3 years	**0.87 g/kg/d of protein**[2]
4–8 years	**0.76 g/kg/d of protein**
9–13 years	**0.76 g/kg/d of protein**

Protein RDA Summary, Ages 1 Through 13 Years

Assuming the variation of maintenance requirements for protein and protein deposition requirements vary, then the RDA is set as indicated at the 97.5th percentile, estimated as follows:

$$RDA = EAR + 2 \ (\sqrt{\ [0.12 \times 0.688 \text{ g protein/kg/d}]^2 + [0.43 \times 1.72 \times Y \text{ g protein/kg/d}]^2}),$$

where Y = 0.104 g for age group 1–3 years, 0.046 g for age group 4–8 years, and 0.043 g for age group 9–13 years. Numbers are rounded to nearest 0.05 g.

Using the reference values for body weight for each age group as shown in Table 1-1, the RDA for protein would be 13 g/d for ages 1–3 years, 19 g/d for 4–8 years, and 34 g/d for 9–13 years.

---

[2]Due to a calculation error in the prepublication copy, the value is changed from 0.88 g/kg/d to 0.87 g/kg/d.

RDA for Boys and Girls
   1–3 years   1.05 g/kg/d or 13 g/d of protein[3]
   4–8 years   0.95 g/kg/d or 19 g/d of protein
   9–13 years   0.95 g/kg/d of 34 g/d of protein

Adolescents Ages 14 Through 18 Years

Since data were not available to determine the maintenance protein requirement in children older than 14 years of age (Table 10-8), and since the maintenance nitrogen requirement of children (110 mg/kg/d) is similar to that for adults (105 mg/kg/d as shown in Table 10-12), the EAR for adolescents 14 through 18 years of age is based on the adult estimates of maintenance requirements from nitrogen balance studies (Rand et al., 2003), plus an additional amount to cover the needs for growth for this age as determined by the factorial method.

Protein EAR Summary, Ages 14 Through 18 Years

The maintenance requirement of adults of 105 mg nitrogen/kg/d or 656 mg protein/kg/d is added to the product of 2.13 (the reciprocal of the slope [0.47], which is the estimate of the efficiency of protein utilization in adults) (Rand et al., 2003), times the mean protein deposition as adjusted for efficiency of protein utilization (0.43), and calculated for boys or girls 14 through 18 years of age using the polynomial equations given in Table 10-9 to estimate protein deposition.

EAR for Boys
   14–18 years   0.73 g/kg/d of protein

EAR for Girls
   14–18 years   0.71 g/kg/d of protein

Protein RDA Summary, Ages 14 Through 18 Years

The RDA for protein for adolescents is set by determining the CV for maintenance and protein deposition. Since the CV of the maintenance requirement could not be calculated from the data shown in Table 10-8, and because of the similarity in maintenance requirements in children (Table 10-8; 110 mg N/kg/d) and adults (105 mg N/kg/d as estimated by

---

[3]Due to a calculation error in the prepublication copy, the value is changed from 1.10 g/kg/d to 1.05 g/kg/d.

Rand et al., [2003]), the CV in adults (12 percent) was also utilized to determine the variation in maintenance requirements for children and adolescents (see section "Protein RDA Summary, Ages 19–50 Years"). A CV of 43 percent for protein deposition was determined in the study of Butte and coworkers (2000), and this varied little with age and gender. Therefore, this value was used as the CV for growth for all ages.

The RDA is set for older adolescents as indicated at the 97.5th percentile, estimated as follows:

$$RDA = EAR + 2 \ (\sqrt{\ [0.12 \times 0.656 \text{ g protein/kg/d}]^2} \\ + [0.43 \times 2.13 \times Y \text{ g protein/kg/d}]^2),$$

where Y = 0.010 g for girls and 0.025 g for boys. Numbers are rounded to nearest 0.05 g.

Using the reference values for body weight shown in Table 1-1, the RDA for protein for girls 14–18 years of age would be 46 g/d, and for boys, 52 g/d.

RDA for Boys
14–18 years   **0. 85 g/kg/d of protein or 52 g/d of protein**

RDA for Girls
14–18 years   **0.85 g/kg/d of protein or 46 g/d of protein**

Adults Ages 19 Through 50 Years

Evidence Considered in Estimating the Average Requirement

In adults, protein requirement estimates have depended on one of two main approaches, namely, the factorial method and nitrogen balance response to different levels of intake of defined quality protein intakes. While the nitrogen balance method for estimation of protein requirements has serious shortcomings (see "Nitrogen Balance Method"), this method remains the primary approach for determining the protein requirement in adults, in large part because there is no validated or accepted alternative.

Nitrogen Balance Studies

Over the last 40 years, a number of analyses of available data on adult nitrogen balance studies have been utilized to estimate adult protein requirements; some reports are listed in Table 10-10. A growing body of data has accumulated that allows a more refined approach to such estimates, as improved techniques for measuring nitrogen output and controlling for

TABLE 10-10 Estimates of Adult Protein Requirements Using Nitrogen Balance Data

Reference	Estimates of Adult Protein Requirements for High Quality Protein (includes estimate of variation in requirements) (g/kg/d)		Estimation of Variation in Requirements (%)
	Men	Women	
FAO/WHO, 1965	0.71	0.71	10
FAO/WHO, 1973	0.60	0.60	15
FAO/WHO/UNU, 1985	0.75	0.75	12.5
Rand et al., 2003	0.80	0.80	12

external variables that impact nitrogen utilization have been implemented, and there has been a move toward standardization of study protocols.

The most recent in-depth analysis conducted at the request of the International Dietary Energy Consultative Group in 1996 and then more recently by the Food and Agriculture Organization, World Health Organization, and the United Nations University (FAO/WHO/UNU) included 19 studies conducted across the globe that measured and published nitrogen balance responses for 235 individuals given at least three levels of nitrogen intake for periods of 10 to 14 days (to be included in the analysis, it was required that individual data be available for at least three levels of intake adapted to by consuming the diet for least 10 days, with urinary and fecal nitrogen collection in the final 5 days of the diet period) (Rand et al., 2003). This was considered important so that estimates of individual requirements could be interpolated. In addition, 9 studies of individuals fed a single level of nitrogen intake or that only provided group data for multiple levels of intake (n = 174 individuals) were used to assess the fit of the analyses conducted (Rand et al., 2003). The studies used were classified on the basis of age of the adults (young: 19 through 52 years of age; old: 53 years of age and older); protein source (animal [animal sources provided > 90 percent of the total protein], vegetable [vegetable sources provided > 90 percent of the total protein], or mixed), as well as gender and climatic origin (temperate or tropical area), and corrected for skin and miscellaneous losses when not included in the nitrogen balance data (Rand et al., 2003). (See Appendix M for data on studies used.)

Analyses have also been made estimating endogenous protein loss in healthy adults when consuming protein-free diets adequate in all other respects. Estimates of endogenous loss from some of the various analyses of protein requirements are included in Table 10-11.

Methods Used to Estimate Individual Requirements

Earlier estimates of adult protein requirements (FAO/WHO, 1965) utilized information from endogenous nitrogen losses as the basis for determining protein requirements, assuming maximal utilization at levels near endogenous losses. However, as discussed in earlier sections, the efficiency of utilization of dietary protein declines as nitrogen equilibrium is reached. More recent approaches have averaged nitrogen balance data obtained from various studies where healthy individuals were given high-quality protein sources so that total nitrogen is considered the limiting dietary component rather than a specific indispensable amino acid (FAO/WHO/UNU, 1985).

With additional data it is possible to estimate requirements using regression analysis. Linear regression of nitrogen balance on nitrogen intake was utilized to estimate the nitrogen intake that would produce zero nitrogen balance in the most recent carefully done analysis available (Rand et al., 2003). In adults, it is generally presumed that the protein requirement is achieved when an individual is in zero nitrogen balance. To some extent, this assumption poses problems that may lead to underestimates of the true protein requirement (see "Nitrogen Balance Method").

Although the authors (Rand et al., 2003) acknowledge that it is known that the nitrogen response curve is nonlinear (because at high intakes the efficiency of nitrogen retention decreases), linear interpolation was utilized because the primary data utilized for the regression were gathered at intake levels close to those that were expected to produce zero balance. In this range there is no indication, either visually or statistically, for the utilization of an interpolation scheme other than linear (Rand et al., 2003). It was also recognized that while the use of more complex models would improve the standard error of fit, these models did not statistically improve the fits, in large part because of the small number of data points (3 to 6) for each individual (Rand et al., 2003).

Estimation of the Median Requirement

Utilizing the recent analysis of nitrogen balance data (Rand et al., 2003), the individual requirement estimates were found to be both significantly skewed and kurtotic, being characterized by more than expected very large or very small requirements (see Figure 10-5) (Rand et al., 2003).

TABLE 10-11 Estimates of Endogenous Loss of Nitrogen

Reference	Estimates of Urinary Losses (mg N/kg/d)		Estimates of Fecal Losses (mg N/kg/d)	Integumental Obligatory and Miscellaneous Losses (mg N/kg/d)	Total Endogenous Loss of Nitrogen (mg N/kg/d)
	Men	Women			
FAO/WHO, 1965	46	46	46	46	~ 100
FAO/WHO, 1973				5	
FAO/WHO/UNU, 1985 (n = 11 studies)	34	27	34	27	Men = 54 Women = 47 All = 52
Rand et al., 2003 (n = 14 studies)				5 temperate 11 tropical	Men = 50 Women = 35 All = 47

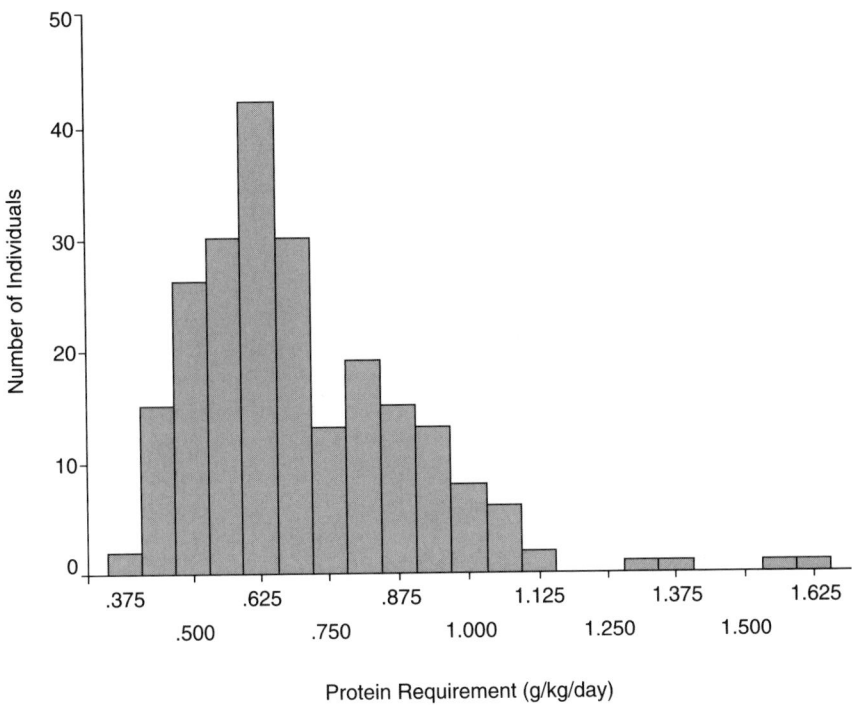

FIGURE 10-5 Distribution of the estimated protein requirements for 225 individuals (Rand et al., 2003) in a trimmed data set showing the skewness of protein requirement.
SOURCE: William Rand, personal communication, 2002.

The median requirement, potentially of use as the EAR, was calculated in two different ways: first as the median of the entire sample of 235 individuals in the primary data set (weighting all individuals the same), and second as the median of the medians of each distinct substudy (weighting each substudy equally) (Rand et al., 2003). In either case, data from all individuals were included in the analysis.

The results of these analyses are included in Table 10-12. Because of the non-normality of the individual data, nonparametric tests were used (Mann-Whitney and Kruskal-Wallis) to compare requirements between the age, gender, diet, and climate subgroups (Table 10-13). Where nonsignificant differences were found, Analysis of Variance was used for power calculations to roughly estimate the differences that could have been found with the data and variability. Separate analyses were conducted for all the

TABLE 10-12 Analyses of Linear Regression Analysis of Nitrogen Requirements in Adults

Data Sets Used	Linear Regression—Median Nitrogen Requirement (mg/kg/d)			Linear Regression—Slope	Intercept at 0 Intake (mg N/kg/d)
	Men	Women	All		
19 Estimation studies (n = 235; men = 181, women = 54)	109	91	105	0.47	–48
95% confidence intervals			(101, 110)	(0.44, 0.50)	(–51, –45)
32 substudies (n = 32 group medians; men = 24, women = 8)	102	102	102	0.49	–47
All individual data (n = 1,593)			103		
Linear regression model (grouped data)			122		
Quadratic regression model (grouped data)			114		
Asymptotic growth exponential (grouped data)			116		
Asymptote			42		
Linear bi-phase			108		
Breakpoint			126		
Asymptote			–7.2		

SOURCE: Rand et al. (2003).

individual requirements and for substudies, both excluding and including secondary estimation data (Rand et al., 2003).

Statistical Analysis of Nitrogen Balance Data to Determine the Protein Requirement

Data Analysis. The relationship between nitrogen balances, corrected for integumental and miscellaneous losses, and nitrogen intake from Rand and coworkers (2003) is shown in Figure 10-6. This figure includes individual data from the linear regression of nitrogen balance in adults examined (Rand et al., 2003). The authors noted that positive nitrogen balance was found in some individuals at nitrogen intakes as low as 60 mg/kg/d, and in other individuals negative balance was noted at nitrogen intakes as high as 200 mg/kg/d. This suggests that at least some of these individuals were not at constant nitrogen balance equilibrium.

In addition, while the nitrogen balance response to increasing nitrogen intake is theoretically expected to be nonlinear, the primary individual data points near the equilibrium balance point demonstrate a linear relationship, which appears to become nonlinear at high intakes. This can be attributed to different study designs in the test data included in Figure 10-6. The data points from only the estimation studies show a linear response over the relatively narrow range of intakes studied, while data points from the test studies also show a response that is not different from linear, although more variable and with a lower slope. Much variability is noted in the response data because the studies differ in methodology, individuals differ from each other, and an individual's response differs from day to day.

Table 10-12, a summary of the nitrogen requirement for all the data points included in the analysis by Rand and coworkers (2003), shows a nitrogen requirement of 105 mg/kg/d or 0.66 g protein/kg/d (105 mg N/kg/d × 6.25), with an approximately 95 percent confidence interval of 101 to 110 mg/kg/d (0.63 to 0.69 g protein/kg/d). When only the individual data points in the primary estimation studies are considered, the nitrogen requirement is 102 mg/kg/d (0.64 g protein/kg/d), and when all of the estimation study data points are considered, the nitrogen requirement is 103 mg/kg/d (0.64 g/kg/d). The median slope of the nitrogen balance response regression was 0.47 mg N/kg/d for all the data points, with a 95 percent confidence interval of 0.44 to 0.50 mg N/kg/d, which is in close agreement with the median slope of the primary estimation studies of 0.49 mg N/kg/d and all estimation studies of 0.47 mg N/kg/d.

Factor Analysis. Since all the data meeting the criteria for the meta-analysis were combined in the regression analysis by the authors (Rand et

TABLE 10-13 Factor Analysis: Estimation of Nitrogen Requirement with Medians and Mann-Whitney or Kruskal-Wallis Testing

Data	Factor	Number of Points	Median Slope	Median Intercept (mg/kg/d)	Median Nitrogen Requirement[a] (mg/kg/d)
Primary estimation studies					
	All	32	0.49	−47.1	102
Climate	Temperate	22	0.45	−43.0	101
	Tropical	10	0.52	−54.8	111
	P-value		0.10	0.020	0.27
Age	Young	30	0.50	−48.9	102
	Old	2	0.31	−36.7	111
	P-value		0.12	0.23	0.97
Gender	Male	24	0.50	−48.9	102
	Female	8	0.46	−42.0	102
	P-value		0.45	0.27	0.62
Diet	Animal	9	0.50	−48.1	101
	Vegetable	11	0.50	−45.9	104
	Mixed	12	0.48	−49.7	102
	P-value		0.88	0.83	0.72
Other estimation studies					
	All	45	0.47	−46.0	103
Climate	Temperate	33	0.42	−41.8	101
	Tropical	12	0.51	−54.5	111
	P-value		0.026	0.002	0.29

		n			
Age	Young	43	0.48	−47.0	103
	Old	2	0.31	−36.7	111
	P-value		0.18	0.27	0.98
Gender	Male	36	0.48	−47.6	103
	Female	9	0.44	−39.2	103
	P-value		0.47	0.40	0.94
Diet	Animal	17	0.46	−40.6	101
	Vegetable	13	0.50	−45.0	108
	Mixed	15	0.47	−50.5	105
	P-value		0.85	0.40	0.64
All data	All	235	0.47	−48.1	105
Climate	Temperate	154	0.45	−45.3	103
	Tropical	81	0.50	−51.9	113
	P-value		0.20	0.011	0.047
Age	Young	221	0.48	−49.4	104
	Old	14	0.31	−36.7	131
	P-value		0.003	0.025	0.401
Gender	Male	181	0.46	−49.4	109
	Female	54	0.47	−43.1	91
	P-value		0.47	0.20	< 0.001
Diet	Animal	64	0.46	−48.8	104
	Vegetable	77	0.47	−49.4	107
	Mixed	94	0.48	−46.6	104
	P-value		0.62	0.81	0.62

[a] Protein requirement = 6.25 × nitrogen requirement.

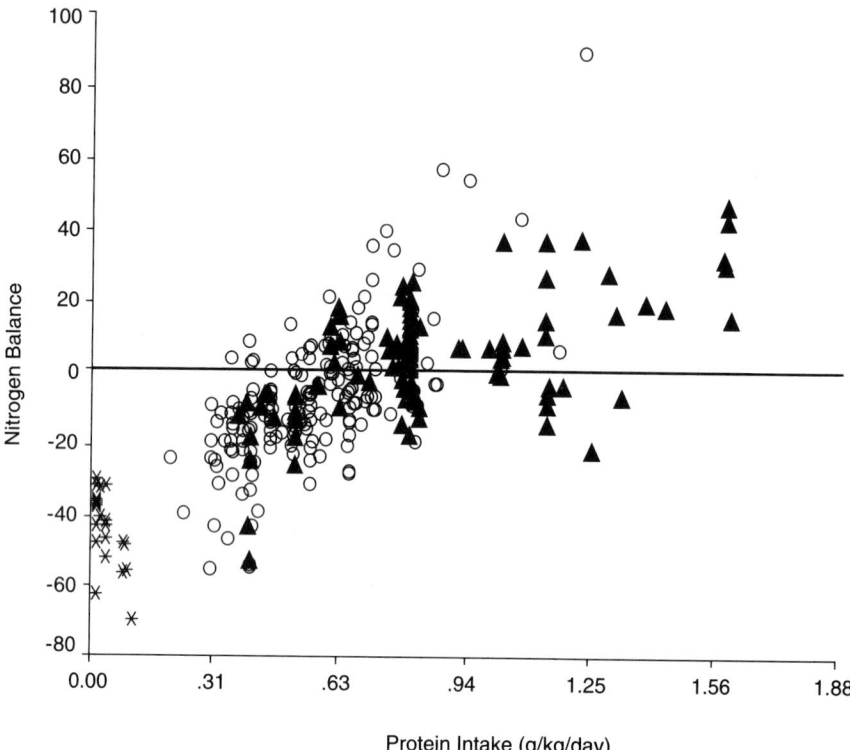

FIGURE 10-6 Relationship between individual nitrogen balances, corrected for integumental and nitrogen losses and nitrogen intake in random selection of data. □ = primary data; ▲ = test data; * = obligatory losses data.
SOURCE: Rand et al. (2003).

al., 2003), a separate analysis was conducted to evaluate the extent to which the four factors thought to have the most influence on protein requirements—climate, age, gender, and dietary protein source—were analyzed. As shown in Table 10-13, expected climate in the country of the study had a significant effect ($p < 0.47$), with differences of the magnitude of about +10 mg N/kg/d (0.06 g protein/kg/d) in tropical climates. The effect of age, as shown in Table 10-13, was a nonsignificant difference of 27 mg N/d (0.17 g protein/d) in the nitrogen requirement between young (19 to 52 years of age) and older (53 years of age and older) individuals per kg of body weight. Although the young individuals had a lower nitrogen requirement than the older individuals, the requirement of young individuals was more variable and more positively skewed than that for the older individuals.

In addition, men had a statistically significant higher median nitrogen requirement by about 18 mg N/kg/d (0.11 g protein/kg/d) than did the women studied, although this difference disappears when medians of the primary estimation studies are compared. Ninety-five percent confidence intervals for these estimates are 104 and 114 mg N/kg/d (0.65 and 0.71 g protein/kg/d) for men and 85 and 104 mg N/kg/d (0.53 and 0.65 g protein/kg/d) for women. Finally, the source of protein (90 percent animal, 90 percent vegetable, or mixed) did not significantly affect the median nitrogen requirement, slope, or intercept. It should be noted that almost all of the studies included as 90 percent vegetable were based on complementary proteins. For further discussion on this aspect of the data analysis and for information on vegetarian diets see later sections on "Protein Quality" and on "Vegetarians."

All of the various estimates of protein requirements (Table 10-10) are confounded by variations in energy intake relative to energy balance and expenditure. It has been estimated that an error of about 10 percent in energy intake as estimated from a diet history or a prediction equation (FAO/WHO/UNU, 1985) would cause the nitrogen balance estimate to be affected by about ± 6 mg/kg/d (Pellett and Young, 1992).

Other Approaches to Determine the Protein Requirement Based on the Recent Meta-Analysis

In addition to the linear statistical approach to determine protein requirements described in detail above, the authors considered three other statistical approaches to the nitrogen balance analysis (Rand et al., 2003). All data from the studies in the meta-analysis were fitted to the following models: linear, quadratic, asymptotic exponential growth and linear biphase (see Table 10-12).

Since the above analyses used all of the available data points without linking the individuals or restricting the range of intakes, the authors made the decision to use nitrogen equilibrium as the criterion and individual linear regressions, using only those individuals in the primary data set to determine the protein requirement (Rand et al., 2003). However, due to the shortcomings of the nitrogen balance method noted earlier, it is recommended that the use of nitrogen balance should no longer be regarded as the "gold standard" for the assessment of the adequacy of protein intake and that alternative means should be sought.

Protein EAR Summary, Ages 19 Through 50 Years

Using the recent meta-analysis of the nitrogen balance studies (Rand et al., 2003), the best estimate of the nitrogen EAR in the healthy adult population is determined to be 105 mg N/kg/d, the median requirement for all data (Table 10-13), or 0.66 g/kg/d of protein (105 mg N/kg/d × 6.25). The criterion of adequacy used for the protein EAR is based on the lowest continuing intake of dietary protein that is sufficient to achieve body nitrogen equilibrium (zero balance). While the data as analyzed in the meta analysis (Rand et al., 2003) do not provide any basis for assuming different requirements for climate, age, or source of protein in the diet, it must be recognized that such a lack of statistically significant differences in this data may well be artifacts of the method and the variability in both its determination and in the individuals measured.

Although the data indicate that women have a lower nitrogen requirement than men per kilogram of body weight, this was only statistically significant when all studies were included, but not when the analysis was restricted to the primary data sets. This difference may be due to differences in body composition between men and women, with women and men having on average 28 and 15 percent fat mass, respectively. When controlled for lean body mass, no gender differences in the protein requirements were found. However, in view of the uncertain significance of the difference between the genders, the same protein EAR on a body weight basis for both men and women is chosen. Based on the reference body weights of 70 kg and 57 kg for men and women, respectively, from Table 1-1, the EAR for protein is 47 g/d for men and 38 g/d for women.

EAR for Men
19–30 years	**0.66 g/kg/d of protein**
31–50 years	**0.66 g/kg/d of protein**

EAR for Women
19–30 years	**0.66 g/kg/d of protein**
31–50 years	**0.66 g/kg/d of protein**

Protein RDA Summary, Ages 19 Through 50 Years

The RDA for protein is set using the nitrogen balance database and methodology detailed by Rand and colleagues (2003) who demonstrated that the natural logarithm of requirement (in mg nitrogen/kg/day) has a normal distribution with a mean of 4.65 and a standard deviation of 0.12. The 97.5th percentile of the log requirement is then calculated as 4.89 (the mean plus 1.96 times the standard deviation) and the RDA is the exponentiation (exp) of this value, 132 mg nitrogen/kg/d, or equivalently, 0.80 g protein/kg/d (rounding to the nearest 0.1 g). It should be noted that protein requirement having a log normal distribution permits the estimation the protein intake adequate for any percentile (P) of a healthy population from the equivalent formulae:

$$\exp[0.12 \times z(P) + 4.65] \text{ for nitrogen (mg/kg/d), or}$$
$$\exp[0.12 \times z(P) - 0.425] \text{ for protein (g/kg/d)}$$

In these equations,

(1) "4.65" and "–0.425" are, respectively, the means of the log requirement distributions in mg nitrogen/kg/d and g protein/kg/d [the EAR in mg nitrogen/kg/d = exp(4.65) = 105, while the EAR in g protein/kg/d = exp(–0.425) = 0.65];

(2) "0.12" is the standard deviation of the log of requirement (note that one feature of log normal distributions is that their standard deviation does not change when the units are changed); and

(3) "z(P)" is the value of the standardized normal distribution associated with P.

For example, the intake that is estimated to be adequate for 80 percent of a healthy population is exp [0.12 × z(0.8) – 0.425] = exp [0.12 × 0.84 – 0.425] = exp[–0.324] = 0.72 g protein/kg/d.

Based on the reference body weights of 70 kg for men and 57 kg for women from Table 1-1, the RDA for protein is 56 g/d for men and 46 g/d for women ages 19 through 50 years.

Because the distribution of individual requirements for protein is log normal, and thus skewed, the calculated standard deviation and coefficient of variation of requirement itself does not have the usual intuitive meaning (that the mean plus two standard deviations exceeds all but about 2.5 percent of the population's requirement). However, because this skewing is not extreme, an approximate standard deviation can be calculated as half the distance from the 16th to the 84th percentile of the protein requirement distribution as estimated from the log normal distribution of requirements. This gives a value of 12.5 mg nitrogen/kg/d (CV = 12 percent) which can be used to estimate the RDA's of other age groups and for individual amino acids where fewer data from the following formula: RDA = EAR + 2 CV, or RDA = 1.24 × EAR.

RDA for Men
19–30 years	**0.80 g/kg/d or 56 g/d of protein**
31–50 years	**0.80 g/kg/d or 56 g/d of protein**

RDA for Women
19–30 years	**0.80 g/kg/d or 46 g/d of protein**
31–50 years	**0.80 g/kg/d or 46 g/d of protein**

Adults Ages 51 Years and Older

Evidence Considered in Estimating the Average Requirement

In the meta-analysis described in Table 10-12 and used as the basis to determine adult protein requirements (Rand et al., 2003), there were six studies to assess the protein requirement of individuals aged 51 years and older. These have been analyzed and evaluated in various publications (Campbell and Evans, 1996; Campbell et al., 1994; Millward and Roberts, 1996; Millward et al., 1997). Table 10-14 shows the value for the EAR derived by the original authors, plus the values obtained in the reassessments of the original data by Campbell's group in 1994 and Millward's group in 1997. The variability among the derived values, and the changes due to reassessment, are the result of the many inadequacies in the original data, which are described below.

Only the study of Cheng and coworkers (1978) involved a direct comparison of old with young adults; however, the authors made no assessment of the miscellaneous nitrogen losses and were not able to show any clear difference in the requirement of older and younger adults. In inter-

TABLE 10-14 Nitrogen Balance Studies in Older Individuals

Reference	Study Population	Protein Intake Levels (g/kg/d)
Cheng et al., 1978	7 men, 60–73 y	0.40, 0.80, 1.60
Uauy et al., 1978	7 men, 7 women	0.57, 0.70, 0.85 0.52, 0.65, 0.80
Zanni et al., 1979	6 men, 63–77 y	0.38, 0.44
Gersovitz et al., 1982	7 men, 70–82 y 8 women, 71–99 y	0.80 0.80
Campbell et al., 1994	8 men, 56–68 y 4 women, 66–80 y	0.80, 1.62 0.80, 1.62
Castaneda et al., 1995b	12 women, 66–79 y	0.45, 0.92

[a] Estimates of average requirements derived from studies on elderly adults by the original authors and in subsequent reanalyses by Millward et al. (1997) and Campbell et al. (1994).

preting the data of Cheng's group, it was suggested that the energy intake of the older Chilean men was too high, 40 kcal/kg/d, as it was the same as that given to the younger men, who would be expected to have higher energy expenditures (Campbell et al., 1994).

Dietary energy excess is believed to give rise to erroneously low estimates of protein requirements (Garza et al., 1976, 1977a). However, the energy requirements of the elderly have been shown to be higher than previously believed (Roberts, 1996). Moreover, the urinary creatinine to body weight ratio reported by Cheng and coworkers (1978) was the same in the old (0.023 g/kg/d) as in the young (0.022 g/kg/d) men, suggesting that the two groups were of similar body composition. This is in contrast to studies in the United States where lower creatinine to body weight ratios were observed in the older adults (0.014 to 0.018 g/kg/d) (Campbell et al., 1994; Uauy et al., 1978; Zanni et al., 1979).

The study of nitrogen balance by Zanni and coworkers (1979) suggested that the average amount of protein intake required to maintain nitrogen balance in older adults was very low (0.46 g/kg/d). This study was performed under almost the same conditions as those used with younger adults in an earlier study from the same laboratory (Calloway and

Energy Intake (kcal/kg/d) [b]	Average Requirement (g protein/kg/d) [a] as calculated by:		
	Authors	Campbell et al. (1994)	Millward et al. (1997)
40 (constant)	0.77	0.93	> 0.4
32	0.70–0.85	0.81	≤ 0.57
28 (varied)	0.83	0.81	Uncertain
31 (varied)	0.46	0.65	Uncertain
32 29 (varied)	> 0.8	—	< 0.8
32 29 (varied)	1.0	1.0	< 0.8
32 (varied)	0.78–0.82	—	< 0.92

[b] Energy intake was either held constant for duration of nitrogen balance period, or varied to maintain body weight; varied levels are average intakes of group as reported by authors.

Margen, 1971) and demonstrated that the amount of protein needed by older adults (0.46 g/kg/d) was quite similar per kg of body weight compared to the younger adults (0.42 g/kg/d). Since the two different diets studied were relatively low in protein (0.38 and 0.44 g/kg/d), Millward and coworkers (1997) suggested that these low protein intakes led to an underestimate of the requirement. Moreover, since the adults were on a protein-free diet for 17 days preceding the two low-protein diets (each fed in random order for 15 days), this could have resulted in significant protein depletion, probably leading to a further underestimate of requirement. On the other hand, the study of Uauy and coworkers (1978) employed energy intakes (30 kcal/kg/d) that may have been too low, suggesting that their estimate of requirement (~0.8 g/kg/d) might have been an overestimate (Millward et al., 1997). It can be seen from Table 10-14 that the reanalysis by Campbell and coworkers (1994) led to overall higher estimates of the requirements of older adults than the original authors, whereas the reanalysis by Millward's group (1997) led to lower estimates.

In studies designed to evaluate the adequacy of diets containing 0.8 g/kg/d of protein (the 1973 FAO/WHO recommendation for a safe level of intake of egg or milk protein in adults [FAO/WHO, 1973]), nitrogen balance was measured in adults given single levels of protein for various periods. Gersovitz and coworkers (1982) showed that almost 50 percent of older men and women were in negative nitrogen balance at this level after 30 days. Similar results were obtained by Campbell and coworkers (1994) in individuals given 0.8 g/kg/d of protein for 11 days, whereas Castaneda and coworkers (1995a) found that the majority of older women were in positive nitrogen balance after 3 and 9 weeks on a diet containing 0.92 g/kg/d of protein.

On the basis of these data and reanalysis of the original data from the studies discussed above, it was suggested that the estimated requirement should be increased (Campbell and Evans, 1996), although Millward and coworkers (1997) were not in agreement with this conclusion. More recent data have shown that elderly adults given 0.8 g/kg/d of protein were in nitrogen balance after 2 weeks, and in positive balance after 8 and 14 weeks (Campbell et al., 2001). However, the thigh muscle area was significantly reduced after 14 weeks compared with 2 weeks, although there were no changes in any other measured indices of body protein composition.

In order to address these problems of interpretation of the relevant literature, the meta-analysis evaluated the data from the studies on elderly adults compared with those from the studies used to evaluate the requirement in younger individuals (Rand et al., 2003). All the data from studies of nitrogen balance in the older adults were included in the regression procedure employed to determine the protein requirement of adults 19 to 50 years of age, and no significant effect of age in terms of the amount of protein required per kilogram of body weight was detected (Table 10-13).

Protein EAR Summary, Ages 51 Years and Older

In summary, no significant effect of age on protein requirement in older adults was detected using the linear regression model by Rand and coworkers (2003) when evaluated in terms of amount needed per kg of body weight, recognizing that lean body mass as a percent of body weight and the protein content of the body both decrease with age. Therefore, for older adults, no additional protein allowance based on body weight beyond that of younger adults is warranted.

EAR for Men
51–70 years	**0.66 g/kg/d of protein**
> 70 years	**0.66 g/kg/d of protein**

EAR for Women
51–70 years	**0.66 g/kg/d of protein**
> 70 years	**0.66 g/kg/d of protein**

Protein RDA Summary, Ages 51 Years and Older

As with younger adults, because the distribution of individual requirements for protein is not a normal distribution and is skewed, its calculated standard deviation and coefficient of variation do not have the usual intuitive meaning (the mean plus two standard deviations exceeding all but about 2.5 percent of the population's requirement). However, an approximate standard deviation can be calculated as half of the distance from the 16th to the 84th percentiles of the protein requirement distribution as estimated from the log normal distribution of requirements. This gives, for comparative purposes, an approximate standard deviation of 12.5 mg N/kg/d (CV = 12 percent). It can thus be assumed as with younger adults percent that the RDA = EAR + 2 CV for protein and individual amino acids, or RDA = 1.24 × EAR. The calculated RDA is rounded to the nearest 0.05.

RDA for Men
51–70 years	**0.80 g/kg/d or 56 g/d of protein**
> 70 years	**0.80 g/kg/d or 56 g/d of protein**

RDA for Women
51–70 years	**0.80 g/kg/d or 46 g/d of protein**
> 70 years	**0.80 g/kg/d or 46 g/d of protein**

Pregnancy

Physiological Adaptations to Protein Metabolism During Pregnancy

Whole body protein turnover, measured by leucine kinetics, is increased in pregnant women at weeks 24 and 35 compared with pregnant women at 13 weeks or with nonpregnant women (Thompson and Halliday, 1992). Similar observations of increased whole body protein turnover during pregnancy have been made using ^{15}N lysine as a tracer (Kalhan and Devapatla, 1999). A significant reduction in urea synthesis has been shown to occur in the first trimester and is sustained throughout pregnancy (Kalhan et al., 1998). There is general agreement that the amount of nitrogen accreted due to a pregnancy involving 12.5 kg of maternal weight gain (which includes a term infant weighing 3.3 kg) is 148 g (equivalent to 925 g protein if using a conversion factor of 6.25) (Hytten and Leitch, 1971; King, 1975). This amount of protein accumulation is predicted by a summation of the protein components of the fetus (440 g), uterus (166 g), expanded maternal blood volume (81 g), placenta (100 g), extracellular fluid (135 g), and amniotic fluid (3 g) (IOM, 1990). There is also evidence from both nitrogen balance studies and whole body potassium counting that there are additional maternal protein-containing tissues that accumulate during pregnancy and are presumed to be in skeletal muscle (Kalhan, 2000; King, 1975; King et al., 1973).

Evidence Considered in Estimating the Average Requirement

Nitrogen and Potassium Balance. King and coworkers (1973) studied 10 adolescent women aged 15 to 19 years during the last trimester of pregnancy. Since all but one of the individuals were more than 4 years beyond menarche, the authors excluded consideration of maternal height growth. Nitrogen retention was linearly related to protein intake when five different nitrogen levels (9.3 to 20.0 g of N/d [58 to 125 g of protein/d]) were fed for 12-day periods, and the slope of the relationship was 0.3 ($r = 0.68$, $p < 0.001$). The average nitrogen retention (corrected for skin and miscellaneous nitrogen losses) was 2.4 g/d.

Nitrogen balance studies in pregnant women that account for skin and miscellaneous losses have shown that nitrogen retention during all periods of pregnancy is double the theoretical factorial gain (Calloway, 1974; King, 1975; King et al., 1973) and as noted previously (see "Nitrogen Balance Methods"), at high nitrogen intakes erroneous positive nitrogen balances have frequently been obtained.

The rate of protein accretion has also been calculated indirectly from the increase in whole body potassium. The average potassium deposition, measured by total body ^{40}potassium counts, was 3.41 mmol/d in the adolescent girls (King et al., 1973), but a review of the literature suggests that this value may be too high. The results of measurements of total body potassium during pregnancy from the study of King's group (1973) and five other reports are shown in Table 10-15, and yield a weighted mean value of 2.48 mmol/d from 120 individuals, most of whom were in their third trimester of pregnancy. To calculate nitrogen deposition, King and coworkers (1973) used the potassium/nitrogen ratio of 2.15 mmol of potassium/g of nitrogen as determined by carcass analysis of 21 whole human infants (Fee and Weil, 1963; Hamilton and Moriarty, 1929; Iob and Swanson, 1934; Widdowson and Dickerson, 1964). Using this ratio, the accumulation of 2.48 mmol/d of potassium is equivalent to a nitrogen deposition of 1.16 g/d (2.48 mmol of potassium/2.15 mmol of potassium/g of nitrogen/d) or 7.2 g protein/d using the factor of 6.25 g of protein/g of nitrogen. This estimates the average amount of protein deposited dur-

TABLE 10-15 Total Body Potassium Content During Pregnancy

Reference	n	Total Body Potassium (mmol/d)	$n \times$ Total Body Potassium (mmol/d)	Average Protein Deposition (g/d)[a]
MacGillivray and Buchanan, 1958	6	3.22	19.3	9.4
King et al., 1973	10	3.41	34.1	9.9
Emerson et al., 1975	5	3.43	17.2	10.0
Pipe et al., 1979	27	1.78	48.1	5.2
Forbes, 1987	50	2.64	132	7.7
Forsum et al., 1988	22	2.13	48.9	6.2
Total	120		297.9	
Mean		2.48[b]		7.2

[a] Protein deposition = Total potassium accumulated (mmol/d) ÷ 2.15 (mmol potassium/g nitrogen) × 6.25.
[b] Mean total body potassium calculated as the sum of column 3 divided by the total number of cases (298 ÷ 120) = 2.48).

ing the third trimester of pregnancy at a total of approximately 670 g of protein.

Calculation of the amount of dietary protein needed for a deposition of 7.2 g of protein/d during the third trimester of pregnancy requires a value for the efficiency of utilization of dietary protein. This was reported as being about 30 percent in a group of adolescent women in the third trimester of pregnancy (King et al., 1973). Closer review of the data indicates that for those six adolescents who demonstrated a positive efficiency at multiple levels of protein intake, the mean of the slope of the positive nitrogen balances was 0.43 ± 0.21 (median = 0.44). Compared with the slope for maintenance of adults of 0.47, which was calculated from a much larger data set (see "Adults Ages 19 Through 50 Years"), it is possible that the paucity of the data for both infants and during pregnancy has obscured the true rate of efficiency of deposition. While other physiological changes occurring in pregnancy appear to enhance nutrient utilization during periods of increased need (e.g., calcium absorption), it would be surprising to find that efficiency of protein utilization during pregnancy is diminished over that of other life stages. However, to ensure adequate intakes, 0.43 was chosen to use based on the six women studied. As calculated in Table 10-16, the average protein deposition was converted to the amount of intake needed to provide this level: 7.2 ÷ 0.43 = 16.7 g of protein/d for accretion during the third trimester.

The protein needed to maintain the new tissue accreted during pregnancy must also be added. The increase of body weight during a full-term pregnancy averages approximately 16 kg, which is the median weight gain of 4,218 women who had good pregnancy outcomes (Carmichael et al., 1997). Weight gain during pregnancy is made up of both additional fat and new lean tissue (including fetus, amniotic fluid, increased plasma volume, etc.), which has been estimated at 91 percent water (van Raaij et al., 1988), compared with the expected 73 percent of water in general nonpregnant lean tissue. The incremental weight gain at the 50th percentile for normal weight individuals with good pregnancy outcomes at the end of the first trimester is 2.2 kg; for the second trimester, 7.3 kg; and for the third trimester, 6.5 kg, which totals 16 kg (Carmichael et al., 1997).

The amount of protein to support additional tissue is calculated in Table 10-16 using a factor of 0.66 g/kg of body weight, the EAR for protein for adults. While it is recognized that pregnancy lean tissue contains a greater amount of water, correction for assumed differences in body composition have not been made given the lack of actual data delineating protein maintenance needs in pregnant women. This results in an average total additional need for protein during the last two trimesters of pregnancy of about 21 g/d over prepregnancy requirements.

653

TABLE 10-16 Derivation of Protein Requirements During Pregnancy

Trimester	[A] Average Additional Body Weight Gained by the End of Trimester (kg)[a]	Total Weight Gain by End of Trimester	Additional Protein to Maintain Increased Body Weight[b] (g/d)	Average Protein Deposition (additional lean tissue)[c] (g/d)	[B] Protein Deposition Corrected for Conversion Efficiency[d] (g/d)	[A + B] Average Total Additional Protein Required (g/d)[e]	RDA (g/d)[f]
1	Δ2.2	2.2	+1.4	~		~	
2	Δ7.3	9.5	+6.3	3.6	8.4	+14.7	
3	Δ6.5	16.0	+10.6	7.2	16.7	+27.3	
Average over 2nd and 3rd trimesters				5.4	12.6	+21.0	+25

a Carmichael et al. (1997); average body weight gain by end of trimester; divided by 2 to get approximate increase mid-trimester.
b End of trimester increase in body weight × 0.66 g/kg/d, the Estimated Average Requirement (EAR) for maintenance of protein in adults.
c From Table 10-15 where protein deposition = total potassium accumulated (mmol/d) ÷ 2.15 (mmol potassium/g nitrogen) × 6.25; and assumption that nitrogen accretion during second trimester is ~ 50% that of third trimester.
d Protein deposition ÷ 0.43, slope of regression line of protein intake versus nitrogen balance (recalculated from King et al., 1973).
e Average required additional amount needed during pregnancy.
f RDA is based on EAR + assumed variation in requirements; amount needed above nonpregnant needs.

Outcome of Food Supplementation Trials. Burke and coworkers (1943) conducted an observational study of 216 mothers giving birth to single infants in Boston and found a significant correlation between average daily protein intake and birth length and birth weight. They concluded that for practical purposes, a protein intake less than 75 g/d was associated with an infant who would be short and light in weight. Studies from the Montreal Diet Dispensary have also shown a relationship between maternal protein-energy intake and birth weight (Higgins, 1976). This study involved 1,736 low-income pregnant women, 20 years of age or more, whose average maternal protein and energy intakes at various stages of pregnancy were 68 g and 2,249 kcal/d during pregnancy, and were increased to an average of 101 g of protein and 2,778 kcal/d by supplementing the mothers with whole milk and eggs during a subsequent pregnancy. Birth weights were significantly higher for siblings with supplemented mothers compared with their older siblings born to the same mothers when they did not receive the supplementary milk and eggs. These data support the value increased intake of foods high in protein and energy during pregnancy and the additional requirements outlined above.

Adolescent Pregnancy. It is well established that both the mother's pre-pregnant weight and weight gain during pregnancy are correlated with the birth weight of the infant (Higgins, 1976; IOM, 1990; Wynn and Wynn, 1979). The problem of adolescent pregnancy is that the mother may still be completing her growth (Frisancho et al., 1983; Hediger et al., 1990; Scholl et al., 1990, 1994). In those pregnancies in which the mother's growth is not yet completed, it appears that there is competition between maternal and fetal growth needs (Hediger et al., 1990; Scholl et al., 1990, 1994).

The Montreal Diet Dispensary studied the effect of supplementing 1,203 low-income pregnant adolescents with whole milk and eggs and compared them with 1,203 pregnant adolescents who did not receive the additional milk and eggs in their diets (Dubois et al., 1997). The adolescents in the intervention group increased their protein intake from 73 g/d to approximately 125 g/d in addition to significantly increasing their energy intake. Participation in the intervention resulted in significantly increased mean birth weights and reduced the rate of low birth weights by 39 percent ($p < 0.001$) in adolescent girls, which again is attributed to the increased consumption of foods rich in protein and energy.

Protein EAR Summary, Pregnancy

Based upon the nitrogen balance study of King and coworkers (1973) and the estimated average protein deposition during pregnancy based on potassium retention in six studies (Table 10-15), the average requirement for additional protein needed for adult pregnant women at the end of the trimester during pregnancy in adult women is calculated and given in Table 10-16. It is composed of two components: the amount needed to maintain the new pregnant tissue and the amount needed for initial deposition. The amount of protein deposition is corrected for the efficiency of protein deposition (using the estimate from the slope of 0.43 from the King and coworkers study [1973], recalculated as described above). Since little weight gain occurs during the first trimester, it is assumed that roughly one-third of the total increase in protein deposition during the 40 weeks of pregnancy (~ 925 g) occurs during the second trimester, with two-thirds occurring during the third trimester.

As described above, by the end of the third trimester, ~17 g/d is needed to allow for adequate protein deposition; it can be assumed that roughly half that amount is needed for growth during the second trimester, or 8 g/d (Table 10-16). Given the small amount of protein accretion expected to occur during the first trimester (as demonstrated by Thompson and Halliday [1992] in protein turnover studies during each trimester), the need for additional protein is rather low at this stage. Thus no additional increase in protein requirements is estimated for the first trimester. Averaging the overall protein needs over the last two trimesters of pregnancy, the EAR is set at 21 g/d above protein needs at the prepregnancy weight. Since this figure includes the protein needs for the additional tissue deposited, when calculating the amount needed per kilogram of body weight to use with pregnant women, only the amount needed for protein deposition is considered. Thus the increased amount on a body-weight basis is +12.6 g of protein/d ÷ 57 kg (reference woman) = +0.22 g of protein/kg/d. This is added to the factor for nonpregnant women of 0.66 g of protein/kg/d, and results in an EAR of 0.88 g of protein/kg/d.

Pregnant individuals who were studied ranged from 15 to 19 years of age (King et al., 1973); however, they were considered mature and physiologically similar to adults, as all but one of the ten young women was 4 to 7 years post-menarche. For adolescents, the additional need for protein during the second and third trimesters is assumed to be the same as for adult women.

EAR for Pregnancy
All age groups   **0.88 g/kg/d of protein or +21 g/d**
                        of additional protein

Protein RDA Summary, Pregnancy

The protein RDA for pregnancy is in addition to the RDA for the nonpregnant woman, which is based on an estimated CV of about 12 percent (see "Protein RDA Summary, Adults 19 Years and Older"). Data for the variability of protein deposition in the fetus and mother was not available. The RDA is thus equal to the EAR + 24 percent. Thus the 1.24 multiplied by the EAR of +21 g protein/d = 26 g; rounded to the nearest 5 g/d, the RDA = +25 g/d.

Again, in considering the amount needed per kilogram of body weight, only that due to protein deposition is considered. The increase in the RDA is thus +12.6 g/d × 1.24 ÷ 57 kg (reference woman) = +0.27 g protein/kg/ d. This is added to the factor for the RDA for non-pregnant women of 0.8 g protein/kg/d = 1.1 g protein/kg/d.

RDA for Pregnancy
  All age groups   **1.1 g/kg/d of protein or +25 g/d**
                         of additional protein

Special Considerations

It is well recognized that multiparous pregnancies are associated with a marked increase in low birth weight and perinatal mortality (Hays and Smeltzer, 1986). Thus, it is logical to assume that a woman supporting the growth of twins has higher protein needs than a woman having a singleton birth. In a study in which the mothers of twins received nutritional intervention (target supplementation was an additional 50 g of protein/d and 1,000 kcal/d) from the 20th week, pregnancy outcome was improved, with a decrease in the low birth weight rate by 25 percent and the very low birth weight rate by 50 percent (Dubois et al., 1991). Although this study did not measure the dietary protein or energy intake of the women bearing twins, they gained 2 kg more than the controls. No study could be found that investigated dietary protein intervention in twin pregnancy. On the basis of these data, it seems prudent to provide women carrying twins with protein intakes of an additional 50 g/d beginning in the second trimester, along with sufficient energy to utilize the protein as efficiently as possible.

Lactation

Evidence Considered in Estimating the Average Requirement

The literature on the relationship between nutritional status and lactation performance is not extensive and suggests that most lactating women, even those who are undernourished with chronically low body mass index, establish adequate lactation (Prentice et al., 1994). While it appears that the concentration of protein in human milk is not influenced by diet or body composition even in undernourished mothers (Lönnerdal 1986), protein intakes of 1 g/kg of body weight/d promoted the conservation of skeletal muscle in order to maintain good milk production in lactating mothers (Motil et al., 1996). Lactating women with these protein intakes appear to adapt by down-regulating protein metabolism (Motil et al., 1996).

The factorial approach is utilized for determining the protein requirement during lactation. In this approach, it is assumed that the process of lactation does not alter the maintenance protein requirement of the nonlactating woman and that the protein and amino acid requirements are increased in proportion to milk production. It is important to emphasize that human milk is characterized by a relatively high concentration of nonprotein nitrogenous substances, which contribute approximately 20 to 27 percent of total milk nitrogen (Butte et al., 1984a, 1984b; Dewey et al., 1996). The quantitatively important component of this fraction of milk is urea. Whether this merely reflects a diversion of urea loss from urine (plus some colonic fermentation) to milk is not known, but in the calculations it is assumed that part of the increased nitrogen needs of the lactating woman will of necessity be derived from her dietary protein. The factor of 6.25, the figure that is utilized to convert nitrogen to protein, was used to convert nonprotein nitrogenous substances to protein.

The additional protein requirement for lactation therefore is defined as the output of total protein and nonprotein nitrogen in milk. Data on the output of protein in human milk are summarized in Table 10-17. This table shows the factorial estimate of the increase in protein requirement associated with lactation and assumes that the incremental efficiency of nitrogen utilization of 0.47 in adults (Table 10-12) and in adolescents (data on the efficiency of nitrogen utilization are not available in this age group) is the same as that noted for the restoration of nitrogen equilibrium in nonlactating women and adolescents. It is assumed that the cost of making protein for maintenance requirements is the same as that for growth and lactation. Whether this assumption is valid is not known.

Protein EAR Summary, Lactation

To estimate the increase in the EAR for lactation, the average protein equivalent of human milk nitrogen output during the first six months of lactation was divided by the average incremental efficiency of dietary protein utilization (0.47 for lactating mothers 19 years of age and older [Table 10-12] and 0.47 for mothers 14 through 18 years of age because data were not available in this age group). The values shown in Table 10-17

TABLE 10-17 Factorial Estimate of the Increment in Protein Requirement Associated with Lactation

Stage (mo)	Protein Content of Human Milk[a] (g protein/d)	Nonprotein Nitrogen Content of Human Milk[a] (g protein/d)	Total Human Milk Nitrogen Output (g protein/d)	Increase in Protein Need[b] (g/d) 14–18 y	Increase in Protein Need[b] (g/d) > 18 y
1	8.93 ± 1.97[a]	2.05 ± 0.4	11.0 ± 2.4	23.4	23.4
2	8.26 ± 1.08[c]	2.02 ± 1.6	10.3 ± 2.7	21.9	21.9
3	8.24 ± 1.54[d]	1.71 ± 1.1	10.0 ± 2.6	21.3	21.3
4–6	7.29 ± 1.27[c]	1.28 ± 0.5	8.6 ± 1.8	18.3	18.3
Mean	8.18	1.76		21.2	21.2

[a] Butte et al. (1984b); Lemons et al. (1982).

[b] The increase in the Estimated Average Requirement (EAR) for protein was calculated by dividing the average protein equivalent of milk nitrogen output by the average incremental efficiency of dietary protein utilization (0.47 for lactating mothers 19 years of age and older [Table 10-12] as well as for lactating mothers 14–18 years of age because data are not available for this age group).

[c] Butte et al. (1984b).

[d] Butte et al. (1984b); Dewey and Lönnerdal (1983); Heinig et al. (1993); Motil et al. (1998); Nommsen et al. (1991).

for the various months of lactation were then averaged to set the amount by which the EAR for nonlactating girls or women should be increased. The result was +21.2 g/d. When the absolute increase was converted to weight-specific intakes by using the reference weights of adolescent girls 14 to 18 years (54 kg) and adult women 19 to 50 years (57 kg) from Chapter 1 (Table 1-1), the numbers were quite close, so the highest value (that for the 14- to 18-year-old category) is provided as the overall recommendation. Adding the average requirement for additional protein needed is calculated as +21.2 ÷ 54 kg (reference weight) = +0.39 g of protein/kg/d. This is added to the recommendation for nonpregnant women of 0.66 g of protein/kg/d to obtain 1.05 g of protein/kg/d.

EAR for Lactation
   All age groups   **1.05 g/kg/d of protein or +21 g/d of additional protein**

Protein RDA Summary, Lactation

The RDA for protein for lactation is set by assuming a CV of 12 percent used for total protein in nonlactating women (see "Protein RDA Summary, Ages 19 Years through 50 Years"). Again, given the closeness of the values, one value is recommended for all age groups. The recommendations are rounded to the nearest +5 g/d and +0.05 g/kg/d of additional protein.

The RDA is thus equal to the EAR plus 24 percent. So, 1.24 multiplied by the EAR of + 21 g of protein/d = +26 g; rounded to the nearest 5 g/d, the RDA = +25 g/d.

Again, in considering the amount needed per kg of body weight, the increase in the RDA is calculated as the EAR of +21 g/d × 1.24 ÷ 54 kg (reference weight) = +0.48 g of protein/kg/d. This is added to the factor for the RDA for nonpregnant women of 0.8 g of protein/kg/d = 1.3 g of protein/kg/d (rounded to nearest 0.1g).

RDA for Lactation
   All age groups   **1.3 g/kg/d of protein or +25 g/d of additional protein[4]**

---

[4]Due to a calculation error in the prepublication copy, the value is changed from 1.1 g/kg/d to 1.3 g/kg/d

Special Considerations

Physical Activity

Although there have been few studies of the requirement for protein by individuals undertaking high levels of physical exercise, it is commonly believed by athletes that a higher than normal protein intake is required to maintain optimum physical performance (Lemon, 1996). Whether or not this is true has significance not only for athletes, but also for those with muscle wasting who wish to preserve muscle mass by training, such as elderly or immobile adults, or those suffering from muscle-wasting diseases. The available literature includes studies of both resistance (bodybuilding) and endurance training.

Endurance Training. Endurance training does not result in muscle building, which would increase muscle protein deposition, but it is well recognized that endurance exercise is accompanied by an increase in the oxidation of branched chain amino acids (Lemon et al., 1982, 1985; Rennie et al., 1981; Wagenmakers, 1998; White and Brooks, 1981), which has been suggested to imply an increased need for dietary protein (Lemon, 1996). However, these were acute studies performed around the time of the exercise itself, and did not take into account the remaining part of the day. An examination of leucine oxidation over a 24-hour period, including exercise during each of the fed and fasting periods, showed that the increase in oxidation, although statistically significant, was small in relation to the total daily amount of oxidation (4 to 7 percent) (El-Khoury et al., 1997). Moreover, the increase in leucine oxidation was proportionally similar with diets containing 1 or 2.5 g/kg/d fed over 7 days prior to the measurement of oxidation during exercise on day 7 (Forslund et al., 1998). Neither leucine nor nitrogen balance was significantly negative, suggesting that the exercise did not compromise body protein homeostasis at either level of protein intake. Although no control group without exercise was studied, the results were similar to those reported previously from individuals at an intake of 1 g/kg/d of protein undergoing the same experimental procedures without exercise (El-Khoury et al., 1994b). Similarly, a study designed to determine the protein requirement of endurance-trained men led to an average requirement estimate in young and older men of 0.94 g/kg/d (Meredith et al., 1989). This value is higher than that derived from the meta-analysis of data from nonexercising individuals (see "Protein EAR Summary, Ages 19 Through 50 Years"). However, as no controls without exercise were included in the study, it is not possible to conclude that the exercise led to a higher protein requirement.

Resistance Training. The effects of resistance training on nitrogen balance have been investigated in older adults (8 men and 4 women, aged 56 to 80 years) at one of two levels of protein intake, 0.8 or 1.6 g/kg/d (Campbell et al., 1995). Before training began, the mean corrected nitrogen balance was not significantly different from zero in the three men and three women receiving the lower protein intake, and was positive in the five men and one woman receiving the higher intake, suggesting a requirement about 0.8 g/kg/d. However, after 12 weeks of resistance training, nitrogen balance became more positive by a similar amount at the two intakes, which the authors suggested was the result of an increased efficiency of protein retention that was more pronounced in those on the lower protein diet as a percent of protein intake. In particular, the improvement in nitrogen balance was independent of the protein intake. However, various aspects of body composition, as well as mid-thigh composition and areas of Type I and II muscle fibers, did not change with resistance training, making the increase in nitrogen retention difficult to interpret.

A similar study was performed by Lemon and coworkers (1992), which compared protein intakes of 1.35 and 2.62 g/kg/d during the first 12 weeks of resistance training in young male strength athletes. Linear interpolation of the nitrogen balances (–3.4 and +8.9 g/d) suggested a protein requirement of 1.4 to 1.5 g/kg/d. However, this estimate of requirement cannot be taken as realistic, because the positive nitrogen balance of 8.9 g/d would correspond to an increase of lean tissue of about 300 g/d. Measurements of body composition showed no changes in lean body mass, creatinine excretion, or biceps muscle nitrogen content in either dietary group. In addition, although there were increases in some measurements of strength, there was no effect attributable to diet. Therefore, the available data do not support the conclusion that the protein requirement for resistance training individuals is greater than that of nonexercising subjects.

Summary. In view of the lack of compelling evidence to the contrary, no additional dietary protein is suggested for healthy adults undertaking resistance or endurance exercise.

Vegetarians

In North America, plant proteins (e.g., those found in cereals, pulses, nuts, starchy roots, vegetables, fruits) account for only about 65 percent of the available food protein per capita (FAO/Agrostat, 1991). Individuals who restrict their diet to plant foods may be at risk of not getting adequate amounts of certain indispensable amino acids because the concentration of lysine, sulfur amino acids, and threonine are sometimes lower in plant food proteins than in animal food proteins (FAO/WHO/UNU, 1985).

However, vegetarian diets that include complementary mixtures of plant proteins can provide the same quality of protein (see "Protein Quality") as that from animal proteins (Young and Pellett, 1994). Plant proteins are generally less digestible than animal proteins; however, digestibility can be altered through processing and preparation. Therefore, consuming a varied diet ensures an adequate intake of protein for vegetarians.

Adult vegetarians consume less protein in their diet than non-vegetarians (Alexander et al., 1994; Ball and Bartlett, 1999; Barr and Broughton, 2000; Haddad et al., 1999; Janelle and Barr, 1995). However, only one of these studies indicated that total protein intakes of 10 of the 25 vegan women were potentially inadequate (Haddad et al., 1999). As was shown in Table 10-13, the nitrogen requirement for adults based on high-quality plant food proteins as determined by regression analysis was not significantly different than the requirement based on animal protein or protein from a mixed diet. In conclusion, available evidence does not support recommending a separate protein requirement for vegetarians who consume complementary mixtures of plant proteins.

FINDINGS BY LIFE STAGE AND GENDER GROUP FOR INDISPENSABLE AMINO ACIDS

The original technique used to determine amino acid requirements in individuals studied with graded levels of intake of the test amino acid was nitrogen balance (see "Nitrogen Balance Method"). Several new methods have been developed and applied in the last few decades. However, nitrogen balance could not be applied to histidine since individuals take 56 days or more to go into negative nitrogen balance on a low histidine or histidine-free diet (Cho et al., 1984), and there haven't been any useful studies on isoleucine, using either nitrogen balance or any of the newer methods.

The amino acid requirements thus developed are used as the basis for recommended protein scoring patterns discussed in a subsequent section.

Infants Ages 0 Through 6 Months

Method Used to Estimate the Adequate Intake

Human milk is recognized as the optimal source of nutrients for infants throughout at least the first year of life and is recommended as the sole nutritional source for infants during the first 4 to 6 months of life (IOM, 1991). Further, there are no reports of healthy full-term infants exclusively and freely fed human milk who manifest any sign of amino acid or protein deficiency (Heinig et al., 1993). Therefore, determination of the adequate intake (AI) for amino acids for infants is based on data from infants fed human milk as the principal source of nutrients during the periods 0 through 6 months of age. The AI is set for ages 0 through 6 months at the mean value of each indispensable amino acid calculated from studies in which the intake of human milk was measured by test weighing volume, and the average concentration of the amino acid in human milk was determined using average values from several reported studies.

Four recent studies on the indispensable amino acid composition of human milk and their mean are shown in Table 10-18. The indispensable amino acid intake on a mg/L basis was calculated from the mean of the amino acid composition of mixed human milk proteins expressed as mg amino acid/g protein (Table 10-18) times the average protein content of human milk of 11.9 g/L from mothers whose infants were 0 through 6 months as assessed by Butte and coworkers (1984a), Dewey and Lönnerdal (1983), Dewey and coworkers (1984), and Nommsen and coworkers (1991) and is in the range of protein content reported in other studies in Table 10-7.

Indispensable Amino Acids AI Summary, Ages 0 Through 6 Months

The AI for infants 0 through 6 months of age is based on the average volume of milk intake of 0.78 L/d (Allen et al., 1991; Heinig et al., 1993), and the mean indispensable amino acid content of human milk (Table 10-18). Multiplying the mean concentration of histidine (274 mg/L), for example, by the average intake of human milk at 0 through 6 months, the AI would be 274 g/L × 0.78 L/d = 214 mg/d. This process was repeated for all the indispensable amino acids. As with the AI for protein, the AIs (which remain essentially the same from 2 weeks to 6 months of age) were converted to weight specific intakes by using the reference weight of 6 kg from Table 1-1.

AI for Infants
0–6 months   214 mg/d or 36 mg/kg/d of histidine
529 mg/d or 88 mg/kg/d of isoleucine
938 mg/d or 156 mg/kg/d of leucine
640 mg/d or 107 mg/kg/d of lysine
353 mg/d or 59 mg/kg/d of methionine + cysteine
807 mg/d or 135 mg/kg/d of phenylalanine + tyrosine
436 mg/d or 73 mg/kg/d of threonine
167 mg/d or 28 mg/kg/d of tryptophan
519 mg/d or 87 mg/kg/d of valine

TABLE 10-18 Amino Acid Content of Human Milk

Amino Acid	Heine et al. (1991) (mg/g protein)	Davis et al. (1994)[a] (mg/g protein)	Villalpando et al. (1998)[a] (mg/g protein)
n	Not given	6	70
Stage of lactation	Not given	> 10 d pp[d]	4 or 6 mo pp
Histidine	23	23 ± 2	21± 2
Isoleucine	58	53 ± 3	64 ± 11
Leucine	101	104 ± 1	105 ± 11
Lysine	62	71 ± 6	79 ± 9
Methionine	18	16 ± 1	14 ± 3
Cysteine	17	20 ± 3	26 ± 3
Phenylalanine	44	37 ± 1	43 ± 15
Tyrosine	47	46 ± 2	58 ± 9
Threonine	46	44 ± 1	47 ± 5
Tryptophan	18	ND[e]	17 ± 2
Valine	60	51 ± 2	63 ± 8

[a] Mean ± Standard Deviation.
[b] Mean ± Standard Error.

Children Ages 7 Months Through 18 Years

Evidence Considered in Estimated the Average Requirement

Nitrogen Balance. The only data derived directly from experiments to determine the indispensable amino acids requirements of children have been obtained by studying nitrogen balance. Pineda and coworkers (1981) conducted nitrogen balance studies in 42 Guatemalan children ranging in age from 21 to 27 months. The children were considered to be in nitrogen balance if all children retained nitrogen in the amount of at least 16 mg/kg/d, the nitrogen requirement for growth in children in this age range derived by FAO/WHO (1973) when given a diet lacking one indispensable amino acid with all other indispensable amino acids at levels considered to be adequate. Their mean amino acid estimates were reported to be: lysine, 66 mg/kg/d; threonine, 37 to 53 mg/kg/d; tryptophan, 13 mg/kg/d; methionine + cysteine, 28 mg/kg/d; isoleucine, 32 mg/kg/d; and valine, 39 mg/kg/d. Unfortunately, with the exception of lysine, no estimates of variance were published.

Darragh and Moughan (1998)[b] (mg/g protein)	Mean (mg/g protein)	Mean[c] (mg/L)
20		
10–14 wk pp		
24 ± 2	23	274
52 ± 4	57	678
94 ± 5	101	1,202
64 ± 4	69	821
14 ± 1	16	190
27 ± 3	22	262
38 ± 9	40	476
38 ± 2	47	559
50 ± 9	47	559
ND[e]	18	214
51 ± 5	56	666

[c] Mean (mg/g total protein) × 11.9 g protein/L of human milk.
[d] pp = Postpartum.
[e] ND = Not determined.

For older children, the only data are those published by Nakagawa and coworkers in the 1960s (1961a, 1961b, 1962, 1963, 1964) on Japanese boys 10 to 12 years of age. Although these data seem to be accurate as there was uniformly negative nitrogen balance when the test amino acid was at zero, the maximum rate of nitrogen retention found when the amino acids were given in adequate quantities was 33 ± 14 mg/kg/d. This is approximately 5-fold higher than that predicted for 11-year-old boys, 7.7 mg/kg/d, as calculated from estimates of the protein deposition for boys this age (48 mg of protein/kg/d ÷ 6.25 mg of protein/mg of nitrogen, from Table 10-9). Thus, it is likely that the values generated in this series of studies are overestimates of the actual requirement. Similar problems of interpreting nitrogen balance studies are apparent in the data for infants aged 0 to 6 months from a number of detailed studies in which infants were given multiple levels of amino acids (Pratt et al., 1955; Snyderman et al., 1955, 1959a, 1959b, 1961a, 1961b, 1963, 1964a, 1964b;). With these studies also, the measured nitrogen balance was higher than what would be expected from the growth rates observed or estimated.

An attempt was made to reanalyze the data from these studies in order to obtain estimates of the mean requirement and its interindividual variance. Nonlinear regression analysis was used to fit the data for nitrogen balance versus amino acid intake to various curves, such as exponential, sigmoid, and bilinear crossover, in order to detect an approach to an asymptote or a breakpoint that could be equated with a requirement. However, these attempts did not lead to interpretable results, which proved to be too sensitive to the specific criteria employed to define the point on the curve that would identify a requirement.

In view of the reservations expressed above, the data from nitrogen balance studies in children were not utilized. Instead, the factorial approach was employed for children from 7 months through 18 years of age.

Factorial Estimate. In view of the doubts about the accuracy of the values generated by the empirical data, the factorial approach using data for growth (and its amino acid composition) and maintenance was utilized to determine requirements. In this model, the growth component was estimated from estimates of the rate of protein deposition at different ages (Table 10-9), the amino acid composition of whole body protein (Table 10-19), and incremental efficiency of protein utilization as derived from the studies in Table 10-8.

The obligatory need for protein deposition (growth) was calculated as the product of the rate of protein deposition (Table 10-9) and the amino acid composition of whole body protein (Table 10-19). This was then converted to a dietary requirement for protein deposition by dividing the need by the incremental efficiency of dietary protein utilization, which is estimated by the average slope of the regression analyses evaluating the protein requirement from studies done in children 7 months through

TABLE 10-19 Indispensable Amino Acid Composition of Whole Body Protein

Amino Acid	mg/g Protein ± 1 Standard Deviation (from interspecies comparison)
Histidine	27 ± 2
Isoleucine	35 ± 3
Leucine	75 ± 2
Lysine	73 ± 3
Methionine + cysteine	35 ± 1
Phenylalanine + tyrosine	73 ± 4
Threonine	42 ± 3
Tryptophan	12 (no extensive data)
Valine	49 ± 4

SOURCE: Davis et al. (1994).

13 years (0.58) from Table 10-8 and in children 14 through 18 years (0.47) from Table 10-12.

It is also necessary to determine a maintenance amino acid requirement since by 7 months of age, the dietary requirement necessary to maintain the body in nitrogen equilibrium accounts for more than 50 percent of the total indispensable amino acid requirement. This was determined in three ways.

First, estimates of the amino acid requirements needed for maintenance were calculated based on estimates of the obligatory nitrogen loss, which is the total rate of loss of nitrogen by all routes (urine, feces, and miscellaneous) in children receiving a protein-free or very low protein intake. Assuming that each individual amino acid contributed to this loss in proportion to its content in body protein, and that this represents the minimal rate of loss for this amino acid, the amount of this amino acid that must be given to replace the loss and achieve nitrogen balance is taken as the maintenance requirement when corrected for the efficiency of nitrogen utilization. Thus, the lysine requirement for maintenance for children 7 months through 13 years of age is calculated by multiplying the obligatory nitrogen loss of 57.4 mg/kg/d (mean intercept from Table 10-8), which is equivalent to 359 mg of protein/kg/d (57.4×6.25), by the estimate of the proportion of lysine in body protein of 0.073 (Table 10-19), to yield a value for lysine of 26.2 mg/kg/d (i.e., 359 mg/kg/d $\times$ 0.073). Then this is divided by the slope of the regression line of protein intake versus nitrogen balance, which represents the efficiency protein utilization of 0.58 (Table 10-8) for children to yield a value of 45 mg/kg/d (i.e., 26.2 mg/kg/d divided by 0.58) for the lysine maintenance requirement. The calculated values for each indispensable amino acid are shown in Table 10-20.

A second method for estimating maintenance requirements is to assume that at nitrogen equilibrium, the relative requirement of each indispensable amino acid is in proportion to its contribution to body protein. Thus, the maintenance protein requirement of 688 mg/kg/d (110 mg of N/kg/d for children through age 13 in Table 10-8 $\times$ 6.25) can be converted into requirements for individual amino acids by multiplying the maintenance protein requirement by the proportional contribution of the amino acid to body protein (Table 10-19). This method is mathematically equivalent to the method described above, but because the values for obligatory loss and maintenance protein requirement were taken from the regression of protein intake against nitrogen balance, for statistical reasons they give slightly different results, and both are given in the Table 10-20.

Since it was noted that the maintenance nitrogen requirement of 110 mg/kg/d (Table 10-8) does not vary with age in children, and the value in children is very similar to that found for adults of 105 mg/kg/d

TABLE 10-20 Factorial Estimates of Maintenance Amino Acid Requirements for Children in Comparison to Adults

Amino Acid	Children		Adults		
	Based on Obligatory Nitrogen Loss (mg/kg/d)[a]	Based on Maintenance Protein Requirement (mg/kg/d)[b]	Based on Maintenance Protein Requirement (mg/kg/d)[c]	Direct Measurement of EAR (mg/kg/d)[d]	Ratio of Maintenance Amino Acid Requirements to EAR
Histidine	17	19	18	ND[e]	—
Isoleucine	22	24	23	ND[e]	—
Leucine	46	52	49	34	1.4
Lysine	45	50	48	31	1.5
Methionine + cysteine	22	24	23	15	1.5
Phenylalanine + tyrosine	45	50	48	27	1.7
Threonine	26	29	28	16	1.7
Tryptophan	7	8	8	4	2.0
Valine	30	34	32	19	1.7

[a] Determined by multiplying the estimated obligatory nitrogen (N) loss in children, 57.4 mg N kg/d × 6.25 (Table 10-8) by the estimates for the amino acid content of whole body protein (Table 10-19) and then dividing by the efficiency of protein utilization, 0.58 for children (slope in Table 10-8) and 0.47 for adults (slope in Table 10-12).

[b] Determined by multiplying the total protein maintenance needs in children aged 7 months through 13 years, 110 mg N/kg/d × 6.25 (Table 10-8) by the amino acid content of whole body protein (Table 10-19).

[c] Determined by multiplying the total protein maintenance needs in adults, 105 mg N/kg/d × 6.25 (Table 10-12) by the amino acid content of whole body protein (Table 10-19).

[d] EAR = Estimated Average Requirement.

[e] ND = Not determined. There have been no direct measurements of isoleucine or histidine requirements in adults.

(Table 10-12), the values for maintenance amino acid requirements were taken to be independent of age in subsequent calculations. However, for adults, who are by definition at maintenance, direct measurements of the estimated average requirement (EAR) for each amino acid have been determined (see "Adults Ages 19 Years and Older"), and are shown in Table 10-20 for comparison with the factorially derived estimates. For all amino acids for adults, the EAR as derived from direct measurements is lower than the factorial approach by a factor of 1.3 to 2.0, depending on the amino acid. This difference is predictable because of the imperfections in the factorial approach. It is likely that the obligatory loss of one amino acid is higher than that for other amino acids in relation to their content in body protein. If this loss cannot be reduced further under basal conditions, then this amino acid will determine the obligatory loss for all other amino acids, which can no longer be used for anabolic processes. In theory, this "limiting" amino acid should be identified as having the lowest ratio between the requirement estimates from maintenance and by direct measurement, which is isoleucine in this report (Table 10-20). However, this is the amino acid with no direct measurements of requirement, as the adult EAR was estimated from its content in egg protein in relation to the other branched chain amino acids.

The important conclusion from the above discussion is that the calculation of the maintenance requirement in adults from the obligatory nitrogen loss gives values in adults that are in general higher than the measured values, and therefore appear to overestimate true maintenance. Moreover, as the maintenance protein requirement is estimated to be the same per kilogram of body weight in adults and children, it is reasonable to conclude that the amino acid values for maintenance needs derived from the obligatory nitrogen loss are likely to be overestimates in children as well as in adults. Therefore, in the factorial calculations to estimate total requirements for indispensable amino acid needs in children, the maintenance requirements for the individual amino acids are those derived on a weight basis from direct measurements or the EAR in adults (Table 10-20).

Indispensable Amino Acid EAR and RDA Summary, Ages 7 Months Through 18 Years

To calculate a factorial estimate of the EAR for individual indispensable amino acids, the amino acid needs for growth or protein deposition are first calculated as the product of the average rate of protein deposition (Table 10-9) and the average amino acid composition of body protein (Table 10-19). Thus, for a 9- through 12-month-old infant depositing on average 242 mg of protein/kg/d (Table 10-9, average of 232 mg/kg/d for girls and 252 mg/kg/d for boys), the obligatory need for lysine (amino acid deposition) is 242 × 0.073 (Table 10-19) = 17.7 mg/kg/d. This is then divided by the partial efficiency of protein deposition (0.58 as shown in Table 10-8 for children aged 7 months through 13 years and 0.47 for children aged 14 through 18 years [see "Adolescents, Ages 14 Through 18 Years"]) to yield a value of 30 mg/kg/d for protein deposition. (The same result would be achieved by multiplying the amino acid deposition figure by 1.72 [reciprocal of 0.58] or 2.13 [reciprocal of 0.47] as indicated in Table 10-21.) This value is then added to the estimated maintenance requirement, which is the same as the EAR in adults on a body weight basis (31 mg/kg/d in Tables 10-20 and 10-21). This gives an EAR for the 9- through 12-month-old infant of 62 mg of lysine/kg/d. In the same way, the EARs for each of the indispensable amino acids at different age groups were calculated and the results are shown in Table 10-21.

The RDA for the indispensable amino acids for children is set by determining the coefficients of variation for maintenance and for protein deposition. Since the maintenance requirement in adults was utilized, the estimate of the coefficient of variation in adults (12 percent) (see "Protein RDA Summary, Ages 19 Through 50 Years") was also utilized to determine the RDA for maintenance requirements for children. A coefficient of variation of 43 percent for protein deposition was determined in the study of Butte and coworkers (2000), and this varied little with age and gender. Therefore, this value was used for variation in growth for all ages. Since the RDA is defined as equal to the EAR plus twice the CV to cover the needs of 97 to 98 percent of the individuals in the group, the protein RDA is equal to the EAR + 2 × square root [(0.12 × Maintenance)^2 + (0.43 × 1.72 for children 7 mo–13 y or 2.13 for children 14–18 y × Protein Deposition)^2]. The RDAs for each indispensable amino acid for each age group are shown in Table 10-21.

Adults Ages 19 Years and Older

Evidence Considered in Estimating the Average Requirement

Several different indicators have been used to determine indispensable amino acid requirements, which include nitrogen balance (N-balance), plasma amino acid concentrations, direct amino acid oxidation (DAAO), 24-hour amino acid balance (AAB), and indicator amino acid oxidation (IAAO). An explanation of each of these indicators is found in the section, "Selection of Indicators for Estimating the Requirement for Individual Amino Acids." In general, the latter three methods, which depend on amino acid kinetic measurements, give higher values for amino acid requirements than do the (classical) nitrogen balance studies.

Resolution of a Controversy. All of the above five methods are based on measuring a change in the particular endpoint in response to graded levels of the test amino acid. A key observation regarding nitrogen balance as an endpoint is that there is a curvilinear relationship between nitrogen balance and test amino acid intake, so that nitrogen retention (nitrogen balance) becomes less efficient as zero balance is approached (Figure 10-7) (Rand and Young, 1999). Furthermore, the earlier work did not include miscellaneous losses in their nitrogen balances. Finally, most studies did not attempt to consider the effect of between-individual variance.

Only two studies were found in which several individuals were studied at four or more different levels of intake of the test amino acid (Jones et al., 1956; Reynolds et al., 1958). Rand and Young (1999) reanalyzed the lysine data of Jones et al. (1956) using regression techniques and found that curvilinear models best fit the data (Figure 10-7). They also examined the effect of adding either 5 or 8 mg/kg/d of miscellaneous nitrogen losses. Whereas Jones and coworkers (1956) had concluded, based on their data, that the lysine requirement was 8 mg/kg/d, the reanalysis by Rand and Young (1999) came to the conclusion that the lysine requirement was in the range of 17 to 36 mg/kg/d, and that the data strongly support a requirement of about 30 mg/kg/d. As shown in Table 10-22, this requirement approximates values derived from DAAO (Meredith et al., 1986), is similar to values derived from 24-hour amino acid balances (Kurpad et al., 2001a, 2002b), and is comparable to values derived from two IAAO studies (Kriengsinyos et al., 2002; Zello et al., 1993).

It is important to note that in growing animals, nitrogen balance and IAAO give comparable values (Zello et al., 1995) as do DAAO and IAAO. All three approaches are based on different assumptions. The reanalysis of the Jones et al. (1956) data by Rand and Young (1999) using nonlinear regression and including miscellaneous losses, has closed the apparent gap between nitrogen balance and the amino acid oxidation techniques.

Twenty-four Hour Amino Acid Balance. As shown in Table 10-22, 24-hour amino acid balance studies have been completed for four amino acids: leucine (El-Khoury et al., 1994a; Kurpad et al., 2001b), lysine (Kurpad et al., 2001a, 2002a), phenylalanine + tyrosine (Basile-Filho et al., 1998), and most recently threonine (Borgonha et al., 2002; Kurpad et al., 2002b). Of the studies, lysine (Kurpad et al., 2001a, 2002a) and threonine (Borgonha et al., 2002; Kurpad et al., 2002b) employed the 24-hour indicator balance method. Furthermore, the initial 24-hour balance study for leucine (El-Khoury et al., 1994b) also included measurement of urea production as further support for the leucine requirement estimate obtained from DAAO (Meguid et al., 1986a). Similarly, the 24-hour lysine balance data lend

TABLE 10-21 Calculations of Estimated Average Requirement (EAR) and Recommended Dietary Allowance (RDA) for Amino Acids for Children Ages 7 Months Through 18 Years

Age and Gender/Amino Acid	Maintenance[a] (mg/kg/d)	Amino Acid Deposition[b] (mg/kg/d)	Total = EAR[c] (mg/kg/d)	RDA[d] (mg/kg/d)
7–12 mo, Boys, Girls				
Histidine	11	7	22	32
Isoleucine	15	9	30	43
Leucine	34	18	65	93
Lysine	31	18	62	89
Methionine + cysteine	15	9	30	43
Phenylalanine + tyrosine	27	18	58	84
Threonine	16	10	34	49
Tryptophan	4	3	9	13
Valine	19	12	39	58
1–3 y, Boys, Girls				
Histidine	11	3	16	21
Isoleucine	15	4	22	28
Leucine	34	8	48	63
Lysine	31	8	45	58
Methionine + cysteine	15	4	22	28
Phenylalanine + tyrosine	27	8	41	54
Threonine	16	5	24	32
Tryptophan	4	1	6	8
Valine	19	5	28	37

continued

4–8 y, Boys, Girls

Histidine	11	1	13	16
Isoleucine	15	2	18	22
Leucine	34	4	40	49
Lysine	31	3	37	46
Methionine + cysteine	15	2	18	22
Phenylalanine + tyrosine	27	3	33	41
Threonine	16	2	19	24
Tryptophan	4	1	5	6
Valine	19	2	23	28

9–13 y, Boys

Histidine	11	1	13	17
Isoleucine	15	2	18	22
Leucine	34	4	40	49
Lysine	31	4	37	46
Methionine + cysteine	15	2	18	22
Phenylalanine + tyrosine	27	4	33	41
Threonine	16	2	19	24
Tryptophan	4	1	5	6
Valine	19	42	23	28

TABLE 10-21 Continued

Age and Gender/Amino Acid	Maintenance[a] (mg/kg/d)	Amino Acid Deposition[b] (mg/kg/d)	Total = EAR[c] (mg/kg/d)	RDA[d] (mg/kg/d)
9–13 y, Girls				
Histidine	11	1	12	15
Isoleucine	15	1	17	21
Leucine	34	2	38	47
Lysine	31	2	35	43
Methionine + cysteine	15	1	17	21
Phenylalanine + tyrosine	27	2	31	38
Threonine	16	1	18	22
Tryptophan	4	< 0.5	5	6
Valine	19	2	22	27
14–18 y, Boys				
Histidine	11	1	12	15
Isoleucine	15	1	17	21
Leucine	34	2	38	47
Lysine	31	2	35	43
Methionine + cysteine	15	1	17	21
Phenylalanine + tyrosine	27	2	31	38
Threonine	16	1	18	22
Tryptophan	4	< 0.5	5	6
Valine	19	1	22	27

14–18 y, Girls				
Histidine	11	< 0.5	12	14
Isoleucine	15	< 0.5	16	19
Leucine	34	1	35	44
Lysine	31	1	32	40
Methionine + cysteine	15	< 0.5	16	19
Phenylalanine + tyrosine	27	1	28	35
Threonine	16	< 0.5	17	21
Tryptophan	4	< 0.5	4	5
Valine	19	1	20	24

[a] Derived from the adult EAR for specified amino acids (from Table 10-20).

[b] Derived using the following equation: Amino acid deposition = mean protein deposition (from Table 10-9) × amino acid composition of whole body protein (from Table 10-19).

[c] EAR for ages 7 mo–13 y = maintenance + amino acid deposition × 1.72. EAR for ages 14–18 y = maintenance + amino acid deposition × 2.13.

[d] RDA for ages 7 mo–13 y = $EAR + 2 \times \sqrt{[(0.12 \times maintenance)^2 + (0.43 \times 1.72 \times mean\ protein\ deposition)^2]}$. RDA for ages 14–18y = $EAR + 2 \times \sqrt{[(0.12 \times maintenance)^2 + (0.43 \times 2.13 \times mean\ protein\ deposition)^2]}$.

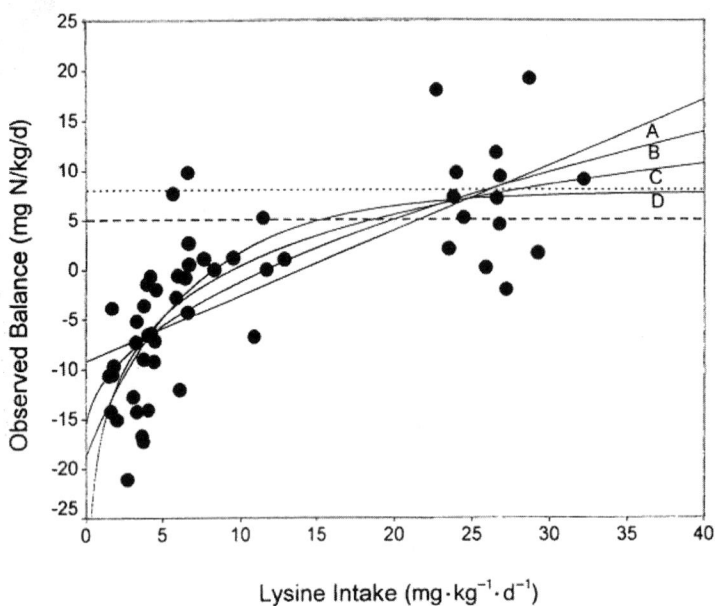

FIGURE 10-7 Relationship between nitrogen balance and test amino acid intake using four different one-fit regression equations: linear (A), square root (B), log (C), and exponential asymptotic (D), superimposed on the original data. Reprinted, with permission, from Rand and Young (1999). Copyright 1999 by the American Society for Nutritional Sciences.

support to the lysine DAAO estimate (Kurpad et al., 2001a; Meredith et al., 1986).

The 24-hour balance model is regarded as being the best from a theoretical point of view, especially when performed with the indicator approach. However, from a practical point of view, the 24-hour amino acid balance studies are very labor intensive with the result that only three or four levels of intake of the test amino acid have been studied for each of leucine, lysine, phenylalanine + tyrosine, and threonine.

Direct Amino Acid Oxidation. The DAAO method has been utilized to investigate six or seven amino acid levels, so it was possible to reanalyze these data using two-phase linear crossover regression analysis and define a breakpoint (which is regarded as the EAR). DAAO can only be used if the carboxyl group of the test amino acid is released to the body bicarbonate pool when the amino acid is committed to degradation. As shown in

TABLE 10-22 Indispensable Amino Acid Studies in Adults

Reference	Amino Acid	Method Used[a] (Number of Levels/ Number of Data Points)	Estimated Average Requirement (mg/kg/d)
Meguid et al., 1986a	Leucine	DAAO reanalyzed (8/52)	24.5
El-Khoury et al., 1994a	Leucine	24-h AAB (3/10)	38.3
Kurpad et al., 2001b	Leucine	24-h AAB (4/40)	40
Meredith et al., 1986	Lysine	DAAO reanalyzed (8/28)	26.6
Zello et al., 1993	Lysine	IAAO (7/42)	36.9
Rand and Young, 1999	Lysine	N-Balance reanalyzed (8/53)	30
Kurpad et al., 2001a	Lysine	24-h IAAB (4/32)	29
Kriengsinyos et al., 2002	Lysine	IAAO (5/60)	35
Kurpad et al., 2002a	Lysine	24-h IAAB (4/36)	29
Reynolds et al., 1958	Methionine + cysteine	N-balance reanalyzed (6/42)	20
Young et al., 1991	Methionine + cysteine	Methionine balance (1/5)	13
Di Buono et al., 2001	Methionine + cysteine	IAAO (6/36)	12.6
Zello et al., 1990	Phenylalanine	DAAO (7/41)	9.1
Roberts et al., 2001	Tyrosine	IAAO (7/42)	6.0
	Phenylalanine + tyrosine		15.1
Basile-Filho et al., 1998	Phenylalanine + tyrosine	24-h AAB	39.0
Zhao et al., 1986	Threonine	DAAO reanalyzed (7/33)	13.5
Wilson et al., 2000	Threonine	IAAO (7/36)	19.0
Borgonha et al., 2002	Threonine	24-h IAAB (3/15)	15.0
Kurpad et al., 2002b	Threonine	24-h IAAB (6/48)	15.0
Lazaris-Brunner et al., 1998	Tryptophan	IAAO (8/36)	4.0
Meguid et al., 1986b	Valine	DAAO reanalyzed (7/37)	19.2

[a] AAB = amino acid balance, DAAO = direct amino acid oxidation, IAAB = indicator amino acid balance and oxidation, IAAO = indicator amino acid oxidation.

Table 10-22, DAAO studies of indispensable amino acid requirements are limited to leucine (Meguid et al., 1986a), lysine (Meredith et al., 1986), phenylalanine (Zello et al., 1990), and valine (Meguid et al., 1986b). DAAO was also utilized to determine the threonine requirement (Zhao et al., 1986). However there are theoretical concerns for this amino acid, since there are two pathways of degradation for threonine; the second pathway, threonine dehydrogenase (TDG), ends in the label being retained in glycine. In practical terms this may not be a serious error since others have shown that the TDG pathway is a minor pathway in adults (Darling et al., 2000).

Indicator Amino Acid Oxidation. IAAO has the advantage that the requirement of any amino acid can be determined, since either phenylalanine (in the presence of an excess of tyrosine to ensure that there is no label retention in the body tyrosine pools) or lysine can and have been used as indicator amino acids in humans and in animals (Bross et al., 2000; Brunton et al., 1998; Zello et al., 1995). A further strength of the IAAO studies is that each adult was fed at six or seven levels of the test amino acid, which has made it possible to define requirements for individuals by two-phase, linear cross-over regression analysis (Brunton et al., 1998; Zello et al., 1995). As shown in Table 10-22, IAAO estimates have been reported for lysine (Kriengsinyos et al., 2002; Zello et al., 1993), methionine + cysteine (Di Buono et al., 2001), tyrosine (Roberts et al., 2001), threonine (Wilson et al., 2000), and tryptophan (Lazaris-Brunner et al., 1998).

As shown in Table 10-22, currently there are amino acid oxidation estimates in which two-phase linear crossover regression analysis has been performed for leucine (DAAO), lysine (both DAAO and IAAO), methionine + cysteine (IAAO), phenylalanine (DAAO), tyrosine (IAAO), threonine (both DAAO and IAAO), tryptophan (IAAO), and valine (DAAO).

Other Indicators. Nonlinear regression was used on two sets of nitrogen balance data as shown by Rand and Young (1999). The first was for lysine in which the original data were in women, each of whom were studied at two to five levels (Jones et al., 1956). This data set was reanalyzed using nonlinear regression, including the addition of 5 or 8 mg of nitrogen/kg/d as miscellaneous losses (Rand and Young, 1999), and these reanalyzed data are included in Table 10-22. Using a similar approach, the data of Reynolds and coworkers (1958) for methionine + cysteine were reanalyzed, and these data are included in Table 10-22. The result is consistent with the data of Zezulka and Calloway (1976a, 1976b), who studied the effect on nitrogen balance of three levels of methionine added to soy protein at a constant and adequate level of total nitrogen. Since there are no direct estimates of the isoleucine requirement, it is estimated from the leucine and valine estimates. The isoleucine requirement was therefore calculated by multiplying the isoleucine requirement calculated from the protein requirement (Table 10-20) by 1.55, the average of the ratios for leucine and valine. Similarly, the requirement for histidine, for which there have also been no direct determinations, is calculated from the protein requirement (Table 10-20) multiplied by 1.7, the average ratio for all amino acids in Table 10-19.

Indispensable Amino Acid EAR Summary, Ages 19 Years and Older

An EAR was derived for each of the indispensable amino acids from the data in Table 10-22. Where more than one EAR was given for an amino acid in Table 10-22, the values were averaged and rounded to the nearest whole number. This approach is weakest with the phenylalanine + tyrosine requirements where there is a large range—from 15.1 to 39 mg/kg/d giving an average value of 27 mg/kg/d. Lysine is the indispensable amino acid with the most estimates (six in all), with the EAR varying from 26.6 to 36.9 mg/kg/d for an average value of 31 mg/kg/d. Given the very few studies available, separate requirements could not be determined for women versus men, or for young and older adults.

EAR for Adults
    19 years and older
          11 mg/kg/d of histidine
          15 mg/kg/d of isoleucine
          34 mg/kg/d of leucine
          31 mg/kg/d of lysine
          15 mg/kg/d of methionine + cysteine
          27 mg/kg/d of phenylalanine + tyrosine
          16 mg/kg/d of threonine
           4 mg/kg/d of tryptophan
          19 mg/kg/d of valine

Indispensable Amino Acid RDA Summary, Ages 19 Years and Older

With protein (see "Protein RDA Summary, Ages 19 Through 50 Years"), because the distribution of individual requirements for protein is not a normal distribution and is skewed, its calculated standard deviation and coefficient of variation do not have the usual intuitive meaning (the mean plus two standard deviations exceeding all but about 2.5 percent of the population's requirement). However, an approximate standard deviation was calculated as half of the distance from the 16th to the 84th percentile of the protein requirement distribution as estimated from the log normal distribution of requirements. This gives, for comparative purposes, an approximate standard deviation of 12.5 mg N/kg/d (a CV = 12 percent). Given the paucity of data, it is assumed that for amino acids a similar deviation should be used; thus the RDA = EAR + 2 CV for amino acids as well as for protein, or RDA = 1.24 × EAR. The calculated RDA is rounded to the nearest whole number.

RDA for Adults

19 years and older

14 mg/kg/d of histidine
19 mg/kg/d of isoleucine
42 mg/kg/d of leucine
38 mg/kg/d of lysine
19 mg/kg/d of methionine + cysteine
33 mg/kg/d of phenylalanine + tyrosine
20 mg/kg/d of threonine
5 mg/kg/d of tryptophan
4 mg/kg/d of valine

Pregnancy

Method Used to Estimate the Average Requirement

There are essentially no data with regard to amino acid requirements during pregnancy, so it is generally assumed that indispensable amino acid needs increase in proportion to the increased protein needs during pregnancy. Since the pregnancy EAR for total protein is 0.88 g/kg/d for women, the amino acid EARs for nonpregnant women were multiplied by 1.33 and rounded to the nearest whole number.

Amino Acid EAR and RDA Summary, Pregnancy

EAR for Pregnancy

For all ages

15 mg/kg/d of histidine
20 mg/kg/d of isoleucine
45 mg/kg/d of leucine
41 mg/kg/d of lysine
20 mg/kg/d of methionine + cysteine
36 mg/kg/d of phenylalanine + tyrosine
21 mg/kg/d of threonine
5 mg/kg/d of tryptophan
25 mg/kg/d of valine

The RDA for amino acids for pregnancy is set by increasing the EAR by the variation in protein derived for adults ages 19 years and older (1.24 × EAR) and rounded to nearest whole number.

RDA for Pregnancy
    For all ages   18 mg/kg/d of histidine
                    25 mg/kg/d of isoleucine
                    56 mg/kg/d of leucine
                    51 mg/kg/d of lysine
                    25 mg/kg/d of methionine + cysteine
                    44 mg/kg/d of phenylalanine + tyrosine
                    26 mg/kg/d of threonine
                     7 mg/kg/d of tryptophan
                    31 mg/kg/d of valine

Lactation

Method Used to Estimate the Average Requirement

There are essentially no data with regard to amino acid requirements during lactation, so it is generally assumed that indispensable amino acid needs will increase over the nonlactating needs by the amount of amino acids found in human milk (Table 10-18).

To estimate the EAR for amino acids for lactation, the average amounts of amino acids in human milk during the first 6 months of lactation expressed as mg/kg/d based on the reference weight of the adult woman in Table 1-1 (see "AI for Infants 0–6 Months"), are added to the EAR for amino acids for the nonlactating woman, expressed as mg/kg/d (see sections "Amino Acids EAR and RDA Summary, Ages 7 Months Through 18 Years" and "Amino Acids EAR and RDA Summary, Ages 19 Years and Older"). The calculated EARs in mg/kg body weight/d are rounded to the nearest whole number.

Amino Acid EAR and RDA Summary, Lactation

EAR for Lactation
    For all ages   15 mg/kg/d of histidine
                    24 mg/kg/d of isoleucine
                    50 mg/kg/d of leucine
                    42 mg/kg/d of lysine
                    21 mg/kg/d of methionine + cysteine
                    41 mg/kg/d of phenylalanine + tyrosine
                    24 mg/kg/d of threonine
                     7 mg/kg/d of tryptophan
                    28 mg/kg/d of valine

The RDA for amino acids for lactation is set by assuming the same (CV) as that for total protein for lactation, 12 percent. The RDA is defined as the EAR plus twice the assumed CV to cover the needs of 97 to 98 percent of the individuals in the group. Therefore, for amino acids the RDA is 124 percent of the EAR for adolescents and adults. The calculated RDA in mg/kg of body weight/d is rounded.

RDA for Lactation
> **For all ages**   **19 mg/kg/d of histidine**
>   **30 mg/kg/d of isoleucine**
>   **62 mg/kg/d of leucine**
>   **52 mg/kg/d of lysine**
>   **26 mg/kg/d of methionine + cysteine**
>   **51 mg/kg/d of phenylalanine + tyrosine**
>   **30 mg/kg/d of threonine**
>   **9 mg/kg/d of tryptophan**
>   **35 mg/kg/d of valine**

INTAKE OF TOTAL PROTEIN AND AMINO ACIDS

Protein Quality

Different sources of protein vary widely in their chemical composition as well as in their nutritional value. The quality of a source of protein (or more specifically the source of nitrogen, since dietary protein is generally measured analytically in terms of nitrogen) is an expression of its ability to provide the nitrogen and amino acid requirements for growth, maintenance, and repair. In practice, protein quality is principally determined by two factors: digestibility and the amino acid composition of the protein in question. In food as opposed to relatively pure protein, the contribution of all of the indispensable amino acids to the total nitrogen content of the food has to be considered in assessing the overall protein quality of the diet.

Digestibility

Nitrogen is excreted in the feces in amounts that usually vary between 10 and 25 percent of the nitrogen intake. As mentioned earlier, only a part of this is derived directly from dietary nitrogen that was not absorbed; the other parts result from protein and other secretions into the gastro-intestinal tract during the process of digestion and from nitrogen contained in fecal bacteria. The unabsorbed part represents mainly proteins that, by reason of their physical characteristics or chemical composition, are resistant to breakdown by the proteolytic digestive enzymes. There is probably a variable contribution of nitrogen contained in other nonabsorbable components, such as amino sugars and other nitrogen-containing materials found in cell walls.

On the other hand, the secretions consist of specific proteins, such as mucins, which represent a loss that is of nutritional importance. These secretions appear to be rich in threonine and cysteine (Roberton et al., 1991), and thus contribute to the requirement for both amino acids. However, both the nonabsorbed and secreted components that make up nitrogen loss are difficult to quantify with any confidence, except in terms of total nitrogen, because of the overwhelming modifying effect of the intestinal microflora. Thus, digestibility (as estimated by nitrogen excretion) is usually determined by measuring the fecal nitrogen (N_{FP}) in individuals consuming the specific nitrogen source and subtracting the fecal nitrogen values obtained when a protein-free diet is given (N_{F0}). This value is then subtracted from the total nitrogen intake (N_I) and expressed as a proportion of the nitrogen intake.

$$\text{True Digestibility} = D_F = (N_I - N_{F\Delta})/N_I,$$

where $N_{FD} = N_{FP} - N_{F0}$.

Fecal nitrogen from a protein-free diet is a measure of the amount of nitrogen from intestinal secretions, on the assumption (probably incorrect) that this component does not vary with different diets (de Lange et al., 1989). The values thus calculated are called "true" digestibility and represent the proportion of the dietary nitrogen that is absorbed. This portion can generally be assumed to be available to the host for meeting the needs for maintenance and growth.

It must be noted that a number of recent studies with isotopically labeled proteins suggest that true digestibility exceeds 90 percent for many common foods such as milk, cereals, and soy and other legumes (Darragh and Hodgkinson, 2000, de Vrese et al., 2000; Mariotti et al., 1999, Gausserès et al., 1997; Gaudichon et al., 1999). It should also be noted that, at present, calculation of the availability (or digestibility) of amino acids from food protein sources is based on the digestibility of total nitrogen as contrasted to that for the individual amino acid. However, there can be quite large differences between the digestibility coefficients for total nitrogen and the individual amino acid. These and other related aspects of protein quality have been reviewed elsewhere (Darragh and Hodgkinson, 2000; Schaafsma, 2000).

The digestive and intestinal phase of dietary protein utilization is currently an active area of research, but it is still, from a practical standpoint, not possible to make major improvements over the estimates of true protein digestibility made some years ago by the Food and Agriculture Organization and the World Health Organization (FAO/WHO, 1991). Therefore, the determination of true digestibility of proteins, diets, and amino acids in this report are based on the approaches and values proposed by FAO/WHO in 1991.

Nitrogen Versus Amino Acids

Absorbed nitrogen is mainly in the form of amino acids, but a proportion is in other compounds such as nucleic acids, creatine, amino sugars, ammonia, and urea. The quantitative extent to which these contribute to nitrogen retention and homeostasis is not known. Creatine can probably be utilized (Metges et al., 1999b), but in general it is unknown to what extent these different compounds can have a sparing effect on the utilization of the amino acids for which they are precursors. However, the major requirement for total nitrogen or protein is for the specific indispensable amino acids (and/or conditionally indispensable amino acids) and an additional source of α-amino nitrogen. At appropriate intakes these maintain protein homeostasis and adequate synthesis of those physiologically important compounds for which amino acids are the obligatory precursors (Table 10-5).

It is conventional to use a value of 6.25 to express the weight ratio of protein to the nitrogen content in foods, which assumes that nitrogen is, on average, 16 percent by weight of mixed protein. However, this factor is in fact quite variable among different proteins. For example, when protein intake is calculated by summing the weight of amino acids as analyzed in a food (less the water of hydrolysis), the protein/nitrogen ratio is 5.38 for egg, 5.62 for whole milk, 4.86 for cooked ham, 5.70 for whole-meal wheat bread, and 6.07 for soymilk. Thus when converting the amount of nitrogen present in a specific foodstuff to total protein, this factor becomes important to use.

These differences in the protein-to-nitrogen ratio of food proteins are not of specific importance in reference to the development of the recommendations for protein requirements given herein. This is because these recommendations have been based initially on nitrogen balance determinations, which in turn were based on analytical measurements of nitrogen intake (from different test proteins or mixtures of proteins). The nitrogen intake values were then converted to protein intakes using the conventional 6.25 factor, irrespective of the protein source used in the various experiments.

However, the protein-to-nitrogen conversion factor does matter in considering the quality of food protein sources when the protein-specific nitrogen conversion factor has been used to convert the chemically determined nitrogen content of the protein to a protein value. In this case, protein intakes and the relation between the amino acid concentrations in the protein should all be referred back to a nitrogen base. For this reason, amino acid requirement patterns delineated below are given in reference to both conventional protein (nitrogen × 6.25) and to a nitrogen basis.

Amino Acids Content of Proteins

The second and generally more important factor that influences the nutritional value of a protein source is the relative content and metabolic availability of the individual indispensable amino acids. If the content of a single indispensable amino acid in the diet is less than the individual's requirement, then it will limit the utilization of other amino acids and thus prevent normal rates of protein synthesis even when the total nitrogen intake level is adequate. Thus, the "limiting amino acid" will determine the nutritional value of the total nitrogen or protein in the diet. This has been illustrated in experiments comparing the relative ability of different protein sources to maintain nitrogen balance. For example, studies have shown, depending on its source and preparation, that more soy protein might be needed to maintain nitrogen balance when compared to egg-white protein, and that the difference may be eliminated by the addition of methionine to the soy diet. This indicates that sulfur amino acids can be limiting in soy (Zezulka and Calloway, 1976a, 1976b). Similarly, the limiting amino acid in wheat protein is lysine (Young et al., 1975a).

The concept of the limiting amino acid has led to the practice of amino acid (or chemical) scoring, whereby the indispensable amino acid composition of the specific protein source is compared with that of a reference amino acid composition profile. Earlier the amino acid composition of a good quality protein such as egg, which is regarded as being well balanced in amino acid content in relation to human needs (FAO/WHO, 1973), was used as a reference or benchmark. Table 10-23 shows the composition of various food protein sources expressed as mg of amino acid per g of protein (nitrogen × 6.25). The composition of amino acids of egg and milk proteins is similar with the exception of the sulfur amino acids methionine and cysteine. However, wheat and beans have lower proportions of indispensable amino acids, especially of lysine and sulfur amino acids, respectively.

The nutritional implications of these differences in the amino acid content of different proteins or mixtures of proteins can be evaluated by

TABLE 10-23 Amino Acid Composition of Major Food Protein Sources (mg/g protein)[a]

Amino Acid	Whole Wheat Flour	Navy Beans	Milk	Eggs
Histidine	22	28	28	24
Isoleucine	40	42	60	63
Leucine	63	76	98	88
Lysine	26	72	79	70
Methionine + cysteine	35	19	34	56
Phenylalanine + tyrosine	81	77	96	98
Threonine	27	39	45	49
Tryptophan	11	10	14	16
Valine	43	46	67	72

[a] Values for protein composition (N × 6.25) are from Young and Pellett (1990).

comparing the amino acid composition of the protein source with a suitable reference amino acid pattern.

Amino Acid Scoring and Protein Quality

In recent years, the amino acid requirement values for humans have been used to develop reference amino acid patterns for purposes of evaluating the quality of food proteins or their capacity to efficiently meet both the nitrogen and indispensable amino acid requirements of the individual. Based on the estimated average requirements for the individual indispensable amino acids presented earlier (Tables 10-20 and 10-21) and for total protein (nitrogen × 6.25) (Tables 10-9 and 10-13), it is possible to establish an amino acid requirement (or scoring) pattern for preschool children and for adults. These are given in Table 10-24 together with the amino acid requirement pattern used for breast-fed infants. It should be noted that this latter pattern is that for human milk and so it is derived quite differently compared to that for the other age groups.

There are three important points that need to be highlighted about the proposed amino acid scoring patterns. First, there are relatively small differences between the amino acid requirement and thus scoring patterns for children and adults, therefore use amino acid requirement pattern for 1 to 3 years of age is recommended as the reference pattern for purposes of assessment and planning of the protein component of diets.

Second, the requirement pattern proposed here for adults is fundamentally different from a number of previously recommended requirement patterns (Table 10-25). The pattern for adults (FAO/WHO/UNU,

TABLE 10-24 Proposed Amino Acid Scoring Patterns for Infants, Preschool Children, and Adults Based on Estimated Requirements for Protein and Indispensable Amino Acids

Amino Acid	Infants[a] (mg/g protein)	Preschool Children (1–3 y) (mg/g protein)[b]	Preschool Children (1–3 y) (mg/g N)[c]	Adults (18+ y) (mg/g protein)[b]	Adults (18+ y) (mg/g N)[c]
Histidine	23	18	114	17	104
Isoleucine	57	25	156	23	142
Leucine	101	55	341	52	322
Lysine	69	51	320	47	294
Methionine + cysteine	38	25	156	23	142
Phenylalanine + tyrosine	87	47	291	41	256
Threonine	47	27	170	24	152
Tryptophan	18	7	43	6	38
Valine	56	32	199	29	180

[a] Pattern based on amino acid composition of human milk (from Table 10-18).
[b] Pattern derived from (EAR for amino acid ÷ EAR for protein); for 1–3 y group, where EAR for protein = 0.88 g/kg/d; for adults, EAR for protein = 0.66 g/kg/d. EAR is Estimated Average Requirement.
[c] Calculated as (mg/g protein) × 6.25.

TABLE 10-25 FNB/IOM Scoring Pattern Compared to Other Proposed Patterns (mg/g protein)

Amino Acid	MIT Pattern[a]	Millward Pattern[b]	FAO/WHO/ UNU Pattern[c]	Recommended FNB/IOM Pattern[d]
Histidine	—	—	—	18
Isoleucine	35	30	13	25
Leucine	65	44	19	55
Lysine	50	31	16	51
Methionine + cysteine	25	27	17	25
Phenylalanine + tyrosine	65	33	19	47
Threonine	25	26	9	27
Tryptophan	10	6	5	7
Valine	35	23	13	32

[a] Young and Pellett (1990).
[b] Millward et al. (1990).
[c] FAO/WHO/UNU (1985).
[d] Based on 1- to 3-year-old Estimated Average Requirements for protein and indispensable amino acids.

1985) has uniformly lower proportions of all the indispensable amino acids, as these requirement values were determined from studies of nitrogen balance, which are now considered to be not as reliable as values derived from metabolic amino acid data (see previous discussion). The other requirement patterns shown in Table 10-25 for adults were published in two recent reviews (Millward, 1999; Young and Borgonha, 2000). The pattern suggested by Millward (1999) is based on a reanalysis of nitrogen balance data that yields values that are generally lower than either the FNB/IOM reference pattern, based on the EARs estimated above, or the MIT pattern (Young and Borgonha, 2000). The MIT pattern includes much of the oxidation and carbon balance data contained in the EAR estimates given in this report, but the reference pattern recommended here is derived from a larger body of data than that used by Young and Borgonha. Thus, the reference amino acid scoring patterns shown in Table 10-24 are designed for use in the evaluation of dietary protein quality.

Third, in generating these amino acid scoring patterns, the EARs for the amino acids and for total protein were used. However, two important statistical considerations need to be raised here: first, the extent to which there is a correlation between nitrogen (protein) and the requirement for a specific indispensable amino acid; second, the impact of the variance for both protein and amino acid requirements on the derived amino acid reference pattern. The extent to which the requirements for specific indispensable amino acids and total protein are correlated is not known. In this report it is assumed that the variance in requirement for each indispensable amino acid is the same as that for the adult protein requirement.

This analysis illustrates one of the uncertainties faced in establishing a reference or scoring pattern and judging the nutritional value of a protein source for an individual. However, on the basis of different experimental studies in groups of subjects, experience shows that a reasonable approximation of the mean value for the relative quality of a protein source or mixture of proteins can be obtained by use of the amino acid scoring pattern proposed in Table 10-26 and a standard amino acid scoring approach, examples of which are given in the following section.

Calculation of Amino Acid Scores for Different Food Proteins

The method for evaluating the relative nutritional quality of different protein sources that is used in this report is based on calculating the protein digestibility corrected amino acid score (PDCAAS) as proposed by FAO/WHO (1991). It is calculated as follows:

TABLE 10-26 Summary FNB/IOM 2002 Amino Acid Scoring Pattern for Use in Children ≥ 1 Year of Age and in All Other Older Age Groups

Amino Acid	mg/g protein[a]	mg/g N
Histidine	18	114
Isoleucine	25	156
Leucine	55	341
Lysine	51	320
Methionine + cysteine	25	156
Phenylalanine + tyrosine	47	291
Threonine	27	170
Tryptophan	7	43
Valine	32	199

[a] Protein = nitrogen × 6.25.

$$\text{PDCAAS (\%)} = \frac{[\text{mg of limiting amino acid in 1-g test protein}]}{\text{mg of same amino acid in 1-g reference protein}} \times [\text{true digestibility } (D_F)(\%)]$$

As mentioned earlier, in comparing the amino acid reference (or scoring) patterns (Table 10-24) for 1- through 3-year-old children and the adult age groups, it would be hard to justify proposing separate amino acid scoring patterns for these populations for practical purposes. Therefore, for calculation of the amino acid score, corrected for digestibility (PDCAAS, %), it is recommended that one scoring pattern be used to cover all ages from 1 year and above, as shown in Table 10-26.

A number of examples of the PDCAAS for different food proteins or diets based on three major protein sources are given in Table 10-27. As shown, wheat (lysine limiting) and chickpea proteins (sulfur amino acid limiting) have a PDCAAS of 44 and 87 percent, respectively. For a diet based on a mixture of wheat, chickpea, and skim milk proteins the PDCAAS is 110 percent, which is truncated to a value of 100, since the relative efficiency of utilization of the limiting amino acid cannot be greater than that of the amino acid scoring pattern at nitrogen intakes sufficient to meet nitrogen needs. Finally, it should be noted that PDCAAS scores have only been calculated here based on four indispensable amino acids (lysine, sulfur amino acids, threonine, and tryptophan). These are

TABLE 10-27 Calculation of PDCAAS[a] for Selected Individual Food Proteins and for a Mixture of These Proteins, Based on the FNB/IOM 2002 Amino Acid Scoring Pattern

Protein	Amino Acid Content (mg/g protein)[b]				Protein Digestibility	PDCAAS (%)
	Lys	SAA	Thr	Trp		
Wheat	25	35	30	11	0.85	42 (Lysine)[c]
Chickpea	70	25	42	13	0.80	80 (SAA)
Milk powder	80	30	37	12	0.95	100 (114—SAA)[d]
Mixture (% of protein) Wheat (19) Chickpea (32) Milk powder (49)						
For combination[e]	64	29	37	12	0.88	100 (102—SAA)

[a] Data for proteins taken from Table 10 of FAO/WHO (1991) using the procedure described therein to determine PDCAAS (Protein Digestibility Corrected Amino Acid Score).
[b] Lys = lysine; SAA = sulfur amino acids; Thr = threonine; Trp = Tryptophan.
[c] Lysine or sulfur amino acid = limiting amino acid.
[d] Where relevant, the nontruncated value for the PDCAAS is given prior to truncation to a value of 100.
[e] Weighted values based on the proportion of the total protein in the mixture that is contributed by each protein source.

the most likely limiting amino acids in common food protein sources and so have been considered here for illustrative purposes.

There have been discussions on ways to improve the PDCAAS procedure and further developments in this context are needed. Until better methods are developed, the foregoing procedure is recommended, using the digestibility values proposed by FAO/WHO (1991).

Comments on Protein Quality for Adults

While the importance of considering protein quality in relation to the protein nutrition of the young has been firmly established and accepted over the years, the significance of protein quality (other than digestibility) of protein sources in adults has been controversial or less clear. The amino acid scoring pattern given in Table 10-24 for adults is not markedly different from that for the preschool age group, implying that protein quality should also be an important consideration in adult protein nutrition.

In the published meta-analysis of nitrogen balance studies by Rand and coworkers (2003), there were no significant differences in the intakes of dietary nitrogen required to meet nitrogen equilibrium between those studies that supplied dietary protein predominantly from animal, vegetable, or mixed protein sources. It is important to realize however, that this aggregate analysis does not suggest that dietary protein quality is of no importance in adult protein nutrition. The examined and aggregated studies included an analysis of those that were designed to compare good quality soy protein (Istfan et al., 1983; Young et al., 1984) as well as one that involved comparison of whole-wheat proteins (Young et al., 1975a) with animal proteins sources using parallel experimental diet groups. The results of these studies showed clearly that the quality of well-processed soy proteins was equivalent to animal protein in the adults evaluated (which would be predicted from the amino acid reference pattern in Table 10-26), while wheat proteins were used with significantly lower efficiency than the animal protein (beef) (again this would be predicted from the procedure above). Similar studies compared rice and egg proteins (Inoue et al., 1973), wheat gluten and egg proteins (Yanez et al., 1982), and lupin and egg proteins (Egana et al., 1992), all demonstrating the higher quality of the animal protein reference sources.

Thus, the aggregate analyses of all available studies analyzed by Rand and coworkers (2003) obscured these results and illustrate the conservative nature of their meta-analysis of the primary nitrogen balance. Moreover, this discussion and presentation of data in Table 10-27 underscores the fact that while lysine is likely to be the most limiting of the indispensable amino acids in diets based predominantly on cereal proteins, the risk of a lysine inadequacy is essentially removed by inclusion of relatively modest amounts of animal or other vegetable proteins, such as those from legumes and oilseeds, or through lysine fortification of cereal flour.

Food Sources

Protein from animal sources such as meat, poultry, fish, eggs, milk, cheese, and yogurt provide all nine indispensable amino acids, and for this reason are referred to as "complete proteins." Proteins from plants, legumes, grains, nuts, seeds, and vegetables tend to be deficient in one or more of the indispensable amino acids and are called "incomplete proteins." Three ounces of lean meat or poultry contain about 25 g of protein, and 3 ounces of fish or 1 cup of soybeans supplies about 20 g of protein. The protein content of 1 cup of yogurt is approximately 8 g, 1 cup of milk is 8 g, and 1 egg or 1 ounce of cheese contains about 6 g. One cup of legumes has approximately 15 g of protein. Cereals, grains, nuts, and vegetables contain about 2 g of protein per serving.

Dietary Intake

Data from nationally representative U.S. and Canadian surveys are available to estimate protein intakes (Appendix Tables E-16 and F-5). In the United States, the median dietary intake of protein by adult men during 1994–1996 and 1998 ranged from 71 to 101 g/d for various age groups (Appendix Table E-16). For women, the median intake ranged from 55 to 62 g/d. For both men and women, protein provided approximately 15 percent of total calories (Appendix Table E-17). Similarly, in Canada, protein provided approximately 15 percent of total calories for adults (Appendix Table F-5).

The amino acids intakes for the U.S. population are found in Appendix Tables D-2 through D-19. The median dietary intake of lysine by adult men during 1988–1994 ranged from 4.65 to 7.50 g/d for various ages (Appendix Table D-11), and by adult women from 3.59 to 4.56 g/d. The median dietary intake of threonine by adult men during 1988–1994 ranged from 2.74 to 4.21 g/d for various ages (Appendix Table D-16) and by adult women from 2.10 to 2.59 g/d. The median dietary intake of tryptophan by adult men and women during 1988–1994 ranged from 0.84 to 1.26 g/d and from 0.65 to 0.78 g/d, respectively (Appendix Table D-17).

TOLERABLE UPPER INTAKE LEVELS FOR PROTEIN

Humans consume a wide range of intakes of protein. As intake is increased, the concentrations of free amino acids and urea in the blood increase postprandially. The nitrogenous substances in the urine also increase, especially urea. These changes are part of the normal regulation of the amino acids and nitrogen and represent no hazards per se, at least within the range of intakes normally consumed by apparently healthy individuals. Nonetheless, a number of adverse effects have been reported, especially at the very high intakes that might be achieved with supplement use, but also at more modest levels.

In addition, some naturally occurring proteins are allergenic to certain sensitive individuals; for example, the glycoprotein fractions of foods have been implicated in allergic responses. However, relatively few protein foods cause most allergic reactions: milk, eggs, peanuts, and soy in children; and fish, shellfish, peanuts, and tree nuts in adults.

Hazard Identification

Adverse Effects

There is little scientific literature on the effects of consuming very high protein diets, but it has been suggested from evidence of the dietary practices of hunter-gatherer populations, both present day and historical, that humans avoid diets that contain too much protein (Cordain et al., 2000; Speth, 1989). Even when meat is the dominant food, diets of a wide range of populations do not usually contain more than about 40 percent of energy as protein (Speth, 1989). Indeed, Eskimos, when eating only meat, maintain a protein intake below 50 percent of energy by eating fat; protein intake estimated from data collected in 1855 was estimated to be about 44 percent (Krogh and Krogh, 1913).

There have been case reports of high levels of intake. Two arctic explorers, Stefansson and Andersen, ate only meat for a whole year while living in New York City (Lieb, 1929; McClellan and Du Bois, 1930; McClellan et al., 1930, 1931). For most of the period, the diet contained 15 to 25 percent of energy as protein, with fat (75 to 85 percent) and carbohydrate (1 to 2 percent) providing the rest, and no ill effects were observed (McClellan and Du Bois, 1930). However, consumption of greater portions of lean meat (45 percent of calories from protein) by one of the two explorers led rapidly to the development of weakness, nausea, and diarrhea, which was resolved when the dietary protein content was reduced to 20 to 25 percent of calories (McClellan and Du Bois, 1930).

If continued, a diet too high in protein results in death after several weeks, a condition known as "rabbit starvation" by early American explorers, as rabbit meat contains very little fat (Speth and Spielmann, 1983; Stefansson, 1944a). Similar symptoms of eating only lean meat were described by Lewis and Clark (McGilvery, 1983). Conversely, an all-meat diet with a protein content between 20 and 35 percent has been reported in explorers, trappers, and hunters during the winters in northern America surviving exclusively on pemmican for extended periods with no adverse effects (McGilvery, 1983; Speth, 1989; Stefansson, 1944b). Pemmican is a concentrated food made by taking lean dried meat that has been pounded finely and then blending it with melted fat. It contains about 20 to 35 percent protein; the remainder is fat (Stefansson, 1944b).

Nitrogen Balance Studies. Nitrogen balance studies at protein intakes of 212 to 300 g/d consistently have shown positive nitrogen balance (Fisher et al. 1967; Oddoye and Margen, 1979; Tarnopolsky et al., 1988), although this is usually attributed to the cumulative errors of the nitrogen balance procedure (Garlick et al., 1999; Hegsted, 1978; Oddoye and Margen, 1979). In particular, no negative nitrogen balances were reported, suggesting that the high protein intake had no detrimental effect on protein homeostasis.

Maximum Urea Synthesis. Rudman and coworkers (1973) studied the effect of meals containing graded levels of protein on the rate of urea production by human liver in vivo. With increasing protein content of the meals, a maximum rate of urea synthesis of 65 mg of urea nitrogen/hour/kg body weight$^{0.75}$ was observed. At higher intakes, the rate was not increased further, but the maximum rate continued longer. In a 70-kg sedentary person, this maximum rate corresponds to about 250 g/d of protein, or about 40 percent of energy. The correspondence of this maximum to the apparent upper level of protein intake (45 percent of energy) described in the earlier section related to the experiences reported by explorers has therefore been suggested as cause and effect (Cordain et al., 2000). However, this interpretation should be made with caution, as there was no period of adaptation to the meal in the study of Rudman's group (1973). It is probable that when high protein diets are given, the capacities to oxidize amino acids and synthesize urea are increased, as has been demonstrated in animals (Das and Waterlow, 1974). However, this does not appear to have been investigated in humans.

Chronic Disease. High protein intakes have also been implicated in chronic diseases such as osteoporosis, renal stones, renal insufficiency, cancer, coronary artery disease, and obesity (see "High Protein Diets" in Chapter 11). However, the current state of the literature does not permit any recommendation of the upper level for protein to be made on the basis of chronic disease risk.

Dose–Response Assessment

The data on the potential for high protein diets to produce gastrointestinal effects, changes in nitrogen balance, maximum urea synthesis, or chronic disease are often conflicting and do not provide dose–response information or clear indications of a lowest-observed-adverse-effect level (LOAEL) or no-observed-adverse-effect level (NOAEL) for these endpoints. Thus, there are insufficient data to establish a Tolerable Upper Intake Level (UL) for total protein. Because of the current widespread use of protein supplements, more research is needed to assess the safety of high protein intakes from supplements; until such information is available, caution is warranted.

The potential implications of high dietary protein for bone and kidney stone metabolism are not sufficiently clear at present to make recommendations for the general population to restrict their protein intake. However, in those who have idiopathic hypercalciuria, the occurrence of kidney stones is much increased, and although there is no evidence to indicate reducing protein intake will decrease the risk of developing kidney stones, these individuals should not be encouraged to consume more protein than the Recommended Dietary Allowance (RDA).

Intake Assessment

Based on distribution data from the 1994–1996, 1998 Continuing Survey of Food Intakes by Individuals (CSFII), the highest mean intake of protein from diet for any gender and life stage group was estimated to be 104 g/d (Appendix Table E-16) for men aged 19 through 30 years of age. For the 70-kg reference man (Table 1-1), this would equate to 1.5 g/kg/d. This life stage group also had the highest reported protein intake at the 99th percentile of intake at 190 g/d, or 2.7 g/kg/d, for the reference 70 kg-man.

Risk Characterization

The risk of adverse effects resulting from excess intakes of protein from foods appears to be very low at the highest intake noted above. Based on distribution data from the 1994–1996, 1998 CSFII (Appendix Table E-17), these 19-30-year-old men would be consuming a mean of 15.2 percent of their energy from protein, and at the 99th percentile, 21.5 percent. Women over the age of 50 had the highest reported percentage of total energy from protein at the 99th percentile of 23.7 percent. Although a UL for protein could not be established, this does not mean that there is not a potential for adverse effects resulting from high protein intakes from food or supplements. Because the data on adverse effects resulting from high protein intakes are limited, caution may be warranted.

TOLERABLE UPPER INTAKE LEVELS FOR INDIVIDUAL AMINO ACIDS

In establishing tolerable upper intake levels (ULs) for amino acids several general points, common to all the amino acids, were noted.

- There is no evidence that amino acids derived from usual or even high intakes of protein from foodstuffs present any risk. Therefore, attention was focused on intakes of amino acids from dietary supplements and when utilized as food ingredients, such as monosodium glutamate in food or aspartic acid and phenylalanine in aspartame.
- This review was confined to those amino acids that are found in dietary protein and only the L-forms of amino acids were considered.
- Recognizing that the ULs are for chronic intake and in keeping with the UL model, only limited emphasis was placed on the results of acute and short-term toxicity studies, while longer-term studies were considered most appropriate for establishing ULs.

- More emphasis was placed on observations of adverse effects in humans than on effects observed in animals. Pharmacokinetic studies were sought to bridge potential differences between animals and humans.
- It was noted that blood concentrations could be considerably higher when amino acids were consumed as supplements as opposed to a component of protein in food, and this was considered in establishing ULs.
- Many animal studies of amino acid toxicity were conducted with diets deficient in protein. Less emphasis was placed on these studies than those with adequate protein diets because of concern over the creation of amino acid imbalances.
- For some well-studied amino acids, there were no adverse effects reported at the highest dose tested in long-term studies. In such cases it was not possible to establish a Lowest-Observed-Adverse-Effect Level (LOAEL) or a No-Observed-Adverse-Effect Level (NOAEL) that was supported by toxicity data. Under these circumstances, it was not possible to establish a UL in keeping with the criteria and procedures required by the UL model.

Alanine

L-Alanine is a dispensable amino acid with glycogenic properties. Studies of food intake, growth, and hematological changes resulting from the oral ingestion of L-alanine in animals and humans reveal little data to suggest a LOAEL or a NOAEL (LSRO, 1992). Based on intake distribution data from the 1988–1994 (NHANES III) mean daily intake for all life stage and gender groups of alanine from food and supplements is approximately 3.6 g/d (Appendix Table D-2). Men 51 through 70 years of age had the highest reported intake at the 99th percentile of 8.5 g/d.

Hazard Identification

Adverse Effects in Animals. In animals, L-alanine exhibits neural inhibitory actions as well as hypothermogenicity (Glyn and Lipton, 1981). There are no adequate data to characterize dose–response relationships for L-alanine in animals.

Adverse Effects in Humans. Oral administration of a single L-alanine dose, up to 50 g/d, increased plasma insulin levels (Genuth, 1973; Genuth and Castro, 1974; Rose et al., 1977). However, there are no chronic studies that can be utilized to establish a UL for supplemental L-alanine in humans.

Dose–Response Assessment

The very limited data on adverse effects of L-alanine intake from dietary supplements (Genuth, 1973; Genuth and Castro, 1974) were considered insufficient for a dose–response assessment and derivation of a UL for L-alanine.

Arginine

L-Arginine is incorporated into tissue proteins, and is required for the synthesis of other amino acids, polyamines, and creatine, as well as for the detoxification of ammonia via the urea cycle (Rodwell, 1990). It is a dispensable glycogenic amino acid, synthesized in adequate amounts from the urea cycle intermediate ornithine. Ornithine, in turn, can be synthesized from proline and possibly from glutamate (Brunton et al., 1999). However, in children with congenital defects of argininosuccinic acid synthetase or argininosuccinase, both urea cycle enzymes, arginine is an indispensable amino acid with daily supplementation required (Brusilow and Horwich, 1989). Based on intake distribution data from the 1988–1994 NHANES III, mean daily intakes for all life stage and gender groups of arginine from food and supplements is approximately 4.2 g/d (Appendix Table D-3). Men 51 through 70 years of age had the highest reported intake at the 99th percentile of 10.1 g/d.

Hazard Identification

Adverse Effects in Animals. Feeding low-protein diets supplemented with 4, 5, or 7.5 percent arginine resulted in depressed body weight gains in rats (Harper et al., 1966; Sauberlich, 1961). However, the growth suppression by excess arginine was lessened when the protein content of the diet was increased and when the quality of protein was improved (Harper et al., 1970).

Oral doses of L-arginine of 0.1, 0.5, and 1.0 g/kg of body weight were given to rats 1 hour before behavioral trials for a period of 5 or 7 days. Avoidance behavior was increased in CDR rats (a strain with poor learning capacity) at the highest dose only. Conditioned avoidance was not affected in Wistar rats, but increased locomotion was reported (Drago et al., 1984).

Studies on the effects of orally administered arginine on the immune system have provided conflicting results. Barbul and coworkers (1980) reported significant increases in thymus weights, thymic lymphocyte content, and in vitro activity of thymic lymphocytes after supplementing the diet of male mice with 0.5, 1, 2, and 3 percent arginine hydrochloride (one-half in the diet and one-half in drinking water) for 6 days. No dose–

response was found, with the maximum stimulation noted at 0.5 percent supplementation of the normal chow diet containing 1.8 percent arginine. Reynolds and coworkers (1990) reported significantly increased thymus weight, spleen cell mitogenesis, and inducible natural killer cell activity in mice after oral arginine (drinking water) doses of 60, 120, or 240 mg/kg of body weight/d. No dose–response was reported with maximum stimulation noted at 60 mg/kg of body weight/d. In young or aged rats, ingestion of diets supplemented with 3 percent L-arginine for 15 days did not result in increased thymus weights and little effect was reported on lymphocyte proliferation or interleukin-2 production as compared to controls (Ronnenberg et al., 1991).

Adverse Effects in Humans. Feeding 30 g of L-arginine hydrochloride/d for 7 days to 21 healthy human volunteers resulted in no changes in liver function, blood urea nitrogen (BUN), creatinine, or blood glucose (Barbul et al., 1981). The nausea and diarrhea reported by two and three adults, respectively, were ameliorated by altering the amount given at any time without decreasing the total daily intake. However, administration of 5 or 10 g of arginine as arginine aspartate for 80 days produced such dose-related reversible effects as increased weight, gastrointestinal disturbances, and somnolence (De Aloysio et al., 1982).

Thirty-six healthy volunteers were divided into 3 equal groups of 12 and orally administered 30 g of arginine hydrochloride (24.8 g of free arginine), 30 g of arginine aspartate (17 g free arginine), or a placebo daily for 14 days (Barbul et al., 1990). Dietary consumption of arginine was not controlled. Supplementation with arginine hydrochloride resulted in the development of mild hyperchloremic acidosis. Side effects of bloating, mild anorexia, and diarrhea were reported by one in the group receiving placebo, three in the group receiving arginine aspartate, and six in the group receiving arginine hydrochloride (Barbul et al., 1990). In another study of 30 elderly adults receiving 17 g of free arginine/d as arginine aspartate for 14 days, no adverse effects were observed (Hurson et al., 1995).

Park and coworkers (1992) administered orally 30 g of arginine free base/d to 10 patients with breast cancer during the three days immediately prior to surgery. A second group of ten cancer patients did not receive arginine supplementation prior to surgery and served as controls. The daily median rate of tumor protein synthesis in arginine-supplemented patients was slightly more than double that found in controls (25.6 percent/d, range 9 to 37 percent/d; 10 percent/d, range 5.5 to 15.8 percent/d, respectively). In addition, in patients receiving arginine supplementation there was a marked stimulation in the expression of the activation antigen Ki67 as measured histologically (~40 percent tumor cells staining with Ki67 compared to ~9 percent in controls). These data indicate that large oral doses of arginine may stimulate tumor growth in humans.

Studies in experimental animals have indicated a suppression of tumor growth after oral administration of arginine (Barbul, 1986; Reynolds et al., 1988; Tachibana, et al., 1985). Paradoxically, there are also published studies showing that arginine can stimulate tumor growth in animal models. Yeatman and coworkers (1991) showed that an arginine-enriched diet stimulated the growth of a murine colon tumor, whereas an arginine-depleted diet inhibited the tumor growth. Arginine was also shown to stimulate tumors in total parenteral nutrition-fed rats, while substitution of ornithine for arginine abolished the effect (Grossie et al., 1992). Moreover, Levy and coworkers (1954) showed that subcutaneous injections of arginine either inhibited or stimulated the tumor, depending on its size at the start of treatment. The mechanism of these effects is unknown, but might in part involve the immune system. Reynolds and coworkers (1988) observed an inhibition of tumor growth with tumors of high immuno-genicity, but stimulation when a tumor of low immunogenicity was used, suggesting that inhibition might only occur when tumors can be recognized and killed by the immune system.

Batshaw and coworkers (1984) treated 17 hyperammonemic infants with 175 to 350 mg L-arginine/kg of body weight/d for 6 to 8 weeks. No adverse effects were reported. Plasma arginine concentrations were approximately twice those in the controls but less than one-third of the minimal concentration postulated to result in neurological effects in hyperargininemia. A follow-up at 18 months of age showed similar IQ scores in all groups. It should be mentioned that Brusilow and coworkers (1984) have used arginine supplements of 210 to 840 mg/kg of body weight/d for 5 years in the treatment of children with inborn errors of urea synthesis. No evidence of intellectual deterioration or visual effects was reported in these patients. In addition, there are several reports regarding patients treated intravenously with arginine hydrochloride for metabolic alkalosis or as a provocative test for growth hormone, where life-threatening hyperkalemia (Bushinsky and Gennari, 1978; Massara et al., 1981) or fatal hyponatremia (Gerard and Luisiri, 1997) were observed. These are acute toxicity reports and thus are not useful to evaluate chronic intakes.

Dose–Response Assessment

Studies of oral administration of supplemental arginine in humans (in excess of normal dietary intakes of approximately 5.4 g/100 g of mixed dietary proteins) were not designed to systematically study the toxicity of chronic oral exposure to this amino acid. They are generally of short duration, do not present dose–response data, and involve small numbers of individuals. Although data from these studies do not support the development of an LOAEL and thus a UL, they do give some indication of the effects from oral arginine intakes of up to 30 g/d. Oral intakes of arginine aspartate providing 5 and 10 g/d of free arginine for 80 days resulted in dose-related weight increases, digestive disturbances, and sleepiness (De Aloysio et al., 1982). Daily intakes of 20 to 30 g of arginine hydrochloride for 7 to 14 days resulted in gastrointestinal disturbances (Barbul et al., 1981, 1990). Such effects were considered mild and responded to lowering the oral dose at various times during the day without affecting the total daily intake.

Although the data appear to indicate minimal effects from arginine supplementation at intakes up to 24.8 g/d of free arginine base, the unconfirmed finding that 30 g/d of arginine for 3 days resulted in a stimulation of tumor growth in breast cancer patients (Park et al., 1992) indicates that dietary supplementation with arginine is not advisable other than in at-risk children with congenital defects of argininosuccinic acid synthetase or argininosuccinase. Therefore, since neither a NOAEL nor LOAEL can be identified for intake of L-arginine from dietary supplements in healthy individuals, a UL could not be determined.

Asparagine

L-Asparagine is a dispensable amino acid, the amide of the dicarboxylic amino acid aspartic acid that is either deaminated during food processing or converted into aspartate by the mucosal cells. Daily human intakes of L-asparagine from dietary protein are about 7.4 g/100 g of dietary protein (LSRO, 1992).

Hazard Identification

There are no data available regarding the toxicity of L-asparagine as a single amino acid supplement, which are relevant for setting an UL.

Dose–Response Assessment

There are no data to characterize a dose–response assessment for supplemental asparagine. However, asparagine is rapidly converted to aspartic acid in the gastrointestinal tract, and the potential adverse health effects from asparagine intake should be considered when developing the UL for aspartic acid.

Aspartic Acid

L-Aspartic acid is a dispensable dicarboxylic amino acid that can be produced by the transamination of oxaloacetic acid arising from glucose breakdown. In the presence of α-ketoglutarate, aspartate is converted to oxaloacetate and glutamate. Based on distribution data from the 1988–1994 NHANES III, mean daily intakes for all life stage and gender groups of aspartic acid from food and supplements are 6.5 g/d (Appendix Table D-4). Men 31 through 50 years of age had the highest intake at the 99th percentile of 15.4 g/d.

Hazard Identification

Adverse Effects in Animals. Neonatal mice (24-hours postpartum) received four subcutaneous injections of L-aspartic acid at 2 g/kg of body weight and were followed for 7 months (Schainker and Olney, 1974). When compared to controls, there was an increase in hypothalmic lesions, obesity, skeletal stunting, and reduced reproductive organ size. Neither blood nor brain concentrations of aspartic acid were measured. Using a similar protocol, Pizzi and coworkers (1978) replicated these findings in mice given gradually increasing doses of monosodium L-aspartic acid (2.2 to 4.4 g/kg of body weight) by subcutaneous injection on days 2 to 11 of life. Animals were followed for 150 days for growth and reproductive behavior and sacrificed between 200 and 300 days of age. Females had reduced litter sizes and fewer pregnancies, and males had reduced fertility. At 190 and 195 days of age, behavioral tests were carried out on the male mice and significant reductions in activity and exploratory behavior were observed in treated animals.

Finkelstein and coworkers (1988) have proposed that some of the adverse effects reported may be the result of insufficient carbohydrate in the diet of mice receiving large acute doses of aspartic acid. When neonatal mice were orally administered 750 mg aspartate/kg of body weight, the characteristic hypothalmic lesions were observed. However, when mice were treated simultaneously by gavage with aspartate and 1 g of Polycose®/kg of body weight, no lesions were found. At a dose of 1 g of aspartate/kg of body weight administered with carbohydrate, there was a reduction of more than 60 percent in the lesions observed compared to the animals treated with aspartate only. Prior injection of insulin (at pharmacological doses) 4 hours before aspartate treatment (750 mg/kg of body weight) reduced, but did not eliminate, the numbers of animals with lesions from 12/12 to 6/10 and decreased the maximum number of necrotic neurons per brain section. This paper reported a threshold dose for a single oral administration of aspartate producing neurotoxicity in infant mice at 650 mg/kg of body weight (Finkelstein et al., 1988).

Finkelstein and coworkers (1983) also conducted an oral exposure study with L-aspartic acid in slightly older infant mice (8 days old). Aspartic acid was administered by oral gavage at a single dose of 0, 250, 500, 650, 750, or 1,000 mg/kg of body weight. Brain regions were assessed at 5 hours after exposure. No hypothalamic neuronal necrosis was observed in animals treated with a single dose of aspartic acid up to and including 500 mg/kg of body weight. Increasing numbers of animals with hypothalamic lesions and severity of lesions (as assessed by numbers of necrotic neurons per brain section) were observed with increasing doses. In contrast, Reynolds and coworkers (1980) gave infant monkeys a single dose of 2 g/kg of body weight of aspartame by gastric tube and found no hypothalamic damage.

None of the above studies on the effects of aspartic acid on hypothalamic structure and function include data on food consumption of the treated animals and the observations of adverse effects have been made in rodents only. The only study in nonhuman primates found no change in the hypothalamus of infant monkeys given an acute dose of aspartame (Reynolds et al., 1980).

Adverse Effects in Humans. Carlson and coworkers (1989) measured the effects of a 10-g bolus dose of L-aspartic acid on pituitary hormone secretion in healthy male and female adults. Aspartic acid had no consistent effect on any hormone measured.

The potassium magnesium salt of aspartic acid (KMA) has been used as a supplement in exercise regimens (Ahlborg et al., 1968; de Haan et al., 1985; Maughan and Sadler, 1983; Sen Gupta and Srivastava, 1973). Acute oral doses in these studies ranged from approximately 75 to 130 mg of KMA/kg of body weight. While no adverse effects were reported, it was not clear from the reports what adverse effects were examined, and plasma aspartic acid concentrations were not reported.

Since the artificial sweetener aspartame contains about 40 percent aspartic acid, studies on the effects of oral administration of this dipeptide provide useful information on the safety of aspartic acid. Twelve normal adults were orally given 34 mg/kg of body weight of aspartame and the equimolar amount of aspartic acid (13 mg/kg of body weight) in a crossover design (Stegink et al., 1977). No increase in plasma or erythrocyte aspartate was found during the 24 hours after dosing. Plasma phenylalanine levels doubled over fasting concentrations 45 to 60 minutes after dosing with aspartame but returned to baseline after 4 hours. Plasma concentrations of other amino acids remained unchanged.

Frey (1976) studied the effects of the oral administration of aspartame to 126 children and adolescents (30 to 77 mg of aspartame/kg body weight/d, equal to 12 to 30 mg of aspartate/kg body weight/d) for 13 weeks in a double-blind study. Each child received a physical examination and special eye examinations before and after the study. In addition, tests for liver and renal function, hematological status, and plasma levels of phenylalanine and tyrosine were conducted. The results of all tests were within normal limits. Using a similar study design and a dose of 36 mg aspartame/kg body weight/d (14 mg aspartate/kg/d) given orally to young adults (mean age 19.3 years), Knopp and coworkers (1976) reported no meaningful effects on plasma triglycerides and cholesterol nor on tests measuring hematological parameters, and liver and renal function.

Dose–Response Assessment

All human studies on the effects of aspartic acid involve acute exposures (Ahlborg et al., 1968; Carlson et al., 1989; de Haan et al., 1985; Maughan and Sadler, 1983; Sen Gupta and Srivastava, 1973). There are some subchronic studies on the oral administration of aspartame to humans (Frey, 1976; Stegink et al., 1977); however, in both studies no dose–response data are available. Although some studies in experimental animals were designed to obtain dose–response data, the effects measured were usually found in all doses studied. Therefore, even if the protocol had used dosing regimens appropriate for the development of a UL, no NOAEL was identified.

The most serious endpoint identified in animal studies was the development of neuronal necrosis in the hypothalamus of newborn rodents after dosing with aspartic acid a few days postpartum. This is a property of dicarboxylic amino acids, since glutamic acid dosing in this animal model results in similar necrotic effects (Stegink, 1976; Stegink et al., 1974). There is still some uncertainty over the relevance to humans of the newborn rodent model for assessing the neuronal necrosis potential of aspartic acid. Neuronal necrosis in the hypothalamus was not found in newborn nonhuman primates with levels of plasma dicarboxylic amino acids 10 times those found in newborn mice with neuronal necrosis (Stegink, 1976; Stegink et al., 1974). In addition, human studies where high doses of aspartic acid or aspartame were given failed to find a significant increase in the plasma level of aspartic acid.

In view of the ongoing scientific debate regarding the sensitivity of newborn animals to the consumption of supplemental dicarboxylic amino acids, it is concluded that aspartic acid dietary supplements are not advisable for infants and pregnant women. Although the scientific data are not sufficient to develop a UL for aspartic acid, it should be noted that dietary supplement doses of up to 8 g/d (approximately 120 mg/kg body weight/d) have not resulted in any documented adverse effects.

Branched-Chain Amino Acids (Leucine, Isoleucine, Valine)

The branched-chain amino acids (BCAA)—leucine, isoleucine, and valine—differ from most other indispensable amino acids in that the enzymes initially responsible for their catabolism are found primarily in extrahepatic tissues. Each undergoes reversible transamination, catalyzed by a branched-chain aminotransferase (BCAT), and yields α-ketoisocaproate (KIC, from leucine), α-keto-β-methylvalerate (KMV, from isoleucine), and α-ketoisovalerate (KIV, from valine). Each of these ketoacids then undergoes an irreversible, oxidative decarboxylation, catalyzed by a branched-chain ketoacid dehydrogenase (BCKAD). The latter is a multienzyme system located in mitochondrial membranes (Danner et al., 1979). The products of these oxidation reactions undergo further transformations to yield acetyl CoA, propionyl CoA, acetoacetate, and succinyl CoA; the BCAA are thus keto- and glucogenic.

Based on distribution data from the 1988–1994 NHANES III, mean daily intakes for all life stage and gender groups of leucine (Appendix Table D-10), isoleucine (Appendix Table D-9) and valine (Appendix Table D-19) from food and supplements are 6.1, 3.6, and 4.0 g/d, respectively. Men 51 through 70 years of age had the highest intakes at the 99th percentile for leucine at 14.1 g/d, isoleucine at 8.2 g/d, and valine at 9.1 g/d.

Hazard Identification

Blood and tissue concentrations of BCAA are altered by several disease and abnormal physiological states, including diabetes mellitus, liver dysfunction, starvation, protein–calorie malnutrition, alcoholism, and obesity. These and other conditions sometimes produce drastic alterations in plasma pools of BCAA (Amen and Yoshimura, 1981). Markedly elevated concentrations of BCAA and branched-chain α-keto acids are associated with maple-syrup urine disease; the latter is caused by an inborn error of metabolism in which BCKAD is low or absent (Hutson and Harper, 1981). BCAA imbalances appear not to cause these various diseases and physiological abnormalities, but rather result from them. Numerous investigations of interrelationships of BCAA in patients having one or more of these conditions have been undertaken; their usefulness for assessing risks to healthy populations is in most cases questionable (LSRO, 1992).

One other set of interactions, in this case concerning BCAA and other amino acids, may be of significance in assessing human risks associated with supplementation. Thus, it has been well established that the BCAA compete with other large neutral amino acids (LNAA, particularly tryptophan and tyrosine) for membrane transport (Anderson and Johnston, 1983). Although the BCAA do not act as direct precursors for neurotransmitters, they can affect transport of certain LNAA across the blood–brain barrier, and thereby influence central nervous system concentrations of certain neurotransmitters. Fernstrom and coworkers (1973) demonstrated, for example, that brain tryptophan levels in rats decrease as the ratio of plasma tryptophan to other LNAA, including the BCAA, declines.

Influences on and Consequences of Metabolism. BCAA-transaminase (BCAAT) exists in at least three different subtypes, and its tissue and cellular distribution varies across species. Differences between rats and humans in this regard raise the possibility that, to the extent that adverse biological effects of the BCAA are dependent upon metabolism, rodent data may not be completely predictive of human responses (Harper et al., 1984). BCKA-dehydrogenase (BCKAD) appears to display similar inter-species variability. It should be noted, however, that in most of the animal studies reported below, it is not entirely clear that these various enzyme activities are critical determinants of the effects seen. Thus, while the animal data must be interpreted with caution, there is no well-established basis for disregarding them entirely.

Among the BCAA, leucine appears to exhibit the highest degree of metabolic activity, although this conclusion may arise at least partially because it has been the subject of more study than isoleucine and valine. Leucine may affect muscle protein turnover (Elia and Livesey, 1983) and stimulate insulin release and tissue sensitivity (Frexes-Steed et al., 1990) as well as somatostatin, glycogen, and zinc release (Danner and Elsas, 1989). It is unclear whether any of these effects have adverse health consequences.

Adverse Effects in Humans. BCAA-enriched protein or amino acid mixtures and, in some cases, BCAA alone, have been used in the treatment of a variety of metabolic disorders. These amino acids have received considerable attention in efforts to reduce brain uptake of aromatic amino acids and to raise low circulating levels of BCAA in patients with chronic liver disease and encephalopathy (LSRO, 1992; Marchesini et al., 1990; Skeie et al., 1990). They have also been used in parenteral nutrition of patients with sepsis and other abnormalities. Although no adverse effects have been reported in these studies, it is not clear that such effects have been carefully monitored (Skeie et al., 1990). Additionally, the data from these studies, because they involved patients with significant and sometimes unusual disease states, are not directly relevant to the problem of assessing risks to normal, healthy humans.

Most studies of the effects of BCAA supplementation involving healthy individuals have been directed at their potential for improving physical or mental performance. It has been hypothesized that BCAA supplementation may reduce muscle catabolism associated with exercise, fasting, or metabolic stress (Hood and Terjung, 1990), and may reduce fatigue associated with increased central nervous system concentrations of serotonin (Newsholme et al., 1991). The first hypothesis is based on the fact that, in humans, the highest concentrations of BCAAT, the catalyst for BCAA oxidation, are found in muscle; the second hypotheses relates to the fact that high circulatory levels of BCAA interfere with the transport of tryptophan, a serotonin precursor, across the blood–brain barrier. Of the individual BCAA, leucine has received the most study, because of its relatively greater rate of oxidation and because it is associated with the rapid release of glucogenic precursors from muscle.

There have been several reports of clinical trials in which groups of healthy humans, in most cases trained athletes, were given high doses of leucine by intravenous infusion (Abumrad et al., 1982; Elia and Livesey, 1983; Eriksson et al., 1983; Hagenfeldt et al., 1980; Tarnopolsky et al., 1991). Most of the studies involved a single dose of the amino acid. These trials measured physical and mental performance, the impact on blood levels of other amino acids, and in one case, of insulin and glucose output. Although some evidence of reduced muscle catabolism and clear evidence of an impact on blood concentrations of other amino acids (most especially, declines in the other BCAA and several other neutral amino acids) can be found in these reports, none of these provides evidence of an adverse effect of leucine. In fact, in one study glutamine output from forearm muscle was significantly increased (Abumrad et al., 1982). It should be noted, however, that possible side effects in all studies were those that might have been recognized subjectively. No potential functional changes were investigated in any of these studies. Thus, although this collection of studies provides no evidence of adverse effects of high doses of leucine, they are of highly limited value in assessing health risks.

Maple Syrup Urine Disease (MSUD). The most common disorder associated with genetic anomalies in BCAA metabolism is Maple Syrup Urine Disease (MSUD), a condition brought about by lack of adequate function in BCKAD. The disorder, which can be diagnosed in the neonatal period, is characterized by very high plasma levels of BCAA, especially leucine. There are six other forms of the condition that have onsets later in life; these different forms are associated with different abnormal subtypes of BCKAD. MSUD is associated with mental retardation and even early death and is treated by dietary control of BCAA. Other less common metabolic disorders are associated with genetic anomalies in specific enzymes involved in BCAA metabolism (LSRO, 1992; Sweetman, 1989). Information on these disorders provides no data helpful to assessing risks in normal populations; the affected populations require medical management involving severe restriction of BCAA consumption.

Adverse Effects in Animals. There have been a relatively large number of studies in rats of high levels of BCAA administration and, in some cases, of individual BCAA (particularly leucine). The largest share of these investigations followed the observation that the BCAA compete with other LNAA (tryptophan, tyrosine) for the blood–brain carrier system (Ashley and Anderson, 1975; Fernstrom et al., 1973). Of particular interest has been the effect of BCAA-induced changes in LNAA/BCAA ratios, and the effects of LNAA and neurotransmitter brain concentrations on food intake and body weight.

Peters and Harper (1987) demonstrated that protein intake was, however, not affected by BCAA-induced changes in neurotransmitter concentrations. In another study, BCAA dosing lowered plasma and brain concentrations of all indispensable amino acids, but there appeared to be no consistent association of these alterations with protein selection (Anderson et al., 1990). Indeed, given a choice, rats adjusted their dietary intakes in response to supplementation with BCAA.

It appears, however, that the creation of imbalances among the BCAA (e.g., by dosing with high levels of any one of them) may sometimes induce reductions in appetite and growth (Block, 1989; Harper et al., 1984). However, these imbalances, which lead to catabolism of muscle, occur only in rats on marginally adequate protein diets (Block, 1989). Thus, for example, Harper et al. (1984) demonstrated that high dietary levels of leucine suppressed the growth of rats fed a low protein diet, and that the growth suppression could be prevented by supplementation with isoleucine and valine. There have been a number of attempts to study BCAA antagonisms in various tissues, and it appears that muscle is the major contributor to the depletion of isoleucine and valine pools in animals consuming high leucine diets. It is not at all clear that induced BCAA imbalances (except possibly in the case of animals on marginally adequate protein diets) have any adverse effects on growth.

The consequences of reduced brain concentrations of neurotransmitters observed in these animal studies that may be associated with high level BCAA supplementation are not entirely clear, nor is their relevance to humans certain, given the known interspecies differences in the activities and tissue distribution of BCAAT and BCKAD.

Kawabe and coworkers (1996) reported on a subchronic feeding study in which L-isoleucine was administered to groups of 10 rats at dietary concentrations of 0, 1.25, 2.5, 5.0, or 8.0 percent for 13 weeks. The amino acid caused no changes in body weights, food consumption, or hematological parameters. At the highest dietary level, increased urine volumes and relative kidney weights and urine pH, together with some alterations in serum electrolytes, were clearly related to treatment. Minimal changes were observed at the 5.0 percent dietary level, although no histopathological alterations were observed in any organs of either gender. No alterations of any type were observed at the 2.5 percent dietary level (corresponding to about 1,800 mg/kg/d).

There is evidence that isoleucine acts as a promoter of urinary bladder carcinogenesis in rats (Kakizoe et al., 1983; Nishio et al., 1986). Thus, Kakizoe and coworkers (1983) exposed 6-week-old rats to low doses of N-butyl-N (4-hydroxybutyl) nitrosamine (BHBN), a known initiator of cancer of the urinary bladder, and supplemented their diets with isoleucine or leucine. After 40 weeks, the incidence of papillomas was significantly elevated in rats receiving isoleucine plus BHBN over that observed in the group receiving BHBN alone. In a follow-up study of similar design, Nishio and coworkers (1986) extended the experimental period to 60 weeks and included diets supplemented with 2 or 4 percent isoleucine or leucine. In this case, both dose levels of both amino acids significantly increased bladder carcinoma incidence over groups receiving BHBN alone or groups receiving amino acids alone (see Table 10-28). It thus appears that both leucine and isoleucine are potent promoters of bladder neoplasms in rats at dietary levels of 2 percent and above; a no-effect level was not identified in either of the above studies. There is no evidence that either amino acid is carcinogenic in the absence of an initiating agent.

Developmental Studies. Persaud (1969) reported that leucine is a teratogen when it is administered by intraperitoneal injection in pregnant female rats at doses as low as 15 mg/kg of body weight. The author suggested that the effects, which were multiple and serious, may have resulted from amino acid imbalances that adversely affected protein synthesis dur-

TABLE 10-28 Incidences of Bladder Carcinomas in Rats After 60 Weeks

Added Substance	Dietary Levels[a]		
	0%	2%	4%
Isoleucine or leucine	0	0	0
BHBN	0		
BHBN and isoleucine		46	77
BHBN and leucine		52	74

[a] Dietary level refers to level of amino acid addition. N-butyl-N (4-hydroxybutyl) nitrosamine (BHNB) was administered at a dose below that known to induce bladder tumors. No papillomas or preneoplastic lesions were observed in the control groups or in the amino acid groups.

ing embryonic development. No attempt has been made to determine whether orally administered BCAA have any such effect.

Matsueda and Niiyama (1982) reported on the effects of dietary supplementation with the individual BCAA on maintenance and outcome of pregnancy in rats. Pregnant rats were fed a low protein (6 percent casein) diet supplemented with 5 percent leucine, isoleucine, or valine. Four control groups were administered the 6 percent casein diet; it was stated (without documentation) that the four control groups were given the 6 percent diets in amounts matching those of pair-fed BCAA groups.

Only 11 out of 20 possible pregnancies were maintained in rats administered leucine and isoleucine (2/10 for the leucine groups and 9/10 for the isoleucine groups). No consistent effects on food intake and maternal body weight gain were observed, except for an increase in both in valine-supplemented dams. All fetal weights in the BCAA groups were less than those in ad libitum controls, and fetal weights in the isoleucine and valine groups (but not the leucine groups) were less than those in pair-fed controls; this same pattern was observed when fetal brain weights were analyzed. In all three BCAA-fed groups, brain concentrations of BCAA, histidine, and arginine were greatly increased relative to ad libitum controls, but no such effects were seen for glutamate or phenylalanine.

This study suggests that BCAA when administered to pregnant rats at high doses (dietary levels of 5 percent, corresponding roughly to a daily dose of 2,000 mg/kg) may reduce fetal body weight and relative brain weights and cause sharp increases in brain concentrations of certain amino acids.

Thoemke and Huether (1984) bred rats for three generations on diets enriched with BCAA at 10 g/kg for each amino acid. They also concurrently studied the effects of tryptophan, tyrosine, and phenylalanine supplementation. Feeding of the supplemented diets commenced in both genders two weeks before mating, and continued through three generations (F1, F2, F3). BCAA caused, as expected, decreases in serum levels of tryptophan and tyrosine in F3 dams, and increases in serum glycine. There were, however, no such differences observed in dams of the F1 and F2 generations and no changes in BCAA levels were observed in any generation. In the F1 generation, diets supplemented with BCAA caused significant decreases in brain weights at days 5 and 10 postpartum, but weights were, in all cases, normal by day 20. In the F2 and F3 generations, however, pup brain weights were reduced at day 5 and did not recover by day 20. The concentrations of neurotransmitters were decreased in the brain in all three generations, with the most significant decrease seen for aspartate; no functional measurements were made to assess the possible effects of these declines in neurotransmitter concentrations.

It is thus clear that alterations in brain chemistry, most especially declines in neurotransmitter concentrations and reductions in brain weight, can be seen in offspring of rats fed supplemental BCAA at 30 g/kg diet (10 g/kg for each amino acid). Assuming that female rats weigh an average of 200 g during gestation and consume about 15 g food/d, then the 30 g/kg level of BCAA corresponds to about 450 mg/d, or a daily dose of 2,250 mg/kg (about 750 mg/kg for each amino acid). This study involved only a single level of supplementation, so a "no-effect" level was not identified.

Summary. There are no reports of adverse health effects associated with normal diets containing BCAA, nor have such effects been reported in healthy persons receiving single, infused supplemental BCAA doses as high as 9.75 g. The several studies in which such large supplemental doses were given are highly limited as a basis for reaching conclusions about safety because most involved only a single dose, and none involved an attempt to assess any functional changes. In some human studies, especially those involving high doses of leucine, metabolic alterations were observed, typically expressed as declines in blood levels of LNAA, including neurotransmitter precursors. In one study, insulin sensitivity was increased by BCAA supplementation.

The effects of BCAA on plasma and whole blood concentrations of amino acids have been convincingly and repeatedly observed under a variety of conditions in experimental animal studies. BCAA compete among themselves and with other LNAA, and these competitive interactions may affect growth and appetite (although significant only in animals on diets marginally adequate in protein). Changes in brain concentrations of neurotransmitters precursors (tryptophan and tyrosine) have also been demonstrated at various levels of supplementation.

Developmental studies in rats also reveal the effect of BCAA supplementation on fetal brain concentrations of neurotransmitters in successive generations of animals. Fetal brain weights are also reduced across generations. Decreases in viable pregnancies have been seen in rats administered supplemental leucine and isoleucine.

Leucine and isoleucine have both been shown to promote bladder carcinogenesis in a two-stage rat model. Neither has been demonstrated to be carcinogenically active in the absence of an initiating agent. A recent 13-week study in rats involving isoleucine provided no evidence that this amino acid could induce pre-neoplastic lesions in the urinary bladder, but did reveal that isoleucine could increase urine volume and pH and relative kidney weights at very high dietary levels. Such effects are generally species specific.

Dose–Response Assessment

There are no adequate dose–response data from human or animal studies upon which to base a UL for BCAA. Tumor promotion data from rat studies cannot be used reliably to assess human risk. It is not at all clear that such two-stage models, involving an initiating agent, are relevant to expected conditions of human exposure (Williams and Whysner, 1996).

Cysteine

L-Cysteine, a dispensable amino acid, is formed metabolically from L-methionine and L-serine. It is interconvertible to cystine, and for purposes of this report, L-cysteine and L-cystine are considered together. Based on distribution data from the 1988–1994 NHANES III, the mean daily intake for all life stage and gender groups of cysteine from food and supplements is 1.0 g/d (Appendix Table D-5). Men 51 through 70 years of age had the highest intakes at the 99th percentile of 2.2 g/d.

Hazard Identification

Acute Adverse Effects in Animals. L-Cysteine is mutagenic in bacteria (Glatt, 1989), but not in mammalian cells (Glatt, 1990). L-Cysteine has been identified as a neuro excitotoxin due to its interaction with N-methyl-D-aspartate (NDMA) receptors (Olney, 1994). Administration to perinatal mice or rats that have an immature blood–brain barrier produces neurotoxicity. Swiss Webster albino mice, 10 to 12 days old, were given a single oral dose of 3 g/kg of body weight of L-cysteine (Olney and Ho, 1970). At 5 hours after treatment, necrosis of hypothalamic neurons was found, as well as retinal lesions.

In male Wistar rats injected intraperitoneally with 1.0 mmol/kg of body weight of cysteine, blood levels of cysteine peaked at about 2 mM at 30 minutes (Calabrese et al., 1997). At 1 hour, exposure produced elevated brain levels of malondialdehyde in the substantia nigra. Subcutaneous injection of 4-day-old Sprague-Dawley rats with L-cysteine 0.5 g/kg of body weight produced no subsequent effect on neurotransmitter or neuropeptide systems in the striatum at 35 days of age (Sivam and Chermak, 1992).

In addition to the report of Olney and Ho (1970) on retinal lesions in mice, subcutaneous injection of 9- to 10-day-old Wistar rats with L-cysteine at 1.2 mg/g body weight produced permanent dystrophy of the inner layers of the retina (Karlsen and Pedersen, 1982).

Acute administration of L-cysteine to rats at a dose of 1.9 g/kg was reported to produce ultrastructural alterations of testicular Sertoli cells and spermatids (Bernacchi et al., 1993).

Acute Adverse Effects in Humans. Single oral doses of 5 and 10 g of L-cysteine have produced nausea and light-headedness in normal humans (Carlson et al., 1989). Reports of chronic administration of L-cysteine to humans were not found.

Dose–Response Assessment

The data on adverse effects of L-cysteine and L-cystine intake from supplements were not considered sufficient for a dose–response assessment and derivation of a UL.

Glutamic Acid, Including Its Sodium Salt

Dietary glutamate is almost totally extracted by the gut and is metabolized rapidly by transamination to α-ketoglutarate, and hence to other intermediary metabolites, notably alanine. The glutamate that escapes capture by the gut is largely taken up by the liver. Glutamate is also synthesized endogenously as a product of transamination of other amino acids during the catabolism of arginine, proline, and histidine, and by the action of glutaminase on glutamine. Its importance in metabolism is that it is a dispensable amino acid that plays a role in the shuttle of nitrogen from amino acid catabolism to urea synthesis through its transamination reamination reactions, and behaves as a neurotransmitter in the brain.

Based on distribution data from the 1988–1994 NHANES III, mean daily intakes for all life stage and gender groups of glutamic acid from food and supplements are approximately 15 g/d (Appendix Table D-6). Men 31 through 50 years of age had the highest intakes at the 99th percentile of 33.7 g/d.

Hazard Identification

Most of the body's free glutamate pool is concentrated in the tissues, especially brain (homogenate, 10 mmol/L; synaptic vesicles, 100 mmol/L) (Meldrum, 2000). By contrast, the concentration of glutamate in the blood is low, typically about 50 μmol/L in the fasting state (Stegink et al., 1982a, 1983a, 1983b). During absorption of a high-protein meal (1g protein/kg/d), there is about a twofold rise in the concentration of glutamic acid in the systemic plasma (Stegink et al., 1982a), returning to baseline 8 hours after the meal. Addition of monosodium glutamate (34 mg/kg) to the meal, which increased the total glutamate intake by 16 percent, did not result in any further increase in glutamate concentration. However, a larger dose of glutamate, 150 mg/kg/d, which increased the total intake by 69 percent, resulted in a larger increase in glutamate level than the meal alone (by about 50 percent) (Stegink et al., 1983b). Both the peak level achieved and the time course of rise in glutamate level have been shown to be highly dependent on the way in which the glutamate is ingested. A single drink of glutamate (150 mg/kg) in water resulted in a large and rapid rise in the plasma level, peaking at about 12 times the basal level at 45 minutes, and falling quickly thereafter (Stegink et al., 1983a). By contrast, a meal consisting of a liquid formula substantially inhibited the rise in glutamate level (Stegink et al., 1983a).

Adverse Effects in Animals. The adverse effects of glutamic acid and its salts have been reviewed in great detail by the Joint FAO/WHO Expert Committee on Food Additives (JECFA) (JECFA, 1988) and the American Institute of Nutrition of the Federation of American Societies for Experimental Biology (FASEB) (Raiten et al., 1995). The acute toxicity has been evaluated in several animal species, with LD_{50} values for the oral route of administration ranging from 16,200 to 19,200 mg/kg of body weight in mice, 10,000 to 19,900 mg/kg of body weight in rats, and greater than 2,300 mg/kg of body weight in rabbits (JECFA, 1988), indicating a low level of acute toxicity. Subchronic studies in mice showed an increase in body fat and female sterility in animals that had been subcutaneously injected with glutamate (2.2 to 4.2 g/kg/d) from day 1 to day 10 of life (Olney, 1969). Mice given subcutaneous injections of glutamate (3 g/kg) at 2 days of age were also found to have higher body weights (Olney, 1969). In similar studies on rats given up to 2.0 g/kg/d of glutamate, no effects on body weight, growth, and the volume and weights of several organs were detected (Hara et al., 1962). Other studies showed no effects of glutamate on learning or recovery from electroconvulsive shock (Porter and Griffin, 1950; Stellar and McElroy, 1948).

Longer-term investigations of the effects of glutamate in animals have revealed few adverse effects. In two studies on mice given glutamate (1 or 4 percent of the diet) for 2 years, no increase in the incidence of malignant tumors was shown, and in other respects the animals were normal (Ebert, 1979b; JECFA, 1988). Similar negative results were reported from chronic studies (2 year) in rats given diets containing 0, 0.1, and 0.4 percent glutamate (JECFA, 1988) and in rats given diets containing 0, 1, 2, and 4 percent glutamate (Owen et al., 1978a). In addition, rats given diets with 0.1 or 0.4 percent glutamate showed no adverse effects on fertility and survival of the young (Ebert, 1979a). Moreover, no adverse effects on body weight gain, food consumption, behavior, electrocardiogram, ophthalmology, hematology, blood chemistry, organ weights, kidney function, or mortality were observed in dogs given diets with 0, 2.5, 5, or 10 percent glutamate (Owen et al., 1978b).

Adverse Effects in Humans. In humans there is a direct relationship between serum glutamate level and nausea and vomiting with concentrations above 1 mmol/L resulting in vomiting in 50 percent of the individuals (Levey et al., 1949). Glutamate has been used for treatment of a variety of medical conditions. For example, arginine glutamate has been given to treat ammonia intoxication, at a dose of 50 g every 8 hours, but no more than 25 g over 1 to 2 hours in order to avoid vomiting (Martindale, 1967). Chronic glutamate treatment of children with approximately 0.3 g/d of glutamic acid for 6 months (Zimmerman and Burgemeister, 1959) and adults with 45 g/d for 10 weeks (Himwich et al., 1954) showed no adverse effects.

Despite the generally low level of toxicity of glutamic acid demonstrated in the studies on animals and humans, there has remained concern over its continued use as a flavor-enhancing agent. This has been fueled by the discovery that high doses of glutamate can under certain circumstances be neurotoxic (Olney, 1969), and by the reported occurrence of distressing symptoms after the consumption of Asian foods, generally known as Chinese restaurant syndrome. As glutamate is an excitatory neurotransmitter, its potential for neurotoxicity has been studied extensively. In 1957 it was shown that injection of glutamate into suckling mice resulted in degeneration of the inner neural layers of the retina (Lucas and Newhouse, 1957). Later work showed that neuronal destruction also occurred in several regions of the brain in mice after glutamate was parenterally administered (Olney, 1969). Neurons are destroyed by excessive activation by glutamate of excitatory receptors located on the dendrosomal surfaces of neurons (Olney, 1989). The most sensitive areas of the brain are those that are relatively unprotected by the blood–brain barrier, notably the arcuate nucleus of the hypothalamus.

In a detailed analysis of the literature on the neurotoxic effects of glutamate in several species, JECFA (1988) concluded that parenteral administration of glutamate results in reproducible lesions in the central nervous system. However, lesions have never been observed in animals taking glutamate with food, although lesions were noted when the glutamate was given as a large dose by gavage. The neonatal mouse is the most sensitive, the sensitivity declining in weanlings through adults. Moreover, the sensitivity is lower in rats, hamsters, guinea pigs, and rabbits, and effects have rarely been detected in nonhuman primates. In addition, there have been a number of reports of behavioral abnormalities in mice and rats given large doses of glutamate in the early neonatal period (Berry et al., 1974; Iwata et al., 1979; Nikoletseas, 1977; Olivo et al., 1986; Pinto-Scognamiglio et al., 1972; Poon and Cameron, 1978; Pradhan and Lynch, 1972). There are also reports of reproductive abnormalities in animals given glutamate as neonates (Lamperti and Blaha, 1976, 1980; Matsuzawa et al., 1979; Pizzi et al., 1977). However, a number of other studies have shown no effect on reproduction (Anantharaman, 1979; Prosky and O'Dell, 1972; Yonetani et al., 1979), and one study reported an enhancement of fertility (Semprini et al., 1971).

No signs of neurological damage have been reported in humans. For example, in adult males given a chemically defined diet in which glutamate was the only source of dispensable nitrogen for periods of 14 to 42 days, no changes in neurologic or hepatic function were detected (Bazzano et al., 1970). However, concern was raised by a report that a large dose of glutamate taken orally stimulated the secretion of prolactin and cortisol (Carlson et al., 1989). Earlier findings that rats injected with 1 g/kg of glutamate showed stimulation in the secretion of luteinizing hormone and testosterone (Olney et al., 1976) were interpreted as indicating that the high concentration of glutamate had penetrated the neuroendocrine parts of the hypothalamus. Similarly, it was shown that the same dose of glutamate stimulated release of prolactin and inhibited the release of growth hormone (Terry et al., 1981). The data of Carlson and coworkers (1989) might therefore be interpreted to imply that the elevated concentration of glutamate was penetrating the hypothalamus in humans, and that neuroendocrine disturbances might be a potential consequence. However, a more recent and more strictly controlled study, employing 12.7 g of monosodium glutamate (160 mg/kg of body weight), failed to show significant changes in prolactin and cortisol or of luteinizing hormone, follicle stimulating hormone, growth hormone, or thyroid stimulating hormone (Fernstrom et al., 1996).

Chinese Restaurant Syndrome. Despite the failure to show any neurological damage in humans resulting from glutamate ingestion, there are many reports of symptoms associated with Chinese Restaurant Syndrome, also called MSG (monosodium glutamate) Symptom Complex (Raiten et al., 1995) and Idiosyncratic Intolerance. These symptoms, which have frequently been reported anecdotally after eating Asian food, have been described as a burning sensation at the back of the neck, forearms, and chest; facial pressure or tightness; chest pain; headache; nausea; upper body tingling and weakness; palpitation; numbness in the back of the neck, arms, and back; and drowsiness. After initial reports of this complaint, the symptoms were attributed to the high concentration of MSG in Asian food (Ambos et al., 1968; Schaumburg and Byck, 1968).

Studies indicated that some of those who reported being susceptible were sensitive to less than 3 g, and that all but one of those studied suffered some symptom at sufficiently high doses (Schaumburg et al., 1969). Later work suggested that as many as 25 to 30 percent of the population might be susceptible (Kenney and Tidball, 1972; Reif-Lehrer, 1976). However, a more recent assessment, using a randomized double-blind crossover design in which the characteristic taste of MSG had been carefully disguised, failed to detect any greater incidence of adverse symptoms after consuming glutamate at a meal (1.5 or 3 g) compared with the placebo (Tarasoff and Kelly, 1993). In fact, a significant negative correlation was found between MSG dose and adverse symptoms. In another study, six adults who believed themselves to be sensitive to MSG were challenged with MSG (6 g) or placebo in a strongly flavored drink to mask the MSG in a double-blind study (Kenney, 1986). Four of the six did not react to either MSG or the placebo, whereas the other two reacted to both. Similarly, 24 individuals, 18 of whom believed themselves to be subject to flushing symptoms after eating Chinese food, were challenged with MSG (3 to 18.5 g), but no cases of flushing occurred (Wilkin, 1986).

Thus in 1988, JECFA concluded that properly conducted and controlled clinical trials had failed to establish a relationship between Chinese Restaurant Syndrome and the ingestion of MSG. Subsequently, the FASEB report (Raiten et al., 1995) concluded that there was no scientifically verifiable evidence of adverse effects in most individuals exposed to high levels of MSG.

FASEB (Raiten et al., 1995) also acknowledged that there was sufficient evidence for the existence of a small subgroup of healthy people that were sensitive to MSG, and that they showed symptoms when exposed to an oral dose of 3 g in the absence of food. A recent double-blind, placebo-controlled study on a self-selected group of individuals who believed themselves to be sensitive to MSG has shown that many have the specific symptoms under experimental conditions that they had previously identified as representing their sensitivity to MSG (Yang et al., 1997). They also identified a dose of 2.5 g as the threshold for the induction of symptoms. A more recent study of similar design confirmed these findings, and also reported that responses did not occur when MSG was given with food (Geha et al., 2000). It was also noted that neither persistent nor serious effects from MSG were observed.

Asthma. Triggering of asthma was another, and potentially more serious, symptom of the MSG Symptom Complex listed by FASEB (Raiten et al., 1995). A recent review by Stevenson (2000) analyzed six studies on asthmatic patients, and has pointed out a number of deficiencies. Two studies indicated that single-blind administration of MSG (1.5 to 2.5 g) was associated with bronchospasm in 14 of 32 (Allen et al., 1987) and 2 of 30 asthmatics (Moneret-Vautrin, 1987). However, the subsequent four studies, employing double-blind approaches, showed no incidence of broncho-spasm after MSG ingestion in a total of 45 asthmatic patients (Germano et al., 1991; Schwartzstein et al., 1987; Woessner et al., 1999; Woods et al., 1998). Clearly there is a need for further study in this area to clarify the inconsistencies, but overall they show no convincing evidence that MSG precipitates asthma attacks.

It has also been suggested that MSG exacerbates urticaria. In a single systematic study of patients with chronic idiopathic urticaria, involving single- and double-blind, placebo-controlled challenges, two patients had positive single-blind, but neither had positive double-blind challenges, suggesting that only a very small proportion of the patients, if any, were sensitive to MSG (Simon, 2000).

Dose–Response Assessment

Despite the large number of studies of glutamate toxicity in animals and humans, there appear to be very few adverse effects of L-glutamate consumption that have significance for humans. The possible involvement of glutamate in the MSG Symptom Complex is not yet established and is of little concern, as there is no evidence that it has any impact on overall health. Although there is no convincing evidence that MSG precipitates asthma attacks, this is an area that needs further study. There is continuing controversy about the potential neurotoxicity of glutamate, but data in this area are conflicting and not sufficient for a dose–response assessment. Thus, a UL for L-glutamate from supplements cannot be established at the present time.

Glutamine

L-Glutamine, a dispensable amino acid, taken orally, is metabolized primarily in the splanchnic tissues. After absorption it is extensively metabolized to citrulline, arginine, glutamate, and proline (Reeds and Burrin, 2001). Extensive metabolism also occurs in lymphocytes, kidney, and liver. However, glutamine is simultaneously being synthesized in many tissues, especially muscle, intestine, brain, and liver (LSRO, 1992). The endogenous rate of production by the adult whole body has been estimated to be 60 to 100 g/d (van Acker et al., 1999). The two enzymes primarily responsible for glutamine metabolism are glutaminase, which converts glutamine to glutamate and ammonia, and glutamine synthetase, which synthesizes glutamine from glutamate and ammonia. Because high concentrations of either glutamic acid or ammonia are known to be neurotoxic, hyperammonemia and hyperglutamic-acidemia are important potential hazards of glutamine consumption.

Hazard Identification

Ziegler and coworkers (1990) performed several individual studies to examine glutamine safety under different circumstances. In the first study, six volunteers were given a single oral dose of glutamine at three different doses (0, 0.1, and 0.3 g/kg of body weight) and monitored for 4 hours. A second study in nine volunteers was performed to investigate the effects of intravenous infusion of glutamine at three doses (0, 0.0125, and 0.025 g/kg body weight/hour) for 4 hours. A third study in seven volunteers was designed to investigate the effects of glutamine-supplemented total parenteral nutrition (TPN) (0, 0.285, and 0.570 g/kg body weight/d) over 5 days. A pharmacokinetic study over 4 hours was also performed in three volunteers. After single oral doses, plasma glutamine concentrations rose in proportion to the dose given, by approximately twofold after 1 hour for the higher dose, and returned to basal within 4 hours. During infusions of glutamine in volunteers, with or without TPN, the plasma glutamine concentration remained elevated by about 30 percent, and no significant changes in plasma glutamate or ammonia were seen. In the two studies of glutamine-supplemented TPN, when serial assessments of mental status were made, there was no evidence of neurotoxicity. Overall, there were no indications of adverse effects at any dose when glutamine was given by either the oral or intravenous route.

Hornsby-Lewis and coworkers (1994) examined the effects of glutamine supplementation in seven patients for up to 4 weeks while receiving TPN plus glutamine at a single dose of 0.285 g/kg body weight/d. There was no significant increase in plasma glutamine concentration, and no other adverse effects were observed, but the authors noted their concern regarding elevations in liver enzymes.

In a randomized, double-blind, controlled study, normal TPN in 60 patients was compared with isonitrogenous TPN including alanyl-glutamine (0.5 g/kg body weight/d, equivalent to 0.34 g/kg/d of glutamine) in 60 patients for 6 days (Jiang et al., 1999). After 6 days the plasma glutamine was increased by 8 percent in the treated group compared with a decrease of 15 percent in the controls. No indications of adverse effects were apparent. Morlion and coworkers (1998) described the results of 28 elective surgery patients given TPN containing alanyl-glutamine (0.3 g/kg/d) or an isonitrogenous control. Plasma glutamine was modestly increased and nitrogen balances were improved compared with the control group. In addition, no adverse effects were observed.

Lacey and coworkers (1996) carried out a randomized, double-blind study of glutamine-supplemented parenteral nutrition (20 percent of amino acids) in 44 preterm neonates for 15 days. On the basis of plasma ammonia and glutamate levels and the absence of clinical signs of neurotoxicity, it was concluded that glutamine at this dose is safe in preterm infants. Also, Roig and coworkers (1996) reported no increases in the concentrations of glutamine, glutamate, and ammonia in very low birth-weight infants given enteral supplements of glutamine (0.3 g/kg/d).

It is notable that despite the substantial number of published investigations in which glutamine has been administered to humans, very few, if any adverse effects have been reported. However, the published studies of toxicity have not fully taken account of a number of important factors, including the chronic consumption of glutamine. Glutamine is an important fuel utilized by most rapidly growing tumors (Kovacevic and Morris, 1972), which may deplete the body's ability to provide glutamine (Chen et al., 1991, 1993; Klimberg and McClellan, 1996). Moreover, tumor cells are dependent on a supply of glutamine for growth (Colquhoun and Newsholme, 1997), and the growth rates correlate with the activity of glutaminase (Knox et al., 1969; Linder-Horowitz et al., 1969). Therefore, although providing supplemental glutamine might restore the body glutamine pool, it is also important to examine the possibility that glutamine supplements may promote cancer. However, the evidence points to the contrary, and in vivo studies have not confirmed this suspicion (Klimberg and McClellan, 1996; Souba, 1993). Oral administration of glutamine did not enhance tumor growth in rats in vivo (Klimberg et al., 1990), and may even depress tumor growth (Fahr et al., 1994; Klimberg and McClellan, 1996).

Dose–Response Assessment

The only reported adverse effect of glutamine was an increase in liver enzymes in patients on TPN supplemented with glutamine (0.285 g/kg body weight/d, corresponding to about 20 g/d), which resolved after cessation of treatment (Hornsby-Lewis et al., 1994). However, in other studies, doses up to 0.57 g/kg/d have been given without any adverse effect being reported. Thus, the data on L-glutamine from supplements are conflicting and are not sufficient for a dose–response assessment and derivation of a UL.

Glycine

Glycine is a dispensable amino acid with glycogenic properties. It is the only amino acid that does not have an asymmetric carbon atom, and its metabolism is linked to that of L-serine. Based on distribution data from the 1988–1994 NHANES III, the mean daily intake for all life stage and gender groups of glycine from food and supplements is 3.2 g/d (Appendix Table D-7). Men 19 through 30 years of age had the highest intakes at the 99th percentile of 7.8 g/d.

Hazard Identification

Adverse Effects in Animals. Growth depression in rats and chicks has been reported after feeding diets containing as much as 10 percent glycine (Harper et al., 1970). Nitrosated glycine can be genotoxic in vitro (Gaspar et al., 1996). It is not, however, mutagenic using a modified Ames test (Hoorn, 1989).

Adverse Effects in Humans. Surgical irrigation solutions of glycine containing 1.5 or 2.2 percent glycine reportedly cause some transient adverse effects (e.g., nausea, diarrhea, and visual disturbances) in patients after transurethral resection of the prostate (Creel et al., 1987; Hahn, 1988; Mizutani et al., 1990; Wang et al., 1989). In patients with schizophrenia, oral doses of approximately 60 g/d of glycine for several weeks failed to reveal adverse effects (Leiderman et al., 1996). There have been no chronic dose–response studies with L-glycine in healthy humans.

Dose–Response Assessment

The data on adverse effects of glycine intake from supplements were considered not sufficient for a dose–response assessment and derivation of a UL.

Histidine

Although histidine is generally regarded as an indispensable amino acid (FAO/WHO/UNU, 1985), removal of histidine from the diet, unlike the eight classical indispensable amino acids, does not induce negative nitrogen balance in the first 10 days (Rose et al., 1951). Further, men fed amino acid-based diets containing 10 g of nitrogen/d devoid of histidine remained in nitrogen balance for up to 2.4 months (Rose, 1957). There were similar reports in women (Reynolds et al., 1958) and children (Nakagawa et al., 1963). Conversely, it has been observed that nitrogen balance becomes gradually negative over a longer period of time and nitrogen balance rapidly became positive upon the reintroduction of histidine (Kopple and Swendseid, 1975).

Histidine is an important component of hemoglobin (8 percent), with the bulk being in the globin portion. The rate of erythropoiesis decreases and hemoglobin falls in adults on a histidine-free diet that is reversed when histidine is restored (Kopple and Swendseid, 1975). In addition, the dipeptide carnosine, found in skeletal muscle, is a large store of histidine and serve as a source of histidine (Christman, 1971). Because of these large body pools of histidine it takes a prolonged period (more than 60 days) to deplete an adult of histidine. Based on distribution data from the 1988–1994 NHANES III, the mean daily intake for all life stage and gender groups of histidine from food and supplements is 2.2 g/d (Appendix Table D-8). Men 51 through 70 years of age had the highest intakes at the 99th percentile of 5.2 g/d.

Hazard Identification

Adverse Effects in Animals. Histidine given acutely by intraperitoneal injection or intravenously has been shown to result in changes in the concentration of brain amino acids (Oishi et al., 1989) and histamine (Schwartz et al., 1972). Young rats (4 to 5 weeks old) treated with an inhibitor of histidinase exhibited reduced locomotor activity after an intraperitoneal injection of histidine (250 mg/kg of body weight) (Dutra-Filho et al., 1989). Pilc and coworkers (1982) reported "bizarre behavior" in rats dosed intraperitoneally with histidine (400 to 800 mg/kg of body weight). These effects have not been examined in rats fed L-histidine and are of minimal use in deriving a UL for the chronic exposure of humans to oral L-histidine.

Feeding low-protein diets supplemented with L-histidine for 3 to 4 weeks resulted in significant body weight losses after only several days in rats. However, the effects became less as increasing levels of high-quality protein were added to the diet (Benevenga and Steele, 1984).

Short-term feeding studies (7 to 46 days) in rats have shown growth retardation, hepatomegaly, and hypercholesterolemia at L-histidine levels of approximately 2 to 4 g/kg body weight/d (Harvey et al., 1981; Hitomi-Ohmura et al., 1992; Ohmura et al., 1986; Solomon and Geison, 1978). Harvey and coworkers (1981) reported significantly reduced concentrations of copper and zinc in the plasma and reduced liver concentrations of copper after feeding diets containing 8 percent L-histidine (~4 g/kg body weight/d) for 46 days. Hypercholesterolemia was eliminated by the simultaneous feeding of an L-histidine- and copper-supplemented diet, supporting the hypothesis that the histidine-induced hypercholesterolemia was a result of changes in copper status. Feeding mice 1.3 g L-histidine/kg body weight/d for 21 days resulted in an increase in the absorption and utilization of zinc with higher concentrations of zinc in liver, muscle, spleen, and pancreas (van Wouwe et al., 1989).

The long-term toxicity and carcinogenicity of L-histidine mono-hydrochloride (HMHC) was studied in 50 male and 50 female rats (Ikezaki et al., 1996). Male rats were fed diets containing 0.47 and 0.96 g/kg body weight/d of HMHC for 104 weeks; female rats were fed 0.56 and 1.1 g/kg body weight/d for the same period. No significant treatment-related increases in any tumors were reported when compared to matched controls. No neoplastic changes were reported in controls or treatment groups. In male rats fed 0.96 g of HMHC/kg body weight/d, increases in red blood cell counts, hemoglobin concentrations, and hematocrit were reported. No evidence of sperm granulomas were observed in male rats fed either 1.6 g of HMHC/kg body weight/d for 13 weeks or 0.97 g/kg body weight/d for 104 weeks (Ikezaki et al., 1994, 1996).

Adverse Effects in Humans. Pinals and coworkers (1977) treated 30 rheumatoid arthritis patients and 30 controls daily with capsules containing 4.5 g of L-histidine for 30 weeks in a double-blind trial followed by 19 patients receiving this dosage for 10 additional months in a period of open treatment. It is not clear which adverse effects were examined; however, the authors concluded that no adverse effects of the histidine therapy were noted. In a similar double-blind treatment design, Blumenkrantz and coworkers (1975) treated 42 patients (16 chronic uremic and 26 undergoing maintenance dialysis) with oral doses of 4 g/d of L-histidine for 17.5 weeks. No adverse effects were reported; however, it was not evident from the report which adverse effects were examined.

Studies on the effects of L-histidine on taste and smell acuity in humans have produced conflicting results. Henkin and coworkers (1975) reported decreased taste and smell acuity in six patients given 8 to 65 g of histidine/d for up to 24 days. In view of the increased urinary excretion of zinc and a decreased concentration of serum zinc, the authors postulated that the effects of histidine administration were due to a zinc-deficient state. In a study of eight healthy men given 4 g/d of histidine for 2 weeks, no effects on smell or taste acuity were reported (Schechter and Prakash, 1979). Similarly, Geliebter and coworkers (1981) failed to find any effect of L-histidine on taste and smell after oral dosing of L-histidine between 24 and 64 g/d for 4 weeks. Even at the lower dose (4 g/d), adverse effects such as headaches, weakness, drowsiness, and nausea were reported, while at the highest doses (24 and 64 g/d) anorexia, painful sensations in the eyes, and changes in visual acuity were reported in two females.

Zlotkin (1989) reported an approximate 70 percent increase in urinary zinc excretion in infants on TPN when the fluid contained 165 mg of histidine/kg body weight/d compared to 95 mg/kg body weight/d in controls. Although the study examined parental administration, it provides further evidence that excess histidine intake in humans can lead to histidine/zinc interactions that might lead to a zinc-deficient state.

Dose–Response Assessment

In experimental animals, the only dose–response study on the chronic oral administration of L-histidine was that of Ikezaki and coworkers (1996). However, this study utilized only two doses, neither of which demonstrated any adverse effects. In addition, no data were reported on the possible effect of the doses on zinc or copper metabolism, an effect reported in both humans and experimental animals.

None of the studies in humans on the effects of L-histidine were designed for developing a UL—they were designed to study the efficacy of utilizing L-histidine as a therapeutic agent in certain disease states. They provide only minimal support for the evaluation of a UL for histidine for apparently healthy individuals. The chronic study on the effects of orally administered histidine in rodents was not considered appropriate for the development of a UL.

There is evidence in humans that doses of L-histidine between 4 and 4.5 g/d over the amounts found in the diet do not result in adverse effects. However, this evidence should be considered tentative given the few individuals studied and lack of dose–response information. There is evidence from studies in experimental animals and humans that intakes of high levels of histidine can alter copper and zinc metabolism. However, the lack of dose–response data precludes identifying the intake concentrations in humans required to elicit such responses.

In conclusion, the available scientific data are not adequate to derive a UL for the chronic oral intake of L-histidine from supplements.

Lysine

L-Lysine, a dibasic amino acid, is indispensable in humans. Lysine, as well as threonine, does not participate in transamination reactions. Carnitine is required for the transport of long-chain fatty acids and is synthesized from lysine and methionine in the liver and kidney (Mayes, 1990). Based on distribution data from the 1988–1994 NHANES III, the mean daily intake for all life stage and gender groups of lysine from food and supplements is 5.3 g/d (Appendix Table D-11). Men 51 through 70 years of age had the highest intakes at the 99th percentile of 12.6 g/d.

Hazard Identification

Acute intake of high levels of lysine interferes with dietary protein metabolism and competes with the transport of arginine, suggesting that adverse effects from high levels of lysine are more likely to occur if protein intake or dietary arginine intake is low. Intravenous L-lysine (16.5 to 41.3 g/d in young men) has been shown to inhibit renal tubular protein reabsorption (Mogensen and Solling, 1977). L-Lysine shares an intestinal transport system with L-arginine (McCarthy et al., 1964; Rosenberg et al., 1966), and competes with L-arginine for reabsorption from renal tubules (Kamin and Handler, 1951; Webber et al., 1961). In addition, increased liver total lipids, triacylglycerol, and cholesterol concentrations were seen in rats fed 5 percent L-lysine and 15 percent casein for 2 weeks (Hevia et al., 1980a), an effect that can be reversed by feeding arginine (Hevia et al., 1980b).

Acute Adverse Effects in Animals. Administration of lysine to pregnant rats does not appear to result in gross morphological changes, but higher fetal mortality and decreases in maternal and fetal body and brain weights have been found (Cohlan and Stone, 1961; Funk et al., 1991, Matsueda and Niiyama, 1982).

Adverse Effects in Humans. Studies of lysine tolerance of human infants have not found adverse effects. In one study, six infants (4 to 11 months of age) were given 60 to 1,080 mg of lysine monohydrochloride per 8 ounces of milk in a series of seven incremental doses for 3 to 4 days at each dose. No behavioral effects were observed, nor was there anorexia, diarrhea, or other signs of gastrointestinal upset, and no evidence of cystinuria (Dubow et al., 1958). Similarly, no adverse effects were reported when 1- to 5-month-old infants were given up to 220 mg/kg body weight of lysine for 15 days (Snyderman et al., 1959b).

Higher plasma and urinary concentrations of carnitine were found in six healthy adult males given a single 5-g oral dose of lysine (Vijayasarathy et al., 1987). In another study of eight healthy males (15 to 20 years of age) given a single oral dose of 1.2 g of L-lysine hydrochloride, growth hormone release was not significantly stimulated and no side effects were reported (Isidori et al., 1981).

Several clinical trials of lysine intakes from 0.6 to 3.0 g/d for 3 to 6 months in people with herpes infections have, in general, not found or reported any adverse effects (DiGiovanna and Blank, 1984, 1985; Griffith et al., 1978, 1987; McCune et al., 1984; Milman et al., 1980; Simon et al., 1985; Thein and Hurt, 1984). The one adverse effect was an upset stomach in 3 of 27 patients given 3 g/d of L-lysine hydrochloride for 6 months and in 1 of the 25 controls (Griffith et al., 1987).

A limitation of these clinical studies is that they were done in humans with a disease. Also, the longest study was only 6 months. Finally, only a limited number of endpoints were investigated. McCune and coworkers (1984) reported no effects on plasma sodium, potassium, and chloride in 41 patients treated for 24 weeks with 1,248 mg/d of L-lysine monohydrochloride.

Dose–Response Assessment

As mentioned above, very few adverse effects of L-lysine have been observed in humans or animals after high, mostly acute, doses. Thus, the data on the adverse effects of L-lysine from supplements were considered not sufficient for a dose–response assessment and derivation of a UL for apparently healthy humans.

Methionine

L-Methionine is an indispensable amino acid with glycogenic properties. In animal studies, it has been described as one of the more toxic amino acids (Health and Welfare Canada, 1990). Humans, as well as other mammals, cannot fix inorganic sulfur into organic molecules and must rely on ingested sulfur amino acids, such as methionine, for the synthesis of protein and biologically active sulfur. Based on distribution data from the 1988–1994 NHANES III, the mean daily intake for all life stage and gender groups of methionine from food and supplements is 1.8 g/d (Appendix Table D-12). Men 51 through 70 years of age had the highest intakes at the 99th percentile of 4.1 g/d.

Hazard Identification

Adverse Effects in Animals. Dietary excesses of L-methionine (2.7 percent of the diet) for 6, 13, or 20 days have been associated with erythrocyte engorgement and accumulation of hemosiderine in rats (Benevenga et al., 1976), and there was a depression of growth and splenic damage. A single dietary dose (2.7 percent of the diet) of L-methionine decreased body growth and also reduced food intake in rats (Steele et al., 1979).

Dietary intakes of 2 to 4 percent of L-methionine caused slight changes in liver cells in rats (Stekol and Szaran, 1962) and slight decreases in liver iron content (Klavins et al., 1963). Darkened spleens caused by increases in iron deposition have been observed in weanling rats fed 1.8 percent methionine diets for 28 days (Celander and George, 1963).

Viau and Leathem (1973) fed pregnant rats 4 percent of their diet as methionine and reported subnormal fetal and placental weights. However, supplemental methionine prevented neural tube defects in rat embryos treated with teratogenic antivisceral yolk sac serum (Fawcett et al., 2000). In the mouse, the administration of methionine reduced experimentally induced spina bifida (Ehlers et al., 1994). Other studies in rodent and primate models support the beneficial effect of methionine supplementation in improving pregnancy outcomes (Chambers et al., 1995; Chatot et al., 1984; Coelho and Klein, 1990; Ferrari et al., 1994; Moephuli et al., 1997).

Adverse Effects in Humans. Single oral doses of about 0.6 g (adults) and 0.08 g (infants) led to increased plasma levels of L-methionine and L-alanine, and decreased plasma concentrations of leucine, isoleucine, valine, tyrosine, tryptophan, and phenylalanine (Stegink et al., 1980, 1982b). Neither report included mention of any adverse effects. Methionine supplements (5 g/d) for periods of weeks were reportedly innocuous in humans (Health and Welfare Canada, 1990). A single oral dose of 7 g has been associated with increased plasma concentrations of methionine and the presence of mixed sulfides (Brattstrom et al., 1984). Single oral doses of 7 g produced lethargy in six individuals and oral administration of 10.5 g of L-methionine to one produced nausea and vomiting (Perry et al., 1965). After an oral administration of 8 g/d of methionine (isomer not specified) for 4 days, serum folate concentrations were decreased in five otherwise healthy adults (Connor et al., 1978).

High doses of methionine (~100 mg/kg of body weight) led to elevated plasma methionine and homocysteine concentrations (Brattstrom et al., 1984, 1990; Clarke et al., 1991; Wilcken et al., 1983). Thus, it was concluded that elevated plasma homocysteine concentrations may be a risk factor for coronary disease (Clarke et al., 1991).

Infants more rapidly metabolized methionine than adults (Stegink et al., 1982b). In women whose average daily intake of methionine was above the lowest quartile of intake (greater than 1.34 g/d), a 30 to 40 percent reduction in neural tube defect-affected pregnancies was observed (Shaw et al., 1997). These reductions were observed for both anencephaly and spina bifida.

Dose–Response Assessment

There are no adequate data to characterize a dose–response relationship for L-methionine. Thus the data on the adverse effects of L-methionine from supplements were considered not sufficient for a dose–response assessment and derivation of a UL for apparently healthy humans.

Phenylalanine

L-Phenylalanine is an indispensable amino acid that has both glycogenic and ketogenic properties. Based on distribution data from the 1988–1994 NHANES III, the mean daily intake for all life stage and gender groups of phenylalanine from food and supplements is 3.4 g/d (Appendix Table D-13). Men 31 through 50 years of age had the highest intakes at the 99th percentile of 7.7 g/d. About 16 percent of the ingested L-phenylalanine is converted to tyrosine in humans (Clarke and Bier, 1982). Unlike most other amino acids, excessive ingestion of L-phenylalanine can be complicated by the coexistence of genetic disorders.

Hazard Identification

Adverse Effects in Animals. Because of major species differences in phenylalanine metabolism between humans and rodents (Clarke and Bier, 1982; Moldawer et al., 1983), studies in which high doses of L-phenylalanine were fed to rodents could not be utilized in developing a UL for L-phenylalanine. There is one study indicating that high concentrations of L-phenylalanine (3 g/kg body weight/d) fed to monkeys from a few days after birth until 2 or 3 years of age can produce irreversible brain damage (Waisman and Harlow, 1965). However, this study does not provide any dose–response data to utilize in determining a UL.

Adverse Effects in Humans. Data are not available on the effects of chronic ingestion of supplemental phenylalanine by apparently healthy adults. Adverse effects were not evident following acute single oral doses of L-phenylalanine as high as 10 g in 13 adult men (Ryan-Harshman et al., 1987).

Most of the literature on the consumption of large doses of L–phenylalanine consists of studies on the effects of large doses of the artificial sweetener aspartame, which is 50 percent by weight phenylalanine. In adults given oral doses of aspartame ranging from 4 to 200 mg/kg of body weight (2 to 100 mg/kg of body weight L-phenylalanine), dose-related increases in plasma phenylalanine were observed (Filer and Stegink, 1988). Ingestion of single doses up to 60 mg/kg of body weight aspartame (30 mg/kg of body weight L-phenylalanine) by normal weight adults had no effect on behavior or cognitive performance (Lieberman et al., 1988; Stokes et al., 1991).

Dose–Response Assessment

The data on the adverse effects of L-phenylalanine intake from supplements were not available for a dose–response assessment and derivation of a UL in apparently healthy humans.

Special Considerations

Phenylketonuria (PKU) is a genetic disorder that impairs phenylalanine hydroxylase (PAH) activity. Impaired PAH activity allows phenylalanine or its catabolic byproducts to accumulate above normal levels in the plasma during critical periods of brain development. Persistently elevated levels of L-phenylalanine in the plasma before and during infancy and childhood can result in irreversible brain damage, growth retardation, and dermatologic abnormalities if dietary phenylalanine is not restricted within 1 month of birth and continued at least through childhood and adolescence (Scriver et al., 1989). Restriction of phenylalanine intake throughout life in PKU patients is necessary to keep plasma phenylalanine levels low and to promote normal growth and brain development (Scriver et al., 1989). If PKU is detected early and treated effectively through strict metabolic control, infants can live a normal life-span (Hellekson, 2001). In the United States, approximately 1 of every 15,000 infants is born with PKU (Hellekson, 2001).

Maternal hyperphenylalaninemia due to deficient phenylalanine hydroxylation is a recognized human teratogen (Lenke and Levy, 1980). Because phenylalanine is actively transported across the placenta (Kudo and Boyd, 1990), a pregnant woman with PKU exposes her developing fetus to potentially harmful levels of phenylalanine. High maternal plasma phenylalanine levels are associated with high incidence of mental retardation, microcephaly, intrauterine growth delay, and congenital heart malformations in the fetus (Scriver et al., 1989). The fetal demand for phenylalanine for protein synthesis is exceeded by the placental supply of L-phenylalanine by only a small amount, suggesting that the safety margin of placental transfer may be small (Chien et al., 1993). Careful maintenance of plasma phenylalanine levels in the mother through dietary control, before conception and throughout her pregnancy, may prevent the teratogenic effects of phenylalanine.

Proline

L-Proline is a dispensable amino acid that can be formed from and converted to glutamic acid. It is incorporated into tissue proteins and can then be hydroxylated to form hydroxproline. Both proline and hydroxyproline are found in large quantities in collagen. Based on distribution data from the 1988–1994 NHANES III, the mean daily intake for all life stage and gender groups of proline from food and supplements is 5.2 g/d (Appendix Table D-14). Boys 14 through 18 years of age had the highest intakes at the 99th percentile of 12.0 g/d.

Hazard Identification

Adverse Effects in Animals. There are minimal data on the adverse effects of L-proline in either experimental animals or humans. Female Sprague Dawley rats given L-proline in drinking water for 1 month (mean dose 50 mg/kg body weight/d) did not exhibit any adverse effects (Kampel et al., 1990).

Genetically hyperprolinemic mice have 6 to 7 times the concentration of proline in the brain as control animals and 10 times the concentration of proline in plasma (Baxter et al., 1985). Hyperprolinemic hybrid mice took longer than control mice to make an initial avoidance response to foot shock in a T-maze and required more trials before learning of the avoidance response (Baxter et al., 1985). No other studies in experimental animals relevant to the evaluation of the toxicity of orally administered L-proline or hydroxyproline could be found.

Adverse Effects in Humans. The only study in humans on the effects of long-term oral administration of proline was a clinical study on the efficacy of proline (isomer not specified) to alter the progression of gyrate atrophy of the choriod and retina (Hayasaka et al., 1985). Four patients (aged 4 to 32 years) were treated with doses of proline between 2 and 10 g/d (mode = 3 g/d) for up to 5 years. No overt adverse effects were reported; however, it was uncertain from the paper which effects were studied.

Dose–Response Assessment

The data on adverse effects of L-proline intake from supplements were not available for a dose–response assessment and derivation of a UL in apparently healthy individuals.

Serine

Serine is a dispensable amino acid that is synthesized endogenously from D-3 phosphoglycerate or glycine. Based on distribution data from the 1988–1994 NHANES III, the mean daily intake for all life stage and gender groups of serine from food and supplements is 3.5 g/d (Appendix

Table D-15). Men 31 through 50 years of age had the highest intakes at the 99th percentile of 7.9 g/d.

Hazard Identification

Adverse Effects in Animals. There are limited data pertaining to the toxicity of supplemental serine. In rats given 100 mg/d of L-serine via stomach tube for 14 days, there was a decrease in food consumption but no other effects were noted (Artom et al., 1945). Other authors (Morehead et al., 1945; Wachstein, 1947) have reported that supplemental L-serine at levels as low as 10 mg/d resulted in decreased appetite, increased mortality, and renal necrosis in rats.

Adverse Effects in Humans. In four healthy adults given a single oral dose of 15 g of serine, no adverse effects were reported (Pepplinkhuizen et al., 1980). There are no studies in humans that would permit an evaluation of the possible adverse effects of repeated administration, thus the safety of repeated dose oral administration of supplemental serine cannot be assessed.

Dose–Response Assessment

The data on the adverse effects of L-serine intake from supplements were not available for a dose–response assessment and derivation of a UL in apparently healthy humans.

Threonine

L-Threonine is a large neutral amino acid that is indispensable. Similar to L-lysine, L-threonine does not take part in transamination reactions. Based on distribution data from the 1988–1994 NHANES III, the mean daily intake for all life stage and gender groups of threonine from food and supplements is 3.0 g/d (Appendix Table D-16). Men 51 through 70 years of age had the highest intakes at the 99th percentile of 7.1 g/d.

Hazard Identification

Adverse Effects in Animals. In rats fed 5 percent threonine added to a 10 percent casein diet, weight gain was reduced compared to controls fed casein alone but there were no changes in liver weight or hepatic DNA, RNA, or protein content (Muramatsu et al., 1971). The evidence indicates that excess threonine is converted to carbohydrate, liver lipids, and carbon dioxide (Yamashita and Ashida, 1971). In weanling pigs, adding 0.5, 1, 2, or 4 percent L-threonine to a 20 percent crude protein diet did not change weight gain, food intake, and gain:feed ratios in comparison to the controls (Edmonds and Baker, 1987; Edmonds et al., 1987).

Adverse Effects in Humans. No data were found on apparently healthy humans given oral L-threonoine supplements. However, L-threonine has been used clinically with the aim of increasing glycine concentrations in the cerebral spinal fluid of patients with spasticity. When given in amounts of 4.5 to 6.0 g/d for 14 days, no adverse clinical effects were noted in such patients (Growdon et al., 1991). Threonine also has been studied in low birth weight infants. In a study of 163 low birth weight infants, threonine serum concentrations were directly related to the threonine concentrations of the formula (Rigo and Senterre, 1980). The authors suggested that threonine intakes should not exceed about 140 mg/kg body weight/d for premature infants.

Dose–Response Assessment

The data on the adverse effects of L-threonine intake from supplements were not available for a dose–response assessment and derivation of a UL in apparently healthy humans.

Tryptophan

L-Tryptophan, an indispensable amino acid, serves as a precursor for several small molecules of functional significance including the vitamin niacin, the neurotransmitter serotonin, the metabolite tryptamine, and the pineal hormone melatonin. Increases in tryptophan have been shown to increase synthesis of the neurotransmitters in brain, blood, and other body organs (Fregly et al., 1989; Leathwood and Fernstrom, 1990; Young, 1986). Based on distribution data from the 1988–1994 NHANES III, the mean daily intake for all life stage and gender groups of tryptophan from food and supplements is 0.9 g/d (Appendix Table D-17). Men 51 through 70 years of age had the highest intakes at the 99th percentile of 2.1 g/d.

Hazard Identification

Adverse Effects in Animals. Several rodent studies have demonstrated that supplementation of low-protein diets with L-tryptophan (5 percent) reduces food intake and weight gain over a 4-day to 4-week period (reviewed by Benevenga and Steele, 1984; Harper et al., 1970). Funk and coworkers (1991) found that rats given a 20 percent casein diet supplemented with 14.3 percent tryptophan for 4 weeks developed scaly tails and thinning hair. However, no adverse effects were seen when the diets contained 1.4 or 2.9 percent L-tryptophan. No cancers were observed over an 80-week period when rats were fed diets containing 2 percent added L-tryptophan (Birt et al., 1987). Addition of 2.5 or 5 percent L-tryptophan to diets of rats and mice for 2 years resulted in decreased body weights of male and female mice and male (but not female) rats (DHEW, 1978). In pigs, supplementation with 0.1 or 1 percent L-tryptophan for up to 40 days did not affect weight gain, but 2 or 4 percent decreased weight gain and 4 percent also decreased food intake (Chung et al., 1991).

Several developmental studies have shown that maternal weight gain is impaired and fetal weight is reduced when maternal rat diets are supplemented with 1.4 to 6 percent L-tryptophan (Funk et al., 1991; Matsueda and Niiyama, 1982). Decreased brain weights were observed when 1 percent L-tryptophan was added to diets of male and female rats beginning 2 weeks before mating (Thoemke and Huether, 1984). Over three successive generations, brain weights decreased with each generation.

Adverse Effects in Humans. Serotonin and its metabolite 5-hydroxy-indoleacetic acid (5-HIAA) in human blood and brain cerebrospinal fluid (CSF) increase after tryptophan loading, which is similar to the effects of L-tryptophan in animals. For example, Young and Gauthier (1981) found elevations in blood and 5-HIAA and CSF serotonin after single doses of 3 or 6 g of L-tryptophan. However, Benedict and coworkers (1983) conducted a double-blind, placebo-controlled trial in six normal men fed 3 g/d of L-tryptophan in divided doses with meals for 3 days, and found a 113 percent elevation in plasma tryptophan, but no changes in platelet or plasma serotonin or in plasma catecholamines. They also found no changes in urinary catecholamines. Additionally, they found no changes in blood pressure, heart rate, plasma sodium levels or 24-hour sodium excretion in urine.

L-Tryptophan administration (2 g) as a single dose before a meal has been found to decrease subjective hunger ratings, food intake, and alertness in men (Hrboticky et al., 1985), but not women (Leiter et al., 1987). Hrboticky and coworkers (1985) also tested 15 humans only once with 0, 1, 2, and 3 g of L-tryptophan. Individuals receiving 2 and 3 g of L-tryptophan had decreased hunger and alertness and increased faintness and dizziness. Administration of 1 g of L-tryptophan with 10 g of carbohydrates before each meal (3 g L-tryptophan/d) for 3 months did not affect body weight of obese humans (Strain et al., 1985). Wurtman and coworkers (1981) found that daily doses of 2.4 g of L-tryptophan for 2 weeks did not produce a significant reduction in the consumption of carbohydrate snacks in the majority of the 24 individuals. Ten healthy adults given 5 g of L-tryptophan in a double-blind, placebo-controlled study reported severe nausea and headache and increased drowsiness soon after ingestion (Greenwood et al., 1975).

Smith and Prockop (1962) reported sustained nystagmus and drowsiness in seven adults given 70 and 90 mg/kg of body weight of L-tryptophan orally in single doses, but found that these effects were absent at 30 or 50 mg/kg. However, Lieberman and coworkers (1985) reported decreased self-ratings of vigor and alertness and increased subjective fatigue in 20 men treated with a single oral dose of 50 mg/kg of tryptophan. Yuwiler and coworkers (1981) also reported that five individuals given 50 or 100 mg/kg/d of L-tryptophan as a single dose or 50 mg/kg/d for 14 days experienced prolonged lethargy and drowsiness within 30 minutes of ingestion under all loading conditions.

Newborns (2 to 3 days of age) given infant formula supplemented with L-tryptophan (about 20 mg) were found to enter active and then quiet sleep sooner than those newborns given unsupplemented formula (Yogman and Zeisel, 1983). In a later study, these same investigators found that low doses of L-tryptophan have sleep-inducing properties in full-term infants (Yogman and Zeisel, 1985).

Finally, retrospective studies covering the time prior to the 1989 eosinophilia-myalgia syndrome (EMS) outbreak—thought to be caused by L-tryptophan contaminated with 1,1-ethylidene-bis[tryptophan] (EBT)—indicate that use of L-tryptophan alone may increase risk of eosinophilic fasciitis. Blauvelt and Falanga (1991) examined the history of L-tryptophan use in 49 patients with cutaneous fibrosis. Eleven of 17 patients reported using L-tryptophan prior to onset of eosinophilic fasciitis, as did two of ten patients with localized scleroderma, but use of L-tryptophan was not reported in any of 22 patients with systemic sclerosis. Intakes of L-tryptophan were from 0.5 to 5 g/d for 1 month to 10 years before the onset of symptoms of eosinophilic fasciitis were noted. L-tryptophan use in individuals with localized scleroderma occurred for 3 or 10 months before onset of symptoms, and intake was 1.5 to 2 g/d. Hibbs and coworkers (1992) found that 9 of 45 patients with eosinophilic fasciitis used 0.5 to 2.5 g/d of L-tryptophan for 1 month to 10 years before symptom onset. It is unknown whether or not these results occurred because of impurities in the L-tryptophan supplements.

Dose–Response Assessment

Taken together, the above studies in humans indicate that relatively short-term (acute and subacute) use of L-tryptophan is associated with appetite suppression, nausea, and drowsiness. However, in the absence of data on the relationship between chronic consumption of L-tryptophan and the potential for adverse effects, and because of continuing uncertainty of the possible role of L-tryptophan in the development of eosinophilic fasciitis, a UL was not established for L-tryptophan.

Tyrosine

L-Tyrosine is considered a conditionally indispensable amino acid because it can be synthesized from L-phenylalanine in the liver. L-Tyrosine is a precursor of several biologically active substances, including catecholamine neurotransmitters, hormones, and melanin skin pigments. Based on distribution data from the 1988–1994 NHANES III, the mean daily intake for all life stage and gender groups of tyrosine from food and supplements is 2.8 g/d (Appendix Table D-18). Men 31 through 50 years of age had the highest intakes at the 99th percentile of 6.4 g/d.

Hazard Identification

Adverse Effects in Animals. In the mouse with elevated tissue concentrations of tyrosine, decarboxylation to tyramine becomes increasingly important, reducing lethality (David et al., 1974). Evidence has been provided that hepatic biotransformation of tyrosine yields a toxic metabolite, possibly an epoxide (David, 1976).

In rodents, feeding studies document the toxicity of large supplements of L-tyrosine (Benevenga and Steele, 1984; Harper et al., 1970). Effects of tyrosine on weight-gain suppression are a function of the protein content of the diet. For example, feeding rats a low-protein diet, 6 or 9 percent casein, retarded weight gain over a 3-week period. This effect of an inadequate protein intake was exacerbated by the addition of 3 to 8 percent L-tyrosine in the diet (Ip and Harper, 1973). With higher protein intakes of 15 or 24 percent, the toxicity of L-tyrosine was reduced, although 8 percent L-tyrosine still resulted in mortality.

Gipson and coworkers (1975) reported corneal lesions in rats fed L-tyrosine. Subsequently, Rich and coworkers (1973) reported that young adult Simonson albino or Long-Evans pigmented rats fed diets containing 5 or 10 percent L-tyrosine for 15 days developed elevated serum tyrosine levels and experienced reduced weight gain. At 10 percent L-tyrosine in the diet, deaths occurred within 10 days. Corneal disease was the first sign of toxicity; keratopathy was evident by 1 day and progressed in severity. The change began as haziness of the cornea, followed by opacities, and vascularization. The corneal changes were accompanied by elevations of tyrosine concentration in the aqueous humor.

Thoemke and Huether (1984) fed 8-week-old rats a diet containing 2.64 percent L-tyrosine. Rats were fed the diet for 2 weeks prior to mating and continually for three generations. No details were reported on overall pregnancy outcomes or behavioral endpoints. Brain weight was measured in all three generations and no differences were seen except at days 15 and 20 postpartum in the F2 generation (92 and 95 percent of controls). Serum concentration of tyrosine of F3 generation rats was increased at postnatal day 5.

Adverse Effects in Humans. No adverse effects have been reported for L-tyrosine from food. Large single doses of L-tyrosine (500 mg/kg/d) or smaller daily doses (100 mg/kg/d) have not been associated with any adverse affects (Al-Damluji et al., 1988; Glaeser et al., 1979; Sole et al., 1985). Nevertheless, the occurrence of corneal and skin lesions in humans with the autosomal recessive genetic disease, tyrosinemia II, in which tyrosine blood levels can be elevated tenfold, suggests that high chronic intakes leading to high-sustained concentrations of tyrosine in plasma and tissues may have adverse effects.

Single oral doses of 100 or 150 mg/kg of L-tyrosine administered to humans lead to a two- to threefold increase in plasma tyrosine concentrations (Cuche et al., 1985; Glaeser et al., 1979) and in urinary excretion of catecholamines and their metabolites (Alonso et al., 1982). Similar amounts given over the day in three equal doses result in similar increments in plasma tyrosine (Benedict et al., 1983; Melamed et al., 1980) and an increase in urinary catecholamines (Agharanya et al., 1981) and their metabolites (Alonso et al., 1982). Tyrosine given at 7.5 g/d decreased both free and conjugated plasma norepinephrine concentrations (Benedict et al., 1983). An increase in the dopamine metabolite, homovanillic acid, has been found in cerebral spinal fluid after L-tyrosine loads (Growdon et al., 1982).

Loads of L-tyrosine of 100 to 150 mg/kg/d have not been found to have any adverse effects on physiological systems (Benedict et al., 1983; Glaeser et al., 1979; Neri et al., 1995). In 13 patients with mild hypertension and given 2.5 g of L-tyrosine for 2 weeks, blood tyrosine was doubled 2 hours after the supplement, but no differences were found in systolic, diastolic, or mean blood pressure, heart rate, or plasma nonepinephrine (Sole et al., 1985). No data on blood concentrations in humans predictive of corneal lesions are available.

Dose–Response Assessment

In the absence of dose response data to describe more fully the relationship of L-tyrosine loads to alteration in catecholamine synthesis, physiological function, and corneal lesions in humans, a UL for L-tyrosine cannot be set for apparently healthy humans.

Intake Assessment

Although no ULs could be set for any of the amino acids, highest median and 99th percentile intakes for the amino acids are found in Table 10-29. All amino acids had their highest median intake for any life stage and gender group in men aged 19 through 30 years. The highest intakes at the 99th percentile were also found in men, with those 51

TABLE 10-29 Highest Median and 99th Percentile of Usual Daily Intake of Amino Acids, United States, Third National Health and Nutrition Examination Survey, 1998–1994

Amino Acid	Highest Median Intake[a] (g/d)	Highest 99th Percentile of Intake (g/d)
Alanine	5.2	8.5[b]
Arginine	5.9	10.1[b]
Aspartic acid	9.2	15.4[c]
Cysteine	1.4	2.2[b]
Glutamic acid	21.1	33.7[c]
Glycine	4.6	7.8[a]
Histidine	3.1	5.2[b]
Isoleucine	4.9	8.2[b]
Leucine	8.5	14.1[b]
Lysine	7.5	12.6[b]
Methionine	2.5	4.1[b]
Phenylalanine	4.8	7.7[c]
Proline	7.2	12.0[d]
Serine	4.8	7.9[c]
Threonine	4.2	7.1[b]
Tryptophan	1.3	2.1[b]
Tyrosine	3.9	6.4[c]
Valine	5.5	9.1[b]

[a] Males, 19–30 y.
[b] Males, 51–70 y.
[c] Males, 31–50 y.
[d] Males, 14–18 y.
NOTE: Data are from Appendix Tables D-2 through D-19.

through 70 years of age consuming the highest intakes for the majority of the amino acids surveyed.

Risk Characterization

Since there is no evidence that amino acids derived from usual or even high intakes of protein from food present any risk, attention was focused on intakes of the L-form of the amino acid found in dietary protein and amino acid supplements. Even from well-studied amino acids, adequate dose–response data from human or animal studies on which to base a UL were not available, but this does not mean that there is no potential for adverse effects resulting from high intakes of amino acids from dietary supplements. Since data on the adverse effects of high levels of amino acids intakes from dietary supplements are limited, caution may be warranted.

RESEARCH RECOMMENDATIONS

- Research is needed on high-protein intakes (>145 mg N/kg/d) in relationship to positive nitrogen balance and requirement estimates, metabolic and possible toxic effects in children and adults, and pathways affected by these high intakes.
- More data are needed on indispensable amino acid requirements for infants, children, and adolescents, as they are very sparse.
- Few studies on additional needs for protein during pregnancy, including estimates of changes in efficiency of conversion of dietary protein for maintenance and tissue accretion, are available. Thus more studies conducted during the length of pregnancy are needed.
- New methods, other than nitrogen balance, need to be validated to determine protein requirements, particularly in regard to long-term health.
- The role of the gastrointestinal system in the metabolism of amino acids, the nature of the amino acid losses, and the extent of synthesis of indispensable amino acids need to be investigated.
- Research on adaptation mechanisms at various intakes of protein is needed.
- Currently protein data for the elderly are sparse and more data are needed. Available data for the very elderly, namely those from 80 to 100 years of age, consists of only two or three adults in their early 80s, and thus studies conducted with this age group need to be done.
- Since ULs could not be established for any of the amino acids (some of which are known to result in toxic effects at high doses) due to insuffi-

cient data on dose–response relationships, more data are needed on adverse effects of high intakes of amino acids.

REFERENCES

Abumrad NN, Robinson RP, Gooch BR, Lacy WW. 1982. The effect of leucine infusion on substrate flux across the human forearm. *J Surg Res* 32:453–463.

Agharanya JC, Alonso R, Wurtman RJ. 1981. Changes in catecholamine excretion after short-term tyrosine ingestion in normally fed human subjects. *Am J Clin Nutr* 34:82–87.

Ahlborg B, Ekelund LG, Nilsson CG. 1968. Effect of potassium-magnesium-aspartate on the capacity for prolonged exercise in man. *Acta Physiol Scand* 74:238–245.

Al-Damluji S, Ross G, Touzel R, Perrett D, White A, Besser GM. 1988. Modulation of the actions of tyrosine by α-2-adrenoceptor blockade. *Br J Pharmacol* 95:405–412.

Alexander D, Ball MJ, Mann J. 1994. Nutrient intake and haematological status of vegetarians and age-sex matched omnivores. *Eur J Clin Nutr* 48:538–546.

Allen DH, Delohery J, Baker G. 1987. Monosodium L-glutamate-induced asthma. *J Allergy Clin Immunol* 80:530–537.

Allen JC, Keller RP, Archer P, Neville MC. 1991. Studies in human lactation: Milk composition and daily secretion rates of macronutrients in the first year of lactation. *Am J Clin Nutr* 54:69–80.

Allison SP. 1992. The uses and limitations of nutritional support. *Clin Nutr* 11:319–330.

Allison SP. 1995. Cost-effectiveness of nutritional support in the elderly. *Proc Nutr Soc* 54:693–699.

Alonso R, Gibson CJ, Wurtman RJ, Agharanya JC, Prieto L. 1982. Elevation of urinary catecholamines and their metabolites following tyrosine administration in humans. *Biol Psychiatry* 17:781–790.

Ambos M, Leavitt NR, Marmorek L, Wolschina SB. 1968. Sin Cib-Syn: Accent on glutamate. *N Engl J Med* 279:105.

Amen RJ, Yoshimura NN. 1981. The pharmacology of branched-chain amino acids. *Nutr Pharmacol* 4:73–116.

Anantharaman K. 1979. In utero and dietary administration of monosodium L-glutamate to mice: Reproductive performance and development in a multigeneration study. In: Filer LJ, ed. *Glutamic Acid: Advances in Biochemistry and Physiology.* Pp. 231–253.

Anderson DM, Williams FH, Merkatz RB, Schulman PK, Kerr DS, Pittard WB. 1983. Length of gestation and nutritional composition of human milk. *Am J Clin Nutr* 37:810–814.

Anderson GH, Johnston JL. 1983. Nutrient control of brain neurotransmitter synthesis and function. *Can J Physiol Pharmacol* 61:271–281.

Anderson GH, Atkinson SA, Bryan MH. 1981. Energy and macronutrient content of human milk during early lactation from mothers giving birth prematurely and at term. *Am J Clin Nutr* 34:258–265.

Anderson SA, Tews JK, Harper AE. 1990. Dietary branched-chain amino acids and protein selection by rats. *J Nutr* 120:52–63.

ARS (Agricultural Research Service). 2001. *USDA Nutrient Database for Standard Reference, Release 14.* Online. U.S. Department of Agriculture. Available at http://www.nal.usda.gov/fnic/foodcomp/Data/SR14/sr14.html. Accessed July 3, 2002.

Artom C, Fishman WH, Morehead RP. 1945. The relative toxicity of l- and dl-serine in rats. *Proc Soc Exp Biol Med* 60:284–287.

Ashley DV, Anderson GH. 1975. Correlation between the plasma tryptophan to neutral amino acid ratio and protein intake in the self-selecting weanling rat. *J Nutr* 105:1412–1421.

Atkinson SA, Anderson GH, Bryan MH. 1980. Human milk: comparison of the nitrogen composition in milk from mothers of premature and full-term infants. *Am J Clin Nutr 33:811-814.*

Ball MJ, Bartlett MA. 1999. Dietary intake and iron status of Australian vegetarian women. *Am J Clin Nutr* 70:353–358.

Barbul A. 1986. Arginine: Biochemistry, physiology, and therapeutic implications. *J Parenter Enteral Nutr* 10:227–238.

Barbul A, Wasserkrug HL, Sisto DA, Seifter E, Rettura G, Levenson SM, Efron G. 1980. Thymic stimulatory actions of arginine. *J Parenter Enteral Nutr* 4:446–449.

Barbul A, Sisto DA, Wasserkrug HL, Efron G. 1981. Arginine stimulates lymphocyte immune response in healthy human beings. *Surgery* 90:244–251.

Barbul A, Lazarou SA, Efron DT, Wasserkrug HL, Efron G. 1990. Arginine enhances wound healing and lymphocyte immune responses in humans. *Surgery* 108:331–337.

Barr SI, Broughton TM. 2000. Relative weight, weight loss efforts and nutrient intakes among health-conscious vegetarian, past vegetarian and nonvegetarian women ages 18 to 50. *J Am Coll Nutr* 19:781–788.

Basile-Filho A, Beaumier L, El-Khoury AE, Yu Y, Kenneway M, Gleason RE, Young VR. 1998. Twenty-four-hour L-[1-^{13}C]tyrosine and L-[3,3-^{2}H$_2$]phenylalanine oral tracer studies at generous, intermediate, and low phenylalanine intakes to estimate aromatic amino acid requirements in adults. *Am J Clin Nutr* 67:640–659.

Batshaw ML, Wachtel RC, Thomas GH, Starrett A, Brusilow SW. 1984. Arginine-responsive asymptomatic hyperammonemia in the premature infant. *J Pediatr* 105:86–91.

Baxter CF, Baldwin RA, Davis JL, Flood JF. 1985. High proline levels in the brains of mice as related to specific learning deficits. *Pharmacol Biochem Behav* 22:1053–1059.

Bazzano G, D'Elia JA, Olson RE. 1970. Monosodium glutamate: Feeding of large amounts in man and gerbils. *Science* 169:1208–1209.

Benabe JE, Martinez-Maldonado M. 1998. The impact of malnutrition on kidney function. *Mineral Electrolyte Metab* 24:20–26.

Benedict CR, Anderson GH, Sole MJ. 1983. The influence of oral tyrosine and tryptophan feeding on plasma catecholamines in man. *Am J Clin Nutr* 38:429–435.

Benevenga NJ, Steele RD. 1984. Adverse effects of excessive consumption of amino acids. *Annu Rev Nutr* 4:157–181.

Benevenga NJ, Yeh M-H, Lalich JJ. 1976. Growth depression and tissue reaction to the consumption of excess dietary methionine and S-methyl-L-cysteine. *J Nutr* 106:1714–1720.

Bergner H, Schwandt H, Kruger U. 1990. Determination of a prececal N-absorption from natural feed by ^{15}N-labeled laboratory rats using the isotope diluation method. *Arch Tierernahr* 40:569–582.

Bernacchi AS, DeFerreyra EC, DeCastro CR, Castro JA. 1993. Ultrastructural alterations in testes from rats treated with cysteine. *Biomed Environ Sci* 6:172–178.

Berry HK, Butcher RE, Elliot LA, Brunner RL. 1974. The effect of monosodium glutamate on the early biochemical and behavioral development of the rat. *Dev Psychobiol* 7:165–173.

Birt DF, Julius AD, Hasegawa R, St. John M, Cohen S. 1987. Effect of L-tryptophan excess and vitamin B_6 deficiency on rat urinary bladder cancer promotion. *Cancer Res* 47:1244–1250.

Bistrian BR. 1990. Recent advances in parenteral and enteral nutrition: A personal perspective. *J Parenteral Enteral Nutr* 14:329–334.

Blauvelt A, Falanga V. 1991. Idiopathic and L-tryptophan-associated eosinophilic fasciitis before and after L-tryptophan contamination. *Arch Dermatol* 127:1159–1166.

Block KP. 1989. Interactions among leucine, isoleucine, and valine with special reference to the branched-chain amino acid antagonism. In: Friedman M, ed. *Absorption and Utilization of Amino Acids*, Vol. 1. Boca Raton, FL: CRC Press. Pp. 229–244.

Blumenkrantz MJ, Shapiro DJ, Swendseid ME, Kopple JD. 1975. Histidine supplementation for treatment of anaemia of uraemia. *Br Med J* 2:530–533.

Borgonha S, Regan MM, Oh SH, Condon M, Young VR. 2002. Threonine requirement of healthy adults, derived with a 24-h indicator amino acid balance technique. *Am J Clin Nutr* 75:698–704.

Brattstrom LE, Hardebo JE, Hultberg BL. 1984. Moderate homocysteinemia—A possible risk factor for arteriosclerotic cerebrovascular disease. *Stroke* 15:1012–1016.

Brattstrom L, Israelsson B, Norrving B, Bergqvist D, Thorne J, Hultberg B, Hamfelt A. 1990. Impaired homocysteine metabolism in early-onset cerebral and peripheral occlusive arterial disease. *Atherosclerosis* 81:51–60.

Bross R, Ball RO, Pencharz PB. 1998. Development of a minimally invasive protocol for the determination of phenylalanine and lysine kinetics in humans during the fed state. *J Nutr* 128:1913–1919.

Bross R, Ball RO, Clarke JTR, Pencharz PB. 2000. Tyrosine requirements in children with classical PKU determined by indicator amino acid oxidation. *Am J Physiol* 278:E195–E201.

Brunton JA, Ball RO, Pencharz PB. 1998. Determination of amino acid requirements by indicator amino acid oxidation: Applications in health and disease. *Curr Opin Clin Nutr Metab Care* 1:449–453.

Brunton JA, Bertolo RF, Pencharz PB, Ball RO. 1999. Proline ameliorates arginine deficiency during enteral but not parenteral feeding in neonatal piglets. *Am J Physiol* 277:E223–E231.

Brusilow SW, Horwich AL. 1989. Urea cycle enzymes. In: Scriver CR, Beaudet AL, Sly WS, Valle D, eds. *The Metabolic Basis of Inherited Disease, 6th ed.* New York: McGraw-Hill. Pp. 629–663.

Brusilow SW, Danney M, Waber LJ, Batshaw M, Burton B, Levitsky L, Roth K, McKeethren C, Ward J. 1984. Treatment of episodic hyperammonemia in children with inborn errors of urea synthesis. *N Engl J Med* 310:1630–1634.

Burke BS, Harding VV, Stuart HC. 1943. Nutrition studies during pregnancy. IV. Relation of protein content of mother's diet during pregnancy to birth length, birth weight, and condition of infant at birth. *J Pediatr* 23:506–515.

Bushinsky DA, Gennari FJ. 1978. Life-threatening hyperkalemia induced by arginine. *Ann Intern Med* 89:632–634.

Butte NF, Garza C, Johnson CA, O'Brian Smith E, Nichols BL. 1984a. Longitudinal changes in milk composition of mothers delivering preterm and term infants. *Early Hum Dev* 9:153–162.

Butte NF, Garza C, O'Brian Smith E, Nichols BL. 1984b. Human milk intake and growth in exclusively breast-fed infants. *J Pediatr* 104:187–195.

Butte NF, Hopkinson JM, Wong WW, Smith EO, Ellis KJ. 2000. Body composition during the first 2 years of life: An updated reference. *Pediatr Res* 47:578–585.

Calabrese V, Rausa N, Antico A, Mangiameli S, Rizza V. 1997. Cysteine-induced enhancement of lipid peroxidation in substantia nigra: Comparative effect with exogenous administration of reduced glutathione. *Drugs Exp Clin Res* 23:25–31.

Calloway DH. 1974. Nitrogen balance during pregnancy. In: Winnick M, ed. *Nutrition and Fetal Development*, Vol. 2. New York: John Wiley and Sons. Pp. 79–94.

Calloway DH, Margen S. 1971. Variation in endogenous nitrogen excretion and dietary nitrogen utilization as determinants of human protein requirement. *J Nutr* 101:205–216.

Calloway DH, Odell AC, Margen S. 1971. Sweat and miscellaneous nitrogen losses in human balance studies. *J Nutr* 101:775–786.

Campbell WW, Evans WJ. 1996. Protein requirements of elderly people. *Eur J Clin Nutr* 50:S180–S185.

Campbell WW, Crim MC, Dallal GE, Young VR, Evans WJ. 1994. Increased protein requirements in elderly people: New data and retrospective reassessments. *Am J Clin Nutr* 60:501–509.

Campbell WW, Crim MC, Young VR, Joseph LJ, Evans WJ. 1995. Effects of resistance training and dietary protein intake on protein metabolism in older adults. *Am J Physiol* 268:E1143–E1153.

Campbell WW, Trappe TA, Wolfe RR, Evans WJ. 2001. The recommended dietary allowance for protein may not be adequate for older people to maintain skeletal muscle. *J Gerontol A Biol Sci Med Sci* 56:M373–M380.

Carlson HE, Miglietta JT, Roginsky MS, Steglink LD. 1989. Stimulation of pituitary hormone secretion by neurotransmitter amino acids in humans. *Metabolism* 38:1179–1182.

Carmichael S, Abrams B, Selvin S. 1997. The pattern of maternal weight gain in women with good pregnancy outcomes. *Am J Public Health* 87:1984–1988.

Castaneda C, Charnley JM, Evans WJ, Crim MC. 1995a. Elderly women accommodate to a low-protein diet with losses of body cell mass, muscle function, and immune response. *Am J Clin Nutr* 62:30–39.

Castaneda C, Dolnikowski GG, Dallal GE, Evans WJ, Crim MC. 1995b. Protein turnover and energy metabolism of elderly women fed a low-protein diet. *Am J Clin Nutr* 62:40–48.

Celander DR, George MJ. 1963. Dietary interrelationships of ethionine and methionine in the weanling rat. *Biochem J* 87:143–146.

Chambers BJ, Klein NW, Nosel PG, Khairallah LH, Romanow JS. 1995. Methionine overcomes neural tube defects in rat embryos cultured on sera from laminin-immunized monkeys. *J Nutr* 125:1587–1599.

Chatot CL, Klein NW, Clapper ML, Resor SR, Singer WD, Russman BS, Holmes GL, Mattson RH, Cramer JA. 1984. Human serum teratogenicity studied by rat embryo culture: Epilepsy, anticonvulsant drugs, and nutrition. *Epilepsia* 25:205–216.

Chen MK, Salloum RM, Austgen TR, Bland JB, Bland KI, Copeland EM, Souba WW. 1991. Tumor regulation of hepatic glutamine metabolism. *J Parenter Enteral Nutr* 15:159–164.

Chen MK, Espat NJ, Bland KI, Copeland EM, Souba WW. 1993. Influence of progressive tumor growth on glutamine metabolism in skeletal muscle and kidney. *Ann Surg* 217:655–667.

Cheng AH, Gomez A, Bergan JG, Lee TC, Monckeberg F, Chichester CO. 1978. Comparative nitrogen balance study between young and aged adults using three levels of protein intake from a combination wheat-soy-milk mixture. *Am J Clin Nutr* 31:12–22.

Chien PFW, Smith K, Watt PW, Scrimgeour CM, Taylor DJ, Rennie MJ. 1993. Protein turnover in the human fetus studied at term using stable isotope tracer amino acids. *Am J Physiol* 265:E31–E35.

Chipponi JX, Bleier JC, Santi MT, Rudman D. 1982. Deficiencies of essential and conditionally essential nutrients. *Am J Clin Nutr* 35:1112–1116.

Cho ES, Anderson HL, Wixom RL, Hanson KC, Krause GF. 1984. Long-term effects of low histidine intake on men. *J Nutr* 114:369–384.

Christman AA. 1971. Determination of anserine, carnosine, and other histidine compounds in muscle extractives. *Anal Biochem* 39:181–187.

Chung TK, Gelberg HB, Dorner JL, Baker DH. 1991. Safety of L-tryptophan for pigs. *J Anim Sci* 69:2955–2960.

Ciechanover A, DiGiuseppe JA, Bercovich B, Orian A, Richter JD, Schwartz AL, Brodeur GM. 1991. Degradation of nuclear oncoproteins by the ubiquitin system in vitro. *Proc Natl Acad Sci USA* 88:139–143.

Clarke JTR, Bier DM. 1982. The conversion of phenylalanine to tyrosine in man. Direct measurement by continuous intravenous tracer infusions of L-[ring-^{2}H$_5$] phenylalanine and L-[1-^{13}C] tyrosine in the postabsorptive state. *Metabolism* 31:999–1005.

Clarke R, Daly L, Robinson K, Naughten E, Cahalane S, Fowler B, Graham I. 1991. Hyperhomocysteinemia: An independent risk factor for vascular disease. *N Engl J Med* 324:1149–1155.

Coelho CN, Klein NW. 1990. Methionine and neural tube closure in cultured rat embryos: Morphological and biochemical analyses. *Teratology* 42:437–451.

Cohlan SQ, Stone SM. 1961. Effects of dietary and intraperitoneal excess of L-lysine and L-leucine on rat pregnancy and offspring. *J Nutr* 74:93–95.

Colquhoun A, Newsholme EA. 1997. Aspects of glutamine metabolism in human tumour cells. *Biochem Mol Biol Int* 41:583–596.

Connor H, Newton DJ, Preston FE, Woods HF. 1978. Oral methionine loading as a cause of acute serum folate deficiency: Its relevance to parental nutrition. *Postgrad Med J* 54:318–320.

Cordain L, Miller JB, Eaton SB, Mann N, Holt SH, Speth JD. 2000. Plant-animal subsistence ratios and macronutrient energy estimations in worldwide hunter-gatherer diets. *Am J Clin Nutr* 71:682–692.

Corish CA, Kennedy NP. 2000. Protein-energy undernutrition in hospital in-patients. *Br J Nutr* 83:575–591.

Creel DJ, Wang JM, Wong KC. 1987. Transient blindness associated with transurethral resection of the prostate. *Arch Ophthalmol* 105:1537–1539.

Cuche JL, Prinseau J, Selz F, Ruget G, Tual JL, Reingeissen L, Devoisin M, Baglin A, Guedon J, Fritel D. 1985. Oral load of tyrosine or L-dopa and plasma levels of free and sulfoconjugated catecholamines in healthy men. *Hypertension* 7:81–89.

Cuervo AM, Dice JF. 1998. Lysosomes, a meeting point of proteins, chaperones, and proteases. *J Mol Med* 76:6–12.

Danner DJ, Elsas LF. 1989. Disorders of branched chain amino acid and keto acid metabolism. In: Scriver CR, Beaudet AL, Sly WS, Valle D, eds. *The Metabolic Basis of Inherited Disease, 6th ed.*, Vol. I. New York: McGraw-Hill. Pp. 671–692.

Danner DJ, Lemmon SK, Besharse JC, Elsas LJ. 1979. Purification and characterization of branched chain alpha-ketoacid dehydrogenase from bovine liver mitochondria. *J Biol Chem* 254:5522–5526.

Darling PB, Grunow J, Rafii M, Brookes S, Ball RO Pencharz PB. 2000. Threonine dehydrogenase is a minor degradative pathway of threonine catabolism in human adults. *Am J Physiol* 278:E877–E884.

Darragh AJ, Hodgkinson SM. 2000. Quantifying the digestibility of dietary protein. *J Nutr* 130:1850S–1856S.

Darragh AJ, Moughan PJ. 1998. The amino acid composition of human milk corrected for amino acid digestibility. *Br J Nutr* 80:25–34.

Das TK, Waterlow JC. 1974. The rate of adaptation of urea cycle enzymes, aminotransferases and glutamic dehydrogenase to changes in dietary protein intake. *Br J Nutr* 32:353–373.

David JC. 1976. Evidence for the possible formation of a toxic tyrosine metabolite by the liver microsomal drug metabolizing system. *Naunyn Schmiedebergs Arch Pharmacol* 292:79–86.

David JC, Dairman W, Udenfriend S. 1974. Decarboxylation to tyramine: A major route of tyrosine metabolism in mammals. *Proc Natl Acad Sci USA* 71:1771–1775.

Davis TA, Nguyen HV, Garcia-Bravo R, Fiorotto ML, Jackson EM, Lewis DS, Lee DR, Reeds PJ. 1994. Amino acid composition of human milk is not unique. *J Nutr* 124:1126–1132.

De Aloysio D, Mantuano R, Mauloni M, Nicoletti G. 1982. The clinical use of arginine aspartate in male infertility. *Acta Eur Fertil* 13:133–167.

de Blaauw I, Deutz NEP, Von Meyenfeldt MF. 1996. In vivo amino acid metabolism of gut and liver during short and prolonged starvation. *Am J Physiol* 270:G298–G306.

de Haan A, van Doorn JE, Westra HG. 1985. Effects of potassium + magnesium aspartate on muscle metabolism and force development during short intensive static exercise. *Int J Sports Med* 6:44–49.

Dekker J, Aelmans PH, Strous GJ. 1991. The oligomeric structure of rat and human gastric mucins. *Biochem J* 277:423–427.

de Lange CFM, Sauer WC, Mosenthin R, Souffrant WB. 1989. The effect of feeding different protein-free diets on the recovery and amino acid composition of endogenous protein collected from the distal ileum and feces in pigs. *J Anim Sci* 67:746–754.

de Vrese M, Frik R, Roos N, Hagemeister H. 2000. Protein-bound D-amino acids, and to a lesser extent lysinoalanine, decrease true ileal protein digestibility in minipigs as determined with ^{15}N-labeling. *J Nutr* 130:2026–2031.

Dewey KG, Lönnerdal B. 1983. Milk and nutrient intake of breast-fed infants from 1 to 6 months: Relation to growth and fatness. *J Pediatr Gastroenterol Nutr* 2:497–506.

Dewey KG, Finley DA, Lönnerdal B. 1984. Breast milk volume and composition during late lactation (7–20 months). *J Pediatr Gastroenterol Nutr* 3:713–720.

Dewey KG, Beaton G, Fjeld C, Lönnerdal B, Reeds P. 1996. Protein requirements of infants and children. *Eur J Clin Nutr* 50:S119–S150.

DHEW (U.S. Department of Health, Education and Welfare). 1978. *Bioassay of L-Tryptophan for Possible Carcinogenicity.* National Cancer Institute Technical Report Series No. 71. Washington, DC: U.S. Government Printing Office.

Di Buono M, Wykes LJ, Ball RO, Pencharz PB. 2001. Total sulfur amino acid requirement in young men determined by indicator amino acid oxidation with L-[1-^{13}C] phenylalanine. *Am J Clin Nutr* 74:756–760.

Diem K. 1962. *Documenta Geigy Scientific Tables, 6th ed.* Ardsley, NY: Geigy Pharmaceuticals. Pp.528.

DiGiovanna JJ, Blank H. 1984. Failure of lysine in frequently recurrent herpes simplex infection. Treatment and prophylaxis. *Arch Dermatol* 120:48–51.

DiGiovanna JJ, Blank H. 1985. Failure of lysine? *Arch Dermatol* 121:21.

Drago F, Continella G, Alloro MC, Auditore S, Pennisi G. 1984. Behavioral effects of arginine in male rats. *Pharmacol Res Commun* 16:899–907.

Dubois S, Dougherty C, Duquette M-P, Hanley JA, Moutquin J-M. 1991. Twin pregnancy: The impact of the Higgins Nutrition Intervention Program on maternal and neonatal outcomes. *Am J Clin Nutr* 53:1397–1403.

Dubois S, Coulombe C, Pencharz P, Pinsonneault O, Duquette M-P. 1997. Ability of the Higgins Nutrition Intervention Program to improve adolescent pregnancy outcome. *J Am Diet Assoc* 97:871–878.

Dubow E, Maher A, Gish D, Erk V. 1958. Lysine tolerance in infants. *J Pediatr* 52:30–37.

Duffy B, Gunn T, Collinge J, Pencharz PB. 1981. The effect of varying protein quality and energy intake on the nitrogen metabolism of parenterally fed very low birthweight (<1600 g) infants. *Pediatr Res* 15:1040–1044.

Dutra-Filho CS, Wannmacher CM, Pires RF, Gus G, Kalil AM, Wajner M. 1989. Reduced locomotor activity of rats made histidinemic by injection of histidine. *J Nutr* 119:1223–1227.

Ebert AG. 1979a. The dietary administration of L-monosodium glutamate, DL-monosodium glutamate, and L-glutamic acid to rats. *Toxicol Lett* 3:71–78.

Ebert AG. 1979b. The dietary administration of monosodium glutamate or glutamic acid to C-57 black mice for 2 years. *Toxicol Lett* 3:65–70.

Edmonds MS, Baker DH. 1987. Amino acid excesses for young pigs: Effects of excess methionine, tryptophan, threonine or leucine. *J Anim Sci* 64:1664–1671.

Edmonds MS, Gonyou HW, Baker DH. 1987. Effect of excess levels of methionine, tryptophan, arginine, lysine or threonine on growth and dietary choice in the pig. *J Anim Sci* 65:179–185.

Egana JI, Fuentes A, Uauy R. 1984. Protein needs of Chilean pre-school children fed milk and soy protein isolate diets. In: Rand WM, Uauy R, Scrimshaw NS, eds. *Protein-Energy Requirement Studies in Developing Countries: Results of International Research.* Tokyo, Japan: United Nations University Press. Pp. 249–257.

Egana JI, Uauy R, Cassorla X, Barrera G, Yanez E. 1992. Sweet lupin protein quality in young men. *J Nutr* 122:2341–2347.

Ehlers K, Drews E, Nau H. 1994. The amino acid methionine reduces the valproic acid-induced spina bifida rate in the mouse. *Teratology* 50:28A.

Elia M, Livesey G. 1983. Effects of ingested steak and infused leucine on forelimb metabolism in man and the fate of the carbon skeletons and amino groups of branched-chain amino acids. *Clin Sci* 64:517–526.

El-Khoury AE, Fukagawa NK, Sanchez M, Tsay RH, Gleason RE, Chapman TE, Young VR. 1994a. The 24-h pattern and rate of leucine oxidation, with particular reference to tracer estimates of leucine requirements in healthy adults. *Am J Clin Nutr* 59:1012–1020.

El-Khoury AE, Fukagawa NK, Sanchez M, Tsay RH, Gleason RE, Chapman TE, Young VR. 1994b. Validation of the tracer-balance concept with reference to leucine: 24-h intravenous tracer studies with L-[1-^{13}C]leucine and [^{15}N-^{15}N]urea. *Am J Clin Nutr* 59:1000–1011.

El-Khoury AE, Forslund A, Olsson R, Branth S, Sjodin A, Andersson A, Atkinson A, Selvaraj A, Hambraeus L, Young VR. 1997. Moderate exercise at energy balance does not affect 24-h leucine oxidation or nitrogen retention in healthy men. *Am J Physiol* 273:E394–E407.

El-Khoury AE, Pereira PC, Borgonha S, Basile-Filho A, Beaumier L, Wang SY, Metges CC, Ajami AM, Young VR. 2000. Twenty-four-hour oral tracer studies with L-[1-^{13}C]lysine at a low (15 mg·kg^{-1}·d^{-1}) and intermediate (29 mg·kg^{-1}·d^{-1}) lysine intake in healthy adults. *Am J Clin Nutr* 72:122–130.

Ellis KJ, Shypailo RJ, Abrams SA, Wong WW. 2000. The reference child and adolescent models of body composition. A contemporary comparison. *Ann NY Acad Sci* 904:374–382.

Emerson K, Poindexter EL, Kothari M. 1975. Changes in total body composition during normal and diabetic pregnancy: Relation to oxygen consumption. *Obstet Gynecol* 45:505–511.

Eriksson LS, Hagenfeldt L, Felig P, Wahren J. 1983. Leucine uptake by splanchnic and leg tissues in man: Relative independence of insulin levels. *Clin Sci* 65:491–498.

Fahr MJ, Kornbluth J, Blossom S, Schaeffer R, Klimberg VS. 1994. Harry M. Vars Research Award. Glutamine enhances immunoregulation of tumor growth. *J Parenter Enteral Nutr* 18:471–476.

FAO (Food and Agriculture Organization). 2000. *The State of Food and Agriculture 2000*. Rome: FAO.

FAO/Agrostat. 1991. *Computerized information series No. 1. Food balance sheets*. Rome: FAO.

FAO/WHO (World Health Organization). 1965. *Protein Requirements*. Report of a Joint FAO/WHO Expert Group. Technical Report Series No. 37. Rome: FAO.

FAO/WHO. 1973. *Energy and Protein Requirements*. Report of a Joint FAO/WHO Ad Hoc Expert Committee. Technical Report Series No. 522. Geneva, Switzerland: WHO.

FAO/WHO. 1991. *Protein Quality Evaluation*. FAO Food and Nutrition Paper 51. Rome: FAO.

FAO/WHO/UNU (United Nations University). 1985. *Energy and Protein Requirements*. Report of a Joint FAO/WHO/UNU Expert Consultation. Technical Report Series No. 724. Geneva, Switzerland: WHO.

Fawcett LB, Pugarelli JE, Brent RL. 2000. Effects of supplemental methionine on antiserum-induced dysmorphology in rat embryos cultured in vitro. *Teratology* 61:332–341.

Fee BA, Weil WB. 1963. Body composition of infants of diabetic mothers by direct analysis. *Ann NY Acad Sci* 110:869.

Fernstrom JD, Larin F, Wurtman RJ. 1973. Correlations between brain tryptophan and plasma neutral amino acid levels following food consumption in rats. *Life Sci* 13:517–524.

Fernstrom JD, Cameron JL, Fernstrom MH, McConaha C, Weltzin TE, Kaye WH. 1996. Short-term neuroendocrine effects of a large oral dose of monosodium glutamate in fasting male subjects. *J Clin Endocrinol Metab* 81:184–191.

Ferrari DA, Gilles PA, Klein NW, Nadler D, Weeks BS, Lammi-Keefe CJ, Hillman RE, Carey SW, Ying Y-K, Maier D, Olsen P, Wemple DW, Greenstein R, Muechler EK, Miller RK, Mariona FG. 1994. Rat embryo development on human sera is related to numbers of previous spontaneous abortions and nutritional factors. *Am J Obstet Gynecol* 170:228–236.

Filer LJ, Stegink LD. 1988. Effect of aspartame on plasma phenylalanine concentration in humans. In: Wurtman RJ, Ritter-Walker E, eds. *Dietary Phenylalanine and Brain Function.* Boston: Birkhauser. Pp. 18–40.

Finkelstein MW, Daabees TT, Stegink LD, Applebaum AE. 1983. Correlation of aspartate dose, plasma dicarboxylic amino acid concentration, and neuronal necrosis in infant mice. *Toxicology* 29:109–119.

Finkelstein MW, Daabees TT, Stegink LD, Applebaum AE. 1988. Aspartate-induced neuronal necrosis in infant mice: Protective effect of carbohydrate and insulin. *J Toxicol Environ Health* 23:395–406.

Fisher H, Brush MK, Griminger P, Sostman ER. 1967. Nitrogen retention in adult man: A possible factor in protein requirements. *Am J Clin Nutr* 20:927–934.

Fomon S. 1991. Requirements and recommended dietary intakes of protein during infancy. *Pediatr Res* 30:391–395.

Forbes GB. 1987. *Human Body Composition: Growth, Aging, Nutrition, and Activity.* New York: Springer-Verlag.

Forslund AH, Hambraeus L, Olsson RM, El-Khoury AE, Yu Y-M, Young VR. 1998. The 24-h whole body leucine and urea kinetics at normal and high protein intakes with exercise in healthy adults. *Am J Physiol* 275:E310–E320.

Forsum E, Sadurskis A, Wager J. 1988. Resting metabolic rate and body composition of healthy Swedish women during pregnancy. *Am J Clin Nutr* 47:942–947.

Fregly MJ, Rowland NE, Sumners C. 1989. Effect of chronic dietary treatment with L-tryptophan on spontaneous salt appetite of rats. *Pharmacol Biochem Behav* 33:401–406.

Frexes-Steed M, Warner ML, Bulus N, Flakoll P, Abumrad NN. 1990. Role of insulin and branched-chain amino acids in regulating protein metabolism during fasting. *Am J Physiol* 258:E907–E917.

Frey GH. 1976. Use of aspartame by apparently healthy children and adolescents. *J Toxicol Environ Health* 2:401–415.

Frisancho AR, Matos J, Flegel P. 1983. Maternal nutritional status and adolescent pregnancy outcome. *Am J Clin Nutr* 38:739–746.

Fuller MF, Garlick PJ. 1994. Human amino acid requirements: Can the controversy be resolved? *Annu Rev Nutr* 14:217–241.

Fuller MF, Reeds PJ. 1998. Nitrogen cycling in the gut. *Annu Rev Nutr* 18:385–411.

Funk DN, Worthington-Roberts B, Fantel A. 1991. Impact of supplemental lysine or tryptophan on pregnancy course and outcome in rats. *Nutr Res* 11:501–512.

Furst P. 1989. Amino acid metabolism in uremia. *J Am Coll Nutr* 8:310–323.

Garlick PJ, Reeds PJ. 1993. Proteins. In: Garrow JS, James WPT, Ralph A, eds. *Human Nutrition and Dietetics.* Edinburgh: Churchill Livingstone. Pp. 56–76.

Garlick PJ, McNurlan MA, Patlak CS. 1999. Adaptation of protein metabolism in relation to limits to high dietary protein intake. *Eur J Clin Nutr* 53:S34–S43.

Garza C, Scrimshaw NS, Young VR. 1976. Human protein requirements: The effect of variations in energy intake within the maintenance range. *Am J Clin Nutr* 29:280–287.

Garza C, Scrimshaw NS, Young VR. 1977a. Human protein requirements: A long-term metabolic nitrogen balance study in young men to evaluate the 1973 FAO/WHO safe level of egg protein intake. *J Nutr* 107:335–352.

Garza C, Scrimshaw NS, Young VR. 1977b. Human protein requirements: Evaluation of the 1973 FAO/WHO safe level of protein intake for young men at high energy intakes. *Br J Nutr* 37:403–420.

Garza C, Scrimshaw NS, Young VR. 1978. Human protein requirements: Interrelationships between energy intake and nitrogen balance in young men consuming the 1973 FAO/WHO safe level of egg protein, with added nonessential amino acids. *J Nutr* 108:90–96.

Gaspar J, Laires A, Va S, Pereira S, Mariano A, Quina M, Rueff J. 1996. Mutagenic activity of glycine upon nitrosation in the presence of chloride and human gastric juice: A possible role in gastric carcinogenesis. *Teratog Carcinog Mutagen* 16:275–286.

Gattas V, Barrera GA, Riumallo JS, Uauy R. 1990. Protein-energy requirements of prepubertal school-age boys determined by using the nitrogen-balance response to a mixed-protein diet. *Am J Clin Nutr* 52:1037–1042.

Gattas V, Barrera GA, Riumallo JS, Uauy R. 1992. Protein-energy requirements of boys 12-14 y old determined by using the nitrogen-balance response to a mixed-protein diet. *Am J Clin Nutr* 56:499–503.

Gaudichon C, Mahe S, Benamouzig R, Luengo C, Fouillet H, Dare S, Van Oycke M, Ferriere F, Rautureau J, Tome D. 1999. Net postprandial utilization of [15N]-labeled milk protein nitrogen is influenced by diet composition in humans. *J Nutr* 129:890–895.

Gausserès N, Mahé S, Benamouzig R, Luengo C, Ferriere F, Rautureau J, Tomé D. 1997. [^{15}N]-Labeled pea flour protein nitrogen exhibits good ileal digestibility and postprandial retention in humans. *J Nutr* 127:1160–1165.

Geha RS, Beiser A, Ren C, Patterson R, Greenberger P, Grammer LC, Ditto AM, Harris KE, Shaughnessy MA, Yarnold PR, Corren J, Saxon A. 2000. Multicenter, double blind, placebo-controlled, multiple-challenge evaluation of reported reactions to monosodium glutamate. *J Allergy Clin Immunol* 106:973–980.

Geliebter AA, Hashim SA, Van Itallie TB. 1981. Oral L-histidine fails to reduce taste and smell acuity but induces anorexia and urinary zinc excretion. *Am J Clin Nutr* 34:119–120.

Genuth SM. 1973. Effects of oral alanine administration in fasting obese subjects. *Metabolism* 22:927–937.

Genuth SM, Castro J. 1974. Effect of oral alanine on blood beta-hydroxybutyrate and plasma glucose, insulin, free fatty acids, and growth hormone in normal and diabetic subjects. *Metabolism* 23:375–386.

Gerard JM, Luisiri A. 1997. A fatal overdose of arginine hydrochloride. *Clin Toxicol* 35:621–625.

Germano P, Cohen SG, Hahn B, Metcalfe DD. 1991. An evaluation of clinical reactions to monosodium glutamate (MSG) in asthmatics, using a blinded placebo-controlled challenge. *J Allergy Clin Immunol* 87:177.

Gersovitz M, Motil K, Munro HN, Scrimshaw NS, Young VR. 1982. Human protein requirements: Assessment of the adequacy of the current Recommended Dietary Allowance for dietary protein in elderly men and women. *Am J Clin Nutr* 35:6–14.

Gipson IK, Burns RP, Wolfe-Lande JD. 1975. Crystals in corneal epithelial lesions of tyrosine-fed rats. *Invest Ophthalmol* 14:937–941.

Glaeser BS, Melamed E, Growdon JH, Wurtman RJ. 1979. Evaluation of plasma tyrosine after a single oral dose of L-tyrosine. *Life Sci* 25:265–271.

Glatt H. 1989. Mutagenicity spectra in *Salmonella typhimurium* strains of glutathione, L-cysteine and active oxygen species. *Mutagenesis* 4:221–227.

Glatt H. 1990. Endogenous mutagens derived from amino acids. *Mutat Res* 238:235–243.

Glyn JR, Lipton JM. 1981. Effects of central administration of alanine on body temperature of the rabbit: Comparisons with the effects of serine, glycine and taurine. *Brain Res Bull* 6:467–472.

Goldberg AL, Rock KL. 1992. Proteolysis, proteasomes and antigen presentation. *Nature* 357:375–379.

Greenwood MH, Lader MH, Kantameneni BD, Curzon G. 1975. The acute effects of oral (–)-tryptophan in human subjects. *Br J Clin Pharmacol* 2:165–172.

Griffith RS, Norins AL, Kagan C. 1978. A multicentered study of lysine therapy in herpes simplex infection. *Dermatologica* 156:257–267.

Griffith RS, Walsh DE, Myrmel KH, Thompson RW, Behforooz A. 1987. Success of L-lysine therapy in frequently recurrent herpes simplex infection. Treatment and prophylaxis. *Dermatologica* 175:183–190.

Grossie VB, Nishioka K, Ajani JA, Ota DM. 1992. Substituting ornithine for arginine in total parenteral nutrition eliminates enhanced tumor growth. *J Surg Oncol* 50:161–167.

Growdon JH, Melamed E, Logue M, Hefti F, Wurtman RJ. 1982. Effects of oral L-tyrosine administration on CSF tyrosine and homovanillic acid levels in patients with Parkinson's disease. *Life Sci* 30:827–832.

Growdon JH, Nader TM, Schoenfeld J, Wurtman RJ. 1991. L-threonine in the treatment of spasticity. *Clin Neuropharmacol* 14:403–412.

Haddad EH, Berk LS, Kettering JD, Hubbard RW, Peters WR. 1999. Dietary intake and biochemical, hematologic, and immune status of vegans compared with nonvegetarians. *Am J Clin Nutr* 70:586S–593S.

Hagenfeldt L, Eriksson S, Wahren J. 1980. Influence of leucine on arterial concentrations and regional exchange of amino acids in healthy subjects. *Clin Sci* 59:173–181.

Hahn RG. 1988. Serum amino acid patterns and toxicity symptoms following the absorption of irrigant containing glycine in transurethral prostatic surgery. *Acta Anaesthesiol Scand* 32:493–501.

Hamilton B, Moriarty M. 1929. Comparison of growth in infancy. *Am J Dis Child* 37:1169.

Hansen RD, Raja C, Allen BJ. 2000. Total body protein in chronic diseases and in aging. *Ann NY Acad Sci* 904:345–352.

Hara S, Shibuya T, Nakakawaji K, Kyu M, Nakamura Y, Hoshikawa H, Takeuchi T, Iwao T, Ino H. 1962. Observations of pharmacological actions and toxicity of sodium glutamate, with comparisons between natural and synthetic products. *J Tokyo Med Coll* 20:69–100.

Harper AE. 1983. Dispensable and indispensable amino acid interrelationships. In: Blackburn GL, Grant JP, Young VR, eds. *Amino Acids. Metabolism and Medical Applications.* Boston: John Wright-PSG. Pp. 105–121.

Harper AE, Becker RV, Stucki WP. 1966. Some effects of excessive intakes of indispensable amino acids. *Proc Soc Exp Biol Med* 121:695–699.

Harper AE, Benevenga NJ, Wohlhueter RM. 1970. Effects of ingestion of disproportionate amounts of amino acids. *Physiol Rev* 50:428–558.

Harper AE, Miller RH, Block KP. 1984. Branched-chain amino acid metabolism. *Annu Rev Nutr* 4:409–454.

Harvey PW, Hunsaker HA, Allen KG. 1981. Dietary L-histidine-induced hypercholesterolemia and hypocupremia in the rat. *J Nutr* 111:639–647.

Hayasaka S, Saito T, Nakajima H, Takahashi O, Mizuno K, Tada K. 1985. Clinical trials of vitamin B$_6$ and proline supplementation for gyrate atrophy of the choroid and retina. *Br J Ophthalmol* 69:283–290.

Hays PM, Smeltzer JS. 1986. Multiple gestation. *Clin Obstet Gynecol* 29:264–285.

Health and Welfare Canada. 1990. *Report of the Expert Advisory Committee on Amino Acids.* Minister of Supply and Services Canada: Ottawa, Canada.

Hediger ML, Scholl TO, Ances IG, Belsky DH, Salmon RW. 1990. Rate and amount of weight gain during adolescent pregnancy: Associations with maternal weight-for-height and birth weight. *Am J Clin Nutr* 52:793–799.

Hegsted DM. 1963. Variation in requirements of nutrients: amino acids. *Fed Proc* 22:1420-1430.

Hegsted DM. 1976. Balance studies. *J Nutr* 106:307–311.

Hegsted DM. 1978. Assessment of nitrogen requirements. *Am J Clin Nutr* 31:1669–1677.

Heine WE, Klein PD, Reeds PJ. 1991. The importance of α-lactalbumin in infant nutrition. *J Nutr* 121:277–283.

Heinig MJ, Nommsen LA, Peerson JM, Lönnerdal B, Dewey KG. 1993. Energy and protein intakes of breast-fed and formula-fed infants during the first year of life and their association with growth velocity: The DARLING Study. *Am J Clin Nutr* 58:152–161.

Heird WC, Driscoll JM, Schullinger JN, Grebin B, Winters RW. 1972. Intravenous alimentation in pediatric patients. *J Pediatr* 80:351–372.

Hellekson KL. 2001. NIH consensus statement on phenylketonuria. *Am Fam Physician* 63:1430–1432.

Henkin RI, Patten BM, Re PK, Bronzert DA. 1975. A syndrome of acute zinc loss. Cerebellar dysfunction, mental changes, anorexia, and taste and smell dysfunction. *Arch Neurol* 32:745–751.

Hershko A, Ciechanover A. 1998. The ubiquiten system. *Ann Rev Biochem* 67:425–479.

Hevia P, Kari FW, Ulman EA, Visek WJ. 1980a. Serum and liver lipids in growing rats fed casein with L-lysine. *J Nutr* 110:1224–1230.

Hevia P, Ulman EA, Kari FW, Visek WJ. 1980b. Serum lipids of rats fed excess L-lysine and different carbohydrates. *J Nutr* 110:1231–1239.

Hibbs JR, Mittleman B, Hill P, Medsger TA. 1992. L-Tryptophan-associated eosinophilic fasciitis prior to the 1989 eosinophilia-myalgia syndrome outbreak. *Arthritis Rheum* 35:299–303.

Higgins AC. 1976. Nutritional status and the outcome of pregnancy. *J Can Diet Assoc* 37:17–35.

Hill GL. 1992. Body composition research: Implications for the practice of clinical nutrition. *J Parenteral Enteral Nutr* 16:197–218.

Himwich WA, Petersen IM, Graves JP. 1954. Ingested sodium glutamate and plasma levels of glutamic acid. *J Appl Physiol* 1:196–199.

Hitomi-Ohmura E, Amano N, Aoyama Y, Yoshida A. 1992. The effect of a histidine-excess diet on cholesterol synthesis and degradation in rats. *Lipids* 27:755–760.

Hood DA, Terjung RL. 1990. Amino acid metabolism during exercise and following endurance training. *Sports Med* 9:23–35.

Hoorn AJ. 1989. Dimethylglycine and chemically related amines tested for mutagenicity under potential nitrosation conditions. *Mutat Res* 222:343–350.

Hornsby-Lewis L, Shike M, Brown P, Klang M, Pearlstone D, Brennan MF. 1994. L-Glutamine supplementation in home total parenteral nutrition patients: Stability, safety, and effects on intestinal absorption. *J Parenteral Enteral Nutr* 18:268–273.

Howat PM, Korslund MK, Abernathy RP, Ritchy SJ. 1975. Sweat losses by and nitrogen balance of preadolescent girls consuming three levels of dietary protein. *Am J Clin Nutr* 28:879–882.

Hrboticky N, Leiter LA, Anderson GH. 1985. Effects of L-tryptophan on short term food intake in lean men. *Nutr Res* 5:595–607.

Huang P-C, Lin CP, Hsu JY. 1980. Protein requirements of normal infants at the age of 1 year: Maintenance nitrogen requirement and obligatory nitrogen losses. *J Nutr* 110:1727–1735.

Hurson M, Regan MC, Kirk SJ, Wasserkrug HL, Barbul A. 1995. Metabolic effects of arginine in a healthy elderly population. *J Parenteral Enteral Nutr* 19:227–230.

Hutson SM, Harper AE. 1981. Blood and tissue branched-chain amino and α-keto acid concentrations: Effect of diet, starvation, and disease. *Am J Clin Nutr* 34:173–183.

Hytten FE, Leitch I. 1971. *The Physiology of Human Pregnancy, 2nd ed.* Oxford: Blackwell.

Ikezaki S, Nishikawa A, Furukawa F, Imazawa T, Enami T, Mitsui M, Takahashi M. 1994. 13-Week subchronic toxicity study of L-histidine monohydrochloride in F344 rats. *Eisei Shikenjo Hokoku* 112:57–63.

Ikezaki S, Nishikawa A, Furukawa F, Enami T, Mitsui M, Tanakamaru Z, Kim HC, Lee IS, Imazawa T, Takahashi M. 1996. Long-term toxicity/carcinogenicity study of L-histidine monohydrochloride in F344 rats. *Food Chem Toxicol* 34:687–691.

Inoue G, Fujita Y, Niiyama Y. 1973. Studies on protein requirements of young men fed egg protein and rice protein with excess and maintenance energy intakes. *J Nutr* 103:1673–1687.

Intengan CL. 1984. Protein requirements of Filipino children 22–29 months old consuming local diets. In: Rand WM, Uauy R, Scrimshaw NS, eds. *Protein-Energy Requirement Studies in Developing Countries: Results of International Research.* Tokyo, Japan: United Nations University Press.

Intengan CL, Roxas BV, Loyola A, Carlos E. 1981. Protein requirements of Filipino children 20 to 29 months old consuming local diets. In: Torun B, Young VR, Rand WM, eds. *Protein-Energy Requirements of Developing Countries: Evaluation of New Data.* Tokyo, Japan: United Nations University Press. Pp. 172–181.

Inubushi T, Shikiji M, Endo K, Kakegawa H, Kishino Y, Katunuma N. 1996. Hormonal and dietary regulation of lysosomal cysteine proteinases in liver under gluconeogenesis conditions. *Biol Chem* 377:539–542.

Iob V, Swanson WW. 1934. Mineral growth of the human fetus. *Am J Dis Child* 47:302.

IOM (Institute of Medicine). 1990. *Nutrition During Pregnancy.* Washington, DC: National Academy Press.

IOM. 1991. *Nutrition During Lactation.* Washington, DC: National Academy Press.

Ip CC, Harper AE. 1973. Effects of dietary protein content and glucagon administration on tyrosine metabolism and tyrosine toxicity in the rat. *J Nutr* 103:1594–1607.

Isidori A, Lo Monaco A, Cappa M. 1981. A study of growth hormone release in man after oral administration of amino acids. *Curr Med Res Opin* 7:475–481.

Istfan N, Murray E, Janghorbani M, Young VR. 1983. An evaluation of the nutritional value of a soy protein concentrate in young adult men using the short-term N-balance method. *J Nutr* 113:2516–2523.

Iwata S, Ichimura M, Matsuzawa Y, Takasaki Y, Sasaoka M. 1979. Behavioural studies in rats treated with monosodium L-glutamate during the early stages of life. *Toxicol Lett* 4:345–357.

Jackson AA. 1989. Optimizing amino acid and protein supply and utilization in the newborn. *Proc Nutr Soc* 48:293–301.

Jackson AA. 1991. The glycine story. *Eur J Clin Nutr* 45:59–65.

Janas LM, Picciano MF, Hatch TF. 1985. Indices of protein metabolism in term infants fed human milk, whey-predominant formula, or cow's milk formula. *Pediatrics* 75:775–784.

Janas LM, Picciano MF, Hatch TF. 1987. Indices of protein metabolism in term infants fed either human milk or formulas with reduced protein concentration and various whey/casein ratios. *J Pediatrics* 10:838–848

Janelle KC, Barr SI. 1995. Nutrient intakes and eating behavior scores of vegetarian and nonvegetarian women. *J Am Diet Assoc* 95:180–186, 189.

Järvenpää AL, Räihä NCR, Rassin DK, Gaull GE. 1982a Milk protein quantity and quality in the term infant. I. Metabolic responses and effect on growth. *Pediatrics* 70:214–220.

Järvenpää AL, Räihä NCR, Rassin DK, Gaull GE. 1982b. Milk protein quantity and quality in the term infant. II. Effects on acidic and neutral amino acids. *Pediatrics* 70:221–230.

JECFA (Joint FAO/WHO Expert Committee on Food Additives). 1988. *Toxicological Evaluation of Certain Food Additives*. WHO Food Additive Series No. 22. Geneva: WHO/FAO.

Jefferson LS, Kimball S. 2001. Amino acid regulation of gene expression. *J Nutr* 131:2460S–2466S.

Jelliffe DB. 1966. The assessment of the nutritional status of the community. WHO Monograph Series No. 53. Geneva: WHO.

Jiang ZM, Cao JD, Zhu XG, Zhao WX, Yu JC, Ma EL, Wang XR, Zhu MW, Shu H, Liu YW. 1999. The impact of alanyl-glutamine on clinical safety, nitrogen balance, intestinal permeability, and clinical outcome in postoperative patients: A randomized, double-blind, controlled study in 120 patients. *J Parenter Enteral Nutr* 23:S62–S66.

Jones EM, Baumann CA, Reynolds MS. 1956. Nitrogen balances of women maintained on various levels of lysine. *J Nutr* 60:549–562.

Jungas RL, Halperin ML, Brosnan JT. 1992. Quantitative analysis of amino acid oxidation and related gluconeogenesis in humans. *Physiol Rev* 72:419–448.

Kakizoe T, Nishio Y, Honma Y, Niijima T, Sugimura T. 1983. L-Isoleucine and L-leucine are promoters of bladder cancer in rats. *Princess Takamatsu Symp* 14:373–380.

Kalhan SC. 2000. Protein metabolism in pregnancy. *Am J Clin Nutr* 71:1249S–1255S.

Kalhan SC, Devapatla S. 1999. Pregnancy, insulin resistance and nitrogen accretion. *Curr Opin Clin Nutr Metab Care* 2:359–363.

Kalhan SC, Rossi KQ, Gruca LL, Super DM, Savin SM. 1998. Relation between transamination of branched-chain amino acid and urea synthesis: Evidence from human pregnancy. *Am J Physiol* 275:E423–E431.

Kamin H, Handler P. 1951. Effect of infusion of single amino acids upon excretion of other amino acids. *Am J Physiol* 164:654–661.

Kampel D, Kupferschmidt R, Lubec G. 1990. Toxicity of D-proline. In: Lubec G, Rosenthal GA, eds. *Amino Acids: Chemistry, Biology, and Medicine*. ESCOM: Leiden, The Netherlands. Pp. 1164–1171.

Karlsen RL, Pedersen OO. 1982. A morphological study of the acute toxicity of L-cysteine on the retina of young rats. *Exp Eye Res* 34:65–69.

Katagiri M, Nakamura K. 2002. Animals are dependent on preformed α-amino nitrogen as an essential nutrient. *Life* 53:125–129.

Kawabe M, Takesada Y, Tamano S, Hagiwara A, Ito N, Shirai T. 1996. Subchronic toxicity study of L-isoleucine in F344 rats. *J Toxicol Environ Health* 47:499–508.

Kenney RA. 1986. The Chinese Restaurant Syndrome: An anecdote revisited. *Food Chem Toxicol* 24:351–354.

Kenney RA, Tidball CS. 1972. Human susceptibility to oral monosodium L-glutamate. *Am J Clin Nutr* 25:140–146.

Khatri IA, Forstner GG, Forstner F. 1998. Susceptibility of the cysteine-rich N-terminal and C-terminal ends of rat intestinal mucin Muc 2 to proteolytic cleavage. *Biochem J* 331:323–330.

Kim KI, McMillan I, Bayley HS. 1983. Determination of amino acid requirements of young pigs using an indicator amino acid. *Br J Nutr* 50:369–382.

King JC. 1975. Protein metabolism during pregnancy. *Clin Perinatol* 2:243–254.

King JC, Calloway DH, Margen S. 1973. Nitrogen retention, total body [40]K and weight gain in teenage pregnant girls. *J Nutr* 103:772–785.

Kirschner M. 1999. Intracellular proteolysis. *Trends Cell Biol* 9:M42–M45.

Klavins JV, Kinney TD, Kaufman N. 1963. Body iron levels and hematologic findings during excess methionine feeding. *J Nutr* 79:101–104.

Klein DG. 1990. Physiologic response to traumatic shock. *AACN Clin Issues Crit Care Nurs* 1:505–521.

Klimberg VS, McClellan J. 1996. Glutamine, cancer, and its therapy. *Am J Surg* 172:418–424.

Klimberg VS, Souba WW, Salloum RM, Plumley DA, Cohen FS, Dolson DJ, Bland KI, Copeland EM. 1990. Glutamine-enriched diets support muscle glutamine metabolism without stimulating tumor growth. *J Surg Res* 48:319–323.

Knopp RH, Brandt K, Arky RA. 1976. Effects of aspartame in young persons during weight reduction. *J Toxicol Environ Health* 2:417–428.

Knox WE, Horowitz ML, Friedell GH. 1969. The proportionality of glutaminase content to growth rate and morphology of rat neoplasms. *Cancer Res* 29:669–680.

Kopple JD. 1987. Uses and limitations of the balance technique. *J Parenter Enteral Nutr* 11:79S–85S.

Kopple JD, Swendseid ME. 1975. Evidence that histidine is an essential amino acid in normal and chronically uremic men. *J Clin Invest* 55:881–891.

Korslund MK, Leung EY, Meiners CR, Crews MG, Taper J, Abernathy RP, Ritchey SJ. 1976. The effects of sweat nitrogen losses in evaluating protein utilization by preadolescent children. *Am J Clin Nutr* 29:600–603.

Kovacevic Z, Morris HP. 1972. The role of glutamine in the oxidative metabolism of malignant cells. *Cancer Res* 32:326–333.

Kriengsinyos W, Wykes LJ, Ball RO, Pencharz PB. 2002. Oral and intravenous tracer protocols of the indicator amino acid oxidation method provide the same estimate of the lysine requirement in healthy men. *J Nutr* 132:2251–2257.

Krogh A, Krogh M. 1913. *A Study of the Diet and Metabolism of Eskimos*. Bianco Luno, Copenhagen.

Kudo Y, Boyd CA. 1990. Transport of amino acids by the human placenta: Predicted effects thereon of maternal hyperphenylalaninaemia. *J Inherit Metab Dis* 13:617–626.

Kurpad AV, Raj T, El-Khoury A, Beaumier L, Kuriyan R, Srivatsa A, Borgonha S, Selvaraj A, Regan MM, Young VR. 2001a. Lysine requirements of healthy adult Indian subjects, measured by an indicator amino acid balance technique. *Am J Clin Nutr* 73:900–907.

Kurpad AV, Raj T, El-Khoury A, Kuriyan R, Maruthy K, Borgonha S, Chandakudlu D, Regan MM, Young VR. 2001b. Daily requirement for and splanchnic uptake of leucine in healthy adult Indians. *Am J Clin Nutr* 74:747–755.

Kurpad AV, Regan MM, Raj T, El-Khoury A, Kuriyan R, Vaz M, Chandakudlu D, Venkataswamy VG, Borgonha S, Young VR. 2002a. Lysine requirements of healthy adult Indian subjects receiving long-term feeding, measured with a 24-h indicator amino acid oxidation and balance technique. *Am J Clin Nutr* 76:404–412.

Kurpad AV, Raj T, Regan MM, Vasudevan J, Caszo B, Nazareth D, Gnanou J, Young VR. 2002b. Threonine requirements of healthy Indian adults, measured by a 24-h indicator amino acid oxidation and balance technique. *Am J Clin Nutr* 76:789–797.

Labow BI, Souba WW. 2000. Glutamine. *World J Surg* 24:1503–1513.

Lacey JM, Crouch JB, Benfell K, Ringer SA, Wilmore CK, Maguire D, Wilmore DW. 1996. The effects of glutamine-supplemented parenteral nutrition in premature infants. *J Parenter Enteral Nutr* 20:74–80.

Laidlaw SA, Kopple JD. 1987. Newer concepts of the indispensable amino acids. *Am J Clin Nutr* 46:593–605.

Lammi-Keefe CJ, Ferris AM, Jensen RG. 1990. Changes in human milk at 0600, 1000, 1400, 1800, and 2200 h. *J Pediatr Gastroenterol Nutr* 11:83–88.

Lamperti A, Blaha G. 1976. The effects of neonatally-administered monosodium glutamate on the reproductive system of adult hamsters. *Biol Reprod* 14:362–369.

Lamperti A, Blaha G. 1980. Further observations on the effects of neonatally administered monosodium glutamate on the reproductive axis of hamsters. *Biol Reprod* 22:687–693.

Lazaris-Brunner G, Rafii M, Ball RO, Pencharz P. 1998. Tryptophan requirement in young adult women as determined by indicator amino acid oxidation with L-[^{13}C]-phenylalanine. *Am J Clin Nutr* 68:303–310.

Leathwood PD, Fernstrom JD. 1990. Effect of an oral tryptophan/carbohydrate load on tryptophan, large neutral amino acid, and serotonin and 5-hydroxyindoleacetic acid levels in monkey brain. *J Neural Transm Gen Sect* 79:25–34.

Leiderman E, Zylberman I, Zukin SR, Cooper TB, Javitt DC. 1996. Preliminary investigation of high-dose oral glycine on serum levels and negative symptoms in schizophrenia: An open-label trial. *Biol Psychiatry* 39:213–215.

Leiter LA, Hrboticky N, Anderson GH. 1987. Effects of L-tryptophan on food intake and selection in lean men and women. *Ann NY Acad Sci* 499:327–328.

Lemon PWR. 1996. Is increased dietary protein necessary or beneficial for individuals with a physically active lifestyle? *Nutr Rev* 54:S169–S175.

Lemon PW, Nagle FJ, Mullin JP, Benevenga NJ. 1982. In vivo leucine oxidation at rest and during two intensities of exercise. *J Appl Physiol* 53:947–954.

Lemon PW, Benevenga NJ, Mullin JP, Nagle FJ. 1985. Effect of daily exercise and food intake on leucine oxidation. *Biochem Med* 33:67–76.

Lemon PW, Tarnopolsky MA, MacDougall JD, Atkinson SA. 1992. Protein requirements and muscle mass/strength changes during intensive training in novice bodybuilders. *J Appl Physiol* 73(2):767-775.

Lemons JA, Moye L, Hall D, Simmons M. 1982. Differences in the composition of preterm and term human milk during early lactation. *Pediatr Res* 16:113–117.

Lenke RR, Levy HL. 1980. Maternal phenylketonuria and hyperphenylalaninemia. An international survey of the outcome of untreated and treated pregnancies. *N Engl J Med* 303:1202–1208.

Lentner C. 1981. *Geigy Scientific Tables, 8th ed.*, Vol. 1. *Units of Measurement, Body Fluids, Composition of the Body, Nutrition.* West Caldwell, NJ: Ciba-Geigy Corporation.

Leverton RM, Gram MR, Brodovsky E, Chaloupka M, Mitchell A, Johnson N. 1956a. The quantitative amino acid requirements of young women. II. Valine. *J Nutr* 58:83–93.

Leverton RM, Gram MR, Chaloupka M, Brodovsky E, Mitchell A. 1956b. The quantitative amino acid requirements of young women. I. Threonine. *J Nutr* 58:59–81.

Leverton RM, Johnson N, Ellison J, Geschwender D, Schmidt F. 1956c. The quantitative amino acid requirements of young women. IV. Phenylalanine, with and without tyrosine. *J Nutr* 58:341–353.

Leverton RM, Johnson N, Pazur J, Ellison J. 1956d. The quantitative amino acid requirements of young women. III. Tryptophan. *J Nutr* 58:219–229.

Levey S, Harroun JE, Smyth CJ. 1949. Serum glutamic acid levels and the occurrence of nausea and vomiting after the intravenous administration of amino acid mixtures. *J Lab Clin Med* 34:1238–1248.

Levy HM, Montanez G, Feaver ER, Murphy EA, Dunn MS. 1954. Effect of arginine on tumor growth in rats. *Cancer Res* 14:198–200.

Lieb CW. 1929. The effects on human beings of a twelve months' exclusive meat diet. *J Am Med Assoc* 93:20–22.

Lieberman HR, Corkin S, Spring BJ, Wurtman RJ, Growdon JH. 1985. The effects of dietary neurotransmitter precursors on human behavior. *Am J Clin Nutr* 42:366–370.

Lieberman HR, Caballero B, Emde GG, Bernstein JG. 1988. The effects of aspartame on human mood, performance, and plasma amino acid levels. In: Wurtman RJ, Ritter-Walker E, eds. *Dietary Phenylalanine and Brain Function.* Boston. Birkhauser. Pp. 198–200.

Linder-Horowitz M, Knox WE, Morris HP. 1969. Glutaminase activities and growth rates of rat hepatomas. *Cancer Res* 29:1195–1199.

Longenecker JB, Hause NL. 1959. Relationship between plasma amino acids and composition of ingested protein. *Arch Bioch Biophys* 84:46.

Longenecker JB, Hause NL. 1961. Relationship between plasma amino acids and composition of ingested protein. II. A shortened procedure to determine plasma amino acid (PAA) ratios. *Am J Clin Nutr* 9:356–362.

Lönnerdal B. 1986. Effects of maternal nutrition in human lactation. In: Hamosh M, Goldman AS, eds. *Human Lactation 2: Maternal and Environmental Factors.* New York: Plenum Press. Pp. 301–323.

Lönnerdal B, Chen CL. 1990. Effects of formula protein level and ration on infant growth, plasma amino acids and serum trace elements I: Cow's milk formula. *Acta Paediatr Scand* 79:257–265.

Lönnerdal B, Woodhouse LR, Glazier C. 1987. Compartmentalization and quantitation of protein in human milk. *J Nutr* 117:1385–1395.

LSRO (Life Sciences Research Office). 1992. *Safety of Amino Acids Used as Dietary Supplements.* Bethesda, MD: LSRO.

Lucas DR, Newhouse JP. 1957. The toxic effect of sodium L-glutamate on the inner layers of the retina. *AMA Arch Ophthalmol* 58:193–201.

Lucas A, Morley R, Cole TJ, Lister G, Leeson-Payne C. 1992. Breast milk and subsequent intelligence quotient in children born preterm. *Lancet* 339:261–264.

MacGillivray I, Buchanan TJ. 1958. Total exchangeable sodium and potassium in non-pregnant women and in normal and pre-eclamptic pregnancy. *Lancet* 2:1090–1093.

Manatt MW, Garcia PA. 1992. Nitrogen balance: Concepts and techniques. In: Nissen S, ed. *Modern Methods in Protein Nutrition and Metabolism.* San Diego: Academic Press. Pp. 9–63.

Marchesini G, Dioguardi FS, Bianchi GP, Zoli M, Bellati G, Roffi L, Martines D, Abbiati R. 1990. Long-term oral branched-chain amino acid treatment in chronic hepatic encephalopathy. A randomized double-blind casein-controlled trial. The Italian Multicenter Study Group. *J Hepatol* 11:92–101.

Mariotti F, Mahe S, Benamouzig R, Luengo C, Dare S, Gaudichon C, Tome D. 1999. Nutritional value of [^{15}N]-soy protein isolate assessed from ileal digestibility and postprandial protein utilization in humans. *J Nutr* 129:1992–1997.

Martindale LW. 1967. *Extra Pharmacopoeia, 25th ed..* London: Pharmaceutical Press.

Massara F, Cagliero E, Bisbocci D, Passarino G, Carta Q, Molinatti GM. 1981. The risk of pronounced hyperkalaemia after arginine infusion in the diabetic subject. *Diabete Metab* 7:149–153.

Matsueda S, Niiyama Y. 1982. The effects of excess amino acids on maintenance of pregnancy and fetal growth in rats. *J Nutr Sci Vitaminol* 28:557–573.

Matsuzawa Y, Yonetani S, Takasaki Y, Iwata S, Sekine S. 1979. Studies on reproductive endocrine function in rats treated with monosodium L-glutamate early in life. *Toxicol Lett* 4:359–371.

Matthews DE. 1999. Proteins and amino acids. In: Shils ME, Olson JA, Shike M, Ross AC, eds. *Modern Nutrition in Health and Disease, 9th ed.* Baltimore: Williams and Wilkins. Pp. 11–48.

Maughan RJ, Sadler DJ. 1983. The effects of oral administration of salts of aspartic acid on the metabolic response to prolonged exhausting exercise in man. *Int J Sports Med* 4:119–123.

Mayes PA. 1990. Oxidation of fatty acids: Ketogenesis. In: Murray RK, Granner DK, Mayes PA, Rodwell VW, eds. *Harper's Biochemistry, 22nd ed.* Norwalk, CT: Appleton and Lange. Pp. 206–217.

McCarthy CF, Borland JL, Lynch HJ, Owen EE, Tyor MP. 1964. Defective uptake of basic amino acids and L-cystine by intestinal mucosa of patients with cystinuria. *J Clin Invest* 43:1518–1524.

McClellan WS, Du Bois EF. 1930. Clinical calorimetry XLV. Prolonged meat diets with a study of kidney function and ketosis. *J Biol Chem* 87:651–668.

McClellan WS, Rupp VR, Toscani V. 1930. Clinical calorimetry XLVI. Prolonged meat diets with a study of the metabolism of nitrogen, calcium and phosphorus. *J Biol Chem* 87:669–680.

McClellan WS, Spencer HJ, Falk EA 1931. Clinical calorimetry XLVII. Prolonged meat diets with a study of the respiratory metabolism. *J Biol Chem* 93:419–434.

McCune MA, Perry HO, Muller SA, O'Fallon WM. 1984. Treatment of recurrent herpes simplex infections with L-lysine monohydrochloride. *Cutis* 34:366–373.

McGilvery RW. 1983. *Biochemistry—A Functional Approach.* Philadelphia: WB Saunders. Pp. 791–793.

McNurlan MA, Garlick PJ. 1980. Contribution of rat liver and gastrointestinal tract to whole-body protein synthesis in the rat. *Biochem J* 186:381–383.

Meakins TS, Jackson AA. 1996. Salvage of exogenous urea nitrogen enhances nitrogen balance in normal men consuming marginally inadequate protein diets. *Clin Sci* 90:215–225.

Meguid MM, Matthews DE, Bier DM, Meredith CN, Soeldner JS, Young VR. 1986a. Leucine kinetics at graded leucine intakes in young men. *Am J Clin Nutr* 43:770–780.

Meguid MM, Matthews DE, Bier DM, Meredith CN, Young VR. 1986b. Valine kinetics at graded valine intakes in young men. *Am J Clin Nutr* 43:781–786.

Melamed E, Glaeser B, Growdon JH, Wurtman RJ. 1980. Plasma tyrosine in normal humans: Effects of oral tyrosine and protein-containing meals. *J Neural Trans* 47:299–306.

Meldrum BS. 2000. Glutamate as a neurotransmitter in the brain: Review of physiology and pathology. *J Nutr* 130:1007S–1015S.

Meredith CN, Wen ZM, Bier DM, Matthews DE, Young VR. 1986. Lysine kinetics at graded lysine intakes in young men. *Am J Clin Nutr* 43:787–794.

Meredith CN, Zackin MJ, Frontera WR, Evans WJ. 1989. Dietary protein requirements and body protein metabolism in endurance-trained men. *J Appl Physiol* 66:2850–2856.

Metges CC, El-Khoury AE, Henneman L, Petzke KJ, Grant I, Bedri S, Pereira PP, Ajami AM, Fuller MF, Young VR. 1999a. Availability of intestinal microbial lysine for whole body lysine homeostasis in human subjects. *Am J Physiol* 277:E597–E607.

Metges CC, Petzke KJ, El-Khoury AE, Henneman L, Grant I, Bedri S, Regan MM, Fuller MF, Young VR. 1999b. Incorporation of urea and ammonia nitrogen into ileal and fecal microbial proteins and plasma free amino acids in normal men and ileostomates. *Am J Clin Nutr* 70:1046–1058.

Millward DJ. 1998. Metabolic demands for amino acids and the human dietary requirement: Millward and Rivers (1988) revisited. *J Nutr* 128:2563S–2576S.

Millward DJ. 1999. The nutritional value of plant-based diets in relation to human amino acid and protein requirements. *Proc Nutr Soc* 58:249–260.

Millward DJ, Roberts SB. 1996. Protein requirements of older individuals. *Nutr Res Rev* 9:67–87.

Millward DJ, Price GM, Pacy PJ, Halliday D. 1990. Maintenance protein requirements: The need for conceptual re-evaluation. *Proc Nutr Soc* 49:473–487.

Millward DJ, Fereday A, Gibson N, Pacy PJ. 1997. Aging, protein requirements, and protein turnover. *Am J Clin Nutr* 66:774–786.

Milman N, Scheibel J, Jessen O. 1980. Lysine prophylaxis in recurrent herpes simplex labialis: A double-blind, controlled crossover study. *Acta Derm Venereol* 60:85–87.

Mizutani AR, Parker J, Katz J, Schmidt J. 1990. Visual disturbances, serum glycine levels and transurethral resection of the prostate. *J Urol* 144:697–699.

Moephuli SR, Klein NW, Baldwin MT, Krider HM. 1997. Effects of methionine on the cytoplasmic distribution of actin and tubulin during neural tube closure in rat embryos. *Proc Natl Acad Sci USA* 94:543–548.

Mogensen CE, Solling K. 1977. Studies on renal tubular protein reabsorption: Partial and near complete inhibition by certain amino acids. *Scand J Clin Lab Invest* 37:477–486.

Moldawer LL, Kawamura I, Bistrian BR, Blackburn GL. 1983. The contribution of phenylalanine to tyrosine in vivo: Studies in the post-absorptive and phenylalanine-loaded rat. *Biochem J* 210:811–817.

Moneret-Vautrin DA. 1987. Monosodium glutamate induced asthma: A study of the potential risk in 30 asthmatics and review of the literature. *Allerg Immunol (Paris)* 19:29–35.

Morehead RP, Fishman WH, Artom C. 1945. Renal injury in the rat following the administration of serine by stomach tube. *Am J Pathol* 21:803–815.

Morlion BJ, Stehle P, Wachtler P, Siedhoff HP, Koller M, Konig W, Furst P, Puchstein C. 1998. Total parenteral nutrition with glutamine dipeptide after major abdominal surgery: A randomised, double-blind, controlled study. *Ann Surg* 227:302–308.

Motil KJ, Opekun AR, Montandon CM, Berthold HK, Davis TA, Klein PD, Reeds PJ. 1994. Leucine oxidation changes rapidly after dietary protein intake is altered in adult women but lysine flux is unchanged as is lysine incorporation into VLDL-apolipoprotein B-100. *J Nutr* 124:41–51.

Motil KJ, Davis TA, Montandon CM, Wong WW, Klein PD, Reeds PJ. 1996. Whole-body protein turnover in the fed state is reduced in response to dietary protein restriction in lactating women. *Am J Clin Nutr* 64:32–39.

Motil KJ, Sheng H-P, Kertz BL, Montandon CM, Ellis KJ. 1998. Lean body mass of well-nourished women is preserved during lactation. *Am J Clin Nutr* 67:292–300.

Munro, HN. 1970. Free amino acid pools and their role in regulation. In: Munro HN, ed. *Mammalian Protein Metabolism*, Vol. IV. New York: Academic Press. Chap 34.

Muramatsu K, Odagiri H, Morishita S, Takeuchi H. 1971. Effect of excess levels of individual amino acids on growth of rats fed casein diets. *J Nutr* 101:1117–1125.

Nakagawa I, Takahashi T, Suzuki T. 1961a. Amino acid requirements of children: Isoleucine and leucine. *J Nutr* 73:186–190.

Nakagawa I, Takahashi T, Suzuki T. 1961b. Amino acid requirements of children: Minimal needs of lysine and methionine based on nitrogen balance method. *J Nutr* 74:401–407.

Nakagawa I, Takahashi T, Suzuki T, Kobayashi K. 1962. Amino acid requirements of children: Minimal needs of threonine, valine and phenylalanine based on nitrogen balance method. *J Nutr* 77:61–68.

Nakagawa I, Takahashi T, Suzuki T, Kobayashi K. 1963. Amino acid requirements of children: Minimal needs of tryptophan, arginine and histidine based on nitrogen balance method. *J Nutr* 80:305–310.

Nakagawa I, Takahashi T, Suzuki T, Kobayashi K. 1964. Amino acid requirements of children: Nitrogen balance at the minimal level of essential amino acids. *J Nutr* 83:115–118.

Neale RJ, Waterlow JC. 1974. The metabolism of ^{14}C-labelled essential amino acids given by intragastric or intravenous infusion to rats on normal and protein-free diets. *Br J Nutr* 32:11–25.

Neri DF, Wiegmann D, Stanny RR, Shappell SA, McCardie A, McKay DL. 1995. The effects of tyrosine on cognitive performance during extended wakefulness. *Aviat Space Environ Med* 66:313–319.

Neville MC, Keller RP, Seacat J, Casey CE, Allen JC, Archer P. 1984. Studies on human lactation. I. Within-feed and between-breast variation in selected components of human milk. *Am J Clin Nutr* 40:635–646.

Newsholme EA, Blomstrand E, Hassmen P, Ekblom B. 1991. Physical and mental fatigue: Do changes in plasma amino acids play a role? *Biochem Soc Trans* 19:358–362.

Nikoletseas MM. 1977. Obesity in exercising, hypophagic rats treated with mono-sodium glutamate. *Physiol Behav* 19:767–773.

Nishio Y, Kakizoe T, Ohtani M, Sato S, Sugimura T, Fukushima S. 1986. L-isoleucine and L-leucine: Tumor promoters of bladder cancer in rats. *Science* 231:843–845.

Nommsen LA, Lovelady CA, Heinig MJ, Lönnerdal B, Dewey KG. 1991. Determinants of energy, protein, lipid, and lactose concentrations in human milk during the first 12 mo of lactation: The DARLING Study. *Am J Clin Nutr* 53:457–465.

Oddoye EA, Margen S. 1979. Nitrogen balance studies in humans: Long-term effect of high nitrogen intake on nitrogen accretion. *J Nutr* 109:363–377.

Ohmura E, Aoyama Y, Yoshida A. 1986. Changes in lipids in liver and serum of rats fed a histidine-excess diet or cholesterol-supplemented diets. *Lipids* 21:748–753.

Oishi R, Furuno K, Gomita Y, Araki Y, Saeki K. 1989. Effect of acute treatment of mice with L-histidine on the brain levels of amino acids. *Jpn J Pharmacol* 49:143–146.

Olivo M, Kitahama K, Valatx JL, Jouvet M. 1986. Neonatal monosodium glutamate dosing alters the sleep-wake cycle of the mature rat. *Neurosci Lett* 67:186–190.

Olney JW. 1969. Brain lesions, obesity, and other disturbances in mice treated with monosodium glutamate. *Science* 164:719–721.

Olney JW. 1989. Glutamate, a neurotoxic transmitter. *J Child Neurol* 4:218–226.

Olney JW. 1994. Excitotoxins in foods. *Neuro Toxicol* 15:535–544.

Olney JW, Ho OL. 1970. Brain damage in infant mice following oral intake of glutamate, aspartate or cysteine. *Nature* 227:609–611.

Olney JW, Cicero TJ, Meyer ER, de Gubareff T. 1976. Acute glutamate-induced elevations in serum testosterone and luteinizing hormone. *Brain Res* 112:420–424.

Owen G, Cherry CP, Prentice DE, Worden AN. 1978a. The feeding of diets containing up to 4% monosodium glutamate to rats for 2 years. *Toxicol Lett* 1:221–226.

Owen G, Cherry CP, Prentice DE, Worden AN. 1978b. The feeding of diets containing up to 10% monosodium glutamate to beagle dogs for 2 years. *Toxicol Lett* 1:217–219.

Park KG, Heys SD, Blessing K, Kelly P, McNurlan MA, Eremin O, Garlick PJ. 1992. Stimulation of human breast cancers by dietary L-arginine. *Clin Sci* 82:413–417.

Patrick J, Pencharz PB, Belmonte M, Ste-Marie M, Boland MP, Issenman RM, Van Aerde JEE, Rousseau-Harsany E. 1994. Undernutrition in children with neurodevelopmental disability. *Can Med Assoc J* 151:753–759.

Pellett PL, Young VR. 1992. The effects of different levels of energy intake on protein metabolism and of different levels of protein intake on energy metabolism: A statistical evaluation from the published literature. In: Scrimshaw NS, Schürch B, eds. *Protein-Energy Interaction.* Lausanne, Switzerland: IDECG, Nestlé Foundation. Pp. 81–121.

Pencharz PB. 1985. Body composition and growth. In: Walker A, ed. *Nutrition in Pediatrics. Basic Science and Clinical Application.* Boston. Little, Brown. Pp. 77–85.

Pencharz PB, Azcue M. 1996. Use of bioelectrical impedance analysis (BIA) measurements in the clinical management of malnutrition. *Am J Clin Nutr* 64:S485–S488.

Pencharz BP, House JD, Wykes LJ, Ball RO. 1996. What are the essential amino acids for the preterm and term infant? In: Bindels JG, Goedhart A, Visser HKA, eds. *Recent Developments in Infant Nutrition. Nutricia Symposia Vol. 9.* Dordrecht, The Netherlands: Kluwer Academic Publishers. Pp. 278–296.

Pepplinkhuizen L, Bruinvels J, Blom W, Moleman P. 1980. Schizophrenia-like psychosis caused by a metabolic disorder. *Lancet* 1:454–456.

Perry TL, Hardwick DF, Dixon GH, Dolman CL, Hansen S. 1965. Hypermethioninemia: A metabolic disorder associated with cirrhosis, islet cell hyperplasia, and renal tubular degeneration. *Pediatrics* 36:236–250.

Persaud TV. 1969. The foetal toxicity of leucine in the rat. *West Indian Med J* 18:34–39.

Peters JC, Harper AE. 1987. Acute effects of dietary protein on food intake, tissue amino acids, and brain serotonin. *Am J Physiol* 252:R902–R914.

Picou D, Halliday D, Garrow JS. 1966. Total body protein, collagen and non-collagen protein in infantile protein malnutrition. *Clin Sci* 30:345–351.

Pilc A, Rogoz Z, Skuza G. 1982. Histidine-induced bizarre behaviour in rats: The possible involvement of central cholinergic system. *Neuropharmacology* 21:781–785.

Pinals RS, Harris ED, Burnett JB, Gerber DA. 1977. Treatment of rheumatoid arthritis with L-histidine: A randomized, placebo-controlled, double-blind trial. *J Rheumatol* 4:414–419.

Pineda O, Torun B, Viteri FE, Arroyave G. 1981. Protein quality in relation to estimates of essential amino acids requirements. In: Bodwell CE, Adkins JS, Hopkins DT, eds. *Protein Quality in Humans: Assessment and In Vitro Estimation.* Westport, CT: AVI Publishing. Pp. 29–42.

Pinto-Scognamiglio W, Amorico L, Gatti GL. 1972. Toxicity and tolerance to monosodium glutamate studied by a conditioned avoidance test. *Farmaco* 27:19–27.

Pipe NGJ, Smith T, Halliday D, Edmonds CJ, Williams C, Coltart TM. 1979. Changes in fat, fat-free mass and body water in human normal pregnancy. *Br J Obstet Gynaecol* 86:929–940.

Pizzi WJ, Barnhart JE, Fanslow DJ. 1977. Monosodium glutamate administration to the newborn reduces reproductive ability in female and male mice. *Science* 196:452–454.

Pizzi WJ, Tabor JM, Barnhart JE. 1978. Somatic, behavioral, and reproductive disturbances in mice following neonatal administration of sodium L-aspartate. *Pharmacol Biochem Behav* 9:481–485.

Pollitt E. 2000. Developmental sequel from early nutritional deficiencies: Conclusive and probability judgements. *J Nutr* 130:350S–353S.

Poon TK, Cameron DP. 1978. Measurement of oxygen consumption and locomotor activity in monosodium glutamate-induced obesity. *Am J Physiol* 234:E532–E534.

Porter PB, Griffin AC. 1950. Effects of glutamic acid on maze learning and recovery from electroconvulsive shocks in albino rats. *J Comp Physiol Psychol* 43:1–15.

Pradhan SN, Lynch JF. 1972. Behavioral changes in adult rats treated with monosodium glutamate in the neonatal stage. *Arch Int Pharmacodyn Ther* 197:301–304.

Pratt EL, Snyderman SE, Cheung MW, Norton P, Holt LE. 1955. The threonine requirement of the normal infant. *J Nutr* 56:231–251.

Prentice AM, Goldberg GR, Prentice A. 1994. Body mass index and lactation performance. *Eur J Clin Nutr* 48:S78–S86.

Prosky L, O'Dell RG. 1972. Biochemical changes of brain and liver in neonatal offspring of rats fed monosodium-L-glutamate. *Experientia* 28:260–263.

Raguso CA, Pereira P, Young VR. 1999. A tracer investigation of obligatory oxidative amino acids losses in healthy, young adults. *Am J Clin Nutr* 70:474–483.

Räihä N, Minoli I, Moro G. 1986a. Milk protein intake in the term infant I: Metabolic responses and effects on growth. *Acta Paediatr Scand* 75:881–886.

Räihä N, Minoli I, Moro G. 1986b. Milk protein intake in the term infant II: Effects on plasma amino acid concentrations. *Acta Paediatr Scand* 75:887–892.

Raiten DJ, Talbot JM, Fisher KD. 1995. *Analysis of Adverse Reactions to Monosodium Glutamate (MSG).* Bethesda, MD: Federation of American Societies for Experimental Biology.

Ramsey BW, Farrell P, Pencharz PB. 1992. Nutritional assessment and management in cystic fibrosis: a consensus report. *Am J Clin Nutr* 55:108–116.

Rand WM, Young VR. 1999. Statistical analysis of nitrogen balance data with reference to the lysine requirement in adults. *J Nutr* 129:1920–1926.

Rand WM, Young VR, Scrimshaw NS. 1976. Change of urinary nitrogen excretion in response to low-protein diets in adults. *Am J Clin Nutr* 29:639–644.

Rand WM, Scrimshaw NS, Young VR. 1981. Conventional ("long-term") nitrogen balance studies for protein quality evaluation in adults: Rationale and limitations. In: Bodwell CE, Adkins JS, Hopkins DT, eds. *Protein Quality in Humans: Assessment and In Vitro Estimation*. Westport, CT: AVI Publishing. Pp. 61–94.

Rand RM, Pellett PL, Young VR. 2003. Meta-analysis of nitrogen balance studies for estimating protein requirements in healthy adults. *Am J Clin Nutr* 77:109–127.

Reeds PJ, Burrin DG. 2001. Glutamine and the bowel. *J Nutr* 131:2505S–2508S.

Reeds PJ, Garlick PJ. 1984. Nutrition and protein turnover in man. *Adv Nutr Res* 6:93–138.

Reeds PJ, Field CR, Jahoor F. 1994. Do the differences between the amino acid compositions of acute-phase and muscle proteins have a bearing on nitrogen loss in traumatic states? *J Nutr* 124:906–910.

Reif-Lehrer L. 1976. Possible significance of adverse reactions to glutamate in humans. *Fed Proc* 35:2205–2211.

Rennie MJ, Edwards RH, Krywawych S, Davies CT, Halliday D, Waterlow JC, Millward DJ. 1981. Effect of exercise on protein turnover in man. *Clin Sci (Lond)* 61:627–639.

Reynolds JV, Thom AK, Zhang SM, Ziegler MM, Naji A, Daly JM. 1988. Arginine, protein malnutrition, and cancer. *J Surg Res* 45:513–522.

Reynolds JV, Daly JM, Shou J, Sigal R, Ziegler MM, Naji A. 1990. Immunologic effects of arginine supplementation in tumor-bearing and non-tumor-bearing hosts. *Ann Surg* 211:202–210.

Reynolds JV, O'Farrelly C, Feighery C, Murchan P, Leonard N, Fulton G, O'Morain C, Keane FB, Tanner WA. 1996. Impaired gut barrier function in malnourished patients. *Br J Surg* 83:1288–1291.

Reynolds MS, Steel DL, Jones EM, Baumann CA. 1958. Nitrogen balances of women maintained on various levels of methionine and cystine. *J Nutr* 64:99–111.

Reynolds WA, Steginck LD, Filer LJ Jr, Renn E. 1980. Aspartame administration to the infant monkey: Hypothalamic morphology and plasma amino acid levels. *Anat Rec* 198:73–85.

Rich LF, Beard ME, Burns RP. 1973. Excess dietary tyrosine and corneal lesions. *Exp Eye Res* 17:87–97.

Rigo J, Senterre H. 1980. Optimal threonine intake for preterm infants fed on oral or parenteral nutrition. *J Parenteral Enteral Nutr* 4:15–17.

Roberton AM, Rabel B, Harding CA, Tasman-Jones C, Harris PJ, Lee SP. 1991. Use of the ileal conduit as a model for studying human small intestinal mucus glycoprotein secretion. *Am J Physiol* 261:G728–G734.

Roberts S. 1996. Energy requirements of older individuals. *Eur J Clin Nutr* 50:S112–S118.

Roberts S, Thorpe JM, Ball RO, Pencharz PB. 2001. Tyrosine requirement of healthy men receiving a fixed phenylalanine intake determined by using indicator amino acid oxidation. *Am J Clin Nutr* 73:276–282.

Rodwell VW. 1990. Conversion of amino acids to specialized products. In: Murray RK, Mayes PA, Granner DK, Rodwell VW, eds. *Harper's Biochemistry*, 22nd ed. Norwalk, CT: Appleton & Lange. Pp. 307–313.

Rogan WJ, Gladen BC. 1993. Breast-feeding and cognitive development. *Early Human Dev* 31:181–193.

Roig JC, Meetze WH, Auestad N, Jasionowski T, Veerman M, McMurray CA, Neu J. 1996. Enteral glutamine supplementation for the very low birthweight infant: Plasma amino acid concentrations. *J Nutr* 126:1115S–1120S.

Ronnenberg AG, Gross KL, Hartman WJ, Meydani SN, Prior RL. 1991. Dietary arginine supplementation does not enhance lymphocyte proliferation or interleukin-2 production in young and aged rats. *J Nutr* 121:1270–1278.

Rose DP, Leklem JE, Fardal L, Baron RB, Shrago E. 1977. Effect of oral alanine loads on the serum triglycerides of oral contraceptive users and normal subjects. *Am J Clin Nutr* 30:691–694.

Rose WC. 1957. The amino acid requirements of adult man. *Nutr Abs Rev* 27:631–647.

Rose WC, Haines WJ, Warner DT, Johnson JE. 1951. The amino acid requirements of man. II. The role of threonine and histidine. *J Biol Chem* 188:49–58.

Rose WC, Borman A, Coon MJ, Lambert GF. 1955a. The amino acid requirements of man. X. The lysine requirement. *J Biol Chem* 214:579–587.

Rose WC, Coon MJ, Lambert GF. 1955b. The amino acid requirements of man. VIII. The metabolic availability of the optical isomers of acetyltryptophan. *J Biol Chem* 212:201–205.

Rose WC, Coon MJ, Lockhart HB, Lambert GF. 1955c. The amino acid requirements of man. XI. The threonine and methionine requirements. *J Biol Chem* 215:101–110.

Rose WC, Eades CH, Coon MJ. 1955d. The amino acid requirements of man. XII. The leucine and isoleucine requirements. *J Biol Chem* 216:225–234.

Rose WC, Leach BE, Coon MJ, Lambert GF. 1955e. The amino acid requirements of man. IX. The phenylalanine requirement. *J Biol Chem* 213:913–922.

Rose WC, Wixom RL, Lockhart HB, Lambert GF. 1955f. The amino acid requirements of man. XV. The valine requirement; Summary and final observations. *J Biol Chem* 217:987–995.

Rosenberg LE, Downing S, Durant JL, Segal S. 1966. Cystinuria: Biochemical evidence for three genetically distinct diseases. *J Clin Invest* 45:365–371.

Rudman D, DiFulco TJ, Galambos JT, Smith RB, Salam AA, Warren WD. 1973. Maximal rates of excretion and synthesis of urea in normal and cirrhotic subjects. *J Clin Invest* 52:2241–2249.

Ryan-Harshman M, Leiter LA, Anderson GH. 1987. Phenylalanine and aspartame fail to alter feeding behavior, mood and arousal in men. *Physiol Behav* 39:247–253.

Said AK, Hegsted DM. 1970. Response of adult rats to low dietary levels of essential amino acids. *J Nutr* 100:1362–1375.

Sauberlich HE. 1961. Studies on the toxicity and antagonism of amino acids for weanling rats. *J Nutr* 75:61–72.

Schaafsma G. 2000. The protein digestibility-corrected amino acid score. *J Nutr* 130:1865S–1867S.

Schainker B, Olney JW. 1974. Glutamate-type hypothalamic-pituitary syndrome in mice treated with aspartate or cysteate in infancy. *J Neural Trans* 35:207–215.

Schaumburg HH, Byck R. 1968. Sin cib-syn: Accent on glutamate. *N Engl J Med* 279:105.

Schaumburg HH, Byck R, Gerstl R, Mashman JH. 1969. Monosodium L-glutamate: Its pharmacology and role in the Chinese restaurant syndrome. *Science* 163:826–828.

Schechter PJ, Prakash NJ. 1979. Failure of oral L-histidine to influence appetite or affect zinc metabolism in man: A double-blind study. *Am J Clin Nutr* 32:1011–1014.

Scholl TO, Hediger ML, Ances IG. 1990. Maternal growth during pregnancy and decreased infant birth weight. *Am J Clin Nutr* 51:790–793.

Scholl TO, Hediger ML, Schall JI, Khoo C-S, Fischer RL. 1994. Maternal growth during pregnancy and the competition for nutrients. *Am J Clin Nutr* 60:183–188.

Schwartz JC, Lampart C, Rose C. 1972. Histamine formation in rat brain in vivo: Effects of histidine loads. *J Neurochem* 19:801–810.

Schwartzstein RM, Kelleher M, Weinberger SE, Weiss JW, Drazen JM. 1987. Airways effects of monosodium glutamate in subjects with chronic stable asthma. *J Asthma* 24:167–172.

Scrimshaw NS, Hussein MA, Murray E, Rand WM, Young VR. 1972. Protein requirements of man: Variations in obligatory urinary and fecal nitrogen losses in young men. *J Nutr* 102:1595–1604.

Scriver CR, Kaufman S, Woo SL. 1989. The hyperphenylalaninemias. In: Scriver CR, Beaudet AL, Sly WS, Valle D, eds. *The Metabolic Basis of Inherited Disease*, 6th ed. New York: McGraw-Hill. Pp. 495–546.

Semprini ME, Frasca MA, Mariani A. 1971. Effects of monosodium glutamate (MSG) administration on rats during the intrauterine life and the neonatal period. *Quaderni delle Nutrizione* 31:85–100.

Sen Gupta J, Srivastava KK. 1973. Effect of potassium-magnesium aspartate on endurance work in man. *Ind J Exp Biol* 11:392–394.

Shaw GM, Velie EM, Schaffer DM. 1997. Is dietary intake of methionine associated with a reduction in risk for neural tube defect-affected pregnancies? *Teratology* 56:295–299.

Simon CA, Van Melle GD, Ramelet AA. 1985. Failure of lysine in frequently recurrent herpes simplex infection. *Arch Dermatol* 121:167–168.

Simon RA. 2000. Additive-induced urticaria: Experience with monosodium glutamate (MSG). *J Nutr* 130:1063S–1066S.

Sivam SP, Chermak T. 1992. Neonatal administration of L-cysteine does not produce long-term effects on neurotransmitter or neuropeptide systems in the rat striatum. *Res Comm Chem Pathol Pharm* 77:219–225.

Skeie B, Kvetan V, Gil KM, Rothkopf MM, Newsholme EA, Askanazi J. 1990. Branch-chain amino acids: Their metabolism and clinical utility. *Crit Care Med* 18:549–571.

Smith B, Prockop DJ. 1962. Central-nervous-system effects of ingestion of L-tryptophan by normal subjects. *N Engl J Med* 267:1338–1341.

Snyderman SE, Pratt EL, Cheung MW, Norton P, Holt LE, Hansen AE, Panos TC. 1955. The phenylalanine requirement of the normal infant. *J Nutr* 56:253–263.

Snyderman SE, Holt LE, Smellie F, Boyer A, Westall RG. 1959a. The essential amino acid requirements of infants: Valine. *Am J Dis Child* 97:186–191.

Snyderman SE, Norton PM, Fowler DI, Holt LE. 1959b. The essential amino acid requirements of infants: Lysine. *Am J Dis Child* 97:175–185.

Snyderman SE, Boyer A, Phansalkar SV, Holt LE. 1961a. Essential amino acid requirements of infants. Tryptophan. *Am J Dis Child* 102:41–45.

Snyderman SE, Roitman EL, Boyer A, Holt LE. 1961b. Essential amino acid requirements of infants. Leucine. *Am J Dis Child* 102:35–40.

Snyderman SE, Boyer A, Roitman E, Holt LE, Prose PH. 1963. The histidine requirement of the infant. *Pediatrics* 31:786–801.

Snyderman SE, Boyer A, Norton PM, Roitman E, Holt LE. 1964a. The essential amino acid requirements of infants. IX. Isoleucine. *Am J Clin Nutr* 15:313–321.

Snyderman SE, Boyer A, Norton PM, Roitman E, Holt LE. 1964b. The essential amino acid requirements of infants. X. Methionine. *Am J Clin Nutr* 15:322–330.

Sole MJ, Benedict CR, Myers MG, Leenen FH, Anderson GH. 1985. Chronic dietary tyrosine supplements do not affect mild essential hypertension. *Hypertension* 7:593–596.

Solomon JK, Geison RL. 1978. Effect of excess dietary L-histidine on plasma cholesterol levels in weanling rats. *J Nutr* 108:936–943.

Souba WW. 1993. Glutamine and cancer. *Ann Surg* 218:715–728.

Speth JD. 1989. Early hominid hunting and scavenging: The role of meat as an energy source. *J Hum Evol* 18:329–343.

Speth JD, Spielmann KA. 1983. Energy source, protein metabolism, and hunter-gatherer subsistence strategies. *J Anthropol Archaeol* 2:1–31.

Stechmiller JK, Treloar D, Allen N. 1997. Gut dysfunction in critically ill patients: A review of the literature. *Am J Crit Care* 6:204–209.

Steele RD, Barber TA, Lalich J, Benevenga NJ. 1979. Effects of dietary 3-methylthiopropionate on metabolism, growth and hematopoiesis in the rat. *J Nutr* 109:1739–1751.

Stefansson V. 1944a. *Arctic Manual.* New York: Macmillan.

Stefansson V. 1944b. Pemmican. *Military Surg* 95:89–98.

Stegink LD. 1976. Absorption, utilization, and safety of aspartic acid. *J Toxicol Environ Health* 2:215–242.

Stegink LD, Shepherd JA, Brummel MC, Murray LM. 1974. Toxicity of protein hydrolysate solutions: Correlation of glutamate dose and neuronal necrosis to plasma amino acid levels in young mice. *Toxicology* 2:285–299.

Stegink LD, Filer LJ, Baker GL. 1977. Effect of aspartame and aspartate loading upon plasma and erythrocyte free amino acid levels in normal adult volunteers. *J Nutr* 107:1837–1845.

Stegink LD, Filer LJ, Baker GL. 1980. Plasma methionine levels in normal adult subjects after oral loading with L-methionine and N-acetyl-L-methionine. *J Nutr* 110:42–49.

Stegink LD, Filer LJ, Baker GL. 1982a. Plasma and erythrocyte amino acid levels in normal adult subjects fed a high protein meal with and without added monosodium glutamate. *J Nutr* 112:1953–1960.

Stegink LD, Filer LJ, Baker GL. 1982b. Plasma and urinary methionine levels in one-year-old infants after oral loading with L-methionine and N-acetyl-L-methionine. *J Nutr* 112:597–603.

Stegink LD, Filer LJ Jr, Baker GL. 1983a. Effect of carbohydrate on plasma and erythrocyte glutamate levels in humans ingesting large doses of monosodium L-glutamate in water. *Am J Clin Nutr* 37:961–968.

Stegink LD, Filer LJ Jr, Baker GL. 1983b. Plasma amino acid concentrations in normal adults fed meals with added monosodium L-glutamate and aspartame. *J Nutr* 113:1851–1860.

Stekol JA, Szaran J. 1962. Pathological effects of excessive methionine in the diet of growing rats. *J Nutr* 77:81–90.

Stellar E, McElroy WD. 1948. Does glutamic acid have any effect on learning? *Science* 108:281–283.

Stephenson LS, Lathan MC, Ottesen EA. 2000. Global malnutrition. *Parasitology* 121:S5–S22.

Stevenson DD. 2000. Monosodium glutamate and asthma. *J Nutr* 130:1067S–1073S.

Stokes AF, Belger A, Banich MT, Taylor H. 1991. Effects of acute aspartame and acute alcohol ingestion upon the cognitive performance of pilots. *Aviat Space Environ Med* 62:648–653.

Stoll B, Henry J, Reeds PJ, Yu H, Jahoor F, Burrin DG. 1998. Catabolism dominates the first-pass intestinal metabolism of dietary essential amino acids in milk protein-fed piglets. *J Nutr* 128:606–614.

Strain GW, Strain JJ, Zumoff B. 1985. L-Tryptophan does not increase weight loss in carbohydrate-craving obese subjects. *Int J Obes* 9:375–380.

Sweetman L. 1989. Branched chain organic acidurias. In: Scriver CR, Beaudet AL, Sly WS, Valle D, eds. *The Metabolic Basis of Inherited Disease*, 6th ed. New York: McGraw-Hill. Pp. 791–819.

Swick RW, Benevenga NJ. 1977. Labile protein reserves and protein turnover. *J Dairy Sci* 60:505–515.

Tachibana K Mukai K, Hiraoka I, Moriguchi S, Takama S, Kishino Y. 1985. Evaluation of the effect of arginine-enriched amino acid solution on tumor growth. *J Parenter Enteral Nutr* 9:428–434.

Tarasoff L, Kelly MF. 1993. Monosodium L-glutamate: A double-blind study and review. *Food Chem Toxicol* 31:1019–1035.

Tarnopolsky MA, MacDougall JD, Atkinson SA. 1988. Influence of protein intake and training status on nitrogen balance and lean body mass. *J Appl Physiol* 64:187–193.

Tarnopolsky MA, Atkinson SA, MacDougall JD, Senor BB, Lemon PW, Schwarcz H. 1991. Whole body leucine metabolism during and after resistance exercise in fed humans. *Med Sci Sports Exerc* 23:326–333.

Taverner MR, Hume ID, Farrell DJ. 1981. Availability to pigs of amino acids in cereal grains. 1. Endogenous levels of amino acids in ileal digesta and faeces of pigs given cereal diets. *Br J Nutr* 46:149–158.

Terry LC, Epelbaum J, Martin JB. 1981. Monosodium glutamate: Acute and chronic effects on rhythmic growth hormone and prolactin secretion, and somatostatin in the undisturbed male rat. *Brain Res* 217:129–142.

Thein DJ, Hurt WC. 1984. Lysine as a prophylactic agent in the treatment of recurrent herpes simplex labialis. *Oral Surg* 58:659–666.

Thoemke F, Huether G. 1984. Breeding rats on amino acid imbalanced diets for three consecutive generations affects the concentrations of putative amino acid transmitters in the developing brain. *Int J Dev Neurosci* 2:567–574.

Thompson GN, Halliday D. 1992. Protein turnover in pregnancy. *Eur J Clin Nutr* 46:411–417.

Torun B, Viteri FE. 1981. Obligatory nitrogen losses and factorial calculations of protein requirements of pre-school children. In: Torun B, Young VR, Rand WM, eds. *Protein-Energy Requirements of Developing Countries: Evaluation of New Data*. Tokyo, Japan: United Nations University Press. Pp. 159–163.

Torun B, Cabrera Santiago M, Viteri FE. 1981. Protein requirements of pre-school children: Milk and soybean protein isolate. In: Torun B, Young VR, Rand WM, eds. *Protein-Energy Requirements of Developing Countries: Evaluation of New Data*. Tokyo, Japan: United Nations University Press. Pp. 182–190.

Uauy R, Scrimshaw NS, Young VR. 1978. Human protein requirements: Nitrogen balance response to graded levels of egg protein in elderly men and women. *Am J Clin Nutr* 31:779–785.

Uauy R, Yanez E, Ballester D, Barrera G, Guzman E, Saitua MT, Zacaris I. 1981. Obligatory urinary and faecal nitrogen losses in young Chilean men fed two levels of dietary energy intake. In: Torun B, Young VR, Rand WM, eds. *Protein-Energy Requirements of Developing Countries: Evaluation of New Data.* Tokyo, Japan: United Nations University Press.

van Acker BA, von Meyenfeldt MF, van der Hulst RR, Hulsewe KW, Wagenmakers AJ, Deutz NE, de Blaauw I, Dejong CH, van Kreel BK, Soeters PB. 1999. Glutamine: The pivot of our nitrogen economy? *J Parenter Enteral Nutr* 23:S45–S48.

van der Schoor SRD, van Goudoever JB, Stoll B, Henry JF, Rosenberger JR, Burrin DG, Reeds PJ. 2001. The pattern of intestinal substrate oxidation is altered by protein restriction in pigs. *Gastroenterology* 121:1167–1175.

van Raaij JMA, Pee MEM, Vermaat-Miedema SH, Schonk CM, Hautvast JGAJ 1988. New equations for estimating body fat mass in pregnancy from body density or total body water. *Am J Clin Nutr* 48:24–29.

van Wouwe JP, Hoogenkamp S, Van den Hamer CJ. 1989. Histidine supplement and Zn status in Swiss random mice. *Biol Trace Elem Res* 22:35–43.

Viau AT, Leathem JH. 1973. Excess dietary methionine and pregnancy in the rat. *J Reprod Fertil* 33:109–111.

Vijayasarathy C, Khan-Siddiqui L, Murthy SN, Bamji MS. 1987. Rise in plasma trimethyllysine levels in humans after oral lysine load. *Am J Clin Nutr* 46:772–777.

Villalpando S, Butte NF, Flores-Huerta S, Thotathuchery M. 1998. Qualitative analysis of human milk produced by women consuming a maize-predominant diet typical of rural Mexico. *Ann Nutr Metab* 42:23–32.

Viteri FE, Martinez C. 1981. Integumental nitrogen losses of pre-school children with different levels and sources of dietary protein intake. In: Torun B, Young VR, Rand WM, eds. *Protein-Energy Requirements of Developing Countries: Evaluation of New Data.* Tokyo, Japan: United Nations University Press.

Wachstein M. 1947. Nephrotoxic action of dl-serine in the rat. II. The protective action of various amino acids and some other compounds. *Arch Pathol* 43:515–526.

Wagenmakers AJ. 1998. Muscle amino acid metabolism at rest and during exercise: Role in human physiology and metabolism. *Exerc Sport Sci Rev* 26:287–314.

Waisman HA, Harlow HF. 1965. Experimental phenylketonuria in infant monkeys: A high phenylalanine diet produces abnormalities simulating those of the hereditary disease. *Science* 147:685–695.

Wang JML, Creel DJ, Wong KC. 1989. Transurethral resection of the prostate, serum glycine levels, and ocular evoked potentials. *Anesthesiology* 70:36–41.

Waterlow JC. 1969. The assessment of protein nutrition and metabolism in the whole animal, with special reference to man. In: Munro HN ed. *Mammalian Protein Metabolism*, Vol III. New York: Academic Press. Pp. 347–348.

Waterlow JC. 1984. Protein turnover with special reference to man. *Quart J Exp Physiol* 69:409–438.

Waterlow JC, Garlick PJ, Millward DJ. 1978. *Protein Turnover in Mammalian Tissues and in the Whole Body.* Amsterdam: North-Holland Publishing.

Webber WA, Brown JL, Pitts RF. 1961. Interactions of amino acids in renal tubular transport. *Am J Physiol* 200:380–386.

White TP, Brooks GA. 1981. [U-14C]glucose, -alanine, and -leucine oxidation in rates at rest and two intensities of running. *Am J Physiol* 240:E155–E165.

Widdowson EM, Dickerson JWT. 1964. Chemical composition of the body. In: Comar CL, Bronner F, eds. *Mineral Metabolism: An Advanced Treatise,* Vol 2. New York: Academic Press.

Wilcken DE, Reddy SG, Gupta VJ. 1983. Homocysteinemia, ischemic heart disease, and the carrier state for homocystinuria. *Metabolism* 32:363–370.

Wilkin JK. 1986. Does monosodium glutamate cause flushing (or merely "glutamania")? *J Am Acad Dermatol* 15:225–230.

Willard MD, Gilsdorf RB, Price RA. 1980. Protein-calorie malnutrition in a community hospital. *J Am Med Assoc* 243:1720–1722.

Williams GM, Whysner J. 1996. Epigenetic carcinogens: Evaluation and risk assessment. *Exp Toxicol Pathol* 48:189–195.

Wilson DC, Pencharz PB. 1997. Nutritional care of the chronically ill. In: Tsang RC, Zlotkin SH, Nichols BL, Hansen JW, eds. *Nutrition During Infancy: Birth to 2 Years.* Cincinnati: Digital Educational Publishing, Inc. Pp. 37–56.

Wilson D, Rafii M, Ball RO, Pencharz PB. 2000. Threonine requirement in young men determined by indicator amino acid oxidation with use of L-[1-^{13}C]-phenylalanine. *Am J Clin Nutr* 71:757–764.

Woessner KM, Simon RA, Stevenson DD. 1999. Monosodium glutamate sensitivity in asthma. *J Allergy Clin Immunol* 104:305–310.

Woods RK, Weiner JM, Thien F, Abramson M, Walters EH. 1998. The effects of monosodium glutamate in adults with asthma who perceive themselves to be monosodium glutamate-intolerant. *J Allergy Clin Immunol* 101:762–771.

Wurtman JJ, Wurtman RJ, Growdon JH, Henry P, Lipscomb A, Zeisel SH. 1981. Carbohydrate craving in obese people: Suppression by treatments affecting serotoninergic transmission. *Int J Eating Disord* 1:2–15.

Wynn M, Wynn A. 1979. *Prevention of Handicap and the Health of Women.* London: Routledge and Kegan Paul. Pp. 43–81.

Yamashita K, Ashida K. 1971. Effect of excessive levels of lysine and threonine on the metabolism of these amino acids in rats. *J Nutr* 101:1607–1614.

Yanez E, Uauy R, Ballester D, Barrera G, Chavez N, Guzman E, Saitua MT, Zacarias I. 1982. Capacity of the Chilean mixed diet to meet the protein and energy requirements of young adult males. *Br J Nutr* 47:1–10.

Yang WH, Drouin MA, Herbert M, Mao Y, Karsh J. 1997. The monosodium glutamate symptom complex: Assessment in a double-blind, placebo-controlled, randomized study. *J Allergy Clin Immunol* 99:757–762.

Yeatman TJ, Risley GL, Brunson ME. 1991. Depletion of dietary arginine inhibits growth of metastatic tumor. *Arch Surg* 126:1376–1382.

Yogman MW, Zeisel SH. 1983. Diet and sleep patterns in newborn infants. *N Engl J Med* 309:1147–1149.

Yogman MW, Zeisel SH. 1985. Nutrients, neurotransmitters and infant behavior. *Am J Clin Nutr* 42:352–360.

Yonetani S, Ishii H, Kirimura J. 1979. Effect of dietary administration of monosodium L-glutamate on growth and reproductive functions in mice. *Oyo Yakuri (Pharmacometrics)* 17:143–152.

Young SN. 1986. The clinical psychopharmacology of tryptophan. In: Wurtman RJ, Wurtman JJ, eds. *Nutrition and the Brain,* Vol. 7. New York: Raven Press. Pp. 49–88.

Young SN, Gauthier S. 1981. Effect of tryptophan administration on tryptophan, 5-hydroxyindoleacetic acid and indoleacetic acid in human lumbar and cisternal cerebrospinal fluid. *J Neurol Neurosurg Psychiatry* 44:323–327.

Young VR. 1987. 1987 McCollum Award Lecture. Kinetics of human amino acid metabolism: Nutritional implications and some lessons. *Am J Clin Nutr* 46:709–725.

Young VR, Borgonha S. 2000. Nitrogen and amino acid requirements: The Massachusetts Institute of Technology Amino Acid Requirement Pattern. *J Nutr* 130:1841S–1849S.

Young VR, Pellett PL. 1990. Current concepts concerning indispensable amino acid needs in adults and their implications for international nutrition planning. *Food Nutr Bull* 12:289–300.

Young VR, Pellett PL. 1994. Plant proteins in relation to human protein and amino acid nutrition. *Am J Clin Nutr* 59:1203S–1212S.

Young VR, Hussein MA, Scrimshaw JS. 1968. Estimate of loss of labile body nitrogen during acute protein deprivation in young adults. *Nature.* 218:568–569.

Young VR, Tontisirin K, Ozalp I, Lakshmanan F, Scrimshaw NS. 1972. Plasma amino acid response curve and amino acid requirements in young men: Valine and lysine. *J Nutr* 102:1159–1169.

Young VR, Taylor YS, Rand WM, Scrimshaw NS. 1973. Protein requirements of man: Efficiency of egg protein utilization at maintenance and sub-maintenance levels in young men. *J Nutr* 103:1164–1174.

Young VR, Fajardo L, Murray E, Rand WM, Scrimshaw NS. 1975a. Protein requirements of man: Comparative nitrogen balance response within the submaintenance-to-maintenance range of intakes of wheat and beef proteins. *J Nutr* 105:534–542.

Young VR, Steffee WP, Pencharz PB, Winterer JC, Scrimshaw NS. 1975b. Total human body protein synthesis in relation to protein requirements at various ages. *Nature* 253:192–194.

Young VR, Puig M, Queiroz E, Scrimshaw NS, Rand WM. 1984. Evaluation of the protein quality of an isolated soy protein in young men: Relative nitrogen requirements and effect of methionine supplementation. *Am J Clin Nutr* 39:16–24.

Young VR, Gucalp C, Rand WM, Matthews DE, Bier DM. 1987. Leucine kinetics during three weeks at submaintenance-to-maintenance intakes of leucine in men: Adaptation and accommodation. *Hum Nutr Clin Nutr* 41:1–18.

Young VR, Bier DM, Pellett PL. 1989. A theoretical basis for increasing current estimates of the amino acid requirements in adult man, with experimental support. *Am J Clin Nutr* 50:80–92.

Young VR, Marchini JS, Cortiella J. 1990. Assessment of protein nutritional status. *J Nutr* 120:1496–1502.

Young VR, Wagner DA, Burini R, Storch KJ. 1991. Methionine kinetics and balance at the 1985 FAO/WHO/UNU intake requirement in adult men studied with L-[^{2}H$_3$-methyl-1-^{13}C]methionine as a tracer. *Am J Clin Nutr* 54:377–385.

Young VR, El-Khoury AE, Raguso CA, Forslund AH, Hambraeus L. 2000. Rates of urea production and hydrolysis and leucine oxidation change linearly over widely varying protein intakes in healthy adults. *J Nutr* 130:761–766.

Yuwiler A, Brammer GL, Morley JE, Raleigh MJ, Flannery JW, Geller E. 1981. Short-term and repetitive administration of oral tryptophan in normal men. Effects on blood tryptophan, serotonin, and kynurenine concentrations. *Arch Gen Psychiatry* 38:619–626.

Zanni E, Calloway DH, Zezulka AY. 1979. Protein requirements of elderly men. *J Nutr* 109:513–524.

Zello GA, Pencharz PB, Ball RO. 1990. Phenylalanine flux, oxidation and conversion to tyrosine in humans studied with L-[1-^{13}C]phenylalanine. *Am J Physiol* 259:E835–E843.

Zello GA, Pencharz PB, Ball RO. 1993. Dietary lysine requirement of young adult males determined by oxidation of L-[1-^{13}C]phenylalanine. *Am J Physiol* 264:E677–E685.

Zello GA, Wykes LJ, Ball RO, Pencharz PB. 1995. Recent advances in methods of assessing dietary amino acid requirements for adult humans. *J Nutr* 125:2907–2915.

Zezulka AY, Calloway DH. 1976a. Nitrogen retention in men fed isolated soybean protein supplemented with L-methionine, D-methionine, N-acetyl-L-methionine, or inorganic sulfate. *J Nutr* 106:1286–1291.

Zezulka AY, Calloway DH. 1976b. Nitrogen retention in men fed varying levels of amino acids from soy protein with or without added L-methionine. *J Nutr* 106:212–221.

Zhao X-H, Wen ZM, Meredith CN, Matthews DE, Bier DM, Young VR. 1986. Threonine kinetics at graded threonine intakes in young men. *Am J Clin Nutr* 43:795–802.

Ziegler TR, Benfell K, Smith RJ, Young LS, Brown E, Ferrari-Baliviera E, Lowe DK, Wilmore DW. 1990. Safety and metabolic effects of L-glutamine administration in humans. *J Parenter Enteral Nutr* 14:137S–146S.

Zimmerman FT, Burgemeister BB. 1959. A controlled experiment of glutamic acid therapy. *AMA Arch Neurol Psych* 81:639–648.

Zlotkin SH. 1989. Nutrient interactions with total parenteral nutrition: Effect of histidine and cysteine intake on urinary zinc excretion. *J Pediatr* 114:859–864.

11

Macronutrients and Healthful Diets

SUMMARY

Acceptable Macronutrient Distribution Ranges (AMDRs) for individuals have been set for carbohydrate, fat, *n*-6 and *n*-3 polyunsaturated fatty acids, and protein based on evidence from interventional trials, with support of epidemiological evidence that suggests a role in the prevention or increased risk of chronic diseases, and based on ensuring sufficient intakes of essential nutrients.

The AMDR for fat and carbohydrate is estimated to be 20 to 35 and 45 to 65 percent of energy for adults, respectively. These AMDRs are estimated based on evidence indicating a risk for coronary heart disease (CHD) at low intakes of fat and high intakes of carbohydrate and on evidence for increased risk for obesity and its complications (including CHD) at high intakes of fat. Because the evidence is less clear on whether low or high fat intakes during childhood can lead to increased risk of chronic diseases later in life, the estimated AMDRs for fat for children are primarily based on a transition from the high fat intakes that occur during infancy to the lower adult AMDR. The AMDR for fat is 30 to 40 percent of energy for children 1 to 3 years of age and 25 to 35 percent of energy for children 4 to 18 years of age. The AMDR for carbohydrate for children is the same as that for adults—45 to 65 percent of energy. The AMDR for protein is 10 to 35 percent of energy for adults and 5 to 20 percent and 10 to 30 percent for children 1 to 3 years of age and 4 to 18 years of age, respectively.

Based on usual median intakes of energy, it is estimated that a lower boundary level of 5 percent of energy will meet the Adequate Intake (AI) for linoleic acid (Chapter 8). An upper boundary for linoleic acid is set at 10 percent of energy for three reasons: (1) individual dietary intakes in the North American population rarely exceed 10 percent of energy, (2) epidemiological evidence for the safety of intakes greater than 10 percent of energy are generally lacking, and (3) high intakes of linoleic acid create a pro-oxidant state that may predispose to several chronic diseases, such as CHD and cancer. Therefore, an AMDR of 5 to 10 percent of energy is estimated for *n*-6 polyunsaturated fatty acids (linoleic acid).

An AMDR for α-linolenic acid is estimated to be 0.6 to 1.2 percent of energy. The lower boundary of the range meets the AI for α-linolenic acid (Chapter 8). The upper boundary corresponds to the highest α-linolenic acid intakes from foods consumed by individuals in the United States and Canada. A growing body of literature suggests that higher intakes of α-linolenic acid, eicosapentaenoic acid (EPA), and docosahexaenoic acid (DHA) may afford some degree of protection against CHD. Because the physiological potency of EPA and DHA is much greater than that for α-linolenic acid, it is not possible to estimate one AMDR for all *n*-3 fatty acids. Approximately 10 percent of the AMDR can be consumed as EPA and/or DHA.

No more than 25 percent of energy should be consumed as added sugars. This maximal intake level is based on ensuring sufficient intakes of certain essential micronutrients that are not present in foods and beverages that contain added sugars. A daily intake of added sugars that individuals should aim for to achieve a healthy diet was not set.

A Tolerable Upper Intake Level (UL) was not set for saturated fatty acids, *trans* fatty acids, or cholesterol (see Chapters 8 and 9). This chapter provides some guidance in ways of minimizing the intakes of these three nutrients while consuming a nutritionally adequate diet.

INTRODUCTION

Unlike micronutrients, macronutrients (fat, carbohydrate, and protein) are sources of body fuel that can be used somewhat interchangeably. Thus, for a certain level of energy intake, increasing the proportion of one macronutrient necessitates decreasing the proportion of one or both of the other macronutrients. The majority of energy is consumed as carbohydrate (approximately 35 to 70 percent, primarily as starch and sugars), and fat (approximately 20 to 45 percent), while the contribution of protein to energy intake is smaller and less varied (10 to 23 percent) (Appendix Tables E-3, E-6, and E-17). Therefore, a high fat diet (high percent of energy from fat) is usually low in carbohydrate and vice versa. In addition to these macronutrients, alcohol can provide on average up to 3 percent of energy of the adult diet (Appendix Table E-18).

A small amount of carbohydrate and as n-6 (linoleic acid) and n-3 (α-linolenic acid) polyunsaturated fatty acids and a number of amino acids that are essential for metabolic and physiological processes, are needed by the brain. The amounts needed, however, each constitute only a small percentage of total energy requirements. Food sources vary in their content of particular macro- and micronutrients. While some nutrients are present in both animal- and plant-derived foods, others are only present or are more abundant in either animal or plant foods. For example, animal-derived foods contain significant amounts of protein, saturated fatty acids, long-chain n-3 polyunsaturated fatty acids, and the micronutrients iron, zinc, and vitamin B_{12}, while plant-derived foods provide greater amounts of carbohydrate, *Dietary Fiber*, linoleic and α-linolenic acids, and micronutrients such as vitamin C and the B vitamins. It may be difficult to achieve sufficient intakes of certain micronutrients when consuming foods that contain very low amounts of a particular macronutrient. Alternatively, if intake of certain macronutrients from nutrient-poor sources is too high, it may also be difficult to consume sufficient micronutrients and still remain in energy balance. Therefore, a diet containing a variety of foods is considered the best approach to ensure sufficient intakes of all nutrients. This concept is not new and has been part of nutrition education programs since the early 1900s. For example, the first U.S. food guide was developed by the U.S. Department of Agriculture in 1916 and suggested consumption of a combination of five different food groups (Guthrie and Derby, 1998). This food guide has evolved to become known as the Food Guide Pyramid (USDA, 1996). Similarly, Canada has developed Canada's Food Guide to Healthy Eating (Health Canada, 1997).

A growing body of evidence indicates that an imbalance in macronutrients (e.g., low or high percent of energy), particularly with certain fatty acids and relative amounts of fat and carbohydrate, can increase risk of several chronic diseases. Much of this evidence is based on epidemiological studies of clinical endpoints such as coronary heart disease (CHD), diabetes, cancer, and obesity. However, these studies demonstrate associations; they do not necessarily infer causality, such as would be derived from controlled clinical trials. Robust clinical trials with specified clinical endpoints are generally lacking for macronutrients. Of importance, factors other than diet contribute to chronic disease, and multifactorial causality of chronic disease can confound the long-term adverse effects of a given macronutrient distribution. It is not possible to determine a defined level of intake at which chronic disease may be prevented or may develop. For example, high fat diets may predispose to obesity, but at what percent of energy intake does this occur? The answer depends on whether energy intake exceeds energy expenditure or is balanced with physical activity.

This chapter reviews the scientific evidence on the role of macronutrients in the development of chronic disease. In addition, the nutrient limitations that can occur with the consumption of too little or too much of a particular macronutrient are discussed. In consideration of the interrelatedness of macronutrients, their role in chronic disease, and their association with other essential nutrients in the diet, Acceptable Macronutrient Distribution Ranges (AMDRs) are estimated and represented as percent of energy intake. These ranges represent (1) intakes that are associated with reduced risk of chronic disease, (2) intakes at which essential dietary nutrients can be consumed at sufficient levels, and (3) intakes based on adequate energy intake and physical activity to maintain energy balance. When intakes of macronutrients fall above or below the AMDR, the risk for development of chronic disease (e.g., diabetes, CHD, cancer) appears to increase.

DIETARY FAT AND CARBOHYDRATE

There are a number of adverse health effects that may result from consuming a diet that is too low or high in fat or carbohydrate (starch and sugars). Furthermore, chronic consumption of a low fat, high carbohydrate or high fat, low carbohydrate diet may result in the inadequate intake of certain essential nutrients.

Low Fat, High Carbohydrate Diets of Adults

The chronic diseases of greatest concern with respect to relative intakes of macronutrients are CHD, diabetes, and cancer. In this section, the relationship between total fat and total carbohydrate intakes are considered. Comparisons are made in terms of *percentage* of total energy intake. For example, a low fat diet signifies a lower percentage of fat relative to total energy. It does not imply that total energy intake is reduced because of consumption of a low amount of fat. The distinction between *hypocaloric* diets and *isocaloric* diets is important, particularly with respect to impact on body weight. Low and high fat diets can still be isocaloric. The failure to identify this distinction has led to considerable confusion in terms of the role of dietary fat in chronic disease.

In the past few decades, the prevalence of overweight and obesity has increased at an alarming rate in many populations, particularly in the United States. Overweight and obesity contribute significantly to various chronic diseases. Consequently, there are two issues to consider for the distribution of fat and carbohydrate intakes in high-risk populations: the distributions that predispose to the development of overweight and obesity, and the distributions that worsen the metabolic consequences in populations that are already overweight or obese. These issues will be considered in the following sections.

Maintenance of Body Weight

A first issue is whether a certain macronutrient distribution interferes with sufficient intake of total energy, that is, sufficient energy to maintain a healthy weight. Sonko and coworkers (1994) concluded that an intake of 15 percent fat was too low to maintain body weight in women, whereas an intake of 18 percent fat was shown to be adequate even with a high level of physical activity (Jéquier, 1999). Moreover, some populations, such as those in Asia, have habitual very low fat intakes (about 10 percent of total energy) and apparently maintain adequate health (Weisburger, 1988). Whether these low fat intakes and consequent low energy consumptions have contributed to a historically small stature in these populations is uncertain.

An issue of more importance for well-nourished but sedentary populations, such as that of the United States, is whether the distribution between intakes of total fat and total carbohydrate influences the risk for weight gain (i.e., for development of overweight or obesity). It has been shown that when men and women were fed isocaloric diets containing 20, 40, or 60 percent fat, there was no difference in total daily energy expenditure (Hill et al., 1991). Similar observations were reported for individuals who consumed diets containing 10, 40, or 70 percent fat, where no change in body weight was observed (Leibel et al., 1992), and for men fed diets containing 9 to 79 percent fat (Shetty et al., 1994). Horvath and colleagues (2000) reported no change in body weight after runners consumed a diet containing 16 percent fat for 4 weeks. These studies contain two important findings: fat and carbohydrate provide similar amounts of metabolic energy predicted from their true energy content, and isocaloric diets provide similar metabolic energy expenditure, regardless of their fat–carbohydrate distribution. In other words, at isocaloric intakes, low fat diets do not produce weight loss.

A number of short- and long-term intervention studies have been conducted on normal-weight or moderately obese individuals to ascertain the effects of altering the fat and energy density content of the diet on body weight (Table 11-1). In general, significant reductions in the percent of

TABLE 11-1 Decreased Fat Intake and Body Weight Change in Normal-Weight or Moderately Obese Individuals

Reference	Study Design	Dietary Fat (% of energy)	Weight Change (kg)	Comments
Short-term studies (< 1 year)				
Boyar et al., 1988	19 women 6-mo intervention Ad libitum diet	34 → 21%	-5.1	Decreased fat intake associated with decreased energy intake
Buzzard et al., 1990	29 postmenopausal women 3-mo parallel Ad libitum diet	38 → 23% 39 → 35%	-2.8 -1.3	Decreased fat intake associated with decreased energy intake
Bloemberg et al., 1991	80 men 26-wk parallel Ad libitum diet	39 → 34% 38 → 37%	-0.94 +0.06	
Kendall et al., 1991	13 women 11-wk crossover Controlled diet	20-25% 35-40%	-2.54 -1.26	Decreased fat intake associated with decreased energy intake Low fat diet, hypocaloric
Leibel et al., 1992	13 men and women 15- to 56-d intervention Controlled diet	0, 40, or 70%	No significant changes in body weight	Isocaloric diets
Westerterp et al., 1996	217 men and women 6-mo parallel Ad libitum diet	35 → 33% 36 → 41%	+0.3 +1.1	

Reference	Study	Fat intake	6 mo	12 mo	Comments
Raben et al., 1997	11 women, 14-d crossover, Ad libitum	46 → 28%	−0.7		Decreased fat intake associated with decreased energy intake
Gerhard et al., 2000	22 women, 4-wk crossover, Controlled diet	20% / 40%	−1.1 / −0.3		Low fat diet, hypocaloric
Saris et al., 2000	398 men and women, 6-mo parallel, Ad libitum diet	36 → 26% / 36 → 28% / 36 → 37%	−0.9 / −1.8 / +0.8		Decreased fat intake associated with decreased energy intake
Long-term studies (≥ 1 year)					
Lee-Han et al., 1988	57 women, 1-y parallel, Ad libitum diet	36 → 23 → 26% / 36 → 34 → 36%	−1.16 / +0.07	−0.93 / +0.62	Decreased fat intake associated with decreased energy intake
Boyd et al., 1990	206 women, 1-y parallel, Ad libitum diet	37 → 21% / 37 → 35%	−1.0 / 0		
Sheppard et al., 1991	276 women, 1- and 2-y parallel, Ad libitum diet	0 to 1 y: 39 → 22% / 39 → 37%; 1 y to 2 y: 22 → 23%	−3.0 / −0.4 / +1.1		Decreased fat intake associated with decreased energy intake

continued

TABLE 11-1 Continued

Reference	Study Design	Dietary Fat (% of energy)			Weight Change (kg)			Comments
Baer, 1993	70 men 1-y parallel Ad libitum diet	38 → 31% 37 → 36%			−5.0 +1.0			Decreased fat intake associated with decreased energy intake
Kasim et al., 1993	72 women 1-y parallel Ad libitum diet	36 → 18% 36 → 34 %			−3.4 −0.8			Decreased fat intake associated with decreased energy intake
Black et al., 1994	76 men and women 2-y parallel Ad libitum diet	40 → 21% 39 → 39%			−2.0 −1.0			
Knopp et al., 1997	137 men 1-y parallel Ad libitum diet	36 → 27% 35 → 22%			−2.9 −2.9			
Stefanick et al., 1998	177 postmenopausal women and 190 men 1-y parallel Ad libitum diet	<u>Women</u> 23% 28%	<u>Men</u> 22% 30%		<u>Women</u> −2.7 +0.8	<u>Men</u> −2.8 +0.5		Decreased fat intake associated with decreased energy intake
Kasim-Karakas et al., 2000	54 postmenopausal women 1-y intervention Controlled diet 4 mo Ad libitum diet 8 mo	34 → 14 → 12%			<u>4 mo</u> −1.3	<u>12 mo</u> −5.9		

energy consumed as fat (greater than 4 percent) resulted in small losses in body weight. The only study that provided isocaloric diets showed no differences in weight gain or loss, despite a wide range in the percent of energy from fat (Leibel et al., 1992). Four meta-analyses of long-term intervention studies associating a low fat diet with body weight concluded that lower fat diets lead to modest weight loss or prevention of weight gain (Astrup et al., 2000; Bray and Popkin, 1998; Hill et al., 2000; Yu-Poth et al., 1999). These studies thus suggest that low fat diets (low percentage of fat) tend to be slightly hypocaloric compared to higher fat diets when compared in outpatient intervention trials.

The finding that higher fat diets are moderately hypercaloric when compared with reduced fat intakes under ad libitum conditions provides a rationale for setting an upper boundary for percentage of fat intake in a population that already has a high prevalence of overweight and obesity. However, a second issue must also be addressed: whether the distribution of fat and carbohydrate modifies the metabolic consequences of overweight and obesity. Two of the more important consequences of obesity are dyslipidemic changes in serum lipoproteins (which predispose to CHD) and changes in glucose and insulin metabolism that accentuate an underlying insulin resistance (which may predispose to both CHD and diabetes). These consequences are discussed in the following sections.

Risk of CHD

Low fat, high carbohydrate diets, compared to higher fat intakes, can induce a lipoprotein pattern called the atherogenic lipoprotein phenotype (Krauss, 2001) or atherogenic dyslipidemia (National Cholesterol Education Program, 2001). In populations where people are routinely physically active and lean, the atherogenic lipoprotein phenotype is minimally expressed. In sedentary populations that tend to be overweight or obese, very low fat, high carbohydrate diets clearly promote the development of this phenotype. Whether this phenotype promotes development of coronary atherosclerosis when it is specifically induced by low fat diets is uncertain, but it is a pattern that is associated with increased risk for CHD when expressed in the general American population. The atherogenic lipoprotein phenotype is characterized by higher triacylglycerol and decreased high density lipoprotein (HDL) cholesterol concentrations and small low density lipoprotein (LDL) particles. A predominance of small LDL particles is associated with a greater risk of CHD (Austin et al., 1990), but it is not known if this association is independent of increased triacylglycerol and decreased HDL cholesterol concentrations.

Table 11-2 and Figures 11-1 and 11-2 show that with decreasing fat and increasing carbohydrate intake, plasma triacylglycerol concentrations

TABLE 11-2 Fat and Carbohydrate Intake and Blood Lipid Concentrations in Healthy Individuals

Reference	Study Design[a]	Total Fat/ Carbohydrate Intake (% of energy)
Coulston et al., 1983	11 men and women 10-d crossover P/S = 1.2–1.3	21 41
Bowman et al., 1988	19 men 10-wk parallel P/S = 0.4	29/60 33/58 45/42 46/42
Borkman et al., 1991	8 men and women 3-wk crossover	20/55 P/S = 0.46 50/31 P/S = 0.22
Kasim et al., 1993	72 women 1-y parallel P/S = 0.68–0.75	18 34
Leclerc et al., 1993	7 men and women 7-d crossover	11/64 30/45 40/45
Krauss and Dreon, 1995	105 men 6-wk crossover P/S = 0.69–0.74	24/60 46/39
O'Hanesian et al., 1996	10 men and women 10-d crossover	17/63 P/S = 0.25 28/57 P/S = 2.2 42/39 P/S = 1.7
Jeppesen et al., 1997	10 postmenopausal women 3-wk crossover P/S = 1.0	25/60 45/40
Kasim-Karakas et al., 1997	14 postmenopausal women 4-mo intervention	14 P/S = 1.2 23 P/S = 1.0 31 P/S = 0.9
Yost et al., 1998	25 men and women 15-d crossover P/S = 0.3	25/55 50/30
Straznicky et al., 1999	14 men 2-wk crossover	25/54 P/S = 1.3 47/36 P/S = 0.1
Kasim-Karakas et al., 2000	54 postmenopausal women 4- to 12-mo crossover P/S = 0.64	12/71 14/69 34/50

Postintervention Blood Lipid Concentration (mmol/L)[b]		
Triacylglycerol	HDL-C	LDL-C
1.51^c	0.98^c	
1.02^d	1.16^d	
0.91^c	1.42^c	2.35^c
1.11^c	1.22^c	2.17^c
0.84^c	1.53^c	2.59^c
1.01^c	1.50^c	2.40^c
0.82^c (+49%)	0.84^c (−24%)	2.88^c (−20%)
0.55^c	1.10^d	3.60^d
1.35^c	1.44^c (−8%)	2.79^c (−10%)
1.25^d	1.56^d	3.09^d
1.11^c	1.03^c	2.29^c
1.29^c	1.15^d	2.47^c
0.87^d	1.32^e	3.05^d
1.59^c	1.09^c	3.26^c
1.13^d	1.27^d	3.69^d
0.8	1.1	2.4
0.8	1.2	2.5
0.8	1.3	3.0
1.97^c	1.38^c	2.74^c
1.29^d	1.49^d	2.81^c
2.47^c	1.24^c	2.61^c
2.10^d	1.32^d	2.93^d
1.85^e	1.34^d	2.89^d
1.14^c	1.22^c	
0.88^d	1.30^d	
0.8^c	1.05^c	2.6^c
0.8^c	1.28^d	3.5^d
1.49^c	1.40^c	3.49^c
2.00^c	1.29^c	3.18^c
1.57^c	1.53^d	3.57^c

continued

TABLE 11-2 Continued

Reference	Study Design[a]	Total Fat/ Carbohydrate Intake (% of energy)
Marckmann et al., 2000	20 women 2-wk crossover	28/59 P/S = 0.7 46/41 P/S = 0.4
Obarzanek et al., 2001b	459 men and women, 8-wk parallel	27/58 P/S = 1.1 37/52 P/S = 0.5

[a] P/S = polyunsaturated/saturated fatty acid ratio.
[b] HDL-C = high density lipoprotein cholesterol, LDL-C = low density lipoprotein cholesterol.

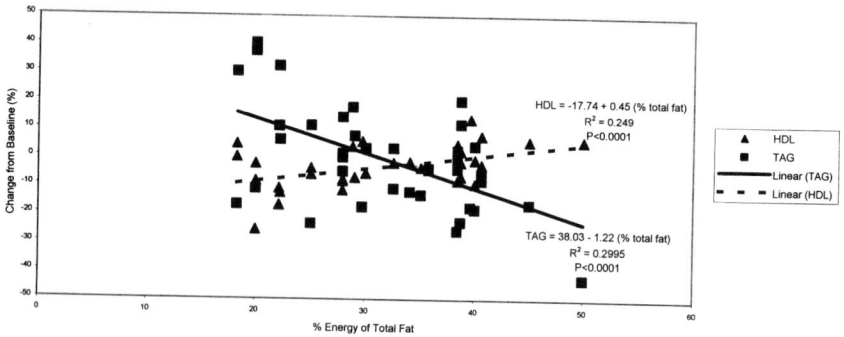

FIGURE 11-1 Relationship between percent of total fat intake and change in triacylglycerol (TAG) (−) and high density lipoprotein (HDL) cholesterol (---) concentrations. Regression equations for percent change in serum TAG and HDL cholesterol predicted by percent total fat in the experimental diets of controlled-feeding studies comparing low fat, high carbohydrate diets to high fat diets. Weighted least-squares regression analyses were performed using the mixed procedure to test for differences in lipid concentrations (SAS Statistical package, version 8.00, SAS Institute, Inc., 1999). Percent of energy from total fat varied from 18.3% to 50%. All diets were low in saturated fat (less than 10% energy). Using these equations, for every 5% decrease in total fat, HDL cholesterol would decrease by 2.2% and triacylglycerol would increase by 6%.

DATA SOURCES: Berry et al. (1992); Curb et al. (2000); Garg et al. (1988, 1992a, 1994); Ginsberg et al. (1990); Grundy (1986); Grundy et al. (1988); Jansen et al. (1998); Kris-Etherton et al. (1999); Lefevre et al., unpublished; Lopez-Segura et al. (1996); Mensink and Katan (1987); Nelson et al. (1995); Parillo et al. (1992); Pelkman et al. (2001); Perez-Jimenez et al. (1995, 1999, 2001).

Postintervention Blood Lipid Concentration (mmol/L)[b]		
Triacylglycerol	HDL-C	LDL-C
0.81[c]	1.34[c]	2.43[c]
0.70[d]	1.56[d]	2.71[d]
+0.4	−0.09	−0.29
−0.09	−0.005	−0.05

[c,d,e] Within each study, LDL-C, HDL-C, or Lp(a) concentrations that are significantly different between treatment groups have a different superscript.

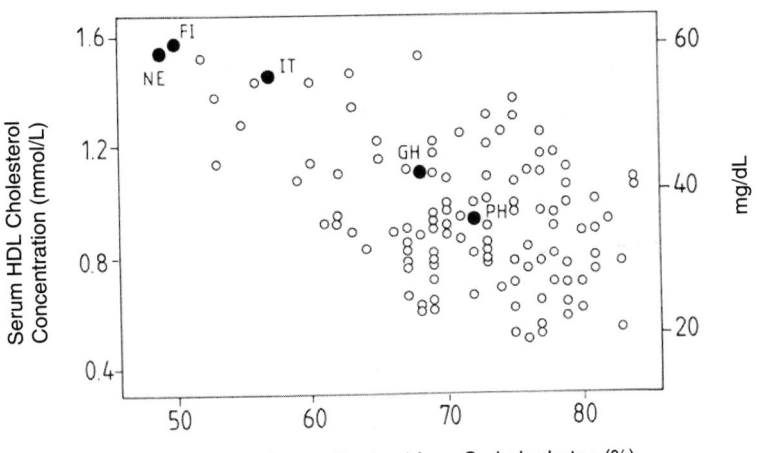

FIGURE 11-2 Relationship between proportion of energy from carbohydrates and serum high density lipoprotein (HDL) cholesterol concentration. • = Mean values for approximately 120 boys from five countries, o = individuals values for boys from the Philippines, FI= Finland, NE = Netherlands, GH = Ghana, IT = Italy, PH = Philippines.

SOURCE: Knuiman et al. (1987).

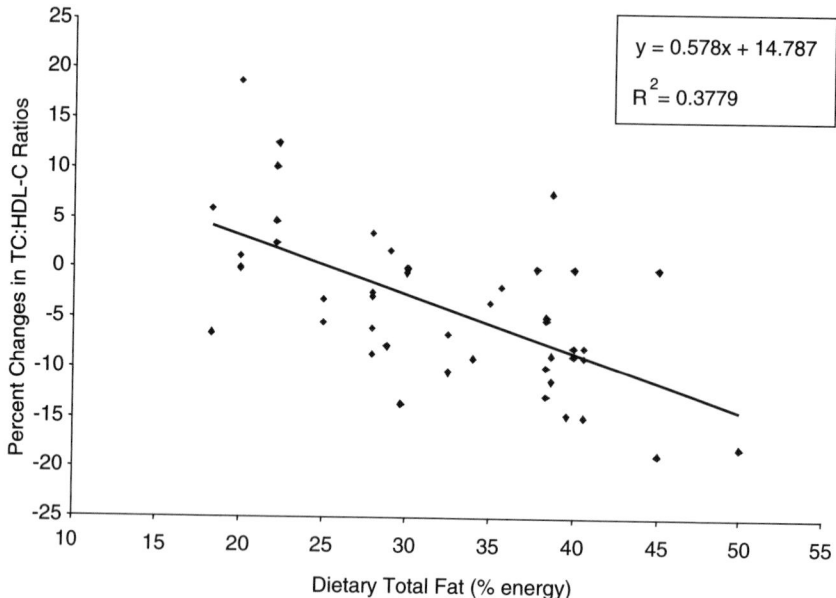

FIGURE 11-3 Relationship between total fat intake and change in total cholesterol (TC):high density lipoprotein (HDL) cholesterol ratio. Weighted least-squares regression analyses were performed using the mixed procedure to test for differences in lipid concentrations (SAS Statistical package, version 8.00, SAS Institute, Inc., 1999).
DATA SOURCES: Berry et al. (1992); Curb et al. (2000); Garg et al. (1988, 1992a, 1994); Ginsberg et al. (1990); Grundy (1986); Grundy et al. (1988); Jansen et al. (1998); Kris-Etherton et al. (1999); Lefevre et al., unpublished; Lopez-Segura et al. (1996); Mensink and Katan (1987); Nelson et al. (1995); Parillo et al. (1992); Pelkman et al. (2001); Perez-Jimenez et al. (1995, 1999, 2001).

increase and plasma HDL cholesterol concentrations decrease. The reduction in HDL cholesterol concentration with low fat intake results in a rise in the total:HDL cholesterol concentration ratio (Figure 11-3). The total:HDL cholesterol ratio has been shown to be an important risk factor for CHD (Castelli et al., 1992; Kannel, 2000). Whether diet-induced changes in the total:HDL cholesterol ratio predispose to CHD remains unclear (Brussard et al., 1982; Jeppesen et al., 1997; Krauss and Dreon, 1995; West et al., 1990; Yost et al., 1998).

In support of the interventional studies, carbohydrate intake is negatively associated with HDL cholesterol concentrations (Table 11-3). Nonetheless, the association between atherogenic lipoprotein phenotype (higher

TABLE 11-3 Epidemiological Studies on Carbohydrate Intake and Blood Lipid Concentrations

Reference	Study Design	Low Density Lipoprotein (LDL) Cholesterol Concentration	High Density Lipoprotein (HDL) Cholesterol Concentration	Triacylglycerol Concentration
Ernst et al., 1980	4,855 men and women Cross-sectional		Inversely related to carbohydrate intake	
Knuiman et al., 1987	Multicountry regression analysis		Inversely related to carbohydrate intake	
Fehily et al., 1988	653 men Cross-sectional regression analysis	No association	Negative association between carbohydrate intake and HDL concentration	No association
West et al., 1990	719 boys Multicountry regression analysis	Decreased with increased carbohydrate intake	Decreased with increased carbohydrate intake	Increased with increased carbohydrate intake
Tillotson et al., 1997	Prospective cohort, 6-y follow-up			
	< 29% carbohydrate	4.18	1.13	2.11
	29–36% carbohydrate	4.13	1.11	2.26
	36–41% carbohydrate	4.13	1.09	2.23
	41–48% carbohydrate	4.11	1.07	2.25
	> 48% carbohydrate	4.14	1.05	2.13

total:HDL cholesterol ratios) and CHD risk provides one rationale for establishing a lower boundary for the Acceptable Macronutrient Distribution Range (AMDR) for high-risk populations.

Risk of Hyperinsulinemia, Glucose Intolerance, and Type 2 Diabetes

Other potential abnormalities accompanying changes in distribution of fat and carbohydrate intakes include increased postprandial responses in plasma glucose and insulin concentrations. These abnormalities are more likely to occur with low fat, high carbohydrate diets. They potentially could be related to the development of both type 2 diabetes and CHD. In particular, repeated daily elevations in postprandial glucose and insulin concentrations could "exhaust" pancreatic β-cells of insulin supply, which could hasten the onset of type 2 diabetes. Some investigators have further suggested these repeated elevations could worsen baseline insulin sensitivity, which could cause susceptible persons to be at increased risk for type 2 diabetes. This form of diabetes, defined by an elevation of fasting serum glucose concentration, is characterized by two defects in glucose metabolism: insulin resistance, a defect in insulin-mediated uptake of glucose by cells, particularly skeletal muscle cells, and a decline in insulin secretory capacity by pancreatic β-cells (Turner and Clapham, 1998). Insulin resistance typically precedes the development of type 2 diabetes by many years. It is known to be the result of obesity, physical inactivity, and genetic factors (Turner and Clapham, 1998). Before the onset of diabetic hyperglycemia, the pancreatic β-cells are able to respond to insulin resistance with an increased insulin secretion, enough to maintain normoglycemia. However, in some persons who are insulin resistant, insulin secretory capacity declines and hyperglycemia ensues (Reaven, 1988, 1995).

The mechanisms for the decline in insulin secretion are not well understood, but one theory is that continuous overstimulation of insulin secretion by the presence of insulin resistance leads to "insulin exhaustion" and hence to decreased insulin secretory capacity (Turner and Clapham, 1998). Whether insulin exhaustion is secondary to a metabolic dysfunction of cellular production of insulin or to a loss of β-cells is uncertain. The accumulation of pancreatic islet-cell amyloidosis may be one mechanism for loss of insulin-secretory capacity (Höppener et al., 2000).

High carbohydrate diets frequently causes greater insulin and plasma glucose responses than do low carbohydrate diets (Chen et al., 1988; Coulston et al., 1987). These excessive responses theoretically could predispose individuals to the development of type 2 diabetes because of prolonged overstimulation of insulin secretion (Grill and Björklund, 2001). The reasoning is similar to that for insulin resistance, namely, excessive stimulation of insulin secretion over a period of many years could result in insulin exhaustion, and hence to hyperglycemia (Turner and Clapham, 1998). This mechanism, although plausible, remains hypothetical. Nonetheless, in the mind of some investigators, it deserves serious consideration.

Other consequences of hyperglycemic responses to high carbohydrate diets might be considered. For example, higher postprandial glucose responses might lead to other changes such as "desensitization" of β-cells for insulin secretion and production of glycated products or advanced glycation end-products, which could either promote atherogenesis or the "aging" process (Lopes-Virella and Virella, 1996). Again, these are hypothetical consequences that need further examination.

Epidemiological Evidence. A number of noninterventional, epidemiological studies have shown no relationship between carbohydrate intake and risk of diabetes (Colditz et al., 1992; Lundgren et al., 1989; Marshall et al., 1991; Meyer et al., 2000; Salmerón et al., 1997), whereas other studies have shown a positive association (Bennett et al., 1984; Feskens et al., 1991a).

Interventional Evidence. Interventional studies in healthy individuals on the influence of high carbohydrate diets on biomarker precursors for type 2 diabetes are lacking and the available data are mixed (Table 11-4) (Beck-Nielsen et al., 1980; Chen et al., 1988; Dunnigan et al., 1970; Fukagawa et al., 1990; Rath et al., 1974; Reiser et al., 1979). Factors such as carbohydrate quality, body weight, exercise, and genetics make the interpretation of such findings difficult. Nonetheless, in overweight and sedentary groups (which carry a heavy burden of insulin resistance and are common in North America), the accentuation of postprandial glucose and insulin concentrations that accompany high carbohydrate diets are factors to consider when setting an upper boundary for AMDRs for dietary carbohydrate (and a lower boundary for dietary fat).

Risk of Nutrient Inadequacy or Excess

Diets Low in Fats. For usual diets that are low in total fat, the intake of essential fatty acids, such as *n*-6 polyunsaturated fatty acids, will be low (Appendix K). In general, with increasing intakes of carbohydrate and decreasing intakes of fat, the intake of *n*-6 polyunsaturated fatty acids decreases. Furthermore, low intakes of fat are associated with low intakes of zinc and certain B vitamins.

The digestion and absorption of fat-soluble vitamins and provitamin A carotenoids are associated with fat absorption. Jayarajan and coworkers (1980) reported that the addition of 5 or 10 g of fat to a low fat (5 g) diet

TABLE 11-4 Intervention Studies on Carbohydrate Intake and Biochemical Indicators of Diabetes

Reference	Study Design
Dunnigan et al., 1970	9 men and women 4-wk crossover 31% sucrose Sucrose-free
Rath et al., 1974	6 men 2- to 5-wk crossover 17% sucrose 52% sucrose
Reiser et al., 1979	19 men and women 6-wk crossover 30% starch 30% sucrose
Beck-Nielsen et al., 1980	7-d intervention Normal diet + 250 g glucose Normal diet + 250 g fructose
Chen et al., 1988	8 men 3- to 5-d crossover 85% carbohydrate 41% carbohydrate 30% carbohydrate
Lundgren et al., 1989	1,462 women, Prospective cohort, 12-y follow-up
Fukagawa et al., 1990	6 men 21- to 28-d intervention 40% carbohydrate 69% carbohydrate

a,b,c Within each study, the indicators of diabetes that are significantly different between treatment groups have a different superscript.

Results

No diet effect on glucose tolerance and plasma insulin

Serum insulin (μg/mL)	Serum glucose (mg/dL)
5.4[a]	87.0[a]
11.8[b]	81.1[b]

Serum insulin (μmunits/mL)	Serum glucose (mg/dL)
9.8[a]	92.5[a]
11.9[b]	94.5[a]

No significant difference in insulin concentrations
The high fructose diet was accompanied by a
significant reduction in insulin binding and insulin
sensitivity

Insulin sensitivity index	Glucose disappearance (%/min)
5.6[a]	2.2[a]
6.1[b]	2.3[b]
3.9[a,c]	1.6[a,c]
5.6[a]	2.2[a]
6.1[b]	2.3[b]
3.9[a,c]	1.6[a,c]

Carbohydrate intake of women who developed
diabetes (212 g/d) was not significantly different
than women who did not develop diabetes (228 g/d)

Serum insulin (pmol/L)	Glucose disposal (μmol/kg/min)
67.4[a]	21.2[a]
50.2[b]	27.8[b]

significantly improved serum vitamin A concentrations. However, the addition of 10 g compared to 5 g did not provide any further benefit. The level of dietary fat has also been shown to improve vitamin K_2 bioavailability (Uematsu et al., 1996). Dose–response data are limited on the amount of dietary fat needed to achieve the optimal absorption of fat-soluble vitamins, but it appears that the level is quite low.

Diets High in Fiber. Most diets that are high in fiber are also high in carbohydrate. High fiber diets have the potential for reduced energy density, reduced energy intake, and poor growth. However, poor growth is unlikely in the United States where most children consume adequate energy and fiber intake is relatively low (Williams and Bollella, 1995). Miles (1992) tested the effects of daily ingestion of 64 g or 34 g of *Dietary Fiber* for 10 weeks in healthy adult males. The ingestion of 64 g/d of *Dietary Fiber* resulted in a reduction in protein utilization from 89.4 to 83.7 percent and in fat utilization from 95.5 to 92.5 percent. Total energy utilization decreased from 94.3 to 91.4 percent. Because most individuals consuming high amounts of fiber would also be consuming high amounts of energy, the slight depression in energy utilization is not significant (Miles, 1992). In other studies, ingestion of high amounts of fruit, vegetable, and cereal fiber (48.3 to 85.6 g/d) also resulted in decreases in apparent digestibilities of energy, crude protein, and fat (Göranzon et al., 1983; Wisker et al., 1988). Again, however, the *Dietary Fiber* intakes were very high, and because the recommendation for *Total Fiber* intake is related to energy intake, the high fiber consumers would also be high energy consumers.

Diets High in Added Sugars. Increased consumption of added sugars can result in decreased intakes of certain micronutrients (Table 11-5). This can occur because of the abundance of added sugars in energy-dense, nutrient-poor foods, whereas naturally occurring sugars are primarily found in fruits, milk, and dairy products that also contain essential micronutrients. Because some micronutrients (e.g., vitamin B_6, vitamin C, and folate), dietary fiber, and phytochemicals were not examined, the association between these nutrients and added sugars intakes is not known. Bowman (1999) used data from Continuing Survey of Food Intakes of Individuals (CSFII) (1994–1996) to assess the relationship between added sugars and intakes of essential nutrients in Americans' diets. The sample ($n = 14,704$) was divided into three groups based on the percentage of energy consumed from added sugars: (1) less than 10 percent of total energy ($n = 5,058$), (2) 10 to 18 percent of total energy ($n = 4,488$), and (3) greater than 18 percent of total energy ($n = 5,158$). Group 3, with a mean of 26.7 percent of energy from added sugars, had the lowest absolute mean intakes of all the micronutrients, especially vitamin A, vitamin C, vitamin B_{12}, folate, calcium, phosphorus, magnesium, and iron. Compared with Groups 1 and 2, a decreased percentage of people in Group 3 met their Recommended Dietary Allowance (RDA) for many micronutrients. The individuals in Group 3 did not meet the 1989 RDA for vitamin E, vitamin B_6, calcium, magnesium, and zinc. In addition, the high sugar consumers (Group 3) had lower intakes of grains, fruits, vegetables, meat, poultry, and fish compared with Groups 1 and 2. At the same time, Group 3 consumed more soft drinks, fruit drinks, punches, ades, cakes, cookies, grain-based pastries, milk desserts, and candies. Similar trends were also reported by Bolton-Smith and Woodward (1995) and Forshee and Storey (2001), but were not observed by Lewis and coworkers (1992). Emmett and Heaton (1995) reported an overall deterioration in the quality of the diet in heavy users of added sugars.

Using 1990–1991 cross-sectional data, Guthrie (1996) found that women whose diets met their RDA for calcium consumed significantly more milk products, fruit, and grains, and less regular soft drinks than women who did not meet their calcium recommendations. Others have shown that intakes of soft drinks are negatively related to intakes of milk (Guenther, 1986; Harnack et al., 1999; Skinner et al., 1999).

To further look at the association between added sugars and certain micronutrient intakes, the median intakes of various micronutrients at every 5th percentile of added sugars intake was determined using data from the Third National Health and Nutrition Examination Survey (NHANES III) (Appendix J). In addition, the prevalence of subpopulations not meeting the Estimated Average Requirement (EAR) or exceeding the Adequate Intake (AI) for these micronutrients was determined. Because not all micronutrients and other nutrients, such as fiber, were evaluated, it is not known what the association is between added sugars and these nutrients. While the trends are not consistent for all age groups, reduced intakes of calcium, vitamin A, iron, and zinc were observed with increasing intakes of added sugars, particularly at intake levels exceeding 25 percent of energy. Although this approach has limitations, it gives guidance for the planning of healthy diets.

Diets High in Total Sugars. In one large dietary survey, linear reductions were observed for certain micronutrients when total sugars intakes increased (Bolton-Smith and Woodward, 1995), whereas no consistent reductions were observed in another survey (Gibney et al., 1995) (Table 11-6). Bolton-Smith (1996) reviewed the literature on the relation of sugars intake to micronutrient adequacy and concluded that, provided consumption of sugars is not excessive (defined as less than 20 percent of total energy intake), no health risks are likely to ensue due to micronutrient inadequacies.

TABLE 11-5 Survey Data on Added Sugars and Micronutrient Intake

Reference	Study Population/Survey	Diet Information
Nelson, 1991	143 children, 11–12 y	7-d weighed diet record
Rugg-Gunn et al., 1991	405 children, 11–14 y	3-d diet record
Lewis et al., 1992	Nationwide Food Consumption Survey (1977–1978)	
Bolton-Smith and Woodward, 1995	11,626 men and women, 25–64 y Scottish Heart Health and MONICA studies	Food frequency questionnaire
Gibson, 1997	1,675 boys and girls, 1.5–4.5 y U.K. National Diet and Nutrition Survey of Children	4-d weighed diet record
Bowman, 1999	Continuing Survey of Food Intakes by Individuals (1994–1996)	Two 24-h recalls
Forshee and Storey, 2001	Continuing Survey of Food Intakes by Individuals (1994–1996)	

Added Sugars Intake (% of energy)	Change in Micronutrient Intake
16 21 27	Decrease in nicotinic acid for girls
10 20	Decrease in vitamin D, protein
Percentile of intake 26th–75th > 75th	Decrease in calcium
Men: 1.0–6.2, 6.3–8.9, 9.0–13.0, 13.1–15.7, 15.8–47.9 Women: 0.8–4.8, 4.9–6.3, 6.4–8.1, 8.2–11.6, 11.7–50.2	Linear reduction in vitamin E, vitamin C, and vitamin A for both men and women
< 12 12–16 16–20 20–25 > 25	Decrease in zinc, calcium, riboflavin Decrease in niacin, thiamin; large decrease in calcium, zinc, riboflavin
< 10 10–18 > 18	Decrease in calcium Decrease in vitamin A, vitamin E, vitamin C, niacin, vitamin B_6, folate, vitamin B_{12}, phosphorus, magnesium, iron, zinc, copper; large decrease in calcium
	Negative correlation between added sugar intake and intake of vitamin A, calcium, and folate

TABLE 11-6 Survey Data on Total Sugar and Micronutrient Intake

Reference	Study Population/Survey	Diet Information
Gibson, 1993	2,705 children Department of Health Survey of British School Children	7-d weighed food record
Bolton-Smith and Woodward, 1995	11,626 men and women, 25–64 y Scottish Heart Health and MONICA studies	Food frequency questionnaire
Gibney et al., 1995	8,296 men and women Nationwide Food Consumption Survey (1987–1988)	3-d food record
Nicklas et al., 1996	568 children, 10 y Bogalusa Heart Study	24-h dietary recall
Farris et al., 1998	568 children, 10 y Bogalusa Heart Study	24-h dietary recall

The impact of total sugar intake on the intake of micronutrients does not appear to be as great as for added sugars. Furthermore, a preliminary analysis of data from NHANES III on the intake of various micronutrients at every 5th percentile of total sugar intake did not reveal any significant associations as was observed for added sugars (Appendix J).

High Fat, Low Carbohydrate Diets of Adults

Risk of Obesity

Epidemiological Evidence. Cross-country epidemiological data of dietary fat intake and obesity have yielded mixed results (Bray and Popkin, 1998;

Total Sugar Intake (% of energy)	Change in Micronutrient Intake
< 20.7	Decrease in iron, nicotinic acid
20.7–25.2	Large decrease in iron, nicotinic acid
> 25.2	No marked changes in micronutrient intake
Men: 2.5–12.0, 12.1–14.7, 14.8–17.2, 17.3–20.7, 20.8–51.4	Linear reduction in vitamin E, retinol, and vitamin A intake
Women: 1.5–11.7, 11.8–14.1, 14.2–16.3, 16.4–19.6, 19.7–52.8	Linear reduction in vitamin E, retinol, carotene, and vitamin A intake
< 10	
10–24	Decrease in riboflavin, thiamin, calcium, iron, zinc, vitamin A
> 24	Decrease in vitamin B_6, vitamin E
18.0	
22.1	
26.4	
31.2	Decrease in percent meeting the Recommended Dietary Allowance for niacin and zinc
16.1	Linear reduction in vitamin B_6, vitamin E,
23.5	thiamin, iron, zinc, and niacin intake with
28.2	increasing total sugar intake
35.6	

Willett, 1998). In some countries, low fat, high carbohydrate diets are associated with a low prevalence of obesity, whereas in others they are not.

Within-country surveys of dietary intake and body mass index (BMI) have also yielded mixed results. Many case-control and prospective studies failed to find a strong correlation between percent of energy intake from fat and body weight (Heitmann et al., 1995; Lissner et al., 2000; Ludwig et al., 1999b; Rissanen et al., 1991; Samaras et al., 1998; Willett, 1998), whereas some did find significant associations (Bray and Popkin, 1998; Dreon et al., 1988; George et al., 1990; Klesges et al., 1992; Miller et al., 1990; Romieu et al., 1988; Tucker and Kano, 1992). Colditz and coworkers (1990) observed no association between fat intake and weight gain prospectively, but did find a positive association between previous weight gain and high fat intake. One statistically well-designed study that included direct measurements of body fat and considered potentially confounding factors such as exercise concluded that total dietary fat was positively correlated with fat mass (adjusted for fat-free mass, $r = 0.22$, $p < 0.0001$) in adults (Larson et al., 1996). Most multiple regression studies found that about 3 percent of the total variance in body fatness was explained by diet, though some studies placed the estimate at 7 to 8 percent (Westerterp et al., 1996). Longitudinal studies generally supported dietary fat as a predictive factor in the development of obesity (Lissner and Heitmann, 1995). However, bias in subject participation, retention, and underreporting of intake may limit the power of these epidemiological studies to assess the relationship between dietary fat and obesity or weight gain (Lissner et al., 2000).

Another line of evidence often cited to indicate that dietary fat is not an important contributor to obesity is that although there has been a reduction in the percent of energy from fat consumed in the United States, there has been an increase in energy intake and a marked gain in average weight (Willett, 1998). Survey data showed an increase in total energy intake over this period (McDowell et al., 1994), so that despite the decline in percent of energy from fat, the total intake of fat (g/d) remained stable. Another study that used food supply data showed that fat intake may indeed be rising in the United States (Harnack et al., 2000).

Mechanisms for Obesity and Interventional Evidence. Several mechanisms have been proposed whereby high fat intakes could lead to excess body accumulation of fat. Foods containing high amounts of fat tend to be energy dense, and the fat is a major contributor to the excess energy consumed by persons who are overweight or obese (Prentice, 2001). The energy density of a food can be defined as the amount of metabolizable energy per unit weight or volume (Yao and Roberts, 2001); water and fat are the main determinants of dietary energy density. Energy density is an issue of interest to the extent that it influences energy intake and thus plays a role in energy regulation, weight maintenance, and the subsequent development of obesity.

Three theoretical mechanisms have been identified by which dietary energy density may affect total energy intake and hence energy regulation (Yao and Roberts, 2001). Some studies suggest that, at least in the short-term, individuals tend to eat in order to maintain a constant volume of food intake because stomach distension triggers vagal signals of fullness (Duncan et al., 1983; Lissner et al., 1987; Seagle et al., 1997; Stubbs et al., 1995a). Thus, consumption of high energy-dense foods could lead to excess energy intake due to the high energy density to small food volume ratio.

A second proposed mechanism is that high energy-dense foods are often more palatable than low energy-dense foods (Drewnowski, 1999; Drewnowski and Greenwood, 1983). A survey of American adults reported that taste is the primary influence for food choice (Glanz et al., 1998). In single-meal studies, high palatability was also associated with increased food consumption (Bobroff and Kissileff, 1986; Price and Grinker, 1973; Yeomans et al., 1997). These results suggest that high energy-dense foods may be overeaten because of effects related to their high palatability.

The third mechanism is that energy-dense foods reduce the rate of gastric emptying (Calbet and MacLean, 1997; Wisen et al., 1993). This reduction, however, does not occur proportionally to the increase in energy density. Although energy-dense foods reduce the rate at which food leaves the stomach, they actually increase the rate at which energy leaves the stomach. Thus, because energy-containing nutrients are digested more quickly, nutrient levels in the blood fall quicker and hunger returns (Friedman, 1995). While a subjective measure, highly palatable meals have also been shown to produce an increased glycemic response compared with less palatable meals that contain the same food items that are combined in different ways (Sawaya et al., 2001). This suggests a generalized link among palatability, gastric emptying, and glycemic response in the underlying mechanisms determining the effects of energy density on energy regulation. Further research on this potential link is needed.

Researchers have used instruments such as visual analogue scales to measure differences in appetite sensations (e.g., hunger and satiety) between treatments in order to examine the effects of altering nutrients that play a major role in energy density, such as dietary fat, on energy regulation (Flint et al., 2000). A number of studies have been conducted in which preloads of differing energy density were given and hunger and satiety were measured either at the subsequent meal or for the remainder of the day. In the studies that administered preloads that had constant volume but different energy content (energy density was altered by changing dietary fat content), there was no consistent difference in subsequent satiety or hunger between the various test meals (Durrant and Royston, 1979; Green et al., 1994; Hill et al., 1987; Himaya et al., 1997; Hulshof et al., 1993; Louis-Sylvestre et al., 1994; Porrini et al., 1995; Rolls et al., 1994). However, in those studies using isoenergetic preloads that differed in volume (energy density was altered by changing dietary fat content), there was consistently increased satiety and reduced hunger after consumption of the low energy-dense preload meals (i.e., those with higher volume) (Blundell et al., 1993; Holt et al., 1995; van Amelsvoort et al., 1989, 1990). It has been reported, however, that diets low in fat and high in carbohydrate may lead to more rapid return of hunger and increased snacking between meals (Ludwig et al., 1999a).

These data suggest that in the short-term, low energy-dense foods appear to increase satiety and decrease hunger compared to high energy-dense foods. Because individuals were blinded to the dietary content of the treatment diets, the results from these studies demonstrate the short-term effects of energy density after controlling for cognitive influences on food intake.

It is important that cognitive factors are taken into account during the interpretation of results of preload studies. When individuals were aware of dietary changes, they generally (Ogden and Wardle, 1990; Shide and Rolls, 1995; Wooley, 1972), but not always (Mattes, 1990; Rolls et al., 1989), compensated for changes in energy density and thus minimized changes in energy intake.

In well-controlled, short-term intervention studies lasting several days or more, high fat diets were consistently associated with higher spontaneous energy intake (Lawton et al., 1993; Proserpi et al., 1997; Thomas et al., 1992). From short- and longer-term studies, volunteers consistently consumed less dietary energy on low fat, low energy dense diets compared to high energy-dense diets (Glueck et al., 1982; Lissner et al., 1987; Poppitt and Swann, 1998; Poppitt et al., 1998; Stubbs et al., 1995b; Thomas et al., 1992; Tremblay et al., 1989, 1991). The extent to which energy intake was reduced on low energy-dense diets was similar for short- and long-term studies.

An alternative way to study the effects of energy density on energy intake in short-term studies has been to compare energy intake between diets of similar energy density that differ in dietary fat content. Using this approach, when fat content was covertly varied between 20 and 60 percent of energy, there was no significant difference in energy intake between groups (Saltzman et al., 1997; Stubbs et al., 1996; van Stratum et al., 1978). These results suggest that energy density plays a more significant role than fat per se in the short-term regulation of food intake.

During overfeeding, fat may be slightly more efficiently used than carbohydrate (Horton et al., 1995), but in one study, no difference was seen (McDevitt et al., 2000). Thus, high fat diets are not intrinsically fattening, calorie for calorie, and will not lead to obesity unless excess total energy is consumed. It is apparent, however, that with the consumption of high fat diets by the free-living population, energy intake does increase, therefore predisposing to increased weight gain and obesity if activity level is not adjusted accordingly (see Table 11-1). While many of the short-term studies showed a more dramatic effect on weight reduction with reduced fat intake, the long-term studies showed weight loss as well.

Conclusions. Epidemiological studies provide mixed results on the question of whether high fat (low carbohydrate) diets predispose to overweight and obesity and promote weight gain. However, a number of short-term studies suggest mechanisms whereby high fat intake could promote weight gain in the long-term. In addition, short- and long-term intervention studies provide evidence that reduced fat intake is accompanied by reduced energy intake and therefore moderate weight reduction or prevention of weight gain. For these reasons, it may be concluded that higher fat intakes are accompanied with increased energy intake and therefore increased risk for weight gain in populations that are already disposed to overweight and obesity, such as that of North America.

Risk of CHD

Epidemiological Evidence. In populations that consume very low fat diets, such as those of rural Asia and Africa, the prevalence of CHD is low (Campbell et al., 1998; Singh et al., 1995; Tao et al., 1989; Walker and Walker, 1978). This fact has led to the concept that low fat diets will protect against CHD. However, this conclusion must be drawn with caution when it is applied to societies in which dietary and exercise habits differ markedly from societies in rural Asia and Africa. In the latter societies, people are highly active and lean (Singh et al., 1995; Walker and Walker, 1978). Both of these factors independently reduce risk for CHD and could offset any potentially detrimental effects of very low fat diets. For this reason, the effects of low fat diets must be viewed in the context of current societal habits in the United States and Canada and of changing habits in developing countries. Furthermore, in more recent years it has become clear that the relationship between fat intake and CHD is related more to the quality of fat than to the quantity. The relationship is clearly shown by cross-population studies. For example, some Mediterranean populations consume diets that are high in total fat and unsaturated fatty acids but low in saturated fatty acids; in these populations, rates of CHD are relatively low (Keys et al., 1980, 1984). In contrast, in northern Europe, where intakes of saturated fatty acids are high, so are rates of CHD (Keys et al., 1980, 1984). Two epidemiological studies showed no relationship between carbohydrate intake and LDL cholesterol concentration (Fehily et al., 1988; Tillotson et al., 1997).

In several recent, long-term prospective studies of diet and chronic disease, rates of CHD did not substantially differ across populations that consumed approximately 25 to 45 percent of energy from fat (Ascherio et al., 1996; Hu et al., 1997). Men who developed CHD were shown to consume a slightly higher percentage of energy from fat (34.7 percent) compared with those who did not develop CHD (33.3 percent); however, this small difference in fat intake may not be significant since intake was based on a

24-hour recall, and the data were not adjusted for energy intake (McGee et al., 1984). Furthermore, Hawaiians, who have a higher incidence of CHD than Japanese living in Hawaii, consumed more energy from fat (35 percent) than the Japanese (31 percent) (Bassett et al., 1969). It has been reported that those who developed CHD consumed slightly less energy from carbohydrate compared to those who did not develop CHD (Kushi et al., 1985; McGee et al., 1984) (Table 11-7). Other studies showed no significant association between risk of CHD and total carbohydrate or sugar intake (Bolton-Smith and Woodward, 1994; Liu et al., 1982, 2000).

Interventional Evidence. Increasing fat intake, as a result of increased saturated fat intake, has been shown to increase LDL cholesterol concentrations (Table 11-2), and therefore risk of CHD. Intervention studies that have investigated the effect of carbohydrate intake on LDL cholesterol concentration have shown mixed results (Table 11-3). Two intervention studies agree with the findings of West and colleagues (1990) in that LDL cholesterol concentration increased when the percent of energy from carbohydrate was decreased from 55 to 31 percent (Borkman et al., 1991) and 59 to 41 percent (Marckmann et al., 2000). However, in other studies in which saturated fatty acids have remained constant, varying the percentage of total fat was found to not alter the LDL cholesterol concentration (Garg et al., 1994; Grundy et al., 1988).

Yu-Poth and colleagues (1999) conducted a meta-analysis on 37 intervention studies that evaluated the effects of the National Cholesterol Education Program's Step I and Step II dietary interventions on various cardiovascular disease risk factors. Reductions in plasma total cholesterol and LDL cholesterol concentrations were significantly correlated with reductions in percentages of total dietary fat, but these also included a decrease in saturated fatty acids. Similarly, individuals who consumed the Dietary Approaches to Stop Hypertension diet, which contains 27 percent of energy from fat and only 7 percent of energy from saturated fat, had reduced total and LDL cholesterol concentrations (Obarzanek et al., 2001b). Singh and colleagues (1992) reported that mortality from CHD and other causes was significantly lower when patients with acute myocardial infarction were fed a reduced fat diet.

The increase in LDL cholesterol concentration observed with increased fat intake is due to the strong positive association between total fat and saturated fat intake and the weak association between total fat and polyunsaturated fat intake (Masironi, 1970; Stamler, 1979). This association is also observed in Appendix Tables K-4, K-5, K-7, and K-8. As shown in many studies, saturated fatty acids raise LDL cholesterol concentrations (see Chapter 8), whereas unsaturated fatty acids do not. In fact, *n*-6 polyunsaturated fatty acids reduce serum LDL cholesterol concentrations somewhat compared with carbohydrate (Hegsted et al., 1993; Mensink and Katan, 1992). The adverse effects of saturated fats are discussed in Chapter 8.

It has been postulated that a high fat intake predisposes to a pro-thrombotic state, which contributes to venous thrombosis, coronary thrombosis, or thrombotic strokes (Barinagarrementeria et al., 1998; Kahn et al., 1997; Salomon et al., 1999). Consumption of diets high in fat (42 or 50 percent) have been shown to increase blood concentrations of the prothrombotic markers, blood coagulation factor VII (VIIc), and activated factor VII (VIIa) (Bladbjerg et al., 1994; Larsen et al., 1997). The concentration of factor VII is associated with increased risk of CHD (Kelleher, 1992). Furthermore, a significant and positive association was found between the level of dietary fat and factor VIIc concentration (Miller et al., 1989).

Relation of Intakes of Saturated Fatty Acids and Total Fat. When fat is consumed in typical foods it contains a mixture of saturated, polyunsaturated, and monounsaturated fatty acids. Even when the content of saturated fatty acids in consumed fats is relatively low, the intakes of these fatty acids can be high with high fat intakes. For example, if all of the dietary fats consumed were low in saturated fatty acids (e.g., 20 percent of fat energy), a total fat intake of 35 percent of total energy would yield a saturated fatty acid intake of 7 percent of total energy. Consumption of a variety of dietary fats would likely result in an even higher percentage of saturated fatty acids. Thus, in practical terms, it would be difficult to avoid high intakes of saturated fatty acids for most persons if total fat intakes exceeded 35 percent of total energy. This fact is revealed by attempts to create a variety of heart-healthy menus (National Cholesterol Education Program, 2001). Moreover, data from CSFII show that with increased fat intake, there tends to be a greater increase in saturated fatty acid intake relative to poly-unsaturated fatty acid intake (Appendix Tables K-4, K-5, K-7, K-8; Masironi, 1970; Stamler, 1979). It should be pointed out, however, that when replacing saturated fatty acid intake with carbohydrate, there is no effect on the total cholesterol:HDL cholesterol ratio (Mensink and Katan, 1992).

Conclusions. A few case-control studies have shown an association between total fat intake and risk for CHD. However, a detailed evaluation of these studies shows that it is not possible to separate total fat intake from saturated fatty acid intake, which is known to raise LDL cholesterol concentrations. Unsaturated fatty acids, which do not raise LDL cholesterol concentrations compared with carbohydrate, have not been implicated in risk for CHD through adverse effects on lipids or other risk factors. Nonetheless, practical efforts to create "heart-healthy" menus reveal that intakes of total fat exceeding 35 percent of total energy result in unacceptably high intakes

TABLE 11-7 Epidemiological Studies on Total Carbohydrate and Sugar Intake and Risk of Coronary Heart Disease (CHD)

Reference	Study Design	Results	Comments
Liu et al., 1982	Multi-country bivariate analysis		No significant association between sugar intake and CHD
McGee et al., 1984	7,088 men Prospective cohort, 10-y follow-up	Mean carbohydrate intake (% of energy) Non-CHD 46.5[a] CHD 45.0[b] Mean sugar intake (% of energy) Non-CHD 8.0[a] CHD 8.1[a]	Those who developed CHD consumed less energy as carbohydrates No association between sugar intake and risk of CHD
Kushi et al., 1985	1,001 men Prospective cohort, 20-y follow-up	Mean carbohydrate intake (% of energy) No CHD death 42.7[a] CHD death 41.2[b] Mean sugar intake (% of energy) No CHD death 17.3[a] CHD death 16.9[a]	Those who died from CHD consumed significantly less total carbohydrate No association between sugar intake and risk of CHD death

Bolton-Smith and Woodward, 1994	11,626 men and women Cross-sectional survey	Mean sugar intake (% of energy)		No association between risk of CHD and either intrinsic or extrinsic sugar intake

Intrinsic sugar	Men	Women
Control	2.06	3.31
CHD	1.89–2.19	3.15–3.31
Added sugar		
Control	11.2	8.55
CHD	10.5–11.4	8.63–9.10

Liu et al., 2000	75,521 women Prospective cohort, 10-y follow-up				No significant association between risk of CHD and total carbohydrate, sucrose, or fructose intake

Relative risk of CHD

Quintile of intake	Carbohydrate	Sucrose	Fructose
1	1.00	1.00	1.00
2	1.02	1.03	0.91
3	1.09	1.16	0.96
4	1.03	1.02	1.11
5	1.23	1.22	1.07

[a,b] Within each study, the mean sugar or carbohydrate intakes that are significantly different between treatment groups have a different superscript.

of saturated fatty acids. Moreover, there is the possibility that high fat intakes may enhance a prothrombotic state, although the evidence to support this mechanism for enhancing CHD risk is not strong enough alone to make solid recommendations.

Risk of Hyperinsulinemia, Glucose Intolerance, the Metabolic Syndrome, and Type 2 Diabetes

The metabolic syndrome (insulin-resistance syndrome) describes a clustering of metabolic abnormalities including insulin resistance (with or without glucose intolerance), an atherogenic lipid profile (high triacylglycerol concentration, low HDL cholesterol concentration, and high small, dense LDL), raised blood pressure, a prothrombotic state, and a proinflammatory state (Reaven, 2001). A prothrombotic state is characterized by elevations of plasminogen activator inhibitor and high fibrinogen concentrations, whereas a proinflammatory state is indicated by high c-reactive protein concentrations and other inflammatory markers. Abdominal obesity (waist circumference > 102 cm in men and 88 cm in women) is highly correlated with the presence of insulin resistance (NHLBI/NIDDK, 1998) and is considered to be one of the clinical components of the metabolic syndrome (National Cholesterol Education Program, 2001). An excess of intra-abdominal fat has been identified as being highly associated with the lipid risk factors of the metabolic syndrome (Després, 1993), although total abdominal fat appears to be even more highly predictive of the insulin resistance component of the syndrome (Abate et al., 1996; Peiris et al., 1988). Many persons with the metabolic syndrome eventually develop type 2 diabetes. Thus, both obesity and weight gain are undisputed as major risk factors for the development of type 2 diabetes (defined as fasting plasma glucose ≥ 7 mmol/L) (American Diabetes Association, 2001).

The contribution of diet per se to the development of type 2 diabetes is less clear. In some laboratory animals (e.g., some species of rodents), a high percentage of fat in the diet will induce insulin resistance (Budohoski et al., 1993; Chisholm and O'Dea, 1987). An important question is whether humans are similarly susceptible to this phenomenon independent of the effects of total fat intake on body fat content. Human studies do not provide a clear answer to this question. Thus, if higher intakes of total fat lead to obesity, this in and of itself will reduce insulin sensitivity and predispose to the metabolic syndrome and type 2 diabetes. Recent studies have demonstrated that reduced fat intake and weight loss result in improved glucose tolerance and reduced risk of type 2 diabetes (Swinburn et al., 2001; Tuomilehto et al., 2001).

Epidemiological Evidence. In several population studies, investigators have attempted to determine the contribution of total fat intake to either insulin sensitivity or diabetes. These analyses are difficult to interpret because of the multiplicity of potential confounding variables. Nevertheless, several studies have reported an association between higher fat intakes and insulin resistance as indicated by high fasting insulin concentration, impaired glucose tolerance, or impaired insulin sensitivity (Lovejoy and DiGirolamo, 1992; Marshall et al., 1991; Mayer et al., 1993), as well as to the development of type 2 diabetes (West and Kalbfleisch, 1971). A number of studies, however, have not shown this association (Coulston et al., 1983; Liu et al., 1983; Salmerón et al., 2001). In the Insulin Resistance Atherosclerosis Study, total fat intake univariately correlated with less insulin sensitivity (Mayer-Davis et al., 1997); however, in multiple regression analyses, the presence of obesity appeared to be a confounding variable. Lovejoy and DiGirolamo (1992) likewise found intercorrelations among insulin resistance, total fat intake, and obesity. In contrast, Larsson and coworkers (1999) found no evidence of independent effects of diet on insulin secretory or sensitivity among 74 postmenopausal women. Although several studies suggest an association between total fat intake and the presence of insulin resistance (Lovejoy, 1999; Vessby, 2000), the degree to which the relationship is mediated by obesity remains uncertain. Decreased physical activity is also a significant predictor of higher postprandial insulin concentrations and may confound some studies (Feskens et al., 1994; Parker et al., 1993).

Interventional Evidence. A number of metabolic and intervention studies have examined the relationships among fat intake, fasting glucose and insulin concentrations, areas under curves for plasma glucose and insulin concentrations, insulin sensitivity, glucose effectiveness, and glucose disposal rates (Table 11-8). Several studies reported that diets containing 35 percent fat were accompanied by more impaired glucose tolerance than diets containing 25 percent fat or less (Fukagawa et al., 1990; Jeppesen et al., 1997; Straznicky et al., 1999; Swinburn et al., 1991). Coulston and coworkers (1983) found that a diet containing 41 percent fat led to significantly higher concentrations of insulin in response to meals compared with a diet containing 21 percent fat, but there were no alterations in fasting concentrations. In other studies, no effect on measures of glucose tolerance were reported when diets varied in fat content from 11 to 30 (Leclerc et al., 1993) or 20 to 50 percent fat (Abbott et al., 1989; Borkman et al., 1991; Howard et al., 1991; Thomsen et al., 1999). When the diet was high in fat (50 percent of energy), the area under the curve for plasma glucose and insulin concentration was lower than when the diet had a low fat content (25 percent of energy) (Yost et al., 1998). In this study, the decreased

TABLE 11-8 Interventional Studies on the Effect of Dietary Fat on the Metabolic Parameters for Glucose and Insulin in Healthy Individuals

Reference	Study Design	Percent of Fat	Fasting Glucose	Fasting Insulin
Coulston et al., 1983	11 men and women 10-d crossover	41–21	NSC[a]	NSC
Chen et al., 1988	8 young men 3- to 5-d crossover	0		
		42	ND	ND
		55	ND	ND
	10 elderly men 3- to 5-d crossover	0–37	ND	ND
Abbott et al., 1989	9 men and women 5-wk crossover	42–21	NSC	NSC
Fukagawa et al., 1990	6 young men 21- to 28-d intervention	42–14	Decreased[b]	Decreased[b]
	6 elderly men and women 21- to 28-d intervention	38–15	Decreased[b]	Decreased[b]
Borkman et al., 1991	8 men and women 3-wk crossover	20–50	NSC	NSC
Howard et al., 1991	7 men and women 5- to 7-wk crossover	42–21	NSC	NSC
	9 men and women 3- to 5-wk longitudinal	42–21	NSC	NSC
	12 Caucasians and 12 Pima Indians 2-wk crossover	15–50	Increased[d]	NSC

Area Under the Curve for Glucose	Area Under the Curve for Insulin	Insulin Sensitivity	Glucose Effectiveness	Glucose Disposal/ Disappearance Rate
NSC	Decreased[b]	ND[c]	ND	ND
ND	ND	Decreased[b]	NSC	ND
ND	ND	Increased[b]	NSC	ND
ND	ND	Decreased[b]	NSC	ND
ND	ND	ND	ND	ND
ND	ND	ND	ND	Increased[b]
ND	ND	ND	ND	NSC
ND	ND	ND	ND	NSC
NSC	ND	ND	ND	ND
ND	ND	ND	ND	ND
Increased[e]	Increased[e]	NSC	Decreased[d]	ND

continued

TABLE 11-8 Continued

Reference	Study Design	Percent of Fat	Fasting Glucose	Fasting Insulin
Swinburn et al., 1991	24 Caucasians and Pima Indians 2-wk crossover	15–50	Increased[d]	NSC
Leclerc et al., 1993	7 men and women 7-d crossover	11–30	NSC	NSC
Jeppesen et al., 1997	10 women 3-wk crossover	25–45	ND	ND
Yost et al., 1998	25 men and women 15-d crossover	25–50	NSC	NSC
Straznicky et al., 1999	14 men 2-wk crossover	25–47	Increased[b]	NSC
Thomsen et al., 1999	16 men and women 4-wk crossover	28–42	NSC	NSC
Kasim-Karakas et al., 2000	54 postmenopausal women 4- to 12-mo crossover	15, 25, and 34	NSC	NSC

[a] NSC = no significant change.
[b] $p < 0.05$.
[c] ND = no data available.
[d] $p < 0.001$.
[e] $p < 0.01$.

fat intake was accompanied by an increased percentage of energy from carbohydrate. Garg and coworkers (1992b) reported that insulin sensitivity, indicated by insulin-mediated glucose disposal, was similar after almost a month of ingestion of either a reduced fat (25 percent of energy) or an increased fat diet (50 percent of energy). However, favorable effects of substituting a monounsaturated fat diet for a saturated fat diet on insulin sensitivity were seen at a total fat intake of up to 37 percent of energy (Vessby et al., 2001). A large, long-term intervention trial in adults showed that reducing total fat intake, in part, reduced the risk of the onset of type 2 diabetes by 58 percent (Tuomilehto et al., 2001). Similarly, the Diabetes Prevention Program Research Group reported that diet modification,

Area Under the Curve for Glucose	Area Under the Curve for Insulin	Insulin Sensitivity	Glucose Effectiveness	Glucose Disposal/ Disappearance Rate
Increased[e]	Increased[e]	NSC	Decreased[d]	ND
NSC	NSC	ND	ND	ND
NSC	Increased[d]	ND	ND	ND
Decreased[e]	Decreased[c]	ND	ND	ND
Increased[e]	NSC	Decreased[b]	ND	ND
ND	NSC	NSC	NSC	ND
ND	ND	ND	ND	ND

including a reduction of total fat intake from 34 to 27 percent of energy reduced the incidence of type 2 diabetes by 58 percent. Thus, there is no definitive evidence from metabolic and interventional studies that higher fat intakes impair insulin sensitivity in humans as they do in various laboratory animals. Any suggestive links between fat intake and either insulin secretion or sensitivity may be mediated through confounding factors, such as body-fat content, making it difficult to detect any independent contribution of total fat intake to insulin sensitivity.

Conclusions. Although high fat diets can induce insulin resistance in rodents, investigations in humans fail to confirm this effect. Moreover, an association between dietary fat intake and risk for diabetes has been reported in some epidemiological studies, but this association is most likely confounded by various factors, such as obesity and glycemic index.

Risk of Cancer

High intakes of dietary fat have been implicated in the development of cancer, especially cancer of the lung, breast, colon, and prostate gland. Early support for this theory comes from laboratory animal and cross-cultural studies. The latter were based largely on international food disappearance data and migrant and time trend studies. In recent years, the theory that a diet high in fat predisposes to certain cancers has been weakened by additional epidemiological studies. Early cross-cultural and case-control studies reported strong associations between total fat intake and breast cancer (Howe et al., 1991; Miller et al., 1978; van't Veer et al., 1990), yet a number of epidemiological studies, most in the last 15 years, have found little or no association between fat intake and breast cancer (Hunter et al., 1996; Jones et al., 1987; Kushi et al., 1992; van den Brandt et al., 1993; Velie et al., 2000; Willett et al., 1987, 1992). A meta-analysis of 23 studies yielded a relative risk of 1.01 and 1.21 from cohort and case-control studies, respectively (Boyd et al., 1993).

Total fat intake in relation to colon cancer has strong support from animal studies (Reddy, 1992). However, evidence from epidemiological studies has been mixed (De Stefani et al., 1997b; Giovannucci et al., 1994; Willett et al., 1990). Howe and colleagues (1997) reported no association between fat intake and risk of colorectal cancer from the combined analysis of 13 case-control studies.

Epidemiological studies tend to suggest that dietary fat intake is not associated with prostate cancer (Ramon et al., 2000; Veierød et al., 1997b). Giovannucci and coworkers (1993), however, reported a positive association between total fat consumption, primarily animal fat, and risk of advanced prostate cancer. Findings on the association between fat intake and lung cancer have been mixed (De Stefani et al., 1997a; Goodman et al., 1988; Veierød et al., 1997a; Wu et al., 1994).

Risk of Nutrient Inadequacy or Excess

Diets High in Fat. With increasing intakes of carbohydrate, and therefore decreasing fat intakes, there is a trend towards reduced consumption of dietary fiber, folate, and vitamin C (Appendix K). With higher fat intakes, it is difficult to create practical high fat menus that do not contain unacceptably high amounts of saturated fatty acids (National Cholesterol Education Program, 2001).

Diets Low in Total Sugars. Micronutrient inadequacy can occur when sugars intake is very low (less than 4 percent of total energy) (Bolton-Smith and Woodward, 1995) because many foods that are abundant in micronutrients, such as fruits and dairy products, also contain naturally occurring sugars. A wide variety of foods from different food groups are needed to meet nutrient requirements. Because sugars are important for the palatability of foods, the complete omission of sugars from the diet could endanger overall nutrient adequacy by leading to low total energy intake, as well as low micronutrient intakes (Bolton-Smith, 1996). Although reduced nutrient intakes have been reported, adverse affects on health have not. Individuals with fructose intolerance, a condition caused by fructose-1-phosphate aldolase deficiency, strictly avoid foods containing fructose and sucrose and yet remain in good health (Burmeister et al., 1991).

AMDRs for Adults

When fat intakes are low and carbohydrate intakes are high, intervention studies, with the support of epidemiological studies, demonstrate a reduction in plasma HDL cholesterol concentration, an increase in the plasma total cholesterol:HDL cholesterol ratio, and an increase in plasma triacylglycerol concentration, which are all consistent with an increased risk of CHD. Conversely, many interventional studies show that when fat intake is high, many individuals consume additional energy, and therefore gain additional weight. Weight gain on high fat diets can be detrimental to individuals already susceptible to obesity and can worsen the metabolic consequences of obesity, particularly the risk of CHD. Moreover, high fat diets are usually accompanied by increased intakes of saturated fatty acids, which can raise plasma LDL cholesterol concentrations and further increase risk for CHD. Based on the apparent risk for CHD that may occur on low fat diets, and the risk for increased energy intake and therefore obesity with the consumption of high fat diets, the AMDR for fat and carbohydrate is estimated to be 20 to 35 and 45 to 65 percent of energy, respectively, for all adults. By consuming fat and carbohydrate within these ranges, the risk for obesity, as well as for CHD and diabetes, can be kept at a minimum. Furthermore, these ranges allow for sufficient intakes of essential nutrients while keeping the intake of saturated fatty acids at moderate levels.

There is no lower limit of intake and no known adverse effects with the chronic consumption of *Dietary Fiber* or *Functional Fiber* (Chapter 7). Therefore, an AMDR is not set for *Dietary, Functional,* or *Total Fiber.*

Maximal Intake Level for Added Sugars

Data from various national surveys show that increasing intakes of added sugars is associated with a decline in the consumption of certain micronutrients, thus increasing the prevalence of those consuming below the EAR or the AI. While such trends exist, it is not possible to determine a defined intake level at which inadequate micronutrient intakes occur. Furthermore, at very low or very high intakes, unusual eating habits most likely exist that allow for other factors to contribute to low micronutrient intakes. Based on the available data, no more than 25 energy from added sugars should be comsumed by adults. A daily intake of added sugars that individuals should aim for to achieve a healthy diet was not set. Total sugars intake can be lowered by consuming primarily sugars that are naturally occurring and present in micronutrient-rich foods, such as milk, dairy products, and fruits, while at the same time limiting consumption of added sugars from foods and beverages that contain minimal amounts of micronutrients, such as soft drinks, fruitades, and candies.

Low Fat, High Carbohydrate Diets of Children

Fat Oxidation

Jones and colleagues (1998) reported a significantly greater fat oxidation in children (aged 5 to 10 years, $n = 12$) than in adults (aged 20 to 30 years, $n = 6$). Breath $^{13}CO_2$ was measured in 12 children and 6 men following an oral bolus dose of [1-^{13}C]palmitic acid (10 mg/kg of body weight) consumed with a test meal. Breath $^{13}CO_2$ excretion was less in the men (35.1 percent of absorbed dose, $P = 0.005$) than in the children (57.0 percent of absorbed dose). The children exhibited greater fat oxidation in the postabsorptive state (2.43 g/h) and postprandial (11.89 g/6 h) states than the men (0.93 g/h postabsorptive, 9.86 g/6 h postprandial). The children also had greater fat oxidation compared with women studied previously by these investigators (0.53 g/h postabsorptive, 0.03 g/6 h postprandial) (Murphy et al., 1995).

Growth

Most studies have reported no effect of the level of dietary fat on growth when energy intake is adequate (Boulton and Magarey, 1995; Fomon et al., 1976; Lagström et al., 1999; Lapinleimu et al., 1995; Niinikoski et al., 1997a, 1997b; Obarzanek et al., 1997; Shea et al., 1993). Two well-controlled trials demonstrated that a diet providing less than 30 percent energy from fat does not result in adverse effects on growth in children up to 8 years of age (Lapinleimu et al., 1995; Niinikoski et al., 1997a, 1997b). A cohort study with a 25-month follow-up showed that there was no difference in stature or growth of children aged 3 to 4 years at baseline across quintiles (27 to 38 percent) of total fat intake (Shea et al., 1993). The Special Turku Coronary Risk Factor Intervention Project showed no difference in growth of children 7 months to 5 years of age when they consumed 21 to 38 percent fat (Lagström et al., 1999). Niinikoski and coworkers (1997a) reported that 1-year-old children who consistently consumed low fat diets (less than 28 percent) grew as well as children with higher fat intakes. A cohort study showed that children aged 2 years in the lower tertile of fat intake (less than 30 percent) had a height and weight similar to that of the higher fat intake groups (Boulton and Magarey, 1995).

A few studies have observed impaired growth among hypercholesterolemic children who were advised to consume 30 percent or less of energy from fat. However, the energy intake was also reduced (Lifshitz and Moses, 1989) or not reported (Hansen et al., 1992). In a group of Canadian children 3 to 6 years of age, a fat intake of less than 30 percent of energy was associated with an odds ratio of 2.3 for weight-for-age below the 50th percentile at 6 years of age (Vobecky et al., 1995). A comprehensive evaluation of the effect of diet-related variables on the growth of children under 6 years of age from 18 Latin American countries (FAO/WHO, 1996) demonstrated that diets providing less than 22 percent energy from fat and with less than 45 percent of total fat from animal fat were related to low birth weight, underweight, and stunting (height-for-age ≤ 2 standard deviations) (Uauy et al., 2000). The dietary determinants that best explained low birth weight were energy, protein, and animal fat, suggesting that high-quality animal protein and associated nutrients are important for growth and development.

Risk of Nutrient Inadequacy or Excess

Diets High in Carbohydrate and Low in Fats. Because the diets of young children are less diversified than that of adults, the risk of inadequate micronutrient intake is increased in these children. A cohort of 500 children aged 3 to 6 years showed that those who consumed less than 30 percent of energy from fat consumed less vitamin A, vitamin D, and vitamin E compared with those who consumed higher intakes of fat (30 to 40 percent) (Vobecky et al., 1995). Calcium intakes decreased by more than 100 mg/d for 4- and 6-year-old children who consumed less than 30 percent of energy from fat (Boulton and Magarey, 1995). Lagström and coworkers (1997, 1999), however, did not observe reduced intakes of micronutrients in children with low fat intakes (26 percent).

The Dietary Intervention Study in Children (DISC), a multi-center, randomized trial of children 8 to 10 years of age, demonstrated that reducing the intake of fat to 28 percent of energy over a 3-year period increased the percentage of children not meeting the RDA for vitamin E and zinc; however, no biochemical evidence of deficiency of these nutrients was found (Obarzanek et al., 1997). Tonstad and Sivertsen (1997) observed no reduced intake of micronutrients with diets providing 25 percent of energy as fat. Nicklas and coworkers (1992) reported reduced intakes of certain micronutrients by 10-year-old children who consumed less than 30 percent of energy as fat; however, this level of fat intake was associated with marked increased intakes of candy. It has been suggested that children who consume a low fat diet can meet their micronutrient recommendation by appropriate selection of certain low fat foods (Peterson and Sigman-Grant, 1997). This is especially true for older children whose diets are typically more diverse.

The tables in Appendix K show the intakes of nutrients at various intake levels of carbohydrate. With increasing intakes of carbohydrate, and therefore decreasing intakes of fat, the intake levels of calcium and zinc markedly decreased in children 1 to 18 years of age (Appendix Tables K-1 through K-3).

Diets High in Added Sugars. Several surveys have evaluated the impact of added sugars intake on micronutrient intakes in children (Table 11-5). Gibson (1997) examined data from the U.K. National Diet and Nutrition Survey of Children Aged 1.5 to 4.5 Years (boys, $n = 848$; girls, $n = 827$) and found evidence of a nutrient dilution effect by nonmilk extrinsic sugars (NMES). Children consuming the highest concentrations of NMES (greater than 24 percent of energy) had intakes of most micronutrients that were between 6 and 20 percent below average. Gibson (1997) concluded that the inverse association of NMES with micronutrient intakes was of most significance for the 20 percent of children with the diets highest in NMES (24.9 percent of energy for boys and 24.5 percent of energy for girls).

In a study of British adolescents, reduced intakes of calcium, phosphorus, iron, vitamin A, vitamin D, and folic acid were associated with increased sugars intakes (mean added sugars intake for the high sugars consumers was 122 g/d for boys and 119 g/d for girls) (Rugg-Gunn et al., 1991). In a smaller survey ($n = 143$), added sugars intakes at levels as high as 27 percent of energy did not have a significant impact on micronutrient intakes (Nelson, 1991).

Similar to that observed for adults using data from NHANES III, increasing the added sugars intake by every 5th percentile tended to be associated with reduced intakes of certain micronutrients, including calcium, vitamin A, iron, and zinc (Appendix Tables J-1 through J-3, J-6, and J-7). This reduction in micronutrient intake was most significant when added sugars intake levels exceeded 25 percent of energy.

From 1989 to 1995, energy intakes increased for U.S. children aged 2 to 17 years primarily due to increased carbohydrate consumption. Beverages, particularly soft drinks, were important contributors to the increased carbohydrate consumption. During this period, micronutrient intakes (except for iron) did not increase and calcium intakes decreased. This was attributed to the fact that increased energy was largely obtained from soft drinks, which do not add nutrients and displace milk in children's diets, with negative consequences for total diet quality (Morton and Guthrie, 1998).

Children who were high consumers of nondiet soft drinks had lower intakes of riboflavin, folate, vitamin A, vitamin C, calcium, and phosphorus in comparison with children who were nonconsumers of soft drinks (Harnack et al., 1999). Several of these nutrients (folate, vitamin A, and calcium) have been identified in national surveys as "shortfall" or "problem" nutrients among various age and gender groups (ARS, 1998). Ballew and colleagues (2000) demonstrated that in U.S. children, milk consumption was positively associated with the likelihood of achieving recommended vitamin A, vitamin B_{12}, folate, calcium, and magnesium intakes in all age groups. Juice (100 percent fruit or vegetable juice) consumption was positively associated with achieving vitamin C and folate recommended intakes in all age groups, as well as magnesium intake among children aged 6 years and older. Soft drink intake was negatively associated with achieving recommended vitamin A intake in all age groups, calcium in children younger than 12 years of age, and magnesium in children 6 years of age and older.

Others have shown that children who consumed milk at the noon meal had the highest daily intakes of vitamin A, vitamin E, calcium, and zinc, whereas the opposite was true for children who consumed soft drinks and tea (Johnson et al., 1998). Hence, beverages that are major contributors of the naturally occurring sugars, such as lactose and fructose, in the diet (e.g., milk and fruit juice) have been positively associated with nutrient adequacy, while beverages that are the principal source of added sugars in the diet (e.g., soft drinks) have been negatively associated with nutrient adequacy in the diets of U.S. children and adolescents (Ballew et al., 2000; Johnson et al., 1998).

Diets High in Total Sugars. The findings from three surveys on the relationship between total sugars intake and micronutrient intake in children are mixed (Table 11-6). Gibson (1993) did not observe reduced micronutrient intakes when total sugars intake exceeded 25 percent of energy. Nicklas and coworkers (1996) reported that the percent of children meeting the RDA for only niacin and zinc was significantly reduced when the intake of total sugars exceeded 31 percent of energy. A linear reduction in several micronutrients was observed with increasing total sugars intake (Farris et al., 1998).

High Fat, Low Carbohydrate Diets of Children

Risk of Obesity

In the United States and Canada, there is evidence that children are becoming progressively overweight (Flegal, 1999; Gortmaker et al., 1987; Tremblay and Willms, 2000; Troiano et al., 1995). Furthermore, Serdula and coworkers (1993) reviewed a number of longitudinal studies with varying cut-off levels for obesity and concluded that 26 to 41 percent of obese preschool children and 42 to 63 percent of obese school-age children became obese adults. Clinical evidence of disease associated with excess body weight, reduced physical activity, or high dietary fat intakes, however, are generally absent. The evidence for a role of dietary fat intakes in promoting higher energy intakes and thus promoting obesity in young children is conflicting.

A positive trend in energy intake was associated with an increased percent of energy from fat for children up to 8 years of age (Boulton and Magarey, 1995). A positive correlation between fat intake and fat mass has been reported for boys 4 to 7 years of age (Nguyen et al., 1996). A lack of effect of dietary fat on BMI and adiposity, however, has been reported for children 1.5 to 4.5 years of age (Atkin and Davies, 2000; Davies, 1997).

The DISC trial found no difference in BMI for children 8 to 10 years of age who consumed diets containing 29 or 33 percent fat over a 3-year period (Lauer et al., 2000). However, several studies showed a positive correlation between dietary fat intake and body fatness in children 8 to 12 years of age (Maffeis et al., 1996; Obarzanek et al., 1994; Ricketts, 1997). The average fat intake of nonobese children was measured to be 31 to 34 percent for children 9 to 11 years old, whereas the average fat intake of obese children was 39 percent of energy (Gazzaniga and Burns, 1993). A positive association between fat intake and several adiposity indices were observed, but only for up to 35 percent of energy (Maillard et al., 2000). Other factors that have been associated with increased BMI include physical activity.

Risk of CHD

Clinical studies have provided some evidence that serum cholesterol concentration is modified in children the same way as in adults, with serum total, LDL, and non-HDL cholesterol concentrations being increased by consuming diets higher in total fat (Lauer et al., 2000; Niinikoski et al., 1996; Obarzanek et al., 2001a; Shannon et al., 1994; Simell et al., 2000; Vartiainen et al., 1986). However, no significant association between dietary fat and LDL cholesterol concentration was observed for boys and girls (aged 8 to 10 years) consuming fat ranging from 10 to 50 percent of energy ($R = -0.04$ to 0.14) (Kwiterovich et al., 1997). Furthermore, a significant positive association between fat intake and total cholesterol concentration was observed in only two of five countries (Knuiman et al., 1983).

Another potential indicator for children's future risk of CHD is the presence of fatty streaks, which are found in the aortas of almost all children over 3 years of age in North America (Holman et al., 1958), and begin to appear in the coronary arteries about 5 to 10 years later than in the aorta (Berenson et al., 1992; McGill, 1968; Stary, 1989; Strong et al., 1992). The prevalence of aortic fatty streaks differs only slightly among children and adolescents of all populations studied, regardless of the frequency of atherosclerosis and coronary artery disease in adults of the respective population (Holman et al., 1958; McGill, 1968). The absence of a relation between aortic fatty streaks and the clinically relevant lesions of atherosclerosis in epidemiological and histological studies has thus raised questions on the clinical significance of fatty streaks in the aorta of young children (Newman et al., 1995; Olson, 2000). The Pathobiological Determinants of Atherosclerosis in Youth Study, however, has provided evidence that an unfavorable lipoprotein pattern (i.e., elevated non-HDL cholesterol and low HDL cholesterol concentrations), obesity, and hyperglycemia are associated with raised fatty streaks in the coronary artery and abdominal aorta in late teenage years (McGill et al., 2000a, 2000b). Similarly, the Bogalusa Heart Study observed a positive association between LDL cholesterol concentration and the percentage of surface with fatty streaks in the aorta (Berenson et al., 1992). These findings are consistent with the hypothesis of the progression of fatty streaks to fibrous plaques under the influence of the prevailing risk factors for coronary artery disease (McGill et al., 2000a, 2000b).

It is still unclear, however, how reduction in serum cholesterol concentration in childhood, if maintained, is associated with risk of CHD in adulthood. In addition, there are still pivotal issues that must be examined further, including the relationship between fatty streaks found in the arteries of young children and the later appearance of raised lesions associated with coronary vascular disease, the effects of dietary total fat modification on predictive risk factors in children, the safety of the diet with respect to total energy and micronutrients for the general population, and the long-term health benefit of establishing healthy dietary patterns early in childhood.

Risk of Nutrient Inadequacy or Excess

Appendix Tables K-1 through K-3 and K-6 provide data from CFSII on the intake of various nutrients based on the level of carbohydrate intake. It can been seen from these tables that as the level of carbohydrate intake decreases, and therefore the level of fat increases, certain nutrients such as folate and vitamin C markedly decrease. Furthermore, with increasing levels of fat intake, the intake of saturated fat relative to linoleic acid intake markedly increases.

AMDRs for Children

The evidence suggests that children have a higher fat oxidation rate compared to adults, and that reduced intake of certain micronutrients can occur with the consumption of low fat diets, whereas there is potential risk of obesity with high fat intakes. High intakes of fat may promote increased risk for CHD and obesity. Dietary fat provides energy, which may be important for younger children with reduced food intakes, particularly during the transition from a diet high in milk to a mixed diet. Thus, there should be a transition from the high fat intake during infancy (55 and 40 percent of energy for the 0- to 6- and 7- to 12-months age groups, respectively) (Chapter 8) to an AMDR for adults (20 to 35 percent of energy). Therefore, it is estimated that the AMDR for fat intake is approximately 30 to 40 percent of energy for children 1 to 3 years of age and 25 to 35 percent of energy for children 4 to 18 years of age. The AMDR for carbohydrate is the same as for adults (45 to 65 percent of energy). The ranges of fat intake include intakes of saturated fat that should be consumed at levels as low as possible while consuming a nutritionally adequate diet.

Maximal Intake Level for Added Sugars

As for adults, no more than 25 percent of energy from added sugars should be consumed by children to ensure adequate micronutrient intakes. For those children whose intake is above this level, added sugars intake can be reduced by consuming sugars that are primarily naturally occurring and present in foods such as milk, dairy products, and fruits, which also contain essential micronutrients.

n-9 MONOUNSATURATED FATTY ACIDS

Approximately 20 to 40 percent of fat is consumed as n-9 mono-unsaturated fatty acids, almost all of which is oleic acid (Appendix Tables E-1 and E-8). Monounsaturated fatty acids are not essential fatty acids, but they may have some benefit in the prevention of chronic disease. Although early research pointed to this potential benefit, most attention has been given to it in the past decade.

Low n-9 Monounsaturated Fatty Acid Diets

Risk of CHD

Epidemiological Evidence. Population data on monounsaturated fatty acid intake and risk of coronary heart disease (CHD) are limited. However, in long-term follow-up studies of the Seven Countries Study, higher intakes of monounsaturated fatty acids were associated with decreased rates of CHD mortality (Keys et al., 1986). Other reports indicate that monounsaturated fatty acids have a neutral or beneficial effect on risk (Hu et al., 1997; Kromhout and de Lezenne Coulander, 1984; Pietinen et al., 1997).

Interventional Evidence. Much work has been conducted and is ongoing to identify the ideal substitute for saturated fat in a blood cholesterol-lowering diet. The effects of a high monounsaturated fatty acid versus a low fat, high carbohydrate diet on serum lipid and lipoprotein concentrations have been a focus of considerable scientific inquiry. Eighteen well-controlled clinical studies that compared the effects of substituting monounsaturated fatty acids versus carbohydrate for saturated fat in a blood cholesterol-lowering diet have recently been reviewed (Kris-Etherton et al., 2000). In these studies, when on both high monounsaturated fat and low fat, high carbohydrate diets, saturated fatty acids contributed to 4 to 12 percent of energy and dietary cholesterol varied from less than 100 up to 410 mg/d. Diets high in monounsaturated fatty acids provided 17 to 33 percent of energy from monounsaturated fatty acids and contained more total fat (33 to 50 percent energy) than the low fat, high carbohydrate diets (18 to 30 percent energy). The low fat, high carbohydrate diets provided 55 to 67 percent of energy from carbohydrate. Compared to baseline values, serum total cholesterol concentrations changed from −17 to +3 percent on the low fat, high carbohydrate diet, whereas it changed from −20 to −3 percent on the high monounsaturated fatty acid diet. The range of decrease in plasma low density lipoprotein (LDL) cholesterol concentration was similar (−22 to +1 percent) among individuals on the two diets. The change in serum triacylglycerol concentrations ranged from −23 to +37 percent for individuals consuming the low fat, high carbohydrate diets and from −43 to +12 percent for diets high in monounsaturated fatty acids. Changes in high density lipoprotein (HDL) cholesterol concentrations ranged from −25 to +2 percent for individuals on the low fat, high carbohydrate diets compared to a −9 to +6 percent change for individuals on diets high in monounsaturated fatty acids.

These data indicate that in weight-stable individuals, a high mono-unsaturated fatty acid, low saturated fatty acid diet results in a more favor-able metabolic profile with respect to total cholesterol, HDL cholesterol, and triacylglycerol concentrations. Figure 11-4 shows that with increased monounsaturated fatty acid intake, there is a favorable reduction in the total cholesterol:HDL cholesterol ratio. Furthermore, a meta-analysis of feeding studies estimated that the regression coefficients for the effects of monounsaturated fatty acids on LDL and HDL cholesterol concentrations were −0.008 and +0.006, respectively, suggesting a slight positive benefit (Clarke et al., 1997).

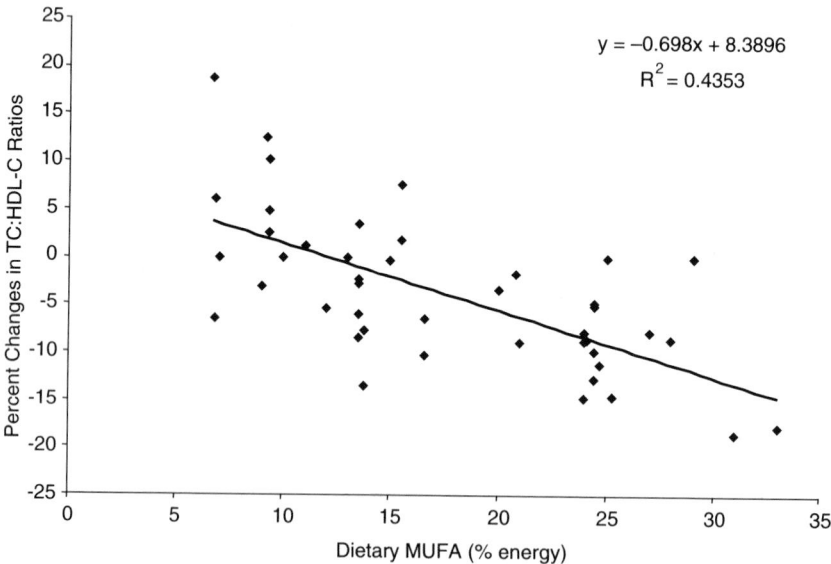

FIGURE 11-4 Relationship between monounsaturated fatty acid (MUFA) intake and total cholesterol (TC):high density lipoprotein cholesterol (HDL-C) concen-tration ratio. Weighted least-squares regression analyses were performed using the mixed procedure to test for differences in lipid concentrations (SAS Statistical package, version 8.00, SAS Institute, Inc., 1999).
DATA SOURCES: Berry et al. (1992); Curb et al. (2000); Garg et al. (1988, 1992a, 1994); Ginsberg et al. (1990); Grundy (1986); Grundy et al. (1988); Jansen et al. (1998); Kris-Etherton et al. (1999); Lefevre et al., unpublished; Lopez-Segura et al. (1996); Mensink and Katan (1987); Nelson et al. (1995); Parillo et al. (1992); Pelkman et al. (2001); Perez-Jimenez et al. (1995, 1999, 2001).

Risk of Diabetes

Epidemiological studies tend to suggest no association between monounsaturated fatty acid intake and risk of indicators for diabetes (Feskens et al., 1995; Marshall et al., 1997). Similarly, some intervention studies showed no effect of monounsaturated fatty acid intake on indicators for risk of diabetes (Fasching et al., 1996; Roche et al., 1998; Thomsen et al., 1999; Vessby et al., 2001). Uusitupa and coworkers (1994), however, reported a significantly lower area under the curve for plasma glucose concentration and a greater glucose disappearance rate when healthy women consumed a diet rich in monounsaturated fatty acids (19 to 20 percent) compared with a diet rich in saturated fatty acids.

Risk of Cancer

Bartsch and colleagues (1999) reported a protective effect of oleic acid on cancer of the breast, colon, and possibly the prostate. A few epidemiological studies have reported an inverse relationship between monounsaturated fatty acid intake and risk of breast cancer (Willett et al., 1992; Wolk et al., 1998), while a number of studies reported no association (Holmes et al., 1999; Hunter et al., 1996; Jones et al., 1987; Kushi et al., 1992; van den Brandt et al., 1993; van't Veer et al., 1990). Increased consumption of olive oil was associated with significantly reduced breast cancer risk (La Vecchia et al., 1995; Martin-Moreno et al., 1994; Trichopoulou et al., 1995).

A diet high in monounsaturated fatty acid-rich vegetable oils, including olive, canola, or peanut oils, has been associated with a protective effect or no risk of prostate cancer (Norrish et al., 2000; Ramon et al., 2000; Schuurman et al., 1999; Veierød et al., 1997b). Some speculate that the apparent protective effects of olive oil (and other vegetable oils) reflect constituents other than monounsaturated fatty acids including squalene (Newmark, 1999), phenolic compounds, antioxidants, and other compounds (Owen et al., 2000).

No significant association has been reported for monounsaturated fatty acid intake and risk of colorectal cancer (Giovannucci et al., 1994; Howe et al., 1997).

Risk of Nutrient Inadequacy

In the United States, monounsaturated fatty acids provide 12 to 13 percent of energy intake. About 50 percent of these fatty acids are consumed via animal products, primarily meat fat (Jonnalagadda et al., 1995). Vegetable oils that are good sources of monounsaturated fatty acids include canola oil and olive oil. Although the major sources of monounsaturated fatty acids (animal fat and vegetable oils) are not required to supply essential nutrients, very low intakes of monounsaturated fatty acids would require increased intakes of other types of fatty acids to achieve recommended fat intakes. Consequently, intakes of saturated and *n*-6 polyunsaturated fatty acids would probably exceed a desirable level of intake (see "*n*-6 Polyunsaturated Fatty Acids" and Chapter 8).

High n-9 Monounsaturated Fatty Acid Diets

There are limited data on the adverse health effects from consuming high levels of *n*-9 monounsaturated fatty acids (see Chapter 8, "Tolerable Upper Intake Levels").

Acceptable Macronutrient Distribution Range

n-9 Monounsaturated fatty acids are not essential in the diet, and the evidence relating low and high intakes of monounsaturated fatty acids and chronic disease is limited. Therefore, an Acceptable Macronutrient Distribution Range (AMDR) for *n*-9 monounsaturated fatty acids is not provided. Nonetheless, practical limits on intakes of monounsaturated fatty acids will be imposed by AMDRs for total fat and other types of fatty acids.

n-6 POLYUNSATURATED FATTY ACIDS

Low n-6 Polyunsaturated Fatty Acid Diets

Risk of CHD

Epidemiological Evidence. Many populations of the world, such as in Crete and Japan, have low total intakes of *n*-6 polyunsaturated fatty acids (e.g., < 4 percent of total energy) without obvious health consequences (Okita et al., 1995; Renaud et al., 1995). However, high intakes of *n*-6 polyunsaturated fats have been associated with blood lipid profiles (e.g., reduced total and low density lipoprotein [LDL] cholesterol, reduced triacylglycerol, and increased high density lipoprotein [HDL] cholesterol concentrations) that are associated with low risk of coronary heart disease (CHD) (Arntzenius et al., 1985; Becker et al., 1983; Sonnenberg et al., 1996). Prospective epidemiological evidence suggests that after controlling for other components of the diet, replacing saturated fats with unsaturated fats decreases risk of CHD (Hu et al., 1997); however, the dose–response relationship between *n*-6 fatty acids and risk of CHD was not adequately established with certainty. An inverse association between linoleic acid intake and risk of coronary death was observed in several prospective studies (Arntzenius et al., 1985; Gartside and Glueck, 1993), while Pietinen and coworkers (1997) did not observe a relationship between linoleic acid intake and risk of CHD. A cross-sectional study showed that linoleic acid was inversely related to the prevalence of CHD, and this effect was stronger with higher intakes of linolenic acid (Djoussé et al., 2001). It is difficult to provide a direct assessment of *n*-6 fatty acids on risk of CHD without taking into consideration the impact of several dietary and nondietary factors, in addition to serum cholesterol concentrations, that lead to CHD and may be modified by the intake of saturated fat and *n*-6 fatty acids.

Interventional Evidence. From the standpoint of blood lipid concentration and CHD, higher *n*-6 polyunsaturated fatty acid intake generally alters blood lipid concentration to result in a decreased risk profile (Katan et al., 1994) (Table 11-9). Controlled trials have examined the effects of substituting *n*-6 fatty acids in the diet to replace carbohydrate or saturated fatty acids (Mensink et al., 1992). In general, any fat that replaces carbohydrate in the diet raises HDL cholesterol and decreases triacylglycerol concentrations, with only small differences between individual fatty acids. *n*-6 Fatty acids decrease LDL cholesterol concentrations to a much greater degree than do saturated fatty acids (Mensink et al., 1992).

Risk of Diabetes

A number of epidemiological studies have been conducted to ascertain whether the quality of fat can affect the risk for diabetes. An inverse relationship was reported for vegetable fats and polyunsaturated fats and risk of diabetes (Colditz et al., 1992; Salmerón et al., 2001; Trevisan et al., 1990). One study reported a positive association between 2-hour glucose concentrations and polyunsaturated fatty acid intake (Mooy et al., 1995). A review of epidemiological studies on this relationship concluded that higher intakes of polyunsaturated fats could be beneficial in reducing the risk for diabetes (Hu et al., 2001).

Risk of Nutrient Inadequacy

Dietary *n*-6 polyunsaturated fatty acids have been reported to contribute approximately 5 to 7 percent of total energy intake of adults (Allison et al., 1999; Fischer et al., 1985), and range up to no more than 10 percent of energy intake (Willett et al., 1987; Appendix Tables E-1 and E-9). The

TABLE 11-9 Interventional Studies on *n*-6 Fatty Acid Intake and Blood Lipid Concentrations

Reference	Study Design	Percent of Energy from Fatty Acid[a]
Becker et al., 1983	12 men 4-wk crossover	4.3 18:2 6.8 18:2 18 18:2
Mattson and Grundy, 1985	20 adults 4-wk crossover	3.9 18:2 29 18:2
McDonald et al., 1989	18 men 18-d parallel	7.9 18:2 and 18.8 18:1 21.3 18:2 and 7.0 18:1
Zock and Katan, 1992	56 men and women 3-wk crossover	3.8 18:2 (*trans* diet) 3.9 18:2 (18:0 diet) 12 18:2 (18:2 diet)
Kris-Etherton et al., 1993	30 and 33 men 26-d crossover	7.2 → 1.7 18:2 7.2 → 2.1 18:2 7.2 → 17.8 18:2 5.7 → 1.6 18:2 5.7 → 1.8 18:2 5.7 → 2.1 18:2
Howard et al., 1995	63 men and women 6-wk crossover	3.0 18:2 4.2 18:2 7.0 18:2 12.8 18:2

[a] 18:2 = linoleic acid, 18:1 = oleic acid.
[b] LDL-C = low density lipoprotein cholesterol, HDL-C = high density lipoprotein cholesterol.

main sources of *n*-6 polyunsaturated fatty acids are vegetable oils (e.g., soybean oil, safflower oil, and corn oil). Linoleic acid, the predominant *n*-6 polyunsaturated fatty acid, is essential in the diet, and therefore an Adequate Intake (AI) is set (see Chapter 8). Based on the estimated energy requirement for each age group, a minimum intake of 5 percent of energy from linoleic acid would be needed to meet the AI.

Postintervention Blood Lipid Concentration (mmol/L)[b]

LDL-C	HDL-C	Total Cholesterol	Triacylglycerol
2.11	1.03	3.44	0.81
1.83	1.12	3.28	0.84
1.68	1.17	3.17	0.79
3.70[c]	1.01[c]	5.80[c]	2.93[c]
3.10[d]	0.91[c]	4.94[d]	2.61[c]
2.52[c]	1.35[c]	3.97[c]	0.82[c]
2.03[d]	1.19[d]	3.39[d]	0.82[c]
3.07[c]	1.37[c]	4.90[c]	1.00[c]
3.00[c]	1.41[c]	4.89[c]	1.04[d]
2.83[d]	1.47[d]	4.74[d]	0.95[c]
2.92[c]	1.16[c]	4.55[c]	0.99[c]
2.66[c]	1.14[c]	4.27[d]	0.98[c]
2.15[d]	1.16[c]	3.59[e]	0.82[d]
3.23[c]	1.34[c]	4.89[c]	0.90[c]
2.79[d]	1.40[c]	4.45[c]	0.79[c]
2.82[d]	1.34[c]	4.40[c]	0.76[c]
4.14	1.16	5.92	1.43
4.14	1.16	5.89	1.41
4.11	1.14	5.87	1.37
4.03	1.16	5.79	1.34

[c,d,e] Within each study, the blood lipid concentrations that are significantly different between treatment groups have a different superscript.

High n-6 Polyunsaturated Fatty Acid Diets

Risk of LDL Oxidation

When exposed to oxidant stress, n-6 fatty acids are vulnerable to attack by free radicals and oxidation into lipid peroxides (Halliwell and Chirico, 1993). An example of lipid peroxidation is LDL oxidation, which plays an important role in the development of atherosclerosis (Steinberg et al.,

1989). Oxidation products of lipids and proteins are found in atherosclerotic plaque and in macrophage foam cells. Compared with monounsaturated fatty acids, in vitro susceptibility of LDLs to undergo oxidative modification has been shown to increase with increased linoleic acid content in LDLs as a result of increased intakes of linoleic acid (Abbey et al., 1993; Berry et al., 1991; Bonanome et al., 1992; Louheranta et al., 1996; Reaven et al., 1991, 1993, 1994).

The mechanism whereby incorporation of polyunsaturated fatty acids into LDLs enhances susceptibility of LDL oxidation has been studied extensively (Chisolm and Steinberg, 2000; Jessup and Kritharides, 2000). Nonetheless, the hypothesis suggesting that a diet rich in polyunsaturated fat increases the polyunsaturated fatty acid content of LDL particles and increases their susceptibility to oxidation, which in turn leads to atherosclerosis and CHD, still needs to be substantiated in human studies before measures of oxidation can be used as adequate indicators of chronic disease.

Risk of Inflammatory Disorders

There has been significant interest in the use of dietary n-6 fatty acids to modulate inflammatory response. γ-Linolenic acid (GLA, 18:3n-6) is the Δ6 desaturase product of linoleic acid and is elongated to dihomo-γ-linolenic acid (DGLA, 20:3n-6). The Δ6 desaturase enzyme is the initial step in desaturation of linoleic acid to arachidonic acid (see Figure 8-1). When given as a dietary supplement, GLA has been found to reduce symptoms of several chronic inflammatory diseases such as rheumatoid arthritis and atopic dermatitis (Andreassi et al., 1997; Leventhal et al., 1993, 1994; Lovell et al., 1981; Tate et al., 1989; Zurier et al., 1996). Even though GLA is the precursor to arachidonic acid, human neutrophils contain an elongase enzyme that converts GLA to DGLA, but they lack the Δ5 desaturase needed to form arachidonic acid. As a result, GLA supplementation results in accumulation of DGLA, but not arachidonic acid, and a reduction in leukotriene B_4 production in neutrophils (Chilton-Lopez et al., 1996; Johnson et al., 1997; Ziboh and Fletcher, 1992). However, plasma arachidonic acid concentrations increase after GLA supplementation (Johnson et al., 1997), and this could have adverse implications for other problems such as platelet aggregation (Rodier et al., 1993).

Risk of Cancer

An 8-year controlled clinical trial of 846 men demonstrated a significant increase in fatal carcinomas when the amount of n-6 polyunsaturated fatty acids fed was 15 percent of energy compared to 4 percent of energy

(Pearce and Dayton, 1971). Epidemiological studies, however, suggest that *n*-6 polyunsaturated fatty acids are not associated (or have an inverse relationship) with cancer. Howe and coworkers (1990) analyzed 12 case-control studies conducted prior to 1990 and determined that the relative risk of breast cancer for an increment of 45 g of polyunsaturated fat per day was only 1.25. More recent case-control and prospective studies further support the minimal effect of *n*-6 polyunsaturated fatty acids on breast cancer risk (Männistö et al., 1999; Toniolo et al., 1994). A similar relationship has been reported for linoleic acid intake and prostate cancer (Giovannucci et al., 1993; Schuurman et al., 1999). A meta-analysis of 7 cohort studies (Hunter et al., 1996) and a combined analysis of 12 case-control studies (Howe et al., 1990) consistently found no relationship between polyunsaturated fats or vegetable fats and risk of breast cancer. The range of intake of polyunsaturated fat was sufficiently large in these combined studies to comfortably conclude that the epidemiological evidence largely contradicts the animal studies; at least to date, no association between polyunsaturated fat, mainly *n*-6 fatty acids, and risk of breast cancer has been detected. Furthermore, in a review of the literature and meta-analyses of case-controlled and prospective epidemiological studies, Zock and Katan (1998) concluded that it was unlikely that high intakes of linoleic acid substantially raise the risk of breast, colorectal, or prostate cancer.

Risk of Nutrient Excess

High intakes of linoleic acid can inhibit the formation of long-chain *n*-3 polyunsaturated fatty acids from α-linolenic acid, which are precursors to the important eicosanoids (see Chapter 8).

Acceptable Macronutrient Distribution Range

Based on the median energy intakes for each age group (Appendix Table E-1), a minimum intake of 5 percent of energy from linoleic acid would be needed to meet the AI (see Chapter 8). An upper boundary of 10 percent of energy is estimated based on the following information: (1) the highest intake of *n*-6 polyunsaturated fatty acids for individuals in North America is approximately 10 percent of energy, (2) there is not a large body of epidemiological evidence that demonstrates the long-term safety of *n*-6 polyunsaturated fatty acid intakes exceeding 10 percent of energy from typical mixed diets, and (3) evidence from human studies demonstrates that enrichment of lipoproteins and cell membranes with *n*-6 polyunsaturated fatty acids contributes to a pro-oxidant state, thus suggesting caution for recommending intakes that exceed 10 percent of energy. For these reasons, an Acceptable Macronutrient Distribution Range (AMDR) is estimated to be 5 to 10 percent of energy for children and adults.

n-3 POLYUNSATURATED FATTY ACIDS

Low n-3 Polyunsaturated Fatty Acid Diets

Risk of CHD and Stroke

Growing evidence suggests that dietary n-3 polyunsaturated fatty acids (eicosapentaenoic acid [EPA] and docosahexaenoic acid [DHA]) reduce the risk of coronary heart disease (CHD) and stroke. n-3 Polyunsaturated fatty acids may reduce CHD risk through a multitude of mechanisms by (1) preventing arrhythmias (Billman et al., 1999; Kang and Leaf, 1996; McLennan, 1993), (2) reducing atherosclerosis (von Schacky et al., 1999), (3) decreasing platelet aggregation by inhibiting the production of thromboxane A_2 (Harker et al., 1993), (4) decreasing plasma triacylglycerol concentration (Harris, 1989), (5) slightly increasing high density lipoprotein (HDL) cholesterol concentration and decreasing triacylglycerol concentration (Harris, 1989, 1997), (6) modulating endothelial function (De Caterina et al., 2000), (7) decreasing proinflammatory eicosanoids (James et al., 2000), and (8) moderately decreasing blood pressure (Morris, 1994).

Epidemiological Evidence. Many of the epidemiological studies used fish or fish oil intake as a surrogate for n-3 polyunsaturated fatty acid intake. The amounts of n-3 fatty acids vary greatly in fish, however, and unless the amounts of n-3 fatty acids are known, any conclusions are open to question. Furthermore, other components in fish may have effects that are similar to n-3 fatty acids and therefore may confound the results. Early epidemiological studies of Greenland Eskimos suggested that diets high in n-3 fatty acids, predominantly EPA and DHA, might protect against CHD (Bang et al., 1976; Dyerberg and Bang, 1979). Subsequent observational epidemiological studies have shown mixed results. In the Zutphen study, eating fish one or two times per week was associated with a significant reduction in CHD mortality (Kromhout et al., 1985). A similar result was found in Rotterdam that compared older people who ate fish with those who did not (Kromhout et al., 1995). In three cohorts from the Seven Countries Study, the consumption of fatty fish, but not total fish or lean fish, was associated with a 34 percent decrease in CHD mortality (Oomen et al., 2000). In the Chicago Western Electric Study, eating more than 35 g/d of fish resulted in decreased CHD mortality, mainly of the nonsudden death type (Daviglus et al., 1997). Utilizing data from 36 countries, an inverse correlation was found between fish consumption and CHD and all-cause mortality (Zhang et al., 1999). In the Multiple Risk Factor Intervention Trial, CHD mortality and intake of *n*-3 fatty acids from fish were significantly and inversely correlated (Dolecek, 1992). In the Physicians' Health Study, eating fish once per week decreased the relative risk of sudden cardiac death by 52 percent compared with eating fish less than once per month (Albert et al., 1998). In this study, although dietary total *n*-3 fatty acid intake correlated inversely with total mortality, no effect on total myocardial infarction, nonsudden cardiac death, or total cardiovascular mortality was observed. The relative risk of sudden death was only 0.58 when 0.3 to 2.6 g/mo of total *n*-3 fatty acids were consumed. Siscovick and colleagues (1995) reported that a mean intake of 2.9 and 5.5 g/mo of long-chain *n*-3 fatty acids reduced the risk of primary cardiac arrest by 30 and 50 percent, respectively. A cross-sectional study showed that α-linolenic acid was inversely related to the prevalence of CHD; this effect was stronger with increasing intakes of linoleic acid (Djoussé et al., 2001).

In contrast to the above studies, the Health Professionals' Follow-up Study showed no significant association between fish intake and risk of CHD (Ascherio et al., 1995). In 16 cohorts from the Seven Countries Study, an inverse association between fish consumption and CHD mortality was found, but after correcting for saturated fat and flavonoid intakes and smoking, this association was not significant (Kromhout et al., 1996). Finally, in the EURAMIC study, adipose tissue biopsy from cases with first myocardial infarction and controls indicated lower α-linolenic acid intake in cases and a relative risk reduction of 58 percent comparing the highest versus lowest quintile of α-linolenic acid intake (Guallar et al., 1999). After adjustment for classical risk factors, the reduction was only 32 percent and no longer significant. In a meta-analysis of 11 prospective cohort studies of fish intake and CHD mortality, the two largest studies found no protective effect and the two smallest found an inverse relationship, with intermediate size studies showing intermediate benefits (Marckmann and Grønbaek, 1999). This analysis suggested that 40 to 60 g/d of fish provided a reduction in CHD mortality in high-risk, but not low-risk, individuals.

There are fewer data with regard to the effects of fish and *n*-3 polyunsaturated fatty acids on stroke. In the Zutphen Study, consumption of more than 20 g/d of fish was associated with a decrease in the risk of stroke (Keli et al., 1994). In the NHANES Epidemiological Follow-up Study, for white women and for black women and men, but not white men, consumption of fish more than once a week was associated with decreased age-adjusted stroke incidence (Gillum et al., 1996). In the Nurses' Health Study, higher consumption of fish and *n*-3 polyunsaturated fatty acids were associated with a reduced risk of total stroke and thrombotic infarction but not hemorrhagic stroke (mainly among women who did not take aspirin regularly) (Iso et al., 2001). In contrast, in the Chicago Western Electric Study and the Physicians' Health Study, fish intake was not significantly associated with decreased stroke risk (Morris et al., 1995; Orencia et al., 1996).

Nonclinical Interventional Evidence. Supplementation with fish oil, which is high in EPA and DHA, reduces triacylglycerol concentrations; low density lipoprotein (LDL) and HDL cholesterol concentrations are either increased or unchanged (Ågren et al., 1996; Axelrod et al., 1994; Bhathena et al., 1991; Bønaa et al., 1992; DeLany et al., 1990; Eritsland et al., 1994a; Haglund et al., 1990; Lungershausen et al., 1994; Mori et al., 1991; Nelson et al., 1997a; Sanders and Hinds, 1992; Saynor and Gillott, 1992; Schmidt et al., 1992).

Data from studies on the effects of EPA and DHA as a percent of energy on blood lipid concentrations in healthy individuals are presented in Table 11-10. In general, EPA+DHA intake is associated with small increases in LDL and HDL cholesterol concentrations and a significant decrease in triacylglycerol concentrations (Harris, 1997).

The consumption of 3.65 to 6 g/d of *n*-3 polyunsaturated fatty acids inhibits platelet aggregation, which in turn prevents the risk of CHD (Mori et al., 1997; Tremoli et al., 1995). Some studies, however, did not show an effect on platelet aggregation after the consumption of 4.5 to 6 g/d of EPA+DHA (Nelson et al., 1997b; Turini et al., 1994).

Randomized, Controlled Clinical Trials Evidence. There are four randomized, controlled clinical trials that show a benefit of fish, fish oils, or α-linolenic acid on CHD prevention. In the Diet and Reinfarction Trial (DART), male myocardial infarction (MI) survivors were encouraged to increase their oily fish intake to 200 to 400 g/wk in order to increase EPA and DHA intake. Over a 2-year period, this resulted in a significant reduction in total mortality, with the greatest benefit in a lower rate of fatal MI (Burr et al., 1989a, 1989b). In the DART trial, of the group randomized to ingest dietary fish, a subgroup chose to ingest 1.5 g/d of fish oil capsules rather than to consume fish. The capsule group had a significant reduction in CHD death and a significant reduction in all-cause mortality, suggesting that the benefits of the fish consumption were in the fish oil fraction (Burr et al., 1994). In the Indian Experiment of Infarct Survival, MI survivors were treated with either fish oil capsules (1.08 g/d of EPA) or mustard oil (2.9 g/d of α-linolenic acid) or placebo for 1 year (Singh et al., 1997). The fish oil and mustard oil groups had decreased total cardiac events, nonfatal infarctions, arrhythmias, left ventricular enlargement, and angina pectoris. The fish oil group, but not the mustard oil group, had decreased cardiac deaths. In the Lyon Diet Heart Study, post-MI patients were randomized into a control group or into an experimental group that received dietary counseling and a special margarine containing α-linolenic acid (de Lorgeril et al., 1994, 1999). The control and experimental groups consumed approximately 0.27 and 0.81 percent of energy as α-linolenic acid, respectively. There was a significant reduction in risk for cardiac death for the experimental group after 27 months, and a reduction after a 4-year follow-up. The extent to which these reductions in risk were due to n-3 fatty acids is uncertain.

In another trial, patients with recent MI were randomized to receive 300 mg of vitamin E, 850 mg of n-3 fatty acids (EPA+DHA), both, or neither (GISSI-Prevenzione Investigators, 1999). After 3.5 years, the n-3 fatty acid group experienced a 15 percent reduction in the primary endpoints of death, nonfatal myocardial infarction, and nonfatal stroke, and a 20 percent reduction in the other primary endpoints of cardiovascular death, nonfatal myocardial infarction, and nonfatal stroke. This group also experienced a 20 percent reduction in all-cause mortality and a 45 percent reduction in sudden deaths compared with the control group. Vitamin E, in contrast to n-3 polyunsaturated fatty acids, had no beneficial effects on cardiovascular endpoints.

n-3 Polyunsaturated fatty acids have also been reported to reduce blood pressure in hypertensive individuals. A meta-analysis of 31 placebo-controlled trials estimated a mean reduction in systolic and diastolic blood pressure of 3.0 and 1.5 mm Hg, respectively (Morris et al., 1993). Furthermore, a statistically significant dose–response effect occurred with the smallest reduction observed with intakes of less than 3 g/d and the largest reduction observed with intakes at 15 g/d.

When 55 individuals were randomized to receive either 5.2 g/d of n-3 fatty acids or a placebo for 12 weeks, heart rate variability (naturally occurring irregular heart beats) significantly increased after supplementation with n-3 fatty acids (Christensen et al., 1997). Because impaired heart rate variability is associated with increased arrhythmic events (Farrell et al., 1991), this finding supports the hypothesis that n-3 polyunsaturated fatty acids have antiarrhythmic effects in humans (Christensen et al., 1997). A more recent study by Christensen and coworkers (1999) reported a dose–response effect on heart rate variability, suggesting antiarrhythmic effects in men but not women, given 3 g/d of EPA plus 2.9 g/d of DHA or 0.9 g/d of EPA plus 0.8 g/d of DHA for 12 weeks. However, the beneficial effect was found only in men with low initial heart rate variability.

TABLE 11-10 *n-3* Fatty Acid (EPA and DHA)[a] Intake and Blood Lipid Concentrations

Reference	Study Design	Percent of Energy from Fatty Acid	Postintervention Blood Lipid Concentration (mmol/L)[b]		
			LDL-C	HDL-C	Triacylglycerol
Flaten et al., 1990	64 men 6-wk parallel	Control diet (0 *n-3*)		1.28[c]	1.71[c]
		Control diet + 2.2 EPA/DHA		1.15[c]	1.23[d]
Kestin et al., 1990	33 men 6-wk parallel	0.6 18:3*n-3*	4.44[c]	1.26[c]	1.62[c]
		2.7 18:3*n-3*	4.55[c]	1.16[c]	1.85[c]
		1.1 EPA/DHA	4.62[d]	1.28[c]	1.24[d]
Bhathena et al., 1991	40 men 10-wk crossover	0 EPA/DHA			1.62[c]
		2.2 EPA/DHA			1.17[d]
Bønaa et al., 1992	144 men and women Cross-sectional	0.28 EPA/DHA/22:5	4.65	1.32	1.95
		0.30 EPA/DHA/22:5	4.71	1.31	1.49
		0.52 EPA/DHA/22:5	4.43	1.36	1.32
		0.72 EPA/DHA/22:5	4.47	1.36	1.34
Eritsland et al., 1994a	511 men and women 9-mo parallel	Control diet	5.03[c]	1.08[c]	2.08[c]
		Control diet + 1.46 EPA/DHA	5.11[c]	1.16[c]	1.57[d]
Eritsland et al., 1994b	57 men and women 6-mo parallel	Control diet	4.84[c]	1.01[c]	1.80[c]
		Control diet + 1.4 EPA/DHA	5.03[c]	0.97[c]	1.71[c]

Ågren et al., 1996	55 men 15-wk parallel	0 n-3 (fish)	2.60^c		1.42^c
		0.36 n-3 (fish)	2.56^c		1.16^d
		0.60 n-3 (DHA oil)	2.42^c		0.97^d
		0.76 n-3 (fish oil)	2.51^c		0.89^d
Grimsgaard et al., 1997	224 men 7-wk parallel	0.19 n-3 (corn oil)	4.10^c	1.40^c	1.33^c
		0.52 n-3 (DHA oil)	4.13^c	1.42^d	1.02^d
		0.55 n-3 (EPA oil)	3.98^c	1.34^c	1.08^d
Sanders et al., 1997	26 men 3-wk crossover	0 EPA/DHA (saturated fat diet)	2.60^c	1.18^c	0.93^c
		0 EPA/DHA (n-6 diet)	2.29^d	1.19^c	0.92^c
		1.5 EPA/DHA (n-3 diet)	2.30^d	1.22^c	0.68^d

[a] EPA = eicosapentaenoic acid, DHA = docosahexaenoic acid.
[b] LDL-C = low density lipoprotein cholesterol, HDL-C = high density lipoprotein cholesterol.
[c,d] Within each study, the blood lipid concentrations that are significantly different between treatment groups have a different superscript.

Risk of Obesity

One study in laboratory mice suggested that diets containing n-3 polyunsaturated fatty acids lead to lower levels of fat accumulation compared with diets containing other fatty acids (Hun et al., 1999). Several studies have examined whether n-3 polyunsaturated fatty acids affect growth of adipose tissue. Parrish and colleagues (1990, 1991) found that rats given a high fat diet supplemented with fish oil had less fat in perirenal and epididymal fat pads and decreased adipocyte volumes compared with rats fed lard. Adipose tissue growth restriction appeared to be the result of limiting the amount of triacylglycerol in each adipose tissue cell rather than by limiting the number of cells. Rustan and colleagues (1993) found similar results using rats fed either lard or lard supplemented with EPA and DHA. Although body weight gain and mean energy expenditure were similar for both groups, the mean respiratory quotient was significantly higher during both fasting and fed periods in rats fed the EPA+DHA supplement. The researchers concluded that the rats supplemented with n-3 fatty acids demonstrated reduced oxidation of fat and increased carbohydrate utilization. Little data exist with respect to the specific effects of dietary n-3 polyunsaturated fatty acids on adiposity in humans; therefore, prevention of obesity cannot be considered an indicator at this time.

Risk of Diabetes

Epidemiological Evidence. While several studies have reported a negative relationship between polyunsaturated fatty acid intake and risk of diabetes (Colditz et al., 1992; Salmerón et al., 2001; Trevisan et al., 1990), fish intake has specifically been reported to have a negative association (Feskens et al., 1991b, 1995). A review of the epidemiological data on this association concluded that polyunsaturated fatty acids, and possibly long-chain n-3 fatty acids, could be beneficial in reducing the risk of diabetes (Hu et al., 2001).

Interventional Evidence. Studies conducted in rodents have shown that administration of fish oil results in increased insulin sensitivity (Chicco et al., 1996) and corrected hyperinsulinemia (Luo et al., 1996). Substituting a proportion of the fat in a high fat diet with fish oil prevented the development of insulin resistance in rats (Storlien et al., 1987) and normalized insulin action in rats experiencing severe insulin resistance (Storlien et al., 1991). Additionally, rats prone to spontaneous diabetes mellitus that were given EPA in doses of 0.1, 0.3, and 1.0 g/kg/d for 8 months had reduced incidences of diabetes (92, 50, and 17 percent, respectively) (Nobukata et al., 2000). Thus, animal evidence suggests that the fatty acid composition of the diet may be an important factor in the effect of dietary fat on insulin action.

Whether a change of dietary fat composition will alter insulin sensitivity in humans remains an open question. Studies in humans have demonstrated a relationship between increased insulin sensitivity and the proportion of long-chain n-3 polyunsaturated fatty acids in skeletal muscle phospholipids (Borkman et al., 1993; Clore et al., 1998). Supplementation with EPA and DHA resulted in improved insulin sensitivity in diabetic individuals (Popp-Snijders et al., 1987) and increased the insulin-stimulated glucose disposal rate in patients with impaired glucose tolerance (Fasching et al., 1991). However, other studies in nondiabetic individuals (Toft et al., 1995) and individuals with type 2 diabetes (Annuzzi et al., 1991; Luo et al., 1998) reported no beneficial effect of n-3 fatty-acid supplementation on insulin action.

Risk of Cancer

Experimental evidence suggests several mechanisms in which n-3 polyunsaturated fatty acids may protect against cancer. n-3 Polyunsaturated fatty acids, particularly DHA and EPA, have been shown to suppress neoplastic transformation (Takahashi et al., 1992), inhibit cell growth and proliferation (Anti et al., 1992; Calviello et al., 1998; Grammatikos et al., 1994), induce apoptosis (Calviello et al., 1998; Lai et al., 1996), and inhibit angiogenesis (Rose and Connolly, 2000), which may occur by suppressing n-6 fatty acid eicosanoid production (see Chapter 8). Animal studies with n-3 fatty acid or fish-oil supplementation have shown inhibition of mammary carcinogenesis and tumor growth (Grammatikos et al., 1994; Karmali et al., 1984), colon carcinogenesis (Deschner et al., 1990; Reddy et al., 1991), and prostate tumorigenesis and tumor cell growth (Karmali et al., 1987).

Across-country epidemiological studies have shown an inverse relationship between dietary fish intake and breast cancer incidence and mortality (Kaizer et al., 1989; Sasaki et al., 1993), but the intakes of n-3 fatty acids in these studies are not well defined. Moreover, despite these results, most case-control and prospective studies have not reported a protective effect of fish consumption on breast cancer (Willett, 1997). Ecological studies have also shown inverse relationships between fish and fish oil intake and colorectal cancer (Caygill and Hill, 1995; Caygill et al., 1996), although some were nonsignificant (Hursting et al., 1990). Results from case-control and prospective studies have been somewhat equivocal (Boutron et al., 1991). However, Willett and colleagues (1990) found that higher fish consumption was associated with less colon cancer in women. No significant associations were reported in the few studies that have examined fish consumption and risk of prostate cancer (Giovannucci et al., 1993; Severson et al., 1989; Talamini et al., 1992).

Risk of Nutrient Inadequacy

Vegetable oils, such as soybean oil, flaxseed oil, and canola oil, contain high amounts of α-linolenic acid. Fatty fishes and fish oils provide a mixture of biologically active EPA and DHA. n-3 Polyunsaturated fatty acids (α-linolenic acid) are essential in the diet and Adequate Intakes (AIs) have been set (see Chapter 8). Intakes of α-linolenic acid range from approximately 0.6 to 1.2 percent of energy (Appendix Tables E-1 and E-11). Low intakes of α-linolenic acid can result in inadequate biosynthesis of the longer-chain n-3 polyunsaturated fatty acids, resulting in an excessive ratio of n-6 polyunsaturated fatty acids (see Chapter 8).

High n-3 Polyunsaturated Fatty Acid Diets

There is evidence to suggest that high intakes of n-3 polyunsaturated fatty acids (EPA and DHA) may have adverse effects on immune function and may increase the risk of excessive bleeding and hemorrhagic stroke (see Chapter 8). High intakes of n-3 polyunsaturated fatty acids (α-linolenic acid) can also result in inadequate biosynthesis of long chain n-6 polyunsaturated fatty acids that are important for prostaglandin and eicosanoid synthesis (see Chapter 8).

Acceptable Macronutrient Distribution Range

α-Linolenic acid is essential in the diet and therefore AIs have been set (see Chapter 8). Up to 10 percent of the AI can be consumed as EPA and/or DHA. The above studies suggest that α-linolenic acid, EPA, and DHA may provide beneficial health effects when consumed at moderate levels. Based on the median energy intake by the various age groups (Appendix Table E-1), it is estimated that approximately 0.6 percent of energy from α-linolenic acid is needed to meet the AI. This level is used as the lower boundary for the Acceptable Macronutrient Distribution Range (AMDR) for α-linolenic acid. The upper boundary of the AMDR for α-linolenic acid is set at 1.2 percent of energy and represents the highest levels of α-linolenic acid consumed in the form of foods by individuals in North America. Data from interventional studies to support the benefit of even higher intakes of α-linolenic acid were not considered strong enough to justify establishing an upper boundary greater than 1.2 percent of energy. Approximately 10 percent of the AMDR for *n*-3 fatty acids (α-linolenic acid) can be consumed as EPA and/or DHA (0.06 to 0.12 percent of energy).

SATURATED FATTY ACIDS, *TRANS* FATTY ACIDS, AND CHOLESTEROL

Low Saturated Fatty Acid, Trans Fatty Acid, and Cholesterol Diets

There are no known risks of chronic disease from consuming low intakes of saturated fatty acids, *trans* fatty acids, or cholesterol. In the United States, saturated fatty acids provided 11 to 12 percent of energy in adult diets and 12.2 to 13.9 percent of energy in the diets of children and adolescents (CDC, 1994). It is estimated that the intake of *trans* fatty acids is approximately 2.6 percent of energy (Allison et al., 1999). The intake of cholesterol by American adults ranges from less than 100 mg/d to just under 770 mg/d (Appendix Table E-15).

It is important to recognize that lower intakes of saturated fatty acids and cholesterol are observed for vegetarians, especially vegans (Janelle and Barr, 1995; Shultz and Leklem, 1983). Because certain micronutrients, saturated fats, and cholesterol are consumed mainly through animal foods, it is possible that diets low in saturated fat and cholesterol are associated with low intakes of these micronutrients. When the micronutrient intakes of Seventh-day Adventist vegetarians and nonvegetarians were measured, there were no significant reductions in micronutrient intakes with the lower saturated fat (7.3 versus 12.6 percent of energy) and cholesterol intakes (186 versus 404 mg/d) of vegetarian compared to nonvegetarian men (12.6 percent of energy and 404 mg/d) (Shultz and Leklem, 1983). Similarly, the intakes of most micronutrients were not significantly lower for vegans, except for vitamin B_{12} (0.51 versus 3.79 mg/d), riboflavin (1.32 versus 1.72 mg/d), and calcium (578 versus 950 mg/d). Vegans had significantly lower intakes of saturated fat (6.9 versus 10.6 percent of energy) and cholesterol (94 versus 231 mg/d) than nonvegetarians (Janelle and Barr, 1995).

Analysis of nutritionally adequate menus indicates that there is a minimum amount of saturated fat that can be consumed so that sufficient levels of linoleic and α-linolenic acid are consumed (as an example see Appendix Tables G-1 and G-2). Other than soy products that are high in *n*-6 and *n*-3 fatty acids, many vegetable-based fat sources are also high in saturated fatty acids, and these differences should be considered in planning menus.

High Saturated Fatty Acid, Trans *Fatty Acid, and Cholesterol Diets*

There is a body of evidence suggesting that saturated and *trans* fatty acids and cholesterol increase blood total and low density lipoprotein cholesterol concentrations, and therefore the risk of coronary heart disease (CHD) (see Chapters 8 and 9). Because the intake of each of these three nutrients and risk of CHD is a positive linear trend, even very low intakes of each may increase risk.

To minimize saturated fatty acid intake requires decreased intake of animal fats (e.g., meat fat and butter fat) and certain oils, such as coconut and palm kernel oil. Saturated fatty acids can be reduced by choosing lean cuts of meat, trimming away visible fat on meats, and eating smaller portions. The amount of butter that is added to foods can be minimized or replaced with vegetable oils or nonhydrogenated vegetable oil spreads. Vegetable oils, such as canola and safflower oil, can be used to replace more saturated oils such as coconut and palm oil. Such changes can reduce saturated fat intake without altering the intake of essential nutrients.

A reduction in the frequency of intake or serving size of certain foods such as liver (375 mg/3 oz slice) and eggs (250 mg/egg) can help reduce the intake of cholesterol, as well as foods that contain eggs, such as cheesecake (170 mg/slice) and custard pie (170 mg/slice). There are a number of meats and dairy products that contain low amounts of cholesterol (e.g., lean meats [30 mg/2 slices] and 2 percent milk [18 mg/cup]). Therefore, there are a variety of foods that are low in saturated fat and cholesterol and also abundant in essential nutrients such as iron, zinc, and calcium.

Trans fatty acids are high in stick margarine and those foods containing vegetable shortenings that have been subjected to hydrogenation. Examples of foods that contain relatively high levels of *trans* fatty acids include cakes, pastries, doughnuts, and french fries (Litin and Sacks, 1993). Therefore, the intake of *trans* fatty acids can be reduced without limiting the intake of most essential nutrients by decreasing the serving size and frequency of intake of these foods, or by using unhardened oil.

CONJUGATED LINOLEIC ACID

Conjugated linoleic acid (CLA) has been shown to play a role in the alteration of body composition in animals (Park et al., 1997), the inhibition of tumor cell growth (Whigham et al., 2000), and the inhibition of experimental atherosclerosis in animals (Lee et al., 1994). The *trans*-10,*cis*-12 CLA isomer appears to be the isomer primarily responsible for the induction of changes in body composition (de Deckere et al., 1999; Park et al., 1999). Several studies suggest that these changes are primarily due to a reduction in lipid uptake by adipocytes (Pariza et al., 2001), which results from the action of CLA on the activities of stearoyl-coenzyme A desaturase (Choi et al., 2000; Lee et al., 1998) and lipoprotein lipase (Park et al., 1997, 1999). The *trans*-10,*cis*-12 CLA isomer has also been reported to inhibit proliferation and differentiation in cultured mouse adipocytes (Brodie et al., 1999) and to induce apoptosis in vivo in the adipose tissue of mice (Tsuboyama-Kasaoka et al., 2000). In addition to body fat reduction, dietary CLA may increase whole body protein accretion in animals, suggesting the enhancement of lean body mass (Ostrowska et al., 1999; Park et al., 1997; Stangl, 2000).

Research on the effects of CLA on body composition in humans has provided conflicting results. Blankson and coworkers (2000) conducted a study in overweight and obese men and women given either placebo or 1.7, 3.4, 5.1, or 6.8 g/d of a CLA preparation consisting of equal parts of the *cis*-9,*trans*-11 and *trans*-10,*cis*-12 isomers. After 12 weeks, none of the groups exhibited significant reductions in body weight or body mass index. However, the groups given 1.7, 3.4, and 6.8 g/d of CLA showed significant decreases in body fat mass compared to the placebo group. No differences in lean body mass were observed. Zambell and coworkers (2000) studied the effects of CLA supplementation in healthy adult women given either placebo or 3 g/d of CLA for 64 days. They found no significant changes in fat-free mass, fat mass, body weight, or percentage of body fat with CLA supplementation.

CLA has been studied for its potential anticancer benefits in numerous animal and in vitro models. CLA mixtures have been shown to exhibit anticarcinogenic properties in skin, lung, forestomach, colorectal, prostate, and mammary tissues (Cesano et al., 1998; Ha et al., 1990; Liew et al., 1995; Schønberg and Krokan, 1995; Shultz et al., 1992), although the majority of the research has been conducted with breast cancer. Ip and Scimeca (1997) conducted a study in female rats chemically induced for mammary tumors and fed a diet containing either 2 percent or 12 percent linoleic acid. The rats were also supplemented with 0, 0.5, 1, 1.5, or 2 percent CLA. The researchers found that increasing CLA from 0.5 to 1 percent resulted in a dose-dependent decrease in both tumor incidence and total number of tumors. No further protection was observed in the groups receiving 1.5 or 2 percent CLA. In addition to inhibiting tumor growth, CLA eliminated the spread of breast cancer cells to the lungs, peripheral bone, and bone marrow of mice supplemented with 1 percent CLA (Visonneau et al., 1997).

Although the exact mechanisms of the anticarcinogenic effects of CLA are not fully understood, several explanations have been offered. It has been suggested that growth inhibition of cancer cells may be due to the ability of CLA to inhibit protein and nucleotide biosynthesis (Ip et al., 1999; Shultz et al., 1992) and to induce cell apoptosis (Ip et al., 1999,

2000). Antioxidant activity of CLA has also been suggested (Ha et al., 1990; Ip et al., 1991); however, this theory has been contradicted by studies showing that CLA does not decrease lipid peroxide formation (Cunningham et al., 1997; van den Berg et al., 1995). Another possible mechanism of cancer cell growth inhibition by CLA includes alteration of eicosanoid metabolism. CLA may compete with linoleic acid in its conversion to arachidonic acid, thereby reducing the biosynthesis of eicosanoids (Banni et al., 1999), which have been associated with the proliferation of cultured breast cancer cells (Karmali, 1986; Noguchi et al., 1995). CLA has been shown to reduce leukotriene B_4 and prostaglandin E_2 levels in animals (Kavanaugh et al., 1999; Sugano et al., 1998). To date, there are insufficient data in humans to recommended a level of CLA at which beneficial health effects may occur.

DIETARY FIBER AND FUNCTIONAL FIBER

Low Fiber Diets

A low fiber diet is often attributed to the intake of a low carbohydrate diet. A number of adverse clinical effects, including impaired laxation and increased risk of cancer, obesity, heart disease, and type 2 diabetes, have been associated with the chronic consumption of low amounts of *Dietary Fiber* or *Functional Fiber*. The studies to support a beneficial role of these fibers are reviewed in Chapter 7.

Certain animal studies have shown that some fibers can actually enhance mineral absorption (Demigné et al., 1989; Levrat et al., 1991a, 1991b). There are several potential mechanisms by which ingestion of *Dietary Fiber* may actually enhance mineral status. For example, a more acidic pH in the colon is produced with fiber fermentation, and this results in more ionized calcium, which is better absorbed (Rémésy et al., 1992). *Dietary Fiber* in the colon can also stimulate bacterial fermentation, which has been associated with increases in calcium, magnesium, and potassium absorption (Demigné et al., 1989; Levrat et al., 1991a). Many fiber sources, such as karaya gum, sugar beet fiber, and coarse bran, are also excellent sources of minerals (Behall et al., 1987; Fairweather-Tait and Wright, 1990; Van Dokkum et al., 1982).

Several investigators have shown that inulin and fructooligosaccharides actually enhance calcium and magnesium absorption (Coudray et al., 1997; Delzenne et al., 1995; Levrat et al., 1991b; Ohta et al., 1995). There is also indirect evidence of this same enhancement with calcium in humans (Trinidad et al., 1993, 1996). A direct effect of fiber on mineral absorption has also been reported in humans where inulin increased the apparent absorption and balance of calcium (Coudray et al., 1997).

High Fiber Diets

There is limited data to suggest that chronic consumption of high fiber diets results in adverse health effects (see Chapter 7). Gastrointestinal distress can occur with the consumption of high fiber diets, but this often subsides with time.

DIETARY PROTEIN

Low Protein Diets

Although uncommon in North America, protein–energy malnutrition (PEM) is one of the most common nutritional diseases in developing countries (Torun and Chew, 1999). The etiology of PEM is complex as there are a number of factors that are attributed to its onset, including insufficient food intake or intake of low protein-containing foods, which in turn is attributed to poverty, unsanitary conditions, and food insecurity. Because PEM is attributed to insufficient food intake, not only are protein and energy limited, but the micronutrients that are often present in protein-containing foods are also limited. Epidemiological analysis from 53 developing countries indicated that 56 percent of deaths in young children were due to the potentiating effects of malnutrition in infectious diseases (Pelletier et al., 1995). The increased duration or susceptibility to infectious diseases such as respiratory infections and diarrhea are due, in part, to the involvement of protein in immune function.

Impaired Immune Function

Chandra (1972) showed that in individuals with PEM, a variety of immune responses were impaired. The major defects observed with severe PEM involve T lymphocytes and the complement system. With PEM, the number of lymphocytes is markedly reduced and delayed cutaneous hypersensitivity responses to both recall and new antigens are depressed (Chandra, 1991), as is the production of several components of the complement system (Keusch et al., 1984). Furthermore, antibody affinity (Chandra et al., 1984) and lysozyme concentrations (Chandra and Newberne, 1977) are decreased.

Impaired Growth

Low protein intake during pregnancy is correlated with a higher incidence of low birth weight (King, 2000). Furthermore, in children, diets low in protein and energy are most frequently associated with a deficit in weight-for-height (wasting) and height-for-age (stunting) (Waterlow, 1976). These deficits can be corrected by the provision of a high protein diet (Badaloo et al., 1999) and with an adequate energy intake to permit catch-up growth. For these reasons, various anthropometric measures are used for diagnosis and monitoring the treatment of PEM.

Low Birth Weight

Rush and coworkers (1980) found decreases in both gestational length and birth weight and increases in very early premature births and mortality with high density protein supplementation (additional 40 g/d) in poor, black pregnant women at risk of having low birth weight infants. In contrast, Adams and coworkers (1978) reported no differences from the controls in mean birth weights of infants of mothers at risk of having a low birth weight infant when these women were supplemented with 40 g/d of protein. No reports were found of protein toxicity in healthy pregnant or lactating women that were not at risk of having a low birth weight infant. Thus, at the present time, low birth weight cannot be utilized to set a Tolerable Upper Intake Level (UL) for protein for women.

Risk of Nutritional Inadequacy

High quality protein is typically consumed via animal products, and therefore vegetarians may consume less high quality protein than omnivores. Because animal foods are the primary sources of certain nutrients, such as calcium, vitamin B_{12}, and bioavailable iron and zinc, low protein intakes may result in inadequate intakes of these micronutrients. As an example, Janelle and Barr (1995) reported significantly lower intakes of riboflavin, vitamin B_{12}, and calcium by vegans who also consumed lower amounts of protein (10 versus 15 percent of energy) compared with nonvegetarians.

Vegetable protein has been shown to decrease plasma cholesterol concentrations in experimental animals and humans (Nagata et al., 1998; Nicolosi and Wilson, 1997; Terpstra et al., 1991). When the ratio of casein:soybean protein in the diet was decreased, there was a reduction in total and non-high density lipoprotein cholesterol concentrations (Fernandez et al., 1999; Teixeira et al., 2000). In laboratory animals, it was shown that the onset of atherosclerosis was significantly reduced when animals were fed a textured vegetable protein diet compared to a beef protein diet (Kritchevsky et al., 1981).

High Protein Diets

Osteoporosis

There is a substantial amount of literature that documents the increase in urinary excretion of calcium with increasing protein intake (Allen et al., 1979; Heaney, 1993; Lemann, 1999). The magnitude of this effect for a doubling of the protein intake, in the absence of change in any other nutrient, is a 50 percent increase in urinary calcium (Heaney, 1993). This has two potential detrimental consequences: loss of bone calcium and increased risk of renal calcium stone formation. Loss of calcium from bone is thought to occur because of bone mineral resorption that provides the buffer for the acid produced by the oxidation of the sulfur amino acids of protein (Barzel and Massey, 1998). However, although increased resorption of bone with increased protein intake has been shown (Kerstetter et al., 1999; Whiting et al., 1997), whether this in practice leads to bone loss and osteoporosis is controversial (Barzel and Massey, 1998; Heaney, 1998). It has recently been concluded that there may be no need to restrain dietary protein intake. Poor protein status itself leads to bone loss, whereas increased protein intake may lead to increased calcium intake, and bone loss does not occur if calcium intake is adequate (Heaney, 1998). In a recent prospective study of men and women aged 55 to 92 years, consumption of animal protein was positively associated with bone mineral density in women, but not in men (Promislow et al., 2002). In contrast, Dawson-Hughes and Harris (2002) reported no association between protein intake and bone mineral density in 342 healthy men and women aged 65 years and older. However, when the individuals were given calcium citrate malate and vitamin D in addition to the high protein intake, there was a favorable change in bone mineral density.

Kidney Stones

It has been estimated that 12 percent of the population in the United States will suffer from a kidney stone at some time (Sierakowski et al., 1978). The most common form of kidney stone is composed of calcium oxalate, and its formation is promoted by high concentrations of calcium and oxalate in the urine. A high animal protein intake in healthy humans increases urinary calcium and oxalate and the overall probability of forming kidney stones by 250 percent (Robertson et al., 1979). Conversely, restricting protein intake improved the lithogenic profile in hypercalciuric patients (Giannini et al., 1999). Also, the incidence of calcium oxalate stones has been shown to be associated with consumption of animal protein (Curhan et al., 1996; Robertson and Peacock, 1982). In contrast, the only long-term prospective trial (4.5 years) of the effect of animal protein restriction on stone formation in newly diagnosed patients with calcium stones gave a negative result (Hiatt et al., 1996). The relative risk factor for recurrent stone formation was 5.6 (confidence interval 1.2–26.1), suggesting that the dietary advice was detrimental. In this study, 50 patients were given low animal protein (56 to 64 g/d) and high fiber, plus adequate fluid and calcium, whereas 49 control patients were only instructed to take adequate water and calcium. However, as protein intake was not the only variable, and in view of the data described above suggesting benefits from lower protein intake, further investigation is necessary.

Renal Failure

Restriction of dietary protein intake is known to lessen the symptoms of chronic renal insufficiency (Walser, 1992). This raises two related, but distinct questions: Do high protein diets have some role in the development of chronic renal failure? Do high protein intakes accelerate the progression of chronic renal failure? The concept that protein restriction might delay the deterioration of the kidney with age was based on studies in rats in which low energy or low protein diets attenuated the development of chronic renal failure (Anderson and Brenner, 1986, 1987). Walser (1992) has argued that this mechanism is unlikely to operate in humans. In particular, the decline in kidney function in the rat is mostly due to glomerulosclerosis, whereas in humans it is due mostly to a decline in filtration by nonsclerotic nephrons. Also, when creatinine clearance was measured in men at 10- to 18-year intervals, the decline with age did not correlate with dietary protein intake (Tobin and Spector, 1986). Correlation of creatinine clearance with protein intake showed a linear relationship with a positive gradient (Lew and Bosch, 1991), suggesting that the low protein intake itself decreased renal function. These factors point to the conclusion that the protein content of the diet is not responsible for the progressive decline in kidney function with age.

Coronary Artery Disease

It is well documented that high dietary protein in rabbits induces hypercholesterolemia and arteriosclerosis (Czarnecki and Kritchevsky, 1993). However, this effect has not been consistently shown in either swine (Luhman and Beitz, 1993; Pfeuffer et al., 1988) or humans. In humans, analysis of data from the Nurses' Health Study showed an inverse relationship between protein intake and risk of cardiovascular disease (Hu et al., 1999). The association was weak but suggests that high protein intake does not increase the risk of cardiovascular disease. Similar conclusions have been reached in observational studies showing an inverse relationship between protein intake and blood pressure (Obarzanek et al., 1996) and that replacement of carbohydrate with protein resulted in lower very low density cholesterol, low density cholesterol, and triglycerides (Wolfe and Piché, 1999).

Obesity

A number of short-term studies indicate that protein intake exerts a more powerful effect on satiety than either carbohydrate or fat (Hill and Blundell, 1990; Rolls et al., 1988; Stubbs et al., 1996). However, some epidemiological studies have shown a positive correlation between protein intake and body fatness, body mass index, and subscapular skinfold (Buemann et al., 1995; Rolland-Cachera et al., 1995). In contrast, a 6-month randomized trial demonstrated that the replacement of some dietary carbohydrate by protein improved weight loss as part of a reduced fat diet (Skov et al., 1999).

Cancer

The fact that the growth of tumor cells in culture is often increased by high amino acid concentrations (Breillout et al., 1990; Collins et al., 1998) raises concern that high dietary protein intake might enhance the incidence or the progression of cancer. Reviews of the literature on colon cancer have concluded that high meat intake may be associated with increased risk, but that high total protein intake is not (Clinton, 1993; Giovannucci and Willett, 1994; Parnaud and Corpet, 1997). A lack of correlation with total protein intake has been found in a case-control study (Slattery et al., 1997), but other studies have reported both increased (Slattery et al., 1994) and decreased (Kato et al., 1997) risk.

For breast cancer, the geographical distribution of incidence is correlated with the availability of dietary protein, especially animal protein (Clinton, 1993). Furthermore, migration to an area with typically higher protein intakes is associated with increased risk of breast cancer (Buell, 1973; Buell and Dunn, 1965). In accord with this, several studies have indicated an association among breast cancer and the intakes of animal protein and fat (Hislop et al., 1986; Lubin et al., 1981, 1986). However, others showed a relationship with fat, but not protein intake (Miller et al., 1978; Phillips, 1975). More recently, a case-control study on 2,569 patients and 2,588 controls showed a slightly negative relationship between total protein and breast cancer (Decarli et al., 1997). Another case-control study on 180 breast-cancer patients and 829 controls also showed no relationship with total protein intake, but there was an increased risk ratio for meat consumption (Toniolo et al., 1994).

For other types of tumors, there also is no clear indication of greater risk with higher protein intakes. Total protein intake was not associated with increased risk of lung cancer (Lei et al., 1996), prostate cancer (Schuurman et al., 1999), endometrial cancer (Barbone et al., 1993; Shu et al., 1993), oral and pharynx cancer (Franceschi et al., 1999), esophogeal cancer (Gao et al., 1994), and non-Hodgkin's lymphoma (Chiu et al., 1996; Ward et al., 1994), although some studies detected a positive relationship with animal protein (Chiu et al., 1996; Shu et al., 1993) or cured meat consumption (Schuurman et al., 1999). Moreover, in some of these studies, there was an inverse relationship with total protein intake (Barbone et al., 1993; Franceschi et al., 1999; Gao et al., 1994). On the other hand, higher protein intake was associated with an increased risk of cancer of the upper digestive tract (De Stefani et al., 1999) and kidney (Chow et al., 1994).

Overall, despite the demonstration of a positive influence of dietary fat and total energy, as well as meat (especially red meat), on some types of tumors, no clear role for total protein has yet emerged. The current state of the literature, therefore, does not permit any recommendation of an upper limit to be made on the basis of cancer risk.

Acceptable Macronutrient Distribution Range

There is no evidence to suggest that the Acceptable Macronutrient Distribution Range (AMDR) for protein should be at levels below the Recommended Dietary Allowance (RDA) for protein (about 10 percent of energy) for adults. There was insufficient evidence to suggest a UL for protein (see Chapter 10) and insufficient data to suggest an upper limit for an AMDR for protein. To complement the AMDRs for fat (20 to 35 percent energy) and carbohydrate (45 to 65 percent energy) for adults, protein intakes may range from 10 to 35 percent of energy intake to ensure a nutritionally adequate diet. For young and older children, the RDA is approximately 5 and 10 percent of energy, respectively. To complement the AMDR for fat (30 to 40 percent of energy) and carbohydrate (45 to 65 percent of energy) for young children and for older children (25 to 35 percent of energy from fat and 45 to 65 percent of energy from carbohydrate), protein intakes may range from 5 to 20 percent for young children and 10 to 30 percent for older children.

REFERENCES

Abate N, Garg A, Peshock RM, Stray-Gundersen J, Adams-Huet B, Grundy SM. 1996. Relationship of generalized and regional adiposity to insulin sensitivity in men with NIDDM. *Diabetes* 45:1684–1693.

Abbey M, Belling GB, Noakes M, Hirata F, Nestel PJ. 1993. Oxidation of low-density lipoproteins: Intraindividual variability and the effect of dietary linoleate supplementation. *Am J Clin Nutr* 57:391–398.

Abbott WGH, Boyce VL, Grundy SM, Howard BV. 1989. Effects of replacing saturated fat with complex carbohydrate in diets of subjects with NIDDM. *Diabetes Care* 12:102–107.

Adams SO, Barr GD, Huenemann RL. 1978. Effect of nutritional supplementation in pregnancy. I. Outcome of pregnancy. *J Am Diet Assoc* 72:144–147.

Ågren JJ, Hänninen O, Julkunen A, Fogelholm L, Vidgren H, Schwab U, Pynnönen O, Uusitupa M. 1996. Fish diet, fish oil and docosahexaenoic acid rich oil lower fasting and postprandial plasma lipid levels. *Eur J Clin Nutr* 50:765–771.

Albert CM, Hennekens CH, O'Donnell CJ, Ajani UA, Carey VJ, Willett WC, Ruskin JN, Manson JE. 1998. Fish consumption and risk of sudden cardiac death. *J Am Med Assoc* 279:23–28.

Allen LH, Oddoye EA, Margen S. 1979. Protein-induced calciuria: A longer term study. *Am J Clin Nutr* 32:741–749.

Allison DB, Egan K, Barraj LM, Caughman C, Infante M, Heimbach J. 1999. Estimated intakes of *trans* fatty and other fatty acids in the US population. *J Am Diet Assoc* 99:166–174.

American Diabetes Association. 2001. Screening for diabetes. *Diabetes Care* 24:S21–S24.

Anderson S, Brenner BM. 1986. Effects of aging on the renal glomerulus. *Am J Med* 80:435–442.

Anderson S, Brenner BM. 1987. The aging kidney: Structure, function, mechanisms, and therapeutic implications. *J Am Geriatr Soc* 35:590–593.

Andreassi M, Forleo P, Di Lorio A, Masci S, Abate G, Amerio P. 1997. Efficacy of γ-linolenic acid in the treatment of patients with atopic dermatitis. *J Int Med Res* 25:266–274.

Annuzzi G, Rivellese A, Capaldo B, Di Marino L, Iovine C, Marotta G, Riccardi G. 1991. A controlled study on the effects of *n*-3 fatty acids on lipid and glucose metabolism in non-insulin-dependent diabetic patients. *Atherosclerosis* 87:65–73.

Anti M, Marra G, Armelao F, Bartoli GM, Ficarelli R, Percesepe A, De Vitis I, Maria G, Sofo L, Rapaccini GL. 1992. Effect of omega-3 fatty acids on rectal mucosal cell proliferation in subjects at risk for colon cancer. *Gastroenterology* 103:883–891.

Arntzenius AC, Kromhout D, Barth JD, Reiber JHC, Bruschke AVG, Buis B, van Gent CM, Kempen-Voogd N, Strikwerda S, van der Velde EA. 1985. Diet, lipoproteins, and the progression of coronary atherosclerosis. The Leiden Intervention Trial. *N Engl J Med* 312:805–811.

ARS (Agricultural Research Service). 1998. *Food and Nutrient Intakes by Individuals in the United States, by Sex and Age, 1994–96*. Washington, DC: U.S. Department of Agriculture.

Ascherio A, Rimm EB, Stampfer MJ, Giovannucci EL, Willett WC. 1995. Dietary intake of marine *n*-3 fatty acids, fish intake, and the risk of coronary disease among men. *N Engl J Med* 332:977–982.

Ascherio A, Rimm EB, Giovannucci EL, Spiegelman D, Stampfer M, Willett WC. 1996. Dietary fat and risk of coronary heart disease in men: Cohort follow up study in the United States. *Br Med J* 313:84–90.

Astrup A, Grunwald GK, Melanson EL, Saris WH, Hill JO. 2000. The role of low-fat diets in body weight control: A meta-analysis of ad libitum dietary intervention studies. *Int J Obes Relat Metab Disord* 24:1545–1552.

Atkin L-M, Davies PSW. 2000. Diet composition and body composition in preschool children. *Am J Clin Nutr* 72:15–21.

Austin MA, King MC, Vranizan KM, Krauss RM. 1990. Atherogenic lipoprotein phenotype: A proposed genetic marker for coronary heart disease risk. *Circulation* 82:495–506.

Axelrod L, Camuso J, Williams E, Kleinman K, Briones E, Schoenfeld D. 1994. Effects of a small quantity of ω-3 fatty acids on cardiovascular risk factors in NIDDM. *Diabetes Care* 17:37–44.

Badaloo A, Boyne M, Reid M, Persaud C, Forrester T, Millward DJ, Jackson AA. 1999. Dietary protein, growth and urea kinetics in severely malnourished children and during recovery. *J Nutr* 129:969–979.

Baer JT. 1993. Improved plasma cholesterol levels in men after a nutrition education program at the worksite. *J Am Diet Assoc* 93:658–663.

Ballew C, Kuester S, Gillespie C. 2000. Beverage choices affect adequacy of children's nutrient intakes. *Arch Pediatr Adolesc Med* 154:1148–1152.

Bang HO, Dyerberg J, Hjørne N. 1976. The composition of food consumed by Greenland Eskimos. *Acta Med Scand* 200:69–73.

Banni S, Angioni E, Casu V, Melis MP, Carta G, Corongiu FP, Thompson H, Ip C. 1999. Decrease in linoleic acid metabolites as a potential mechanism in cancer risk reduction by conjugated linoleic acid. *Carcinogenesis* 20:1019–1024.

Barbone F, Austin H, Partridge EE. 1993. Diet and endometrial cancer: A case-control study. *Am J Epidemiol* 137:393–403.

Barinagarrementeria F, González-Duarte A, Cantú-Brito C. 1998. Prothrombic states and cerebral ischemia. *Rev Neurol* 26:85–91.

Bartsch H, Nair J, Owen RW. 1999. Dietary polyunsaturated fatty acids and cancers of the breast and colorectum: Emerging evidence for their role as risk modifiers. *Carcinogenesis* 20:2209–2218.

Barzel US, Massey LK. 1998. Excess dietary protein can adversely affect bone. *J Nutr* 128:1051–1053.

Bassett DR, Abel M, Moellering RC, Rosenblatt G, Stokes J. 1969. Coronary heart disease in Hawaii: Dietary intake, depot fat, "stress," smoking, and energy balance in Hawaiian and Japanese men. *Am J Clin Nutr* 22:1483–1503.

Becker N, Illingworth R, Alaupovic P, Connor WE, Sundberg EE. 1983. Effects of saturated, monounsaturated, and ω-6 polyunsaturated fatty acids on plasma lipids, lipoproteins, and apoproteins in humans. *Am J Clin Nutr* 37:355–360.

Beck-Nielsen H, Pedersen O, Lindskov HO. 1980. Impaired cellular insulin binding and insulin sensitivity induced by high-fructose feeding in normal subjects. *Am J Clin Nutr* 33:273–278.

Behall KM, Scholfield DJ, Lee K, Powell AS, Moser PB. 1987. Mineral balance in adult men: Effect of four refined fibers. *Am J Clin Nutr* 46:307–314.

Bennett PH, Knowler WC, Baird HR, Butler WJ, Pettitt DJ, Reid JM. 1984. Diet and the development of noninsulin-dependent diabetes mellitus: An epidemiological perspective. In: Pozza G, ed. *Diet, Diabetes, and Atherosclerosis.* New York: Raven Press. Pp. 109–119.

Berenson GS, Wattigney WA, Tracy RE, Newman WP, Srinivasan SR, Webber LS, Dalferes ER, Strong JP. 1992. Atherosclerosis of the aorta and coronary arteries and cardiovascular risk factors in persons aged 6 to 30 years and studied at necropsy (The Bogalusa Heart Study). Am J Cardiol 70:851–858.

Berry EM, Eisenberg S, Haratz D, Friedlander Y, Norman Y, Kaufmann NA, Stein Y. 1991. Effects of diets rich in monounsaturated fatty acids on plasma lipo-proteins—The Jerusalem Nutrition Study: High MUFAs vs high PUFAs. Am J Clin Nutr 53:899–907.

Berry EM, Eisenberg S, Friedlander Y, Harats D, Kaufmann NA, Norman Y, Stein Y. 1992. Effects of diets rich in monounsaturated fatty acids on plasma lipopro-teins—The Jerusalem Nutrition Study. II. Monounsaturated fatty acids vs car-bohydrates. Am J Clin Nutr 56:394–403.

Bhathena SJ, Berlin E, Judd JT, Kim YC, Law JS, Bhagavan HN, Ballard-Barbash R, Nair PP. 1991. Effects of ω3 fatty acids and vitamin E on hormones involved in carbohydrate and lipid metabolism in men. Am J Clin Nutr 54:684–688.

Billman GE, Kang JX, Leaf A. 1999. Prevention of sudden cardiac death by dietary pure ω-3 polyunsaturated fatty acids in dogs. Circulation 99:2452–2457.

Black HS, Herd JA, Goldberg LH, Wolf JE, Thornby JI, Rosen T, Bruce S, Tschen JA, Foreyt JP, Scott LW, Jaax S, Andrews K. 1994. Effect of a low-fat diet on the incidence of actinic keratosis. N Engl J Med 330:1272–1275.

Bladbjerg EM, Marckmann P, Sandström B, Jespersen J. 1994. Non-fasting factor VII coagulant activity (FVII:C) increased by high fat diet. Thromb Haemost 71:755–758.

Blankson H, Stakkestad JA, Fagertun H, Thom E, Wadstein J, Gudmundsen O. 2000. Conjugated linoleic acid reduces body fat mass in overweight and obese humans. J Nutr 130:2943–2948.

Bloemberg BPM, Kromhout D, Goddijn HE, Jansen A, Obermann-de Boer GL. 1991. The impact of the Guidelines for a Healthy Diet of the Netherlands Nutrition Council on total and high density lipoprotein cholesterol in hyper-cholesterolemic free-living men. Am J Epidemiol 134:39–48.

Blundell JE, Burley VJ, Cotton JR, Lawton CL. 1993. Dietary fat and the control of energy intake: Evaluating the effects of fat on meal size and postmeal satiety. Am J Clin Nutr 57:772S–778S.

Bobroff EM, Kissileff HR. 1986. Effects of changes in palatability on food intake and the cumulative food intake curve in man. Appetite 7:85–96.

Bolton-Smith C. 1996. Intake of sugars in relation to fatness and micronutrient adequacy. Int J Obes Relat Metab Disord 20:S31–S33.

Bolton-Smith C, Woodward M. 1994. Coronary heart disease: Prevalence and dietary sugars in Scotland. J Epidemiol Community Health 48:119–122.

Bolton-Smith C, Woodward M. 1995. Antioxidant vitamin adequacy in relation to consumption of sugars. Eur J Clin Nutr 49:124–133.

Bønaa KH, Bjerve KS, Nordøy A. 1992. Habitual fish consumption, plasma phospholipid fatty acids, and serum lipids: The Tromsø Study. Am J Clin Nutr 55:1126–1134.

Bonanome A, Pagnan A, Biffanti S, Opportuno A, Sorgato F, Dorella M, Maiorino M, Ursini F. 1992. Effect of dietary monounsaturated and polyunsaturated fatty acids on the susceptibility of plasma low density lipoproteins to oxidative modification. Arterioscler Thromb 12:529–533.

Borkman M, Campbell LV, Chisholm DJ, Storlien LH. 1991. Comparison of the effects on insulin sensitivity of high carbohydrate and high fat diets in normal subjects. J Clin Endocrinol Metab 72:432–437.

Borkman M, Storlien LH, Pan DA, Jenkins AB, Chisholm DJ, Campbell LV. 1993. The relation between insulin sensitivity and the fatty-acid composition of skeletal-muscle phospholipids. *N Engl J Med* 328:238–244.

Boulton TJC, Magarey AM. 1995. Effects of differences in dietary fat on growth, energy and nutrient intake from infancy to eight years of age. *Acta Paediatr* 84:146–150.

Boutron MC, Wilpart M, Faivre J. 1991. Diet and colorectal cancer. *Eur J Cancer Prev* 1:13–20.

Bowman MP, Van Doren J, Taper LJ, Thye FW, Ritchey SJ. 1988. Effect of dietary fat and cholesterol on plasma lipids and lipoprotein fractions in normolipidemic men. *J Nutr* 118:555–560.

Bowman SA. 1999. Diets of individuals based on energy intakes from added sugars. *Fam Econ Nutr Rev* 12:31–38.

Boyar AP, Rose DP, Loughridge JR, Engle A, Palgi A, Laakso K, Kinne D, Wynder EL. 1988. Response to a diet low in total fat in women with postmenopausal breast cancer: A pilot study. *Nutr Cancer* 11:93–99.

Boyd NF, Cousins M, Beaton M, Kriukov V, Lockwood G, Tritchler D. 1990. Quantitative changes in dietary fat intake and serum cholesterol in women: Results from a randomized, controlled trial. *Am J Clin Nutr* 52:470–476.

Boyd NF, Martin LJ, Noffel M, Lockwood GA, Tritchler DL. 1993. A meta-analysis of studies of dietary fat and breast cancer risk. *Br J Cancer* 68:627–636.

Bray GA, Popkin BM. 1998. Dietary fat intake does affect obesity! *Am J Clin Nutr* 68:1157–1173.

Breillout F, Antoine E, Poupon MF. 1990. Methionine dependency of malignant tumors: A possible approach for therapy. *J Natl Cancer Inst* 82:1628–1632.

Brodie AE, Manning VA, Ferguson KR, Jewell DE, Hu CY. 1999. Conjugated linoleic acid inhibits differentiation of pre- and post-confluent 3T3-L1 preadipocytes but inhibits cell proliferation only in preconfluent cells. *J Nutr* 129:602–606.

Brussaard JH, Katan MB, Groot PHE, Havekes LM, Hautvast JGAJ. 1982. Serum lipoproteins of healthy persons fed a low-fat diet or a polyunsaturated fat diet for three months. A comparison of two cholesterol-lowering diets. *Atherosclerosis* 42:205–219.

Budohoski L, Panczenko-Kresowska B, Langfort J, Z̆ernicka E, Dubaniewicz A, Ziemlan'ski S`, Challiss RAJ, Newsholme WA. 1993. Effects of saturated and polyunsaturated fat enriched diet on the skeletal muscle insulin sensitivity in young rats. *J Physiol Pharmacol* 44:391–398.

Buell P. 1973. Changing incidence of breast cancer in Japanese-American women. *J Natl Cancer Inst* 51:1479–1483.

Buell P, Dunn JE. 1965. Cancer mortality among Japanese Issei and Nisei of California. *Cancer* 18:656–664.

Buemann B, Tremblay A, Bouchard C. 1995. Social class interacts with the association between macronutrient intake and subcutaneous fat. *Int J Obes Relat Metab Disord* 19:770–775.

Burmeister LA, Valdivia T, Nuttal FQ. 1991. Adult hereditary fructose intolerance. *Arch Intern Med* 151:773–776.

Burr ML, Fehily AM, Gilbert JF, Rogers S, Holliday RM, Sweetnam PM, Elwood PC, Deadman NM. 1989a. Effects of changes in fat, fish, and fibre intakes on death and myocardial reinfarction: Diet and Reinfarction Trial (DART). *Lancet* 2:757–761.

Burr ML, Fehily AM, Rogers S, Welsby E, King S, Sandham S. 1989b. Diet and Reinfarction Trial (DART): Design, recruitment, and compliance. *Eur Heart J* 10:558–567.

Burr ML, Sweetnam PM, Fehily AM. 1994. Diet and reinfarction. *Eur Heart J* 15:1152–1153.

Buzzard IM, Asp EH, Chlebowski RT, Boyar AP, Jeffery RW, Nixon DW, Blackburn GL, Jochimsen PR, Scanlon EF, Insull W, Elashoff RM, Butram R, Wynder EL. 1990. Diet intervention methods to reduce fat intake: Nutrient and food group composition of self-selected low-fat diets. *J Am Diet Assoc* 90:42–50, 53.

Calbet JA, MacLean DA. 1997. Role of caloric content on gastric emptying in humans. *J Physiol* 498:553–559.

Calviello G, Palozza P, Piccioni E, Maggiano N, Frattucci A, Franceschelli P, Baroli GM. 1998. Dietary supplementation with eicosapentaenoic and docosahexaenoic acid inhibits growth of Morris hepatocarcinoma 3924A in rats: Effects on proliferation and apoptosis. *Int J Cancer* 75:699–705.

Campbell TC, Parpia B, Chen J. 1998. Diet, lifestyle, and the etiology of coronary artery disease: The Cornell China Study. *Am J Cardiol* 82:18T–21T.

Castelli WP, Anderson K, Wilson PWF, Levy D. 1992. Lipids and risk of coronary heart disease. The Framingham Study. *Ann Epidemiol* 2:23–28.

Caygill CPJ, Hill MJ. 1995. Fish, *n*-3 fatty acids and human colorectal and breast cancer mortality. *Eur J Cancer Prev* 4:329–332.

Caygill CPJ, Charlett A, Hill MJ. 1996. Fat, fish, fish oil and cancer. *Br J Cancer* 74:159–164.

CDC (Centers for Disease Control and Prevention). 1994. Daily dietary fat and total food-energy intakes—Third National Health and Nutrition Examination Survey, Phase 1, 1988–91. *Morb Mortal Wkly Rep* 43:116–117, 123–125.

Cesano A, Visonneau S, Scimeca JA, Kritchevsky D, Santoli D. 1998. Opposite effects of linoleic acid and conjugated linoleic acid on human prostatic cancer in SCID mice. *Anticancer Res* 18:833–838.

Chandra RK. 1972. Immunocompetence in undernutrition. *J Pediatr* 81:1194–1200.

Chandra RK. 1991. 1990 McCollum Award lecture. Nutrition and immunity: Lessons from the past and new insights into the future. *Am J Clin Nutr* 53:1087–1101.

Chandra RK, Newberne PM. 1977. *Nutrition, Immunity, and Infection: Mechanisms of Interactions*. New York: Plenum Press.

Chandra RK, Chandra S, Gupta S. 1984. Antibody affinity and immune complexes after immunization with tetanus toxoid in protein-energy malnutrition. *Am J Clin Nutr* 40:131–134.

Chen M, Bergman RN, Porte D. 1988. Insulin resistance and β-cell dysfunction in aging: The importance of dietary carbohydrate. *J Clin Endocrinol Metab* 67:951–957.

Chicco A, D'Alessandro ME, Karabatas L, Gutman R, Lombardo YB. 1996. Effect of moderate levels of dietary fish oil on insulin secretion and sensitivity, and pancreas insulin content in normal rats. *Ann Nutr Metab* 40:61–70.

Chilton-Lopez T, Surette ME, Swan DD, Fonteh AN, Johnson MM, Chilton FH. 1996. Metabolism of gammalinolenic acid in human neutrophils. *J Immunol* 156:2941–2947.

Chisholm KW, O'Dea K. 1987. Effect of short-term consumption of a high fat diet on glucose tolerance and insulin sensitivity in the rat. *J Nutr Sci Vitaminol* 3:377–390.

Chisolm GM, Steinberg D. 2000. The oxidative modification hypothesis of athero-genesis: An overview. *Free Radic Biol Med* 28:1815–1826.

Chiu BC, Cerhan JR, Folsom AR, Sellers TA, Kushi LH, Wallace RB, Zheng W, Potter JD. 1996. Diet and risk of non-Hodgkin lymphoma in older women. *J Am Med Assoc* 275:1315–1321.

Choi Y, Kim Y-C, Han Y-B, Park Y, Pariza M, Ntambi JM. 2000. The *trans*-10,*cis*-12 isomer of conjugated linoleic acid downregulates stearoyl-CoA desaturase 1 gene expression in 3T3-L1 adipocytes. *J Nutr* 130:1920–1924.

Chow WH, Gridley G, McLaughlin JK, Mandel JS, Wacholder S, Blot WJ, Niwa S, Fraumeni JF. 1994. Protein intake and risk of renal cell cancer. *J Natl Cancer Inst* 86:1131–1139.

Christensen JH, Gustenhoff P, Korup E, Aarøe J, Møller JM, Rasmussen K, Dyerberg J, Schmidt EB. 1997. *n*-3 Polyunsaturated fatty acids, heart rate variability and ventricular arrhythmias in patients with previous myocardial infarcts. *Ugeskr Laeger* 159:5525–5529.

Christensen JH, Christensen MS, Dyerberg J, Schmidt EB. 1999. Heart rate variability and fatty acid content of blood cell membranes: A dose-response study with *n*-3 fatty acids. *Am J Clin Nutr* 70:331–337.

Clarke R, Frost C, Collins R, Appleby P, Peto R. 1997. Dietary lipids and blood cholesterol: Quantitative meta-analysis of metabolic ward studies. *Br Med J* 314:112–117.

Clinton SK. 1993. Dietary protein and the origins of human cancer. In: Liepa GU, Beitz DC, Beynen AC, Gorman MA, eds. *Dietary Proteins: How They Alleviate Disease and Promote Better Health*. Champaign, IL: American Oil Chemists' Society. Pp. 84–122.

Clore JN, Li J, Gill R, Gupta S, Spencer R, Azzam A, Zuelzer W, Rizzo WB, Blackard WG. 1998. Skeletal muscle phosphatidylcholine fatty acids and insulin sensitivity in normal humans. *Am J Physiol* 275:E665–E670.

Colditz GA, Willett WC, Stampfer MJ, London SJ, Segal MR, Speizer FE. 1990. Patterns of weight change and their relation to diet in a cohort of healthy women. *Am J Clin Nutr* 51:1100–1105.

Colditz GA, Manson JE, Stampfer MJ, Rosner B, Willett WC, Speizer FE. 1992. Diet and risk of clinical diabetes in women. *Am J Clin Nutr* 55:1018–1023.

Collins CL, Wasa M, Souba WW, Abcouwer SF. 1998. Determinants of glutamine dependence and utilization by normal and tumor-derived breast cell lines. *J Cell Physiol* 176:166–178.

Coudray C, Bellanger J, Castiglia-Delavaud C, Rémésy C, Vermorel M, Rayssignuier Y. 1997. Effect of soluble or partly soluble dietary fibres supplementation on absorption and balance of calcium, magnesium, iron and zinc in healthy young men. *Eur J Clin Nutr* 51:375–380.

Coulston AM, Liu GC, Reaven GM. 1983. Plasma glucose, insulin and lipid responses to high-carbohydrate low-fat diets in normal humans. *Metabolism* 32:52–56.

Coulston AM, Hollenbeck CB, Swislocki AL, Chen YD, Reaven GM. 1987. Deleterious metabolic effects of high-carbohydrate, sucrose-containing diets in patients with non-insulin-dependent diabetes mellitus. *Am J Med* 82:213–220.

Cunningham DC, Harrison LY, Shultz TD. 1997. Proliferative responses of normal human mammary and MCF-7 breast cancer cells to linoleic acid, conjugated linoleic acid and eicosanoid synthesis inhibitors in culture. *Anticancer Res* 17:197–204.

Curb JD, Wergowske G, Dobbs JC, Abbott RD, Huang B. 2000. Serum lipid effects of a high-monounsaturated fat diet based on macadamia nuts. *Arch Intern Med* 160:1154–1158.

Curhan GC, Willet WC, Rimm EB, Stampfer MJ. 1996. A prospective study of dietary calcium and other nutrients and the risk of kidney stones in men: 8 Year follow-up. In: Pak CY, Resnick MI, Preminger GM, eds. *Urolithiasis.* Dallas, TX: Millet. Pp. 164–166.

Czarnecki SK, Kritchevsky D. 1993. Dietary protein and atherosclerosis. In: Liepa GU, Beitz DC, Beynen AC, Gorman MA, eds. *Dietary Proteins: How They Alleviate Disease and Promote Better Health.* Champaign, IL: American Oil Chemists' Society. Pp. 42–56.

Davies PS. 1997. Diet composition and body mass index in pre-school children. *Eur J Clin Nutr* 51:443–448.

Daviglus ML, Stamler J, Orencia AJ, Dyer AR, Liu K, Greenland P, Walsh MK, Morris D, Shekelle RB. 1997. Fish consumption and the 30-year risk of fatal myocardial infarction. *N Engl J Med* 336:1046–1053.

Dawson-Hughes B, Harris SS. 2002. Calcium intake influences the association of protein intake with rates of bones loss in elderly men and women. *Am J Clin Nutr* 75:773–779.

Decarli A, Favero A, La Vecchia C, Russo A, Ferraroni M, Negri E, Franceschi S. 1997. Macronutrients, energy intake, and breast cancer risk: Implications from different models. *Epidemiology* 8:425–428.

De Caterina R, Liao JK, Libby P. 2000. Fatty acid modulation of endothelial activation. *Am J Clin Nutr* 71:213–223.

de Deckere EAM, van Amelsvoort JMM, McNeill GP, Jones P. 1999. Effects of conjugated linoleic acid (CLA) isomers on lipid levels and peroxisome proliferation in the hamster. *Br J Nutr* 82:309–317.

DeLany JP, Vivian VM, Snook JT, Anderson PA. 1990. Effects of fish oil on serum lipids in men during a controlled feeding trial. *Am J Clin Nutr* 52:477–485.

de Lorgeril M, Renaud S, Mamelle N, Salen P, Martin J-L, Monjaud I, Guidollet J, Touboul P, Delaye J. 1994. Mediterranean alpha-linolenic acid-rich diet in secondary prevention of coronary heart disease. *Lancet* 343:1454–1459.

de Lorgeril M, Salen P, Martin J-L, Monjaud I, Delaye J, Mamelle N. 1999. Mediterranean diet, traditional risk factors, and the rate of cardiovascular complications after myocardial infarction. Final report of the Lyon Diet Heart Study. *Circulation* 99:779–785.

Delzenne N, Aertssens J, Verplaetse H, Roccaro M, Roberfroid M. 1995. Effect of fermentable fructo-oligosaccharides on mineral, nitrogen and energy digestive balance in the rat. *Life Sci* 57:1579–1587.

Demigné C, Levrat M-A, Rémésy C. 1989. Effects of feeding fermentable carbohydrates on the cecal concentrations of minerals and their fluxes between the cecum and blood plasma in the rat. *J Nutr* 119:1625–1630.

Deschner EE, Lytle JS, Wong G, Ruperto JF, Newmark HL. 1990. The effect of dietary omega-3 fatty acids (fish oil) on azoxymethanol-induced focal areas of dysplasia and colon tumor incidence. *Cancer* 66:2350–2356.

Després J-P. 1993. Abdominal obesity as important component of insulin-resistance syndrome. *Nutrition* 9:452–459.

De Stefani E, Deneo-Pellegrini H, Mendilaharsu M, Carzoglio JC, Ronco A. 1997a. Dietary fat and lung cancer: A case-control study in Uruguay. *Cancer Causes Control* 8:913–921.

De Stefani E, Mendilaharsu M, Deneo-Pellegrini H, Ronco A. 1997b. Influence of dietary levels of fat, cholesterol, and calcium on colorectal cancer. *Nutr Cancer* 29:83–89.

De Stefani E, Ronco A, Mendilaharsu M, Deneo-Pellegrini H. 1999. Diet and risk of cancer of the upper aerodigestive tract. II. Nutrients. *Oral Oncol* 35:22–26.

Djoussé L, Pankow JS, Eckfeldt JH, Folsom AR, Hopkins PN, Province MA, Hong Y, Ellison RC. 2001. Relation between dietary linolenic acid and coronary artery disease in the National Heart, Lung, and Blood Institute Family Heart Study. *Am J Clin Nutr* 74:612–619.

Dolecek TA. 1992. Epidemiological evidence of relationships between dietary poly-unsaturated fatty acids and mortality in the Multiple Risk Factor Intervention Trial. *Proc Soc Exp Med Biol* 200:177–182.

Dreon DM, Frey-Hewitt B, Ellsworth N, Williams PT, Terry RB, Wood PD. 1988. Dietary fat:carbohydrate ratio and obesity in middle-aged men. *Am J Clin Nutr* 47:995–1000.

Drewnowski A. 1999. Intense sweeteners and energy density of foods: Implications for weight control. *Eur J Clin Nutr* 53:757–763.

Drewnowski A, Greenwood MR. 1983. Cream and sugar: Human preferences for high-fat foods. *Physiol Behav* 30:629–633.

Duncan KH, Bacon JA, Weinsier RL. 1983. The effects of high and low energy density diets on satiety, energy intake, and eating time of obese and nonobese subjects. *Am J Clin Nutr* 37:763–767.

Dunnigan MG, Fyfe T, McKiddie MT, Crosbie SM. 1970. The effects of isocaloric exchange of dietary starch and sucrose on glucose tolerance, plasma insulin and serum lipids in man. *Clin Sci* 38:1–9.

Durrant M, Royston P. 1979. Short-term effects of energy density on salivation, hunger and appetite in obese subjects. *Int J Obes* 3:335–347.

Dyerberg J, Bang HO. 1979. Haemostatic function and platelet polyunsaturated fatty acids in Eskimos. *Lancet* 2:433–435.

Emmett PM, Heaton KW. 1995. Is extrinsic sugar a vehicle for dietary fat? *Lancet* 345:1537–1540.

Eritsland J, Arnesen H, Seljeflot I, Høstmark AT. 1994a. Long-term metabolic effects of *n*-3 polyunsaturated fatty acids in patients with coronary artery dis-ease. *Am J Clin Nutr* 61:831–836.

Eritsland J, Seljeflot I, Abdelnoor M, Arnesen H, Torjesen PA. 1994b. Long-term effects of *n*-3 fatty acids on serum lipids and glycaemic control. *Scand J Clin Lab Invest* 54:273–280.

Ernst N, Fisher M, Smith W, Gordon T, Rifkind BM, Little JA, Mishkel MA, Williams OD. 1980. The association of plasma high-density lipoprotein cholesterol with dietary intake and alcohol consumption. The Lipid Research Clinics Program Prevalence Study. *Circulation* 62:IV41–IV52.

Fairweather-Tait SM, Wright AJA. 1990. The effects of sugar-beet fibre and wheat bran on iron and zinc absorption in rats. *Br J Nutr* 64:547–552.

FAO/WHO (Food and Agricultural Organization/World Health Organization). 1996. *Sixth World Food and Nutrition Survey*. Rome: FAO.

Farrell TG, Bashir Y, Cripps T, Malik M, Poloniecki J, Bennett ED, Ward DE, Camm AJ. 1991. Risk stratification for arrhythmic events in postinfarction patients based on heart rate variability, ambulatory electrocardiographic vari-ables and the signal-averaged electrocardiogram. *J Am Coll Cardiol* 18:687–697.

Farris RP, Nicklas TA, Myers L, Berenson GS. 1998. Nutrient intake and food group consumption of 10-year-olds by sugar intake level: The Bogalusa Heart Study. *J Am Coll Nutr* 17:579–585.

Fasching P, Ratheiser K, Waldhäusl W, Rohac M, Osterrode W, Nowotny P, Vierhapper H. 1991. Metabolic effects of fish-oil supplementation in patients with impaired glucose tolerance. *Diabetes* 40:583–589.

Fasching P, Ratheiser K, Schneeweiss B, Rohac M, Nowotny P, Waldhausl W. 1996. No effect of short-term dietary supplementation of saturated and poly- and monounsaturated fatty acids on insulin secretion and sensitivity in healthy men. *Ann Nutr Metab* 40:116–122.

Fehily AM, Yarnell JWG, Bolton CH, Butland BK. 1988. Dietary determinants of plasma lipids and lipoproteins: The Caerphilly Study. *Eur J Clin Nutr* 42:405–413.

Fernandez ML, Wilson TA, Conde K, Vergara-Jimenez M, Nicolosi RJ. 1999. Hamsters and guinea pigs differ in their plasma lipoprotein cholesterol distribution when fed diets varying in animal protein, soluble fiber, or cholesterol content. *J Nutr* 129:1323–1332.

Feskens EJM, Bowles CH, Kromhout D. 1991a. Carbohydrate intake and body mass index in relation to the risk of glucose tolerance in an elderly population. *Am J Clin Nutr* 54:136–140.

Feskens EJ, Bowles CH, Kromhout D. 1991b. Inverse association between fish intake and risk of glucose intolerance in normoglycemic elderly men and women. *Diabetes Care* 14:935–941.

Feskens EJM, Loeber JG, Kromhout D. 1994. Diet and physical activity as determinants of hyperinsulinemia: The Zutphen Elderly Study. *Am J Epidemiol* 140:350–360.

Feskens EJM, Virtanen SM, Räsänen L, Tuomilehto J, Stengard J, Pekkanen J, Nissinen A, Kromhout D. 1995. Dietary factors determining diabetes and impaired glucose tolerance: A 20-year follow-up of the Finnish and Dutch cohorts of the Seven Countries Study. *Diabetes Care* 18:1104–1112.

Fischer DR, Morgan KJ, Zabik ME. 1985. Cholesterol, saturated fatty acids, poly-unsaturated fatty acids, sodium, and potassium intakes of the United States population. *J Am Coll Nutr* 4:207–224.

Flaten H, Høstmark AT, Kierulf P, Lystad E, Trygg K, Bjerkedal T, Osland A. 1990. Fish-oil concentrate: Effects on variables related to cardiovascular disease. *Am J Clin Nutr* 52:300–306.

Flegal KM. 1999. The obesity epidemic in children and adults: Current evidence and research issues. *Med Sci Sports Exerc* 31:S509–S514.

Flint A, Raben A, Blundell JE, Astrup A. 2000. Reproducibility, power and validity of visual analogue scales in assessment of appetite sensations in single test meal studies. *Int J Obes Relat Metab Disord* 24:3–48.

Fomon SJ, Thomas LN, Filer LJ, Anderson TA, Nelson SE. 1976. Influence of fat and carbohydrate content of diet on food intake and growth of male infants. *Acta Paediatr Scand* 65:136–144.

Forshee RA, Storey ML. 2001. The role of added sugars in the diet quality of children and adolescents. *J Am Coll Nutr* 20:32–43.

Franceschi S, Levi F, Conti E, Talamini R, Negri E, Dal Maso L, Boyle P, Decarli A, La Vecchia C. 1999. Energy intake and dietary pattern in cancer of the oral cavity and pharynx. *Cancer Causes Control* 10:439–444.

Friedman MI. 1995. Control of energy intake by energy metabolism. *Am J Clin Nutr* 62:1096S–1100S.

Fukagawa NK, Anderson JW, Hageman G, Young VR, Minaker KL. 1990. High-carbohydrate, high-fiber diets increase peripheral insulin sensitivity in healthy young and old adults. *Am J Clin Nutr* 52:524–528.

Gao YT, McLaughlin JK, Gridley G, Blot WJ, Ji BT, Dai Q, Fraumeni JF. 1994. Risk factors for esophageal cancer in Shanghai, China. II. Role of diet and nutrients. *Int J Cancer* 58:197–202.

Garg A, Bonanome A, Grundy SM, Zhang Z-J, Unger RH. 1988. Comparison of a high-carbohydrate diet with a high-monounsaturated-fat diet in patients with non-insulin-dependent diabetes mellitus. *N Engl J Med* 319:829–834.

Garg A, Grundy SM, Koffler M. 1992a. Effect of high carbohydrate intake on hyperglycemia, islet function, and plasma lipoproteins in NIDDM. *Diabetes Care* 15:1572–1580.

Garg A, Grundy SM, Unger RH. 1992b. Comparison of effects of high and low carbohydrate diets on plasma lipoproteins and insulin sensitivity in patients with mild NIDDM. *Diabetes* 41:1278–1285.

Garg A, Bantle JP, Henry RR, Coulston AM, Griver KA, Raatz SK, Brinkley L, Chen Y-DI, Grundy SM, Huet BA, Reaven GM. 1994. Effects of varying carbohydrate content of diet in patients with non-insulin-dependent diabetes mellitus. *J Am Med Assoc* 271:1421–1428.

Gartside PS, Glueck CJ. 1993. Relationship of dietary intake to hospital admission for coronary heart and vascular disease: The NHANES II National Probability Study. *J Am Coll Nutr* 6:676–684.

Gazzaniga JM, Burns TL. 1993. Relationship between diet composition and body fatness, with adjustment for resting energy expenditure and physical activity, in preadolescent children. *Am J Clin Nutr* 58:21–28.

George V, Tremblay A, Després JP, Leblanc C, Bouchard C. 1990. Effect of dietary fat content on total and regional adiposity in men and women. *Int J Obes* 14:1085–1094.

Gerhard GT, Connor SL, Wander RC, Connor WE. 2000. Plasma lipid and lipoprotein responsiveness to dietary fat and cholesterol in premenopausal African American and white women. *Am J Clin Nutr* 72:56–63.

Giannini S, Nobile M, Sartori L, Dalle Carbonare L, Ciuffreda M, Corro P, D'Angelo A, Calo L, Crepaldi G. 1999. Acute effects of moderate dietary protein restriction in patients with idiopathic hypercalciuria and calcium nephrolithiasis. *Am J Clin Nutr* 69:267–271.

Gibney M, Sigman-Grant M, Stanton JL, Keast DR. 1995. Consumption of sugars. *Am J Clin Nutr* 62:178S–194S.

Gibson SA. 1993. Consumption and sources of sugars in the diets of British school-children: Are high-sugar diets nutritionally inferior? *J Hum Nutr Diet* 6:355–371.

Gibson SA. 1997. Non-milk extrinsic sugars in the diets of pre-school children: Association with intakes of micronutrients, energy, fat and NSP. *Br J Nutr* 78:367–378.

Gillum RF, Mussolino ME, Madans JH. 1996. The relationship between fish consumption and stroke incidence. The NHANES I epidemiologic follow-up study. *Arch Intern Med* 156:537–542.

Ginsberg HN, Barr SL, Gilbert A, Karmally W, Deckelbaum R, Kaplan K, Ramakrishnan R, Holleran S, Dell RB. 1990. Reduction of plasma cholesterol levels in normal men on an American Heart Association Step 1 diet or a Step 1 diet with added monounsaturated fat. *N Engl J Med* 322:574–579.

Giovannucci E, Willet WC. 1994. Dietary factors and risk of colon cancer. *Ann Med* 26:443–452.

Giovannucci E, Rimm EB, Colditz GA, Stampfer MJ, Ascherio A, Chute CC, Willett WC. 1993. A prospective study of dietary fat and risk of prostate cancer. *J Natl Cancer Inst* 85:1571–1579.

Giovannucci E, Rimm EB, Stampfer MJ, Colditz GA, Ascherio A, Willett WC. 1994. Intake of fat, meat, and fiber in relation to risk of colon cancer in men. *Cancer Res* 54:2390–2397.

GISSI-Prevenzione Investigators. 1999. Dietary supplementation with n-3 poly-unsaturated fatty acids and vitamin E after myocardial infarction: Results of the GISSI-Prevenzione trial. *Lancet* 354:447–455.

Glanz K, Basil M, Maibach E, Goldberg J, Snyder D. 1998. Why Americans eat what they do: Taste, nutrition, cost, convenience, and weight control concerns as influences on food consumption. *J Am Diet Assoc* 98:1118–1126.

Glueck CJ, Hastings MM, Allen C, Hogg E, Baehler L, Gartside PS, Phillips D, Jones M, Hollenbach EJ, Braun B, Anastasia JV. 1982. Sucrose polyester and covert caloric dilution. *Am J Clin Nutr* 35:1352–1359.

Goodman MT, Kolonel LN, Yoshizawa CN, Hankin JH. 1988. The effect of dietary cholesterol and fat on the risk of lung cancer in Hawaii. *Am J Epidemiol* 128:1241–1255.

Göranzon H, Forsum E, Thilén M. 1983. Calculation and determination of metabolizable energy in mixed diets to humans. *Am J Clin Nutr* 38:954–963.

Gortmaker SL, Dietz WH, Sobol AM, Wehler CA. 1987. Increasing pediatric obesity in the United States. *Am J Dis Child* 141:535–540.

Grammatikos SI, Subbaiah PV, Victor TA, Miller WM. 1994. n-3 and n-6 Fatty acid processing and growth effects in neoplastic and non-cancerous human mammary epithelial cell lines. *Br J Cancer* 70:219–227.

Green SM, Burley VJ, Blundell JE. 1994. Effect of fat- and sucrose-containing foods on the size of eating episodes and energy intake in lean males: Potential for causing overconsumption. *Eur J Clin Nutr* 48:547–555.

Grill V, Björklund A. 2001. Overstimulation and beta-cell function. *Diabetes* 50:S122–S124.

Grimsgaard S, Bønaa KH, Hansen J-B, Nordøy A. 1997. Highly purified eicosapentaenoic acid and docosahexaenoic acid in humans have similar triacylglycerol-lowering effects but divergent effects on serum fatty acids. *Am J Clin Nutr* 66:649–659.

Grundy SM. 1986. Comparison of monounsaturated fatty acids and carbohydrates for lowering plasma cholesterol. *N Engl J Med* 314:745–748.

Grundy SM, Florentin L, Nix D, Whelan MF. 1988. Comparison of monounsaturated fatty acids and carbohydrates for reducing raised levels of plasma cholesterol in man. *Am J Clin Nutr* 47:965–969.

Guallar E, Aro A, Jiménez FJ, Martín-Moreno JM, Salminen I, van't Veer P, Kardinaal AFM, Gómez-Aracena J, Martin BC, Kohlmeier L, Kark JD, Mazaev VP, Ringstad J, Guillén J, Riemersma RA, Huttunen JK, Thamm M, Kok FJ. 1999. Omega-3 fatty acids in adipose tissue and risk of myocardial infarction. The EURAMIC Study. *Arterioscler Thromb Vasc Biol* 19:1111–1118.

Guenther PM. 1986. Beverages in the diets of American teenagers. *J Am Diet Assoc* 86:493–499.

Guthrie JF. 1996. Dietary patterns and personal characteristics of women consuming recommended amounts of calcium. *Fam Econ Nutr Rev* 9:33–49.

Guthrie JF, Derby B. 1998. Changes in consumers' knowledge of food guide recommendations, 1990–91 versus 1994–95. *Fam Econ Nutr Rev* 11:42–48.

Ha YL, Storkson J, Pariza MW. 1990. Inhibition of benzo(a)pyrene-induced mouse forestomach neoplasia by conjugated dienoic derivatives of linoleic acid. *Cancer Res* 50:1097–1101.

Haglund O, Wallin R, Luostarinen R, Saldeen T. 1990. Effects of a new fluid fish oil concentrate, ESKIMO-3, on triglycerides, cholesterol, fibrinogen and blood pressure. *J Intern Med* 227:347–353.

Halliwell B, Chirico S. 1993. Lipid peroxidation: Its mechanism, measurement, and significance. *Am J Clin Nutr* 57:715S–725S.

Hansen D, Michaelsen KF, Skovby F. 1992. Growth during treatment of familial hypercholesterolemia. *Acta Paediatr* 81:1023–1025.

Harker LA, Kelly AB, Hanson SR, Krupski W, Bass A, Osterud B, Fitzgerald GA, Goodnight SH, Connor WE. 1993. Interruption of vascular thrombus formation and vascular lesion formation by dietary *n*-3 fatty acids in fish oil in non-human primates. *Circulation* 87:1017–1029.

Harnack L, Stang J, Story M. 1999. Soft drink consumption among US children and adolescents: Nutritional consequences. *J Am Diet Assoc* 99:436–441.

Harnack LJ, Jeffery RW, Boutelle KN. 2000. Temporal trends in energy intake in the United States: An ecologic perspective. *Am J Clin Nutr* 71:1478–1484.

Harris WS. 1989. Fish oils and plasma lipid and lipoprotein metabolism in humans: A critical review. *J Lipid Res* 30:785–807.

Harris WS. 1997. *n*-3 Fatty acids and serum lipoproteins: Human studies. *Am J Clin Nutr* 65:1645S–1654S.

Health Canada. 1997. *Canada's Food Guide to Healthy Eating.* Ottawa: Minister of Public Works and Government Services Canada.

Heaney RP. 1993. Protein intake and the calcium economy. *J Am Diet Assoc* 93:1259–1260.

Heaney RP. 1998. Excess dietary protein may not adversely affect bone. *J Nutr* 128:1054–1057.

Hegsted DM, Ausman LM, Johnson JA, Dallal GE. 1993. Dietary fat and serum lipids: An evaluation of the experimental data. *Am J Clin Nutr* 57:875–883.

Heitmann BL, Lissner L, Sørensen TIA, Bengtsson C. 1995. Dietary fat intake and weight gain in women genetically predisposed for obesity. *Am J Clin Nutr* 61:1213–1217.

Hiatt RA, Ettinger B, Caan B, Quesenberry CP, Duncan D, Citron JT. 1996. Randomized controlled trial of a low animal protein, high fiber diet in the prevention of recurrent calcium oxalate kidney stones. *Am J Epidemiol* 144:25–33.

Hill AJ, Blundell JE. 1990. Sensitivity of the appetite control system in obese subjects to nutritional and serotoninergic challenges. *Int J Obes* 14:219–233.

Hill AJ, Leathwood PD, Blundell JE. 1987. Some evidence for short-term caloric compensation in normal weight human subjects: The effects of high- and low-energy meals on hunger, food preference and food intake. *Hum Nutr Appl Nutr* 41:244–257.

Hill JO, Peters JC, Reed GW, Schlundt DG, Sharp T, Greene HL. 1991. Nutrient balance in humans: Effects of diet composition. *Am J Clin Nutr* 54:10–17.

Hill JO, Melanson EL, Wyatt HT. 2000. Dietary fat intake and regulation of energy balance: Implications for obesity. *J Nutr* 130:284S–288S.

Himaya A, Fantino M, Antoine JM, Bronel L, Louis-Sylvestre J. 1997. Satiety power of dietary fat: A new appraisal. *Am J Clin Nutr* 65:1410–1418.

Hislop TG, Coldman AJ, Elwood JM, Brauer G, Kan L. 1986. Childhood and recent eating patterns and risk of breast cancer. *Cancer Detect Prev* 9:47–58.

Holman RL, McGill HC, Strong JP, Greer JC. 1958. The natural history of athero-sclerosis. The early aortic lesions as seen in New Orleans in the middle of the 20th century. *Am J Pathol* 34:209–235.

Holmes MD, Hunter DJ, Colditz GA, Stampfer MJ, Hankinson SE, Speizer FE, Rosner B, Willett WC. 1999. Association of dietary intake of fat and fatty acids with risk of breast cancer. *J Am Med Assoc* 281:914–920.

Holt SH, Miller JC, Petocz P, Farmakalidid E. 1995. A satiety index of common foods. *Eur J Clin Nutr* 49:675–690.

Höppener JWM, Ahrén B, Lips CJM. 2000. Islet amyloid and type 2 diabetes mellitus. *N Engl J Med* 343:411–419.

Horton TJ, Drougas H, Brachey A, Reed GW, Peters JC, Hill JO. 1995. Fat and carbohydrate overfeeding in humans: Different effects on energy storage. *Am J Clin Nutr* 62:19–29.

Horvath PJ, Eagen CK, Fisher NM, Leddy JJ, Pendergast DR. 2000. The effects of varying dietary fat on performance and metabolism in trained male and female runners. *J Am Coll Nutr* 19:52–60.

Howard BV, Abbott WGH, Swinburn BA. 1991. Evaluation of metabolic effects of substitution of complex carbohydrates for saturated fat in individuals with obesity and NIDDM. *Diabetes Care* 14:786–795.

Howard BV, Hannah JS, Heiser CC, Jablonski KA, Paidi MC, Alarif L, Robbins DC, Howard WJ. 1995. Polyunsaturated fatty acids result in greater cholesterol lowering and less triacylglycerol elevation than do monounsaturated fatty acids in a dose–response comparison in a multiracial study group. *Am J Clin Nutr* 62:392–402.

Howe GR, Hirohata T, Hislop TG, Iscovich JM, Yuan J-M, Katsouyanni K, Lubin F, Marubini E, Modan B, Rohan T, Toniolo P, Shunzhang Y. 1990. Dietary factors and risk of breast cancer: Combined analysis of 12 case-control studies. *J Natl Cancer Inst* 82:561–569.

Howe GR, Friedenreich CM, Jain M, Miller AB. 1991. A cohort study of fat intake and risk of breast cancer. *J Natl Cancer Inst* 83:336–340.

Howe GR, Aronson KJ, Benito E, Castelleto R, Cornée J, Duffy S, Gallagher RP, Iscovich JM, Deng-ao J, Kaaks R, Kune GA, Kune S, Lee HP, Lee M, Miller AB, Peters RK, Potter JD, Riboli E, Slattery ML, Trichopoulos D, Tuyns A, Tzonou A, Watson LF, Whittemore AS, Wu-Willimas AH, Shu Z. 1997. The relationship between dietary fat intake and risk of colorectal cancer: Evidence from the combined analysis of 13 case-control studies. *Cancer Causes Control* 8:215–228.

Hu FB, Stampfer MJ, Manson JE, Rimm E, Colditz GA, Rosner BA, Hennekens CH, Willett WC. 1997. Dietary fat intake and the risk of coronary heart disease in women. *N Engl J Med* 337:1491–1499.

Hu FB, Stampfer MJ, Manson JE, Rimm E, Colditz GA, Speizer FE, Hennekens CH, Willett WC. 1999. Dietary protein and risk of ischemic heart disease in women. *Am J Clin Nutr* 70:221–227.

Hu FB, van Dam RM, Liu S. 2001. Diet and risk of type II diabetes: The role of types of fat and carbohydrate. *Diabetologia* 44:805–817.

Hulshof T, De Graaf C, Weststrate JA. 1993. The effects of preloads varying in physical state and fat content on satiety and energy intake. *Appetite* 21:273–286.

Hun CS, Hasegawa K, Kawabata T, Kato M, Shimokawa T, Kagawa Y. 1999. Increased uncoupling protein2 mRNA in white adipose tissue, and decrease in leptin, visceral fat, blood glucose, and cholesterol in KK-A^y mice fed with eicosapentaenoic and docosahexaenoic acids in addition to linolenic acid. *Biochem Biophys Res Comm* 259:85–90.

Hunter DJ, Spiegelman D, Adami H-O, Beeson L, van den Brandt PA, Folsom AR, Fraser GE, Goldbohn A, Graham S, Howe GR, Kushi LH, Marshall JR, McDermott A, Miller AB, Speizer FE, Wolk A, Yaun S-S, Willett W. 1996. Cohort studies of fat intake and the risk of breast cancer—A pooled analysis. *N Engl J Med* 334:356–361.

Hursting SD, Thornquist M, Henderson MM. 1990. Types of dietary fat and the incidence of cancer at five sites. *Prev Med* 19:242–253.

Ip C, Scimeca JA. 1997. Conjugated linoleic acid and linoleic acid are distinctive modulators of mammary carcinogenesis. *Nutr Cancer* 27:131–135.

Ip C, Chin SF, Scimeca JA, Pariza MW. 1991. Mammary cancer prevention by conjugated dienoic derivative of linoleic acid. *Cancer Res* 51:6118–6124.

Ip C, Ip MM, Loftus T, Shoemaker S, Shea-Eaton W. 2000. Induction of apoptosis by conjugated linoleic acid in cultured mammary tumor cells and premalignant lesions of the rat mammary gland. *Cancer Epidemiol Biomarkers Prev* 9:689–696.

Ip MM, Masso-Welch PA, Shoemaker SF, Shea-Eaton WK, Ip C. 1999. Conjugated linoleic acid inhibits proliferation and induces apoptosis of normal rat mammary epithelial cells in primary culture. *Exp Cell Res* 250:22–34.

Iso H, Rexrode KM, Stampfer MJ, Manson JE, Colditz GA, Speizer FE, Hennekens CH, Willett WC. 2001. Intake of fish and omega-3 fatty acids and risk of stroke in women. *J Am Med Assoc* 285:304–312.

James MJ, Gibson RA, Cleland LG. 2000. Dietary polyunsaturated fatty acids and inflammatory mediator production. *Am J Clin Nutr* 71:343S–348S.

Janelle KC, Barr SI. 1995. Nutrient intakes and eating behavior scores of vegetarian and nonvegetarian women. *J Am Diet Assoc* 95:180–196.

Jansen S, Lopez-Miranda J, Salas J, Castro P, Paniagua JA, Lopez-Segura F, Ordovas JM, Jimenez-Pereperez JA, Blanco A, Perez-Jimenez F. 1998. Plasma lipid response to hypolipidemic diets in young healthy non-obese men varies with body mass index. *J Nutr* 128:1144–1149.

Jayarajan P, Reddy V, Mohanram M. 1980. Effect of dietary fat on absorption of β carotene from green leafy vegetables in children. *Indian J Med Res* 71:53–56.

Jeppesen J, Schaaf P, Jones C, Zhou M-Y, Chen Y-DI, Reaven GM. 1997. Effects of low-fat, high-carbohydrate diets on risk factors for ischemic heart disease in postmenopausal women. *Am J Clin Nutr* 65:1027–1033.

Jéquier E. 1999. Response to and range of acceptable fat intake in adults. *Eur J Clin Nutr* 53:S84–S93.

Jessup W, Kritharides L. 2000. Metabolism of oxidized LDL by macrophages. *Curr Opin Lipidol* 11:473–481.

Johnson MM, Swan DD, Surette ME, Stegner J, Chilton T, Fonteh AN, Chilton FH. 1997. Dietary supplementation with γ-linolenic acid alters fatty acid content and eicosanoid production in healthy humans. *J Nutr* 127:1435–1444.

Johnson RK, Panely C, Wang MQ. 1998. The association between noon beverage consumption and the diet quality of school-age children. *J Child Nutr Manage* 22:95–100.

Jones AE, Murphy JL, Stolinski M, Wootton SA. 1998. The effect of age and gender on the metabolic disposal of [1-^{13}C]palmitic acid. *Eur J Clin Nutr* 52:22–28.

Jones DY, Schatzkin A, Green SB, Block G, Brinton LA, Ziegler RG, Hoover R, Taylor PR. 1987. Dietary fat and breast cancer in the National Health and Nutrition Examination Survey. I. Epidemiologic follow-up study. *J Natl Cancer Inst* 79:465–471.

Jonnalagadda SS, Egan SK, Heimbach JT, Harris SS, Kris-Etherton PM. 1995. Fatty acid consumption pattern of Americans: 1987–1988 USDA Nationwide Food Consumption Survey. *Nutr Res* 15:1767–1781.

Kahn SR, Solymoss S, Flegel KM. 1997. Nonvalvular atrial fibrillation: Evidence for a prothrombic state. *Can Med Assoc J* 157:673–681.

Kaizer L, Boyd NF, Kriukov V, Tritchler D. 1989. Fish consumption and breast cancer risk: An ecologic study. *Nutr Cancer* 12:61–68.

Kang JX, Leaf A. 1996. Antiarrhythmic effects of polyunsaturated fatty acids: Recent studies. *Circulation* 94:1774–1780.

Kannel WB. 2000. The Framingham Study: Its 50-year legacy and future promise. *J Atheroscler Thromb* 6:60–66.

Karmali RA. 1986. Eicosanoids and cancer. *Prog Clin Biol Res* 222:687–697.

Karmali RA, Marsh J, Fuchs C. 1984. Effect of omega-3 fatty acids on growth of a rat mammary tumor. *J Natl Cancer Inst* 73:457–461.

Karmali RA, Reichel P, Cohen LA, Terano T, Hirai A, Tamura Y, Yoshida S. 1987. The effects of dietary omega-3 fatty acids on the DU-145 transplantable human prostatic tumor. *Anticancer Res* 7:1173–1179.

Kasim SE, Martino S, Kim P-N, Khilnani S, Boomer A, Depper J, Reading BA, Heilbrun LK. 1993. Dietary and anthropometric determinants of plasma lipoproteins during a long-term low-fat diet in healthy women. *Am J Clin Nutr* 57:146–153.

Kasim-Karakas SE, Lane E, Almario R, Mueller W, Walzem R. 1997. Effects of dietary fat restriction on particle size of plasma lipoproteins in postmenopausal women. *Metabolism* 46:431–436.

Kasim-Karakas SE, Almario RU, Mueller WM, Peerson J. 2000. Changes in plasma lipoproteins during low-fat, high-carbohydrate diets: Effects of energy intake. *Am J Clin Nutr* 71:1439–1447.

Katan MB, Zock PL, Mensink RP. 1994. Effects of fats and fatty acids on blood lipids in humans: An overview. *Am J Clin Nutr* 60:1017S–1022S.

Kato I, Akhmedkhanov A, Koenig K, Toniolo PG, Shore RE, Riboli E. 1997. Prospective study of diet and female colorectal cancer: The New York University Women's Health Study. *Nutr Cancer* 28:276–281.

Kavanaugh CJ, Liu K-L, Belury MA. 1999. Effect of dietary conjugated linoleic acid on phorbol ester-induced PGE_2 production and hyperplasia in mouse epidermis. *Nutr Cancer* 33:132–138.

Keli SO, Feskens EJ, Kromhout D. 1994. Fish consumption and risk of stroke. The Zutphen Study. *Stroke* 25:328–332.

Kelleher CC. 1992. Plasma fibrinogen and factor VII as risk factors for cardiovascular disease. *Eur J Epidemiol* 8:79–82.

Kendall A, Levitsky DA, Strupp BJ, Lissner L. 1991. Weight loss on a low-fat diet: Consequence of the imprecision of the control of food intake in humans. *Am J Clin Nutr* 53:1124–1129.

Kerstetter JE, Mitnick ME, Gundberg CM, Caseria DM, Ellison AF, Carpenter TO, Insogna KL. 1999. Changes in bone turnover in young women consuming different levels of dietary protein. *J Clin Endocrinol Metab* 84:1052–1055.

Kestin M, Clifton P, Belling GB, Nestel PJ. 1990. *n*-3 Fatty acids of marine origin lower systolic blood pressure and triglycerides but raise LDL cholesterol compared with *n*-3 and *n*-6 fatty acids from plants. *Am J Clin Nutr* 51:1028–1034.

Keusch GT, Torun B, Johnson RB, Urrutia JJ. 1984. Impairment of hemolytic complement activation by both classical and alternative pathways in serum from patients with kwashiorkor. *J Pediatr* 105:434–436.

Keys A, Aravanis C, Blackburn H, Buzina R, Djordević BS, Dontas AS, Fidanza F, Karvonen MJ, Kimura N, Menotti A, Mohaček I, Nedeljković S, Puddu V, Punsar S, Taylor HL, van Buchem FSP. 1980. *Seven Countries. A Multivariate Analysis of Death and Coronary Heart Disease.* Cambridge, MA: Harvard University Press.

Keys A, Menotti A, Aravanis C, Blackburn H, Djordević BS, Buzinz R, Dontas AS, Fidanza F, Karvonen MJ, Kimura N, Mohaček I, Nedeljković S, Puddu V, Punsar S, Taylor HL, Conti S, Kromhout D, Toshima H. 1984. The Seven Countries Study: 2,289 deaths in 15 years. *Prev Med* 13:141–154.

Keys A, Menotti A, Karvonen MJ, Aravanis C, Blackburn H, Buzina R, Djordjević BS, Dontas AS, Fidanza F, Keys MH. 1986. The diet and 15-year death rate in the Seven Countries Study. *Am J Epidemiol* 124:903–915.

King JC. 2000. Physiology of pregnancy and nutrient metabolism. *Am J Clin Nutr* 71:1218S–1225S.

Klesges RC, Klesges LM, Haddock CK, Eck LH. 1992. A longitudinal analysis of the impact of dietary intake and physical activity on weight change in adults. *Am J Clin Nutr* 55:818–822.

Knopp RH, Walden CE, Retzlaff BM, McCann BS, Dowdy AA, Albers JJ, Gey GO, Cooper MN. 1997. Long-term cholesterol-lowering effects of 4 fat-restricted diets in hypercholesterolemic and combined hyperlipidemic men. *J Am Med Assoc* 278:1509–1515.

Knuiman JT, Westenbrink S, van der Heyden L, West CE, Burema J, De Boer J, Hautvast JGAJ, Räsänen L, Virkkunen L, Viikari J, Lokko P, Pobee JOM, Ferro-Luzzi A, Ferrini AM, Scaccini C, Sette S, Villavieja GM, Bulatao-Jayme J. 1983. Determinants of total and high density lipoprotein cholesterol in boys from Finland, the Netherlands, Italy, the Philippines and Ghana with special reference to diet. *Hum Nutr Clin Nutr* 37:237–254.

Knuiman JT, West CE, Katan MB, Hautvast JGAJ. 1987. Total cholesterol and high density lipoprotein cholesterol levels in populations differing in fat and carbohydrate intake. *Arteriosclerosis* 7:612–619.

Krauss RM. 2001. Atherogenic lipoprotein phenotype and diet-gene interactions. *J Nutr* 131:340S–343S.

Krauss RM, Dreon DM. 1995. Low-density-lipoprotein subclasses and response to a low-fat diet in healthy men. *Am J Clin Nutr* 62:478S–487S.

Kris-Etherton PM (for the DELTA Investigators). 1996. Effects of replacing saturated fat (SFA) with monounsaturated fat (MUFA) or carbohydrate (CHO) on plasma lipids and lipoproteins in individuals with markers for insulin resistance. *FASEB J* 10:2666.

Kris-Etherton PM, Derr J, Mitchell DC, Mustad VA, Russell ME, McDonnell ET, Salabsky D, Pearson TA. 1993. The role of fatty acid saturation on plasma lipids, lipoproteins, and apolipoproteins: I. Effects of whole food diets high in cocoa butter, olive oil, soybean oil, dairy butter, and milk chocolate on the plasma lipids of young men. *Metabolism* 42:121–129.

Kris-Etherton PM, Pearson TA, Wan Y, Hargrove RL, Moriarty K, Fishell V, Etherton TD. 1999. High-monounsaturated fatty acid diets lower both plasma cholesterol and triacylglycerol concentrations. *Am J Clin Nutr* 70:1009–1015.

Kris-Etherton PM, Zhao G, Pelkman CL, Fishell VK, Coval SM. 2000. Beneficial effects of a diet high in monounsaturated fatty acids on risk factors for cardiovascular disease. *Nutr Clin Care* 3:153–162.

Kritchevsky D, Tepper SA, Czarnecki SK, Klurfeld DM, Story JA. 1981. Experimental atherosclerosis in rabbits fed cholesterol-free diets. Part 9. Beef protein and textured vegetable protein. *Atherosclerosis* 39:169–175.

Kromhout D, de Lezenne Coulander C. 1984. Diet, prevalence and 10-year mortality from coronary heart disease in 871 middle-aged men. *Am J Epidemiol* 119:733–741.

Kromhout D, Bosschieter EB, de Lezenne Coulander C. 1985. The inverse relation between fish consumption and 20-year mortality from coronary heart disease. *N Engl J Med* 312:1205–1209.

Kromhout D, Feskens EJM, Bowles CH. 1995. The protective effect of a small amount of fish on coronary heart disease mortality in an elderly population. *Int J Epidemiol* 24:340–345.

Kromhout D, Bloemberg BPM, Feskens EJM, Hertog MGL, Menotti A, Blackburn H. 1996. Alcohol, fish, fibre and antioxidant vitamins intake do not explain population differences in coronary heart disease mortality. *Int J Epidemiol* 25:753–759.

Kushi LH, Lew RA, Stare FJ, Ellison CR, el Lozy M, Bourke G, Daly L, Graham I, Hickey N, Mulcahy R, Kevaney J. 1985. Diet and 20-year mortality from coronary heart disease. The Ireland–Boston Diet–Heart Study. *N Engl J Med* 312:811–888.

Kushi LH, Sellers TA, Potter JD, Nelson CL, Munger RG, Kaye SA, Folsom AR. 1992. Dietary fat and postmenopausal breast cancer. *J Natl Cancer Inst* 84:1092–1099.

Kwiterovich PO, Barton BA, McMahon RP, Obarzanek E, Hunsberger S, Simons-Morton D, Kimm SYS, Friedman LA, Lasser N, Robson A, Lauer R, Stevens V, Van Horn L, Gidding S, Snetselaar L, Hartmuller VW, Greenlick M, Franklin F. 1997. Effects of diet and sexual maturation on low-density lipoprotein cholesterol during puberty. The Dietary Intervention Study in Children (DISC). *Circulation* 96:2526–2533.

Lagström H, Jokinen E, Seppänen R, Rönnemaa T, Viikari J, Välimäki I, Venetoklis J, Myyrinmaa A, Niinikoski H, Lapinleimu H, Simell O. 1997. Nutrient intakes by young children in a prospective randomized trial of a low-saturated fat, low-cholesterol diet. The STRIP Baby Project. *Arch Pediatr Adolesc Med* 151:181–188.

Lagström H, Seppänen R, Jokinen E, Niinikoski H, Rönnemaa T, Viikari J, Simell O. 1999. Influence of dietary fat on the nutrient intake and growth of children from 1 to 5 y of age: The Special Turku Coronary Risk Factor Intervention Project. *Am J Clin Nutr* 69:516–523.

Lai PBS, Ross JA, Fearson KCH, Anderson JD, Carter DC. 1996. Cell cycle arrest and induction of apoptosis in pancreatic cancer cells exposed to eicosapentaenoic acid in vitro. *Br J Cancer* 74:1375–1383.

Lapinleimu H, Viikari J, Jokinen E, Salo P, Routi T, Leino A, Rönnemaa R, Seppänen R, Välimäki I, Simell O. 1995. Prospective randomised trial in 1062 infants of diet low in saturated fat and cholesterol. *Lancet* 345:471–476.

Larsen LF, Bladbjerg E-M, Jespersen J, Marckmann P. 1997. Effects of dietary fat quality and quantity on postprandial activation of blood coagulation factor VII. *Arterioscler Thromb Vasc Biol* 17:2904–2909.

Larson DE, Hunter GR, Williams MJ, Kekes-Szabo T, Nyikos I, Goran MI. 1996. Dietary fat in relation to body fat and intraabdominal adipose tissue: A cross-sectional analysis. *Am J Clin Nutr* 64:677–684.

Larsson H, Elmståhl S, Berglund G, Ahrén B. 1999. Habitual dietary intake versus glucose tolerance, insulin sensitivity and insulin secretion in postmenopausal women. *J Intern Med* 245:581–591.

Lauer RM, Obarzanek E, Hunsberger SA, Van Horn L, Hartmuller VW, Barton BA, Stevens VJ, Kwiterovich PO, Franklin FA, Kimm SYS, Lasser NL, Simons-Morton DG. 2000. Efficacy and safety of lowering dietary intake of total fat, saturated fat, and cholesterol in children with elevated LDL cholesterol: The Dietary Intervention Study in Children. *Am J Clin Nutr* 72:1332S–1342S.

La Vecchia C, Negri E, Franceschi S, Decarli A, Giacosa A, Lipworth L. 1995. Olive oil, other dietary fats, and the risk of breast cancer (Italy). *Cancer Causes Control* 6:545–550.

Lawton CL, Burley VJ, Wales JK, Blundell JE. 1993. Dietary fat and appetite control in obese subjects: Weak effects on satiation and satiety. *Int J Obes Relat Metab Disord* 17:409–416.

Leclerc I, Davignon I, Lopez D, Garrel DR. 1993. No change in glucose tolerance and substrate oxidation after a high-carbohydrate, low-fat diet. *Metabolism* 42:365–370.

Lee KN, Kritchevsky D, Pariza MW. 1994. Conjugated linoleic acid and athero-sclerosis in rabbits. *Atherosclerosis* 108:19–25.

Lee KN, Pariza MW, Ntambi JM. 1998. Conjugated linoleic acid decreases hepatic stearoyl-CoA desaturase mRNA expression. *Biochem Biophys Res Comm* 248:817–821.

Lee-Han H, Cousins M, Beaton M, McGuire V, Kriukov V, Chipman M, Boyd N. 1988. Compliance in a randomized clinical trial of dietary fat reduction in patients with breast dysplasia. *Am J Clin Nutr* 48:575–586.

Lei YX, Cai WC, Chen YZ, Du YX. 1996. Some lifestyle factors in human lung cancer: A case control study of 792 lung cancer cases. *Lung Cancer* 14:S121–S136.

Leibel RL, Hirsch J, Appel BE, Checani GC. 1992. Energy intake required to maintain body weight is not affected by wide variation in diet composition. *Am J Clin Nutr* 55:350–355.

Lemann J. 1999. Relationship between urinary calcium and net acid excretion as determined by dietary protein and potassium: A review. *Nephron* 81:18–25.

Leventhal LJ, Boyce EG, Zurier RB. 1993. Treatment of rheumatoid arthritis with gammalinolenic acid. *Ann Intern Med* 119:867–873.

Leventhal LJ, Boyce EG, Zurier RB. 1994. Treatment of rheumatoid arthritis with blackcurrant seed oil. *Br J Rheumatol* 33:847–852.

Levrat M-A, Behr SR, Rémésy C, Demigné C. 1991a. Effects of soybean fiber on cecal digestion in rats previously adapted to a fiber-free diet. *J Nutr* 121:672–678.

Levrat M-A, Rémésy C, Demigné C. 1991b. High propionic acid fermentations and mineral accumulation in the cecum of rats adapted to different levels of inulin. *J Nutr* 121:1730–1737.

Lew SQ, Bosch JP. 1991 Effect of diet on creatinine clearance and excretion in young and elderly healthy subjects and in patients with renal disease. *J Am Soc Nephrol* 2:856–865.

Lewis CL, Park YK, Dexter PB, Yetley EA. 1992. Nutrient intakes and body weights of persons consuming high and moderate levels of added sugars. *J Am Diet Assoc* 92:708–713.

Liew C, Schut HAJ, Chin SF, Pariza MW, Dashwood RH. 1995. Protection of conjugated linoleic acids against 2-amino-3-methylimidazo[4,5-*f*]quinoline-induced colon carcinogenesis in the F344 rat: A study of inhibitory mechanisms. *Carcinogenesis* 16:3037–3043.

Lifshitz F, Moses N. 1989. Growth failure. A complication of dietary treatment of hypercholesterolemia. *Am J Dis Child* 143:537–542.

Lissner L, Heitmann BL. 1995. Dietary fat and obesity: Evidence from epidemiology. *Eur J Clin Nutr* 49:79–90.

Lissner L, Levitsky DA, Strupp BJ, Kalkwarf HJ, Roe DA. 1987. Dietary fat and the regulation of energy intake in human subjects. *Am J Clin Nutr* 46:886–892.

Lissner L, Heitmann BL, Bengtsson C. 2000. Population studies of diet and obesity. *Br J Nutr* 83:S21–S24.

Litin L, Sacks F. 1993. Trans-fatty-acid content of common foods. *N Engl J Med* 329:1969–1970.

Liu GC, Coulston AM, Reaven GM. 1983. Effect of high-carbohydrate-low-fat diets on plasma glucose, insulin and lipid responses in hypertriglyceridemic humans. *Metabolism* 32:750–753.

Liu K, Stamler J, Trevisan M, Moss D. 1982. Dietary lipids, sugar, fiber, and mortality from coronary heart disease. Bivariate analysis of international data. *Arteriosclerosis* 2:221–227.

Liu S, Willett WC, Stampfer MJ, Hu FB, Franz M, Sampson L, Hennekens CH, Manson JE. 2000. A prospective study of dietary glycemic load, carbohydrate intake, and risk of coronary heart disease in US women. *Am J Clin Nutr* 71:1455–1461.

Lopes-Virella MF, Virella G. 1996. Modified lipoproteins, cytokines and macrovascular disease in non-insulin-dependent diabetes mellitus. *Ann Med* 28:347–354.

Lopez-Segura F, Velasco F, Lopez-Miranda J, Castro P, Lopez-Pedrera R, Blanco A, Jimenez-Pereperez J, Torres A, Trujillo J, Ordovas JM, Perez-Jiminez F. 1996. Monounsaturated fatty acid-enriched diet decreases plasma plasminogen activator inhibitor type 1. *Ateriosacler Thromb Vasc Biol* 16:82–88.

Louheranta AM, Porkkala-Sarataho EK, Nyyssonen MK, Salonen RM, Salonen JT. 1996. Linoleic acid intake and susceptibility of very-low-density and low density lipoproteins to oxidation in men. *Am J Clin Nutr* 63:698–703.

Louis-Sylvestre J, Tournier A, Chapelot D, Chabert M. 1994. Effect of a fat-reduced dish in a meal on 24-h energy and macronutrient intake. *Appetite* 22:165–172.

Lovejoy JC. 1999. Dietary fatty acids and insulin resistance. *Curr Atheroscler Rep* 1:215–220.

Lovejoy J, DiGirolamo M. 1992. Habitual dietary intake and insulin sensitivity in lean and obese adults. *Am J Clin Nutr* 55:1174–1179.

Lovell CR, Burton JL, Horrobin DF. 1981. Treatment of atopic eczema with evening primrose oil. *Lancet* 1:278.

Lubin F, Wax Y, Modan B. 1986. Role of fat, animal protein, and dietary fiber in breast cancer etiology: A case-control study. *J Natl Cancer Inst* 77:605–612.

Lubin JH, Burns PE, Blot WJ, Ziegler RG, Lees AW, Fraumeni JF. 1981. Dietary factors and breast cancer risk. *Int J Cancer* 28:685–689.

Ludwig DS, Majzoub JA, Al-Zahrani A, Dallal GE, Blanco I, Roberts SB. 1999a. High glycemic index foods, overeating, and obesity. *Pediatrics* 103:E26.

Ludwig DS, Pereira MA, Kroenke CH, Hilner JE, Van Horn L, Slattery ML, Jacobs DR. 1999b. Dietary fiber, weight gain, and cardiovascular disease risk factors in young adults. *J Am Med Assoc* 282:1539–1546.

Luhman CM, Beitz DC. 1993. Dietary protein and blood cholesterol homeostasis. In: Liepa GU, Beitz DC, Beynen AC, Gorman MA, eds. *Dietary Proteins: How They Alleviate Disease and Promote Better Health.* Champaign, IL: American Oil Chemists' Society. Pp. 57–76.

Lundgren H, Bengtsson C, Blohmé G, Isaksson B, Lapidus L, Lenner RA, Saaek A, Winther E. 1989. Dietary habits and incidence of noninsulin-dependent diabetes mellitus in a population study of women in Gothenburg, Sweden. *Am J Clin Nutr* 49:708–712.

Lungershausen YK, Abbey M, Nestel PJ, Howe PRC. 1994. Reduction of blood pressure and plasma triglycerides by omega-3 fatty acids in treated hypertensives. *J Hypertens* 12:1041–1045.

Luo J, Rizkalla SW, Boillot J, Alamowitch C, Chaib H, Bruzzo F, Desplanque N, Dalix A-M, Durand G, Slama G. 1996. Dietary (*n*-3) polyunsaturated fatty acids improve adipocyte insulin action and glucose metabolism in insulin-resistant rats: Relation to membrane fatty acids. *J Nutr* 126:1951–1958.

Luo J, Rizkalla SW, Vidal H, Oppert J-M, Colas C, Boussari A, Guerre-Millo M, Chapuis A-S, Chevalier A, Durand G, Slama G. 1998. Moderate intake of *n*-3 fatty acids for 2 months has no detrimental effect on glucose metabolism and could ameliorate the lipid profile in type 2 diabetic men: Results of a controlled study. *Diabetes Care* 21:717–724.

Maffeis C, Pinelli L, Schutz Y. 1996. Fat intake and adiposity in 8 to 11-year-old obese children. *Int J Obes Relat Metab Disord* 20:170–174.

Maillard G, Charles MA, Lafay L, Thibult N, Vray M, Borys J-M, Basdevant A, Eschwège E, Romon M. 2000. Macronutrient energy intake and adiposity in non obese prepubertal children aged 5–11 y (the Fleurbaix Laventie Ville Santé Study). *Int J Obes Relat Metab Disord* 24:1608–1617.

Männistö S, Pietinen P, Virtanen M, Kataja V, Uusitupa M. 1999. Diet and the risk of breast cancer in a case-control study: Does the threat of disease have an influence on recall bias? *J Clin Epidemiol* 52:429–439.

Marckmann P, Grønbaek M. 1999. Fish consumption and coronary heart disease mortality. A systematic review of prospective cohort studies. *Eur J Clin Nutr* 53:585–590.

Marckmann P, Raben A, Astrup A. 2000. Ad libitum intake of low-fat diets rich in either starchy foods or sucrose: Effects on blood lipids, factor VII coagulant activity, and fibrinogen. *Metabolism* 49:731–735.

Marshall JA, Hamman RF, Baxter J. 1991. High-fat, low-carbohydrate diet and the etiology of non-insulin-dependent diabetes mellitus: The San Luis Valley Diabetes Study. *Am J Epidemiol* 134:590–603.

Marshall JA, Bessesen DH, Hamman RF. 1997. High saturated fat and low starch and fibre are associated with hyperinsulinemia in a non-diabetic population: The San Luis Valley Diabetes Study. *Diabetologia* 40:430–438.

Martin-Moreno JM, Willett WC, Gorgojo L, Banegas JR, Rodriguez-Artalejo F, Fernandez-Rodriguez JC, Maisonneuve P, Boyle P. 1994. Dietary fat, olive oil intake and breast cancer risk. *Int J Cancer* 58:774–780.

Masironi R. 1970. Dietary factors and coronary heart disease. *Bull World Health Organ* 42:103–114.

Mattes R. 1990. Effects of aspartame and sucrose on hunger and energy intake in humans. *Physiol Behav* 47:1037–1044.

Mattson FH, Grundy SM. 1985. Comparison of effects of dietary saturated, monounsaturated, and polyunsaturated fatty acids on plasma lipids and lipoproteins in man. *J Lipid Res* 26:194–202.

Mayer EJ, Newman B, Quesenberry CP, Selby JV. 1993. Usual dietary fat intake and insulin concentrations in healthy women twins. *Diabetes Care* 16:1459–1469.

Mayer-Davis EJ, Monaco JH, Hoen HM, Carmichael S, Vitolins MZ, Rewers MJ, Haffner SM, Ayad MF, Bergman RN, Karter AJ. 1997. Dietary fat and insulin sensitivity in a triethnic population: The role of obesity. The Insulin Resistance Atheroscelrosis Study (IRAS). *Am J Clin Nutr* 65:79–87.

McDevitt RM, Poppitt SD, Murgatroyd PR, Prentice AM. 2000. Macronutrient disposal during controlled overfeeding with glucose, fructose, sucrose, or fat in lean and obese women. *Am J Clin Nutr* 72:369–377.

McDonald BE, Gerrard JM, Bruce VM, Corner EJ. 1989. Comparison of the effect of canola oil and sunflower oil on plasma lipids and lipoproteins and on in vivo thromboxane A_2 and prostacyclin production in healthy young men. *Am J Clin Nutr* 50:1382–1388.

McDowell MA, Briefel RR, Alaimo K, Bischof AM, Caughman CR, Carroll MD, Loria CM, Johnson CL. 1994. Energy and macronutrient intakes of persons ages 2 months and over in the United States: Third National Health and Nutrition Examination Survey, Phase 1, 1988–91. *Adv Data* 255:1–24.

McGee DL, Reed DM, Yano K, Kagan A, Tillotson J. 1984. Ten-year incidence of coronary heart disease in the Honolulu Heart Program. Relationship to nutrient intake. *Am J Epidemiol* 119:667–676.

McGill HC. 1968. Fatty streaks in the coronary arteries and aorta. *Lab Invest* 18:100–104.

McGill HC, McMahan CA, Zieske AW, Sloop GD, Walcott JV, Troxclair DA, Malcom GT, Tracy RE, Oalmann MC, Strong JP. 2000a. Associations of coronary heart disease risk factors with the intermediate lesion of atherosclerosis in youth. *Arterioscler Thromb Vasc Biol* 20:1998–2004.

McGill HC, McMahan CA, Zieske AW, Tracy RE, Malcom GT, Herderick EE, Strong JP. 2000b. Association of coronary heart disease risk factors with microscopic qualities of coronary atherosclerosis in youth. *Circulation* 102:374–379.

McLennan PL. 1993. Relative effects of dietary saturated, monounsaturated, and polyunsaturated fatty acids on cardiac arrhythmias in rats. *Am J Clin Nutr* 57:207–212.

Mensink RP, Katan MB. 1987. Effect of monounsaturated fatty acids versus complex carbohydrates on high-density lipoproteins in healthy men and women. *Lancet* 1:122–125.

Mensink RP, Katan MB. 1992. Effect of dietary fatty acids on serum lipids and lipoproteins. A meta-analysis of 27 trials. *Arterioscler Thromb* 12:911–919.

Mensink RP, Zock PL, Katan MB, Hornstra G. 1992. Effect of dietary *cis* and *trans* fatty acids on serum lipoprotein[a] levels in humans. *J Lipid Res* 33:1493–1501.

Meyer KA, Kushi LH, Jacobs DR, Slavin J, Sellers TA, Folsom AR. 2000. Carbohydrates, dietary fiber, and incident of type 2 diabetes in older women. *Am J Clin Nutr* 71:921–930.

Miles CW. 1992. The metabolizable energy of diets differing in dietary fat and fiber measured in humans. *J Nutr* 122:306–311.

Miller AB, Kelly A, Choi NW, Matthews V, Morgan RW, Munan L, Burch JD, Feather J, Howe GR, Jain M. 1978. A study of diet and breast cancer. *Am J Epidemiol* 107:499–509.

Miller GJ, Cruickshank JK, Ellis LJ, Thompson RL, Wilkes HC, Stirling Y, Mitropoulos KA, Allison JV, Fox TE, Walker AO. 1989. Fat consumption and factor VII coagulant activity in middle-aged men. An association between a dietary and thrombogenic coronary risk factor. *Atherosclerosis* 78:19–24.

Miller WC, Lindeman AK, Wallace J, Niederpruem M. 1990. Diet composition, energy intake, and exercise in relation to body fat in men and women. *Am J Clin Nutr* 52:426–430.

Mooy JM, Grootenhuis PA, de Vries H, Valkenburg HA, Bouter LM, Kostense PJ, Heine RJ. 1995. Prevalence and determinants of glucose intolerance in a Dutch Caucasian population. The Hoorn Study. *Diabetes Care* 18:1270–1273.

Mori TA, Vandongen R, Masarei JRL, Rouse IL, Dunbar D. 1991. Comparison of diets supplemented with fish oil or olive oil on plasma lipoproteins in insulin-dependent diabetics. *Metabolism* 40:241–246.

Mori TA, Beilin LJ, Burke V, Morris J, Ritchie J. 1997. Interactions between dietary fat, fish, and fish oils and their effects on platelet function in men at risk of cardiovascular disease. *Arterioscler Thromb Vasc Biol* 17:279–286.

Morris MC. 1994. Dietary fats and blood pressure. *J Cardiovasc Risk* 1:21–30.

Morris MC, Sacks F, Rosner B. 1993. Does fish oil lower blood pressure? A meta-analysis of controlled trials. *Circulation* 88:523–533.

Morris MC, Manson JE, Rosner B, Buring JE, Willett WC, Hennekens CH. 1995. Fish consumption and cardiovascular disease in the Physicians' Health Study: A prospective study. *Am J Epidemiol* 142:166–175.

Morton JF, Guthrie JF. 1998. Changes in children's total fat intakes and their food group sources of fat, 1989–91 versus 1994–95: Implications for diet quality. *Fam Econ Nutr Rev* 11:44–57.

Murphy JL, Jones A, Brookes S, Wootton SA. 1995. The gastrointestinal handling and metabolism of [1-^{13}C]palmitic acid in healthy women. *Lipids* 30:291–298.

Nagata C, Takatsuka N, Kurisu Y, Shimizu H. 1998. Decreased serum total cholesterol concentration is associated with high intake of soy products in Japanese men and women. *J Nutr* 128:209–213.

National Cholesterol Education Program. 2001. *Third Report of the National Cholesterol Education Program (NCEP) Expert Panel on Detection, Evaluation, and Treatment of High Blood Cholesterol in Adults (Adult Treatment Panel III)*. NIH Publication No. 01-3670. Bethesda, MD: National Institutes of Health.

Nelson GJ, Schmidt PC, Kelly DS. 1995. Low-fat diets do not lower plasma cholesterol levels in healthy men compared to high-fat diets with similar fatty acid composition at constant caloric intake. *Lipids* 30:969–976.

Nelson GJ, Schmidt PC, Bartolini GL, Kelley DS, Kyle D. 1997a. The effect of dietary docosahexaenoic acid on plasma lipoproteins and tissue fatty acid composition in humans. *Lipids* 32:1137–1146.

Nelson GJ, Schmidt PS, Bartolini GL, Kelley DS, Kyle D. 1997b. The effect of dietary docosahexaenoic acid on platelet function, platelet fatty acid composition, and blood coagulation in humans. *Lipids* 32:1129–1136.

Nelson M. 1991. Food, vitamins and IQ. *Proc Nutr Soc* 50:29–35.

Newman TB, Garber AM, Holtzman NA, Hulley SB. 1995. Problems with the report of the Expert Panel on blood cholesterol levels in children and adolescents. *Arch Pediatr Adolesc Med* 149:241–247.

Newmark HL. 1999. Squalene, olive oil, and cancer risk: Review and hypothesis. *Ann NY Acad Sci* 889:193–203.

Nguyen VT, Larson DE, Johnson RK, Goran MI. 1996. Fat intake and adiposity in children of lean and obese parents. *Am J Clin Nutr* 63:507–513.

NHLBI/NIDDK (National Heart, Lung, and Blood Institute/National Institute of Diabetes and Digestive and Kidney Diseases). 1998. *Clinical Guidelines on the Identification, Evaluation, and Treatment of Overweight and Obesity in Adults. The Evidence Report.* NIH Publication No. 98-4083. Bethesda, MD: National Institutes of Health.

Nicklas TA, Webber LS, Koschak M, Berenson GS. 1992. Nutrient adequacy of low fat intakes for children: The Bogalusa Heart Study. *Pediatrics* 89:221–228.

Nicklas TA, Myers L, Farris RP, Srinivasan SR, Berenson GS. 1996. Nutritional quality of a high carbohydrate diet as consumed by children: The Bogalusa Heart Study. *J Nutr* 126:1382–1388.

Nicolosi RJ, Wilson TA. 1997. The anti-atherogenic effect of dietary soybean protein concentrate in hamsters. *Nutr Res* 17:1457–1467.

Niinikoski H, Viikari J, Rönnemaa T, Lapinleimu H, Jokinen E, Salo P, Seppänen R, Leino A, Tuominen J, Välimäki I, Simell O. 1996. Prospective randomized trial of low-saturated-fat, low-cholesterol diet during the first 3 years of life. The STRIP Baby Project. *Circulation* 94:1386–1393.

Niinikoski H, Lapinleimu H, Viikari J, Rönnemaa T, Jokinen E, Seppänen R, Terho P, Tuominen J, Välimäki I, Simell O. 1997a. Growth until 3 years of age in a prospective, randomized trial of a diet with reduced saturated fat and cholesterol. *Pediatrics* 99:687–694.

Niinikoski H, Viikari J, Rönnemaa T, Helenius H, Jokinen E, Lapinleimu H, Routi T, Lagström H, Seppänen R, Välimäki I, Simell O. 1997b. Regulation of growth of 7- to 36-month-old children by energy and fat intake in the prospective, randomized STRIP baby trial. *Pediatrics* 100:810–816.

Nobukata H, Ishikawa T, Obata M, Shibutani Y. 2000. Long-term administration of highly purified eicosapentaenoic acid ethyl ester prevents diabetes and abnormalities of blood coagulation in male WBN/Kob rats. *Metabolism* 49:912–919.

Noguchi M, Rose DP, Earashi M, Miyazaki I. 1995. The role of fatty acids and eicosanoid synthesis inhibitors in breast carcinoma. *Oncology* 52:265–271.

Norrish AE, Jackson RT, Sharpe SJ, Skeaff CM. 2000. Men who consume vegetable oils rich in monounsaturated fat: Their patterns and risk of prostate cancer (New Zealand). *Cancer Causes Control* 11:609–615.

Obarzanek E, Schreiber GB, Crawford PB, Goldman SR, Barrier PM, Frederick MM, Lakatos E. 1994. Energy intake and physical activity in relation to indexes of body fat: The National Heart, Lung, and Blood Institute Growth and Health Study. *Am J Clin Nutr* 60:15–22.

Obarzanek E, Velletri PA, Cutler JA. 1996. Dietary protein and blood pressure. *J Am Med Assoc* 275:1598–1603.

Obarzanek E, Hunsberger SA, Van Horn L, Hartmuller VV, Barton BA, Stevens VJ, Kwiterovich PO, Franklin FA, Kimm SYS, Lasser NL, Simons-Morton DG, Lauer RM. 1997. Safety of a fat-reduced diet: The Dietary Intervention Study in Children (DISC). *Pediatrics* 100:51–59.

Obarzanek E, Kimm SYS, Barton BA, Van Horn L, Kwiterovich PO, Simons-Morton DG, Hunsberger SA, Lasser NL, Robson AM, Franklin FA, Lauer RM, Stevens VJ, Friedman LA, Dorgan JF, Greenlick MR. 2001a. Long-term safety and efficacy of a cholesterol-lowering diet in children with elevated low-density lipoprotein cholesterol: Seven-year results of the Dietary Intervention Study in Children (DISC). *Pediatrics* 107:256–264.

Obarzanek E, Sacks FM, Vollmer WM, Bray GA, Miller ER, Lin P-H, Karanja NM, Most-Windhauser MM, Moore TJ, Swain JF, Bales CW, Proschan MA. 2001b. Effects on blood lipids of a blood pressure-lowering diet: The Dietary Approaches to Stop Hypertension (DASH) Trial. *Am J Clin Nutr* 74:80–89.

Ogden J, Wardle J. 1990. Cognitive restraint and sensitivity to cues for hunger and satiety. *Physiol Behav* 47:477–481.

O'Hanesian MA, Rosner B, Bishop LM, Sacks FM. 1996. Effects of inherent responsiveness to diet and day-to-day diet variation on plasma lipoprotein concentrations. *Am J Clin Nutr* 64:53–59.

Ohta A, Ohtsuki M, Baba S, Adachi T, Sakata T, Sakaguchi E. 1995. Calcium and magnesium absorption from the colon and rectum are increased in rats fed fructooligosaccharides. *J Nutr* 125:2417–2424.

Okita M, Yoshida S, Yamamoto J, Suzuki K, Kaneyuki T, Kubota M, Sasagawa T. 1995. *n*-3 and *n*-6 Fatty acid intake and serum phospholipid fatty acid composition in middle-aged women living in rural and urban areas in Okayama Prefecture. *J Nutr Sci Vitaminol* 41:313–323.

Olson RE. 2000. Is it wise to restrict fat in the diets of children? *J Am Diet Assoc* 100:28–32.

Oomen CM, Feskens EJM, Räsänen L, Fidanza F, Nissinen AM, Menotti A, Kok FJ, Kromhout D. 2000. Fish consumption and coronary heart disease mortality in Finland, Italy, and the Netherlands. *Am J Epidemiol* 151:999–1006.

Orencia AJ, Daviglus ML, Dyer AR, Shekelle RB, Stamler J. 1996. Fish consumption and stroke in men. 30-Year findings of the Chicago Western Electric Study. *Stroke* 27:204–209.

Ostrowska E, Muralitharan M, Cross RF, Bauman DE, Dunshea FR. 1999. Dietary conjugated linoleic acids increase lean tissue and decrease fat deposition in growing pigs. *J Nutr* 129:2037–2042.

Owen RW, Giacosa A, Hull WE, Haubner R, Spiegelhalder B, Bartsch H. 2000. The antioxidant/anticancer potential of phenolic compounds isolated from olive oil. *Eur J Cancer* 36:1235–1247.

Parillo M, Rivellese AA, Ciardullo AV, Capaldo B, Giacco A, Genovese S, Riccardi G. 1992. A high-monounsaturated-fat/low-carbohydrate diet improves peripheral insulin sensitivity in non-insulin-dependent diabetic patients. *Metabolism* 41:1373–1378.

Pariza MW, Park Y, Cook ME. 2001. The biologically active isomers of conjugated linoleic acid. *Prog Lipid Res* 40:283–298.

Park Y, Albright KJ, Liu W, Storkson JM, Cook ME, Pariza MW. 1997. Effect of conjugated linoleic acid on body composition in mice. *Lipids* 32:853–858.

Park Y, Storkson JM, Albright KJ, Liu W, Pariza MW. 1999. Evidence that the *trans*-10,*cis*-12 isomer of conjugated linoleic acid induces body composition changes in mice. *Lipids* 34:235–241.

Parker DR, Weiss ST, Troisi R, Cassano PA, Vokonas PS, Landsberg L. 1993. Relationship of dietary saturated fatty acids and body habitus to serum insulin concentrations: The Normative Aging Study. *Am J Clin Nutr* 58:129–136.

Parnaud G, Corpet DE. 1997. Colorectal cancer: Controversial role of meat consumption. *Bull Cancer* 84:899–911.

Parrish CC, Pathy DA, Angel A. 1990. Dietary fish oils limit adipose tissue hypertrophy in rats. *Metabolism* 39:217–219.

Parrish CC, Pathy DA, Parkes JG, Angel A. 1991. Dietary fish oils modify adipocyte structure and function. *J Cell Physiol* 148:493–502.

Pearce ML, Dayton S. 1971. Incidence of cancer in men on a diet high in poly-unsaturated fat. *Lancet* 1:464–467.

Peiris AN, Struve MF, Mueller RA, Lee MB, Kissebah AH. 1988. Glucose metabo-lism in obesity: Influence of body fat distribution. *J Clin Endocrinol Metab* 67:760–767.

Pelkman CL, Coval SM, Mauger DT, Zhao G, Kris-Etherton PM. 2001. A meta-analysis of low-fat versus high-MUFA diets. *FASEB J* 15:394.

Pelletier DL, Frongillo EA, Schroeder DG, Habicht J-P. 1995. The effects of mal-nutrition on child mortality in developing countries. *Bull World Health Organ* 73:443–448.

Perez-Jimenez F, Espino A, Lopez-Segura F, Blanco J, Ruiz-Gutierrez V, Prada JL, Lopez-Miranda J, Jimenez-Pereperez J, Ordovas JM. 1995. Lipoprotein con-centrations in normolipidemic males consuming oleic acid-rich diets from two different sources: Olive oil and oleic acid-rich sunflower oil. *Am J Clin Nutr* 62:769–775.

Perez-Jimenez F, Catrso P, Lopez-Miranda J, Paz-Rojas E, Blanco A, Lopez-Segura F, Velasco F, Marin C, Fuentes F, Ordovas JM. 1999. Circulating levels of endothelial function are modulated by dietary monounsaturated fat. *Athero-sclerosis* 145:351–358.

Perez-Jimenez F, Lopez-Miranda J, Pinillos MD, Gomez P, Pas-Rojas E, Montilla P, Marin C, Velasco MJ, Blanco-Molina A, Jimenez Pereperez JA, Ordovas JM. 2001. A Mediterranean and a high-carbohydrate diet improves glucose metabolism in healthy young persons. *Diabetologica* 44:2038–2043.

Peterson S, Sigman-Grant M. 1997. Impact of adopting lower-fat food choices on nutrient intake of American children. *Pediatrics* 100:E4.

Pfeuffer M, Ahrens F, Hagemeister H, Barth CA. 1988. Influence of casein versus soy protein isolate on lipid metabolism of minipigs. *Ann Nutr Metab* 32:83–89.

Phillips RL. 1975. Role of life-style and dietary habits in risk of cancer among Seventh-Day Adventists. *Cancer Res* 35:3513–3522.

Pietinen P, Ascherio A, Korhonen P, Hartman AM, Willett WC, Albanes D, Virtamo J. 1997. Intake of fatty acids and risk of coronary heart disease in a cohort of Finnish men. The Alpha-Tocopherol, Beta-Carotene Cancer Prevention Study. *Am J Epidemiol* 145:876–887.

Poppitt SD, Swann DL. 1998. Dietary manipulation and energy compensation: Does the intermittent use of low-fat items in the diet reduce total energy intake in free-feeding lean men? *Int J Obes Relat Metab Disord* 22:1024–1031.

Poppitt SD, Swann DL, Murgatroyd PR, Elia M, McDevitt RM, Prentice AM. 1998. Effect of dietary manipulation on substrate flux and energy balance in obese women taking the appetite suppressant dexfenfluramine. *Am J Clin Nutr* 68:1012–1021.

Popp-Snijders C, Schouten JA, Heine RJ, van der Meer J, van der Veen EA. 1987. Dietary supplementation of omega-3 polyunsaturated fatty acids improves insulin sensitivity in non-insulin-dependent diabetes. *Diabetes Res* 4:141–147.

Porrini M, Crovetti R, Riso P, Santangelo A, Testolin G. 1995. Effects of physical and chemical characteristics of food on specific and general satiety. *Physiol Behav* 57:461–468.

Prentice AM. 2001. Overeating: The health risks. *Obes Res* 9:234S–238S.

Price JM, Grinker J. 1973. Effects of degree of obesity, food deprivation, and palatability on eating behavior of humans. *J Comp Physiol Psychol* 85:265–271.

Promislow JHE, Goodman-Gruen D, Slymen DJ, Barrett-Conner E. 2002. Protein consumption and bone mineral density in the elderly. The Rancho Bernardo Study. *Am J Epidemiol* 155:636–644.

Proserpi C, Sparti A, Schutz Y, Di Vetta V, Milon H, Jéquier E. 1997. Ad libitum intake of a high-carbohydrate or high-fat diet in young men: Effects on nutrient balances. *Am J Clin Nutr* 66:539–545.

Raben A, Macdonald I, Astrup A. 1997. Replacement of dietary fat by sucrose or starch: Effects on 14 d ad libitum energy intake, energy expenditure and body weight in formerly obese and never-obese subjects. *Int J Obes Relat Metab Disord* 21:846–859.

Ramon JM, Bou R, Romea S, Alkiza ME, Jacas M, Ribes J, Oromi J. 2000. Dietary fat intake and prostate cancer risk: A case-control study in Spain. *Cancer Causes Control* 11:679–685.

Rath R, Mašek J, Kujalová V, Slabochová Z. 1974. Effect of a high sugar intake on some metabolic and regulatory indicators in young men. *Nahrung* 18:343–353.

Reaven GM. 1988. Banting lecture 1988. Role of insulin resistance in human disease. *Diabetes* 37:1595–1607.

Reaven GM. 1995. Pathophysiology of insulin resistance in human disease. *Physiol Rev* 75:473–486.

Reaven GM. 2001. Insulin resistance, compensatory hyperinsulinemia, and coronary heart disease: Syndrome X revisited. In: Jefferson LS, Cherrington AD, Goodman HM, eds. *Handbook of Physiology. Section 7: The Endocrine System. Volume II: The Endocrine Pancreas and Regulation of Metabolism.* Oxford: Oxford University Press. Pp. 1169–1197.

Reaven P, Parthasarathy S, Grasse BJ, Miller E, Almazan F, Mattson FH, Khoo JC, Steinberg D, Witztum JL. 1991. Feasibility of using an oleate-rich diet to reduce the susceptibility of low-density lipoprotein to oxidative modification in humans. *Am J Clin Nutr* 54:701–706.

Reaven P, Parthasarathy S, Grasse BJ, Miller E, Steinberg D, Witztum JL. 1993. Effects of oleate-rich and linoleate-rich diets on the susceptibility of low density lipoprotein to oxidative modification in mildly hypercholesterolemic subjects. *J Clin Invest* 91:668–676.

Reaven PD, Grasse BJ, Tribble DL. 1994. Effects of linoleate-enriched and oleate-enriched diets in combination with alpha-tocopherol on the susceptibility of LDL and LDL subfractions to oxidative modification in humans. *Arterioscler Thromb* 14:557–566.

Reddy BS. 1992. Dietary fat and colon cancer: Animal model studies. *Lipids* 27:807–813.

Reddy BS, Burill C, Rigotty J. 1991. Effect of diets high in ω-3 and ω-6 fatty acids on initiation and postinitiation stages of colon carcinogenesis. *Cancer Res* 51:487–491.

Reiser S, Handler HB, Gardner LB, Hallfrisch JG, Michaelis OE, Prather ES. 1979. Isocaloric exchange of dietary starch and sucrose in humans. II. Effect on fasting blood insulin, glucose, and glucagon and on insulin and glucose response to a sucrose load. *Am J Clin Nutr* 32:2206–2216.

Rémésy C, Behr SR, Levrat M-A, Demigné C. 1992. Fiber fermentability in the rat cecum and its physiological consequences. *Nutr Res* 12:1235–1244.

Renaud S, de Lorgeril M, Delaye J, Guidollet J, Jacquard F, Mamelle N, Martin JL, Monjaud I, Salen P, Toubol P. 1995. Creten Mediterranean diet for prevention of coronary heart disease. *Am J Clin Nutr* 61:1360S–1367S.

Ricketts CD. 1997. Fat preferences, dietary fat intake and body composition in children. *Eur J Clin Nutr* 51:778–781.

Rissanen AM, Heliövaara M, Knekt P, Reunanen A, Aromaa A. 1991. Determinants of weight gain and overweight in adult Finns. *Eur J Clin Nutr* 45:419–430.

Robertson WG, Peacock M. 1982. The pattern of urinary stone disease in Leeds and in the United Kingdom in relation to animal protein intake during the period 1960–1980. *Urol Int* 37:394–399.

Robertson WG, Heyburn PJ, Peacock M, Hanes FA, Swaminathan R. 1979. The effect of high animal protein intake on the risk of calcium stone-formation in the urinary tract. *Clin Sci* 57:285–288.

Roche HM, Zampelas A, Jackson KG, Williams CM, Gibney MJ. 1998. The effect of test meal monounsaturated fatty acid:saturated fatty acid ratio on postprandial lipid metabolism. *Br J Nutr* 79:419–424.

Rodier M, Colette C, Crastes de Paulet P, Crastes de Paulet A, Monnier L. 1993. Relationships between serum lipids, platelet membrane fatty acid composition and platelet aggregation in type 2 diabetes mellitus. *Diabete Metab* 19:560–565.

Rolland-Cachera MF, Deheeger M, Akrout M, Bellisle F. 1995. Influence of macronutrients on adiposity development: A follow up study of nutrition and growth from 10 months to 8 years of age. *Int J Obes Relat Metab Disord* 19:573–578.

Rolls BJ, Hetherington M, Burley VJ. 1988. The specificity of satiety: The influence of foods of different macronutrient content on the development of satiety. *Physiol Behav* 43:145–153.

Rolls BJ, Laster LJ, Summerfelt A. 1989. Hunger and food intake following consumption of low-calorie foods. *Appetite* 13:115–127.

Rolls BJ, Kim-Harris S, Fischman MW, Foltin RW, Moran TH, Stoner SA. 1994. Satiety after preloads with different amounts of fat and carbohydrate: Implications for obesity. *Am J Clin Nutr* 60:476–487.

Romieu I, Willett WC, Stampfer MJ, Colditz GA, Sampson L, Rosner B, Hennekens CH, Speizer FE. 1988. Energy intake and other determinants of relative weight. *Am J Clin Nutr* 47:406–412.

Rose DP, Connolly JM. 2000. Regulation of tumor angiogenesis by dietary fatty acids and eicosanoids. *Nutr Cancer* 37:119–127.

Rugg-Gunn AJ, Hackett AF, Jenkins GN, Appleton DR. 1991. Empty calories? Nutrient intake in relation to sugar intake in English adolescents. *J Hum Nutr Diet* 4:101–111.

Rush D, Stein Z, Susser M. 1980. A randomized controlled trial of prenatal nutrition supplementation in New York City. *Pediatrics* 65:683–697.

Rustan AC, Hustvedt B-E, Drevon CA. 1993. Dietary supplementation of very long-chain *n*-3 fatty acids decreases whole body lipid utilization in the rat. *J Lipid Res* 34:1299–1309.

Salmerón J, Manson JE, Stampfer MJ, Colditz GA, Wing AL, Willett WC. 1997. Dietary fiber, glycemic load, and risk of non-insulin-dependent diabetes mellitus in women. *J Am Med Assoc* 277:472–477.

Salmerón J, Hu FB, Manson JE, Stampfer MJ, Colditz GA, Rimm EB, Willett WC. 2001. Dietary fat intake and risk of type 2 diabetes in women. *Am J Clin Nutr* 73:1019–1026.

Salomon O, Steinberg DM, Zivelin A, Gitel S, Dardik R, Rosenberg N, Berliner S, Inbal A, Many A, Lubetsky A, Varon D, Martinowitz U, Seligsohn U. 1999. Single and combined prothrombic factors in patients with idiopathic venous thromboembolism. Prevalence and risk assessment. *Arterioscler Thromb Vasc Biol* 19:511–518.

Saltzman E, Dallal GE, Roberts SB. 1997. Effect of high-fat and low-fat diets on voluntary energy intake and substrate oxidation: Studies in identical twins consuming diets matched for energy density, fiber, and palatability. *Am J Clin Nutr* 66:1332–1339.

Samaras K, Kelly PJ, Chiano MN, Arden N, Spector TD, Campbell LV. 1998. Genes versus environment. The relationship between dietary fat and total and central abdominal fat. *Diabetes Care* 21:2069–2076.

Sanders TAB, Hinds A. 1992. The influence of a fish oil high in docosahexaenoic acid on plasma lipoprotein and vitamin E concentrations and haemostatic function in healthy male volunteers. *Br J Nutr* 68:163–173.

Sanders TAB, Oakley FR, Miller GJ, Mitropoulos KA, Crook D, Oliver MF. 1997. Influence of n-6 versus n-3 polyunsaturated fatty acids in diets low in saturated fatty acids on plasma lipoproteins and hemostatic factors. *Arterioscler Thromb Vasc Biol* 17:3449–3460.

Saris WHM, Astrup A, Prentice AM, Zunft HJF, Formiguera X, Verboeket-van de Venne WPHG, Raben A, Poppitt SD, Seppelt B, Johnston S, Vasilaras TH, Keogh GF. 2000. Randomized controlled trial of changes in dietary carbohydrate/fat ratio and simple vs complex carbohydrates on body weight and blood lipids: The CARMEN study. *Int J Obes Relat Metab Disord* 24:1310–1318.

Sasaki S, Horacsek M, Kesteloot H. 1993. An ecological study of the relationship between dietary fat intake and breast cancer mortality. *Prev Med* 22:187–202.

Sawaya AL, Fuss PJ, Dallal GE, Tsay R, McCrory MA, Young V, Roberts SB. 2001. Meal palatability, substrate oxidation and blood glucose in young and older men. *Physiol Behav* 72:5–12.

Saynor R, Gillott T. 1992. Changes in blood lipids and fibrinogen with a note on safety in a long term study on the effects of n-3 fatty acids in subjects receiving fish oil supplements and followed for seven years. *Lipids* 27:533–538.

Schmidt EB, Lervang H-H, Varming K, Madsen P, Dyerberg J. 1992. Long-term supplementation with n-3 fatty acids. I: Effect on blood lipids, haemostasis and blood pressure. *Scand J Clin Lab Invest* 52:221–228.

Schønberg S, Krokan HE. 1995. The inhibitory effect of conjugated dienoic derivates (CLA) of linoleic acid on the growth of human tumor cell lines is in part due to increased lipid peroxidation. *Anticancer Res* 15:1241–1246.

Schuurman AG, van den Brandt PA, Dorant E, Brants HAM, Goldbohm RA. 1999. Association of energy and fat intake with prostate carcinoma risk. Results from the Netherlands Cohort Study. *Cancer* 86:1019–1027.

Seagle HM, Davy BM, Grunwald G, Hill JO. 1997. Energy density of self-reported food intake: Variation and relationship to other food components. *Obes Res* 5:78S.

Serdula MK, Ivery D, Coates RJ, Freedman DS, Williamson DF, Byers TE. 1993. Do obese children become obese adults? A review of the literature. *Prev Med* 22:167–177.

Severson RK, Nomura AMY, Grove JS, Stemmermann GN. 1989. A prospective study of demographics, diet, and prostate cancer among men of Japanese ancestry in Hawaii. *Cancer Res* 49:1857–1860.

Shannon BM, Tershakovec AM, Martel JK, Achterberg CL, Cortner JA, Smiciklas-Wright HS, Stallings VA, Stolley PD. 1994. Reduction of elevated LDL-cholesterol levels of 4- to 10-year-old children through home-based dietary education. *Pediatrics* 94:923–927.

Shea S, Basch CE, Stein AD, Contento IR, Irigoyen M, Zybert P. 1993. Is there a relationship between dietary fat and stature or growth in children three to five years of age? *Pediatrics* 92:579–586.

Sheppard L, Kristal AR, Kushi LH. 1991. Weight loss in women participating in a randomized trial of low-fat diets. *Am J Clin Nutr* 54:821–828.

Shetty PS, Prentice AM, Goldberg GR, Murgatroyd PR, McKenna APM, Stubbs RJ, Volschenk PA. 1994. Alterations in fuel selection and voluntary food intake in response to isoenergetic manipulation of glycogen stores in humans. *Am J Clin Nutr* 60:534–543.

Shide DJ, Rolls BJ. 1995. Information about the fat content of preloads influences energy intake in healthy women. *J Am Diet Assoc* 95:993–998.

Shu XO, Zheng W, Potischman N, Brinton LA, Hatch MC, Gao YT, Fraumeni JF. 1993. A population-based case-control study of dietary factors and endometrial cancer in Shanghai, People's Republic of China. *Am J Epidemiol* 137:155–165.

Shultz TD, Leklem JE. 1983. Dietary status of Seventh-day Adventists and non-vegetarians. *J Am Diet Assoc* 83:27–33.

Shultz TD, Chew BP, Seaman WR, Luedecke LO. 1992. Inhibitory effect of conjugated dienoic derivates of linoleic acid and β-carotene on the in vitro growth of human cancer cells. *Cancer Lett* 63:125–133.

Sierakowski R, Finlayson B, Landes RR, Finlayson CD, Sierakowski N. 1978. The frequency of urolithiasis in hospital discharge diagnoses in the United States. *Invest Urol* 15:438–441.

Simell O, Niinikoski H, Rönnemaa T, Lapinleimu H, Routi T, Lagström H, Salo P, Jokinen E, Viikari J. 2000. Special Turku Coronary Risk Factor Intervention Project for Babies (STRIP). *Am J Clin Nutr* 72:1316S–1331S.

Singh RB, Rastogi SS, Verma R, Laxmi B, Singh R, Ghosh S, Niaz MA. 1992. Randomised controlled trial of cardioprotective diet in patients with recent acute myocardial infarction: Results of one year follow up. *Br Med J* 304:1015–1019.

Singh RB, Ghosh S, Niaz AM, Gupta S, Bishnoi I, Sharma JP, Agarwal P, Rastogi SS, Beegum R, Chibo H. 1995. Epidemiologic study of diet and coronary risk factors in relation to central obesity and insulin levels in rural and urban populations of north India. *Int J Cardiol* 47:245–255.

Singh RB, Niaz MA, Sharma JP, Kumar R, Rastogi V, Moshiri M. 1997. Randomized, double-blind, placebo-controlled trial of fish oil and mustard oil in patients with suspected acute myocardial infarction: The Indian Experiment of Infarct Survival—4. *Cardiovasc Drugs Ther* 11:485–491.

Siscovick DS, Raghunathan TE, King I, Weinmann S, Wicklund KG, Albright J, Bovbjerg V, Arbogast P, Smith H, Kushi LH, Cobb LA, Copass MK, Psaty BM, Lemaitre R, Retzlaff B, Childs M, Knopp RH. 1995. Dietary intake and cell membrane levels of long-chain *n*-3 polyunsaturated fatty acids and the risk of primary cardiac arrest. *J Am Med Assoc* 274:1363–1367.

Skinner JD, Carruth BR, Moran J, Houck K, Coletta F. 1999. Fruit juice intake is not related to children's growth. *Pediatrics* 103:58–64.

Skov AR, Toubro S, Ronn B, Holm L, Astrup A. 1999. Randomized trial on protein vs carbohydrate in ad libitum fat reduced diet for the treatment of obesity. *Int J Obes Relat Metab Disord* 23:528–536.

Slattery ML, Potter JD, Sorenson AW. 1994. Age and risk factors for colon cancer (United States and Australia): Are there implications for understanding differences in case-control and cohort studies? *Cancer Causes Control* 5:557–563.

Slattery ML, Caan BJ, Potter JD, Berry TD, Coates A, Duncan D, Edwards SL. 1997. Dietary energy sources and colon cancer risk. *Am J Epidemiol* 145:199–210.

Sonko BJ, Prentice AM, Poppitt SD, Prentice A, Jequier E, Whitehead RG. 1994. Could dietary fat intake be an important determinant of seasonal weight changes in a rural subsistence farming community in The Gambia? In: *Nestlé Foundation for the Study of the Problems of Nutrition in the World. Annual Report 1994.* Lausanne, Switzerland: Nestlé Foundation. Pp. 74–87.

Sonnenberg LM, Quatromoni PA, Gagnon DR, Cupples LA, Franz MM, Ordovas JM, Wilson PWF, Schaefer EJ, Millen BE. 1996. Diet and plasma lipids in women. II. Macronutrients and plasma triglycerides, high-density lipoprotein, and the ratio of total to high-density lipoprotein cholesterol in women: The Framingham Nutrition Studies. *J Clin Epidemiol* 49:665–672.

Stamler J. 1979. Population studies. In: Levy R, Rifkind B, Dennis B, Ernst N, eds. *Nutrition, Lipids, and Coronary Heart Disease.* New York: Raven Press. Pp. 25–88.

Stangl GI. 2000. Conjugated linoleic acids exhibit a strong fat-to-lean partitioning effect, reduce serum VLDL lipids and redistribute tissue lipids in food-restricted rats. *J Nutr* 130:1140–1146.

Stary HC. 1989. Evolution and progression of atherosclerotic lesions in coronary arteries of children and young adults. *Arteriosclerosis* 9:I19–I32.

Stefanick ML, Mackey S, Sheehan M, Ellsworth N, Haskell WL, Wood PD. 1998. Effects of diet and exercise in men and postmenopausal women with low levels of HDL cholesterol and high levels of LDL cholesterol. *N Engl J Med* 339:12–20.

Steinberg D, Parthawarathy S, Carew TE, Khoo JC, Witztum JL. 1989. Beyond cholesterol. Modifications of low-density lipoprotein that increase its atherogenicity. *N Engl J Med* 320:915–924.

Storlien LH, Kraegen EW, Chisholm DJ, Ford GL, Bruce DG, Pascoe WS. 1987. Fish oil prevents insulin resistance induced by high-fat feeding. *Science* 237:885–888.

Storlien LH, Jenkins AB, Chisholm DJ, Pascoe WS, Khouri S, Kraegen EW. 1991. Influence of dietary fat composition on development of insulin resistance in rats. Relationship to muscle triglyceride and ω-3 fatty acids in muscle phospholipid. *Diabetes* 40:280–289.

Straznicky NE, O'Callaghan CJ, Barrington VE, Louis WJ. 1999. Hypotensive effect of low-fat, high-carbohydrate diet can be independent of changes in plasma insulin concentrations. *Hypertension* 34:580–585.

Strong JP, Malcom GT, Newman WP, Oalmann MC. 1992. Early lesions of atherosclerosis in childhood and youth: Natural history and risk factors. *J Am Coll Nutr* 11:51S–54S.

Stubbs RJ, Harbron CG, Murgatroyd PR, Prentice AM. 1995a. Covert manipulation of dietary fat and energy density: Effect on substrate flux and food intake in men eating ad libitum. *Am J Clin Nutr* 62:316–329.

Stubbs RJ, Ritz P, Coward WA, Prentice AM. 1995b. Covert manipulation of the ratio of dietary fat to carbohydrate and energy density: Effect on food intake and energy balance in free-living men eating ad libitum. *Am J Clin Nutr* 62:330–337.

Stubbs RJ, Harbron CG, Prentice AM. 1996. Covert manipulation of the dietary fat to carbohydrate ratio of isoenergetically dense diets: Effect on food intake in feeding men ad libitum. *Int J Obes Relat Metab Disord* 20:651–660.

Sugano M, Tsujita A, Yamasaki M, Noguchi M, Yamada K. 1998. Conjugated linoleic acid modulates tissue levels of chemical mediators and immunoglobulins in rats. *Lipids* 33:521–527.

Swinburn BA, Boyce VL, Bergman RN, Howard BV, Bogardus C. 1991. Deterioration in carbohydrate metabolism and lipoprotein changes induced by modern, high fat diet in Pima Indians and Caucasians. *J Clin Endocrinol Metab* 73:156–165.

Swinburn BA, Metcalf PA, Ley SJ. 2001. Long-term (5-year) effects of a reduced-fat diet intervention in individuals with glucose intolerance. *Diabetes Care* 24:619–624.

Takahashi M, Przetakiewicz M, Ong A, Borek C, Lowenstein JM. 1992. Effect of omega 3 and omega 6 fatty acids on transformation of cultured cells by irradiation and transfection. *Cancer Res* 52:154–162.

Talamini R, Franceschi S, La Vecchia C, Serraino D, Barra S, Negri E. 1992. Diet and prostatic cancer: A case-control study in Northern Italy. *Nutr Cancer* 18:277–286.

Tao SC, Huang ZD, Wu XG, Zhou BF, Xiao ZK, Hao JS, Li YH, Cen RC, Rao XX. 1989. CHD and its risk factors in the People's Republic of China. *Int J Epidemiol* 18:S159–S163.

Tate G, Mandell BF, Laposata M, Ohliger D, Baker DG, Schumacher HR, Zurier RB. 1989. Suppression of acute and chronic inflammation by dietary gamma linolenic acid. *J Rheumatol* 16:729–733.

Teixeira SR, Potter SM, Weigel R, Hannum S, Erdman JW, Hasler CM. 2000. Effects of feeding 4 levels of soy protein for 3 and 6 wk on blood lipids and apolipoproteins in moderately hypercholesterolemic men. *Am J Clin Nutr* 71:1077–1084.

Terpstra AHM, Holmes JC, Nicolosi RJ. 1991. The hypocholesterolemic effect of dietary soybean protein vs. casein in hamsters fed cholesterol-free or cholesterol-enriched semipurified diets. *J Nutr* 121:944–947.

Thomas CD, Peters JC, Reed GW, Abumrad NN, Sun M, Hill JO. 1992. Nutrient balance and energy expenditure during ad libitum feeding of high-fat and high-carbohydrate diets in humans. *Am J Clin Nutr* 55:934–942.

Thomsen C, Rasmussen O, Christiansen C, Pedersen E, Vesterlund M, Storm H, Ingerslev J, Hermansen K. 1999. Comparison of the effects of a monounsaturated fat diet and a high carbohydrate diet on cardiovascular risk factors in first degree relatives to type-2 diabetic subjects. *Eur J Clin Nutr* 52:818–823.

Tillotson JL, Grandits GA, Bartsch GE, Stamler J. 1997. Relation of dietary carbohydrates to blood lipids in the special intervention and usual care groups in the Multiple Risk Factor Intervention Trial. *Am J Clin Nutr* 65:314S–326S.

Tobin J, Spector D. 1986. Dietary protein has no effect on future creatinine clearance (Ccr). *Gerontologist* 26:59A.

Toft I, Bønaa KH, Ingebretsen OC, Nordøy A, Jenssen T. 1995. Effects of *n*-3 polyunsaturated fatty acids on glucose homeostasis and blood pressure in essential hypertension. A randomized, controlled trial. *Ann Intern Med* 123:911–918.

Toniolo P, Riboli E, Shore RE, Pasternack BS. 1994. Consumption of meat, animal products, protein, and fat and risk of breast cancer: A prospective cohort study in New York. *Epidemiology* 5:391–397.

Tonstad S, Sivertsen M. 1997. Relation between dietary fat and energy and micronutrient intakes. *Arch Dis Child* 76:416–420.

Torun B, Chew F. 1999. Protein-energy malnutrition. In: Shils ME, Olson JA, Shike M, Ross AC, eds. *Modern Nutrition in Health and Disease*, 9th ed. Baltimore, MD: Williams and Wilkins. Pp. 963–988.

Tremblay A, Plourde G, Despres J-P, Bouchard C. 1989. Impact of dietary fat content and fat oxidation on energy intake in humans. *Am J Clin Nutr* 49:799–805.

Tremblay A, Lavallee N, Almeras N, Allard L, Despres J-P, Bouchard C. 1991. Nutritional determinants of the increase in energy intake associated with a high-fat diet. *Am J Clin Nutr* 53:1134–1137.

Tremblay MS, Willms JD. 2000. Secular trends in the body mass index of Canadian children. *Can Med Assoc J* 163:1429–1433.

Tremoli E, Maderna P, Marangoni F, Colli S, Eligini S, Catalano I, Angeli MT, Pazzucconi F, Gainfranceschi G, Davi G, Stragliotto E, Sirtori CR, Galli C. 1995. Prolonged inhibition of platelet aggregation after *n*-3 fatty acid ethyl ester ingestion by healthy volunteers. *Am J Clin Nutr* 61:607–613.

Trevisan M, Krogh V, Freudenheim J, Blake A, Muti P, Panico S, Farinaro E, Mancini M, Menotti A, Ricci G. 1990. Consumption of olive oil, butter, and vegetable oils and coronary heart disease risk factors. The Research Group ATS-RF2 of the Italian National Research Council. *J Am Med Assoc* 263:688–692.

Trichopoulou A, Katsouyanni K, Stuver S, Tzala L, Gnardellis C, Rimm E, Trichopoulos D. 1995. Consumption of olive oil and specific food groups in relation to breast cancer risk in Greece. *J Natl Cancer Inst* 87:110–116.

Trinidad TP, Wolever TMS, Thompson LU. 1993. Interactive effects of Ca and SCFA on absorption in the distal colon of men. *Nutr Res* 13:417–425.

Trinidad TP, Wolever TMS, Thompson LU. 1996. Effect of acetate and propionate on calcium absorption from the rectum and distal colon of humans. *Am J Clin Nutr* 63:574–578.

Troiano RP, Flegal KM, Kuczmarski RJ, Campbell SM, Johnson CL. 1995. Overweight prevalence and trend for children and adolescents: The National Health and Nutrition Examination Surveys, 1963 to 1991. *Arch Pediatr Adolesc Med* 149:1085–1091.

Tsuboyama-Kasaoka N, Takahashi M, Tanemura K, Kim H-J, Tange T, Okuyama H, Kasai M, Ikemoto S, Ezaki O. 2000. Conjugated linoleic acid supplementation reduces adipose tissue by apoptosis and develops lipodystrophy in mice. *Diabetes* 49:1534–1542.

Tucker LA, Kano MJ. 1992. Dietary fat and body fat: A multivariate study of 205 adult females. *Am J Clin Nutr* 56:616–622.

Tuomilehto J, Lindström J, Eriksson JG, Valle TT, Hämäläinen H, Ilanne-Parikka P, Keinänen-Kiukaanniemi S, Laakso M, Louheranta A, Rastas M, Salminen V, Uusitupa M. 2001. Prevention of type 2 diabetes mellitus by changes in lifestyle among subjects with impaired glucose tolerance. *N Eng J Med* 344:1343–1350.

Turini ME, Powell WS, Behr SR, Holub BJ. 1994. Effects of a fish-oil and vegetable-oil formula on aggregation and ethanolamine-containing lysophospholipid generation in activated human platelets and on leukotriene production in stimulated neutrophils. *Am J Clin Nutr* 60:717–724.

Turner NC, Clapham JC. 1998. Insulin resistance, impaired glucose tolerance and non-insulin-dependent diabetes, pathologic mechanisms and treatment: Current status and therapeutic possibilities. *Prog Drug Res* 51:33–94.

Uauy R, Mize CE, Castillo-Duran C. 2000. Fat intake during childhood: Metabolic responses and effects on growth. *Am J Clin Nutr* 72:1354S–1360S.

Uematsu T, Nagashima S, Niwa M, Kohno K, Sassa T, Ishii M, Tomono Y, Yamato C, Kanamaru M. 1996. Effect of dietary fat content on oral bioavailability of menatetrenone in humans. *J Pharm Sci* 85:1012–1016.

USDA (U.S. Department of Agriculture). 1996. *The Food Guide Pyramid.* Home and Garden Bulletin No. 252. Washington, DC: U.S. Government Printing Office.

Uusitupa M, Schwab U, Mäkimattila S, Karhapää P, Sarkkinen E, Maliranta H, Ågren J, Penttilä I. 1994. Effects of two high-fat diets with different fatty acid compositions on glucose and lipid metabolism in healthy young women. *Am J Clin Nutr* 59:1310–1316.

van Amelsvoort JM, van Stratum P, Kraal JH, Lussenburg RN, Houtsmuller UMT. 1989. Effects of varying the carbohydrate:fat ratio in a hot lunch on postprandial variables in male volunteers. *Br J Nutr* 61:267–283.

van Amelsvoort JM, van Stratum P, Dubbelman GP, Lussenburg RN. 1990. Effects of meal size reduction on postprandial variables in male volunteers. *Ann Nutr Metab* 34:163–174.

van den Berg JJM, Cook NE, Tribble DL. 1995. Reinvestigation of the antioxidant properties of conjugated linoleic acid. *Lipids* 30:599–605.

van den Brandt PA, van't Veer P, Goldbohm RA, Dorant E, Volovics A, Hermus RJJ, Sturmans F. 1993. A prospective cohort study on dietary fat and the risk of postmenopausal breast cancer. *Cancer Res* 53:75–82.

Van Dokkum W, Wesstra A, Schippers FA. 1982. Physiological effects of fibre-rich types of bread. 1. The effect of dietary fibre from bread on the mineral balance of young men. *Br J Nutr* 47:451–460.

van Stratum P, Lussenburg RN, van Wezel LA, Vergroesen AJ, Cremer HD. 1978. The effect of dietary carbohydrate:fat ratio on energy intake by adult women. *Am J Clin Nutr* 31:206–212.

van't Veer P, Kok FJ, Brants HAM, Ockhuizen T, Sturmans F, Hermus RJJ. 1990. Dietary fat and the risk of breast cancer. *Int J Epidemiol* 19:12–18.

Vartiainen E, Puska P, Pietinen P, Nissinen A, Leino U, Uusitalo U. 1986. Effects of dietary fat modifications on serum lipids and blood pressure in children. *Acta Paediatr Scand* 75:396–401.

Veierød MB, Laake P, Thelle DS. 1997a. Dietary fat intake and risk of lung cancer: A prospective study of 51,452 Norwegian men and women. *Eur J Cancer Prev* 6:540–549.

Veierød MB, Laake P, Thelle DS. 1997b. Dietary fat intake and risk of prostate cancer: A prospective study of 25,708 Norwegian men. *Int J Cancer* 73:634–638.

Velie E, Kulldorff M, Schairer C, Block G, Albanes D, Schatzkin A. 2000. Dietary fat, fat subtypes, and breast cancer in postmenopausal women: A prospective cohort study. *J Natl Cancer Inst* 92:833–839.

Vessby B. 2000. Dietary fat and insulin action in humans. *Br J Nutr* 83:S91–S96.

Vessby B, Uusitupa M, Hermansen K, Riccardi G, Rivellese AA, Tapsell LC, Nälsén C, Berglund L, Louheranta A, Rasmussen BM, Calvert GD, Maffetone A, Pedersen E, Gustafsson I-B, Storlien LH. 2001. Substituting dietary saturated for monounsaturated fat impairs insulin sensitivity in healthy men and women: The KANWU study. *Diabetologia* 44:312–319.

Visonneau S, Cesano A, Tepper SA, Scimeca JA, Santoli D, Kritchevsky D. 1997. Conjugated linoleic acid suppresses the growth of human breast adenocarcinoma cells in SCID mice. *Anticancer Res* 17:969–974.

Vobecky JS, Vobecky J, Normand L. 1995. Risk and benefit of low fat intake in childhood. *Ann Nutr Metab* 39:124–133.

von Schacky C, Angerer P, Kothny W, Theisen K, Mudra H. 1999. The effect of dietary ω-3 fatty acids on coronary atherosclerosis. A randomized, double-blind, placebo-controlled trial. *Ann Intern Med* 130:554–562.

Walker AR, Walker BF. 1978. High high-density-lipoprotein cholesterol in African children and adults in a population free of coronary heart disease. *Br Med J* 2:1336–1337.

Walser M. 1992. The relationship of dietary protein to kidney disease. In: Liepa GU, Beitz DC, Beynen AC, Gorman MA, eds. *Dietary Proteins: How They Alleviate Disease and Promote Better Health.* Champaign, IL: American Oil Chemists' Society. Pp. 168–178.

Ward MH, Zahm SH, Weisenburger DD, Gridley G, Cantor KP, Saal RC, Blair A. 1994. Dietary factors and non-Hodgkin's lymphoma in Nebraska (United States). *Cancer Causes Control* 5:422–432.

Waterlow JC. 1976. Classification and definition of protein-energy malnutrition. *Monogr Ser World Health Organ* 62:530–555.

Weisburger JH. 1988. Comparison of nutrition as customary in the Western World, the Orient, and northern populations (Eskimos) in relation to specific disease risk. *Arctic Med Res* 47:110–120.

West CE, Sullivan DR, Katan MB, Halferkamps IL, van der Torre HW. 1990. Boys from populations with high-carbohydrate intake have higher fasting triglyceride levels than boys from populations with high-fat intake. *Am J Epidemiol* 131:271–282.

West KM, Kalbfleisch JM. 1971. Influence of nutritional factors on prevalence of diabetes. *Diabetes* 20:99–108.

Westerterp KR, Verboeket-van de Venne WPHG, Westerterp-Plantenga MS, Velthuis-te Wierik EJM, de Graaf C, Weststrate JA. 1996. Dietary fat and body fat: An intervention study. *Int J Obes Relat Metab Disord* 20:1022–1026.

Whigham LD, Cook ME, Atkinson RL. 2000. Conjugated linoleic acid: Implications for human health. *Pharmacol Res* 42:503–510.

Whiting SJ, Anderson DJ, Weeks SJ. 1997. Calciuric effects of protein and potassium bicarbonate but not of sodium chloride or phosphate can be detected acutely in adult women and men. *Am J Clin Nutr* 65:1465–1472.

Willett WC. 1997. Specific fatty acids and risks of breast and prostate cancer: Dietary intake. *Am J Clin Nutr* 66:1557S–1563S.

Willett WC. 1998. Is dietary fat a major determinant of body fat? *Am J Clin Nutr* 67:556S–562S.

Willett WC, Stampfer MJ, Colditz GA, Rosner BA, Hennekens CH, Speizer FE. 1987. Dietary fat and the risk of breast cancer. *N Engl J Med* 316:22–28.

Willett WC, Stampfer MJ, Colditz GA, Rosner BA, Speizer FE. 1990. Relation of meat, fat, and fiber intake to the risk of colon cancer in a prospective study among women. *N Engl J Med* 323:1664–1672.

Willett WC, Hunter DJ, Stampfer MJ, Colditz G, Manson JE, Spiegelman D, Rosner B, Hennekens CH, Speizer FE. 1992. Dietary fat and fiber in relation to risk of breast cancer. An 8-year follow-up. *J Am Med Assoc* 268:2037–2044.

Williams CL, Bollella M. 1995. Is a high-fiber diet safe for children? *Pediatrics* 96:1014–1019.

Wisen O, Hellstrom PM, Johansson C. 1993. Meal energy density as a determinant of postprandial gastrointestinal adaptation in man. *Scand J Gastroenterol* 28:737–743.

Wisker E, Maltz A, Feldheim W. 1988. Metabolizable energy of diets low or high in dietary fiber from cereals when eaten by humans. *J Nutr* 118:945–952.

Wolfe BMJ, Piché LA. 1999. Replacement of carbohydrate by protein in a conventional-fat diet reduced cholesterol and triglyceride concentrations in healthy normolipidemic subjects. *Clin Invest Med* 22:140–148.

Wolk A, Bergström R, Hunter D, Willett W, Ljung H, Holmberg L, Bergkvist L, Bruce Å, Adami H-O. 1998. A prospective study of association of mono-unsaturated fat and other types of fat with risk of breast cancer. *Arch Intern Med* 158:41–45.

Wooley SC. 1972. Physiologic versus cognitive factors in short term food regulation in the obese and nonobese. *Psychosom Med* 34:62–68.

Wu Y, Zheng W, Sellars TA, Kushi LH, Bostick RM, Potter JD. 1994. Dietary cholesterol, fat, and lung cancer incidence among older women: The Iowa Women's Health Study (United States). *Cancer Causes Control* 5:395–400.

Yao M, Roberts SB. 2001. Dietary energy density and weight regulation. *Nutr Rev* 59:247–258.

Yeomans MR, Gray RW, Mitchell CJ, True S. 1997. Independent effects of palatability and within-meal pauses on intake and appetite ratings in human volunteers. *Appetite* 29:61–76.

Yost TJ, Jensen DR, Haugen BR, Eckel RH. 1998. Effect of dietary macronutrient composition on tissue-specific lipoprotein lipase activity and insulin action in normal-weight subjects. *Am J Clin Nutr* 68:296–302.

Yu-Poth S, Zhao G, Etherton T, Naglak M, Jonnalagadda S, Kris-Etherton PM. 1999. Effects of the National Cholesterol Education Program's Step I and Step II dietary intervention programs on cardiovascular disease risk factors: A meta-analysis. *Am J Clin Nutr* 69:632–646.

Zambell KL, Keim NL, Van Loan MD, Gale B, Benito P, Kelley DS, Nelson GJ. 2000. Conjugated linoleic acid supplementation in humans: Effects of body composition and energy expenditure. *Lipids* 35:777–782.

Zhang J, Sasaki S, Amano K, Kesteloot H. 1999. Fish consumption and mortality from all causes, ischemic heart disease, and stroke: An ecological study. *Prev Med* 28:520–529.

Ziboh VA, Fletcher MP. 1992. Dose-response effects of dietary γ-linolenic acid-enriched oils on human polymorphonuclear-neutrophil biosynthesis of leukotriene B_4. *Am J Clin Nutr* 55:39–45.

Zock PL, Katan MB. 1992. Hydrogenation alternatives: Effects of *trans* fatty acids and stearic acid versus linoleic acid on serum lipids and lipoproteins in humans. *J Lipid Res* 33:399–410.

Zock PL, Katan MB. 1998. Linoleic acid intake and cancer risk: A review and meta-analysis. *Am J Clin Nutr* 68:142–153.

Zurier RB, Rossetti RG, Jacobson EW, DeMarco DM, Liu NY, Temming JE, White BM, Laposata M. 1996. Gamma-linolenic acid treatment of rheumatoid arthritis. A randomized, placebo-controlled trial. *Arthritis Rheum* 39:1808–1817.

12

Physical Activity

SUMMARY

Physical activity promotes health and vigor. Cross-sectional data from a doubly labeled water database were used to define a recommended level of physical activity, based on the physical activity level (PAL) associated with a normal body mass index (BMI) range of 18.5 to 25 kg/m². In addition to the activities identified with a sedentary lifestyle, an average of 60 minutes of daily moderate intensity physical activity (e.g., walking/jogging at 3 to 4 miles/hour) or shorter periods of more vigorous exertion (e.g., jogging for 30 minutes at 5.5 miles/hour) was associated with a normal BMI and therefore is recommended for normal-weight individuals. This amount of physical activity leads to an "active" lifestyle, corresponding to a PAL greater than 1.6 (see Chapter 5). Because the Dietary Reference Intakes are provided for the general healthy population, recommended levels of physical activity for weight loss of obese individuals are not provided.

For children, the physical activity recommendation is also an average of 60 minutes of moderate intensity daily activity. Increasing the energy expenditure of physical activity (EEPA) needs to be considered in determining the energy intake to achieve energy balance in weight stable adults, and adequate growth and development in children (Chapter 5). Body weight serves as the ultimate indicator of adequate energy intake. Increasing EEPA, or maintaining an active lifestyle provides an important means for individuals to balance food energy intake with total energy expenditure.

BACKGROUND INFORMATION

A distinction is made between physical activity[1] and exercise;[2] the latter is considered more vigorous and leads to improvements in physical fitness.[3] In qualitative terms, exercise can be defined as activity sufficiently vigorous to raise breathing to a level where conversation is labored and sweating is noticeable on temperate days. As indicated in Table 5-10, cross-sectional data indicated that the average physical activity level (PAL) among adults participating in the doubly labeled water (DLW) studies included in the DLW Database (Appendix I) was about 1.7, reflecting physical activity habits equivalent to walking 5 to 7 miles/day at 3 to 4 mph, in addition to the activities required by a sedentary lifestyle. Also regular physical activity may improve mood by reducing depression and anxiety, thereby enhancing the quality of life. The beneficial outcomes of regular physical activity and exercise appear to pertain to persons of all ages, and both women and men of diverse ethnic groups.

Throughout history, balancing dietary energy intake and total energy expenditure (TEE) has been accomplished unconsciously by most individuals because of the large component of occupation-related energy expenditure. Today, despite common knowledge that regular physical activity is healthful, more than 60 percent of Americans are not regularly physically active, and 25 percent are not active at all (HHS, 1996). It seems reasonable to anticipate continuation of the current trend for reductions in occupational physical activity and other energy expending activities of daily life. If this is to be offset by deliberately increasing voluntary physical activity, it needs to be kept in mind that in previously sedentary individuals adding periods of mild to moderate intensity exercise can unconsciously be compensated for by reducing other activities during the remainder of the day, so that TEE may be less affected than expected (Epstein and Wing, 1980; van Dale et al., 1989). Hence, to increase physical activity and to thereby facilitate weight control, recreational activities and physical training programs need to add, and not substitute for, other physical activities of daily life.

The trend for decreased activity by adults is similar to trends seen in children who are less active in and out of school (HHS, 1996). As both lack of physical activity and obesity are now recognized as risk factors for

---

[1]Physical activity—Bodily movement that is produced by the contraction of muscle and that substantially increases energy expenditure (HHS, 1996).

[2]Exercise (exercise training)—Planned structured and repetitive bodily movement done to promote or maintain one or more components of physical fitness.

[3]Physical fitness—A set of attributes that people have that relates to the ability to perform physical activity.

several chronic diseases, logic requires that activity recommendations accompany dietary recommendations.

History of Physical Activity Recommendations

United States

In 1953, Kraus and Hirschland (1953) alerted health and fitness professionals, the general public, and President Dwight D. Eisenhower to the relatively poor physical condition of American youth. Their paper and other events led to the formation of the President's Council on Youth Fitness (HHS, 1996). Under President John F. Kennedy, the council was renamed the President's Council on Physical Fitness, and in 1965 it established five levels of physical fitness for adult men and women. Subsequently, the word "sports" was added to the title of the organization, making it the President's Council on Physical Fitness and Sports (HHS, 1996).

Recognizing relationships among blood lipids, diet, and physical activity, the American Heart Association (AHA) issued in 1972 the first of its handbooks and statements on the use of endurance exercise training and exercise testing for the diagnosis and prevention of heart disease (AHA, 1972). In 1978, the American College of Sports Medicine (ACSM) issued its position statement on cardio-respiratory fitness and body composition titled "The Recommended Quantity and Quality of Exercise for Developing and Maintaining Fitness in Healthy Adults" (ACSM, 1978). Subsequently, ACSM issued a series of guidelines for exercise testing and prescription (ACSM, 1980).

In 1979, agencies of the federal government became involved when the United States Department of Heath, Education, and Welfare (DHEW) issued *Healthy People: The Surgeon General's Report on Health Promotion and Disease Prevention*, which recommended endurance exercise training (DHEW, 1979). In 1988, the U.S. Department of Heath and Human Services (HHS) issued *The Surgeon General's Report on Nutrition and Health*, which promoted endurance exercise as a means of weight control (HHS, 1988). Activities such as walking, jogging, and bicycling three times a week for 20 minutes were recommended.

That report was followed in 1990 by the U.S. Department of Agriculture (USDA)/Department of Health and Human Services *Dietary Guidelines for Americans*, which evaluated the role of activity in energy balance but did not offer specific exercise recommendations (USDA/HHS, 1990). In 1995, HHS issued the report *Healthy People 2000*, which listed health objectives for the nation, including an objective for physical activity and fitness (HHS, 1995). That same year, USDA and HHS updated *Dietary Guidelines for Americans* and recommended 30 minutes or more of moderate-intensity physical activity preferably on all days of the week (USDA/HHS, 1995). In 1996 the HHS report *Physical Activity and Health: A Report of the Surgeon General* was published and offered specific recommendations for physical activity: a minimum of 30 minutes of moderate intensity on most, if not all, days of the week.

The 2000 *Dietary Guidelines for Americans* recommends that adults accumulate at least 30 minutes and children 60 minutes of moderate physical activity most days of the week, preferably daily (USDA/HHS, 2000). In addition, that report recommended combining sensible eating with regular physical activity and acknowledged that physical activity and nutrition work together for better health. Physical activity and fitness objectives of *Healthy People 2010* seek to increase the proportion of Americans that engage in daily physical activity to improve health, fitness, and quality of life (HHS, 2000).

Canada

In Canada, similar recommendations have been proposed. An early initiative was the Toronto International Conference on Physical Activity and Cardiovascular Health in 1966. Toronto was also the site of the 1988 International Consensus Conference on Exercise, Fitness and Health. In 1992, coinciding with Canada's 125th birthday, the Second International Conference on Physical Activity, Fitness, and Health was held. That meeting resulted in publication of the report, *Physical Activity, Fitness, and Health* (Bouchard et al., 1994).

Most recently, in cooperation with Health Canada and the Canadian Society of Exercise Physiology, *Canada's Physical Activity Guide to Healthy Active Living* has been published (Health Canada, 1998). This guide describes the benefits of regular physical activity and makes specific recommendations to improve fitness and achieve particular health-related outcomes such as decreasing the risk of premature death from chronic diseases (heart disease, obesity, high blood pressure, type II diabetes, osteoporosis, stroke, colon cancer, and depression). The recommendations include 60 minutes of "light effort" exercises (e.g., light walking, easy gardening), 30 to 60 minutes of "moderate effort" exercises (e.g., brisk walking, biking, swimming, water aerobics, leaf raking), or 20 to 30 minutes of "vigorous effort" exercises (e.g., aerobics, jogging, hockey, fast swimming, fast dancing, basketball). For moderate and vigorous activities, the Canadian recommendations are for 4 or more days per week and also include participation in flexibility activities (4–7 days per week) and strength activities (4–7 days per week).

PHYSICAL ACTIVITY LEVEL AND ENERGY BALANCE

Aside from dietary energy intake, energy expenditure of physical activity (EEPA) is the variable that a person can control, in contrast to age, height, and gender (Chapter 5). Energy expenditure can rise many times over resting rates during exercise, and the effects of an exercise bout on energy expenditure persist for hours, if not a day or longer (Benedict and Cathcart, 1913; Van Zant, 1992). Thus, changing activity level can have major impacts on total energy expenditure (TEE) and on energy balance. Further, exercise does not automatically increase appetite and energy intake in direct proportion to activity-related changes in energy expenditure (Blundell and King, 1998; Hubert et al., 1998; King et al., 1997). In humans and other mammals, energy intake is closely related to physical activity level when body mass is in the ideal range, but too little or too much exercise may disrupt hypothalamic and other mechanisms that regulate body mass (Mayer et al., 1954, 1956).

Impact of Physical Activity on Energy Expenditure and on PAL

Metabolic Equivalents (METs)

The impact of various physical activities is often described and compared in terms of METs (i.e., multiples of an individual's resting oxygen uptake), and one MET is defined as a rate of oxygen (O_2) consumption of 3.5 ml/kg/min in adults. Taking the oxygen energy equivalent of 5 kcal/L consumed, this corresponds to 0.0175 kcal/minute/kg (3.5 mL/min/kg × 0.005 kcal/mL). A rate of energy expenditure of 1.0 MET thus corresponds to 1.2 kcal/min in a man weighing 70 kg (0.0175 kcal/kg/minute × 70 kg) and to 1.0 kcal/minute in a woman weighing 57 kg (0.0175 kcal/kg/min × 57 kg) based on the reference body weights for adults in Table 1-1.

Knowing the intensity of a type of physical activity in terms of METs (see Table 12-1 for the METs for various activities) allows a simple assessment of its impact on the energy expended while the activity is performed (number of METs × minutes × 0.0175 kcal/kg/minute). However, as mentioned in Chapter 5, the increase in daily energy expenditure is somewhat greater because exercise induces an additional small increase in expenditure for some time after the exertion itself has been completed. This "excess post-exercise oxygen consumption" (EPOC) (Gaesser and Brooks, 1984) depends on exercise intensity and duration as well as other factors, such as the types and durations of activities in normal living; EPOC has been estimated at about 15 percent of the increment in expenditure that occurs during the exertion itself (Bahr et al., 1987). The thermic effect of food (TEF), which needs to be consumed to cover the expenditure associated

TABLE 12-1 Intensity and Impact of Various Activities on Physical Activity Level (PAL) in Adults[a]

Activity	Metabolic Equivalents (METs)[b]	ΔPAL/10 min[c]	ΔPAL/h[c]
Leisure			
Mild			
Billiards	2.4	0.013	0.08
Canoeing (leisurely)	2.5	0.014	0.09
Dancing (ballroom)	2.9	0.018	0.11
Golf (with cart)	2.5	0.014	0.09
Horseback riding (walking)	2.3	0.012	0.07
Playing			
Accordion	1.8	0.008	0.05
Cello	2.3	0.012	0.07
Flute	2.0	0.010	0.06
Piano	2.3	0.012	0.07
Violin	2.5	0.014	0.09
Volleyball (noncompetitive)	2.9	0.018	0.11
Walking (2 mph)	2.5	0.014	0.09
Moderate			
Calisthenics (no weight)	4.0	0.029	0.17
Cycling (leisurely)	3.5	0.024	0.14
Golf (without cart)	4.4	0.032	0.19
Swimming (slow)	4.5	0.033	0.20
Walking (3 mph)	3.3	0.022	0.13
Walking (4 mph)	4.5	0.033	0.20
Vigorous			
Chopping wood	4.9	0.037	0.22
Climbing hills (no load)	6.9	0.056	0.34
Climbing hills (5-kg load)	7.4	0.061	0.37
Cycling (moderately)	5.7	0.045	0.27
Dancing			
Aerobic or ballet	6.0	0.048	0.29
Ballroom (fast) or square	5.5	0.043	0.26
Jogging (10-min miles)	10.2	0.088	0.53
Rope skipping	12.0	0.105	0.63
Skating			
Ice	5.5	0.043	0.26
Roller	6.5	0.052	0.31
Skiing (water or downhill)	6.8	0.055	0.33
Squash	12.1	0.106	0.63
Surfing	6.0	0.048	0.29
Swimming	7.0	0.057	0.34
Tennis (doubles)	5.0	0.038	0.23
Walking (5 mph)	8.0	0.067	0.40

continued

TABLE 12-1 Continued

Activity	Metabolic Equivalents (METs)[b]	ΔPAL/10 min[c]	ΔPAL/h[c]
Activities of daily living			
Gardening (no lifting)	4.4	0.032	0.19
Household tasks, moderate effort	3.5	0.024	0.14
Lifting items continuously	4.0	0.029	0.17
Light activity while sitting	1.5	0.005	0.03
Loading/unloading car	3.0	0.019	0.11
Lying quietly	1.0	0.000	0.00
Mopping	3.5	0.024	0.14
Mowing lawn (power mower)	4.5	0.033	0.20
Raking lawn	4.0	0.029	0.17
Riding in a vehicle	1.0	0.000	0.00
Sitting	0.0	0.000	0.00
Taking out trash	3.0	0.019	0.11
Vacuuming	3.5	0.024	0.14
Walking the dog	3.0	0.019	0.11
Walking from house to car or bus	2.5	0.014	0.09
Watering plants	2.5	0.014	0.09

[a] PAL is the physical activity level that is the ratio of the total energy expenditure to the basal energy expenditure.

[b] METs are multiples of an individual's resting oxygen uptakes, defined as the rate of oxygen (O_2) consumption of 3.5 mL of O_2/min/kg body weight in adults.

[c] In the PAL shown here, an allowance has been made to include the delayed effect of physical activity in causing excess postexercise O_2 consumption and the dissipation of some of the food energy consumed through the thermic effect of food.

SOURCE: Adapted from Fletcher et al. (2001).

with a given activity, must also be taken into account. The TEF dissipates about 10 percent of the food energy consumed. The impact of a given activity on daily energy expenditure under conditions of energy balance thus includes the intensity of the physical activity in terms of METS, the EPOC, and the TEF and expressed as:

$$\text{\# of METs} \times \text{min} \times 0.022 \text{ kcal/kg/min} \times \text{kg body weight,}$$

where 0.022 kcal/kg/min = 0.0175 kcal/kg/min × 1.15 percent (EPOC) ÷ 0.9 percent (TEF).

Bijnen and coworkers (1998) found that activities with METs greater than 4 are more effective than less intensive activities in reducing cardiovascular mortality. A rate of energy expenditure of 4.5 METs corresponds to the upper boundary for moderate activities (Table 12-1) and elicits an exertion that falls into the upper range of the percent of Vo_2max considered to reflect light physical activity intensity for 20- to 39-year-old adults, but falls into the lower range of moderate intensities in 40- to 64-year-old adults (Fletcher et al., 2001). A rate of exertion of 4.5 METs is reached, for example, by walking at a speed of 4 mph (Table 12-1).

Physical Activity Level (PAL)

While METs describe activity intensities relative to a resting metabolic rate (RMR), the physical activity level (PAL) is defined as the ratio of total energy expenditure (TEE) to basal energy expenditure (BEE). Thus, the actual impact on PAL depends to some extent on body size and age, as these are determinants of the BEE (Figure 12-1). The impact of these factors can be judged by examining the ratio of MET (extrapolated to 24 hours) to BEE. It is noteworthy that the errors that this introduces in the calculation of PAL values, at least over the normal range of body weights, is of minor importance in comparison to the very large uncertainties generally inherent in the assessment of the duration and intensity of physical activities in individuals and populations.

For a typical 30-year-old reference man and woman 1.77 m and 1.63 m in height and weighing 70 kg and 57 kg (Chapter 1, Table 1-1), BEEs are 1,684 and 1,312 kcal/day, respectively (calculated from the predictive BEE equations in Chapter 5. These correspond to 0.95 and 0.91 times the 1,764 and 1,436 kcal/day obtained by extrapolating a rate of 1.0 MET[4] to 24 hours for reference men and women (1,764 kcal/day = 1 MET × 1,440 min × 0.0175 kcal/kg/min × 70 kg and 1,436 kcal/day = 1 MET × 1,440 min × 0.0175 kcal/kg/min × 57 kg). The following equations, derived for reference body weights of 70 kg for men and 57 kg for women, were utilized to determine the change in PAL for each of the activities in Table 12-1.

Men: ΔPAL = (# of METs − 1) × 1.34 × (min/1,440 min),

where 1.34 = 1.15 percent (EPOC) ÷ 0.9 percent (TEF) ÷ 0.95 percent.[5]

Women: ΔPAL = (# of METs − 1) × 1.42 × (min/1,440 min),

where 1.42 = 1.15 percent (EPOC) ÷ 0.9 percent (TEF) ÷ 0.91.[5]

---

[4]Defined as 0.0175 kcal/kg/min.
[5]Correction to cover EPOC and TEF.

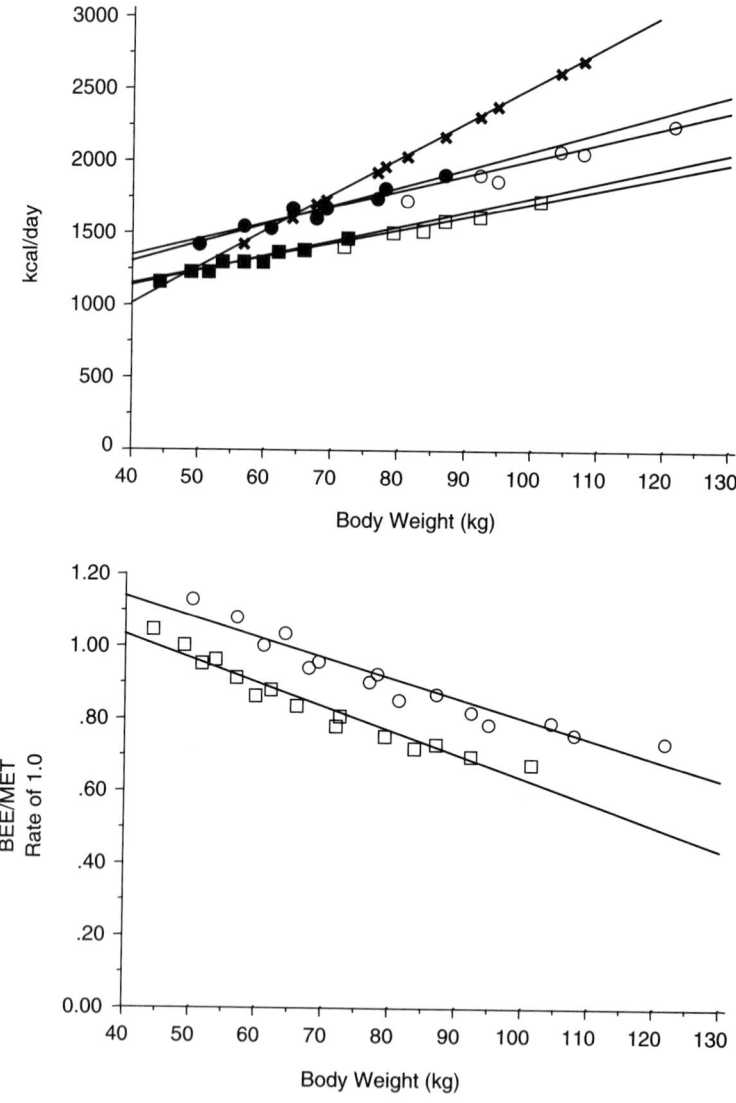

FIGURE 12-1 Relationship of basal energy expenditure (BEE), metabolic equivalents rate and body weight in 30-year-old adults. The upper panel shows the impact of body weight on BEE in men (○) and women (□) and on a MET-rate of 1.0 (×) extrapolated to 24 h. Points with body mass indexes (BMIs) from 18.5 up to 25 kg/m² are filled in. The lower panel shows the ratio of BEE divided by an MET rate of 1.0 for a given body weight for men (○) with reference heights of 1.75 m or reference height ± 1 standard deviation (i.e., 1.64 or 1.86 m), and for women (□) with reference heights of 1.62 m or reference height ± 1 standard deviation (i.e., 1.55 or 1.70 m), and BMI of 18.5, 22.5 (men) or 21.5 (women), 25, 30, and 35 kg/m².

The coefficients given in Table 12-1 can then be used to arrive at an estimate of an individual's PAL by cumulating the effects of the various activities performed on the basis of their duration and intensities (see below, "Physical Activity for Adults").

Because it is the most significant physical activity in the life of most individuals, walking/jogging is taken as the reference activity, and the impact of other activities can be considered in terms of exertions equivalent to walking/jogging, to the extent that these activities are weight bearing and hence involve costs proportional to body weight. The effect of walking/jogging on energy expenditure at various speeds is given in Table 12-1 in terms of METs and is also shown in the upper panel of Figure 12-2. The middle panel describes the energy expended in kcal/hour for walking or jogging at various speeds by individuals weighing 70 or 57 kg (the reference body weights for men and women, respectively from Table 1-1. The figure's lower panel describes the total cost of walking or jogging one mile at various speeds, including the increments in energy expenditure above the resting rate during and after walking or jogging plus a commensurate increase in TEF. The energy expended per mile walked or jogged is essentially constant at speeds ranging from 2 to 4 miles/hour (1 kcal/mile/kg for a man [70 kcal/mile/70 kg] to 1.1 kcal/mile/kg for a woman [65 kcal/mile/57 kg], or approximately 1.1 kcal/mile/kg body weight; lower panel, Figure 12-2), but increases progressively at higher speeds.

According to the formulas shown above, walking at a speed of 4 mph (4.5 METs, upper panel, Figure 12-2) for 60 minutes causes an increase in the daily ΔPAL of 0.195 ([4.5 METs – 1] × 1.34 × 60 min/1,440 min) in men and 0.204 ([4.5 METs – 1] × 1.42 × 60 min/1,440 min) in women, or a ΔPAL of approximately 0.20 as given in Table 12-1. Walking or jogging at speeds of 4.5 mph raises the metabolic rate to 6 METS (upper panel, Figure 12-2), increasing the impact on changing the daily PAL by half to 0.30 for sixty minutes (ΔPAL in men = [6 METs – 1] × 1.34 × 60 min/1,440 min = 0.279, ΔPAL in women = [6 METs – 1] × 1.42 × 60 min/1,440 min = 0.296). Indeed, walking or jogging to cover 4.5 miles in 60 minutes, at a cost of 107 kcal/mile (lower panel, Figure 12-2) or 1.53 kcal/mile/kg (107 kcal/mile ÷ 70 kg) in men, or performing some equally demanding activity for 60 minutes, will cause an increase in PAL of approximately 0.30.

Impact of Body Weight on Energy Expenditure

The impact of body weight on energy expenditure while walking at various speeds is illustrated in Figure 12-3, while Figure 12-4 describes how body weight affects the total increase in energy expenditure caused by

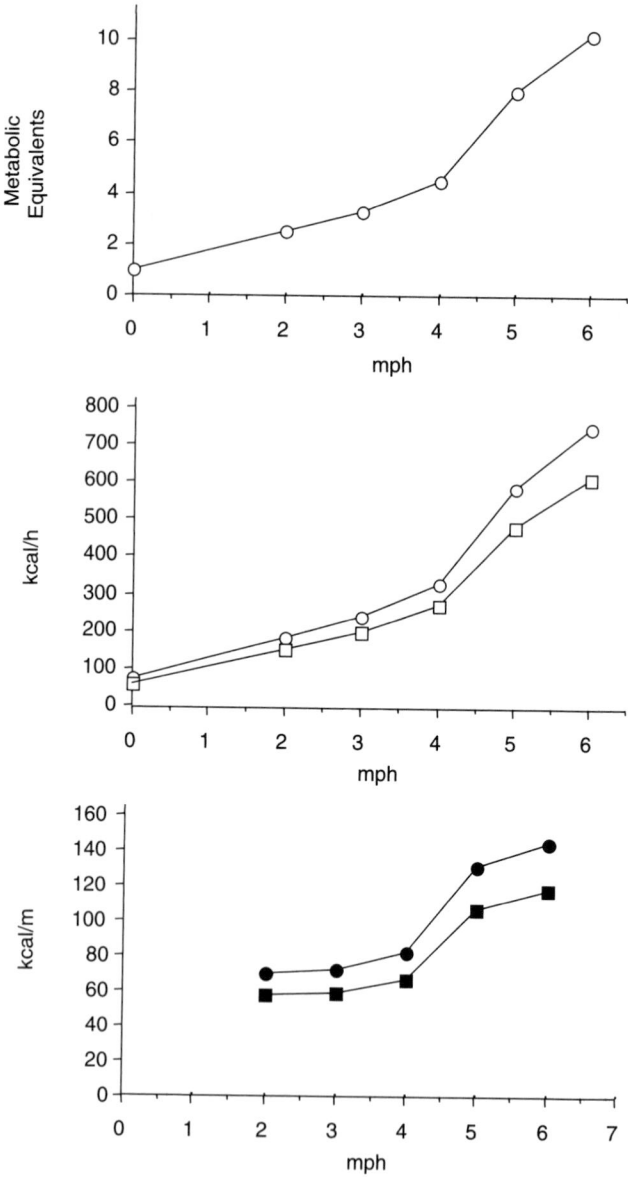

FIGURE 12-2 Relationships of energy expenditure and walking/jogging speeds. The upper panel shows the rate of energy expenditure as a function of walking/jogging speed. The middle panel shows the energy expended by a 70-kg man (○) and by a 57-kg woman (□) while walking/jogging 1 h at various speeds. The lower panel shows the increase in daily energy expenditure induced by walking/jogging 1 m at various speeds for a 70-kg man (●) and a 57-kg woman (■).

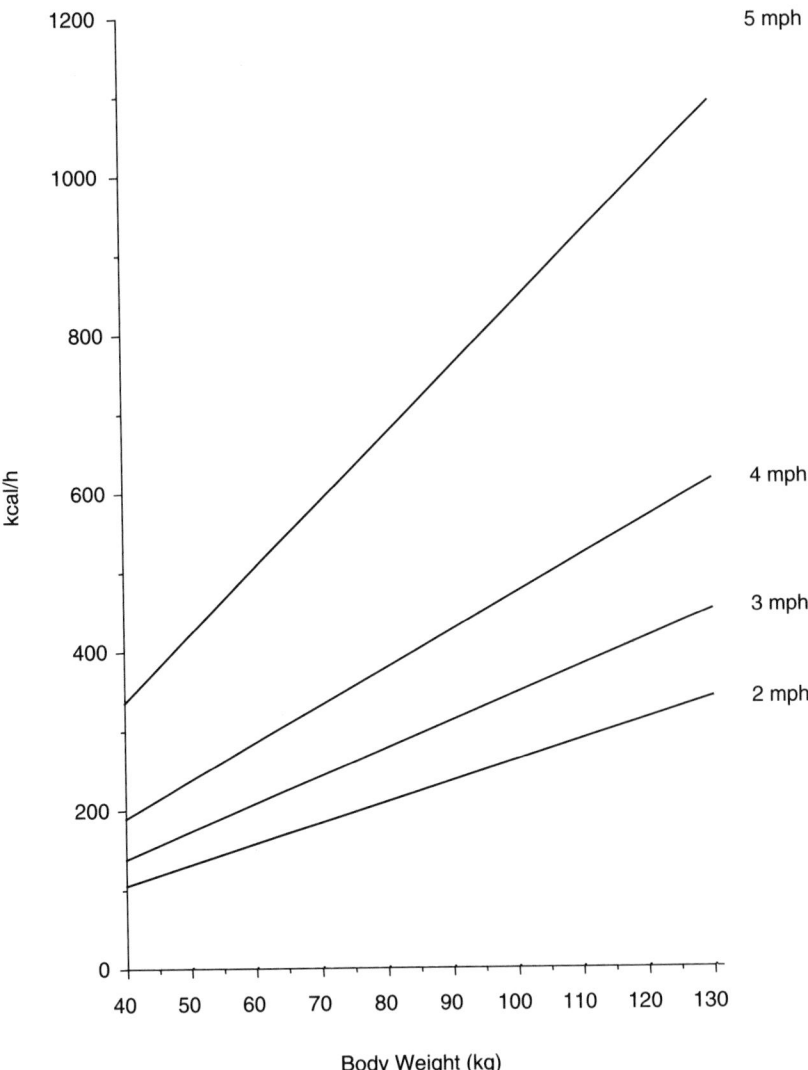

FIGURE 12-3 Impact of body weight on energy expenditure while walking at speeds of 2, 3, 4, or 5 mph.

walking one mile at various speeds. Figures 12-5 for men and 12-6 for women show how body weight influences how far and for how many minutes adults must walk at speeds of 2, 3, 4, or 5 mph (or to engage in activities rated as MET = 2.5, 3.3, 4.5, or 8.0) to raise the PAL level by 0.10. These figures also describe the effect of more demanding physical activity,

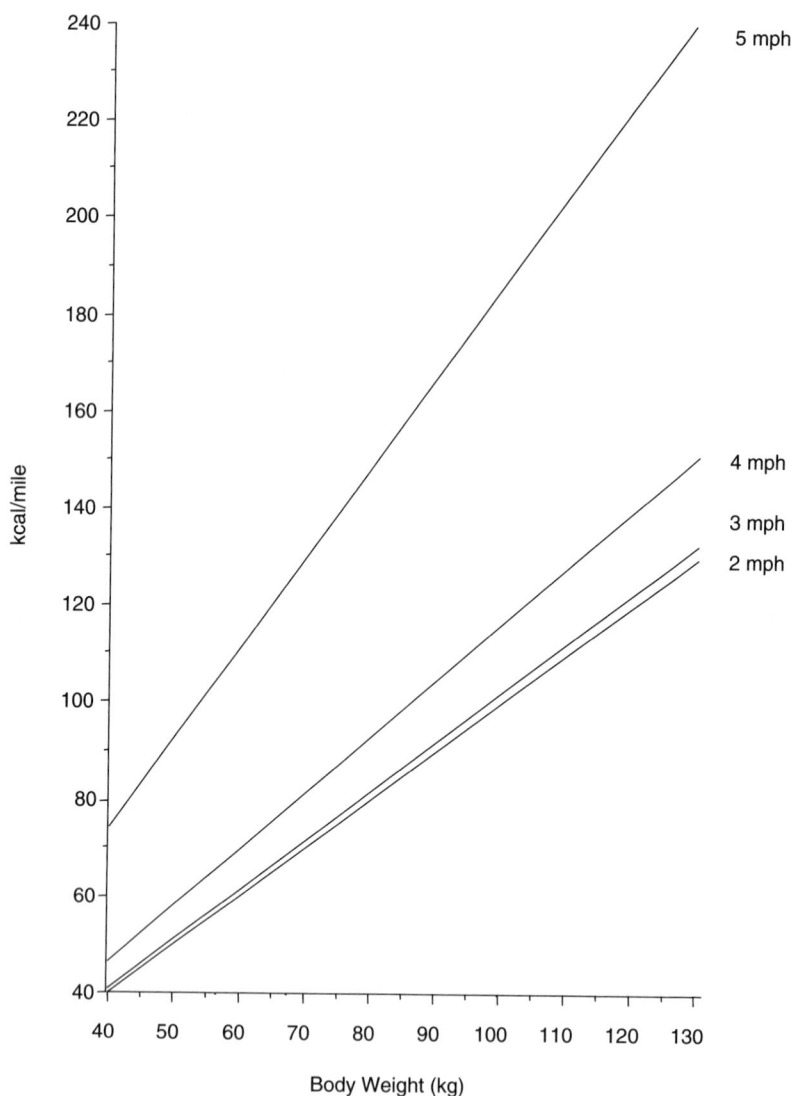

FIGURE 12-4 Impact of body weight on energy cost of walking 1 mile at speeds of 2, 3, 4, or 5 mph in men and women.

such as running at speeds of 6 or 8 mph, corresponding to exertions at 10.2 or 13.5 METs. While the effect on TEE/miles covered does not increase substantially as fast walking (5 mph) changes to jogging (6 mph) and running (8 mph) (upper panels of Figures 12-5 and 12-6), the time required for a given impact on PAL is reduced. This illustrates that high

MEN

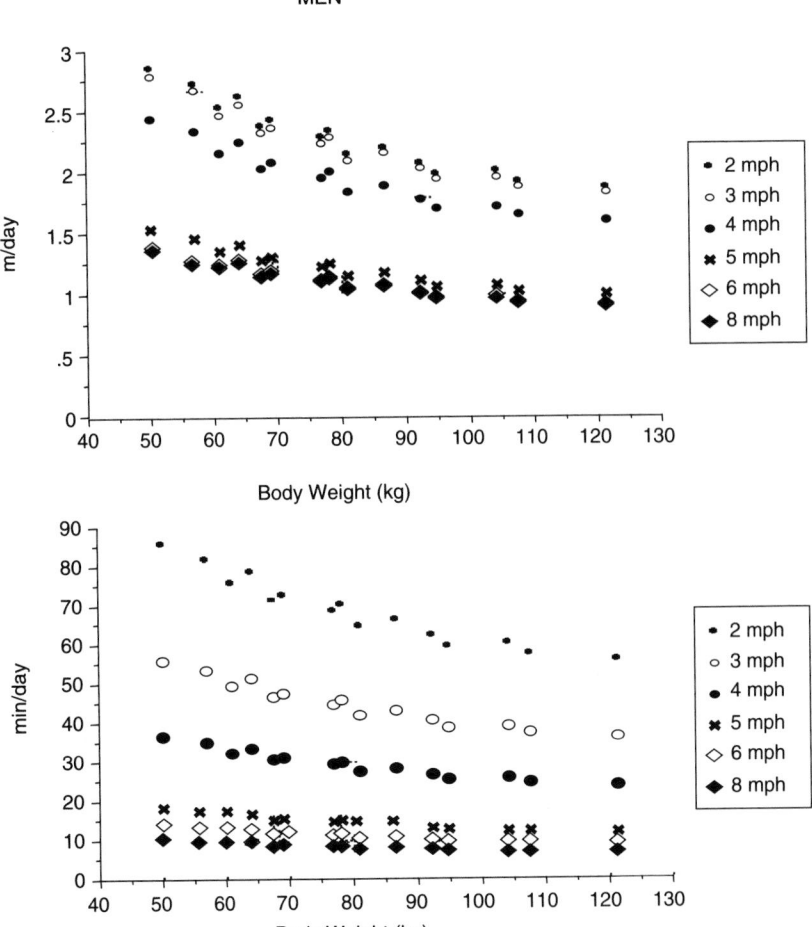

FIGURE 12-5 Distance to cover per day for men to raise physical activity level (PAL) value by 0.10 while walking or running at various speeds (upper panel) and time required to do so (lower panel). The points shown are for men with reference heights of 1.75 m or reference heights ± 1 standard deviation (i.e., 1.64 m or 1.86 m) and body mass index of 18.5, 22.5, 25, 30, or 35 kg/m^2. Energy expenditures while walking or running at speeds of 2, 3, 4, 5, or 8 mph are 2.5, 3.3, 4.5, 8.0, 10.2, and 13.5 metabolic equivalents (METs), respectively (Fletcher et al., 2001). The impact on ΔPAL was calculated as (MET − 1.0) × minutes × 1.15 ÷ 0.9 (where 1.15 accounts for excess [~15%] post-exercise oxygen consumption [Bahr et al., 1987] and 0.9 accounts for a 10% dissipation of food energy consumed by the thermic effect of food) and related to predicted basal energy expenditures for 30-year-old men calculated from the predictive basal energy expenditure equations in Chapter 5; see "Estimation of Energy Expenditure in Normal and Overweight/Obese Adults."

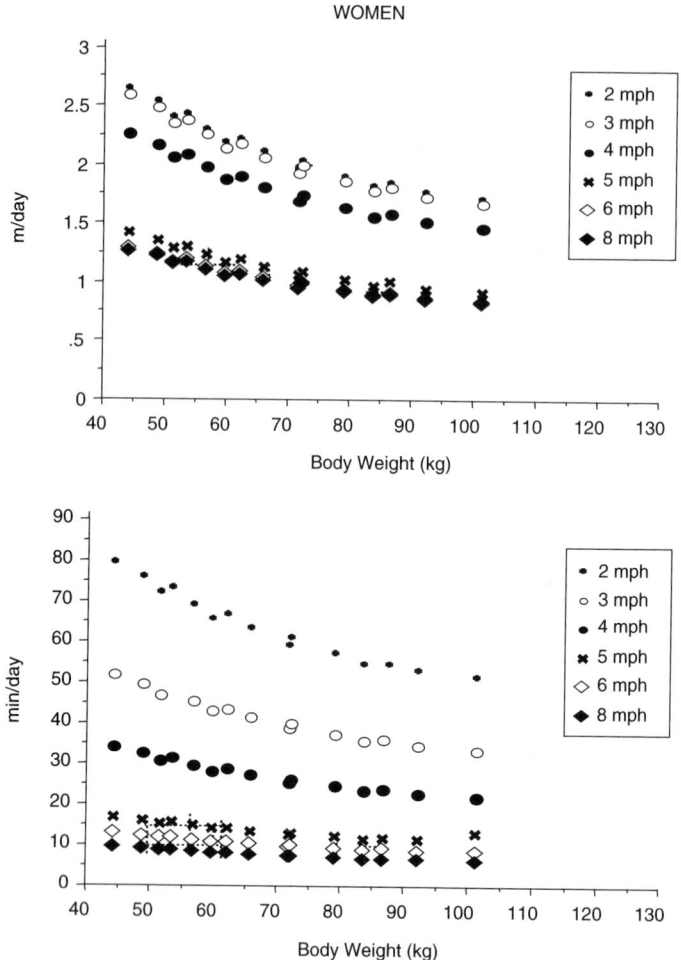

FIGURE 12-6 Distance to cover per day for women to raise physical activity level (PAL) value by 0.10 while walking or running at various speeds (upper panel) and time required to do so (lower panel). The points shown are for women with reference heights of 1.62 m or reference heights ± 1 standard deviation (i.e., 1.55 m or 1.70 m) and a body mass index of 18.5, 22.5, 25, 30, or 35 kg/m². Energy expenditures while walking or running at speeds of 2, 3, 4, 5, or 8 mph are 2.5, 3.3, 4.5, 8.0, 10.2, and 13.5 metabolic equivalents (METs), respectively (Fletcher et al., 2001). The impact on ΔPAL was calculated as (MET − 1.0) × minutes × 1.15 ÷ 0.9 (where 1.15 accounts for excess [~15%] post-exercise oxygen consumption [Bahr et al., 1987] and 0.9 accounts for a 10 percent dissipation of food energy consumed by the thermic effect of food) and related to predicted basal energy expenditures for 30-year-old women calculated from the predictive basal energy expenditure (BEE) equations in Chapter 5; see "Estimation of Energy Expenditure in Normal and Overweight/Obese Adults."

intensity activities must be included to achieve high PAL levels if the time spent exercising is to remain within a certain range. Cross-sectional data from a doubly labeled water database indicate that the PALs are similar for normal weight and obese individuals (Tables 5-10 and 5-11). While this is true, because energy expenditure increases with increasing body weight, there is a greater total daily energy expenditure in obese subjects (Table 5-10 and 5-11).

Physical Activity for Adults

The rationale for categorizing the cross-sectional data on adults in the doubly labeled water (DLW) database by PAL (Appendix Table I-3), as sedentary (PAL ≥ 1.0 < 1.4), low active (PAL ≥ 1.4 < 1.6), active (PAL ≥ 1.6 < 1.9), and very active (PAL ≥ 1.9 < 2.5) categories is provided in Chapter 5. Ideally, PAL of an individual can be determined from DLW studies; however, in nonexperimental situations, heart rate monitors, accelerometers, and other devices as well as activity inventories can be used. As explained earlier, the PAL coefficients in Tables 12-1 to 12-3 are based on rates of energy expenditure during physical activity reported in terms of METs, with an allowance for the EPOC induced by physical activities and the TEF that needs to be consumed to cover the overall cost of these activities.

Table 12-2 shows how adults can use the information presented in Table 12-1 to evaluate their PAL based on their daily activities. In the example shown in Table 12-2, the "sedentary" column illustrates the impact of an adult's typical daily living activities on the PAL ratio of TEE:BEE. This activity-induced increase in PAL of 0.29 is to be added to a base value of 1.1, which represents the BEE of 1.0 to which 10 percent has been added to account for the dissipation of energy due to the TEF that needs to be consumed to cover BEE. This adds up to a sedentary PAL value of 1.39, which corresponds to a sedentary lifestyle (PAL ≥ 1.0 < 1.4). Incorporating a 30 min/day walk at a speed of 4 mph raises the PAL to 1.49 ("low active" column), which corresponds to a low active lifestyle (PAL ≥ 1.4 < 1.6). If in addition to walking 30 min/day at a speed of 4 mph, an adult cycled moderately for another 25 minutes and played tennis for 40 minutes, the PAL would increase to 1.75 (the first "active" column), which reflects an active lifestyle (PAL ≥ 1.6 < 1.9). The second "active" column illustrates a mix of activities as reflected by the average time spent per day on various forms of activity and exercise. Finally, the "very active" column describes a level of activity corresponding to a PAL of 2.06, indicative of a very active lifestyle (PAL ≥ 1.9 < 2.5).

Because activities vary greatly from day to day, a person's PAL can be more accurately evaluated from a meticulous activity log maintained over a period of a week or more. The example in Table 12-3 describes an adult

TABLE 12-2 Intensity and Impact of Various Activities on Physical Activity Level (PAL) Estimations (Daily Example)

Activity	METs[a]	ΔPAL/ 10 min	ΔPAL/h
Leisure			
Mild			
Billiards	2.4	0.013	0.08
Canoeing (leisurely)	2.5	0.014	0.09
Dancing (ballroom)	2.9	0.018	0.11
Golf (with cart)	2.5	0.014	0.09
Horseback riding (walking)	2.3	0.012	0.07
Playing			
Accordion	1.8	0.008	0.05
Cello	2.3	0.012	0.07
Flute	2.0	0.01	0.06
Piano	2.3	0.012	0.07
Violin	2.5	0.014	0.09
Volleyball (noncompetitive)	2.9	0.018	0.11
Walking (2 mph)	2.5	0.014	0.09
Moderate			
Calisthenics (no weight)	4.0	0.029	0.17
Cycling (leisurely)	3.5	0.024	0.14
Golf (without cart)	4.4	0.032	0.19
Swimming (slow)	4.5	0.033	0.20
Walking (3 mph)	3.3	0.022	0.13
Walking (4 mph)	4.5	0.033	0.20
Vigorous			
Chopping wood	4.9	0.037	0.22
Climbing hills (no load)	6.9	0.056	0.34
Climbing hills (5-kg load)	7.4	0.061	0.37
Cycling (moderately)	5.7	0.045	0.27
Dancing			
Aerobic or ballet	6.0	0.048	0.29
Ballroom (fast) or square	5.5	0.043	0.26
Jogging (10-min miles)	10.2	0.088	0.53
Rope skipping	12.0	0.105	0.63
Skating			
Ice	5.5	0.043	0.26
Roller	6.5	0.052	0.31
Skiing (water or downhill)	6.8	0.055	0.33
Squash	12.1	0.106	0.63
Surfing	6.0	0.048	0.29
Swimming	7.0	0.057	0.34
Tennis (doubles)	5.0	0.038	0.23
Walking (5 mph)	8.0	0.067	0.40

Sedentary[b]	Low Active[b]	Active[b]	Active (Mix)[b] Avg	Very Active[b]
Min ΔPAL	Min ΔPAL	Min ΔPAL	Min ΔPAL	Min ΔPAL
			10 0.014	
			10 0.012	
			10 0.012	
			10 0.029	
			10 0.032	
			10 0.022	
30 0.099		30 0.099	10 0.033	
		25 0.113		45 0.203
			10 0.088	15 0.132
				10 0.105
			10 0.057	
		40 0.152	20 0.076	60 0.228

continued

TABLE 12-2 Continued

Activity	METs[a]	ΔPAL/ 10 min	ΔPAL/h
Activities of daily living			
Gardening (no lifting)	4.4	0.032	0.19
Household tasks, moderate effort	3.5	0.024	0.14
Lifting items continuously	4.0	0.029	0.17
Light activity while sitting	1.5	0.005	0.03
Loading/unloading car	3.0	0.019	0.11
Lying quietly	1.0	0	0
Mopping	3.5	0.024	0.14
Mowing lawn (power mower)	4.5	0.033	0.20
Raking lawn	4.0	0.029	0.17
Riding in a vehicle	1.0	0	0
Taking out trash	3.0	0.019	0.11
Vacuuming	3.5	0.024	0.14
Walking the dog	3.0	0.019	0.11
Walking from house to car or bus	2.5	0.014	0.09
Watering plants	2.5	0.014	0.09

ΔPAL/day due to activities of daily living

Sedentary PAL = basal energy expenditure (BEE) + thermic effect
  of food (0.1 × BEE) + sedentary activities =

ΔPAL due to exercise and leisure activities ΔPAL /day

                                                PAL =

[a] METs are multiples of an individual's resting oxygen (O_2) uptake, defined as a rate of O_2 consumption of 3.5 mL of O_2/min/kg body weight in adults.

whose activities of daily living raises energy expenditure to a sedentary PAL of 1.39 (PAL $\geq$ 1.0 < 1.4). If the individual recorded all additional activities over the week and added all of the ΔPALs for each of the activities performed as shown in Table 12-3, the adult would have had a mean increase in PAL of 0.65/day above basal expenditure. Thus, when added to the PAL of 1.1 (representing a base BEE value of 1.0 + 10 percent for TEF), this individual would move into the "active" category with a PAL of 1.75 (PAL $\geq$ 1.6 < 1.9).

A somewhat simplified approach, instead of recording all activities, would be to evaluate whether the level of daily living activities is comparable to that depicted in Tables 12-2 and 12-3. If they are, then a log of daily activities may be kept, and their average ΔPAL could be added to the PAL value (1.39) corresponding to that for a sedentary lifestyle in the example in Tables 12-2 and 12-3.

Sedentary[b]		Low Active[b]		Active[b]		Active (Mix)[b] Avg		Very Active[b]	
Min	ΔPAL	Min	ΔPAL	Min	ΔPAL	Min	ΔPAL	Min	ΔPAL
25	0.060	25	0.060	25	0.060	25	0.060	25	0.060
120	0.060	120	0.060	120	0.060	120	0.060	120	0.060
5	0.010	5	0.010	5	0.010	5	0.010	5	0.010
10	0.024	10	0.024	10	0.024	10	0.024	10	0.024
10	0.029	10	0.029	10	0.029	10	0.029	10	0.029
5	0.010	5	0.010	5	0.010	5	0.010	5	0.010
10	0.024	10	0.024	10	0.024	10	0.024	10	0.024
15	0.029	15	0.029	15	0.029	15	0.029	15	0.029
20	0.028	20	0.028	20	0.028	20	0.028	20	0.028
12	0.017	12	0.017	12	0.017	12	0.017	12	0.017
	0.29		0.29		0.29		0.29		0.29
	1.39		1.39		1.39		1.39		1.39
			0.10		0.36		0.38		0.67
	1.39		**1.49**		**1.75**		**1.77**		**2.06**

[b] PAL levels are Sedentary: PAL ≥ 1.0 < 1.4; Low Active: PAL ≥ 1.4 < 1.6; Active: PAL ≥ 1.6 < 1.9; Active (Mix): PAL ≥ 1.6 < 1.9; Very Active: PAL ≥ 1.9 < 2.5.

The factorial approach summations of various estimates of activities and durations applied in Tables 12-2 and 12-3 to evaluate energy turnover is more convenient than previous procedures inasmuch as it is applicable without making reference to body weight, as required, though often ignored, in estimating increments in energy expenditure in terms of their cost in kcal. Furthermore, the ΔPAL coefficients in Table 12-1 include an appropriate allowance for EPOC and TEF, whose effects are commonly disregarded when evaluating energy turnover. However, it must be remembered that the reliability of evaluations of overall energy expenditure and ΔPALs depends greatly on the accuracy of the activity estimates or activity logs and on whether they were obtained during a period representative of the habitual lifestyle. Because intentional and spontaneous activities are interrelated, assessing ΔPALs of individuals and populations can be more difficult. From the standpoint of energetics, any activity raises metabolic

TABLE 12-3 Weekly Activities and Their Impact on Physical Activity Level (PAL) in an Active Individual (Weekly Activity Log)

Activity	METs[a]	ΔPAL/ 10 min	ΔPAL/h
Leisure			
Mild			
Billiards	2.4	0.013	0.08
Canoeing (leisurely)	2.5	0.014	0.09
Dancing (ballroom)	2.9	0.018	0.11
Golf (with cart)	2.5	0.014	0.09
Horseback riding (walking)	2.3	0.012	0.07
Playing			
Accordion	1.8	0.008	0.05
Cello	2.3	0.012	0.07
Flute	2.0	0.010	0.06
Piano	2.3	0.012	0.07
Violin	2.5	0.014	0.09
Volleyball (noncompetitive)	2.9	0.018	0.11
Walking (2 mph)	2.5	0.014	0.09
Moderate			
Calisthenics (no weight)	4.0	0.029	0.17
Cycling (leisurely)	3.5	0.024	0.14
Golf (without cart)	4.4	0.032	0.19
Swimming (slow)	4.5	0.033	0.2
Walking (3 mph)	3.3	0.022	0.13
Walking (4 mph)	4.5	0.033	0.2
Vigorous			
Chopping wood	4.9	0.037	0.22
Climbing hills (no load)	6.9	0.056	0.34
Climbing hills (5-kg load)	7.4	0.061	0.37
Cycling (moderately)	5.7	0.045	0.27
Dancing			
Aerobic or ballet	6.0	0.048	0.29
Ballroom (fast) or square	5.5	0.043	0.26
Jogging (10-min miles)	10.2	0.088	0.53
Rope skipping	12.0	0.105	0.63
Skating			
Ice	5.5	0.043	0.26
Roller	6.5	0.052	0.31
Skiing (water or downhill)	6.8	0.055	0.33
Squash	12.1	0.106	0.63
Surfing	6.0	0.048	0.29
Swimming	7.0	0.057	0.34
Tennis (doubles)	5.0	0.038	0.23
Walking (5 mph)	8.0	0.670	0.40

Weekly Activity Log

Day 1 (min)	Day 2 (min)	Day 3 (min)	Day 4 (min)	Day 5 (min)	Day 6 (min)	Day 7 (min)	Total Minutes	ΔPAL
				20			20	0.036
	30					60	90	0.105
15					10		25	0.030
				50			50	0.092
					80		80	0.253
60							60	0.130
		50					50	0.167
						100	100	0.617
			40				40	0.180
		20		10			30	0.265
		30					30	0.170
	60				60		120	0.460

continued

TABLE 12-3 Continued

Activity	METs[a]	ΔPAL/ 10 min	ΔPAL/h
Activities of daily living			
Gardening (no lifting)	4.4	0.032	0.19
Household tasks, moderate effort	3.5	0.024	0.14
Lifting items continuously	4.0	0.029	0.17
Light activity while sitting	1.5	0.005	0.03
Loading/unloading car	3.0	0.019	0.11
Lying quietly	1.0	0	0
Mopping	3.5	0.024	0.14
Mowing lawn (power mower)	4.5	0.033	0.2
Raking lawn	4.0	0.029	0.17
Riding in a vehicle	1.0	0	0
Taking out trash	3.0	0.019	0.11
Vacuuming	3.5	0.024	0.14
Walking the dog	3.0	0.019	0.11
Walking from house to car or bus	2.5	0.014	0.09
Watering plants	2.5	0.014	0.09

Min spent on daily living activities
Min spent on daily leisure activities and exercise

[a] METs are multiples of an individual's resting oxygen (O_2) uptake, defined as a rate of O_2 consumption of 3.5 mL of O_2/min/kg body weight in adults.

rate over basal and thus helps in raising energy expenditure. Some activities, such as fidgeting, are spontaneous and can have variable effects on TEE (see Chapter 5 "Spontaneous Non-Exercise Activity"). In room calorimeters, the metabolic costs of unintentional, nondirected activities can be quantified (Ravussin et al., 1986).

Physical Activity for Children

Measurements of the energy expended in various activities are much more limited in children than adults. Torun (1990) compiled the energy expenditure of several common activities in children from 28 studies and expressed the data as multiples of basal metabolic rate (BMR). The activities

Weekly Activity Log

Day 1 (min)	Day 2 (min)	Day 3 (min)	Day 4 (min)	Day 5 (min)	Day 6 (min)	Day 7 (min)	Total Minutes	ΔPAL
10	30	20	40	10	20	20	150	0.350
160	160	180	160	160	90	90	1,000	0.500
				10	10	20	40	0.073
	20			10		10	40	0.093
			50				50	0.165
20					20		40	0.113
					20		20	0.038
30				30			60	0.140
	30			45		30	105	0.193
30	30	30	30	30	20	20	190	0.285
			30			20	50	0.075
250	270	230	310	295	180	210	1,745	2.025
75	90	100	40	80	150	160	695	2.505

$$\Delta PAL/week = 2.025 + 2.505 = 4.530$$
$$mean\ \Delta PAL/day = 4.53/7 = 0.65$$
$$\textbf{mean PAL = 1.1 + mean } \Delta\textbf{PAL/day = 1.75}$$

were classified into 10 categories as shown in Tables 12-4 (Boys) and 12-5 (Girls). When the data are expressed as multiples of BMR, the values are similar for boys and girls. There are no age-related differences for sedentary activities (lying awake, sitting), but the values for walking and moving around increases from early childhood to adolescence. Kimm and colleagues (2002) reported a decline in physical activity in girls during adolescence. The impact of performing various activities for 10 and 60 minutes on PAL also are shown for children in Tables 12-4 and 12-5. The use of MET values for various activities measured in adults leads to errors that increase with decreasing age in children.

To classify children into PAL categories, judgment must be made on their PAL. In Tables 12-6 and 12-7, the differences in energy expenditure

TABLE 12-4 Various Activities: Intensity and Impacts on Physical Activity Level (PAL) in Children (Boys)

Age (y) Activity	Energy Expenditure (kcal/kg/min)					Energy expenditure of categories of activity at different ages expressed as multiples of BMR (Torun, 1990)				
	1.5–6	7–12	13–14	15–16	17–19	1.5–6	7–12	13–14	15–16	17–19
Lying awake	0.046	0.035	0.026	0.024	0.020	1.1	1.1	1.0	1.1	1.1
Sitting quietly	0.047	0.037	0.028	0.028	0.026	1.2	1.2	1.1	1.2	1.4
Standing quietly			0.029	0.033	0.027			1.3	1.5	1.5
Standing, moderate movement		0.069	0.052	0.052			2.2	2.1	2.4	
Walking, free velocity, level ground	0.078	0.078	0.066	0.066	0.053	2.1	2.9	2.8	3.3	3.1
Walking, fast, uphill or with load	0.098	0.110	0.103	0.094		2.6	3.4	3.8	4.4	
At school or light work		0.055–0.084			0.030		1.9–3.0			1.7
Light and moderate housework										
Leisure and moderate play	0.073–0.094	0.061–0.126	0.056–0.075	0.054		1.9–2.5	2.3–4.7	2.5–3.3	2.5	
Running, exercise sports			0.068–0.132	0.067	0.072–0.099			3.1–5.6	3.6	3.9–5.4

TABLE 12-5 Various Activities: Intensity and Impacts on Physical Activity Level (PAL) in Children (Girls)

Age (y) Activity	Energy Expenditure (kcal/kg/min)					Energy expenditure of categories of activity at different ages expressed as multiples of BMR (Torun, 1990)				
	1.5–6	7–12	13–14	15–16	17–19	1.5–6	7–12	13–14	15–16	17–19
Lying awake	0.046			0.018	0.018	1.1			1.1	1.1
Sitting quietly	0.047	0.032	0.027	0.021	0.021	1.2	1.2	1.4	1.2	1.2
Standing quietly			0.028	0.024	0.024			1.4	1.4	1.4
Standing, moderate movement										
Walking, free velocity, level ground	0.078	0.068	0.059	0.057	0.057	2.1	2.7	3.2	3.4	3.4
Walking, fast, uphill or with load	0.098					2.6				
At school or light work				0.026–0.031	0.026–0.031				1.6–1.8	1.6–1.8
Light and moderate housework				0.046–0.058	0.046–0.058				2.9–3.6	2.9–3.6
Leisure and moderate play	0.073–0.094			0.032–0.050	0.032–0.050	1.9–2.5			1.9–3.1	1.9–3.1
Running, exercise sports				0.067–0.100	0.067–0.100				3.9–5.9	3.9–5.9

ΔPAL/10 min					ΔPAL/60 min				
1.5–6	7–12	13–14	15–16	17–19	1.5–6	7–12	13–14	15–16	17–19
0.0009	0.0009	0.0000	0.0009	0.0009	0.0053	0.0053	0.0000	0.0053	0.0053
0.0018	0.0018	0.0009	0.0018	0.0036	0.0107	0.0107	0.0053	0.0107	0.0213
		0.0027	0.0044	0.0044			0.0160	0.0266	0.0266
	0.0107	0.0098	0.0124			0.0639	0.0586	0.0746	
0.0098	0.0169	0.0160	0.0204	0.0186	0.0586	0.1012	0.0959	0.1225	0.1118
0.0142	0.0213	0.0249	0.0302			0.0852	0.1278	0.1491	0.1811
	0.008–0.018			0.0062		0.048–0.108			0.0373
0.008–0.013	0.012–0.033	0.013–0.020	0.0133		0.048–0.078	0.072–0.198	0.078–0.120	0.0799	
		0.019–0.041	0.0231	0.026–0.039			0.114–0.246	0.1385	

ΔPAL/10 min					ΔPAL/60 min				
1.5–6	7–12	13–14	15–16	17–19	1.5–6	7–12	13–14	15–16	17–19
0.0009			0.0009	0.0009	0.0053			0.0053	0.0053
0.0018	0.0018	0.0036	0.0018	0.0018	0.0107	0.0107	0.0213	0.0107	0.0107
		0.0036	0.0036	0.0036			0.0213	0.0213	0.0213
0.0098	0.0151	0.0195	0.0213	0.0213	0.0586	0.0905	0.1172	0.1278	0.1278
0.0142					0.0852				
			0.005–0.007	0.005–0.007				0.030–0.042	0.030–0.042
			0.017–0.023	0.017–0.023				0.102–0.138	0.102–0.138
0.008–0.013			0.008–0.019	0.008–0.019	0.048–0.078			0.048–0.114	0.048–0.114
			0.026–0.043	0.026–0.043				0.156–0.258	0.156–0.258

TABLE 12-6 Total Energy Expenditure (TEE) in Boys and Walking Times at Speeds of 2.5 mph to Move to the Next Higher Physical Activity Level (PAL)

Age (y)	Weight (kg)[a]	Height (m)[a]	BEE (kcal/d)[b]	BEE METs (kcal/kg/ min)[c]	BEE METs (kcal/ kg/hr)	TEE (kcal/d) Sedentary PAL[d]	Low Active PAL[d]	Active PAL[d]	Very Active PAL[d]	PAL Low Active PAL[e]
3	14.3	0.95	889	0.043	2.59	1,142	1,304	1,465	1,663	1.47
4	16.2	1.02	935	0.040	2.40	1,195	1,370	1,546	1,763	1.47
5	18.4	1.09	985	0.037	2.23	1,255	1,446	1,638	1,874	1.47
6	20.7	1.15	1,030	0.035	2.07	1,308	1,515	1,722	1,977	1.47
7	23.1	1.22	1,084	0.033	1.95	1,373	1,597	1,820	2,095	1.47
8	25.6	1.28	1,132	0.031	1.84	1,433	1,672	1,911	2,205	1.48
9	28.6	1.34	1,187	0.029	1.73	1,505	1,762	2,018	2,334	1.48
10	31.9	1.39	1,240	0.027	1.62	1,576	1,850	2,124	2,461	1.49
11	35.9	1.44	1,303	0.025	1.51	1,666	1,960	2,254	2,615	1.50
12	40.5	1.49	1,376	0.024	1.42	1,773	2,088	2,403	2,792	1.52
13	45.6	1.56	1,471	0.022	1.34	1,910	2,251	2,593	3,013	1.53
14	51.0	1.64	1,578	0.021	1.29	2,065	2,434	2,804	3,258	1.54
15	56.3	1.70	1,669	0.021	1.23	2,198	2,593	2,988	3,474	1.55
16	60.9	1.74	1,734	0.020	1.19	2,295	2,711	3,127	3,638	1.56
17	64.6	1.75	1,764	0.019	1.14	2,341	2,771	3,201	3,729	1.57
18	67.2	1.76	1,777	0.018	1.10	2,358	2,798	3,238	3,779	1.57

[a] From Chapter 5, Table 5-8.

[b] BEE = Basal Energy Expenditure, calculated from equations in Chapter 5; see "TEE Equations for Normal-Weight Children."

[c] MET = Metabolic Equivalents as calculated from BEE/weight (kg)/1,440 minutes (1 day).

[d] From Chapter 5, Table 5-20.

[e] PAL = Physical Activity Level = TEE/BEE.

above the sedentary level for the low active, active, and very active PAL categories have been expressed in terms of minutes walking at 2.5 mph. Because the BEE and walking energy expenditure (kcal/kg/min) decrease with age differentially, the MET equivalent for walking is not constant and actually increases with age (see Tables 12-6 and 12-7). Thus, the energy cost of walking 2.5 mph decreases from 0.92–0.75 to 0.04–0.05 kcal/kg/min from early childhood to adolescence, and the corresponding MET values increase from ~2.0 to ~3.0.

Examining the number of minutes of walking that would be required to go from the sedentary to the low active (~120 minutes), active (~230 minutes), and very active (~400 minutes) categories, it is clear that children in the active and very active categories are most likely participating in moderate and vigorous activities, in addition to walking at 2.5 mph. With

Active PAL[e]	Very Active PAL[e]	Difference in energy expenditure from sedentary level (kcal/d)			Energy cost of walking 2.5 mph (kcal/kg/ 2.5 min)[f]	METs of walking mph[g]	Walking equivalent (min)[h]		
		Low Active– Sedentary	Active– Sedentary	Very Active– Sedentary			Low Active– Sedentary	Active– Sedentary	Very Active– Sedentary
1.65	1.87	162	323	521	0.092	2.13	123	246	396
1.65	1.89	175	351	568	0.089	2.23	121	242	392
1.66	1.90	191	383	619	0.087	2.34	119	239	387
1.67	1.92	207	414	669	0.084	2.44	118	237	383
1.68	1.93	224	447	722	0.082	2.52	118	236	381
1.69	1.95	239	478	772	0.079	2.59	118	235	380
1.70	1.97	257	513	829	0.077	2.67	117	233	377
1.71	1.98	274	548	885	0.074	2.76	115	231	373
1.73	2.01	294	588	949	0.072	2.85	114	228	367
1.75	2.03	315	630	1,019	0.069	2.94	112	224	362
1.76	2.05	341	683	1,103	0.067	2.99	112	224	361
1.78	2.06	369	739	1,193	0.064	3.00	112	225	363
1.79	2.08	395	790	1,276	0.062	3.01	113	227	366
1.80	2.10	416	832	1,343	0.059	3.01	115	230	371
1.81	2.11	430	860	1,388	0.057	3.00	117	234	377
1.82	2.13	440	880	1,421	0.054	2.96	120	241	388

f Determined from treadmill testing (Puyau et al., 2002; Treuth et al., 1998; Treuth et al., 2000; Treuth et al. (2003).

g Calculated as energy cost of walking 2.5 mph (kcal/kg/min) divided by BEE MET (kcal/kg/min).

h Calculated by dividing the difference in energy expenditure from sedentary level (kcal/d) by the energy cost of walking 2.5 mph (kcal/kg/min) × weight (kg).

information on the number of minutes children spend in moderate and vigorous play and work, the appropriate PAL category can be assigned.

Physical Activity for Pregnant Women

For women who have been previously physically active, continuation of physical activities during pregnancy and postpartum can be advantageous (Mottola and Wolfe, 2000). Unfortunately, too much or improper activity can be injurious to the woman and fetus. Regular exercise during pregnancy counteracts the effects of deconditioning that lead to fatigue, loss of muscle tone, poor posture, joint laxity, back pain, and muscle cramping (Brooks et al., 2000). Likewise, physical fitness improves glucose tolerance and insulin action, improves emotional well-being and helps

TABLE 12.7 Total Energy Expenditure (TEE) in Girls and Walking Times at Speeds of 2.5 mph to Move to the Next Higher Physical Activity Level (PAL)

Age (y)	Weight (kg)[a]	Height (m)[a]	BEE (kcal/d)[b]	BEE METs (kcal/kg/ min)[c]	BEE METs (kcal/ kg/hr)	TEE (kcal/d) Sedentary PAL[d]	TEE (kcal/d) Low Active PAL[d]	TEE (kcal/d) Active PAL[d]	TEE (kcal/d) Very Active PAL[d]	PAL Low Active PAL[e]
3	13.9	0.94	879	0.044	2.63	1,060	1,223	1,375	1,629	1.39
4	15.8	1.01	910	0.040	2.40	1,113	1,290	1,455	1,730	1.42
5	17.9	1.08	943	0.037	2.20	1,169	1,359	1,537	1,834	1.44
6	20.2	1.15	979	0.034	2.02	1,227	1,431	1,622	1,941	1.46
7	22.8	1.21	1,014	0.031	1.85	1,278	1,495	1,699	2,038	1.47
8	25.6	1.28	1,056	0.029	1.72	1,340	1,573	1,790	2,153	1.49
9	29.0	1.33	1,094	0.026	1.57	1,390	1,635	1,865	2,248	1.49
10	32.9	1.38	1,139	0.024	1.44	1,445	1,704	1,947	2,351	1.50
11	37.2	1.44	1,193	0.022	1.34	1,513	1,788	2,046	2,475	1.50
12	41.6	1.51	1,253	0.021	1.26	1,592	1,884	2,158	2,615	1.50
13	45.8	1.57	1,306	0.020	1.19	1,659	1,967	2,256	2,737	1.51
14	49.4	1.60	1,337	0.019	1.13	1,693	2,011	2,309	2,806	1.50
15	52.0	1.62	1,351	0.018	1.08	1,706	2,032	2,337	2,845	1.50
16	53.9	1.63	1,352	0.017	1.05	1,704	2,034	2,343	2,858	1.50
17	55.1	1.63	1,340	0.017	1.01	1,685	2,017	2,328	2,846	1.51
18	56.2	1.63	1,327	0.016	0.98	1,665	1,999	2,311	2,833	1.51

[a] From Chapter 5, Table 5-9.
[b] BEE = Basal Energy Expenditure, calculated from equations in Chapter 5; see "TEE Equations for Normal-Weight Children."
[c] MET = Metabolic Equivalents as calculated from BEE/weight (kg)/1,440 minutes (1 day).
[d] From Chapter 5, Table 5-21.
[e] PAL = Physical Activity Level = TEE/BEE.

prevent excessive weight gain. Fitness promotes faster delivery, which is considered beneficial to mother and baby, and hastens recovery from pregnancy. Moreover, resumption of physical activity after pregnancy is important for restoration of normal body weight. Women who gain more than the recommended weight during pregnancy and who fail to lose this weight 6 months after giving birth are at much higher risk of being obese nearly a decade later (Rooney and Schauberger, 2002). Professional organizations such as the American College of Obstetricians and Gynecologists (ACOG) have published guidelines and specific recommendations for exercise by women before, during, and after pregnancy (ACOG, 1994).

A full description of the benefits and hazards of exercise for the pregnant woman and fetus is beyond the scope of this report. Physically active

Active PAL[e]	Very Active PAL[e]	Difference in energy expenditure from sedentary level (kcal/d)			Energy cost of walking 2.5 mph (kcal/kg/2.5 min)[f]	METs of walking mph[g]	Walking equivalent (min)[h]		
		Low Active–Sedentary	Active–Sedentary	Very Active–Sedentary			Low Active–Sedentary	Active–Sedentary	Very Active–Sedentary
1.57	1.85	163	315	569	0.095	2.16	124	239	432
1.60	1.90	177	342	617	0.091	2.28	123	237	428
1.63	1.94	190	368	665	0.088	2.40	121	234	423
1.66	1.98	204	395	714	0.085	2.51	119	231	418
1.68	2.01	217	421	760	0.081	2.63	117	228	411
1.70	2.04	233	450	813	0.078	2.72	117	226	408
1.70	2.05	245	475	858	0.074	2.84	114	220	398
1.71	2.06	259	502	906	0.071	2.96	111	215	388
1.72	2.07	275	533	962	0.068	3.04	109	212	382
1.72	2.09	292	566	1,023	0.064	3.07	109	212	383
1.73	2.10	308	597	1,078	0.061	3.07	110	214	387
1.73	2.10	318	616	1,113	0.058	3.06	112	217	392
1.73	2.11	326	631	1,139	0.054	3.00	116	224	405
1.73	2.11	330	639	1,154	0.051	2.91	121	234	422
1.74	2.12	332	643	1,161	0.047	2.81	127	246	445
1.74	2.13	334	646	1,168	0.044	2.68	135	261	472

f Determined from treadmill testing (Puyau et al., 2002; Treuth et al., 1998; Treuth et al., 2000; Treuth et al. (2003).

g Calculated as energy cost of walking 2.5 mph (kcal/kg/min) divided by BEE MET (kcal/kg/min).

h Calculated by dividing the difference in energy expenditure from sedentary level (kcal/d) by the energy cost of walking 2.5 mph (kcal/kg/min) × weight (kg).

TABLE 12-8 Target Heart Rate Zones for Healthy Pregnant Women

Age (y)	Heart Rate (beats/min)
< 20	140–155
20–29	135–150
30–39	130–145
> 40	125–140

SOURCE: Mottola and Wolfe, 2000.

and fit women should consult with their physician on how to exercise safely during pregnancy, and probably no pregnant woman should begin an exercise-training program without medical evaluation and exercise instruction. To an extent, anatomy and physiology protect the fetus from injury because the uterus provides a protective environment, the placenta can use alternative energy fuels (e.g., lactate), and fetal blood has a higher affinity of oxygen than does adult hemoglobin (Mottola and Wolfe, 2000). However, excessive exercise or incorrect exercise could compromise placental blood flow, expose the fetus to hypoxemia (low blood oxygen), hypoglycemia (low blood sugar), or hyperthermia (high body temperature), or increase risk of trauma to woman and fetus. Excessive exercise could increase the risk of preterm delivery and lower birth weight (ACOG, 1994).

Education, common sense, and the feeling of body wellness that comes from regular physical activity can be important in guiding a pregnant woman who wants to retain the health benefits of physical activity. For instance, moderate-intensity, rhythmical activities (walking, cycling, swimming, jogging, and dancing) are recommended, whereas activities such as water skiing, surfing, scuba diving, and mountaineering at high altitudes pose unknown risks to the fetus and are not recommended at any time during pregnancy (ACOG, 1995). Similarly, intense physical activity and exercising for extended periods while dehydrated, under hot environmental conditions, and while fasted may increase the risk of hyperthermia and hypoglycemia. Usually, as pregnancy progresses, women instinctively alter exercise activity patterns. Women also need be aware to change or enhance exercise equipment, such as switching from supine to upright cycling. ACOG publishes several texts (e.g., *Encyclopedia of Women's Health*) and brochures (e.g., "Wellness Exercise During Pregnancy") that provide advice for the general public and health professionals.

Historically, concern has been that intense physical activity could result in low birth weight infants and preterm delivery, but this concern needs to be balanced against the need to control body weight during pregnancy and afterward and current evidence that prudent physical activity performed at moderate intensities within current guidelines has no adverse effects on fetal development (Mottola and Wolfe, 2000). Exercise prescriptions for pregnant women are not dissimilar to those for other adults. Exercise sessions should be preceded by a 5- to 15-minute warm-up, and followed by a similar cool-down period. Training duration should be 15 to 30 minutes. Exercise frequency should be 3 to 5 times per week, and not increase in frequency during first or third trimesters because of fatigue and an evaluation of risks to benefits. Exercise intensity should be moderate and elicit 60 to 70 percent Vo_2max, which can be monitored by the maternal heart rate response as shown in Table 12-8. Alternatively, on the 20-point

Borg Rating of Perceived Exertion Scale, women should be exercising at an intensity between 12 and 14 ("somewhat hard"). And finally, intensity can be gauged by the talk test, or exercise intensity where lactic acidosis drives pulmonary minute ventilation so that the pregnant woman is out of breath and cannot carry on a conversation.

Physical Activity Level Consistent with a Normal Body Mass Index

Based on Table 12-2, 30 minutes of moderately intensive physical activity (ΔPAL = 0.099 for walking at 4 mph) would be sufficient to raise the PAL of a person doing only the activities of daily living (PAL = 1.39) from the "sedentary" category (PAL $\geq$ 1.0 < 1.4), to the "low active" category (PAL $\geq$ 1.4 < 1.6), but insufficient to raise the PAL to the "active" category (PAL $\geq$ 1.6 < 1.9), the average PAL category of normal weight adults in the DLW database with BMIs from 18.5 up to 25 kg/m^2 (Table 5-10). One hour of moderately intensive physical activity (ΔPAL = 0.2 for walking at 4 mph) would raise the PAL from 1.39 to 1.59, the upper range of the low active category (PAL $\geq$ 1.4 < 1.6). Thus on the average, an energy expenditure equivalent to at least 60 minutes of moderate intensity physical activity is required to raise the PAL from the "sedentary" to the "active" category (PAL $\geq$ 1.6 < 1.9).

Physical Activity Recommendations for Adults and Children

Cross-sectional data from the DLW database were used to define a recommended level of physical activity for adults and children, based on the PAL associated with a normal BMI range of 18.5 to 25 kg/m^2 (Chapter 5). Factors known to affect body weight were controlled for in the DLW studies, allowing for a reliable assessment of the level of physical activity consistent with a normal weight. Because an average of 60 min/day of moderate intensity physical activity provides a PAL that is associated with a normal BMI range, this is the amount of activity that is recommended for normal weight adults. As stated in Chapter 4, the Dietary Reference Intakes are provided for the apparently healthy population, therefore recommended levels of physical activity that would result in weight loss of overweight or obese individuals are not provided.

In terms of making a realistic physical activity recommendation for busy individuals to maintain their weight, it is important to recognize that exercise and activity recommendations consider "accumulated" physical activity. This involves consideration of EEPAs of both low intensity activities of daily life (e.g., taking the stairs at work) as well as participating in more vigorous activities (e.g., taking an aerobics class). Recognition of the value of accumulated physical activity in raising TEE makes reasonable activity patterns and sedentary occupations compatible by including significant amounts of moderate intensity activity (e.g., 60 minutes/day of brisk walking) or exercises requiring high intensities (e.g., jogging or running) performed regularly (4–7 days/week).

It is difficult to determine a quantifiable recommendation for physical activity based on reduced risk of chronic disease. Meeting the 60 minute/day physical activity recommendation, however, offers additional benefits in reducing risk of chronic diseases, for example, by favorably altering blood lipid profiles, changing body composition by decreasing body fat and increasing muscle mass, or both (Eliakim et al., 1997; Schwartz et al., 1991; Wei et al., 1997; Wilbur et al., 1999).

EVIDENCE FOR HEALTHFUL EFFECTS OF PHYSICAL ACTIVITY

Epidemiological Evidence for Reduced Risk of Chronic Diseases and Mortality

Men and women with moderate to high levels of physical activity or cardio-respiratory fitness have lower mortality rates than sedentary individuals with low fitness (Blair et al., 1993; Colditz and Coakley, 1997; Myers et al., 2002; Paffenbarger et al., 1994; Sandvik et al., 1993). For instance, in a study of Harvard alumni, mortality rates for men walking on average less than 9 miles each week were 15 percent higher than in men walking more than 9 miles a week (Paffenbarger et al., 1994). Moreover, in the same study, men who took up vigorous sports activities lowered their risk of death by 23 percent compared to those who remained sedentary (Paffenbarger et al., 1993). Similar favorable effects were observed in the Aerobics Center Longitudinal Study as men in the lowest quintile of fitness who improved their fitness to a moderate level, reduced mortality risk by 44 percent, an extent comparable to that achieved by smoking cessation (Blair et al., 1995). Results from observational and experimental studies of humans and laboratory animals provide biologically plausible insights into the benefits of regular physical activity on the delayed progression of several chronic diseases. The interrelationships between physical activity and cancer, cardiovascular disease, type 2 diabetes mellitus, obesity, and skeletal health are detailed in Chapter 3.

Table 12-9 shows seven prospective studies that associated varying ranges of leisure time energy expenditure (kcal/day or kcal/week) with the risk of chronic diseases and/or associated mortality. Assuming an average of 150 kcal expended per 30 minutes of moderate physical activity (Leon et al., 1987), the amount (minutes/day) of physical activity associated with risk was determined. The required amount of physical activity depended on the endpoint being evaluated. The minimum amount of physical activity that provided a health benefit ranged from 15 to 60 minutes/day. The amount of physical activity that provided the lowest risk of morbidity and/or mortality was 60 to greater than 90 minutes/day.

The proposed recommendation for a daily energy expenditure equivalent to that expended during 60 minutes of brisk walking is consistent with those recommendations in *Physical Activity and Health: A Report of the Surgeon General* (HHS, 1996). This recommendation is also consistent with Canada's "Physical Activity Guide to Healthy Living" (Health Canada, 1998), and the World Health Organization technical report on obesity (2000). Specifically, recommendation number 3 in Chapter 2 of the Surgeon General's report states: "Recommendations from experts agree that for better health, physical activity should be performed regularly. The most recent recommendations advise people of all ages to include a minimum of 30 minutes of physical activity of moderate intensity (such as brisk walking) on most, if not all, days of the week. It is also acknowledged that for most people, greater health benefits can be obtained by engaging in physical activity of more vigorous intensity or of longer duration."

Since the articulation of the HHS recommendation for a minimum 30 minutes/day of physical activity (HHS, 1996), evidence from epidemiological, observational and intervention studies continue to support the quoted statement above. Recently, the Women's Health Initiative Observational Study reported that 2.5 hours/week of vigorous exercise was associated with significantly reduced risk of cardiovascular disease in postmenopausal women (Manson et al., 2002). Moreover, they showed that more vigorous exercise was associated with an increased degree of protection. Conversely, physical inactivity, noted by prolonged sitting, was shown to be a significant risk factor for cardiovascular disease.

Similarly, reporting on treadmill evaluations of over 6,000 men studied over a 6-year period, Myers and coworkers (2002) concluded that "exercise capacity is a more powerful predictor of mortality among men than other established risk factors for cardiovascular disease." Recently, Kraus and colleagues (2002) demonstrated favorable effects of jogging for 6 months on blood lipoprotein profiles in overweight men and women, and the extent of changes were related to the amount and intensity of exercise.

Mental Health

Regular exercise has historically been associated with physical health and vigor (HHS, 1996), but exercise may also contribute to the sense of overall well-being and improved mood state. Mental health variables have

TABLE 12-9 Prospective Studies on the Level of Physical Activity in Reducing the Risk of Chronic Disease and Mortality

Reference	Subjects	Study Design[a]
Paffenbarger et al., 1978	16,936 Harvard male alumni, 35–74 y	Questionnaire on leisure-time physical activity, 6- to 10-y follow-up on risk of first heart attack
Paffenbarger et al., 1986	16,936 Harvard male alumni, 35–74 y	Questionnaire on leisure-time physical activity, 12- to 16-y follow-up on all-cause mortality
Leon et al., 1987	12,866 men, 35–57 y	Multiple Risk Factor Intervention Trial using Minnesota questionnaire of leisure-time physical activity, 7-y follow-up on CHD, other and all-cause mortality
Slattery et al., 1989	3,043 U.S. male railroad workers	Leisure-time physical activity questionnaire, 17- to 20-y follow-up on CHD and all-cause mortality
Helmrich et al., 1991	5,990 men, 39–68 y	Questionnaire on leisure-time physical activity, 14-y follow-up on development of type 2 diabetes
Haapanen et al., 1996	1,072 Finnish men, 35–63 y	Questionnaire on leisure-time physical activity, 10-y follow-up on the incidence of all-cause mortality and CVD mortality

Findings[b]	Analysis of Findings
The *minimum* amount of time associated with a reduction in a first heart attack was > 500 kcal/wk The *maximum* reduction in risk of a first heart attack was associated with leisure-time energy expenditure of 2,000–2,999 kcal/wk	The *minimum* amount of physical activity associated with a reduction in a first heart attack was > 15 min/d The *maximum* reduction in risk of a fatal heart attack was at 60–90 min/d
All-cause mortality declined steadily as ranges of energy expenditure from physical activity increased from 500–999 to 3,000–3,500 kcal/wk, beyond which rates slightly increased	The *minimum* amount of physical activity associated with reduced mortality was 30–60 min/d The amount of physical activity associated with *maximum* reduction in mortality was 85–100 min/d The *minimum* amount of physical activity associated with reduced CHD and all-cause mortality was 30–60 min/d. The amount of physical activity associated with the *maximum* reduced CHD and all-cause mortality was 30–60 min/d
The *minimum* amount of total leisure physical activity associated with reduced CHD, CVD and all-heart mortality was 251–1,000 kcal/wk Risk from death was the lowest when total leisure-time physical activity (light to moderate) was 1,001–1,999 kcal/wk	The *minimum* amount of total leisure time physical activity associated with reduced mortality was 10–30 min/d 30–60 min/d of total leisure time physical activity was associated with the *maximum* reduced risk of mortality
The *minimum* amount of mild/moderate physical activity associated with a reduced incidence of type 2 diabetes was 1,000–1,499 kcal/wk The incidence of type 2 diabetes declined as energy expenditure increased from < 500 (rr = 1) to > 3,500 kcal/wk (rr = 0.48)	The *minimum* range of mild/moderate physical activity associated with a reduced risk of type 2 diabetes was 30–45 min/d The amount of mild/moderate physical activity associated with the *maximum* reduction in type 2 diabetes was > 90 min/d
The *minimum* amount of physical activity associated with a reduced risk of CVD and all-cause mortality was 800–1,500 kcal/wk The amount of physical activity associated with the *maximum* reduction in all-cause mortality was > 2,100 kcal/wk and 800–1,500 kcal/wk for CVD mortality	The *minimum* amount of physical activity associated with reduced mortality was 23–45 min/d The amount of physical activity associated with the *maximum* reduction in all-cause mortality was > 60 min/d and 23–45 min/d for CVD mortality

continued

TABLE 12-9 Continued

Reference	Subjects	Study Design[a]
Rockhill et al., 2001	121,701 female nurses, 30–55y	Questionnaire on physical activity, 20-y follow-up of all-cause mortality, and death from various diseases

[a] CHD = coronary heart disease, CVD = cardiovascular disease.
[b] rr = relative risk.

been related to various forms of exercise, particularly acute and chronic aerobic exercise. The research evidence now supports stronger conclusions than presented in the *Physical Activity and Health: A Report of the Surgeon General* (HHS, 1996). The vast majority of review articles have concluded that acute or chronic aerobic exercise is related to favorable changes in anxiety, depression, stress reactivity, positive mood, self-esteem, and cognitive functioning (Anthony, 1991; Craft and Landers, 1998; Landers and Arent, 2001; Mutrie, 2000; North et al., 1990; Paluska and Schwenk, 2000; Salmon, 2001). Although one reviewer (Mutrie, 2000) has argued for a causal relationship between exercise and the reduction of clinical depression, others suggest that there are not enough clinical trial studies to support a causal interpretation (Landers and Arent, 2001). Examination of the meta-analyses indicates that the overall magnitude of the effect of exercise on anxiety, depression, stress reactivity, and cognitive functioning ranges from small to moderate, but in all cases, these effects are statistically significant (Landers and Arent, 2001).

These results are encouraging, but there is still much to learn before the relationship between physical activity and mental health can be fully understood. Recent reviews on endorphins (Hoffman, 1997), serotonin (Chaouloff, 1997), and norepinephrine (Dishman, 1997) have provided experimental evidence for potential mechanisms by which exercise can produce calming effects and mood enhancements.

Findings[b]	Analysis of Findings
The *minimum* amount of physical activity associated with a reduced risk of all-cause mortality and specific causes or mortality was 1–1.9 h/wk The *maximum* reduction in risk (rr = 0.71) of all-cause mortality was observed for those who expended > 7 h/wk of physical activity; those specific causes of death that were most affected were respiratory deaths (rr = 0.23) and noncancer, non-CVD, and nondiabetes deaths (rr = 0.46)	The *minimum* amount of physical activity associated with a reduced risk of mortality was 15–30 min/d A minimum amount of physical activity associated with the *maximum* reduction in mortality was 60 min/d

NOTE: 150 kcal = 30 min of a combination of light, moderate, and some vigorous physical activity (Leon et al., 1987).

BALANCE OF CARBOHYDRATE AND LIPID OXIDATION DURING EXERCISE AND RECOVERY

The balance of carbohydrate and lipid used by an individual during exercise depends mainly on relative intensity, or level of effort as related to the individual's maximal rate of oxygen consumption (Vo_2max) the greatest oxygen consumption that can be attained during an all out physical effort). In general, Vo_2max is related to body muscle mass and is a relatively constant value for a given individual but it can be altered by various factors, particularly aerobic training, which will induce a change of 10 to 20 percent. Thus, on an absolute basis, bigger individuals tend to have a larger Vo_2max (measured in liters of O_2 consumed/minute) than do smaller individuals. However, Vo_2max is also related to the size of the body and the heart. Hence, for purposes of comparison, Vo_2max is frequently considered in terms of mL/kg/min. Some examples are illustrative. An unfit man of average weight (70 kg) might have an absolute Vo_2max of 2.8 L/min, corresponding to 40 mL/kg/min (2.8 L/70 kg/min). If the man's resting metabolic rate (RMR) is 250 mL/min, he would be expected to be capable of 11.5 MET (40 mL/kg/min divided by 1 MET defined as 3.5 mL O_2/kg/min). However, a heart disease patient of the same body size might be capable of only a Vo_2max of 0.50 to 0.75 L/min, corresponding to 7 mL/kg/min (0.5 L/70 kg/min) to 10 mL/kg/min (0.75 L/70 kg/min). This would be equivalent to 2 (7 mL/kg/min divided by 3.5 mL O_2/kg/min) or 3 METs (10 mL/kg/min divided by 3.5 mL O_2/kg/min), while an Olympic-class middle distance runner of the same weight may be capable of achieving a

Vo_2max of 6 L/min, which is equivalent to 85 mL O_2/kg/min (6 L/70 kg/min), or 24 METs (85 mL O_2/kg/min divided by 3.5 mL O_2/kg/min).

Lipid is the main energy source in muscle and at the whole-body level during rest and mild intensity activity (Brooks and Mercier, 1994). As intensity increases, a shift from the predominant use of lipid to carbohydrate occurs. Figure 12-7 describes this crossover concept and, as can be seen in the figure, the relative use of fat is greatest at relatively low exercise intensities, particularly when individuals are fasting. Training slightly increases the relative use of fat as the energy source during low to moderate exercise intensities, particularly in the fasted state. In regard to the amount of fat oxidized, it must be considered that the energy output for a given percent of Vo_2max is proportionally higher (in this case 50 percent) in trained rather than in untrained cyclists. However, at relatively high power outputs, substrate use crosses over to predominant use of carbohydrate energy sources regardless of training state or recent carbohydrate nutrition.

To be used for energy generation, protein must first be degraded to amino acids before the carbon-hydrogen-oxygen skeleton can be used as an energy source through the pathways of carbohydrate and lipid metabolism, while the amino acid nitrogen is transferred and eliminated, primarily in the form of urea. The rate at which amino acids contribute to energy generation is fairly constant and does not increase nearly as much as glucose and fatty acid oxidation during periods of physical exertion. While the rate of oxidation of particular amino acids (e.g., leucine) may rise significantly during exercise, not all amino acids respond in the same way, and amino acids diminish in relative importance as fuels when power output rises during exercise (Brooks et al., 2000), providing only a small percentage of the energy used during physical activity (Brooks, 1987). Indeed, using amino acids as a major energy source would be wasteful, since protein is the most limited energy yielding nutrient. Beyond the overriding effect of relative exercise intensity, other factors such as exercise duration, gender, training status, and dietary history play important, but secondary, roles in determining the pattern of substrate utilization (Brooks et al., 2000). Therefore, the same general relationships among relative exercise intensity, duration, and pattern of substrate utilization hold for most persons, including endurance athletes.

Intensity of Physical Activity

Oxidation of lipid provides most of the energy (~ 60 percent) for non-contracting skeletal muscle and overall for the body at rest in people who have not eaten for 10 to 12 hours (i.e., postabsorptive conditions) (Brooks, 1997). Glucose released from the liver into the circulation provides the remainder of the energy for the body overall, particularly the brain, kidneys,

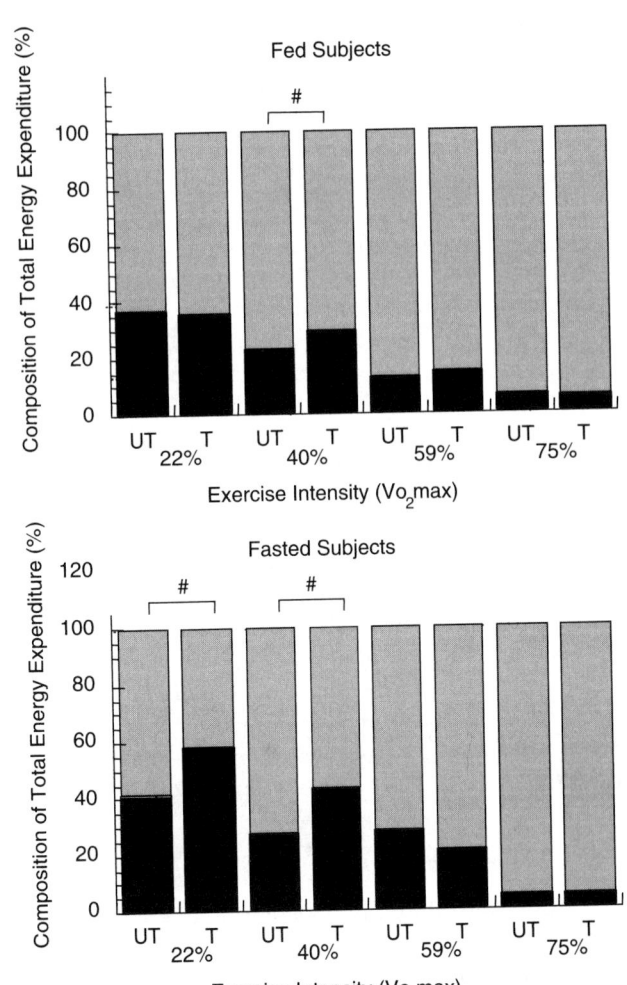

FIGURE 12-7 Illustration of the effects of relative exercise intensity, recent carbo-hydrate feeding, and training status on the relative use of carbohydrate (CHO) and lipid (black) energy sources as determined by indirect calorimetry. Untrained men (UT) and trained (T) male cyclists were studied after being recently fed (3–4 h after a 550-kcal meal [87% CHO, 11% protein, 2% fat]) or after an overnight (12-h) fast, during continuous cycling at graded relative exercise intensities over peri-ods of 120 min (22% and 40% Vo_2max), 90 min (59% Vo_2max), and 45 min (75% Vo_2max). Exercise intensity expressed as a percentage of maximal oxygen con-sumption (Vo_2max), which averaged 39 and 58 mL of oxygen/min/kg body weight among the UT and T cyclists. $p < 0.05$ for #. Reprinted, with permission, from Bergman and Brooks (1999). Copyright 1999 by the American Physiological Soci-ety.

and blood. During mild exercise, the use of lipid increases, but if the level of effort increases, carbohydrate energy sources are used to a relatively greater extent (Figure 12-7). Peak rate of lipid oxidation is achieved at approximately 45 percent of Vo_2max. For exercises intensities greater than 50 percent of Vo_2max, the oxidation of free fatty acids declines in muscle, both as a percentage of total energy as well as on an absolute basis. In other words, there is crossover from prevalence of lipid oxidation at rest and during mild exercise to predominance of carbohydrate energy sources during moderate and greater efforts. The main carbohydrate energy source is muscle glycogen, and this is supplemented to some extent by glucose and lactate—glucose mobilized from the liver and lactate produced by muscle glycogen breakdown. If exercise persists beyond 60 to 90 minutes, lipid use will rise as carbohydrate fuel sources become depleted. In this case, the intensity of exercise must drop because of the depletion of muscle glycogen, decreasing levels of blood glucose, and other fatiguing consequences of the effort (Graham and Adamo, 1999).

Dietary carbohydrate is relatively rapidly assimilated compared to fat and protein, thus raising blood glucose and insulin levels. The increments in blood glucose and insulin in response to carbohydrate intake are less in trained than in untrained individuals (Dela et al., 1991; King et al., 1987). Still, carbohydrate feeding stimulates carbohydrate oxidation, raising the respiratory exchange ratio $(RER = R = Vco_2/Vo_2)$ in all individuals. Hence, as shown in Figure 12-7 for fed individuals, crossover to predominant carbohydrate oxidation occurs already during mild (22% Vo_2max) exercise, even in trained individuals, if they have recently consumed carbohydrates.

Duration of Physical Activity

Within seconds after initiation of even mild exercise, muscle glycogen stores are mobilized to provide energy for muscle work. Over the next few minutes, as circulatory oxygen supply rises to meet demand and muscle cell energy homeostasis is restored, the use of muscle glycogen subsides and free fatty acids (FFA) as well as lipid previously stored within muscle cells (intramuscular triacylglycerol) are activated and used. After the transition period in which glycogen is primarily used, the fuel mix used during sustained mild intensity exercise returns toward the mix used at rest, in which FFA predominate. Such mild intensities correspond to easy walking and household chores. As exercise intensity increases, FFA oxidation increases, achieving a peak at about 45 percent Vo_2max; thereafter, use of carbohydrate fuel sources (i.e., muscle glycogen, blood glucose, lactate) rises exponentially and lipid oxidation declines (Figure 12-7). Depending on the person, the change from fat to carbohydrate dependence occurs at different levels of exertion. In some individuals, this may happen during activities such as brisk walking. When labored breathing accompanies exercise, crossover to carbohydrate dependence has generally occurred.

In most cases, relationships between activity duration and intensity will be inversely related—harder intensity physical activities will necessarily be of less duration than easier ones. Extreme effort is made possible in part by the use of preformed high-energy bonds in the form of creatine-phosphate, in addition to energy generation by glycogen and glucose catabolism, with very little use of fat, leading to fatigue within seconds or minutes. Thus, the energy flux rate will be high, but total energy liberated small. In contrast, activities of mild to moderate intensity, performed over periods of hours, can result in large increments of energy expenditure with a substantial contribution coming from lipid stores (Brooks et al., 2000). Therefore, in order to use physical activity to enhance body fat utilization, sustained activity that causes substantial increases in energy expenditure is more important than the peak rate of substrate oxidation. Even in highly fit athletes, glycogen reserves will become largely depleted after maintaining high rates of exertion for several hours, so that increasing amounts of lipid will be oxidized. As a result of such physical activity, increased lipid oxidation will also take place during recovery from exercise (Chad and Quigley, 1991; Kiens and Richter, 1998).

Gender

In general, metabolic responses of women and men are similar, but women oxidize more lipid than men during exercise and when performing a task at a given level of intensity (Friedlander et al., 1998a, 1998b, 1999; Tarnopolsky et al., 1990). Paradoxically, women depend more on blood glucose and less on muscle glycogen than do men. The effects of menstrual variations on substrate utilization are under investigation, but the effects are likely to be small, because estrogen and progesterone appear to have antagonistic effects on substrate utilization (Campbell et al., 2001; Suh et al., 2002). In contrast to the effects of menstrual cycle variations in endogenous ovarian sex steroids, high levels of exogenous synthetic ovarian steroid analogs, such as contained in oral contraceptives, cause a mild insulin resistance and decrease use of blood glucose in women at rest (Yen and Vela, 1968). Consequently, men and women may possibly differ subtly in patterns of substrate utilization during physical activity, but overall patterns of carbohydrate and lipid use are similar. The effect of menopause on substrate utilization during exercise has not been studied in sufficient detail to establish if it leads to significant changes in substrate utilization. However, changes in body fat content and distribution after menopause suggest that patterns of activity and energy substrate utilization change after menopause (Poehlman et al., 1995).

Age

Maximal oxygen consumption is typically stable in the third decade of life, but then declines approximately 1 percent/year (0.5 ml/kg/min) after age 30 (Raven and Mitchell, 1980). This age-related decline is associated with the decline in muscle mass and maximal heart rate that decreases approximately 1 beat/min/year (Suominen et al., 1977). As a result, fat oxidation during physical activity is decreased and carbohydrate oxidation is increased in elderly adults (Sial et al., 1996). Recognizing that Vo_2max declines with age, any given task is likely to be accomplished at relatively greater exercise intensity, and consequently greater dependence on carbohydrate-derived energy sources. However, if relative exercise intensity is considered, many older individuals are capable of prolonged exercise at 50 to 60 percent of Vo_2max, and accordingly can oxidize significant quantities of carbohydrate and lipid (Sial et al., 1996) to favorably affect physiological systems as well as change energy balance and body composition.

Sedentary older individuals who become active through resumption of outdoor activities, gymnasium exercises, or other forms of occupational or recreational activities respond much like younger individuals (Hagberg et al., 1989; Hagerman et al., 2000). While the extent of adaptation is obviously limited in older ages, relative changes in muscle strength and aerobic capacity can be comparable or even greater than in younger adults (Hagberg et al., 1989; Hagerman et al., 2000). It must be noted that acute illness resulting in bed rest can result in a notable (~10 percent) decline in Vo_2max in 1 week, but the decline is transient and recovery occurs in a similar time frame after resumption of regular physical activities (Greenleaf and Kozlowski, 1982).

Growth and Development

In general, in children maximal oxygen consumption is higher per unit of body weight and higher in boys than girls, although the difference is small until the pubertal growth. The growth spurt usually comes earlier in girls than boys, so maximal oxygen consumption in 12- to 13-year-old girls may match or surpass that of age-matched boys. However, in boys, puberty results in much larger increments in total muscle mass, blood volume, and lung and heart size than girls. Girls acquire more fat mass than do boys and boys frequently lose body fat during the pubertal growth spurt. Consequently, puberty results in a large increment in Vo_2max whether expressed in absolute or relative terms in boys. In girls, the relative rise in Vo_2max during the pubertal growth spurt is smaller, since the absolute increase in muscle mass is less and the relative rise in fat mass (FM) is greater than in boys. Regular endurance exercise can result in a significant increment in the Vo_2max of boys and girls (Brown et al., 1972; Mahon and Vaccaro, 1989, 1994; Vaccaro and Clarke, 1978) as well as in adults (Gallo et al., 1989; Maciel et al., 1985; Tabata et al., 1996).

It is generally assumed that the pattern of substrate utilization in children during rest and exercise is similar to that in adults. However, the data on effect of exercises of graded intensities and duration on the balance of substrate utilization in children are scarce. Compared to adults, the capacity of glycogenolysis in non–fully differentiated skeletal muscle is less in children, and they are generally less capable of speed and power-related activities (Krahenbuhl and Williams, 1992).

Physical activity levels in children vary widely, as they are capable of large amounts of spontaneous, self-directed physical activity (Blaak et al., 1992). The effects of exercise on body composition in children are likely greater than in adults, because of the much greater levels of growth hormone in children (Borer, 1995). Because growth hormone has both anabolic (tissue-building) and lipolytic (fat-mobilizing) effects (Bengtsson et al., 1990), it is not surprising that physically active children are stronger and leaner than their obese counterparts (Owens et al., 1999).

Results from the 1999 Youth Risk Behavior Study (CDC, 2000) indicate that only 29 percent of high school students attend physical education classes daily, and participation declines to 20 percent by grade 12 (Table 12-10). Furthermore, not only is there a decline in the frequency of physical education participation by high school students, but there is also a steady decline in the vigor of participation, as estimated by length of time engaging in physical activity/exercise during class.

PHYSICAL FITNESS

Endurance (Aerobic) Exercise

Traditionally, the types of activities recommended for cardiovascular fitness are those of a prolonged endurance nature, such as bicycling, hiking, jogging, and swimming. Sometimes the word "aerobic" is used as an alternative to describe such activities because integrated functions of lungs, heart, cardiovascular system, and associated muscles are involved. Because of the energy demands associated with aerobic activity, such activities have the potential to impact body fat mass (FM) (Grund et al., 2001). By decreasing FM and preserving fat free mass (FFM), prolonged mild to moderate intensity endurance exercise can change body composition.

TABLE 12-10 Percentage of Students in Grades 9 Through 12 Who Reported Enrollment in Physical Education Classes, Attendance in Physical Education Classes Daily, and Spending More Than 20 Minutes Exercising During Class, by Demographic Group[a]

Demographic Group	Enrolled in Physical Education Classes	Attended Physical Education Classes Daily	Exercised More Than 20 Min per Class[b]
Overall total	56.1 (48.9–63.3)	29.1 (19.7–38.5)	76.3 (72.6–80.0)
Gender			
Females	51.5 (43.8–59.2)	26.3 (17.3–35.3)	69.6 (65.6–73.6)
Males	60.7 (53.7–67.7)	31.9 (21.9–41.9)	82.1 (77.5–86.7)
Race/ethnicity			
White, non-Hispanic			
Total	56.1 (46.3–65.9)	28.3 (15.5–41.1)	78.7 (74.3–83.1)
Females	51.7 (40.5–62.9)	25.8 (13.3–38.3)	72.4 (67.0–77.8)
Males	60.2 (51.0–69.4)	30.8 (17.5–41.1)	83.8 (79.3–88.3)
Black, non-Hispanic			
Total	52.9 (39.1–66.7)	29.2 (19.3–39.1)	67.8 (64.3–71.3)
Females	47.1 (34.1–60.1)	25.5 (17.0–34.0)	55.8 (50.2–61.4)
Males	59.2 (43.4–75.0)	33.1 (20.4–45.8)	78.4 (74.3–82.5)
Hispanic			
Total	59.3 (52.3–66.3)	40.4 (31.5–49.3)	75.5 (70.5–80.5)
Females	53.6 (44.5–62.7)	36.2 (25.9–46.5)	70.8 (63.9–77.7)
Males	65.1 (58.1–72.1)	44.6 (35.9–53.3)	79.6 (73.5–85.7)
Grade in school			
9th			
Total	78.9 (73.0–84.8)	42.1 (29.6–54.6)	78.7 (74.5–82.9)
Females	75.6 (69.0–82.2)	40.3 (28.1–52.5)	72.5 (65.6–79.4)
Males	82.3 (76.4–88.2)	44.0 (30.8–57.2)	84.4 (80.1–88.7)
10th			
Total	60.9 (49.0–72.8)	30.4 (20.7–40.1)	75.1 (69.9–80.3)
Females	56.6 (43.1–70.1)	27.9 (17.7–38.1)	70.2 (64.6–75.8)
Males	65.3 (54.1–76.5)	32.8 (22.6–43.0)	79.4 (72.8–86.0)
11th			
Total	40.7 (31.5–49.9)	20.0 (11.7–28.3)	75.7 (70.9–80.5)
Females	36.8 (27.6–46.0)	16.6 (8.2–25.0)	68.0 (61.2–74.8)
Males	44.6 (34.5–54.7)	23.5 (15.0–32.0)	82.0 (76.0–88.0)
12th			
Total	36.6 (25.6–47.6)	20.1 (10.2–30.0)	73.4 (63.3–83.5)
Females	29.4 (17.6–41.2)	16.6 (8.5–24.7)	60.1 (51.9–68.3)
Males	43.8 (32.7–54.9)	23.6 (11.4–35.8)	82.3 (71.1–93.5)

[a] 95% confidence interval.
[b] Among students enrolled in physical education classes.
SOURCE: CDC. 2000. 1999 Youth Risk Behavior Survey.

Resistance Exercise and General Physical Fitness

Initial efforts by health professionals to reduce FM involved endurance exercise protocols mainly because of the large impact on total energy expenditure and links to coronary heart disease risk amelioration. More recent efforts using resistance exercise training, or combinations of resistance and endurance exercises, have been tried to maintain the interest of participants as well as to positively affect body composition through stimulation of anabolic stimuli (Grund et al., 2001). Practitioners of speed, power, and resistance exercises can change body composition by means of the muscle-building effects of such exertions. Moreover, exercises that strengthen muscles, bones, and joints stimulate muscle and skeletal development in children, as well as assist in balance and locomotion in the elderly, thereby minimizing the incidence of falls and associated complications of trauma and bed rest (Evans, 1999). While resistance training exercises have not yet been shown to have the same effects on risks of chronic diseases, their effects on muscle strength are an indication to include them in exercise prescriptions, in addition to activities that promote cardiovascular fitness and flexibility.

Supplementation of Water and Nutrients

As noted earlier, carbohydrate is the preferred energy source for working human muscle (Figure 12-7) and is often utilized in preference to body fat stores during exercise (Bergman and Brooks, 1999). However, over the course of a day, the individual is able to appropriately adjust the relative uses of glucose and fat, so that recommendations for nutrient selection for very active people, such as athletes and manual laborers, are generally the same as those for the population at large. With regard to the impact of activity level on energy balance, modifications in the amounts, type, and frequency of food consumption may need to be considered within the context of overall health and fitness objectives. Such distinct objectives may be as varied as: adjustment in body weight to allow peak performance in various activities, replenishment of muscle and liver glycogen reserves, accretion of muscle mass in growing children and athletes in training, or loss of body fat in overweight individuals. However, dietary considerations for active persons need to be made with the goal of assuring adequate overall nutrition.

Following the recently released joint position statement of the American College of Sports Medicine, American Dietetics Association, and Dietitians of Canada (ACSM et al., 2000), water and fluids containing carbohydrates and electrolytes may be consumed immediately prior to, during, and after physical activity. For instance, a collegiate swimmer arriving on an empty stomach at the training site should be provided with fluids during and immediately after training as well as food after training. Similarly, following competition or training for competition, athletes should rehydrate and consume a high carbohydrate meal (ACSM, 2000). For the healthy individual, the amount and intensity of exercise recommended is unlikely to lead to glycogen depletion, dehydration, or water intoxication. Nonetheless, timing of post-exercise meals to promote restoration of glycogen reserves and other anabolic processes can benefit resumption of normal daily activities.

ADVERSE EFFECTS OF EXCESSIVE PHYSICAL ACTIVITY

Adverse Effects

Overuse Injuries

Physical exercise has the potential to cause overuse injuries to muscles, bones, and joints as well as injuries caused by accidents. Additionally, preexisting conditions can be aggravated upon initiation of a physical activity program, and chronic, repetitive activities can result in injuries. For instance, running can result in injuries to muscles and joints of the lower limbs and back, swimming can cause or irritate shoulder injuries, and cycling can cause or worsen problems to the hands, back, or buttocks. Fortunately, the recommendation in this report to accumulate a given amount of activity does not depend on any particular exercise or sports form. Hence, the activity recommendation can be implemented in spite of possible mild, localized injuries by varying the types of exercise (e.g., walking instead of jogging). Recalling the dictum of "do no harm," the physical activity recommendations in this report are intended to be healthful and invigorating. Activity-related injuries are always frustrating and often avoidable, but they do occur and need to be resolved in the interest of long-term general health and short-term physical fitness.

Dehydration and Hyperthermia

Physical activity results in conversion of the potential chemical energy in carbohydrates and fats to mechanical energy, but in this process most (~ 75 percent) of the energy released appears as heat (Brooks et al., 2000). Evaporative heat loss from sweat is the main mechanism by which humans prevent hyperthermia and heat injuries during exercise. Unfortunately, the loss of body water as sweat during exercise may be greater than what can be replaced during the activity, even if people drink ad libitum or are on a planned diet. Hence, exercise may result in dehydration that increases the stress and relative difficulty of subsequent activity. This can be aggravated by environmental conditions that increase fluid losses, such as heat, humidity, and lack of wind (Barr, 1999). Therefore, as already described, people should consume water before, during (if possible), and after exercise (ACSM et al., 2000).

A weight loss of 1 to 2 percent of body weight on a day following exercise cannot be attributed to a loss of body fat, but reflects some degree of hypohydration that needs to be compensated for by the consumption of fluids (ACSM et al., 2000). Individuals who have lost more than 2 percent of body weight are to be considered physiologically impaired (Naghii, 2000) and should not exercise, but rehydrate.

Hypothermia

Hypothermia can result from water exposure and during winter sports. Even exposure to cool, damp environments can be dangerous to inadequately clothed and physically exhausted individuals. Accidental immersion due to capsizing of boats, poor choice of clothing during skiing, change in weather, or physical exhaustion leading to an inability to generate adequate body heat to maintain core body temperature can all lead to death, even when temperatures are above freezing. Prevention of hypothermia and its treatment are beyond this report; however, hypothermia is unlikely to accrue from attempts to fulfill the physical activity recommendation. Because water and winter sports are gaining popularity and do provide means to enjoyably follow the physical activity recommendation, safe participation in such activities needs special instruction and supervision.

Cardiac Events

While regular physical activity promotes cardiovascular fitness and reduces risks associated with cardiovascular diseases (CVD), heavy physical exertion can trigger the development of arrhythmias or myocardial infarctions (Mittleman et al., 1993; Thompson, 1982; Willich et al., 1993) or, in some instances, can lead to sudden death (Kohl et al., 1992; Koplan, 1979; Siscovick et al., 1984; Thompson, 1982). Thus, while it is true that compared to the population at large, individuals who exercise regularly have reduced risk of CVD and sudden cardiac death, there is a transient increase in risk in this group during and immediately after vigorous exercise (Kohl et al., 1992; Siscovick et al., 1984). However, Manson and colleagues (2002) recently reported that both walking and vigorous activity were associated with marked reductions in the incidence of cardiovascular events.

Female Athlete Triad

Although loading the skeleton through resistance (e.g., weight training, weight-bearing exercises) and impact activities (e.g., jumping) increases bone mineral density (BMD) (Fuchs et al., 2001; Welten et al., 1994), athletic women who undereat and/or overtrain can develop a condition, or cluster of conditions (disordered eating, amenorrhea, and osteoporosis) termed the "female athlete triad" (ACSM, 1997; Thrash and Anderson, 2000; West, 1998). In this triad, disordered eating and chronic energy deficits can disrupt the hypothalamic-pituitary axis, leading to loss of menses, osteopenia, and premature osteoporosis (Loucks et al., 1998), increasing the possibility of hip, spine, and forearm fractures. While dangerous in themselves, skeletal injuries can predispose victims to a cascade of events including thromboses, infections, and physical deconditioning.

Prevention of Adverse Effects

The possibility that exercise can result in overuse injuries, dehydration, and heart problems has been noted above. Consequently, a prudent approach to initiating physical activity or exercise by previously sedentary individuals is recommended. Men over 40 years of age and women over 50 years of age, those with pre-existing conditions, known or suspected risk factors or symptoms of cardiovascular and other chronic diseases (physical inactivity being a known risk factor) should seek medical evaluation as well as clinical exercise testing, clearance, and advice prior to initiating an exercise program (ACSM, 2000). The evaluation should include a stress electrocardiogram and blood pressure evaluation. Ideally, respiratory measurements should be performed to evaluate Vo_2max.

For all individuals initiating an exercise program, emphasis should be placed on the biological principle of stimulus followed by response. Hence, easy exercises must be performed regularly before more vigorous activities are conducted. Similarly, exercise participants need to rest and recover from previous activities prior to resuming or increasing training load. Also, as already noted, conditions of chronic soreness or acute pain and insomnia could be symptoms of over-training. Hence, activity progression should be discontinuous with adequate recovery periods to minimize chances of injury and permit physiological adaptations to occur. Those adaptations are elicited during exercise but occur during recovery. Thus, physical activity recommendations for healthful living, whether a minimum of 30 minutes for most days, as recommended in the Surgeon General's report (HHS, 1996), or 60 minutes a day, should not be construed as the starting point for an adult wishing to change from a sedentary lifestyle to a more active form of living. Depending on the individual, as little as 5 to

10 minutes a day may represent an appropriate starting point, undertaken under professional supervision for those with cardiovascular risk or orthopedic problems. Attention also needs to be given to stretching and strengthening activities as part of the physical activity core to healthful living.

RESEARCH RECOMMENDATIONS

- More information is needed on the effect of exercise (i.e., endurance, resistance, other), frequency, intensity, and duration on body fatness in young and elderly adults and children.
- More information is needed on the effects of exercise on substrate utilization and the roles of various energy depots (liver glycogen, muscle glycogen, adipose triacylglycerol, intramuscular triacylglycerol) in exercise and recovery in children, adults, and the elderly.
- Research is needed to determine whether the timing of meals and exercise can be used to optimize changes in, or to maintain favorable Body Mass Indexes and body compositions of moderately and very active individuals.
- Research is needed to determine whether there are dietary compositions that optimize accretion of lean tissue in growing children and physically active adults.
- More information is needed to identify the mechanisms by which acute and chronic physical activity alter substrate utilization and body composition.
- Efforts need to be undertaken to develop reliable, noninvasive, and clinically appropriate measurements of body composition, cardiovascular function, and physical fitness.
- Efforts should be directed at developing practical, yet reliable methods to assess habitual levels of physical activity.

REFERENCES

ACOG (American College of Obstetricians and Gynecologists).1994. Exercise during pregnancy and the postpartum period. *Tech Bull* 189. Washington DC.

ACOG (American College of Obstetricians and Gynecologists). 1995. Planning for pregnancy, birth and beyond. *Tech Bull.* Washington, DC.

ACSM (American College of Sports Medicine). 1978. The recommended quantity and quality of exercise for developing and maintaining fitness in healthy adults. *Med Sci Sports* 10:vii–x.

ACSM. 1980. *Guidelines for Graded Exercise Testing and Prescription*, 2nd ed. Philadelphia: Lea and Febiger.

ACSM. 1997. Position Stand: The female athlete triad. *Med Sci Sports Exercise* 29:I-xi.

ACSM. 2000. *ACSM's Guidelines for Exercise Testing and Prescription*, 6th ed. Philadelphia: Lippincott, Williams and Wilkins.

ACSM, American Dietetic Association, Dietitians of Canada. 2000. Joint position statement. Nutrition and athletic performance. *Med Sci Sports Exerc* 32:2130–2145.

AHA (American Heart Association). 1972. *Exercise Testing and Training of Apparently Healthy Individuals: A Handbook for Physicians.* New York: AHA.

Anthony J. 1991. Psychologic aspects of exercise. *Clin Sports Med* 10:171–180.

Bahr R, Ingnes I, Vaage O, Sejersted OM, Newsholme EA. 1987. Effect of duration of exercise on excess postexercise O_2 consumption. *J Appl Physiol* 62:485–490.

Barr SI. 1999. Effects of dehydration on exercise performance. *Can J Appl Physiol* 24:164–172.

Benedict FG, Cathcart EP. 1913. *Muscular Work: A Metabolic Study with Special Reference to the Efficiency of the Human Body as a Machine.* Publication No. 187. Washington, DC: Carnegie Institution of Washington.

Bengtsson B-Å, Brummer R-J, Bosaeus I. 1990. Growth hormone and body composition. *Horm Res* 33:19–24.

Bergman B, Brooks GA. 1999. Respiratory gas-exchange ratios during graded exercise in fed and fasted trained and untrained men. *J Appl Physiol* 86:479–487.

Bijnen FCH, Caspersen CJ, Feskens EJM, Saris WHM, Mosterd WL, Kromhout D. 1998. Physical activity and 10-year mortality from cardiovascular diseases and all causes: The Zutphen Elderly Study. *Arch Intern Med* 158:1499–1505.

Blaak EE, Westerterp KR, Bar-Or R, Wouters LJM, Saris WHM. 1992. Total energy expenditure and spontaneous activity in relation to training in obese boys. *Am J Clin Nutr* 55:777–782.

Blair SN, Kohl HW, Barlow CE. 1993. Physical activity, physical fitness, and all-cause mortality in women: Do women need to be active? *J Am Coll Nutr* 12:368–371.

Blair SN, Kohl HW, Barlow CE, Paffenbarger RS, Gibbons LW, Macera CA. 1995. Changes in physical fitness and all-cause mortality. A prospective study of healthy and unhealthy men. *J Am Med Assoc* 273:1093–1098.

Blundell JE, King NA. 1998. Effects of exercise on appetite control: Loose coupling between energy expenditure and energy intake. *Int J Obes Relat Metab Disord* 22:S22–S29.

Borer KT. 1995. The effects of exercise on growth. *Sports Med* 26:375–397.

Bouchard C, Shephard RJ, Stephens T. 1994. *Physical Activity, Fitness, and Health: International Proceedings and Consensus Statement.* Champaign, IL: Human Kinetics.

Brooks GA. 1987. Amino acid and protein metabolism during exercise and recovery. *Med Sci Sports Exerc* 19:S150–S156.

Brooks GA. 1997. Importance of the 'crossover' concept in exercise metabolism. *Clin Exp Pharmacol Physiol* 24:889–895.

Brooks GA, Mercier J. 1994. Balance of carbohydrate and lipid utilization during exercise: The 'crossover' concept. *J Appl Physiol* 76:2253–2261.

Brooks GA, Fahey TD, White TP, Baldwin KM. 2000. *Exercise Physiology: Human Bioenergetics and Its Applications,* 3rd ed. Mountain View, CA: Mayfield Publishing.

Brown CH, Harrower JR, Deeter MF. 1972. The effects of cross-country running on pre-adolescent girls. *Med Sci Sports* 4:1–5.

Campbell SE, Angus DJ, Febbraio MA. 2001. Glucose kinetics and exercise performance during phases of the menstrual cycle: Effect of glucose ingestion. *Am J Physiol* 281:E817–E825.

CDC (Centers for Disease Control and Prevention). 2000. Youth risk behavior surveillance—United States, 1999. *Mor Mortal Wkly Rep CDC Surveill Summ* 49(SS-5):1–96.

Chad KE, Quigley BM. 1991. Exercise intensity: Effect on postexercise O_2 uptake in trained and untrained women. *J Appl Physiol* 70:1713–1719.

Chaouloff F. 1997. The serotonin hypothesis. In: Morgan WP, ed. *Physical Activity and Mental Health*. Washington, DC: Taylor and Francis. Pp. 179–198.

Colditz GA, Coakley E. 1997. Weight, weight gain, activity, and major illnesses: The Nurses' Health Study. *Int J Sports Med* 18:S162–S170.

Craft LL, Landers DM. 1998. The effect of exercise on clinical depression and depression resulting from mental illness: A meta-analysis. *J Sport Exerc Psychol* 20:339–357.

Dela F, Mikines KJ, Von Linstow M, Galbo H. 1991. Twenty-four-hour profile of plasma glucose and glucoregulatory hormones during normal living conditions in trained and untrained men. *J Clin Endocrinol Metab* 73:982–989.

DHEW (U.S. Department of Health, Education, and Welfare). 1979. *Healthy People: The Surgeon General's Report on Health Promotion and Disease Prevention*. DHEW (PHS) Publication No. 79-55071. Rockville, MD: Public Health Service.

Dishman RK. 1997. The norephinephrine hypothesis. In: Morgan WP, ed. *Physical Activity and Mental Health*. Washington, DC: Taylor and Francis. Pp. 199–212.

Eliakim A, Burke GS, Cooper DM. 1997. Fitness, fatness, and the effect of training assessed by magnetic resonance imaging and skinfold-thickness measurements in healthy adolescent females. *Am J Clin Nutr* 66:223–231.

Epstein LH, Wing RR. 1980. Aerobic exercise and weight. *Addict Behav* 5:371–388.

Evans WJ. 1999. Exercise training guidelines for the elderly. *Med Sci Sports Exerc* 31:12–17.

Fletcher GF, Balady GJ, Amsterdam EA, Chaitman B, Eckel R, Fleg J, Froelicher VF, Leon AS, Piña IL, Rodney R, Simons-Morton DG, Williams MA, Bazzarre T. 2001. Exercise standards for testing and training. A statement for healthcare professionals from the American Heart Association. *Circulation* 104:1694–1740.

Friedlander AL, Casazza GA, Horning MA, Buddinger TF, Brooks GA. 1998a. Effects of exercise intensity and training on lipid metabolism in young women. *Am J Physiol* 275:E853–E863.

Friedlander AL, Casazza GA, Horning MA, Huie MJ, Piacentini MF, Trimmer JK, Brooks GA. 1998b. Training-induced alterations of carbohydrate metabolism in women: Women respond differently from men. *J Appl Physiol* 85:1175–1186.

Friedlander AL, Casazza GA, Horning MA, Usaj A, Brooks GA. 1999. Endurance training increases fatty acid turnover, but not fat oxidation, in young men. *J Appl Physiol* 86:2097–2105.

Fuchs RK, Bauer JJ, Snow CM. 2001. Jumping improves hip and lumbar spine bone mass in prepubescent children: A randomized controlled trial. *J Bone Miner Res* 16:148–156.

Gaesser GA, Brooks GA. 1984. Metabolic bases of excess post-exercise oxygen consumption: A review. *Med Sci Sports Exerc* 16:29–43.

Gallo L, Maciel BC, Marin-Neto JA, Martins LEB. 1989. Sympathetic and parasympathetic changes in heart rate control during dynamic exercise induced by endurance training in man. *Braz J Med Biol Res* 22:631–643.

Graham TE, Adamo KB. 1999. Dietary carbohydrate and its effects on metabolism and substrate stores in sedentary and active individuals. *Can J Appl Physiol* 24:393–415.

Greenleaf JE, Kozlowski S. 1982. Physiological consequences of reduced physical activity during bed rest. *Exerc Sport Sci Rev* 10:84–119.

Grund A, Krause H, Kraus M, Siewers M, Rieckert H, Müller MJ. 2001. Association between different attributes of physical activity and fat mass in untrained, endurance- and resistance-trained men. *Eur J Appl Physiol* 84:310–320.

Hagberg JM, Graves JE, Limacher M, Woods DR, Leggett SH, Cononie C, Gruber JJ, Pollock ML. 1989. Cardiovascular responses of 70- to 79-yr-old men and women to exercise training. *J Appl Physiol* 66:2589–2594.

Hagerman FC, Walsh SJ, Staron RS, Hikida RS, Gilders RM, Murray TF, Toma K, Ragg KE. 2000. Effects of high-intensity resistance training on untrained older men. I. Strength, cardiovascular, and metabolic responses. *J Gerontol A Biol Sci Med Sci* 55:B336–B346.

Haapanen N, Miilunpaio S, Vuori I, Oja P, Pasanen M. 1996. Characteristics of leisure time physical activity associated with decreased risk of premature all-cause and cardiovascular disease mortality in middle-aged men. *Am J Epidemiol* 143:870-880.

Health Canada. 1998. *Canada's Physical Activity Guide to Healthy Active Living.* Ottawa, Canada: Health Canada, Canadian Society for Exercise Physiology.

Helmrich SP, Ragland DR, Leung RW, Paffenbarger RS. 1991. Physical activity and reduced occurrence of non-insulin-dependent diabetes mellitus. *N Engl J Med* 325:147-152.

HHS (U.S. Department of Health and Human Services). 1988. *The Surgeon General's Report on Nutrition and Health.* HHS (PHS) Publication No. 88-50210. Washington, DC: Public Health Service.

HHS. 1995. *Healthy People 2000: Midcourse Review and 1995 Revisions.* Washington, DC: Public Heath Service.

HHS. 1996. *Physical Activity and Health: A Report of the Surgeon General.* Atlanta, GA: Centers for Disease Control and Prevention.

HHS. 2000. *Healthy People 2010: Understanding and Improving Health,* 2nd ed. Washington, DC: U.S. Department of Health and Human Services.

Hoffman P. 1997. The endorphin hypothesis. In: Morgan WP, ed. *Physical Activity and Mental Health.* Washington, DC: Taylor and Francis. Pp. 163–177.

Hubert P, King NA, Blundell JE. 1998. Uncoupling the effects of energy expenditure and energy intake: Appetite response to short-term energy deficit induced by meal omission and physical activity. *Appetite* 31:9–19.

Kiens B, Richter EA. 1998. Utilization of skeletal muscle triacylglycerol during postexercise recovery in humans. *Am J Physiol* 275:E332–E337.

Kimm SYS, Glynn NW, Kriska AM, Barton BA, Kronsberg SS, Daniels SR, Crawford PB, Sabry ZI, Liu K. 2002. Decline in physical activity in black girls and white girls during adolescence. *N Engl J Med* 347:709-715.

King DS, Dalsky GP, Staten MA, Clutter WE, Van Houten DR, Holloszy JO. 1987. Insulin action and secretion in endurance-trained and untrained humans. *J Appl Physiol* 63:2247–2252.

King NA, Lluch A, Stubbs RJ, Blundell JE. 1997. High dose exercise does not increase hunger or energy intake in free living males. *Eur J Clin Nutr* 51: 478–483.

Kohl HW, Powell KE, Gordon NF, Blair SN, Paffenbarger RS. 1992. Physical activity, physical fitness, and sudden cardiac death. *Epidemiol Rev* 14:37–58.

Koplan JP. 1979. Cardiovascular deaths while running. *J Am Med Assoc* 242:2578–2579.

Krahenbuhl GS, Williams TJ. 1992. Running economy: Changes with age during childhood and adolescence. *Med Sci Sports Exerc* 24:462–466.

Kraus H, Hirschland RP. 1953. Muscular fitness and health. *J Health Phys Ed Rec* 24:17–19.

Kraus WE, Houmard JA, Duscha BD, Knetzger KJ, Wharton MB, McCartney JS, Bales CW, Henes S, Samsa GP, Otvos JD, Kulkarni KR, Slentz CA. 2002. Effects of the amount and intensity of exercise on plasma lipoproteins. *N Engl J Med* 347:1483-1492.

Landers DM, Arent SM. 2001. Physical activity and mental health. In: Singer RN, Hausenblas HA, Janelle CM, eds. *Handbook of Sport Psychology*, 2nd ed. New York: John Wiley and Sons. Pp. 740–765.

Leon AS, Connett J, Jacobs DR, Rauramaa R. 1987. Leisure-time physical activity levels and risk of coronary heart disease and death. *JAMA* 258:2388-2395.

Loucks AB, Verdun M, Heath EM. 1998. Low energy availability, not stress of exercise, alters LH pulsatility in exercising women. *J Appl Physiol* 84:37–46.

Maciel BC, Gallo L, Marin-Neto JA, Lima-Filho EC, Terra-Filho J, Manco JC. 1985. Parasympathetic contribution to bradycardia induced by endurance training in man. *Cardiovasc Res* 19:642–648.

Mahon AD, Vaccaro P. 1989. Ventilatory threshold and Vo$_2$max changes in children following endurance training. *Med Sci Sports Exerc* 21:425–431.

Mahon AD, Vaccaro P. 1994. Cardiovascular adaptations in 8- to 12-year-old boys following a 14-week running program. *Can J Appl Physiol* 19:139–150.

Manson JE, Greenland P, LaCroix AZ, Stefanick ML, Moutton CP, Oberman A, Perri MG, Sheps DS, Pettinger MB, Siscovick DS. 2002. Walking compared with vigorous exercise for the prevention of cardiovascular events in women. *N Engl J Med* 347:716–725.

Mayer J, Marshall NB, Vitale JJ, Christensen JH, Mashayekhi MB, Stare FJ. 1954. Exercise, food intake and body weight in normal rats and genetically obese adult mice. *Am J Physiol* 177:544–548.

Mayer J, Roy P, Mitra KP. 1956. Relation between caloric intake, body weight, and physical work: Studies in an industrial male population in West Bengal. *Am J Clin Nutr* 4:169–175.

Mittleman MA, Maclure M, Tofler GH, Sherwood JB, Goldberg RJ, Muller JE. 1993. Triggering of acute myocardial infarction by heavy physical exertion. Protection against triggering by regular exertion. *N Engl J Med* 329:1677–1683.

Mottola MF, Wolfe LA. 2000. The pregnant athlete. In: Drinkwater BL, ed. *Women in Sport*. Oxford: Backwell Science. Pp. 194-207.

Mutrie N. 2000. The relationship between physical activity and clinically defined depression. In: Biddle JH, Fox KR, Boutcher SH, eds. *Physical Activity and Psychological Well-Being*. London: Routledge. Pp. 46–62.

Myers J, Prakash M, Froelicher V, Do D, Partington S, Atwood JE. 2002. Exercise capacity and mortality among men referred for exercise testing. *N Engl J Med* 346:793–801.

Naghii MR. 2000. The significance of water in sport and weight control. *Nutr Health* 14:127–132.

North TC, McCullagh P, Tran ZV. 1990. Effect of exercise on depression. *Exerc Sport Sci Rev* 18:379–415.

Owens S, Gutin B, Allison J. 1999. Effect of physical training on total and visceral fat in obese children. *Med Sci Sports Exerc* 31:143–148.

Paffenbarger RS, Wing AL, Hyde RT. 1978. Chronic disease in former college students. XVI. Physical activity as an index of heart attack risk in college alumni. *Am J Epidemiol* 108:161-175.

Paffenbarger RS, Hyde RT, Wing AL, Hsieh CC. 1986. Physical activity, all-cause mortality, longevity of college alumni. *N Engl J Med* 314:605-613.

Paffenbarger RS, Hyde RT, Wing AL, Lee I-M, Jung DL, Kampert JB. 1993. The association of changes in physical-activity level and other lifestyle characteristics with mortality among men. *N Engl J Med* 328:538–545.

Paffenbarger RS, Kampert JB, Lee I-M, Hyde RT, Leung RW, Wing AL. 1994. Changes in physical activity and other lifeway patterns influencing longevity. *Med Sci Sports Exerc* 26:857–865.

Paluska SA, Schwenk TL. 2000. Physical activity and mental health. Current concepts. *Sports Med* 29:167–180.

Poehlman ET, Toth MJ, Gardner AW. 1995. Changes in energy balance and body composition at menopause: A controlled longitudinal study. *Ann Intern Med* 123:673–675.

Puyau MR, Adolph AL, Vohra FA, Butte NF. 2002. Validation and calibration of physical activity monitors in children. *Obes Res* 10:150–157.

Raven PB, Mitchell J. 1980. The effect of aging on the cardiovascular response to dynamic and static exercise. In: Weisfeldt ML, ed. *The Aging Heart: Its Function and Response to Stress.* New York: Raven Press. Pp. 269–296.

Ravussin E, Lillioja S, Anderson TE, Christin L, Bogardus C. 1986. Determinants of 24-hour energy expenditure in man. Methods and results using a respiratory chamber. *J Clin Invest* 78:1568–1578.

Rockhill B, Willett WC, Manson JE, Leitzmann MF, Stampfer MJ, Hunter DJ, Colditz GA. 2001. Physical activity and mortality: a prospective study among women. *Am J Pub Health.* 91:578-583.

Rooney BL, Schauberger, CW. 2002. Excess pregnancy weight gain and long-term obesity: One decade later. *Obstet and Gynecol* 100: 245–252.

Salmon P. 2001. Effects of physical exercise on anxiety, depression, and sensitivity to stress: A unifying theory. *Clin Psychol Rev* 21:33–61.

Sandvik L, Erikssen J, Thaulow E, Erikssen G, Mundal R, Rodahl K. 1993. Physical fitness as a predictor of mortality among healthy, middle-aged Norwegian men. *N Engl J Med* 328:533–537.

Schwartz RS, Shuman WP, Larson V, Cain KC, Fellingham GW, Beard JC, Kahn SE, Stratton JR, Cerqueira MD, Abrass IB. 1991. The effect of intensive endurance exercise training on body fat distribution in young and older men. *Metabolism* 40:545–551.

Sial S, Coggan AR, Carroll R, Goodwin J, Klein S. 1996. Fat and carbohydrate metabolism during exercise in elderly and young subjects. *Am J Physiol* 271:E983–E989.

Siscovick DS, Weiss NS, Fletcher RH, Lasky T. 1984. The incidence of primary cardiac arrest during vigorous exercise. *N Engl J Med* 311:874–877.

Slattery ML, Jacobs DR, Nichman MZ. 1989. Leisure time physical activity and coronary heart disease death. The US Railroad Study. *Circulation* 79:304-311.

Suh SH, Casazza GA, Horning MA, Miller BF, Brooks GA. 2002. Luteal and follicular glucose fluxes during rest and exercise in 3-h postabsorptive women. *J Appl Physiol* 93:42–50.

Suominen H, Heikkinen E, Parkatti T, Forsberg S, Kiiskinen A. 1977. Effects of "lifelong" physical training on functional aging in men. *Scand J Soc Med Suppl* 14:225–240.

Tabata I, Nishimura K, Kouzaki M, Hirai Y, Ogita F, Miyachi M, Yamamoto K. 1996. Effects of moderate-intensity endurance and high-intensity intermittent training on anaerobic capacity and Vo_{2max}. *Med Sci Sports Exerc* 28:1327–1330.

Tarnopolsky LJ, MacDougall JD, Atkinson SA, Tarnopolsky MA, Sutton JR. 1990. Gender differences in substrate for endurance exercise. *J Appl Physiol* 68:302–308.

Thompson PD. 1982. Cardiovascular hazards of physical activity. *Exerc Sport Sci Rev* 10:208–235.

Thrash LE, Anderson JJB. 2000. The female athlete triad: Nutrition, menstrual disturbances, and low bone mass. *Nutr Today* 35:168–174.

Torun B. 1990. Energy cost of various physical activities in healthy children. In: Schurch B, Scrimshaw NS, eds. *Activity, Energy Expenditure and Energy Requirements of Infants and Children.* Switzerland: IDECG. Pp. 139–183.

Treuth MS, Adolph AL, Butte NF. 1998. Energy expenditure in children predicted from heart rate and activity calibrated against respiration calorimetry. *Am J Physiol* 275:E12–E18.

Treuth MS, Butte NF, Puyau M, Adolph A. 2000. Relations of parental obesity status to physical activity and fitness of prepubertal girls. *Pediatrics* 106:e49.

Treuth MS, Sunehag AL, Trautwein LM, Bier DM, Haymond MW, Butte NF. (2003). Metabolic adaptation to high-fat and high-carbohydrate diets in children. *Am J Clin Nutr* 77:479–489.

USDA/HHS (U.S. Department of Agriculture/Department of Health and Human Services). 1990. *Nutrition and Your Health: Dietary Guidelines for Americans,* 3rd ed. Home and Garden Bulletin No. 232. Washington, DC: U.S. Government Printing Office.

USDA/HHS. 1995. *Nutrition and Your Health: Dietary Guidelines for Americans,* 4th ed. Home and Garden Bulletin No. 232. Washington, DC: U.S. Government Printing Office.

USDA/HHS. 2000. *Nutrition and Your Health: Dietary Guidelines for Americans,* 5th ed. Home and Garden Bulletin No. 232. Washington, DC: U.S. Government Printing Office.

Vaccaro P, Clarke DH. 1978. Cardiorespiratory alterations in 9 to 11 year old children following a season of competitive swimming. *Med Sci Sports* 10:204–207.

van Dale D, Schoffelen PFM, ten Hoor F, Saris WHM. 1989. Effects of addition of exercise to energy restriction on 24-hour energy expenditure, sleeping metabolic rate and daily physical activity. *Eur J Clin Nutr* 43:441–451.

Van Zant RS. 1992. Influence of diet and exercise on energy expenditure—A review. *Int J Sport Nutr* 2:1–19.

Wei M, Macera CA, Hornung CA, Blair SN. 1997. Changes in lipids associated with change in regular exercise in free-living men. *J Clin Epidemiol* 50:1137–1142.

Welten DC, Kemper HCG, Post GB, Van Mechelen W, Twisk J, Lips P, Teule GJ. 1994. Weight-bearing activity during youth is a more important factor for peak bone mass than calcium intake. *J Bone Miner Res* 9:1089–1096.

West RV. 1998. The female athlete. The triad of disordered eating, amenorrhoea and osteoporosis. *Sports Med* 26:63–71.

Wilbur J, Naftzger-Kang L, Miller AM, Chandler P, Montgomery A. 1999. Women's occupations, energy expenditure, and cardiovascular risk factors. *J Women's Health* 8:377–387.

Willich SN, Lewis M, Löwel H, Arntz H-R, Schubert F, Schröder R. 1993. Physical exertion as a trigger of acute myocardial infarction. *N Engl J Med* 329:1684–1690.

World Health Organization (WHO). 2000. *Obesity: Preventing and Managing the Global Epidemic.* Geneva:WHO.

Yen SSC, Vela P. 1968. Effects of contraceptive steroids on carbohydrate metabolism. *J Clin Endocrinol* 28:1564–1570.

13

Applications of Dietary Reference Intakes for Macronutrients

This chapter presents a general discussion of the appropriate uses of the Dietary Reference Intakes (DRIs) in the assessment and planning of diets for individuals and for groups. It also provides guidance for the use of the DRIs developed for the nutrients presented in this report, including specific examples and special considerations.

OVERVIEW

The Dietary Reference Intakes (DRIs) may be used for many purposes, most of which fall into two broad categories: assessing current nutrient intakes and planning for future nutrient intakes. Each category may be further subdivided into uses for individual diets and for group diets (Figure 13-1).

For example, the Recommended Dietary Allowance (RDA), Estimated Average Requirement (EAR), and Tolerable Upper Intake Level (UL) may be used in assessing the diet of an individual as one aspect of a nutritional status assessment. The RDA and Adequate Intake (AI) may be used as a basis for planning a diet for the same individual. Likewise, the EAR and UL are used to assess the nutrient intakes of a group, such as persons participating in dietary surveys conducted as part of the National Nutrition Monitoring System. The EAR and UL can also be used to plan nutritionally adequate diets for groups, such as people receiving meals in nursing homes, schools, prisons, and other group settings.

In the past, RDAs in the United States and Recommended Nutrient Intakes (RNIs) in Canada were the primary reference standards available

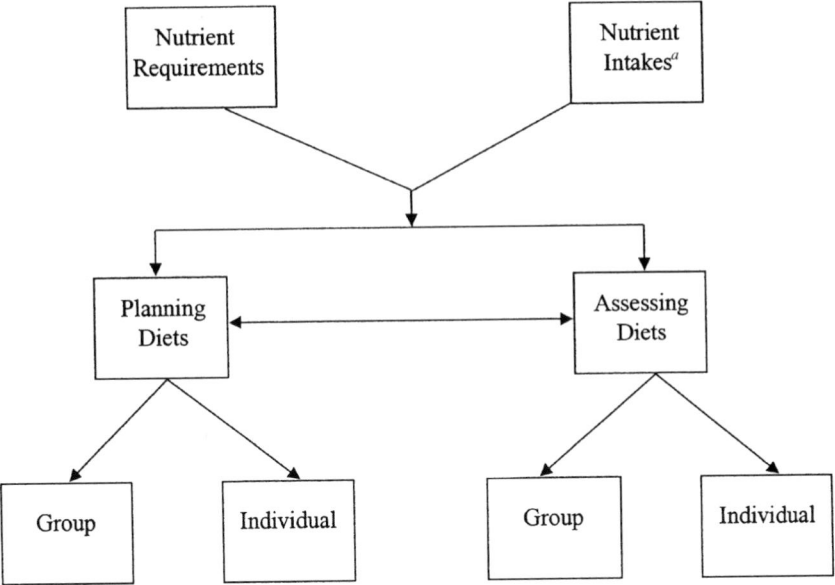

FIGURE 13-1 Conceptual framework—uses of Dietary Reference Intakes.
a Food plus supplements.

to health professionals for assessing and planning diets of individuals and groups and for making judgments about inadequate and excessive intake. However, neither the former RDAs nor the RNIs were ideally suited for many of these purposes (IOM, 1994). The DRIs provide a more complete set of reference values. The transition from using the former RDAs and RNIs to using all of the DRIs appropriately will require time and effort by health professionals and others.

Appropriate uses of each of the new DRIs are described briefly in this chapter and in more detail in a report on the application of the DRIs in assessment (IOM, 2000) and in a forthcoming report on their uses in planning. Included in this chapter are specific applications to the nutrients discussed in this report. Details on how the DRIs are set with reference to specific life stage and gender groups, and the primary criterion that defines adequacy for each of these nutrients are given in Chapters 5 through 10.

ASSESSING NUTRIENT INTAKES OF INDIVIDUALS

Dietary assessment methods have several inherent inaccuracies. One is that individuals underreport their intakes (Mertz et al., 1991; Schoeller,

1995; Schoeller et al., 1990), and it appears that obese individuals often do so to a greater extent than do normal-weight individuals (Heitmann and Lissner, 1995). There is no method to adjust intakes to account for under-reporting by individuals and much work is needed to develop an acceptable method. Another inherent inaccuracy is the quality of food composition databases.

Furthermore, large day-to-day variations in intake, which are exhibited by almost all individuals, mean that it often takes a prohibitively large number of days of intake measurement to approximate usual intake (Basiotis et al., 1987). As a result, caution is indicated when interpreting nutrient assessments based on self-reported dietary data covering only a few days of intake. Data on nutrient intakes should be interpreted in combination with information on typical food usage patterns to determine if the recorded intakes are representative of that individual's usual intake.

Finally, because there is considerable variation in intakes both within and between individuals, as well as variation associated with the requirement estimate, other factors must be evaluated in conjunction with the diet. The Dietary Reference Intakes (DRIs) should be used in conjunction with other data in assessing the adequacy of the diet of a specific individual. The nutritional status of an individual can be definitively determined only by a combination of dietary, anthropometric, physiological and biochemical data.

Using the Estimated Average Requirement and the Recommended Dietary Allowance

The Estimated Average Requirement (EAR) estimates the median of a distribution of requirements for a specific life stage and gender group, but it is not possible to know where an individual's requirement falls within this distribution without further anthropometric, physiological, or biochemical measures. Thus from dietary data alone, it is only possible to estimate the *likelihood* of nutrient adequacy or inadequacy. Furthermore, only rarely are precise and representative data on the usual intake of an individual available, adding additional uncertainty to the evaluation of an individual's dietary adequacy.

An approach for using data from dietary records or recalls to estimate the likelihood that an individual's nutrient intake is adequate is presented in *Dietary Reference Intakes: Applications in Dietary Assessment* (IOM, 2000). This approach is appropriate for nutrients with symmetrical requirement distributions, which is thought to be true for all macronutrients in this report for which EARs have been established. The following data are required:

- individual's mean nutrient intake over a given number of days
- day-to-day standard deviation (SD) of intakes for each nutrient of interest, as estimated from larger data sets for the appropriate life stage and gender group
  - EAR
  - SD of the nutrient requirement in the individual's life stage and gender group.

From this information a ratio is computed that compares the magnitude of difference between the individual's intake and the EAR to an estimate of variability of intake and requirements. The bigger the difference between intake and EAR and the lower the variability of intakes and requirements, the greater is the degree of certainty in assessing whether the individual's nutrient intake is adequate, inadequate, or excessive. This approach is quantitative and should be used only when the data listed above are available.

However, in the more common situation where the estimate of usual intake is not based on actual 24-hour recalls or records, but on dietary history or food frequency questionnaires, a qualitative interpretation of intakes can be used. For example, many practitioners use the diet history method to construct a likely usual day's intake, but the error structure associated with this method is unknown. While the error associated with food frequency questionnaires has been evaluated (Carroll et al., 1996; Liu, 1994), use of these tools for quantitative nutrient assessment is still not possible due to lack of accurate portion size estimates and grouping of food items (IOM, 2000). Thus, a practitioner should be cautious when using this method to approximate usual intakes.

Users of the DRIs may find it useful to consider that observed intakes below the EAR probably need to be improved (because the probability of adequacy is 50 percent or less) and those between the EAR and the Recommended Dietary Allowance (RDA) probably need to be improved (because the probability of adequacy is less than 97 to 98 percent). Only if intakes have been observed for a large number of days and are at the RDA, or observed intakes for fewer days are well above the RDA, should one have a high level of confidence that the intake is adequate. Such considerations are not applicable in the case of energy intake, which should match energy expenditure in individuals maintaining desirable body weight (see later section, "Planning Nutrient Intakes of Individuals," and Chapter 5).

Using the Adequate Intake

Adequate Intakes (AIs) have been set for infants younger than 7 months of age for n-3 and n-6 polyunsaturated fatty acids and protein. By definition, infants born at term who are exclusively fed human milk by healthy mothers consume an adequate nutrient intake. Infants who consume formulas with a nutrient profile similar to human milk (after adjustment for differences in bioavailability) are also assumed to consume adequate levels of nutrients. When an infant formula contains nutrient levels that are lower than those found in human milk, the likelihood of nutrient adequacy for infants who consume this formula cannot be determined because data on infants fed lower concentrations of nutrients are not available. AIs have also been established for infants 7 to 12 months of age for all nutrients covered in this report except protein, and for all individuals for *Total Fiber* and the *n*-3 and *n*-6 polyunsaturated fatty acids.

Equations that can be used to estimate the degree of confidence that an individual's usual intake meets or exceeds the AI are presented (IOM, 2000). The data required include the individual's reported intake over a given number of days, the AI for the age/gender group, and the day-to-day (within-person) SD for the nutrient of interest, as estimated from larger data sets for the appropriate life stage and gender group. Usual individual intakes that are equal to or above the AI can be assumed to be adequate. However, the likelihood of inadequacy of usual intakes below the AI cannot be determined.

Using the Tolerable Upper Intake Level

The Tolerable Upper Intake Level (UL) is used to examine the possibility of over-consumption of a nutrient. Equations have been developed to determine the degree of confidence that an individual's intake is below the UL (IOM, 2000). If an individual's usual nutrient intake remains below the UL, there is no risk of adverse effects from excessive intake. At intakes above the UL, the potential for risk of adverse effects increases. However, the intake at which a given individual will develop adverse effects as a result of taking large amounts of one or more nutrients is not known with certainty. No ULs were set for the macronutrients in this report. However, there is no established benefit to almost all healthy individuals who consume amounts of nutrients that exceed the RDA or AI.

Equations that can be used to estimate the degree of confidence that an individual's usual intake equals or exceeds the UL are presented in *Dietary Reference Intakes: Applications in Dietary Assessment* (IOM, 2000). The data required include the individual's reported intake over a given number of days, the UL for the life stage and gender group, and the day-to-day (within-person) SD for the nutrient of interest, as estimated from larger data sets for the appropriate life stage and gender group.

Using the Acceptable Macronutrient Distribution Range

In addition to presenting DRIs for macronutrients, this report also presents Acceptable Macronutrient Distribution Ranges (AMDRs) for individuals as a proportion of total energy intake. The AMDRs represent intakes that minimize the potential for chronic disease over the long-term, permit essential nutrients to be consumed at adequate levels, and should be associated with adequate energy intake and physical activity to maintain energy balance. The AMDRs for adults are 20 to 35 percent of energy from fat (including 0.6 to 1.2 percent of energy from *n*-3 polyunsaturated fatty acids and 5 to 10 percent of energy from *n*-6 polyunsaturated fatty acids), 45 to 65 percent of energy from carbohydrate, and 10 to 35 percent of energy from protein. For children, the AMDRs for total fat are 30 to 40 percent between the ages of 1 and 3 years, and 25 to 35 percent between the ages of 4 and 18 years. AMDRs for protein and carbohydrate do not vary with age.

To estimate the degree of confidence that an individual's diet falls within the AMDR, the equations developed could be used to estimate the degree of confidence that the individual's intake exceeds the AI or remains below the UL (IOM, 2000). The equation for the AI could be used to determine the degree of confidence that intake is above the lower end of the AMDR, and the equation for the UL could be used to determine the degree of confidence that intake is below the upper end of the AMDR. The data required include the individual's average intake of the macronutrient of interest as a percent of energy intake over a given number of days, the boundaries of the AMDR, and the day-to-day (within-person) SD of percent energy intake, as estimated from larger data sets for the appropriate life stage and gender group.

ASSESSING NUTRIENT INTAKES OF GROUPS

The assessment of nutrient adequacy for groups of people requires unbiased, quantitative information on the intake of the nutrient of interest by individuals in the group. Care must be taken to ensure the quality of the information upon which assessments are made so that they are not underestimates or overestimates of total nutrient intake. Estimates of total nutrient intake, including amounts from supplements, should be obtained. It is also important to use appropriate food composition tables with accurate nutrient values for the foods as consumed.

Several steps must be taken to assess the intake of a group. First, the intake distribution must be adjusted to remove the effect of day-to-day variation of individual intake. This can be accomplished either by collect-

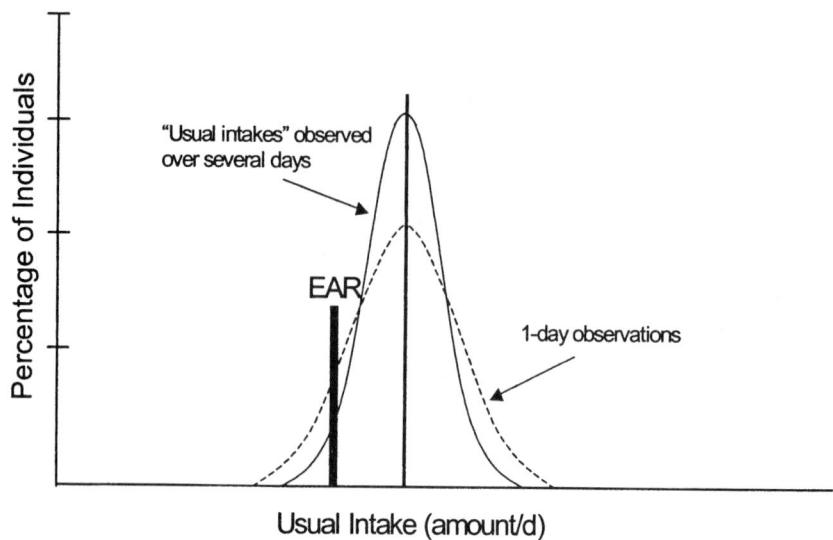

FIGURE 13-2 Comparison of 1-day and usual intakes for estimating the proportion of a group consuming below the Estimated Average Requirement (EAR).

ing dietary data for each individual over a large number of days or by statistical adjustments to the intake distribution. The statistical adjustments are based on assumptions about the day-to-day variation derived from repeat measurements of a representative subset of the group under study (Nusser et al., 1996). When this adjustment is performed and observed intakes are thus more representative of the usual diet, the intake distribution narrows, giving a more precise estimate of the proportion of the group with usual intakes below requirements (Figure 13-2). An explanation of this adjustment procedure has been presented in two previous reports (IOM, 2000; NRC, 1986).

A statistical approach is then used to combine the information on nutrient intakes with the information on nutrient requirements in order to determine the apparent percent prevalence of nutrient inadequacy in the group. Two approaches are briefly described below and in detail elsewhere (IOM, 2000; NRC, 1986).

The Probability Approach

Using the probability approach requires knowledge of both the distribution of requirements and the distribution of usual intakes for the population of interest. As described previously (IOM, 2000; NRC, 1986), the probability approach involves: (1) determining the risk of inadequacy for each individual in the population and then (2) averaging the individual probabilities of inadequacy across the group. Appendix C of *Dietary Reference Intakes: Applications in Dietary Assessment* (IOM, 2000) demonstrates how to carry out the necessary calculations to obtain a prevalence estimate for a group. Statistical programs (e.g., SAS or similar software) can be used to carry out these procedures.

The EAR Cut-Point Method

In most situations a cut-point method using the Estimated Average Requirement (EAR) may be used to estimate the prevalence of inadequate intakes. This cut-point method is a simplification of the full probability approach of calculating the prevalence of inadequacy described by the National Research Council (NRC, 1986). The cut-point method allows the prevalence of inadequate intakes in a population to be approximated by determining the percentage of individuals in the group whose usual intakes are less than the EAR for the nutrient of interest. This method assumes that the intake and requirement distributions are independent, an assumption that is not valid for the energy requirements addressed in this report because energy intakes are highly correlated to energy expenditure. The cut-point method further assumes that the variability of intakes among individuals within the group under study is at least as large as the variability of their requirements. This assumption is usually warranted in free-living populations. Finally, it assumes that the requirement distribution is symmetrical. This is thought to be true for all of the macronutrients discussed in this report.

Using the Estimated Average Requirement

If the assumptions for the EAR cut-point method are met, the prevalence of inadequate intakes may be estimated by the proportion of the distribution of usual intakes that falls below the EAR. An example of using the EAR cut-point method to assess the dietary carbohydrate adequacy of women aged 31 to 50 years follows. Dietary intake data are available from the 1994–1996 Continuing Survey of Food Intakes by Individuals. Estimated intakes are based on respondents' intakes, which were adjusted to remove within-person variability using the Iowa State University method (Appendix Table E-2). The EAR for women in this age group is 100 g/day. Examination of the distribution of usual carbohydrate intake reveals that intakes at the 1st and 5th percentiles are 87 and 118 g/day, respectively. Thus, fewer than 5 percent of women in this age group appear to have inadequate carbohydrate intakes.

Overestimates of the prevalence of inadequate intakes could result if the data used are based on intakes that are systematically underreported or if foods rich in the nutrient of interest are underreported. Such underreporting is common in national surveys (Briefel et al., 1997). Currently, a method for adjusting intakes to compensate for underreporting by individuals is not available, and much work is needed to develop an acceptable method. Conversely, underestimates of the prevalence of inadequacy could result if foods rich in the nutrient of interest were overreported. A more extensive discussion of potential sources of error in self-reported dietary data can be found in the report *Dietary Reference Intakes: Applications in Dietary Assessment* (IOM, 2000).

Comparison of Assessments Using the Probability Approach and Biochemical Assessment

If requirement estimates are correct, dietary intake data are reliable estimates of true usual intake, and biochemical measures reflect the same functional criterion used to set the requirement of a nutrient for the same population, then the prevalence of apparently inadequate dietary intakes and biochemical deficiencies or indicators of inadequacy should be similar.

Using the Recommended Dietary Allowance

The Recommended Dietary Allowances are not useful in estimating the prevalence of inadequate intakes for groups. As described above, the EAR should be used for this purpose.

Using the Adequate Intake

In this report Adequate Intakes (AIs) are assigned for all nutrients for infants through the age of 6 months and reflect the average intake of infants receiving human milk. Human milk and formulas with the same nutrient composition as human milk (after adjustment for bioavailability) provide the appropriate levels of nutrients for full-term infants of healthy, well-nourished mothers. For infants ages 7 to 12 months, AIs are set for carbohydrate and n-3 and n-6 polyunsaturated fatty acids and reflect the average intakes of infants receiving human milk and complementary foods. Groups of infants consuming formulas with lower levels of nutrients than that found in human milk may be at some risk of inadequacy, although the prevalence of inadequacy cannot be quantified.

This report provides AIs for all life stage and gender groups for *Total Fiber* and n-3 and n-6 polyunsaturated fatty acids. Groups with median intakes equal to or above the AI for *Total Fiber* and n-3 and n-6 polyunsaturated fatty acids can be assumed to have a low prevalence of inadequacy (provided that intake variability does not exceed that of the healthy group used to establish the AI). However, when the AI is not set as a mean intake of a healthy group (e.g., fiber), confidence in this assessment should be less than it would be if the AI represents the median intake of a healthy group. It is important to note that group median intakes below the AI cannot be assumed to be inadequate.

Using the Tolerable Upper Intake Level

The proportion of the population with usual intakes below the Tolerable Upper Intake Level (UL) is likely to be at no risk of adverse effects due to overconsumption. However, the proportion of the population consuming above the UL may potentially be at some risk.

The mean intake of a population cannot be used to evaluate the prevalence of intakes above the UL. A distribution of usual intakes, including intakes from supplements, is required to assess the proportion of the population that might be at risk of over-consumption. However, if the mean or median intake is equal to or greater than the UL, it suggests that the number of individuals with excessive intake is high and warrants further investigation.

Using the Acceptable Macronutrient Distribution Range

Although primarily directed at individuals, the Acceptable Macronutrient Distribution Range (AMDR) also permits assessment of populations. By determining the proportion of the group that falls below, within, and above the AMDR, it is possible to assess population adherence to recommendations and to determine the proportion of the population that is outside the range. If significant proportions of the population fall outside the range, concern could be heightened for possible adverse consequences. Planning and public health messages can then be instituted to attempt to attain a low prevalence of intakes below or above the AMDR.

For example, the AMDR for total fat intake of children 4 to 18 years of age is 25 to 35 percent of energy. Appendix Table E-6 presents data on the usual daily intake of total fat as a percentage of energy intake and indicates that for all groups of children and adolescents, the 5th percentile of intake is at least 25 percent. Thus, fewer than 5 percent of children have intakes below the AMDR for total fat. The 75th percentiles of intake are close to 35 percent, suggesting that approximately 25 percent of children and adolescents have intakes above the AMDR for total fat. Intakes of the remaining 70 to 75 percent fall within the AMDR.

PLANNING NUTRIENT INTAKES OF INDIVIDUALS

Using the Recommended Dietary Allowance

Individuals should use the Recommended Dietary Allowance (RDA) as the target for their intakes for those nutrients for which RDAs have been established. Intakes at this level ensure that the risk to individuals of not meeting their requirements is very low (2 to 3 percent). For example, the RDA for protein for adults is 0.8 g/kg/day, or 56 and 46 g/day for reference men and women weighing 70 kg and 57 kg, respectively. For a small adult weighing 45 kg, the recommended protein intake would be 36 g/day, while for a larger adult weighing 90 kg, the RDA would be 72 g/day.

Using the Adequate Intake

Adequate Intakes (AIs) are set for infants younger than 7 months of age for all nutrients, and for all nutrients except protein and indispensable amino acids for infants 7 through 12 months of age. Human milk, by definition, supplies the AI for a nutrient for term infants; it is not necessary to plan additional sources of intake for infants exclusively fed human milk. Likewise, an infant formula with a nutrient profile similar to human milk (after adjustment for differences in bioavailability) should supply adequate nutrients for an infant.

In this report AIs are also set for children, adolescents, and adults for *Total Fiber* and *n*-3 and *n*-6 polyunsaturated fatty acids. Accordingly, individuals should use the AI as their goal for intake of these nutrients.

Using the Tolerable Upper Intake Level

Tolerable Upper Intake Levels (Uls) were not set for the macronutrients covered in this report.

Using the Acceptable Macronutrient Distribution Range

In addition to meeting the RDA or AI and remaining below the UL, an individual's intake of macronutrients should be planned so that carbohydrate, total fat, *n*-3 and *n*-6 polyunsaturated fatty acids, and protein are within their respective Acceptable Macronutrient Distribution Ranges.

PLANNING NUTRIENT INTAKES OF GROUPS

Using the Estimated Average Requirement and the Tolerable Upper Intake Level

For those nutrients with Estimated Average Requirements (EAR), the EAR may be used as a basis for planning or making recommendations for the nutrient intakes of groups. The mean intake of a group should be high enough so that only a small percentage of the group would have intakes below the EAR, thus indicating a low prevalence of dietary inadequacy. The approach to planning for a low prevalence of inadequacy differs depending on whether or not the distributions of intake and requirements are normally distributed. Additional details are provided in the forthcoming Institute of Medicine report on dietary planning.

For example, assume that the goal of planning was to target a 2 to 3 percent prevalence of inadequacy for a nutrient for which both requirement and intake distributions were statistically normal. This would be attained by planning a group mean intake equal to the EAR plus 2 standard deviations (SD) of the *intake* distribution. Because the variability of intakes generally exceeds the variability of requirements, this target group mean intake will usually exceed the Recommended Dietary Allowance (which equals the EAR plus 2 SDs of the *requirement* distribution). Prevalence of inadequacy more or less than 2 to 3 percent could also be considered. Mean intakes needed to attain the desired prevalence would be estimated by determining the number of SDs of intake added to the EAR that would result in the desired percentage prevalence below the EAR. This can be done by consulting tables that list areas under the curve of the standard normal distribution in relation to SD scores (z-scores).

When the distribution of intakes is skewed (as is true for intakes of most nutrients), a low prevalence of inadequacy can be attained by planning to position the intake distribution such that only the targeted proportion is below the EAR. Finally, when it is known that requirements for a nutrient are not normally distributed and one wants to ensure a low group prevalence of inadequacy, it is necessary to examine both the intake and requirement distributions to determine a median intake at which the proportion of individuals with intakes below requirements is likely to be low.

In addition to planning for an acceptably low group prevalence of intakes below the EAR, the planned distribution also needs to be examined to ensure that the prevalence of intakes above the Tolerable Upper Intake Level (UL) is also acceptably low.

Using the EAR and UL in planning intakes of groups involves the analysis of data and a number of key considerations such as:

- determination of the current usual nutrient intake distribution of the group of interest expressed in the same unit as the EAR (e.g., g/day, g/kg/day, percent of energy);
- selection of the degree of risk that can be tolerated when planning for the group (e.g., a 2 to 3 percent prevalence versus a higher or lower prevalence); and
- consideration of various possible interventions to shift the current distribution, if necessary, to produce an acceptably low prevalence of intakes below the EAR, as well as an acceptably low prevalence of intakes above the UL; some targeted interventions may increase the intake of only those most at risk, while other interventions (e.g., fortification of the food supply) may increase the intake, to varying degrees, of the majority of the population.

Using the Adequate Intake in Planning for Groups

As indicated previously, Adequate Intakes (AIs) have been established for some of the nutrients discussed in this report. Planning a median group intake that meets the AI should, by definition, be associated with a low prevalence of inadequacy, if the AI was set as the median intake of a healthy group and the group being planned for has similar characteristics to the group used to establish the AI. If the AI was not set as the median intake of a healthy group (e.g., the AI for *Total Fiber*), there is less confidence that the prevalence of inadequacy would be low if the group's median intake met the AI.

Using the Acceptable Macronutrient Distribution Range

In addition to ensuring that the group prevalence of intakes below the EAR or above the UL is acceptably low, an additional goal of planning is to achieve a macronutrient distribution in which the intakes of most of the group fall within the Acceptable Macronutrient Distribution Ranges (AMDRs). There may be a tendency for planners to develop menus and patterns in which the mean population intakes are at the midpoint of the AMDRs; this is one method to plan for low prevalence of intakes below or above the AMDR. For example, a meal program for a university dormitory might be planned using the midpoint of the ranges for carbohydrate and fat (for adults, these would be 55 and 28 percent of energy, respectively). The remaining 17 percent of energy would come from protein. Assessment would be needed to determine whether intakes of most members of the group fell within the AMDR, or whether interventions were required to target one end of the distribution (e.g., those with fat intakes above 35 percent). However, planning for the midpoint of a range is not the only way that the AMDR can be used to plan for groups. Using the university dormitory example, a dietary pattern might be planned in which the mean intake from fat was 30 percent of energy. Assessment conducted following implementation of the program might reveal that actual fat intakes of the students ranged from about 25 percent to about 35 percent of energy. In other words, the prevalence of intakes outside the acceptable range is low, despite a mean fat intake that is higher than the midpoint of the range. While the AMDR can be used as a general quantitative guideline for planning and evaluating diets, qualitative considerations, such as a menu low in saturated fats, may be at least as important as these quantitative guidelines (see Chapter 11).

NUTRIENT-SPECIFIC CONSIDERATIONS

Energy

Planning Energy Intakes for Individuals

The underlying objective of planning for energy is similar to planning for nutrients—to attain an acceptably low risk of inadequacy and of excess. The approach to planning for energy, however, differs substantially from planning for other nutrients. When planning for an individual's intake of nutrient such as vitamins and minerals, the goal is a low risk of inadequacy by meeting the Recommended Dietary Allowance (RDA) or Adequate Intake (AI), and a low risk of excess by remaining below the Tolerable Upper Intake Level (UL). Even though intakes at or above the RDA or AI are almost certainly above an individual's requirement, there are no adverse effects to the individual of consuming an intake above his or her requirement, provided intake remains below the UL; however there are also no documented benefits.

The situation for energy is quite different. There are adverse effects to individuals who consume energy above their requirements—over time, weight gain will occur. This difference is reflected in the fact that there is no RDA for energy, as it would be inappropriate to recommend an intake that exceeded the requirement (and would lead to weight gain) of 97 to 98 percent of individuals. The requirement for energy for individuals of normal weight is expressed as an Estimated Energy Requirement (EER), which reflects the energy expenditure associated with an individual's sex, age, height, weight, and physical activity level.

Equations are presented to estimate an individual's energy expenditure, with separate equations for normal (body mass index [BMI] > 18.5 and < 25) and overweight (BMI ≥ 25) individuals, as well as for all individuals with BMI > 18.5 (i.e., including normal, overweight, and obese subjects).

For overweight individuals, these equations estimate Total Energy Expenditure (TEE), rather than the EER, which is reserved for normal weight individuals. In all cases, however, the equations estimate the energy expenditure associated with maintaining current body weight and activity level. They were not developed, for example, to lead to weight loss in overweight individuals. However, just as is the case with other nutrients, energy expenditures vary from one individual to another, even though their characteristics may be similar. This variability is reflected in the standard deviation (SD), which allows for estimation of the range within which the individual's energy expenditure could vary. Note that this does not imply that an individual would maintain energy balance at any intake within this range; it simply indicates how variable requirements could be among those with similar characteristics.

For example, the equation for the EER of women ages 19 years and older with a BMI > 18.5 and < 25 is:

$$\text{Energy (kcal)} = 354.1 - (6.91 \times \text{age [y]}) + \text{physical activity coefficient} \times (9.36 \times \text{weight [kg]} + 726 \times \text{height [m]})$$

The SD is 160 kcal. Therefore, the EER for a normal-weight, 33-year-old low-active woman (i.e., with a physical activity level (PAL) between 1.4 and 1.59, for whom the physical activity coefficient is 1.12), with a height of 1.63 m and a weight of 55 kg would be:

$$\text{Energy (kcal)} = 354.1 - (6.91 \times 33) + 1.12 \times (9.36 \times 55 + 726 \times 1.63) = 2{,}028$$

The 95 percent confidence interval for this equation reflects the range within which a given individual's energy expenditure likely falls, and in this example, it would be $2{,}028 \pm (2 \times 160)$, or between 1,708 and 2,348 kcal/day. It must be realized that considerable uncertainties are inherent in making such predictions, notably because of possible misclassification of individuals into the various PAL categories (i.e., sedentary, low active, active, and very active).

Usual energy intakes are highly correlated with expenditure when considered over periods of weeks or months. This means that most people who have access to enough food will, on average, consume amounts of energy very close to the amounts that they expend, and as a result, maintain their weight over extended periods of time. Any changes in weight that do occur usually reflect small imbalances accumulated over a long period of time. For normal individuals who are weight-stable, at a healthy weight, and performing at least the minimal recommended amount of activity, their energy requirement (and recommended intake) is their usual energy intake. Thus, if an individual's usual energy intake were known, the plan would be to maintain it rather than use the EER (or if overweight, the TEE). In many situations, however, the usual energy intake of an individual is not known, and the estimated energy requirement equations are useful planning tools.

Using the EER (or TEE) to Maintain Body Weight. When the goal is to maintain body weight in an individual with specified characteristics (age, height, weight, and activity level), an initial estimate for energy intake is provided by the equation for the energy expenditure of an individual with those characteristics. By definition, the estimate would be expected to underestimate the true energy expenditure 50 percent of the time and to overestimate it 50 percent of the time, leading to corresponding changes in body weight. This indicates that monitoring of body weight would be required when implementing intakes based on the equations that predict individual energy requirements. For example, if subjects were enrolled in a study in which it was important to maintain body weight, each individual would be fed the amount of energy estimated to be needed based on the EER equation. Body weight would be closely monitored over time, and the amount of energy provided to each individual would be adjusted up or down from the EER (or TEE) as required to maintain body weight.

Using the EER (or TEE) to Plan to Prevent Weight Loss. In some situations the goal of planning might be to prevent weight loss in an individual with specified characteristics. In this situation, the EER or TEE equation could be used to derive the average energy expenditure for the individual, and then an amount equal to two times the SD added. This would lead to an intake that would be expected to exceed the actual energy expenditure of all but 2 to 3 percent of the individuals with similar characteristics. Using the above example for the 33-year-old, low-active woman, one would provide 2,028 + (2 × 160) kcal, or 2,348 kcal. This intake would prevent weight loss in almost all individuals with similar characteristics. Of course, this level of intake would lead to weight gain in most of these individuals.

Using the EER (or TEE) to Plan to Prevent Weight Gain. If the goal of planning is to prevent weight gain in an individual with specified characteristics, the appropriate EER equation could be used to derive the average energy expenditure for the individual, and then subtract an amount equal to two times the SD. This would lead to an intake that would be expected to fall below the actual energy requirements of all but 2.5 percent of the individuals with similar characteristics. Using the above example for the 33-year-old, low-active woman, the energy requirement would be 2,028 − (2 × 160) kcal, or 1,708 kcal. This intake would prevent weight gain in almost all individuals with similar characteristics. Of course, this level of intake would lead to weight loss in most of these individuals.

Planning for Energy for Groups

As is true for individuals, the underlying objective in planning the energy intake of a group is similar to planning intakes for other nutrients—to attain an acceptably low prevalence of inadequacy and of potential excess. The approach to planning for energy, however, differs substantially from planning for other nutrients. When the Estimated Average Requirement (EAR) cut-point method is used to plan for a group's intake of nutrients such as vitamins and minerals, a low prevalence of inadequacy is obtained by positioning the intake distribution such that an acceptably low proportion of the group has an intake below the EAR. A low prevalence of potential risk of excess is obtained by positioning the intake distribution such that an acceptably low proportion of the group has an intake above the UL. Even though the planned distribution of intakes would exceed the actual requirements of all but the designated proportion of the group (in many cases, by a considerable margin), there are no known adverse effects to the group of consuming vitamins and minerals in amounts that exceed requirements, provided the proportion above the UL also remains low.

In the case of energy, however, there *are* adverse effects for the individuals in the group whose intakes are above their requirements, as weight gain is bound to occur over time. Therefore, the EAR cut-point method to plan for group intakes of energy is clearly inappropriate. In addition, the assumptions required to apply this method, as well as for the probability approach, do not hold for energy. Most notably, the methods assume that intakes are essentially uncorrelated with requirements. In the case of energy, however, intakes are very highly correlated with requirements.

What, then, can be done to plan for energy intakes of groups? There are two possible approaches: estimate energy requirements for the reference person or obtain an average of estimated maintenance energy needs for group members.

Estimate Energy Requirements for the Reference Person. One approach is to use the EER for the reference person who represents the group. For example, to plan for a large group of men ages 19 to 30 years, estimate the EER for the reference male with a weight of 70 kg and a height of 1.76 m and who is considered low active, and use this number (~2,700 kcal) as the target for the group. This approach would require the assumption that all members of the group were similar to the reference person, or that the reference individual accurately represented group average values for age, height, weight, and activity level, and that these variables were symmetrically distributed. If either assumption held, the resulting EER would approximate the group mean energy requirement.

However, if the assumptions did not hold true, as is likely in many situations, the estimates would be incorrect. At a practical level, it is likely that the estimate obtained would be less than the true average energy expenditure of the group, since for most life stage and gender groups the reference person weighs less than the average person.

Obtain an Average of Estimated Maintenance Energy Needs for Group Members. The preferred approach would be to plan for an intake equal to the average energy expenditure for the group. For example, using the same group of 19- to 30-year-old men from the previous section, the energy expenditure for each individual in the group would be estimated (assuming access to data on height, weight, age, and activity level). The average of these values would be used as the planning goal for maintenance of current weight and activity level. Table 13-1 shows an example of how this is done for a small group of six healthy men with a BMI < 25. If the group included men with a BMI > 25, the equations developed to estimate the Total Energy Expenditure for overweight individuals would be used for those individuals with BMI > 25.

In this hypothetical example, the average planned intake exceeds the EER of five of the men, and is below the EER of one large, very active man (in a larger, more homogeneous group, the estimate would be expected to

TABLE 13-1 Obtaining an Average Estimated Energy Requirement (EER) for a Group

Subject	Age (y)	Height (m)	Weight (kg)	Physical Activity Level	Physical Activity Level Coefficient	EER[a] (kcal)
1	21	1.83	95	Sedentary	1.0	2,961
2	27	1.77	75	Low active	1.12	2,811
3	25	1.69	60	Active	1.27	2,794
4	19	1.80	75	Low active	1.12	2,905
5	30	1.73	80	Very active	1.45	3,575
6	25	1.75	75	Low active	1.12	2,818
Mean	24.5	1.76	76.7	—	1.18	2,977

[a] Energy (kcal) = 661.8 − 9.53 × age (y) + physical activity coefficient × [15.91 × weight (kg) + 539.6 × height (m)]. Physical activity level coefficient = 1.0 (sedentary), 1.12 (active), 1.45 (very active).

be inadequate for half the men and above the requirement for the other half). However, because intakes and expenditures are highly correlated, and assuming that all members of the group have free access to food, most members of the group will consume an amount of energy equal to their expenditure. Thus, planning for an intake that approximates the mean energy expenditure should allow the group to meet energy needs for weight maintenance and current activity levels.

Caveats. As with other planning applications, it should be emphasized that the planning goal is for energy intakes. The above approach requires the assumption that free access to food is available, that each member of the group consumes an amount of energy that approximates their individual expenditure, and that food is not wasted or spoiled. As with other planning examples, food waste and to what extent the amount of energy offered would need to exceed the target median intake need to be considered. Assessing the plan following its implementation would lead to further refinements.

Assessing Energy Intakes

As was true for planning, the approach to assessing the adequacy of energy intakes differs from that described for other nutrients. This arises in part from theoretical considerations. Perhaps more importantly though, it is related to the fact that for energy, unlike most nutrients, a readily observable, accurate biological indicator—body weight—can be used to assess the long-term adequacy of energy intake. An individual or group with a BMI above the desirable range reflects long-term excess energy intake, while the converse is true when BMI is below the desirable range.

The availability of a biological indicator to assess the adequacy of energy intake becomes particularly critical because of the effect of dietary underreporting on the assessment of adequacy. It is now widely accepted, and supported by a large body of literature, that underreporting of food intake is pervasive in dietary surveys (Black et al., 1993). Underreporters can constitute anywhere from 10 to 45 percent of the total sample, depending on the age, gender, and body composition of the sample. Underreporting tends to increase in prevalence as children age (Livingstone et al., 1992), and is greater among women than among men (Johnson et al., 1994). Both the prevalence and severity of underreporting is greater among obese individuals compared with lean individuals (Bandini et al., 1999; Lichtman et al., 1992; Prentice et al., 1986). In addition, those of low socioeconomic status (characterized by low incomes, low educational attainment, and low literacy levels) are more likely to report low energy intakes (Johnson et al., 1998; Kristal et al., 1997; Pryer et al., 1997). Therefore, self-reported energy intakes do not reflect actual energy intakes, and other methods must be used to determine their adequacy. Relative body weight (as reflected by BMI) is a preferred indicator of energy adequacy for individuals and for groups.

Assessing Adequacy of Energy Intakes of Individuals. Theoretically, one could compare the usual energy intake of an individual to his or her requirement to maintain current weight and activity level, as estimated using the equations developed to estimate energy expenditure. However, as noted above, the EER (or TEE) equation provides an estimate that is the midpoint of the range within which the expenditure of an individual with specified characteristics could vary, and the individual's actual expenditure could be considerably above or below the midpoint. Accordingly, comparing the individual's intake to the calculated average expenditure is essentially meaningless. For example, the EER for a 33-year-old, low-active woman with a height of 1.63 m and a weight of 55 kg would be calculated at 2,028 kcal, but expenditure for a woman with these characteristics could vary between 1,708 and 2,348 kcal. If the woman's actual energy intake averaged 2,200 kcal, her actual intake could be inadequate, adequate, or excessive.

BMI, in contrast, provides a useful indicator of the adequacy of usual energy intake in relation to usual energy expenditure. If the woman in the above example had a BMI of 22 (i.e., within the healthy range of > 18.5 and < 25), her usual energy intake would be assessed as adequate relative to her usual expenditure. If her BMI was 17 (below the healthy range), then she would be assessed as having an inadequate energy intake; if it was 33 (above the healthy range), her intake would be assessed as excessive.

Assessing Adequacy of Energy Intakes of Groups. Instead of assessing the adequacy of energy intake by comparing reported intakes (which are almost always affected by considerable underreporting) to estimated expenditure, relying on BMI as a biological indicator is preferable. The distribution of BMI within a population group can be assessed, and the proportions of the group with BMI below, within, and above the desirable range would reflect the proportions with inadequate, adequate, and excessive energy intakes. When this approach is applied to body-weight data of adults ages 19 to 50 years obtained in the Continuing Survey of Food Intakes by Individuals, 59 percent of men and 44 percent of women are found to have a BMI ≥ 25, reflecting excessive energy intake; 40 percent of men and 52 percent of women have a BMI within the ideal range, reflecting adequacy; and 0.9 percent of men and 4.6 percent of women have a BMI below 18.5, reflecting inadequacy.

Although the above discussion refers to the adequacy of energy intake, it should be reiterated that intake is just one component of energy balance. Excessive intake must be interpreted as being excessive *in relation to energy expenditure*. In many cases, intake may not be excessive in absolute terms; instead, inadequate energy expenditure may be the primary factor in contributing to long-term positive energy balance. This has important implications for how this issue is best addressed at the population level. There are a number of reasons why increased energy expenditure may be a more appropriate solution than decreased energy intake to long-term positive energy balance (i.e., overweight). First, restricting energy intake also decreases the ability to meet requirements of many nutrients. Second, evidence exists to support the concept that much of the health risk attributed to an increased BMI is associated with poor fitness. Increasing physical activity, thereby improving fitness, improves health outcomes of overweight individuals irrespective of changes in relative weight (Blair et al., 1993, 1995).

Implications of Underreporting for Other Macronutrients. In addition to the major impact of underreporting on assessment of the adequacy of energy intake, it also has potential implications for other macronutrients. If it is assumed that underreporting of macronutrients occurs in proportion to underreporting of energy intake, macronutrients expressed as a percentage of energy would be relatively accurate. Accordingly, there would be little impact on the estimated proportions of those whose intakes fall outside the Acceptable Macronutrient Distribution Ranges (AMDRs) for carbohydrate, protein, total fat, and *n*-3 and *n*-6 polyunsaturated fatty acids. Underreporting would, however, overestimate the prevalence of dietary inadequacy for protein, indispensable amino acids, and carbohydrate. Conversely, it has been suggested that underreporting of nutrients may not occur in proportion to underreporting of energy (IOM, 2000). If, for example, fat intake is preferentially underreported, this would lead to an underestimate of the proportion of those whose intakes are above the upper end of the AMDRs for total fat and for *n*-3 and *n*-6 polyunsaturated fatty acids. It could also lead to an overestimate of the percentage of energy derived from carbohydrate.

Total Carbohydrate

The Dietary Reference Intakes (DRIs) for total carbohydrate (starches and sugars) are set in this report as EARs and RDAs, expressed as absolute amounts (g/day) that support brain glucose utilization. The RDA for carbohydrate (130 g/day) is an average minimum requirement and is lower than what most North Americans consume (Appendix Table E-2). A UL is not established for total carbohydrate. Most people can meet their requirement for carbohydrate without difficulty by consuming a varied diet containing breads, rice, other grain products, potatoes, fruits, vegetables, milk products, and (in moderate amounts) starch- or sugar-based snack foods.

As discussed in Chapter 11, to achieve a healthful balance of the macronutrients that supply energy, the AMDR for total carbohydrate is 45 to 65 percent of energy. This range allows for intakes of carbohydrate that exceeds the RDA of 130 g/day. The carbohydrate content of most U.S. diets is either less than or within this range (see Appendix Table E-3), but it is more likely to be within this range if food selections emphasize grains, fruits, and vegetables prepared with minimal or modest amounts of fat.

Added Sugars

Added sugars are defined as sugars and syrups that are added to foods during processing or preparation. Major sources of added sugars include soft drinks, cakes, cookies, pies, fruitades, fruit punch, dairy desserts, and candy (USDA/HHS, 2000). Specifically, added sugars include white sugar, brown sugar, raw sugar, corn syrup, corn-syrup solids, high-fructose corn syrup, malt syrup, maple syrup, pancake syrup, fructose sweetener, anhydrous dextrose, and crystal dextrose. Since added sugars provide only energy when eaten alone and lower nutrient density when added to foods, it is suggested that added sugars in the diet should not exceed 25 percent of total energy intake. Usual intakes above this level place an individual at potential risk of not meeting micronutrient requirements. Nutrient data on added sugars has only recently become available in the U.S. Department of Agriculture's (USDA) Pyramid Servings Database, which includes data on added sugars for over 7,000 foods. Appendix Table D-1 describes the Third National Health and Nutrition Examination Survey (NHANES III) results on the distribution of intakes of added sugar.

To assess the sugar intakes of groups requires knowledge of the distribution of usual added sugar intake as a percent of energy intake. Once this is determined, the percentage of the population exceeding the maximum suggested level can be evaluated. Because the criterion for the suggested maximum intake level of added sugars is the risk of associated inadequate intakes of micronutrients, such an evaluation would be complemented by assessing micronutrient intakes, as described in the DRI report for those nutrients (IOM, 2001) and the report on dietary assessment (IOM, 2000).

Dietary, Functional, and Total Fiber

Dietary Fiber is defined in this report as nondigestible carbohydrates and lignin that are intrinsic and intact in plants. *Functional Fiber* is defined as isolated, nondigestible carbohydrates that have beneficial physiological effects in humans. *Total Fiber* is the sum of *Dietary Fiber* and *Functional Fiber*. Fiber includes viscous forms that lower serum cholesterol concentrations (i.e., soluble fiber: oat bran, beans) and the bulking agents that improve laxation (i.e., insoluble fiber: wheat bran). The AI for *Total Fiber* is 38 and 25 g/day for 19- to 50-year-old men and women, respectively, based on a reduced risk of coronary heart disease for those within the highest quintiles of dietary fiber consumption (g/1,000 kcal) in several epidemiological studies and the median energy intake (Appendix Table E-1). Unlike the AI for some nutrients, this AI does not describe the median *Total Fiber* intake of a healthy population. Instead, it is based on health benefits associated with consuming foods that are rich in fiber. Based on CSFII data (Appendix Table E-4), the median *Dietary Fiber* intakes are 16.5 to 17.9 g/day for men and 12.1 to 13.3 g/day for women. Thus, it is evident that to meet the AI, most people will need to substantially increase their *Total Fiber* intake. Usual intakes that meet or exceed the AI can be assumed adequate, but the likelihood of inadequacy of usual intakes below the AI cannot be determined.

Fiber consumption can be increased by substituting whole grain or products with added cereal bran for more refined bakery, cereal, pasta, and rice products; by choosing whole fruits instead of fruit juices; by consuming fruits and vegetables without removing edible membranes or peels; and by eating more legumes, nuts, and seeds. For example, whole wheat bread contains three times as much *Dietary Fiber* as white bread, and the fiber content of a potato doubles if the peel is consumed. The soluble and insoluble fiber components of 228 U.S. foods have been published by Marlett and Cheung (1997).

Dietary fiber data are listed for a wide range of foods in the USDA Nutrient Database for Standard Reference (USDA, 2001). The dietary fiber values in the USDA database represent *Total Fiber* (including both dietary and functional fiber) as defined in this report. For most diets (those that have not been fortified with *Functional Fiber* that was isolated and added for health purposes), the contribution of *Functional Fiber* is minor relative to the naturally occurring *Dietary Fiber*. For example, the *Functional Fiber* content for foods such as fat-free yogurts and ice creams that contain added guar gums and carrageenan is so low that the USDA database generally indicates zero dietary fiber for these foods. Although the AI is set for *Total Fiber*, this AI is generally based upon the fibers present in foods, and until these terms are further incorporated into nutrient databases, it is appropriate to apply the *Dietary Fiber* data from the USDA database to the AI for *Total Fiber*.

Because there is insufficient evidence of deleterious effects of high *Dietary Fiber* as part of an overall healthy diet, a Tolerable Upper Intake Level has not been established.

Total Fat and n-3 and n-6 Polyunsaturated Fatty Acids

Total Fat

No RDAs or AIs are set for total fat, but an AMDR of 20 to 35 percent of energy is recommended for adults (Chapter 11). Thus, when planning diets for individuals, it is necessary to first calculate the individual's estimated energy expenditure, determine 20 and 35 percent of this number in kilocalories, and then divide by 9 kcal/g to get the range of fat intake in grams per day. For example, a person whose energy expenditure was 2,300 kcal/day should aim for an energy intake from fat of 460 to 805 kcal/day. In grams of total fat, intake should be between 51 and 89 g/day.

Likewise, when assessing fat intakes of individuals, the goal is to determine if usual energy intake from total fat is between 20 and 35 percent. As illustrated above, this is a relatively simple calculation assuming both usual fat intake and usual energy intake are known. However, because dietary data are typically based on a small number of days of records or recalls, it may not be possible to state with confidence that a diet is within this range. As explained in the DRI dietary assessment report (IOM, 2000), an adjustment can be made for the likelihood that these are not representative days, based on the day-to-day variation in fat intake and the number of days of dietary data.

When planning fat intakes for groups, the goal is to minimize the intakes of total fat that are outside the AMDR of 20 to 35 percent of energy from fat. If planning is for a confined population, a procedure similar to the one described for individuals may be used: determine the necessary energy intake from the planned meals and plan for a fat intake that provides between 20 and 35 percent of this value. If the group is not confined, then planning intakes is more complex and ideally begins with knowledge of the distribution of usual energy intake from fat. Then the distribution can be examined, and feeding and education programs designed to either increase, or more likely, decrease the percent of energy from fat.

Assessing the fat intake of a group requires knowledge of the distribution of usual fat intake as a percent of energy intake. Once the distribution is described, the percent of the population outside the AMDR can be calculated. For example, Appendix Table E-6 shows that in the CSFII, less than 1 percent of the population was below 20 percent of energy from fat, while over 50 percent consumed greater than 35 percent of energy from fat.

n-3 and n-6 Polyunsaturated Fatty Acids

n-3 and n-6 Polyunsaturated fatty acids have an AI based on median intakes of linoleic acid and α-linolenic acid from CFSII, respectively. In addition to an AI, an AMDR is provided for n-3 and n-6 fatty acids. The suggested range is 0.6 to 1.2 percent of energy from n-3 fatty acids and 5 to 10 percent of energy from n-6 fatty acids. Thus, there are several considerations when planning and evaluating n-3 and n-6 fatty acid intakes. Usual intakes that meet or exceed the AI can be assumed adequate, but the likelihood of inadequacy of usual intakes below the AI cannot be determined. Assessing n-3 and n-6 fatty acid intakes of groups against the AMDR requires knowledge of the distribution of usual fatty acid intake as a percentage of energy intake. Once the distribution is described, the percentage of the population outside the AMDR can be calculated.

Saturated Fatty Acids, Trans Fatty Acids, and Cholesterol

No RDAs, AIs, or AMDRs are provided for saturated fatty acids, *trans* fatty acids, and cholesterol. However, with increasing intakes of either of these three nutrients, there is an increased risk of coronary heart disease. Chapter 11 provides some dietary guidance on ways to reduce the intake of saturated fatty acids, *trans* fatty acids, and cholesterol. For example, when planning diets, it is desirable to replace saturated fat with either monounsaturated or polyunsaturated fats to the greatest extent possible.

Protein and Amino Acids

The EARs and RDAs for protein and amino acids have been expressed as grams per kilogram per day, the first DRIs to be expressed in this way. This implies that requirements and recommended intakes vary among individuals of different sizes, and should be individualized when used for dietary assessment or planning. The potential implications of this are discussed below.

Dietary Assessment

For most nutrients for which EARs have been defined, the prevalence of inadequate intakes can be estimated as the proportion of the distribution of usual intakes that falls below the EAR using the EAR cut-point method (IOM, 2000). However, this method requires a number of assumptions, including that the individual requirement for the nutrient in question has a symmetric distribution. As described in Chapter 10, the distribution of the individual requirement for protein for adults is skewed, however, this skewing appears to be slight and the EAR cut-point method is expected to provide a good approximation to prevalence.

However, if more accuracy is needed, the "probability approach" can be used. This approach has been described elsewhere (IOM, 2000; NRC, 1986), and its application for assessing the prevalence of inadequacy of iron intakes has been illustrated (IOM, 2002). The probability approach for assessing the adequacy of protein intakes is identical to that outlined for iron, with the simplification that percentiles of protein requirement can be explicitly calculated from the formula given in Chapter 10 ("RDA Summary, Ages 19–50 Years").

Planning the Diet

When planning a diet for an individual, recommended intakes can be determined on the basis of the individual's body weight. Although the RDA for the reference adult male is 56 g/day of protein (based on 0.8 g/kg/day for a 70-kg person), the recommended intakes for men weighing 60 kg and 90 kg would be 48 and 72 g/day, respectively.

It should be noted that the DRIs are intended to apply to healthy individuals. Thus, determining a recommended protein intake based on current body weight may not be appropriate for those who are significantly underweight or overweight. For example, a medical professional might choose to specify a protein intake for a malnourished, underweight patient based on what the patient's body weight would be if he were healthy. A patient weighing 40 kg, whose body weight when healthy was 55 kg, could thus have a recommended protein intake of 44 g/day (55 kg × 0.8 g/kg), rather than the 32 g/day that would be determined based on current weight. Conversely, protein intakes recommended for individuals who are morbidly obese could be based on the amounts recommended for those with more normal body weights.

Are Planning and Assessing Intakes of Indispensable Amino Acids Necessary?

The previous RDAs and Recommended Nutrient Intakes did not include recommended intakes for indispensable amino acids; it was assumed that individuals consuming a mixed diet with recommended amounts of protein would obtain required amounts of indispensable amino acids. In other words, it was not necessary to assess or plan for intakes of indispensable amino acids. Now that EARs and RDAs have been provided for indispensable amino acids, it is important to re-examine the question: Is it necessary to consider indispensable amino acids when conducting dietary planning and assessment, or is it sufficient to consider only total protein?

The simplest scenario for answering this question relates to dietary planning for individuals. When planning for individuals, the objective is to meet the RDA, as doing so ensures a very low risk of inadequacy. Thus, do diets that provide the RDA for protein also provide the RDAs for indispensable amino acids? It appears that this may not necessarily occur, at least for the amino acid lysine. Data in Table 13-2 suggest that although most protein sources provide recommended amounts of threonine, tryptophan, and sulfur-containing amino acids, this is not true for lysine. Animal protein sources provide recommended intakes of lysine, but it is clear that individuals who do not consume animal protein sources, or who consume limited amounts, would be unlikely to obtain the recommended amounts of lysine when total protein intake is equal to the RDA, unless their diets were usually high in beans or other legumes. Even then, diets could be marginal, as the data in Table 13-2 regarding amino acid composition do not account for the apparent lower digestibility of some plant protein sources. Beans, for example, have a digestibility of 82 percent relative to milk and meat. Thus, it appears that, in addition to assessing and planning total protein intakes, it is also necessary to assess and plan for intakes of the amino acid lysine in individuals consuming proteins with low levels of lysine.

TABLE 13-2 Selected Indispensable Amino Acid Content of Protein Sources Compared with Recommended Levels

| | Indispensable Amino Acid (mg/g protein) | | | |
	Lysine	Threonine	Tryptophan	Sulfur Amino Acids
Scoring pattern, adult	47	24	6	23
FNB/IOM Recommended Protein Scoring Pattern (Child 1–3 y)	51	27	7	25
Canadian diet, 1984	61	38	12	34
U.S. diet, 1977	68	39	12	35
Wheat bread	28[a]	30	13	39
Garbanzo beans	67	37	10	26[a]
Beef	83	44	11	37
Cheddar cheese	76	33	12	29
Tofu	66	41	16	27
Brown rice	38[a]	37	13	35
Almonds	29[a]	32	15	25[a]
Peanut butter	36[a]	34	10	33
Cornmeal	28[a]	38	7	39

[a] The amino acid content in these foods is lower than the proportion recommended for the proper balance of indispensable amino acids in the total diet, based on the FNB/IOM Recommended Protein Scoring Pattern (Table 10-26). Thus a mixed diet containing a variety of protein sources is recommended.

As alluded to above, the need to plan and assess intakes of lysine is likely of greatest importance for individuals whose diets emphasize plant foods and are relatively low in total protein. For example, consider a woman who weighs 57 kg and follows a plant-based diet that provides the RDA for total protein (in her case, 57 × 0.8 g/kg = 45 g/day). She would be unlikely to meet her RDA for lysine (2.2 g/day) unless 50 percent or more of her dietary protein was provided from beans or tofu (rich sources of lysine). To be specific, 23 g of protein from beans and tofu would provide about 1.5 g of lysine, and 22 grams of protein from other sources, such as wheat, rice and nuts, would provide about 0.7 g of lysine. However, if her total protein intake was higher, (e.g., about 63 g/day, close to the median protein intake of women reported in the CSFII survey [Appendix Table E-16]), she could meet her RDA for lysine with much smaller amounts of beans and tofu.

INTEGRATED EXAMPLE

The preceding discussion illustrates that there are many considerations involved in dietary assessment and planning for energy and macronutrients. The example that follows illustrates how these considerations might be addressed in planning the macronutrient intake of an individual. Let us assume that the individual is a 35-year-old woman, 1.68 m in height, and weighing 69 kg. Her job is not physically active, and she does little planned exercise, so it might appear that activity level would be classified as sedentary. However, to provide a more reliable indication of her activity level, she keeps a 7-day record of her activities using a chart similar to that provided in Chapter 12 (Table 12-3), and this also confirms that she is sedentary.

Energy

Because recommended intakes of at least some nutrients relate to energy requirements, the first step would be to estimate her energy expenditure. Her BMI is 24.4, so the equation for normal-weight adults would be used. Assuming it was appropriate to maintain her current weight and activity level, the Estimated Energy Requirement for a woman with her characteristics would be about 2,000 kcal/day. Of course, her individual energy expenditure could be above or below this amount, but it provides a starting point. An additional consideration would be that her current activity level is less than the recommended of "active." If her energy needs were estimated based on being "active," the estimate would be 2,150 kcal, and other values listed below would change proportionally.

Fatty Acids

The AI for n-3 polyunsaturated fatty acid (α-linolenic acid) is 1.1 g/day, and the AI for n-6 polyunsaturated fatty acid (linoleic acid) is 12 g/day. Therefore, her diet should provide these levels of fatty acids, which would provide 9.9 and 108 kcal/day from n-3 and n-6 fatty acids, respectively, toward her total energy intake. Longer-chain polyunsaturated n-3 (approximately 10 percent) and n-6 fatty acids can contribute toward this AI.

Protein

The RDA for protein is 0.8 g/kg/day, so her recommended intake would be 55 g/day (69 kg × 0.8 g/kg), which would provide 220 kcal/day. In addition, she would need to meet recommended intakes of indispensable amino acids, of which lysine is most likely to be limiting. Her recommended lysine intake would be 38 mg/kg/day, or approximately 2.6 g/day.

Carbohydrate and Total Fiber

The RDA for carbohydrate for adult women is 120 g/day, which is equivalent to 480 kcal/day. More than 120 g/day will probably be needed to assure adequate energy consumption within the AMDR for carbohydrate. The AI for *Total Fiber* is 25 g/day and her diet should be planned to provide for this level of intake. The contribution of *Total Fiber* to energy (kcal/g) intake is still unclear.

Energy Distribution

The amount of energy provided by the recommended intakes of essential fatty acids, protein, and carbohydrate totals only 818 kcal/day, yet her estimated requirement is approximately 2,000 kcal/day. Her energy intake might be allocated among macronutrients as shown in Table 13-3 for an overall healthy diet.

Because the estimated energy expenditure of 2,000 kcal/day may differ from actual energy expenditure (and lead to changes in weight that may not be desirable), her weight should be monitored over time and energy intake adjusted as appropriate.

SUMMARY

The Dietary Reference Intakes (DRIs) may be used to assess nutrient intakes as well as to plan nutrient intakes. Box 13-1 summarizes the appropriate uses of the DRIs for individuals and groups.

TABLE 13-3 Example of Macronutrients in a 2,000 kcal Diet

Nutrient	AMDR[a] (%)	Range for 2,000 kcal (g)	Selected Amount (% of energy)	Amount for 2,000 kcal (g)	Energy for 2,000 kcal
Fat	20–35%	44–78	30	67 g	600 kcal
n-3 PUFA[b]	0.6–1.2%	1.3–2.7	0.8	1.8 g	16 kcal
(as part of total fat)					(as part of total fat)
n-6 PUFA	5–10%	11–22	7	16 g	144 kcal
(as part of total fat)					(as part of total fat)
Protein	10–35%	50–175	15	75 g	300 kcal
Carbohydrate	45–65%	225–325	55	275 g	1,100 kcal

[a] AMDR = Acceptable Macronutrient Distribution Range.
[b] PUFA = polyunsaturated fatty acid.

REFERENCES

Bandini LG, Vu D, Must A, Cyr H, Goldberg A, Dietz WH. 1999. Comparison of high-calorie, low-nutrient-dense food consumption among obese and non-obese adolescents. *Obes Res* 7:438–443.

Basiotis PP, Welsh SO, Cronin FJ, Kelsay JL, Mertz W. 1987. Number of days of food intake records required to estimate individual and group nutrient intakes with defined confidence. *J Nutr* 117:1638–1641.

Black AE, Prentice AM, Goldberg GR, Jebb SA, Bingham SA, Livingstone MBE, Coward WA. 1993. Measurements of total energy expenditure provide insights into the validity of dietary measurements of energy intake. *J Am Diet Assoc* 93:572–579.

Blair SN, Kohl HW, Barlow CE. 1993. Physical activity, physical fitness, and all-cause mortality in women: Do women need to be active? *J Am Coll Nutr* 12:368–371.

Blair SN, Kohl HW, Barlow CE, Paffenbarger RS, Gibbons LW, Macera CA. 1995. Changes in physical fitness and all-cause mortality. A prospective study of healthy and unhealthy men. *J Am Med Assoc* 273:1093–1098.

Briefel RR, Sempos CT, McDowell MA, Chien S, Alaimo K. 1997. Dietary methods research in the Third National Health and Nutrition Examination Survey: Underreporting of energy intake. *Am J Clin Nutr* 65:1203S–1209S.

Carroll RJ, Freedman LS, Hartman AM. 1996. Use of semiquantitative food frequency questionnaires to estimate the distribution of usual intake. *Am J Epidemiol* 143:392–404.

Heitmann BL, Lissner L. 1995. Dietary underreporting by obese individuals—Is it specific or non-specific? *Br Med J* 311:986–989.

IOM (Institute of Medicine). 1994. *How Should the Recommended Dietary Allowances Be Revised?* Washington, DC: National Academy Press.

IOM. 2000. *Dietary Reference Intakes: Applications in Dietary Assessment.* Washington, DC: National Academy Press.

BOX 13-1
Uses of Dietary Reference Intakes for Healthy Individuals and Groups

Type of Use	*For the Individual*[a]	*For a Group*[b]
Assessment	**EAR**[c]: Use to examine the probability that usual intake is inadequate.	**EAR:** Use to estimate the prevalence of inadequate intakes within a group.
	RDA: Usual intake at or above this level has a low probability of inadequacy.	**RDA:** Do not use to assess intakes of groups
	AI[d]: Usual intake at or above this level has a low probability of inadequacy.	**AI**[d]: Mean usual intake at this level implies a low prevalence of inadequate intakes.
	UL: Intake above this level has a potential risk of adverse effects.	**UL:** Use to estimate the percentage of the population at potential risk of adverse effects from excess nutrient intake.
Planning	**RDA**[e]: Aim for this intake.	**EAR**[e]: Use to plan an intake distribution with a low prevalence of inadequate intakes.
	AI[d]: Aim for this intake.	
	UL: Use as a guide to limit intake; chronic intake of higher amounts may increase the potential risk of adverse effects.	**AI**[d]: Use to plan mean intakes.
		UL: Use to plan intake distributions with a low prevalence of intakes potentially at risk of adverse effects.

[a] Requires accurate measure of usual intake. Evaluation of true status requires clinical, biochemical, and anthropometric data.

[b] Requires statistically valid approximation of distribution of usual intakes.

[c] Requires information on the variability of day-to-day intake and the variability of the requirement.

[d] For the nutrients in this report, AIs are set for infants for all nutrients, and for other age groups for *Total Fiber* and for *n*-3 and *n*-6 polyunsaturated fatty acids. The AI may be used as a guide for infants as it reflects the average intake from human milk. Infants consuming formulas with the same nutrient composition as human milk consume an adequate amount after adjustments are made for differences in bioavailability. In the context of assessing groups, when the AI for a nutrient is not based on mean intakes of a healthy population, this assessment is made with less confidence.

[e] In the case of energy, an Estimated Energy Requirement (EER) is provided; it is the dietary energy intake that is predicted (with variance) to maintain energy balance in a healthy adult of defined age, gender, weight, height, and level of physical activity, consistent with good health. In children and pregnant and lactating women, the EER is taken to include the needs associated with the deposition of tissues or the secretion of milk at rates consistent with good health. For individuals, the EER represents the midpoint of a range within which an individual's energy requirement is likely to vary. As such, it is below the needs of half the individuals with specified characteristics and exceeds the needs of the other half. Body weight should be monitored and energy intake adjusted accordingly.

NOTE: RDA = Recommended Dietary Allowance, EAR = Estimated Average Requirement, AI = Adequate Intake, UL = Tolerable Upper Intake Level.

IOM. 2001. *Dietary Reference Intakes for Vitamin A, Vitamin K, Arsenic, Boron, Chromium, Copper, Iodine, Iron, Manganese, Molybdenum, Nickel, Silicon, Vanadium, and Zinc.* Washington, DC: National Academy Press.

Johnson RK, Goran MI, Poehlman ET. 1994. Correlates of over- and under-reporting of energy intake in healthy older men and women. *Am J Clin Nutr* 59:1286–1290.

Johnson RK, Soultanakis RP, Matthews DE. 1998. Literacy and body fatness are associated with underreporting of energy intake in US low-income women using the multiple-pass 24-hour recall: A doubly labeled water study. *J Am Diet Assoc* 98:1136–1140.

Kristal AR, Feng Z, Coates RJ, Oberman A, George V. 1997. Associations of race/ethnicity, education, and dietary intervention with the validity and reliability of a food frequency questionnaire: The Women's Health Trial Feasibility Study in Minority Populations. *Am J Epidemiol* 146:856–869.

Lichtman SW, Pisarska K, Berman ER, Pestone M, Dowling H, Offenbacher E, Weisel H, Heshka S, Matthews DE, Heymsfield SB. 1992. Discrepancy between self-reported and actual caloric intake and exercise in obese subjects. *N Engl J Med* 327:1893–1898.

Liu K. 1994. Statistical issues related to semiquantitative food-frequency questionnaires. *Am J Clin Nutr* 59:262S–265S.

Livingstone MB, Prentice AM, Coward WA, Strain JJ, Black AE, Davies PS, Stewart CM, McKenna PG, Whitehead RG. 1992. Validation of estimates of energy intake by weighed dietary record and diet history in children and adolescents. *Am J Clin Nutr* 56:29–35.

Marlett JA, Cheung TF. 1997. Database and quick methods of assessing typical dietary fiber intakes using data for 228 commonly consumed foods. *J Am Diet Assoc* 97:1139–1148.

Mertz W, Tsui JC, Judd JT, Reiser S, Hallfrisch J, Morris ER, Steele PD, Lashley E. 1991. What are people really eating? The relation between energy intake derived from estimated diet records and intake determined to maintain body weight. *Am J Clin Nutr* 54:291–295.

NRC (National Research Council). 1986. *Nutrient Adequacy. Assessment Using Food Consumption Surveys.* Washington, DC: National Academy Press.

Nusser SM, Carriquiry AL, Dodd KW, Fuller WA. 1996. A semiparametric transformation approach to estimating usual daily intake distributions. *J Am Stat Assoc* 91:1440–1449.

Prentice AM, Black AE, Coward WA, Davies HL, Goldberg GR, Murgatroyd PR, Ashford J, Sawyer M, Whitehead RG. 1986. High levels of energy expenditure in obese women. *Br Med J* 292:983–987.

Pryer JA, Vrijheid M, Nichols R, Kiggins M, Elliott P. 1997. Who are the 'low energy reporters' in the dietary and nutritional survey of British adults? *Int J Epidemiol* 26:146–154.

Schoeller DA. 1995. Limitations in the assessment of dietary energy by self-report. *Metabolism* 44:18–22.

Schoeller DA, Bandini LG, Dietz WH. 1990. Inaccuracies in self-reported intake identified by comparison with the doubly labelled water method. *Can J Physiol Pharmacol* 68:941–949.

USDA (U.S. Department of Agriculture). 2001. *USDA Nutrient Database for Standard Reference, Release 14.* Online. Nutrient Data Laboratory. Available at http://www.nal.usda.gov/fnic/foodcomp. Accessed April 2, 2002.

USDA/HHS (U.S. Department of Health and Human Services). 2000. *Nutrition and Your Health: Dietary Guidelines for Americans.* Home and Garden Bulletin No. 232. Washington, DC: U.S. Government Printing Office.

14

A Research Agenda

The Panel on Macronutrients and the Standing Committee on the Scientific Evaluation of Dietary Reference Intakes were charged with developing a research agenda to provide a basis for public-policy decisions related to recommended intakes of energy, fat, carbohydrate, and protein. This chapter describes the approach used to develop the research agenda, briefly summarizes gaps in knowledge, and presents a prioritized research agenda. Sections at the end of Chapters 5 through 10 and Chapter 12 presented prioritized lists of research topics.

APPROACH

The following approach resulted in the research agenda identified in this chapter.

1. Identify gaps in knowledge to understand the role of macronutrients in human health, functional and biochemical indicators to assess macronutrient requirements, methodological problems related to the assessment of intake of these macronutrients and to the assessment of adequacy of intake, relationships of nutrient intake to chronic disease, and adverse effects of macronutrients.

2. Examine data to identify major discrepancies between intake and recommended intakes and consider possible reasons for such discrepancies.

3. Consider the need to protect individuals with extreme or distinct vulnerabilities due to genetic predisposition or disease conditions.

4. Weigh the alternatives and set priorities based on expert judgment.

968

MAJOR KNOWLEDGE GAPS

Requirements

To derive an Estimated Average Requirement (EAR), the criterion must be known for a particular status indicator or combination of indicators that is consistent with impaired status as defined by some clinical consequence. For some of the macronutrients considered in this report, such as *n*-6 and *n*-3 polyunsaturated fatty acids, there is a dearth of information on the biochemical values that reflect abnormal function. A priority should be to determine if there is a correlation between existing status indicators and clinical endpoints in the same subjects. For some macronutrients, such as indispensable amino acids, more data are needed using clinical endpoints or intermediate endpoints of impaired function to determine their requirements in regard to long-term health. For determining energy requirements, more information is needed on the form, frequency, intensity, and duration of exercise that is consistent with a healthy body weight for all age groups. The number of doubly labeled water studies for the determination of total energy expenditure in certain life stage and gender categories is limited and should be expanded.

For many of the essential macronutrients, useful data are seriously lacking for setting requirements for infants, children, adolescents, pregnant and lactating women, and the elderly. As an example, more information is needed on the role of *n*-3 polyunsaturated fatty acids in the neurodevelopment of term infants. Studies should use graded levels of nutrient intake and a combination of response indexes, and they should consider other points raised above. For some of the macronutrients, studies should examine whether the requirement varies substantially by trimester of pregnancy. Data are lacking about gender issues with respect to metabolism and requirements of macronutrients.

Methodology

For some macronutrients, serious limitations exist in the methods available to analyze laboratory values indicative of energy balance and macronutrient status. For instance, biological markers of risk of excess weight gain in children and young adults are needed, as are the standardization and validation of indicators in relation to functional outcome. As an example, to better understand the relationship between fiber and colon cancer, there needs to be increased validation of intermediate markers such as polyp recurrence and the assessment of functional markers (e.g., fecal bulk) of fiber intake. These methodological limitations have slowed progress in conducting or interpreting studies of energy and macronutrient requirements.

Potential sources of error in self-reported intake data include under-reporting of portion sizes and frequency of intake, omission of foods, and inaccuracies related to the use of food composition tables. It is not possible to adjust intakes based on underreporting, and much work is needed to develop an acceptable method to do so. Reliable methods to track dietary energy intakes of populations need to be developed. Furthermore, expansion and revision of food composition tables are needed to allow for further understanding of the relationship between macronutrient intake and health. As an example, a comprehensive database for the *trans* fatty acid content and glycemic index of foods consumed in North America is needed.

Relationships of Intake to Chronic Disease

There are major gaps in knowledge linking the intake of some macro-nutrients and the prevention and retardation of certain chronic diseases common in North America. Because the relationship between macronutrient intake and risk of chronic disease is a trend, it is difficult to ascertain the optimal range of intake for each macronutrient. Long-term, multi-dose clinical trials are needed to ascertain, for instance, the optimal range of total, saturated, and unsaturated fatty acids intake to best prevent chronic diseases such as coronary heart disease, obesity, cancer, and diabetes. Dose–response studies are also needed to determine the intake level of fiber to promote optimum laxation. To resolve whether or not fiber is protective against colon cancer in individuals or a subset of individuals, genotyping and phenotyping of individuals in fiber/colon cancer trials is needed. Long-term clinical trials are needed to further understand the role of glycemic index in the prevention of chronic disease.

Adverse Effects

There is a body of evidence to suggest that high intakes of total fat, saturated fatty acids, *trans* fatty acids, and cholesterol increase the risk of adverse health effects (e.g., elevated low-density lipoprotein [LDL] choles-terol concentration); however, a Tolerable Upper Intake Level could not be established for any of the fats or cholesterol because of the linear trend that often exists between intake and degree of adverse effect. Therefore, more clinical research is needed to ascertain clearly defined intake levels at which significant risk can occur for adverse health effects. In addition, further information is needed on the various factors that contribute to the wide inter-individual variation in LDL cholesterol response to dietary cholesterol. There is some animal data to suggest that high intakes of *n*-6 polyunsaturated fatty acids can increase the risk of certain types of cancer.

This information is lacking in humans and is much needed. Research is needed to identify intake levels at which adverse effects begin to occur with the chronic consumption of high levels of protein and of the long-chain *n*-3 polyunsaturated fatty acids: eicosapentaenoic acid and docosahexaenoic acid.

THE RESEARCH AGENDA

Four major types of information gaps were noted: (1) a lack of data designed specifically to estimate average requirements in presumably healthy humans, (2) a lack of data on the nutrient needs of infants, children, adolescents, the elderly, and pregnant women, (3) a lack of multi-dose, long-term studies to determine the role of macronutrients in reducing the risk of certain chronic diseases, and (4) a lack of studies designed to detect adverse effects of chronic high intakes of these nutrients.

Highest priority is given to research that has the potential to prevent or retard human disease processes and to prevent deficiencies with functional consequences. The following five areas for research were assigned the highest priority (other research recommendations are found at the ends of Chapters 5 through 10 and Chapter 12):

- Dose–response studies to help identify the requirements of macronutrients that are essential in the diet (e.g., indispensable amino acids and *n*-6 and *n*-3 polyunsaturated fatty acids) for all life-stage and gender groups. It is recognized that it is not possible to identify a defined intake level of fat for optimal health; however, it is recognized that further information is needed to identify acceptable ranges of intake for fat, as well as for protein and carbohydrate based on prevention of chronic disease and optimal nutrition;
- Studies to further understand the beneficial roles of *Dietary* and *Functional Fibers* in human health;
- Information on the form, frequency, intensity, and duration of exercise that is successful in managing body weight in children and adults;
- Long-term studies on the role of glycemic index in preventing chronic diseases, such as diabetes and coronary heart disease, in healthy individuals, and;
- Studies to investigate the levels at which adverse effects occur with chronic high intakes of carbohydrate, fiber, fat, and protein. For nutrients such as saturated fatty acids, *trans* fatty acids, and cholesterol, biochemical indicators of adverse effects can occur at very low intakes. Thus, more information is needed to ascertain defined levels of intakes at which relevant health risks may occur.

APPENDIXES A THROUGH M

Pages 973-1257 are not printed in this book but are on the CD-ROM attached to the inside back cover.

Biographical Sketches of Panel and Subcommittee Members

TANYA D. AGURS-COLLINS, Ph.D., R.D., is an assistant professor in the Department of Community Health and Family Practice and a nutritional epidemiologist in the Division of Epidemiology and Biostatistics at the Howard University Cancer Center in Washington, D.C. Dr. Agurs-Collins' primary research interests include the role of nutrition in cancer and diabetes, nutrition and aging, and disease prevention in minority populations. She has worked at the D.C. Office on Aging as a nutrition consultant, at the U.S. Department of Agriculture's Human Nutrition Education Division, the American Dietetic Association, and the District of Columbia Department of Human Services' WIC program. Dr. Agurs-Collins was the president of the District of Columbia Metropolitan Area Dietetic Association in 1998–1999. She is a member of the Mayoral-appointed Board of Dietetics and Nutrition of the District of Columbia Government, where she developed licensing rules, regulations, and the state nutrition examination. Dr. Agurs-Collins was the 1999–2000 recipient of the American Association for Cancer Research, Historically Black Colleges and Universities Faculty Award in Cancer Research and the 1999–2000 Outstanding Dietitian of the Year Award, District of Columbia Metropolitan Area Dietetic Association. She earned her Ph.D. in nutrition from the Pennsylvania State University.

G. HARVEY ANDERSON, Ph.D., is a professor of nutritional sciences, physiology, and medical sciences at the University of Toronto. At the University, he is also codirector of the Program in Food Safety, Nutritional and Regulatory Affairs. His research centers on food selection and intake regulation, diet and behavior, metabolism and pharmacologic effects of amino acids, infant nutrition, and dietary patterns and chronic disease. Dr. Anderson received his Ph.D. in nutritional sciences from the University of Illinois.

SUSAN I. BARR, Ph.D., is a professor of nutrition at the University of British Columbia. Her research interests focus on the associations among nutrition, physical activity, and bone health in women and she has authored over 75 publications. Dr. Barr served as vice president of the Canadian Dietetic Association (now Dietitians of Canada) and is a fellow of both the Dietitians of Canada and the American College of Sports Medicine. She is currently a member of the Scientific Advisory Board of the Osteoporosis Society of Canada and the Medical Advisory Board of the Milk Processors Education Program. Dr. Barr received a Ph.D. in human nutrition from the University of Minnesota and is a registered dietitian in Canada.

GEORGE C. BECKING, Ph.D., is an associate with Phoenix OHC, Inc. in Kingston, Canada, specializing in toxicology and risk assessment related to human health effects of chemicals. Previously, he was a scientist with the World Health Organization (WHO), working in the International Programme on Chemical Safety, where his responsibilities included the evaluation of human health risks from metals including copper and zinc. He also was a research scientist and scientific manager at Health Canada, where he worked in the areas of biochemistry, pharmacology, nutrition toxicology, and toxicology of food-borne and environmental contaminants. He has published over 60 papers and book chapters in the fields of biochemistry, toxicology, and risk assessment methodology. Dr. Becking earned his Ph.D. in biochemistry from Queen's University in Kingston, Ontario.

GEORGE A. BROOKS, Ph.D., is a professor of integrative biology at the University of California at Berkeley and specializes in the areas of exercise physiology and metabolism. His research is intended to elaborate the pathways and controls of lactic acid formation and removal during and after exercise and to study the integration of carbohydrates, lipids, and amino and fatty acids into the carbon flux sustaining exercise. To study these problems in detail, isotope tracer, biochemical, and molecular techniques have been developed and are used extensively. Additionally, the effects of acute and chronic bouts of exercise, gender, hypoxia, and perturbations in oxygen transport on energy fluxes and associated cellular organelles, membranes, and enzyme systems are under investigation. Dr. Brooks is responsible for articulating the "Crossover Concept" describing the balance of carbohydrate and lipid used during physical exercise, as well as for discovery of the "Cell-Cell" and "Intracellular Lactate Shuttles" that describe the pivotal role of lactate in intermediary metabolism.

NANCY F. BUTTE, Ph.D., M.P.H., is a professor of pediatrics at the U.S. Department of Agriculture/Agricultural Research Center Children's Nutrition Research Center, Department of Pediatrics, Baylor College of Medicine, Houston, Texas. Her memberships include the American Society of Clinical Nutrition (Budgetary Committee, 1998–present), the International Society for Research on Human Milk and Lactation (Executive Committee, 1996–present and Secretary/Treasurer, 1990–1992), the Society for International Nutrition Research (Executive Committee, 1996–present), and the International Dietary Energy Consultancy Group Steering Committee (1994–present). Her areas of expertise are energy requirements of infants, children, and women during pregnancy and lactation. Dr. Butte received her Ph.D. in nutrition and her M.P.H. in public health nutrition at the University of California at Berkeley.

BENJAMIN CABALLERO, M.D., Ph.D., is a professor and director of the Center for Human Nutrition and Division of Human Nutrition, Department of International Health, Johns Hopkins Bloomberg School of Public Health, and a professor of pediatrics at the Johns Hopkins School of Medicine. He is currently president of the Society for International Nutrition Research and a member of the American Society of Nutritional Sciences, the American Society for Clinical Nutrition, the North American Society for the Study of Obesity, and the North American Society of Pediatric Gastroenterology and Nutrition. He is a member of the editorial board of the *American Journal of Clinical Nutrition* and the editor of the *Encyclopedia of Human Nutrition*. Dr. Caballero's expertise is childhood obesity and amino acid and protein metabolism. He received his M.D. from the University of Buenos Aires, Argentina, and his Ph.D. (in neuroendocrine regulation and metabolism) from the Massachusetts Institute of Technology.

ALICIA L. CARRIQUIRY, Ph.D., is an associate professor in the Department of Statistics at Iowa State University. Since 1990, Dr. Carriquiry has been a consultant for the U.S. Department of Agriculture (USDA) Human Nutrition Information Service. She has also consulted to the U.S. Environmental Protection Agency and the National Pork Producers Council and is an affiliate for the Law and Economics Consulting Group. At present, Dr. Carriquiry is investigating the statistical issues associated with the Third National Health and Nutrition Examination Survey (NHANES III) and she has recently completed reports on improving USDA's food intake surveys and methods to estimate adjusted intake, and biochemical measurement distributions for NHANES III. Dr. Carriquiry is the current president of the International Society for Bayesian Analysis and is an elected member of the International Statistical Institute. She is editor of *Statistical Science* and serves on the Executive Committee of the Board of Directors of the National Institute of Statistical Science and of the Institute of Mathematical Statistics. She was elected fellow of the American Statistical Association in 1999. Dr. Carriquiry's research interests include nutrition and dietary assessment, Bayesian methods and applications, mixed models and variance component estimation, environmental statistics, stochastic volatility, and linear and nonlinear filtering. She received her Ph.D. in statistics and animal science from Iowa State.

ANN M. COULSTON, M.S., R.D., F.A.D.A., is an established expert in clinical nutrition and research. Currently, she is a partner at Hattner-Coulston Nutrition Associates, LLC, where she serves as a nutrition consultant to public relation firms and the food and nutrition industry. She is also a nutrition consultant at Stanford University School of Medicine. She is a past president of the American Dietetic Association and of the California Dietetic Association. She has more than a 20-year history of clinical research at Stanford University where her research centered on the nutritional needs of adults and the elderly. Her special research interest is in the nutritional management of diabetes and dyslipidemias, particularly in the role of dietary carbohydrates. Ms. Coulston has been recognized by the American Dietetic Association (ADA) Foundation for Excellence in the practice of clinical nutrition and research and has also received the ADA's Medallion Award for leadership and the Distinguished Service and Outstanding Member Award of the California Dietetic Association.

BARBARA L. DEVANEY, Ph.D., is an economist and senior fellow at Mathematica Policy Research in Princeton, New Jersey. Her substantive expertise is in the areas of food assistance and nutrition policy and child health policy and programs. She has conducted several studies of the school nutrition programs, the Food Stamp Program, and the Special Supplemental Nutrition program for Women, Infants and Children. Dr. Devaney also serves on the advisory board for the Maternal and Child Health Nutrition Leadership Training Program and was a visiting professor at the University of California at Los Angeles, where she taught classes on food and nutrition assistance policy.

GEORGE C. FAHEY JR., Ph.D., is a professor of animal sciences and nutritional sciences at the University of Illinois and assistant dean in the Office of Research, Agricultural Experiment Station. Dr. Fahey earned his Ph.D. at West Virginia University. His current research interests are the effects of different fiber sources on nutrient digestibility, and gastrointestinal tract health in humans and companion animals.

ELAINE FAUSTMAN, Ph.D., is a professor of environmental health, toxicology program director at the Institute for Risk Analysis and Risk Communication, and director of the Center for Child Environmental Health Risks at the University of Washington. The long-range objective of Dr. Faustman's research is to identify biochemical mechanisms of developmental toxicity and to develop new methods for the evaluation of health risks from environmental agents. Her research in risk assessment includes an effort to combine results derived from laboratory experiments to develop mechanistically-based toxikinetic and toxicodynamic models of developmental toxicity. Dr. Faustman received her Ph.D. in toxicology and pharmacology from Michigan State University.

JEAN-PIERRE FLATT, Ph.D., is a professor emeritus in the Department of Biochemistry and Molecular Biology at the University of Massachusetts Medical Center. His research expertise relates to the regulation of energy and macronutrient balances, and on the roles of dietary fat, carbohydrate balance, and exercise on body weight regulation and obesity. Dr. Flatt serves on the Nestlé Foundation for the Study of Nutritional Problems in the World. He earned his Ph.D. at the University of Lausanne, Switzerland, and his postdoctoral training was at Harvard Medical School.

SUSAN K. FRIED, Ph.D., is a professor in the Department of Nutritional Sciences at Rutgers University. Dr. Fried joined the faculty at Rockefeller University as an assistant professor in the Laboratory of Human Metabolism and Behavior in 1986, before moving to Rutgers in 1990. She has been the director of the Graduate Program in Nutritional Sciences at Rutgers since 1996. Dr. Fried's research concerns the regulation of adipose tissue metabolism, with a focus on the mechanisms underlying depot differences in human adipocyte metabolism. Her research program utilizes in vitro and in vivo methods to undercover the nutritional and hormonal mechanisms regulating the production of leptin and other cytokines by human adipose tissue from lean and obese subjects. Dr. Fried currently serves on the editorial boards of the *Journal of Nutrition, Obesity Research,* and the *Biochemical Journal.* She has served on a number of national scientific advisory panels and is currently a member of the Nutrition Study Section of the National Institutes of Health. Dr. Fried is a member of the American Society for Nutritional Sciences, the American Society for Clinical Nutrition, the American Physiological Society, and the North American Association for the Study of Obesity. She earned an A.B. in biology at Barnard College and a Ph.D. in nutritional biochemistry at Columbia University. She was a post-doctoral fellow in endocrinology and metabolism at Emory University and in lipid biochemistry at the Medical College of Pennsylvania.

PETER J. GARLICK, Ph.D., is a professor in the Department of Surgery and director of the Core Laboratory of the General Clinical Research Center at the State University of New York at Stony Brook. He served 13 years in the Department of Nutrition of the London School of Hygiene and Tropical Medicine, followed by 10 years at the Rowett Research Institute in Aberdeen, Scotland. His research has concentrated on the nutritional control of protein and amino acid metabolism in health and disease, especially on studies in humans employing stable isotope tracers, leading to 140 original scientific articles. Dr. Garlick is a foreign adjunct professor of the Karolinska Institute, Sweden, and has served on several editorial boards. He earned his Ph.D. at London University, England.

SCOTT M. GRUNDY, M.D., Ph.D., is director of the Center for Human Nutrition and chairman of the Department of Clinical Nutrition at the University of Texas Southwestern Medical Center at Dallas. Dr. Grundy's major research area is in cholesterol and lipoprotein metabolism. He has published over 200 original papers as well as numerous solicited articles and book chapters. Dr. Grundy served as editor-in-chief of the *Journal of Lipid Research* for five years and is on the editorial boards of the *American Journal of Physiology: Endocrinology and Metabolism, Arteriosclerosis,* and *Circulation.* He serves on numerous national and international committees and serves as chairman of the Cholesterol Education Program Adult Treatment Panel II for the National Institutes of Health. Dr. Grundy's numerous awards and honors include The Award of Merit from the American Heart Association, an honorary degree in medicine from the University of Helsinki, Finland, the Roger J. Williams Award in preventive nutrition, and the Bristol Myers Squibb/Mead Johnson Award for Distinguished Achievement in Nutrition Research. He was elected to the Institute of Medicine in 1995. Dr. Grundy received his M.D. from Baylor University Medical School and his Ph.D. from Rockefeller University.

SUZANNE HENDRICH, Ph.D., is a professor of food science and human nutrition and associate dean in the College of Family and Consumer Sciences at Iowa State University. Her research is focused on the bioavailability and health effects of soy isoflavones and other naturally occurring, potentially health-protective food components and foodborne toxicants, such as fumonisins. Dr. Hendrich received her Ph.D. in nutrition from the University of California at Berkeley and was a postdoctoral trainee at the University of Wisconsin before moving to Iowa State.

JANET HUNT, Ph.D., R.D., is a research nutritionist and scientist at the U.S. Department of Agriculture/Agricultural Research Service (USDA/ARS)

Human Nutrition Research Center in Grand Forks, ND, and an adjunct professor of nutrition and dietetics at the University of North Dakota. Her responsibilities at USDA/ARS include leading a Mineral Utilization Research Management Unit, conducting research on human trace elements requirements and bioavailability, and overseeing dietary and whole body counting services to support human nutrition research. Dr. Hunt has extensively published on the topics of zinc absorption and iron status. She serves on the editorial board for the *Journal of the American Dietetic Association* and authored the association's Position Statement on Vitamin and Mineral Supplements. She is also a member of the American Society for Clinical Nutrition and the American Society for Nutritional Sciences. She received her Ph.D. in nutrition from the University of Minnesota.

SHEILA M. INNIS, Ph.D., is a professor in the Department of Pediatrics at the University of British Columbia. Memberships include the Canadian Society for Nutritional Sciences and the Canadian Federation of Biological Societies (counsellor, 1983–1986; regional correspondent for British Columbia, 1982–1987; vice-president, 1987–1988; president, 1988–1989), the International Society for the Study of Fatty Acids and Lipids (Scientific Advisory Committee), the American Institute of Nutrition, and the American Pediatric Society. Her awards include the University of British Columbia Postdoctoral Research Prize, American Institute of Nutrition Travel Award, Borden Award, and Faculty of Medicine Distinguished Medical Lecturer. Dr. Innis' research expertise is n-3 and n-6 fatty acid transport and formula fat composition.

DAVID J.A. JENKINS, M.D., Ph.D., D.Sc., is a Canada Research Chair in Nutritional Metabolism and a professor in both the Departments of Medicine and of Nutritional Sciences, Faculty of Medicine, University of Toronto; a staff physician in the Division of Endocrinology and Metabolism; and director of the Clinical Nutrition and Risk Factor Modification Center at St. Michael's Hospital. Dr. Jenkins has served on committees in Canada and the United States that have formulated nutritional guidelines for the treatment of diabetes. Awards include the Borden Award of the Canadian Society of Nutritional Sciences, the Goldsmith Award for Clinical Research of the American College of Nutrition, the Vahouny Medal for distinction in research in dietary fiber, and the McHenry Award of the Canadian Society of Nutritional Sciences. His research area is the use of diet in the prevention and treatment of hyperlipidemia and diabetes. He was educated at Oxford University, where he obtained his M.D. and Ph.D.

RACHEL K. JOHNSON, Ph.D., M.P.H., R.D., is Acting Dean of the College of Agriculture and Life Sciences, Professor of Nutrition, and a University

Scholar at the University of Vermont. Memberships include the Dietary Guidelines Scientific Advisory Committee (1998–2000), the U.S. Food and Drug Administration Food Advisory Committee/Additives and Ingredients Subcommittee (2001-present), American Dietetic Association Board of Directors (2002-2004), and the American Society for Nutritional Sciences. Dr. Johnson testified before the United States Senate Agriculture, Nutrition, and Forestry Committee Hearing on Senate Bill S.1614, "The Better Nutrition and Health for Children Act of 1993." Dr. Johnson's research expertise is national nutrition policy, pediatric nutrition, dietary intake methodology, and energy metabolism. She has published numerous scholarly papers on these and other topics. Dr. Johnson earned a Ph.D. in nutrition from the Pennsylvania State University and an M.P.H. from the University of Hawaii. She completed a dietetic internship at the Indiana University Medical Center.

RONALD M. KRAUSS, M.D., is Senior Scientist in the Life Sciences Division of Lawrence Berkeley National Laboratory, and Adjunct Professor in the Department of Nutritional Sciences, University of California at Berkeley. He received his undergraduate and medical degrees from Harvard University with honors and served his internship and residency on the Harvard Medical Service of Boston City Hospital. He then joined the staff of the National Heart, Lung and Blood Institute in Bethesda, Maryland, first as a Clinical Associate and then as a Senior Investigator in the Molecular Disease Branch. Dr. Krauss is board-certified in internal medicine, endocrinology and metabolism, and is a member of the American Society for Clinical Investigation, the American Federation for Clinical Research, and the American Society of Clinical Nutrition. He has received a number of awards including the American Heart Association Scientific Councils Distinguished Achievement Award. Dr. Krauss has been a Senior Advisor to the National Cholesterol Education Program, and is actively involved with the American Heart Association (AHA), having served as Chairman of the Nutrition Committee. He is founder and Chair of the AHA Council on Nutrition, Physical Activity, and Metabolism. His research involves studies on genetic, dietary, and hormonal effects on plasma lipoproteins and coronary disease risk.

PENNY KRIS-ETHERTON, Ph.D., R.D., is a distinguished professor of nutrition in the Department of Nutrition and ADA Plan V Program Director at Pennsylvania State University. Memberships include the American Dietetic Association (ADA representative to WOMENHEART and to the American Heart Association Nutrition Committee), the American Society for Nutritional Sciences, the American Society of Clinical Nutrition, and the Society for Nutrition Education. She is a recipient of the Lederle Award for Human Nutrition Research of the American Society for Nutritional Sciences and ADA's Foundation Award for Excellence in Research. Dr. Kris-Etherton's expertise is in the areas of diet and coronary heart disease risk factors, nutritional regulation of lipoprotein, and cholesterol metabolism. She earned her Ph.D. at the University of Minnesota.

ALICE H. LICHTENSTEIN, D.Sc., is a senior scientist and director of the Cardiovascular Nutrition Research Laboratory at the Jean Mayer U.S. Department of Agriculture Human Nutrition Research Center on Aging at Tufts University and the Stanley N. Gershoff professor of nutrition science and policy at the Gerald J. & Dorothy R. Friedman School of Nutrition Science & Policy at Tufts University. Dr. Lichtenstein earned her D.Sc. at Harvard University and received her postdoctoral training at the Cardiovascular Institute at Boston University School of Medicine. Dr. Lichtenstein has served on many committees of the American Society of Nutritional Sciences and the American Heart Association, where she currently serves as vice-chair of the Nutrition Committee. She is on the editorial boards of *Atherosclerosis* and *Journal of Lipid Research* and on the editorial advisory boards of *Nutrition in Clinical Care* and the *Tufts University Health & Nutrition*. She recently served on the 2000 Dietary Guidelines Advisory Committee. Her research interesting include the areas of plasma lipoprotein response to dietary modification with respect to fatty acids, protein, phytoestrogens, and plant sterols, and the effect of diet on lipoprotein kinetic behavior. She is specifically interested in the response of older, moderately hypercholesterolemic individual to dietary modification with the intent to decrease risk of developing cardiovascular disease.

JOANNE R. LUPTON, Ph.D., is a regent's professor and holds the William W. Allen Endowed Chair in Human Nutrition at Texas A&M University. Dr. Lupton has served on the Nutrition Study Section at the National Institutes of Health and is associate editor of the *Journal of Nutrition* and *Nutrition and Cancer*. She has won several teaching awards, including the U.S. Department of Agriculture (Southern Region) award, and was the recipient of the Vice Chancellor's Award for Research at Texas A&M. Dr. Lupton is also the Associate Program Leader for Nutrition and Exercise Physiology for the National Space Biomedical Research Institute. Her expertise is the effect of dietary fibers on colonic lumenal contents, colonic cell proliferation, signal transduction, and colon carcinogenesis.

JUDITH MARLETT, Ph.D., R.D., is a professor in the College of Agricultural and Life Sciences, University of Wisconsin, Madison. Her principal research interests are the role of dietary fiber in human nutrition and in the human gastrointestinal tract and nutrient bioavailability.

SANDFORD A. MILLER, Ph.D., is a senior fellow at the Center for Food and Nutrition Policy, Virginia Polytechnic Institute and State University. He previously was the dean of the Graduate School of Biomedical Sciences and a professor in the Departments of Biochemistry and Medicine at The University of Texas Health Sciences Center at San Antonio. He is the former director of the Center for Food Safety and Applied Nutrition at the Food and Drug Administration. Prior to that, he was a professor of nutritional biochemistry at the Massachusetts Institute of Technology. Dr. Miller has served on many national and international government and professional society advisory committees, including the Federation of American Societies for Experimental Biology Expert Committee on GRAS Substances, the National Advisory Environmental Health Sciences Council of the National Institutes of Health, the Joint World Health Organization/Food and Agriculture Organization (WHO/FAO) Expert Advisory Panel on Food Safety (chairman), and the steering committees of several WHO/FAO panels. He also served as chair of the Joint FAO/WHO Expert Consultation on the Application of Risk Analysis to Food Standards Issues. He is author or coauthor of more than 200 original scientific publications. Dr. Miller received his B.S. in chemistry from the City College of New York and his M.S. and Ph.D. from Rutgers University in physiology and biochemistry.

IAN C. MUNRO, Ph.D., is a leading authority on toxicology and has over 30 years of experience in dealing with complex regulatory issues related to product safety. He has in excess of 150 scientific publications in the fields of toxicology and risk assessment. Dr. Munro formerly held senior positions at Health and Welfare Canada as director of the Bureau of Chemical Safety and director general of the Food Directorate, Health Protection Branch. He was responsible for research and standard setting activities related to microbial and chemical hazards in food and the nutritional quality of the Canadian food supply. He has contributed significantly to the development of risk assessment procedures in the field of public health, both nationally and internationally, through membership on various committees dealing with the regulatory aspects of risk assessment and risk management of public health hazards. Dr. Munro is a fellow of the Royal College of Pathologists, London. He is a graduate of McGill University in biochemistry and nutrition and holds a Ph.D. from Queen's University in pharmacology and toxicology.

SUZANNE MURPHY, Ph.D., R.D., is a researcher at the Cancer Research Center of Hawaii at the University of Hawaii, Honolulu. Previously, she was an adjunct associate professor in the Department of Nutritional Sciences at the University of California at Berkeley and director of the

California Expanded Food and Nutrition Program at the University of California at Davis. Dr. Murphy's research interests include dietary assessment methodology, development of food composition databases, and nutritional epidemiology. She served as a member of the National Nutrition Monitoring Advisory Council and the 2000 Dietary Guidelines Advisory Committee, and is currently on editorial boards for the *Journal of Food Composition and Analysis* and *Nutrition Today*. Dr. Murphy is a member of numerous professional organizations including the American Dietetic Association, the American Society for Nutritional Sciences, the American Public Health Association, the American Society for Clinical Nutrition, and the Society for Nutrition Education. She has over 50 publications on dietary assessment methodology and has lectured nationally and internationally on this subject. She received her B.S. in mathematics from Temple University and her Ph.D. in nutrition from the University of California at Berkeley.

FRANK Q. NUTTALL, M.D., Ph.D., is a professor of internal medicine at the University of Minnesota School of Medicine and chief of the Metabolism/Endocrine and Nutrition Section of the Veterans Affairs Medical Center in Minneapolis, a position he has held since 1970. Dr. Nuttall is a member of the American Diabetes Association, the Endocrine Society, and the American Society of Biological Chemists and is a fellow of the American College of Physicians and the American College of Nutrition. His research interests include diabetes mellitus, control of glycogen metabolism, and glycogen synthase and phosphorylase systems. He received his M.D. from the University of Utah and his Ph.D. in biochemistry from the University of Minnesota.

HARRIS PASTIDES, Ph.D., is dean of the University of South Carolina's School of Public Health and a professor in the Department of Epidemiology and Biostatistics. Previously, he was chair and a professor of the Department of Biostatistics and Epidemiology at the School of Public Health and Health Sciences at the University of Massachusetts at Amherst. Dr. Pastides is a consultant to the World Health Organization's Program in Environmental Health and is a fellow of the American College of Epidemiology. He was a Fulbright Senior Research Fellow and visiting professor at the University of Athens Medical School in Greece from 1987 to 1988. Dr. Pastides has been a principal investigator or coinvestigator on over 30 externally-funded research grants, results of which have been published in numerous peer-reviewed journals. Dr. Pastides earned his M.P.H. and Ph.D. from Yale University.

PAUL PENCHARZ, M.D., is a professor of pediatrics and nutritional sciences at the University of Toronto. Dr. Pencharz is also a senior scientist at the Research Institute Hospital for Sick Children in Toronto as well as a member of the Division of Gastroenterology and Nutrition at the Hospital for Sick Children. He is the recipient of several prestigious awards such as the Borden Award in Nutrition of the Canadian Society for Nutritional Sciences, the Sandoz Award of the Clinical Research Society of Toronto, the Agnes Higgins Award of the March of Dimes, the Osborne Mendel Award of the American Society for Nutrition Sciences, and the Nutrition Award of the American Academy of Pediatrics. Dr. Pencharz has served on the grant review boards for the Medical Research Council, the National Institutes of Health, the U.S. Department of Agriculture, and the Canadian Diabetes Association. His research expertise is protein, amino acid, and energy metabolism in neonates and young adults, especially in patients suffering from cystic fibrosis.

F. XAVIER PI-SUNYER, M.D., M.P.H., is director of the Obesity Research Center and chief of Endocrinology, Diabetes and Nutrition at St. Luke's–Roosevelt Hospital Center, and a professor of medicine at the College of Physicians and Surgeons, Columbia University. His research interests are in the hormonal control of carbohydrate metabolism, diabetes mellitus, obesity, and food intake regulation. Dr. Pi-Sunyer is a past president of the American Diabetes Association, the American Society for Clinical Nutrition, and the North American Association for the Study of Obesity. He has served on the National Institute of Digestive Disorders and Kidney Diseases' Task Force for the Prevention and Treatment of Obesity and has been a member of numerous National Institutes of Health (NIH) study sections and review groups. He was chairman of the National Heart and Lung Institute Task Force that produced the NIH clinical guidelines on *the Identification, Evaluation, and Treatment of Obesity*. Dr. Pi-Sunyer is editor-in-chief of *Obesity Research* and associate editor of the *International Journal of Obesity*. He holds a B.A. in chemistry from Oberlin College, an M.D. from Columbia University College of Physicians and Surgeons, and an M.P.H. from Harvard University.

WILLIAM M. RAND, Ph.D., is a professor (biostatistics) in the Department of Family Medicine and Community Health, Tufts University School of Medicine and also is a professor at the Tufts Schools of Veterinary Medicine and of Dental Medicine. Prior to his appointment at Tufts he was in the Nutrition and Food Science Department at the Massachusetts Institute of Technology (MIT). While at MIT he helped develop, and served as the first director of, INFOODS (International Network of Food Data systems) as well as directing the United Nations University research efforts in the area of protein requirements. He was a member of the 1981 FAO/WHO/UNU Consultation of Energy and Protein Requirements, and is a member of the current FAO/WHO/UNU Consultation on Protein and Amino Acid Requirements. Dr. Rand's general expertise is in statistical modeling and application of statistics to biomedical problems. He received his Ph.D. in biostatistics from the University of California at Los Angeles.

PETER J. REEDS (deceased), Ph.D., was a professor of pediatrics at Baylor College of Medicine and chief of the Nutrient Metabolism Program at the U.S. Department of Agriculture (USDA)/Agricultural Research Service Children's Nutrition Research Center. He was the recipient of several honors and awards and has served on many journal editorial boards. Dr. Reeds served as a permanent member of the Nutrition Study Section, National Institutes of Health and the International Review Panel, United Kingdom Agricultural and Food Research Council. In addition, he served as chairman of the Human Nutrient Requirements for Optimal Health Panel, National Research Initiative, USDA. Dr. Reeds' research expertise was protein metabolism and amino acid requirements, specifically the regulation of growth and protein deposition by diet and other environmental variables such as stress and infection.

ERIC B. RIMM, Sc.D., is an associate professor of epidemiology and nutrition at the Harvard School of Public Health. Dr. Rimm is project director of a National Heart, Lung, and Blood Institute- and National Cancer Institute-funded prospective study of diet and chronic disease among men, as well as the principal investigator of a National Institute on Alcoholism and Alcohol Abuse study. Memberships include the Executive Committee of the Epidemiology and Prevention Council of the American Heart Association and the Society for Epidemiologic Research. He has authored over 150 papers with a main research focus on the associations between diet and other lifestyle characteristics and the risk of obesity, diabetes, and cardiovascular disease.

SUSAN B. ROBERTS, Ph.D., is chief of the Energy Metabolism Laboratory of the Jean Mayer U.S. Department of Agriculture Human Nutrition Research Center on Aging at Tufts University. She is also a professor of nutrition in the School of Nutrition Science and Policy at Tufts and a professor of psychiatry and a scientific staff member in the Department of Pediatrics at Tufts University Medical School. Her research focus is infant and adult obesity, infant nutrient requirements, breastfeeding, and nutrition and aging. She chairs national meetings on dietary prevention of obesity and sits on international committees for evaluation of nutritional requirements. Dr. Roberts has recently published a book that provides dietary guidance for children and serves as an advisor to the Center for

Science in the Public Interest on nutrition-related issues. She received her Ph.D. from the University of Cambridge.

JOSEPH V. RODRICKS, Ph.D., is one of the founding principals of the ENVIRON Corporation, with internationally recognized expertise in assessing the risks to human health of exposure to toxic substances. He is certified as a diplomate of the American Board of Toxicology. Before working as a consultant, he spent fifteen years at the Food and Drug Administration (FDA). In his final three years at FDA, he was Deputy Associate Commissioner for Science, with special responsibility for risk assessment. He has more than 100 scientific publications on food safety and risk assessment and has lectured nationally and internationally on these subjects. Dr. Rodricks is the author of *Calculated Risks*, a nontechnical introduction to toxicology and risk assessment. He received his B.S. from the Massachusetts Institute of Technology and his Ph.D. in biochemistry from the University of Maryland.

JOANNE L. SLAVIN, Ph.D., is a professor in the Department of Food and Nutrition Sciences at University of Minnesota. She earned her B.S., M.S., and Ph.D. in nutrition from the University of Wisconsin-Madison. Her laboratory is actively involved in research on dietary fiber, phytoestrogens from flax and soy, and whole grains. Dr. Slavin has published more than 100 reviewed research articles and has given hundreds of nutrition seminars for professional and lay audiences. She is a science communicator for the Institute of Food Technologists and a member of numerous scientific societies, including the America Dietetic Association, the American Society for Nutritional Sciences, and the American Association for Cancer Research. She is a frequent source for the media on topics ranging from functional foods to sports nutrition. Her research interests are human nutrition, dietary fiber, nutrient bioavailability, sports nutrition, carbohydrate metabolism, and the role of diet in cancer prevention.

JON A. STORY, Ph.D., is a professor of nutritional physiology in the Department of Foods and Nutrition and associate dean of the Graduate School at Purdue University. He has served on the editorial board of the *Journal of Nutrition*, as program manager of the U.S. Department of Agriculture (USDA) Competitive Grants Program in Human Nutrition, as chairman of a FASEB Summer Conference on dietary fiber, and on the USDA Human Nutrition Board of Scientific Counselors. His research interests are dietary fiber and cholesterol and bile acid metabolism.

VALERIE TARASUK, Ph.D., is an associate professor of the Faculty of Medicine at the University of Toronto's Departments of Nutritional Sciences and Public Health Sciences. Her primary research interests are in domestic food insecurity and hunger and dietary assessment. Her specialties within these areas are in social and economic determinates of health and nutrition, population-level indicators of risk, evaluation of public policies in response to food insecurity, and the statistical analysis of dietary intake data at the individual and population levels. Dr. Tarasuk has served on several committees and advisory groups including the Nutrition Expert Advisory Group of the Canadian Community Health Survey, the External Advisory Panel for Food Directorate Review of Policies on the Addition of Vitamins and Minerals to Foods, the Expert Scientific Workshop to Evaluate the Integrated National Food and Nutrition Survey, the Advisory Baseline Study Group for the Canada Prenatal Nutrition Program, and the Nutrition Expert Group for the National Population Health Survey. She chaired the Data Review Panel for the Saskatchewan Nutrition Survey. She earned her Ph.D. in nutritional sciences with minors in epidemiology and biostatistics at the University of Toronto.

JOHN A. THOMAS, Ph.D., is an emeritus professor in the Department of Pharmacology, University of Texas Health Science Center, and served as the Center's vice president from 1988 to 1998. Previously, he was Vice President for Corporate Research at Baxter-International and associate dean of the School of Medicine at West Virginia University. He has held professorships in the departments of pharmacology and toxicology in several medical schools including Iowa, Virginia, and West Virginia. He has authored over 12 textbooks and research monographs and has published over 350 scientific articles in the areas of endocrine pharmacology and reproductive toxicology. He is the recipient of several national awards including the Merit Award from the Society of Toxicology, Certificate of Scientific Services from the U.S. Environmental Protection Agency, and Distinguished Lecturer in Medical Sciences from the American Medical Association. Dr. Thomas serves as a specialty editor for *Toxicology and Applied Pharmacology* and is on the editorial board of *Food and Chemical Toxicology*. He is an elected foreign member of the Russian Academy of Medical Sciences. Dr. Thomas earned his M.A. and Ph.D. from the University of Iowa.

CHRISTINE L. WILLIAMS, M.D., M.P.H., is director of the Children's Cardiovascular Health Center and professor of clinical pediatrics at Columbia University, College of Physicians and Surgeons. She received her M.D. from the University of Pittsburgh, her M.P.H. from Harvard University, and completed residences at the Johns Hopkins University and the Medical College of Pennsylvania. She is the current chair of the American Heart Association's Committee on Atherosclerosis, Hypertension and Obesity in Youth. Dr. Williams is a specialist in child nutrition and preventive cardiology, and her research interests include the effects of fiber consumption in the pediatric population.

GARY M. WILLIAMS, M.D., is a professor of pathology, Department of Pathology, director of Environmental Pathology and Toxicology, and head of the Program on Medicine, Food and Chemical Safety at New York Medical College, Valhalla. He received the *Arnold J. Lehman Award* from the Society of Toxicology in 1982, the Ambassador in Toxicology Award from the Mid-Atlantic Chapter of the Society of Toxicology in 2001, and the Enhancement of Animal Welfare Award from the Society of Toxicology in 2002. Dr. Williams has served on numerous editorial boards and currently is a member of the boards of *Archives of Toxicology, European Journal of Cancer Prevention,* and *Drug and Chemical Toxicology.* He has also served on numerous working groups and committees of the National Research Council, U.S. Environmental Protection Agency, International Agency for Research on Cancer, and World Health Organization. His research focuses in mechanisms of chemical genotoxicity and carcinogenicity. He is author or co-author of over 465 scientific publications. Dr. Williams received his B.A. from Washington and Jefferson College and his M.D. from the University of Pittsburgh School of Medicine and trained as an intern and resident in pathology at Massachusetts General Hospital.

Index

Summary Tables,
Dietary Reference Intakes

Dietary Reference Intakes (DRIs): Recommended Intakes for Individuals, Vitamins
Food and Nutrition Board, Institute of Medicine, National Academies

Life Stage Group	Vitamin A (µg/d)[a]	Vitamin C (mg/d)	Vitamin D (µg/d)[b,c]	Vitamin E (mg/d)[d]	Vitamin K (µg/d)	Thiamin (mg/d)
Infants						
0–6 mo	400*	40*	5*	4*	2.0*	0.2*
7–12 mo	500*	50*	5*	5*	2.5*	0.3*
Children						
1–3 y	**300**	**15**	5*	**6**	30*	**0.5**
4–8 y	**400**	**25**	5*	**7**	55*	**0.6**
Males						
9–13 y	**600**	**45**	5*	**11**	60*	**0.9**
14–18 y	**900**	**75**	5*	**15**	75*	**1.2**
19–30 y	**900**	**90**	5*	**15**	120*	**1.2**
31–50 y	**900**	**90**	5*	**15**	120*	**1.2**
51–70 y	**900**	**90**	10*	**15**	120*	**1.2**
> 70 y	**900**	**90**	15*	**15**	120*	**1.2**
Females						
9–13 y	**600**	**45**	5*	**11**	60*	**0.9**
14–18 y	**700**	**65**	5*	**15**	75*	**1.0**
19–30 y	**700**	**75**	5*	**15**	90*	**1.1**
31–50 y	**700**	**75**	5*	**15**	90*	**1.1**
51–70 y	**700**	**75**	10*	**15**	90*	**1.1**
> 70 y	**700**	**75**	15*	**15**	90*	**1.1**
Pregnancy						
14–18 y	**750**	**80**	5*	**15**	75*	**1.4**
19–30 y	**770**	**85**	5*	**15**	90*	**1.4**
31–50 y	**770**	**85**	5*	**15**	90*	**1.4**
Lactation						
14–18 y	**1,200**	**115**	5*	**19**	75*	**1.4**
19–30 y	**1,300**	**120**	5*	**19**	90*	**1.4**
31–50 y	**1,300**	**120**	5*	**19**	90*	**1.4**

NOTE: This table (taken from the DRI reports, see www.nap.edu) presents Recommended Dietary Allowances (RDAs) in **bold type** and Adequate Intakes (AIs) in ordinary type followed by an asterisk (*). RDAs and AIs may both be used as goals for individual intake. RDAs are set to meet the needs of almost all (97 to 98 percent) individuals in a group. For healthy breastfed infants, the AI is the mean intake. The AI for other life stage and gender groups is believed to cover needs of all individuals in the group, but lack of data or uncertainty in the data prevent being able to specify with confidence the percentage of individuals covered by this intake.

[a] As retinol activity equivalents (RAEs). 1 RAE = 1 µg retinol, 12 µg β-carotene, 24 µg α-carotene, or 24 µg β-cryptoxanthin. The RAE for dietary provitamin A carotenoids is twofold greater than retinol equivalents (RE), whereas the RAE for preformed vitamin A is the same as RE.

[b] As cholecalciferol. 1 µg cholecalciferol = 40 IU vitamin D.

[c] In the absence of adequate exposure to sunlight.

[d] As α-tocopherol. α-Tocopherol includes *RRR*-α-tocopherol, the only form of α-tocopherol that occurs naturally in foods, and the *2R*-stereoisomeric forms of α-tocopherol (*RRR*-, *RSR*-, *RRS*-, and *RSS*-α-tocopherol) that occur in fortified foods and supplements. It does not include the *2S*-stereoisomeric forms of α-tocopherol (*SRR*-, *SSR*-, *SRS*-, and *SSS*-α-tocopherol), also found in fortified foods and supplements.

[e] As niacin equivalents (NE). 1 mg of niacin = 60 mg of tryptophan; 0–6 months = preformed niacin (not NE).

[f] As dietary folate equivalents (DFE). 1 DFE = 1 µg food folate = 0.6 µg of folic acid

Riboflavin (mg/d)	Niacin (mg/d)[e]	Vitamin B_6 (mg/d)	Folate (µg/d)[f]	Vitamin B_{12} (µg/d)	Pantothenic Acid (mg/d)	Biotin (µg/d)	Choline (mg/d)[g]
0.3*	2*	0.1*	65*	0.4*	1.7*	5*	125*
0.4*	4*	0.3*	80*	0.5*	1.8*	6*	150*
0.5	6	0.5	150	0.9	2*	8*	200*
0.6	8	0.6	200	1.2	3*	12*	250*
0.9	12	1.0	300	1.8	4*	20*	375*
1.3	16	1.3	400	2.4	5*	25*	550*
1.3	16	1.3	400	2.4	5*	30*	550*
1.3	16	1.3	400	2.4	5*	30*	550*
1.3	16	1.7	400	2.4[h]	5*	30*	550*
1.3	16	1.7	400	2.4[h]	5*	30*	550*
0.9	12	1.0	300	1.8	4*	20*	375*
1.0	14	1.2	400[i]	2.4	5*	25*	400*
1.1	14	1.3	400[i]	2.4	5*	30*	425*
1.1	14	1.3	400[i]	2.4	5*	30*	425*
1.1	14	1.5	400	2.4[h]	5*	30*	425*
1.1	14	1.5	400	2.4[h]	5*	30*	425*
1.4	18	1.9	600[j]	2.6	6*	30*	450*
1.4	18	1.9	600[j]	2.6	6*	30*	450*
1.4	18	1.9	600[j]	2.6	6*	30*	450*
1.6	17	2.0	500	2.8	7*	35*	550*
1.6	17	2.0	500	2.8	7*	35*	550*
1.6	17	2.0	500	2.8	7*	35*	550*

from fortified food or as a supplement consumed with food = 0.5 µg of a supplement taken on an empty stomach.

g Although AIs have been set for choline, there are few data to assess whether a dietary supply of choline is needed at all stages of the life cycle, and it may be that the choline requirement can be met by endogenous synthesis at some of these stages.

h Because 10 to 30 percent of older people may malabsorb food-bound B_{12}, it is advisable for those older than 50 years to meet their RDA mainly by consuming foods fortified with B_{12} or a supplement containing B_{12}.

i In view of evidence linking folate intake with neural tube defects in the fetus, it is recommended that all women capable of becoming pregnant consume 400 µg from supplements or fortified foods in addition to intake of food folate from a varied diet.

j It is assumed that women will continue consuming 400 µg from supplements or fortified food until their pregnancy is confirmed and they enter prenatal care, which ordinarily occurs after the end of the periconceptional period—the critical time for formation of the neural tube.

SOURCES: *Dietary Reference Intakes for Calcium, Phosphorous, Magnesium, Vitamin D, and Fluoride* (1997); *Dietary Reference Intakes for Thiamin, Riboflavin, Niacin, Vitamin B6, Folate, Vitamin B12, Pantothenic Acid, Biotin, and Choline* (1998); *Dietary Reference Intakes for Vitamin C, Vitamin E, Selenium, and Carotenoids* (2000); *Dietary Reference Intakes for Vitamin A, Vitamin K, Arsenic, Boron, Chromium, Copper, Iodine, Iron, Manganese, Molybdenum, Nickel, Silicon, Vanadium, and Zinc* (2001); *and Dietary Reference Intakes for Water, Potassium, Sodium, Chloride, and Sulfate* (2005). These reports may be accessed via http://www.nap.edu.

Dietary Reference Intakes (DRIs): Recommended Intakes for Individuals, Elements
Food and Nutrition Board, Institute of Medicine, National Academies

Life Stage Group	Calcium (mg/d)	Chromium (µg/d)	Copper (µg/d)	Fluoride (mg/d)	Iodine (µg/d)	Iron (mg/d)	Magnesium (mg/d)
Infants							
0–6 mo	210*	0.2*	200*	0.01*	110*	0.27*	30*
7–12 mo	270*	5.5*	220*	0.5*	130*	11	75*
Children							
1–3 y	500*	11*	340	0.7*	90	7	80
4–8 y	800*	15*	440	1*	90	10	130
Males							
9–13 y	1,300*	25*	700	2*	120	8	240
14–18 y	1,300*	35*	890	3*	150	11	410
19–30 y	1,000*	35*	900	4*	150	8	400
31–50 y	1,000*	35*	900	4*	150	8	420
51–70 y	1,200*	30*	900	4*	150	8	420
> 70 y	1,200*	30*	900	4*	150	8	420
Females							
9–13 y	1,300*	21*	700	2*	120	8	240
14–18 y	1,300*	24*	890	3*	150	15	360
19–30 y	1,000*	25*	900	3*	150	18	310
31–50 y	1,000*	25*	900	3*	150	18	320
51–70 y	1,200*	20*	900	3*	150	8	320
> 70 y	1,200*	20*	900	3*	150	8	320
Pregnancy							
14–18 y	1,300*	29*	1,000	3*	220	27	400
19–30 y	1,000*	30*	1,000	3*	220	27	350
31–50 y	1,000*	30*	1,000	3*	220	27	360
Lactation							
14–18 y	1,300*	44*	1,300	3*	290	10	360
19–30 y	1,000*	45*	1,300	3*	290	9	310
31–50 y	1,000*	45*	1,300	3*	290	9	320

NOTE: This table presents Recommended Dietary Allowances (RDAs) in **bold type** and Adequate Intakes (AIs) in ordinary type followed by an asterisk (*). RDAs and AIs may both be used as goals for individual intake. RDAs are set to meet the needs of almost all (97 to 98 percent) individuals in a group. For healthy breastfed infants, the AI is the mean intake. The AI for other life stage and gender groups is believed to cover needs of all individuals in the group, but lack of data or uncertainty in the data prevent being able to specify with confidence the percentage of individuals covered by this intake.

Manganese (mg/d)	Molybdenum (µg/d)	Phosphorus (mg/d)	Selenium (µg/d)	Zinc (mg/d)	Potassium (g/d)	Sodium (g/d)	Chloride (g/d)
0.003*	2*	100*	15*	2*	0.4*	0.12*	0.18*
0.6*	3*	275*	20*	3	0.7*	0.37*	0.57*
1.2*	17	460	20	3	3.0*	1.0*	1.5*
1.5*	22	500	30	5	3.8*	1.2*	1.9*
1.9*	34	1,250	40	8	4.5*	1.5*	2.3*
2.2*	43	1,250	55	11	4.7*	1.5*	2.3*
2.3*	45	700	55	11	4.7*	1.5*	2.3*
2.3*	45	700	55	11	4.7*	1.5*	2.3*
2.3*	45	700	55	11	4.7*	1.3*	2.0*
2.3*	45	700	55	11	4.7*	1.2*	1.8*
1.6*	34	1,250	40	8	4.5*	1.5*	2.3*
1.6*	43	1,250	55	9	4.7*	1.5*	2.3*
1.8*	45	700	55	8	4.7*	1.5*	2.3*
1.8*	45	700	55	8	4.7*	1.5*	2.3*
1.8*	45	700	55	8	4.7*	1.3*	2.0*
1.8*	45	700	55	8	4.7*	1.2*	1.8*
2.0*	50	1,250	60	12	4.7*	1.5*	2.3*
2.0*	50	700	60	11	4.7*	1.5*	2.3*
2.0*	50	700	60	11	4.7*	1.5*	2.3*
2.6*	50	1,250	70	13	5.1*	1.5*	2.3*
2.6*	50	700	70	12	5.1*	1.5*	2.3*
2.6*	50	700	70	12	5.1*	1.5*	2.3*

SOURCES: *Dietary Reference Intakes for Calcium, Phosphorous, Magnesium, Vitamin D, and Fluoride* (1997); *Dietary Reference Intakes for Thiamin, Riboflavin, Niacin, Vitamin B6, Folate, Vitamin B12, Pantothenic Acid, Biotin, and Choline* (1998); *Dietary Reference Intakes for Vitamin C, Vitamin E, Selenium, and Carotenoids* (2000); *Dietary Reference Intakes for Vitamin A, Vitamin K, Arsenic, Boron, Chromium, Copper, Iodine, Iron, Manganese, Molybdenum, Nickel, Silicon, Vanadium, and Zinc* (2001); and *Dietary Reference Intakes for Water, Potassium, Sodium, Chloride, and Sulfate* (2005). These reports may be accessed via http://www.nap.edu.

Dietary Reference Intakes (DRIs): Recommended Intakes for Individuals, Total Water and Macronutrients

Food and Nutrition Board, Institute of Medicine, National Academies

Life Stage Group	Total Water[a] (L/d)	Carbo-hydrate (g/d)	Total Fiber (g/d)	Fat (g/d)	Linoleic Acid (g/d)	α-Linolenic Acid (g/d)	Protein[b] (g/d)
Infants							
0–6 mo	0.7*	60*	ND	31*	4.4*	0.5*	9.1*
7–12 mo	0.8*	95*	ND	30*	4.6*	0.5*	11.0+
Children							
1–3 y	1.3*	130	19*	ND[c]	7*	0.7*	13
4–8 y	1.7*	130	25*	ND	10*	0.9*	19
Males							
9–13 y	2.4*	130	31*	ND	12*	1.2*	34
14–18 y	3.3*	130	38*	ND	16*	1.6*	52
19–30 y	3.7*	130	38*	ND	17*	1.6*	56
31–50 y	3.7*	130	38*	ND	17*	1.6*	56
51–70 y	3.7*	130	30*	ND	14*	1.6*	56
> 70 y	3.7*	130	30*	ND	14*	1.6*	56
Females							
9–13 y	2.1*	130	26*	ND	10*	1.0*	34
14–18 y	2.3*	130	26*	ND	11*	1.1*	46
19–30 y	2.7*	130	25*	ND	12*	1.1*	46
31–50 y	2.7*	130	25*	ND	12*	1.1*	46
51–70 y	2.7*	130	21*	ND	11*	1.1*	46
> 70 y	2.7*	130	21*	ND	11*	1.1*	46
Pregnancy							
14–18 y	3.0*	175	28*	ND	13*	1.4*	71
19–30 y	3.0*	175	28*	ND	13*	1.4*	71
31–50 y	3.0*	175	28*	ND	13*	1.4*	71
Lactation							
14–18 y	3.8*	210	29*	ND	13*	1.3*	71
19–30 y	3.8*	210	29*	ND	13*	1.3*	71
31–50 y	3.8*	210	29*	ND	13*	1.3*	71

NOTE: This table presents Recommended Dietary Allowances (RDAs) in **bold type** and Adequate Intakes (AIs) in ordinary type followed by an asterisk (*). RDAs and AIs may both be used as goals for individual intake. RDAs are set to meet the needs of almost all (97 to 98 percent) individuals in a group. For healthy breastfed infants, the AI is the mean intake. The AI for other life stage and gender groups is believed to cover the needs of all individuals in the group, but lack of data or uncertainty in the data prevent being able to specify with confidence the percentage of individuals covered by this intake. The plus (+) symbol indicates a change from the prepublication copy due to a calculation error.

[a] Total water includes all water contained in food, beverages, and drinking water.

[b] Based on g protein per kg of body weight for the reference body weight, e.g., for adults 0.8 g/kg body weight for the reference body weight.

[c] Not determined.

SOURCES: *Dietary Reference Intakes for Energy, Carbohydrate, Fiber, Fat, Fatty Acids, Cholesterol, Protein, and Amino Acids* (2002/2005); *Dietary Reference Intakes for Water, Potassium, Sodium, Chloride, and Sulfate* (2005). These reports may be accessed via http://www.nap.edu.

Dietary Reference Intakes (DRIs): Acceptable Macronutrient Distribution Ranges
Food and Nutrition Board, Institute of Medicine, National Academies

	Range (percent of energy)		
Macronutrient	Children, 1–3 y	Children, 4–18 y	Adults
Fat	30–40	25–35	20–35
n-6 Polyunsaturated fatty acids[a] (linoleic acid)	5–10	5–10	5–10
n-3 Polyunsaturated fatty acids[a] (α-linolenic acid)	0.6–1.2	0.6–1.2	0.6–1.2
Carbohydrate	45–65	45–65	45–65
Protein	5–20	10–30	10–35

[a] Approximately 10 percent of the total can come from longer-chain n-3 or n-6 fatty acids.

SOURCE: *Dietary Reference Intakes for Energy, Carbohydrate, Fiber, Fat, Fatty Acids, Cholesterol, Protein, and Amino Acids* (2002/2005).

Dietary Reference Intakes (DRIs): Additional Macronutrient Recommendations
Food and Nutrition Board, Institute of Medicine, National Academies

Macronutrient	Recommendation
Dietary cholesterol	As low as possible while consuming a nutritionally adequate diet
Trans fatty acids	As low as possible while consuming a nutritionally adequate diet
Saturated fatty acids	As low as possible while consuming a nutritionally adequate diet
Added sugars	Limit to no more than 25% of total energy

SOURCE: *Dietary Reference Intakes for Energy, Carbohydrate, Fiber, Fat, Fatty Acids, Cholesterol, Protein, and Amino Acids* (2002/2005).

Dietary Reference Intakes (DRIs): Tolerable Upper Intake Levels (UL[a]), Vitamins
Food and Nutrition Board, Institute of Medicine, National Academies

Life Stage Group	Vitamin A (µg/d)[b]	Vitamin C (mg/d)	Vitamin D (µg/d)	Vitamin E (mg/d)[c,d]	Vitamin K	Thiamin
Infants						
0–6 mo	600	ND[f]	25	ND	ND	ND
7–12 mo	600	ND	25	ND	ND	ND
Children						
1–3 y	600	400	50	200	ND	ND
4–8 y	900	650	50	300	ND	ND
Males, Females						
9–13 y	1,700	1,200	50	600	ND	ND
14–18 y	2,800	1,800	50	800	ND	ND
19–70 y	3,000	2,000	50	1,000	ND	ND
> 70 y	3,000	2,000	50	1,000	ND	ND
Pregnancy						
14–18 y	2,800	1,800	50	800	ND	ND
19–50 y	3,000	2,000	50	1,000	ND	ND
Lactation						
14–18 y	2,800	1,800	50	800	ND	ND
19–50 y	3,000	2,000	50	1,000	ND	ND

[a] UL = The highest level of daily nutrient intake that is likely to pose no risk of adverse health effects to almost all individuals in the general population. Unless otherwise specified, the UL represents total intake from food, water, and supplements. Due to lack of suitable data, ULs could not be established for vitamin K, thiamin, riboflavin, vitamin B_{12}, pantothenic acid, biotin, and carotenoids. In the absence of ULs, extra caution may be warranted in consuming levels above recommended intakes.

[b] As preformed vitamin A only.

[c] As α-tocopherol; applies to any form of supplemental α-tocopherol.

[d] The ULs for vitamin E, niacin, and folate apply to synthetic forms obtained from supplements, fortified foods, or a combination of the two.

[e] β-Carotene supplements are advised only to serve as a provitamin A source for individuals at risk of vitamin A deficiency.

Ribo-flavin	Niacin (mg/d)[d]	Vitamin B_6 (mg/d)	Folate (μg/d)[d]	Vitamin B_{12}	Pantothenic Acid	Biotin	Choline (g/d)	Carote-noids[e]
ND	ND	ND	ND	ND	ND	ND	ND	ND
ND	ND	ND	ND	ND	ND	ND	ND	ND
ND	10	30	300	ND	ND	ND	1.0	ND
ND	15	40	400	ND	ND	ND	1.0	ND
ND	20	60	600	ND	ND	ND	2.0	ND
ND	30	80	800	ND	ND	ND	3.0	ND
ND	35	100	1,000	ND	ND	ND	3.5	ND
ND	35	100	1,000	ND	ND	ND	3.5	ND
ND	30	80	800	ND	ND	ND	3.0	ND
ND	35	100	1,000	ND	ND	ND	3.5	ND
ND	30	80	800	ND	ND	ND	3.0	ND
ND	35	100	1,000	ND	ND	ND	3.5	ND

f ND = Not determinable due to lack of data of adverse effects in this age group and concern with regard to lack of ability to handle excess amounts. Source of intake should be from food only to prevent high levels of intake.

SOURCES: *Dietary Reference Intakes for Calcium, Phosphorous, Magnesium, Vitamin D, and Fluoride* (1997); *Dietary Reference Intakes for Thiamin, Riboflavin, Niacin, Vitamin B_6, Folate, Vitamin B_{12}, Pantothenic Acid, Biotin, and Choline* (1998); *Dietary Reference Intakes for Vitamin C, Vitamin E, Selenium, and Carotenoids* (2000); and *Dietary Reference Intakes for Vitamin A, Vitamin K, Arsenic, Boron, Chromium, Copper, Iodine, Iron, Manganese, Molybdenum, Nickel, Silicon, Vanadium, and Zinc* (2001). These reports may be accessed via http://www.nap.edu.

Dietary Reference Intakes (DRIs): Tolerable Upper Intake Levels (UL[a]), Elements
Food and Nutrition Board, Institute of Medicine, National Academies

Life Stage Group	Arse-nic[b]	Boron (mg/d)	Calci-um (g/d)	Chro-mium	Copper (µg/d)	Fluo-ride (mg/d)	Iodine (µg/d)	Iron (mg/d)	Magne-sium (mg/d)[c]
Infants									
0–6 mo	ND[f]	ND	ND	ND	ND	0.7	ND	40	ND
7–12 mo	ND	ND	ND	ND	ND	0.9	ND	40	ND
Children									
1–3 y	ND	3	2.5	ND	1,000	1.3	200	40	65
4–8 y	ND	6	2.5	ND	3,000	2.2	300	40	110
Males, Females									
9–13 y	ND	11	2.5	ND	5,000	10	600	40	350
14–18 y	ND	17	2.5	ND	8,000	10	900	45	350
19–70 y	ND	20	2.5	ND	10,000	10	1,100	45	350
> 70 y	ND	20	2.5	ND	10,000	10	1,100	45	350
Pregnancy									
14–18 y	ND	17	2.5	ND	8,000	10	900	45	350
19–50 y	ND	20	2.5	ND	10,000	10	1,100	45	350
Lactation									
14–18 y	ND	17	2.5	ND	8,000	10	900	45	350
19–50 y	ND	20	2.5	ND	10,000	10	1,100	45	350

[a] UL = The highest level of daily nutrient intake that is likely to pose no risk of adverse health effects to almost all individuals in the general population. Unless otherwise specified, the UL represents total intake from food, water, and supplements. Due to lack of suitable data, ULs could not be established for arsenic, chromium, silicon, potassium, and sulfate. In the absence of ULs, extra caution may be warranted in consuming levels above recommended intakes.

[b] Although the UL was not determined for arsenic, there is no justification for adding arsenic to food or supplements.

[c] The ULs for magnesium represent intake from a pharmacological agent only and do not include intake from food and water.

[d] Although silicon has not been shown to cause adverse effects in humans, there is no justification for adding silicon to supplements.

[e] Although vanadium in food has not been shown to cause adverse effects in humans,

Manga-nese (mg/d)	Molyb-denum (µg/d)	Nickel (mg/d)	Phos-phorus (g/d)	Potas-sium	Sele-nium (µg/d)	Sili-con[d]	Sul-fate	Vana-dium (mg/d)[e]	Zinc (mg/d)	Sodi-um (g/d)	Chlo-ride (g/d)
ND	ND	ND	ND	ND	45	ND	ND	ND	4	ND	ND
ND	ND	ND	ND	ND	60	ND	ND	ND	5	ND	ND
2	300	0.2	3.0	ND	90	ND	ND	ND	7	1.5	2.3
3	600	0.3	3.0	ND	150	ND	ND	ND	12	1.9	2.9
6	1,100	0.6	4.0	ND	280	ND	ND	ND	23	2.2	3.4
9	1,700	1.0	4.0	ND	400	ND	ND	ND	34	2.3	3.6
11	2,000	1.0	4.0	ND	400	ND	ND	1.8	40	2.3	3.6
11	2,000	1.0	3.0	ND	400	ND	ND	1.8	40	2.3	3.6
9	1,700	1.0	3.5	ND	400	ND	ND	ND	34	2.3	3.6
11	2,000	1.0	3.5	ND	400	ND	ND	ND	40	2.3	3.6
9	1,700	1.0	4.0	ND	400	ND	ND	ND	34	2.3	3.6
11	2,000	1.0	4.0	ND	400	ND	ND	ND	40	2.3	3.6

there is no justification for adding vanadium to food and vanadium supplements should be used with caution. The UL is based on adverse effects in laboratory animals and this data could be used to set a UL for adults but not children and adolescents.

ƒND = Not determinable due to lack of data of adverse effects in this age group and concern with regard to lack of ability to handle excess amounts. Source of intake should be from food only to prevent high levels of intake.

SOURCES: *Dietary Reference Intakes for Calcium, Phosphorous, Magnesium, Vitamin D, and Fluoride* (1997); *Dietary Reference Intakes for Thiamin, Riboflavin, Niacin, Vitamin B6, Folate, Vitamin B12, Pantothenic Acid, Biotin, and Choline* (1998); *Dietary Reference Intakes for Vitamin C, Vitamin E, Selenium, and Carotenoids* (2000); *Dietary Reference Intakes for Vitamin A, Vitamin K, Arsenic, Boron, Chromium, Copper, Iodine, Iron, Manganese, Molybdenum, Nickel, Silicon, Vanadium, and Zinc* (2001); *and Dietary Reference Intakes for Water, Potassium, Sodium, Chloride, and Sulfate* (2005). These reports may be accessed via http://www.nap.edu.

Dietary Reference Intakes (DRIs): Estimated Average Requirements for Groups
Food and Nutrition Board, Institute of Medicine, National Academies

Life Stage Group	CHO (g/d)	Protein (g/kg/d)	Vit A (µg/d)[a]	Vit C (mg/d)	Vit E (mg/d)[b]	Thiamin (mg/d)	Ribo-flavin (mg/d)	Niacin (mg/d)[c]	Vit B$_6$ (mg/d)
Infants									
7–12 mo		1.0							
Children									
1–3 y	100	0.87	210	13	5	0.4	0.4	5	0.4
4–8 y	100	0.76	275	22	6	0.5	0.5	6	0.5
Males									
9–13 y	100	0.76	445	39	9	0.7	0.8	9	0.8
14–18 y	100	0.73	630	63	12	1.0	1.1	12	1.1
19–30 y	100	0.66	625	75	12	1.0	1.1	12	1.1
31–50 y	100	0.66	625	75	12	1.0	1.1	12	1.1
51–70 y	100	0.66	625	75	12	1.0	1.1	12	1.4
> 70 y	100	0.66	625	75	12	1.0	1.1	12	1.4
Females									
9–13 y	100	0.76	420	39	9	0.7	0.8	9	0.8
14–18 y	100	0.71	485	56	12	0.9	0.9	11	1.0
19–30 y	100	0.66	500	60	12	0.9	0.9	11	1.1
31–50 y	100	0.66	500	60	12	0.9	0.9	11	1.1
51–70 y	100	0.66	500	60	12	0.9	0.9	11	1.3
> 70 y	100	0.66	500	60	12	0.9	0.9	11	1.3
Pregnancy									
14–18 y	135	0.88	530	66	12	1.2	1.2	14	1.6
19–30 y	135	0.88	550	70	12	1.2	1.2	14	1.6
31–50 y	135	0.88	550	70	12	1.2	1.2	14	1.6
Lactation									
14–18 y	160	1.05	885	96	16	1.2	1.3	13	1.7
19–30 y	160	1.05	900	100	16	1.2	1.3	13	1.7
31–50 y	160	1.05	900	100	16	1.2	1.3	13	1.7

NOTE: This table presents Estimated Average Requirements (EARs), which serve two purposes: for assessing adequacy of population intakes and as the basis for calculating Recommended Dietary Allowances (RDAs) for individuals. EARs have not been established for vitamin D, vitamin K, pantothenic acid, biotin, choline, calcium, chromium, fluoride, manganese, or other nutrients not yet evaluated via the DRI process.

[a] As retinol activity equivalents (RAEs). 1 RAE = 1 µg retinol, 12 µg β-carotene, 24 µg α-carotene, or 24 µg β-cryptoxanthin. The RAE for dietary provitamin A carotenoids is twofold greater than retinol equivalents (RE), whereas the RAE for preformed vitamin A is the same as RE.

[b] As α-tocopherol. α-Tocopherol includes *RRR*-α-tocopherol, the only form of α-tocopherol that occurs naturally in foods, and the *2R*-stereoisomeric forms of α-tocopherol (*RRR*-, *RSR*-, *RRS*-, and *RSS*-α-tocopherol) that occur in fortified foods and supplements. It does not include the *2S*-stereoisomeric forms of α-tocopherol (*SRR*-, *SSR*-, *SRS*-, and *SSS*-α-tocopherol), also found in fortified foods and supplements.

Folate (µg/d)[a]	Vit B$_{12}$ (µg/d)	Copper (µg/d)	Iodine (µg/d)	Iron (mg/d)	Magnesium (mg/d)	Molybdenum (µg/d)	Phosphorus (mg/d)	Selenium (µg/d)	Zinc (mg/d)
				6.9					2.5
120	0.7	260	65	3.0	65	13	380	17	2.5
160	1.0	340	65	4.1	110	17	405	23	4.0
250	1.5	540	73	5.9	200	26	1,055	35	7.0
330	2.0	685	95	7.7	340	33	1,055	45	8.5
320	2.0	700	95	6	330	34	580	45	9.4
320	2.0	700	95	6	350	34	580	45	9.4
320	2.0	700	95	6	350	34	580	45	9.4
320	2.0	700	95	6	350	34	580	45	9.4
250	1.5	540	73	5.7	200	26	1,055	35	7.0
330	2.0	685	95	7.9	300	33	1,055	45	7.3
320	2.0	700	95	8.1	255	34	580	45	6.8
320	2.0	700	95	8.1	265	34	580	45	6.8
320	2.0	700	95	5	265	34	580	45	6.8
320	2.0	700	95	5	265	34	580	45	6.8
520	2.2	785	160	23	335	40	1,055	49	10.5
520	2.2	800	160	22	290	40	580	49	9.5
520	2.2	800	160	22	300	40	580	49	9.5
450	2.4	985	209	7	300	35	1,055	59	10.9
450	2.4	1,000	209	6.5	255	36	580	59	10.4
450	2.4	1,000	209	6.5	265	36	580	59	10.4

[c] As niacin equivalents (NE). 1 mg of niacin = 60 mg of tryptophan.

[d] As dietary folate equivalents (DFE). 1 DFE = 1 µg food folate = 0.6 µg of folic acid from fortified food or as a supplement consumed with food = 0.5 µg of a supplement taken on an empty stomach.

SOURCES: *Dietary Reference Intakes for Calcium, Phosphorous, Magnesium, Vitamin D, and Fluoride* (1997); *Dietary Reference Intakes for Thiamin, Riboflavin, Niacin, Vitamin B$_6$, Folate, Vitamin B$_{12}$, Pantothenic Acid, Biotin, and Choline* (1998); *Dietary Reference Intakes for Vitamin C, Vitamin E, Selenium, and Carotenoids* (2000); *Dietary Reference Intakes for Vitamin A, Vitamin K, Arsenic, Boron, Chromium, Copper, Iodine, Iron, Manganese, Molybdenum, Nickel, Silicon, Vanadium, and Zinc* (2001), and *Dietary Reference Intakes for Energy, Carbohydrate, Fiber, Fat, Fatty Acids, Cholesterol, Protein, and Amino Acids* (2002/2005). These reports may be accessed via www.nap.edu.

Table 17-1   The Planets

Planet	Symbol	Mean Distance from Sun, Earth = 1 [a]	Diameter, Thousands of km	Mass, Earth = 1 [b]	Mean Density, Water = 1 [c]	Surface Gravity, Earth = 1 [d]	Escape Speed, km/s [e]	Period of Rotation on Axis	Period of Revolution around Sun	Eccentricity of Orbit [h]	Inclination of Orbit to Ecliptic [i]	Known Satellites [j]
Mercury	☿	0.39	4.9	0.055	5.4	0.38	4.3	59 days	88 days	0.21	7°00'	0
Venus	♀	0.72	12.1	0.82	5.25	0.90	10.4	243 days[f]	225 days	0.01	3°34'	0
Earth	⊕	1.00	12.7	1.00	5.52	1.00	11.2	24 h	365 days	0.02	—	1
Mars	♂	1.52	6.8	0.11	3.93	0.38	5.0	24.5 h	687 days	0.09	1°51'	2
Jupiter	♃	5.20	143	318	1.33	2.6	60	10 h	11.9 yr	0.05	1°18'	63
Saturn	♄	9.54	120	95	0.71	1.2	36	10 h	29.5 yr	0.06	2°29'	60
Uranus	♅	19.2	51	15	1.27	1.1	22	16 h[g]	84 yr	0.05	0°46'	27
Neptune	♆	30.1	50	17	1.70	1.2	24	16 h	165 yr	0.01	1°46'	13

[a]The mean earth-sun distance is called the astronomical unit, where 1 AU = 1.496 × 10⁸ km.

[b]The earth's mass is 5.98 × 10²⁴ kg.

[c]The density of water is 1 g/cm³ = 10³ kg/m³.

[d]The acceleration of gravity at the earth's surface is 9.81 m/s².

[e]Speed needed for permanent escape from the planet's gravitational field.

[f]Venus rotates in the opposite direction from the other planets.

[g]The axis of rotation of Uranus is only 8° from the plane of its orbit.

[h]The difference between the minimum and maximum distances from the sun divided by the average distance.

[i]The ecliptic is the plane of the earth's orbit.

[j]Probably more small ones around Jupiter, Saturn, and Uranus.

The Physical Universe

Fourteenth Edition

Konrad B. Krauskopf
*Late Professor Emeritus of Geochemistry,
Stanford University*

Arthur Beiser

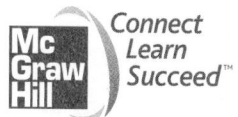

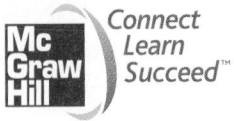

THE PHYSICAL UNIVERSE, FOURTEENTH EDITION

Published by McGraw-Hill, a business unit of The McGraw-Hill Companies, Inc., 1221 Avenue of the Americas, New York, NY 10020. Copyright © 2012 by The McGraw-Hill Companies, Inc. All rights reserved. Previous editions © 2010, 2008, and 2006. No part of this publication may be reproduced or distributed in any form or by any means, or stored in a database or retrieval system, without the prior written consent of The McGraw-Hill Companies, Inc., including, but not limited to, in any network or other electronic storage or transmission, or broadcast for distance learning.

Some ancillaries, including electronic and print components, may not be available to customers outside the United States.

 This book is printed on recycled, acid-free paper containing 10% postconsumer waste.

1 2 3 4 5 6 7 8 9 0 QDB/QDB 1 0 9 8 7 6 5 4 3 2 1

ISBN 978-0-07-351216-7
MHID 0-07-351216-8

Vice President, Editor-in-Chief: *Marty Lange*
Vice President, EDP: *Kimberly Meriwether David*
Senior Director of Development: *Kristine Tibbetts*
Publisher: *Ryan Blankenship*
Senior Sponsoring Editor: *Debra B. Hash*
Senior Developmental Editor: *Mary E. Hurley*
Executive Marketing Manager: *Lisa Nicks*
Senior Project Manager: *April R. Southwood*
Senior Buyer: *Kara Kudronowicz*
Lead Media Project Manager: *Stacy A. Vath*
Senior Designer: *David W. Hash*
Cover/Interior Designer: *Rokusek Design*
Cover Image: *Surfer riding large wave, Maui, Hawaii, USA, ©David Fleetham/Photographer's Choice/Getty Images*
Senior Photo Research Coordinator: *John C. Leland*
Photo Research: *Mary Reeg*
Compositor: *Laserwords Private Limited*
Typeface: *10/12 New Aster*
Printer: *Quad/Graphics*

Library of Congress Cataloging-in-Publication Data

Krauskopf, Konrad B. (Konrad Bates), 1910-2003.
  The physical universe / Konrad B. Krauskopf, Arthur Beiser. — 14th ed.
      p. cm.
  Includes index.
  ISBN 978-0-07-351216-7 — ISBN 0-07-351216-8 (hard copy : alk. paper) 1. Physical sciences—
Textbooks. I. Beiser, Arthur. II. Title.
  Q161.2.K7 2012
  500.2—dc22
                                                                    2010032243

www.mhhe.com

Brief Contents

v

Contents

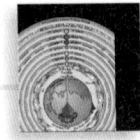
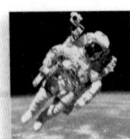
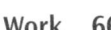
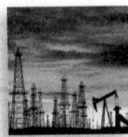

5 Matter and Heat 141

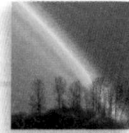

6 Electricity and Magnetism 181

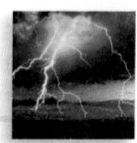

7 Waves 221

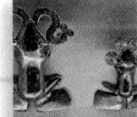

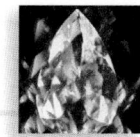
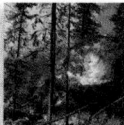
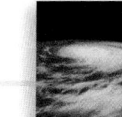

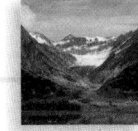
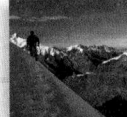
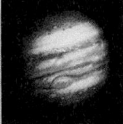
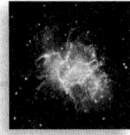

Preface

Creating Informed Citizens

The aim of *The Physical Universe* is to present, as simply and clearly as possible, the essentials of physics, chemistry, earth science, and astronomy to students whose main interests lie elsewhere.

Because of the scope of these sciences and because we assume minimal preparation on the part of the reader, our choice of topics and how far to develop them had to be limited. The emphasis throughout is on the basic concepts of each discipline. We also try to show how scientists approach problems and why science is a never-ending quest rather than a fixed set of facts.

The book concentrates on those aspects of the physical sciences most relevant to a nonscientist who wants to understand how the universe works and to know something about the connections between science and everyday life. We hope to equip readers to appreciate major developments in science as they arrive and to be able to act as informed citizens on matters that involve science and public policy. In particular, there are serious questions today concerning energy supply and use and the contribution of carbon dioxide emissions to global warming. Debates on these questions require a certain amount of scientific literacy, which this book is intended to provide, in order that sensible choices be made that will determine the welfare of generations to come. Past choices have not always benefited our planet and its inhabitants: it is up to us to see that future choices do.

> *"[Krauskopf/Beiser's* The Physical Universe *provides] a good coverage of the basic physical sciences. It gives the basic principles of the different physical sciences and builds real content knowledge. (In contrast, so many texts now tend to "discuss" topics rather than developing an understanding of basic principles.) It has sufficient real-world applications to make the text interesting to the students. I like the way timely, controversial topics are discussed."*
>
> —Linda Arney Wilson, *Middle Tennessee State University*

Scope and Organization

There are many possible ways to organize a book of this kind. We chose the one that provides the most logical progression of ideas, so that each new subject builds on the ones that came before.

> *"This textbook has more of what we teach in Physical Science than any other book on the market. The improvement of each revision is great. . . . I have used 4 editions of this textbook because it is well written; the multiple choice questions and the end-of-the-chapter questions and problems provide numerous opportunities for the student to apply concepts discussed in each chapter. Numerous illustrations are provided for the more visual learner."*
>
> —Etta C. Gravely, *NC A&T University*

Our first concern in *The Physical Universe* is the scientific method, using as illustration the steps that led to today's picture of the universe and the earth's place in it. Next we consider motion and the influences that affect moving bodies. Gravity, energy, and momentum are examined, and the theory of relativity is introduced. Then we examine the many issues associated with the energy that today's world consumes in ever-increasing amounts and the accompanying environmental consequences. Matter in its three states now draws our attention, and we pursue this theme from the kinetic-molecular model to the laws of thermodynamics and the significance of entropy. A grounding in electricity and magnetism follows, and then an exploration of wave phenomena that includes the electromagnetic theory of light. We go on from there to the atomic nucleus and elementary particles, followed by a discussion of the quantum theories of light and of matter that lead to the modern view of atomic structure.

> *"This was my favorite chapter [Chapter 1]. It was also my students' favorite. It generated a great deal of discussion and it motivated the students. . . . I was extremely impressed with how this text introduced the scientific method and then used that methodology to discuss one of the "Great Debates" in scientific history, Geocentric vs. Heliocentric. My students not only learned how the method is applied, but they enjoyed the banter of which view made sense. In fact, I received a number of emails where students went out on their own to do further investigation. . . . It also set the stage for more engaging conversation about the world around them."*
>
> —Leroy Salary, Jr., *Norfolk State University*

The transition from physics to chemistry is made via the periodic table. A look at chemical bonds and how they act to hold together molecules, solids, and liquids is followed by a survey of chemical reactions, organic chemistry, and the chemistry of life.

> *"The authors do a great job of explaining the historical relevance of the periodic table and they give an excellent introduction of the definition of what is chemistry by painting a clear picture of how to relate atoms and elements to compounds and chemical reactions."*
>
> —Antonie H. Rice, *University of Arkansas at Pine Bluff*

Our concern next shifts to the planet on which we live, and we begin by inquiring into the oceans of air and water that cover it. From there we proceed to the materials of the earth, to its ever-evolving crust, and to its no-longer-mysterious interior. After a survey of the main events in the earth's geological history we go on to what we know about our nearest neighbors in space—planets and satellites, asteroids, meteoroids, and comets.

Now the sun, the monarch of the solar system and the provider of nearly all our energy, claims our notice. We go on to broaden our astronomical sights to include the other stars, both individually and as members of the immense assemblies called galaxies. The evolution of the universe starting from the big bang is the last major subject, and we end with the origin of the earth and the likelihood that other inhabited planets exist in the universe and how we might communicate with them.

> *"This is one of the best chapters [Chapter 18] on stars in a text of this level that I have read. It addresses the various aspects of the stars (size, distance, evolution, etc.) in an easy to understand manner. It also provides information concerning the history of the current knowledge of stars."*
>
> —Wilda Pounds, *Northeast Mississippi Community College*

Mathematical Level

The physical sciences are quantitative, which has both advantages and disadvantages. On the plus side, the use of mathematics allows many concepts to be put in the form of clear, definite statements that can be carried further by reasoning and whose predictions can be tested objectively. Less welcome is the discomfort many of us feel when faced with mathematical discussions.

The mathematical level of *The Physical Universe* follows Albert Einstein's prescription for physical theories: "Everything should be as simple as possible, but not simpler." A modest amount of mathematics enables the book to show how science makes sense of the natural world and how its findings led to the technological world of today. In general, the more complicated material supplements rather than dominates the presentation, and full mastery is not needed to understand the rest of the book. The basic algebra needed is reviewed in the Math Refresher. Powers-of-ten notation for small and large numbers is carefully explained there. This section is self-contained and can provide all the math background needed.

How much mathematics is appropriate for a given classroom is for each individual instructor to decide. To this end, a section is included in the thirteenth edition Instructor's Manual that lists the slightly more difficult computational material in the text. This material can be covered as wished or omitted without affecting the continuity or conceptual coverage of a course.

> *"The author has done a wonderful job balancing the verbal and mathematical explanations. The clear, well-labeled diagrams included to assist understanding mathematical expressions are excellent."*
>
> —Paul A. Withey, *Northwestern State University of Louisiana*

New To This Edition

Because the organization of the previous edition worked well in the classroom, it was not altered. The book now has a new, larger format and the text has been divided into many more subsections, both steps that should make the student's task easier. In addition, a website (www.mhhe.com/krauskopf) has been established that contains additional material of various kinds, such as more complex examples and expansions of some topics treated only briefly in the book. The glossary is now in the website, and important new developments in the physical sciences will be described there as they are reported. The entire book was brought up to date and various changes were made to increase its clarity. There are 35 new sidebars and 355 new or revised exercises. Answers to end-of-chapter multiple choice questions were moved to the end of the book. Revised and expanded topics include, among others, power, heat transfer, electric power grids and DC transmission, radiation hazards, nuclear fusion, blackbody radiation, atomic states and orbitals, chemical energy, electrochemical cells, atmospheric energy, the solar system, solar emissions, and exoplanets. Sections with major changes are indicated below.

Chapter 1 The Scientific Method   Sections 1.1 Scientific Method and 1.2 Why Science Is Successful revised.

Chapter 2 Motion   Section 2.14 Artificial Satellites updated.

Chapter 3 Energy   Section 3.2 Power revised.

Chapter 4 Energy and the Future   Entire chapter rewritten with much new material. New and revised topics include global warming; the greenhouse effect; tar sands oil; electric and fuel cell cars; new sources of natural gas; carbon capture and storage; pollution from fossil fuel use; nuclear, solar, and wind energies; geothermal energy and earthquake risk; energy storage; biofuels; conservation; geoengineering; and international efforts to control greenhouse gases.

Chapter 5 Matter and Heat   New section 5.10 Heat Transfer.

Chapter 6 Electricity and Magnetism   New material on electric power grid and on DC power transmission.

Chapter 8 The Nucleus   Sections 8.5 Radiation Hazards and 8.12 Nuclear Fusion revised.

Chapter 9 The Atom   Sections 9.2 Photons, 9.13 Quantum Numbers, and 9.14 Exclusion Principle revised with new material on atomic states and atomic orbitals.

Chapter 10 The Periodic Law   Sections 10.9 Shells and Subshells and 10.10 Explaining the Periodic Table revised.

Chapter 11 Crystals, Ions, and Solutions   Sections 11.8 Water and 11.9 Water Pollution revised.

Chapter 12 Chemical Reactions   Sections 12.6 Chemical Energy and Stability and 12.13 Electrochemical Cells revised.

Chapter 14 Atmosphere and Hydrosphere   Section 14.4 Atmospheric Energy revised.

Chapter 15 The Rock Cycle   Section 15.6 Earthquakes revised and updated.

Chapter 16 The Evolving Earth   Section 16.18 Human History revised.

Chapter 17 The Solar System   Sections 17.6 Mars, 17.8 Asteroids, and subsections on dwarf planets and the moon revised.

Chapter 18 The Stars   Sections 18.1 The Telescope, 18.6 Sunspots, and 18.13 Stellar Evolution revised.

Chapter 19 The Universe   Section 19.11 Exoplanets revised and many small changes elsewhere.

"Chapter 4 is a now-necessary application of what these students are learning about energy, chemistry, and the evolving earth and our responsible use of scientific knowledge and technological enhancements to human life."

—Roxanne R. Lane, *Northwestern State University of Louisiana, Natchitoches*

The Learning System

A variety of aids are provided in *The Physical Universe* to help the reader master the text.

Chapter Opener   An outline provides a preview of major topics, showing at a glance what the chapter covers. A list of goals, in order by section, helps to focus the reader on what is most important in the chapter.

Illustrations   The illustrations, both line drawings and photographs, are full partners to the text and provide a visual pathway to understanding scientific observations and principles for students unaccustomed to abstract argument.

Worked Examples   A full grasp of physical and chemical ideas includes an ability to solve problems based on these ideas. Some students, although able to follow the discussions in the book, nevertheless may have trouble putting

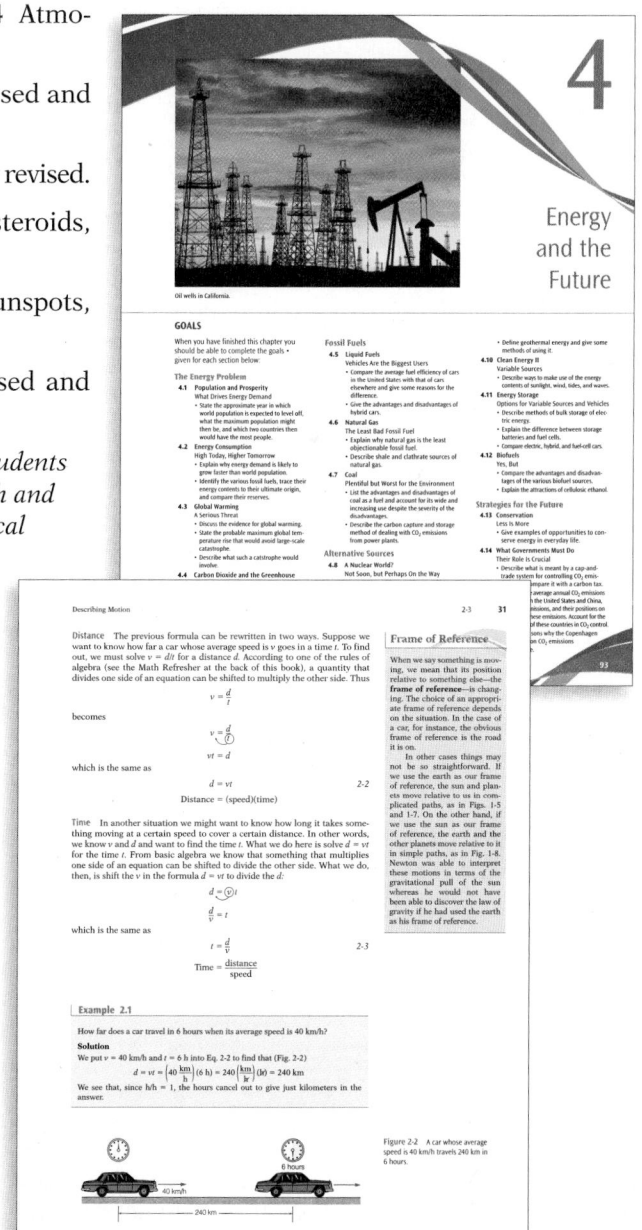

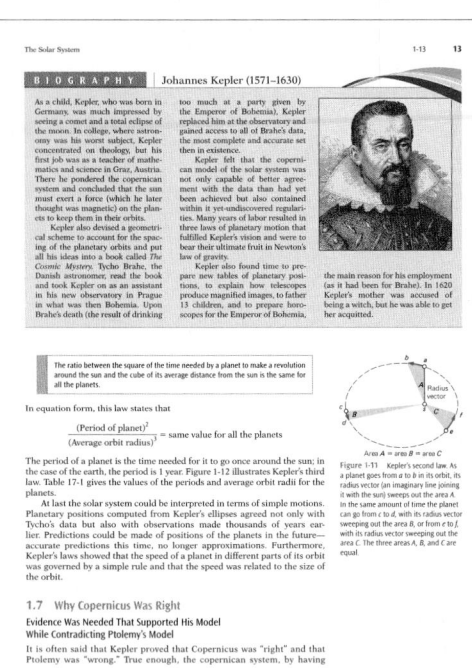

their knowledge to use in this way. To help them, detailed solutions of typical problems are provided that show how to apply formulas and equations to real-world situations. Besides the worked examples, answers and outline solutions for half the end-of-chapter exercises are given at the end of the text. Thinking through the model solutions should bring the unsolved even-numbered problems within reach. In addition to its role in reinforcing the understanding of physical and chemical ideas, solving problems can provide great pleasure, and it would be a shame to miss out on this pleasure. The worked examples in the text are not limited to problems—nearly half of them show how basic ideas can be used to answer serious questions that do not involve calculations.

Bringing Science to Life

Biographies   Brief biographies of 40 major figures in the development of the physical sciences appear where appropriate throughout the text. The biographies provide human and historical perspectives by attaching faces and stories to milestones in these sciences.

Sidebars   These are brief accounts of topics related to the main text. A sidebar may provide additional information on a particular subject, comment on its significance, describe its applications, consider its historical background, or present recent findings. Thirty-five new ones have been added for this edition.

"The textbook does a nice job of covering contemporary topics, which is a way to keep non-science majors interested. I also like the biographies and have sometimes assigned students to go deeper into someone's biography and report to class. Somehow, making these scientists become 'real' for the students makes them enjoy the course more. I also like to show them how some of the topics covered in the course are fairly recent, how there are things we still do not understand. It is important for them to know that science is alive and continues to develop its body of knowledge."

—Ana Ciereszko, *Miami Dade College*

End-of-Chapter Features

Important Terms and Ideas   Important terms introduced in the chapter are listed together with their meanings, which serves as a chapter summary. A list of the **Important Formulas** needed to solve problems based on the chapter material is also given where appropriate.

Exercises   An average of over a hundred exercises on all levels of difficulty follow each chapter, almost a fifth of them new. They are of three kinds, multiple choice, questions, and problems:

- **Multiple Choice** An average chapter has 41 Multiple-Choice exercises (with answers at the back of the book) that act as a quick, painless check on understanding. Correct answers provide reinforcement and encouragement; incorrect ones identify areas of weakness.

- **Exercises** Exercises consist of both questions and problems arranged according to the corresponding text section. Each group begins with questions and goes on to problems. Some of the questions are meant to find out how well the reader has understood the chapter material. Others ask the reader to apply what he or she has learned to new situations. Answers to the odd-numbered questions are given at the back of the book. The physics and chemistry chapters include problems that range from quite easy to moderately challenging. The ability to work out such problems signifies a real understanding of these subjects. Outline solutions (not just answers) for the odd-numbered problems are given at the back of the book.

"The multiple-choice exercises and the questions and problems are a very nice feature of this book and it is definitely above average. . . . There is a good balance between the conceptual versus computational questions."

—Omar Franco Guerrero, *University of Delaware*

McGraw-Hill ConnectPlus™ Physics

ConnectPlus offers an innovative and inexpensive electronic textbook integrated within the Connect online homework platform. ConnectPlus Physics provides students with online assignments and assessments and 24/7 online access to an eBook—an online edition of the *The Physical Universe* text.

With ConnectPlus Physics, instructors can deliver assignments, quizzes, and tests online.

- All of the Exercises from *The Physical Universe* 14E text are presented in an auto-gradable format and tied to the text's learning objectives. Exercises are formatted in either multiple-choice or open-ended numeric entry, with a variety of static and randomized, algorithmic versions.
- Questions and Interactive Problems from the Student Study Guide are also available in an auto-gradable format.

Instructors can edit existing questions or author entirely new problems. Track individual student performance—by question, assignment or in relation to the class overall—with detailed grade reports. Integrate grade reports easily with Learning Management Systems (LMS) such as WebCT and Blackboard. And much more.

By choosing ConnectPlus Physics, instructors are providing their students with a powerful tool for improving academic performance and truly mastering course material. ConnectPlus Physics allows students to practice important skills at their own pace and on their own schedule. Importantly, students' assessment results and instructors' feedback are all saved online—so students can continually review their progress and plot their course to success.

As part of the ehomework process, instructors can assign chapter and section readings from the text. With ConnectPlus, links to relevant text topics are also provided where students need them most—accessed directly from the ehomework problem!

The ConnectPlus eBook:

- Provides students with an online eBook, allowing for anytime, anywhere access to *The Physical Universe* textbook to aid them in successfully completing their work, wherever and whenever they choose.
- Includes Community Notes for student-to-student or instructor-to-student note sharing to greatly enhance the user learning experience.
- Allows for insertion of lecture discussions or instructor-created additional examples using Tegrity (see page xxi) to provide additional clarification or varied coverage on a topic.
- Merges media and assessments with the text's narrative to engage students and improve learning and retention. The eBook includes animations and inline assessment questions.
- Pinpoints and connects key physical science concepts in a snap using the powerful eBook search engine.
- Manages notes, highlights, and bookmarks in one place for simple, comprehensive review.

With the ConnectPlus companion site, instructors also have access to Power Point lecture outlines, the Instructor's Manual, PowerPoint files with electronic images from the text, clicker questions, quizzes, animations, and many other resources directly tied to text-specific materials in *The Physical Universe*.

Students have access to a variety of self-quizzes, key term matching exercises, animations, web links, additional worked examples, and expansions of some topics treated only briefly in the text. The Glossary is now on the website and important new developments in the physical sciences will be described on the website as they are reported.

See www.mhhe.com/krauskopf to learn more and register.

Blackboard   Do More

McGraw- Hill Higher Education and Blackboard have teamed up.

Blackboard, the Web-based course-management system, has partnered with McGraw-Hill to better allow students and faculty to use online materials and activities to complement face-to-face teaching. Blackboard features exciting social learning and teaching tools that foster more logical, visually impactful and active learning opportunities for students. You'll transform your closed-door classrooms into communities where students remain connected to their educational experience 24 hours a day.

This partnership allows you and your students access to McGraw-Hill's Connect™ and Create™ right from within your Blackboard course—all with one single sign-on.

Not only do you get single sign-on with Connect™ and Create™, you also get deep integration of McGraw-Hill content and content engines right in Blackboard. Whether you're choosing a book for your course or building Connect™ assignments, all the tools you need are right where you want them—inside of Blackboard.

Gradebooks are now seamless. When a student completes an integrated Connect™ assignment, the grade for that assignment automatically (and instantly) feeds your Blackboard grade center.

McGraw-Hill and Blackboard can now offer you easy access to industry leading technology and content, whether your campus hosts it, or we do. Be sure to ask your local McGraw-Hill representative for details.

CourseSmart eBook

CourseSmart is a new way for faculty to find and review eBooks. It's also a great option for students who are interested in accessing their course materials digitally and saving money. *CourseSmart* offers thousands of the most commonly adopted textbooks across hundreds of courses from a wide variety of higher education publishers. It is the only place for faculty to review and compare the full text of a textbook online, providing immediate access without the environmental impact of requesting a print exam copy. At *CourseSmart*, students can save up to 50% off the cost of a print book, reduce their impact on the environment, and gain access to powerful Web tools for learning including full text search, notes and highlighting, and email tools for sharing notes between classmates. For further details, contact your sales representative or go to www.coursesmart.com.

Create

Visit www.mcgrawhillcreate.com *today to register and experience how McGraw-Hill Create™ empowers you to teach your students your way.*

With McGraw-Hill Create™, www.mcgrawhillcreate.com, instructors can easily rearrange text chapters, combine material from other content sources, and quickly upload their own content, such as course syllabus or teaching notes. Content can be found in Create by searching through thousands of leading McGraw-Hill textbooks. Create allows instructors to arrange texts to fit their teaching style. Create also allows users to personalize a book's appearance by selecting the cover and adding the instructor's name, school, and course information. With Create, instructors can receive a complimentary print review copy in 3–5 business days or a complimentary electronic review copy (eComp) via email in minutes.

Complete Set of Assets for Instructors and Students

Presentation Center

Build instructional materials wherever, whenever, and however you want!

Accessed from your textbook's website, an online digital library containing photos, artwork, animations, and other media types can be used to create customized lectures, visually enhanced tests and quizzes, compelling course websites, or attractive printed support materials. All assets are copyrighted by McGraw-Hill Higher Education, but can be used by instructors for classroom purposes. The visual resources in this collection include:

- **Art** Full-color digital files of all illustrations in the book can be readily incorporated into lecture presentations, exams, or custom-made classroom materials. In addition, all files are pre-inserted into PowerPoint slides for ease of lecture preparation.
- **Photos** The photos collection contains digital files of photographs from the text, which can be reproduced for multiple classroom uses.
- **Tables and Worked Examples** Tables and Worked Examples that appear in the text have been saved in electronic form for use in classroom presentations and/or quizzes.
- **Animations** Numerous full-color animations illustrating important processes are also provided. Harness the visual impact of concepts in motion by importing these files into classroom presentations or online course materials.

Also residing on your textbook's website are:

- **PowerPoint Lecture Outlines** Ready-made presentations that combine art, animation, and lecture notes are provided for each chapter of the text.
- **PowerPoint Slides** For instructors who prefer to create their lectures from scratch, illustrations, photos, tables, and worked examples from the text are pre-inserted by chapter into blank PowerPoint slides.

Computerized Test Bank Online

A comprehensive bank of test questions is provided within a computerized test bank powered by McGraw-Hill's flexible electronic testing program EZ Test Online (www.eztestonline.com). EZ Test Online allows you to create paper and online tests or quizzes in this easy to use program!

Imagine being able to create and access your test or quiz anywhere, at any time without installing the testing software. Now, with EZ Test Online, instructors can select questions from multiple McGraw-Hill test banks or author their own, and then either print the test for paper distribution or give it online.

Test Creation

- Author/edit questions online using the 14 different question type templates.
- Create printed tests or deliver online to get instant scoring and feedback.
- Create questions pools to offer multiple versions online—great for practice.
- Export your tests for use in WebCT, Blackboard, PageOut, and Apple's iQuiz.

- Compatible with EZ Test Desktop tests you've already created.
- Sharing tests with colleagues, adjuncts, TAs is easy.

Online Test Management

- Set availability dates and time limits for your quiz or test.
- Control how your test will be presented.
- Assign points by question or question type with drop down menu.
- Provide immediate feedback to students or delay until all finish the test.
- Create practice tests online to enable student mastery.
- Your roster can be uploaded to enable student self-registration.

Online Scoring and Reporting

- Automated scoring for most of EZ Test's numerous question types.
- Allows manual scoring for essay and other open-response questions.
- Manual rescoring and feedback is also available.
- EZ Test's grade book is designed to easily export to your grade book.
- View basic statistical reports.

Support and Help

- User's Guide and built-in page-specific help.
- Flash tutorials for getting started on the support site.
- Support Website—www.mhhe.com/eztest.
- Product specialist available at 1-800-331-5094.
- Online Training: http://auth.mhhe.com/mpss/workshops/.

Personal Response Systems

Personal Response Systems ("Clickers") can bring interactivity into the classroom or lecture hall. Wireless response systems give the instructor and students immediate feedback from the entire class. Wireless response pads are essentially remotes that are easy to use and engage students, allowing instructors to motivate student preparation, interactivity, and active learning. Instructors receive immediate feedback to assess which concepts students understand. Questions covering the content of *The Physical Universe* text and formatted in PowerPoint are available on *The Physical Universe* website.

> *"I require students to use eInstruction's remotes. I use the remotes to measure whether students have mastered some of the important concepts. . . . I find them very useful—they give me immediate feedback—they allow daily attendance to be taken quickly and rather painlessly."*
>
> —Robert J. Backes, *Pittsburg State University*

> *"I use the website materials to prepare all my lectures in PowerPoint, since I develop my lectures to my liking. All tests are prepared using the test bank provided by the publisher. . . . These materials have tremendously lightened my workload. I haven't had to re-invent the wheel so to speak. I can change my exams every semester and shuffle my answers from class to class. Well done."*
>
> —Colley Baldwin, *Medgar Evers College, CUNY*

Student Study Guide

Another helpful resource can be found in *The Physical Universe* Student Study Guide. With this study guide, students will maximize their use of *The Physical Universe* text package. It supplements the text with additional, self-directed activities and complements the text by focusing on the important concepts, theories, facts, and processes presented by the authors. Questions and Interactive Problems from the Student Study Guide are also assignable in ConnectPlus in an auto-gradable format.

Tegrity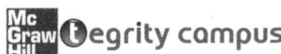

Tegrity Campus is a service that makes class time available all the time by automatically capturing every lecture in a searchable format for students to review when they study and complete assignments. With a simple one-click start-and-stop process, instructors capture all computer screens and corresponding audio. Students replay any part of any class with easy-to-use browser-based viewing on a PC or Mac. Educators know that the more students can see, hear, and experience class resources, the better they learn. With Tegrity Campus, students quickly recall key moments by using Tegrity Campus's unique search feature. This search helps students efficiently find what they need, when they need it across an entire semester of class recordings. Help turn all students' study time into learning moments immediately supported by the class lecture.

To learn more about Tegrity, watch a 2 minute Flash demo at http://tegritycampus.mhhe.com.

Disclaimer

McGraw-Hill offers various tools and technology products to support *The Physical Universe* textbook. Students can order supplemental study materials by contacting their campus bookstore, calling 1-800-262-4729, or online at www.shopmcgraw-hill.com. Instructors can obtain teaching aids by calling the McGraw-Hill Customer Service Department at 1-800-338-3987, visiting our online catalog at www.mhhe.com, or by contacting their local McGraw-Hill sales representative.

As a full-service publisher of quality educational products, McGraw-Hill does much more than just sell textbooks. We create and publish an extensive array of print, video, and digital supplements to support instruction. Orders of new (versus used) textbooks help us to defray the cost of developing such supplements, which is substantial. Local McGraw-Hill representatives can be consulted to learn about the availability of the supplements that accompany *The Physical Universe*. McGraw-Hill representatives can be found by using the tab labeled "My Sales Rep" at www.mhhe.com.

Acknowledgments

Comments from users have always been of much help in revising *The Physical Universe*. Detailed reviews of its thirteenth edition by the following teachers were especially valuable and are much appreciated:

Massimo Bertino, *Virginia Commonwealth University*

Muhammad Bhatti, *University of Texas Pan American*

Debra Burris, *University of Central Arkansas*

Francis Cobbina, *Columbus State Community College*

Mahmoud Gassem, *South Texas College*

Shubo Han, *Fayetteville State University*

Gregg Jaeger, *Boston University CGS*

Kari Lavalli, *Boston University*

Hector Leal, *University of Texas Pan American*

Ari Maller, *New York City College of Technology*

Larry Mattix, *Norfolk State University*

Terud Morishige, *University of Central Oklahoma*

Edgar Newman, *Coastal Carolina University*

James Pazun, *Pfeiffer University*

Galen Pickett, *California State University, Long Beach*

Tchao Podona, *Miami Dade College—North*

Kent Price, *Morehead State University*

Bruce Schulte, *Pulaski Technical College*

Maria Tarafa, *Miami-Dade College, Interamerica*

Rhonda Thompson, *North Carolina A&T State University*

Nancy Woods of Des Moines Area Community College compiled the Videolists in the Instructor's Manual for *The Physical Universe*. Steven Carey of the University of Mobile helped prepare the Goals for each chapter. Linda Kondrick of Arkansas Tech University was of great help in checking the exercises and their answers while preparing the online homework versions of the exercises. I am grateful to all of them.

Thanks are due to the various ancillary authors. Steven Carey of the University of Mobile wrote the Student Study Guide to accompany the text. The following contributed to the many online resources: Charles Hughes of the University of Central Oklahoma wrote the daily concept quizzes; Robert Schoch of Boston University authored the multiple-choice quizzes; S. Raj Chaudhury of Christopher Newport University contributed the clicker questions; and Tony Sauncy of Angelo State University authored the PowerPoint lecture outlines.

Finally, I want to thank my friends at McGraw-Hill, especially Mary Hurley and April Southwood, for their skilled and dedicated help in producing this edition.

Arthur Beiser

Meet the Authors

Konrad B. Krauskopf was born and raised in Madison, Wisconsin, and earned a B.S. in chemistry from University of Wisconsin in 1931. He then earned a Ph.D. in chemistry at the University of California in Berkeley. When the Great Depression made jobs in chemistry scarce, Professor Krauskopf decided to study geology, which had long fascinated him. Through additional graduate work at Stanford University, he earned a second Ph.D. and eventually a position on the Stanford faculty. He remained at Stanford until his retirement in 1976. During his tenure, Professor Krauskopf also worked at various times with the U.S. Geological Survey, served with the U.S. Army in occupied Japan, and traveled to Norway, France, and Germany on sabbatical leaves. His research interests included field work on granites and metamorphic rocks and laboratory study on applications of chemistry to geologic problems, especially the formation of ore deposits. In later years, Professor Krauskopf spent time working with various government agencies on the problem of radioactive waste disposal. Professor Krauskopf passed away on May 8, 2003.

Arthur Beiser, a native of New York City, received B.S., M.S., and Ph.D. degrees in physics from New York University, where he later served as Associate Professor of Physics. He then was Senior Research Scientist at the Lamont Geological Observatory of Columbia University. His research interests were chiefly in cosmic rays and in magnetohydrodynamics as applied to geophysics and astrophysics. In addition to theoretical work, he participated in a cosmic-ray expedition to an Alaskan peak and directed a search for magnetohydrodynamic waves from space in various Pacific locations. A Fellow of The Explorers Club, Dr. Beiser was the first chairman of its Committee on Space Exploration. He is the author or coauthor of 36 books, mostly college texts on physics and mathematics, 14 of which have been translated into a total of 26 languages. Two of his books are on sailing, *The Proper Yacht* and *The Sailor's World*. Figure 13-1 is a photograph of Dr. Beiser at the helm of his 58-ft sloop; he and his wife Germaine have sailed over 130,000 miles, including two Atlantic crossings and a rounding of Cape Horn. Germaine Beiser, who has degrees in physics from the Massachusetts Institute of Technology and New York University, is the author or coauthor of 7 books on various aspects of physics and has contributed to *The Physical Universe*. She is the editor of a cruising guide to the Adriatic Sea.

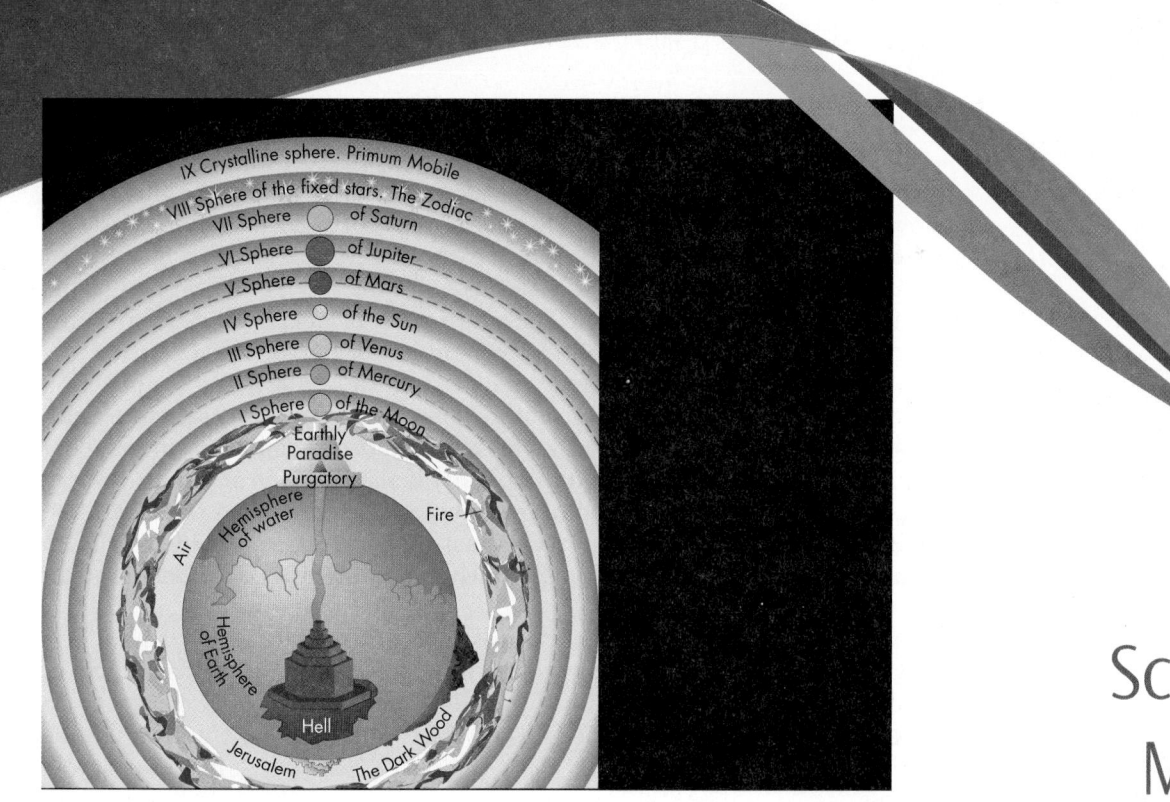

Medieval picture of the universe.

The Scientific Method

GOALS

When you have finished this chapter you should be able to complete the goals given for each section below:

How Scientists Study Nature

1.1 The Scientific Method
Four Steps
- Outline the scientific method.
- Distinguish between a law and a theory.
- Discuss the role of a model in formulating a scientific theory.

1.2 Why Science Is Successful
Science Is a Living Body of Knowledge, Not a Set of Frozen Ideas
- Explain why the scientific method has been more successful than other approaches to understanding the natural world.

The Solar System

1.3 A Survey of the Sky
Everything Seems to Circle the North Star
- Give the reason why Polaris is the heavenly body that remains most nearly stationary in the sky.
- Define constellation.

- Tell how to distinguish planets from stars by observations of the night sky made several weeks or months apart.

1.4 The Ptolemaic System
The Earth as the Center of the Universe

1.5 The Copernican System
A Spinning Earth That Circles the Sun
- Compare how the ptolemaic and copernican systems account for the observed motions of the sun, moon, planets, and stars across the sky.
- Define day and year.

1.6 Kepler's Laws
How the Planets Actually Move
- Explain the significance of Kepler's laws.

1.7 Why Copernicus Was Right
Evidence Was Needed That Supported His Model While Contradicting Ptolemy's Model
- State why the copernican system is considered correct.

Universal Gravitation

1.8 What Is Gravity?
A Fundamental Force
- Define fundamental force.

1.9 Why the Earth Is Round
The Big Squeeze
- Explain why the earth is round but not a perfect sphere.

1.10 The Tides
Up and Down Twice a Day
- Explain the origin of tides.
- Account for the difference between spring and neap tides.

1.11 The Discovery of Neptune
Another Triumph for the Law of Gravity
- Explain in terms of the scientific method why the discovery of Neptune was so important in confirming the law of gravity.

How Many of What

1.12 The SI System
All Scientists Use These Units
- Change the units in which a quantity is expressed from those of one system of units to those of another system.
- Use metric prefixes for small and large numbers.
- Use significant figures correctly in a calculation.

All of us belong to two worlds, the world of people and the world of nature. As members of the world of people, we take an interest in human events of the past and present and find such matters as politics and economics worth knowing about. As members of the world of nature, we also owe ourselves some knowledge of the sciences that seek to understand this world. It is not idle curiosity to ask why the sun shines, why the sky is blue, how old the earth is, why things fall down. These are serious questions, and to know their answers adds an important dimension to our personal lives.

We are made of atoms linked together into molecules, and we live on a planet circling a star—the sun—that is a member of one of the many galaxies of stars in the universe. It is the purpose of this book to survey what physics, chemistry, geology, and astronomy have to tell us about atoms and molecules, stars and galaxies, and everything in between. No single volume can cover all that is significant in this vast span, but the basic ideas of each science can be summarized along with the raw material of observation and reasoning that led to them.

Like any other voyage into the unknown, the exploration of nature is an adventure. This book records that adventure and contains many tales of wonder and discovery. The search for knowledge is far from over, with no end of exciting things still to be found. What some of these things might be and where they are being looked for are part of the story in the chapters to come.

How Scientists Study Nature

Every scientist dreams of lighting up some dark corner of the natural world—or, almost as good, of finding a dark corner where none had been suspected. The most careful observations, the most elaborate calculations will not be fruitful unless the right questions are asked. Here is where creative imagination enters science, which is why many of the greatest scientific advances have been made by young, nimble minds.

Scientists study nature in a variety of ways. Some approaches are quite direct: a geologist takes a rock sample to a laboratory and, by inspection and analysis, finds out what it is made of and how and when it was probably formed. Other approaches are indirect: nobody has ever visited the center of the earth or ever will, but by combining a lot of thought with clues from different sources, a geologist can say with near certainty that the earth has a core of molten iron.

No matter what the approaches to particular problems may be, however, the work scientists do always fits into a certain pattern of steps. This pattern, a general scheme for gaining reliable information about the universe, has become known as the **scientific method.**

1.1 The Scientific Method

Four Steps

We can think of the scientific method in terms of four steps: (1) formulating a problem, (2) observation and experiment, (3) interpreting the data, and (4) testing the interpretation by further observation and experiment to check its predictions. These steps are often carried out by different scientists, sometimes many years apart and not always in this order. Whatever way it is carried out, though, the scientific method is not a mechanical process but a human activity that needs creative thinking in all its steps. Looking at the natural world is at the heart of the scientific method, because the results

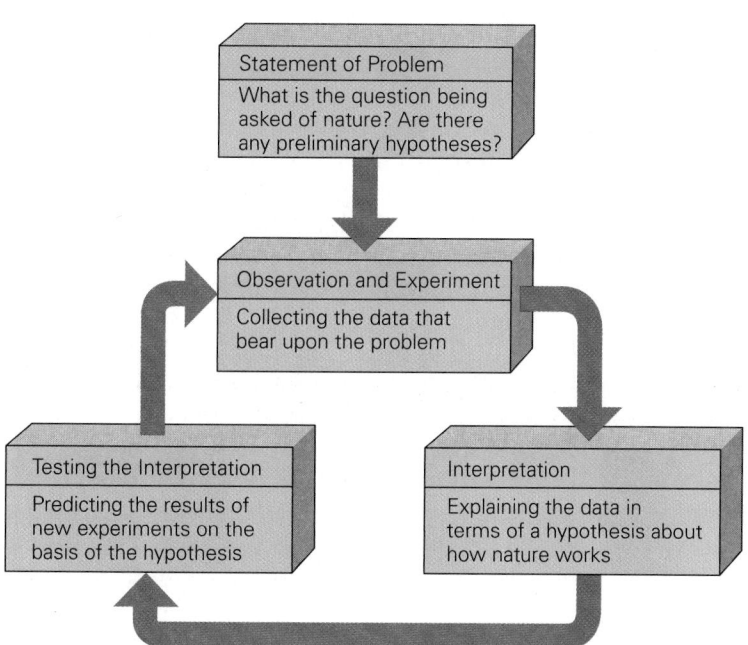

Figure 1-1 The scientific method. No hypothesis is ever final because future data may show that it is incorrect or incomplete. Unless it turns out to be wrong, a hypothesis never leaves the loop of experiment, interpretation, testing. Of course, the more times the hypothesis goes around the loop successfully, the more likely it is to be a valid interpretation of nature. Experiment and hypothesis thus evolve together, with experiment having the final word. Although a hypothesis may occur to a scientist as he or she studies experimental results, often the hypothesis comes first and relevant data are sought afterward to test it.

of observation and experiment serve not only as the foundations on which scientists build their ideas but also as the means by which these ideas are checked (Fig. 1-1).

1. **Formulating a problem** may mean no more than choosing a certain field to work in, but more often a scientist has in mind some specific idea he or she wishes to investigate. In many cases formulating a problem and interpreting the data overlap. The scientist has a speculation, perhaps only a hunch, perhaps a fully developed **hypothesis,** about some aspect of nature but cannot come to a definite conclusion without further study.
2. **Observation and experiment** are carried out with great care. Facts about nature are the building blocks of science and the ultimate test of its results. This insistence on accurate, objective data is what sets science apart from other modes of intellectual endeavor.
3. **Interpretation** may lead to a general rule or **law** to which the data seem to conform. Or it may be a **theory,** which is a more ambitious attempt to account for what has been found in terms of how nature works. In any case, the interpretation must be able to cover new data obtained under different circumstances. As put forward orginally, a scientific interpretation is usually called a hypothesis.
4. **Testing the interpretation** involves making new observations or performing new experiments to see whether the interpretation correctly predicts the results. If the results agree with the predictions, the scientist is clearly on the right track. The new data may well lead to refinements of the original idea, which in turn must be checked, and so on indefinitely.

The Laws of Nature The laws of a country tell its citizens how they are supposed to behave. Different countries have different laws, and even in one country laws are changed from time to time. Furthermore, though he or she may be caught and punished for doing so, anybody can break any law at any time.

The laws of nature are different. Everything in the universe, from atoms to galaxies of stars, behaves in certain regular ways, and these regularities

Finding the Royal Road

Hermann von Helmholtz, a German physicist and biologist of a century ago, summed up his experience of scientific research in these words: "I would compare myself to a mountain climber who, not knowing the way, ascends slowly and toilsomely and is often compelled to retrace his steps because his progress is blocked; who, sometimes by reasoning and sometimes by accident, hits upon signs of a fresh path, which leads him a little farther; and who, finally, when he has reached his goal, discovers to his annoyance a royal road which he might have followed if he had been clever enough to find the right starting point at the beginning."

Experiment Is the Test

A master of several sciences, Michael Faraday, who lived a century and a half ago, is best remembered for his discoveries in electricity and magnetism (see biography in Sec. 6.18). This statement appears in the entry for March 19, 1849 in his laboratory notebook: "Nothing is too wonderful to be true if it be consistent with the laws of nature, and . . . experiment is the best test of such consistency."

Faraday was a Fellow of Britain's Royal Society, which was founded in 1660 to promote the use of observation and experiment to study the natural world. The oldest scientific organization in the world, the Royal Society has as its motto *Nullus in Verba*—Latin for "Take nobody's word for it." On its 350th anniversary, the Royal Society held a celebration of "the joy and vitality of science, its importance to society and culture, and its role in shaping who we are and who we will become."

are the laws of nature. To be considered a law of nature, a given regularity must hold everywhere at all times within its range of applicability.

The laws of nature are worth knowing for two reasons apart from satisfying our curiosity about how the universe works. First, we can use them to predict phenomena not yet discovered. Thus Isaac Newton's law of gravity was applied over a century ago to apparent irregularities in the motion of the planet Uranus, then the farthest known planet from the sun. Calculations not only showed that another, more distant planet should exist but also indicated where in the sky to look for it. Astronomers who looked there found a new planet, which was named Neptune.

Second, the laws of nature can give us an idea of what goes on in places we cannot examine directly. We will never visit the sun's interior (much too hot) or the interior of an atom (much too small), but we know a lot about both regions. The evidence is indirect but persuasive.

Theories   A **law** tells us *what*; a **theory** tells us *why*. A theory explains why certain events take place and, if they obey a particular law, how that law originates in terms of broader considerations. For example, Albert Einstein's general theory of relativity interprets gravity as a distortion in the properties of space and time around a body of matter. This theory not only accounts for Newton's law of gravity but goes further, including the prediction—later confirmed—that light should be affected by gravity.

As the French mathematician Henri Poincaré once remarked, "Science is built with facts just as a house is built with bricks, but a collection of facts is not a science any more than a pile of bricks is a house."

Models   It may not be easy to get a firm intellectual grip on some aspect of nature. Therefore a **model**—a simplified version of reality—is often part of a hypothesis or theory. In developing the law of gravity, Newton considered the earth to be perfectly round, even though it is actually more like a grapefruit than like a billiard ball. Newton regarded the path of the earth around the sun as an oval called an **ellipse**, but the actual orbit has wiggles no ellipse ever had. By choosing a sphere as a model for the earth and an ellipse as a model for its orbit, Newton isolated the most important features of the earth and its path and used them to arrive at the law of gravity.

If Newton had started with a more realistic model—a somewhat squashed earth moving somewhat irregularly around the sun—he probably would have made little progress. Once he had formulated the law of gravity, Newton was then able to explain how the spinning of the earth causes it to become distorted into the shape of a grapefruit and how the attractions of the other planets cause the earth's orbit to differ from a perfect ellipse.

Theory

In science a *theory* is a fully developed logical structure based on general principles that ties together a variety of observations and experimental findings and permits as-yet-unknown phenomena and connections to be predicted. A theory may be more or less speculative when proposed, but the point is that it is a large-scale framework of ideas and relationships.

To people ignorant of science, a theory is a suggestion, a proposal, what in science is called a hypothesis. For instance, believers in creationism, the unsupported notion that all living things simultaneously appeared on earth a few thousand years ago, scorn Darwin's theory of evolution (see Sec. 16.8) as "just a theory" despite the wealth of evidence in its favor and its bedrock position in modern biology. In fact, few aspects of our knowledge of the natural world are as solidly established as the theory of evolution.

1.2   Why Science Is Successful

Science Is a Living Body of Knowledge, Not a Set of Frozen Ideas

What has made science such a powerful tool for investigating nature is the constant testing and retesting of its findings. As a result, science is a living body of information and not a collection of dogmas. The laws and theories of science are not necessarily the final word on a subject: they are valid only as long as no contrary evidence comes to light. If such contrary evidence does turn up, the law or theory must be modified or even discarded. To rock the boat is part of the game; to overturn it is one way to win. Thus science is a self-correcting search for better understanding of the natural world, a search with no end in sight.

Scientists are open about the details of their work, so that others can follow their thinking and repeat their experiments and observations. Nothing is accepted on anybody's word alone, or because it is part of a religious or political doctrine. "Common sense" is not a valid argument, either; if common sense were a reliable guide, we would not need science. What counts are definite measurements and clear reasoning, not vague notions that vary from person to person.

The power of the scientific approach is shown not only by its success in understanding the natural world but also by the success of the technology based on science. It is hard to think of any aspect of life today untouched in some way by science. The synthetic clothing we wear, the medicines that lengthen our lives, the cars and airplanes we travel in, the telephone, internet, radio, and television by which we communicate—all are ultimately the products of a certain way of thinking. Curiosity and imagination are part of that way of thinking, but the most important part is that nothing is ever taken for granted but is always subject to test and change.

Religion and Science   In the past, scientists were sometimes punished for daring to make their own interpretations of what they saw. Galileo, the first modern scientist (see biography in Sec. 2.5), was forced by the Roman Catholic Church in 1633 under threat of torture to deny that the earth moves about the sun. Even today, attempts are being made to compel the teaching of religious beliefs—for instance, the story of the Creation as given in the Bible—under the name of science. But "creation science" is a contradiction in terms. The essence of science is that its results are open to change in the light of new evidence, whereas the essence of creationism is that it is a fixed doctrine with no basis in observation. The scientific method has been the means of liberating the world from ignorance and superstition. To discard this method in favor of taking at face value every word in the Bible is to replace the inquiring mind with a closed mind.

Those who wish to believe that the entire universe came into being in 6 days a few thousand years ago are free to do so. What is not proper is for certain politicians (whom Galileo would recognize if he were alive today) to try to turn back the intellectual clock and compel such matters of faith to be taught in schools alongside or even in place of scientific concepts, such as evolution (Sec. 16.8), that have abundant support in the world around us. To anyone with an open mind, the evidence that the universe and its inhabitants have developed over time and continue to do so is overwhelming, as we shall see in later chapters. Nothing stands still. The ongoing evolution of living things is central to biology; the ongoing evolution of the earth is central to geology; the ongoing evolution of the universe is central to astronomy.

Many people find religious beliefs important in their lives, but such beliefs are not part of science because they are matters of faith with ideas that are meant to be accepted without question. Skepticism, on the other

Degrees of Doubt

Although in principle everything in science is open to question, in practice many ideas are not really in doubt. The earth is certainly round, for instance, and the planets certainly revolve around the sun. Even though the earth is not a perfect sphere and the planetary orbits are not perfect ellipses, the basic models will always be valid.

Other beliefs are less firm. An example is the current picture of the future of the universe. Quite convincing data suggest that the universe has been expanding since its start in a "big bang" about 13.7 billion years ago. What about the future? It seems likely from the latest measurements that the expansion will continue forever, but this conclusion is still tentative and is under active study by astronomers today.

hand, is at the heart of science. Science follows where evidence leads; religion has fixed principles. It is entirely possible—and indeed most religious people do this—to consult sacred texts for inspiration and guidance while accepting that observation and reason represent the path to another kind of understanding. But religion and science are not interchangeable because their routes and destinations are different—which means that science classrooms are not the place to teach religion. To mix the religious and the scientific ways of looking at the world is good for neither, particularly if compulsion is involved.

Advocates of intelligent design assert that evolution is an atheistic concept. Yet religious leaders of almost all faiths see no conflict between evolution and religious belief. According to Cardinal Paul Poupard, head of the Roman Catholic Church's Pontifical Council for Culture, "we . . . know the dangers of a religion that severs its links with reason and becomes prey to fundamentalism. The faithful have the obligation to listen to that which secular modern science has to offer."

The Solar System

What the Constitution Says

The founders of the United States of America insisted on the separation of church and state, a separation that is part of the Constitution. What happens in countries with no such separation, in the past and in the present, testifies to the wisdom of the founders. In 1987 the U.S. Supreme Court ruled that teaching creationism in the public schools is illegal because it is a purely religious doctrine. In response, the believers in creationism changed its name to "intelligent design" without specifying who the designer was or how the design was put into effect. Their sole argument is that life is too complex and diverse to be explained by evolution, when in fact this is precisely what evolution does with overwhelming success. Nevertheless attempts have continued to be made to include intelligent design in science classes in public schools. All such attempts have been ruled illegal by the courts. (For more, see Sec. 1.2 at www.mmhe.com/krauskopf.)

Each day the sun rises in the east, sweeps across the sky, and sets in the west. The moon, planets, and most stars do the same. These heavenly bodies also move relative to one another, though more slowly.

There are two ways to explain the general east-to-west motion. The most obvious is that the earth is stationary and all that we see in the sky revolves around it. The other possibility is that the earth itself turns once a day, so that the heavenly bodies only appear to circle it. How the second alternative came to be seen as correct and how this finding led to the discovery of the law of gravity are important chapters in the history of the scientific method.

1.3   A Survey of the Sky

Everything Seems to Circle the North Star

One star in the northern sky seems barely to move at all. This is the North Star, or **Polaris,** long used as a guide by travelers because of its nearly unchanging position. Stars near Polaris do not rise or set but instead move around it in circles (Fig. 1-2). These circles carry the stars under Polaris from west to east and over it from east to west. Farther from Polaris the circles get larger and larger, until eventually they dip below the horizon. Sun, moon, and stars rise and set because their circles lie partly below the horizon. Thus, to an observer north of the equator, the whole sky appears to revolve once a day about this otherwise ordinary star.

Why does Polaris occupy such a central position? The earth rotates once a day on its axis, and Polaris happens by chance to lie almost directly over the North Pole. As the earth turns, everything else around it seems to be moving. Except for their circular motion around Polaris, the stars appear fixed in their positions with respect to one another. Stars of the Big Dipper move halfway around Polaris between every sunset and sunrise, but the shape of the Dipper itself remains unaltered. (Actually, as discussed later, the stars *do* change their relative positions, but the stars are so far away that these changes are not easy to detect.)

Constellations   Easily recognized groups of stars, like those that form the Big Dipper, are called **constellations** (Fig. 1-3). Near the Big Dipper is the less

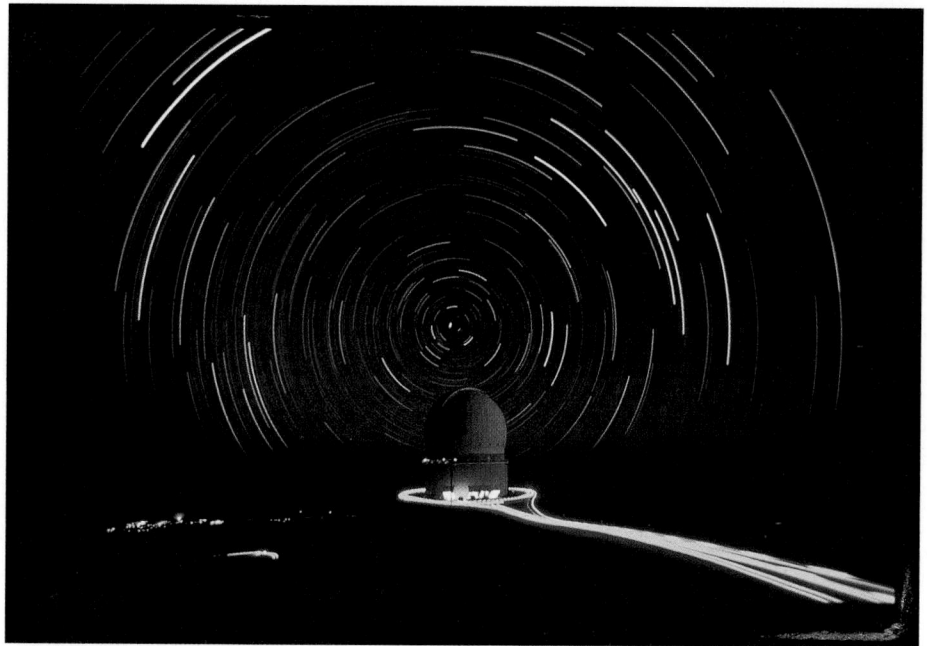

Figure 1-2 Time exposure of stars in the northern sky. The trail of Polaris is the bright arc slightly to the left of the center of the larger arcs. The dome in the foreground houses one of the many telescopes on the summit of Mauna Kea, Hawaii. This location is favored by astronomers because observing conditions are excellent there. The lights of cars that moved during the exposure are responsible for the yellow traces near the dome.

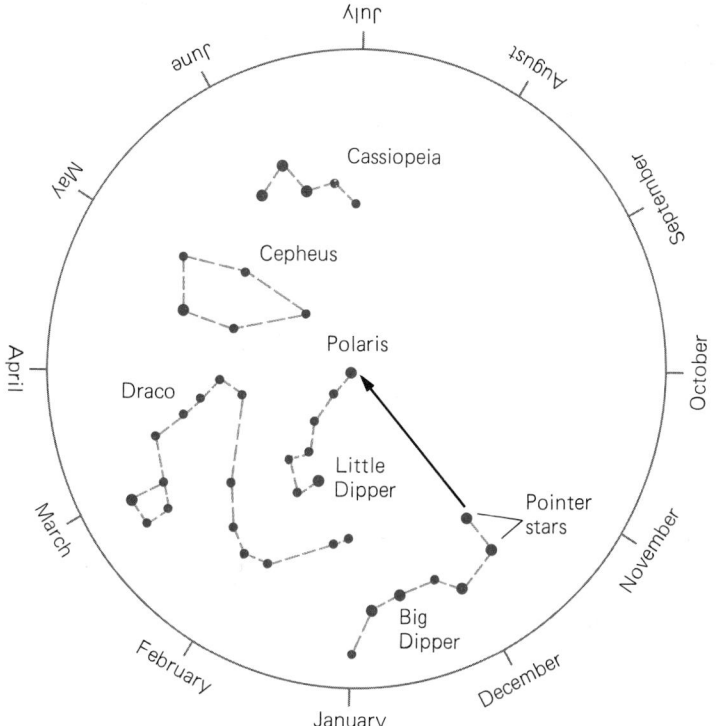

Figure 1-3 Constellations near Polaris as they appear in the early evening to an observer who faces north with the figure turned so that the current month is at the bottom. Polaris is located on an imaginary line drawn through the two "pointer" stars at the end of the bowl of the Big Dipper. The brighter stars are shown larger in size.

conspicuous Little Dipper with Polaris at the end of its handle. On the other side of Polaris from the Big Dipper are Cepheus and the W-shaped Cassiopeia, named for an ancient king and queen of Ethiopia. Next to Cepheus is Draco, which means dragon.

Elsewhere in the sky are dozens of other constellations that represent animals, heroes, and beautiful women. An especially easy one to recognize on winter evenings is Orion, the mighty hunter of legend. Orion has four stars, three of them quite bright, at the corners of a warped rectangle with a

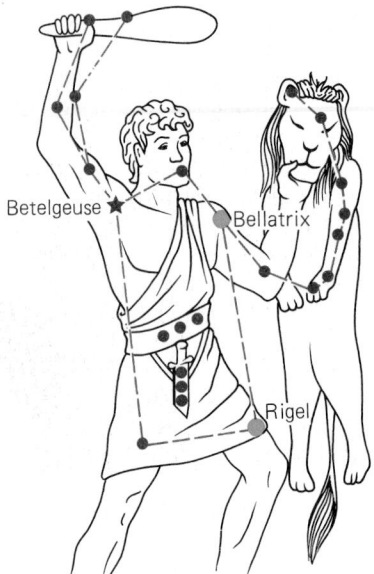

Figure 1-4 Orion, the mighty hunter. Betelgeuse is a bright red star, and Bellatrix and Rigel are bright blue stars. Stars that seem near one another in the sky may actually be far apart in space. The three stars in Orion's belt, for instance, are in reality at very different distances from us.

belt of three stars in line across its middle (Fig. 1-4). Except for the Dippers, a lot of imagination is needed to connect a given star pattern with its corresponding figure, but the constellations nevertheless are useful as convenient labels for regions of the sky.

Sun and Moon   In their daily east-west crossing of the sky, the sun and moon move more slowly than the stars and so appear to drift eastward relative to the constellations. In the same way, a person on a train traveling west who walks toward the rear car is moving east relative to the train although still moving west relative to the ground. In the sky, the apparent eastward motion is most easily observed for the moon. If the moon is seen near a bright star on one evening, by the next evening it will be some distance east of that star, and on later nights it will be farther and farther to the east. In about 4 weeks the moon drifts eastward completely around the sky and returns to its starting point.

The sun's relative motion is less easy to follow because we cannot observe directly which stars it is near. But if we note which constellations appear where the sun has just set, we can estimate the sun's location among the stars and follow it from day to day. We find that the sun drifts eastward more slowly than the moon, so slowly that the day-to-day change is scarcely noticeable. Because of the sun's motion each constellation appears to rise about 4 min earlier each night, and so, after a few weeks or months, the appearance of the night sky becomes quite different from what it was when we started our observations.

By the time the sun has migrated eastward completely around the sky, a year has gone by. In fact, the **year** is defined as the time needed for the sun to make such an apparent circuit of the stars.

Planets   Five other celestial objects visible to the naked eye also shift their positions with respect to the stars. These objects, which themselves resemble stars, are **planets** (Greek for "wanderer") and are named for the Roman gods Mercury, Venus, Mars, Jupiter, and Saturn. Like the sun and moon, the planets shift their positions so slowly that their day-to-day motion is hard to detect. Unlike the sun, they move in complex paths. In general, each planet drifts eastward among the stars, but its relative speed varies and at times the planet even reverses its relative direction to head westward briefly. Thus the path of a planet appears to consist of loops that recur regularly, as in Fig. 1-5.

1.4   The Ptolemaic System

The Earth as the Center of the Universe

Although the philosophers of ancient Greece knew that the apparent daily rotation of the sky could be explained by a rotation of the earth, most of them preferred to regard the earth as stationary. The scheme most widely accepted

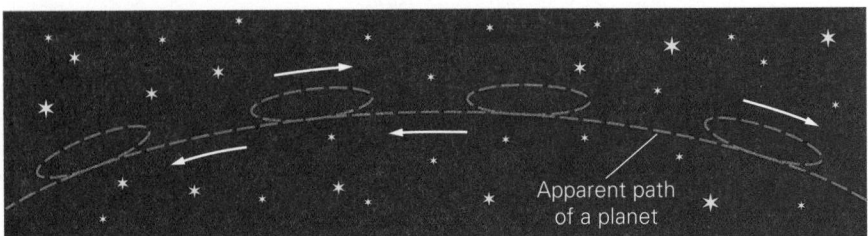

Figure 1-5 Apparent path of a planet in the sky looking south from the northern hemisphere of the earth. The planets seem to move eastward relative to the stars most of the time, but at intervals they reverse their motion and briefly move westward.

was originally the work of Hipparchus. Ptolemy of Alexandria (Fig. 1-6) later included Hipparchus's ideas into his *Almagest*, a survey of astronomy that was to be the standard reference on the subject for over a thousand years. This model of the universe became known as the **ptolemaic system.**

The model was intricate and ingenious (Fig. 1-7). Our earth stands at the center, motionless, with everything else in the universe moving about it either in circles or in combinations of circles. (To the Greeks, the circle was the only "perfect" curve, hence the only possible path for a celestial object.) The fixed stars are embedded in a huge crystal sphere that makes a little more than a complete turn around the earth each day. Inside the crystal sphere is the sun, which moves around the earth exactly once a day. The difference in speed between sun and stars is just enough so that the sun appears to move eastward past the stars, returning to a given point among them once a year. Near the earth in a small orbit is the moon, revolving more slowly than the sun. The planets Venus and Mercury come between moon and sun, the other planets between sun and stars.

To account for irregularities in the motions of the planets, Ptolemy imagined that each planet moves in a small circle about a point that in turn follows a large circle about the earth. By a combination of these circular motions a planet travels in a series of loops. Since we observe these loops edgewise, it appears to us as if the planets move with variable speeds and sometimes even reverse their directions of motion in the sky.

From observations made by himself and by others, Ptolemy calculated the speed of each celestial object in its assumed orbit. Using these speeds he could then figure out the location in the sky of any object at any time, past or future. These calculated positions checked fairly well, though not perfectly, with positions that had been recorded centuries earlier, and the predictions also agreed at first with observations made in later years. So Ptolemy's

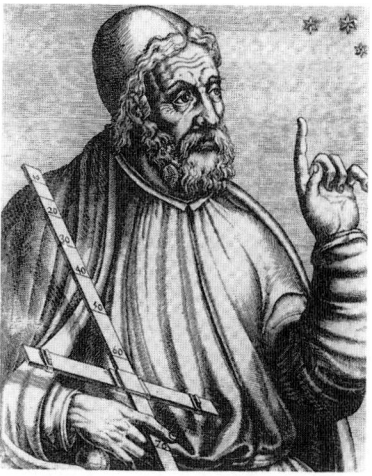

Figure 1-6   Ptolemy (A.D. 100–170).

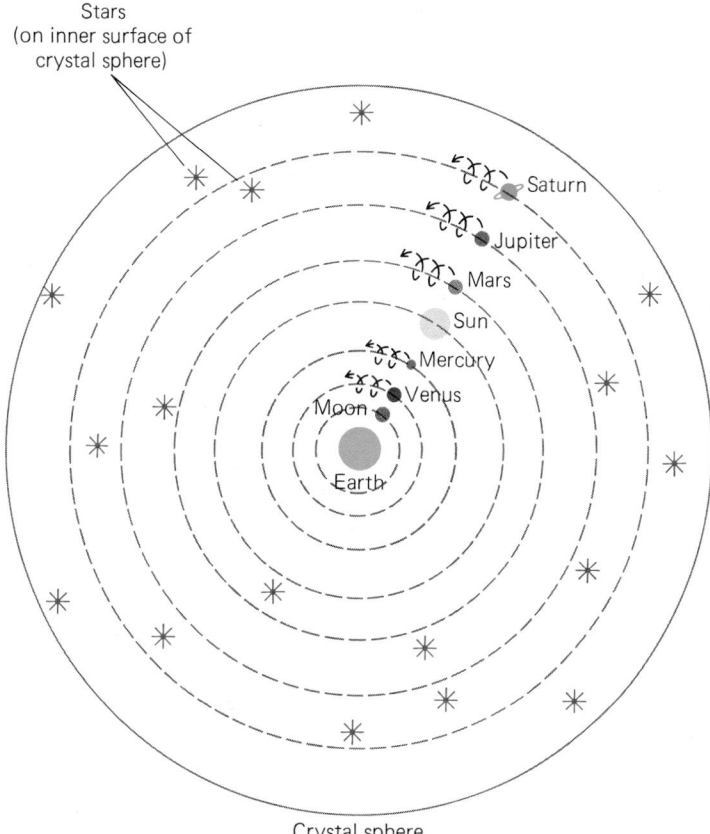

Stars
(on inner surface of
crystal sphere)

Saturn

Jupiter

Mars

Sun

Mercury

Venus

Moon

Earth

Crystal sphere
with earth at center

Figure 1-7   The ptolemaic system, showing the assumed arrangement of the members of the solar system within the celestial sphere. Each planet is supposed to travel around the earth in a series of loops, while the orbits of the sun and moon are circular. Only the planets known in Ptolemy's time are shown. The stars are all supposed to be at the same distance from the earth.

The Temple of the Sun

Here is how Copernicus summed up his picture of the solar system: "Of the moving bodies first comes Saturn, who completes his circuit in 30 years. After him Jupiter, moving in a twelve-year revolution. Then Mars, who revolves biennially. Fourth in order an annual cycle takes place, in which we have said is contained the earth, with the lunar orbit as an epicycle, that is, with the moon moving in a circle around the earth. In the fifth place Venus is carried around in 9 months. Then Mercury holds the sixth place, circulating in the space of 80 days. In the middle of all dwells the Sun. Who indeed in this most beautiful temple would place the torch in any other or better place than one whence it can illuminate the whole at the same time?"

system fulfilled all the requirements of a scientific theory: it was based on observation, it accounted for the celestial motions known in his time, and it made predictions that could be tested in the future.

1.5 The Copernican System

A Spinning Earth That Circles the Sun

By the sixteenth century it had become clear that something was seriously wrong with the ptolemaic model. The planets were simply not in the positions in the sky predicted for them. The errors could be removed in two ways: either the ptolemaic system could be made still more complicated, or it could be replaced by a different model of the universe.

Nicolaus Copernicus, a versatile and energetic Pole of the early sixteenth century, chose the second approach. Let us consider the earth, said Copernicus, as one of the planets, a sphere rotating once a day on its axis. Let us imagine that all the planets, including the earth, circle the sun (Fig. 1-8), that the moon circles the earth, and that the stars are all far away. In this model, it is the earth's rotation that explains the daily rising and setting of celestial objects, not the motions of these objects. The apparent shifting of the sun among the stars is due to the earth's motion in its orbit. As the earth swings around the sun, we see the sun changing its position against the background of the stars. The moon's gradual eastward drift is mainly due to its orbital motion. Apparently irregular movements of the planets are really just combinations of their motions with our own shifts of position as the earth moves.

The **copernican system** offended both Protestant and Catholic religious leaders, who did not want to see the earth taken from its place at the hub of the universe. The publication of Copernicus's manuscript began a long and bitter argument. To us, growing up with the knowledge that the earth moves, it seems odd that this straightforward idea was so long and so violently opposed. But in the sixteenth century good arguments were available to both sides.

Consider, said supporters of Ptolemy, how fast the earth's surface must move to complete a full turn every 24 h. Would not everything loose be flung into space by this whirling ball, just as mud is thrown from the rim of a carriage wheel? And would not such dizzying speeds produce a great wind

Figure 1-8 The copernican system. The planets, including the earth, are supposed to travel around the sun in circular orbits. The earth rotates daily on its axis, the moon revolves around the earth, and the stars are far away. All planets in the solar system are shown here. There are also a number of dwarf planets, such as Pluto; see Sec. 17.11. The actual orbits are ellipses and are not spaced as shown here, though they do lie in approximately the same plane.

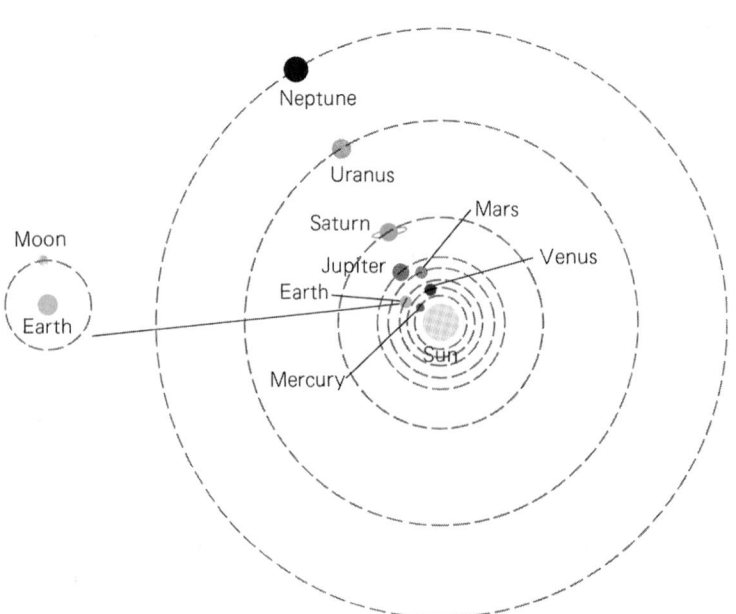

BIOGRAPHY | Nicolaus Copernicus (1473–1543)

When Columbus made his first voyage to the New World Copernicus was a student in his native Poland. In the years that followed intellectual as well as geographical horizons receded before eager explorers. In 1496 Copernicus went to Italy to learn medicine, theology, and astronomy. Italy was then an exciting place to be, a place of business expansion and conflicts between rival cities, great fortunes and corrupt governments, brilliant thinkers and inspired artists such as Leonardo da Vinci and Michelangelo.

After 10 years in Italy Copernicus returned to Poland where he practiced medicine, served as a canon in the cathedral of which his uncle was the bishop, and became

involved in currency reform, but much of his time was devoted to developing the idea that the planets move around the sun rather than around the earth. The idea was not new—the ancient Greeks were aware of it—but Copernicus went further and worked out the planetary orbits and speeds in detail. Although a summary of his results had been circulated in manuscript form earlier, not until a few weeks before his death was Copernicus's *De Revolutionibus Orbium Coelestium* published in book form.

Today *De Revolutionibus* is recognized as one of the foundation stones of modern science, but soon after its appearance it was condemned by the Catholic Church (which did not lift its ban until 1835)

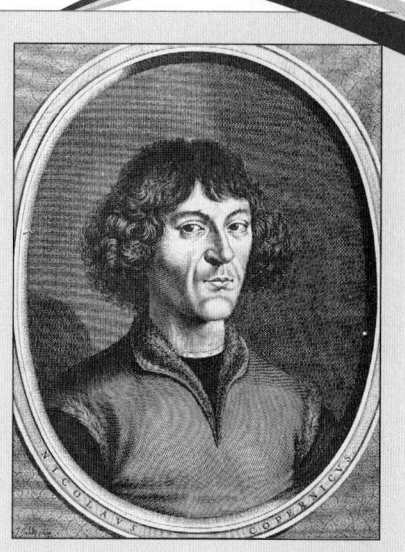

and had little impact on astronomy until Kepler further developed its concepts over a half century later.

to blow down buildings, trees, plants? The earth does spin rapidly, replied the followers of Copernicus, but the effects are counterbalanced by whatever force it is that holds our feet to the ground. Besides, if the speed of the earth's rotation is a problem, how much more of a problem would be the tremendous speeds of the sun, stars, and planets if they revolve, as Ptolemy thought, once a day around a fixed earth?

1.6 Kepler's Laws

How the Planets Actually Move

Fortunately, improvements in astronomical measurements—the first since the time of the Greeks—were not long in coming. Tycho Brahe (1546–1601), an astronomer working for the Danish king, built an observatory on the island of Hven near Copenhagen in which the instruments were remarkably precise (Fig. 1-9). With the help of these instruments, Tycho, blessed with exceptional eyesight and patience, made thousands of measurements, a labor that occupied much of his life. Even without the telescope, which had not yet been invented, Tycho's observatory was able to determine celestial angles to better than $\frac{1}{100}$ of a degree.

At his death in 1601, Tycho left behind his own somewhat peculiar model of the solar system, a body of superb data extending over many years, and an assistant named Johannes Kepler. Kepler regarded the copernican scheme "with incredible and ravishing delight," in his words, and fully expected that Tycho's improved figures would prove Copernicus correct once and for all. But this was not the case; after 4 years of work on the orbit of Mars alone, Kepler could not get Tycho's data to fit any of the models of the solar system that had by then been proposed.

If the facts do not agree with the theory, then the scientific method requires that the theory, no matter how attractive, must be discarded. Kepler then began to look for a new cosmic design that would fit Tycho's observations better.

Leap Years

A day is the time needed for the earth to make a complete turn on its axis, and a year is the time it needs to complete an orbit around the sun. The length of the year is slightly less than 365 days and 6 hours. Thus adding an extra day to February every 4 years (namely those years evenly divisible by 4, which are accordingly called **leap years**) keeps the seasons from shifting around the calendar.

The remaining discrepancy adds up to a full day too much every 128 years. To take care of most of this discrepancy, century years not divisible by 400 will not be leap years; thus 2000 was a leap year but 2100 will not be one.

Figure 1-9 A 1598 portrait of Tycho Brahe in his observatory. The man at the right is determining the position of a celestial body by shifting a sighting vane along a giant protractor until the body is visible through the aperture at upper left. There were four of each kind of instrument in the observatory, which were used simultaneously for reliable measurements.

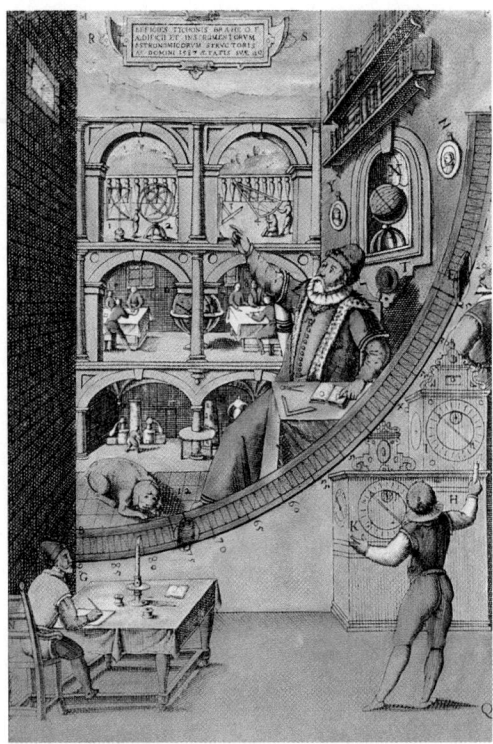

The First Law After considering every possibility, which meant years of drudgery in making calculations by hand, Kepler found that circular orbits for the planets were out of the question even when modified in various ways. He abandoned circular orbits reluctantly, for he was something of a mystic and believed, like Copernicus and the Greeks, that circles were the only fitting type of path for celestial bodies. Kepler then examined other geometrical figures, and here he found the key to the puzzle (Fig. 1-10). According to **Kepler's first law:**

> The paths of the planets around the sun are ellipses with the sun at one focus.

The Second Law Even this crucial discovery was not enough, as Kepler realized, to establish the courses of the planets through the sky. What was needed next was a way to relate the speeds of the planets to their positions in their elliptical orbits. Kepler could not be sure a general relationship of this kind even existed, and he was overjoyed when he had figured out the answer, known today as **Kepler's second law:**

> A planet moves so that its radius vector sweeps out equal areas in equal times.

The radius vector of a planet is an imaginary line between it and the sun. Thus in Fig. 1-11 each of the shaded areas is covered in the same period of time. This means that each planet travels faster when it is near the sun than when it is far away. The earth, for instance, has a speed of 30 km/s when it is nearest the sun and 29 km/s when it is farthest away, a difference of over 3 percent.

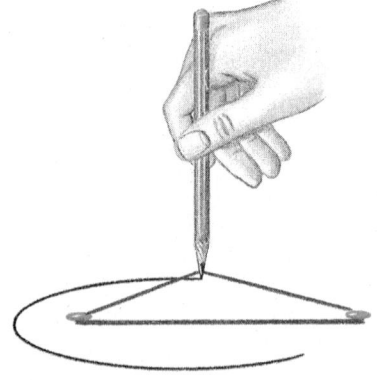

Figure 1-10 To draw an ellipse, place a loop of string over two tacks a short distance apart. Then move a pencil as shown, keeping the string taut. By varying the length of the string, ellipses of different shapes can be drawn. The points in an ellipse corresponding to the positions of the tacks are called **focuses;** the orbits of the planets are ellipses with the sun at one focus, which is Kepler's first law.

The Third Law A great achievement, but Kepler was not satisfied. He was obsessed with the idea of order and regularity in the universe, and spent 10 more years making calculations. It was already known that, the farther a planet is from the sun, the longer it takes to orbit the sun. **Kepler's third law** of planetary motion gives the exact relationship:

| Johannes Kepler (1571–1630)

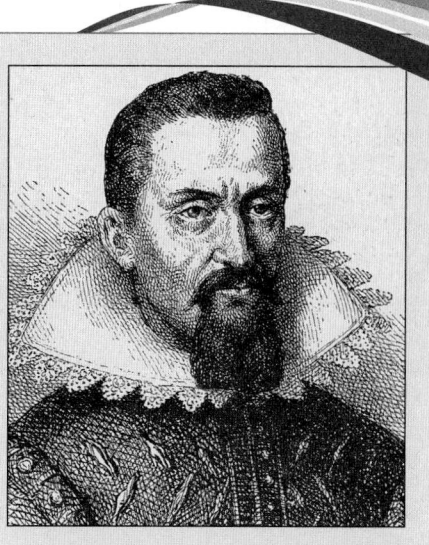

As a child, Kepler, who was born in Germany, was much impressed by seeing a comet and a total eclipse of the moon. In college, where astronomy was his worst subject, Kepler concentrated on theology, but his first job was as a teacher of mathematics and science in Graz, Austria. There he pondered the copernican system and concluded that the sun must exert a force (which he later thought was magnetic) on the planets to keep them in their orbits.

Kepler also devised a geometrical scheme to account for the spacing of the planetary orbits and put all his ideas into a book called *The Cosmic Mystery*. Tycho Brahe, the Danish astronomer, read the book and took Kepler on as an assistant in his new observatory in Prague in what was then Bohemia. Upon Brahe's death (the result of drinking

too much at a party given by the Emperor of Bohemia), Kepler replaced him at the observatory and gained access to all of Brahe's data, the most complete and accurate set then in existence.

Kepler felt that the copernican model of the solar system was not only capable of better agreement with the data than had yet been achieved but also contained within it yet-undiscovered regularities. Many years of labor resulted in three laws of planetary motion that fulfilled Kepler's vision and were to bear their ultimate fruit in Newton's law of gravity.

Kepler also found time to prepare new tables of planetary positions, to explain how telescopes produce magnified images, to father 13 children, and to prepare horoscopes for the Emperor of Bohemia,

the main reason for his employment (as it had been for Brahe). In 1620 Kepler's mother was accused of being a witch, but he was able to get her acquitted.

> The ratio between the square of the time needed by a planet to make a revolution around the sun and the cube of its average distance from the sun is the same for all the planets.

In equation form, this law states that

$$\frac{(\text{Period of planet})^2}{(\text{Average orbit radius})^3} = \text{same value for all the planets}$$

The period of a planet is the time needed for it to go once around the sun; in the case of the earth, the period is 1 year. Figure 1-12 illustrates Kepler's third law. Table 17-1 gives the values of the periods and average orbit radii for the planets.

At last the solar system could be interpreted in terms of simple motions. Planetary positions computed from Kepler's ellipses agreed not only with Tycho's data but also with observations made thousands of years earlier. Predictions could be made of positions of the planets in the future— accurate predictions this time, no longer approximations. Furthermore, Kepler's laws showed that the speed of a planet in different parts of its orbit was governed by a simple rule and that the speed was related to the size of the orbit.

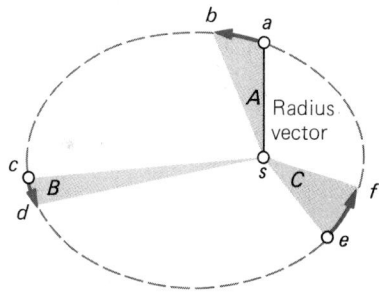

Area **A** = area **B** = area **C**

Figure 1-11 Kepler's second law. As a planet goes from *a* to *b* in its orbit, its radius vector (an imaginary line joining it with the sun) sweeps out the area A. In the same amount of time the planet can go from *c* to *d*, with its radius vector sweeping out the area B, or from *e* to *f*, with its radius vector sweeping out the area C. The three areas A, B, and C are equal.

1.7   Why Copernicus Was Right

Evidence Was Needed That Supported His Model
While Contradicting Ptolemy's Model

It is often said that Kepler proved that Copernicus was "right" and that Ptolemy was "wrong." True enough, the copernican system, by having

Occam's Razor

In science, as a general rule, the simplest explanation for a phenomenon is most likely to be correct: less is more. This principle was first clearly expressed by the medieval philosopher William of Occam (or Ockham), who was born in England in 1280. In 1746 the French philosopher Etienne de Condillac called the principle **Occam's razor,** an elegant metaphor that suggests cutting away unnecessary complications to get at the heart of the matter. Copernicus was one of many successful users of Occam's razor. To be sure, as when shaving with an actual razor, it is possible to go too far; as the mathematician Alfred Whitehead said, "Seek simplicity, and distrust it."

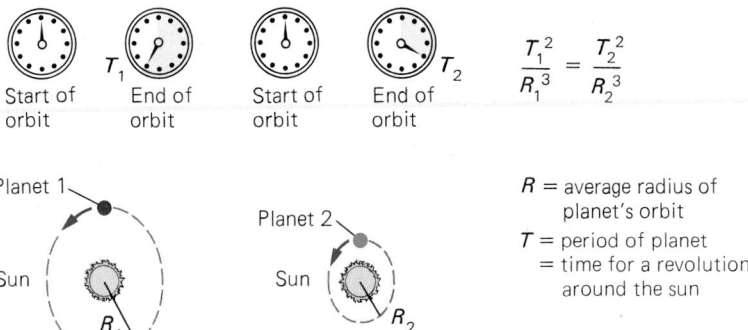

Figure 1-12   Kepler's third law states that the ratio T^2/R^3 is the same for all the planets.

Example 1.1

Kepler's laws should be obeyed by all satellite systems, not just the solar system. In the seventeenth century the French astronomer Cassini discovered four of Saturn's satellites (more have been discovered since). The names, periods, and orbit radii of these satellites are as follows:

Tethys	1.89 days	Rhea	4.52 days
	2.95×10^5 km		5.27×10^5 km
Dione	2.74 days	Iapetus	79.30 days
	3.77×10^5 km		35.60×10^5 km

Verify that Kepler's third law holds for these satellites.

Solution

What we must do is calculate the ratio T^2/R^3 for each satellite. The result for Tethys is

$$\frac{(1.89 \text{ days})^2}{(2.95 \times 10^5 \text{ km})^3} = 1.40 \times 10^{-16} \text{ days}^2/\text{km}^3$$

The ratio turns out to be the same for the other satellites as well, so we conclude that Kepler's third law holds for this satellite system. [Calculations that involve powers of ten are discussed in the Math Refresher at the end of this book. We note that $(10^5)^3 = 10^{3(5)} = 10^{15}$ and $1/10^{15} = 10^{-15}$.]

---

the planets move around the sun rather than around the earth, was simpler than the ptolemaic system. As modified by Kepler, the copernican system was also more accurate. However, the ptolemaic system could also be modified to be just as accurate, though in a very much more complicated way. Astronomers of the time squared themselves both with the practical needs of their profession and with the Church by using the copernican system for calculations while asserting the truth of the ptolemaic system.

The copernican system is attractive because it accounts in a straightforward way for many aspects of what we see in the sky. However, only observations that contradict the ptolemaic system can prove it wrong. The copernican system is today considered correct because there is direct evidence of various kinds for the motions of the planets around the sun and for the rotation of the earth. An example of such evidence is the change in apparent position of nearby stars relative to the background of distant ones as the earth revolves around the sun (Fig. 1-13), an effect called **parallax;** see Sec. 18.8. Shifts of this kind are small because all stars are far away, but they have been found.

Astrology

To our ancestors of thousands of years ago, things happened in the world because gods caused them to happen. Famine and war, earthquake and eclipse—any conceivable catastrophe—all occurred under divine control. In time the chief gods were identified with the sun, the moon, and the five planets visible to the naked eye: Mercury, Venus, Mars, Jupiter, and Saturn. Early observers of the sky were primarily interested in finding links between celestial events and earthly ones, a study that became known as **astrology.**

Until only a few hundred years ago, astronomy was almost entirely in the service of astrology. The wealth of precise astronomical measurements that ancient civilizations compiled had as their purpose interpreting the ways of the gods.

Almost nobody today takes seriously the mythology of old. Although the basis of the connection has disappeared, however, some people still believe that the position in the sky of various celestial bodies at certain times controls the world we live in and our individual destinies as well.

It does not seem very gracious for contemporary science to dismiss astrology in view of the great debt astronomy owes its practitioners of long ago. However, it is hard to have confidence in a doctrine that, for all its internal consistency and often delightful notions, nevertheless lacks any basis in scientific theory or observation and has proved no more useful in predicting the future than a crystal ball.

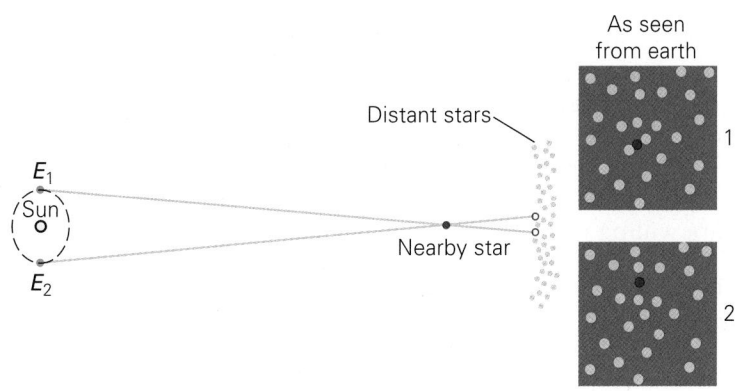

Figure 1-13   As a consequence of the earth's motion around the sun, nearby stars shift in apparent position relative to distant stars. The effect is known as parallax.

Universal Gravitation

As we know from everyday experience, and as we shall learn in a more precise way in Chap. 2, a force is needed to cause something to move in a curved path (Fig. 1-14). The planets are no exception to this rule: a force of some kind must be acting to hold them in their orbits around the sun. Three centuries ago Isaac Newton had the inspired idea that this force must have the same character as the familiar force of gravity that pulls things to the earth's surface.

1.8   What Is Gravity?

A Fundamental Force

Perhaps, thought Newton, the moon revolves around the earth much as the ball in Fig. 1-14 revolves around the hand holding the string, with gravity taking the place of the pull of the string. In other words, perhaps the moon is a falling object, pulled to the earth just as we are, but moving so fast in its orbit that the earth's pull is just enough to keep the moon from flying off (Fig. 1-15). The earth and its sister planets might well be held in their orbits by a stronger gravitational pull from the sun. These notions turned out to be true, and Newton was able to show that his detailed theory of gravity accounts for Kepler's laws.

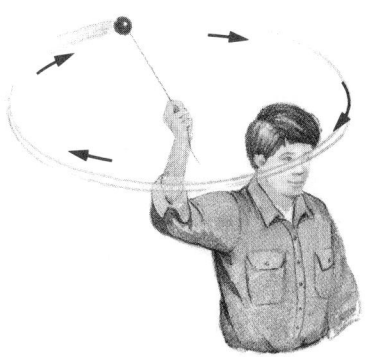

Figure 1-14   An inward force is needed to keep an object moving in a curved path. The force here is provided by the string. If no force acts on it, a moving object will continue moving in a straight line at constant speed. (This is Newton's first law of motion and is discussed in Sec. 2.7.)

Figure 1-15   The gravitational pull of the earth on the moon causes the moon to move in an orbit around the earth. If the earth exerted no force on the moon, the moon would fly off into space. If the moon had no orbital motion, it would fall directly to the earth.

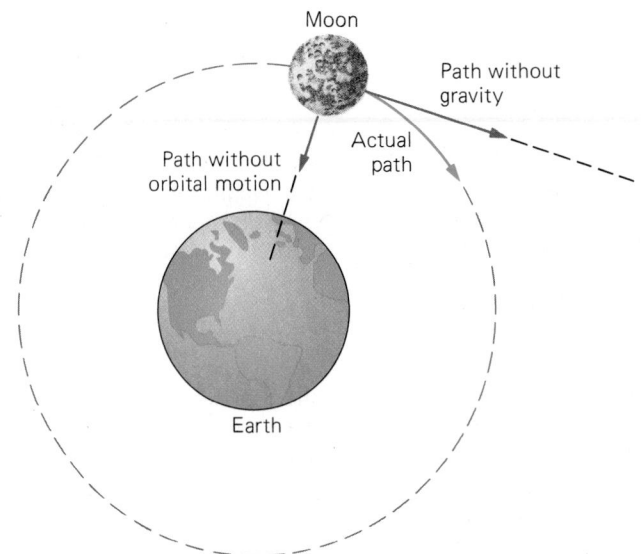

It is worth noting that Newton's discovery of the **law of gravity** depended on the copernican model of the solar system. "Common sense" tells us that the earth is the stationary center of the universe, and people were once severely punished for believing otherwise. Clearly the progress of our knowledge about the world we live in depends upon people, like Copernicus, who are able to look behind the screen of appearances that make up everyday life and who are willing to think for themselves.

Fundamental Forces   Gravity is a **fundamental force** in the sense that it cannot be explained in terms of any other force. Only four fundamental forces are known: gravitational, electromagnetic, weak, and strong. These forces are responsible for everything that happens in the universe. Gravitational forces act between all bodies everywhere and hold together planets, stars, and the giant groups of stars called galaxies. Electromagnetic forces, which (like gravity) are unlimited in range, act between electrically charged particles and govern the structures and behavior of atoms, molecules, solids, and liquids. When a bat hits a ball, the interaction between them can be traced to electromagnetic forces. The weak and strong forces have very short ranges and act inside atomic nuclei. (Fundamental forces are further discussed in Sec. 8.14.)

The Law of Gravity Is the Same Everywhere   How can we be sure that Newton's law of gravity, which fits data on the solar system, also holds throughout the rest of the universe? The evidence for this generalization is indirect but persuasive. For instance, many double stars are known in which each member of the pair revolves around the other, which means some force holds them together. Throughout the universe stars occur in galaxies, and only gravity could keep them assembled in this way.

But is the gravity that acts between stars the same as the gravity that acts in the solar system? Analyzing the light and radio waves that reach us from space shows that the matter in the rest of the universe is the same as the matter found on the earth. If we are to believe that the universe contains objects that do not obey Newton's law of gravity, we must have evidence for such a belief—and there is none. This line of thought may not seem as positive as we might prefer, but taken together with various theoretical arguments, it has convinced nearly all scientists that gravity is the same everywhere.

BIOGRAPHY | Isaac Newton (1642–1727)

Although his mother wanted him to stay on the family farm in England, the young Newton showed a talent for science and went to Cambridge University for further study. An outbreak of plague led the university to close in 1665, the year Newton graduated, and he returned home for 18 months.

In that period Newton came up with the binomial theorem of algebra; invented calculus, which gave science and engineering a new and powerful mathematical tool; discovered the law of gravity, thereby not only showing why the planets move as they do but also providing the key to understanding much else about the universe; and demonstrated that white light is a composite of light of all colors—an amazing list. As Newton later wrote, "In those days I was in the prime of my age for invention, and minded mathematics and philosophy more than at any time since."

Legend has it that Newton's interest turned to gravity when he was struck on the head by a failing apple. Newton's own recollection was given to a visiting friend: "We went

into the garden and drank tea, under some apple trees . . . he told me he was just in the same situation when the notion of gravitation came into his mind. 'Why should that apple always descend perpendicularly to the ground,' thought he to himself."

When Cambridge University reopened, Newton went back and 2 years later became professor of mathematics there. He lived quietly and never married, carrying out experimental as well as theoretical research in many areas of physics; a reflecting telescope he made with his own hands was widely admired.

Especially significant was Newton's development of the laws of motion (see Chap. 2), which showed exactly how force and motion are related, and his application of them to a variety of problems. Newton collected the results of his work on mechanics in the *Principia*, a scientific classic that was published in 1687. A later book, *Opticks*, summarized his efforts in this field. Newton also spent much time on chemistry, though here with little success.

After writing the *Principia*, Newton began to drift away from science.

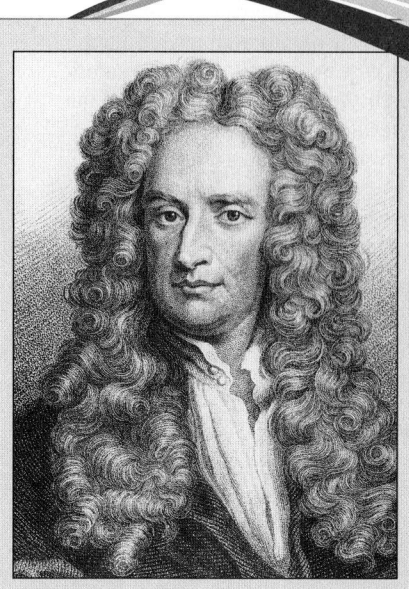

He became a member of Parliament in 1689 and later an official, eventually the Master, of the British Mint. At the Mint Newton helped reform the currency (one of Kepler's interests, too) and fought counterfeiters. Newton's spare time in his last 30 years was mainly spent in trying to date events in the Bible. He died at 85, a figure of honor whose stature remains great to this day.

1.9   Why the Earth Is Round

The Big Squeeze

A sign of success of any scientific theory is its ability to account for previously mysterious findings. One such finding is the roundness of the earth (Fig. 1-16), which was known by the Greeks as long ago as the fifth century B.C. (Fig. 1-17). Early thinkers believed the earth was round because a sphere is the only "perfect" shape, a vague idea that actually explains nothing. In fact, the earth is round because gravity squeezes it into this shape.

As shown in Fig. 1-18, if any part of the earth were to stick out very much, the gravitational attraction of the rest of the earth would pull downward on the projection. The material underneath would then flow out sideways until the projection became level or nearly so. The downward forces around the rim of a deep hole would similarly cause the surrounding material to flow into it. The same argument applies to the moon, the sun, and the stars.

Such irregularities as mountains and ocean basins are on a very small scale compared with the earth's size. The total range from the Pacific depths to the summit of Everest is less than 20 km, not much compared with the earth's radius of 6400 km.

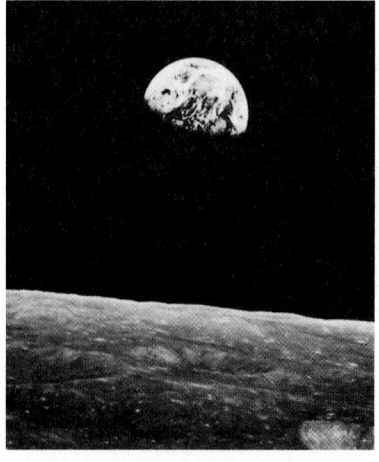

Figure 1-16   Astronauts in the Apollo 11 spacecraft saw this view of the earth as they orbited the moon, part of whose bleak landscape appears in the foreground. The earth is indeed round.

Figure 1-17   In the distant past evidence for the spherical shape of the earth came from travelers who found that, when they went north, more stars stayed above the horizon all night, and that, when they went south, additional stars became visible. Eratosthenes (276–194 B.C.) determined the earth's size with remarkable accuracy by comparing the length of the sun's shadow at noon on the same day in two places on the same north-south line.

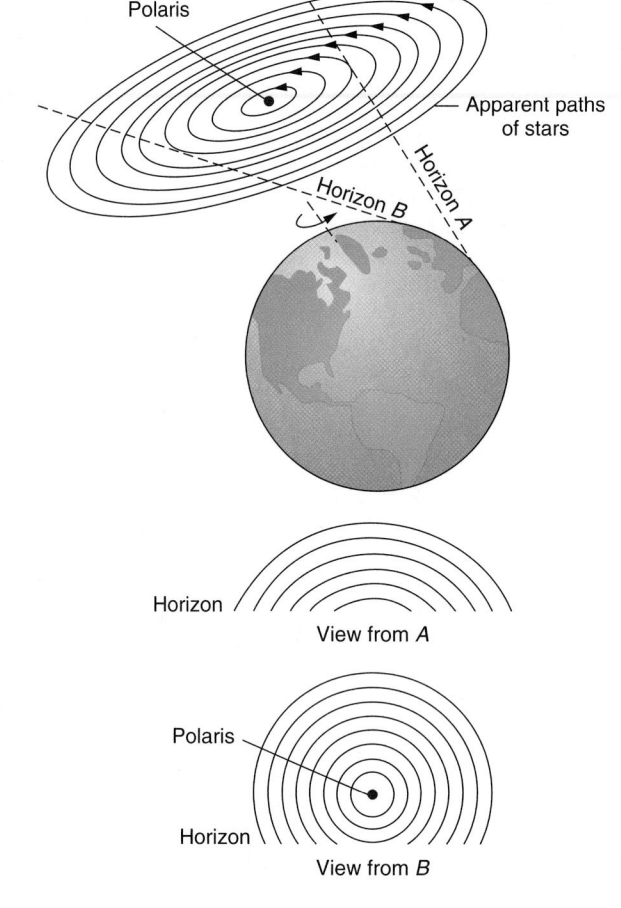

Figure 1-18   Gravity forces the earth to be round. *(a)* How a large bump would be pulled down. *(b)* How a large hole would be filled in.

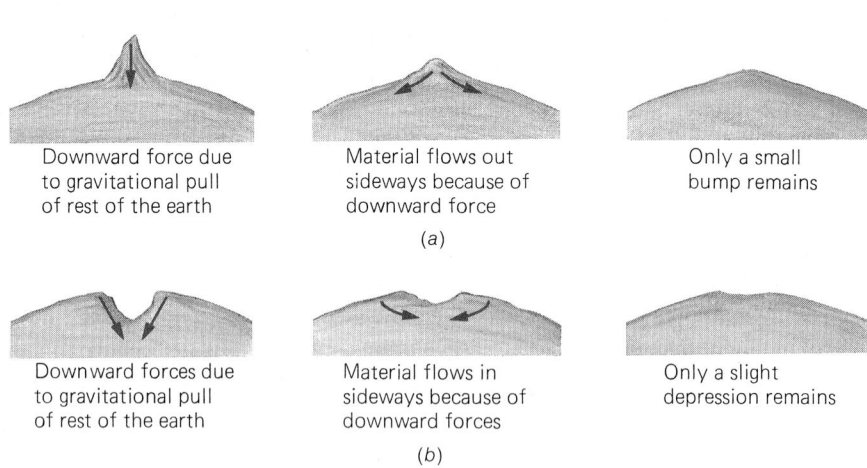

The earth is not a perfect sphere. The reason was apparent to Newton: since the earth is spinning rapidly, inertia causes the equatorial portion to swing outward, just as a ball on a string does when it is whirled around. As a result the earth bulges slightly at the equator and is slightly flattened at the poles, much like a grapefruit. The total distortion is not great, for the earth is only 43 km wider than it is high (Fig. 1-19). Venus, whose "day" is 243 of our days, turns so slowly that it has almost no distortion. Saturn, at the other extreme, spins so rapidly that it is almost 10 percent out of round.

1.10   The Tides

Up and Down Twice a Day

Those of us who live near an ocean know well the rhythm of the tides, the twice-daily rise and fall of water level. Usually the change in height is no more than a few meters, but in some regions—the Bay of Fundy in eastern Canada is one—the total range can be over 20 m. What causes the advance and retreat of the oceans on such a grand scale?

One factor is that the moon gravitationally attracts different parts of the earth to different extents. In Fig. 1-20 the moon's tug is strongest at *A*, which is closest, and weakest at *B*, which is farthest away. Also, the rotation of the moon around the earth is too simple a picture—what actually happens is that both bodies rotate around the center of mass (CM) of the earth-moon system. (Think of the earth and the moon as opposite ends of a dumbbell. The CM is the balance point of the dumbbell; it is inside the earth 4700 km from its center.)

As it wobbles around the CM, the solid earth is pulled away from the water at *B*, where the moon's tug is weakest, to leave the water there heaped up in a tidal bulge. At *A*, the greater tug of the moon dominates to cause a tidal bulge there as well. The bulges stay in place as the earth revolves under them to produce two high tides and two low tides at a given place every day (Fig. 1-21).

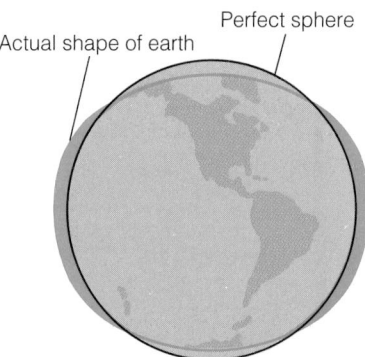

Figure 1-19   The influence of its rotation distorts the earth. The effect is greatly exaggerated in the figure; the equatorial diameter of the earth is actually only 43 km (27 mi) more than its polar diameter.

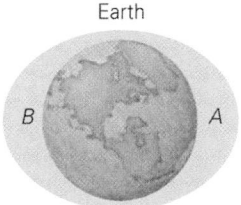
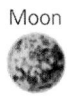

Figure 1-20   The origin of the tides. The moon's attraction for the waters of the earth is greatest at *A*, least at *B*. As the earth and moon rotate around the center of mass of the earth-moon system, which is located inside the earth, water is heaped up at *A* and *B*. The water bulges stay in place as the earth turns on its axis to produce two high and two low tides every day. As the earth turns under the bulges, friction between the oceans and the ocean floors slows down the earth's rotation. As a result the tidal bulges lag slightly behind the earth-moon line. The effect of tidal friction is thus to lengthen the day. The rate of increase is a mere 1 s per day in every 43,500 years, but it adds up. Measurements of the daily growth markings on fossil corals show that the day was only 22 h long 380 million years ago.

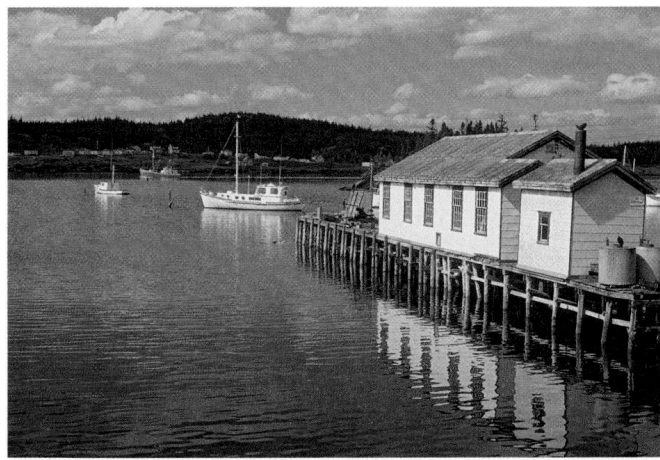
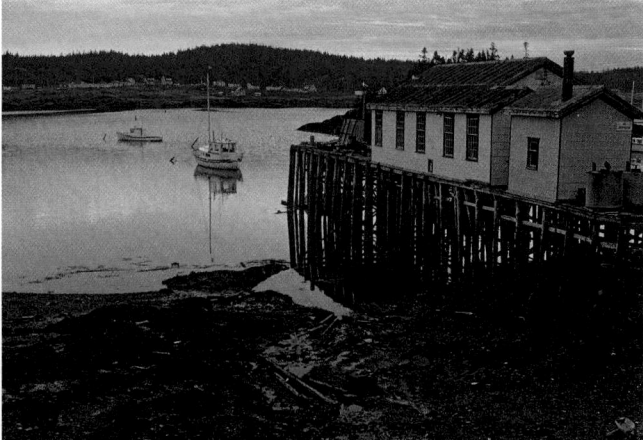

Figure 1-21   High and low water in the Bay of Fundy at Blacks Harbour in New Brunswick, Canada. Two tidal cycles occur daily.

Figure 1-22   Variation of the tides. Spring tides are produced when the moon is at M_1 or M_2, neap tides when the moon is at M_3 or M_4. The range between high and low water is greatest for spring tides.

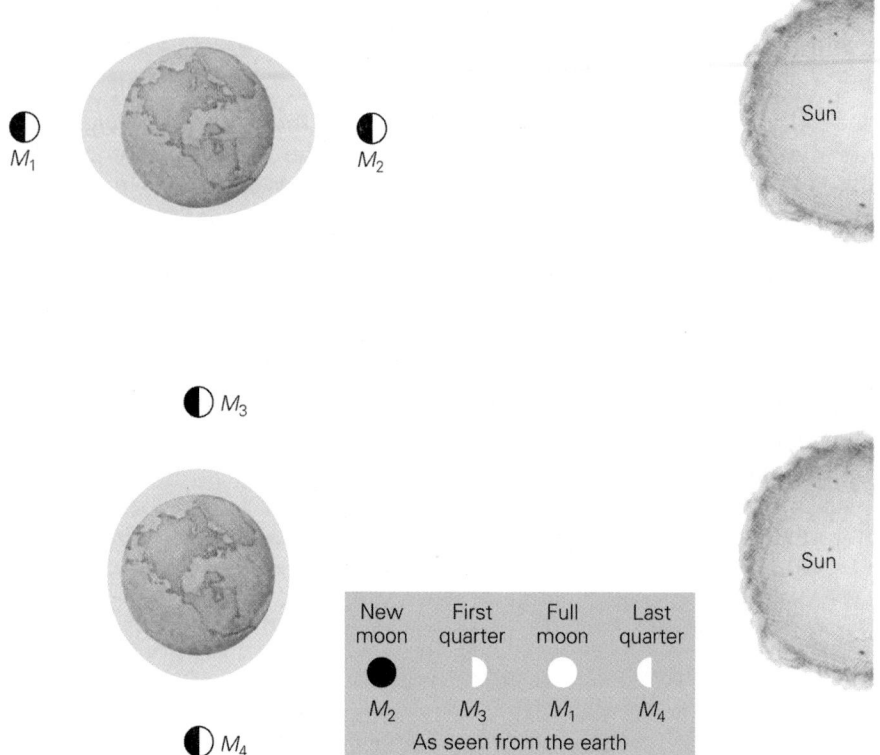

New moon	First quarter	Full moon	Last quarter
●	◖	○	◗
M_2	M_3	M_1	M_4

As seen from the earth

Spring and Neap Tides

There is more to the story. The sun also affects the waters of the earth, but to a smaller extent than the moon even though the gravitational tug of the sun exceeds that of the moon. The reason is that what is involved in the tides is the *difference* between the attractions on the near and far sides of the earth, and this difference is greater for the moon because it is closer to the earth than the sun. About twice a month—when the sun, moon, and earth are in a straight line—solar tides add to lunar tides to give the especially high (and low) **spring tides;** see Fig. 1-22. When the line between moon and earth is perpendicular to that between sun and earth, the tide-raising forces partly cancel to give **neap tides,** whose range is smaller than average.

1.11   The Discovery of Neptune

Another Triumph for the Law of Gravity

In Newton's time, as in Ptolemy's, only six planets were known: Mercury, Venus, Earth, Mars, Jupiter, and Saturn. In 1781 a seventh, Uranus, was identified. Measurements during the next few years enabled astronomers to work out details of the new planet's orbit and to predict its future positions in the sky. To make these predictions, not only the sun's attraction but also the smaller attractions of the nearby planets Jupiter and Saturn had to be considered. For 40 years, about half the time needed for Uranus to make one complete revolution around the sun, calculated positions of the planet agreed well with observed positions.

Then a discrepancy crept in. Little by little Uranus moved away from its predicted path among the stars. The calculations were checked and rechecked, but no mistake could be found. There were two possibilities: either the law of gravity, on which the calculations were based, was wrong, or else some unknown body was pulling Uranus away from its predicted path.

So firmly established was the law of gravitation that two young men, Urbain Leverrier in France and John Couch Adams in England, set themselves the task of calculating the orbit of an unknown body that might be responsible for the discrepancies in Uranus's position. Adams sent a sketchy account of his studies to George Airy, England's Astronomer Royal. Because the calculations were incomplete, although later found to be correct as far as they went, Airy asked for further details. Adams (who later blamed habitual lateness and a dislike of writing) did not respond.

A year later, in 1846, Leverrier, with no knowledge of Adams's work, went further and proposed an actual position in the sky where the new planet should be found. He sent his result to a German astronomer, Johan Gottlieb Galle, who turned his telescope to the part of the sky where the new planet should appear. Very close to the position predicted by Leverrier, Galle found a faint object, which had moved slightly by the following night. This was indeed the eighth member of the sun's family and was called Neptune. The theory of gravity had again successfully gone around the loop of the scientific method shown in Fig. 1-1.

How Many of What

When we say that the distance between Chicago and Minneapolis is 405 miles, what we are really doing is comparing this distance with a certain standard length called the mile. Standard quantities such as the mile are known as **units.** The result of every measurement thus has two parts. One is a number (405 for the Chicago-Minneapolis distance) to answer the question "How many?" The other is a unit (the mile in this case) to answer the question "Of what?"

1.12   The SI System

All Scientists Use These Units

The most widely used units today are those of the International System, abbreviated **SI** after its French name Système International d'Unités. Examples of SI units are the **meter** (m) for length, the **second** (s) for time, the **kilogram** (kg) for mass, the **joule** (J) for energy, and the **watt** (W) for power. SI units are used universally by scientists and in most of the world in everyday life as well. Although the British system of units, with its familiar foot and pound, remains in common use only in a few English-speaking countries, it is on the way out and eventually will be replaced by the SI. Since this is a book about science, only SI units will be used from here on.

The great advantage of SI units is that their subdivisions and multiples are in steps of 10, 100, 1000, and so on, in contrast to the irregularity of British units. In the case of lengths, for instance (Fig. 1-23),

$$1 \text{ meter (m)} = 100 \text{ centimeters (cm)}$$
$$1 \text{ kilometer (km)} = 1000 \text{ meters}$$

whereas

$$1 \text{ foot (ft)} = 12 \text{ inches (in.)}$$
$$1 \text{ mile (mi)} = 5280 \text{ feet}$$

Meter, Kilogram, Second

SI units are derived from the units of the older **metric system.** This system was introduced in France two centuries ago to replace the hodgepodge of traditional units, often different in different countries and even in different parts of the same country, that was making commerce and industry difficult.

The **meter,** the standard of length, was originally defined as one ten-millionth of the distance from the equator to the North Pole. The **gram,** the standard of mass, was defined as the mass of 1 cubic centimeter (cm^3) of water; 1 cm^3 is the volume of a cube 1 cm (0.01 m) on each edge, and 1 kilogram = 1000 grams. The

meter and gram were new units. The ancient division of a day into 24 hours, an hour into 60 minutes, and a minute into 60 seconds was kept for the definition of the second as $1/(24)(60)(60) = 1/86{,}400$ of a day.

As more and more precision became needed, these definitions were modified several times. Today the second is specified in terms of the microwave radiation given off under certain circumstances by one type of cesium atom, ^{133}Cs: 1 s equals the time needed for 9,192,631,770 cycles of this radiation to be emitted.

The meter, which for convenience had become the distance between two scratches on a

platinum-iridium bar kept at Sèvres, France, is now the distance traveled in 1/299,792,458 s by light in a vacuum. There are approximately 3.28 feet in a meter.

The kilogram is the mass of a platinum-iridium cylinder 39 mm in diameter and 39 mm high at Sèvres. Despite much effort, a unit of mass based on a physical property measurable anywhere has not proved practical as yet. As discussed in Sec. 2.10, mass and weight are not the same. The weight of a given mass is the force with which gravity attracts it to the earth; the weight of 1 kg is 2.2 pounds on the earth's surface and decreases with altitude (see Fig. 2-38).

Figure 1-23 There are 1000 meters in a kilometer and 100 centimeters in a meter.

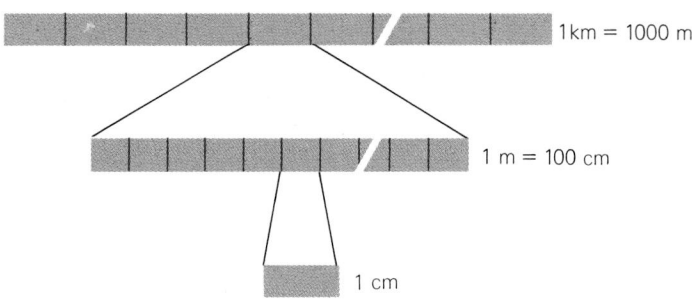

1 km = 1000 m

1 m = 100 cm

1 cm

Table 1-1	Subdivisions and Multiples of SI Units (The Symbol μ Is the Greek Letter "mu")			
Prefix	**Power of 10**	**Abbreviation**	**Pronunciation**	**Common Name**
Pico-	10^{-12}	p	pee' koe	Trillionth
Nano-	10^{-9}	n	nan' oe	Billionth
Micro-	10^{-6}	μ	my' kroe	Millionth
Milli-	10^{-3}	m	mil' i	Thousandth
Centi-	10^{-2}	c	sen' ti	Hundredth
Hecto-	10^{2}	h	hec' toe	Hundred
Kilo-	10^{3}	k	kil' oe	Thousand
Mega-	10^{6}	M	meg' a	Million
Giga-	10^{9}	G	ji' ga	Billion
Tera-	10^{12}	T	ter' a	Trillion

Table 1-1 lists the most common subdivisions and multiples of SI units. Each is designated by a prefix according to the corresponding power of 10. (Powers of 10 are widely used in science. What they mean and how to make calculations with them are reviewed in the Math Refresher at the back of the book starting on p. A-1.)

Example 1.2

How many nanometers are in a kilometer?

Solution

A nanometer is a billionth (10^{-9}) of a meter and a kilometer is a thousand (10^3) meters. Hence

$$\frac{\text{kilometer}}{\text{nanometer}} = \frac{10^3 \text{ m}}{10^{-9} \text{ m}} = 10^{12}$$

There are 10^{12}—a trillion—nanometers in a kilometer. [We note from the Math Refresher that $10^n/10^m = 10^{n-m}$, so here $10^3/10^{-9} = 10^{3-(-9)} = 10^{3+9} = 10^{12}$.]

Table 1-2	Conversion Factors for Length	
Multiply a Length Expressed in	**By**	**To Get the Same Length Expressed in**
Centimeters	$0.394 \, \frac{\text{in.}}{\text{cm}}$	Inches
Meters	$39.4 \, \frac{\text{in.}}{\text{m}}$	Inches
Meters	$3.28 \, \frac{\text{ft}}{\text{m}}$	Feet
Kilometers	$0.621 \, \frac{\text{mi}}{\text{km}}$	Miles
Inches	$2.54 \, \frac{\text{cm}}{\text{in.}}$	Centimeters
Feet	$30.5 \, \frac{\text{cm}}{\text{ft}}$	Centimeters
Feet	$0.305 \, \frac{\text{m}}{\text{ft}}$	Meters
Miles	$1.61 \, \frac{\text{km}}{\text{mi}}$	Kilometers

Table 1-2 contains conversion factors for changing a length expressed in one system to its equivalent in the other. (More conversion factors are given inside the back cover of this book.) We note from the table that there are about $2\frac{1}{2}$ centimeters in an inch, so a centimeter is roughly the width of a shirt button; a meter is a few inches longer than 3 feet; and a kilometer is nearly $\frac{2}{3}$ mile.

Significant Figures   In Example 1-3 the distance expressed in centimeters is 8.78×10^4 cm. Does this mean that $d = 87,800$ cm exactly?

The answer is, not necessarily. We are only sure of the three digits 8, 7, and 8, which are the **significant figures** here. By writing $d = 8.78 \times 10^4$ cm we can see just how precisely the distance is being expressed. If we needed less precision, we could round off the value of d to 8.8×10^4 cm. However, we could *not* write $d = 8.780 \times 10^4$ cm, which contains four significant figures, because the original distance was given as 878 m, which has only three such figures.

In part (b) of Example 1-3, the actual result of the calculation is

$$d = (0.878 \text{ km})(0.621 \text{ mi/km}) = 0.545238 \text{ mi}$$

Because both the initial numbers had only three significant figures, the result can only have three also, so it was given as $d = 0.545$ mi.

Example 1.3

A few years ago a NASA official quoted a distance of 878 m to a reporter and added, "I don't know what this is in terms of kilometers or miles." Let us help him.

Solution

(a) Since 1 km = 10^3 m = 1000 m, the distance in kilometers is

$$d = \frac{878 \text{ m}}{1000 \text{ m/km}} = 0.878 \text{ km}$$

We note that

$$\frac{1}{\text{m/km}} = \frac{\text{km}}{\text{m}}$$

and therefore

$$\frac{\text{m}}{\text{m/km}} = \frac{(\cancel{\text{m}})(\text{km})}{\cancel{\text{m}}} = \text{km}$$

If instead we wanted this distance in centimeters, we would proceed in this way:

$$d = (878 \text{ m})(10^2 \text{ cm/m}) = 878 \times 10^2 \text{ cm} = (8.78 \times 10^2)(10^2) \text{ cm}$$
$$= 8.78 \times 10^{2+2} \text{ cm} = 8.78 \times 10^4 \text{ cm}$$

This is the usual way such a quantity would be expressed. The Math Refresher at the end of the book might come in handy here.

(b) From Table 1-2 the conversion factor we need is 0.621 mi/km, so

$$d = (0.878 \text{ \cancel{km}})\left(0.621 \frac{\text{mi}}{\cancel{\text{km}}}\right) = 0.545 \text{ mi}$$

When a calculation has several steps, it is a good idea to keep an extra digit in the intermediate steps. Then, at the end, the final result can be rounded off to the correct number of significant figures.

For simplicity, in this book zeros after the decimal point have usually been omitted from values given in problems. For instance, it should be assumed that when a length of 7 m is stated, what is really meant is 7.000 . . . m.

Important Terms and Ideas

The **scientific method** of studying nature has four steps: (1) formulating a problem; (2) observation and experiment; (3) interpreting the results; (4) testing the interpretation by further observation and experiment. When first proposed, a scientific interpretation is called a **hypothesis**. After thorough checking, it becomes a **law** if it states a regularity or relationship, or a **theory** if it uses general considerations to account for specific phenomena.

Polaris, the North Star, lies almost directly above the North Pole. A **constellation** is a group of stars that form a pattern in the sky. The **planets** are heavenly bodies that shift their positions regularly with respect to the stars.

In the **ptolemaic system,** the earth is stationary at the center of the universe. In the **copernican system,** the earth rotates on its axis and, with the other planets, revolves around the sun. Observational evidence supports the copernican system.

Kepler's laws are three regularities that the planets obey as they move around the sun.

Newton's **law of gravity** describes the attraction all bodies in the universe have for one another. The gravitational forces the sun exerts on the planets are what hold them in their orbits. Kepler's laws are explained by the law of gravity.

The **tides** are periodic rises and falls of sea level caused by differences in the gravitational pulls of the moon and sun. Water facing the moon is attracted to it more than the earth itself is, and the earth moves away from water on its far side. The corresponding effect of the sun is smaller than that of the moon and acts to increase or decrease tidal ranges, depending on the relative positions of the moon and sun.

To measure something means to compare it with a standard quantity of the same kind called a **unit.** The **SI** system of units is used everywhere by scientists and in most of the world in everyday life as well. The SI unit of length is the **meter** (m).

The **significant figures** in a number are its accurately known digits. When numbers are combined arithmetically, the result has as many significant figures as those in the number with the fewest of them.

Multiple Choice

1. The "scientific method" is
   a. a continuing process
   b. a way to arrive at ultimate truth
   c. a laboratory technique
   d. based on accepted laws and theories

2. A scientific law or theory is valid
   a. forever
   b. for a certain number of years, after which it is retested
   c. as long as a committee of scientists says so
   d. as long as it is not contradicted by new experimental findings

3. A hypothesis is
   a. a new scientific idea
   b. a scientific idea that has been confirmed by further experiment and observation
   c. a scientific idea that has been discarded because it disagrees with further experiment and observation
   d. a group of linked scientific ideas

4. The ongoing evolution of living things
   a. is one of the basic concepts of biology
   b. is one of the basic concepts of Intelligent Design
   c. has no basis in observation
   d. is in conflict with all religions

5. The object in the sky that apparently moves least in the course of time is
   a. Polaris   **c.** the sun
   b. Venus   **d.** the moon

6. A constellation is
   a. an especially bright star
   b. an apparent pattern of stars in the sky
   c. a group of stars close together in space
   d. a group of planets close together in space

7. Which of the following is no longer considered valid?
   a. the ptolemaic system
   b. the copernican system
   c. Kepler's laws of planetary motion
   d. Newton's law of gravity

8. A planet not visible to the naked eye is
   a. Mars   **c.** Mercury
   b. Venus   **d.** Neptune

9. The planet closest to the sun is
   a. earth   **c.** Mars
   b. Venus   **d.** Mercury

10. Leap years are needed because
    a. the earth's orbit is not a perfect circle
    b. the length of the day varies
    c. the length of the year varies
    d. the length of the year is not a whole number of days

11. Kepler modified the copernican system by showing that the planetary orbits are
    a. ellipses
    b. circles

    c. combinations of circles forming looped orbits
    d. the same distance apart from one another

12. The speed of a planet in its orbit around the sun
    a. is constant
    b. is highest when the planet is closest to the sun
    c. is lowest when the planet is closest to the sun
    d. varies, but not with respect to the planet's distance from the sun

13. According to Kepler's third law, the time needed for a planet to complete an orbit around the sun
    a. is the same for all the planets
    b. depends on the planet's size
    c. depends on the planet's distance from the sun
    d. depends on how fast the planet spins on its axis

14. The law of gravity
    a. applies only to large bodies such as planets and stars
    b. accounts for all known forces
    c. holds only in the solar system
    d. holds everywhere in the universe

15. The earth bulges slightly at the equator and is flattened at the poles because
    a. it spins on its axis
    b. it revolves around the sun
    c. of the sun's gravitational pull
    d. of the moon's gravitational pull

16. The usual tidal pattern in most parts of the world consists of
    a. a high tide one day and a low tide on the next
    b. one high tide and one low tide daily
    c. two high tides and two low tides daily
    d. three high tides and three low tides daily

17. Tides are caused
    a. only by the sun
    b. only by the moon
    c. by both the sun and the moon
    d. sometimes by the sun and sometimes by the moon

18. High tide occurs at a given place
    a. only when the moon faces the place
    b. only when the moon is on the opposite side of the earth from the place
    c. both when the moon faces the place and when the moon is on the opposite side of the earth from the place
    d. when the place is halfway between facing the moon and being on the opposite side of the earth from the moon

19. The prefix micro stands for
    a. 1/10   **c.** 1/1000
    b. 1/100   **d.** 1/1,000,000

20. A centimeter is
    a. 0.001 m   **c.** 0.1 m
    b. 0.01 m   **d.** 10 m

21. Of the following, the shortest is
    a. 1 mm   **c.** 0.001 m
    b. 0.01 in.   **d.** 0.001 ft

22. Of the following, the longest is
    a. 1000 ft   **c.** 1 km
    b. 500 m   **d.** 1 mi

23. A person is 180 cm tall. This is equivalent to
    a. 4 ft 6 in.   **c.** 5 ft 11 in.
    b. 5 ft 9 in.   **d.** 7 ft 1 in.

24. The measurements of a room are given as length = 5.28 m and width = 3.1 m. Since (5.28)(3.1) = 16.368, the room's area is correctly expressed as
    a. 16 m^2 **c.** 16.4 m^2
    b. 16.0 m^2 **d.** 16.368 m^2

Exercises

1.2 Why Science Is Successful

1. What role does "common sense" play in the scientific method?

2. What is the basic distinction between the scientific method and other ways of looking at the natural world?

3. What is the difference between a hypothesis and a law? Between a law and a theory?

4. Scientific models do not correspond exactly to reality. Why are they nevertheless so useful?

5. According to the physicist Richard Feynman, "Science is the culture of doubt." Does this mean that science is an unreliable guide to the natural world?

1.3 A Survey of the Sky

6. What does a year correspond to in terms of observations of the sun and stars?

7. You are lost in the northern hemisphere in the middle of nowhere on a clear night. How could you tell the direction of north by looking at the sky?

8. In terms of what you would actually observe, what does it mean to say that the moon apparently moves eastward among the stars?

9. What must be your location if the stars move across the sky in circles centered directly overhead?

1.5 The Copernican System

10. How do leap years fit into the ptolemaic system? Into the copernican system?

11. From observations of the moon, why would you conclude that it is a relatively small body revolving around the earth rather than another planet revolving around the sun?

12. The sun, moon, and planets all follow approximately the same path from east to west across the sky. What does this suggest about the arrangement of these members of the solar system in space?

13. What is the basic difference between the ptolemaic and copernican models? Why is the ptolemaic model considered incorrect?

14. Ancient astronomers were troubled by variations in the brightnesses of the various planets with time. Does the ptolemaic or the copernican model account better for these variations?

15. Compare the ptolemaic and copernican explanations for (a) the rising and setting of the sun; (b) the eastward drift of the sun relative to the stars that takes a year for a complete circuit; (c) the eastward drift of the moon relative to the stars that takes about 4 weeks for a complete circuit.

16. What do you think is the reason scientists use an ellipse rather than a circle as the model for a planetary orbit?

17. The average distance from the earth to the sun is called the astronomical unit (AU). If an asteroid is 4 AU from the sun and its period of revolution around the sun is 8 years, does it obey Kepler's third law?

1.7 Why Copernicus Was Right

18. As the earth revolves around the sun, some stars seem to shift their positions during the year relative to other stars. How is this effect (called parallax) explained in the ptolemaic system? In the copernican system?

1.8 What Is Gravity?

19. Why is gravity considered a fundamental force whereas the force a bat exerts on a ball is not?

1.9 Why The Earth Is Round

20. What, if anything, would happen to the shape of the earth if it were to rotate on its axis faster than it does today?

1.10 The Tides

21. What is the difference between spring and neap tides? Under what circumstances does each occur?

22. The length of the day has varied. When did the longest day thus far occur?

23. The earth takes almost exactly 24 h to make a complete turn on its axis, so we might expect each high tide to occur 12 h after the one before. However, the actual time between high tides is 12 h 25 min. Can you account for the difference?

24. Does the sun or the moon have the greater influence in causing tides?

1.12 The SI System

25. In the following pairs of length units, which is the shorter: inch, centimeter? Yard, meter? Mile, kilometer?

26. A European driving from Paris to Brussels finds she has covered 291 km. How many miles is this?

27. The world's tallest tree is a sequoia in California 368 ft high. How high is this in meters? In kilometers?

28. The diameter of an atom is roughly 10^4 times the diameter of its nucleus. If the nucleus of an atom were 1 mm across, how many feet across would the atom be?

29. How many square feet are there in an area of 1.00 square meters? Use the proper number of significant figures in the answer.

30. A swimming pool is exactly 20 m long, 7 m wide, and 2 m deep. What is its volume in cubic feet to 3 significant figures?

31. The speedometer of a European car gives its speed in kilometers per hour. What is the car's speed in miles per hour when the speedometer reads 80?

32. A horse galloped a mile in 2 min 35 s. What was its average speed in km/h?

33. How many microphones are there in a megaphone?

34. Use the proper number of significant figures to express the values of

　a. $47.2 + 9.11 - 14$

　b. $(3.58 \times 10^2)(2.1 \times 10^3)$

　c. $\dfrac{7.8 \times 10^3}{3.21 \times 10^{-2}} + 5.4 \times 10^4$

　d. $\sqrt{68}$

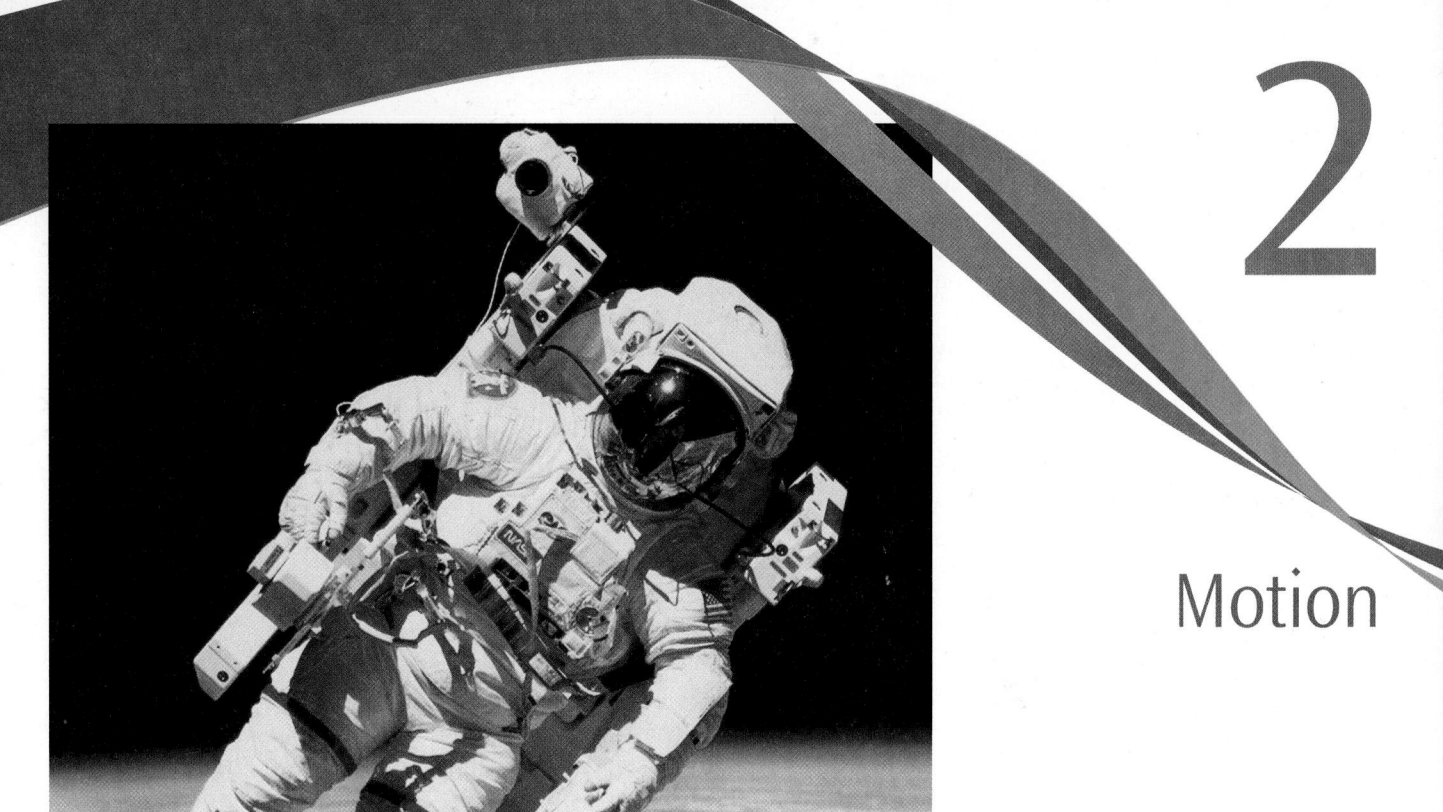

Astronaut Bruce McCandless near the orbiting Space Shuttle *Challenger*.

GOALS

When you have finished this chapter you should be able to complete the goals given for each section below:

Describing Motion

2.1 Speed
How Fast Is Fast
- Distinguish between instantaneous and average speeds.
- Use the formula $v = d/t$ to solve problems that involve distance, time, and speed.

2.2 Vectors
Which Way as Well as How Much
- Distinguish between scalar and vector quantities and give several examples of each.
- Use the Pythagorean theorem to add two vector quantities of the same kind that act at right angles to each other.

2.3 Acceleration
Vroom!
- Define acceleration and find the acceleration of an object whose speed is changing.
- Use the formula $v_2 = v_1 + at$ to solve problems that involve speed, acceleration, and time.

2.4 Distance, Time, and Acceleration
How Far?
- Use the formula $d = v_1t + \frac{1}{2}at^2$ to solve problems that involve distance, time, speed, and acceleration.

Acceleration Due to Gravity

2.5 Free Fall
A Downward Acceleration
- Explain what is meant by the acceleration of gravity.
- Separate the velocity of an object into vertical and horizontal components in order to determine its motion.

2.6 Air Resistance
Why Raindrops Don't Kill
- Describe the effect of air resistance on falling objects.

Force and Motion

2.7 First Law of Motion
Constant Velocity Is as Natural as Being at Rest
- Define force and indicate its relationship to the first law of motion.

2.8 Mass
A Measure of Inertia

2.9 Second Law of Motion
Force and Acceleration
- Discuss the significance of the second law of motion, $F = ma$.
- Use $F = ma$ to solve problems that involve force.

2.10 Mass and Weight
Weight Is a Force

- Distinguish between mass and weight and find the weight of an object of given mass.

2.11 Third Law of Motion
Action and Reaction
- Use the third law of motion to relate action and reaction forces.

Gravitation

2.12 Circular Motion
A Curved Path Requires an Inward Pull
- Explain the significance of centripetal force in motion along a curved path.
- Relate the centripetal force on an object moving in a circle to its mass, speed, and the radius of the circle.

2.13 Newton's Law of Gravity
What Holds the Solar System Together
- State Newton's law of gravity and describe how gravitational forces vary with distance.

2.14 Artificial Satellites
Thousands Circle the Earth
- Account for the ability of a satellite to orbit the earth without either falling to the ground or flying off into space.
- Define escape speed.

Everything in the universe is in nonstop movement. Whatever the scale of size, from the tiny particles inside atoms to the huge galaxies of stars far away in space, motion is the rule, not the exception. In order to understand the universe, we must begin by understanding motion and the laws the scientific method shows it to obey.

The laws of motion that govern the behavior of atoms and stars apply just as well to the objects of our daily lives. Engineers need these laws to design cars and airplanes, machines of all kinds, even roads—how steeply to bank a highway curve is calculated from the same basic formula that Newton combined with Kepler's findings to arrive at the law of gravity. Terms such as speed and acceleration, force and weight, are used by everyone. Let us now see exactly what these terms mean and how the quantities they refer to are related.

Describing Motion

When an object goes from one place to another, we say it moves. If the object gets there quickly, we say it moves fast; if the object takes a long time, we say it moves slowly. The first step in analyzing motion is to be able to say just how fast is fast and how slow is slow.

2.1 Speed

How Fast Is Fast

The **speed** of something is the rate at which it covers distance. The higher the speed, the faster it travels and the more distance it covers in a given period of time.

If a car goes through a distance of 40 kilometers in a time of 1 hour, its speed is 40 kilometers per hour, usually written 40 km/h.

What if the time interval is not exactly 1 hour? For instance, the car might travel 60 km in 2 hours on another trip. The general formula for speed is distance divided by time:

$$\text{Speed} = \frac{\text{distance}}{\text{time}}$$

Hence the car's speed in the second case is

$$\text{Speed} = \frac{\text{distance}}{\text{time}} = \frac{60 \text{ km}}{2 \text{ h}} = 30 \text{ km/h}$$

The same formula works for times of less than a full hour. The speed of a car that covers 24 km in half an hour is, since $\frac{1}{2}$ h = 0.5 h,

$$\text{Speed} = \frac{\text{distance}}{\text{time}} = \frac{24 \text{ km}}{0.5 \text{ h}} = 48 \text{ km/h}$$

These speeds are all **average speeds,** because we do not know the details of how the cars moved during their trips. They probably went slower than the average during some periods, faster at others, and even came to a stop now and then at traffic lights. What the speedometer of a car shows is the car's **instantaneous speed** at any moment, that is, how fast it is going at that moment (Fig. 2-1).

For the sake of convenience, quantities such as distance, time, and speed are often abbreviated and printed in italics:

$$d = \text{distance} \qquad t = \text{time} \qquad v = \text{speed}$$

In terms of these symbols the formula for speed becomes

$$v = \frac{d}{t} \qquad \textit{Speed} \qquad \qquad \textit{2-1}$$

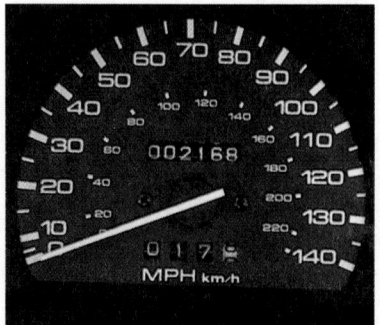

Figure 2-1 The speedometer of a car shows its instantaneous speed. This speedometer is calibrated in both mi/h (here MPH) and km/h.

Distance The previous formula can be rewritten in two ways. Suppose we want to know how far a car whose average speed is v goes in a time t. To find out, we must solve $v = d/t$ for a distance d. According to one of the rules of algebra (see the Math Refresher at the back of this book), a quantity that divides one side of an equation can be shifted to multiply the other side. Thus

$$v = \frac{d}{t}$$

becomes

$$v = \frac{d}{t}$$

$$vt = d$$

which is the same as

$$d = vt \qquad \qquad \text{2-2}$$

$$\text{Distance} = (\text{speed})(\text{time})$$

Time In another situation we might want to know how long it takes something moving at a certain speed to cover a certain distance. In other words, we know v and d and want to find the time t. What we do here is solve $d = vt$ for the time t. From basic algebra we know that something that multiplies one side of an equation can be shifted to divide the other side. What we do, then, is shift the v in the formula $d = vt$ to divide the d:

$$d = v\,t$$

$$\frac{d}{v} = t$$

which is the same as

$$t = \frac{d}{v} \qquad \qquad \text{2-3}$$

$$\text{Time} = \frac{\text{distance}}{\text{speed}}$$

Frame of Reference

When we say something is moving, we mean that its position relative to something else—the **frame of reference**—is changing. The choice of an appropriate frame of reference depends on the situation. In the case of a car, for instance, the obvious frame of reference is the road it is on.

In other cases things may not be so straightforward. If we use the earth as our frame of reference, the sun and planets move relative to us in complicated paths, as in Figs. 1-5 and 1-7. On the other hand, if we use the sun as our frame of reference, the earth and the other planets move relative to it in simple paths, as in Fig. 1-8. Newton was able to interpret these motions in terms of the gravitational pull of the sun whereas he would not have been able to discover the law of gravity if he had used the earth as his frame of reference.

Example 2.1

How far does a car travel in 6 hours when its average speed is 40 km/h?

Solution

We put $v = 40$ km/h and $t = 6$ h into Eq. 2-2 to find that (Fig. 2-2)

$$d = vt = \left(40\,\frac{\text{km}}{\text{h}}\right)(6\text{ h}) = 240\left(\frac{\text{km}}{\text{h}}\right)(\text{h}) = 240\text{ km}$$

We see that, since h/h = 1, the hours cancel out to give just kilometers in the answer.

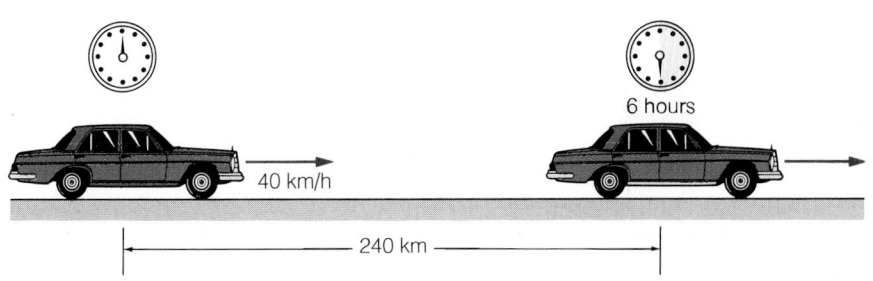

Figure 2-2 A car whose average speed is 40 km/h travels 240 km in 6 hours.

Example 2.2

You are standing 100 m north of your car when an alligator appears 20 m north of you and begins to run toward you at 8 m/s, as in Fig. 2-3. At the same moment you start to run toward your car at 5 m/s. Will you reach the car before the alligator reaches you?

Solution

You are 100 m from your car and so would need

$$t_1 = \frac{d_1}{v_1} = \frac{100 \text{ m}}{5 \text{ m/s}} = 20 \text{ s}$$

to reach it. The alligator is 120 m from the car but would need only

$$t_2 = \frac{d_2}{v_2} = \frac{120 \text{ m}}{8 \text{ m/s}} = 15 \text{ s}$$

to reach it. Hence the alligator would overtake you before you get to the car. Too bad.

Figure 2-3 Watch out for alligators.

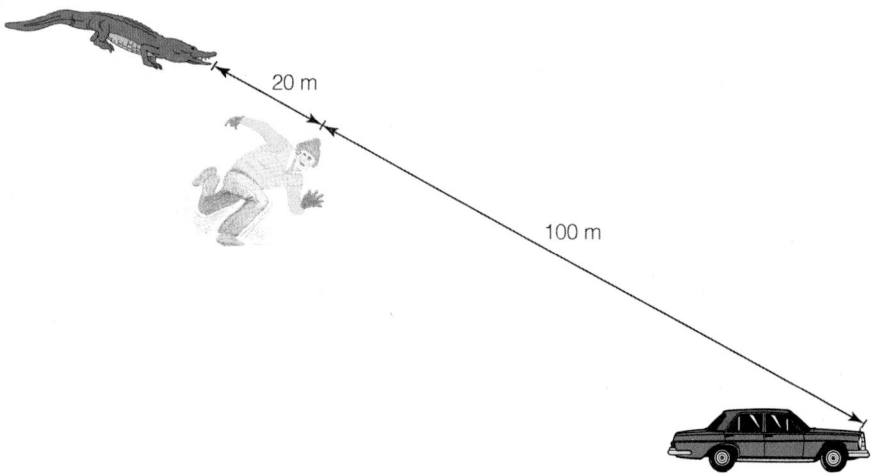

2.2 Vectors

Which Way as Well as How Much

Some quantities need only a number and a unit to be completely specified. It is enough to say that the area of a farm is 600 acres, that the frequency of a sound wave is 440 cycles per second, that a lightbulb uses electric energy at the rate of 75 watts. These are examples of **scalar quantities.** The **magnitude** of a quantity refers to how large it is. Thus the magnitudes of the scalar quantities given above are respectively 600 acres, 440 cycles per second, and 75 watts.

A **vector quantity,** on the other hand, has a direction as well as a magnitude associated with it, and this direction can be important. Displacement (change in position) is an example of a vector quantity. If we drive 1000 km north from Denver, we will end up in Canada; if we drive 1000 km south, we will end up in Mexico.

Force is another example of a vector quantity. Applying enough upward force to this book will lift it from the table. Applying a force of the same magnitude downward on the book will press it harder against the table, but the book will not move.

Speed and Velocity   The **speed** of a moving object tells us only how fast the object is going, regardless of its direction. Speed is therefore a scalar quantity. If we are told that a car has a speed of 40 km/h, we do not know where it is headed, or even if it is moving in a straight line—it might well be going in

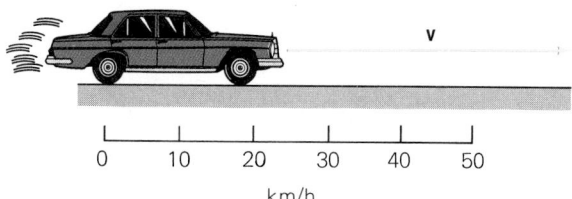

Figure 2-4 The vector **v** represents a velocity of 40 km/h to the right. The scale is 1 cm = 10 km/h.

a circle. The vector quantity that includes both speed and direction is called **velocity.** If we are told that a car has a constant velocity of 40 km/h toward the west, we know all there is to know about its motion and can easily figure out where it will be in an hour, or 2 hours, or at any other time.

Vectors   A handy way to represent a vector quantity on a drawing is to use a straight line called a **vector** that has an arrowhead at one end to show the direction of the quantity. The length of the line is scaled according to the magnitude of the quantity. Figure 2-4 shows how a velocity of 40 km/h to the right is represented by a vector on a scale of 1 cm = 10 km/h. All other vector quantities can be pictured in a similar way.

Vector quantities are usually printed in boldface type (**F** for force, **v** for velocity). Italic type is used for scalar quantities (*f* for frequency, *V* for volume). Italic type is also used for the magnitudes of vector quantities: *F* is the magnitude of the force **F**; *v* is the magnitude of the velocity **v.** For instance, the magnitude of a velocity **v** of 40 km/h to the west is the speed *v* = 40 km/h. A vector quantity is usually indicated in handwriting by an arrow over its symbol, so that $\vec{F}$ means the same thing as **F.**

Adding Vectors   To add scalar quantities of the same kind, we just use ordinary arithmetic. For example, 5 kg of onions plus 3 kg of onions equals 8 kg of onions. The same method holds for vector quantities of the same kind whose directions are the same. If we drive north for 5 km and then continue north for another 3 km, we will go a total of 8 km to the north.

What if the directions are different? If we drive north for 5 km and then east for 3 km, we will not end up 8 km from our starting point. The vector diagram of Fig. 2-5 provides the answer. To add the vectors **A** and **B,** we draw **B** with its tail at the head of **A.** Connecting the tail of **A** with the head of **B** gives us the vector **C,** which corresponds to our net displacement from the start of our trip to its finish. The length of **C** tells us that our displacement was slightly less than 6 km. Any number of vectors of the same kind can be added in this way by stringing them together tail to head and then joining the tail of the first with the head of the last one.

Pythagorean Theorem   A **right triangle** is one in which two of its sides are perpendicular, that is, meet at a 90° angle. The **Pythagorean theorem** is a useful relationship that holds in such a triangle. This theorem states that the sum of the squares of the short sides of a right triangle is equal to the square of its hypotenuse (longest side). For the triangle of Fig. 2-5,

$$A^2 + B^2 = C^2 \qquad \textit{Pythagorean theorem} \qquad 2\text{-}4$$

where *A, B,* and *C* are the respective magnitudes of the vectors **A, B,** and **C.**

We can therefore express the length of any of the sides of a right triangle in terms of the other sides by solving Eq. 2-4 accordingly:

$$A = \sqrt{C^2 - B^2} \qquad\qquad 2\text{-}5$$

$$B = \sqrt{C^2 - A^2} \qquad\qquad 2\text{-}6$$

$$C = \sqrt{A^2 + B^2} \qquad\qquad 2\text{-}7$$

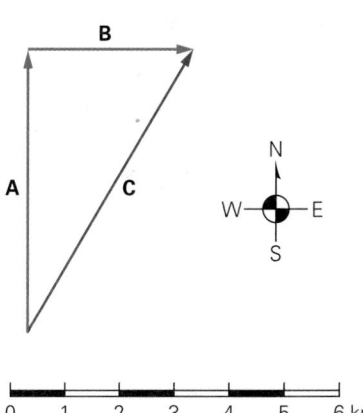

Figure 2-5 Adding vector **B** (3 km east) to vector **A** (5 km north) gives vector **C** whose length corresponds to 5.83 km. According to the Pythagorean theorem, $A^2 + B^2 = C^2$ in any right triangle.

Example 2.3

Use the Pythagorean theorem to find the displacement of a car that goes north for 5 km and then east for 3 km, as in Fig. 2-5.

Solution

Here we let $A = 5$ km and $B = 3$ km. From Eq. 2-7 we have

$$C = \sqrt{A^2 + B^2} = \sqrt{(5 \text{ km})^2 + (3 \text{ km})^2} = \sqrt{(25 + 9) \text{ km}^2}$$
$$= \sqrt{34 \text{ km}^2} = 5.83 \text{ km}$$

This method evidently gives a more accurate result than using a scale drawing.

Figure 2-6 Three cases of accelerated motion, showing successive positions of a body after equal periods of time. (*a*) The intervals between the positions of the body increase in length because the body is traveling faster and faster. (*b*) The intervals decrease in length because the body is slowing down. (*c*) Here the intervals are the same in length because the speed is constant, but the direction of motion is constantly changing.

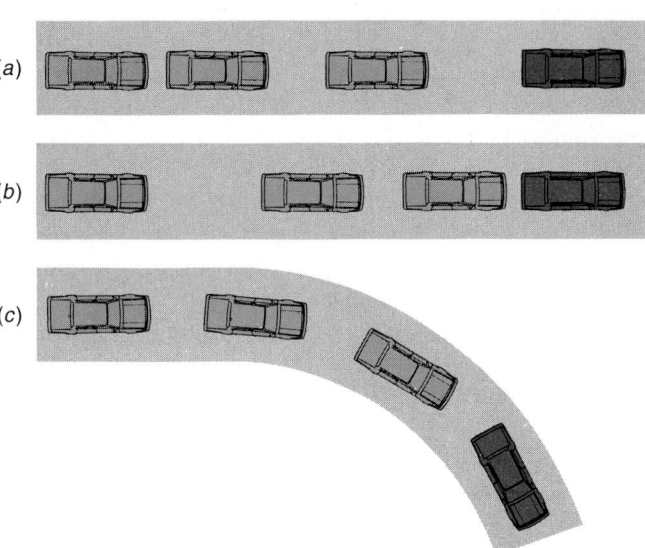

(a)

(b)

(c)

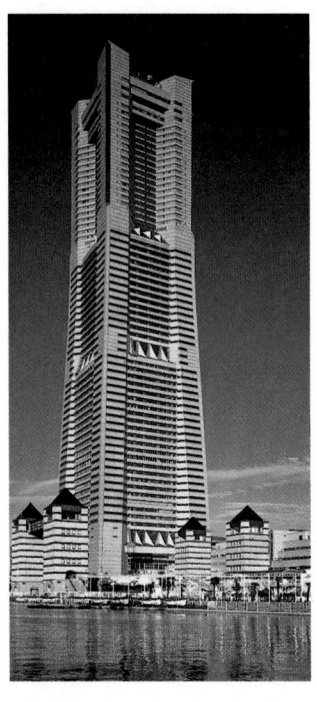

Figure 2-7 Express elevators in tall buildings have accelerations of no more than 1 m/s² to prevent passenger discomfort. One of the world's fastest elevators, in the Yokohama Landmark Tower (Japan's highest building), climbs 69 floors in 40 s, but only 5 s is spent at its top speed of 12.5 m/s (28 mi/h). The elevator reaches this speed at the 27th floor and then begins to slow down at the 42nd floor.

2.3   Acceleration

Vroom!

An **accelerated** object is one whose velocity is changing. As in Fig. 2-6, the change can be an increase or a decrease in speed—the object can be going faster and faster, or slower and slower (Fig. 2-7). A change in direction, too, is an acceleration, as discussed later. Acceleration in general is a vector quantity. For the moment, though, we will stick to straight-line motion, where acceleration is the rate of change of speed. That is,

$$a = \frac{v_2 - v_1}{t} \qquad \textit{Straight-line motion} \qquad 2\text{-}8$$

$$\text{Acceleration} = \frac{\text{change in speed}}{\text{time interval}}$$

where the symbols mean the following:

a = acceleration
t = time interval
v_1 = speed at start of time interval = initial speed
v_2 = speed at end of time interval = final speed

Not all accelerations are constant, but a great many are very nearly so. In what follows all accelerations are assumed to be constant. In Sec. 2-7 we will see why acceleration is such an important quantity in physics.

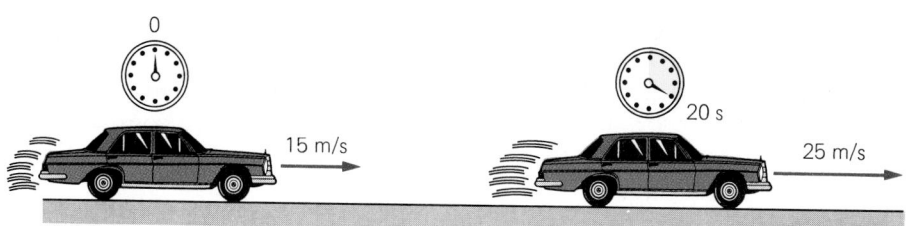

Figure 2-8 A car whose speed increases from 15 m/s to 25 m/s in 20 s has an acceleration of 0.5 m/s².

Example 2.4

The speed of a car changes from 15 m/s (about 34 mi/h) to 25 m/s (about 56 mi/h) in 20 s when its gas pedal is pressed hard (Fig. 2-8). Find its acceleration.

Solution
Here

$$v_i = 15 \text{ m/s} \quad v_f = 25 \text{ m/s} \quad t = 20 \text{ s}$$

and so the car's acceleration is

$$a = \frac{v_f - v_i}{t} = \frac{25 \text{ m/s} - 15 \text{ m/s}}{20 \text{ s}} = \frac{10 \text{ m/s}}{20 \text{ s}} = \frac{0.5 \text{ m/s}}{\text{s}} = 0.5 \text{ m/s}^2$$

This result means that the speed of the car increases by 0.5 m/s during each second the acceleration continues. It is customary to write (m/s)/s (meters per second per second) as just m/s² (meters per second squared) since

$$\frac{\text{m/s}}{\text{s}} = \frac{\text{m}}{(\text{s})(\text{s})} = \frac{\text{m}}{\text{s}^2}$$

Example 2.5

A car whose brakes can produce an acceleration of −6 m/s² is traveling at 30 m/s when its brakes are applied. (a) What is the car's speed 2 s later? (b) What is the total time needed for the car to come to a stop?

Solution

(a) From Eq. 2-9,

$$v_2 = v_1 + at = 30 \text{ m/s} + (-6 \text{ m/s}^2)(2 \text{ s})$$

$$= (30 - 12) \text{ m/s} = 18 \text{ m/s}$$

(b) Now $v_2 = 0 = v_1 + at$, so $at = -v_1$ and

$$t = -\frac{v_1}{a} = -\frac{30 \text{ m/s}}{-6 \text{ m/s}^2} = 5 \text{ s}$$

Suppose we know the acceleration of a car (or anything else) and want to know its speed after it has been accelerated for a time t. What we do is first rewrite Eq. 2-8 in the form

$$at = v_2 - v_1$$

which gives us what we want,

$$v_2 = v_1 + at \qquad \textit{Final speed} \qquad 2\text{-}9$$

$$\frac{\text{Final}}{\text{speed}} = \frac{\text{initial}}{\text{speed}} + \text{change in speed}$$

Not all accelerations increase speed. Something whose speed is decreasing is said to have a **negative acceleration.** For instance, when the brakes of a car are applied, its acceleration might be -6 m/s^2, which means that its speed drops by 6 m/s in each second that the acceleration continues (see Example 2.5). (Sometimes a negative acceleration is called a **deceleration.**)

2.4   Distance, Time, and Acceleration

How Far?

An interesting question is, how far does something, say a car, go when it is accelerated from speed v_1 to speed v_2 in the time t?

To find out, we begin by noting that the car's *average* speed $\bar{v}$ during the acceleration (assumed uniform) is

$$\bar{v} = \frac{v_1 + v_2}{2} \qquad \textit{Average speed} \qquad 2\text{-}10$$

The car moves exactly as far in the time t as if it had the constant speed v equal to its average speed $\bar{v}$. Therefore the distance the car covers in the time t is

$$d = \bar{v}t = \left(\frac{v_1 + v_2}{2}\right)t = \frac{v_1 t}{2} + \frac{v_2 t}{2}$$

The value of v_2, the car's final speed, is given by Eq. 2-9, which means that

$$d = \frac{v_1 t}{2} + \left(\frac{v_1 + at}{2}\right)t = \frac{v_1 t}{2} + \frac{v_1 t}{2} + \frac{at^2}{2}$$

$$d = v_1 t + \tfrac{1}{2} at^2 \qquad \textit{Distance under constant} \atop \textit{acceleration} \qquad 2\text{-}11$$

If the car is stationary at the start of the acceleration, $v_1 = 0$, and

$$d = \tfrac{1}{2} at^2 \qquad \textit{Distance starting from rest} \qquad 2\text{-}12$$

Example 2.6

How far did the car of Example 2-5 go while coming to a stop?

Solution

Here $v_1 = 30$ m/s, $a = -6$ m/s^2, and $t = 5$ s, so

$$d = v_1 t + \tfrac{1}{2} at^2 = (30 \text{ m/s})(5 \text{ s}) + \tfrac{1}{2}(-6 \text{ m/s}^2)(5 \text{ s})^2$$

$$= 150 \text{ m} - 75 \text{ m} = 75 \text{ m}$$

Example 2.7

An airplane needed 20 s to take off from a runway 500 m long. What was its acceleration? Its final speed?

Solution

Since the airplane started from rest, $v_1 = 0$ and $d = \tfrac{1}{2} at^2$. Therefore its acceleration was

$$a = \frac{2d}{t^2} = \frac{2(500 \text{ m})}{(20 \text{ s})^2} = 2.5 \text{ m/s}^2$$

The airplane's final speed was

$$v_2 = v_1 + at = 0 + (2.5 \text{ m/s}^2)(20 \text{ s}) = 50 \text{ m/s}$$

As we can see, by defining certain quantities (here speed and acceleration) and relating them to each other and to directly measurable quantities (here distance and time) we can build up a structure of equations that enables us to answer questions with a pencil and paper that otherwise would need separate, perhaps difficult, observations on real objects.

Acceleration Due to Gravity

Drop a stone, and it falls. Does the stone fall at a constant speed, or does it go faster and faster? Does the stone's motion depend on its weight, or its size, or its shape?

Before Galileo, philosophers tried to answer such questions in terms of supposedly self-evident principles, concepts so seemingly obvious that there was no need to test them. This was the way in which Aristotle (384–322 B.C.), the famous thinker of ancient Greece, approached the subject of falling bodies. To Aristotle, every kind of material had a "natural" place where it belonged and toward which it tried to move. Thus fire rose "naturally" toward the sun and stars, whereas stones were "earthy" and so fell downward toward their home in the earth. A big stone was more earthy than a small one and so, Aristotle thought, ought to fall faster.

The trouble with these ideas, and many others like them, is that they are wrong—only the scientific method, not unsupported speculation, can provide reliable information about how the universe works.

2.5 Free Fall

A Downward Acceleration

Almost two thousand years later the Italian physicist Galileo, the first modern scientist, found that the higher a stone is when it is dropped, the greater its speed when it reaches the ground (Figs. 2-9 and 2-10). This means the stone is accelerated. Furthermore, the acceleration is the same for *all* stones, big and small. For more accuracy with the primitive instruments of his time, Galileo measured the accelerations of balls rolling down an inclined plane rather than their accelerations in free fall, but his conclusions were perfectly general; modern experiments have verified them to at least 1 part in 10^{12} (a trillion!).

Galileo's experiments showed that, if there were no air for them to push their way through, all falling objects near the earth's surface would have the same acceleration of 9.8 m/s². This acceleration is usually abbreviated g:

$$\textbf{Acceleration due to gravity} = g = 9.8 \text{ m/s}^2$$

Ignoring for the moment the effect of air resistance, something that drops from rest has a speed of 9.8 m/s at the end of the first second, a speed of (9.8 m/s²)(2 s) = 19.6 m/s at the end of the next second, and so on (Fig. 2-11). In general, under these circumstances

$$v_{\text{downward}} = gt \qquad \textit{Object falling from rest} \qquad 2\text{-}13$$

How Far Does a Falling Object Fall?   Equation 2-9 tells us the speed of a falling object at any time t after it has been dropped from rest (and before it hits the ground, of course). To find out how far h the object has fallen in the time t, we refer back to Eq. 2-12 for accelerated motion starting from rest. Here the distance is $d = h$ and the acceleration is that of gravity, so $a = g$, which gives

$$h = \tfrac{1}{2} gt^2 \qquad \textit{Object falling from rest} \qquad 2\text{-}14$$

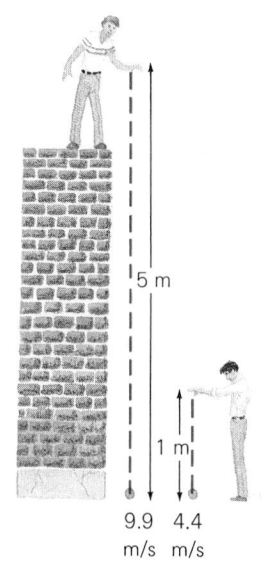

Figure 2-9 Falling bodies are accelerated downward. A stone dropped from a height of 5 m strikes the ground with a speed more than double that of a stone dropped from a height of 1 m.

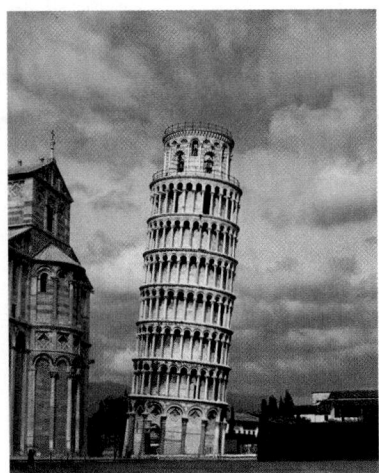

Figure 2-10 The Leaning Tower of Pisa, which is 58 m high, was begun in 1174 and took over two centuries to complete. During its construction the tower started to sink into the clay soil under its south side, and corrections were made to the upper floors to try to make them level. Today the tilt is 5.5° and continues to increase, leaving the tower in danger of collapse if efforts to stabilize the ground under it fail. According to legend, Galileo dropped a bullet and a cannonball from the tower to show that all objects fall with the same acceleration.

The t^2 factor means that h increases with time much faster than the object's speed v, which is given by $v = gt$. Figure 2-12 shows h and v for various times of fall. At $t = 10$ s, the object's speed is 10 times its speed at $t = 1$ s, but the distance it has fallen is 100 times the distance it fell during the first second.

Thrown Objects   The downward acceleration g is the same whether an object is just dropped or is thrown upward, downward, or sideways. If a ball is held in the air and dropped, it goes faster and faster until it hits the ground. If the

Figure 2-11   All falling objects near the earth's surface have a downward acceleration of 9.8 m/s². (The distance an object will have fallen in each time interval is not shown to scale here.)

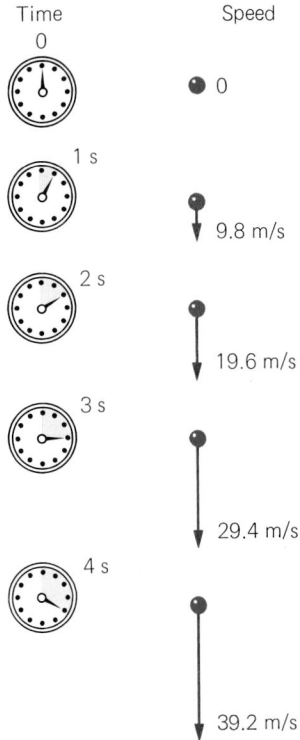

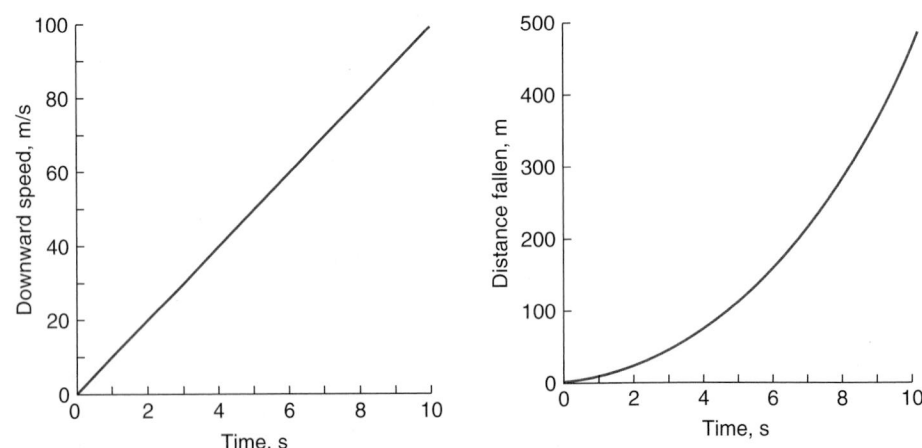

Figure 2-12   Downward speed and distance fallen in the first 10 seconds after an object is dropped from rest. Air resistance (Sec. 2.6) is ignored here. The distance fallen increases with time at a greater rate than the downward speed. For instance, 1 s after being dropped, an object has fallen through 4.9 m and has a speed of 9.8 m/s, but 10 s after being dropped, it has fallen through 490 m but its speed has increased to only 98 m/s.

BIOGRAPHY Galileo Galilei (1564–1642)

Galileo fathered modern science by clearly stating the central idea of the scientific method: the study of nature must be based on observation and experiment. He also pioneered the use of mathematical reasoning to interpret and generalize his findings.

Galileo was born in Pisa, Italy; following a local custom, his given name was a variation of his family name. Although his father thought that medicine would be a more sensible career choice, Galileo studied physics and mathematics and soon became a professor at Pisa and afterward at Padua. His early work was on accelerated motion, falling bodies, and the paths taken by projectiles.

Later, with a telescope he had built, Galileo was the first person to see sunspots, the phases of Venus, the four largest satellites of Jupiter, and the mountains of the moon. Turning his telescope to the Milky Way, he found that it consisted of individual stars. To Galileo, as to his contemporaries, these discoveries were "infinitely stupendous."

By then famous, in 1610 Galileo went to Florence as court mathematician to Cosimo, Duke of Tuscany. Here Galileo expounded the copernican model of the universe and pointed out that his astronomical observations supported this model. Galileo discovered Jupiter's four largest satellites in 1610 and concluded from his observations, shown here, that they revolve around Jupiter.

Because the ptolemaic model with the earth as the stationary center of the universe was part of the doctrine of the Catholic Church,

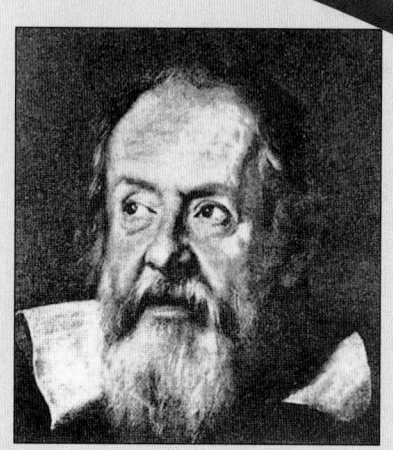

the Holy Office told Galileo to stop advocating the contrary, and he obeyed. Then, when a friend of his became pope in 1631, Galileo resumed teaching the merits of the copernican system. But the pope turned against him, and in 1633, when he was 70, Galileo was convicted of heresy by the Inquisition. Although he escaped being burnt at the stake, the fate of other heretics, Galileo was sentenced to house arrest for the remainder of his life and was forced to publicly deny that

the earth moves. (According to legend, Galileo then muttered, "Yet it does move.")

Even in 1992, the 350th anniversary of Galileo's death, a Vatican commission did not mention, let alone regret, the Church's role in silencing Galileo. Pope John Paul II spoke of Galileo's condemnation, which almost extinguished Italian science for over a century, as merely a matter of "mutual incomprehension."

It would be nice to think that today, four centuries after Galileo's time, the age of reason has become firmly established. But religious fundamentalists who seek to replace the findings of science by their own particular interpretations of the Bible are again on the march. Do we really want a return to the blind ignorance of the past? Evolution in biology, geology, and astronomy is now under attack, and a movement to return to "Biblical astronomy," with the earth at the center of the universe, has actually started. The struggle to keep reason in the life of the mind is neverending, but it is an essential struggle.

ball is thrown horizontally, we can imagine its velocity as having two parts, a horizontal one that stays constant and a vertical one that is affected by gravity. The result, as in Fig. 2-13, is a curved path that becomes steeper as the downward speed increases.

When a ball is thrown upward, as in Fig. 2-14, the effect of the downward acceleration of gravity is at first to reduce the ball's upward speed. The upward speed decreases steadily until finally it is zero. The ball is then at the

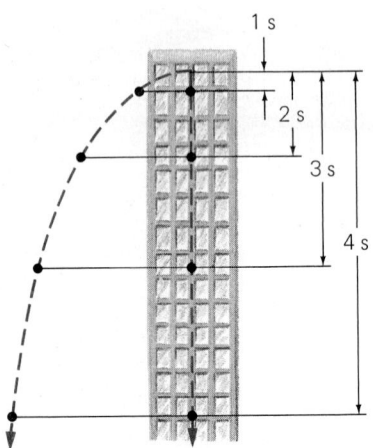

Figure 2-13   The acceleration of gravity does not depend upon horizontal motion. When one ball is thrown horizontally from a building at the same time that a second ball is dropped vertically, the two reach the ground at the same time because both have the same downward acceleration.

Example 2.8

A stone dropped from a bridge strikes the water 2.2 s later. How high is the bridge above the water?

Solution

Substituting in Eq. 2-14 gives

$$h = \tfrac{1}{2} g t^2 = \tfrac{1}{2} (9.8 \text{ m/s}^2)(2.2 \text{ s})^2 = 24 \text{ m}$$

Example 2.9

An apple is dropped from a window 20 m above the ground. (a) How long does it take the apple to reach the ground? (b) What is its final speed?

Solution

(a) Since $h = \tfrac{1}{2} g t^2$,

$$t = \sqrt{\frac{2h}{g}} = \sqrt{\frac{(2)(20 \text{ m})}{9.8 \text{ m/s}^2}} = 2.0 \text{ s}$$

(b) From Eq. 2-13 the ball's final speed is

$$v = gt = 19.6 \text{ m/s}$$

Example 2.10

An airplane is in level flight at a velocity of 150 m/s and an altitude of 1500 m when a wheel falls off. What horizontal distance will the wheel travel before it strikes the ground?

Solution

The horizontal velocity of the wheel does not affect its vertical motion. The wheel therefore reaches the ground at the same time as a wheel dropped from rest at an altitude of 1500 m, which is

$$t = \sqrt{\frac{2h}{g}} = \sqrt{\frac{(2)(1500 \text{ m})}{9.8 \text{ m/s}^2}} = 17.5 \text{ s}$$

In this time the wheel will travel a horizontal distance of

$$d = v_{\text{horiz}} t = (150 \text{ m/s})(17.5 \text{ s}) = 2625 \text{ m} = 2.63 \text{ km}$$

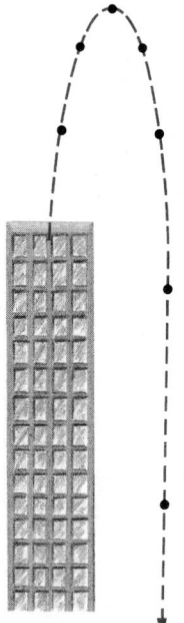

Figure 2-14   When a ball is thrown upward, its downward acceleration reduces its original speed until it comes to a momentary stop. At this time the ball is at the top of its path, and it then begins to fall as if it had been dropped from there. The ball is shown after equal time intervals.

top of its path, when the ball is at rest for an instant. The ball next begins to fall at ever-increasing speed, exactly as though it had been dropped from the highest point.

Interestingly enough, something thrown upward at a certain speed will return to its starting point with the same speed, although the object is now moving in the opposite direction.

What happens when a ball is thrown downward? Now the ball's original speed is steadily increased by the downward acceleration of gravity. When the ball reaches the ground, its final speed will be the sum of its original speed and the speed increase due to the acceleration.

When a ball is thrown upward at an angle to the ground, the result is a curved path called a **parabola** (Fig. 2-15). The maximum range (horizontal distance) for a given initial speed occurs when the ball is thrown at an angle

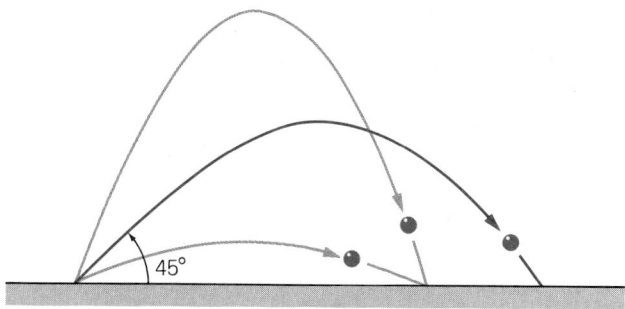

Figure 2-15 In the absence of air resistance, a ball travels farthest when it is thrown at an angle of 45°.

| **Example 2.11**

A stone thrown upward reaches its highest point 2.2 s later. (a) How high did it go? (b) What was its initial speed?

Solution

(a) The height h is the same as that from which the stone would have been dropped to reach the ground in 2.2 s. Hence

$$h = \frac{1}{2}gt^2 = \frac{(9.8 \text{ m/s}^2)(2.2 \text{ s})^2}{2} = 23.7 \text{ m}$$

(b) The upward speed was the same as the downward speed the stone would have had 2.2 s after being dropped, so

$$v = gt = (9.8 \text{ m/s}^2)(2.2 \text{ s}) = 21.6 \text{ m/s}$$

---

of 45° above the ground. At higher and lower angles, the range will be shorter. As the figure shows, for every range up to the maximum there are two angles at which the ball can be thrown and land in the same place.

2.6   Air Resistance

Why Raindrops Don't Kill

Air resistance keeps falling things from developing the full acceleration of gravity. Without this resistance raindrops would reach the ground with bullet-like speeds and even a light shower would be dangerous.

In air, a stone falls faster than a feather because air resistance affects the stone less. In a vacuum, however, there is no air, and the stone and feather fall with the same acceleration of 9.8 m/s² (Fig. 2-16).

The faster something moves, the more the air in its path resists its motion. At 100 km/h (62 mi/h), the drag on a car due to air resistance is about 5 times as great as the drag at 50 km/h (31 mi/h). In the case of a falling object, the air resistance increases with speed until it equals the force of gravity on the object. The object then continues to drop at a constant **terminal speed** that depends on its size and shape and on how heavy it is (Table 2-1). A person in free fall has a terminal speed of about 54 m/s (120 mi/h), but with an open parachute the terminal speed of only about 6.3 m/s (14 mi/h) permits a safe landing (Fig. 2-17).

Air resistance reduces the range of a projectile. Figure 2-18 shows how the path of a ball is affected. In a vacuum, as we saw in Fig. 2-15, the ball goes farthest when it is thrown at an angle of 45°, but in air (that is, in real life), the maximum range occurs for an angle of less than 45°. For a baseball struck hard by a bat, an angle of 40° will take it the greatest distance.

Table 2-1	**Some Terminal Speeds (1 m/s = 2.2 mi/h)**
Object	**Terminal Speed**
16-lb shot	145 m/s
Baseball	42
Golf ball	40
Tennis ball	30
Basketball	20
Large raindrop	10
Ping-Pong ball	9

Figure 2-16   In a vacuum all bodies fall with the same acceleration.

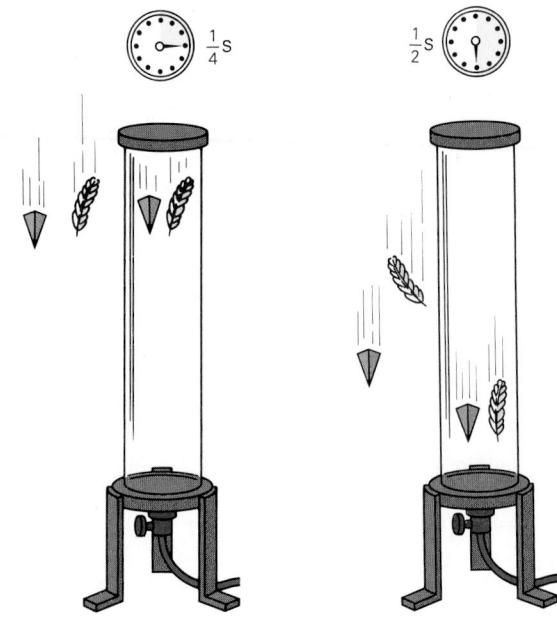

Figure 2-17   The terminal speeds of sky divers are greatly reduced when their parachutes open, which permits them to land safely.

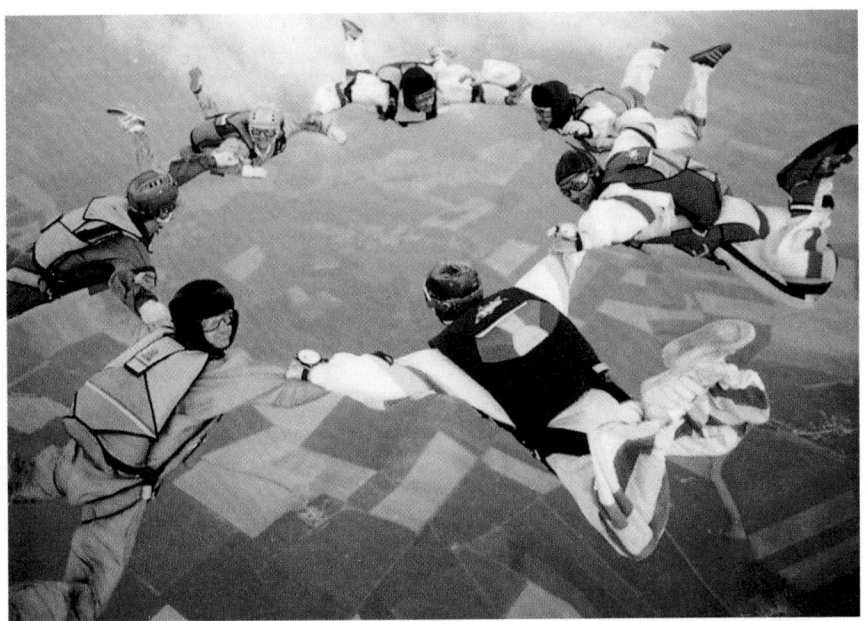

Figure 2-18   Effect of air resistance on the path of a thrown ball. An angle of less than 45° now gives the greatest range.

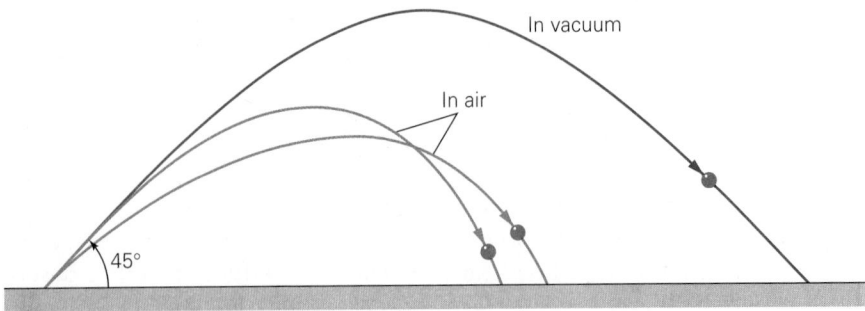

Force and Motion

What can make something originally at rest begin to move? Why do some things move faster than others? Why are some accelerated and others not? Questions like these led Isaac Newton to formulate three principles that summarize so much of the behavior of moving bodies that they have become known as the **laws of motion.** Based on observations made by Newton and others, these laws are as valid today as they were when they were set down about three centuries ago.

2.7   First Law of Motion

Constant Velocity Is as Natural as Being at Rest

Imagine a ball lying on a level floor. Left alone, the ball stays where it is. If you give it a push, the ball rolls a short way and then comes to a stop. The smoother the floor, the farther the ball rolls before stopping. With a perfectly round ball and a perfectly smooth and level floor, and no air to slow down its motion, would the ball ever stop rolling?

There will never be a perfect ball and a perfect surface for it to roll on, of course. But we can come close. The result is that, as the resistance to its motion becomes less and less, the ball goes farther and farther for the same push. We can reasonably expect that, under ideal conditions, the ball would keep rolling forever.

This conclusion was first reached by Galileo. Later it was stated by Newton as his **first law of motion:**

> If no net force acts on it, an object at rest remains at rest and an object in motion remains in motion at constant velocity (that is, at constant speed in a straight line).

According to this law, an object at rest never begins to move all by itself—a force is needed to start it off. If it is moving, the object will continue going at constant velocity unless a force acts to slow it down, to speed it up, or to change its direction. Motion at constant velocity is just as "natural" as staying at rest.

Force   In thinking about **force,** most of us think of a car pulling a trailer or a person pushing a lawn mower or lifting a crate. Also familiar are the force of gravity, which pulls us and things about us downward, the pull of a magnet on a piece of iron, and the force of air pushing against the sails of a boat. In these examples the central idea is one of pushing, pulling, or lifting. Newton's first law gives us a more precise definition:

> A force is any influence that can change the speed or direction of motion of an object.

When we see something accelerated, we know that a force must be acting upon it.

Although it seems simple and straightforward, the first law of motion has far-reaching implications. For instance, until Newton's time most people believed that the orbits of the moon around the earth and of the planets around the sun were "natural" ones, with no forces needed to keep these bodies moving as they do. However, because the moon and planets move in curved paths, their velocities are not constant, so according to the first law, forces of some kind *must* be acting on them. The search for these forces led Newton to the law of gravitation.

It is worth emphasizing that just applying a force to an object at rest will not necessarily set the object in motion. If we push against a stone wall, the wall is not accelerated as a result. Only if a force is applied to an object that

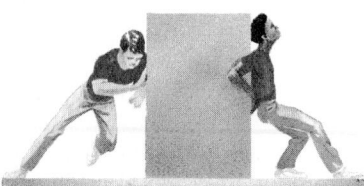

Figure 2-19   When several forces act on an object, they may cancel one another out to leave no net force. Only a net (or **unbalanced**) force can accelerate an object.

is able to respond will the state of rest or motion of the object change. On the other hand, *every* acceleration can be traced to the action of a force.

An object continues to be accelerated only as long as a **net force**—a force not balanced out by one or more other forces—acts upon it (Fig. 2-19). An ideal car on a level road would therefore need its engine only to be accelerated to a particular speed, after which it would keep moving at this speed forever with the engine turned off. Actual cars are not so cooperative because of the retarding forces of friction and air resistance, which require counteracting by a force applied by the engine to the wheels.

2.8   Mass

A Measure of Inertia

The reluctance of an object to change its state of rest or of uniform motion in a straight line is called **inertia.**

When you are in a car that starts to move, you feel yourself pushed back in your seat (Fig. 2-20). What is actually happening is that your inertia tends to keep your body where it was before the car started moving. When the car stops, on the other hand, you feel yourself pushed forward. What is actually happening now is that your inertia tends to keep your body moving while the car comes to a halt.

The name **mass** is given to the property of matter that shows itself as inertia. The inertia of a bowling ball exceeds that of a basketball, as you can tell by kicking them in turn, so the mass of the bowling ball exceeds that of the basketball. Mass may be thought of as quantity of matter: the more mass something has, the greater its inertia and the more matter it contains (Fig. 2-21).

Figure 2-20   (*a*) When a car suddenly starts to move, the inertia of the passengers tends to keep them at rest relative to the earth, and so their heads move backward relative to the car. (*b*) When the car comes to a sudden stop, inertia tends to keep the passengers moving, and so their heads move forward relative to the car.

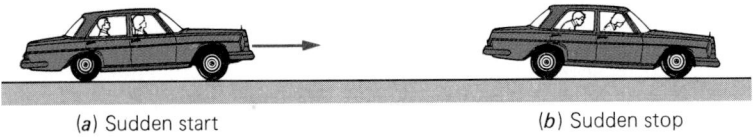

(*a*) Sudden start   (*b*) Sudden stop

Figure 2-21   The more mass an object has, the greater its resistance to a change in its state of motion, as this shot-putter knows.

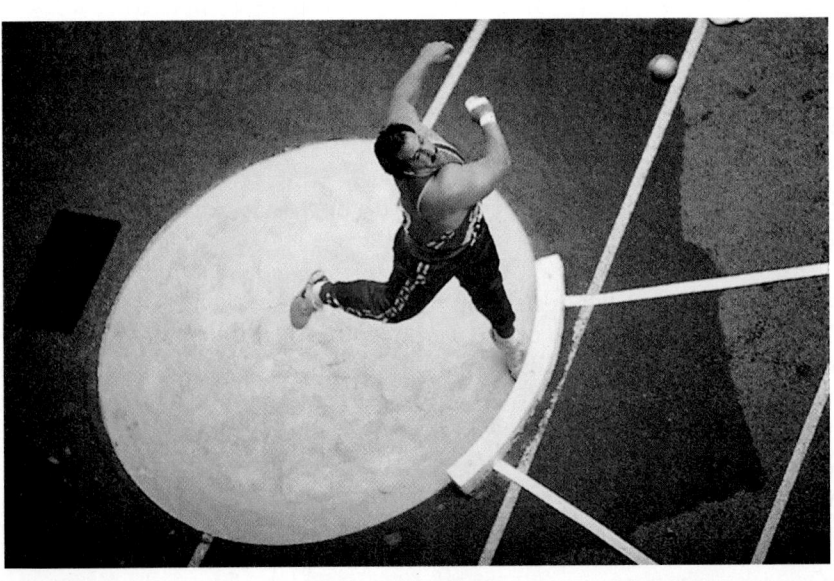

Friction

Friction is a force that acts to oppose the motion of an object past another object with which it is in contact. The harder the objects are pressed together, the stronger the frictional force.

Friction is an actual force, unlike inertia. Even a small net force can accelerate an object despite its inertia, but friction may prevent a small force from pushing one object across another.

Friction has two chief causes. One is the interlocking of irregularities in the two surfaces, which prevents one surface from sliding smoothly past the other. The second cause is the tendency for materials in very close contact to stick together because of attractive forces between their respective atoms and molecules, as described in Sec. 11.3.

Sometimes friction is welcome. The fastening ability of nails and screws and the resistive action of brakes depend on friction, and walking would be impossible without it. In other cases friction means wasted effort, and to reduce it lubricants (oil and grease) and rollers or wheels are commonly used. About half the power of a car's engine is lost to friction in the engine itself and in its drive train. The joints of the human body are lubricated by a substance called synovial fluid, which resembles blood plasma.

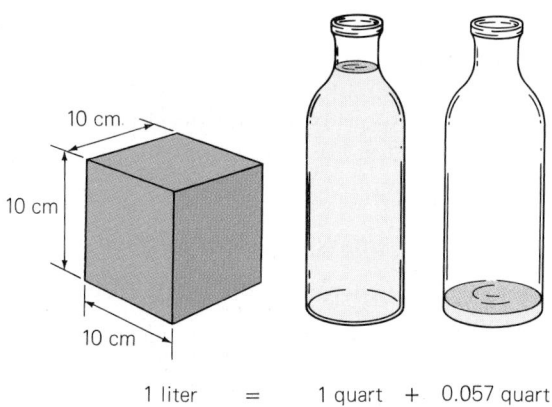

1 liter   =   1 quart   +   0.057 quart

Figure 2-22   A liter, which is equal to 1.057 quarts, represents a volume of 1000 cubic centimeters (cm^3). One liter of water has a mass of 1 kg.

The SI unit of mass is the **kilogram** (kg). A liter of water, which is a little more than a quart, has a mass of 1 kg (Fig. 2-22). Table 2-2 lists a range of mass values.

2.9   Second Law of Motion

Force and Acceleration

Throw a baseball hard, and it leaves your hand going faster than if you toss it gently. This suggests that the greater the force, the greater the acceleration while the force acts. Experiments show that doubling the net force doubles the acceleration, tripling the net force triples the acceleration, and so on (Fig. 2-23).

Do all balls you throw with the same force leave your hand with the same speed? Heave an iron shot instead, and it is clear that the more mass something has, the less its acceleration for a given force. Experiments make the relationship precise: for the same net force, doubling the mass cuts the acceleration in half, tripling the mass cuts the acceleration to one-third its original value, and so on.

Table 2-2	Some Approximate Mass Values
The sun	2×10^{30} kg
The earth	6×10^{24}
Large tanker	4×10^8
747 airliner (at takeoff)	4×10^5
Large car	2×10^3
165-lb person	75
This book	1.4
Pencil	3×10^{-3}
Postage stamp	3×10^{-5}
Smallest known bacterium	1×10^{-19}
Oxygen molecule	5×10^{-26}
Electron	9×10^{-31}

Muscular Forces

The forces an animal exerts result from contractions of its skeletal muscles, which occur when the muscles are electrically stimulated by nerves. The maximum force a muscle can exert is proportional to its cross-sectional area and can be as much as 70 N/cm² (100 lb/in.²).

An athlete might have a biceps muscle in his arm 8 cm across, so it could produce up to 3500 N (790 lb) of force. This is a lot, but the geometry of an animal's skeleton and muscles favors range of motion over force. As a result the actual force a person's arm can exert is much smaller than the forces exerted by the arm muscles themselves, but the person's arm can move through

a much greater distance than the amount the muscles contract.

An animal whose length is L has muscles that have cross-sectional areas and hence strengths roughly proportional to L^2. But the mass of the animal depends on its volume, which is roughly proportional to L^3. Therefore the larger an animal is, in general, the weaker it is relative to its mass. This is obvious in nature. For instance, even though insect muscles are intrinsically weaker than human muscles, many insects can carry loads several times their weights, whereas animals the size of humans are limited to loads comparable with their weights.

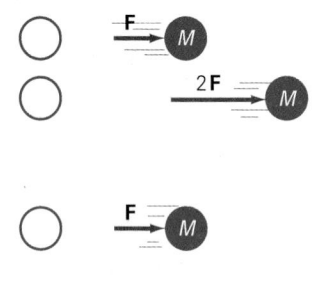

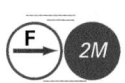

Figure 2-23   Newton's second law of motion. When different forces act upon identical masses, the greater force produces the greater acceleration. When the same force acts upon different masses, the greater mass receives the smaller acceleration.

Newton's **second law of motion** is a statement of these findings. If we let F = net force and m = mass, this law states that

$$a = \frac{F}{m} \qquad \text{Second law of motion} \qquad 2\text{-}15$$

$$\text{Acceleration} = \frac{\text{force}}{\text{mass}}$$

Another way to express the second law of motion is in the form of a definition of force:

$$F = ma \qquad\qquad 2\text{-}16$$

$$\text{Force} = (\text{mass})(\text{acceleration})$$

The second law of motion was experimentally verified down to an acceleration of 5×10^{-14} m/s² in 2007.

An important aspect of the second law concerns direction. The direction of the acceleration is always the same as the direction of the net force. A car is going faster and faster—therefore the net force on it is in the same direction as that in which the car is headed. The car then slows down—therefore the net force on it is now in the direction *opposite* that in which it is headed (Fig. 2-24).

Thus we can say that

> The net force on an object equals the product of the mass and the acceleration of the object. The direction of the force is the same as that of the acceleration.

Figure 2-24   The direction of a force is significant. A force applied to a car in the direction in which it is moving (for instance by giving more fuel to its engine) produces a positive acceleration, which increases the speed of the car. A force applied opposite to the direction of motion (for instance by using the brakes) produces a negative acceleration, which decreases the speed of the car until it comes to a stop. An acceleration that reduces the speed of a moving object is sometimes called a deceleration.

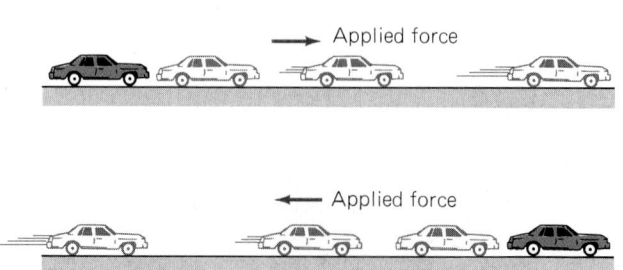

The second law of motion is the key to understanding the behavior of moving objects because it links cause (force) and effect (acceleration) in a definite way (Fig. 2-25). When we speak of force from now on, we know exactly what we mean, and we know exactly how an object free to move will respond when a given force acts on it.

The Newton   The second law of motion shows us how to define a unit for force. If we express mass m in kilograms and acceleration a in m/s^2, force F is given in terms of (kg)(m/s^2). This unit is given a special name, the **newton** (N). Thus

$$1 \text{ newton} = 1 \text{ N} = 1 \text{ (kg)(m/s}^2)$$

When a force of 1 N is applied to a 1-kg mass, the mass is given an acceleration of 1 m/s^2 (Fig. 2-26).

In the British system, the unit of force is the **pound** (lb). The pound and the newton are related as follows:

$$1 \text{ N} = 0.225 \text{ lb}$$
$$1 \text{ lb} = 4.45 \text{ N}$$

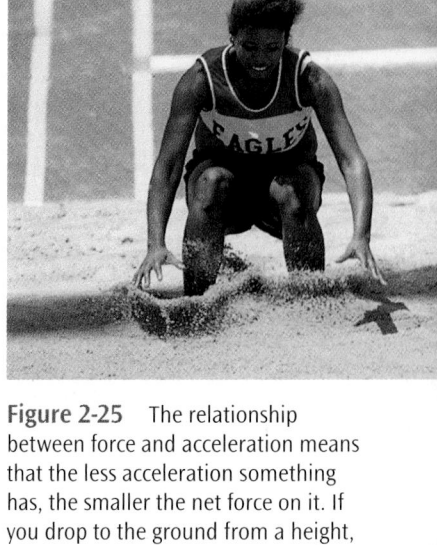

Figure 2-25   The relationship between force and acceleration means that the less acceleration something has, the smaller the net force on it. If you drop to the ground from a height, as this jumper has, you can reduce the force of the impact by bending your knees as you hit the ground so you come to a stop gradually instead of suddenly. The same reasoning can be applied to make cars safer. If a car's body is built to crumple progressively in a crash, the forces acting on the passengers will be smaller than if the car were rigid.

Example 2.12

When a tennis ball is served, it is in contact with the racket for a time that is typically 0.005 s, which is 5 thousandths of a second. Find the force needed to serve a 60-g tennis ball at 30 m/s.

Solution
Since the ball starts from rest, $v_1 = 0$, and its acceleration when struck by the racket is, from Eq. 2-8,

$$a = \frac{v_2 - v_1}{t} = \frac{30 \text{ m/s} - 0}{0.005 \text{ s}} = 6000 \text{ m/s}^2$$

Because the ball's mass is 60 g = 0.06 kg, the force the racket must exert on it is

$$F = ma = (0.06 \text{ kg})(6000 \text{ m/s}^2) = 360 \text{ N}$$

In more familiar units, this force is 81 lb. Of course, it does not seem so great to the person serving because the duration of the impact is so brief (Fig. 2-27).

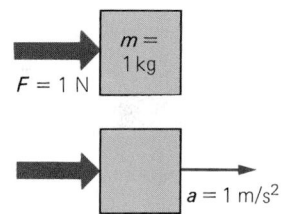

Figure 2-26   A force of 1 newton gives a mass of 1 kilogram an acceleration of 1 m/s^2.

Figure 2-27   A person serving a tennis ball must exert a force of 360 N on it for the ball to have a speed of 30 m/s if the racket is in contact with the ball for 0.005 s.

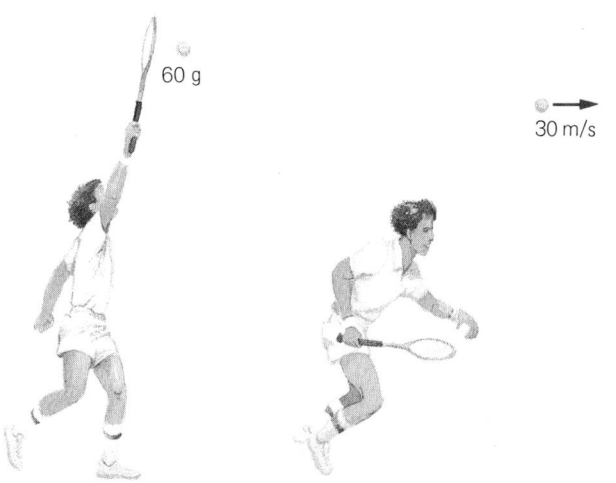

60 g

30 m/s

Your Weight Elsewhere in the Solar System

The more mass a planet has and the smaller it is, the greater the acceleration of gravity g at its surface. The values of g for the various planets are listed in Table 17-1. From these values, if you know your mass you can figure out your weight on any planet using the formula $w = mg$. In familiar units, if you weigh 150 lb on the earth, here is what you would weigh on the planets and the moon:

Mercury	57 lb	Saturn	180 lb
Venus	135	Uranus	165
Earth	150	Neptune	180
Mars	57	Moon	25
Jupiter	390		

2.10   Mass and Weight

Weight Is a Force

The **weight** of an object is the force with which it is attracted by the earth's gravitational pull. If you weigh 150 lb (668 N), the earth is pulling you down with a force of 150 lb. Weight is different from mass, which refers to how much matter something contains. There is a very close relationship between weight and mass, however.

Let us look at the situation in the following way. Whenever a net force F is applied to a mass m, Newton's second law of motion tells us that the acceleration a of the mass will be in accord with the formula

$$F = ma$$
$$\text{Force} = \text{(mass)(acceleration)}$$

In the case of an object at the earth's surface, the force gravity exerts on it is its weight w. This is the force that causes the object to fall with the constant acceleration $g = 9.8 \text{ m/s}^2$ when no other force acts. We may therefore substitute w for F and g for a in the formula $F = ma$ to give

$$w = mg \qquad \textit{Weight and mass} \qquad \text{2-17}$$
$$\text{Weight} = \text{(mass)(acceleration of gravity)}$$

The weight w of an object and its mass m are always proportional to each other: twice the mass means twice the weight, and half the mass means half the weight.

In the SI system, mass rather than weight is normally specified. A customer in a French grocery might ask for a kilogram of bread or 5 kg of potatoes. To find the weight in newtons of something whose mass in kilograms is known, we simply turn to $w = mg$ and set $g = 9.8 \text{ m/s}^2$. Thus the weight of 5 kg of potatoes is

$$w = mg = (5 \text{ kg})(9.8 \text{ m/s}^2) = 49 \text{ N}$$

This is the force with which the earth attracts a mass of 5 kg.

At the earth's surface, the weight of a 1-kg mass in British units is 2.2 lb. The weight in pounds of 5 kg of potatoes is therefore 5(2.2 lb) = 11 lb. The mass that corresponds to a weight of 1 lb is 454 g.

Example 2.13

An elevator whose total mass is 600 kg is suspended by a cable that can exert a maximum upward force of $F_{max} = 15,000$ N. What is the greatest upward acceleration the elevator can have? The greatest downward acceleration?

Solution

When the elevator is stationary (or moving at constant speed) the upward force the cable exerts is just the elevator's weight of

$$w = mg = (600 \text{ kg})(9.8 \text{ m/s}^2) = 5880 \text{ N}$$

To accelerate the elevator upward, an additional upward force F is needed (Fig. 2-28), where

$$F = F_{max} - w = 15,000 \text{ N} - 5880 \text{ N} = 9120 \text{ N}$$

The elevator's upward acceleration when this net force acts on it is

$$a = \frac{F}{m} = \frac{9120 \text{ N}}{600 \text{ kg}} = 15.2 \text{ m/s}^2$$

For the elevator to have a downward acceleration of more than the acceleration of gravity g, a downward force besides its own weight is needed. The cable cannot push the elevator downward, so its greatest downward acceleration is $g = 9.8 \text{ m/s}^2$.

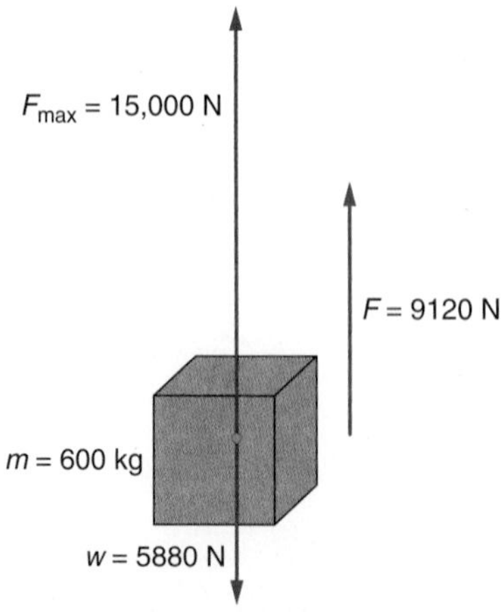

$F_{max} = 15,000$ N

$F = 9120$ N

$m = 600$ kg

$w = 5880$ N

Figure 2-28   The net upward force on an elevator of mass 600 kg is 9120 N when its supporting cable exerts a total upward force of 15,000 N.

Weight Varies with Location

The mass of something is a more basic property than its weight because the pull of gravity on it is not the same everywhere. This pull is less on a mountaintop than at sea level and less at the equator than near the poles because the earth bulges slightly at the equator. A person who weighs 200 lb in Lima, Peru, would weigh nearly 201 lb in Oslo, Norway. On the surface of Mars the same person would weigh only 76 lb, and he or she would be able to jump much higher than on the earth. However, the person would not be able to throw a ball any faster: because the force F the person exerts on the ball and the ball's mass m are the same on both planets, the acceleration a would be the same, too.

2.11 Third Law of Motion

Action and Reaction

Suppose you push against a heavy table and it does not move. This must mean that the table is resisting your push on it. The table stays in place because your force on it is matched by the opposing force of friction between the table legs and the floor. You don't move because the force of the table on you is matched by a similar opposing force between your shoes and the floor.

Now imagine that you and the table are on a frozen lake whose surface is so slippery on a warm day that there is no friction. Again you push on the table, which this time moves away as a result (Fig. 2-29). But you can stick to the ice no better than the table can, and you find yourself sliding backward. No matter what you do, pushing on the table always means that the table pushes back on you.

Considerations of this kind led Newton to his **third law of motion:**

> When one object exerts a force on a second object, the second object exerts an equal force in the opposite direction on the first object.

No force ever occurs singly. A chair pushes downward on the floor; the floor presses upward on the chair (Fig. 2-30). The firing of a rifle exerts a force on the bullet; at the same time the firing exerts a backward push (recoil) on the rifle. A pear falls from a tree because of the earth's pull on the pear; there is an equal upward pull on the earth by the pear that is not apparent because the earth has so much more mass than the pear, but this upward force is nevertheless present.

Action and Reaction Forces Newton's third law always applies to two different forces on two different objects—the **action force** that the first object exerts on the second, and the opposite **reaction force** the second exerts on the first.

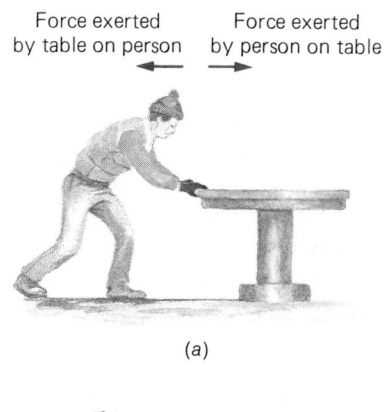

Force exerted by table on person   Force exerted by person on table

(a)

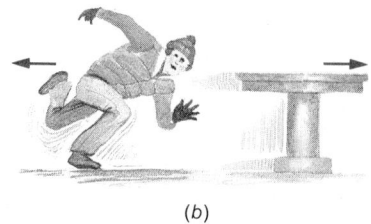

(b)

Figure 2-29 Action and reaction forces act on different bodies. Pushing a table on a frozen lake results in person and table moving apart in opposite directions.

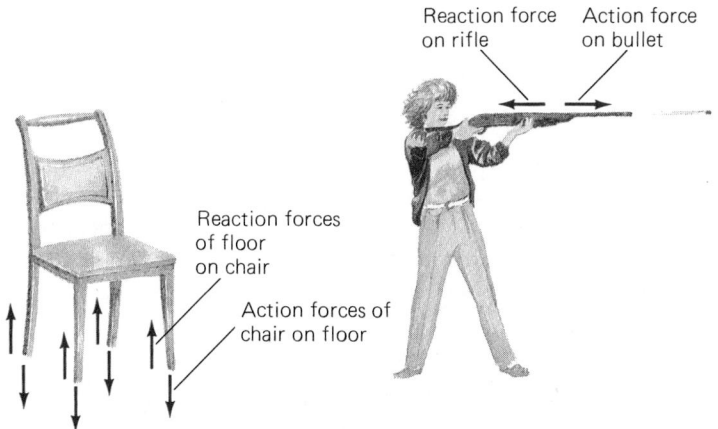

Reaction forces of floor on chair

Action forces of chair on floor

Reaction force on rifle   Action force on bullet

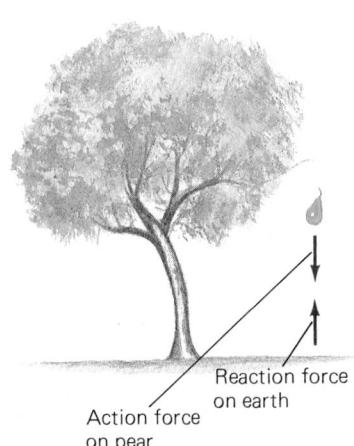

Reaction force on earth

Action force on pear

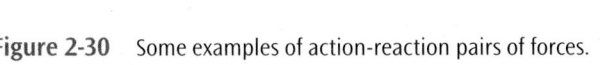

Figure 2-30 Some examples of action-reaction pairs of forces.

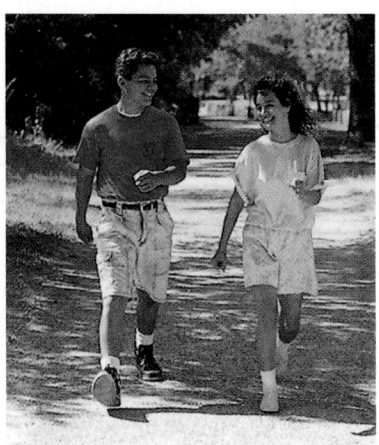

Figure 2-31   When these people push backward on the ground with their feet, the ground pushes forward on them. The latter reaction force is what leads to their forward motion.

The third law of motion permits us to walk. When you walk, what is actually pushing you forward is not your own push on the ground but instead the reaction force of the ground on you (Fig. 2-31). As you move forward, the earth itself moves backward, though by too small an amount (by virtue of its enormous mass) to be detected.

Sometimes the origin of the reaction force is not obvious. A book lying on a table exerts the downward force of its weight; but how can an apparently rigid object like the table exert an upward force on the book? If the tabletop were made of rubber, we would see the book push it down, and the upward force would result from the elasticity of the rubber. A similar explanation actually holds for tabletops of wood or metal, which are never perfectly rigid, although the depressions made in them may be extremely small.

It is sometimes arbitrary which force of an action-reaction pair to consider action and which reaction. For instance, we can't really say that the gravitational pull of the earth on a pear is the action force and the pull of the pear on the earth is the reaction force, or the other way around. When you push on the ground when walking, however, it is legitimate to call this force the action force and the force with which the earth pushes back on you the reaction force.

Gravitation

Left to itself, a moving object travels in a straight line at constant speed. Because the moon circles the earth and the planets circle the sun, forces must be acting on the moon and planets. As we learned in Chap. 1, Newton discovered that these forces are the same in nature as the gravitational force that holds us to the earth. Before we consider how gravity works, we must look into exactly how curved paths come about.

2.12   Circular Motion

A Curved Path Requires an Inward Pull

Tie a ball to the end of a string and whirl the ball around your head, as in Fig. 2-32. What you will find is that your hand must pull on the string to keep the ball moving in a circle. If you let go of the string, there is no longer an inward force on the ball, and it flies off to the side.

Centripetal Force   The force that has to be applied to make something move in a curved path is called **centripetal** ("toward the center") **force:**

> Centripetal force = inward force on an object moving in a curved path

The centripetal force always points toward the center of curvature of the object's path, which means the force is at right angles to the object's direction of motion at each moment. In Fig. 2-32 the ball is moving in a circle, so its velocity vector **v** is always tangent to the circle and the centripetal force vector **F**$_c$ is always directed toward the center of the circle.

A detailed calculation shows that the centripetal force **F**$_c$ needed for something of mass m and speed v to travel in a circle of radius r has the magnitude

$$F_c = \frac{mv^2}{r} \qquad \textit{Centripetal force} \qquad 2\text{-}18$$

This formula tells us three things about the force needed to cause an object to move in a circular path: (1) the greater the object's mass, the greater the force; (2) the faster the object, the greater the force; and (3) the smaller the circle, the greater the force (Fig. 2-33).

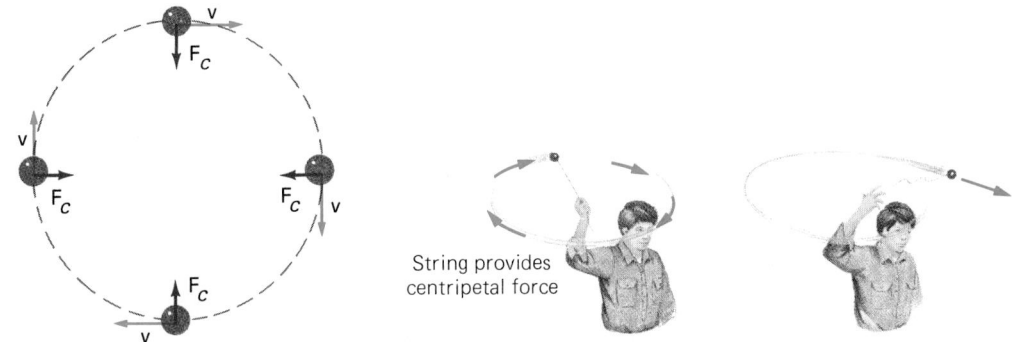

Figure 2-32   A centripetal force is necessary for circular motion. An inward centripetal force **F**$_c$ acts upon every object that moves in a curved path. If the force is removed, the object continues moving in a straight line tangent to its original path.

String provides
centripetal force

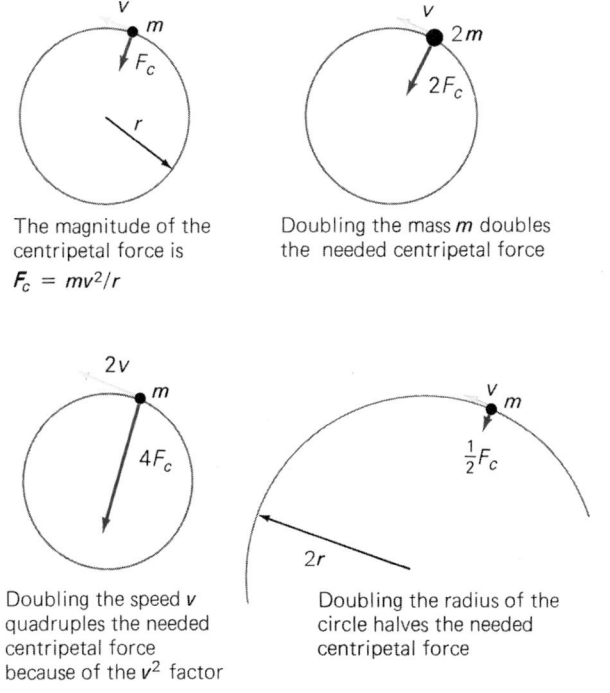

The magnitude of the
centripetal force is

F$_c$ = mv^2/r

Doubling the mass m doubles
the needed centripetal force

Doubling the speed v
quadruples the needed
centripetal force
because of the v^2 factor

Doubling the radius of the
circle halves the needed
centripetal force

Figure 2-33   The centripetal force needed to keep an object moving in a circle depends upon the mass and speed of the object and upon the radius of the circle. The direction of the force is always toward the center of the circle. (Centripetal force is the name given to any force that is always directed toward a center of motion. It is not a distinct type of force, such as gravity or friction.)

Example 2.14

Find the centripetal force needed by a 1000-kg car moving at 5 m/s to go around a curve 30 m in radius, as in Fig. 2-34.

Solution

The centripetal force needed to make the turn is

$$F_c = \frac{mv^2}{r} = \frac{(1000 \text{ kg})(5 \text{ m/s})^2}{30 \text{ m}} = 833 \text{ N}$$

This force (184 lb) is easily transferred from the road to the car's tires if the road is dry and in good condition. However, if the car's speed were 20 m/s, the force needed would be 16 times as great, and the car would probably skid outward.

To reduce the chance of skids, particularly when the road is wet and therefore slippery, highway curves are often **banked** so that the roadbed tilts inward. A car going around a banked curve has an inward reaction force on it provided by the road itself, apart from friction (Fig. 2-35).

[For another example, see Sec. 2.12 at www.mhhe.com/krauskopf.]

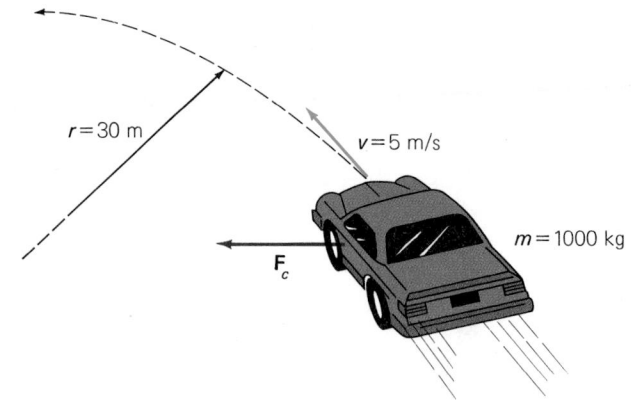

Figure 2-34 A centripetal force of 833 N is needed by this car to make the turn shown.

Figure 2-35 A wall of snow provides this bobsled with the centripetal force it needs to round the turn.

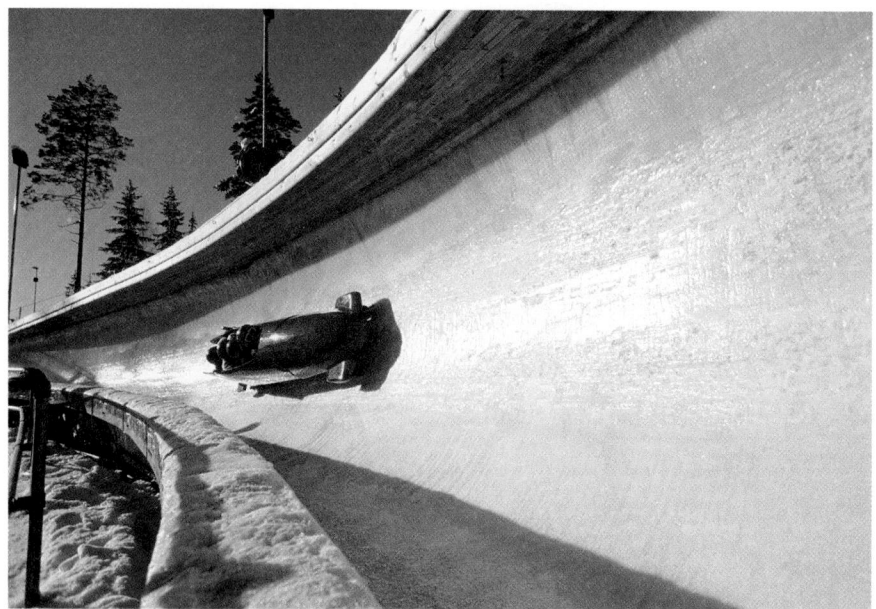

From the formula for F_c we can see why cars rounding a curve are so difficult to steer when the curve is sharp (small r) or the speed is high (a large value for v means a very large value for v^2). On a level road, the centripetal force is supplied by friction between the car's tires and the road. If the force needed to make a particular turn at a certain speed is more than friction can supply, the car skids outward.

2.13 Newton's Law of Gravity

What Holds the Solar System Together

Newton used Kepler's laws of planetary motion and Galileo's findings about falling bodies to establish how the gravitational force between two objects depends on their masses and on the distance between them. His conclusion was this:

> Every object in the universe attracts every other object with a force proportional to both of their masses and inversely proportional to the square of the distance between them.

In equation form, **Newton's law of gravity** states that the force F that acts between two objects whose masses are m_1 and m_2 is

$$\text{Gravitational force} = F = \frac{Gm_1m_2}{R^2} \qquad \textit{Law of gravity} \qquad 2\text{-}19$$

Here R is the distance between the objects and G is a constant of nature, the same number everywhere in the universe. The value of G is $6.670 \times 10^{-11} \text{ N} \cdot \text{m}^2/\text{kg}^2$.

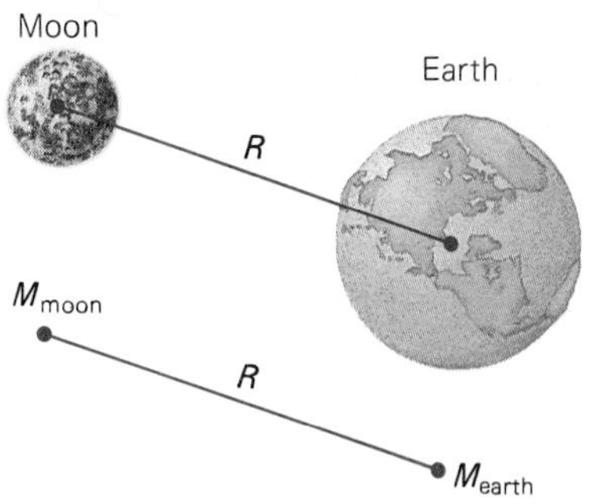

Center of Mass The point in an object from which R is to be measured depends on the object's shape and on the way in which its mass is distributed. The **center of mass** of a uniform sphere is its geometric center (Fig. 2-36).

The inverse square—$1/R^2$—variation of gravitational force with distance R means that this force drops off rapidly with increasing R (Fig. 2-37).

Figure 2-38 shows how this variation affects the weight of a 61-kg astronaut who leaves the earth on a spacecraft. At the earth's surface she weighs 600 N (135 lb); that is, the gravitational attraction of the earth on her is 600 N. When she is 100 times farther from the center of the earth, her weight is $1/100^2$ or $\frac{1}{10,000}$ as great, only 0.06 N—the weight of a cigar on the earth's surface.

Figure 2-36 For computing gravitational effects, spherical bodies (such as the earth and moon) may be regarded as though their masses are located at their geometrical centers, provided that they are uniform spheres or consist of concentric uniform spherical shells.

2.14 Artificial Satellites

Thousands Circle the Earth

The first artificial satellite, Sputnik I, was launched by the Soviet Union in 1957. Since then thousands of others have been put into orbits around the earth, most of them by the United States and the former Soviet Union. Men

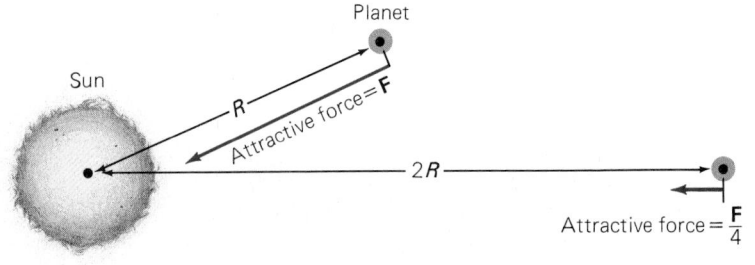

Figure 2-37 The gravitational force between two bodies depends upon the square of the distance between them. The gravitational force on a planet would drop to one-fourth its usual amount if the distance of the planet from the sun were to be doubled. If the distance is halved, the force would increase to 4 times its usual amount.

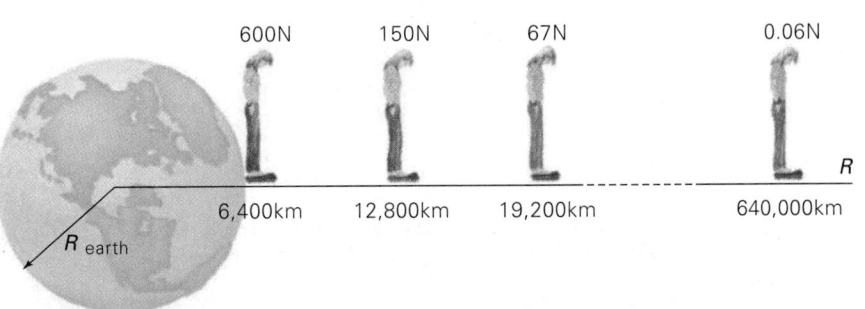

Figure 2-38 The weight of a person near the earth is the gravitational force the earth exerts upon her. As she goes farther and farther away from the earth's surface, her weight decreases inversely as the square of her distance from the earth's center. The mass of the person here is 61 kg.

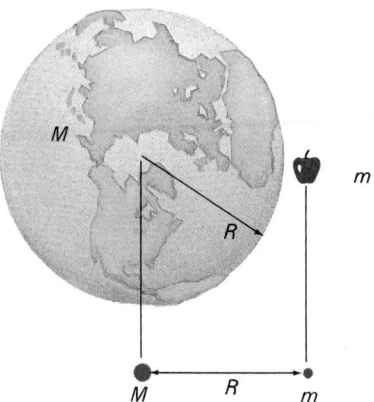

Figure 2-39 The gravitational force of the earth on an apple at the earth's surface is the same as the force between masses M and m the distance R apart. This force equals the weight of the apple.

Example 2.15

On the basis of what we know already, we can find the mass of the earth. This sounds, perhaps, like a formidable job, but it is really fairly easy to do. It is worth following as an example of the indirect way in which scientists go about performing such seemingly impossible feats as "weighing" the earth, the sun, other planets, and even distant stars.

Solution

Let us focus our attention on an apple of mass m on the earth's surface. The downward force of gravity on the apple is its weight of mg:

$$\text{Weight of apple} = F = mg$$

We can also use Newton's law of gravity to find F, with the result

$$\text{Gravitational force on apple} = F = \frac{GmM}{R^2}$$

Here M is the earth's mass and R is the distance between the apple and the center of the earth, which is the earth's radius of 6400 km $= 6.4 \times 10^6$ m (Fig. 2-39). The two ways to find F must give the same result, so

$$\text{Gravitational force on apple} = \text{weight of apple}$$

$$\frac{GmM}{R^2} = mg$$

We note that the apple's mass m appears on both sides of this equation, hence it cancels out. Solving for the earth's mass M gives

$$M = \frac{gR^2}{G} = \frac{(9.8 \ m/s^2)(6.4 \times 10^6 \ m)^2}{6.67 \times 10^{-11} \ N \cdot m^2/kg^2} = 6 \times 10^{24} \ \text{kg}$$

The number 6×10^{24} is 6 followed by 24 zeros! Enormous as it is, the earth is one of the least massive planets: Saturn has 95 times as much mass, and Jupiter 318 times as much. The sun's mass is more than 300,000 times that of the earth.

and women have been in orbit regularly since 1961, when a Soviet cosmonaut circled the globe at an average height of 240 km (Fig. 2-40).

Almost a thousand active satellites are now in orbit. (Over 2000 more are inactive.) About half belong to the United States, 10 percent to Russia, and 4 percent to China, with the rest distributed among two dozen other

Figure 2-40 An earth satellite is always falling toward the earth. As a result, an astronaut inside feels "weightless," just as a person who jumps off a diving board feels "weightless." But a gravitational force does act on both people—what is missing is the upward reaction force of the ground, the diving board, the floor of a room, the seat of a chair, or whatever each person would otherwise be pressing on. In the case of an astronaut, the floor of the satellite falls just as fast as he or she does instead of pushing back.

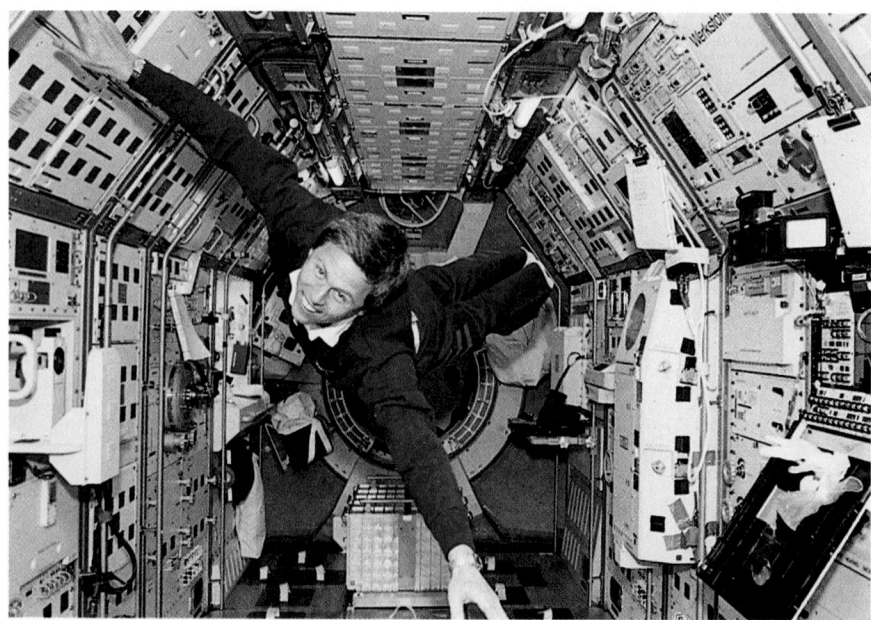

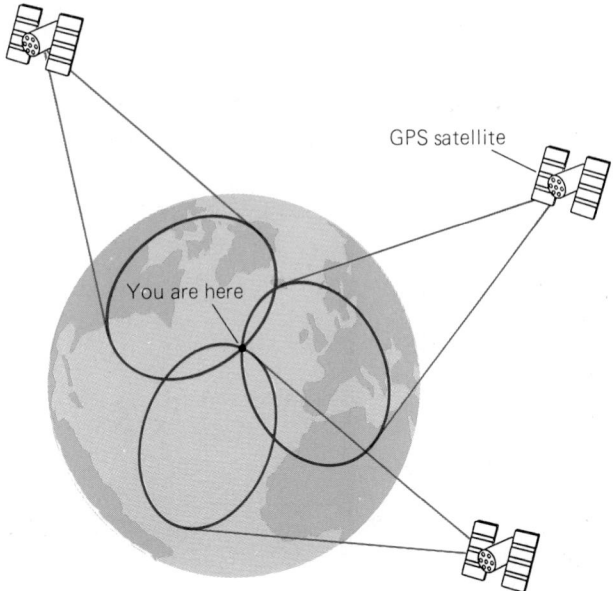

GPS satellite

You are here

Figure 2-41 In the Global Positioning System (GPS), each of a fleet of orbiting satellites sends out coded radio signals that enable a receiver on the earth to determine both the exact position of the satellite in space and its exact distance from the receiver. Given this information, a computer in the receiver then calculates the circle on the earth's surface on which the receiver must lie. Data from three satellites give three circles, and the receiver must be located at the one point where all three intersect.

countries. The closest satellites, from 80 to 2000 km above the earth, are mostly "eyes in the sky" that map the earth's surface; survey it for military purposes; provide information on weather and resources such as mineral deposits, crops, and water; and carry out various scientific studies. A group of 66 satellites in low-earth orbit supports the worldwide Iridium telephone system.

Twenty-seven satellites (3 of them spares) at an altitude of 20,360 km are used in the Global Positioning System (GPS) developed by the United States (Fig. 2-41). GPS receivers, some hardly larger than a wristwatch, enable users to find their positions, including altitude, anywhere in the world at any time with uncertainties of only a few meters (Fig. 2-42). A similar system, called Glonass, is operated by Russia; China has begun work on a system called Baldu ("Big Dipper"); and the European Union is developing yet another system, called Galileo.

The most distant satellites, nearly half the total, circle the equator exactly once a day, so they remain in place indefinitely over a particular location on the earth. A satellite in such a geostationary orbit can "see" a large area of

Seeing Satellites

On a dark night many satellites, even quite small ones, are visible to the naked eye because of the sunlight they reflect. The best times to look are an hour or so before sunrise and an hour or so after sunset. High-altitude satellites can be seen for longer periods because they spend more time outside the earth's shadow. When conditions are just right, the as-yet-incomplete International Space Station is about as bright as the brightest stars. When it is finished, the ISS may rival Venus, except for the moon the most brilliant object in the night sky.

Space Junk

A remarkable amount of debris is in orbit around the earth, relics of the 5000 or so rockets that have thus far gone into space. Most of the debris orbits are 700 to 1000 km above the earth. The U.S. Space Surveillance Network uses radar to track more than 20,000 objects over 10 cm across, which range from dropped astronaut tools all the way up to discarded rocket stages and "dead" satellites, that might collide catastrophically with spacecraft. Unfortunately this system, together with a private one that supplements it, cannot foresee every potential collision, even two satellites smashing together. In 2009 such a catastrophe actually occurred between two communications satellites at an altitude of 780 km, adding over 1500 more pieces of debris to those already in orbit.

In addition, millions of smaller bits and pieces are out there, many of them able to damage spacecraft windows, solar cells, and other relatively fragile components. Even encountering something the size of a pea would be an unwelcome event when its impact speed is 15 to 45 times the speed of a bullet. This is no idle worry: in 2009, the three astronauts in the International Space Station had to temporarily retreat into its "lifeboat," a Russian Soyuz spacecraft, when warned that a 9-mm metal fragment might be on a collision course. In fact, the fragment, whose relative speed was about 32,000 km/h, missed, but by less than 4.5 km. The warning came too late for the ISS to move out of the way, as it had eight times before in its 8 years in orbit.

Figure 2-42 An automobile navigation system uses GPS data to show the location of a car on a displayed map and can give visual or verbal directions to a destination. The map can be a normal top-down view or, in some models, a perspective view.

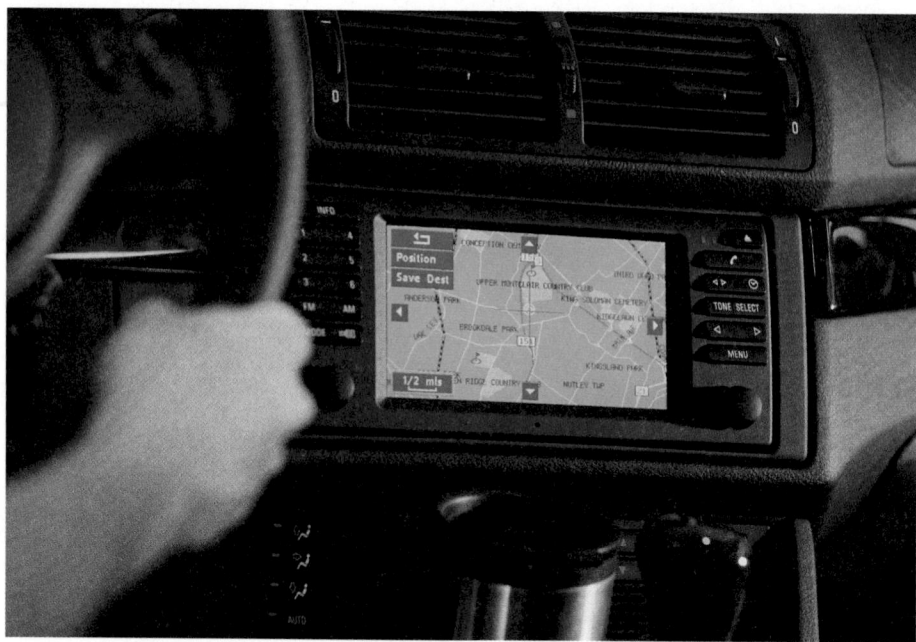

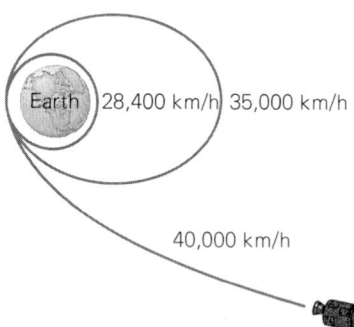

Earth | 28,400 km/h | 35,000 km/h

40,000 km/h

Figure 2-43 The minimum speed an earth satellite can have is 28,400 km/h. The escape speed from the earth is 40,000 km/h.

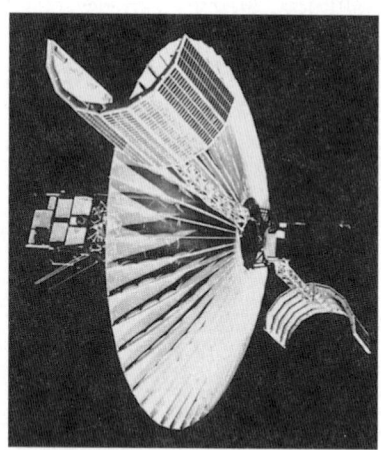

Figure 2-44 This Landsat satellite circles the earth at an altitude of 915 km. The satellite carries a television camera and a scanner system that provides images of the earth's surface in four color bands. The data radioed back provide information valuable in geology, water supply, agriculture, and land-use planning. Today the cost of placing a satellite in earth orbit is between about $10,000 and $20,000 per kg of payload, but new rocket designs are hoped to do this for as little as $2000 per kg.

the earth's surface. Most satellites in geostationary orbits are used to relay communications of all kinds from one place to another, which is often cheaper than using cables between them.

Why Satellites Don't Fall Down What keeps all these satellites up there? The answer is that a satellite *is* actually falling down but, like the moon (which is a natural satellite), at exactly such a rate as to circle the earth in a stable orbit. "Stable" is a relative term, to be sure, since friction due to the extremely thin atmosphere present at the altitudes of actual satellites will eventually bring them down. Satellite lifetimes in orbit range from a matter of days to hundreds of years.

Let us think about a satellite in a circular orbit. The gravitational force on the satellite is its weight mg, where g is the acceleration of gravity at the satellite's altitude (the value of g decreases with increasing altitude). The centripetal force a satellite of speed v needs to circle the earth at the distance r from the earth's center is mv^2/r. Since the earth's gravity is providing this centripetal force,

$$\text{Centripetal force} = \text{gravitational force}$$
$$\frac{mv^2}{r} = mg$$
$$v^2 = rg$$
$$\text{Satellite speed} = v = \sqrt{rg}$$

The mass of the satellite does not matter.

For an orbit a few kilometers above the earth's surface, the satellite speed turns out to be about 28,400 km/h. Anything sent off around the earth at this speed will become a satellite of the earth. (Of course, at such a low altitude air resistance will soon bring it down.) At a lower speed than this an object sent into space would simply fall to the earth, while at a higher speed it would have an elliptical rather than a circular orbit (Fig. 2-43). A satellite initially in an elliptical orbit can be given a circular orbit if it has a small rocket motor to give it a further push at the required distance from the earth (Fig. 2-44).

Escape Speed   If its original speed is high enough, at least 40,000 km/h, a spacecraft can escape entirely from the earth. The speed required for something to leave the gravitational influence of an astronomical body permanently is called the **escape speed.** Readers of *Through the Looking Glass* may recall the Red Queen's remark, "Now, here, you see, it takes all the running you can do to stay in the same place. If you want to get somewhere else, you must run at least twice as fast as that!" The ratio between escape speed and minimum orbital speed is actually $\sqrt{2}$, about 1.41. Escape speeds for the planets are listed in Table 17-1.

It is worth keeping in mind that escape speed is the initial speed needed for something to leave a planet (or other astronomical body, such as a star) permanently when there is no further propulsion. A spacecraft whose motor runs continuously can go out into space without ever reaching the escape speed—even a snail's pace would be enough, given sufficient time.

Important Terms and Ideas

When we say something is moving, we mean that its position relative to something else—the **frame of reference**—is changing. The choice of an appropriate frame of reference depends on the situation.

The **speed** of an object is the rate at which it covers distance relative to a frame of reference. The object's **velocity** specifies both its speed and the direction in which it is moving. The **acceleration** of an object is the rate at which its speed changes. Changes in direction are also accelerations.

A **scalar quantity** has magnitude only; mass and speed are examples. A **vector quantity** has both magnitude and direction; force and velocity are examples. An arrowed line that represents the magnitude and direction of a quantity is called a **vector.**

The **acceleration of gravity** is the downward acceleration of a freely falling object near the earth's surface. Its value is $g = 9.8$ m/s^2.

The **inertia** of an object is the resistance the object offers to any change in its state of rest or motion. The property of matter that shows itself as inertia is called **mass;** mass may be thought of as quantity of matter. The unit of mass is the **kilogram** (kg).

A **force** is any influence that can cause an object to be accelerated. The unit of force is the **newton** (N). The **weight** of an object is the gravitational force with which the earth attracts it.

Newton's **first law of motion** states that, if no net force acts on it, every object continues in its state of rest or uniform motion in a straight line. Newton's **second law of motion** states that when a net force F acts on an object of mass m, the object is given an acceleration of F/m in the same direction as that of the force. Newton's **third law of motion** states that when one object exerts a force on a second object, the second object exerts an equal but opposite force on the first. Thus for every **action force** there is an equal but opposite **reaction force.**

The **centripetal force** on an object moving along a curved path is the inward force needed to cause this motion. Centripetal force acts toward the center of curvature of the path.

Newton's law of gravity states that every object in the universe attracts every other object with a force directly proportional to both their masses and inversely proportional to the square of the distance separating them.

Important Formulas

Pythagorean theorem for right triangle (C is longest side): $A^2 + B^2 = C^2$

$$\text{Speed: } v = \frac{d}{t}$$

$$\text{Acceleration: } a = \frac{v_2 - v_1}{t}$$

$$d = v_1 t + \tfrac{1}{2}at^2$$

$$h = \tfrac{1}{2}gt^2$$

$$\text{Second law of motion: } F = ma$$

$$\text{Weight: } w = mg$$

$$\text{Centripetal force: } F_c = \frac{mv^2}{r}$$

$$\text{Law of gravity: } F = \frac{Gm_1 m_2}{R^2}$$

Multiple Choice

1. Which of the following quantities is not a vector quantity?
   a. velocity
   b. acceleration
   c. mass
   d. force

2. Which of the following statements is incorrect?
   a. All vector quantities have directions.
   b. All vector quantities have magnitudes.
   c. All scalar quantities have directions.
   d. All scalar quantities have magnitudes.

3. A box suspended by a rope is pulled to one side by a horizontal force. The tension in the rope
   a. is less than before
   b. is unchanged
   c. is greater than before
   d. may be any of the above, depending on how strong the force is

4. The sum of two vectors is a minimum when the angle between them is
   a. 0
   b. 45°
   c. 90°
   d. 180°

5. In which of the following examples is the motion of the car not accelerated?
   a. A car turns a corner at the constant speed of 20 km/h.
   b. A car climbs a steep hill with its speed dropping from 60 km/h at the bottom to 15 km/h at the top.
   c. A car climbs a steep hill at the constant speed of 40 km/h.
   d. A car climbs a steep hill and goes over the crest and down on the other side, all at the same speed of 40 km/h.

6. Two objects have the same size and shape but one of them is twice as heavy as the other. They are dropped simultaneously from a tower. If air resistance is negligible,
   a. the heavy object strikes the ground before the light one
   b. they strike the ground at the same time, but the heavy object has the higher speed
   c. they strike the ground at the same time and have the same speed
   d. they strike the ground at the same time, but the heavy object has the lower acceleration because it has more mass

7. The acceleration of a stone thrown upward is
   a. greater than that of a stone thrown downward
   b. the same as that of a stone thrown downward
   c. less than that of a stone thrown downward
   d. zero until it reaches the highest point in its path

8. You are riding a bicycle at constant speed when you throw a ball vertically upward. It will land
   a. in front of you
   b. on your head
   c. behind you
   d. any of the above, depending on the ball's speed

9. When an object is accelerated,
   a. its direction never changes
   b. its speed always increases
   c. it always falls toward the earth
   d. a net force always acts on it

10. If we know the magnitude and direction of the net force on an object of known mass, Newton's second law of motion lets us find its
    a. position
    b. speed
    c. acceleration
    d. weight

11. The weight of an object
    a. is the quantity of matter it contains
    b. is the force with which it is attracted to the earth
    c. is basically the same quantity as its mass but is expressed in different units
    d. refers to its inertia

12. Compared with her mass and weight on the earth, an astronaut on Venus, where the acceleration of gravity is 8.8 m/s^2, has
    a. less mass and less weight
    b. less mass and the same weight
    c. less mass and more weight
    d. the same mass and less weight

13. The earth and the moon exert equal and opposite forces on each other. The force the earth exerts on the moon
    a. is the action force
    b. is the reaction force
    c. can be considered either as the action or as the reaction force
    d. cannot be considered as part of an action-reaction pair because the forces act in opposite directions

14. A car that is towing a trailer is accelerating on a level road. The magnitude of the force the car exerts on the trailer is
    a. equal to the force the trailer exerts on the car
    b. greater than the force the trailer exerts on the car
    c. equal to the force the trailer exerts on the road
    d. equal to the force the road exerts on the trailer

15. When a boy pulls a cart, the force that causes him to move forward is
    a. the force the cart exerts on him
    b. the force he exerts on the cart
    c. the force he exerts on the ground with his feet
    d. the force the ground exerts on his feet

16. In order to cause something to move in a circular path, it is necessary to provide
    a. a reaction force
    b. an inertial force
    c. a centripetal force
    d. a gravitational force

17. An object is moving in a circle with a constant speed. Its acceleration is constant in
  a. magnitude only
  b. direction only
  c. both magnitude and direction
  d. neither magnitude nor direction

18. A car rounds a curve on a level road. The centripetal force on the car is provided by
  a. inertia
  b. gravity
  c. friction between the tires and the road
  d. the force applied to the steering wheel

19. The centripetal force that keeps the earth in its orbit around the sun is provided
  a. by inertia
  b. by the earth's rotation on its axis
  c. partly by the gravitational pull of the sun
  d. entirely by the gravitational pull of the sun

20. The gravitational force with which the earth attracts the moon
  a. is less than the force with which the moon attracts the earth
  b. is the same as the force with which the moon attracts the earth
  c. is more than the force with which the moon attracts the earth
  d. varies with the phase of the moon

21. The speed needed to put a satellite in orbit does not depend on
  a. the mass of the satellite
  b. the radius of the orbit
  c. the shape of the orbit
  d. the value of g at the orbit

22. An astronaut inside an orbiting satellite feels weightless because
  a. he or she is wearing a space suit
  b. the satellite is falling toward the earth just as fast as the astronaut is, so there is no upward reaction force on him or her
  c. there is no gravitational pull from the earth so far away
  d. the sun's gravitational pull balances out the earth's gravitational pull

23. A bicycle travels 12 km in 40 min. Its average speed is
  a. 0.3 km/h   **c.** 18 km/h
  b. 8 km/h   **d.** 48 km/h

24. Which one or more of the following sets of displacements might be able to return a car to its starting point?
  a. 5, 5, and 5 km   **c.** 5, 10, and 10 km
  b. 5, 5, and 10 km   **d.** 5, 5, and 20 km

25. An airplane whose airspeed is 200 km/h is flying in a wind of 80 km/h. The airplane's speed relative to the ground is between
  a. 80 and 200 km/h   **c.** 120 and 200 km/h
  b. 80 and 280 km/h   **d.** 120 and 280 km/h

26. A ship travels 200 km to the south and then 400 km to the west. The ship's displacement from its starting point is
  a. 200 km   **c.** 450 km
  b. 400 km   **d.** 600 km

27. How long does a car whose acceleration is 2 m/s^2 need to go from 10 m/s to 30 m/s?
  a. 10 s   **c.** 40 s
  b. 20 s   **d.** 400 s

28. A ball is thrown upward at a speed of 12 m/s. It will reach the top of its path in about
  a. 0.6 s   **c.** 1.8 s
  b. 1.2 s   **d.** 2.4 s

29. A car that starts from rest has a constant acceleration of 4 m/s^2. In the first 3 s the car travels
  a. 6 m   **c.** 18 m
  b. 12 m   **d.** 172 m

30. A car traveling at 10 m/s begins to be accelerated at 12 m/s^2. The distance the car covers in the first 5 s after the acceleration begins is
  a. 15 m   **c.** 53 m
  b. 25 m   **d.** 65 m

31. A car with its brakes applied has an acceleration of -1.2 m/s^2. If its initial speed is 10 m/s, the distance the car covers in the first 5 s after the acceleration begins is
  a. 15 m   **c.** 35 m
  b. 32 m   **d.** 47 m

32. The distance the car of Multiple Choice 31 travels before it comes to a stop is
  a. 6.5 m   **c.** 21 m
  b. 8.3 m   **d.** 42 m

33. A bottle falls from a blimp whose altitude is 1200 m. If there was no air resistance, the bottle would reach the ground in
  a. 5 s   **c.** 16 s
  b. 11 s   **d.** 245 s

34. When a net force of 1 N acts on a 1-kg body, the body receives
  a. a speed of 1 m/s
  b. an acceleration of 0.1 m/s^2
  c. an acceleration of 1 m/s^2
  d. an acceleration of 9.8 m/s^2

35. When a net force of 1 N acts on a 1-N body, the body receives
  a. a speed of 1 m/s
  b. an acceleration of 0.1 m/s^2
  c. an acceleration of 1 m/s^2
  d. an acceleration of 9.8 m/s^2

36. A car whose mass is 1600 kg (including the driver) has a maximum acceleration of 1.20 m/s^2. When a certain passenger is also in the car, its maximum acceleration becomes 1.13 m/s^2. The mass of the passenger is
  a. 100 kg   **c.** 112 kg
  b. 108 kg   **d.** 134 kg

37. A 300-g ball is struck with a bat with a force of 150 N. If the bat was in contact with the ball for 0.020 s, the ball's speed is
   a. 0.01 m/s   **c.** 2.5 m/s
   b. 0.1 m/s   **d.** 10 m/s

38. A bicycle and its rider together have a mass of 80 kg. If the bicycle's speed is 6 m/s, the force needed to bring it to a stop in 4 s is
   a. 12 N   **c.** 120 N
   b. 53 N   **d.** 1176 N

39. The weight of 400 g of onions is
   a. 0.041 N   **c.** 3.9 N
   b. 0.4 N   **d.** 3920 N

40. A salami weighs 3 lb. Its mass is
   a. 0.31 kg   **c.** 6.6 kg
   b. 1.36 kg   **d.** 29.4 kg

41. An upward force of 600 N acts on a 50-kg dumbwaiter. The dumbwaiter's acceleration is
   a. 0.82 m/s^2 **c.** 11 m/s^2
   b. 2.2 m/s^2 **d.** 12 m/s^2

42. The upward force the rope of a hoist must exert to raise a 400-kg load of bricks with an acceleration of 0.4 m/s^2 is
   a. 160 N   **c.** 3760 N
   b. 1568 N   **d.** 4080 N

43. The radius of the circle in which an object is moving at constant speed is doubled. The required centripetal force is
   a. one-quarter as great as before
   b. one-half as great as before

   c. twice as great as before
   d. 4 times as great as before

44. A car rounds a curve at 20 km/h. If it rounds the curve at 40 km/h, its tendency to overturn is
   a. halved   **c.** tripled
   b. doubled   **d.** quadrupled

45. A 1200-kg car whose speed is 6 m/s rounds a turn whose radius is 30 m. The centripetal force on the car is
   a. 48 N   **c.** 240 N
   b. 147 N   **d.** 1440 N

46. If the earth were 3 times as far from the sun as it is now, the gravitational force exerted on it by the sun would be
   a. 3 times as large as it is now
   b. 9 times as large as it is now
   c. one-third as large as it is now
   d. one-ninth as large as it is now

47. A woman whose mass is 60 kg on the earth's surface is in a spacecraft at an altitude of one earth's radius above the surface. Her mass there is
   a. 15 kg   **c.** 60 kg
   b. 30 kg   **d.** 120 kg

48. A man whose weight is 800 N on the earth's surface is also in the spacecraft of Multiple Choice 47. His weight there is
   a. 200 N   **c.** 800 N
   b. 400 N   **d.** 1600 N

Exercises

2.1 Speed

1. A woman standing before a cliff claps her hands, and 2.8 s later she hears the echo. How far away is the cliff? The speed of sound in air at ordinary temperatures is 343 m/s.

2. The starter of a race stands at one end of a line of runners. What is the difference in time between the arrival of the sound of his pistol at the nearest runner and at the most distant runner 10 m farther away? (In a sprint, 0.01 s can mean the difference between winning and coming in second.)

3. In 1977 Steve Weldon ate 91 m of spaghetti in 29 s. At the same speed, how long would it take Mr. Weldon to eat 5 m of spaghetti?

4. A snake is slithering toward you at 1.5 m/s. If you start walking when it is 5 m away, how fast must you go so that the snake will not overtake you when you have gone 100 m?

5. A woman jogs for 2 km at 8 km/h and then walks for 2 km at 6 km/h. What is her average speed for the entire trip?

2.2 Vectors

6. Three forces, each of 10 lb, act on the same object. What is the maximum total force they can exert on the object? The minimum total force?

7. Is it correct to say that scalar quantities are abstract, idealized quantities with no precise counterparts in the physical world, whereas vector quantities properly represent reality because they take directions into account?

8. A man is rowing at 8 km/h in a river 1.5 km wide in which the current is 5 km/h. (a) In what direction should he head in order to get across the river in the shortest possible time? (b) How much time will he take if he goes in this direction? (c) How far downstream will the boat have gone when it reaches the opposite side?

9. A woman walks 70 m to an elevator and then rises upward 40 m. What is her displacement from her starting point?

10. Two tugboats are towing a ship. Each exerts a horizontal force of 5 tons and the angle between their towropes is 90°. What net force is exerted on the ship?

2.3 Acceleration

11. Can a rapidly moving object have the same acceleration as a slowly moving one?

12. The acceleration of a certain moving object is constant in magnitude and direction. Must the path of the object be a straight line? If not, give an example.

13. A car whose acceleration is constant reaches a speed of 80 km/h in 20 s starting from rest. How much more time is required for it to reach a speed of 130 km/h?

14. The brakes of a car are applied to give it an acceleration of -3 m/s^2. The car comes to a stop in 5 s. What was its speed when the brakes were applied?

15. A car starts from rest and reaches a speed of 40 m/s in 10 s. If its acceleration remains the same, how fast will it be moving 5 s later?

16. The brakes of a car moving at 14 m/s are applied, and the car comes to a stop in 4 s. (a) What was the car's acceleration? (b) How long would the car take to come to a stop starting from 20 m/s with the same acceleration? (c) How long would the car take to slow down from 20 m/s to 10 m/s with the same acceleration?

2.4 Distance, Time, and Acceleration

17. A car is moving at 10 m/s when it begins to be accelerated at 2.5 m/s^2. (a) How long does the car take to reach a speed of 25 m/s? (b) How far does it go during this period?

18. The driver of a train moving at 20 m/s applies the brakes when it passes an amber signal. The next signal is 1 km down the track and the train reaches it 75 s later. Find the train's acceleration and its speed at the next signal.

19. A car starts from rest and covers 400 m (very nearly $\frac{1}{4}$ mi) in 20 s. Find the average acceleration of the car and its final speed.

2.5 Free Fall

20. Is it true that something dropped from rest falls three times farther in the second second after being let go than it does in the first second?

21. A rifle is aimed directly at a squirrel in a tree. Should the squirrel drop from the tree at the instant the rifle is fired or should it remain where it is? Why?

22. The acceleration of gravity on the surface of Venus is 8.9 m/s^2. Would a ball thrown upward on Venus return to the ground sooner or later than a ball thrown upward with the same speed on the earth?

23. When a football is thrown, it follows a curved path through the air like the ones shown in Fig. 2-18. Where in its path is the ball's speed greatest? Where is it least?

24. A crate is dropped from an airplane flying horizontally at constant speed. How does the path

of the crate appear to somebody on the airplane? To somebody on the ground?

25. A stone is thrown horizontally from a cliff and another, identical stone is dropped from there at the same time. Do the stones reach the ground at the same time? How do their speeds compare when they reach the ground? Their accelerations?

26. (a) Imagine that Charlotte drops a ball from a window on the twentieth floor of a building while at the same time Fred drops another ball from a window on the nineteenth floor of that building. As the balls fall, what happens to the distance between them (assuming no air resistance)? (b) Next imagine that Charlotte and Fred are at the same window on the twentieth floor and that Fred drops his ball a few seconds after Charlotte drops hers. As the balls fall, what happens to the distance between them now (again assuming no air resistance)?

27. A person in a stationary elevator drops a coin and the coin reaches the floor of the elevator 0.6 s later. Would the coin reach the floor in less time, the same time, or more time if it were dropped when the elevator was (a) falling at a constant speed? (b) falling at a constant acceleration? (c) rising at a constant speed? (d) rising at a constant acceleration?

28. How fast must a ball be thrown upward to reach a height of 12 m?

29. A person dives off the edge of a cliff 33 m above the surface of the sea below. Assuming that air resistance is negligible, how long does the dive last and with what speed does the person enter the water?

30. A ball dropped from the roof of a building takes 4 s to reach the street. How high is the building?

31. A ball is thrown downward at 12 m/s. What is its speed 1.0 s later?

32. When will a stone thrown vertically upward at 9.8 m/s reach the ground?

33. A ball is thrown upward from the edge of a cliff with an initial speed of 6 m/s. (a) How fast is it moving 0.5 s later? In what direction? (b) How fast is it moving 2 s later? In what direction? (Consider upward as + and downward as −; then $v_1 = +6$ m/s and $g = -9.8$ m/s^2.)

34. The air resistance experienced by a falling object is not an important factor until a speed of about half its terminal speed is reached. The terminal speed of a golf ball is 40 m/s. How much time is needed for a dropped golf ball to reach a speed of half this? How far does it fall in this time?

35. A ball is thrown vertically upward with an initial speed of 30 m/s. (a) How long will it take the ball to reach the highest point in its path? (b) How long will it take the ball to return to its starting place? (c) What will the ball's speed be there?

36. A rifle is aimed directly at the bull's-eye of a target 50 m away. If the bullet's speed is 350 m/s, how far below the bull's-eye does the bullet strike the target?

37. An airplane is in level flight at a speed of 100 m/s and an altitude of 1200 m when a windshield wiper falls off. What will the wiper's speed be when it reaches the ground? (Hint: A vector calculation is needed.)

38. A ball is thrown horizontally from the roof of a building 20 m high at 30 m/s. At what speed will the ball strike the ground?

39. A bullet is fired horizontally from a rifle at 200 m/s from a cliff above a plain below. The bullet reaches the plain 5 s later. (a) How high was the cliff? (b) How far from the cliff did the bullet reach the plain? (c) What was the bullet's speed when it reached the plain?

40. An airplane whose speed is 60 m/s is flying at an altitude of 500 m over the ocean toward a stationary sinking ship. At what horizontal distance from the ship should the crew of the airplane drop a pump into the water next to the ship?

41. A person at the masthead of a sailboat moving at constant speed in a straight line drops a wrench. The masthead is 20 m above the boat's deck and the stern of the boat is 10 m behind the mast. Is there a minimum speed the sailboat can have so that the wrench will not land on the deck? If there is such a speed, what is it?

2.9   Second Law of Motion

42. Compare the tension in the coupling between the first two cars of a train with the tension in the coupling between the last two cars when (a) the train's speed is constant and (b) the train is accelerating.

43. In accelerating from a standing start to a speed of 300 km/h (186 mi/h—not its top speed!), the 1900-kg Bugatti Veyron sports car exerts an average force on the road of 9.4 kN. How long does the car take to reach 300 km/h?

44. A 12,000-kg airplane launched by a catapult from an aircraft carrier is accelerated from 0 to 200 km/h in 3 s. (a) How many times the acceleration due to gravity is the airplane's acceleration? (b) What is the average force the catapult exerts on the airplane?

45. The brakes of a 1200-kg car exert a force of 4 kN. How long will it take for them to slow the car to a stop from an initial speed of 24 m/s?

46. A force of 20 N gives an object an acceleration of 5 m/s². (a) What force would be needed to give the same object an acceleration of 1 m/s²? (b) What force would be needed to give it an acceleration of 10 m/s²?

47. A bicycle and its rider together have a mass of 80 kg. If the bicycle's speed is 6 m/s, how much force is needed to bring it to a stop in 4 s?

48. A 430-g soccer ball at rest on the ground is kicked with a force of 600 N and flies off at 15 m/s. How long was the toe of the person kicking the ball in contact with it?

49. A car and driver with a total mass of 1600 kg has a maximum acceleration of 1.2 m/s². If the car picks up three 80-kg passengers, what is its maximum acceleration now?

50. Before picking up the passengers, the driver of the car of Exercise 49 shifts into neutral when the car is moving at 80 km/h and finds that its speed has dropped to 65 km/h after 10 s. What was the average drag force acting on the car?

2.10   Mass and Weight

51. Consider the statement: Sara weighs 55 kg. What is wrong with the statement? Give two ways to correct it.

52. When a force equal to its weight is applied to an object free to move, what is its acceleration?

53. A person weighs 85 N on the surface of the moon and 490 N on the surface of the earth. What is the acceleration of gravity on the surface of the moon?

54. A mass of 8 kg and another of 12 kg are suspended by a string on either side of a frictionless pulley. Find the acceleration of each mass.

55. An 80-kg man slides down a rope at constant speed. (a) What is the minimum breaking strength the rope must have? (b) If the rope has precisely this strength, will it support the man if he tries to climb back up?

56. How much force is needed to give a 5-kg box an upward acceleration of 2 m/s²?

57. A parachutist whose total mass is 100 kg is falling at 50 m/s when her parachute opens. Her speed drops to 6 m/s in 2 s. What is the total force her harness had to withstand? How many times her weight is this force?

58. A person in an elevator suspends a 1-kg mass from a spring balance. What is the nature of the elevator's motion when the balance reads 9.0 N? 9.8 N? 10.0 N?

59. A person stands on a scale in an elevator. When the elevator is at rest, the scale reads 700 N. When the elevator starts to move, the scale reads 600 N. (a) Is the elevator going up or down? (b) Is it accelerated? If so, what is the acceleration?

60. A 60-kg person stands on a scale in an elevator. How many newtons does the scale read (a) when the elevator is ascending with an acceleration of 1 m/s²; (b) when it is descending with an acceleration of 1 m/s²; (c) when it is ascending at a constant speed of 3 m/s; (d) when it is descending at a constant speed of 3 m/s; (e) when the cable has broken and the elevator is descending in free fall?

2.11   Third Law of Motion

61. Since the opposite forces of the third law of motion are equal in magnitude, how can anything ever be accelerated?

62. What is the relationship, if any, between the first and second laws of motion? Between the second and third laws of motion?

63. A book rests on a table. (a) What is the reaction force to the force the book exerts on the table? (b) To the force gravity exerts on the book?

64. A car with its engine running and in forward gear goes up a hill and then down on the other side. What forces cause it to move upward? Downward?

65. An engineer designs a propeller-driven spacecraft. Because there is no air in space, the engineer includes a supply of oxygen as well as a supply of fuel for the motor. What do you think of the idea?

66. Two children wish to break a string. Are they more likely to succeed if each takes one end of the string and they pull against each other, or if they tie one end of the string to a tree and both pull on the free end? Why?

67. When a 5-kg rifle is fired, the 9-g bullet is given an acceleration of 30 km/s while it is in the barrel. (a) How much force acts on the bullet? (b) Does any force act on the rifle? If so, how much and in what direction?

2.12 Circular Motion

68. Where should you stand on the earth's surface to experience the most centripetal force? The least?

69. Under what circumstances, if any, can something move in a circular path without a centripetal force acting on it?

70. A person swings an iron ball in a vertical circle at the end of a string. At what point in the circle is the string most likely to break? Why?

71. A car makes a clockwise turn on a level road at too high a speed and overturns. Do its left or right wheels leave the road first?

72. When you whirl a ball at the end of a string, the ball seems to be pulling outward away from your hand. When you let the string go, however, the ball moves along a straight path perpendicular to the direction of the string at the moment you let go. Explain each of these effects.

73. A 40-kg crate is lying on the flat floor of a truck moving at 15 m/s. A force of 150 N is needed to slide the crate against the friction between the bottom of the crate and the floor. What is the minimum radius of a turn the station wagon can make if the box is not to slip?

74. The greatest force a level road can exert on the tires of a certain 2000-kg car is 4 kN. What is the highest speed the car can round a curve of radius 200 m without skidding?

75. Find the minimum radius at which an airplane flying at 300 m/s can make a U-turn if the centripetal force on it is not to exceed 4 times the airplane's weight.

76. Some people believe that aliens from elsewhere in the universe visit the earth in spacecraft that travel faster than jet airplanes and can turn in their own lengths. Calculate the centripetal force on a 100-kg alien in a spacecraft moving at 500 m/s (1120 mi/h) while it is making a turn of radius 30 m. How many times the weight of the alien is this force? Do you think such stories can be believed?

77. The 200-g head of a golf club moves at 40 m/s in a circular arc of 1.2 m radius. How much force must the player exert on the handle of the club to prevent it from flying out of her hands at the bottom of the swing? Ignore the mass of the club's shaft.

78. An airplane flying at a constant speed of 160 m/s pulls out of a dive in a circular arc. The 80-kg pilot presses down on his seat with a force of 3000 N at the bottom of the arc. What is the radius of the arc?

2.13 Newton's Law of Gravity

79. A track team on the moon could set new records for the high jump or pole vault (if they did not need space suits, of course) because of the smaller gravitational force. Could sprinters also improve their times for the 100-m dash?

80. If the moon were half as far from the earth as it is today, how would the gravitational force it exerts on the earth compare with the force it exerts today?

81. Compare the weight and mass of an object at the earth's surface with what they would be at an altitude of two earth's radii.

82. A hole is bored to the center of the earth and a stone is dropped into it. How do the mass and weight of the stone at the earth's center compare with their values at the earth's surface?

83. Is the sun's gravitational pull on the earth the same at all seasons of the year? Explain.

84. The centripetal force that keeps the moon in its orbit around the earth is provided by the gravitational pull of the earth. This force accelerates the moon toward the earth at 2.7×10^{-3} m/s^2, so that the moon is continually "falling" toward the earth. How far does the moon fall toward the earth per second? Per year? Why doesn't the moon come closer and closer to the earth?

85. According to Kepler's second law, the earth travels fastest when it is closest to the sun. Is this consistent with the law of gravitation? Explain.

86. A 2-kg mass is 1 m away from a 5-kg mass. What is the gravitational force (a) that the 5-kg mass exerts on the 2-kg mass, and (b) that the 2-kg mass exerts on the 5-kg mass? (c) If both masses are free to move, what are their respective accelerations if no other forces are acting?

87. A dishonest grocer installs a 100-kg lead block under the pan of his scale. How much gravitational force does the lead exert on 2 kg of cheese placed on the pan if the centers of mass of the lead and cheese are 0.3 m apart? Compare this force with the weight of 1 g of cheese to see if putting the lead under the scale was worth doing.

88. A bull and a cow elephant, each of mass 2000 kg, attract each other gravitationally with a force of 2×10^{-5} N. How far apart are they?

2.14 Artificial Satellites

89. An airplane makes a vertical circle in which it is upside down at the top of the loop. Will the passengers fall out of their seats if there is no belt to hold them in place?

90. Two satellites are launched from Cape Canaveral with the same initial speeds relative to the earth's surface. One is sent toward the west, the other toward the east. Will there be any difference in their orbits? If so, what will the difference be and why?

91. Is an astronaut in an orbiting spacecraft actually "weightless"?

92. With the help of the data in Table 17-1, find the minimum speed artificial satellites must have to pursue stable orbits about Mars.

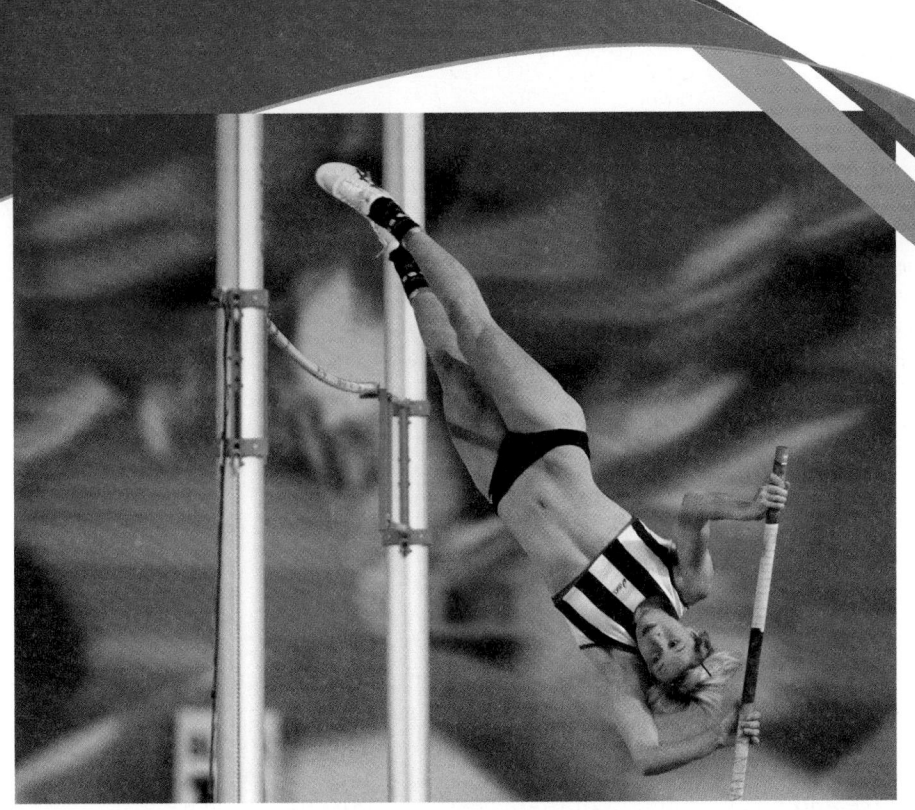

In a pole vault, the athlete's energy of motion while running is first transformed into energy of position at the top of the vault, then back into energy of motion while falling, and finally into work done when landing.

3

Energy

GOALS

When you have finished this chapter you should be able to complete the goals given for each section below:

Work

3.1 The Meaning of Work
A Measure of the Change a Force Produces
- Explain why work is an important quantity.

3.2 Power
The Rate of Doing Work
- Relate work, power, and time.

Energy

3.3 Kinetic Energy
The Energy of Motion

3.4 Potential Energy
The Energy of Position
- Distinguish between kinetic energy and potential energy.
- Give several examples of potential energy.

3.5 Energy Transformations
Easy Come, Easy Go

3.6 Conservation of Energy
A Fundamental Law of Nature
- State the law of conservation of energy and give several examples of energy transformations.
- Use the principle of conservation of energy to analyze events in which work and different forms of energy are transformed into one another.

3.7 The Nature of Heat
The Downfall of Caloric
- Discuss why heat is today regarded as a form of energy rather than as an actual substance.

Momentum

3.8 Linear Momentum
Another Conservation Law
- Define linear momentum and discuss its significance.

3.9 Rockets
Momentum Conservation Is the Basis of Space Travel
- Use the principle of conservation of lin-ear momentum to analyze the motion

of objects that collide with each other or push each other apart, for instance, when a rocket is fired.

3.10 Angular Momentum
A Measure of the Tendency of a Spinning Object to Continue to Spin
- Explain how conservation of angular momentum is used by skaters to spin faster and by footballs to travel farther.

Relativity

3.11 Special Relativity
Things Are Seldom What They Seem
- Describe several relativistic effects and indicate why they are not conspicuous in the everyday world.

3.12 Rest Energy
Matter Is a Form of Energy
- Explain what is meant by rest energy and be able to calculate the rest energy of an object of given mass.

3.13 General Relativity
Gravity Is a Warping of Spacetime
- Describe how gravity is interpreted in Einstein's general theory of relativity.

The word energy has become part of everyday life. We say that an active person is energetic. We hear a candy bar described as being full of energy. We complain about the cost of the electric energy that lights our lamps and turns our motors. We worry about some day running out of the energy stored in coal and oil. We argue about whether nuclear energy is a blessing or a curse. Exactly what is meant by energy?

In general, energy refers to an ability to accomplish change. When almost anything happens in the physical world, energy is somehow involved. But "change" is not a very precise notion, and we must be sure of exactly what we are talking about in order to go further. Our procedure will be to begin with the simpler idea of work and then use it to relate change and energy in the orderly way of science.

Work

Changes that take place in the physical world are the result of forces. Forces are needed to pick things up, to move things from one place to another, to squeeze things, to stretch things, and so on. However, not all forces act to produce changes, and it is the distinction between forces that accomplish change and forces that do not that is central to the idea of work.

3.1   The Meaning of Work

A Measure of the Change a Force Produces

Suppose we push against a wall. When we stop, nothing has happened even though we exerted a force on the wall. But if we apply the same force to a stone, the stone flies through the air when we let it go (Fig. 3-1). The difference is that the wall did not move during our push but the stone did. A physicist would say that we have done work on the stone, and as a result it was accelerated and moved away from our hand.

Or we might try to lift a heavy barbell. If we fail, the world is exactly the same afterward. If we succeed, though, the barbell is now up in the air, which represents a change (Fig. 3-2). As before, the difference is that in the second case an object moved while we exerted a force on it, which means that work was done on the object.

To make our ideas definite, **work** is defined in this way:

> The work done by a force acting on an object is equal to the magnitude of the force multiplied by the distance through which the force acts when both are in the same direction.

If nothing moves, no work is done, no matter how great the force. And even if something moves, work is not done on it unless a force is acting on it.

What we usually think of as work agrees with this definition. However, we must be careful not to confuse becoming tired with the amount of work done. Pushing against a wall for an afternoon in the hot sun is certainly tiring, but we have done no work because the wall didn't move.

In equation form,

$$W = Fd \qquad Work \qquad\qquad 3\text{-}1$$

Work done = (applied force)(distance through which force acts)

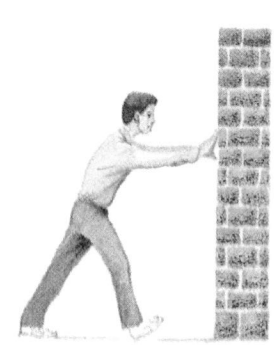

No work done

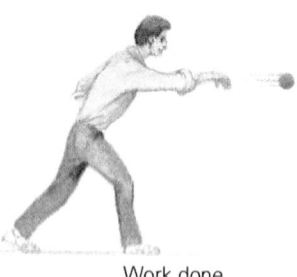

Work done

Figure 3-1 Work is done by a force when the object it acts on moves while the force is applied. No work is done by pushing against a stationary wall. Work is done when throwing a ball because the ball moves while being pushed during the throw.

Direction   The direction of the force **F** is assumed to be the same as the direction of the displacement **d.** If not, for example in the case of a child pulling a wagon with a rope not parallel to the ground, we must use for F the magnitude F_d of the projection of the applied force **F** that acts in the direction of motion (Fig. 3-3).

A force that is perpendicular to the direction of motion of an object can do no work on the object. Thus gravity, which results in a downward force on everything near the earth, does no work on objects moving horizontally along the earth's surface. However, if we drop an object, work is definitely done on it as it falls to the ground.

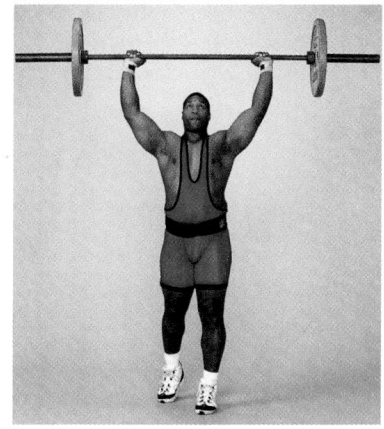

The Joule   The SI unit of work is the **joule** (J), where one joule is the amount of work done by a force of one newton when it acts through a distance of one meter. That is,

$$1 \text{ joule (J)} = 1 \text{ newton-meter (N} \cdot \text{m)}$$

Figure 3-2   Work is done when a barbell is lifted, but no work is done while it is being held in the air even though this can be very tiring.

The joule is named after the English scientist James Joule and is pronounced "jool." To raise an apple from your waist to your mouth takes about 1 J of work. Since $1 \text{ N} = 1 \text{ kg} \cdot \text{m/s}^2$, the joule can also be expressed as $1 \text{ J} = 1 \text{ N m} = 1 \text{ kg} \cdot \text{m}^2/\text{s}^2$, which is more convenient in some problems.

Work Done Against Gravity   It is easy to find the work done in lifting an object against gravity. The force of gravity on the object is its weight of mg. In order to raise the object to a height h above its original position (Fig. 3-4*a*), we need to apply an upward force of $F = mg$. With $F = mg$ and $d = h$, Eq. 3-1 becomes

$$W = mgh \qquad \textit{Work done against gravity} \qquad 3\text{-}2$$
$$\text{Work} = (\text{weight})(\text{height})$$

Only the total height h is involved here: the particular route upward taken by the object is not significant. Excluding friction, exactly as much work must be done when you climb a flight of stairs as when you go up to the same floor in an elevator (Fig. 3-5)—though the source of the work is not the same, to be sure.

If an object of mass m at the height h falls, the amount of work done *by* gravity on it is given by the same formula, $W = mgh$ (Fig. 3-4*b*).

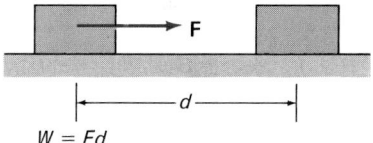

$$W = Fd$$

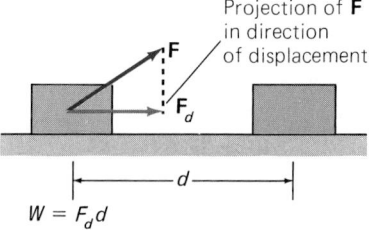

Projection of **F** in direction of displacement

$$W = F_d d$$

Figure 3-3   When a force and the distance through which it acts are parallel, the work done is equal to the product of F and d. When they are not in the same direction, the work done is equal to the product of d and the magnitude F_d of the projection of **F** in the direction of **d.**

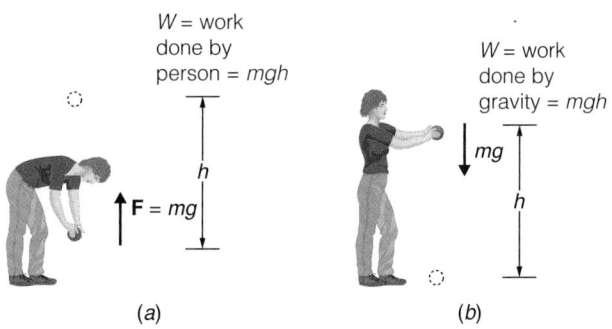

$W = $ work done by person $= mgh$

$W = $ work done by gravity $= mgh$

(*a*)   (*b*)

Figure 3-4   (*a*) The work a person does to lift an object to a height h is mgh. (*b*) If the object falls through the same height, the force of gravity does the work mgh.

Figure 3-5 Neglecting friction, the work needed to raise a person to a height *h* is the same regardless of the path taken.

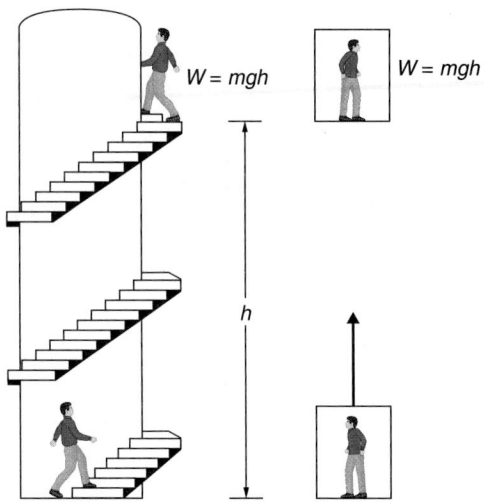

Example 3.1

(a) A horizontal force of 100 N is used to push a 20-kg box across a level floor for 10 m. How much work is done? (b) How much work is needed to raise the same box by 10 m?

Solution

(a) The work done in pushing the box is

$$W = Fd = (100 \text{ N})(10 \text{ m}) = 1000 \text{ J}$$

The mass of the box does not matter here. What counts is the applied force, the distance through which it acts, and the relative directions of the force and the displacement of the box.

(b) Now the work done is

$$W = mgh = (20 \text{ kg})(9.8 \text{ m/s}^2)(10 \text{ m}) = 1960 \text{ J}$$

The work done in this case does depend on the mass of the box.

3.2 Power

The Rate of Doing Work

The time needed to carry out a job is often as important as the amount of work needed. If we have enough time, even the tiny motor of a toy train can lift an elevator as high as we like. However, if we want the elevator to take us up fairly quickly, we must use a motor whose output of work is rapid in terms of the total work needed. Thus the rate at which work is being done is significant. This rate is called **power:** The more powerful something is, the faster it can do work.

If the amount of work *W* is done in a period of time *t*, the power involved is

$$P = \frac{W}{t} \qquad \textit{Power} \qquad \text{3-3}$$

$$\text{Power} = \frac{\text{work done}}{\text{time interval}}$$

The SI unit of power is the **watt** (W), where

$$1 \text{ watt (W)} = 1 \text{ joule/second (J/s)}$$

Example 3.2

A 15-kW electric motor provides power for the elevator of a building. What is the minimum time needed for the elevator to rise 30 m to the sixth floor when its total mass when loaded is 900 kg?

Solution

The work that must be done to raise the elevator is $W = mgh$. Since $P = W/t$, the time needed is

$$t = \frac{W}{P} = \frac{mgh}{P} = \frac{(900 \text{ kg})(9.8 \text{ m/s}^2)(30 \text{ m})}{15 \times 10^3 \text{ W}} = 17.6 \text{ s}$$

The Horsepower

The **horsepower** (hp) is the traditional unit of power in engineering. The origin of this unit is interesting. In order to sell the steam engines he had perfected two centuries ago, James Watt had to compare their power outputs with that of a horse, a source of work his customers were familiar with.

After various tests, Watt found that a typical horse could perform work at a rate of 497 W for as much as 10 hours per day. To avoid any disputes, he increased this figure by one-half to establish the unit he called the horsepower. Watt's horsepower therefore represents a rate of doing work of 746 W:

1 horsepower (hp) = 746 W
= 0.746 kW
1 kilowatt (kW) = 1.34 hp

Few horses can develop this much power for very long. The early steam engines ranged from 4 to 100 hp, with the 20-hp model being the most popular.

Thus a motor with a power output of 500 W is capable of doing 500 J of work per second. The same motor can do 250 J of work in 0.5 s, 1000 J of work in 2 s, 5000 J of work in 10 s, and so on. The watt is quite a small unit, and often the **kilowatt** (kW) is used instead, where 1 kW = 1000 W.

A person in good physical condition is usually capable of a continuous power output of about 75 W, which is 0.1 horsepower. A runner or swimmer during a distance event may have a power output 2 or 3 times greater. What limits the power output of a trained athlete is not muscular development but the supply of oxygen from the lungs through the bloodstream to the muscles, where oxygen is used in the metabolic processes that enable the muscles to do work. However, for a period of less than a second, an athlete's power output may exceed 5 kW, which accounts for the feats of weightlifters and jumpers.

Force, Speed, and Power   Often a force performs work on an object moving at constant speed in the same direction as that of the force. The work done is $W = Fd$ when the force F acts over the distance d in the time t, so that in this situation Eq. 3-3 becomes

$$P = \frac{W}{t} = \frac{Fd}{t}$$

But d/t equals v, the object's constant speed, so

$$P = Fv \qquad\qquad 3\text{-}4$$

$$\text{Power} = (\text{force})(\text{speed})$$

Suppose we want to know how much thrust a 5000-kW (6700 hp) aircraft engine produces when the speed of the airplane it powers is 240 m/s (537 mi/h). The answer comes in one step: $F = P/v = 21$ kN (2.3 tons).

Energy

We now go from the straightforward idea of work to the complex and many-sided idea of **energy:**

> Energy is that property something has that enables it to do work.

When we say that something has energy, we mean it is able, directly or indirectly, to exert a force on something else and perform work. When work is done on something, energy is added to it. Energy is measured in the same unit as work, the joule.

3.3   Kinetic Energy

The Energy of Motion

Energy occurs in several forms. One of them is the energy a moving object has because of its motion. Every moving object has the capacity to do work. By striking something else, the moving object can exert a force and cause the second object to shift its position, to break apart, or to otherwise show the effects of having work done on it. It is this property that defines energy, so we conclude that all moving things have energy by virtue of their motion.

The energy of a moving object is called **kinetic energy** (KE). ("Kinetic" is a word of Greek origin that suggests motion is involved.)

The kinetic energy of a moving thing depends upon its mass and its speed. The greater the mass and the greater the speed, the more the KE. A train going at 30 km/h has more energy than a horse galloping at the same speed and more energy than a similar train going at 10 km/h. The exact way KE varies with mass m and speed v is given by the formula

$$KE = \tfrac{1}{2}mv^2 \qquad \textit{Kinetic energy} \qquad\qquad 3\text{-}5$$

Energy and Speed   The v^2 factor means the kinetic energy increases very rapidly with increasing speed. At 30 m/s a car has 9 times as much KE as at 10 m/s—and requires 9 times as much force to bring to a stop in the same distance (Fig. 3-6). The fact that KE, and hence the ability to do work (in this case, damage), depends upon the square of the speed is what is responsible for the severity of automobile accidents at high speeds. The variation of KE with mass is less marked: a 2000-kg car going at 10 m/s has just twice the KE of a 1000-kg car with the same speed. (For a derivation of Eq. 3-5 and a sidebar on running speeds, see Sec. 3.3 at www.mhhe.com/krauskopf.)

3.4   Potential Energy

The Energy of Position

When we drop a stone, it falls faster and faster and finally strikes the ground. If we lift the stone afterward, we see that it has done work by making a

Figure 3-6   Kinetic energy is proportional to the square of the speed. A car traveling at 30 m/s has 9 times the KE of the same car traveling at 10 m/s.

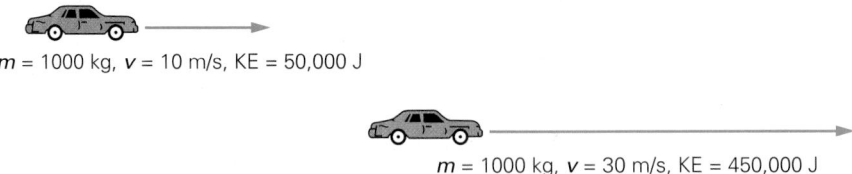

m = 1000 kg, v = 10 m/s, KE = 50,000 J

m = 1000 kg, v = 30 m/s, KE = 450,000 J

Example 3.3

Find the kinetic energy of a 1000-kg car when its speed is 10 m/s.

Solution

From Eq. 3-5 we have

$$KE = \tfrac{1}{2}mv^2 = \left(\tfrac{1}{2}\right)(1000 \text{ kg})(10 \text{ m/s})^2$$

$$= \left(\tfrac{1}{2}\right)(1000 \text{ kg})(10 \text{ m/s})(10 \text{ m/s}) = 50,000 \text{ J} = 50 \text{ kJ}$$

In order to bring the car to this speed from rest, 50 kJ of work had to be done by its engine. To stop the car from this speed, the same amount of work must be done by its brakes.

Example 3.4

Have you ever wondered how much force a hammer exerts on a nail? Suppose you hit a nail with a hammer and drive the nail 5 mm into a wooden board (Fig. 3-7). If the hammer's head has a mass of 0.6 kg and it is moving at 4 m/s when it strikes the nail, what is the average force on the nail?

Solution

The KE of the hammer head is $\frac{1}{2}mv^2$, and this amount of energy becomes the work Fd done in driving the nail the distance $d = 5$ mm $= 0.005$ m into the board. Hence

$$\text{KE of hammer head} = \text{work done on nail}$$

$$\tfrac{1}{2}mv^2 = Fd$$

and
$$F = \frac{mv^2}{2d} = \frac{(0.6 \text{ kg})(4 \text{ m/s})^2}{2(0.005 \text{ m})} = 960 \text{ N}$$

This is 216 lb—watch your fingers!

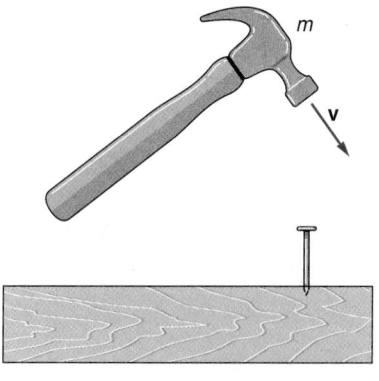

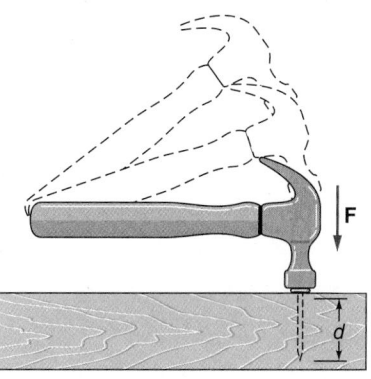

Figure 3-7 When a hammer strikes this nail, the hammer's kinetic energy is converted into the work done to push the nail into the wooden board.

shallow hole in the ground. In its original raised position, the stone must have had the capacity to do work even though it was not moving at the time and therefore had no KE.

The amount of work the stone could do by falling to the ground is called its **potential energy** (PE). Just as kinetic energy may be thought of as energy of motion, potential energy may be thought of as energy of position (Fig. 3-8).

Examples of potential energy are everywhere. A book on a table has PE since it can fall to the floor. A skier at the top of a slope, water at the top of a waterfall, a car at the top of the hill, anything able to move toward the earth under the influence of gravity has PE because of its position. Nor is the earth's gravity necessary: a stretched spring has PE since it can do work when it is let go, and a nail near a magnet has PE since it can do work in moving to the magnet (Fig. 3-9).

Gravitational Potential Energy When an object of mass m is raised to a height h above its original position, its gravitational potential energy is equal to the work that was done against gravity to bring it to that height (Fig. 3-10). According to Eq. 3-2 this work is $W = mgh$, and so

$$\text{PE} = mgh \qquad \textit{Gravitational potential energy} \qquad 3\text{-}6$$

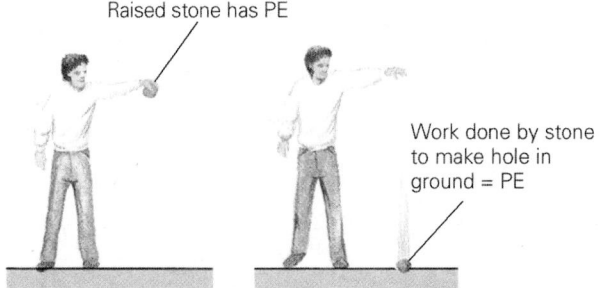

Figure 3-8 A raised stone has potential energy because it can do work on the ground when dropped.

Figure 3-9   Two examples of potential energy.

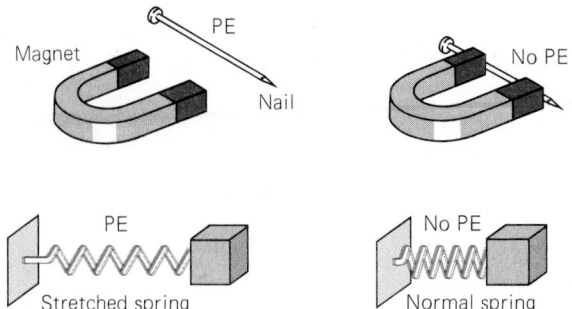

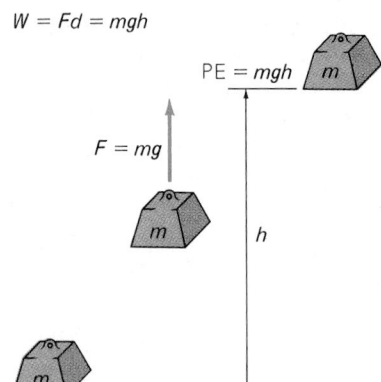

$W = Fd = mgh$

$PE = mgh$

$F = mg$

h

Figure 3-10   The increase in the potential energy of a raised object is equal to the work *mgh* used to lift it.

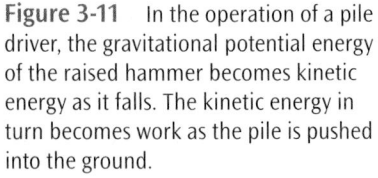

Example 3.5

Find the potential energy of a 1000-kg car when it is on top of a 45-m cliff.

Solution

From Eq. 3-6 the car's potential energy is

$$PE = mgh = (1000 \text{ kg})(9.8 \text{ m/s}^2)(45 \text{ m}) = 441,000 \text{ J} = 441 \text{ kJ}$$

This is less than the KE of the same car when it moves at 30 m/s (Fig. 3-6). Thus a crash at 30 m/s into a wall or tree will yield more work—that is, do more damage—than dropping the car from a cliff 45 m high.

This result for PE agrees with our experience. Consider a pile driver (Fig. 3-11), a simple machine that lifts a heavy weight (the "hammer") and allows it to fall on the head of a pile, which is a wooden or steel post, to drive the pile into the ground. From the formula *PE = mgh* we would expect the effectiveness of a pile driver to depend on the mass *m* of its hammer and the height *h* from which it is dropped, which is exactly what experience shows.

PE Is Relative   It is worth noting that the gravitational PE of an object depends on the level from which it is reckoned. Often the earth's surface is convenient, but sometimes other references are more appropriate.

Figure 3-11   In the operation of a pile driver, the gravitational potential energy of the raised hammer becomes kinetic energy as it falls. The kinetic energy in turn becomes work as the pile is pushed into the ground.

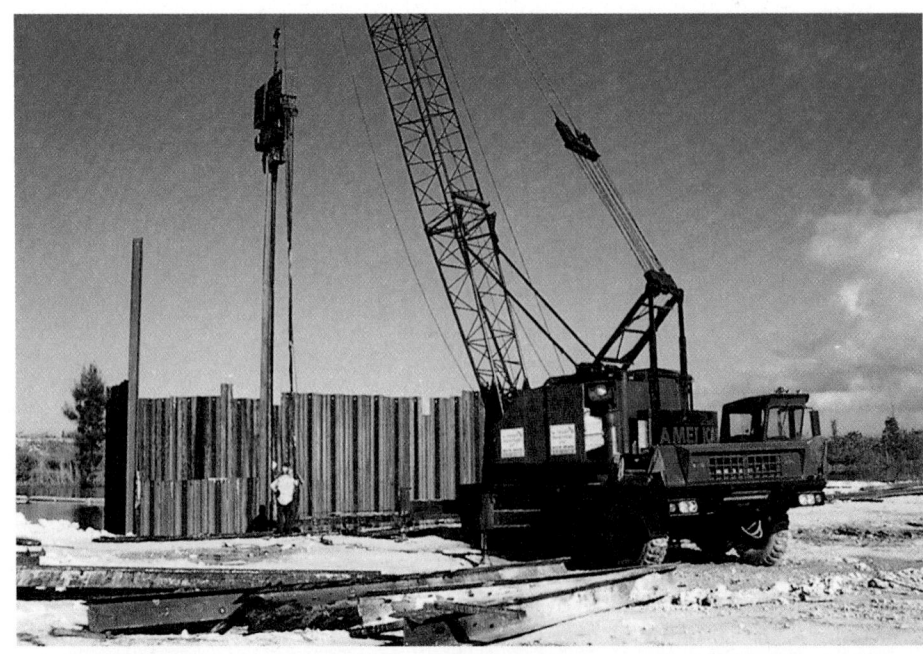

Suppose you lift this book as high as you can above the table while remaining seated. It will then have a PE *relative to the table* of about 12 J. But the book will have a PE *relative to the floor* of about twice that, or 24 J. And if the floor of your room is, say, 50 m above the ground, the book's PE *relative to the ground* will be about 760 J.

What is the book's true PE? The answer is that there is no such thing as "true" PE. Gravitational PE is a relative quantity. However, the *difference* between the PEs of an object at two points *is* significant, since it is this difference that can be changed into work or KE.

3.5 Energy Transformations

Easy Come, Easy Go

Nearly all familiar mechanical processes involve interchanges among KE, PE, and work. Thus when the car of Fig. 3-12 is driven to the top of a hill, its engine must do work in order to raise the car. At the top, the car has an amount of PE equal to the work done in getting it up there (neglecting friction). If the engine is turned off, the car can still coast down the hill, and its KE at the bottom of the hill will be the same as its PE at the top.

Changes of a similar nature, from kinetic energy to potential and back, occur in the motion of a planet in its orbit around the sun (Fig. 3-13) and in the motion of a pendulum (Fig. 3-14). The orbits of the planets are ellipses with the sun at one focus (Fig. 1-10), and each planet is therefore at a constantly varying distance from the sun. At all times the total of its potential and kinetic energies remains the same. When close to the sun, the PE of a planet is low and its KE is high. The additional speed due to increased KE keeps the planet from being pulled into the sun by the greater gravitational force on it at this point in its path. When the planet is far from the sun, its PE is higher and its KE lower, with the reduced speed exactly keeping pace with the reduced gravitational force.

A pendulum (Fig. 3-14) consists of a ball suspended by a string. When the ball is pulled to one side with its string taut and then released, it swings back and forth. When it is released, the ball has a PE relative to the bottom of its path of mgh. At its lowest point all this PE has become kinetic energy $\frac{1}{2}mv^2$. After reaching the bottom, the ball continues in its motion until it rises to the same height h on the opposite side from its initial position. Then, momentarily at rest since all its KE is now PE, the ball begins to retrace its path back through the bottom to its initial position.

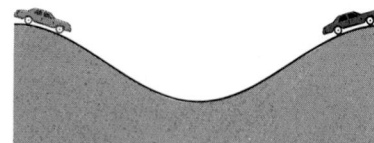

Figure 3-12 In the absence of friction, a car can coast from the top of one hill into a valley and then up to the top of another hill of the same height as the first. During the trip the initial potential energy of the car is converted into kinetic energy as the car goes downhill, and this kinetic energy then turns into potential energy as the car climbs the next hill. The total amount of energy (KE + PE) remains unchanged.

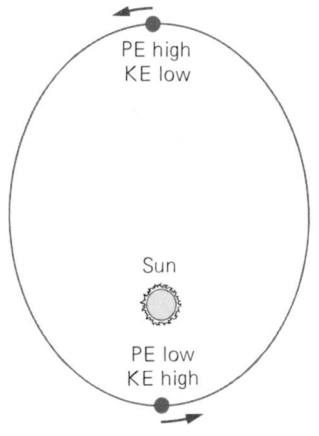

Figure 3-13 Energy transformations in planetary motion. The total energy (KE + PE) of the planet is the same at all points in its orbit. (Planetary orbits are much more nearly circular than shown here.)

Example 3.6

A girl on a swing is 2.2 m above the ground at the ends of her motion and 1.0 m above the ground at the lowest point. What is the girl's maximum speed?

Solution

The maximum speed v will occur at the lowest point where her potential energy above this point has been entirely converted to kinetic energy. If the difference in height is $h = (2.2 \text{ m}) - (1.0 \text{ m}) = 1.2 \text{ m}$ and the girl's mass is m, then

$$\text{Kinetic energy} = \text{change in potential energy}$$

$$\tfrac{1}{2}mv^2 = mgh$$

$$v = \sqrt{2gh} = \sqrt{2(9.8 \text{ m/s}^2)(1.2 \text{ m})} = 4.8 \text{ m/s}$$

The girl's mass does not matter here.

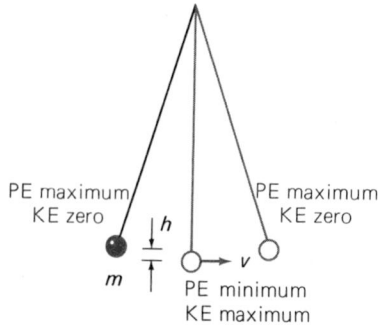

Figure 3-14 Energy transformations in pendulum motion. The total energy of the ball stays the same but is continuously exchanged between kinetic and potential forms.

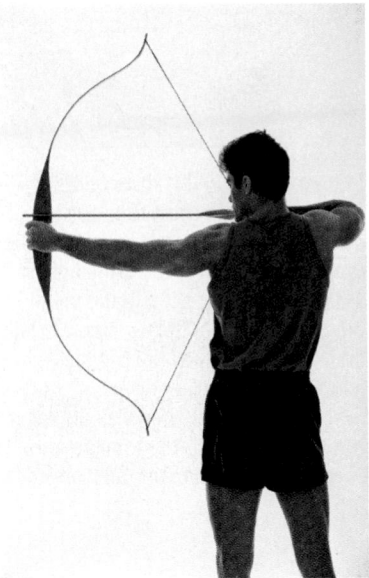

Figure 3-15   The elastic potential energy of the bent bow becomes kinetic energy of the arrow when the bowstring is released.

Transformations to and from kinetic energy may involve potential energies other than gravitational. An example is the elastic potential energy of a bent bow, as in Fig. 3-15.

Other Forms of Energy   Energy can exist in a variety of forms besides kinetic and potential. The *chemical energy* of gasoline is used to propel our cars and the chemical energy of food enables our bodies to perform work. *Heat energy* from burning coal or oil is used to form the steam that drives the turbines of power stations. *Electric energy* turns motors in home and factory. *Radiant energy* from the sun performs work in causing water from the earth's surface to rise and form clouds, in producing differences in air temperature that cause winds, and in promoting chemical reactions in plants that produce foods.

Just as kinetic energy can be converted to potential energy and potential to kinetic, so other forms of energy can readily be transformed. In the cylinders of a car engine, for example, chemical energy stored in gasoline and air is changed first to heat energy when the mixture is ignited by the spark plugs, then to kinetic energy as the expanding gases push down on the pistons. This kinetic energy is in large part transmitted to the wheels, but some is used to turn the generator and thus produce electric energy for charging the battery, and some is changed to heat by friction in bearings. Energy transformations go on constantly, all about us.

3.6   Conservation of Energy

A Fundamental Law of Nature

A skier slides down a hill and comes to rest at the bottom. What became of the potential energy he or she had at the top? The engine of a car is shut off while the car is allowed to coast along a level road. Eventually the car slows down and comes to a stop. What became of its original kinetic energy?

All of us can give similar examples of the apparent disappearance of kinetic or potential energy. What these examples have in common is that heat is always produced in an amount just equivalent to the "lost" energy (Fig. 3-16). One kind of energy is simply being converted to another; no energy is lost, nor is any new energy created. Exactly the same is true when electric, magnetic, radiant, and chemical energies are changed into one another or into heat. Thus we have a law from which no deviations have ever been found:

> Energy cannot be created or destroyed, although it can be changed from one form to another.

This generalization is the **law of conservation of energy.** It is the principle with the widest application in science, applying equally to distant stars and to biological processes in living cells.

We shall learn later in this chapter that matter can be transformed into energy and energy into matter. The law of conservation of energy still applies, however, with matter considered as a form of energy.

3.7   The Nature of Heat

The Downfall of Caloric

Although it comes as little surprise to us today to learn that heat is a form of energy, in earlier times this was not so clear. Less than two centuries ago most scientists regarded heat as an actual substance called **caloric.** Absorbing caloric caused an object to become warmer; the escape of caloric caused

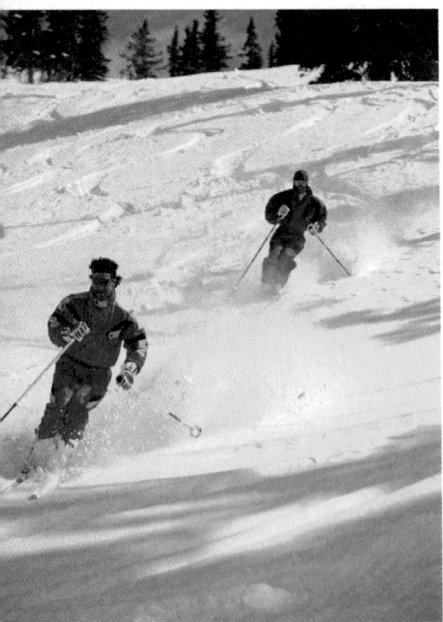

Figure 3-16   The potential energy of these skiers at the top of the slope turns into kinetic energy and eventually into heat as they slide downhill.

it to become cooler. Because the weight of an object does not change when the object is heated or cooled, caloric was considered to be weightless. It was also supposed to be invisible, odorless, and tasteless, properties that, of course, were why it could not be observed directly.

Actually, the idea of heat as a substance was fairly satisfactory for materials heated over a flame, but it could not account for the unlimited heat that could be generated by friction. One of the first to appreciate this difficulty was the American Benjamin Thompson (Fig. 3-17), who had supported the British during the Revolutionary War and thought it wise to move to Europe afterward, where he became Count Rumford.

One of Rumford's many occupations was supervising the making of cannon for a German prince, and he was impressed by the large amounts of heat given off by friction in the boring process. He showed that the heat could be used to boil water and that heat could be produced again and again from the same piece of metal. If heat was a fluid, it was not unreasonable that boring a hole in a piece of metal should allow it to escape. However, even a dull drill that cut no metal produced a great deal of heat. Also, it was hard to imagine a piece of metal as containing an infinite amount of caloric, and Rumford accordingly regarded heat as a form of energy.

Joule   James Prescott Joule (Fig. 3-18) was an English brewer who performed a classic experiment that settled the nature of heat once and for all. Joule's experiment used a small paddle wheel inside a container of water (Fig. 3-19). Work was done to turn the paddle wheel against the resistance of the water, and Joule measured exactly how much heat was supplied to the water by friction in this process. He found that a given amount of work always produced exactly the same amount of heat. This was a clear demonstration that heat is energy and not something else.

Joule also carried out chemical and electrical experiments that agreed with his mechanical ones, and the result was his announcement of the law of conservation of energy in 1847, when he was 29. Although Joule was a modest man ("I have done two or three little things, but nothing to make a fuss about," he later wrote), many honors came his way, including naming the SI unit of energy after him.

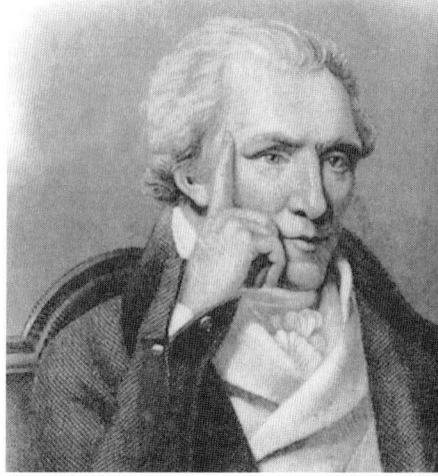

Figure 3-17   Count Rumford (1753–1814).

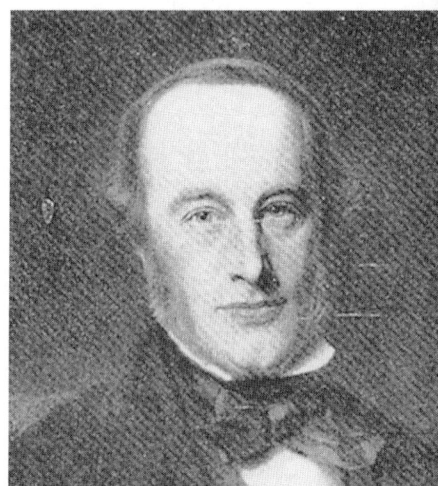

Figure 3-18   James Prescott Joule (1818–1889).

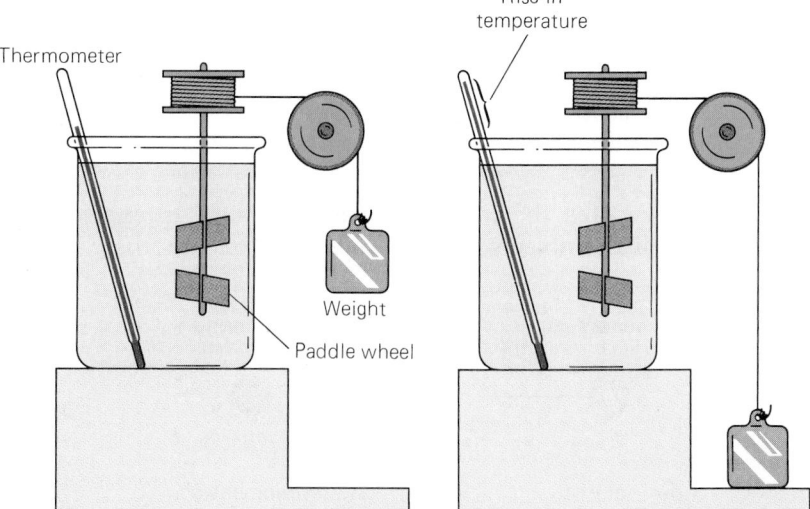

Figure 3-19   Joule's experimental demonstration that heat is a form of energy. As the weight falls, it turns the paddle wheel, which heats the water by friction. The potential energy of the weight is converted first into the kinetic energy of the paddle wheel and then into heat.

What is Heat?

As we shall learn in Chap. 5, the heat content of a body of matter consists of the KE of random motion of the atoms and molecules of which the body consists. The greater the average KE of each of its atoms and molecules, the higher the temperature of the body.

Momentum

Because the universe is so complex, a variety of different quantities besides the basic ones of length, time, and mass are useful to help us understand its many aspects. We have already found velocity, acceleration, force, work, and energy to be valuable, and more are to come. The idea behind defining each of these quantities is to single out something that is involved in a wide range of observations. Then we can boil down a great many separate findings about nature into a brief, clear statement, for example, the law of conservation of energy. Now we shall learn how the concepts of linear and angular momenta can give us further insights into the behavior of moving things.

3.8   Linear Momentum

Another Conservation Law

As we know (Sec. 2.7), a moving object tends to continue moving at constant speed along a straight path. The **linear momentum** of such an object is a measure of this tendency. The more linear momentum something has, the more effort is needed to slow it down or to change its direction. Another kind of momentum is **angular momentum,** which reflects the tendency of a spinning body to continue to spin. When there is no question as to which is meant, linear momentum is usually referred to simply as momentum.

The linear momentum **p** of an object of mass m and velocity **v** (we recall that velocity includes both speed and direction) is defined as

$$\mathbf{p} = m\mathbf{v} \qquad \textit{Linear momentum} \qquad \qquad 3\text{-}7$$

Linear momentum = (mass)(velocity)

The greater m and **v** are, the more difficult it is to change the object's speed or direction.

This definition of momentum is in accord with our experience. A baseball hit squarely by a bat (large **v**) is more difficult to stop than a baseball thrown gently (small **v**). The heavy iron ball used for the shotput (large m) is more difficult to stop than a baseball (small m) when their speeds are the same (Fig. 3-20).

Conservation of Momentum   Momentum considerations are most useful in situations that involve explosions and collisions. When outside forces do not act on the objects involved, their combined momentum (taking directions into account) is conserved, that is, does not change:

> In the absence of outside forces, the total momentum of a set of objects remains the same no matter how the objects interact with one another.

This statement is called the **law of conservation of momentum.** What it means is that, if the objects interact only with one another, each object

Figure 3-20   The linear momentum $m\mathbf{v}$ of a moving object is a measure of its tendency to continue in motion at constant velocity. The symbol > means "greater than."

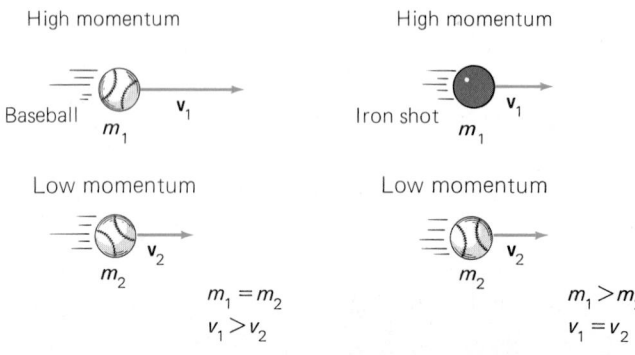

Total momentum $= m_1 \mathbf{v}_1 = (m_1 + m_2) \mathbf{v}_2$

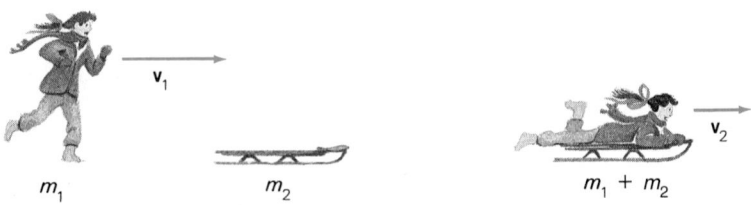

$\mathbf{v}_1$

m_1 m_2 $m_1 + m_2$

$\mathbf{v}_2$

Figure 3-21   When a running girl jumps on a stationary sled, the combination moves off more slowly than the girl's original speed. The total momentum of girl + sled is the same before and after she jumps on it.

can have its momentum changed in the interaction, provided that the total momentum after it occurs is the same as it was before.

Momentum is conserved when a running girl jumps on a stationary sled, as in Fig. 3-21. Even if there is no friction between the sled and the snow, the combination of girl and sled moves off more slowly than the girl's running speed. The original momentum, which is that of the girl alone, had to be shared between her and the sled when she jumped on it. Now that the sled is also moving, the new speed must be less than before in order that the total momentum stays the same.

Example 3.7

Let us see what happens when an object breaks up into two parts. Suppose that an astronaut outside a space station throws away a 0.5-kg camera in disgust when it jams (Fig. 3-22). The mass of the spacesuited astronaut is 100 kg, and the camera moves off at 6 m/s. What happens to the astronaut?

Solution

The total momentum of the astronaut and camera was zero originally. According to the law of conservation of momentum, their total momentum must therefore be zero afterward as well. If we call the astronaut A and the camera C, then

$$\text{Momentum before} = \text{momentum afterward}$$
$$0 = m_A v_A + m_C v_C$$

Hence

$$m_A v_A = -m_C v_C$$

where the minus sign signifies that $\mathbf{v}_A$ is opposite in direction to $\mathbf{v}_C$. Throwing the camera away therefore sets the astronaut in motion as well, with camera and astronaut moving in opposite directions. Newton's third law of motion (action-reaction) tells us the same thing, but conservation of momentum enables us to find the astronaut's speed at once:

$$v_A = -\frac{m_C v_C}{m_A} = -\frac{(0.5 \text{ kg})(6 \text{ m/s})}{100 \text{ kg}} = -0.03 \text{ m/s}$$

After an hour, which is 3600 s, the camera will have traveled $v_C t = 21,600 \text{ m} = 21.6$ km, and the astronaut will have traveled $v_A t = 108$ m in the opposite direction if not tethered to the space station.

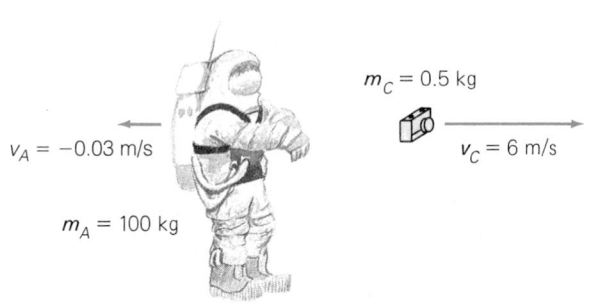

$m_C = 0.5$ kg

$v_A = -0.03$ m/s $v_C = 6$ m/s

$m_A = 100$ kg

Figure 3-22   The momentum $m_C v_C$ to the right of the thrown camera is equal in magnitude to the momentum $m_A v_A$ to the left of the astronaut who threw it away.

Collisions

Applying the law of conservation of momentum to collisions gives some interesting results. These are shown in Fig. 3-23 for an object of mass m and speed v that strikes a stationary object of mass M and does not stick to it. Three situations are possible:

1. The target object has more mass, so that $M > m$. What happens here is that the incoming object bounces off the heavier target one and they move apart in opposite directions.
2. The two objects have the same mass, so that $M = m$. Now the incoming object stops and the target object moves off with the same speed v the incoming one had.
3. The target object has less mass, so that $m > M$. In this case the incoming object continues in its original direction after the impact but with reduced speed while the target object moves ahead of it at a faster pace. The greater m is compared with M, the closer the target object's final speed is to $2v$.

The third case corresponds to a golf club striking a golf ball (Fig. 3-24). This suggests that the more mass the clubhead has for a given speed, the faster the ball will fly off when struck. However, a heavy golf club is harder to swing fast than a light one, so a compromise is necessary. Experience has led golfers to use clubheads with masses about 4 times the 46-g mass of a golf ball when they want maximum distance. A good golfer can swing a clubhead at over 50 m/s.

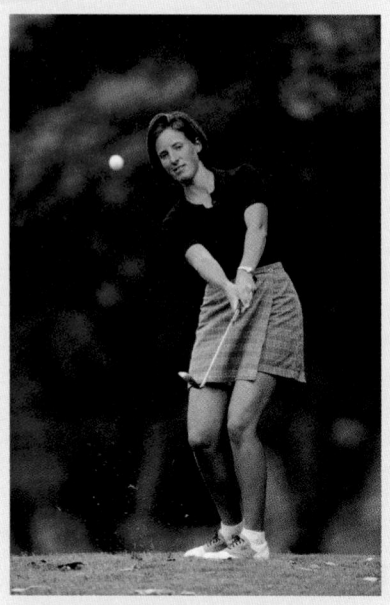

Figure 3-24   The speed of a golf ball is greater than the speed of the clubhead that struck it because the mass of the ball is smaller than that of the clubhead.

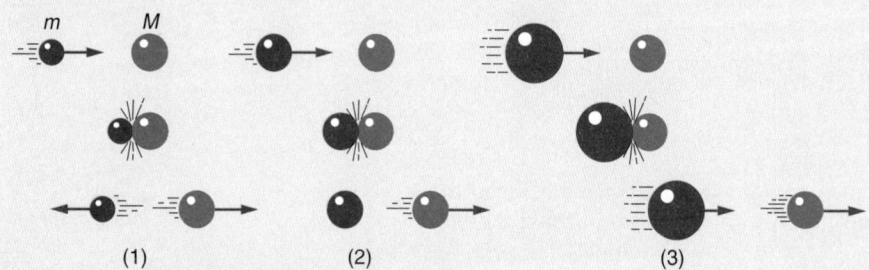

(1)   (2)   (3)

Figure 3-23   How the effects of a head-on collision with a stationary target object depend on the relative masses of the two objects.

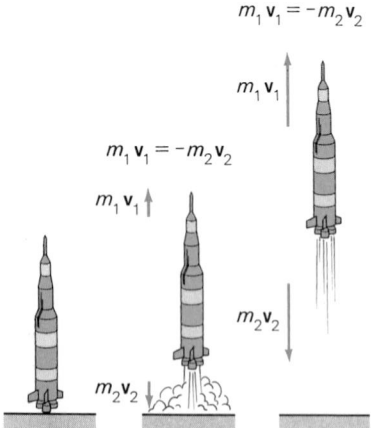

$m_1 \mathbf{v}_1 = -m_2 \mathbf{v}_2$

$m_1 \mathbf{v}_1$

$m_1 \mathbf{v}_1 = -m_2 \mathbf{v}_2$

$m_1 \mathbf{v}_1$

$m_2 \mathbf{v}_2$

$m_2 \mathbf{v}_2$

Figure 3-25   Rocket propulsion is based upon conservation of momentum. If gravity is absent, the downward momentum of the exhaust gases is equal in magnitude and opposite in direction to the upward momentum of the rocket at all times.

3.9   Rockets

Momentum Conservation Is the Basis of Space Travel

The operation of a rocket is based on conservation of linear momentum. When the rocket stands on its launching pad, its momentum is zero. When it is fired, the momentum of the exhaust gases that rush downward is balanced by the momentum in the other direction of the rocket moving upward. The total momentum of the entire system, gases and rocket, remains zero, because momentum is a vector quantity and the upward and downward momenta cancel (Fig. 3-25).

Thus a rocket does not work by "pushing" against its launching pad, the air, or anything else. In fact, rockets function best in space where no atmosphere is present to interfere with their motion.

The ultimate speed a rocket can reach is governed by the amount of fuel it can carry and by the speed of its exhaust gases. Because both these quantities are limited, **multistage rockets** are used in the exploration of space. The first stage is a large rocket that has a smaller one mounted in front of it. When the fuel of the first stage has burnt up, its motor and empty fuel tanks are cast off. Then the second stage is fired. Since the second stage is already moving rapidly and does not have to carry the motor and empty fuel tanks of the first stage, it can reach a much higher final speed than would otherwise be possible.

Depending upon the final speed needed for a given mission, three or even four stages may be required. The Saturn V launch vehicle that carried the Apollo 11 spacecraft to the moon in July 1969 had three stages. Just before takeoff the entire assembly was 111 m long and had a mass of nearly 3 million kg (Fig. 3-26).

3.10   Angular Momentum

A Measure of the Tendency of a Spinning Object to Continue to Spin

We have all noticed the tendency of rotating objects to continue to spin unless they are slowed down by an outside agency. A top would spin indefinitely but for friction between its tip and the ground. Another example is the earth, which has been turning for billions of years and is likely to continue doing so for many more to come.

The rotational quantity that corresponds to linear momentum is called **angular momentum,** and **conservation of angular momentum** is the formal way to describe the tendency of spinning objects to keep spinning.

The precise definition of angular momentum is complicated because it depends not only upon the mass of the object and upon how fast it is turning, but also upon how the mass is arranged in the body. As we might expect, the greater the mass of a body and the more rapidly it rotates, the more angular momentum it has and the more pronounced is its tendency to continue to spin. Less obvious is the fact that, the farther away from the axis of rotation the mass is distributed, the more the angular momentum.

An illustration of both the latter fact and the conservation of angular momentum is a skater doing a spin (Fig. 3-28). When the skater starts the spin, she pushes against the ice with one skate to start turning. Initially both arms and one leg are extended, so that her mass is spread as far as possible from the axis of rotation. Then she brings her arms and the outstretched leg in tightly against her body, so that now all her mass is as close as possible to the axis of rotation. As a result, she spins faster. To make up for the change in the mass distribution, the speed must change as well to conserve angular momentum.

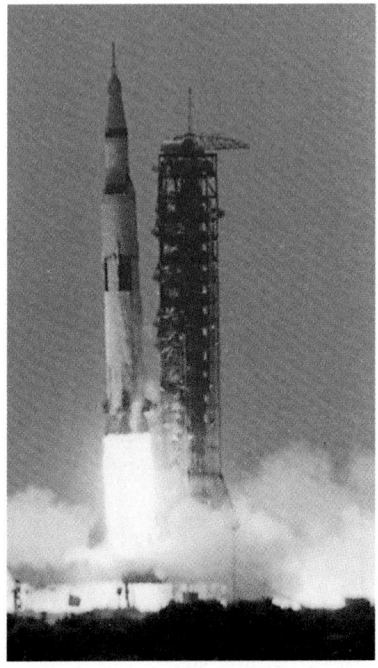

Figure 3-26   Apollo 11 lifts off its pad to begin the first human visit to the moon. The spacecraft's final speed was 10.8 km/s, which is equivalent to 6.7 mi/s. Conservation of linear momentum underlies rocket propulsion.

Conservation Principles

The conservation principles of energy, linear momentum, and angular momentum are useful because they are obeyed in all known processes. They are significant for another reason as well. In 1917 the German mathematician Emmy Noether (Fig. 3-27) proved that:

1. If the laws of nature are the same at all times, past, present, and future, then energy must be conserved.
2. If the laws of nature are the same everywhere in the universe, then linear momentum must be conserved.
3. If the laws of nature do not depend on direction, then angular momentum must be conserved.

All other conservation principles in physics, for instance conservation of electric charge (Sec. 6.2), can also be traced to similar general regularities in the universe. Thus the existence of these principles testifies to a profound order in the universe, despite the irregularities and randomness of many aspects of it, a truly remarkable finding. In 1933 Noether moved to the United States where, after a period at the Institute for Advanced Study in Princeton, she became a professor at Bryn Mawr.

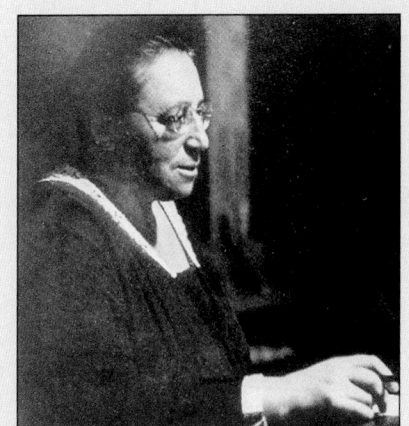

Figure 3-27   Emmy Noether (1882–1935).

Figure 3-28 Conservation of angular momentum. Angular momentum depends upon both the speed of turning and the distribution of mass. When the skater pulls in her arms and extended leg, she spins faster to compensate for the change in the way her mass is distributed.

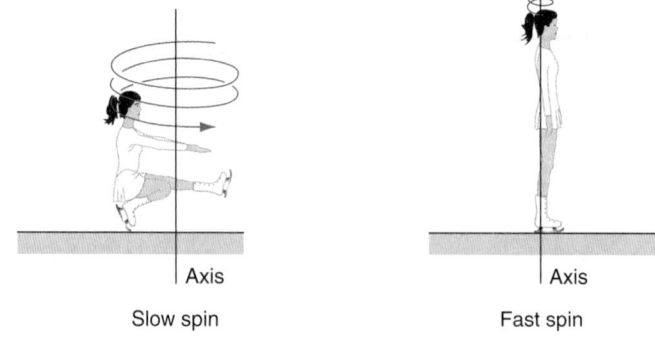

Slow spin   Fast spin

Planetary Motion

Kepler's second law of planetary motion (Fig. 1-11) has an origin similar to that of the changing spin rate of a skater. A planet moving around the sun has angular momentum, which must be the same everywhere in its orbit. As a result the planet's speed is greatest when it is close to the sun, least when it is far away.

Spin Stabilization Like linear momentum, angular momentum is a vector quantity with direction as well as magnitude. Conservation of angular momentum therefore means that a spinning body tends to maintain the *direction* of its spin axis in addition to the amount of angular momentum it has. A stationary top falls over at once, but a rapidly spinning top stays upright because its tendency to keep its axis in the same orientation by virtue of its angular momentum is greater than its tendency to fall over (Fig. 3-29). Footballs and rifle bullets are sent off spinning to prevent them from tumbling during flight, which would increase air resistance and hence shorten their range (Fig. 3-30).

Figure 3-29 The faster a top spins, the more stable it is. When all its angular momentum has been lost through friction, the top falls over.

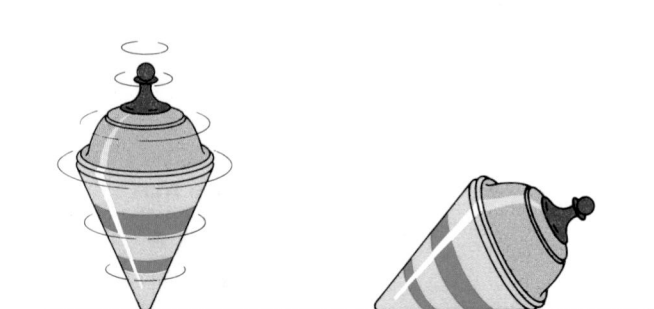

Figure 3-30 Conservation of angular momentum keeps a spinning football from tumbling end-over-end, which would slow it down and reduce its range.

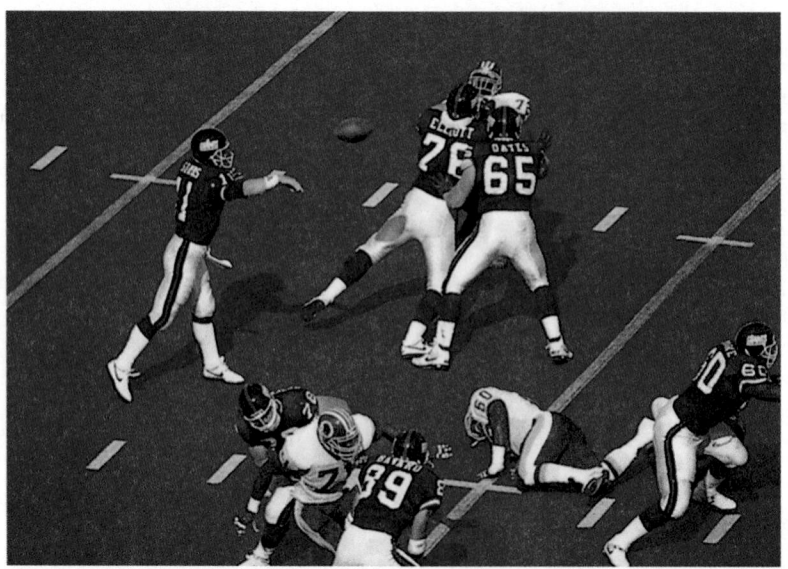

Relativity

In 1905 a young physicist of 26 named Albert Einstein published an analysis of how measurements of time and space are affected by motion between an observer and what he or she is studying. To say that Einstein's **theory of relativity** revolutionized science is no exaggeration.

Relativity links not only time and space but also energy and matter. From it have come a host of remarkable predictions, all of which have been confirmed by experiment. Eleven years later Einstein took relativity a step further by interpreting gravity as a distortion in the structure of space and time, again predicting extraordinary effects that were verified in detail.

3.11 Special Relativity

Things Are Seldom What They Seem

Thus far in this book no special point has been made about how such quantities as length, time, and mass are measured. In particular, who makes a certain measurement would not seem to matter—everybody ought to get the same result. Suppose we want to find the length of an airplane when we are on board. All we have to do is put one end of a tape measure at the airplane's nose and look at the number on the tape at the airplane's tail.

But what if we are standing on the ground and the airplane is in flight? Now things become more complicated because the light that carries information to our instruments travels at a definite speed. According to Einstein, our measurements from the ground of length, time, and mass in the airplane would differ from those made by somebody moving with the airplane.

Postulates of Relativity   Einstein began with two postulates. The first concerns **frames of reference,** which were mentioned in Sec. 2.1. Motion always implies a frame of reference relative to which the location of something is changing. A passenger walking down the aisle moves relative to an airplane, the airplane moves relative to the earth, the earth moves relative to the sun, and so on (Fig. 3-31).

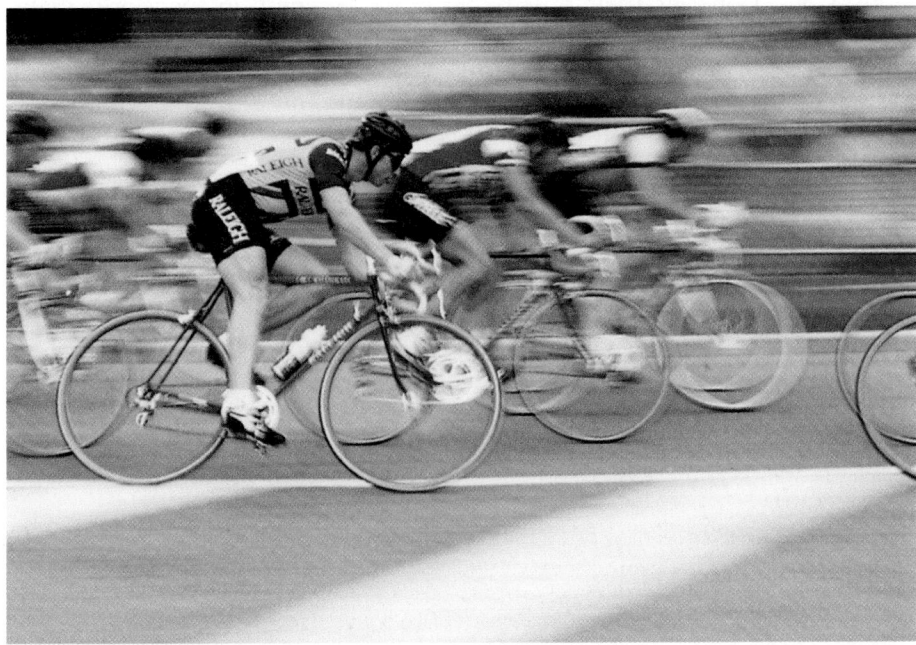

Figure 3-31 All motion is relative to a chosen frame of reference. Here the photographer has turned the camera to keep pace with one of the cyclists. Relative to him, both the road and the other cyclists are moving. There is no fixed frame of reference in nature, and therefore no such thing as "absolute motion"; all motion is relative.

If we are in the windowless cabin of a cargo airplane, we cannot tell whether the airplane is in flight at constant velocity or is at rest on the ground, since without an external frame of reference the question has no meaning. To say that something is moving always requires a frame of reference. From this follows Einstein's first postulate:

> The laws of physics are the same in all frames of reference moving at constant velocity with respect to one another.

If the laws of physics were different for different observers in relative motion, the observers could find from these differences which of them were "stationary" in space and which were "moving." But such a distinction does not exist, hence the first postulate.

The second postulate, which follows from the results of a great many experiments, states that

> The speed of light in free space has the same value for all observers.

The speed of light in free space is always $c = 3 \times 10^8$ m/s, about 186,000 mi/s.

Length, Time, and Kinetic Energy   Let us suppose I am in an airplane moving at the constant velocity **v** relative to you on the ground. I find that the airplane is L_0 long, that it has a mass of m, and that a certain time interval (say an hour on my watch) is t_0. Einstein showed from the above postulates that you, on the ground, would find that

1. The length L you measure is shorter than L_0.
2. The time interval t you measure is longer than t_0.
3. The kinetic energy KE you determine is greater than $\frac{1}{2}mv^2$.

That is, to you on the ground, the airplane appears shorter than to me and to have more KE, and to you, my watch appears to tick more slowly.

The differences between L and L_0, t and t_0, and KE and $\frac{1}{2}mv^2$ depend on the ratio v/c between the relative speed v of the frames of reference (here the speed of the airplane relative to the ground) and the speed of light c. Because c is so great, these differences are too small to detect at speeds like those of airplanes. However, they must be taken into account in spacecraft flight. And, at speeds near c, which often occur in the subatomic world of such tiny particles as electrons and protons, relativistic effects are conspicuous. Although at speeds much less than c the formula $\frac{1}{2}mv^2$ for kinetic energy is still valid, at high speeds the theory of relativity shows that the KE of a moving object is higher than $\frac{1}{2}mv^2$ (Fig. 3-32).

Figure 3-32   The faster an object moves relative to an observer, the more the object's kinetic energy KE exceeds $\frac{1}{2}mv^2$. This effect is only conspicuous at speeds near the speed of light $c = 3 \times 10^8$ m/s, which is about 186,000 mi/s. Because an object would have an infinite KE if $v = c$, nothing with mass can ever move that fast or faster.

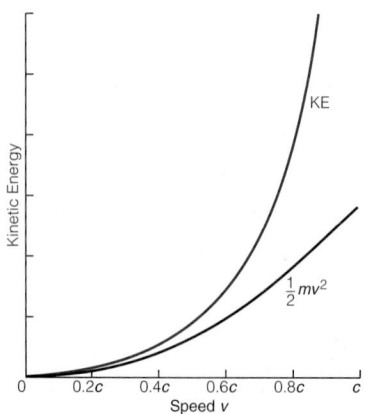

The Ultimate Speed Limit   As we can see from the graph, the closer v gets to c, the closer KE gets to infinity. Since an infinite kinetic energy is impossible, this conclusion means that nothing can travel as fast as light or faster: c is the absolute speed limit in the universe. The implications of this limit for space travel are discussed in Chap. 19.

Einstein's 1905 theory, which led to the above results among others, is called **special relativity** because it is restricted to constant velocities. His later theory of **general relativity,** which deals with gravity, includes accelerations.

3.12   Rest Energy

Matter Is a Form of Energy

The most far-reaching conclusion of special relativity is that mass and energy are related to each other so closely that matter can be converted into energy and energy into matter. The **rest energy** of a body is the energy equivalent of its mass. If a body has the mass m, its rest energy is

$$E_0 = mc^2 \qquad \text{Rest energy} \qquad\qquad 3\text{-}8$$

$$\text{Rest energy} = (\text{mass})(\text{speed of light})^2$$

Experiments show that this formula is accurate to at least 0.00004 percent.

The rest energy of a 1.4-kg object, such as this book, is

$$E_0 = mc^2 = (1.4\ \text{kg})(3 \times 10^8\ \text{m/s})^2 = 1.26 \times 10^{17}\ \text{J}$$

quite apart from any kinetic or potential energy it might have. If liberated, this energy would be more than enough to send a million tons to the moon. By contrast, the PE of this book on top of Mt. Everest, which is 8850 m high, relative to its sea-level PE is 1.21×10^5 J, about 10^{12}—a trillion—times smaller.

How is it possible that so much energy can be bottled up in even a little bit of matter without anybody having known about it until Einstein's work? In fact, we do see matter being converted into energy around us all the time. We just do not normally think about what we find in these terms. All the energy-producing reactions of chemistry and physics, from the lighting of a match to the nuclear fusion that powers the sun and stars, involve the disappearance of a small amount of matter and its reappearance as energy. The simple formula $E_0 = mc^2$ has led not only to a better understanding of how

---

Example 3.8

How much mass is converted into energy per day in a 100-MW nuclear power plant?

Solution
There are $(60)(60)(24) = 86{,}400$ s/day, so the energy liberated per day is

$$E_0 = Pt = (10^2)(10^6\ \text{W})(8.64 \times 10^4\ \text{s}) = 8.64 \times 10^{12}\ \text{J}$$

From Eq. 3-8 the corresponding mass is

$$m = \frac{E_0}{c^2} = \frac{8.64 \times 10^{12}\ \text{J}}{(3 \times 10^8\ \text{m/s})^2} = 9.6 \times 10^{-5}\ \text{kg}$$

This is less than a tenth of a gram—not much. To liberate the same amount of energy from coal, about 270 tons would have to be burned.

BIOGRAPHY | Albert Einstein (1879–1955)

Bitterly unhappy with the rigid discipline of the schools of his native Germany, Einstein went to Switzerland at 16 to complete his education and later got a job examining patent applications at the Swiss Patent Office in Berne. Then, in 1905, ideas that had been in his mind for years when he should have been paying attention to other matters (one of his math teachers called Einstein a "lazy dog") blossomed into three short papers that were to change decisively the course of not only physics but modern civilization as well.

The first paper proposed that light has a dual character with particle as well as wave properties. This work is described in Chap. 9 together with the quantum theory of the atom that flowed from it.

The subject of the second paper was brownian motion, the irregular zigzag motion of tiny bits of suspended matter such as pollen grains in water (Fig. 3-33). Einstein arrived at a formula that related brownian motion to the bombardment of the particles by randomly moving molecules of the fluid in which they were suspended. Although the molecular theory of matter had been proposed many years before, this formula was the long-awaited definite link with experiment that convinced the remaining doubters that molecules actually exist. The third paper introduced the theory of relativity.

Although much of the world of physics was originally either indifferent or skeptical, even the most

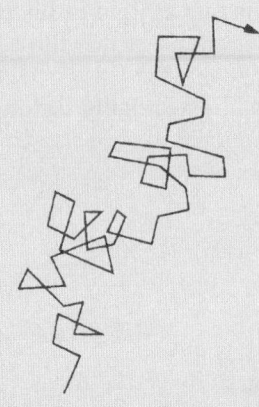

Figure 3-33   The irregular path of a microscopic particle bombarded by molecules. The line joins the positions of a single particle observed at constant intervals. This phenomenon is called brownian movement and is direct evidence of the reality of molecules and their random motions. It was discovered in 1827 by the British botanist Robert Brown.

unexpected of Einstein's conclusions were soon confirmed and the development of what is now called modern physics began in earnest. After university posts in Switzerland and Czechoslovakia, in 1913 Einstein took up an appointment at the Kaiser Wilhelm Institute in Berlin that left him able to do research free of financial worries and routine duties. His interest was now mainly in gravity, and he began where Newton had left off more than 200 years earlier.

The general theory of relativity that resulted from Einstein's work provided a deep understanding of

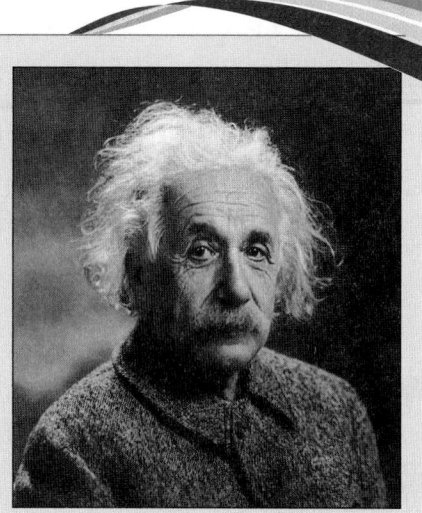

gravity, but his name remained unknown to the general public. This changed in 1919 with the dramatic discovery that gravity affects light exactly as Einstein had predicted. He immediately became a world celebrity, but his well-earned fame did not provide security when Hitler and the Nazis came to power in Germany in the early 1930s. Einstein left in 1933 and spent the rest of his life at the Institute for Advanced Study in Princeton, New Jersey, thereby escaping the fate of millions of other European Jews at the hands of the Germans.

Einstein's last years were spent in a fruitless search for a "unified field theory" that would bring together gravitation and electromagnetism in a single picture. The problem was worthy of his gifts, but it remains unsolved to this day although progress is being made.

nature works but also to the nuclear power plants—and nuclear weapons—that are so important in today's world.

The discovery that matter and energy can be converted into each other does not affect the law of conservation of energy provided we include mass as a form of energy. Table 3-1 lists the basic features of the various quantities introduced in this chapter.

3.13   General Relativity

Gravity Is a Warping of Spacetime

Einstein's general theory of relativity, published in 1916, related gravitation to the structure of space and time. What is meant by "the structure of

Table 3-1	**Energy, Power, and Momentum**				
Quantity	**Type**	**Symbol**	**Unit**	**Meaning**	**Formula**
Work	Scalar	W	Joule (J)	A measure of the change produced by a force that acts on something	$W = Fd$
Power	Scalar	P	Watt (W)	The rate at which work is being done	$P = W/t$
Kinetic energy	Scalar	KE	Joule (J)	Energy of motion	$KE = \frac{1}{2}mv^2$
Potential energy	Scalar	PE	Joule (J)	Energy of position	$PE_{gravitational} = mgh$
Rest energy	Scalar	E_0	Joule (J)	Energy equivalent of the mass of an object	$E_0 = mc^2$
Linear momentum	Vector	**p**	Kg · m/s	A measure of the tendency of a moving object to continue moving in the same straight line at the same speed	$\mathbf{p} = m\mathbf{v}$
Angular momentum	Vector	—	—	A measure of the tendency of a rotating object to continue rotating about the same axis at the same speed	—

space and time" can be given a quite precise meaning mathematically, but unfortunately no such precision is possible using ordinary language. All the same, we can legitimately think of the force of gravity as arising from a warping of spacetime around a body of matter so that a nearby mass tends to move toward the body, much as a marble rolls toward the bottom of a saucer-shaped hole (Fig. 3-34). In an apt formulation, "Matter tells spacetime how to curve, and spacetime tells matter how to move."

It may seem as though one abstract concept is merely replacing another, but in fact the new point of view led Einstein and other scientists to a variety of remarkable discoveries that could not have come from the older way of thinking.

Gravity and Light   Perhaps the most spectacular of Einstein's results was that light ought to be subject to gravity. The effect is very small, so a large mass, such as that of the sun, is needed to detect the influence of its gravity on light. If Einstein was right, light rays that pass near the sun should be bent toward it by 0.0005°—the diameter of a dime seen from a mile away. To check this prediction, photographs were taken of stars that appeared in the sky near the sun during an eclipse in 1919, when they could be seen because the moon obscured the sun's disk (see Chap. 17). These photographs were then compared with photographs of the same region of the sky taken when the sun was far away (Fig. 3-35), and the observed changes in the apparent positions of the stars matched Einstein's calculations. Other predictions based on general relativity have also been verified, and the theory remains today without serious rival. (For more, see Sec. 3.13 at www.mhhe.com/krauskopf.)

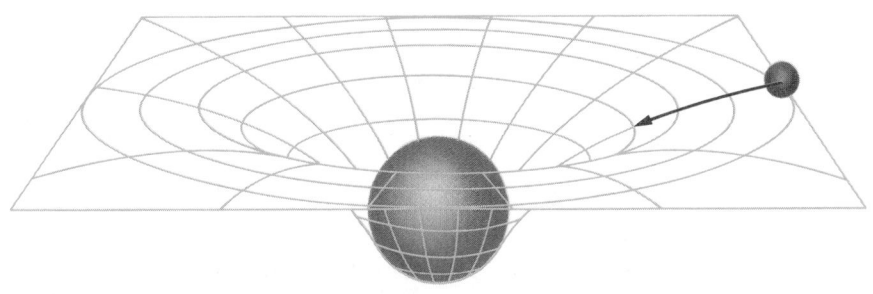

Figure 3-34   General relativity pictures gravity as a warping of the structure of space and time due to the presence of a body of matter. An object nearby experiences an attractive force as a result of this distortion in spacetime, much as a marble rolls toward the bottom of a saucer-shaped hole in the ground.

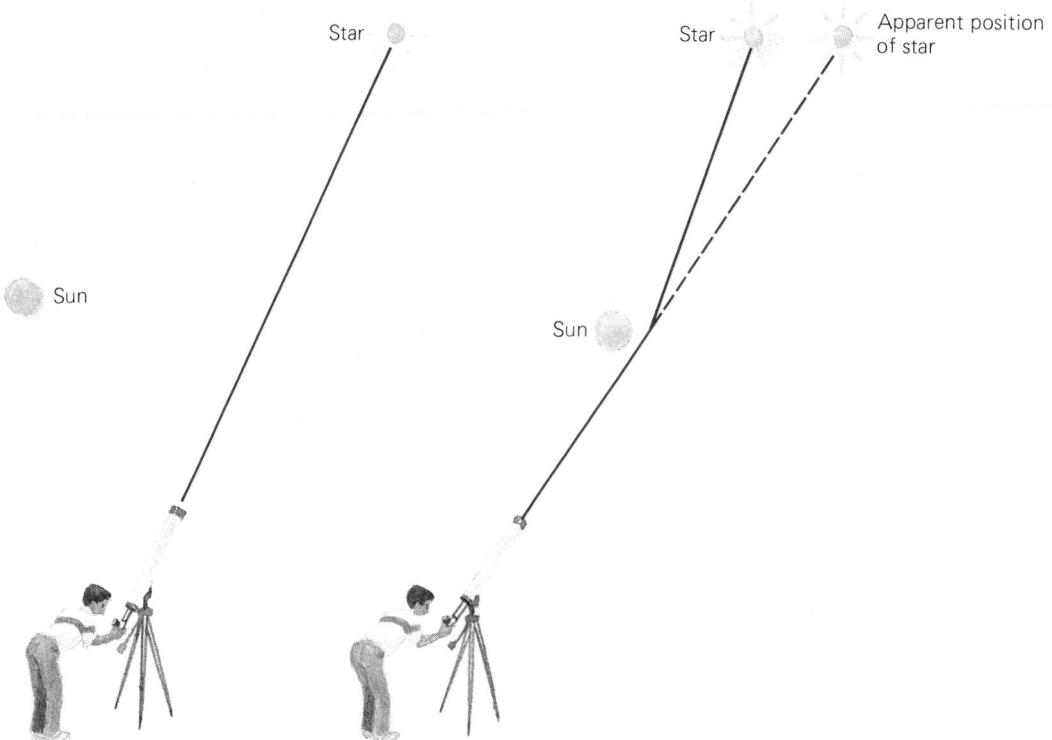

Figure 3-35   Starlight that passes near the sun is deflected by its strong gravitational pull. The deflection, which is very small, can be measured during a solar eclipse when the sun's disk is obscured by the moon.

Important Terms and Ideas

Work is a measure of the change, in a general sense, that a force causes when it acts upon something. The work done by a force acting on an object is the product of the magnitude of the force and the distance through which the object moves while the force acts on it. If the direction of the force is not the same as the direction of motion, the projection of the force in the direction of motion must be used. The unit of work is the **joule** (J).

Power is the rate at which work is being done. Its unit is the **watt** (W).

Energy is the property that something has that enables it to do work. The unit of energy is the joule. The three broad categories of energy are **kinetic energy,** which is the energy something has by virtue of its motion, **potential energy,** which is the energy something has by virtue of its position, and **rest energy,** which is the energy something has by virtue of its mass. According to the **law of conservation of energy,** energy cannot be created or destroyed, although it can be changed from one form to another (including mass).

Linear momentum is a measure of the tendency of a moving object to continue in motion along a straight line. **Angular momentum** is a measure of the tendency of a rotating object to continue spinning about the same axis. Both are vector quantities. If no outside forces act on a set of objects, then their linear and angular momenta are **conserved,** that is, remain the same regardless of how the objects interact with one another.

According to the **special theory of relativity,** when there is relative motion between an observer and what is being observed, lengths are shorter than when at rest, time intervals are longer, and kinetic energies are greater. Nothing can travel faster than the speed of light.

The **general theory of relativity,** which relates gravitation to the structure of space and time, correctly predicts that light should be subject to gravity.

Important Formulas

Work: $W = Fd$

Power: $P = \dfrac{W}{t} = Fv$

Kinetic energy: $KE = \frac{1}{2}mv^2$

Gravitational potential energy: $PE = mgh$

Linear momentum: $\mathbf{p} = m\mathbf{v}$

Rest energy: $E_0 = mc^2$

Multiple Choice

1. Which of the following is not a unit of work?
   a. newton-meter
   b. joule
   c. kilogram-meter
   d. watt-hour

2. An object at rest may have
   a. velocity
   b. momentum
   c. kinetic energy
   d. potential energy

3. A moving object must have which one or more of the following?
   a. potential energy
   b. kinetic energy
   c. rest energy
   d. momentum

4. When the momentum of a moving object is increased, there must also be an increase in which one or more of the following of the object's properties?
   a. speed
   b. acceleration
   c. kinetic energy
   d. potential energy

5. The total amount of energy (including the rest energy of matter) in the universe
   a. cannot change
   b. can decrease but not increase
   c. can increase but not decrease
   d. can either increase or decrease

6. When the speed of a moving object is halved,
   a. its KE is halved
   b. its PE is halved
   c. its rest energy is halved
   d. its momentum is halved

7. Two balls, one of mass 5 kg and the other of mass 10 kg, are dropped simultaneously from a window. When they are 1 m above the ground, the balls have the same
   a. kinetic energy
   b. potential energy
   c. momentum
   d. acceleration

8. A bomb dropped from an airplane explodes in midair.
   a. Its total kinetic energy increases
   b. Its total kinetic energy decreases
   c. Its total momentum increases
   d. Its total momentum decreases

9. The operation of a rocket is based upon
   a. pushing against its launching pad
   b. pushing against the air
   c. conservation of linear momentum
   d. conservation of angular momentum

10. A spinning skater whose arms are at her sides then stretches out her arms horizontally.
    a. She continues to spin at the same rate
    b. She spins more rapidly
    c. She spins more slowly
    d. Any of the choices could be correct, depending on how heavy her arms are

11. According to the principle of relativity, the laws of physics are the same in all frames of reference
    a. at rest with respect to one another
    b. moving toward or away from one another at constant velocity
    c. moving parallel to one another at constant velocity
    d. all of these

12. The formula $\frac{1}{2}mv^2$ for kinetic energy
    a. is the correct formula if v is properly interpreted
    b. always gives too high a value
    c. is the low-speed approximation to the correct formula
    d. is the high-speed approximation of the correct formula

13. A spacecraft has left the earth and is moving toward Mars. An observer on the earth finds that, relative to measurements made when the spacecraft was at rest, its
    a. length is shorter
    b. KE is less than $\frac{1}{2}mv^2$
    c. clocks tick faster
    d. rest energy is greater

14. The upper limit to the speed of an object with mass
    a. depends on the mass
    b. corresponds to a KE equal to its rest energy
    c. is the speed of sound
    d. is the speed of light

15. It is not true that
    a. light is affected by gravity
    b. the mass of a moving object depends upon its speed
    c. the maximum speed anything can have is the speed of light
    d. momentum is a form of energy

16. Albert Einstein did not discover that
    a. the length of a moving object is less than its length at rest
    b. the acceleration of gravity g is a universal constant
    c. light is affected by gravity
    d. gravity is a warping of spacetime

17. The work done in holding a 50-kg object at a height of 2 m above the floor for 10 s is
    a. 0   c. 1000 J
    b. 250 J   d. 98,000 J

18. The work done in lifting 30 kg of bricks to a height of 20 m is
    a. 61 J   c. 2940 J
    b. 600 J   d. 5880 J

19. A total of 4900 J is used to lift a 50-kg mass. The mass is raised to a height of
   a. 10 m   **c.** 960 m
   b. 98 m   **d.** 245 km

20. The work a 300-W electric grinder can do in 5.0 min is
   a. 1 kJ
   b. 1.5 kJ
   c. 25 kJ
   d. 90 kJ

21. A 150-kg yak has an average power output of 120 W. The yak can climb a mountain 1.2 km high in
   a. 25 min
   b. 4.1 h
   c. 13.3 h
   d. 14.7 h

22. A 40-kg boy runs up a flight of stairs 4 m high in 4 s. His power output is
   a. 160 W   **c.** 40 W
   b. 392 W   **d.** 1568 W

23. Car A has a mass of 1000 kg and is moving at 60 km/h. Car B has a mass of 2000 kg and is moving at 30 km/h. The kinetic energy of car A is
   a. half that of car B
   b. equal to that of car B
   c. twice that of car B
   d. 4 times that of car B

24. A 1-kg object has a potential energy of 1 J relative to the ground when it is at a height of
   a. 0.102 m   **c.** 9.8 m
   b. 1 m   **d.** 98 m

25. A 1-kg object has kinetic energy of 1 J when its speed is
   a. 0.45 m/s   **c.** 1.4 m/s
   b. 1 m/s   **d.** 4.4 m/s

26. The 2-kg blade of an ax is moving at 60 m/s when it strikes a log. If the blade penetrates 2 cm into the log as its KE is turned into work, the average force it exerts is
   a. 3 kN   **c.** 72 kN
   b. 90 kN   **d.** 180 kN

27. A 1-kg ball is thrown in the air. When it is 10 m above the ground, its speed is 3 m/s. At this time most of the ball's total energy is in the form of
   a. kinetic energy
   b. potential energy relative to the ground
   c. rest energy
   d. momentum

28. A 10,000-kg freight car moving at 2 m/s collides with a stationary 15,000-kg freight car. The two cars couple together and move off at
   a. 0.8 m/s   **c.** 1.3 m/s
   b. 1 m/s   **d.** 2 m/s

29. A 30-kg girl and a 25-kg boy are standing on frictionless roller skates. The girl pushes the boy, who moves off at 1.0 m/s. The girl's speed is
   a. 0.45 m/s   **c.** 0.83 m/s
   b. 0.55 m/s   **d.** 1.2 m/s

30. An object has a rest energy of 1 J when its mass is
   a. 1.1×10^{-17} kg   **c.** 1 kg
   b. 3.3×10^{-9} kg   **d.** 9×10^{16} kg

31. The smallest part of the total energy of the ball of Multiple Choice 27 is
   a. kinetic energy
   b. potential energy relative to the ground
   c. rest energy
   d. momentum

32. The lightest particle in an atom is an electron, whose rest mass is 9.1×10^{-31} kg. The energy equivalent of this mass is approximately
   a. 10^{-13} J   **c.** 3×10^{-23} J
   b. 10^{-15} J   **d.** 10^{-47} J

Exercises

3.1   The Meaning of Work

1. Is it correct to say that all changes in the physical world involve energy transformations of some sort? Why?

2. Under what circumstances (if any) is no work done on a moving object even though a net force acts upon it?

3. The sun exerts a gravitational force of 4.0×10^{28} N on the earth, and the earth travels 9.4×10^{11} m in its yearly orbit around the sun. How much work is done by the sun on the earth each year?

4. A crate is pushed across a horizontal floor at constant speed by a horizontal force of 140 N, which is just enough to overcome the friction between the crate and the floor. (a) How much work is done in pushing the crate through 10 m? (b) Rollers are then used under the crate to reduce friction and the same force is applied over the next 10 m. What happens to the work done now? (c) Will there be any change in the speed of the crate?

5. A total of 490 J of work is needed to lift a body of unknown mass through a height of 10 m. What is its mass?

6. A woman eats a cupcake and proposes to work off its 400-kJ energy content by exercising with a 15-kg barbell. If each lift of the barbell from chest height to overhead is through 60 cm and the efficiency of her body under these circumstances is 10 percent, how many times must she lift the barbell?

7. The acceleration of gravity on the surface of Mars is 3.7 m/s^2. If an astronaut in a space suit can jump upward 20 cm on the earth's surface, how high could he jump on the surface of Mars?

3.2   Power

8. The kilowatt-hour is a unit of what physical quantity or quantities?

9. The motor of a boat develops 60 kW when the boat's speed is 15 km/h. With how much force does the water resist the motion of the boat?

10. How much power must the legs of a 70-kg man develop in order to run up a staircase 5 m high in 9 s?

11. A weightlifter raises a 70-kg barbell from the floor to a height of 2.2 m in 1.2 s. What was his average power output during the lift?

12. An escalator 14 m long is carrying a 70-kg person from one floor to another 8 m higher. The escalator has a speed of 1.0 m/s. (a) How much work does the escalator do in carrying the person to the top? (b) What is its power output while doing so?

13. A 700-kg horse whose power output is 1.0 hp is pulling a sled over the snow at 3.5 m/s. Find the force the horse exerts on the sled.

14. A person's metabolic processes can usually operate at a power of 6 W/kg of body mass for several hours at a time. If a 60-kg woman carrying a 12-kg pack is walking uphill with an energy-conversion efficiency of 20 percent, at what rate, in meters/hour, does her altitude increase?

15. A crane whose motor has a power input of 5.0 kW lifts a 1200-kg load of bricks through a height of 30 m in 90 s. Find the efficiency of the crane, which is the ratio between its output power and its input power.

16. A total of 10^4 kg of water per second flows over a waterfall 30 m high. If half of the power this flow represents could be converted into electricity, how many 100-W lightbulbs could be supplied?

3.3   Kinetic Energy

17. Which of these energies might correspond to the KE of a person riding a bicycle on a road? 10 J; 1 kJ; 100 kJ

18. What is the speed of an 800-kg car whose KE is 250 kJ?

19. A moving object whose initial KE is 10 J is subject to a frictional force of 2 N that acts in the opposite direction. How far will the object move before coming to a stop?

20. Is the work needed to bring a car's speed from 0 to 10 km/h less than, equal to, or more than the work needed to bring its speed from 10 to 20 km/h? If the amounts of work are different, what is the ratio between them?

21. A 1-kg salmon is hooked by a fisherman and it swims off at 2 m/s. The fisherman stops the salmon in 50 cm by braking his reel. How much force does the fishing line exert on the fish?

22. During a circus performance, John Tailor was fired from a compressed-air cannon whose barrel was 20 m long. Mr. Tailor emerged from the cannon (twice on weekdays, three times on Saturdays and Sundays) at 40 m/s. If Mr. Tailor's mass was 60 kg, what was the average force on him when he was inside the cannon's barrel?

23. How long will it take a 1000-kg car with a power output of 20 kW to go from 10 m/s to 20 m/s?

3.4   Potential Energy

24. Does every moving body possess kinetic energy? Does every stationary body possess potential energy?

25. As we will learn in Chap. 6, electric charges of the same kind (both positive or both negative) repel each other, whereas charges of opposite sign (one positive and the other negative) attract each other. (a) What happens to the PE of a positive charge when it is brought near another positive charge? (b) When it is brought near a negative charge?

26. A 60-kg woman jumps off a wall 80 cm high and lands on a concrete road with her knees stiff. Her body is compressed by 8 cm at the moment of impact. (a) What was the average force the road exerted on her body? (b) If the woman bent her knees on impact so that she came to a stop over a distance of 40 cm, what would the average force on her body be?

3.5   Energy Transformations

27. In what part of its orbit is the earth's potential energy greatest with respect to the sun? In what part of its orbit is the earth's kinetic energy greatest? Explain your answers.

28. A 3-kg stone is dropped from a height of 100 m. Find its kinetic and potential energies when it is halfway to the ground.

29. Two identical balls move down a tilted board. Ball A slides down without friction and ball B rolls down. Which ball reaches the bottom first? Why?

30. (a) A yo-yo is swung in a vertical circle in such a way that its total energy KE + PE is constant. At what point in the circle is its speed a maximum? A minimum? Why? (b) If the yo-yo has a speed of 3 m/s at the top of the circle, whose radius is 80 cm, what is its speed at the bottom?

31. A ball is dropped from a height of 1 m and loses 10 percent of its kinetic energy when it bounces on the ground. To what height does it then rise?

32. A person sitting under a coconut palm is struck by a 1-kg coconut that fell from a height of 20 m. (a) Find the kinetic energy of the coconut when it reaches the person. (b) Find the average force exerted by the coconut if its impact is absorbed over a distance of 5 cm. (c) What is this force in pounds? Is it a good idea to sit under a coconut palm?

33. A skier is sliding downhill at 8 m/s when she reaches an icy patch on which her skis move freely

with negligible friction. The difference in altitude between the top of the icy patch and its bottom is 10 m. What is the speed of the skier at the bottom of the icy patch? Do you have to know her mass?

34. A force of 10 N is used to lift a 600-g ball from the ground to a height of 1.8 m, when it is let go. What is the speed of the ball when it is let go?

3.6 Conservation of Energy

3.7 The Nature of Heat

35. Why does a nail become hot when it is hammered into a piece of wood?

36. A man skis down a slope 90 m high. If 80 percent of his initial potential energy is lost to friction and air resistance, what is his speed at the bottom of the slope?

37. In an effort to lose weight, a person runs 5 km per day at a speed of 4 m/s. While running, the person's body processes consume energy at a rate of 1.4 kW. Fat has an energy content of about 40 kJ/g. How many grams of fat are metabolized during each run?

38. An 80-kg crate is raised 2 m from the ground by a man who uses a rope and a system of pulleys. He exerts a force of 220 N on the rope and pulls a total of 8 m of rope through the pulleys while lifting the crate, which is at rest afterward. (a) How much work does the man do? (b) What is the change in the potential energy of the crate? (c) If the answers to these questions are different, explain why.

39. An 800-kg car coasts down a hill 40 m high with its engine off and the driver's foot pressing on the brake pedal. At the top of the hill the car's speed is 6 m/s and at the bottom it is 20 m/s. How much energy was converted into heat on the way down?

3.8 Linear Momentum

40. (a) When an object at rest explodes into two parts that fly apart, must they move in exactly opposite directions? (b) When a moving object strikes a stationary one, must they move off in exactly opposite directions?

41. A golf ball and a Ping-Pong ball are dropped in a vacuum chamber. When they have fallen halfway to the bottom, how do their speeds compare? Their kinetic energies? Their potential energies? Their momenta?

42. Is it possible for an object to have more kinetic energy but less momentum than another object? Less kinetic energy but more momentum?

43. What happens to the momentum of a car when it comes to a stop?

44. The speed of an airplane doubles in flight. (a) How is the law of conservation of momentum obeyed in this situation? (b) The law of conservation of energy?

45. When the kinetic energy of an object is doubled, what happens to its momentum?

46. What, if anything, happens to the speed of a fighter plane when it fires a cannon at an enemy plane in front of it?

47. A ball of mass m rolling on a smooth surface collides with a stationary ball of mass M. (a) Under what circumstances will the first ball come to a stop while the second ball moves off? (b) Under what circumstances will the first ball reverse its direction while the second ball moves off in the original direction of the first ball? (c) Under what circumstances will both balls move off in the original direction of the first ball?

48. A railway car is at rest on a frictionless track. A man at one end of the car walks to the other end. (a) Does the car move while he is walking? (b) If so, in which direction? (c) What happens when the man comes to a stop?

49. An empty dump truck coasts freely with its engine off along a level road. (a) What happens to the truck's speed if it starts to rain and water collects in it? (b) The rain stops and the accumulated water leaks out. What happens to the truck's speed now?

50. A boy throws a 4-kg pumpkin at 8 m/s to a 40-kg girl on roller skates, who catches it. At what speed does the girl then move backward?

51. A 30-kg girl who is running at 3 m/s jumps on a stationary 10-kg sled on a frozen lake. How fast does the sled with the girl on it then move?

52. A 70-kg man and a 50-kg woman are in a 60-kg boat when its motor fails. The man dives into the water with a horizontal speed of 3 m/s in order to swim ashore. If he changes his mind, can he swim back to the boat if his swimming speed is 1 m/s? If not, can the woman change the boat's motion enough by diving off it at 3 m/s in the opposite direction? Could she then return to the boat herself if her swimming speed is also 1 m/s?

53. The 176-g head of a golf club is moving at 45 m/s when it strikes a 46-g golf ball and sends it off at 65 m/s. Find the final speed of the clubhead after the impact, assuming that the mass of the club's shaft can be neglected.

54. A 40-kg skater moving at 4 m/s overtakes a 60-kg skater moving at 2 m/s in the same direction and collides with her. The two skaters stick together. (a) What is their final speed? (b) How much kinetic energy is lost?

55. The two skaters of Exercise 54 are moving in opposite directions when they collide and stick together. Answer the same questions for this case.

56. A 1000-kg car moving east at 80 km/h collides head-on with a 1500-kg car moving west at 40 km/h, and the two cars stick together. (a) Which way does the wreckage move and with what initial speed? (b) How much KE is lost in the collision?

3.10 Angular Momentum

57. As the polar ice caps melt, the length of the day increases. Why?

58. All helicopters have two rotors. Some have both rotors on vertical axes but rotating in opposite directions, and the rest have one rotor on a horizontal axis perpendicular to the helicopter body at the tail. Why is a single rotor never used?

59. The earthquake that caused the Indian Ocean tsunami of 2004 (see Fig. 14.38) led to changes in the earth's crust that reduced its diameter slightly. What effect, if any, do you think this reduction had on the length of the day?

3.11 Special Relativity

60. What are the two postulates from which Einstein developed the special theory of relativity?

61. The theory of relativity predicts a variety of effects that disagree with our everyday experience. Why do you think this theory is universally accepted by scientists?

62. What physical quantity will all observers always find the same value for?

63. The length of a rod is measured by several observers, one of whom is stationary with respect to the rod. What must be true of the value obtained by the stationary observer?

64. Under what circumstances does it become conspicuous that the formula $KE = \frac{1}{2}mv^2$ understates the kinetic energy of a moving object of speed v?

65. Why is it impossible for an object to move faster than the speed of light?

3.12 Rest Energy

66. The potential energy of a golf ball in a hole is negative with respect to the ground. Under what circumstances (if any) is the ball's kinetic energy negative? Its rest energy?

67. What is the effect on the law of conservation of energy of the discovery that matter and energy can be converted into each other?

68. A certain walking person uses energy at an average rate of 300 W. All of this energy has its ultimate origin in the sun. How much matter is converted to energy in the sun per hour to supply this person?

69. One kilogram of water at 0°C contains 335 kJ of energy more than 1 kg of ice at 0°C. What is the mass equivalent of this amount of energy?

70. When 1 g of gasoline is burned in an engine, about 48 kJ of heat is produced. How much mass is lost in the process? Do you think this mass change could be directly measured?

71. Approximately 5.4×10^6 J of chemical energy is released when 1 kg of dynamite explodes. What fraction of the total energy of the dynamite is this?

72. Approximately 4×10^9 kg of matter is converted into energy in the sun per second. Express the power output of the sun in watts.

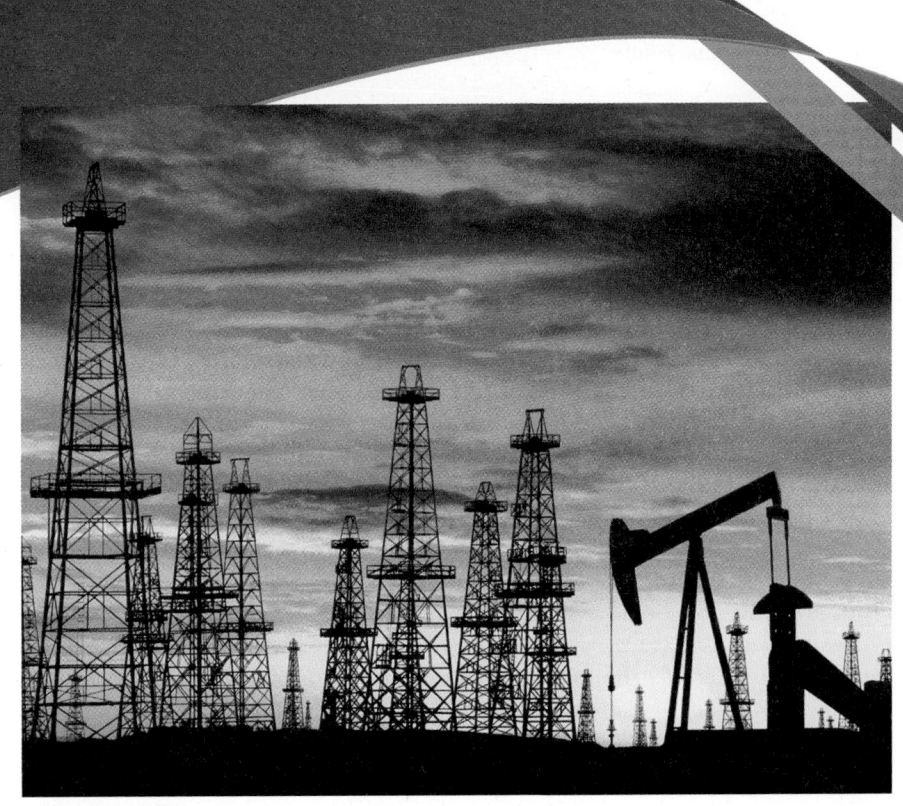

Oil wells in California.

4

Energy and the Future

GOALS

When you have finished this chapter you should be able to complete the goals • given for each section below:

The Energy Problem

4.1 Population and Prosperity
What Drives World Energy Demand
- State the approximate year in which world population is expected to level off, what the maximum population might then be, and which two countries then would have the most people.

4.2 Energy Consumption
High Today, Higher Tomorrow
- Explain why energy demand is likely to grow faster than world population.
- Identify the various fossil fuels, trace their energy contents to their ultimate origin, and compare their reserves.

4.3 Global Warming
A Serious Threat
- Discuss the evidence for global warming.
- State the probable maximum global temperature rise that would avoid large-scale catastrophe.
- Describe what such a catstrophe would involve.

4.4 Carbon Dioxide and the Greenhouse Effect
The Cause of Global Warming
- Explain the greenhouse effect and how it acts to heat the atmosphere.
- State the role of carbon dioxide in global warming and give examples of other greenhouse gases.
- Outline the role of deforestation in global warming.

Fossil Fuels

4.5 Liquid Fuels
Vehicles Are the Biggest Users
- Compare the average fuel efficiency of cars in the United States with that of cars elsewhere and give some reasons for the difference.
- Give the advantages and disadvantages of hybrid cars.

4.6 Natural Gas
The Least Bad Fossil Fuel
- Explain why natural gas is the least objectionable fossil fuel.
- Describe shale and clathrate sources of natural gas.

4.7 Coal
Plentiful but Worst for the Environment
- List the advantages and disadvantages of coal as a fuel and account for its wide and increasing use despite the severity of the disadvantages.
- Describe the carbon capture and storage method of dealing with CO_2 emissions from power plants.

Alternative Sources

4.8 A Nuclear World?
Perhaps On the Way
- Compare nuclear fission and nuclear fusion as energy sources.
- State the approximate percentage of electricity in the United States that comes from nuclear energy and explain why no new nuclear plants have been built for many years.

4.9 Clean Energy I
Continuous Sources
- Define geothermal energy and give some methods of using it.

4.10 Clean Energy II
Variable Sources
- Describe ways to make use of the energy contents of sunlight, wind, tides, and waves.

4.11 Energy Storage
Options for Variable Sources and Vehicles
- Describe methods of bulk storage of electric energy.
- Explain the difference between storage batteries and fuel cells.
- Compare electric, hybrid, and fuel-cell cars.

4.12 Biofuels
Yes, But
- Compare the advantages and disadvantages of the various biofuel sources.
- Explain the attractions of cellulosic ethanol.

Strategies for the Future

4.13 Conservation
Less Is More
- Give examples of opportunities to conserve energy in everyday life.

4.14 What Governments Must Do
Their Role Is Crucial
- Describe what is meant by a cap-and-trade system for controlling CO_2 emissions and compare it with a carbon tax.
- Compare the average annual CO_2 emissions per person in the United States and China, their total emissions, and their positions on controlling these emissions. Account for the importance of these countries in CO_2 control.
- Give the reasons why the Copenhagen conference on CO_2 emissions was a failure.

The rise of modern civilization would have been impossible without the discovery of vast resources of energy and the development of ways to transform it into useful forms. All that we do requires energy. The more energy we have at our command, the better we can satisfy our desires for food, clothing, shelter, warmth, light, transport, communication, and manufactured goods.

Unfortunately oil and natural gas, the most convenient fuels, although currently abundant, have become expensive, have limited reserves, and, together with the more plentiful coal, are largely responsible for global warming through the carbon dioxide their burning produces. Other energy sources have handicaps of one kind or another, some serious, as well as good features. Nuclear fusion, the ultimate energy source, remains a technology of the future at best.

At the same time, world population is increasing and people everywhere seek better lives, both factors that bring a need for more and more energy. The Industrial Revolution of the nineteenth century was powered largely by coal; in the twentieth century oil and gas became the leading fuels. Nothing is more important today than the choice and implementation of an appropriate energy strategy for the twenty-first century.

This is an unusual chapter for this book both because it is nontechnical and because it covers some of the essential social, economic, and even political dimensions of its subject, which does not exist in a vacuum. The decisions that businesses and governments make now and in the future are critical, and it is essential that they be made in full view of an informed public. In this chapter the energy problem in all its complexity is considered in one place so how its various parts fit together is clear. Even though scientific elements that cannot be properly discussed this early in the book are left for later chapters, the basic ideas are all here so that those who do not cover the entire text can view the situation as a whole and appreciate how it affects them (and how they affect it).

The Energy Problem

The energy problem has three elements:

1. Ever-increasing demand for energy driven by an expanding world population and its growing prosperity.
2. Inevitable decline in the economical supply of fossil fuels, which now furnish about 85 percent of the world's energy.
3. Carbon dioxide from the burning of fossil fuels is the chief contributor to the global warming that affects life on earth.

We will look at these matters in turn before going on to examine present and future sources of energy and then considering how best to secure the future while continuing to meet the most essential of our needs.

4.1 Population and Prosperity

What Drives World Energy Demand

For most of the hundred thousand or so years that modern humans have existed there were too few of them to have much effect on their resources or environments. Twelve thousand years ago, when agriculture began, the world's human population was probably about 5 million. It was perhaps 500 million in 1650, 1 billion in 1850, and 1.6 billion as recently as 1900. It is about 7 billion today and is climbing rapidly (Fig. 4-1). The current rate of population increase is a little over 230,000 per day—another United States every 4 years, another China every 18 years.

Future Population   It is obvious that the world's population cannot keep growing at the present rate, and indeed must decrease. Already, according to the U.N. Environment Program, "the human population is now so large that the amount of resources needed to sustain it exceeds what is available at current consumption patterns." An average fertility rate of 2.1 children per woman (the 0.1 takes into account girls who do not live to adulthood) means a constant population. Over 60 countries have already reached this rate or even less; it is 2.05 in the United States, 1.2 in Japan and South Korea, 1.3 in Spain and Italy. In other countries, however, fertility rates are higher. In sub-Saharan Africa, the overall fertility rate is 5.4. Africa's population is expected to quadruple before stabilizing, the last region to do so.

The annual rate of unintended pregnancies worldwide is thought to be comparable to the rate of population increase. Poverty, low status of women, ignorance, tradition, and the doctrines of some religions all contribute to rising populations by obstructing access to the safe and efficient family planning methods already used in much of the world. Nevertheless, a global shift to smaller families, with every child a wanted child, has begun. In China, whose population is now 1.3 billion, fertility halved between 1970 and 1996; in Bangladesh, with 150 million people, a similar reduction took even less time.

As Fig. 4-1 shows, hopeful but plausible estimates of world population suggest a leveling off at around 9.2 billion by 2050, 1½ more Chinas for the earth to support than today. (If current fertility rates were unchanged, there would be over a billion more of us than that.) By 2050 India is likely to have passed China as the most populous nation and might then have more people than there were in the entire world in 1900. After peaking in 2050 the curve of Fig. 4-1 is projected to turn downward. If that happens, an eventual population fall to a stable size that permits comfortable lives for everybody might then occur.

What would a sustainable population count for the earth be? Half of today's figure? A third? Even less? Nobody knows because any estimate must involve a wide variety of factors, many without reliable numbers attached. What is clear, however, is that there are too many people today for the world to support for much longer both their demands on natural resources and their assaults on the environment in which they live.

Prosperity   In parallel with a ballooning population is a broad rise in prosperity. In 1990 nearly 30 percent of the world's people lived on less than the equivalent of $1/day; today the proportion (still a disgrace) is down to half that, which means more energy use per person. Higher up the economic ladder, life is also getting better, which has the same effect. As an example of what this implies for the future, we can compare car ownership in China (1.3 billion people) with that in the United States (310 million people). These were recently about 40 and 800 cars/1000 people, respectively. Incomes in China are increasing by 9 to 10 percent/year (China expects to expand its middle class to at least half its population by 2020) and in 2009 it became the world's largest car market. Even if China never catches up with the car ownership rate of the United States, in time there will be hundreds of millions more cars there gobbling up fuel of some kind. In India (1.1 billion largely poor people), whose population and economy are both growing steadily, car sales are increasing by over 20 percent each year; some new cars there cost as little as $2500. The world's automotive fleet, now over 900 million cars, is expected to grow to 2 billion by 2050.

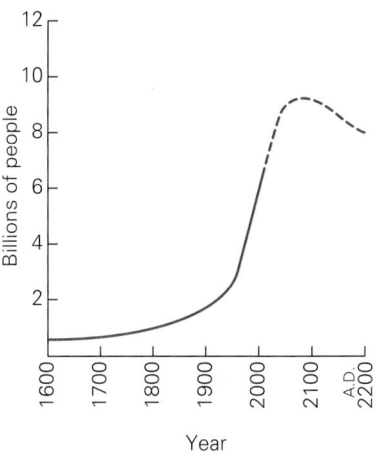

Figure 4-1   World population according to United Nations figures—currently about 7 billion. Estimates for future population vary widely. Shown is an optimistic projection with a peak of about 9.2 billion in 2050. An eventual decrease in population would be the first since the Black Death of the fourteenth century. Unless the decrease occurs in time, resources of all kinds will give out and the environment, already under threat, will turn hostile.

4.2 Energy Consumption

High Today, Higher Tomorrow

As the world economy expands, so does its consumption of energy. In the advanced countries, the standard of living is already high and their populations are stable, so their need for energy is unlikely to grow very much. Indeed, this need may even decline as their energy use becomes more efficient. Elsewhere, rates of energy consumption are still low, less than 1 kW per person for more than half the people of the world compared with about 10.5 kW per person in the United States (Fig. 4-2). These people seek better lives, which means more energy, and their numbers are swelling, which means still more energy. About a tenth of all spending in the United States goes to energy.

Figure 4-3 shows world energy consumption from 1980 to the present together with three projections for the future. The middle curve assumes an average annual rise in energy use of 1 percent in the advanced countries and a 3 percent rise in other countries, figures thought to be realistic. The bottom curve corresponds to a lower rate of economic growth than anticipated and the top curve to a higher rate. The midrange estimate for 2030 is nearly one and a half times today's energy consumption.

Almost all the energy available to us today has a single source—the sun. Light and heat reach us directly from the sun; food and wood owe their energy content to photosynthesis (Sec. 13.12) powered by sunlight falling on plants; water power exists because the sun's heat evaporates water from the oceans that falls later as rain and snow on high ground; wind power comes

Figure 4-2   Energy use per person in various countries. The energy needs of the huge populations at the lower end of the list are increasing. China alone has a population of 1.3 billion and its energy consumption is growing at over four times the world average; it has accounted for 80 percent of the world's new power plants in recent years and is expected to continue doing so for years to come. The United Kingdom consists of England, Scotland, Wales, and Northern Ireland. Senegal is a fairly typical African country.

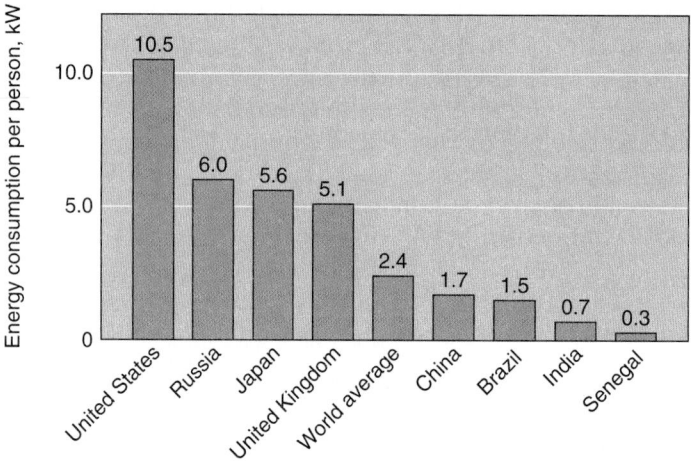

Figure 4-3   Annual world energy consumption 1980–2030. The energy unit is the exojoule (EJ), where 1 EJ = 10^{18} J = 24 million tons of oil equivalent. Most of the future increase in energy consumption is expected to come from developing countries with large populations, mainly China and India.

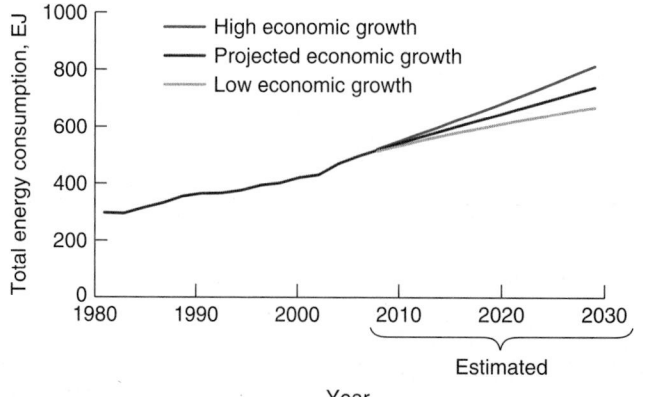

from motions in the atmosphere due to unequal heating of the earth's surface by the sun. The fossil fuels coal, oil, and natural gas were formed from the remains of plants and animals that contain energy derived from sunlight millions of years ago. Only nuclear energy, tidal energy, and heat from sources inside the earth cannot be traced to the sun's rays (Figs. 4-4 and 4-5).

Future Sources Fossil fuels, which today furnish by far the greatest part of the world's energy, cannot last forever. As their reserves decline, their prices will go up accordingly, which is already happening. The increased cost of energy will burden all economies, especially those of developing countries, which use energy less efficiently. For instance, China needs over twice as much energy as the United States does per unit of output.

The Stone Age did not end because the world ran out of stones but because superior technologies came into being. The same will be true for fossil fuels: well before they actually run out, they will be replaced because they have become too expensive, both in terms of money and in terms of the harm they cause to the environment. Then renewable and nuclear (fission and, perhaps, fusion) energies will become the principal energy sources.

Petroleum—more familiarly, oil—will be the first fossil fuel whose trend in Fig. 4-5 will begin to turn downward. At present, the world uses over 85 million barrels of oil per day (a quarter of that by the United States) and demand is still rising. And at least 3.5 million barrels of oil per day of new production capacity is needed each year to offset the declining flow from old wells. Where will all this oil come from? More oil is still being found and methods exist to extract some of the oil that remains in old wells, though at more expense per barrel. However, the last year in which more oil was discovered than consumed was more than a quarter of a century ago, and by now two barrels of oil are burned for every barrel discovered.

Sooner or later—probably before 2030, possibly as soon as 2020—oil production will reach a peak and start to decline. The flow of oil will not stop then, of course, but its price will soar. This will bring about a drastic change in the world's patterns of energy use that will be hard to adjust to because oil burns efficiently and is easy to extract, process, store, and transport. Seventy percent of the oil used today goes into fuels that power ships, trains, aircraft, cars, and trucks, and oil is a valued feedstock for synthetic material of all kinds.

Natural gas fuels the power stations that generate a fifth of the electricity used in the United States (Fig. 4-6) and provides heat for more than half its homes. Reserves of natural gas far exceed those of oil, though new technology will be required to exploit the largest deposits (Sec. 4.6). But it, too, will not last forever.

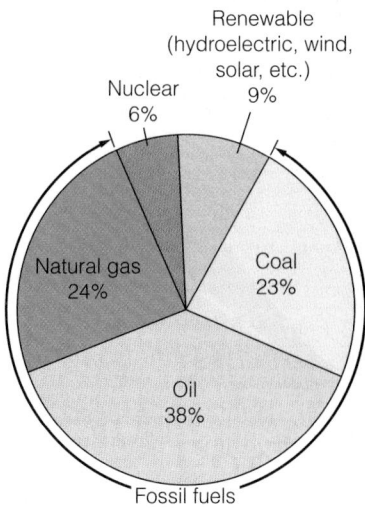

Figure 4-4 Sources of commercial energy production worldwide. Fossil fuels are responsible for 85 percent of the world's energy consumption (apart from firewood, still widely used, which is not included here). The percentages for energy sources in the United States are not very different from those of the world as a whole. However, China's figures are quite different: coal provides $2\frac{1}{2}$ times as much of its energy as the world average with correspondingly smaller proportions for other sources. The world total is around 12 billion tons of oil equivalent. (An average family car burns about 1 ton of oil equivalent per year.)

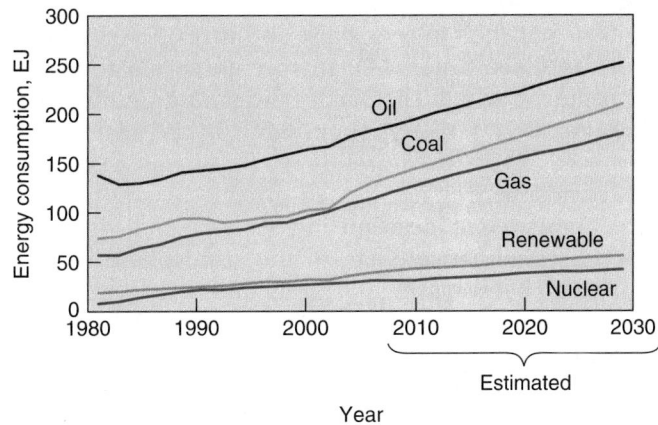

Figure 4-5 Annual world energy consumption from various sources. Serious international action to moderate global warming would reduce the projected rises in fossil-fuel use and increase the others.

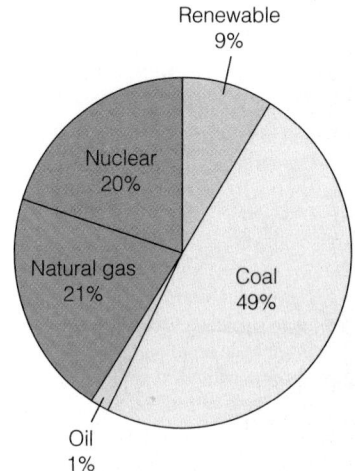

Figure 4-6 Sources of electric energy in the United States. In Europe, the contribution of renewable sources is 16 percent, a level not expected to be reached in the United States until at least 2030.

Even though the coal we consume every year took about 2 million years to accumulate, apparently—the data are not entirely reliable—enough remains for perhaps a century at the present rate of consumption, less if coal use continues to increase at its current rate. Coal reserves are equivalent in energy content to several times oil reserves. Coal is the cheapest fossil fuel. Before 1941, coal was the world's chief fuel, and it is likely to return to first place when oil and gas run out. As with them, coal prices are headed upward, more than tripling in the past decade, and will increase even faster as production declines.

Nonfossil Sources   Nuclear fuel reserves exceed those of fossil fuels. Besides having an abundant fuel supply, a properly built and properly operating nuclear plant is in many respects an excellent energy source. Nuclear energy is already responsible for about a fifth of the electricity generated in the United States, and in a number of other countries the proportion is even higher; in France it is three-quarters. After a period of being largely out of favor, nuclear energy is about to come into wider use, as discussed in Sec. 4.8.

What about the energy of direct sunlight, of winds and tides, of falling water, of trees and plants, of the earth's own internal heat? After all, the technologies needed to exploit these renewable resources already exist and are steadily improving. Though their contributions will certainly help, it is unlikely that such sources will supply a large part of the world's energy needs for decades to come. In every case, the required installation is either expensive (though decreasingly so) for the energy obtained, or practical only in favorable locations, or both. Some cannot provide energy reliably all the time, and most of them need a lot of space.

Although fossil fuels clearly cannot cope indefinitely with expected energy demand, with the help of nuclear and renewable technologies there are sufficient reserves of fossil fuels to last at least much of the rest of this century. But there is another consideration: the billions of tons of carbon dioxide produced each year by the burning of fossil fuels are mainly responsible for the warming of the atmosphere that is going on today, a warming that seems sure to have serious consequences for our planet. To continue burning fossil fuels at the ever-increasing rates of Fig. 4-5 is a recipe for disaster, as we shall see next.

4.3   Global Warming

A Serious Threat

The average temperature of the earth's surface and the atmosphere just above it has varied throughout the earth's history. Warm spells and cold ones have alternated, including ice ages in which immense sheets of ice blanketed much of the globe, but the changes back and forth occurred over relatively long periods of time (see Chap. 14). In recent years a totally new pattern of change has begun in which the earth is warming up much faster than it ever has before (Fig. 4-7), a rise of about 0.5°C in the past 30 years and still climbing.

The earth's atmosphere is not heated directly by sunlight but indirectly through the greenhouse effect described in Secs. 4.4 and 14.4. The chief agent responsible for the greenhouse effect in the atmosphere is the gas carbon dioxide (CO_2), and global warming is chiefly due to its growing CO_2 content. (The symbol CO_2 means that each carbon dioxide molecule consists of two oxygen atoms bonded to a carbon atom.)

Some consequences of increasing world temperatures are already obvious. Sea ice in the Arctic is melting steadily and in 20 years or so the North Pole is likely to be free of ice in the summer, for the first time in 3 million years. Similar melting is taking place around the Antarctic continent (Fig. 4-8).

Signs of Warming

Increasing air temperatures, shrinking glaciers, and rising seas are not the only signs that the world is getting hotter. The oceans store far more heat than the atmosphere, so changes in their temperatures are more significant—and they, too, are climbing. Hurricanes and other tropical storms, whose energy comes from warm ocean water, are becoming stronger. Storms elsewhere are becoming more frequent and more severe.

Climate patterns are changing as well, with record rainfalls in some areas and record droughts in others. Deserts in Africa and central Asia are spreading. Wildfires are more and more common worldwide. In the United States, the Atlantic and Pacific coastal regions are becoming wetter while some of the central states can expect to be increasingly starved of water.

Not all is bad for now: spring comes earlier every year, which lengthens the growing season in the high latitudes to increase food production there. But some plants and animals are already having trouble keeping up with their new environments, and a quarter of all species may die out by 2100. Overall crop yields sooner or later will decline as temperatures go up and droughts occur more frequently, unwelcome tidings for the still-swelling world population.

Also ominous is the effect of rising temperatures on the spread of disease. Previously safe parts of the Mediterranean Sea now host toxic warm-water algae. Milder winters have allowed the ticks that carry Lyme disease to spread farther across North America and Scandinavia. Mosquitoes, which are vectors of such maladies as malaria and dengue fever, range over a larger part of the world than before, and because their metabolism goes up with temperature, they also feed more often. There are many more examples.

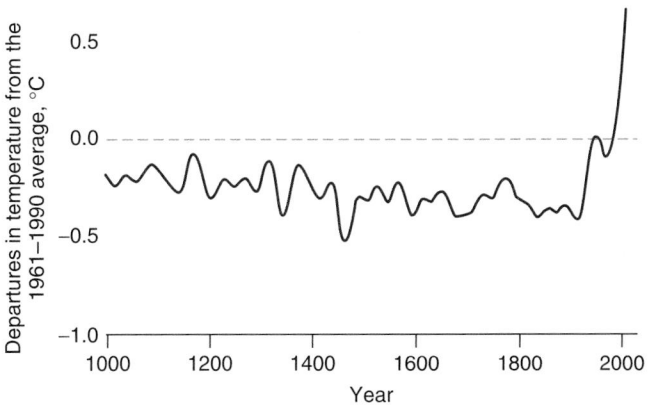

Figure 4-7   Average global surface temperatures for the past thousand years. Temperatures are continuing to rise sharply.

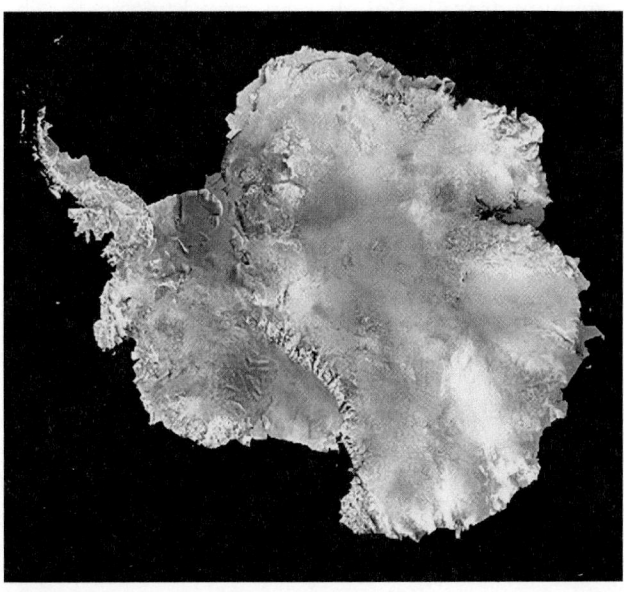

Figure 4-8   Much of Antarctica is surrounded by giant ice shelves fed by glaciers on shore. Global warming has led to the breakup of large sections of the ice shelves, which drift out to sea as icebergs and eventually melt. Because the shelves are floating to start with, their melting does not raise sea level, but meltwater from the Antarctic ice cap itself will continue to do so as global warming proceeds. If the Antarctic and Greenland ice caps were to melt, sea level would rise by at least 10 m, which would drastically change the map of the world's land areas. Complete melting would take a long time, but once well under way it would be irreversible because seawater and bare ground absorb sunlight more efficiently than ice, an excellent reflector, does.

Conflicts to Come

The large-scale disruptions of normal life that global warming seems to be on the way to bringing about are not likely to be met passively by those involved. It is entirely possible that within the lifetimes of many people alive today, hundreds of millions of Latin Americans, Africans, and Asians will run short of freshwater and food. Rising seas made worse by storm surges will add to the misery.

How will the rest of the world, by then already near or at the limit of its ability to support its own populations, react to the refugees swarming in, desperate to survive? We all know the answer. An alarmist view? Not according to the U.N. Panel on Climate Change, the U.N. Security Council, the Pentagon, and other worried observers. Only if both global population and CO_2 emissions begin to fall very soon is there any prospect of a peaceful world of thriving people in the future.

Sea Level   The melting of sea ice does not affect sea level, just as the melting of an ice cube in a glass of water does not change the water level, but the melting of ice on land is another story. Global warming is causing sea level to rise at 3.4 mm/year today, almost twice as fast as a decade ago and still accelerating. Although much of the rise is due to water expanding as it is heated, as most substances do, the melting of the vast glaciers of Greenland and Antarctica is responsible for a growing proportion.

The polar icecaps are on the way to melting on a scale large enough to inundate coastal regions everywhere. This will leave huge numbers of people to be resettled on higher ground; nearly half the world's population now lives on or near coasts, a proportion expected to be three-quarters in the not-too-distant future. Even before gondolas fill the flooded streets of coastal cities, the underground water deposits that supply most of their freshwater will have been contaminated by seawater.

How much higher will sea level go? If present trends in carbon dioxide emissions continue, a minimum sea-level rise of 1 m by 2100 can be expected, possibly as much as twice that. Even a 1-m rise would displace at least 140 million coastal dwellers. If all the proposed programs to reduce world carbon dioxide emissions are actually carried out, the rise would still be around 0.75 m. In any case, the melting will not stop in 2100 but will persist as long as elevated temperatures do, raising sea level yet more in centuries to come.

Future Temperatures   The average surface temperature since 1880 has gone up by about 0.83°C. Sunlight is reflected back into space by ice, and the loss of ice means much more solar energy absorbed by the land and sea that it once covered. The result is a feedback loop that accelerates global warming. This means that time is not on our side: action taken now would make a bigger difference than the same action taken later.

It is generally agreed that a global temperature increase of 2°C beyond preindustrial values is the most that can be tolerated without catastrophic impacts on human (and all other) life. A rise of 2°C may not seem like much, but to keep it from being exceeded would mean drastic changes in the world's ways of producing and using energy. Such changes would be very expensive and affect the lives of almost everybody.

At the other extreme, most calculations of the result of doing nothing beyond the measures already being taken suggest a global temperature rise of over 4°C by 2100. The earth would then be warmer than it has been for 55 million years with environmental changes on a huge scale. The middle and tropical latitudes would be too hot and dry to support the variety of living things they now do, with surviving humans crowded together in the polar regions. How many people could such a planet support? Maybe a billion or two, certainly far less than the projected 9.2 billion of Fig. 4-1, which does not take global warming into account.

In the rest of this chapter, we will see what is responsible for global warming and what can—must—be done to prevent such a nightmare future.

4.4   Carbon Dioxide and the Greenhouse Effect

The Cause of Global Warming

Every body of matter radiates light regardless of its temperature; the hotter it is, the more it gives off (see Fig. 5-6). The radiation from something very hot, such as the sun, is obvious because its glow is mainly visible light. The radiation from something at room temperature, however, is chiefly infrared light to which the eye is not sensitive. The interior of a greenhouse is warmer than the outside air because the glass of its windows is transparent to visible light from the sun whereas the infrared light given off by its contents is absorbed by the glass, so that the incoming energy is trapped.

As discussed in Sec. 14.4, this **greenhouse effect** is largely responsible for heating the earth's atmosphere and its surface. The visible light from the sun that reaches the surface is reradiated as infrared light that is readily absorbed by several gases in the atmosphere. One of the most important of these gases is carbon dioxide. As a result, the atmosphere is heated mainly from below by the earth and only to a smaller extent from above by the sun, as shown in Fig. 14-12. Without the greenhouse effect, the earth's surface would average $-18°C$ instead of its current average of $15°C$.

Atmospheric CO_2 Is Increasing

In the past, the total energy that the earth and its atmosphere reradiated back into space equalled the total energy they received from the sun. However, the CO_2 content of the atmosphere is steadily increasing, which means that the earth and its atmosphere are absorbing energy at a greater rate than before and are heating up. The result is global warming.

Even if the CO_2 content of the atmosphere were to stop rising, there would still be a time lag until the earth's surface reached a final temperature at which the energy input and output flows were in balance. The temperature surge in recent years shown in Fig. 4-7 is only about half of what is needed to equalize the energy flows, so global warming will continue until that happens no matter what action is taken. Because CO_2 persists in the atmosphere for about a century after entering it, global temperatures would then fall very gradually. Time is not on our side.

Analyzing air bubbles trapped in Greenland and Antarctic ice shows that the CO_2 concentration in the atmosphere is currently 27 percent higher than at any time in the past 650,000 years. The chief cause in recent times is the burning of fossil fuels to generate electricity; heat our homes; propel our cars, trains, ships, and airplanes; and power various industrial processes. All but 15 percent of the world's energy comes from carbon-based fuels. Each kilogram of carbon burned yields 3.7 kg of CO_2, and at present our chimneys and exhaust pipes pour out about 30 billion tons of CO_2 per year.

The United States and China are by far the largest emitters of CO_2 (Figs. 4-9 and 4-10). In 2000, total Chinese emissions, then half those of the United States, were expected to catch up around 2025. They actually did so

Soot

Although an enhanced greenhouse effect is the chief contributor to global warming, recent studies show that another important factor is soot, which consists of black carbon particles produced when various fuels are incompletely burned. Soot may be responsible for as much as 18 percent of global warming. A good deal of soot enters the atmosphere from old, inefficient diesel engines, but most apparently comes from primitive cooking stoves widely used in parts of Africa and Asia with wood and dung as fuel. As the soot particles absorb sunlight, they heat up and warm the air around them.

Because soot particles stay aloft for only a few weeks and so do not accumulate in the atmosphere the way greenhouse gases do, replacing the primitive stoves with efficient ones (about $20 each) would have an immediate effect. If, say, 20 million stoves were replaced with help from developed countries (the stove users themselves have incomes of only about $2/day), the cost would be $400 million, an extremely modest sum to slow global warming by a useful amount.

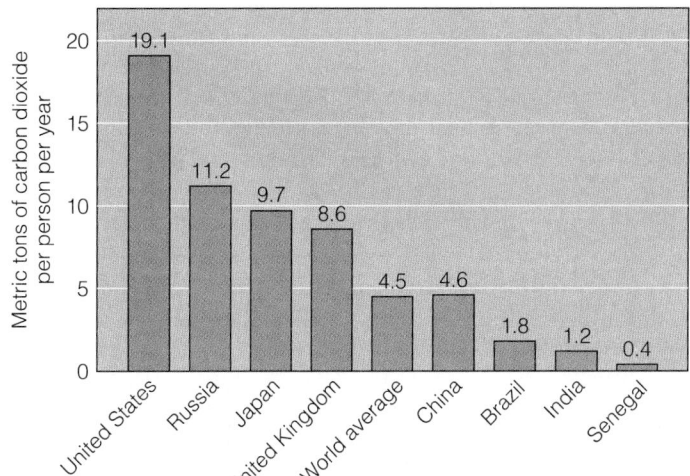

Figure 4-9 Annual carbon dioxide emissions from fossil fuels per person in various countries in 2007. (1 metric ton = 1000 kg)

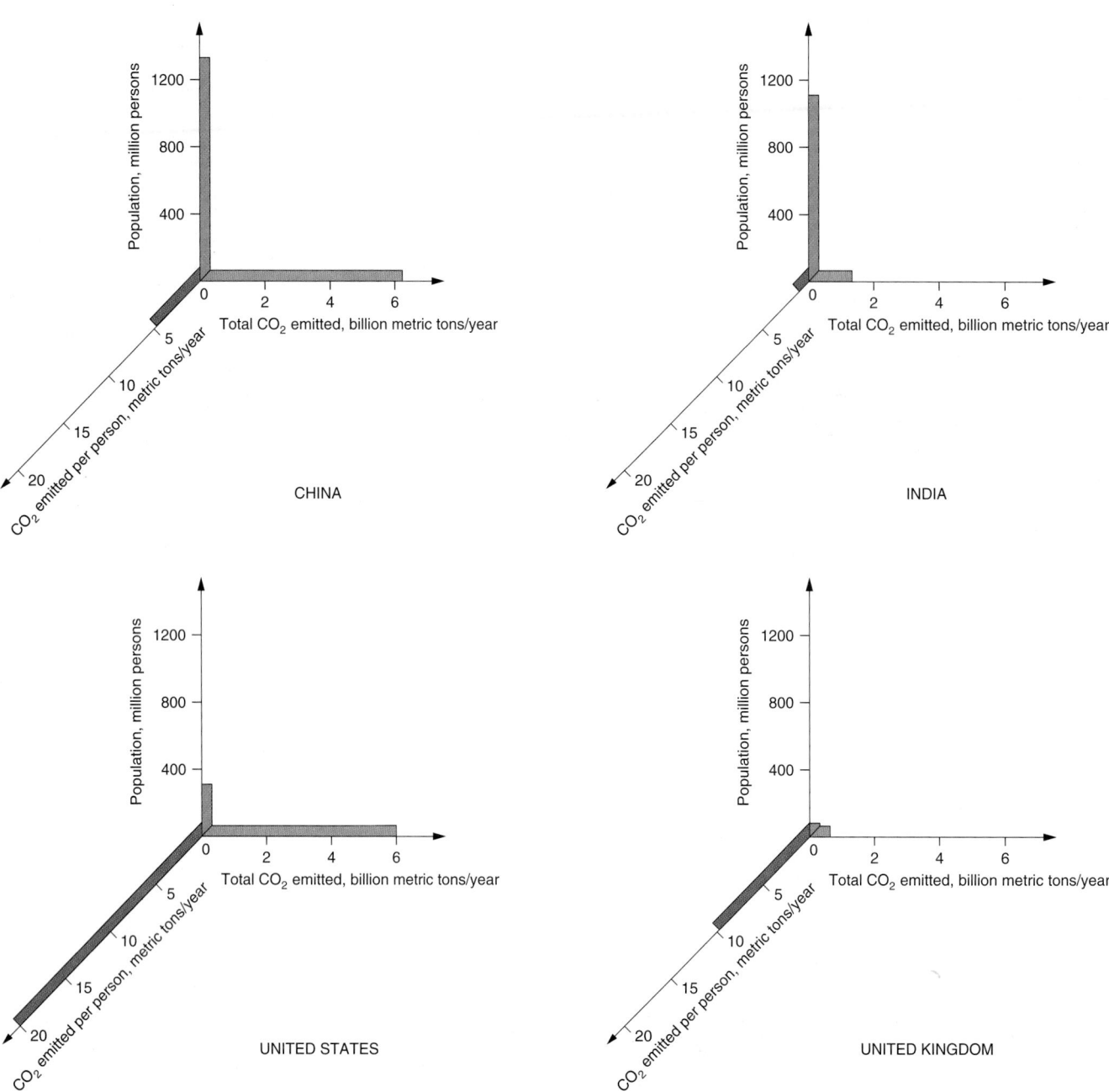

Figure 4-10   Population and annual CO_2 emissions from fossil fuels of four countries in 2007. China and India have the largest populations, with three out of eight of the world's people between them. For now India emits less than a fifth as much CO_2 per person as China does. China and the United States each account for a fifth of the world's CO_2 emissions, but there are over four times as many Chinese. The United Kingdom, whose CO_2 emissions per person are about twice China's and half those of the United States, is a fairly typical industrialized country. CO_2 emissions from most less-developed countries are very small, only about 400 kg per person per year in Africa's Senegal, for example, but because such countries are largely agricultural they will suffer most from global warming.

in 2007 and are still rising much more rapidly than those of the United States as China continues its dash to industrialize.

As we can see from Fig. 4-11, the CO_2 content of the atmosphere, now around 390 ppm, has gone up by over 35 percent since 1860 and is currently growing at 2 ppm/year. The increase represents about half the CO_2 from burning fossil fuels; the rest is absorbed by the oceans, soils, and forests. As fossil fuels continue to be burned at a high rate, the greenhouse "window" becomes a better and better trap for heat and the ultimate temperature of

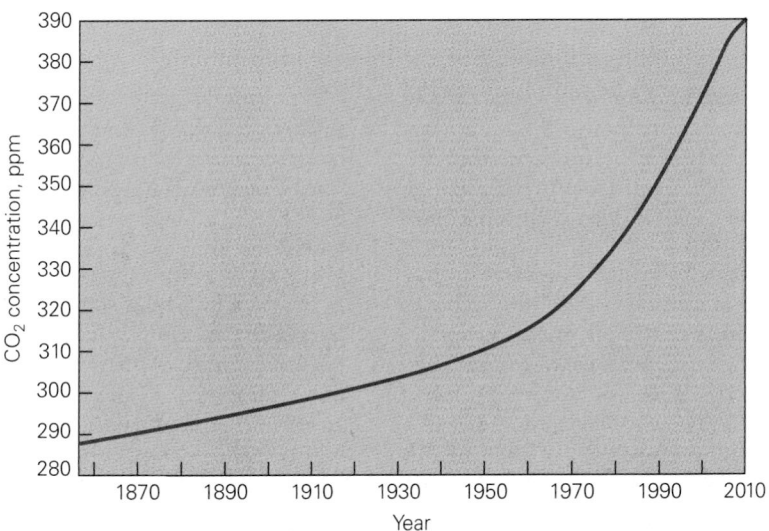

Figure 4-11 Carbon dioxide concentration in the atmosphere since 1860, in parts per million (ppm). The total today is nearly 3 trillion tons. There was little change in CO_2 concentration in the 10 thousand years before 1860. If CO_2 emissions do not fall significantly, its concentration is expected to climb to at least 500 ppm in this century. The resulting enhanced greenhouse effect will then push global temperatures past the threshold for severe and long-lasting environmental damage.

the earth's surface will continue to go up. If nothing is done, by 2100 atmospheric CO_2 is projected to reach 965 ppm with a disastrous temperature rise of perhaps 4.8°C.

Many climate scientists think that the CO_2 concentration in the atmosphere should not exceed 450 ppm to prevent global temperatures from

Other Greenhouse Gases

Although CO_2 is the most important of the **greenhouse gases** human activities are responsible for, it is not the only one (Fig. 4-12). Following it in significance are the CFCs and HCFCs, a group of artificially made gases mainly used in refrigeration and air-conditioning (Sec. 14.1). They leak into the atmosphere in much smaller amounts than Fig. 4-12 suggests, but are highly efficient as greenhouse gases—1 kg of most of them is equivalent to several tons of CO_2—and remain active for several decades. The quoted figure of 24 percent corresponds to their contribution to global warming.

Next in its impact on global warming is **methane,** the chief constituent of natural gas. A methane molecule consists of four hydrogen atoms bonded to a carbon atom, so its chemical formula is CH_4. Methane is 23 times as efficient as CO_2 in trapping heat but fortunately has the short lifetime in the atmosphere of about a dozen years. About 600 million tons of methane are released annually into the atmosphere from

wetlands, in the production of fossil fuels, in the decay of organic matter (for instance in landfills), in rice growing, and, in surprising quantities, as by-products of the digestion of food by cattle, sheep, and termites. A cow belches 200 liters or so of methane every day.

Methane in vast quantities—perhaps 50 billion tons—from the decomposition of organic remains has been locked into the frozen lands of Siberia and northern Canada for thousands of years. Now global warming is melting the permafrost and methane is bubbling out—an estimated 100,000 tons every summer day from Siberia's peat bogs alone. Like the increased absorption of sunlight by newly ice-free areas of polar lands and sea, this is another feedback loop that accelerates global warming. The methane concentration in the atmosphere today from all sources is over twice what it was in preindustrial times.

Nitrous oxide, N_2O, is 310 times as potent a greenhouse gas as CO_2 and has an average lifetime in

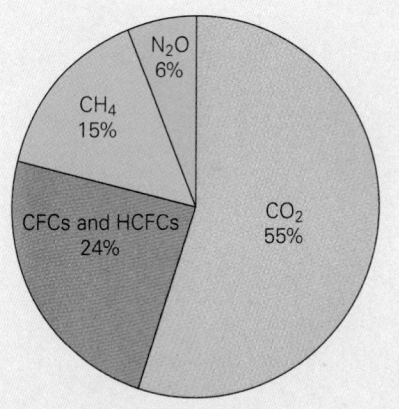

Figure 4-12 The contributions to global warming of the chief greenhouse gases.

the atmosphere of around 120 years. It is given off when fossil fuels and organic matter are burned, when fertilizers are used (3 to 5 percent of the nitrogen added by them to the soil ends up as N_2O), and in various industrial processes. Rainforests and the oceans also emit some N_2O. The N_2O concentration in the atmosphere, now 18 percent over its preindustrial level, is also on the way up.

Deforestation

Every year 50,000 square miles of rainforest are destroyed, for the most part to create farmland. About half the tropical forests that the world once had are now gone, which has reduced the diversity of living things. As a rule, the soil under a tropical forest is poor and wears out after only a few crops, and additional forest is then cleared. Trees are about half carbon, and cutting them down to rot or be burned adds an estimated 3 billion tons of CO_2 annually into the atmosphere, almost a fifth of total CO_2 emissions.

Another unfortunate aspect of deforestation comes from the fact that CO_2 and water are the raw materials from which trees, like all plants, manufacture carbohydrates with the help of sunlight (Sec. 13.12). A typical rainforest tree (one of around 200 billion) removes 22 kg of CO_2 from the atmosphere every year, a process that stops when the tree is cut down. Today forest growth absorbs about as much CO_2 as China emits—more than all the world's cars, trucks, trains, aircraft, and ships emit.

Indonesia releases more CO_2 through deforestation than any other country, which puts it into third place, behind the United States and China, as a source of CO_2 emissions due to human activity. Large-scale deforestation continues in Brazil, which gains it fourth place in this list. Many tropical countries have lost most of their rainforests: the Philippines, 90 percent; Madagascar, 95 percent; Haiti, 99 percent. Figure 4-13 shows how large the contribution of deforestation is to overall greenhouse gas emissions.

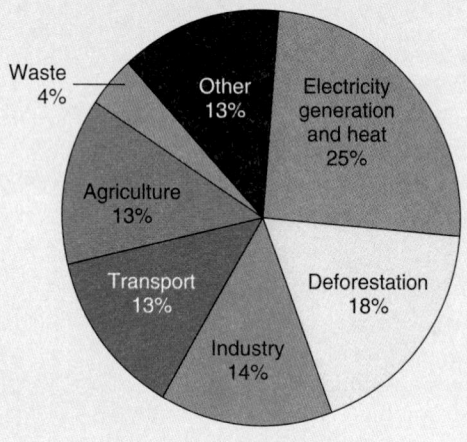

Figure 4-13   Origins of greenhouse gas emissions.

rising beyond 2°C, which might permit civilized human life, not just mere survival at best. This would require CO_2 emissions to peak in this decade and then drop to less than half of their present rate by 2050.

In December 2009, representatives, including many leaders, of 193 countries met in Copenhagen to come up with definite plans to accomplish this goal. They could not agree on almost anything, but many promised to take various measures to moderate the increase in emissions. An assessment of these promises suggests a CO_2 concentration in 2100 of 755 ppm, nearly double today's value, which implies in turn a temperature rise of 3.8°C. Even adding in more-or-less vague measures that a number of countries said they would consider only reduces these figures to 590 ppm and 2.9°C—still too much. Section 4.14 considers the kinds and extents of the actions (not words) governments would have to take to avoid foreseeable disaster.

Fossil Fuels

Coal, oil, and natural gas are called **fossil fuels** because they were formed millions of years ago by the partial decay of the remains of swamp plants (coal) and marine organisms such as algae and plankton (oil and natural gas); see Sec. 16.15. Coal consists mainly of carbon, oil and natural gas consist of both carbon and hydrogen. Burning coal liberates energy as its carbon combines chemically with oxygen from the air to form carbon dioxide. Burning natural gas and fuels such as gasoline liberates more energy per gram (Fig. 4-14) as their carbon and hydrogen combine with oxygen to form carbon dioxide and water vapor, respectively. Figure 4-15 shows the recent and projected CO_2 emissions traceable to the various fossil fuels.

Fossil fuels today provide about 85 percent of world energy consumption (Fig. 4-4). Oil and natural gas are versatile and convenient to transport and use, but they are growing increasingly expensive as they become harder to extract from declining reserves. Oil prices have more than tripled in the past decade. Coal is relatively cheap and its widely distributed reserves are greater, but burning coal does the most damage to the environment. Various schemes have been proposed to utilize fossil fuels more efficiently and cleanly. Some of these schemes are more practical than others, but in the long run the role of fossil fuels in energy production will have to decline.

Another consideration in the case of the United States is that, because it imports two-thirds of the oil it uses (and has only 3 percent of world reserves), it is vulnerable to disruptions in its oil supply such as the 1973

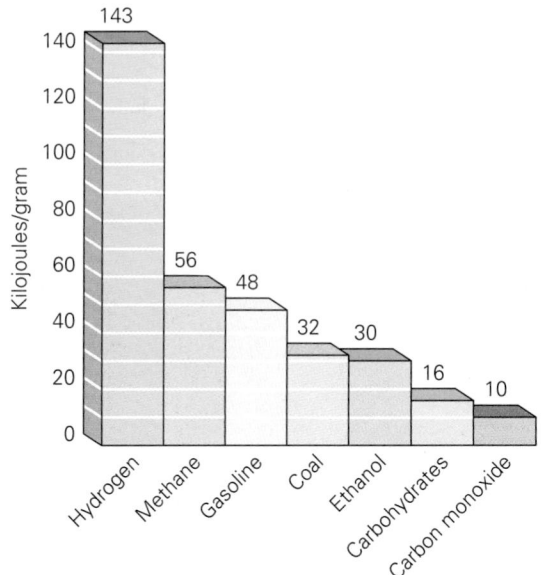

Figure 4-14   Energy contents of various fuels. Shown are the number of kilojoules of energy liberated when 1 g of each fuel is burned. Carbohydrates provide much of the energy in our diets (see Sec. 13.11). These fuels produce carbon dioxide (coal), water (hydrogen), or both when burned.

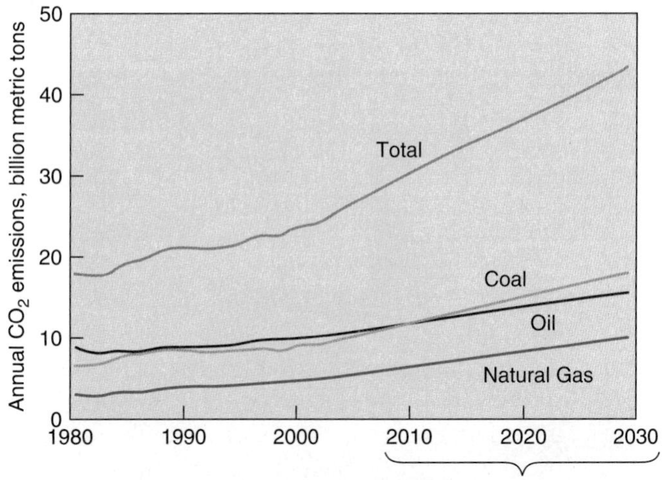

Figure 4-15   World carbon dioxide emissions from fossil fuels (1 metric ton = 1000 kg). The projections are based on current trends continuing and predict a total rise of 2.1 percent per year to give 44 billion metric tons of CO_2 given off in 2030, $1\frac{1}{2}$ times as much as today. To reverse the upward sweep of these curves and keep the earth habitable will require immediate effective action to keep population growth down, to use energy more efficiently, and to replace fossil fuels with nuclear and renewable sources.

Arab oil embargo. Making do with less oil would make the country more self-sufficient in energy supply as well as benefitting the environment.

4.5   Liquid Fuels

Vehicles Are the Biggest Users

The world's largest producers of crude oil are Saudi Arabia, Russia, the United States, Iran, and China, in that order. Smaller but still substantial amounts come from a number of other countries, as shown in Fig. 4-16. Most new oil wells nowadays are located offshore (Fig. 4-17). The United States, which uses over 20 million barrels per day, is by far the largest consumer of oil, followed by China, Japan, India, and Russia.

Transport fuels make up 70 percent of oil products. Gasoline and diesel fuel are the most common transport fuels and consist of mixtures of various hydrocarbons—chemical compounds of carbon and hydrogen—derived from oil, as described in Chap. 13. In a vehicle engine, the gaseous products of burning fuel, mainly H_2O (water) and CO_2, expand rapidly because of the intense heat generated by the reaction. This expansion forces down the pistons of the engine, which in turn causes the crankshaft to rotate and provide power to the vehicle wheels (see Sec. 5-13). For every gallon of gasoline burned, over 8 kg of CO_2 are produced. A typical sport utility vehicle (SUV) can put 20 kg of CO_2 into the atmosphere in a 40-mile commute (Fig. 4.18).

Figure 4-16   The chief oil and gas deposits in the world.

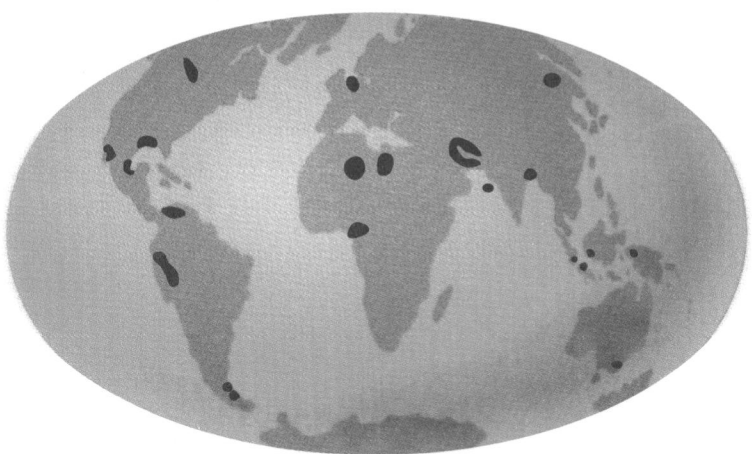

Figure 4-17   Oil drilling rig in the Gulf of Mexico off the Louisiana coast. It is more and more difficult to find new oil deposits to satisfy the world's increasing appetite.

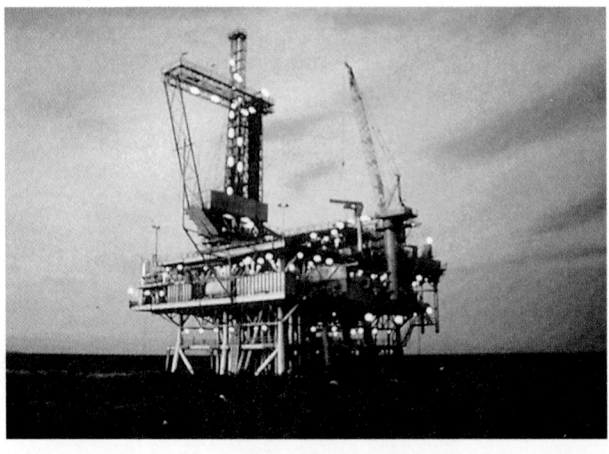

Tar Sands Oil

As the cost of oil increases, previously uneconomical sources are beginning to be exploited, none of them ideal. The most important are the tar sands (mixtures of a tarlike material known as bitumen, sand, and clay) found over a vast area—the size of Florida—in Canada's province of Alberta; other large deposits are in Venezuela with smaller ones elsewhere, including Utah. Tar sands worldwide contain more oil than there is in reserves of ordinary crude oil, but only some of it is practical to extract. Tar sands oil costs far more than crude oil per barrel to produce, in part because converting tar sands to usable oil needs a lot of energy, several times as much as crude oil; most of this energy comes from natural gas. Even so, producing oil from tar sands is a profitable business in Canada.

The CO_2 emissions that accompany extracting oil from tar sands range from 1.4 to 4 times the emissions in the case of crude oil. They add up to about 3.6 million tons of CO_2 per year now, which is expected to double by 2015. There is more bad news: mining the tar sands has thus far churned up 160 square miles of land, of which only a sixth is being reclaimed at present. And the three to five barrels of water that go into the steam needed to produce each barrel of tar sands oil, too contaminated afterward for further use, end up stored in toxic ponds that already cover 50 square miles.

Over 100 billion dollars has already been invested in Canadian tar sands projects with more on the way. Current oil output from tar sands there is 1.3 million barrels per day, expected to reach 3.3 million in 2020. U.S. law bans federal agencies from buying fuel from alternative sources, such as tar sands, if their production and use result in more greenhouse gas emissions than in the case of ordinary sources. But nongovernmental consumers are under no such restrictions, and half the oil Canada ships to the United States (9 percent of total imports) comes from tar sands.

Saving Fuel Increasing the fuel efficiency of cars and trucks will save money, reduce pollution and global warming, and postpone the day when oil runs out. One approach is to minimize air resistance by designing more streamlined vehicle shapes. SUVs are especially bad in this respect. Engines can be improved; one method is to have several cylinders shut down when less power is needed, others involve direct fuel injection and variable valve timing. Better transmissions would also help, and reducing vehicle weight would pay big dividends.

In most of the world, gasoline and diesel fuel are expensive (in Europe, at least twice American prices), so fuel economy is prized and efficient cars are normal. In the United States, where fuel until recently was relatively cheap, fuel economy was ignored by car makers until legislation in 1975 required a minimum of 27.5 mi/gal averaged over a maker's range of ordinary cars. However, SUVs, vans, and pickups—over half the cars on the road—were not covered by this requirement. As a result, the actual average mileage in the United States is today the lowest in the world, not much over half the current European average of about 40 mi/gal (expected to reach 50 mi/gal in a few years; in Japan it is nearly that high already). Forty percent of the oil consumed in the United States is used by its cars. Hence improving their mileage, fought bitterly by American car makers (just as they did seat belts and pollution controls earlier, showing the same kind of misplaced priorities that later led two of them into bankruptcy) but finally required by a 2007 law will make a welcome difference. The eventual average to be met by new cars and light trucks by 2016 is set at 35.5 mi/gal (still less than today's European average). Additional regulations set limits on greenhouse gas emission by these vehicles.

The fuel economy of American cars is low not only because of their unnecessary size and weight and gas-guzzling engines but also because 97 percent of them use gasoline engines whereas the more efficient diesel cars are in the majority elsewhere. The latest diesel engines (unlike older ones) are quiet, produce little pollution, and are 20 to 40 percent more efficient than gasoline engines. If only a third of American cars and light trucks were diesels (the heavy trucks are already), the savings would amount to the equivalent of all the oil imported from Saudi Arabia. Performance is not an issue: a diesel car won the classic 24-h Le Mans race in France recently.

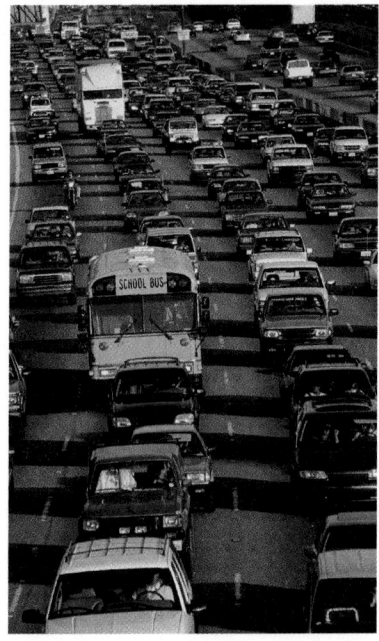

Figure 4-18 Traffic jam on a multilane highway. Although water vapor and carbon dioxide are the chief components of vehicle exhausts, they also contain carbon monoxide (CO) and various hydrocarbons, which are poisonous, and nitrogen oxides, which contribute to acid rain (see Sec. 4.7) through the nitric acid they form. The hazard of CO comes from its tendency to combine permanently with the hemoglobin in the blood in place of oxygen. This deprives the body of some of the oxygen it needs and leads to brain damage or death if too much CO is inhaled; no other poison injures or kills as many people as CO.

Hybrid Cars

A **hybrid car** has both a gasoline engine and one or more electric motors, which under computer control are used separately or together as driving circumstances require (Fig. 4-19). When not much power is needed, the engine stops and the motors take over. The motors obtain their energy from a set of batteries that are charged both by the engine and by "regenerative braking"—slowing the car is done by using its motors as generators to convert its KE of motion to electric energy for storage. Regenerative braking reduces the energy cost of city driving by around 20 percent. A smaller than usual gasoline engine, which is more economical with fuel, can be used because the electric motors can supplement it for extra power when accelerating or climbing steep hills.

Hybrid cars average twice the mileage of ordinary cars; if all cars in the United States were hybrids, 1.5 billion barrels of oil would be saved each year. Carbon dioxide emissions from conventional American cars average 452 g per mile, hybrids average 294 g. A new version of hybrids, called "plug-in hybrids," can have their batteries recharged from ordinary household outlets and so act as purely electric cars for short distances such as most commutes. If the household electricity comes from coal-burning power plants, as about half of American electricity does (Fig. 4-6), the total CO_2 emitted per mile rises to an estimated 326 g; if natural gas is the fuel, the total falls to 256 g; if alternative sources (nuclear, hydroelectric, wind, solar) are involved, the total falls even farther,

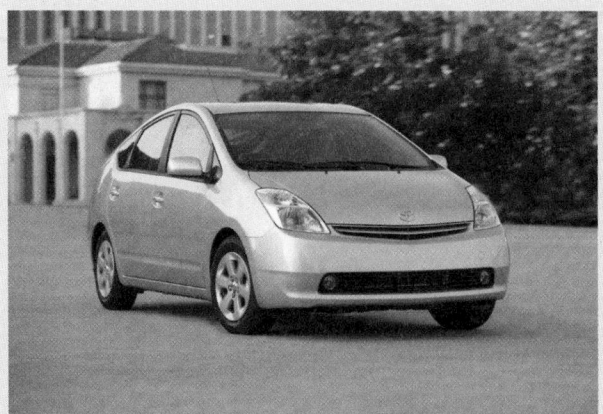

Figure 4-19   The Toyota Prius, the pioneer hybrid gasoline-electric car, has had sales of over 2 million since it first appeared in 1997 and kept more than 10 million tons of CO_2 out of the atmosphere. Other car makers have begun producing hybrids as well. Plug-in hybrids, the next generation, have batteries that can be recharged from household outlets as well as by their engines and by regenerative braking. Half of all new cars may be plug-in hybrids by 2025.

typically to 150 g, a third as much as in the case of ordinary cars. This matters because CO_2 emissions from American cars add up to about 20 percent of the country's total.

4.6   Natural Gas

The Least Bad Fossil Fuel

When burned, natural gas combines with oxygen to give carbon dioxide and water vapor, as liquid fuels derived from oil do, but with less pollution. Natural gas consists of the lighter hydrocarbons, chiefly methane. Natural gas is cheaper than oil per unit of energy content, though coal is still cheaper. It is more efficient than other fossil fuels in producing electricity, and its share of world generating capacity, now over 30 percent (21 percent in the United States) is steadily increasing. A gas-fired power plant typically gives off only about half as much CO_2 per unit of energy as a conventional coal-fired plant. Also widely used for heating, natural gas is expected to eventually replace oil as the world's chief energy source until it, too, begins to run out. Natural gas is an important feedstock for manufacturing chemicals of many kinds.

The largest producers of natural gas are Russia, the United States, Canada, Iran, and Norway, in that order. The United States imports 17 percent of the natural gas it uses, most of it by pipeline from Canada but some by sea from elsewhere as LNG—liquified natural gas (Fig. 4-20). The LNG is regasified at nine special coastal terminals and then carried by pipeline to consumers. China is building a number of such terminals to receive LNG, in its case that originate in undersea fields off the west coast of Australia.

New Sources   Until now almost all commercial natural gas came from wells drilled down to porous underground rock formations (Sec. 16.15). Over half the world's gas reserves in such formations are in the three countries

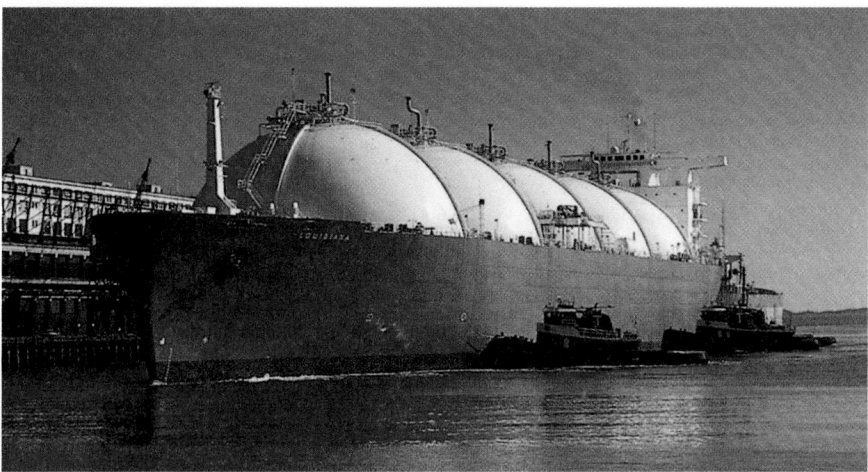

Figure 4-20   Natural gas, which is mainly methane, is carried in liquid form at low temperature (methane boils at −161°C) in tankers such as this as well as in pipelines. Liquid methane occupies about 600 times less volume than methane gas. The tanks are spherical to minimize heat flow into them: a sphere has the least surface area for a given volume. The liquid natural gas (LNG) is kept cold by being allowed to evaporate continuously, which absorbs the heat that passes through the tank walls. The gas that comes off is used to power the ship's engines, so it is not wasted. Perhaps 250 million tons of LNG is shipped around the world each year.

of Russia, Iran, and Qatar (a small Arab state in the Middle East). Less than 5 percent is in the United States. Recently, improved methods have been developed to extract natural gas trapped in shale beds in the United States and elsewhere; shale is a type of rock (Fig. 15-16). Adding in the gas from these beds increases world gas reserves by an as-yet imprecise amount but perhaps 50 percent, conceivably even more. Already gas from shale beds in Texas, Louisiana, and Pennsylvania is on the market, and shale projects are starting in Europe, India, and China. About 7 percent of the natural gas in the United States comes from the Barnett shale field in Texas. The giant Marcellus field underlies almost two-thirds of Pennsylvania as well as parts of adjacent states.

Shale gas production begins by drilling down to a deposit of gas-filled rock and then forcing in a mix of chemicals and water to break up the rock. Next the water is pumped out and methane, now free, escapes through the bore hole. Many such wells are needed, which can be a problem in populated areas. Another problem is contamination of nearby water supplies by liberated methane and the chemicals in the fracturing water. Plans to drill for shale gas in New York State had to be abandoned because of water purity fears. Still, so much shale gas apparently can be extracted in the United States in environmentally acceptable ways that there is even the possibility that its LNG terminals may eventually be converted from methane import to methane export.

Under certain circumstances, methane can be trapped inside ice crystals (see Fig. 11-18) to form a methane-rich substance usually called **methane clathrate** (sometimes methane hydrate or methane ice). Within the earth, natural gas, which is mostly methane, is a product of the decomposition of organic matter by bacteria, as described in Sec. 16.15. Most clathrates are formed when such methane comes in contact with extremely cold water underground where pressures are high. Deposits have turned out to be common under the seabeds of the continental shelves of oceans (Fig. 14-36) and inside and beneath permafrost in such places as Alaska and Siberia. More rarely they occur elsewhere, for instance in sediments on the seabed itself; some years ago a large piece was picked up by a fishing net off the west coast of Canada. Methane clathrates resemble dirty ice, have the consistency of sherbet, and burst into flames when lit by a match.

An immense amount of methane is locked up in clathrates; estimates vary from 2 to 10 times the amount of methane in ordinary sources of natural gas. Thus clathrates may contain more energy than that in the reserves of those sources plus the reserves of oil and coal. Unfortunately, collecting the methane in clathrates economically will not be easy because it is not sufficiently concentrated. But the prospect of so much energy almost within reach is so attractive that prospecting for accessible deposits and developing technology to extract their methane are racing ahead. An optimistic but not absurd forecast has commercial exploitation starting somewhere as soon as 2015.

4.7 Coal

Plentiful but Worst for the Environment

Until it was overtaken by oil, coal was the chief energy source under human control. Coal is cheap and its reserves are large. The energy in a dollar's worth of coal typically costs around $3 in the form of natural gas and $6 in the form of fuel oil. Coal is widely distributed as well as abundant; the United States has a quarter of the world's reserves—the coal in Illinois alone contains more energy than all the oil in Saudi Arabia (Fig. 4-21). The chief producers of coal are China (40 percent of the world's total), the United States, India, and Australia (which exports most of the output of its mines). (For information on underground coal fires see Sec. 4.7 at www.mhhe.com/krauskopf.)

The United States uses 90 percent of its mined coal to generate half its electricity in about 600 power plants (Fig. 4-22). China, which relies on coal for two-thirds of its energy, over twice the world average, already burns more coal than the United States, Europe, and Japan combined; by 2030 it will have more than doubled its current usage. Every week one or two new coal-fired power plants open somewhere in China. In all, over a thousand such plants are either newly built or under construction around the world. About 150 of them are in the United States.

Unfortunately coal is not an ideal fuel. For the same energy output, coal produces nearly a third more CO_2 than oil fuels and about twice as much as natural gas. Burning coal is responsible for 40 percent of the 30 billion tons of CO_2 released into the atmosphere per year by human activities (see Fig. 4-15), a proportion that will grow as coal use widens. During the normal 60-year lifespan of a 500 MW coal-fired power plant, it will emit 200 million tons of CO_2.

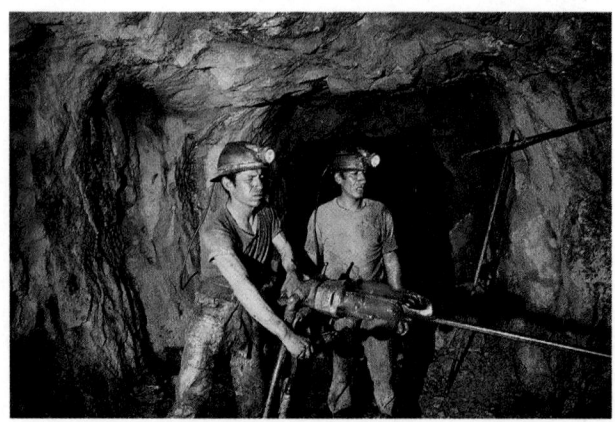

Figure 4-21 About half the coal extracted in the United States comes from underground mines such as this one. The rest is gouged in the open from deposits that lie near the surface after the overlying soil has been stripped away. Most of the underground mines are in the eastern part of the country; most of the surface mines are in the western part. The coal currently consumed in the world each year took about 2 million years to accumulate.

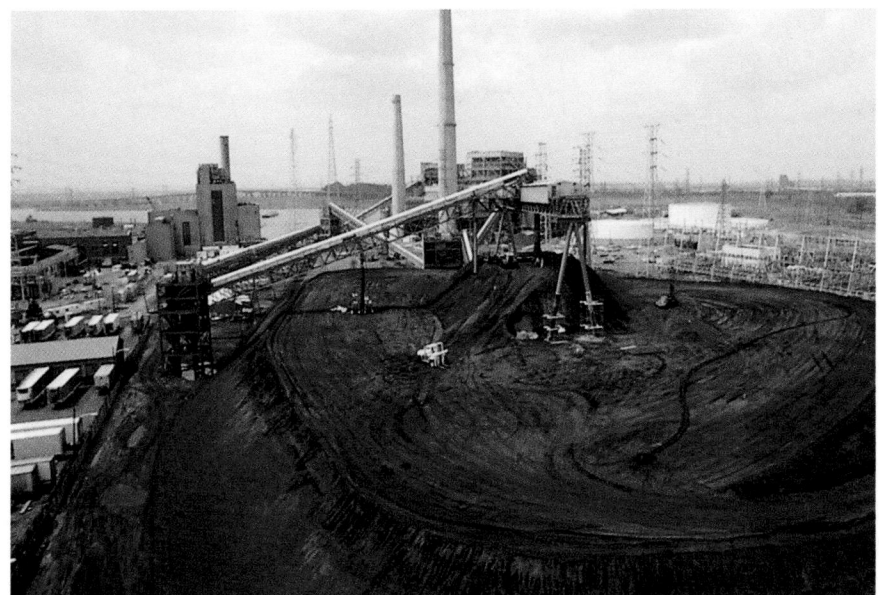

Figure 4-22   Coal, shown here piled next to an electric power plant in Newark, New Jersey, is the most abundant fossil fuel and is used to produce over half the electric energy generated in the United States. Coal is responsible for more CO_2 and other pollutants per unit of energy released than any other source.

Concerns about the environmental impact of coal-fired power plants, together with high construction costs and reduced prices for the cleaner natural gas, have led to the cancellation in the past decade of plans for over one hundred such plants in the United States. Several dozen more projected plants await final decisions. If any are approved, they may be along the last built without carbon storage and capture, as described below.

Cogeneration   As discussed in Sec. 5.14, a basic physical principle called the second law of thermodynamics states that it is impossible to take heat from a source (such as a furnace or a nuclear reactor) and convert all of it to mechanical energy or work (for instance in a steam turbine connected to an electric generator). Some heat, usually a lot, must go to waste. In the case of an electric power station, the actual efficiency is less than half—only about 3–4 J of every 10 J of heat input becomes electric energy.

Older power stations just discharge the leftover heat into nearby bodies of water or into the atmosphere via cooling towers. Nowadays combined heat and power stations are being built that capture the excess heat and use it for domestic heat and in various industrial applications. Such cogeneration conserves fuel and thereby cuts CO_2 emissions as well. This is not a technology of the future but a practical way of getting the most out of every ton of fossil fuel burned in a power station and every ton of CO_2 it releases. The main obstacle to wider use of cogeneration is that, although the heat is cheap, the piping needed to distribute it is not.

Carbon Capture and Storage   Because coal, whose use is expected to climb 40 percent by 2030, is going to remain a major energy source for a long time, it is essential to find ways to eliminate, or at least severely reduce, the CO_2 that using coal dumps into the atmosphere. A straightforward method is to pump the CO_2 from coal-burning plants deep underground for permanent burial. Suitable geological formations are widely available, and if necessary the captured CO_2 can be carried by pipeline as much as hundreds of kilometers from its source to a storage site.

Such **carbon capture and storage** (CCS) is now being done on a small scale with CO_2 liberated in other processes. In Europe's North Sea, where natural gas from Norwegian wells is contaminated with excessive CO_2, a million tons of CO_2 each year are stripped from the natural gas and injected into porous rocks a kilometer below the seabed where it displaces seawater. No CO_2

Figure 4-23　At this facility in Algeria in the Sahara Desert, carbon dioxide found mixed with natural gas is separated out and then pumped 2 km underground. Such sequestration keeps the carbon dioxide from entering the atmosphere where it would contribute to global warming by enhancing the greenhouse effect.

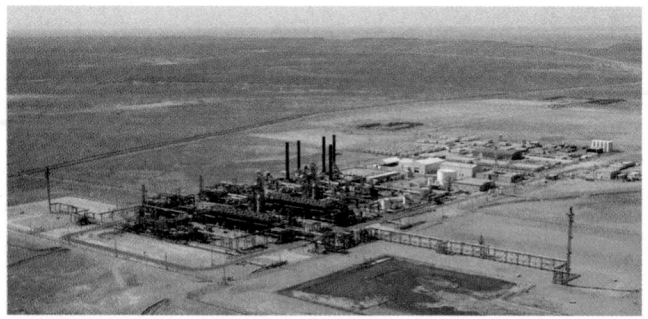

has been found to be leaking out in over a decade of operation. A similar carbon capture and storage is being carried out at a gas field in Algeria (Fig. 4-23).

Various pilot operations around the world are under way to further develop the technology involved, some of it new. One of them involves taking CO_2 produced by an Illinois corn-processing plant and injecting a million tons of it to a depth of 7500 m. In West Virginia, the first CCS trial to involve an actual coal-fired power plant will inject 100,000 tons of liquid CO_2 annually (about 1.5 percent of the plant's emissions) into a sandstone layer 2400 m below the surface. Work on larger-scale experimental CCS projects, usually with government support, has either started or will start soon in China, Canada, Australia, and several European countries.

Unfortunately, to separate CO_2 from the other flue gases spewed out by a coal-fired power plant and then to bury it might double the cost of the required installation and use a quarter or more of the energy produced. CCS will inevitably be a very expensive way to reduce CO_2 emissions. Too expensive? At present, other low-carbon energy sources, such as nuclear, wind, solar, and certain biofuels, seem so much more attractive economically that CCS will have a hard time being widely adopted without major government involvement of some kind, carrot (subsidies) and/or stick (a heavy CO_2 emissions tax, a severe cap-and-trade system; see Sec. 4.14).

There is another consideration, but nobody knows yet how serious it is: can CCS induce earthquakes? The buried liquid CO_2 exerts high pressures on the porous rock of its reservoir, and in certain geologic formations it is conceivable this could be enough to trigger earthquakes. A small earthquake in 2008 near the North Sea CO_2 reservoir, mentioned on the previous page, may—or may not—have been triggered by the injected CO_2. Had the quake been stronger, it could have led to a tsunami (Sec. 14.12).

Coal Gasification　A more economical approach to keeping the CO_2 from coal burning out of the atmosphere is the integrated gasification combined cycle (IGCC), in which coal is first turned into a mixture of gases. An artificial gas fuel—syngas (for "synthesis gas")—can be made by passing very hot steam over coal to yield a mixture of carbon monoxide and hydrogen. Contaminants such as sulfur and mercury are readily removed, and the result is a gas fuel that can be burned in a power plant as cleanly as natural gas. Hydrogen could be separated out for use as the energy source for vehicles whose only emissions would be water vapor, H_2O. The CO_2 from burning syngas is easier to capture than the CO_2 from burning coal directly, which makes injecting it underground a more practical proposition. Several syngas power plants have been built and more are on the way, though not yet with provision for CCS.

Syngas can be the starting point for a variety of products. One is methane, the chief constituent of natural gas, and indeed a plant in North Dakota has been making methane for use as a fuel from coal since 1984 (Fig. 4-24). Syngas can also be used to create liquid fuels such as gasoline and diesel fuel. This was done on a large scale in oil-short Germany during World War II.

Coal Ash

Burning coal leaves behind solid residues in the form of ash. Coal ash contains significant amounts of heavy metals such as arsenic, lead, mercury, and selenium, which can cause cancer, neurological problems, and birth defects if absorbed by the body. About 130 million tons of coal ash are produced each year in the United States, and most of it is simply dumped in 1300 or so locations in 46 states. The rest is used in construction and some (unbelievably) is even added to soil to improve its ability to hold water.

Radioactive elements, notably uranium and thorium, are also present in coal ash. Some ash contains so much uranium that recovering it for use as nuclear fuel may be an economic proposition. A trial program for this purpose is under way in China.

The disposal of coal ash is seldom effectively regulated, for instance by requiring the deposit sites to have impermeable linings and the ash to be stored as dry as possible. These measures would help prevent the heavy metals from leaching into nearby groundwater, lakes, rivers, and streams. Recently 77 areas in the United States were found to have water contaminated by heavy metals from ash dumps. The Environmental Protection Agency has been studying the issue for over 30 years, including a finding that the concentration of arsenic to which people might be exposed by drinking water contaminated by coal ash could increase the risk of cancer by several hundred times. However, it has yet to take any action.

In 2008, an earthen dike around a pond filled with a mixture of ash and water at a Tennessee Valley Authority generating plant gave way and a billion gallons of toxic sludge flooded 300 acres of land around it. Cleanup costs are an estimated $1 billion. Such events on a smaller scale are not unusual wherever coal ash is dumped. Outside the coal industry, which opposes regulation or even monitoring of ash dumps, the long-term effects on the health of local human and animal populations of introducing heavy metals from coal ash, both in spills and by gradual leaching, are a source of concern.

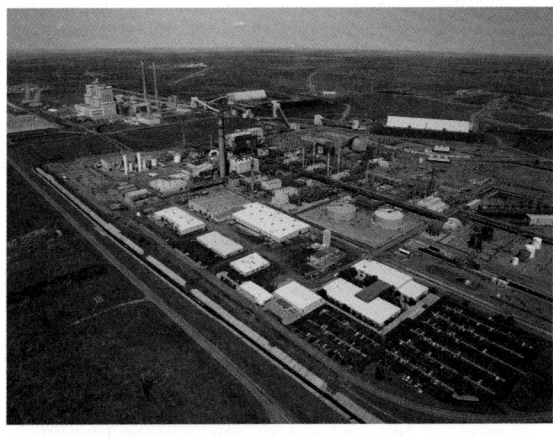

Figure 4-24   The Great Plains Synfuels plant near Beulah, North Dakota, in operation since 1984, produces 4.5 million m^3 of syngas per day from 18,000 tons of coal. A by-product is CO_2, which is sent through a pipeline to Canadian oil fields where it is buried in old wells after helping to recover oil from them. Other profitable by-products include ingredients for fertilizers and raw materials for plastics.

However, manufacturing and using these artificial fuels in place of ordinary gasoline and diesel fuel is quite expensive and doubles the overall amount of CO_2 produced. With global warming a reality, coal-to-liquid fuels do not seem the way to go.

Pollution   Even apart from its role in global warming, coal is far from being a desirable fuel. Not only is mining it dangerous and usually leaves large tracts of land unfit for further use, but also the air pollution due to coal burning adversely affects the health of millions of people. The National Academy of Sciences estimates that the cost of health damage due to coal burning in the United States is around $60 billion per year. Toxic substances in coal smoke include mercury, arsenic, beryllium, cadmium, and dioxins. Interestingly enough, coal-fired power plants expose people living around them to more radioactivity—from traces of uranium, thorium, and radium in their smoke—than do normally operating nuclear plants.

Mercury, which attacks the nervous system and is particularly harmful to unborn children, is an especially unfortunate component of coal smoke. Coal-fired plants in the United States discharge 48 tons of mercury each year,

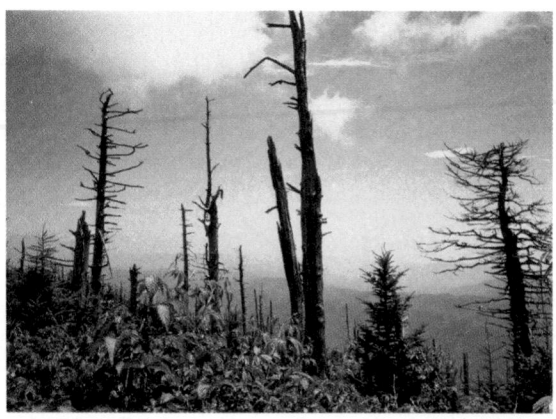

Figure 4-25   Acid rain, together with atmospheric sulfur dioxide (which attacks chlorophyll), led to the destruction of this forest in North Carolina. Healthy and abundant forests are needed not only for timber but also because they absorb CO_2 from the atmosphere, protect soil from erosion, help prevent floods, furnish habitats for most kinds of land plants and animals, and participate in the water cycle.

a major reason why 6 percent of women of childbearing age in this country have enough mercury in their bloodstreams to put a fetus at risk of developmental damage. Nearly all states warn their residents about mercury contamination in their waters and in fish caught there.

Although the Clean Air Act of 1990 required power companies to control mercury emissions, the industry objected that the expense would be too great (according to the Government Accountability Office, it would be pennies per month per consumer of electricity) and very few plants were ever equipped for this. Needless nervous system damage in the country was the result. Finally, a lawsuit by environmental and public-health groups led to a 2009 federal court order that obliged the Environmental Protection Agency to begin enforcing the Act, which it agreed to start doing at the end of 2011 by setting limits for toxic power plant emissions.

Acid Rain   Coal contains several percent of sulfur, and when coal is burned, the sulfur combines with oxygen to form sulfur dioxide, SO_2. Every year 50 to 60 million tons of SO_2 are released into the atmosphere from this source. Some nitrogen from the air also combines with oxygen in furnaces to form nitrogen oxides; vehicle exhausts also contain nitrogen oxides. The sulfur and nitrogen oxides react with atmospheric moisture to give sulfuric and nitric acids. The result is acid rain (and acid snow) that can be as much as 60 times more acidic than normal rainwater.

Acid rain has two main effects on soils. One is to dissolve and carry away valuable plant nutrients. The other is to convert ordinarily harmless aluminum compounds, abundant in many soils, to toxic varieties. As a result, forests are dying (Fig. 4-25) and fish have disappeared from many lakes and rivers due to aluminum washed into them. Drinking water has been contaminated in a number of regions by metals released by acidified water, such as cadmium and copper besides aluminum. The technology exists for "scrubbing" sulfur and nitrogen oxides from exhaust gases, and coal-fired power plants built or upgraded after 1977 are supposed to limit emissions of them. However, lax enforcement allowed over 30 upgraded plants to violate the law. Legal action finally began in 2009 to compel the owners of these plants to behave responsibly. In China, by far the largest emitter of sulfur dioxide, acid rain falls on a third of the country, with serious ecological consequences.

Alternative Sources

We now look at the sources responsible for the 15 percent of commercial energy production that does not involve burning fossil fuels. Although each of these sources has limitations of various kinds, it may be a good choice in certain situations. If the full potential of these sources is realized, the world will depend much less, perhaps very little, on fossil fuels with all their shortcomings. Of the available alternatives, the only one that can replace fossil fuels on a major scale in the relatively near future is nuclear energy. But other technologies are rapidly advancing, and eventually it will become clear which paths are the best to follow toward a sustainable energy supply for the world.

Today energy derived from fossil fuels is cheaper than energy from most alternative sources. There are two reasons. The first is that damage to the environment is not reflected in the prices of fossil fuels. If this factor is taken into account, the present cost advantage of fossil fuels disappears. The second reason is that the technologies based on fossil fuels benefit from long experience with them together with economies of scale. As alternative sources mature, these advantages will fade away.

4.8 A Nuclear World?

Perhaps on the Way

A nuclear reactor obtains its energy from the **fission** (breaking apart) of the nuclei of a certain kind of uranium atoms, as described in Chap. 8. In a nuclear power plant, steam from boilers heated by such a reactor runs turbines connected to electric generators. In 1951, in Idaho, electricity was produced for the first time from a nuclear plant.

Today 443 reactors in 31 countries generate about 450 GW of electric power, a sixth of the world total. Without them over 20 million barrels of oil (or their equivalent in coal or natural gas) would have to be burned every day. France, Belgium, and Taiwan obtain more than half their electricity from nuclear plants, with several other countries close behind (Fig. 4-26). In the United States, nuclear energy is responsible for about 20 percent of its electricity, somewhat more than the world average of 16 percent; there are 104 reactors in 31 states that produce a total of about 100 GW.

How Much Land?

A problem for land-based renewable energy sources is that they need a lot of land. To serve a medium-sized city takes somewhere around 1 GW of electric power capacity, which could be provided by a single large fossil-fuel or nuclear plant. How much land would a renewable source require for the same capacity? Solar cells would have to cover about 5000 acres (including rooftops), wind turbines over twice that. A 1-GW hydroelectric installation would have to be fed from at least a 40-square-mile reservoir or lake, and crops for conversion to biofuel would have to spread across 200 square miles of farmland to give 1 GW averaged over a year.

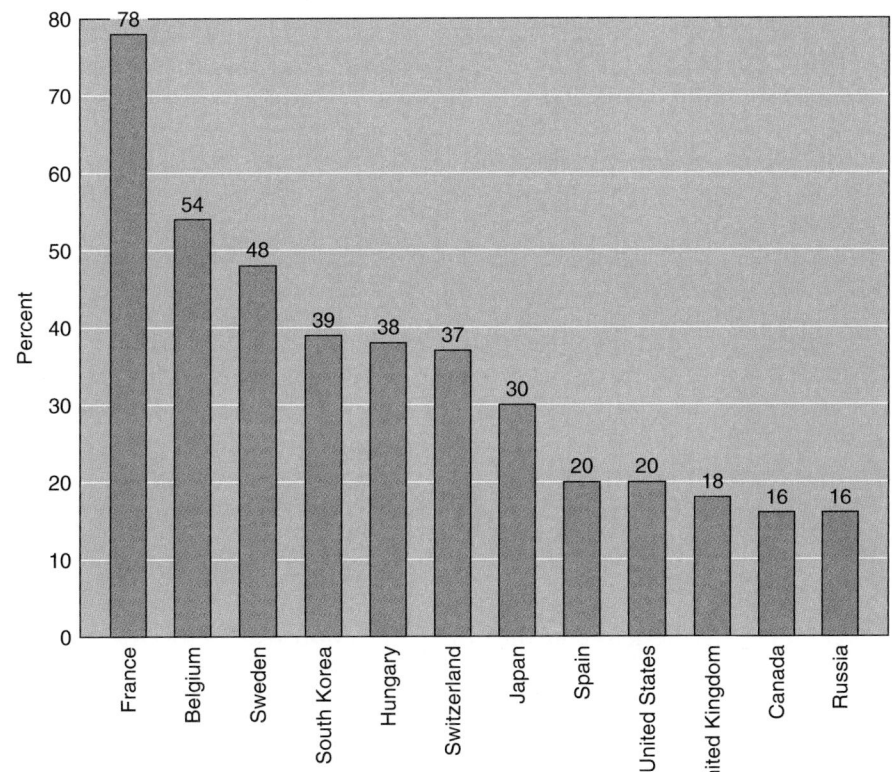

Figure 4-26 Percentage of electric energy in various countries that comes from nuclear power stations. France is more dependent on nuclear energy than any other country; it has 59 nuclear power plants. As a result, its emissions of CO_2 per kWh of electricity are extremely low. The United States, with five times the population of France, has 104 such plants.

Nuclear Weapons

Natural uranium consists of two varieties, ^{238}U and ^{235}U, of which only ^{235}U can undergo fission (see Secs. 8.9–8.11). Natural uranium contains only 0.7 percent of ^{235}U and must have this proportion increased to about 3 percent to make reactor fuel. The process by which natural uranium is enriched in ^{235}U can be continued further until the proportion is over 90 percent, and the result is the active ingredient of one kind of nuclear weapon, or "atomic bomb." Furthermore, in its operation a nuclear reactor produces another element, plutonium, that can be separated out from used fuel rods. Like ^{235}U, plutonium can also be used in nuclear weapons.

At present nine countries are known to possess a total of nearly 23,000 of both kinds of these weapons of mass destruction, sufficient to wipe out all human life many times over, and other countries could develop them if they wished. The threat of nuclear weapons proliferation is one of the reasons why not everybody welcomes the expansion of nuclear energy.

The uranium that fuels nuclear plants, fairly abundant in the earth's crust, should be able to support a large expansion of nuclear energy in the decades to come, and is not unduly expensive to mine and purify. The price of nuclear energy is determined mainly by construction costs, not fuel costs, which may well decrease from their present heights as more plants are built. Nuclear plants do not emit CO_2 and so do not contribute to global warming; if the present ones were fossil-fuel plants, nearly 3 billion more tons of CO_2 would be released each year into the atmosphere.

Yet for all the success of nuclear technology, construction has not begun on any new nuclear power stations in the United States since 1979. Why not?

Three Mile Island and Chernobyl   In March 1979 failures in its cooling system disabled one of the reactors at Three Mile Island in Pennsylvania, and a certain amount of radioactive material escaped. Although a reactor cannot explode in the way an atomic bomb does, breakdowns due to poor design, shoddy construction, inadequate maintenance, and errors in operation—all present at Three Mile Island—can occur that put large populations at risk. Although a true catstrophe was narrowly avoided, the Three Mile Island incident made it clear that the hazards associated with nuclear energy are real, and the lack of candor, then and later, by industry and government about these hazards was even more worrying.

After 1979 it was inevitable that greater safety would have to be built into new reactors, adding to their already high cost. In addition, the demand for electricity in the United States was not increasing as fast as expected, partly because of efforts toward greater efficiency and partly because of a decline in some of the industries (such as steel, cars, and chemicals) that are heavy users. As a result, new reactors made less economic sense than before, which together with widespread public unease led to a halt in the expansion of nuclear energy in the United States.

Elsewhere the situation was different. Nuclear reactors still seemed the best way to meet the energy needs of many countries without adequate fossil fuel resources. Then, in April 1986, a badly planned test caused a severe accident that destroyed a 1-GW reactor at Chernobyl in Ukraine, then part of the Soviet Union. This was the worst environmental disaster of technological origin in history and contributed to the collapse of the Soviet Union.

The lack of a containment shell, normal elsewhere, allowed nearly 200 tons of radioactive material to escape and be carried around the world by winds. Ukraine, Belarus, and parts of Russia were most affected. The radioactivity in the fallout was 400 times that produced by the Hiroshima atomic bomb. Radiation levels in many parts of Europe rose well above usual and are still high enough to represent a hazard in a large area that was downwind of Chernobyl.

About 350,000 residents of the Chernobyl vicinity were permanently evacuated from their homes, leaving behind ghost towns and villages. Thousands of people became ill, including about 4000 children who developed thyroid cancer. Because cancer and leukemia also have causes other than radiation, the death toll from these maladies due to Chernobyl will never be known; estimates range from thousands to tens of thousands.

As in the United States after Three Mile Island, public anxiety over the safety of nuclear programs grew abroad after Chernobyl. Some countries, for instance Italy, then abandoned plans for new reactors and closed down some existing ones. (Italy today has the most expensive electricity in Europe and has begun to build reactors again.) In other countries, for instance France, the logic behind their nuclear programs remained strong enough for them to continue despite Chernobyl.

Nuclear Energy Today   The latest designs for nuclear plants promise major improvements in efficiency and reliability over previous ones, which makes

Nuclear Wastes

Quite apart from the safety of the reactors themselves is the issue of what to do with the radioactive wastes they produce. Although a lot of the radioactivity is gone in a few months and much of the rest in a few hundred years, some will continue to be dangerous for millions of years. At present there are no long-term repositories for nuclear wastes anywhere in the world. Over 60,000 tons of spent nuclear fuel are being stored in the United States alone in cooling ponds (to prevent overheating) at 72 reactor installations where they may leak and are vulnerable to terrorist attack.

Burying nuclear wastes deep underground would seem to be the best long-term way to dispose of them. The right location is easy to specify but not easy to find: it must be stable geologically with no earthquakes likely, no nearby population centers, a type of rock that does not disintegrate in the presence of heat and radiation but is easy to drill into, and little groundwater that might become contaminated.

In 1987 the United States government chose Yucca Mountain in Nevada as the most suitable site it could find for storing nuclear wastes indefinitely, but further studies that cost over $6 billion brought to light various serious objections and in 2010 the project was abandoned. A new approach is to adapt existing oil-industry technology to drill holes 5 km deep into hard rock. The lowest 2 km of each hole would be filled with containers of spent fuel and then securely capped. At such depths, there is little chance that groundwater would be contaminated, unlike the case of Yucca Mountain where the burial would have been only about 300 m below the surface.

modern plants cheaper to run per unit of output than their fossil-fuel cousins. They are also safer than before. Together with increasing demand for energy, the result is an international boom in nuclear plants with new ones currently being built in 13 countries. In the United States, over two dozen new nuclear plants are being considered, each of which would cost billions of dollars and take at least 7 years to build. The International Atomic Energy Agency thinks global nuclear capacity might quadruple by 2050 if renewable sources and carbon capture technology are not successful on large enough scales. But even if the enormous costs could be met, the speed of nuclear expansion could be limited by shortages of skilled workers, of the needed construction materials, and of manufacturing capacity; for instance, Japan has the only steelworks anywhere able to forge reactor containment vessels ($150 million each), and its waiting list is years long.

Nuclear Fusion   Enormous as the energy produced by splitting a large atomic nucleus into smaller ones is, the joining together of small nuclei to form larger ones gives off even more energy for the same amount of starting materials (see Sec. 8.12). Such **nuclear fusion** is the energy source of the sun and stars. Here on earth, there are what seem to be realistic hopes that fusion will take over the lead as a source of energy at some time in the future—safe, no greenhouse gases, very little radioactive waste, and abundant fuel, much of it from the oceans.

In laboratories, fusion reactors have been built that liberate energy for short periods as predicted by theory. In order to operate continuously and to yield energy on a commercial scale, the reactors must be much larger (a planned experimental reactor called ITER will weigh 23,000 tons), but no fundamental reason is known why such reactors should not be successful. Of course, a technical success is not necessarily an economic success, but if it becomes one before environmental disaster intervenes, fusion energy may be the ultimate solution to our energy problems.

4.9   Clean Energy I

Continuous Sources

An ideal energy source should not deplete resources or harm the environment. A number of sources meet these criteria and, despite issues of cost and location in some cases, electricity is starting to come from them in serious amounts: about 5 percent of total electricity in the United States, twice that in Europe. Just what proportion of global energy demand these sources will eventually provide remains to be seen, as does the timescale of their adoption, but their increasing popularity is a sign of hope.

"Clean" and sustainable energy sources fall into two categories that depend on whether they can supply energy continuously (hydroelectric, geothermal) or only at rates that vary with the time of day (solar, tidal) or with weather conditions (wind, waves). We will first look at the two main continuous sources, moving water and geothermal heat.

Hydroelectricity   The kinetic energy of moving water has been used by mills and factories for centuries, and has powered electric generators since 1870 (Fig. 4-27). Hydropower now provides 2.2 percent of the world's energy with capacity up by over 40 percent since 1980. Norway obtains 99 percent of its electricity from falling water, Brazil 84 percent, Canada 58 percent, and 13 African countries 60 percent or more each.

The United States has a total hydroelectric capacity of 96 GW; its largest installation, at the Grand Coulee Dam, produces 6.8 GW. The largest hydroelectric plant now operating anywhere is on the Brazil-Paraguay border and is rated at 14 GW. When completed, the Three Gorges Dam in China, on which work began in 1994, will take the lead with a capacity of 22.4 GW. This dam is the world's biggest civil engineering project and, together with other such projects there, will increase China's total hydroelectric output to half again its current 129 GW. Major hydroelectric installations are also under construction or having plans finalized elsewhere, mainly in Asia (a total of 14 GW in India alone) and South America (6.5 GW in Brazil). In Africa, too, more such installations are projected—with a sixth of the world's population it produces only 4 percent of the world's electricity.

Even when the new dams are completed, only about a third of the world's hydroelectric potential will have been utilized. But many of the remaining sites cannot be exploited economically for a variety of reasons. Furthermore,

Figure 4-27   This hydroelectric installation on the Niagara River in New York State has a capacity of 2.2 GW of electric power. The ultimate source of this power is sunlight, which evaporates water that later falls as rain or snow that drains into the river upstream of the dam.

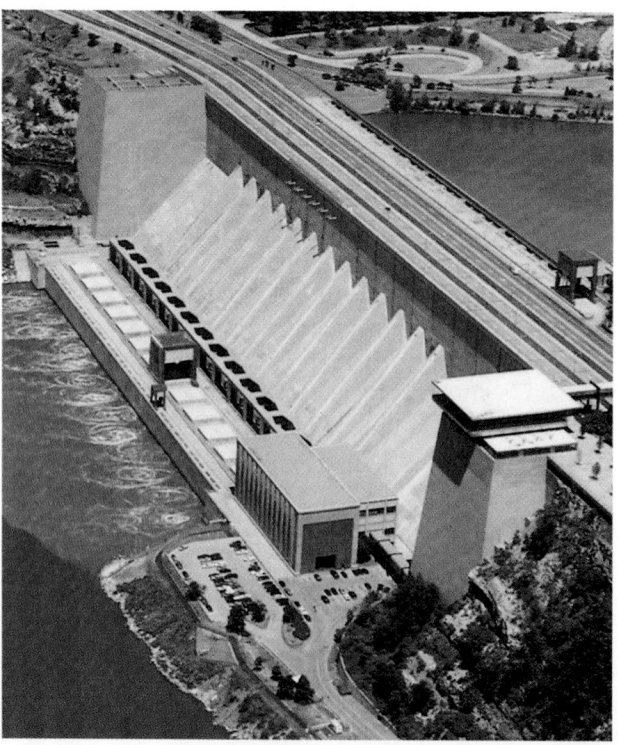

Geothermal Heat Pumps

Temperatures at the earth's surface are affected by solar radiation and by cold and warm air masses carried by winds (see Chap. 14). As a result, they may vary a great deal between day and night, from one day to the next, and as seasons change. If we dig down only a meter or two, though, we will find a fairly steady year-round temperature of 7°C to 21°C (45°F to 75°F), depending on location. In much of the world, the underground temperature is higher in winter and lower in summer than the aboveground one. This means that, compared with conventional heating and air-conditioning methods, a huge amount of energy would be saved—and a lot less CO_2 emitted—with systems that could heat and cool buildings by transferring heat from the ground in winter and to the ground in summer.

Such systems not only exist but are in use in 33 countries; in the United States, about a million have already been installed with more added every year. The systems are based on **geothermal heat pumps** that are like the heat pump described in Sec. 5.13 except that they use the earth as the heat reservoir instead of the outside air. A geothermal heat pump is extremely efficient and can transfer as much as 5 joules of heat for each joule of input energy. In winter, the system absorbs heat from the ground by means of a fluid, usually water, that flows through buried pipes. The heat pump in effect then concentrates the heat and uses it to raise the temperature of air that is circulated inside the building in ducts. In summer, the system is operated in reverse to extract heat from the hot air in the building and discharge it to the cooler earth below the surface.

Geothermal heat pump systems are not cheap to install, but the reduced energy needed means that they pay for themselves in a few years. Since they last for 20 years or more with little maintenance, the long-term savings are considerable, not to mention the benefits to the environment.

an increasingly significant problem with hydropower installations is the social and environmental damage they may cause, for instance by flooding wide areas and turning once fertile river valleys into wastelands unfit for agriculture. The Three Gorges Dam, which created a lake 643 km (about 400 miles) long, has already displaced 1.4 million people. The Chinese government expects that 3–4 million more people will have to be relocated in years to come as the Three Gorges project causes the bed of the Yangtze River to silt up, its banks to erode, and its waters and those of the lake to become polluted. Environmental concerns have even led to the dismantling of a number of existing hydropower dams—nearly a hundred in the United States in the past few years.

Geothermal   Temperature increases with depth in the earth. As we shall learn in Sec. 15.8, the earth's heat partly comes from the decay of radioactive minerals in its interior and partly is heat remaining from the earth's early history when it was much hotter than today. In many places water below the surface is hot enough for useful energy to be extracted. One such place is at The Geysers north of San Francisco where turbines powered by natural steam drive generators that produce 750 MW of electricity (Fig. 4-28). Even where suitable hot water or steam is not present underground, water from the surface can be pumped into cracks in deep rock formations and then recovered as hot water or steam from wells drilled nearby. Carbon dioxide under pressure can also be used to extract such **geothermal heat.** Over their respective lifetimes, geothermal power plants produce electricity at less cost than coal-fired plants, the cheapest conventional sources.

At present 24 countries have geothermal power plants with a total capacity of almost 9 GW, and more are being built. Iceland and the Philippines obtain over a quarter of their electricity from such plants. Indonesia hopes to achieve a similar proportion by 2025. Although its current share of the world's energy supply is only 0.4 percent, a recent study found that geothermal energy has enormous potential. In the United States, the world's largest producer of geothermal energy with 2.8 GW of capacity at present and 4 GW more being developed, hot rocks less than 10 km underground could satisfy all of the country's electrical needs for the foreseeable future.

Figure 4-28 This power station at The Geysers, California, runs on geothermal energy. It has been operating since 1960.

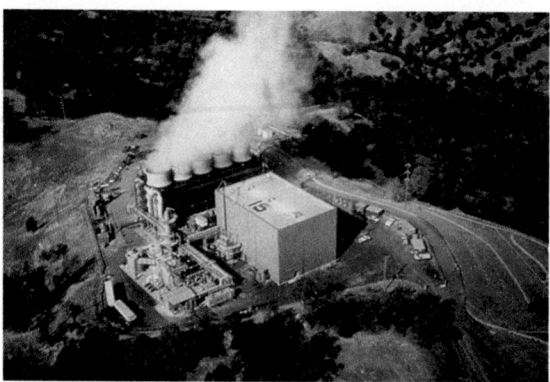

Besides a role in generating electricity, hot subsurface water is widely used for heating purposes, mainly in buildings (nearly all of Iceland's buildings are heated in this way) but also in agriculture to lengthen the growing season for crops.

Earthquake Hazards   For all its promise, geothermal energy has at least one cloud shadowing its future. Mention was made in Sec. 4.7 of the possibility that earthquakes could occur when CO_2 from fossil-fuel power plants is injected into underground reservoirs for storage. Such a risk is even more worrying in geothermal projects that force water at high pressure into hot (over 150°C), dry rocks to fracture them into a network of cracks. Then water is pumped down a bore hole to the network, where it boils. The resulting steam comes to the surface via another hole to drive a steam turbine that powers an electric generator or for district heating. Progress on an installation of this kind in Basel, Switzerland, was stopped in 2006 when a series of small earthquakes was triggered that shook the city; they continued for months afterward.

Unaware of the Basel earthquakes, the U.S. Energy Department approved and provided some of the financing for a number of similar projects in this country. The first was to be located in northern California, one of the most earthquake-prone parts of the world. In 2009, when officials finally learned of the Basel events, which they said had not been fully disclosed in the project's application (although the company involved disputes this), they ordered work halted. Conventional geothermal plants that use naturally heated water are not usually sources of concern, but clearly the water-injection method requires greater care in the choice of suitable geological regions than has been given thus far.

4.10 Clean Energy II

Variable Sources

Now we consider clean energy sources whose output is not constant. This is not necessarily a major disadvantage because, when available, their electricity can replace that from fossil-fuel sources even if only intermittently. And, as mentioned later, several methods exist for storing the energy of variable sources until needed.

Solar Cells   Sunlight is a form of energy in motion and it can deliver a surprising amount of power to each square meter on which it falls. In the United States, the average ranges from 87 W/m^2 in Alaska to 248 W/m^2 in Hawaii. In Chicago, it is 155 W/m^2, and at this rate a tennis court there receives solar energy equivalent to that in a gallon of gasoline every hour and a half.

Photovoltaic (PV) cells are available that convert the energy in sunlight directly to electricity. Although the supply of sunlight varies with location, time of day, season, and weather, such **solar cells** have the advantage of no moving parts and almost no maintenance. For a given power output solar cells are quite a bit more expensive than fossil-fuel plants, but they have no fuel or operating costs. Improving technology is steadily increasing the efficiency of solar cells, now as much as 20 percent for commercial cells and over 40 percent for experimental ones, and dropping their price.

Although solar cells now provide less than 0.2 percent of the world's electricity, installed capacity is growing and should at least reach 4 percent of the total by 2020. Some countries are leaders: Germany, for instance, despite its often cloudy skies, has 3 GW of solar cells, over half the world's solar-cell capacity, on the roofs of 300,000 homes and businesses. China is installing 2 GW of solar cells on a desert site larger than Manhattan in Inner Mongolia. By 2020, this project and others are expected to have enlarged the country's solar capacity to 20 GW (which is still only half the capacity of the coal-fired power plants that are being built there every year). India has the same 20 GW target for 2020, rising to 200 GW for 2050; the United States is expected to exceed 15 GW of solar capacity by 2020. But if the new ideas currently being studied for cheaper, more efficient technology succeed, these projections may turn out to be serious underestimates—the advances in computer technology in the recent past also outran reasonable expectations.

A big advantage of solar cells is that they can be placed close to where their electricity is to be used, for instance on rooftops (Fig. 4-29). This can mean major savings because it eliminates distribution costs in rural areas where power lines would otherwise have to be built. In Kenya, more households get their electricity from solar cells than from power plants. Even when electricity grids exist, rooftop solar cells are becoming common. As part of California's efforts to have more of its energy needs come from renewable sources, the "One Million Solar Roofs" program will have 3 GW of partly subsidized solar panels installed by 2018.

Concentrated Solar Power   In another approach, called **concentrated solar power (CSP),** solar energy is first converted into heat, which is then used to produce steam for turbines that drive electric generators. Such installations cost much less than PV ones of the same capacity but are practical only where there is open land with reliable sunshine. In one CSP method, curved mirrors form troughs that focus sunlight on pipes filled with oil that becomes very hot as a result. The hot oil then turns water into steam in a boiler; it can be stored in an insulated tank and can release its heat during the night. Nine

Solar Water Heating

Exposing pipe arrays filled with water to sunlight is a simple and cheap way to capture solar energy for household hot water and space heating. About 90 GW of solar energy is exploited in this way every year worldwide. Two-thirds of this energy is collected in China, where by replacing fossil-fuel burning, CO_2 emissions are reduced by several hundred million tons annually.

In other countries such direct solar water heating is less common, only 1.8 percent of the world total in the United States, for instance. Solar water heaters are now mandatory on new buildings in Hawaii, as they have been since 2006 in parts of Spain.

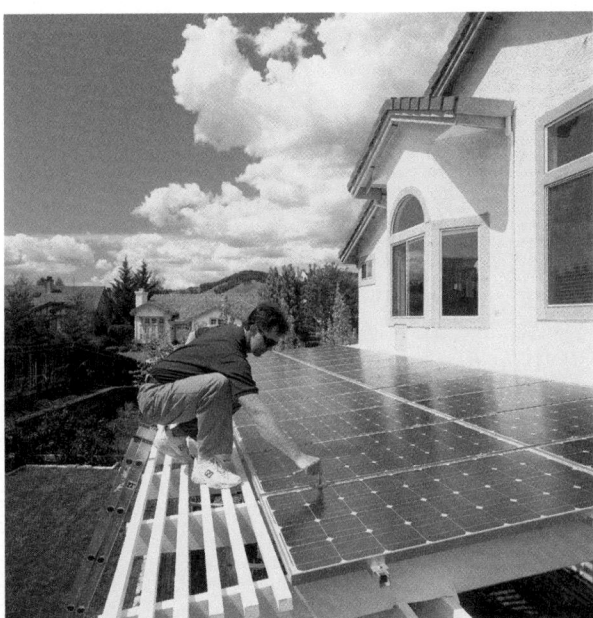

Figure 4-29   Array of solar cells being installed over the back porch of a house in California.

arrays of this kind in the Mohave Desert in California have been furnishing 354 MW of electricity for over 20 years (Fig. 4-30). An array in Nevada, with 19,300 4-m pipes, yields 64 MW.

Instead of using fixed curved mirrors, another CSP system has a large number of movable flat mirrors that track the sun to direct sunlight on a receiver atop a central tower. In the receiver, sunlight heats molten salt that goes to a boiler. This arrangement produces steam at a much higher temperature than trough-type ones do, which improves turbine efficiency (Sec. 5.14). The hot molten salt can be stored to enable electricity to be generated at night, which is done in a 17-MW plant in Spain. New large-scale CSP projects of both kinds are under way around the world, including a $2 billion, 500-MW facility in California.

Wind Windmills are nothing new and were once widely used for such tasks as grinding grain and pumping water. Holland alone had 9000 of them. Now windmills are back in fashion for generating electricity, and although they are practical only where winds are powerful and reliable, such winds are found in many parts of the world (Fig. 4-31). Today somewhat over

Figure 4-30 This concentrated solar power (CSP) installation in the Mohave Desert uses thousands of curved mirrors to direct sunlight to heat oil that then generates steam to power turbine generators.

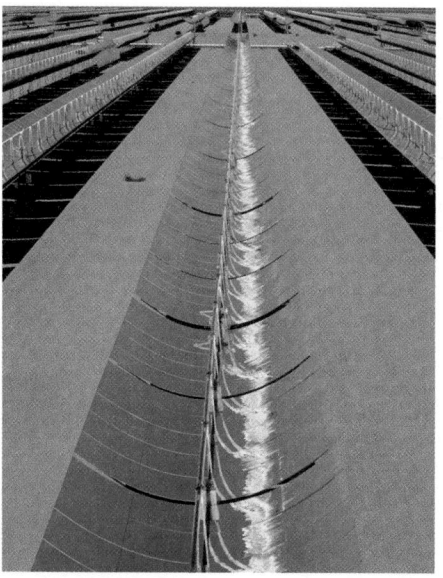

Figure 4-31 Wind turbine "farm" near Palm Springs, California. Such farms consist of as many as several hundred turbines and can supply energy to tens of thousands of homes and businesses. The largest wind farm in the United States is in Texas and has a capacity of 780 MV. As in the case of solar power, the wind power potential in the United States will exceed its needs for the foreseeable future.

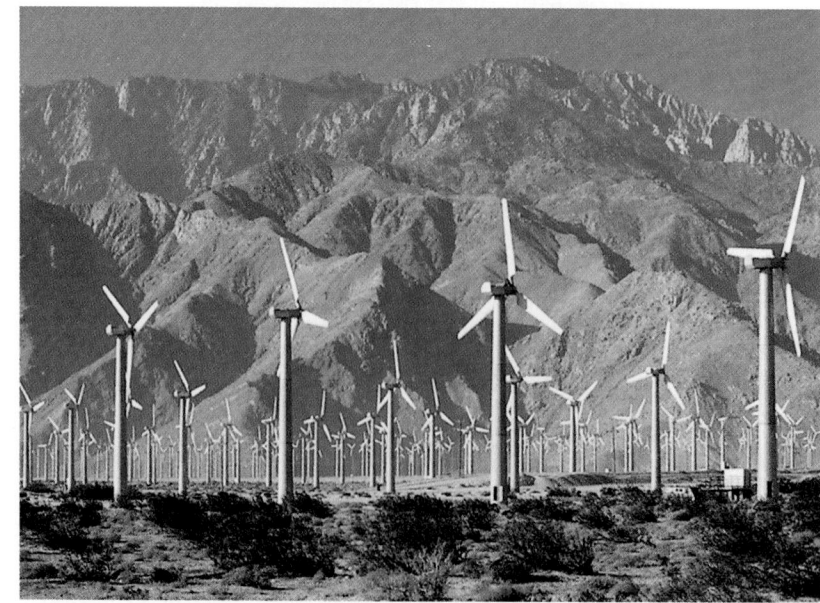

A Solar Future?

How much land would be needed for solar collectors to provide all of the 3 TW of power the United States consumes? This will tell us whether there is a fundamental limit to the potential for solar energy in the country. If we consider land in the sunny Southwest and assume an overall efficiency of 10 percent for a system of collectors plus overnight energy storage facilities, the answer is roughly 52,000 square miles. This is 1.5 percent of the total area of the United States; 10 percent of the combined areas of Nevada, Arizona, and New Mexico; less than half the area of America's national parks. So there is enough land for any desired amount of solar energy, especially since any realistic scenario for the future would have other renewable sources—and perhaps nuclear fusion reactors as well—carrying part of the load.

From a global perspective, the picture changes. Europe, for instance, has an average population density of 319 people per square mile whereas the United States averages only 82. There is little open land in Europe as well as less sunshine than in the United States. But not far away lie the empty deserts of North Africa and the Middle East, which have enough area for CSP installations that could satisfy the whole world's electrical appetite, let alone Europe's. A group of 12 European industrial, utility, and financial companies is organizing a bold $580 billion project called Desertec that would use CSP collectors in these deserts to produce 15 percent of Europe's electricity by 2050. Twenty high-voltage, direct-current power lines (Sec. 6.19) would carry the electricity under the Mediterranean Sea to Europe. Is this a better idea than planting more PV panels on European rooftops? Not everybody thinks so.

2 percent of the world's electricity comes from wind, slightly more than the proportion in the United States.

A typical large modern turbine has three fiberglass- or carbon fiber-reinforced blades 60 m long that turn up to 22 times per minute to generate up to 5 MW. Such a turbine starts to produce electricity at a wind speed of about 9 mi/h, reaches full power at about 31 mi/h, and is shut down to prevent damage in storm winds of 56 mi/h or more. Its average output naturally depends on the usual winds at its location, with 40 percent of the maximum considered good. Because turbine efficiency increases with size, 10-MW turbines with 75-m blades are in prospect, which would bring the cost of wind electricity closer to those of fossil-fuel or nuclear power plants without their disadvantages.

Wind is the world's fastest-growing (over 20 percent per year) source of renewable emission-free energy; its potential remains barely tapped. Wind turbines have been installed in 80 countries thus far. The global total of wind energy capacity is over 160 GW, up from 59 GW in 2005; the United States has the most, over 50 GW, closely followed by China with Germany, Spain, and India farther behind. In the United States, Texas produces by far the most wind energy, with Iowa, California, and Minnesota next. The country hopes to have 300 GW of wind capacity by 2030, which would provide a fifth of its electrical demand. China, too, is marching ahead, with six giant wind farms planned of 10–20 GW capacity each, plus smaller ones.

More and more turbine farms are being sited in shallow offshore waters where they have minimal environmental impact and can take advantage of the stronger and steadier winds there. Such farms are about twice as expensive as onshore ones. Denmark (the largest builder of wind turbines) expects to generate half of its electricity by 2025 from offshore turbines; it is over a third of the way there already. Contracts have been signed for nine wind farms with about 6000 giant turbines to be installed off the British coast starting in 2013 at an estimated cost of $120 billion. With a total capacity of 30 GW, the turbines will help the U.K. meet its target of obtaining 40 percent of its electricity from renewable sources by 2020. In the United States, a wind farm of 130 turbines with a total capacity of 468 MW proposed for an offshore location south of Cape Cod in Massachusetts finally received federal approval in 2010 after 9 years of opposition from local residents. The farm, which would be the first of its kind in the country, is planned to cover 24 square miles and cost $1 billion. It is expected to be followed by at least half a dozen other wind farms in the shallow waters off the U.S. East Coast and in the Great Lakes. In Europe's North Sea, which has a great many oil and gas production platforms already in place, wind turbines are beginning to sprout atop them to power their operations; using existing platforms saves a third of the cost.

Tides   The twice daily rise and fall of the tides (Sec. 1.10) is accompanied by corresponding flows of water into and out of bays and river mouths. Harnessing the considerable energy involved is another old idea: in Europe, tide mills go back to the twelfth century. Tidal power is reliable and has low operating costs. On the other hand, the tidal cycle means that there is no energy output for two periods of a few hours per day, which leaves a large investment idle for that part of the time.

There are two main approaches to extracting energy from the tides. One of them involves spanning a narrow inlet on a coast that has a large—over 5 m—tidal range with a dam that traps water on a rising tide and then directs it to turbine generators when the water level outside has dropped. An installation of this kind in the Rance River in northern France has supplied 240 MW of peak electric power since 1966 (Fig. 4-32). In South Korea a new 254 MW tidal power installation, for the time being the world's largest, will be followed in 2014 by another one whose capacity will be 812 MW and cost $1.9 billion. Even bigger tidal plants are being contemplated elsewhere, for instance in England's Severn Estuary, where the tidal range of over 13 m is second only to the range in the Bay of Fundy in eastern Canada. Turbine generators set in a 16-km barrage would furnish 8.6 GW of peak power, 5 percent of the country's needs. On the downside of tidal power, apart from its expense ($30 billion or so for the Severn installation), there is the risk that altering tidal flow patterns may harm local ecosystems.

The other approach is to use submerged turbines to drive generators as tidal currents run back and forth past their blades. An undersea tidal farm of this kind can be on a small scale that avoids the cost and environmental issues of a dam. Such farms have been installed off the Norwegian coast and in New York's East River; locations for others in the United States and elsewhere are being studied.

Waves   As anybody who has stood in the surf or watched waves dash against a rocky shore knows, waves carry energy in abundance. A number of schemes have been thought up to capture this energy, which ultimately comes from the sun whose uneven heating of the atmosphere causes the winds that ruffle the seas. In one of them ocean waves run up a sloping funnel-like channel to a reservoir above. Water from the reservoir then powers a turbine generator on its way back down to the ocean. But this simple system is feasible only where the seabed is so shaped that wave energy is focused on a particular spot on a coast and where the winds that drive the waves are usually onshore.

A wave energy converter that can be used anywhere, called Pelamis (after a species of sea serpent), employs a series of semisubmerged cylindrical sections 180 m long and 4 m in diameter that are hinged together. The sections swing back and forth relative to one another when waves pass by, and these motions drive pumps that force oil at high pressure to hydraulic motors coupled to electric generators. Each section has a maximum output of 750 W. Several Pelamis arrays have been operated in tests off the British and Portuguese coasts. A number of other wave energy conversion schemes are under development. If all goes well, the future may see 30-MW arrays that would each be spread over a square kilometer of ocean near many of the world's coasts.

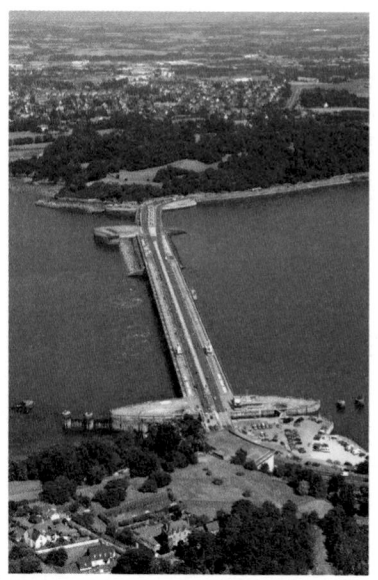

Figure 4-32   This 1966 barrage across the Rance River in France uses tidal flows to drive turbine generators that supply 240 MW of peak electric power.

4.11   Energy Storage

Options for Variable Sources and Vehicles

Effective ways to store energy on a large scale to even out its supply from variable sources are clearly desirable. In addition, to replace oil-based vehicle fuels will require improved or entirely new forms of portable energy storage. Storage systems for both purposes are already in limited use, and a great deal of work is going on to improve them and to try to come up with better new ones.

Bulk Storage   Electric energy from a variable source not needed at a particular time can be stored as gravitational potential energy by using it to pump water up to a high reservoir. Then, at night when there is no sunshine, or when the wind stops, or when the tide is not running, the water is allowed to fall through turbine generators. Four such systems have been installed in Britain and one in California, with two more planned there. In a variant of this arrangement, Denmark sends surplus electricity from its wind farms to Norway to be used instead of electricity from Norwegian hydroelectric plants, thereby conserving water in the reservoirs to use for returning electricity to Denmark when winds there are light.

In another scheme, air can be pumped into a sealed underground cavern, an abandoned mine, or an exhausted natural-gas well and the compressed air later released to power a generator. An advantage here is that suitable caverns are more common than elevated sites for water reservoirs. Compressed air storage facilities have been operating in Germany since 1978 and in Alabama since 1991, and a large new one is being developed in California.

In a storage battery, electric energy is converted into chemical energy that can subsequently be converted back into electric energy (Sec. 12.13). The rechargeable batteries familiar in cars and in electronic devices of many kinds are not suitable for the substantial amounts of energy involved in commercial power generation. However, "flow batteries" have been devised in which the energy-rich chemicals of the charged battery do not have to remain there but can be pumped out into separate tanks while fresh starting chemicals replace them. Reversing the flow allows the stored energy to return to its original electric form for withdrawal. Flow batteries are more complex than conventional ones and their technology is still being improved. Still, various kinds have been on the market for some time and their capacities are going up; a 432-GJ flow battery is being built for a 15-MW power system in the United Kingdom.

Electric Cars   Hybrids that use electric motors powered by storage batteries to supplement gasoline engines, as described in Sec. 4.5, were introduced as far back as 1997. All-electric cars (Fig. 4.33) have recently joined hybrids on the road thanks to better storage batteries that can deliver ranges adequate for commuting and journeys of modest length. All storage batteries have the handicap of low energy densities (energy content per kilogram) compared with gasoline and diesel fuel, only 1/300 as much in the case of traditional lead-acid batteries. Lithium-ion batteries of the kind used in electronic equipment such as laptop computers have up to six times higher energy densities than lead-acid batteries, but even they are heavy: the Tesla Roadster, the first all-electric car with a range of over 200 miles, is powered by 6831 lithium-ion cells that weigh almost half a ton and take 3.5 h to charge. (The car is named after the electricity pioneer Nikola Tesla.)

The overall energy efficiency of an all-electric car, starting from the source of the grid electricity used to charge its batteries, is considerably higher than that of an ordinary car, with the cost per mile a quarter as much. The saving is even greater when the charging is done at night at lower off-peak electricity

Figure 4-33   The all-electric Tesla S sedan has a range of up to 300 miles, depending on the battery pack chosen. If the electricity supply is suitable, its batteries can be recharged in 45 min. Discharged batteries can be swapped for fully charged ones in 5 min.

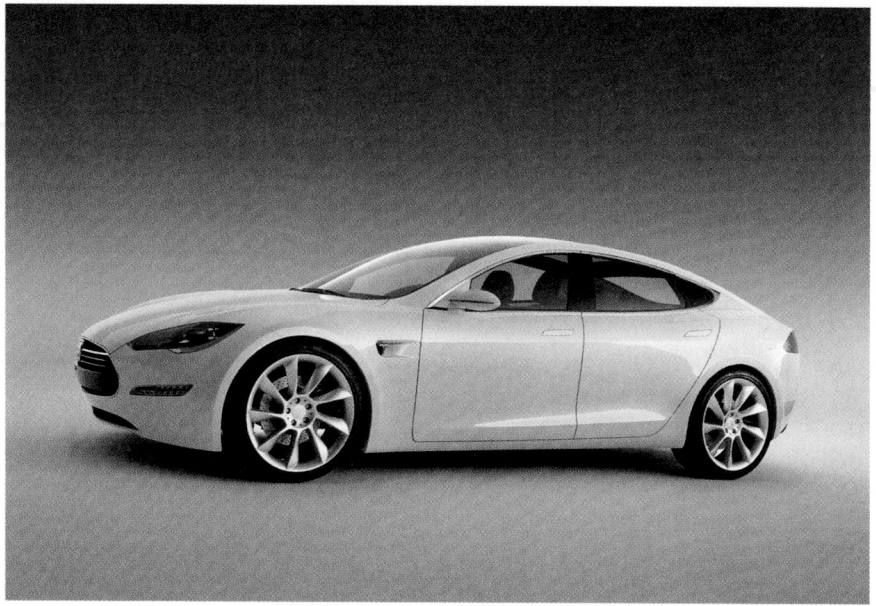

rates. An electric car emits no CO_2 itself, of course, and the CO_2 from the generating plants that produce the electricity used to charge its batteries is less than half that emitted by an ordinary car. Electric cars will be even greener in the future as alternative sources replace fossil-fuel plants.

Most of the world's major car companies are starting to build electric cars, which they expect to take a larger and larger share of the car market. Germany is supporting a program to have a million electric cars on its roads by 2020, and the United States government is helping to finance efforts to improve batteries for electric cars. Thirteen of China's largest cities will have all-electric bus fleets by 2014.

For most driving, the limited range of an electric car is acceptable, especially as charging stations are already being installed in parking lots and garages in the United States and Europe. Two-thirds of American commutes are 15 miles or less each way. Charging times of 3–5 hours are being brought down; the batteries of the Tesla S sedan can be charged in 45 minutes from 480-V outlets, and as little as 10 minutes does not seem impossible for future batteries.

To get around the problem of long trips, some manufacturers provide their plug-in electric cars with gasoline-driven generators (or even gasoline propulsion engines), so the result is really a hybrid, not an electric car. The Chevrolet Volt is a hybrid of this kind whose range under battery alone is 40 miles. Another approach is to establish networks of stations that can recharge or even replace batteries low on charge rapidly. Such networks are now being installed in a number of countries by a company called A Better Place; its name comes from what it hopes the world will be if its efforts succeed.

Hydrogen and Fuel Cells   As we can see in Fig. 4-14, mass for mass, hydrogen liberates more energy when it combines with oxygen than any of the other fuels listed—three times as much as gasoline, for instance. It is a clean fuel as well: the only product of its use is water, with no carbon dioxide or harmful pollutants. Unfortunately, although hydrogen is by far the most abundant element in the universe, on earth it is found only in compounds with other elements (notably with oxygen in water, H_2O) and must be separated out from them. Therefore hydrogen is really a storage and delivery medium and not a primary fuel in itself.

Nowadays, hydrogen is usually produced by reacting natural gas with steam, with CO_2 as a by-product. This process depletes a resource and contributes to global warming. Another, more expensive method called **electrolysis** (Sec. 10.17) involves passing electric current through water to break up its H_2O molecules into their hydrogen and oxygen components. Electrolysis requires as much input energy as the energy obtained by recombining the hydrogen and oxygen later. If the input energy comes from fossil-fuel plants, as it would today, resources are again not conserved and CO_2 is added to the atmosphere. In the long run, to be sure, alternative sources could supply clean energy and perhaps bacteria or algae will be found that can liberate hydrogen on a commercial basis from plant materials or during photosynthesis; they already do so in the laboratory, but inefficiently.

Hydrogen can be used to provide energy in two ways. One is simply by burning it, which is done in welding torches and in spacecraft propulsion engines. Under development are cars that use hydrogen in place of gasoline in similar engines.

The other approach employs **fuel cells,** devices in which hydrogen and oxygen react directly to produce water and electricity rather than water and heat. Unlike batteries, which also obtain electric current directly from chemical reactions, fuel cells can provide current indefinitely without having to be replaced or recharged because the working substances are fed in continuously.

The electricity output from a hydrogen fuel cell can be used to power an electric vehicle just as electricity from a battery can (Fig. 4-34). As a vehicle fuel, however, hydrogen has a major storage problem because under ordinary conditions it is a gas that takes up far too much volume for the energy a car needs. In liquid form, it is compact enough, but to liquify hydrogen means cooling it below $-253°C$, which takes up to 40 percent of its energy content. Hydrogen can also be squeezed into a suitably smaller space by a pressure about 700 times that of the atmosphere—which means 5 tons per square inch—which also takes energy. In either case, the required tank is quite heavy, though not as heavy as batteries that hold equivalent energy.

But even if the problems of fuel-cell technology and of practical hydrogen production and storage are solved, there is also the chicken-and-egg situation in which nobody wants to install a vastly expensive supply system (the United States has about 160,000 gasoline stations) before cars exist to use

Not a New Idea

In his 1874 novel *The Mysterious Island*, one of Jules Verne's characters predicts that "water one day will be employed as fuel, that hydrogen and oxygen which constitute it . . . will furnish an inexhaustible source of heat and light . . . Water will be the coal of the future." Another character responds (as do we all), "I should like to see that."

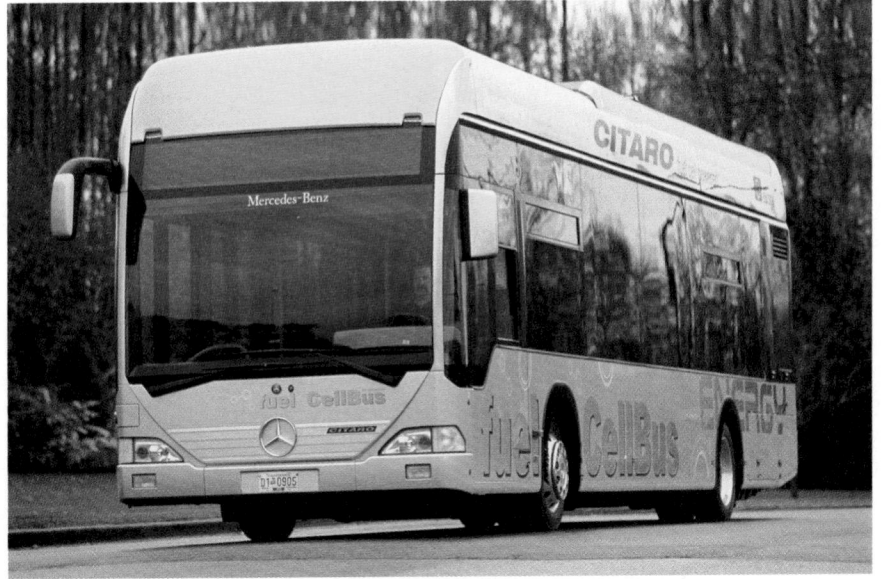

Figure 4-34 This prototype bus is powered by fuel cells that operate on hydrogen. Similar technology is used in cars from other manufacturers, which are undergoing road tests, but commercial models are not expected for some time. Such vehicles are more efficient than gasoline- or diesel-fueled ones, and in their operation only water vapor is given off. However, they are more expensive to build and operate than battery-powered electric vehicles, which are expected to be in the majority in the future.

them, and nobody wants to buy a fuel-cell car before there are filling stations for it everywhere. The advantages of battery-powered electric cars over their fuel-cell cousins make them by far the favorites to take over the world's roads.

4.12   Biofuels

Yes, But

Biofuels made from plant matter are obviously renewable and have the advantage that the CO_2 given off when they are burned will be absorbed afterward during photosynthesis by the next crop to be grown (Sec. 13.12). Under the right circumstances they could bring energy independence closer in many countries. However, it is not at all clear that biofuels as a class have yet made much, if any, progress toward reducing greenhouse gas emissions even as they replace fossil fuels. When the entire life cycles of their production and use are considered, today the only commercial biofuels environmentally superior to fossil fuels are ethanol from sugar cane and biodiesel from used cooking oil. Government subsidies for biofuels have cost huge sums, and because most current biofuels are made from food crops, food prices have increased in a number of regions. Fortunately, new biofuel technologies are on the way that will not compete with food crops.

The simplest way to use crops—and organic wastes such as municipal garbage, manure, scrap paper, and so on—for energy is just to burn them, either by themselves to make steam to heat buildings and generate electricity or in coal-fired power plants alongside coal. More and more installations of both kinds are coming into use, waste disposal being an especial attraction in many cities. However, a number of problems, such as supply limitations and pollution control, make this approach unlikely to provide more than a relatively small fraction of the world's total energy needs.

Biofuels for vehicles are a different story. Ethanol—the alcohol in beverages such as wine, beer, and whiskey—yields almost two-thirds as much energy when burned as gasoline and can be added to or even be used instead of gasoline in car engines. Henry Ford's first Model T cars, introduced in 1908, could run on either ethanol or gasoline. Diesel engines cannot run on ethanol, but "biodiesel" made from various plant oils and animal fats can similarly supplement or replace diesel fuel derived from petroleum.

Vehicle biofuels are receiving more and more attention with over 40 countries encouraging their use by various subsidies and requirements. Worldwide ethanol production has more than tripled since 2000 and biodiesel even more. The United States, the European Union, and China have set ambitious targets for vehicle biofuels, in the case of the United States a four-fold increase in alternatives to gasoline by 2022. Currently biofuels provide about 2 percent of the energy used globally for transport.

Ethanol   Fuel ethanol in the United States, the world's leading producer, comes from corn; in Brazil, in second place, it comes from sugar cane. The two countries share 90 percent of the total market.

Sugar cane is about 10 times as efficient as most other plants in utilizing solar energy. The sugar in its juice can be directly fermented by yeasts into ethanol, which is then extracted by distillation. In Brazil, which has large areas of land suitable for sugar cane cultivation, all cars use ethanol, either by itself or blended with gasoline. This has cut Brazil's consumption of gasoline in half and lowered its CO_2 emissions considerably. There is less air pollution in Brazilian cities as well. China is a customer of Brazilian ethanol in the hope of similarly reducing the pollution of its urban air, among the world's worst.

Algae to the Rescue?

Certain algae can produce an oil whose conversion to various biofuels is straightforward. This approach was studied in the 1970s and 1980s but experiments stopped when crude oil became cheaper. In new work to carry the idea further, suitable algae, some genetically modified for the purpose, are being grown in ponds that have CO_2 bubbled up through them for the algae to use with water and sunlight in the photosynthesis that nourishes them. If the CO_2 is piped in from fossil-fuel plants, their CO_2 emissions would be used productively, a better alternative to just releasing them into the atmosphere or even to burying them underground.

An acre of soybeans can yield 60 gallons of biofuel per year and an acre of corn 260 gallons, whereas an acre of algae might be able to yield more than 2000 gallons without using agricultural land. If deriving biofuel from algae proves practical on the scale required, which is not certain, all the transport fuel needs of the United States could perhaps be supplied from ponds whose area would correspond to only a few percent of the area used for the country's agriculture.

Another method being tried has the algae confined to water-filled plastic containers exposed to sunlight, with CO_2 circulated through them (Fig. 4-35). In both cases, it seems possible for sewage or fertilizer-laden agricultural runoff water to provide the other nutrients algae require, another plus.

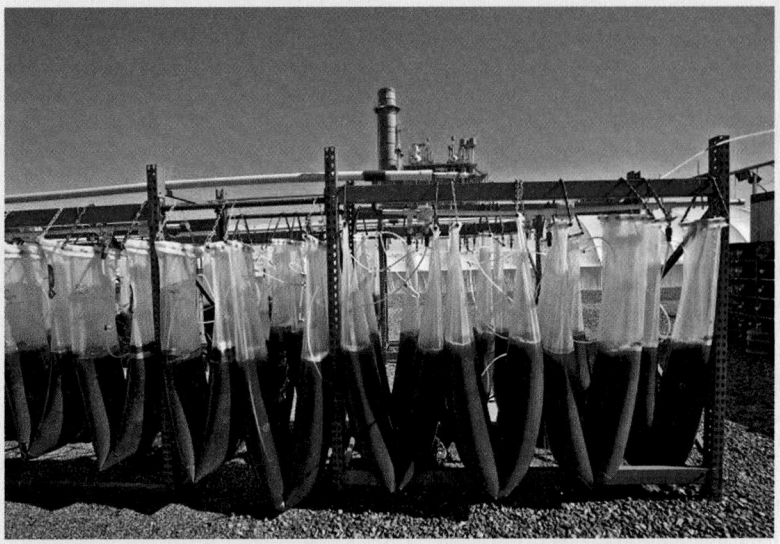

Figure 4-35 Reactors at the 1.04-GW Redhawk gas-fired power plant in Arizona use algae to convert some of its CO_2 emissions to biodiesel with the help of water and sunlight.

In the United States, a lot of fossil-fuel energy is needed to grow corn and to process it into ethanol (the starch in the corn must first be converted into sugars). As a result, each gallon of corn ethanol takes five to eight times the energy to produce as a gallon of cane ethanol and is accordingly more expensive. Using corn ethanol instead of gasoline does little to reduce net CO_2 emissions; if coal is one of the fossil fuels used to produce the ethanol, the result is an increase in CO_2 emissions. (Using cane ethanol gives a reduction of 90 percent.) When forests and grasslands are cleared to grow corn, around a century may be needed before there is any CO_2 benefit.

Then what are the attractions of corn ethanol in the United States? To begin with, there are generous subsidies to corn farmers and a tax credit for converting corn to ethanol that costs taxpayers over $5 billion per year. Second, a 2007 law requires that increasing minimum amounts of corn ethanol be used in vehicle fuels, so there is a guaranteed market for it. Third, the government maintains the price of sugar too high for it to be an economical source of ethanol, and a substantial tariff keeps out cheap cane ethanol from Brazil. Finally, high oil prices make ethanol more competitive with gasoline (though oil prices tend to vary considerably and when they come down, ethanol production does too).

As the problematic aspects of corn ethanol come into focus, a number of countries are reducing or eliminating the subsidies and other inducements for its use that once seemed like good ideas. The United States, the largest producer and user by far, is studying ways to reduce the environmental costs of biofuels, especially those of corn ethanol.

Food Versus Fuel

Increasingly worrying is the use of agricultural land for fuel rather than for food in a time of expanding population (see Fig. 4-1): 230,000 new mouths every day. The corn needed for the ethanol to fill an SUV's fuel tank would feed a person for a year. Over a fifth of the corn harvest in the United States—which produces 40 percent of the world's corn—already goes to make ethanol, a proportion still climbing.

The diversion of corn to fuel has helped drive its price sharply upward everywhere, as has happened with other crops that farmers are replacing with corn. With animal feed more expensive, meat and dairy products also cost more. For the world's poor, many of them in Africa, this is bad news that is getting worse as corn ethanol production rises. Both of the U.N.'s food agencies regard biofuel production warily; a report to one of them concluded that using food crops for biofuels is "a crime against humanity."

Cellulosic Ethanol   Fortunately the drawbacks to corn ethanol apply with much less force to cellulosic ethanol. Cellulose is the main constituent of all plants (Sec. 13.11) and agricultural waste, wood, and certain grasses are cheap and abundant sources; municipal waste contains a great deal of cellulose. Some grasses yield several times as much ethanol per acre as corn and can grow on poor agricultural land. Furthermore obtaining ethanol from cellulose involves far less fossil-fuel energy than in the case of corn ethanol, and up to a 70 percent reduction in CO_2 emissions. Starting from sugar cane is even better, but there is far more cellulose available and at less cost. The trouble is that, while going from cellulose to ethanol has been done in the laboratory, it is not quite practical to do so on an industrial scale. But sooner or later workable methods will inevitably be found, and cellulosic ethanol is likely to push aside corn ethanol on its way to becoming a major vehicle fuel. Some think cellulosic ethanol rather than electricity will power the cars of the future. Ethanol is not the only biofuel that can be made from cellulosic raw materials, of which over 1.3 billion tons annually are thought to be available in the United States without affecting the food supply.

Biodiesel   A century ago some of Rudolf Diesel's first engines ran on peanut oil. Vegetable oils, now in processed form, are once again powering such engines either by themselves or in blends with ordinary diesel fuel. Soy, palm, rapeseed (canola), cottonseed, and sunflower oils are all feedstocks for biodiesel. Vegetable oils and animal fats that have already been used for cooking, charmingly known in the trade as "yellow grease," are a cheaper source of biodiesel but their supply is more limited. Soybeans are responsible for most of the biodiesel produced in the United States, with an energy yield of 2 J for each joule of input. Other oils have even better yields and need considerably less land. On an overall basis, biodiesel use involves less CO_2 emission—the amount of reduction depends on the source—than the use of conventional diesel fuel or of ethanol from corn. Biodiesel is at present more expensive to produce than conventional diesel fuel, but, as with ethanol, its sale is subsidized or required, or both, in many countries, including the United States, and its share of the market is going up. In the United States, biodiesel use is expected to increase by 50 percent to 630 million gallons per year by 2020, about a sixth of it coming from yellow grease and the rest from soybeans.

Although biodiesel is a relatively green fuel in itself, growing the crops from which it comes may not be. For instance, the rapeseed that is the primary oil source in Europe often needs so much fertilizer made using natural gas that overall CO_2 emissions remain high. Even worse are destructive farming practices in some countries. In a notorious case, Indonesian swamps are being drained and the peat under them burned to make room for palm-oil plantations. The result is 2 billion tons of CO_2 entering the atmosphere annually, 8 percent of global CO_2 emissions from burning fossil fuels—far more CO_2 than using the palm oil grown there could ever save in the future. The European Union now bans the import of biofuels whose production involves degrading the environment in ways such as this.

Strategies for the Future

Clearly no simple solution to the problem of providing safe, clean, cheap, and abundant energy is possible in the near future. But there is much that can be done, first of all by improving the efficiency of energy use, which gives a much better return on investment than any form of energy generation. A serious effort could probably save the United States at least half of the electricity it now consumes, for instance. This would mean changes in how we live: technology alone could not do the job. Also essential is to sensibly utilize the various available renewable sources and to expand the production of fission nuclear energy, all the while trying to make fusion energy practical as soon as possible. If the world's population also stabilizes or, better, decreases, social disaster (starvation, war) and environmental catastrophe (a planet unfit for life) may well be avoided even if fusion never becomes practical.

4.13 Conservation

Less Is More

Our children and grandchildren will have to live with the results of what is done (and not done) today about the energy problem and the global warming and resource depletion that are part of it. Is there anything we, as users of energy in our personal lives and in our work, can do that will earn their respect? The answer is yes, taking conservation seriously can make a real difference if enough of us participate, and our pocketbooks will benefit as well. As the saying goes, not to be part of the solution is to be part of the problem.

Major opportunities to save energy during their years of use come in the intelligent design and careful construction of new buildings, both residential and commercial. The best new buildings need less than 20 percent as much energy as older ones for heating, cooling, and lighting. Existing homes almost always benefit from better insulation (including double glazing) and attention to excluding drafts. Upgrading to more efficient space and water heaters, kitchen and laundry appliances, and so forth usually pay for themselves in lower running costs while helping the planet by reducing energy use. Simply painting roofs white can cut the electricity consumed by air-conditioning by as much as 20 percent; a move to "cool roofs" is under way in many warm parts of the world (Fig. 4-36). (In fact, roads cover so much area that using light-colored surfaces instead of black ones would reflect enough sunlight back into space to moderate global warming by a useful amount.)

In everyday life, replacing ordinary lightbulbs with energy-saving ones, loading dishwashers full, not using hot water in clothes washers, and hanging laundry out to dry all help, as does setting thermostats for heating lower than usual in winter and for air-conditioning higher than usual in summer. Buying fuel-efficient cars, driving them at moderate speeds, and sharing

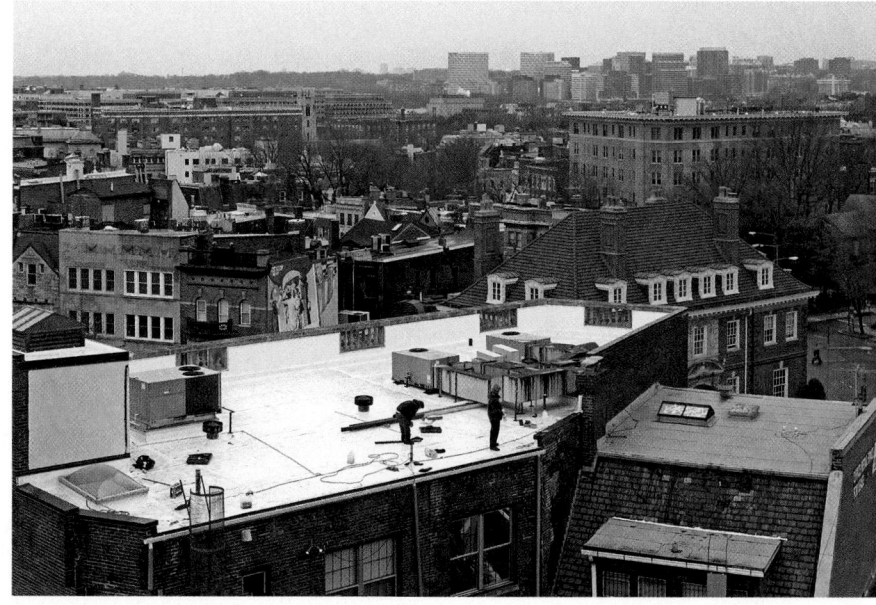

Figure 4-36 Rooftops painted white, such as this one in Washington, D.C., reflect rather than absorb sunlight and so reduce the energy consumed by air-conditioning in summer.

New Lightbulbs

In an ordinary incandescent light-bulb a tungsten filament glows when heated by the passage of an electric current. Such bulbs are very inefficient; about 95 percent of the energy they consume becomes heat, and there are billions of them—perhaps 4 billion in the United States alone, using 9 percent of all its electricity. They last around 1000 hours.

In a fluorescent tube an electric discharge causes the atoms in a mercury vapor to emit invisible ultraviolet light. A coating of a material called a phosphor on the inside of the glass tube absorbs the ultraviolet light and, in a process called fluorescence, gives off visible light. Fluorescent lamps are about 5 times as efficient as incandescent ones and last up to 10 times

longer. A compact fluorescent light-bulb (CFL), like the ones shown in Fig. 4-37, that replaces an ordinary bulb of the same brightness saves several times its additional cost each year in electricity bills and hundreds of pounds of CO_2 emitted by a fossil-fuel power plant.

A 2007 law calls for phasing out 100-W incandescent bulbs in the United States in stages between 2012 and 2014 in favor of energy-saving bulbs such as CFLs. The result will be to cut $18 billion per year from electricity charges and reduce CO_2 emissions by about 160 million tons, equivalent to taking tens of millions of cars off the roads or shutting down as many as 80 coal-fired power plants. Phasing out incandescent bulbs is under way in Europe and elsewhere, and

has been completed in some countries, for instance Australia and Brazil.

Eventually light-emitting diodes (LEDs) may well take over the lighting market. LEDs employ microchip technology like that used in modern electronic devices and are compact, rugged, and versatile. The best current ones are two to three times as efficient as CFLs and last 50,000 hours, with room for improvement on both counts. Another advantage is that, unlike CFLs, they have no mercury to dispose of safely when discarded. LEDs are already widely used in instrument lighting, flashlights, traffic signals, street lights, and car headlights—a few among an increasing list of applications—but are still too expensive for general lighting.

Figure 4-37   A compact fluorescent bulb uses much less power for a given light output than an ordinary incandescent bulb.

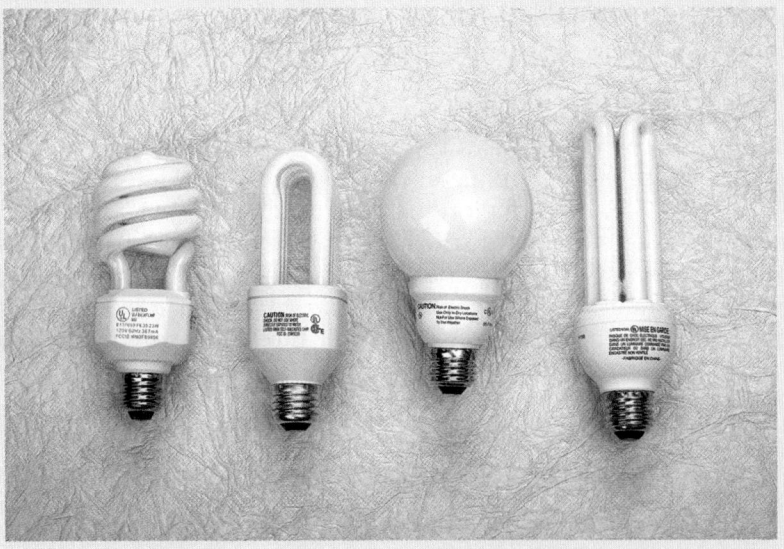

rides instead of going alone have always been good ideas, as is keeping in mind that buses and trains average as little as a tenth as much energy per passenger-mile as cars do. Everything counts: just switching computers, audio and video equipment, coffeemakers, and other devices off instead of leaving them on standby at night would eliminate at least 5 percent of residential energy use in the United States, equivalent to the output of 18 typical power stations.

Recycling can help: to recycle aluminum uses less than 9 percent as much energy as to refine it from its ores, and billions of aluminum cans are discarded every year. Recycling other metals, glass, plastic bottles, paper, and cardboard also conserves energy and raw materials and is kinder to the environment than burial in landfills or burning in incinerators. San Francisco's recycling rate of 70 percent, well above the U.S. average of 33 percent, shows what can be done.

Industry, too, cannot continue with business as usual. As with individuals, those companies that have adopted better practices have often found them to save money as well as contributing to a healthy planet. Thus DuPont has cut CO_2 emissions severely in recent years while saving billions of dollars in energy costs through greater efficiency. General Electric is another convert and has brought its CO_2 emissions down despite an expansion that otherwise would have increased them. GE is sure that clean and energy-efficient technologies are its future.

These are not isolated examples: environmental awareness is now more and more accepted as part of good corporate citizenship. A recent survey of business leaders around the world put environmental concerns at the top of a list of the issues that will be most important to their companies in the near future. Even the oil giant ExxonMobil, once a leading skeptic of global warming and of the need for alternative energy sources, is now spending $300 million to develop biofuels from algae; it also supports taxing CO_2 emissions and is reducing its own.

The U.S. Climate Action Partnership consists of several dozen major firms in a variety of fields that find global warming no idle threat and intend to work together to help combat it. They have called for "strong" federal action. But plenty of business interests, including the 3-million-member U.S. Chamber of Commerce (which has an annual war chest of $200 million), are fighting against all global warming legislation. A number of Chamber members have left it over this issue, including Apple and the utilities Pacific Gas and Electric, Exelon, and PNM Resources ("we see climate change as the most pressing environmental and economic issue of our time").

4.14   What Governments Must Do

Their Role Is Crucial

Governments everywhere have become aware of the gravity of the energy problem and of the need for them to respond, though few are acting with the urgency required. An obvious step is to impose the highest feasible efficiency standards for appliances, buildings, and vehicles. As long ago as 1975, California began to introduce regulations that required greater efficiencies in energy use, with the result that average energy consumption per person there has changed little since then although in the rest of the United States it has increased by 50 percent. California consumers are saving $6 billion per year in energy costs.

A key element in California's strategy was to decouple utility profits from electricity sales—the profits of utilities there depend on the success of their energy efficiency programs. Elsewhere, because they profit from waste, utilities have no interest in energy efficiency. California pioneered efficiency standards for appliances, which helped the entire country because it is not economical for manufacturers to have separate product lines for different states. As an example of the result, the average energy used by refrigerators in the United States declined by 75 percent even as their sizes increased and their prices fell. A more recent measure worth being copied requires that, by 2020, all new residential buildings consume zero net energy; for commercial buildings, the deadline is 2030.

Another step is to use both incentives and regulations to promote solar, wind, geothermal, cellulosic ethanol, and other renewable clean energy sources while avoiding such blind alleys as corn ethanol. Nuclear energy should similarly be encouraged to expand. Above all, every effort should be made to phase out fossil fuels, especially coal. Because coal will nevertheless

Smart Meters

A "smart" electric meter in a home tells its residents at any time how much electricity is being consumed (in some cases by which circuits) so they can manage its use efficiently. A local utility's cost of electricity increases with demand above a certain base level, and its rates to large businesses are changed accordingly during each day. Smart meters enable the utility to vary its rates to homes that have them in the same way. Thus, home customers can reduce their bills by running power-hungry appliances during off-peak periods, of which the utility informs them. This benefits the utility industry as well because, by evening out demand, less reserve capacity is needed. The meters also let customers avoid waste whose amount they may not have been aware of, and allow utilities to detect service interruptions as they occur. In 2009, the U.S. Energy Department provided $3.4 billion to help pay for 18 million smart meters, with utilities putting in $4.7 billion of their own.

continue to be burned in quantity for a long time to come, developing ways to capture and bury the resulting CO_2 must be accelerated. Subsidies that encourage the production and use of fossil fuels, still common in the world (the United States spends over $10 billion per year on them), cannot continue. The International Energy Agency calculates that, if such subsidies were scrapped, this step alone would eventually reduce overall greenhouse gas emissions by around 10 percent.

A different facet of the energy problem is deforestation, which as we saw in Fig. 4-13 gives rise to 18 percent of worldwide greenhouse gas emissions. A U.N. program called REDD—for Reducing Emissions from Deforestation and Forest Degradation in Developing Countries—is under way to do what its name suggests by having rich countries subsidize poor ones to invest in low-emission paths to development instead of plundering their forests.

The most cost-effective means of helping to curb global warming is to provide family planning aid to people who want it but have little or no access for the reasons given in Sec. 4.1. According to one careful study, each dollar spent on family planning results in nearly five times the reduction in greenhouse gas emissions as the same dollar spent on technological fixes such as those based on solar and wind energies. Although religious leaders who oppose family planning have managed to keep the subject taboo in public discussions, population growth is becoming more and more recognized as a significant factor in global warming. The U.N. Population Fund, for instance, has made clear the link, and in a letter urging the U.S. administration to increase funding for family planning, a group of members of Congress stated that it "should be part of larger strategies for climate change mitigation and adaptation."

Carbon Tax   Subsidizing alternative energy sources to shrink the gaps between their costs and those of fossil fuels and setting mandatory targets for their use in place of fossil sources both have roles to play in reducing CO_2 emissions. However, most economists feel that a more direct approach is also needed.

The simplest, fairest, most transparent, and most effective such approach is to levy a tax—usually called a **carbon tax** for short—on the amount of CO_2 emitted in the production and use of a fossil fuel. In this way polluters would pay for the harm they do to the environment, which would encourage them to reduce their emissions. A carbon tax would be easy to administer and hard to avoid, and its rate could be adjusted from time to time to achieve the desired total CO_2 reduction. Several countries already have carbon taxes, and others are considering them. Sweden has had a carbon tax since 1991, which has lowered CO_2 emissions by 20 percent while allowing its economy to grow by 44 percent. Because in the United States voting for a new tax is regarded as political suicide, a carbon tax stands little chance of being enacted despite its obvious advantages. Perhaps the chance would be greater if the tax money were distributed among the country's citizens, as has been proposed.

Cap-and-Trade   Another approach is to use a **cap-and-trade system** in which a regionwide total (the cap) is set for annual CO_2 emissions. The government then auctions or gives away permits to emit CO_2 that add up to the overall ceiling. Companies that do not use their entire quotas can sell the leftover permits to companies whose emissions exceed their quotas. A proper choice of the cap would make the price of traded permits high enough to serve as an incentive to big emitters such as power companies to invest in greater efficiency, carbon capture and storage, and clean technologies. If the permits are auctioned, the government receives money that can be used to help ease the transition to clean alternative energy. If permits are free, there is the problem of distributing them fairly. This can easily result in a large cap being set so that all emitters are satisfied with their quotas—and emissions are reduced by little or nothing. Either way the price of traded permits, unlike a tax, would vary with general economic conditions and other unpredictable factors, which would add a new element of uncertainty for businesses planning future investments.

The European Union's Emission Trading System (ETS), the world's largest, began operating in 2005 and illustrates the problems that can arise in such a scheme. Free permits were issued, but many polluting industries were exempted and the caps were set so high that companies in the system received generous quotas. As a result, CO_2 emissions rose, not fell, in the ETS and electric utilities found it cheaper to continue to fuel their furnaces with coal than to switch to less-polluting natural gas. Even though their permits were free and they did not have to buy others, utilities in various countries raised their charges to consumers, for which they blamed the ETS. The German utility RWE, the largest CO_2 emitter in Europe, collected about $6.5 billion in this way before being forced to stop. The ETS was so poorly designed and run that in one 18-month period outright fraud cost it $7.4 billion before being discovered.

Starting in 2013, ETS permits will be auctioned, not free, in the hope of finally making fossil-fuel use sufficiently expensive to encourage investments in reducing CO_2 emissions. Meeting a 2020 target of a 20 percent reduction might increase elecricity bills by 10–15 percent, considered a fair price for the expected benefits. However, the new system, like the old, has important loopholes. One of them is that some member countries, for instance Poland and Germany, both heavy coal users, were given exemptions for much of their emissions. Another is that carbon offsets (see sidebar) also will continue to be allowed.

Copenhagen   There is general agreement that global temperatures should not increase by more than 2°C if environmental catastrophe is to be avoided. To keep temperatures below this figure, the world's greenhouse gas emissions have to be rolled back to perhaps half their 1990 level. The tools that governments have for the purpose are the direct regulation of fossil-fuel use, subsidies for clean energy sources, carbon taxes, and cap-and-trade systems. Each country or region must choose for itself which one or more of these tools fit its situation best.

The big question is how much each country should contribute to the overall reduction needed, whose total cost is estimated at between $500 billion and $1 trillion annually. This seems like a lot, but it is only around 1 percent of world economic output. In December 2009, a two-week conference of 193 countries in Copenhagen considered the matter but could not agree on how the total cost should be apportioned among the various countries. The conference concluded with a statement of broad general principles that should govern such an apportionment, but no details or numbers. However, one of the principles, initially opposed by China and other developing countries, did represent a real step forward: any firm promises of emission cuts would eventually be subject to international monitoring and reporting.

On one side of the basic division in Copenhagen were the developed countries, which as a group are rich and responsible for most of the CO_2 emissions, past and present, that have led to global warming. On the other side were the developing countries, which as a group contain 85 percent of the world's population, are poor, and have CO_2 emissions well below those of the developed countries (see Fig. 4-9). The developing countries are in the

Carbon Offsets

A **carbon offset** is a credit to emit CO_2 that a company in a cap-and-trade system receives in exchange for financing an emission-reduction project in a poor country. For example, the CO_2 emissions saved by building a hydroelectric installation in, say, India could be sold as offsets to coal-burning companies elsewhere to allow them to emit a corresponding amount of CO_2. In principle, such projects would not go ahead without the offset money, but in practice many have turned out to already exist (a third in the case of hydroelectric ones) or would be developed in any case. Even worse, carbon offsets have been sold for planting trees while existing forests in the same country are cut down, so the result is again a net increase in emissions as the buyer gets cheap credits to pour CO_2 into the atmosphere. Although carbon offset programs are widely considered to be failures, the companies that profit from them have managed to keep them in cap-and-trade systems.

Plan B

What if cuts in CO_2 emissions made in the future turn out to be too little and too late? Is there a Plan B in that event, which is all too possible? In fact, a number of schemes have been suggested to tackle a hyperactive greenhouse effect. They fall into two categories. The first involves removing excess CO_2 from the atmosphere, for example by fertilizing areas of the oceans with iron sulfate to stimulate algae (for whom iron is a crucial nutrient often in short supply) to flourish and absorb atmospheric CO_2. When the algae die, their remains, it is assumed, would sink to the sea floor taking the carbon with them.

The other Plan B category involves reducing the amount of sunlight that reaches the earth's surface. One suggestion for this is to spray seawater into the atmosphere over the oceans. Evaporation would leave tiny salt particles to act as condensation nuclei for smaller than usual water droplets. The result would be clouds that would reflect more sunlight back into space than normal clouds.

Unfortunately there is much doubt about how practical such geoengineering projects would be. Thus calculations show that no less than 1.4 billion tons of seawater would have to be sprayed aloft each year to stop global warming, and a trial of the algae method gave disappointing results: predators lost no time in gobbling up the algae. There is also the serious matter of the side effects of such manipulations of the global environment, some foreseeable and others that may come as unwelcome surprises. While Plan B studies should certainly continue, there seems to be no sure substitute in sight for drastically reducing worldwide CO_2 emissions while there is still time.

process of raising their standards of living, today relatively low. This means that, as the economies of developing countries grow, so will the amount of energy they use. Since fossil fuels (especially coal) are the cheapest energy sources, their CO_2 emissions will also grow.

The position in Copenhagen of the developing countries started with a refusal to do anything that would impede their rising prosperity. If the developed countries, already extremely prosperous, want them to curb their CO_2 emissions, the developed countries should pay for substituting clean energy for fossil-fuel energy. The developed countries themselves, as the chief emitters of CO_2, should also take most or all of the burden of decreasing its worldwide total. Furthermore, since the developed countries are responsible for most of the CO_2 poured into the atmosphere since the start of the Industrial Revolution, these countries should help the others adapt to changing climates.

It was not surprising that the developed countries were unhappy with these demands. They were especially disheartened when China and India, with over a third of the world's population and modernizing fast, would not accept any limits on their future CO_2 emissions. (By 2030, China's economy will have passed that of the United States with India, now eleventh, in third place.) In view of this, the United States would not give a specific target for its own efforts. Since China and the United States, each with 20 percent of the total (Fig. 4-10), are the largest producers of CO_2, no other countries would make a firm commitment either. In fact, much of the world is already investing in clean energy projects and expects to continue doing so, but the existing efforts, as mentioned in Sec. 4.4, are far from what is needed to keep temperature rises below 2°C.

Although the Copenhagen conference was a disappointment, so important is its objective of worldwide binding agreements to curb global warming that efforts to this end are sure to continue. Unfortunately, there is no time to spare: the later effective action comes, the more it will cost, both in money and in hardships for affected parts of the world. John Holdren, the White House science advisor, sums up the situation in this way: "We're driving in a car with bad brakes in a fog and heading for a cliff. We know for sure that the cliff is out there. We just don't know exactly where it is. Prudence would suggest that we should start putting on the brakes."

Important Terms and Ideas

The **fossil fuels** coal, oil, and natural gas were formed by the partial decay of the remains of plants and marine organisms that lived millions of years ago.

Methane, the main constituent of natural gas, is a compound of carbon and hydrogen with the chemical formula CH_4.

The **greenhouse effect** refers to the process by which a greenhouse is heated: sunlight can enter through its windows, but the infrared radiation the warm interior gives off is absorbed by glass, so the incoming energy is trapped. The earth's atmosphere is heated in a similar way by absorbing infrared radiation from the warm earth. **Greenhouse gases** are gases that absorb infrared radiation; the chief ones in the atmosphere are carbon dioxide (CO_2), methane, nitrous oxide (N_2O), and a group of gases used in refrigeration called CFCs and HCFCs.

Carbon capture and storage (CCS) involves pumping CO_2 emitted by power plants or other sources into underground reservoirs.

In **nuclear fission,** a large atomic nucleus (notably a nucleus of one kind of uranium atom) splits into smaller ones, a process that gives off considerable energy. A nuclear reactor produces energy from nuclear fissions that occur at a controlled rate.

In **nuclear fusion,** two small nuclei unite to form a larger one, a process that also gives off considerable energy. The sun and stars obtain their energy from nuclear fusion, but fusion technology for power plants is still under development.

Geothermal energy comes from the heat of the earth's interior.

A **photovoltaic cell,** also called a **solar cell,** converts the energy in sunlight directly to electric energy.

In a **concentrated solar power** (**CSP**) installation, solar energy is first converted into heat and then into electric energy.

In a **fuel cell,** electric current is produced by means of chemical reactions.

Biofuels made from plant matter can supplement or replace gasoline and diesel fuel.

In a **cap-and-trade** system for controlling CO_2 emissions, an overall cap on them is set for a region and companies there are given or buy at auction permits to emit CO_2 whose total equals the cap. Companies that do not use their full quotas can sell the leftover permits to companies that exceed their quotas.

Multiple Choice

1. The number of people in the world may reach a maximum in 2050 of about
   - **a.** 1 billion
   - **b.** 2.5 billion
   - **c.** 6.7 billion
   - **d.** 9.2 billion

2. Arrange these sources in the order of the energy they supply to the world today, starting with the source of the most energy.
   - **a.** coal
   - **b.** oil
   - **c.** renewable
   - **d.** nuclear

3. Of the following, the energy source likely to be used up first is
   - **a.** coal
   - **b.** oil
   - **c.** natural gas
   - **d.** nuclear

4. Of the following, the energy source likely to last the longest is
   - **a.** coal
   - **b.** oil
   - **c.** natural gas
   - **d.** nuclear

5. Energy use per person in the United States today is
   - **a.** about the same as the world average
   - **b.** about 10 percent more than the world average
   - **c.** about one and a half times the world average
   - **d.** about four times the world average

6. World energy use in 2030 is expected to be
   - **a.** less than today
   - **b.** about the same as today
   - **c.** about one and a half times what it is today
   - **d.** about four times what it is today

7. Energy not ultimately derived from solar radiation is found in
   - **a.** tides
   - **b.** waves
   - **c.** falling water
   - **d.** wind

8. If present trends continue, an optimistic average global temperature increase by 2100 might be about
   - **a.** 1°C
   - **b.** 2°C
   - **c.** 4°C
   - **d.** 10°C

9. The source that produces the most carbon dioxide per joule of energy liberated is
   - **a.** coal
   - **b.** oil
   - **c.** natural gas
   - **d.** nuclear

10. The average amount of CO_2 emitted each year per person in the United States is about
    - **a.** 1 ton
    - **b.** 2 tons
    - **c.** 5 tons
    - **d.** 20 tons

11. The radiation from an object at room temperature is mainly in the form of
    - **a.** infrared light
    - **b.** visible light
    - **c.** ultraviolet light
    - **d.** any of the above, depending on its color

12. The earth's atmosphere is primarily heated by
    - **a.** direct sunlight
    - **b.** sunlight reflected by the earth's surface
    - **c.** infrared light radiated by the earth's surface
    - **d.** carbon dioxide emissions

13. A gas that does not contribute to global warming is
   a. methane
   c. nitrous oxide
   b. nitrogen
   d. carbon dioxide

14. Arrange these countries in increasing order of their CO_2 emissions per person.
   a. China
   c. United Kingdom
   b. United States
   d. India

15. The country or countries each responsible for about one-fifth of the total of the world's CO_2 emissions is (are)
   a. China
   c. Russia
   b. India
   d. United States

16. Of the following fuels, the one that gives off the most heat per gram when burned is
   a. hydrogen
   c. gasoline
   b. methane
   d. coal

17. Of the following fuels, the one that gives off the least heat per gram when burned is
   a. hydrogen
   c. gasoline
   b. methane
   d. coal

18. Which of the following is not a fossil fuel?
   a. hydrogen
   c. oil
   b. natural gas
   d. coal

19. The proportion of world energy supplied by sources other than fossil fuels is about
   a. 15 percent
   c. 50 percent
   b. 25 percent
   d. 85 percent

20. The proportion of oil used by the United States that is imported is about
   a. 1/10
   c. 1/2
   b. 1/5
   d. 2/3

21. Most oil today is used for
   a. transportation
   c. electricity
   b. heating
   d. lubrication

22. In the United States, coal is chiefly used
   a. for heating
   b. to generate electricity
   c. to make syngas
   d. to manufacture plastics

23. Natural gas consists largely of
   a. hydrogen
   c. nitrogen
   b. oxygen
   d. methane

24. The least polluting of the following fuels is
   a. coal
   c. diesel fuel
   b. gasoline
   d. natural gas

25. Which of these statements about carbon capture and storage (CCS) is true?
   a. CCS has never been tried, even on a small scale.
   b. Earthquakes are a potential hazard for CCS.
   c. CCS is relatively cheap.
   d. There are few underground rock formations suitable for CCS.

26. The impurity in coal that contributes to acid rain is
   a. nitrogen
   c. carbon
   b. sulfur
   d. chlorine

27. The worst emitters of mercury, which damages the nervous system, are power plants that use
   a. coal
   c. natural gas
   b. oil
   d. nuclear energy

28. Syngas is made from
   a. coal
   c. natural gas
   b. oil
   d. carbon dioxide

29. Of the following countries, the one that obtains the largest proportion of its electricity from nuclear energy is
   a. France
   c. Japan
   b. China
   d. United States

30. The proportion of electricity generated in the United States that comes from nuclear energy is roughly
   a. 1 percent
   c. 20 percent
   b. 5 percent
   d. 50 percent

31. In the relatively near future, the technology most able to replace fossil fuels on a large scale is
   a. nuclear
   c. solar
   b. wind
   d. biofuels

32. Of the following problems associated with various energy sources, the least significant for nuclear fission is
   a. waste disposal
   b. fuel reserves
   c. diversion to weapons manufacture
   d. construction expense

33. Bright sunlight might deliver energy to an area of 1 square meter at a rate of
   a. 1 W
   c. 100 W
   b. 10 W
   d. 1000 W

34. The output of which of the following renewable energy sources varies least?
   a. wind
   c. geothermal
   b. waves
   d. solar

35. Of the following renewable energy sources, the one that currently produces more of the world's electricity than any of the others is
   a. wind
   c. geothermal
   b. waves
   d. solar

36. Of the following technologies, the one that may eventually become the chief energy source in the world involves the use of
   a. nuclear fission
   c. fuel cells
   b. nuclear fusion
   d. biofuels

37. Of the following technologies, the one farthest from being a commercial energy source in the near future involves the use of
   a. nuclear fission
   c. fuel cells
   b. nuclear fusion
   d. biofuels

38. Biofuels based on which of the following seem to have the most promise for the future?
   a. corn
   c. soybeans
   b. cellulose
   d. algae

39. Of the following, the strategy for coping with future energy shortages with the most in its favor is to
   a. burn more coal
   b. produce more oil from tar sands
   c. divert more agricultural land to making biofuels
   d. increase energy efficiency and energy conservation

40. The least helpful government approach to controlling greenhouse gas emissions is
   a. a carbon tax
   b. a cap-and-trade system
   c. to require increasing use of clean technologies
   d. to subsidize biofuels

Exercises

4.1 Population and Prosperity

1. What are the three main factors that will require changes in today's patterns of energy production and consumption?

4.2 Energy Consumption

2. Even if the developed countries stabilize or reduce their energy consumption in years to come, worldwide energy consumption will increase. What are the two main reasons for this?

3. The average rate of energy consumption per person in the United States is about how many times the average in China: twice, three times, four times, six times?

4. List the fossil fuels in the order in which they will probably be used up.

5. Explain how sunlight is responsible for these energy sources: food, wood, water power, wind power, fossil fuels.

6. What energy sources cannot be traced to sunlight falling on the earth?

4.3 Global Warming

7. Approximately what proportion of the world's population lives on or near coasts and so may be under future threat from rising sea level?

8. (a) Give two reasons why global warming is causing sea level to rise. (b) What is the minimum sea-level rise expected by 2100: 10 cm, 50 cm, 1 m, 10 m?

9. Once the polar ice sheets have melted beyond a certain amount, melting will continue even if CO_2 emissions stop rising. Why?

10. The oceans as well as the atmosphere are growing warmer. What does this imply for tropical storms such as hurricanes?

11. When was the last time world temperatures were as high as they are likely to be in 2100 if current rates of CO_2 emission continue: hundreds of years ago, thousands of years ago, millions of years ago?

4.4 Carbon Dioxide and the Greenhouse Effect

12. Every body of matter radiates light. What is characteristic of light radiated by something very hot, such as the sun? Of light radiated by something at ordinary temperatures, such as the earth's surface?

13. What is the nature of the greenhouse effect in the earth's atmosphere?

14. List the chief greenhouse gases in the atmosphere. What property do they share?

15. About half the CO_2 from burning fossil fuels enters the atmosphere. What becomes of the rest?

16. (a) Why is deforestation so important in global warming? (b) In round numbers, which proportion of worldwide greenhouse gas emissions is due to deforestation: 5 percent, 10 percent, 20 percent, 40 percent?

17. List the fossil fuels in the order in which they contribute to world CO_2 emissions.

4.5 Liquid Fuels

18. What fuel liberates the most energy per gram when it burns? What is produced when it burns?

19. Most of the world's oil is used as a fuel for what purpose?

20. How do the oil reserves in tar sands compare with the reserves of ordinary crude oil? What are some of the disadvantages of tar sand oil?

21. What is regenerative braking and what kinds of cars can make use of it? What is the advantage of regenerative braking?

22. What are some of the reasons why the average fuel efficiency of cars in the United States is the lowest in the world?

4.6 Natural Gas

23. The amount of CO_2 emitted per kilowatt-hour of electricity by a gas-fired power plant is about half that emitted by a coal-fired plant. What do you think is the reason that coal-fired plants are much more common?

24. Why is natural gas rarely used as a vehicle fuel?

25. What is shale gas? Methane clathrate? Where are they found and why is great interest being shown in them?

4.7 Coal

26. What are the chief advantages of coal as a fuel? The chief disadvantage?

27. Coal is responsible for approximately which proportion of the electricity generated in the United States: one-quarter, one-half, three-quarters?

28. Coal smoke contains sulfur and mercury. Why are they harmful?

29. Why do you think that, per joule of energy liberated when they are burned, coal produces more carbon dioxide than the other fossil fuels?

30. (a) List the desirable aspects of coal gasification, the process in which coal is turned into a mixture of gases called syngas. (b) Is there any way to prevent the CO_2 emitted when coal is burned from entering the atmosphere? If so, why is it not widely used?

4.8 A Nuclear World?

31. What is the basic difference between nuclear fission and nuclear fusion? In what way are they similar?

32. What role does uranium play in nuclear energy production? What is the uranium supply situation?

33. How does a nuclear power plant produce electricity?

34. Explain why no nuclear power plants were planned in the United States between 1979 and now but are currently being considered for construction.

35. List the potential advantages of fusion energy.

36. What stands in the way of the immediate use of nuclear fusion as a commercial energy source?

37. Is there anywhere outside of laboratories where fusion energy is produced today?

4.9 Clean Energy I

4.10 Clean Energy II

38. Give examples of clean sources that can supply energy continuously and examples of others whose output varies with time of day and weather conditions.

39. Of the various clean energy sources, which provides the most energy worldwide today?

40. Give several reasons why fossil-fuel energy is cheaper than energy from most renewable sources.

41. What does a photovoltaic cell do? What is another name for it?

42. What advantages do photovoltaic cells have for installation in remote regions?

43. Instead of a new 500-MW coal-fired power plant, a wind farm of turbines rated at 2 MW maximum output each is to be installed. If the average turbine output is 40 percent of the maximum, how many turbines are needed?

44. Explain how tide and wave energies can be captured.

45. (a) What major advantage does geothermal energy have over solar, wind, tidal, and wave energies? (b) What is its chief disadvantage?

46. List four practical ways to store energy from noncontinuous energy sources.

4.11 Hydrogen and Fuel Cells

47. When hydrogen combines with oxygen, a great deal of energy is liberated with only water as the product. What are the two main factors that hold back wider use of hydrogen as a fuel?

48. What are the advantages and disadvantages of hydrogen fuel cells?

4.12 Biofuels

49. (a) Why is corn not regarded as an ideal choice for producing ethanol? (b) Cellulose is apparently a better choice. Why is it not in wide use?

50. Why are algae so interesting as a way of producing biodiesel fuel?

4.13 Conservation

51. A long-term goal for energy efficiency envisions an average use of 65 GJ per person per year. To what continuous power in kilowatts does this correspond?

4.14 What Governments Must Do

52. A major obstacle to a worldwide agreement on reducing greenhouse gas emissions is that the developing countries want the developed ones to do what three things?

53. Explain the cap-and-trade system for controlling CO_2 emissions. Is there an alternative means of control?

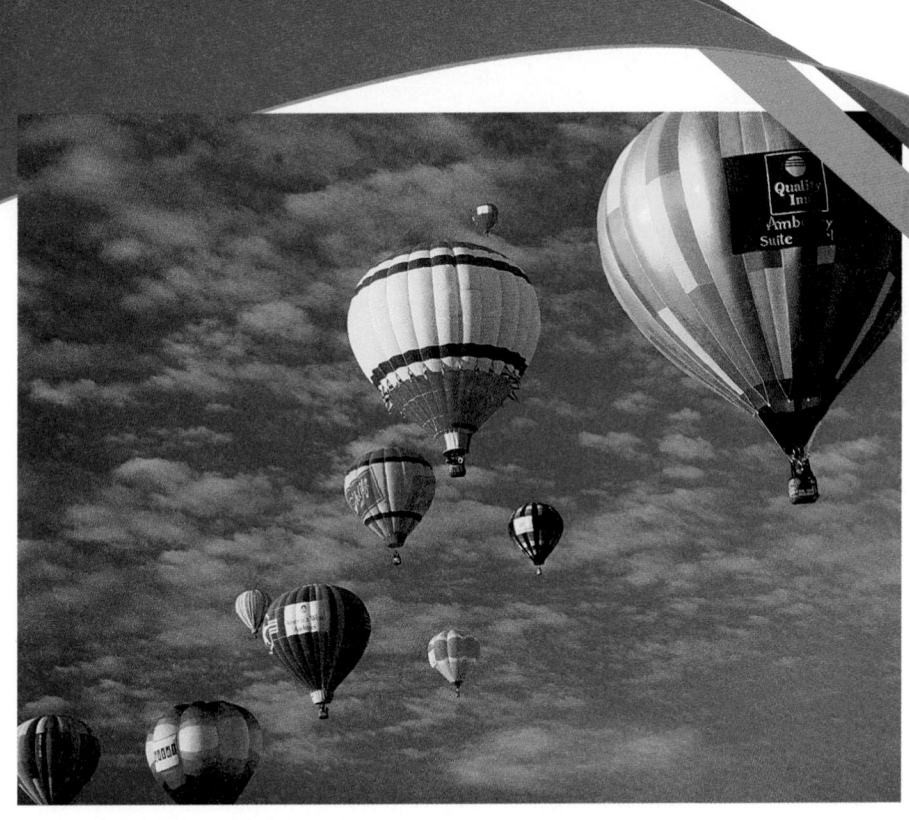

In 1999, a hot-air balloon circled the earth nonstop.

5

Matter and Heat

GOALS

When you have finished this chapter you should be able to complete the goals • given for each section below:

Temperature and Heat

5.1 Temperature
Putting Numbers to Hot and Cold
• Distinguish between temperature and heat.
• Describe how various thermometers work.
• Convert temperatures from the celsius to the fahrenheit scale and vice versa.

5.2 Heat
Different Substances Need Different Amounts of Heat for the Same Temperature Change
• Define the specific heat capacity of a substance and use it to relate the heat added to or removed from a given mass of the substance to a temperature change it undergoes.

5.3 Metabolic Energy
The Energy of People and Animals
• Discuss the significance of the metabolic rate of an animal and how to convert between kilocalories and kilojoules.

Fluids

5.4 Density
A Characteristic Property of Every Material
• Define density and calculate the mass of a body of matter given its density and volume.

5.5 Pressure
How Much of a Squeeze

• Define pressure and account for the increase in pressure with depth in a liquid or gas.

5.6 Buoyancy
Sink or Swim
• State Archimedes' principle and explain its origin.

5.7 The Gas Laws
Ideal Gases Obey Them
• Use Boyle's law to relate pressure and volume changes in a gas at constant temperature.
• Use Charles's law to relate temperature and volume changes in a gas at constant pressure.
• Show how the ideal gas law is related to Boyle's law and Charles's law.

Kinetic Theory of Matter

5.8 Kinetic Theory of Gases
Why Gases Behave as They Do
• State the three basic assumptions of the kinetic theory of gases.

5.9 Molecular Motion and Temperature
The Faster the Molecules, the Higher the Temperature
• Discuss the connection between temperature and molecular motion.
• Explain the significance of the absolute temperature scale and the meaning of absolute zero.

5.10 Heat Transfer
Three Mechanisms
• Describe the three different ways by which heat can be transferred from one place to another.

Changes of State

5.11 Liquids and Solids
Intermolecular Forces Hold Them Together
• Account for the differences of gases, liquids, and solids in terms of the forces between their molecules.

5.12 Evaporation and Boiling
Liquid into Gas
• Distinguish between evaporation and boiling and between a gas and a vapor.
• Explain what is meant by heat of vaporization.

5.13 Melting
Solid into Liquid
• Explain what is meant by heat of fusion and discuss why it is less than heat of vaporization for the same substance.
• State the meaning of sublimation.

Energy Transformations

5.14 Heat Engines
Turning Heat into Work
• Discuss why heat engines cannot be perfectly efficient.
• Compare heat engines and refrigerators.

5.15 Thermodynamics
You Can't Win
• State the two laws of thermodynamics.

5.16 Fate of the Universe
Order into Disorder

5.17 Entropy
The Arrow of Time
• Relate entropy to the second law of thermodynamics.

Suppose our microscopes had no limit to their power, so that we could examine a drop of water at any magnification we like. What would we find if the drop were enlarged a million or more times? Would we still see a clear, structureless liquid? If not, what else?

The answer is that, on a very small scale of size, our drop of water consists of billions of tiny separate particles. Indeed, *all* matter does, whether in the form of a solid, a liquid, or a gas. This much was suspected over 2000 years ago in ancient Greece. Modern science has not only confirmed this suspicion but extended it: the particles that make up all matter are in constant random motion, and the kinetic energy of this motion is what constitutes heat. In everyday life, matter shows no direct sign of either the particles or their motion. However, plenty of indirect signs support this picture, and we shall consider some of them in this chapter.

Temperature and Heat

Temperature and heat are easy to confuse. Certainly the higher its temperature, the more heat something contains. But we cannot say that an object at one temperature contains more heat than another object at a lower temperature just because of the temperature difference. A cup of boiling water is at a higher temperature than a pailful of cool water, but the pailful of cool water would melt more ice (Fig. 5-1). And the same masses of different substances at the same temperature contain different amounts of heat. A kilogram of boiling water can melt 32 times as much ice as 1 kg of gold at the temperature of the water, for instance.

5.1   Temperature

Putting Numbers to Hot and Cold

Temperature, like force, is a physical quantity that means something to us in terms of our sense impressions. And, as with force, a certain amount of discussion is needed before a statement of exactly what temperature signifies can be given. Such a discussion appears later in this chapter. For the time being, we can simply regard temperature as that which gives rise to sensations of hot and cold.

A **thermometer** is a device that measures temperature. Most substances expand when heated and shrink when cooled (Fig. 5-2), and the thermometers we use in everyday life are designed around this property of matter.

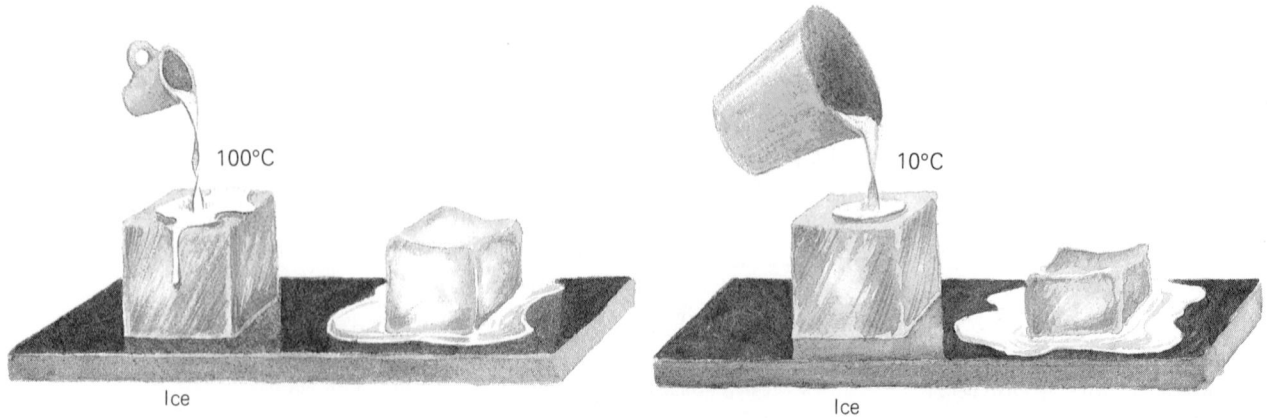

Figure 5-1   The heat content of a given substance depends upon both its mass and its temperature. A pail of cool water contains more heat than a cup of boiling water.

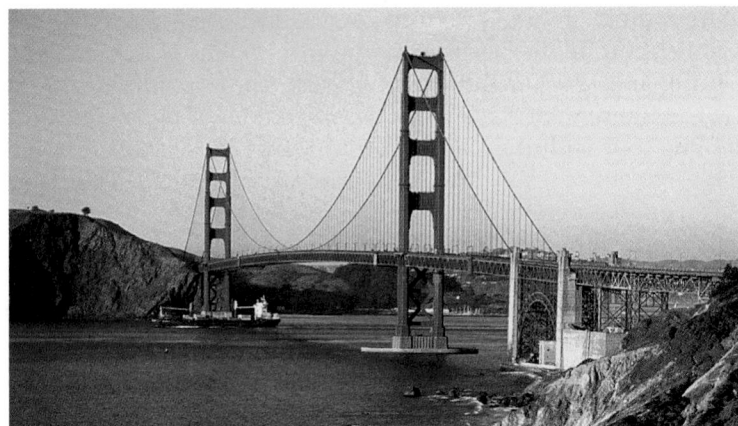

Figure 5-2 Allowance must be made in the design of a bridge for its expansion and contraction as the temperature changes. The Golden Gate Bridge in San Francisco varies by over a meter in length between summer and winter.

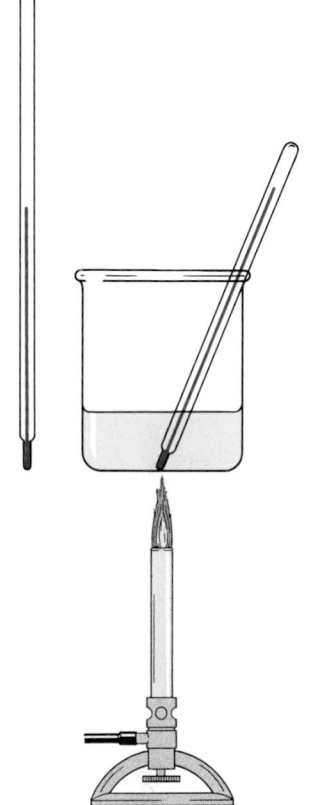

More precisely, they are based upon the fact that different materials react to a given temperature change to different extents. The familiar liquid-in-glass thermometer (Fig. 5-3) works because a liquid expands more than glass when heated and contracts more than glass when cooled. Thus the length of the liquid column in the glass tube provides a measure of the temperature around the bulb.

Another common thermometer used for high temperatures, such as in ovens and furnaces, makes use of the different rates of expansion of different kinds of metals. Two straight strips of dissimilar metals are joined together at a particular temperature (Fig. 5-4). At higher temperatures the bimetallic strip bends so that the metal with the greater expansion is on the outside of the curve, and at lower temperatures it bends in the opposite direction. In each case the exact amount of bending depends upon the temperature. Bimetallic strips of this kind are used in the **thermostats** that switch on and off heating systems, refrigerators, and freezers at preset temperatures.

Thermal expansion is not the only property of matter that can be used to make a thermometer. As another example, the color and amount of light emitted by an object vary with its temperature. A poker thrust into a fire first glows dull red, then successively bright red, orange, and yellow. Finally, if the poker achieves a high enough temperature, it becomes "white hot." The color of the light given off by a glowing object is thus a measure of its temperature (Figs. 5-5 and 5-6). This property is used by astronomers to determine the temperatures of stars.

Figure 5-3 A liquid-in-glass thermometer. Mercury or a colored alcohol solution responds to temperature changes to a greater extent than glass does, and so the length of the liquid column is a measure of the temperature of the thermometer bulb.

Figure 5-4 A bimetallic strip thermometer. No matter on which side the heat is applied, the bend is away from the more expansive metal. The higher the temperature, the greater the deflection. At low temperatures the deflection is in the opposite direction. Steel and copper are often used in bimetallic strips; the steel expands less when heated.

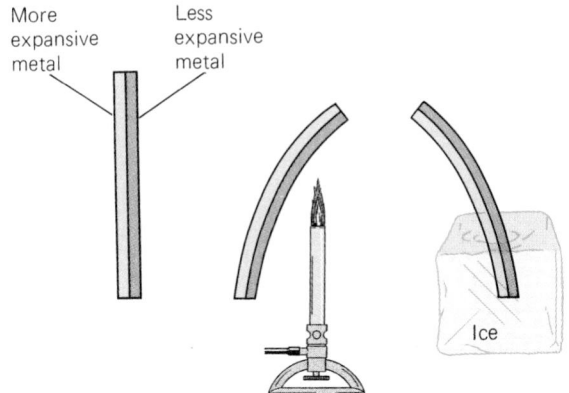

More expansive metal   Less expansive metal

Ice

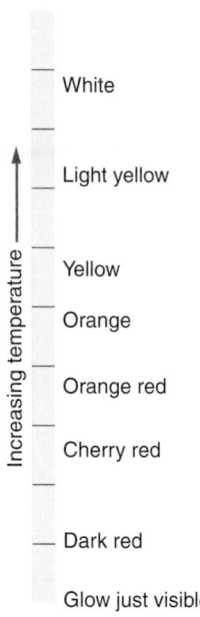

White

Light yellow

Yellow

Orange

Orange red

Cherry red

Dark red

Glow just visible

Increasing temperature →

Figure 5-5   The color of an object hot enough to glow varies with its temperature as shown here.

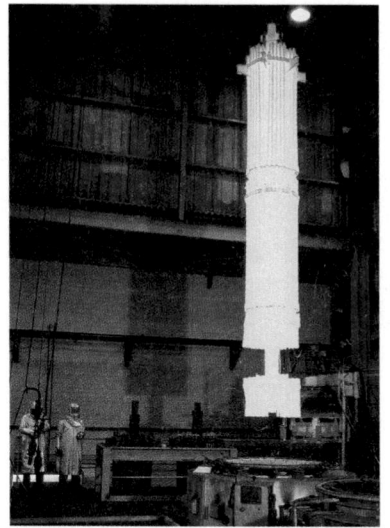

Figure 5-6   The color and brightness of an object heated until it glows, such as this steel beam, depends on its temperature. An object that glows white is hotter than one that glows red and gives off more light as well.

Temperature Scales   Two temperature scales are used in the United States. On the **Fahrenheit scale** the freezing point of water is 32° and the boiling point of water is 212°. On the **Celsius scale** these points are 0° and 100° (Fig. 5-7). The Fahrenheit scale is used only in a few English-speaking countries that cling to it with the same obstinacy that preserves the equally awkward British system of units. The rest of the world, and all scientists, use the more convenient Celsius (or centigrade) scale.

To go from a Fahrenheit temperature T_F to a Celsius temperature T_C, and vice versa, we note that 180°F separates the freezing and boiling points of water on the Fahrenheit scale. On the Celsius scale, however, the difference is 100°C. Therefore Fahrenheit degrees are $\frac{100}{180}$, or $\frac{5}{9}$, as large as Celsius degrees:

5 Celsius degrees = 9 Fahrenheit degrees

Taking into account that the freezing point of water is 0°C = 32°F, we see that

$$\text{Fahrenheit temperature} = T_F = \tfrac{9}{5}T_C + 32° \qquad 5\text{-}1$$

$$\text{Celsius temperature} = T_C = \tfrac{5}{9}(T_F - 32°) \qquad 5\text{-}2$$

Thus the Celsius equivalent of the normal body temperature of 98.6°F is

$$T_C = \tfrac{5}{9}(98.6° - 32.0°) = \tfrac{5}{9}(66.6°) = 37.0°C$$

5.2   Heat

Different Substances Need Different Amounts of Heat for the Same Temperature Change

The **heat** in a body of matter is the sum of the kinetic energies of all the separate particles that make up the body. The more energy these particles have, the more heat the body contains, and the higher its temperature. Thus the heat content of a body can also be called its **internal energy.**

Since heat is a form of energy, the joule is the proper unit for it. The amount of heat needed to raise or lower the temperature of 1 kg of a substance by 1°C depends on the nature of the substance. In the case of water, 4.2 kJ of heat is required per kilogram per °C (Fig. 5-8). To heat 1 kg of water from, say, 20°C to 60°C means raising its temperature by 40°C. The amount of heat that must be added is therefore (1 kg)(4.2 kJ/ kg · °C) (40°C) = 168 kJ.

For a given temperature change, liquid water must have more heat added to or taken away from it per kilogram than nearly all other materials. For instance, to change the temperature of 1 kg of ice by 1°C, we must transfer to

---

Example 5.1

In 1983 a temperature of −89°C was measured at a Russian research station in Antarctica, a record low for the earth's surface. What is the Fahrenheit equivalent of this temperature?

Solution
From Eq. 5-1

$$T_F = \tfrac{9}{5}(-89°C) + 32° = -160° + 32° = -128°F$$

On both scales, brrr.

or from it 2.1 kJ, about half as much as for water. To do the same for 1 kg of gold takes only 0.13 kJ.

Specific Heat   The **specific heat capacity** (or just **specific heat**) of a substance is the amount of heat that must be added to or removed from 1 kg of the substance in order to change its temperature by 1°C. The symbol of specific heat is c and its unit is the kJ/kg · °C. Thus the specific heat of water is c_{water} = 4.2 kJ/kg · °C. Table 5-1 gives the specific heats of various substances. We note that metals have fairly low specific heats, as we saw for gold, which means that relatively little heat is needed to change their temperatures by a given amount compared with other materials of the same mass.

When an amount of heat Q is added to or removed from a mass m of a substance whose specific heat is c, the resulting temperature change ΔT (Δ is the Greek capital letter "delta" and in physics usually means "change in") is related to Q, m, and ΔT by the formula

$$Q = mc\,\Delta T \qquad\qquad 5\text{-}3$$

Heat transferred = (mass)(specific heat)(temperature change)

The examples show how Eq. 5-3 can be used.

Example 5.2

A person decides to lose weight by eating only cold food. A 100-g piece of apple pie yields about 1500 kJ of energy when eaten. If its specific heat is 1.7 kJ/kg · °C, how much less is its energy content at 5°C than at 25°C?

Solution

Since ΔT here is 25°C − 5°C = 20°C, the energy difference is

$$Q = mc\Delta T = (0.1\ \text{kg})(1.7\ \text{kJ/kg} \cdot °\text{C})(20°\text{C}) = 3.4\ \text{kJ}$$

The saving amounts to (3.4 kJ)/(1500 kJ) = 0.0023 = 0.23 percent of the total energy provided by eating the pie—this is not really a practical path to becoming thin.

Btu

In the United States, though no longer in Great Britain, the **British Thermal Unit** (Btu) is sometimes used as a unit of heat. The Btu is defined as the heat needed to raise the temperature of 1 lb of water by 1°F; 1 Btu = 1.054 kJ. Another common heat unit, the kilocalorie, is discussed in Sec. 5.3.

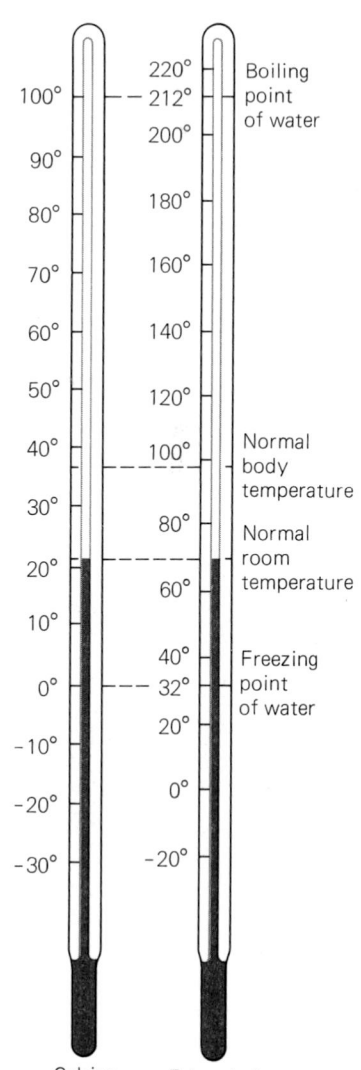

Figure 5-7   Comparison of the Celsius and Fahrenheit temperature scales.

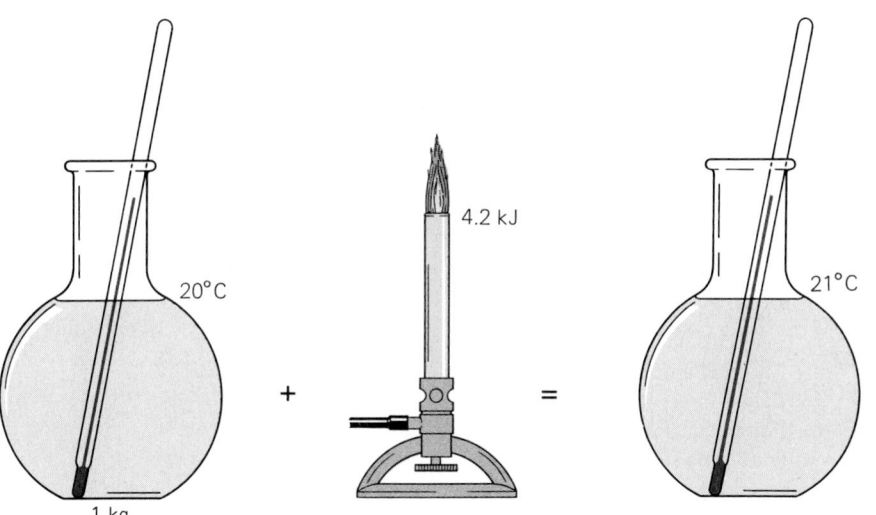

Figure 5-8   To raise the temperature of 1 kg of water by 1°C, 4.2 kJ of heat must be added to it. The same amount of heat must be removed to cool the water by 1°C.

Table 5-1	Some Specific Heats
Substance	**Specific Heat, kJ/kg · °C**
Alcohol (ethyl)	2.4
Aluminum	0.92
Concrete	2.9
Copper	0.39
Glass	0.84
Gold	0.13
Human body	3.5
Ice	2.1
Iron	0.46
Steam	2.0
Water	4.2
Wood	1.8

Example 5.3

Find the difference in temperature between the water at the top and at the bottom of a waterfall 50 m high. Assume that all the potential energy lost by the water in falling goes into heat.

Solution

The potential energy of a mass m of water at the top of the waterfall is PE = mgh, where h = 50 m is the height of the waterfall. If this energy is converted into the heat Q, then, since for water c = 4.2 kJ/kg · °C = 4200 J/kg · °C,

$$PE = Q$$
$$mgh = mc \, \Delta T$$

$$\Delta T = \frac{gh}{c} = \frac{(9.8 \text{ m/s}^2)(50 \text{ m})}{4200 \text{ J/kg} \cdot °C} = 0.12°C$$

Example 5.4

How long will a 1.2-kW electric kettle take to heat 0.8 kg of water from 20°C to 100°C?

Solution

The heat supplied by the kettle in the time t is $Pt = Q$, where P is the kettle's power of 1.2 kW. We proceed as follows, with ΔT = 100°C − 20°C = 80°C:

$$Pt = Q = mc \, \Delta T$$

$$t = \frac{mc \, \Delta T}{P} = \frac{(0.8 \text{ kg})(4.2 \text{ kJ/kg} \cdot °C)(80°C)}{1.2 \text{ kW}} = 224 \text{ s} = 3.7 \text{ min}$$

5.3   Metabolic Energy

The Energy of People and Animals

Metabolism refers to the biochemical processes by which the energy content of the food an animal eats is liberated. Table 5-2 lists the energy contents of some common foods. The unit is the **kilocalorie** (kcal), which is the amount

Table 5-2	Energy Contents of Some Common Foods (1 kcal = 4.2 kJ)
Food	**kcal**
1 raw onion	5
1 dill pickle	15
6 asparagus	20
1 gum drop	35
1 poached egg	75
8 raw oysters	100
1 banana	120
1 cupcake	130
1 broiled hamburger patty	150
1 glass milk	165
1 cup bean soup	190
$\frac{1}{2}$ cup tuna salad	220
1 ice cream soda	325
$\frac{1}{2}$ broiled chicken	350
1 lamb chop	420

Metabolism and Size

A large animal has more surface area than a small one and so is capable of a higher power output. However, a large animal also has more mass than a small one, and because an animal's mass goes up faster with its size than its skin area does, its metabolic rate per kilogram decreases. Typical basal metabolic rates, which correspond to an animal resting, are 5.2 W/kg for a pigeon, 1.2 W/kg for a person, and 0.67 W/kg for a cow. African elephants partly overcome the limitation of the small surface/ mass ratio of their huge bodies by their enormous ears, which help them get rid of metabolic heat. Most birds are small because, with increasing size, a bird's metabolic rate (and hence power output) per kilogram decreases while the work it must perform per kilogram to fly stays the same. Large birds such as ostriches and emus are not notable for their flying ability (Fig. 5-9).

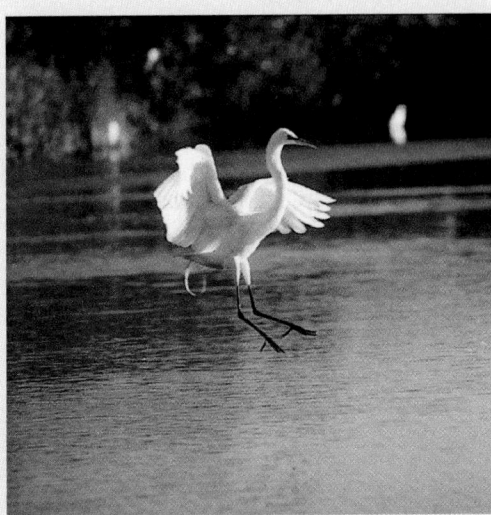

Figure 5-9 Egret coming in for a landing in the Florida Everglades. Birds are limited in size because the larger an animal is, the less is its ability to dissipate waste metabolic energy per unit of body mass.

Example 5.5

A 50-kg girl eats a banana and she then proposes to work off its 120 kcal energy content by climbing a hill. If her body is 10 percent efficient, how high must she climb?

Solution

From Sec. 3-1 we know that the amount of work needed to raise something whose mass is m through the height h is $W = mgh$. Here the available energy is 10 percent of (120 kcal)(4.2 kJ/kcal) = 504 kJ, so $W = (0.10)(504 \text{ kJ}) = 50.4 \text{ kJ} = 50.4 \times 10^3$ J, and the height is

$$h = \frac{W}{mg} = \frac{50.4 \times 10^3 \text{ J}}{(50 \text{ kg})(9.8 \text{ m/s}^2)} = 102 \text{ m}$$

of heat needed to change the temperature of 1 kg of water by 1°C. Thus 1 kcal = 4.2 kJ. The "calorie" used by dieticians is actually the kilocalorie.

The proportion of metabolic energy that is converted to mechanical work by muscular activity is not very high, only 10 or 20 percent. (An electric motor with the same power output as a person is typically 50 percent efficient, and larger electric motors are more efficient still.) The rest of the energy goes into heat, most of which escapes through the animal's skin. The maximum power output an animal is capable of depends upon its maximum metabolic rate, which in turn depends upon its ability to dissipate the resulting heat, and therefore upon its surface area.

When an animal is active, its metabolic rate may be much greater than its basal rate. A 70-kg person, to give an example, has a basal metabolic rate of around 80 W. When the person is reading or doing light work while sitting, the rate will go up to perhaps 125 W. Walking means a metabolic rate of 300 W or so, and running hard increases it to as much as 1200 W. The highest known metabolic rates per kilogram are those of the flight muscles of insects.

An animal's brain as well as its muscles uses energy to function. Your brain, with only 2 percent of your body's mass, uses 20 to 25 percent of your metabolic energy—thinking is hard work! The proportion is only about 9 percent for monkeys and 5 percent for cats and dogs.

When the intake of energy from food exceeds a person's metabolic needs, the excess goes into additional tissue: muscle if there is enough physical activity, otherwise fat. The energy stored in fat is available should metabolic needs not be provided by food at a later time.

Fluids

The particles of matter in a solid vibrate around fixed positions, so the solid has a definite size and shape (Fig. 5-10). In a liquid, the particles are about as far apart as those in a solid but are able to move about. Hence a liquid sample has a definite volume but flows to fit its container. In a gas, the particles can move freely, so a gas has neither a definite volume nor shape but fills whatever container it is in.

Liquids and gases are together called **fluids** because they flow readily. This ability has some interesting consequences. One is buoyancy, which permits objects to float in a fluid under certain conditions—a balloon in air, a ship in water. In order to understand how buoyancy comes about, we must first look into the ideas of density and pressure.

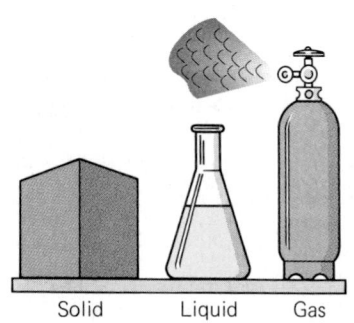

Solid   Liquid   Gas

Figure 5-10   Solids, liquids, and gases. A solid maintains its shape and volume no matter where it is placed; a liquid assumes the shape of its container while maintaining its volume; a gas expands indefinitely unless stopped by the walls of a container.

5.4   Density

A Characteristic Property of Every Material

The **density** of a material is its mass per unit volume:

$$d = \frac{m}{V} \quad \textit{Density} \qquad 5\text{-}4$$

$$\text{Density} = \frac{\text{mass}}{\text{volume}}$$

When we say that lead is a "heavy" metal and aluminum a "light" one, what we really mean is that lead has a higher density than aluminum: the density

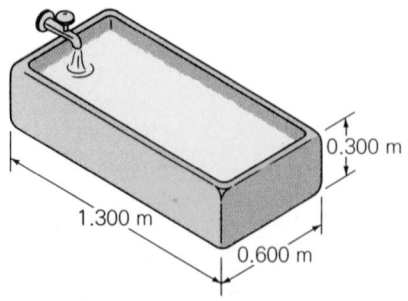

Figure 5-11   The volume of water in this bathtub is equal to the product (length)(width)(height).

Example 5.6

Find the mass of the water in a bathtub whose interior is 1.300 m long and 0.600 m wide and that is filled to a height of 0.300 m (Fig. 5-11).

Solution
The water's volume is

$$V = (\text{length})(\text{width})(\text{height})$$

$$= (1.300 \text{ m})(0.600 \text{ m})(0.300 \text{ m}) = 0.234 \text{ m}^3$$

According to Table 5-3 the density of water is 1000 kg/m^3. Rewriting $d = m/V$ as $m = dV$ gives

$$\text{Mass} = (\text{density})(\text{volume})$$

$$m = dV = \left(1000\frac{\text{kg}}{\text{m}^3}\right)(0.234 \text{ m}^3) = 234 \text{ kg}$$

The weight of this amount of water is a little over 500 lb.

Table 5-3	Densities of Various Substances at Room Temperature and Atmospheric Pressure		
Substance	**Density, kg/m³**	**Substance**	**Density, kg/m³**
Air	1.3	Hydrogen	0.09
Alcohol (ethyl)	7.9×10^2	Ice	9.2×10^2
Aluminum	2.7×10^3	Iron and steel	7.8×10^3
Balsa wood	1.3×10^2	Lead	1.1×10^4
Concrete	2.3×10^3	Mercury	1.4×10^4
Gasoline	6.8×10^2	Oak	7.2×10^2
Gold	1.9×10^4	Water, pure	1.00×10^3
Helium	0.18	Water, sea	1.03×10^3

of lead is 11,300 kg per cubic meter (kg/m³) whereas that of aluminum is only 2700 kg/m³, a quarter as much.

Although the proper SI unit of density is the kg/m³, densities are often given instead in g/cm³ (grams per cubic centimeter), where 1 g/cm³ = 1000 kg/m³ = 10^3 kg/m³. Thus the density of lead can also be expressed as 11.3 g/cm³. Table 5-3 lists the densities of some common substances.

5.5 Pressure

How Much of a Squeeze

We next look into what is meant by **pressure**. When a force F acts perpendicular to a surface whose area is A, the pressure acting on the surface is the ratio between the force and the area:

$$p = \frac{F}{A} \quad \textit{Pressure} \qquad 5\text{-}5$$

$$\text{Pressure} = \frac{\text{force}}{\text{area}}$$

The SI unit of pressure is the **pascal** (Pa), where

$$1 \text{ pascal} = 1 \text{ Pa} = 1 \text{ newton/meter}^2$$

This unit honors the French scientist and philosopher Blaise Pascal (1623–1662). The pascal is a very small unit: the pressure exerted by pushing really hard on a table with your thumb is about a million pascals. For this reason the **kilopascal** (kPa) is often used, where 1 kPa = 1000 Pa = 10^3 Pa = 0.145 lb/in².

Example 5.7

A 60-kg woman balances on the heel of one shoe, whose area is 0.5 cm² (Fig. 5-12). How much pressure does she exert on the floor?

Solution

The force exerted by the heel of the woman's shoe is her weight, so $F = mg = (60 \text{ kg})$ $(9.8 \text{ m/s}^2) = 588 \text{ N}$. Since 1 cm = 10^{-2} m, the area of the heel is $A = (0.5 \text{ cm}^2)$ $(10^{-4} \text{ m}^2/\text{cm}^2) = 5 \times 10^{-5}$ m², and the pressure on the floor is

$$p = \frac{F}{A} = \frac{588 \text{ N}}{5 \times 10^{-5} \text{ m}^2} = 1.2 \times 10^7 \text{ N/m}^2 = 12 \text{ MPa}$$

This is 40 times the pressure the feet of the 35-ton dinosaur apatosaurus are estimated to have exerted on the ground.

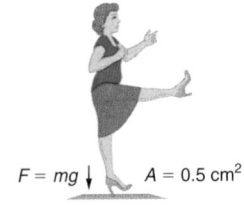

$F = mg \downarrow \qquad A = 0.5 \text{ cm}^2$

Figure 5-12 Pressure is force per unit area. The heel of this 60-kg woman exerts a pressure of 12 MPa on the floor. Being stepped on by such a heel is not recommended.

Blood Pressure

The pressures that force blood through the lungs and the rest of the body are produced by the heart (Fig. 5-13). The heart consists of two pumps, called **ventricles.** The contraction and relaxation of the muscular walls of the ventricles take the place of the piston strokes of an ordinary pump. The right ventricle pumps blood from the veins through the lungs, where it absorbs oxygen from the air that has been breathed in and gives up carbon dioxide. The oxygenated blood then goes to the more powerful left ventricle, which pumps it via the aorta and the arteries to the rest of the body. A typical rate of blood flow in a resting person is 6 L/min.

Arterial blood pressures are measured by using an inflatable cuff that is pumped up until the flow of blood stops, as monitored by a stethoscope (Fig. 5-14). Air is then let out of the cuff until the flow just begins again, which is recognized by a gurgling sound in the stethoscope. The pressure at this point is called **systolic** and corresponds to the maximum pressure the heart produces in the arteries. Next, more air is let out until the gurgling stops, which corresponds to normal blood flow. The pressure now, called **diastolic,** corresponds to the arterial pressure between strokes of the heart.

Blood pressures are usually expressed in *torr,* which is the pressure exerted by a column of mercury 1 mm high; 1 torr = 133 Pa. In a healthy person the systolic and diastolic blood pressures are about 120 and 80 torr, respectively.

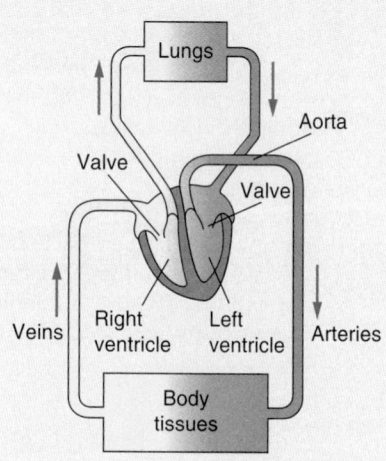

Figure 5-13   The human circulatory system.

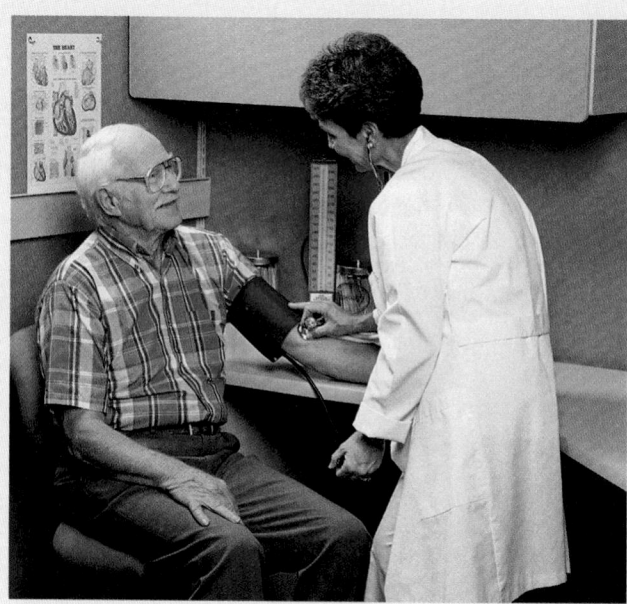

Figure 5-14   Measuring blood pressure.

Example 5.8

Before a storm people in a house closed its doors and windows so tightly that the air pressure inside remained at 101 kPa even when the outside pressure fell to 98 kPa. How much force acted on a window 80 cm high and 120 cm wide?

Solution

The area of the window is $A = (0.80 \text{ m})(1.2 \text{ m}) = 0.96 \text{ m}^2$. The net pressure on the window was the difference Δp between the inside pressure (which gives rise to an outward force) of 101 kPa and the outside pressure (which gives rise to an inward force) of 98 kPa, so $\Delta p = 3 \text{ kPa} = 3 \times 10^3 \text{ Pa}$. Therefore the outward force on the window was

$$F = \Delta pA = (3 \times 10^3 \text{ Pa})(0.96 \text{ m}^2) = 2880 \text{ N}$$

which corresponds to 636 lb! This may well have been enough to break the window or push it out of its frame. Evidently a building should not be sealed when a large change in pressure due to a storm is forecast.

Pressure in a Fluid   Pressure is a useful quantity where fluids are concerned for these reasons:

1. The forces that a fluid exerts on the walls of its container, and those that the walls exert on the fluid, always act perpendicular to the walls.
2. The force exerted by the pressure in a fluid is the same in all directions at a given depth.
3. An external pressure exerted on a fluid is transmitted uniformly throughout the fluid.

These properties mean that we can transmit a force from one place to another by applying pressure with a pump to a fluid at one end of a tube and then allowing the fluid at the other end of the tube to push against a movable piston. Machines in which forces are transmitted by liquids are called **hydraulic** (Fig. 5-15), and those that use compressed air are called **pneumatic.**

Pressure and Depth   The pressure in a fluid increases with depth because of the weight of the overlying fluid. The amount of the increase is proportional to both the depth and the fluid density: the greater these are, the greater the pressure. In a tire pump, the air inside is under greater pressure at the bottom of the cylinder than at the top because of the weight of the air in the cylinder. In the case of a tire pump, the pressure difference is very small, of course, but elsewhere it can be significant. At sea level on the earth, for instance, the pressure due to the weight of the air above us averages 101 kPa, nearly 15 lb/in^2. This corresponds to a force of 10.1 N on every square centimeter of our bodies. We are not aware of this pressure because the pressures inside our bodies are the same. Atmospheric pressures are measured with instruments called **barometers,** one type of which is shown in Fig. 5-16.

Because pressure increases with depth, most submarines cannot go down more than a few hundred meters without the danger of collapsing. At a depth of 10 km in the ocean, the pressure is about 1000 times sea-level atmospheric pressure, enough to compress water by 3 percent of its volume. Fish that live at such depths are not crushed for the same reason we can survive the pressure at the bottom of our ocean of air: pressures inside their bodies are kept equal to pressures outside.

Scuba divers carry tanks of compressed air with regulator valves that provide air at the same pressure as the water around them (Fig. 5-17). ("Scuba" stands for *s*elf-*c*ontained *u*nderwater *b*reathing *a*pparatus.) When a diver returns to the surface, he or she must breathe out continuously to allow the air pressure in the lungs to decrease at the same rate as the external pressure decreases. If this is not done, the pressure difference may burst the lungs. When brought to the surface quickly, deep-sea fish sometimes explode because of their high internal pressures.

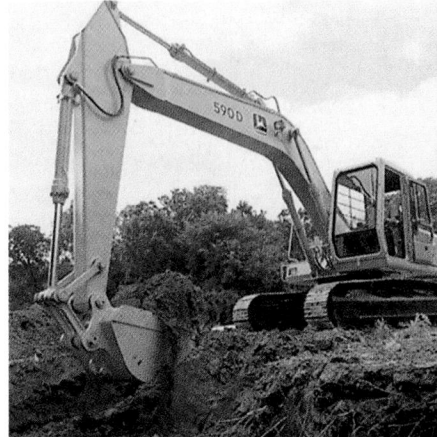

Figure 5-15   A hydraulic ram converts pressure in a liquid into an applied force. The pressure is provided by an engine-driven pump.

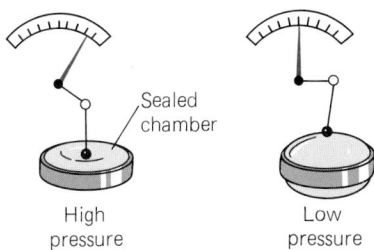

Figure 5-16   An aneroid barometer. The flexible ends of a sealed metal chamber are pushed in by a high atmospheric pressure. Under low atmospheric pressure, the air inside the chamber pushes the ends out.

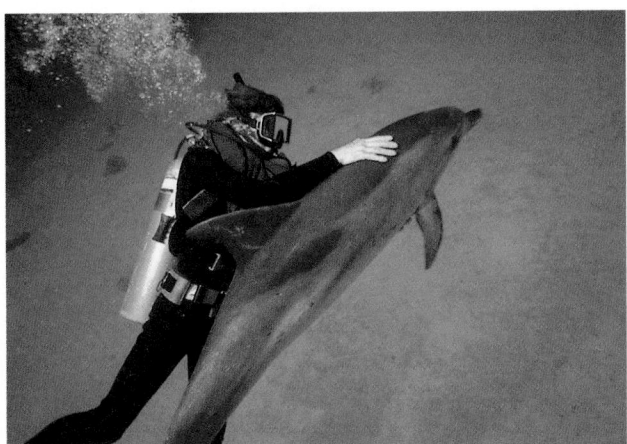

Figure 5-17   Air at high pressure in the tank of a scuba diver is reduced by a regulator valve to the pressure at the depth of the water. The diver must wear lead weights to overcome his or her buoyancy. The deeper the diver goes, the greater the water pressure, and the faster the air in the tank is used up.

5.6 Buoyancy

Sink or Swim

An object immersed in a fluid is acted upon by an upward force that arises because pressures in a fluid increase with depth. Hence the upward force on the bottom of the object is greater than the downward force on its top. The difference between the two forces is the **buoyant force.**

Buoyancy enables balloons to float in the air and ships to float in the sea. If the buoyant force on an immersed object is equal to or greater than its weight, the object floats; if the force is less than its weight, the object sinks.

Imagine a solid object of any kind whose volume is V that is in a tank of water (Fig. 5-18). A body of water of the same size and shape in the tank is supported by a buoyant force F_b equal to its weight of $w_{water} = dVg$. The buoyant force is the result of all of the forces that the rest of the water in the tank exert on this particular body of water. This force is always upward because the pressure underneath the body of water is greater than the pressure above it. The pressures on the sides cancel one another out, as shown in the figure.

If we now replace the body of water by the solid object, the forces on the object are the same as before. The buoyant force therefore remains dVg so that

$$F_b = dVg \qquad \textit{Buoyant force} \qquad 5\text{-}6$$

In this formula, d is the density of the fluid (which need not be water, of course), V is the volume of fluid displaced by the solid object, and g is the acceleration of gravity, 9.8 m/s^2.

Archimedes' Principle Thus we have **Archimedes' principle:**

> Buoyant force on an object in a fluid = weight of fluid displaced by the object.

Archimedes' principle holds whether the object floats or sinks. If the object's weight w_{object} is greater than the buoyant force F_b, it sinks. If its weight is equal to or less than the buoyant force, it floats, in which case the volume V refers only to the part of the object that is in the fluid.

The condition for an object to float in a given fluid is that its average density be the same as or lower than the density of the fluid (Fig. 5-19). Why does a steel ship float when the density of steel is nearly 8 times that of water? The

Figure 5-18 Archimedes' principle. The buoyant force F_b on an object immersed in water (or other fluid) is equal to the weight of the body of water displaced by the object.

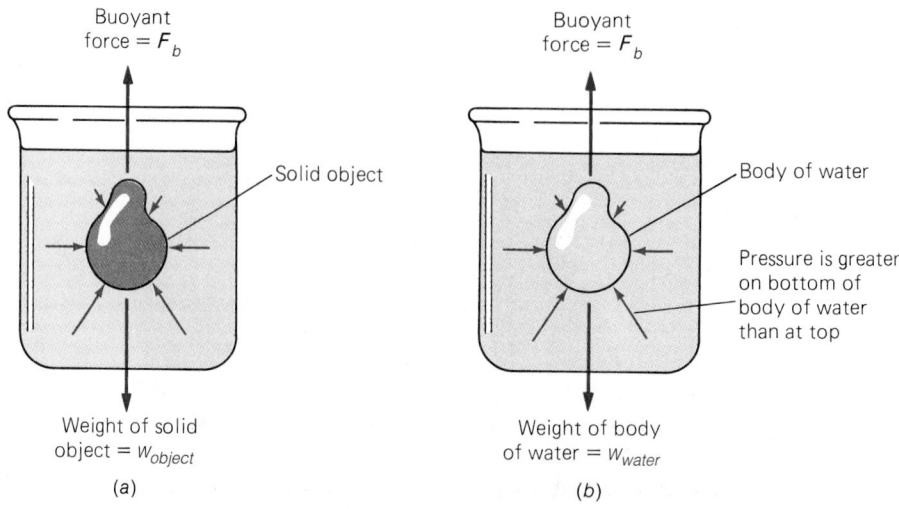

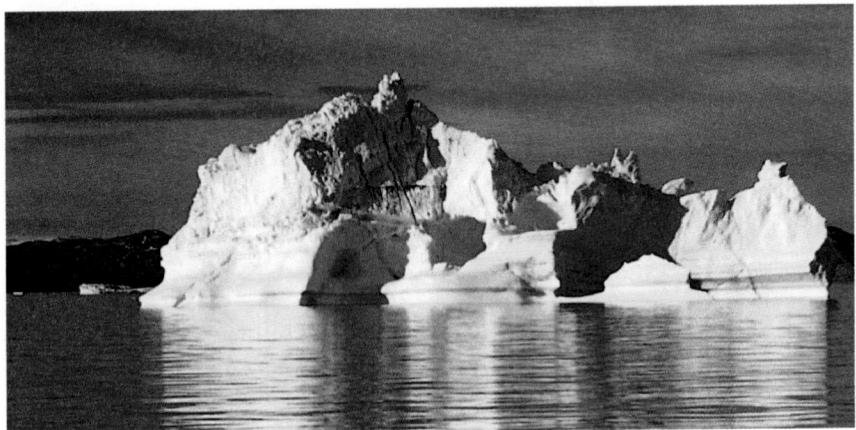

Figure 5-19 Because water expands when it freezes, ice floats. Nearly 90 percent of the volume of this iceberg near Greenland lies below the surface. An iceberg is a chunk of freshwater ice that has broken off from an ice cap, such as those that cover Greenland and Antarctica, or from a glacier at the edge of the sea.

| Example 5.9

The density of a person is slightly less than that of pure water (which is why people can float). Assuming that these densities are the same, find the buoyant force of the atmosphere on a 60-kg person.

Solution

The first step is to find the person's volume. Since $d = m/V$ (density = mass/volume) and $d_{water} = 1.00 \times 10^3$ kg/m^3 from Table 5-3, we have

$$V = \frac{m}{d_{water}} = \frac{60 \text{ kg}}{1.00 \times 10^3 \text{ kg/m}^3}$$
$$= 0.06 \text{ m}^3$$

(Since 1 m = 3.28 ft, 1 m^3 = 35.3 ft^3, and 0.06 m^3 = 2.1 ft^3.)

The buoyant force is equal to the weight $w = m_{air}g = d_{air}Vg$ of the air displaced by the person, so

$$F_b = d_{air}Vg$$
$$= (1.3 \text{ kg/m}^3)(0.06 \text{ m}^3)(9.8 \text{ m/s}^2)$$
$$= 0.76 \text{ N}$$

This is about 2.7 ounces.

answer is that the ship is a hollow shell, so its average density is less than that of water even when loaded with cargo. If the ship springs a leak and fills with water, its average density goes up, and the ship sinks. The purpose of a life jacket is to reduce the average density of a person in the water so that she floats higher and is less likely to get water in her lungs and drown as a result.

5.7 The Gas Laws

Ideal Gases Obey Them

In many ways the gaseous state is the one whose behavior is the easiest to describe and account for. As an important example, the pressures, volumes, and temperatures of gas samples are related by simple formulas that have no counterpart in the cases of liquids and solids. The discovery of these formulas led to a search for their explanation in terms of the basic nature of gases, a search that resulted in the kinetic theory of matter.

Boyle's Law Suppose that a sample of some gas is placed in the cylinder of Fig. 5-20, and a pressure of 100 kPa is applied. The final volume of the sample is 1 m^3. If we double the pressure to 200 kPa, the piston will move down until the gas volume is 0.5 m^3, half its original amount, provided the

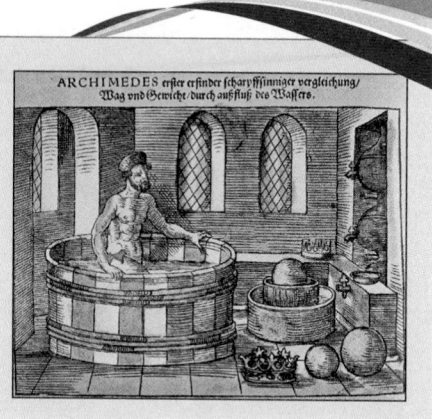

The pre-eminent scientist/mathematician of the ancient world, Archimedes was born in Syracuse, Sicily, at that time a Greek colony. He went to Alexandria, Egypt, to study under a former pupil of Euclid and then returned to Syracuse where he spent the rest of his life.

Many stories have come down through the ages about Archimedes, some of them possibly true. The principle named after him, that the buoyant force on a submerged object equals the weight of the fluid it displaces, is supposed to have come to him while in his bath, whereupon he rushed naked into the street crying "Eureka!" ("I've got it!"). He had been trying to think of a way to determine whether a new crown made for King Hieron of Sicily was pure gold without damaging

it and used his discovery to show that it was not; the goldsmith was then executed.

Archimedes worked out the theory of the lever and remarked (so it is said), "Give me a place to stand and I can move the world." King Hieron then challenged him to move something really large, even if not the world, and Archimedes responded by using a system of pulleys, which are developments of the lever, to haul a laden ship overland all by himself.

Archimedes was an able mathematician, and among his other accomplishments he calculated that the value of π lay between 223/71 and 220/70, an extremely good approximation. Archimedes is given credit for keeping the Roman fleet that attacked Syracuse in 215 B.C. at bay for 3 years by a variety of clever

devices, including giant lenses that focused sunlight on the ships and set them afire.

Finally the Romans did conquer Syracuse, and a Roman soldier found Archimedes bent over a mathematical problem scratched in the sand. When Archimedes would not stop work immediately, the soldier killed him.

gas temperature is kept unchanged. If the pressure is made 10 times greater, the piston will move down farther, until the gas occupies a volume of 0.1 m³, again if the gas temperature is kept unchanged.

These findings can be summarized by saying that the volume of a given quantity of a gas at constant temperature is inversely proportional to the pressure applied to it. (By "inversely proportional" is meant that as the pressure increases, the volume decreases by the same proportion.) If the volume of the gas is V_1 when the pressure is p_1 and the volume changes to V_2 when the pressure is changed to p_2, the relationship among the various quantities is

$$\frac{p_1}{p_2} = \frac{V_2}{V_1} \qquad \text{(at constant temperature)} \qquad \textit{Boyle's law} \qquad 5\text{-}7$$

Figure 5-20 Boyle's law: At constant temperature, the volume of a sample of any gas is inversely proportional to the pressure applied to it. Here $p_1V_1 = p_2V_2 = p_3V_3$.

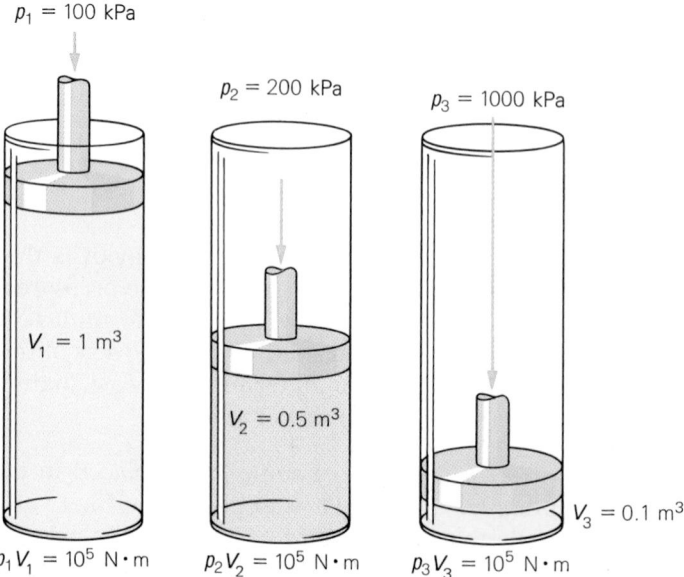

p_1 = 100 kPa

p_2 = 200 kPa

p_3 = 1000 kPa

V_1 = 1 m³

V_2 = 0.5 m³

V_3 = 0.1 m³

$p_1V_1 = 10^5$ N·m $p_2V_2 = 10^5$ N·m $p_3V_3 = 10^5$ N·m

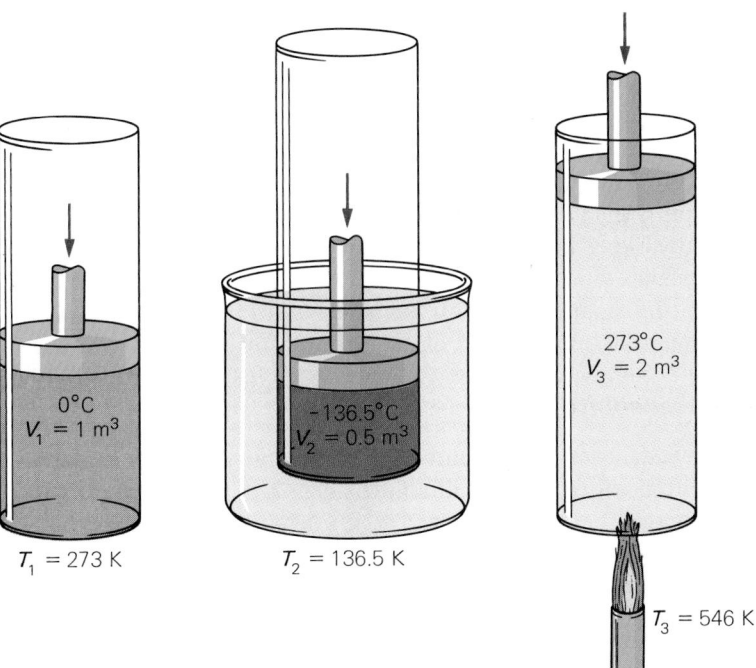

Figure 5-21 Charles's law: At constant pressure, the volume of a gas sample is directly proportional to its absolute temperature T_K, where $T_K = T_C + 273\,°$. Here $V_1/T_1 = V_2/T_2 = V_3/T_3$.

This relationship is called **Boyle's law,** in honor of the English physicist who discovered it. It is often written in the equivalent form $p_1V_1 = p_2V_2$.

Example 5.10

When water is boiled in a pot, the bubbles of steam increase in size as they rise through the water. Why?

Solution
The pressure in the water decreases toward the top, hence the steam bubbles expand.

Example 5.11

A scuba diver whose 12-liter (L) tank is filled with air at a pressure of 150 atmospheres (atm) is swimming at a depth of 15 m where the water pressure is 2.5 atm. If she uses 30 L of air per minute at the same pressure as the water pressure, how long can she stay at that depth?

Solution
We begin by using Boyle's law to determine the volume V_2 of air available at a pressure of $p_2 = 2.5$ atm:

$$V_2 = \frac{p_1V_1}{p_2} = \frac{(150\ \text{atm})(12\ \text{L})}{2.5\ \text{atm}}$$
$$= 720\ \text{L}$$

However, 12 L of air remains in the tank, so only 708 L is usable and will last for

$$\frac{708\ \text{L}}{30\ \text{L/min}} = 23.6\ \text{min}$$

Charles's Law Changes in the volume of a gas sample are also related to temperature changes in a simple way. If a gas is cooled steadily, starting at 0°C, while its pressure is maintained constant, its volume decreases by $\frac{1}{273}$ of its volume at 0°C for every degree the temperature falls. If the gas is heated, its volume increases by the same fraction (Figs. 5-21 and 5-22). If volume

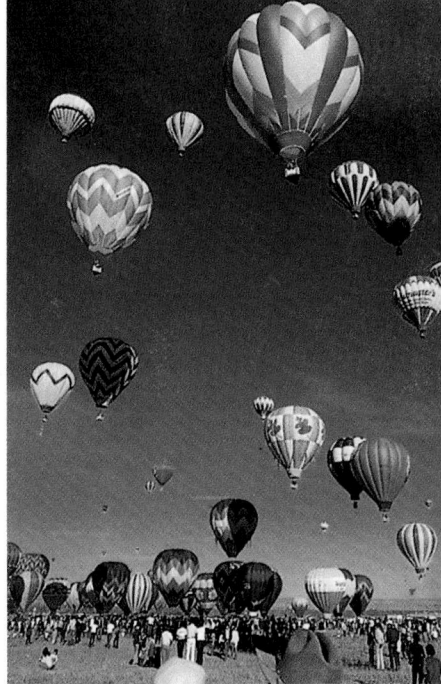

Figure 5-22 At constant pressure, heating a gas causes it to expand. The density of hot air therefore is less than the density of cool air at the same pressure, which is why a hot-air balloon is buoyant. These balloons have propane burners in their gondolas to supply the needed heat.

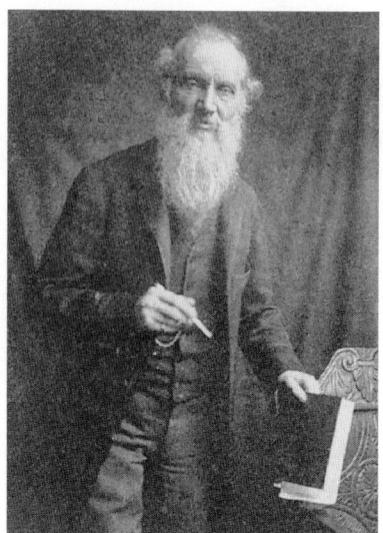

Figure 5-23 Lord Kelvin (1824 – 1907). A notable physicist but a poor prophet, he announced in 1900 that "there is nothing new to be discovered in physics now."

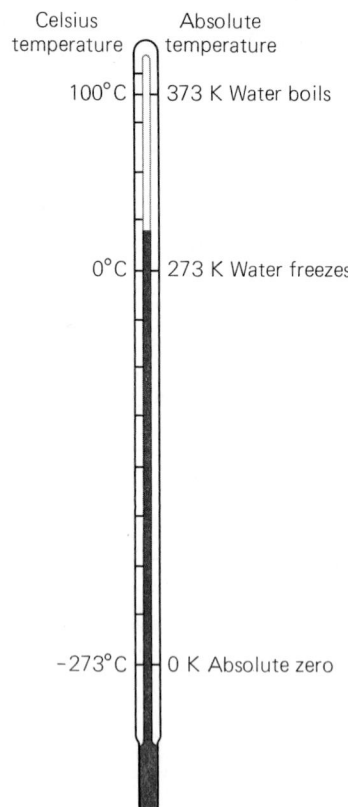

Figure 5-24 The absolute temperature scale.

rather than pressure is kept fixed, the pressure increases with rising temperature and decreases with falling temperature, again by the fraction $\frac{1}{273}$ of its 0°C value for every degree change.

These figures suggest an obvious question: What would happen to a gas if we could lower its temperature to −273°C? If we kept the gas at constant volume, the pressure at this temperature ought to fall to zero. If the pressure stayed constant, the volume ought to fall to zero.

It is hardly likely, however, that our experiments would have such results. In the first place, we should find it impossible to reach quite so low a temperature. In the second place, all known gases turn into liquids before that temperature is reached. Nevertheless, a temperature of −273°C has a special significance, a significance that will become clearer shortly. This temperature is called **absolute zero.**

Absolute Temperature   For many scientific purposes it is convenient to begin the temperature scale at absolute zero. Temperatures on such a scale, given as the number of degrees Celsius above absolute zero, are called **absolute temperatures.** Thus the freezing point of water is 273° absolute, written as 273 K ("273 kelvins") in honor of the English physicist Lord Kelvin (Fig. 5-23), and the boiling point of water is 373 K. Any Celsius temperature T_C can be changed to its equivalent absolute temperature T_K by adding 273 (Fig. 5-24):

$$T_K = T_C + 273 \qquad\qquad 5\text{-}8$$

Absolute temperature = Celsius temperature + 273

Using the absolute scale, we can express the relationship between gas volumes and temperatures quite simply: the volume of a gas is directly proportional to its absolute temperature (Fig. 5-25). This relation may be expressed in the form

$$\frac{V_1}{V_2} = \frac{T_1}{T_2} \qquad \text{(at constant pressure)} \qquad \textit{Charles's law} \qquad 5\text{-}9$$

where the T's are absolute temperatures. Discovered by two eighteenth-century French physicists, Jacques Alexandre Charles and Joseph Gay-Lussac, this relation is commonly known as **Charles's law.** Charles's law can also be written $V_1/T_1 = V_2/T_2$.

Ideal Gas Law   Boyle's and Charles's laws can be combined in a single formula known as the **ideal gas law:**

$$\frac{p_1 V_1}{T_1} = \frac{p_2 V_2}{T_2} \qquad \textit{Ideal gas law} \qquad 5\text{-}10$$

At constant temperature, $T_1 = T_2$ and we have Boyle's law. At constant pressure, $p_1 = p_2$ and we have Charles's law. Another way to write the ideal gas law is

$$\frac{pV}{T} = \text{constant} \qquad \textit{Ideal gas law} \qquad 5\text{-}11$$

since this particular combination of quantities does not change in value for a gas sample even though the individual quantities p, V, and T may vary.

The ideal gas law is obeyed approximately by all gases. The significant thing is not that the agreement with experiment is never quite perfect but that *all* gases behave almost identically.

An **ideal gas** is defined as one that obeys Eq. 5-11 exactly. Although no ideal gases actually exist, they do provide a target for a theory of the gaseous state to aim at. As we shall see, the kinetic theory of gases is indeed

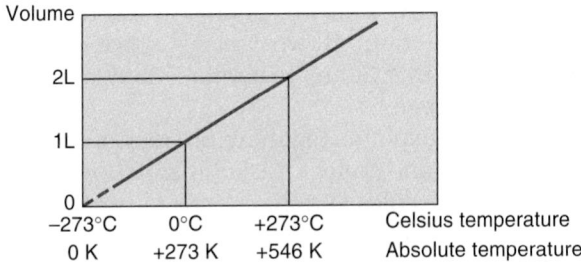

Figure 5-25   Graphic representation of Charles's law, showing the proportionality between volume and absolute temperature for a gas at constant pressure. If the temperature of the gas could be reduced to absolute zero, its volume would fall to zero. Actual gases liquefy at temperatures above absolute zero.

able to explain the ideal gas law, which means that it is a valid guide to the essential nature of gases. [For an example, see Sec. 5.7 www.mhhe.com/krauskopf.]

Kinetic Theory of Matter

The **kinetic theory of matter** accounts for a wide variety of physical and chemical properties of matter in terms of a simple model. According to this model, all matter is composed of tiny particles. In the case of a gas, the particles are usually **molecules** that consist of two or more atoms. In liquids and solids, the particles may be molecules, atoms, or ions, as discussed in Chap. 10. In this chapter, for simplicity, the basic particles characteristic of any substance will be called molecules.

5.8   Kinetic Theory of Gases

Why Gases Behave as They Do

Today we know a great deal about the sizes, speeds, even shapes of the molecules in various kinds of matter.

For example, a molecule of nitrogen, the chief constituent of air, is about 0.18 billionth of a meter (1.8×10^{-10} m) across and has a mass of 4.7×10^{-26} kg. It travels (at 0°C) at an average speed of 500 m/s, about the speed of a rifle bullet, and in each second collides with more than a billion other molecules. Of similar dimensions and moving with similar speeds in each cubic centimeter of air are 2.7×10^{19} other molecules. If all the molecules in such a thimbleful of air were divided equally among the 6.7 billion people on the earth, each person would receive several billion molecules.

Assumptions of Kinetic Theory   The three basic assumptions of the kinetic theory for gas molecules, which have been verified by experiment, are these:

1. Gas molecules are small compared with the average distance between them.
2. Gas molecules collide without loss of kinetic energy.
3. Gas molecules exert almost no forces on one another, except when they collide.

A gas, then, is mostly empty space, with its isolated molecules moving helter-skelter like a swarm of angry bees in a closed room (Fig. 5-26). Each molecule collides with others perhaps billions of times a second, changing its speed and direction at each collision but unaffected by its neighbors between collisions. If a series of collisions brings it momentarily to a stop, new collisions will set it in motion. If its speed becomes greater than the average,

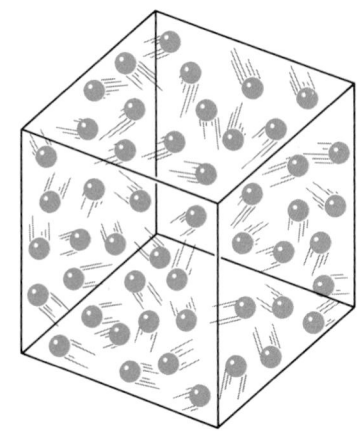

Figure 5-26   The molecules of a gas are in constant random motion.

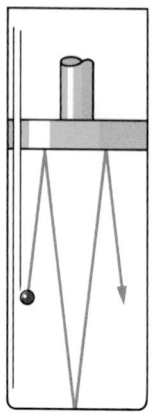

Figure 5-27   Gas pressure is the result of molecular bombardment. For simplicity, only vertical molecular motions are shown.

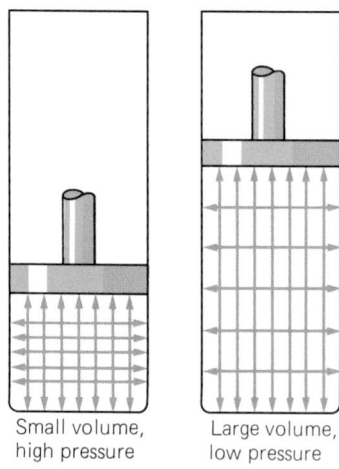

Small volume, high pressure

Large volume, low pressure

Figure 5-28   Origin of Boyle's law. Expanding a gas sample means that its molecules must travel farther between successive impacts on the container wall and that their blows are spread over a larger area, so the gas pressure drops.

successive collisions will slow it down. There is no order in the motion, no uniformity of speed or direction. All we can say is that the molecules have a certain average speed and that at any instant as many molecules are moving in one direction as in another.

This animated picture explains the more obvious properties of gases. The ability of a gas to expand and to leak through small openings follows from the rapid motion of its molecules and their lack of attraction for one another. Gases are easily compressed because the molecules are, on the average, widely separated. One gas mixes with another because the spaces between molecules leave plenty of room for others. Because a given volume of a gas consists mainly of empty space, the mass of that volume is much less than that of the same volume of a liquid or a solid.

Origin of Boyle's Law   The pressure of a gas on the walls of its container is the result of bombardment by billions and billions of molecules, the same bombardment that causes brownian movement (Fig. 5-27). The many tiny, separate blows affect our senses and our measuring instruments as a continuous force.

The kinetic theory accounts nicely for Boyle's law, $p_1V_1 = p_2V_2$ (at constant temperature). As in Fig. 5-28, we can think of the molecules of a gas in a cylinder as moving in a regular manner, some of them vertically between the piston and the base of the cylinder and the others horizontally between the cylinder walls. If the piston is raised so that the gas volume is doubled, the vertically moving molecules have twice as far to go between collisions with top and bottom and hence will strike only half as often. The horizontally moving molecules must spread their blows over twice as great an area, and hence the number of impacts per unit area will be cut in half. Thus the pressure in all parts of the cylinder is exactly halved, as Boyle's law predicts. It is not hard to extend this reasoning to a real gas whose molecules move at random.

5.9   Molecular Motion and Temperature

The Faster the Molecules, the Higher the Temperature

To account for the effect of a temperature change on a gas, the kinetic theory requires a further concept:

4. The absolute temperature of a gas is proportional to the average kinetic energy of its molecules.

This concept was used by Einstein to explain brownian motion (see Einstein biography in Sec. 3.12).

That temperature should be related to molecular energies and thus to molecular speeds follows from the increase in the pressure of a confined gas as its temperature rises. Increases in pressure must mean that the molecules are striking the walls of their container more forcefully and so must be moving faster.

What Absolute Zero Means   Earlier in this chapter we learned that the pressure of a gas approaches zero as its temperature falls toward 0 K, which is −273°C. For the pressure to become zero, molecular bombardment must stop. Thus absolute zero is interpreted as the temperature at which gas molecules would lose their kinetic energies completely, as shown in Fig. 5-29. (This is a simplification of the actual situation: in reality, even at 0 K a molecule will have a very small amount of KE that cannot be reduced.) There can be no lower temperature, simply because there can be no smaller amount of energy. The regular increase of gas pressure with absolute temperature if the volume is constant and the similar increase of volume if the pressure is constant (Charles's law) follow from this definition of absolute zero.

Origin of Charles's Law   If temperature is a measure of average molecular energy, then compressing a gas in a cylinder ought to cause its temperature to rise. While the piston of Fig. 5-30 is moving down, molecules rebound from it with increased energy just as a baseball rebounds with increased energy from a moving bat. To verify this prediction, all we have to do is pump up a bicycle tire and notice how hot the pump becomes after the air in it has been compressed a few times. On the other hand, if a gas is expanded by pulling a piston outward, its temperature falls, since each molecule that strikes the retreating piston gives up some of its kinetic energy (Fig. 5-31).

The cooling effect of gas expansion explains the formation of clouds from rising moist air, as discussed in Chap. 14. Atmospheric pressure decreases with altitude, and the water vapor in the moist air cools as it moves upward until it condenses into the water droplets that constitute clouds.

5.10   Heat Transfer

Three Mechanisms

Heat can be transferred from one place to another in the three ways shown in Fig. 5-32.

If we put one end of a poker into a fire, the other end becomes warm as heat flows through the poker. Such **conduction** is a consequence of the kinetic behavior of matter. Molecules at the hot end of a solid object vibrate faster and faster as the temperature there increases, and when these molecules collide with their less energetic neighbors, some KE transfers to them. Heat flows through a liquid by conduction in a similar way. Gases are poor conductors because their molecules are relatively far apart and so do not collide as often.

Metals are exceptionally good at conducting heat (copper is 3000 times better than wood) because some of the electrons in them are able

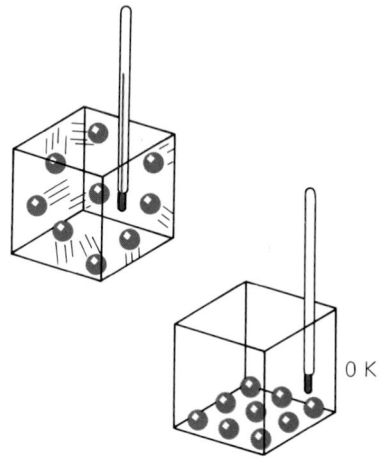

Figure 5-29   According to the kinetic theory of gases, at absolute zero the molecules of a gas would not move. More advanced theories show that even at 0 K a very slight movement will persist.

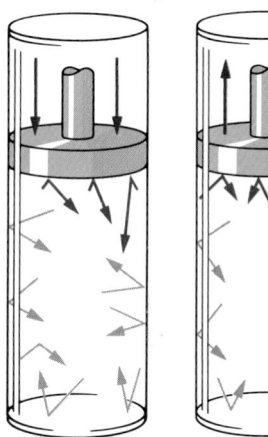

Molecular energy increases   Molecular energy decreases

Figure 5-30   Compressing a gas causes its temperature to rise because molecules rebound from the piston with more energy. Expanding a gas causes its temperature to drop because molecules rebound from the piston with less energy.

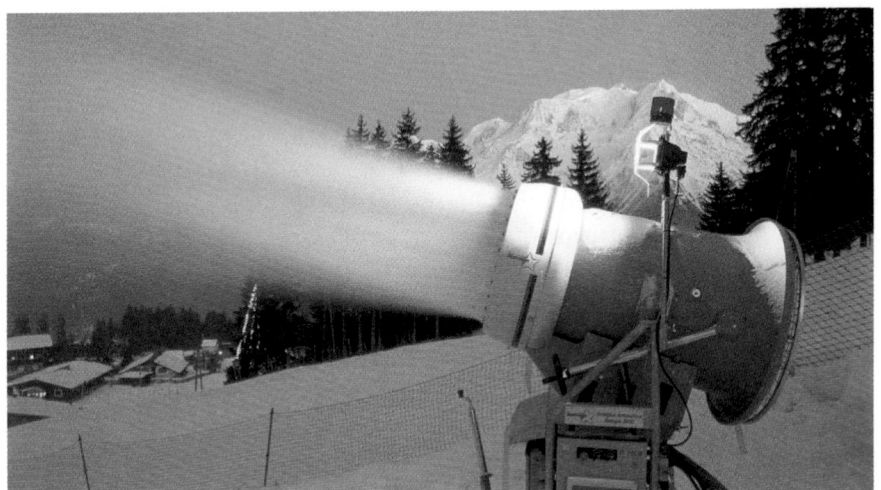

Figure 5-31   In the operation of a snowmaking machine, a mixture of compressed air and water is blown through a set of nozzles. The expansion of the air cools the mixture sufficiently to freeze the water into the ice crystals of snow.

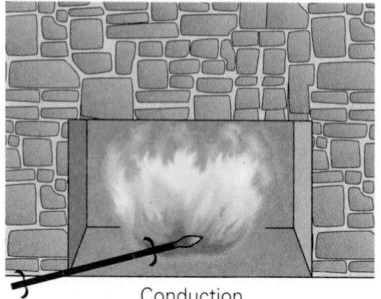

Conduction

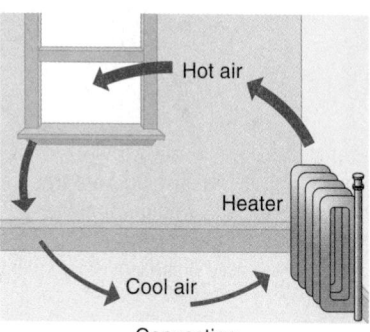

Convection

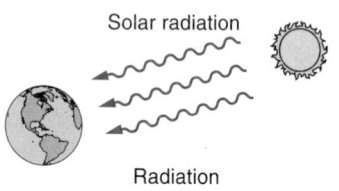

Radiation

Figure 5-32   Examples of the three mechanisms of heat transfer.

to move freely instead of being bound to particular atoms (see Sec. 11.2). Picking up KE at the hot end of a metal object, the free electrons travel past many atoms before finally giving up their added KE in collisions. Heat conduction by free electrons in a metal compares with heat conduction in other materials as travel by express train compares with travel by local train.

Conduction is inefficient in air, and a heater warms a room through the actual movement of hot air. When a portion of a fluid (a gas or a liquid) is heated, it expands so that it becomes lighter—that is, less dense—than the cooler fluid around it, and its resulting buoyancy causes it to move upward ("heat rises"). This process is called **convection.** Fig. 14-16 shows how convection in the atmosphere can lead to winds.

Radiation   In space, which is virtually empty, neither conduction nor convection can occur to any real extent. Instead, the earth receives heat from the sun in the form of radiation, which consists of electromagnetic waves; light and radio waves are examples of such radiation (see Secs. 7.8 and 7.9). The earth in turn radiates energy to space (see Sec. 14.4).

Waves are the subject of Chap. 7, but we can jump ahead here to mention that one of their properties is wavelength, the distance between the crest of one wave and the crest of the next. Every object radiates electromagnetic waves of all wavelengths: the hotter it is, the more energy it radiates and the shorter the predominant wavelength. Because the color of what we see depends on the chief wavelength in the light that reaches our eyes, the color of an object hot enough to glow depends on its temperature, as we saw in Fig. 5-5.

An object need not be so hot that it emits visible light for it to be radiating. The radiation from something at room temperature, for example, is mainly infrared light that our eyes do not respond to (but which our instruments can detect; see Fig. 9-4).

Changes of State

The kinetic theory of matter is clearly a success in explaining the behavior of gases. Let us now see what this theory has to say about liquids and solids. In particular, changes of state between gas and liquid and between liquid and solid are extremely interesting in molecular terms.

5.11   Liquids and Solids

Intermolecular Forces Hold Them Together

If a gas is like a swarm of angry bees, the molecules in a liquid are more like bees in a hive, crawling over one another constantly. Liquids flow because their molecules slide past one another easily, but they flow less readily than gases because of intermolecular attractions that act over short distances.

The forces between the molecules of a solid are stronger than those in a liquid, so strong that the molecules are not free to move about (Fig. 5-33). They are hardly at rest, however. Held in position as if by springs attached to its neighbors, each molecule vibrates back and forth rapidly (Fig. 5-34). Each spring represents a bond between two adjacent molecules. Such bonds are electrical in nature. A solid is elastic because its molecules return to their normal separations after being pulled apart or pushed together when a moderate force is applied. If the force is great, the solid may be permanently deformed. In this process, the molecules shift to new positions and find new

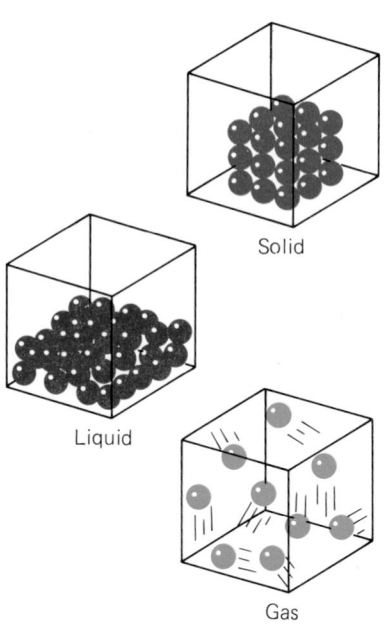

Solid

Liquid

Gas

Figure 5-33 Molecular models of a solid, a liquid, and a gas. The molecules of a solid are attached to one another; those of a liquid can slide past one another; those of a gas move freely except when they collide with one another or with the walls of a container.

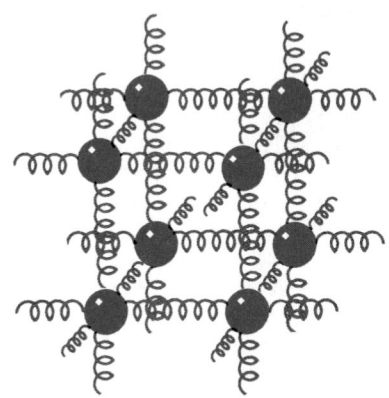

Figure 5-34 The particles of a solid can be imagined as being held together by tiny springs that permit them to vibrate back and forth. The higher the temperature, the more energetic the vibrations. When a solid is squeezed, the springs are (so to speak) pushed together; when it is stretched, the springs are pulled apart.

partners for their attractive forces. Too much applied force, of course, may break the solid apart.

5.12   Evaporation and Boiling

Liquid into Gas

Suppose we have two liquids, water and alcohol, in open dishes (Fig. 5-35). Molecules in each dish are moving in all directions, with a variety of speeds. At any instant some molecules are moving fast enough upward to escape into the air in spite of the attractions of their slower neighbors. By this loss of its faster molecules each liquid gradually evaporates. Since the remaining molecules are the slower ones, evaporation leaves cool liquids behind. The alcohol evaporates more quickly than the water and cools itself more noticeably because the attraction of its particles for one another is smaller and a greater number can escape.

When we add heat to a liquid, eventually a temperature is reached at which even molecules of average speed can overcome the forces binding them together. Now bubbles of gas form throughout the liquid, and it begins to boil. This temperature is accordingly called the **boiling point** of the liquid. As we would expect, the boiling point of alcohol (78°C) is lower than that of water (100°C).

Thus evaporation differs from boiling in two ways:

1. Evaporation occurs only at a liquid surface; boiling occurs in the entire volume of liquid.
2. Evaporation occurs at all temperatures; boiling occurs only at the boiling point or higher temperatures.

Heat of Vaporization   Whether evaporation takes place by itself from an open dish or is aided by heating, forming a gas from a liquid requires energy. In the first case energy is supplied from the heat content of the liquid itself (since the liquid grows cooler), in the other case from the outside source of heat. For water at its boiling point of 100°C, 2260 kJ (the **heat of vaporization**) is needed to change each kilogram of liquid into gas (Fig. 5-36). With no difference in temperature between liquid and gas, there is no difference in their average molecular kinetic energies. If not into kinetic energy, into what form of molecular energy does the 2260 kJ of heat go?

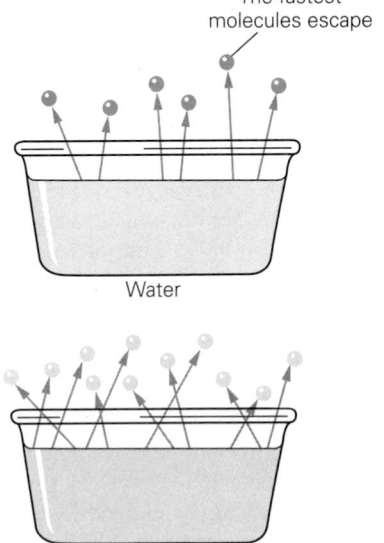

The fastest molecules escape

Water

Alcohol

Figure 5-35 Evaporation. Alcohol evaporates more rapidly than water because the attractive forces between its molecules are smaller. In each case, the faster molecules escape. Hence the average kinetic energy of the remaining molecules is lower and the liquid temperature drops.

Figure 5-36 The heat of vaporization of water is 2260 kJ/kg.

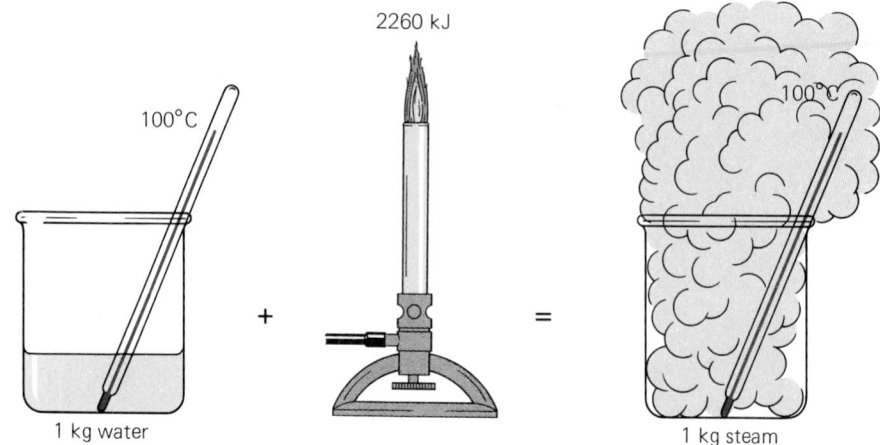

Gas and Vapor

A gas is a substance whose molecules are too far apart to attract one another except in collisions. As a result, a gas will expand indefinitely unless stopped by the walls of a container or, in the case of a planet's atmosphere, is prevented from leaving the planet by gravity.

However, even a substance that is normally a liquid or solid at a certain temperature may lose molecules from its surface. These molecules make up a **vapor.** Under ordinary conditions water is a liquid, but enough water molecules escape (mainly from the oceans) for water vapor to comprise up to 4 percent of the earth's atmosphere. When hot enough, water becomes steam, which is a gas.

Pressure Cookers

Boiling points vary with pressure: the higher the pressure, the higher the boiling point. At twice sea-level atmospheric pressure, for instance, water boils at 120°C. The pressure cooker is based on this observation (Fig. 5-37).

When water is heated in a closed container, the pressure in the container increases, and the temperature at which the water inside boils will be correspondingly higher than 100°C. In this way food can be cooked faster than in an open pan. Similarly, lowering the pressure reduces the boiling point. Atmospheric pressure decreases with altitude (see Fig. 14-1), so the boiling point of water in Denver, which is well above sea level, is 96°C; on top of the even higher Pikes Peak it is only 88°C.

Intermolecular forces provide the answer. In a liquid these forces are strong because the molecules are close together. To tear the molecules apart, to separate them by the wide distances that exist in the gas, requires that these strong forces be overcome. Each molecule must be moved, against the pull of its neighbors, to a new position in which their attraction for it is very small. Just as a stone thrown upward against the earth's gravity gains potential energy, so molecules moved apart in this way gain potential energy—potential energy with respect to intermolecular forces. When a gas becomes a liquid, the process is reversed. The molecules "fall" toward one another under the influence of their mutual attractions, and their potential energy is taken up as heat by the surroundings.

5.13 Melting

Solid into Liquid

Just as heat must be added at its boiling point to turn a liquid into a gas, so heat at its melting point is needed to turn a solid into a liquid. The heat required to change 1 kg of a solid at its melting point into a liquid is called the **heat of fusion** of the substance. The same amount of heat must be given

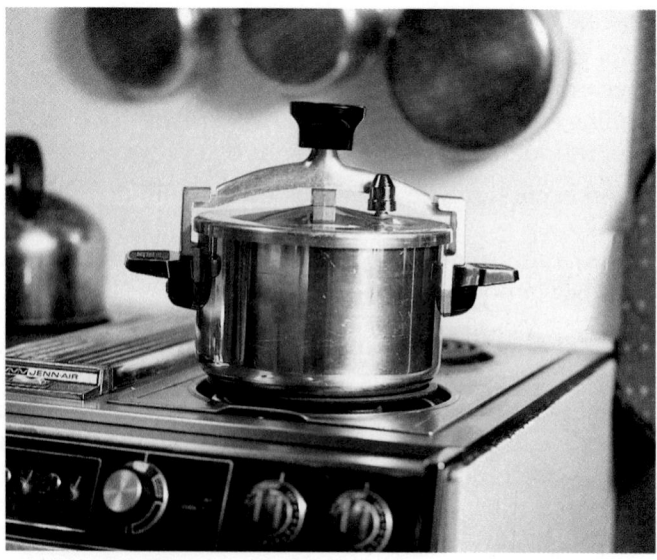

Figure 5-37 Because the boiling point of water increases with pressure, a pressure cooker such as this one enables food to be cooked at a higher temperature than in an open pan.

Example 5.12

The high heat of vaporization of water is what makes steam dangerous (Fig. 5-38). Compare the heat given to a person's skin when 1 g (about a third of a teaspoonful) of water at 100°C falls on it with the heat given by 1 g of steam at 100°C. Assume that the skin is at the normal body temperature of 37°C.

Solution

Since the specific heat of water is c = 4.2 kJ/kg · °C and here ΔT = (100°C − 37°C) = 63°C, the heat given up by the hot water in cooling is

$$Q_1 = mc\,\Delta T = (0.001 \text{ kg})(4.2 \text{ kJ/kg} \cdot {}°\text{C})(63°\text{C}) = 0.26 \text{ kJ}$$

The heat given up by the steam is this amount plus the heat Q_2 given up as the steam at 100°C condenses into water at 100°C, which is

$$Q_2 = (0.001 \text{ kg})(2260 \text{ kJ/kg} \cdot {}°\text{C}) = 2.26 \text{ kJ}$$

The total is $Q_1 + Q_2$ = 2.52 kJ—nearly 10 times as much as in the case of the hot water.

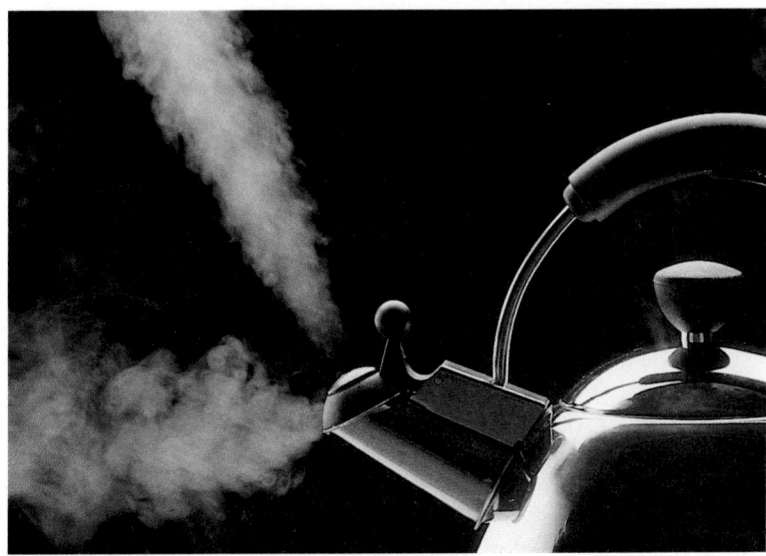

Figure 5-38 Great care must always be taken near steam because the heat of vaporization of water is so great.

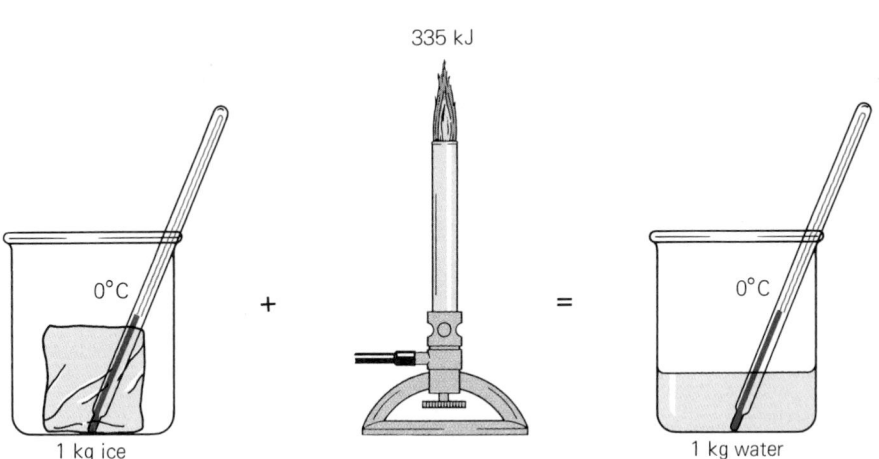

335 kJ

0°C

1 kg ice

0°C

1 kg water

Figure 5-39 The heat of fusion of water is 335 kJ/kg.

off by 1 kg of the substance when it is a liquid at its melting point for it to harden into a solid. The heat of fusion of water is 335 kJ/kg (Fig. 5-39). Most other substances have lower heats of fusion (Table 5-4).

Table 5-4	Some Heats of Fusion and Vaporization			
	Melting point, °C	Heat of fusion, kJ/kg	Boiling point, °C	Heat of vaporization, kJ/kg
Copper	1083	134	1187	5069
Ethanol[1]	−114	105	78	854
Lead	330	25	1170	870
Mercury	−39	12	358	297
Nitrogen	−210	26	−196	201
Oxygen	−219	14	−183	213
Water	0	335	100	2260

[1]Ethanol is also known as ethyl alcohol.

Figure 5-40 The orderly arrangement of particles in a crystalline solid changes to the random arrangement of particles in a liquid when enough energy is supplied to the solid to overcome the bonding forces within it.

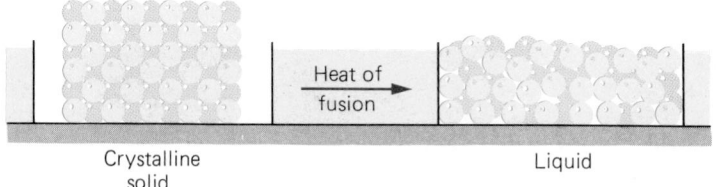

Crystalline solid   Liquid

The heat of fusion of a substance is always much smaller than its heat of vaporization. The molecules of a solid are arranged in a fixed pattern such that the forces holding each one to its neighbors are as large as possible. To overcome these forces and give the molecules the random, constantly shifting arrangement of a liquid, additional energy must be given to them (Fig. 5-40). However, the molecules still stick together sufficiently to give a liquid sample a definite volume. To turn a liquid into a gas, enough energy must be added to pull the molecules permanently apart, a much harder job. The molecules of the gas can then move about freely, and the gas expands. At atmospheric pressure 1 L of water becomes 1680 L of steam; in a vacuum, it would expand indefinitely.

Figure 5-41 shows what happens as we supply heat to 1 kg of ice originally at −50°C. The ice warms up until it reaches 0°C, when it begins to melt. Then the temperature remains steady at 0°C until all the ice has melted. When all the ice has become water, the temperature rises again. When the water reaches 100°C, it starts to turn into steam, which takes a lot of heat, much more than the ice needed to melt. Finally all the water has become

Example 5.13

An ice cube at 0°C is dropped to the ground and melts into water at 0°C. If all the original potential energy of the ice above the ground went into melting the ice, from what height did the ice cube fall?

Solution

If L is the heat of fusion of water, $Q = mL = PE = mgh$ and

$$h = \frac{L}{g} = \frac{335 \text{ kJ/kg}}{9.8 \text{ m/s}^2} = 34 \text{ km}$$

We did not have to know the mass of the ice cube.

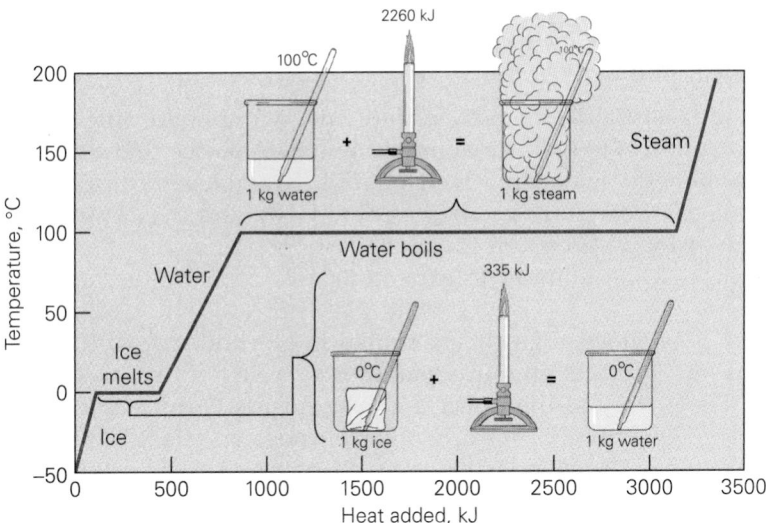

Figure 5-41   A graph of the temperature of 1 kg of water, originally ice at −50°C, as heat is added to it.

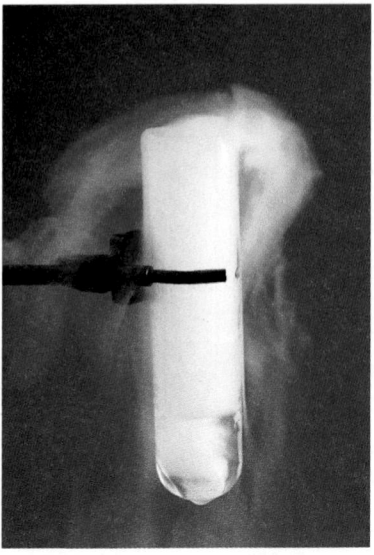

Figure 5-42   Solid carbon dioxide ("dry ice") vaporizes into a gas at atmospheric pressure, a process called sublimation.

steam at 100°C and the temperature of the steam now increases as more heat is added.

Sublimation   Most substances change directly from the solid to the vapor state, a process called **sublimation,** under the right conditions of temperature and pressure. Usually pressures well under atmospheric pressure are needed for sublimation. A familiar exception is solid carbon dioxide ("dry ice"), which turns into a gas without first becoming a liquid, at temperatures above −79°C, even at atmospheric pressure (Fig. 5-42). Figure 5-43 summarizes all the changes of state we have been discussing.

The best instant coffee is prepared with the help of sublimation. The brewed coffee is first frozen and then put in a vacuum chamber. The ice in the frozen coffee sublimes to water vapor, which is pumped away. Freeze drying affects the flavor of coffee much less than drying it by heating. The same process is also used to preserve other materials of biological origin, such as blood plasma.

Energy Transformations

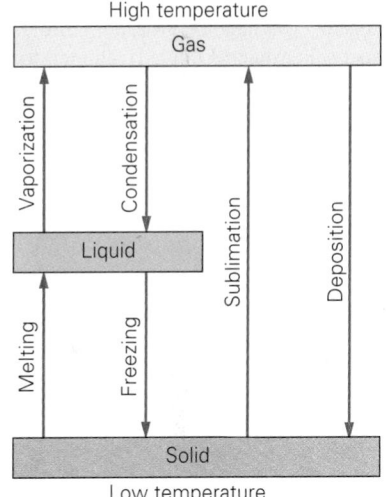

Figure 5-43   The various changes of state.

Any form of energy, including heat, can be converted to any other form. But heat is unusual in that it cannot be converted *efficiently.* We routinely obtain mechanical energy from the heat given off by burning coal and oil in engines of various types, but a large part of the heat is always wasted—about two-thirds in the case of electric power stations, for example. The losses are serious because nearly all the "raw" energy available to modern civilization is liberated from its sources as heat.

The basic inefficiency of all engines whose energy input is heat was discovered in the nineteenth century, at the start of the Industrial Revolution. It is not a question of poor design or construction; the transformation of heat simply will not take place without such losses. Research both by engineers trying to get as much mechanical energy as possible from each ton of fuel and by scientists whose interest was in the properties of heat eventually brought to light why such transformations are so wasteful. As we shall see, the ultimate reason is that what we call heat is actually the kinetic energy of random molecular motion.

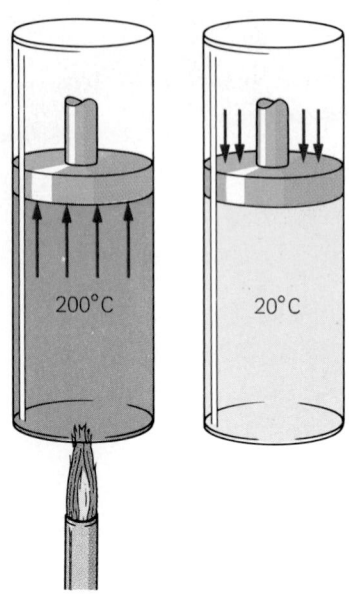

Figure 5-44 An idealized heat engine. A gas at 200°C gives out more energy in expanding than is required to compress the gas at 20°C. This excess energy is available for doing work.

5.14 Heat Engines

Turning Heat into Work

Heat is the easiest and cheapest form of energy to obtain, since all we have to do to obtain it is to burn an appropriate fuel. A device that turns heat into mechanical energy is called a **heat engine.** Examples are the gasoline and diesel engines of cars, the jet engines of aircraft, and the steam turbines of ships and power stations. All these engines operate in the same basic way: a gas is heated and allowed to expand against a piston or the blades of a turbine.

Figure 5-44 shows a gas being heated in a cylinder. As the temperature of the gas increases, its pressure increases as well, and the piston is pushed upward. The energy of the upward-moving piston can be used to propel a car or turn a generator or for any other purpose we wish. When the piston reaches the top of the cylinder, however, the conversion of heat into mechanical energy stops. In order to keep the engine working, we must now push the piston back down again in order to begin another energy-producing expansion.

If we push the piston down while the gas in the cylinder is still hot, we will find that we have to do exactly as much work as the energy provided by the expansion. Thus there will be no net work done at all. To make the engine perform a net amount of work in each cycle, we must now cool the gas so that less work is needed to compress it. It is in this cooling process that heat is lost. There is no way to avoid throwing away some of the heat added to the gas in the expansion if the engine is to continue to work. The wasted heat usually ends up in the atmosphere around the engine, in the water of a nearby river, or in the ocean.

What happens in a complete cycle, then, is that heat flows in and out of the engine, and during the flow we manage to change some of the heat into mechanical energy, as in Fig. 5-45. Heat flows by itself from a hot reservoir to a cold one, so we need *both* reservoirs for a heat engine to operate. In a gasoline or diesel engine the hot reservoir is the burning gases of the power stroke and the cold reservoir is the atmosphere.

Refrigerators   A vast amount of heat is contained in the molecular motions of the atmosphere, the oceans, and the earth itself, but only rarely can we use it because we need a colder reservoir nearby to which the heat can flow. What about using a refrigerator as the cold reservoir? A **refrigerator** is the

Figure 5-45 A heat engine converts part of the heat flowing from a hot reservoir to a cold one into work. A refrigerator extracts heat from a cold reservoir and delivers it to a hot one by doing work that is converted into heat.

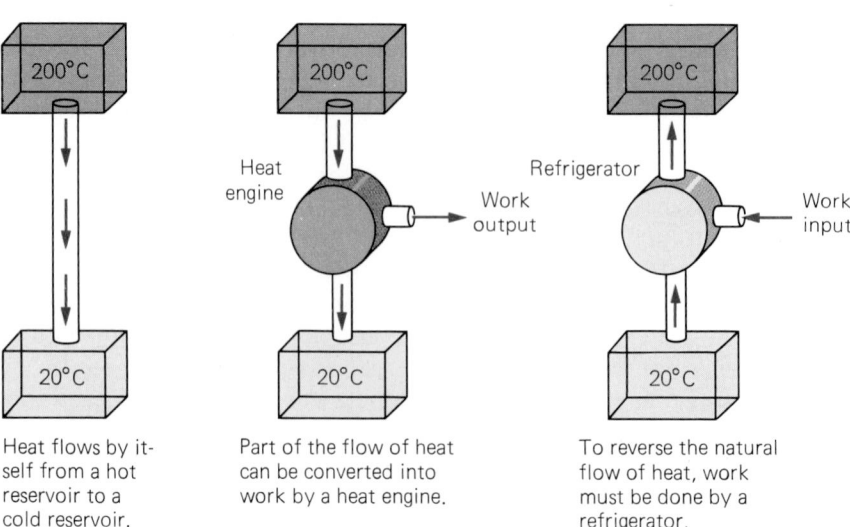

Heat flows by itself from a hot reservoir to a cold reservoir.

Part of the flow of heat can be converted into work by a heat engine.

To reverse the natural flow of heat, work must be done by a refrigerator.

Gasoline and Diesel Engines

The operating cycle of a four-stroke gasoline engine is shown in Fig. 5-46. In the intake stroke, a mixture of gasoline and air from the carburetor is sucked into the cylinder as the piston moves downward. In the compression stroke, the fuel-air mixture is compressed to one-seventh or one-eighth of its original volume. At the end of the compres-sion stroke the spark plug is fired, which ignites the fuel-air mixture. The expanding gases force the piston downward in the power stroke. Finally the piston moves upward again to force the spent gases out through the exhaust valve.

In a diesel engine, only air is drawn into the cylinder in the intake stroke. At the end of the compression stroke, diesel fuel is injected into the cylinder and is ignited by the high temperature of the compressed air. No spark plug is needed. Diesel engines are more efficient because they have higher compression ratios than gasoline engines but are also heavier and more expensive.

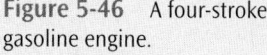

Figure 5-46 A four-stroke gasoline engine.

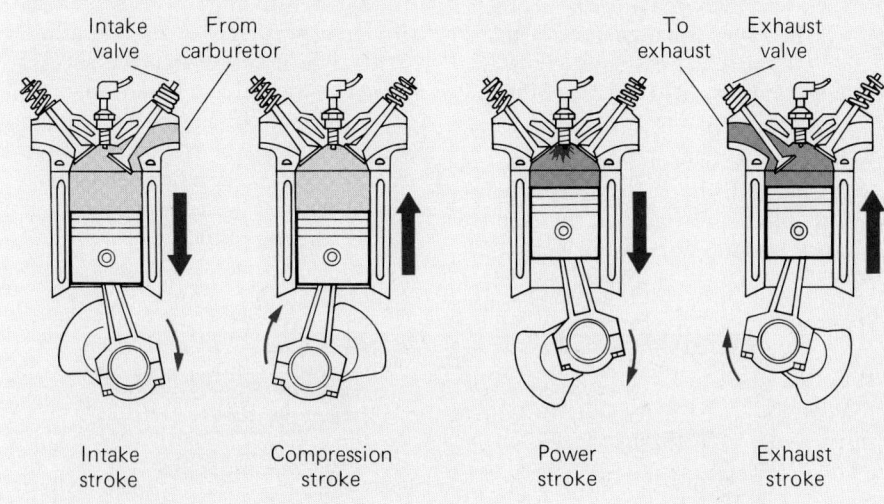

reverse of a heat engine, as we see in Fig. 5-45. It uses mechanical energy to push heat "uphill" from a cold reservoir (the inside of the refrigerator) to a warm reservoir (the air of the kitchen), a path opposite to the normal direction of heat flow. Because of the energy needed to drive a refrigerator, using one as the cold reservoir for a heat engine would be a losing proposition.

5.15 Thermodynamics

You Can't Win

Thermodynamics is the science of heat transformation, and it has two fundamental laws:

> 1. Energy cannot be created or destroyed, but it can be converted from one form to another.
> 2. It is impossible to take heat from a source and change all of it to mechanical energy or work; some heat must be wasted.

The first law of thermodynamics is the same as the law of conservation of energy discussed in Chap. 3. What it means is that we can't get something for nothing. The second law singles out heat from other kinds of energy and recognizes that all conversions of heat into any of the others must be inefficient.

Engine Efficiency   Thermodynamics is able to specify the maximum efficiency of a heat engine, ignoring losses to friction and other practical difficulties. The maximum efficiency turns out to depend only on the absolute

How a Refrigerator Works

A refrigerator takes in heat at a low temperature and exhausts it at a higher one. Figure 5-47 shows a refrigerator whose working substance is an easily liquefied gas called a **refrigerant.** The operation of the refrigeration system of Fig. 5-47 proceeds as follows:

1. The **compressor,** usually driven by an electric motor, brings the refrigerant to a high pressure, which raises its temperature as well.
2. The hot refrigerant passes through the **condenser,** an array of thin tubes that give off heat from the refrigerant to the atmosphere. The condenser is on the back of most household refrigerators. As it cools, the refrigerant becomes a liquid under high pressure.
3. The liquid refrigerant now goes into the **expansion valve,** from which it emerges at a lower pressure and temperature.
4. In the **evaporator** the cool liquid refrigerant absorbs heat from the storage chamber and vaporizes. Farther along in the evaporator the refrigerant vapor absorbs more heat and becomes warmer. The warm vapor then goes back to the compressor to begin another cycle.

In step 4 of this cycle, heat is extracted from the storage chamber by the refrigerant. In step 1, work is done on the refrigerant by the compressor. In step 2, heat from the refrigerant leaves the system. A refrigerator might remove two or more times as much heat from its storage chamber as the amount of work done.

A **heat pump** is a refrigeration system that takes heat from the cold outdoors in winter and delivers it to the interior of a house (see Sec. 4.9). The advantage of a heat pump is that it transfers more heat than the energy it uses in its operation. Thus a heat pump may be several times more efficient than an ordinary furnace. In summer the same heat pump can be used in reverse to serve as an air conditioner to take heat from the house and exhaust it to the warmer outdoors.

Figure 5-47   A typical refrigeration system. Heat is absorbed by the refrigerant from the storage chamber in the evaporator and is given up by the refrigerant in the condenser.

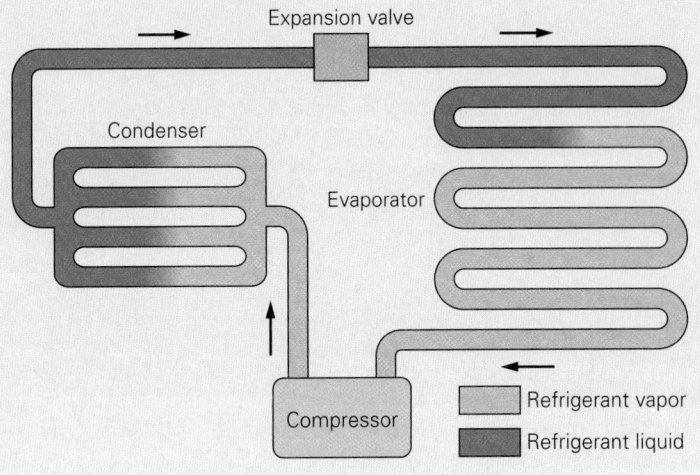

temperatures T_{hot} and T_{cold} of the hot and cold reservoirs between which the engine operates:

$$\text{Maximum efficiency} = \left(\frac{\text{work output}}{\text{energy input}}\right)_{\text{maximum}}$$

$$\text{Eff(max)} = 1 - \frac{T_{\text{cold}}}{T_{\text{hot}}} \qquad \textit{Engine efficiency} \qquad 5\text{-}12$$

The greater the ratio between the two temperatures, the less heat is wasted and the more efficient the engine.

Figure 5-48 shows the basic design of a steam turbine. In a power station, the steam comes from a boiler heated by a coal, oil, or gas furnace or by a nuclear reactor, and the turbine shaft is connected to an electric generator (Fig. 5-49). In a typical power station, steam enters a turbine at about 570°C and leaves at about 95°C into a partial vacuum. The corresponding absolute temperatures are 843 K and 368 K, so the maximum efficiency of such a turbine is

$$\text{Eff(max)} = 1 - \frac{T_{\text{cold}}}{T_{\text{hot}}} = 1 - \frac{368\text{ K}}{843\text{ K}} = 0.56$$

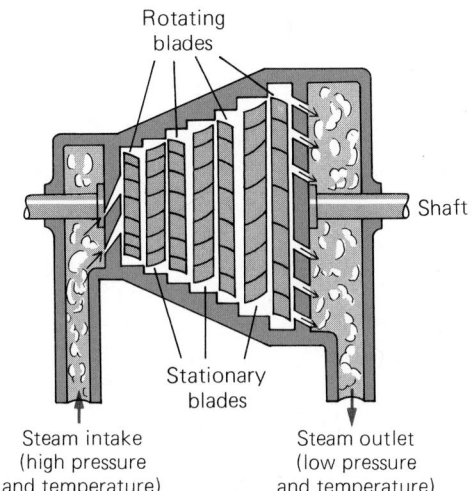

Rotating
blades

Shaft

Stationary
blades

Steam intake
(high pressure
and temperature)

Steam outlet
(low pressure
and temperature)

Figure 5-48   In a steam turbine, steam moves past several sets of rotating blades on the same shaft to obtain as much power as possible. The stationary blades direct the flow of steam in the most effective way.

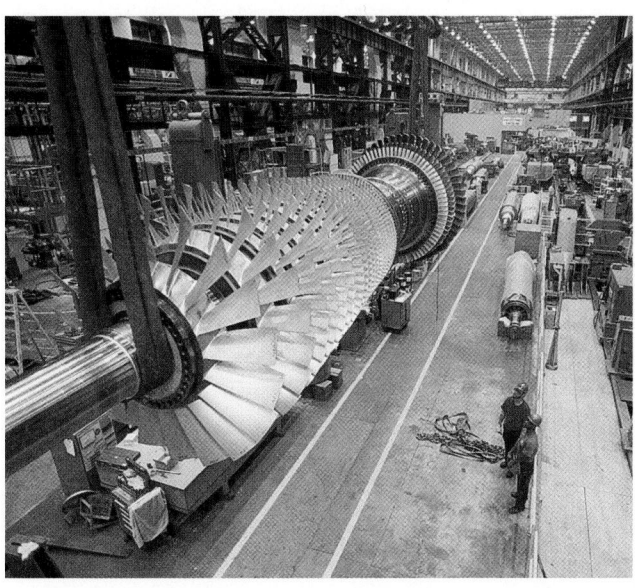

Figure 5-49   The rotor of a steam turbine. Such a rotor might turn at 3600 revolutions per minute to produce perhaps 200 MW of power.

which is 56 percent. The actual efficiency is less than 40 percent because of friction and other sources of energy loss (Fig. 5-50).

Why a Heat Engine Must Be Inefficient   On a molecular level, it is not hard to see why heat resists being changed into other forms of energy. When heat is added to the gas of a heat engine, its molecules increase their average speeds. But the molecules are moving in random directions, whereas the engine can draw upon the increased energies of only those molecules that are moving in more or less the same direction as the piston or turbine blades. If we could line up the molecules and aim them all, like miniature bullets, right at the piston or turbine blades, all the added energy could be turned into mechanical energy. Because this is impossible, only a fraction of any heat given to a gas can be extracted as energy of orderly motion. The nature of heat is responsible for the inefficiency of heat engines, and there is no way around it.

5.16   Fate of the Universe

Order into Disorder

Other kinds of energy can be entirely converted into heat, whereas only part of a given amount of heat can be converted the other way. As a result,

Figure 5-50 Energy flow in electric generating plants. A large part of the energy waste is due to the unavoidable thermodynamic inefficiency of the turbine.

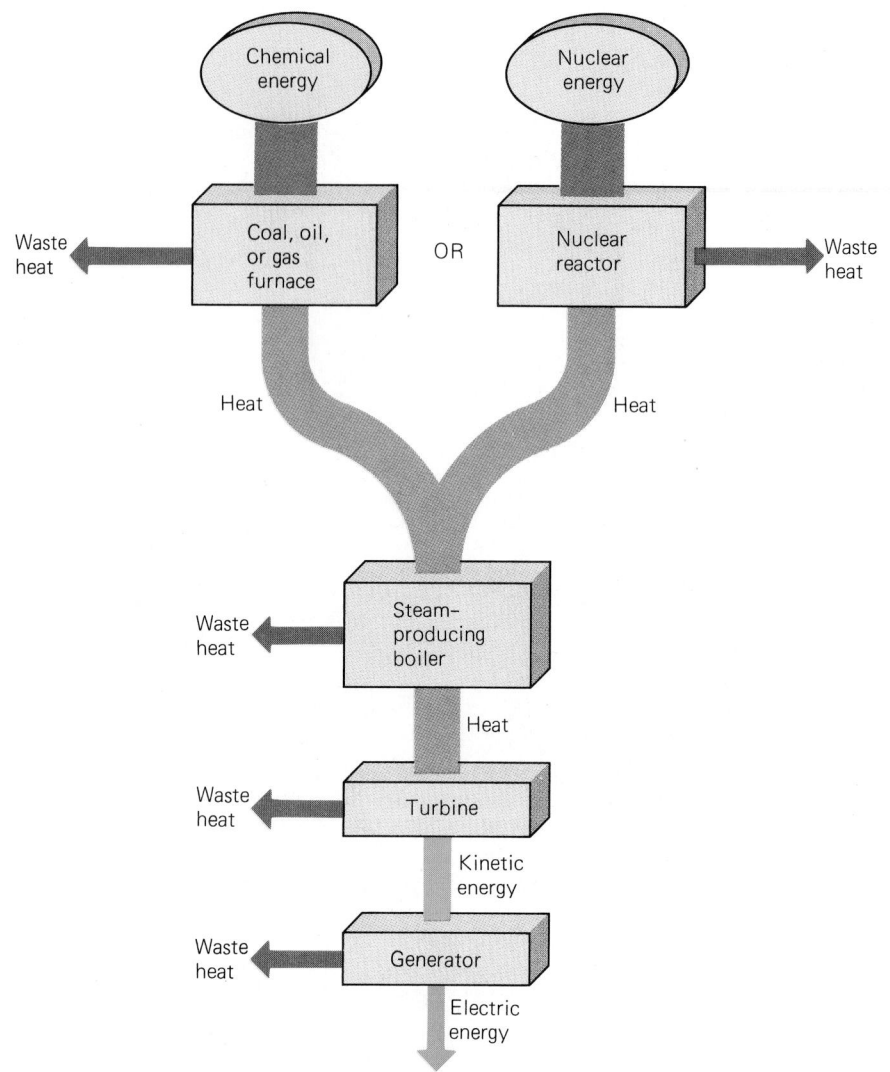

there is an overall tendency toward an increase in the heat energy of the universe at the expense of the other kinds it contains. We see this tendency all around us in everyday life. When coal or oil burns in an engine, much of its chemical energy becomes heat; when any kind of machine is operated, friction turns some of its energy into heat; an electric lightbulb emits heat as well as light; and so on. Most of the lost energy is dissipated in the atmosphere, the oceans, and the earth itself where it is largely unavailable for recovery.

In the world of nature a similar steady degradation of energy into unusable heat occurs. In the universe as a whole, the stars (for instance, the sun) constitute the hot reservoir and everything else (for instance, the earth) constitutes the cold reservoir from a thermodynamic point of view. As time goes on, the stars will grow cooler and the rest of the universe will grow warmer, so that less and less energy will be available to power the further evolution of the universe. On a molecular level, order will become disorder. If this process continues indefinitely, the entire universe will be at the same temperature and all its particles will have the same average energy. This condition is sometimes called the "heat death" of the universe. However, as we shall see in Sec. 19.9, this is not the only possible fate of the universe.

5.17   Entropy

The Arrow of Time

Although "disorder" may not seem a very precise concept, a quantity called **entropy** can be defined that is a measure of the disorder of the molecules that make up any body of matter. For instance, the entropy of liquid water is nearly three times that of ice, which reflects the more random arrangement of the molecules in the liquid state than in the solid state. The entropy of steam is still greater.

In terms of entropy, the second law of thermodynamics becomes

> The entropy of a system of some kind isolated from the rest of the universe cannot decrease.

If a puddle of water were to rise from the ground by itself while turning into ice, the process could conserve energy (and so obey the first law of thermodynamics) as the heat lost by the water becomes kinetic energy of the ice (Fig. 5-51). However, such an event would decrease the entropy of the water, and so cannot occur. The advantage of expressing the second law in terms of entropy is that, because entropy can be determined for a variety of systems, this law can be applied in an exact way to such systems.

Biological systems might seem to violate the second law. Certainly entropy decreases when a plant turns carbon dioxide and water into leaves and flowers. But this transformation of disorder into order needs the energy of sunlight to take place. If we take into account the increase in the entropy of the sun as it produces the required sunlight, the net result is an increase in the entropy of the universe. There is no way to avoid the second law.

An Unusual Principle   The second law is an unusual physical principle in several respects. It does not apply to individual particles, only to assemblies of many particles. It does not say what can occur, only what cannot occur. And it is unique in that it is closely tied to the direction of time.

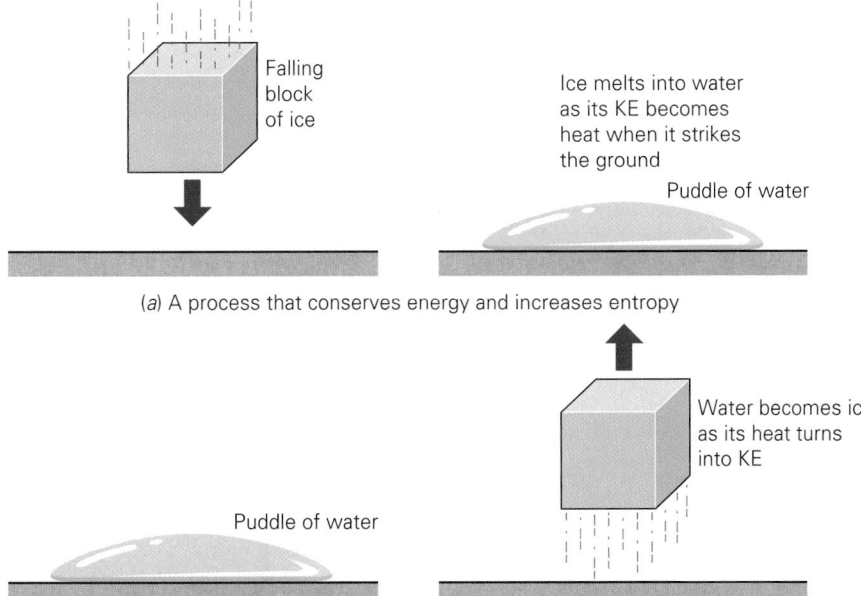

(a) A process that conserves energy and increases entropy

Falling block of ice

Ice melts into water as its KE becomes heat when it strikes the ground

Puddle of water

Puddle of water

Water becomes ice as its heat turns into KE

(b) A process that conserves energy and decreases entropy

Figure 5-51   The second law of thermodynamics provides a way to distinguish between processes that conserve energy and (a) increase entropy, hence are possible, and those that (b) decrease entropy, hence are impossible.

Ludwig Boltzmann (1844–1906)

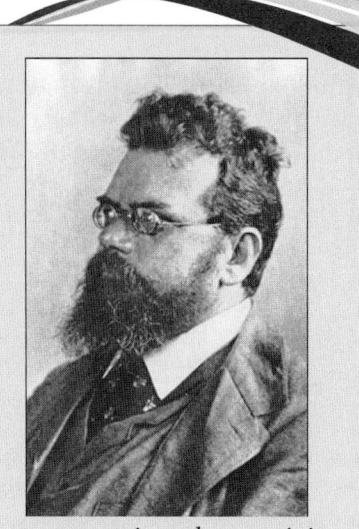

A native of Vienna, Boltzmann attended the university there. He then taught and carried out research at a number of institutions in Austria and Germany, moving from one to another every few years. Boltzmann was interested in poetry, music, and travel, and visited the United States three times, something unusual in those days.

Of Boltzmann's many contributions to physics, the most important were to the kinetic theory of gases and to the foundations of thermodynamics. The constant k in the formula $KE_{av} = \frac{3}{2}kT$ for the average molecular energy in a gas at the absolute temperature T is called Boltzmann's constant in

honor of his work. The mathematical relationship between molecular disorder and entropy was developed by Boltzmann; a monument to him in Vienna is inscribed with this relationship.

Boltzmann was a champion of the atomic theory of matter, still controversial in the late nineteenth century because there was then only indirect evidence for the existence of atoms and molecules. Battles with nonbelieving scientists deeply upset Boltzmann, and in his later years asthma, headaches, and poor eyesight further depressed his spirits. He committed suicide in 1906, not long after Albert Einstein published a paper on brownian motion

that was to convince the remaining doubters of the correctness of the atomic theory.

Events that involve only a few individual particles are always reversible. Nobody can tell whether a film of a billiard ball bouncing around is being run forward or backward. But events that involve many-particle systems are not always reversible. The film of an egg breaking when dropped makes no sense when run backward. The arrow of time always points in the direction of entropy increase. Time never runs backward; a broken egg never reassembles itself; in the universe as a whole, entropy—and the disorder it mirrors—marches on.

Important Terms and Ideas

Temperature is that property of a body of matter that gives rise to sensations of hot and cold; it is a measure of average molecular kinetic energy. **Heat** is molecular kinetic energy.

A **thermometer** is a device for measuring temperature. In the **Celsius scale,** the freezing point of water is given the value 0°C and the boiling point of water the value 100°C. In the **Fahrenheit scale,** these temperatures are given the values 32°F and 212°F.

The **specific heat** of a substance is the amount of heat needed to change the temperature of 1 kg of the substance by 1°C.

The **density** of a substance is its mass per unit volume.

The **pressure** on a surface is the perpendicular force per unit area acting on the surface. The unit of pressure is the **pascal,** which is equal to the newton/meter². The pressure at any point in a fluid depends on the weight of the fluid above the point as well as on any applied pressure.

According to **Archimedes' principle,** the upward **buoyant force** on an object immersed in a fluid is equal to the weight of fluid displaced by the object.

Boyle's law states that, at constant temperature, the volume of a gas sample is inversely proportional to its pressure.

The **absolute temperature scale** has its zero point at −273°C; temperatures in this scale are designated K. **Absolute zero** is 0 K = −273°C. **Charles's law** states that, at constant pressure, the volume of a gas sample is directly proportional to its absolute temperature.

The **ideal gas law**—which states that pV/T = constant for a gas sample regardless of changes in p, V, and T—is a combination of Boyle's and Charles's laws and is approximately obeyed by all gases.

According to the **kinetic theory of matter,** all matter consists of tiny individual **molecules** that are in constant random motion. The ideal gas law can be explained by the kinetic theory on the basis that the absolute temperature of a gas is proportional to the average kinetic energy of its molecules. At absolute zero, gas molecules would have no kinetic energy.

In **conduction,** heat is carried from one place to another by molecular collisions. In **convection,** the transport is by the motion of a volume of hot fluid. **Radiation** transfers heat by means of **electromagnetic waves,** which require no material medium for their passage.

The **heat of vaporization** of a substance is the amount of heat needed to change 1 kg of it at its boiling point from the liquid to the gaseous state. The **heat of fusion** of a substance is the amount of heat needed to change 1 kg of it at its melting point from the solid to the liquid state.

Sublimation is the direct conversion of a substance from the solid to the vapor state without it first becoming a liquid.

A **heat engine** is a device that converts heat into mechanical energy or work. The **first law of thermodynamics** is the law of conservation of energy. The **second law of thermodynamics** states that some of the heat input

to a heat engine must be wasted in order for the engine to operate.

A **refrigerator** uses mechanical energy to transfer heat from a cold reservoir to a hot one, a path opposite to the normal direction of heat flow. It is the reverse of a heat engine.

Entropy is a measure of the disorder of the particles that make up a body of matter. In a system of any kind isolated from the rest of the universe, entropy cannot decrease.

Important Formulas

Temperature scales: $T_F = \frac{9}{5} T_C + 32°$

$$T_C = \frac{5}{9}(T_F - 32°)$$

Amount of heat: $Q = mc\,\Delta T$

Density: $d = \frac{m}{V}$

Pressure: $p = \frac{F}{A}$

Boyle's law: $\frac{p_1}{p_2} = \frac{V_2}{V_1}$ (at constant temperature)

Absolute temperature scale: $T_K = T_C + 273$

Charles's law: $\frac{V_1}{V_2} = \frac{T_1}{T_2}$ (at constant pressure; temperatures on absolute scale)

Ideal gas law: $\frac{p_1 V_1}{T_1} = \frac{p_2 V_2}{T_2}$ (temperatures on absolute scale)

Maximum efficiency of heat engine:

$$\text{Eff(max)} = 1 - \frac{T_{\text{cold}}}{T_{\text{hot}}} \quad \text{(temperatures on absolute scale)}$$

Multiple Choice

1. Two thermometers, one calibrated in °F and the other in °C, are used to measure the same temperature. The numerical reading on the Fahrenheit thermometer
   a. is less than that on the Celsius thermometer
   b. is equal to that on the Celsius thermometer
   c. is greater than that on the Celsius thermometer
   d. may be any of these, depending on the temperature

2. One gram of steam at 100°C causes a more serious burn than 1 g of water at 100°C because the steam
   a. is less dense
   b. strikes the skin with greater force
   c. has a higher specific heat
   d. contains more energy

3. Heat transfer in a gas can occur by
   a. radiation only
   b. convection only
   c. radiation and convection only
   d. radiation, convection, and conduction

4. Heat transfer in a vacuum can occur by
   a. radiation only
   b. convection only
   c. radiation and convection only
   d. radiation, convection, and conduction

5. The fluid at the bottom of a container is
   a. under less pressure than the fluid at the top
   b. under the same pressure as the fluid at the top

c. under more pressure than the fluid at the top
   d. any of these, depending upon the circumstances

6. The pressure of the earth's atmosphere at sea level is due to
   a. the gravitational attraction of the earth for the atmosphere
   b. the heating of the atmosphere by the sun
   c. the fact that most living things constantly breathe air
   d. evaporation of water from the seas and oceans

7. Buoyancy occurs because, as the depth in a fluid increases, the fluid's
   a. pressure increases
   b. pressure decreases
   c. density increases
   d. density decreases

8. The density of freshwater is 1.00 g/cm³ and that of seawater is 1.03 g/cm³. A ship will float
   a. higher in freshwater than in seawater
   b. lower in freshwater than in seawater
   c. at the same level in freshwater and seawater
   d. any of the above, depending on the shape of its hull

9. An ice cube whose center consists of liquid water is floating in a glass of water. When the ice melts, the level of water in the glass
   a. rises
   b. remains the same

c. falls

d. any of the above, depending on the relative volume of water inside the ice cube

10. A person stands on a very sensitive scale and inhales deeply. The reading on the scale
    a. increases
    b. does not change
    c. decreases
    d. any of the above, depending on how the expansion of the person's chest compares with the volume of air inhaled

11. At constant pressure, the volume of a gas sample is directly proportional to
    a. the size of its molecules
    b. its Fahrenheit temperature
    c. its Celsius temperature
    d. its absolute temperature

12. Which of the following statements is not correct?
    a. Matter is composed of tiny particles called molecules.
    b. These molecules are in constant motion, even in solids.
    c. All molecules have the same size and mass.
    d. The differences between the solid, liquid, and gaseous states of matter lie in the relative freedom of motion of their respective molecules.

13. Molecular motion is not responsible for
    a. the pressure exerted by a gas
    b. Boyle's law
    c. evaporation
    d. buoyancy

14. Absolute zero may be regarded as that temperature at which
    a. water freezes
    b. all gases become liquids
    c. all substances become solid
    d. molecular motion in a gas would be the minimum possible

15. On the molecular level, heat is
    a. kinetic energy
    b. potential energy
    c. rest energy
    d. all of these, in proportions that depend on the circumstances

16. At a given temperature
    a. the molecules in a gas all have the same average speed
    b. the molecules in a gas all have the same average energy
    c. light gas molecules have lower average energies than heavy gas molecules
    d. heavy gas molecules have lower average energies than light gas molecules

17. The temperature of a gas sample in a container of fixed volume is raised. The gas exerts a higher pressure on the walls of its container because its molecules
    a. lose more PE when they strike the walls
    b. lose more KE when they strike the walls

c. are in contact with the walls for a shorter time

d. have higher average velocities and strike the walls more often

18. The volume of a gas sample is increased while its temperature is held constant. The gas exerts a lower pressure on the walls of its container because its molecules strike the walls
    a. less often
    b. with lower velocities
    c. with less energy
    d. with less force

19. When evaporation occurs, the liquid that remains is cooler because
    a. the pressure on the liquid decreases
    b. the volume of the liquid decreases
    c. the slowest molecules remain behind
    d. the fastest molecules remain behind

20. When a vapor condenses into a liquid,
    a. its temperature rises
    b. its temperature falls
    c. it absorbs heat
    d. it gives off heat

21. Food cooks more rapidly in a pressure cooker than in an ordinary pot with a loose lid because
    a. the pressure forces heat into the food
    b. the high pressure lowers the boiling point of water
    c. the high pressure raises the boiling point of water
    d. the tight lid keeps the heat inside the cooker

22. A heat engine takes in heat at one temperature and turns
    a. all of it into work
    b. some of it into work and rejects the rest at a lower temperature
    c. some of it into work and rejects the rest at the same temperature
    d. some of it into work and rejects the rest at a higher temperature

23. In any process, the maximum amount of heat that can be converted to mechanical energy
    a. depends on the amount of friction present
    b. depends on the intake and exhaust temperatures
    c. depends on whether kinetic or potential energy is involved
    d. is 100 percent

24. In any process, the maximum amount of mechanical energy that can be converted to heat
    a. depends on the amount of friction present
    b. depends on the intake and exhaust temperatures
    c. depends on whether kinetic or potential energy is involved
    d. is 100 percent

25. A frictionless heat engine can be 100 percent efficient only if its exhaust temperature is
    a. equal to its input temperature
    b. less than its input temperature

c. 0°C

d. 0 K

26. The physics of a refrigerator most closely resembles the physics of

  a. a heat engine

  b. the melting of ice

  c. the freezing of water

  d. the evaporation of water

27. The working substance (or refrigerant) used in most refrigerators is a

  a. gas that is easy to liquify

  b. gas that is hard to liquify

  c. liquid that is easy to solidify

  d. liquid that is hard to solidify

28. Heat is absorbed by the refrigerant in a refrigerator when it

  a. melts

  b. vaporizes

  c. condenses

  d. is compressed

29. A refrigerator gives off

  a. less heat than it absorbs from its contents

  b. the same amount of heat it absorbs from its contents

  c. more heat than it absorbs from its contents

  d. Any of these choices could be correct, depending on the circumstances

30. The second law of thermodynamics does not lead to the conclusion that

  a. on a molecular level, order will eventually become disorder in the universe

  b. all the matter in the universe will eventually end up at the same temperature

  c. no heat engine can convert heat into work with 100 percent efficiency

  d. the total amount of energy in the universe, including rest energy, is constant

31. The greater the entropy of a system of particles,

  a. the less the energy of the system

  b. the more the energy of the system

  c. the less the order of the system

  d. the more the order of the system

32. The Celsius equivalent of a temperature of 120°F is

  a. 35°C

  b. 49°F

  c. 67°C

  d. 88°C

33. Oxygen boils at −183°C. The Fahrenheit equivalent of this temperature is

  a. −215°F

  b. −297°F

  c. −329°F

  d. −361°F

34. When 400 kJ of heat is added to 12 kg of water at 2°C, its final temperature is

  a. 5.9°C

  b. 7.9°C

c. 11.7°C

d. 17.9°C

35. When 1 kg of steam at 200°C loses 3 MJ of heat, the result is

  a. ice

  b. water and ice

  c. water

  d. water and steam

36. When 20 kJ of heat are removed from 1.2 kg of ice originally at −5°C, its new temperature is

  a. −18°C

  b. −23°C

  c. −26°C

  d. −35°C

37. A 3-kg pine board is 20 cm wide, 2 cm thick, and 2 m long. The density of the board is

  a. 240 kg/m^3

  b. 267 kg/m^3

  c. 375 kg/m^3

  d. 469 kg/m^3

38. A 2-kg brick has the dimensions 7.5 cm × 15 cm × 30 cm. The pressure the brick exerts when standing on its smallest face is

  a. 0.0178 Pa

  b. 0.0225 Pa

  c. 178 Pa

  d. 225 Pa

39. An object suspended from a spring scale is lowered into a pail filled to the brim with water, and 4 N of water overflows. The scale shows that the object weighs 6 N in the water. The weight in air of the object is

  a. 2 N

  b. 4 N

  c. 6 N

  d. 10 N

40. A wooden plank 200 cm long, 30 cm wide, and 40 mm thick floats in water with 10 mm of its thickness above the surface. The mass of the board is

  a. 1.8 kg

  b. 18 kg

  c. 24 kg

  d. 176 kg

41. If the pressure on 10 m^3 of air is increased from 200 kPa to 800 kPa, the new volume of air will be

  a. 1.25 m^3

  b. 1.67 m^3

  c. 2.5 m^3

  d. 40 m^3

42. Lead melts at 330°C. On the absolute scale this temperature corresponds to

  a. 57 K

  b. 362 K

  c. 571 K

  d. 603 K

43. At which of the following temperatures would the molecules of a gas have twice the average kinetic energy they have at room temperature, 20°C?

  a. 40°C

  b. 80°C

  c. 313°C

  d. 586°C

44. An ideal frictionless engine absorbs heat at 400 K and exhausts heat at 300 K. Its efficiency is

  a. 25 percent

  b. 33 percent

  c. 75 percent

  d. 133 percent

45. If a heat engine that exhausts heat at 400 K is to have an efficiency of 33 percent, it must take in heat at a minimum of

  a. 133 K

  b. 449 K

  c. 532 K

  d. 600 K

Exercises

5.1   Temperature

1. Running hot water over the metal lid of a glass jar makes it easier to open the jar. Why?

2. When a mercury-in-glass thermometer is heated, its mercury column goes down briefly before rising. Why?

3. Three iron bars are heated in a furnace to different temperatures. One of them glows white, another yellow, and the third red. Which is at the highest temperature? The lowest?

4. Why do you think the Celsius temperature scale is sometimes called the centigrade scale?

5. Normal room temperature is about 20°C. What is this temperature on the Fahrenheit scale?

6. What is the Celsius equivalent of a temperature of 160°F?

7. Dry ice (solid carbon dioxide) starts to vaporize into a gas at −112°F. What is this temperature on the Celsius scale?

8. You have a Fahrenheit thermometer in your left hand and a Celsius thermometer in your right hand. Both thermometers show the same reading in degrees. What is the temperature?

5.2   Heat

9. Why is a piece of ice at 0°C more effective in cooling a drink than the same mass of cold water at 0°C?

10. Would it be more efficient to warm your bed on a cold night with a hot water bottle that contains 1 kg of water at 50°C or with a 1-kg gold bar at 50°C? Why?

11. A cup of hot coffee can be cooled by placing a cold spoon in it. A spoon of which of the following materials would be most effective for this purpose? Assume the spoons all have the same mass: aluminum, copper, iron, glass.

12. A 150-L water heater is rated at 8 kW. If 20 percent of its heat escapes, how long does the heater take to raise the temperature of 150 L of water from 10°C to 60°C?

13. How many kJ of heat are needed to raise the temperature of 200 g of water from 20°C to 100°C in preparing a cup of coffee?

14. The specific heat of granite is 0.80 kJ/kg · °C. If 1.6 MJ of heat are added to a 100-kg granite statue of James Prescott Joule that is originally at 18°C, what is the final temperature of the statue?

15. The diet of a 60-kg person provides 12,000 kJ daily. If this amount of energy were added to 60 kg of water, by how much would its temperature be increased?

16. Ninety kilojoules of heat were added to a 2.0-kg piece of wood whose temperature then rose from 20°C to 48°C. What was the specific heat of the wood?

17. The average specific heat of a certain 25-kg storage battery is 0.84 kJ/kg · °C. When it is fully charged, the battery contains 1.4 MJ of electric energy. If all of this energy were dissipated inside the battery, by how much would its temperature increase?

18. An essential part of a home solar heating system is a way to store heat for use at night and on cloudy days. In a certain system, the water used for storage is initially at 75°C and it is required to provide an average of 6.0 kW to keep the house at an average of 18°C for 3 days. How much water is needed?

19. A 10-kg stone is dropped into a pool of water from a height of 100 m. How much energy in joules does the stone have when it strikes the water? If all this energy goes into heat and if the pool contains 10 m³ of water, by how much is its temperature raised? (The mass of 1 m³ of water is 10³ kg.)

5.4   Density

20. Why do tables of densities always include the temperature for which the listed values hold? What would be true of the densities of most solids and liquids at a temperature higher than the quoted one?

21. A room is 5 m long, 4 m wide, and 3 m high. What is the mass of the air it contains?

22. A 156-kg coil of sheet steel is 0.80 mm thick and 50 cm wide. How long is the steel in the coil?

23. A 50-g bracelet is suspected of being gold-plated lead instead of pure gold. It is dropped into a full glass of water and 4 cm³ of water overflows. Is the bracelet pure gold?

24. A 1200-kg concrete slab that measures 2 m × 1 m × 20 cm is delivered to a building under construction. Does the slab contain steel reinforcing rods or is it plain concrete?

25. Mammals have approximately the same density as freshwater. (a) Find the volume in liters of a 55-kg woman and (b) the volume in cubic meters of a 140,000-kg blue whale. (Note: 1 liter = 10^{-3} m^3 = 0.001 m^3.)

26. A cube of gold 30 mm long on each edge (the size of an ice cube) is usually worth at least $18,000. If that is its value, how much is a gram of gold worth?

27. The radius of the earth is 6.37×10^6 m and its mass is 5.98×10^{24} kg. (a) Find the average density of the earth. (b) The average density of the rocks at the earth's surface is 2.7×10^3 kg/m^3. What must be true of the matter of which the earth's interior is composed? Is it likely that the earth is hollow and peopled by another species, as the ancients believed? (Note: The volume of a sphere of radius R is $\frac{4}{3}\pi R^3$.)

5.5 Pressure

28. Some water is boiled briefly in an open metal can. The can is then sealed while still hot. Why does the can collapse when it cools?

29. When a person drinks a soda through a straw, where does the force come from that causes the soda to move upward?

30. A U-shaped tube contains water and an unknown liquid separated by mercury, as in Fig. 5-52. How does the density of the liquid compare with the density of water? How do the pressures at *A* and *B* compare?

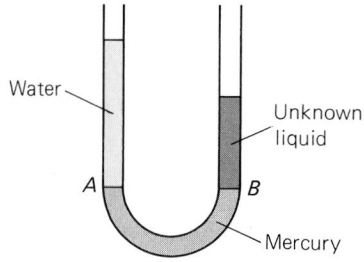

Figure 5-52

31. The three containers shown in Fig. 5-53 are filled with water to the same height. Compare the pressures at the bottoms of the containers.

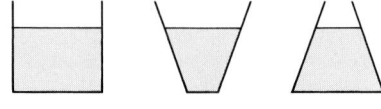

Figure 5-53

32. A 60-kg swami lies on a bed of nails with his body supported by 4000 nails. The area of the point of each nail is 1 mm^2. If the threshold pressure for pain is 1 MPa, how unpleasant is the experience for the swami? What if the point area is 0.1 mm^2?

33. A tire pump has a piston whose cross-sectional area is 0.001 m^2. If a force of 150 N is applied to the piston, find the pressure on the air in the pump.

34. A nail whose cross-sectional area is 3 mm^2 is embedded in a tire in which the air pressure is 1.8 bar. How much force tends to push the nail out?

35. A 1200-lb car is equally supported by its 4 tires, which are inflated to a pressure of 2 bar. What area of each tire is in contact with the road?

36. The smallest bone in the index finger of a 75-kg circus acrobat has a cross-sectional area of 0.5 cm^2 and breaks under a pressure of 1.7×10^8 Pa. Is it safe for the acrobat to balance his entire weight on this finger?

37. A hypodermic syringe whose cylinder has a cross-sectional area of 60 mm^2 is used to inject a liquid medicine into a patient's vein in which the blood pressure is 2 kPa. (a) What is the minimum force needed on the plunger of the syringe? (b) Why is the cross-sectional area of the needle irrelevant?

38. At the distance of the earth from the sun, the pressure exerted by sunlight is about 10^{-5} Pa. How much force does this pressure exert on a 10 m^2 array of solar cells on a satellite when the array is perpendicular to the direction of the sunlight? If the satellite has a mass of 300 kg, what acceleration does this force give it?

5.6 Buoyancy

39. Why does buoyancy occur? Under what circumstances does an object float in a fluid?

40. Two balls of the same size but of different mass are dropped from a tower. If the air resistance is the same for both, will they reach the ground together? If not, which will arrive first? Why?

41. A wooden block is submerged in a tank of water and pressed down against the bottom of the tank so that there is no water underneath it. The block is released. Will it rise to the surface or stay where it is?

42. A jar is filled to the top with water, and a piece of cardboard is slid over the opening so that there is only water in the jar. If the jar is turned over, will the cardboard fall off? What will happen if there is any air in the jar?

43. A ship catches fire, and its steel hull expands as it heats up. What happens to the volume of water the ship displaces? What happens to the height of the ship's deck above the water?

44. A bridge in Sweden carries the Göta Canal over a highway. What, if anything, happens to the load on the bridge when a boat passes across it in the canal?

45. As Table 5-3 shows, ice has a lower density than water, which is why ice floats. What will happen when an ice cube floating in a glass of water filled to the brim begins to melt?

46. An ice cube with an air bubble inside it is floating in a glass of water. Compare what happens to the water level in the glass when the ice melts with what would happen if the cube had no bubble in it.

47. A sailboat has a lead or iron keel to keep it upright despite the force wind exerts on its sails. What

difference, if any, is there between the stability of a sailboat in freshwater and in seawater?

48. An aluminum canoe is floating in a swimming pool. After a while it begins to leak and sinks to the bottom of the pool. What, if anything, happens to the water level in the pool?

49. How much force is needed to support a 100-kg iron anchor when it is submerged in seawater? (Hint: First find the anchor's volume.)

50. A 40-kg girl dives off a raft whose area is 3 m² that is floating in a freshwater lake. By how much does the raft rise?

51. A raft 3 m long, 2 m wide, and 30 cm thick, made from solid balsa wood, is floating in a freshwater lake. How many 65-kg people can it support?

52. As global warming proceeds, sea level is rising, partly because of thermal expansion and partly because of meltwater from disappearing icecaps and glaciers. Coastal cities are expected to be flooded as a result. By how much would sea level go down if all the ships in the oceans are removed? The world's oceans have a surface area of about 3.5×10^{14} m² and the mass of all the ships afloat is roughly 1.8×10^{12} kg.

53. A 200-L iron tank has a mass of 36 kg. (a) Will it float in seawater when empty? (b) When filled with freshwater? (c) When filled with gasoline?

5.7 The Gas Laws

54. What are the equivalents of 0 K, 0°C, and 0°F in the other temperature scales?

55. A certain quantity of hydrogen occupies a volume of 1000 cm³ at 0°C (273 K) and ordinary atmospheric pressure. (a) If the pressure is tripled but the temperature is held constant, what will the volume of the hydrogen be? (b) If the temperature is increased to 273°C but the pressure is held constant, what will the volume of the hydrogen be?

56. A tire contains air at a pressure of 2.8 bar at 10°C. If the tire's volume is unchanged, what will the air pressure in it be when the tire warms up to 35°C as the car is driven?

57. An oxygen cylinder used for welding contains 40 L of oxygen at 20°C and a pressure of 17 MPa. The density of oxygen is 1.4 kg/m³ at 20°C and atmospheric pressure of 101 kPa. Find the mass of the oxygen in the cylinder.

58. A weather balloon carries instruments that measure temperature, pressure, and humidity as it rises through the atmosphere. Suppose such a balloon has a volume of 1.2 m³ at sea level where the pressure is 1 atm and the temperature is 20°C. When the balloon is at an altitude of 11 km (36,000 ft) the pressure is down to 0.5 atm and the temperature is about −55°C. What is the volume of the balloon then?

59. To what Celsius temperature must a gas sample initially at 20°C be heated if its volume is to double while its pressure remains the same?

60. The propellant gas that remains in an empty can of spray paint is at atmospheric pressure. If such a can at 20°C is thrown into a fire and is heated to 600°C, how many times atmospheric pressure is the new pressure inside the can? (The higher pressure may burst the can, which is why such cans should not be thrown into a fire.)

61. An air tank used for scuba diving has a safety valve set to open at a pressure of 28 MPa. The normal pressure of the full tank at 20°C is 20 MPa. If the tank is heated after being filled to 20 MPa, at what temperature will the safety valve open?

5.8 Kinetic Theory of Gases

5.9 Molecular Motion and Temperature

62. A glass of water is stirred and then allowed to stand until the water stops moving. What becomes of the KE of the moving water?

63. Is it meaningful to say that an object at a temperature of 200°C is twice as hot as one at 100°C?

64. Gas molecules have speeds comparable with those of rifle bullets, yet it is observed that a gas with a strong odor (ammonia, for instance) takes a few minutes to diffuse through a room. Why?

65. At absolute zero, a sample of an ideal gas would have zero volume. Why would this not be true of an actual gas at absolute zero?

66. The pressure on a sample of hydrogen is doubled, while its temperature is kept unchanged. What happens to the average speed of the hydrogen molecules?

67. When they are close together, molecules attract one another slightly. As a result of this attraction, are gas pressures higher or lower than expected from the ideal gas law?

68. Temperatures in both the Celsius and Fahrenheit scales can be negative. Why is a negative temperature impossible on the absolute scale?

69. How can the conclusion of kinetic theory that molecular motion occurs in solids be reconciled with the observation that solids have definite shapes and volumes?

70. A 1-L tank holds 1 g of hydrogen at 0°C and another 1-L tank holds 1 g of oxygen at 0°C. The mass of an oxygen molecule is 16 times the mass of a hydrogen molecule. (a) Do the tanks hold the same number of molecules? If not, which holds more? (b) Do the gases exert the same pressure? If not, which exerts the greater pressure? (c) Do the molecules in the tanks have the same average energy? If not, in which are the average energies greater? (d) Do the molecules in the tanks have the same average speeds? If not, in which are the average speeds greater?

71. To what temperature must a gas sample initially at 27°C be raised in order for the average energy of its molecules to double?

72. A tank holds 1 kg of nitrogen at 25°C and a pressure of 100 kPa. What happens to the pressure when 4 kg of nitrogen are added to the tank at the same

temperature? Explain your answer in terms of kinetic theory of gases.

73. A mixture of the gases hydrogen and carbon dioxide (CO_2) is at 20°C. A CO_2 molecule has about 22 times the mass of a hydrogen molecule, whose average speed at 20°C is about 1.6 km/s. What is the average speed of a CO_2 molecule in the mixture?

5.10 Heat Transfer

74. You can safely put your hand inside a hot oven for a short time, but even a momentary contact with the metal walls of the oven will cause a burn. Explain.

75. Outdoors in winter, why does the steel blade of a shovel feel colder than its wooden handle?

76. A thermos bottle consists of two glass vessels, one inside the other, with air removed from the space between them. The vessels are both coated with thin metal films. Why is this device so effective in keeping its contents at a constant temperature?

77. What is the advantage of installing the heating element of an electric kettle near its bottom?

5.12 Evaporation and Boiling

78. Why does evaporation cool a liquid?

79. Why does blowing across hot coffee cool it down?

80. If you wish to speed up the rate at which potatoes are cooking in a pan of boiling water, would it be better to turn up the gas flame or use a pressure cooker?

81. Give as many methods as you can think of that will increase the rate of evaporation of a liquid sample. Explain why each method will have this effect.

82. How much heat is given off when 1 kg of steam at 100°C condenses and cools to water at 20°C?

83. A total of 500 kJ of heat are added to 1 kg of water at 20°C. What is the final temperature of the water? If it is 100°C, how much steam, if any, is produced?

84. Many power stations get rid of their waste heat by using it to boil water and allowing the resulting steam to escape into the atmosphere via a cooling tower. How much water would a power station need per second to dispose of 1000 MW of waste heat? Consider only the vaporization of the water; the heat used to raise the water to the boiling point is much less.

85. Solar energy arrives at a rate of 1.2 kW at a reflecting dish with an area of 1 m^2 that focuses the light on a jar that contains 100 g of water initially at 20°C. How long will it take the water to reach 100°C and then boil away if no energy is lost?

5.13 Melting

86. A lead bullet at 100°C strikes a steel plate and melts. What was its minimum speed? The specific heat of lead is 0.13 kJ/kg · °C.

87. Water at 50°C can be obtained by mixing together which one or more of the following? Which of the others would have final temperatures higher than 50°C and which lower than 50°C?

 a. 1 kg of ice at 0°C and 1 kg of steam at 100°C

 b. 1 kg of ice at 0°C and 1 kg of water at 100°C

 c. 1 kg of water at 0°C and 1 kg of steam at 100°C

 d. 1 kg of water at 0°C and 1 kg of water at 100°C

5.14 Heat Engines
5.15 Thermodynamics

88. Why are both a hot and a cold reservoir needed for a heat engine to operate?

89. The oceans contain an immense amount of heat energy. Why can a submarine not make use of this energy for propulsion?

90. A person tries to cool a kitchen by switching on an electric fan and closing the kitchen door and windows. What will happen?

91. In another attempt to cool the kitchen, the person leaves the refrigerator door open, again with the kitchen door and windows closed. Now what will happen?

92. Is it correct to say that a refrigerator "produces cold"? If not, why not?

93. The first law of thermodynamics is the same as the law of conservation of energy. Is there any law of nature that is the same as the second law of thermodynamics?

94. An engine is proposed that is to operate between 250°C and 60°C with an efficiency of 40 percent. Will the engine perform as predicted? If not, what would its maximum efficiency be?

95. An engine that operates between 2000 K and 700 K has an efficiency of 40 percent. What percentage of its maximum possible efficiency is this?

96. An engine that operates at the maximum efficiency possible takes in 6.0 MJ of heat at 327°C and exhausts waste heat at 127°C. How much work does it perform?

97. Surface water in a tropical ocean is typically at 27°C whereas at a depth of a kilometer or more it is at only about 5°C. It has been proposed to operate heat engines using surface water as the hot reservoir and deep water (pumped to the surface) as the cold reservoir. What would the maximum efficiency of such an engine be? Why might such an engine eventually be a practical proposition even with so low an efficiency?

98. Three designs for an engine to operate between 450 K and 300 K are proposed. Design *A* is claimed to require a heat input of 800 J for each 1000 J of work output, design *B* a heat input of 2500 J, and design *C* a heat input of 3500 J. Which design would you choose and why?

5.16 Entropy

99. The evolution of today's animals from their primitive ancestors of billions of years ago represents a large increase in order, which corresponds to a decrease in entropy. How can this be reconciled with the second law of thermodynamics?

100. When salt is dissolved in water, do you think the entropy of the system of salt + water increases or decreases? Why?

Electricity and Magnetism

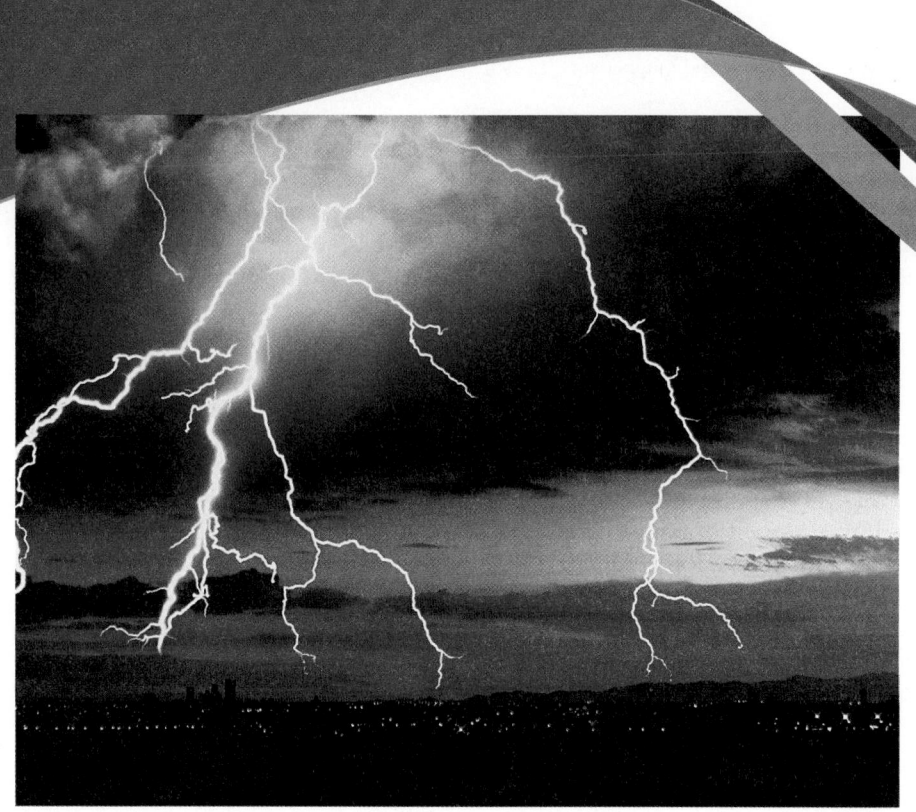

Lightning is an electrical discharge in the atmosphere.

GOALS

When you have finished this chapter you should be able to complete the goals
• given for each section below:

Electric Charge

6.1 Positive and Negative Charge
Opposites Attract

6.2 What Is Charge?
Protons, Electrons, and Neutrons
• Discuss what is meant by electric charge.
• Describe the structure of an atom.

6.3 Coulomb's Law
The Law of Force for Electric Charges
• State Coulomb's law for electric force and compare it with Newton's law of gravity.

6.4 Force on an Uncharged Object
Why a Comb Can Attract Bits of Paper
• Account for the attraction between a charged object and an uncharged one.

Electricity and Matter

6.5 Matter in Bulk
Gravity versus Electricity

6.6 Conductors and Insulators
How Charge Flows from One Place to Another
• Distinguish among conductors, semiconductors, and insulators.
• Define ion and give several ways of producing ionization.

6.7 Superconductivity
A Revolution in Technology May Be Near
• Define superconductivity and discuss its potential importance.

Electric Current

6.8 The Ampere
The Unit of Electric Current
• Discuss what is meant by the direction of an electric current.

6.9 Potential Difference
The Push behind a Current
• Describe electric current and potential difference (voltage) by analogy with the flow of water in a pipe.

6.10 Ohm's Law
Current, Voltage, and Resistance
• Use Ohm's law to solve problems that involve the current in a circuit, the resistance of the circuit, and the voltage across the circuit.
• Explain the consequences of open and short circuit faults and the function of fuses and circuit breakers.

6.11 Electric Power
Current Times Voltage
• Relate the power consumed by an electrical appliance to the current in it and the voltage across it.
• Discuss series and parallel connections of circuit elements.

Magnetism

6.12 Magnets
Attraction and Repulsion
• State what is meant by the poles of a magnet and distinguish between its north and south poles.

6.13 Magnetic Field
How Magnetic Forces Act

• Describe what is meant by a magnetic field and discuss how it can be pictured by field lines.

6.14 Oersted's Experiment
Magnetic Fields Originate in Moving Electric Charges
• State the connection between electric charges and magnetic fields.
• Use the right-hand rule to find the direction of the magnetic field around an electric current.

6.15 Electromagnets
How to Create a Strong Magnetic Field
• Explain how an electromagnet works.

Using Magnetism

6.16 Magnetic Force on a Current
A Sidewise Push
• Describe the force a magnetic field exerts on an electric current.

6.17 Electric Motors
Mechanical Energy from Electric Energy
• Discuss the operation of an electric motor.

6.18 Electromagnetic Induction
Electric Energy from Mechanical Energy
• Describe electromagnetic induction and explain how a generator makes use of it to produce an electric current.

6.19 Transformers
Stepping Voltage Up or Down
• Explain how a transformer changes the voltage of an alternating current and why this is useful.

We have now learned about force and motion, mass and energy, the law of gravity, and the concept of matter as being made up of tiny moving molecules. With the help of these ideas we have been able to make sense of a wide variety of observations, from the paths of the planets across the sky to the melting of ice and the boiling of water. Is this enough for us to understand how the entire physical universe works?

For an answer all we need do is run a hard rubber comb through our hair on a dry day. Little sparks occur, and the comb then can pick up small bits of dust and paper. What is revealed in this way is an **electrical** phenomenon, something that neither gravity nor the kinetic theory of matter can account for.

In everyday life electricity is familiar as that which causes our lightbulbs to glow, many of our motors to turn, our telephones and radios to bring us sounds, our television screens to bring us images. But there is more to electricity than its ability to transport energy and information. All matter turns out to be electrical in nature, and electric forces are what bind electrons to nuclei to form atoms and what hold atoms together to form molecules, liquids, and solids. Most of the properties of the ordinary matter around us—an exception is mass—can be traced to electrical forces.

Electric Charge

The first recorded studies of electricity were made in Greece by Thales of Miletus about 2500 years ago. Thales experimented with amber, called *electron* in Greek, and fur. The name **electric charge** is today given to whatever it is that a piece of amber (or hard rubber) possesses as a result of being rubbed with fur. It is this charge that causes sparks to occur and that attracts light objects such as bits of paper.

6.1 Positive and Negative Charge

Opposites Attract

Let us begin by hanging a small plastic ball from a thread, as in Fig. 6-1. We touch the ball with a hard rubber rod and find that nothing happens. Next we stroke the rod with a piece of fur and again touch the plastic ball with the rod. This time the ball flies away from the rod. What must have occurred is that some of the electric charge on the rod has flowed to the ball, and the fact that the ball then flies away from the rod means that charges of the same kind repel each other (Fig. 6-2).

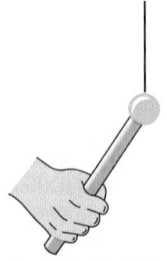

1. A plastic ball held by a string is touched by a hard rubber rod. Nothing happens.

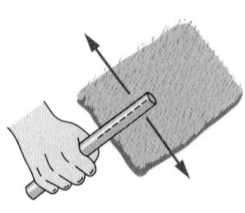

2. The rubber rod is stroked against a piece of fur.

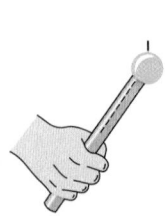

3. The plastic ball is again touched by the rubber rod.

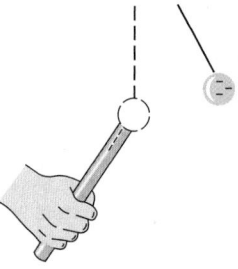

4. After the touch, the plastic ball flies away from the rod.

Figure 6-1   A rubber rod stroked with fur becomes negatively charged. When it is touched against a plastic ball, some of the negative charge flows to the ball. The plastic ball then flies away because like charges repel each other.

BIOGRAPHY | Benjamin Franklin (1706–1790)

Although best known for his role in establishing the United States as an independent country (he helped draft the Declaration of Independence and the Constitution), Franklin was also the first notable American scientist and inventor. The Franklin stove, the lightning rod, and bifocal eyeglasses were products of his ingenuity. By analyzing the records of Atlantic voyages in the sailing ships of his time, he inferred the existence of the Gulf Stream (see Sec. 14.13).

Franklin was especially interested in electricity, and he interpreted what was then known about it in terms of a fluid: a positive charge meant an excess of the fluid, and a negative charge a deficiency. In this picture an electric current involves the motion of the fluid from a positively charged object to a negatively charged object where it is absorbed. If the excess in one object matches the deficiency in the other, both become neutral as a result. Even today electricians regard electric currents in this way, although it is now known that what moves are negatively charged electrons in the opposite direction.

In the most famous of his experiments, Franklin produced sparks from the end of the wet string of a kite flown in a thunderstorm, from which he concluded that lightning is an electrical phenomenon. (He was careful not to touch the string directly; an imitator who did was electrocuted.)

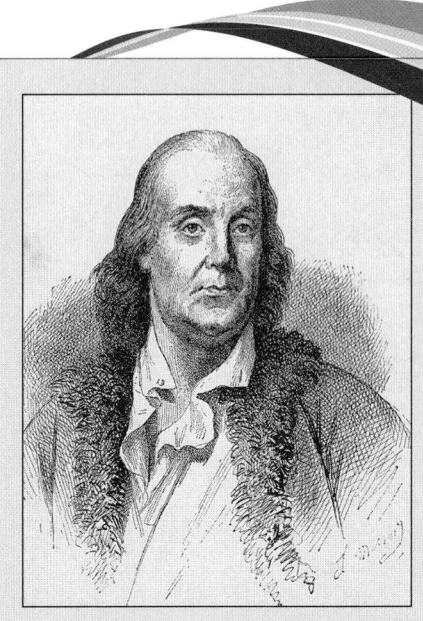

Is there only one kind of electric charge? To find out, we try other combinations of materials and see what happens when the various charged plastic balls are near each other. Figure 6-3 shows the result when one ball has been charged by a rubber rod stroked with fur and the other ball has been charged by a glass rod stroked with silk: the two balls fly together. We conclude that the charges on the rods are somehow different and that different charges attract each other.

Comprehensive experiments show that *all* electric charges fall into one of these two types. Regardless of origin, charges always behave as though they came either from a rubber rod rubbed with fur or from a glass rod rubbed with silk. Benjamin Franklin suggested names for these two basic kinds of electricity. He called the charge produced on the rubber rod **negative charge** and the charge produced on the glass rod **positive charge.** These definitions are still used today.

These experiments can be summarized very simply:

> All electric charges are either positive or negative. Like charges repel one another; unlike charges attract one another.

Charge Separation We have thus far been paying attention to the positive charge of the glass and the negative charge of the rubber. However, we do not produce only positive charge by rubbing glass with silk or only negative charge by stroking rubber with fur. If the fur used with the rubber is brought near a negatively charged plastic ball, the ball is attracted. Thus the fur must have a positive charge (Fig. 6-4). Similarly the silk used with the glass turns out to have a negative charge. Whenever electric charge is produced by contact between two objects of different materials, one of them ends up with a positive charge and the other a negative charge. Which is which depends on the particular materials used.

The rubbing process does not *create* the electric charges that appear as a result. All "uncharged" objects actually contain equal amounts of positive

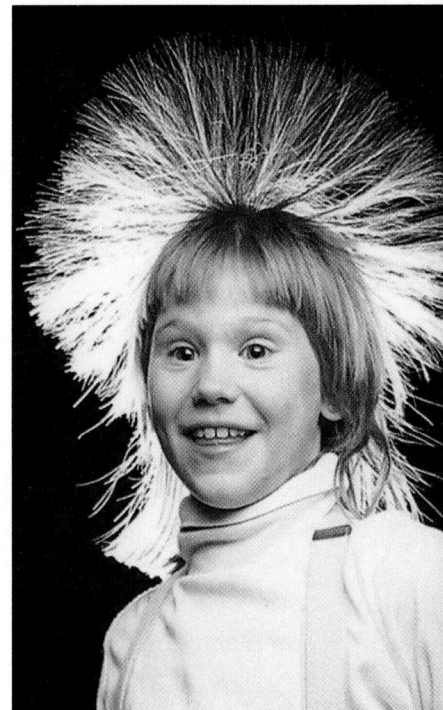

Figure 6-2 This girl has been given an electric charge by touching the terminal of a static electric generator. Because all her hairs have charge of the same sign, they repel one another.

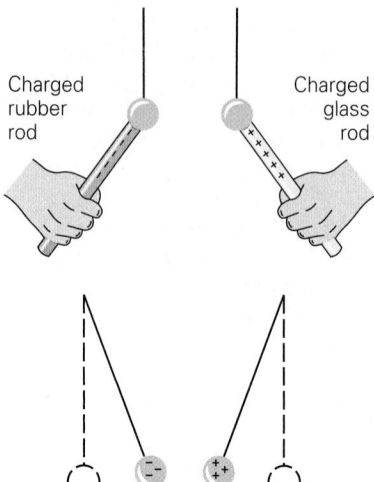

Figure 6-3 A glass rod stroked with silk becomes positively charged. When one plastic ball is touched with a negatively charged rubber rod and another plastic ball is touched with a positively charged glass rod, the two balls fly together because unlike charges attract each other.

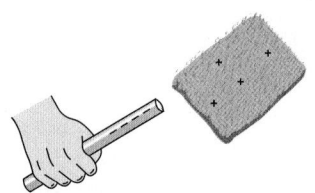

Figure 6-4 When a rubber rod is stroked against a piece of fur, charges that were originally mixed together evenly become separated so that the rod becomes negatively charged and the fur becomes positively charged.

Conservation of Charge

We have already met the laws of conservation of energy (with mass considered as a form of energy), momentum, and angular momentum. Here is another, the **law of conservation of charge:**

> The net electric charge in an isolated system remains constant.

"Net charge" means the algebraic sum of the charges present in the system, that is, the total with negative charges canceling out positive charges of the same magnitude (and vice versa if there is more negative charge present). Net charge can be positive, negative, or zero. Every known physical process in the universe conserves electric charge. Separating or bringing together charges does not affect their magnitudes, so such rearrangements leave the net charge the same.

and negative charge. For some pairs of materials, as we have seen, mere rubbing is enough to separate some of the charges from each other. In most cases, however, the charges are firmly held in place and more elaborate treatment is needed to pull them apart.

An object whose positive and negative charges exactly balance out is said to be electrically **neutral.**

6.2 What Is Charge?

Protons, Electrons, and Neutrons

In our own experience, matter and electric charge seem continuous, so that we can imagine dividing them into smaller and smaller portions without limit. But there is another level beyond reach of our senses, though not beyond reach of our instruments, on which every substance is revealed as being composed of tiny bits of matter called **atoms.** (Atoms are discussed in detail in later chapters along with how they join together to form molecules, liquids, and solids.) Over 100 varieties of atoms are known, but each of them is made up of just three kinds of **elementary particles;** nature is very economical. Two of the particles carry electric charges, so that charge, like mass, comes in small parcels of definite size. The third particle has no charge.

Atomic Structure   The three elementary particles found in atoms are

1. The **proton,** which has a mass of 1.673×10^{-27} kg and is positively charged
2. The **electron,** which has a mass of 9.11×10^{-31} kg and is negatively charged
3. The **neutron,** which has a mass of 1.675×10^{-27} kg and is uncharged

The proton and electron have exactly the same amounts of charge, although of opposite sign. Protons and neutrons have almost equal masses, which are nearly 2000 times greater than the electron mass.

Every atom has a small, central **nucleus** of protons and neutrons with its electrons moving about the nucleus some distance away (Fig. 6-5). Different types of atoms have different combinations of protons and neutrons in their nuclei. For instance, the most common carbon atom has a nucleus that contains six protons and six neutrons; the most common uranium atom has a nucleus that contains 92 protons and 146 neutrons. The electrons in an atom are normally equal in number to the protons, so the atom is electrically neutral unless disturbed in some way.

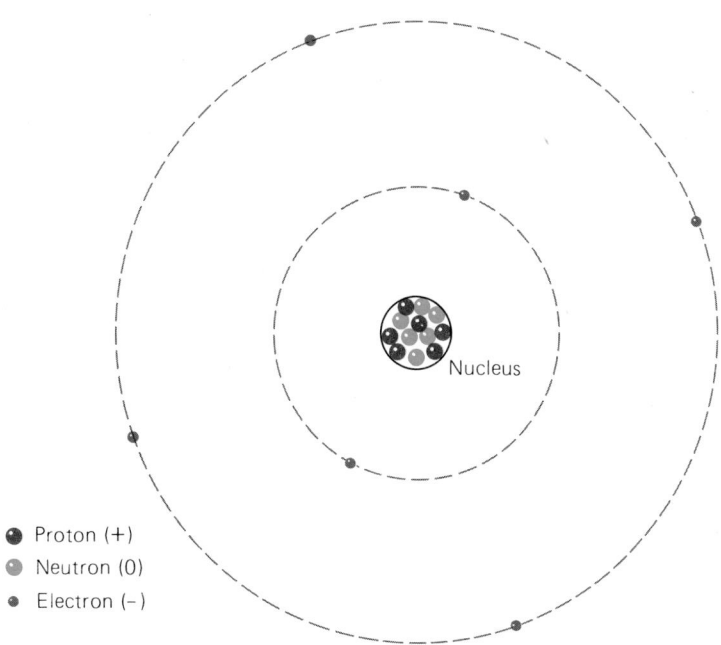

Figure 6-5   An atom consists of a central nucleus of protons and neutrons with electrons moving around it some distance away. Shown is a schematic diagram (not to scale) of the most common type of carbon atom, which has six protons, six neutrons, and six electrons. Two of the electrons are relatively near the nucleus, the others are farther away. A more realistic way to think of atomic structure is discussed in Sec. 9.13.

Nucleus

● Proton (+)
● Neutron (0)
● Electron (−)

What actually *is* charge? All that can be said is that electric charge, like mass, is a fundamental property of certain elementary particles of which all matter is composed. Their masses give rise to gravitational forces; their charges give rise to electric forces. Elementary particles have other attributes, too, that affect their behavior. Much about elementary particles is understood at present, as we shall learn in Secs. 8.13 to 8.15. However, just why the properties of these particles exist and have the magnitudes they do is still the subject of much study. One thing is clear, though: there is no simple answer to the question, "What is charge?"

The Coulomb   The unit of electric charge is the **coulomb** (C). The proton has a charge of $+1.6 \times 10^{-19}$ C and the electron has a charge of -1.6×10^{-19} C. All charges, both positive and negative, are therefore found only in multiples of 1.6×10^{-19} C. This basic quantity of charge is abbreviated e:

$$e = 1.6 \times 10^{-19} \text{ C} \qquad \textit{Basic unit of charge in nature}$$

Electric charge appears continuous outside the laboratory because e is such a small quantity. A charge of -1 C, for example, corresponds to more than 6 billion billion electrons (Fig. 6-6). Atoms are small, too: coal is almost pure carbon, and 6 billion billion carbon atoms would make a piece of coal only about the size of a pea.

6.3   Coulomb's Law

The Law of Force for Electric Charges

The forces between electric charges can be studied in rather simple experiments, such as that shown in Fig. 6-7. What we find is that the force between a charged rod and a charged plastic ball depends on two things: how close the rod is to the ball, and how much charge each one has.

Precise measurements show that the force between charges follows the same inverse-square variation with distance that the gravitational force between two masses does (see Sec. 2.13). For instance, when the charges are 2 cm apart, the force between them is $\frac{1}{4}$ as great as the force when they are 1 cm apart; it is 4 times greater when they are $\frac{1}{2}$ cm apart (Fig. 6-8a). If R is

Figure 6-6 Electric charge is not continuous but occurs in multiples of $\pm e = \pm1.6 \times 10^{-19}$ coulomb. (These pictures are not to be taken literally, of course: the mutual repulsion of the particles would prevent their assembly in this way.)

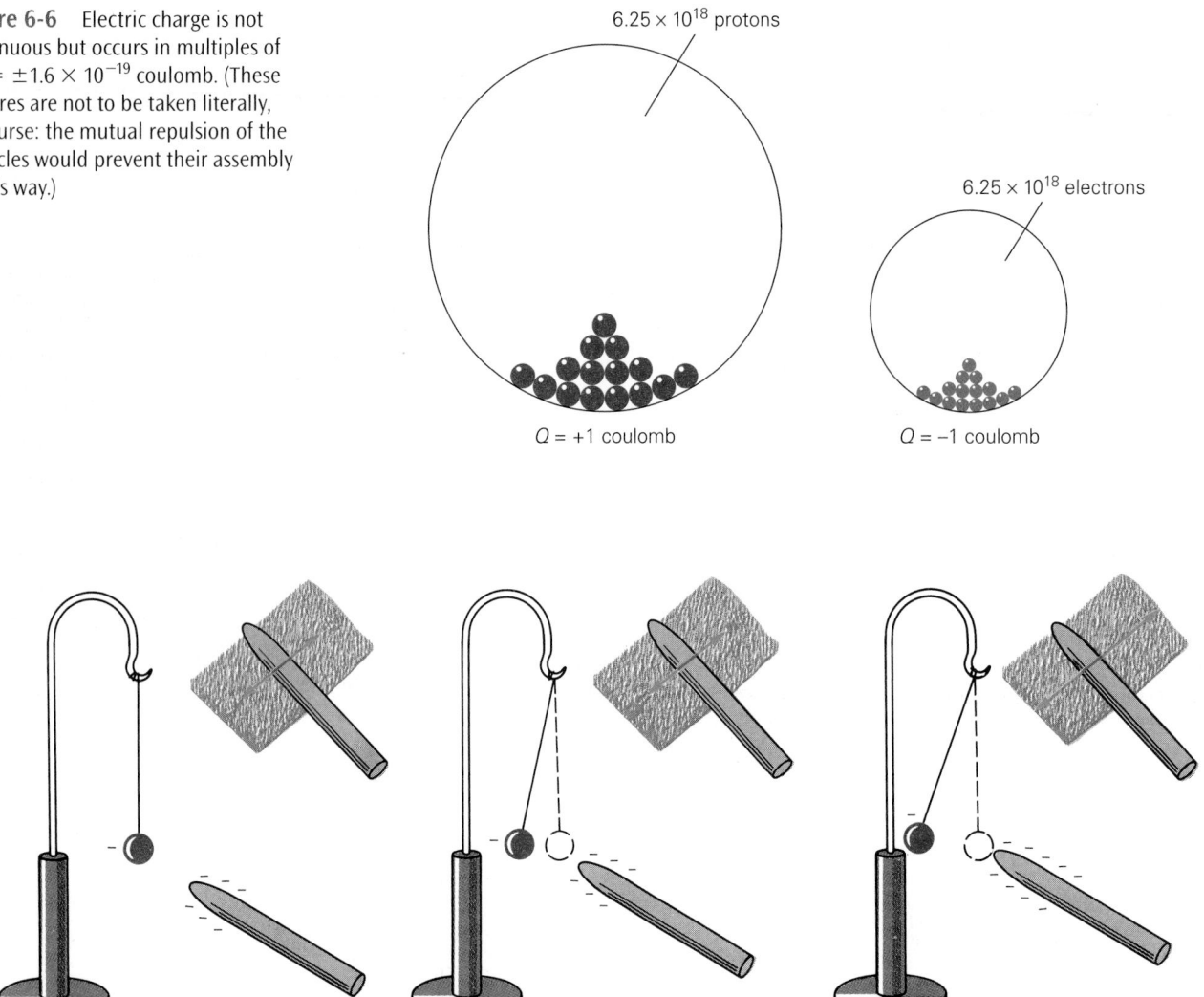

6.25 × 10¹⁸ protons

$Q = +1$ coulomb

6.25 × 10¹⁸ electrons

$Q = -1$ coulomb

Rod brought closer

After stroking vigorously with fur

Figure 6-7 The forces between electric charges. When a rubber rod that has been stroked with fur is brought near a negatively charged plastic ball, the force on the ball is greater when the rod is held close to it and also greater when the rod has been vigorously stroked.

the distance between the charges, we can say that the force between them is proportional to $1/R^2$.

The force also depends on the magnitude of each charge: if either charge is doubled, the force doubles too, and if both charges are doubled, the force increases fourfold (Fig. 6-8*b*). If the charges have the respective magnitudes Q_1 and Q_2, then the force varies as their product Q_1Q_2.

These results are summarized in **Coulomb's law:**

$$F = \frac{KQ_1Q_2}{R^2} \qquad \textit{Electric force} \qquad 6\text{-}1$$

which is named in honor of Charles Coulomb, who helped develop it (Fig. 6-9). The quantity K is a constant whose value is almost exactly

$$K = 9 \times 10^9 \text{ N} \cdot \text{m}^2/\text{C}^2 \qquad \textit{Electric force constant}$$

The Coulomb Is a Large Unit.   Just by looking at this formula we can see that the force between two charges of 1 C each that are separated by 1 m is 9×10^9 N, 9 billion newtons. This is an enormous force, equal to about

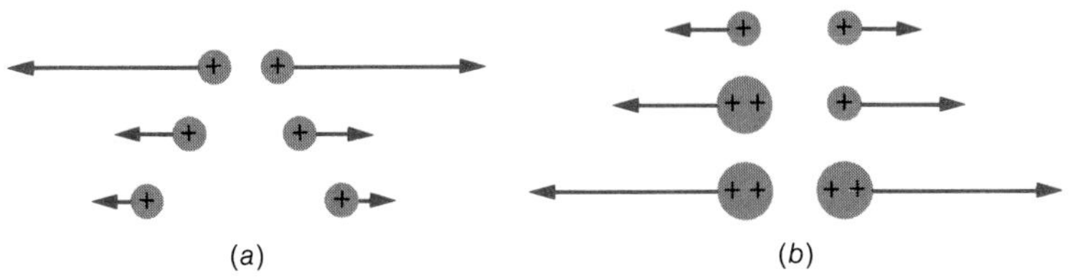

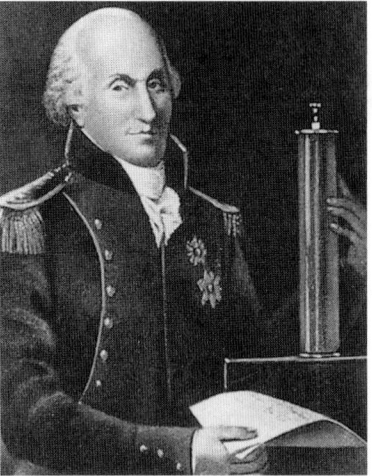

Figure 6-8 (*a*) The force between two charges varies inversely as the square of their separation; increasing the distance reduces the force. (*b*) The force is proportional to the product of the charges. Attractive forces behave the same way.

2 billion lb! We conclude that the coulomb is a very large unit indeed, and that even the most highly charged objects that can be produced cannot contain more than a small fraction of a coulomb of net charge of either sign.

The concept of a force field, described in Sec. 6.13, is a useful way to think about how electric charges interact with one another.

6.4 Force on an Uncharged Object

Why a Comb Can Attract Bits of Paper

One sign that a body has an electric charge is that it causes small, uncharged objects such as dust particles, bits of paper, and suspended plastic balls to move toward it. Where does the force come from?

The explanation comes from the fact that the electrons in a solid have some freedom of movement. In a metal this freedom is considerable, but even in other substances the electrons can shift around a little without leaving their parent atoms or molecules. When a comb is given a negative charge by being run through our hair, electrons in a nearby bit of paper are repelled by the negative charge and move away as far as they can (Fig. 6-10). The side

Figure 6-9 Charles Coulomb (1736–1806).

Example 6.1

How far apart should two electrons be if the force each exerts on the other is to equal the weight of an electron at sea level?

Solution

The weight of an electron at sea level is $m_e g$, $Q_1 = Q_2 = e$ here, so from Eq. 6-1

$$m_e g = \frac{KQ_1Q_2}{R^2} = \frac{Ke^2}{R^2}$$

Solving for R gives

$$R = \sqrt{\frac{Ke^2}{m_e g}} = \sqrt{\frac{(9 \times 10^9 \text{ N} \cdot \text{m}^2/\text{C}^2)(1.6 \times 10^{-19} \text{ C})^2}{(9.1 \times 10^{-31} \text{ kg})(9.8 \text{ m/s}^2)}} = 5.1 \text{ m}$$

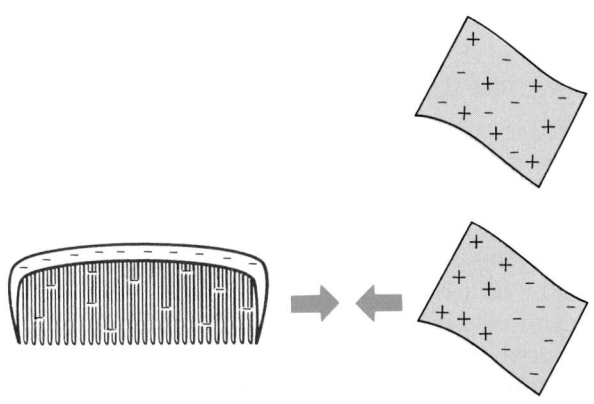

Figure 6-10 A charged object attracts an uncharged one by first causing a separation of charge in the latter. The effect is much exaggerated here; except in metals, the charge displacement takes place within individual atoms and molecules.

of the paper near the comb is left with a positive charge, and the paper is accordingly attracted to the comb.

If the comb is removed without actually touching the paper, the disturbed electrons resume their normal positions. Only a small amount of charge separation actually occurs, and so, with little force available, only very light things can be picked up this way.

Electricity and Matter

Let us now look into some aspects of the electrical behavior of matter.

6.5   Matter in Bulk

Gravity Versus Electricity

Coulomb's law for the force between charges is one of the fundamental laws of physics, in the same category as Newton's law of gravity. The latter, as we know, is written in equation form as

$$F = \frac{Gm_1m_2}{R^2} \qquad \textit{Gravitational force} \qquad 2\text{-}19$$

Coulomb's law resembles the law of gravity with the difference that gravitational forces are always attractive but electric forces may be either attractive or repulsive.

This last fact has an important consequence. Because one lump of matter always attracts another lump gravitationally, matter in the universe tends to come together into large masses. Even though dispersive influences of various kinds exist, they must fight against this steady attraction. Galaxies, stars, and planets, which condensed from matter that was originally spread out in space, bear witness to this cosmic herd instinct.

To collect much electric charge of either sign, however, is far more of a feat. Charges of opposite sign attract each other strongly, so it is hard to separate neutral matter into differently charged portions. And charges of the same sign repel each other, so putting together a large amount of charge of one sign is difficult.

To sum up, we can say that a system of electrically neutral particles is most stable (that is, has a minimum potential energy) when the particles make up a single body, while a system of electric charges is most stable when charges of opposite signs pair off to cancel each other out. Hence on a cosmic scale gravitational forces are significant and electric ones are not.

On an atomic scale, however, the reverse is true. The masses of subatomic particles are too small for them to interact gravitationally to any appreciable extent, whereas their electric charges are large enough for electric forces to exert marked effects.

6.6   Conductors and Insulators

How Charge Flows from One Place to Another

A substance through which electric charge can flow readily is called a **conductor.** Metals are the only solid conductors at room temperature, copper being an especially good one. In a metal, each atom gives up one or more electrons to a "gas" of electrons that can move relatively freely inside the metal. The atoms themselves stay in place and are not involved in the movement of charge. Metals are also the most efficient conductors of heat.

In an **insulator,** charge can flow only with great difficulty. Nonmetallic solids are insulators because all their electrons are tightly bound to particular atoms or groups of atoms. Glass, rubber, and plastics are good insulators.

Example 6.2

The hydrogen atom, the simplest of all, consists of a single proton as its nucleus with an electron an average of 5.3×10^{-11} m away. Compare the electric and gravitational forces between the proton and the electron in this atom.

Solution

The electric force between the proton and electron is, from Eq. 6-1,

$$F_{elec} = \frac{KQ_1Q_2}{R^2} = \frac{Ke^2}{R^2}$$

and the gravitational force between them is, from Eq. 2-19,

$$F_{grav} = \frac{Gm_1m_2}{R^2} = \frac{Gm_pm_e}{R^2}$$

Since both forces vary with distance as $1/R^2$, their ratio will be the same regardless of how far apart the proton and electron are. This ratio is

$$\frac{F_{elec}}{F_{grav}} = \frac{Ke^2/R^2}{Gm_pm_e/R^2} = \frac{Ke^2}{Gm_pm_e}$$

$$= \frac{(9 \times 10^9 \text{ N} \cdot \text{m/C}^2)(1.6 \times 10^{-19} \text{ C})^2}{(6.7 \times 10^{-11} \text{ N} \cdot \text{m}^2/\text{kg}^2)(1.7 \times 10^{-27} \text{ kg})(9.1 \times 10^{-31} \text{ kg})}$$

$$= 2.2 \times 10^{39}$$

The electric force is over 10^{39} times the gravitational force! Clearly, gravitational effects are negligible within atoms compared with electric effects.

Electrical Grounding

The earth as a whole, at least that part of it beneath the outer dry soil, is a fairly good electrical conductor. Hence if a charged object is connected with the earth by a piece of metal, the charge is conducted away from the object to the earth. This convenient method of removing the charge from an object is called **grounding** the object. As a safety measure, the metal shells of electrical appliances are grounded through special wires that give electric charges in the shells paths to the earth. The round post in the familiar three-prong electric plug is the ground connection.

A few substances, called **semiconductors,** are between conductors and insulators in their ability to let charge move through them. Semiconductors have made possible devices called **transistors,** whose ability to transmit charge can be changed at will. Transistors are widely used in modern electronics, notably in portable telephones and in radio and television receivers. A computer contains millions of transistors that act as miniature switches to perform arithmetic and carry out logical operations. Semiconductor memories are also used in computers, with huge numbers of memory elements built into a "chip" smaller than a fingernail (Fig. 6-11).

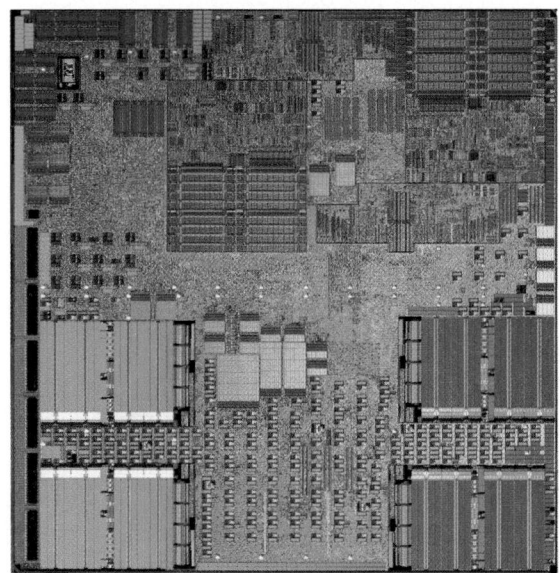

Figure 6-11 Enlargement of a semiconductor "chip" that contains the millions of circuit elements that make up a microprocessor used in a supercomputer.

Ions   The conduction of electricity through gases and liquids—in a neon sign, for instance, or in the acid of a storage battery—involves the movement of charged atoms and molecules called **ions.** An atom or molecule gains a positive charge (becomes a positive ion) when it loses one or more electrons, and it gains a negative charge (becomes a negative ion) when electrons in excess of its normal number become attached to it.

The process of forming ions, or **ionization,** can take place in a number of ways. A gas like ordinary air, which is normally a poor conductor, becomes ionized when x-rays, ultraviolet light, or radiation from a radioactive material pass through it, when an electric spark is produced, or even when a flame burns in it. Air molecules are sufficiently disturbed by these processes that electrons are torn loose from some of them. The electrons thus set free may attach themselves to adjacent molecules, so both positive and negative ions are formed (Fig. 6-12).

Eventually oppositely charged ions come together, whereupon the extra electrons on negative ions shift to positive ions to give neutral molecules again. At normal atmospheric pressure and temperature the ions last no more than a few seconds.

In the upper part of the earth's atmosphere, air molecules are so far apart on the average that the ionization produced by x-rays and ultraviolet light from the sun tends to persist. The ability of these ions to reflect radio waves makes possible long-range radio communication (see Sec. 7-9).

In contrast with gases, certain liquids may be permanently ionized to a greater or lesser extent (see Chap. 11). The conductivity of pure water itself is extremely small, but even traces of some impurities increase its conductivity enormously. Since most of the water we use in daily life is somewhat impure, it is usually considered a fair conductor of electricity.

6.7   Superconductivity

A Revolution in Technology May Be Near

Even the best conductors resist to some extent the flow of charge through them at ordinary temperatures. However, when extremely cold, some substances lose all electrical resistance. This phenomenon, called **superconductivity,** was discovered by Kamerlingh Onnes in the Netherlands in 1911. For example, aluminum is a superconductor below 1.2 K, which is −272°C. Such temperatures are difficult and expensive to reach, and as a result superconductivity has not been exploited commercially to any great extent.

If electrons are set in motion in a closed wire loop at room temperature, they will come to a stop in less than a second even in a good conductor such

Figure 6-12   A gas such as air becomes ionized when x-rays disrupt its molecules. A molecule losing an electron becomes a positive ion; a molecule gaining an electron becomes a negative ion. Ultraviolet light, radiation from radioactive substances, sparks, and flames also cause ionization to occur.

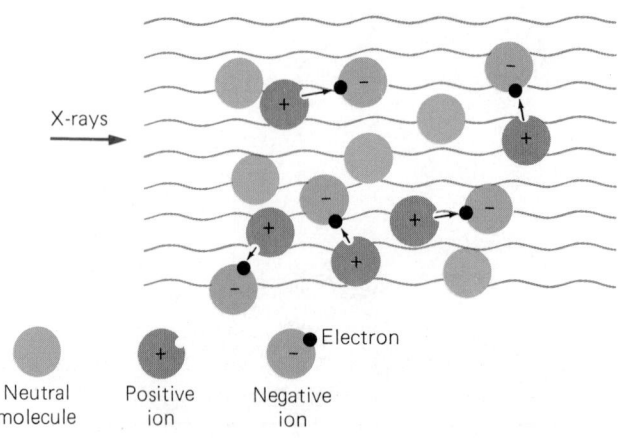

BIOGRAPHY | John Bardeen (1908–1991)

In 1945 John Bardeen, who was born in Wisconsin and educated there and at Princeton, joined a research group at Bell Telephone Laboratories led by William Shockley. In 1948 the group produced the first transistor, for which Shockley, Bardeen, and their collaborator Walter Brattain received a Nobel Prize in 1956. Bardeen later said, "I knew the transistor was important, but I never foresaw the revolution in electronics it would bring."

In 1951 Bardeen left Bell Labs for the University of Illinois where, together with Leon Cooper and J. Robert Schrieffer, he developed the theory of superconductivity. Compared with his earlier work on the transistor, "Superconductivity was

more difficult to solve, and it required some radically new concepts."

According to the theory, the motions of two electrons can become correlated through their interactions with the atoms in a crystal, which enables the pair to move with complete freedom through the crystal. Bardeen received his second Nobel Prize in 1972 for this theory along with Cooper and Schrieffer; he was the first person to receive two such prizes in the same field.

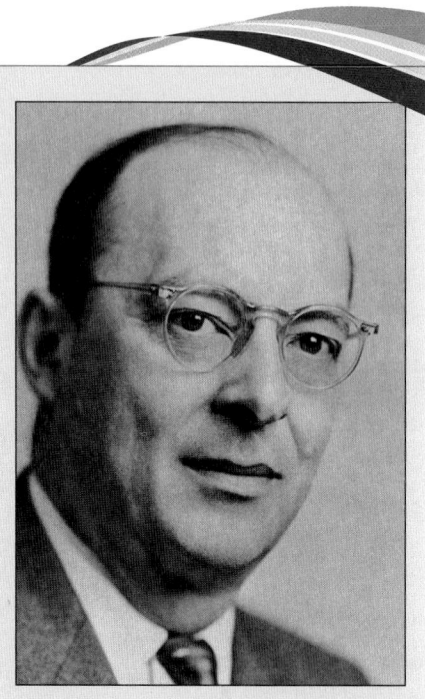

as copper. In a superconducting wire loop, on the other hand, electrons have circulated for years with no outside help.

Superconductivity is important because electric currents—flows of charge—are the means by which electric energy is carried from one place to another. Electric currents are also the means by which magnetic fields are produced in such devices as electric motors, as we shall learn later in this chapter. In an ordinary conductor, some of the energy of a current is lost as heat. Where long distances or large currents are involved, quite a bit of energy can be wasted in this way. About 8 percent of the electric energy generated in the United States is lost as heat in transmission lines.

High-Temperature Superconductors   Despite much effort, until 1986 no substance was known that was superconducting above 23 K. In that year Alex Müller and Georg Bednorz, working in Switzerland, discovered a ceramic that was superconducting up to 35 K. Soon afterward others extended their approach to produce superconductivity at temperatures as high as 164 K. Although still extremely cold ($-109°C$) by everyday standards, such temperatures are above the 77 K boiling point of liquid nitrogen, which is cheap (cheaper than milk) and readily available.

Despite being difficult to manufacture, more complicated to install, and costlier, superconducting cables cooled with liquid nitrogen can be attractive when large currents must be transmitted. For instance, in many places existing underground ducts are already filled with copper wires, leaving no room to expand electricity supply. Using superconducting cables in such situations may be less expensive than putting in new ducts. Electromagnets in MRI medical scanners and in some particle accelerators use superconducting wires, and electric motors, generators, and transformers using them are being developed.

A room-temperature superconductor would truly revolutionize the world's technology. As just one example, all trains would run suspended above the ground by magnetic forces, resulting in better fuel efficiency and high speeds. In general, less waste of electric energy would mean a lower rate of depletion of fuel resources and reduced pollution. A room-temperature superconductor, though still a dream, does not seem quite so hopeless a dream as it did not so long ago.

Electric Current

A flow of charge from one place to another constitutes an **electric current.** Currents and not stationary charges are involved in nearly all the practical applications of electricity.

6.8 The Ampere

The Unit of Electric Current

A battery changes chemical energy into electric energy. If we connect a wire between the terminals of a battery to make a complete conducting path, or **circuit,** electrons will flow into the wire from the negative terminal and out of the wire into the positive terminal. Chemical reactions in the battery keep the electrons moving. We do not say, "The electrons carry the current," or "The motion of the electrons produces a current"; the moving electrons *are* the current.

The flow of electricity along a wire is a lot like the flow of water in a pipe (Fig. 6-13). When we describe the rate at which water moves through a pipe, we give the flow in terms of, say, liters per second. If 5 liters of water passes through a given pipe each second, the flow is 5 liters/s.

The description of electric current, symbol I, follows the same pattern. As we know, quantity of electric charge is measured in coulombs, as quantity of water is measured in liters. The natural way to refer to a flow of charge in a wire, then, is in terms of the number of coulombs per second that go past any point in the wire:

$$I = \frac{Q}{t} \qquad \textit{Electric current} \qquad\qquad 6\text{-}2$$

$$\text{Electric current} = \frac{\text{charge transferred}}{\text{time interval}}$$

The unit of electric current is called the **ampere** (A), after the French physicist André Marie Ampère. That is,

$$1 \text{ ampere} = 1\,\frac{\text{coulomb}}{\text{second}}$$

$$1 \text{ A} = 1 \text{ C/s}$$

The current in the lightbulb of most desk lamps is a little less than 1 A.

Example 6.3

Since electric current is a flow of charge, why are two wires, not just one, needed to connect a battery or generator to an appliance such as a motor or lightbulb?

Solution

If a single wire were used, charge of one sign or the other (depending on the situation) would be permanently transferred from the source of current to the appliance. In a short time so much charge would have been transferred that the source would be unable to shift further charge against the repulsive force of the charge piled up at the appliance. Thus a single wire cannot carry a current continuously. With two wires, however, charge can be circulated from source to appliance and back, which permits a steady flow of energy to the appliance.

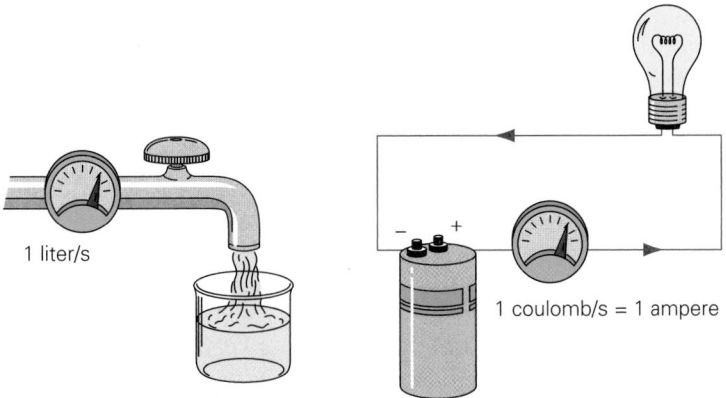

Figure 6-13   The ampere is the unit of electric current. The flow of charge in a circuit is like the flow of water in a pipe except that a return wire is needed in order to have a complete conducting path. An electric current is always assumed to go from the + terminal of a battery or generator to its − terminal through the external circuit.

Direction of Current

It is customary to regard an electric current as consisting of positive charges in motion. Thus a current is assumed to go from the positive terminal of a battery or generator to its negative terminal through the external circuit, as in Fig. 6-13.

In reality, an electric current in a metal is a flow of electrons, which are negatively charged. However, a current of negative charges going one way is electrically the same as a current of positive charges going the other way. Since it makes no difference in practice, this book will follow the usual convention of considering current as a flow of positive charge.

Example 6.4

How many electrons per second flow past a point in a wire carrying a current of 1 A?

Solution
The electron charge is $Q = e = 1.6 \times 10^{-19}$ C, and so a current of 1 A = 1 C/s corresponds to a flow of

$$\frac{\text{Electrons}}{\text{time}} = \frac{Q/t}{Q/\text{electron}} = \frac{1 \text{ C/s}}{1.6 \times 10^{-19} \text{ C/electron}}$$
$$= 6.3 \times 10^{18} \text{ electrons/s}$$

6.9   Potential Difference

The Push behind a Current

Consider a liter of water at the top of a waterfall. The water has potential energy there, since it can move downward under the pull of gravity. When the water drops, its PE decreases. As we learned in Chap. 3, the work that can be obtained from the liter of water during its fall is equal to its decrease in PE.

Now consider a coulomb of negative charge on the − terminal of a battery. It is repelled by the − terminal and attracted by the + terminal, and so it has a certain amount of PE. When the coulomb of charge has moved along a wire to the + terminal, its PE is gone. The work the coulomb of charge can perform while flowing from the − to the + terminal of the battery is equal to this decrease in PE.

The decrease in its PE brought about by the motion of 1 C of charge from the − to the + terminal is called the **potential difference** between the two terminals. It is analogous to the difference in height in the case of water (Fig. 6-14). The potential difference V between two points is equal to the corresponding energy difference W per coulomb:

$$V = \frac{W}{Q} \qquad \textit{Potential difference} \qquad 6-3$$

$$\text{Potential difference} = \frac{\text{potential energy difference}}{\text{charge transferred}}$$
$$= \frac{\text{work done to transfer charge } Q}{\text{charge transferred}}$$

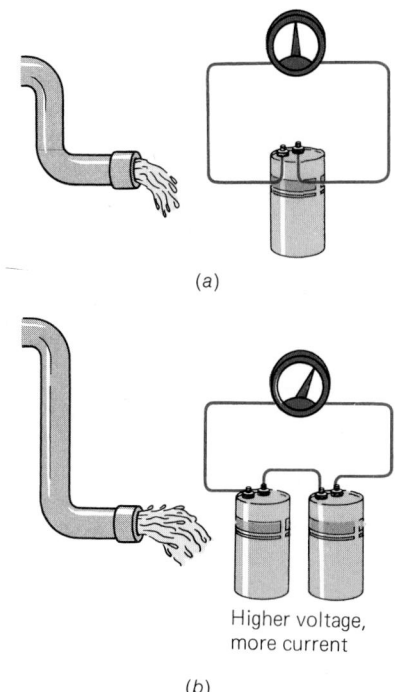

Higher voltage,
more current

(b)

Figure 6-14   The flow of electric charge in a wire is analogous to the flow of water in a pipe. Thus having the water fall through a greater height at (b) than at (a) yields a greater flow of water, which corresponds to using two batteries to obtain a higher potential difference and thereby a greater current.

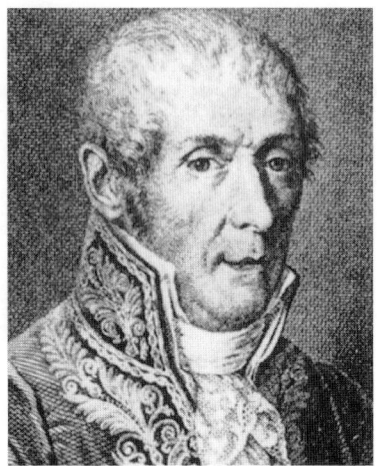

Figure 6-15   Alessandro Volta (1745–1827).

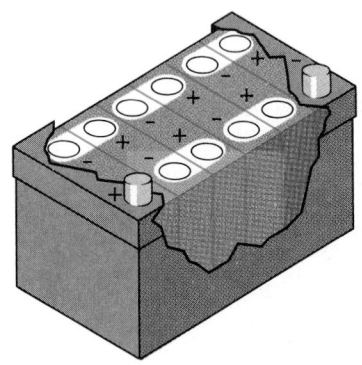

Figure 6-16   A 12-V storage battery consists of six 2-V cells connected in series.

The Volt   We measure difference of height in meters; we measure difference of potential in **volts,** named for the Italian physicist Alessandro Volta (Fig. 6-15). When 1 coulomb of charge travels through 1 volt of potential difference, the work that it does is equal to 1 joule. By definition:

$$1 \text{ volt} = 1 \frac{\text{joule}}{\text{coulomb}}$$

$$1 \text{ V} = 1 \text{ J/C}$$

Potential difference is often called simply **voltage.**

Batteries   The normal potential difference between the terminals of a car's storage battery is about 12 V, in the case of a dry cell about 1.5 V. Every coulomb of electricity at the negative terminal of the storage battery can do 8 times as much work as a coulomb at the negative terminal of a dry cell—just as a liter of water at the top of a waterfall 12 m high can do 8 times as much work as a liter at the top of a 1.5-m fall. If a storage battery and a dry cell are connected in identical circuits, the battery will push 8 times as many electrons around its circuit in a given time as the dry cell, giving a current 8 times as great.

We may think of the potential difference between two points as the amount of "push" available to move charge between the points.

If we connect two or more batteries together as shown in Fig. 6-14b, the available voltage is increased. The method of connection, called **series,** is − terminal to + terminal, so that each battery in turn supplies its "push" to electrons flowing through the set. The voltage of a particular cell depends on the chemical reactions that take place in it. In the case of the lead-acid storage battery of a car, each cell has a voltage of 2 V, and six of them are connected together to give the 12 V needed to run the car's electrical equipment (Fig. 6-16).

As its name suggests, a storage battery can be **recharged** when the energy it contains is used up. Ordinary dry-cell batteries, such as those used in flashlights and various devices, have voltages of 1.5 V and cannot be recharged. (How batteries work is described in Sec. 12.13.)

Example 6.5

How much energy is stored in a 12-V, 60 A · h battery when it is fully charged? If the mass of the battery is 20 kg and all the energy stored in it is used to raise it from the ground, how high would it go?

Solution

Since 1 A = 1 C/s and 1 h = 3600 s, the amount of charge the battery can transfer from one of its terminals to the other is

$$Q = (60 \text{ A} \cdot \text{h})\left(1 \frac{\text{C/s}}{\text{h}}\right)\left(3600 \frac{\text{s}}{\text{h}}\right) = 2.16 \times 10^5 \text{ C}$$

and the stored energy is, from Eq. 6-3,

$$W = QV = (2.16 \times 10^5 \text{ C})(12 \text{ V}) = 2.59 \times 10^6 \text{ J}$$

The potential energy of the battery at the height h is PE = mgh. Hence $W = mgh$ and

$$h = \frac{W}{mg} = \frac{2.59 \times 10^6 \text{ J}}{(20 \text{ kg})(9.8 \text{ m/s}^2)} = 1.32 \times 10^4 \text{ m} = 13.2 \text{ km}$$

Mt. Everest is only 8.85 km high—a charged battery can contain a lot of energy.

Lightning

Charge separation occurs in a thunderstorm when water droplets and ice crystals in a cloud collide, and the separation grows in scale through convectional updrafts and downdrafts. The result is a region of positive charge in the upper part of the cloud with a region of negative charge below it. By the mechanism shown in Fig. 6-10, the latter region induces a charge separation in the ground under the cloud, with positive charge uppermost facing the negative charge in the cloud (Fig. 6-17).

Potential differences inside a thundercloud and between the cloud and the ground range up to millions of volts and result in electric discharges (which are really giant sparks) that appear as lightning strokes along the paths where charges flow (Fig. 6-18). Exactly what triggers a lightning stroke is not completely understood, but a promising idea is that cosmic-ray particles from space (see Sec. 19.5) are responsible.

Although cloud-to-ground strokes are the most familiar, lightning is actually much more frequent inside thunderclouds, where it is hidden from our view by the clouds although we can hear the thunder it causes. Thunder is the result of the heating of the air along the path of a lightning stroke, whose sudden expansion gives rise to intense sound waves. "Sheet lightning" is a luminosity in the sky due to a lightning stroke that is behind a cloud or occurs below the horizon.

Lightning usually strikes the highest point in an area, such as a tall tree or a ship offshore. The safest place to be in a thunderstorm is inside a building or a car. If caught in the open, one should crouch down but not lie flat, because strong horizontal currents flow in the ground near where lightning strikes.

Airplanes are regularly struck by lightning, and indeed often trigger lightning when flying through charged clouds. Most airplanes have aluminum skins that conduct the currents of lightning strokes harmlessly around their interiors. The reinforced plastic skins of other aircraft incorporate metal fibers for such shielding.

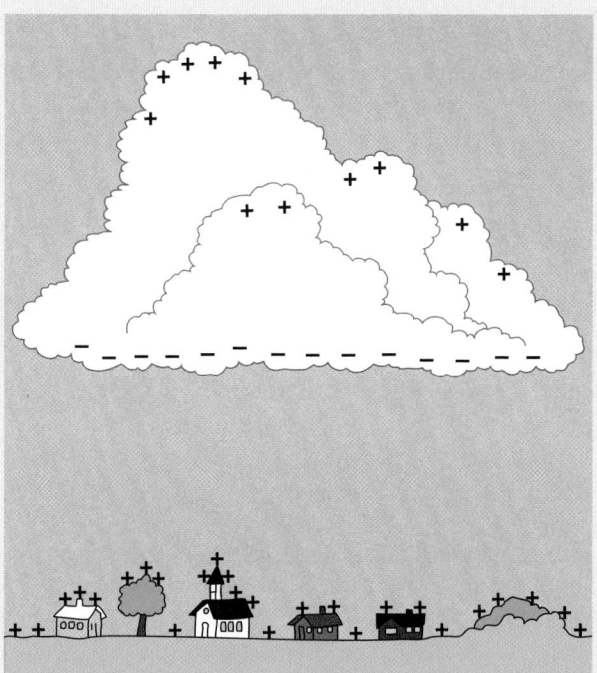

Figure 6-17   The negative charge on the bottom of a thundercloud induces a positive charge in the ground under it.

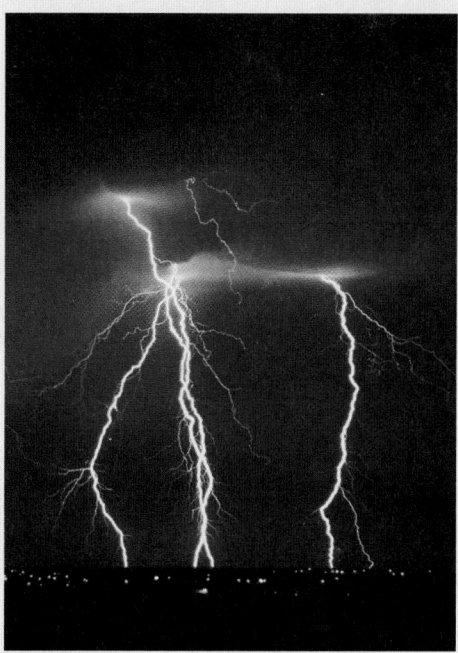

Figure 6-18   About 20 million lightning strokes reach the ground in the United States each year, killing several hundred people and causing much property damage.

Ampere-hours   A battery is rated according to the total amount of charge it can transfer from one terminal to the other, expressed in ampere-hours (A · h). A typical car battery has a capacity of 60 A · h, which means it can supply a current of 60 A for 1 h, a current of 30 A for 2 h, a current of 1 A for 60 h, and so on. The less the current, the longer the battery can supply it.

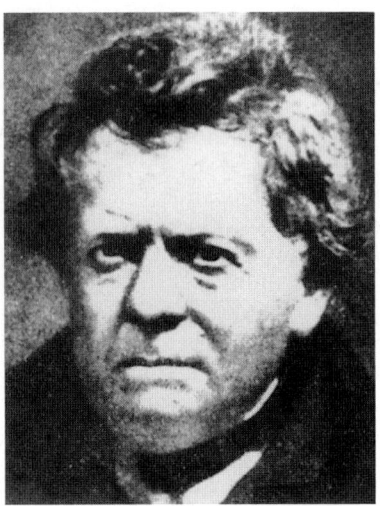

Figure 6-19   Georg Ohm
(1787–1854).

6.10 Ohm's Law

Current, Voltage, and Resistance

When different voltages are applied to the ends of the same piece of wire, we find that the current in the wire is proportional to the potential difference. Doubling the voltage doubles the current. This generalization is called **Ohm's law** after its discoverer, the German physicist Georg Ohm (Fig. 6-19).

The property of a conductor that opposes the flow of charge in it is called **resistance.** We can think of resistance as a kind of friction. The more the resistance in a circuit, the less the current for a given applied voltage (Fig. 6-20). If we write I for current, V for voltage, and R for resistance, Ohm's law says that

$$I = \frac{V}{R} \qquad Ohm's\ law \qquad 6\text{-}4$$

$$\text{Current} = \frac{\text{voltage}}{\text{resistance}}$$

The unit of resistance is the **ohm,** whose abbreviation is Ω, the Greek capital letter "omega." Hence 1 A = 1 V/Ω and

$$1\ \text{ohm} = 1\ \frac{\text{volt}}{\text{ampere}}$$

$$1\ \Omega = 1\ \text{V/A}$$

The resistance of a wire or other metallic conductor depends on the material it is made of (an iron wire has 7 times the resistance of a copper wire of the

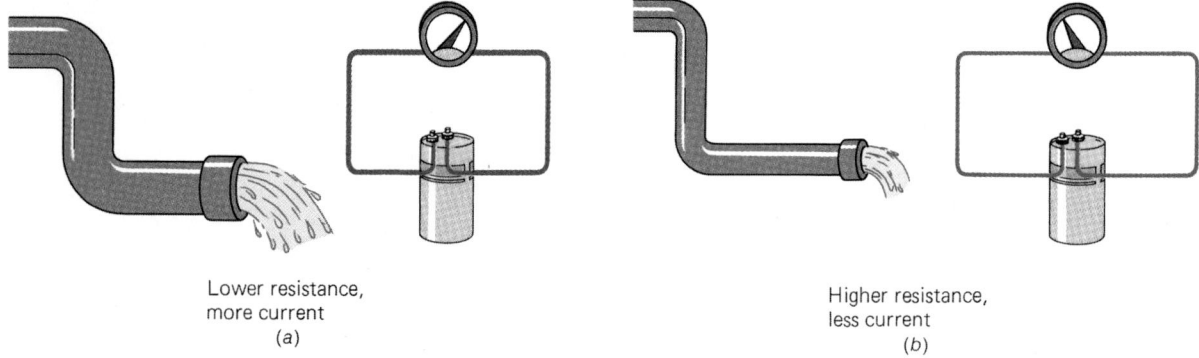

Lower resistance,
more current
(a)

Higher resistance,
less current
(b)

Figure 6-20   (a) A short, wide pipe yields a large flow of water, which corresponds to using a short, thick wire that offers less resistance to the flow of charge. (b) A long, narrow pipe yields a small flow of water, which corresponds to using a long, thin wire that offers more resistance to the flow of charge.

Circuit Faults

An electric circuit basically consists of a source of electric energy, such as a battery or generator, a load—for instance, a lightbulb or motor—and wires that connect them. There are two common modes of failure in actual circuits. In one, a wire breaks or comes loose from its terminal. The resulting **open circuit** does not provide a complete conducting path and no current flows.

In a **short circuit,** the connecting wires either accidentally touch each other or are joined by a stray conductor such as a misplaced screwdriver. The current now has an alternate path of very low resistance and, because $I = V/R$, a high current flows. A short circuit is dangerous because the high current produces a lot of heat, which can start a fire or even melt the wires involved.

Fuses and circuit breakers are designed to open electric circuits whenever unsafe amounts of current pass through them, and so they provide protection from the results of a short circuit. All power lines have fuses or circuit breakers for this reason, and many individual electric appliances are so equipped as well.

same size); its length (the longer the wire, the more its resistance); its cross-sectional area (the greater this area, the less the resistance); and the temperature (the higher the temperature, the more the resistance).

The Nature of Ohm's Law　Despite its name, Ohm's law is not a basic physical principle such as the law of conservation of energy. Ohm's law is obeyed only by metallic conductors, not by gaseous or liquid conductors and not by such electronic devices as transistors.

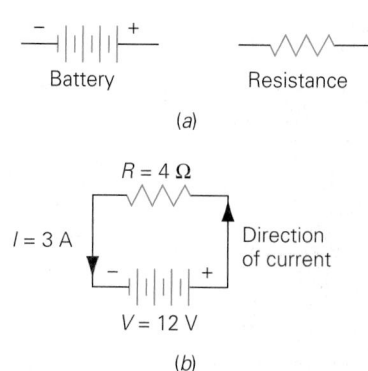

Figure 6-21　(*a*) Symbols for a battery and a resistance. (*b*) A current of 3 A flows in a circuit whose resistance is 4 Ω when a potential difference of 12 V is applied. The current direction is from the + terminal of the battery to the − terminal.

Example 6.6

A car has a 12-V battery whose capacity is 60 A · h. If the car's headlights and taillights have a total resistance of 4 Ω (Fig. 6-21), how long can they be left on before the battery runs down? Assume that the car's engine is not running, so its generator is not recharging the battery.

Solution

The first step is to find the current. From Eq. 6-4,

$$I = \frac{V}{R} = \frac{12 \text{ V}}{4 \text{ }\Omega} = 3 \text{ A}$$

Because the battery's capacity is 60 A · h, the lights can be left on for

$$t = \frac{60 \text{ A} \cdot \text{h}}{3 \text{ A}} = 20 \text{ h}$$

before the battery runs down.

Example 6.7

Find the resistance of a 120-V electric toaster that draws a current of 4 A.

Solution

To find the resistance, we rewrite Ohm's law, Eq. 6-4, in the form $R = V/I$ and substitute the given values:

$$R = \frac{V}{I} = \frac{120 \text{ V}}{4 \text{ A}} = 30 \text{ }\Omega$$

The resistance of the toaster is 30 Ω.

6.11　Electric Power

Current Times Voltage

Electric energy is so useful both because it is conveniently carried by wires and because it is easily converted into other kinds of energy. Electric energy in the form of electric current becomes radiant energy in a lightbulb, chemical energy when a storage battery is charged, kinetic energy in an electric motor, heat in an electric oven. In each case the current performs work on the device it passes through, and the device then turns this work into another kind of energy.

　　As in the case of the energy lost due to friction, the energy lost due to the resistance of a conductor becomes heat. This is the basis of electric heaters and stoves. In a lightbulb, the filament is so hot that it glows white. In electric circuits it is obviously important to use wires large enough in diameter, and hence small enough in resistance, to prevent the wires becoming so hot that they melt their insulation and start fires. A thin extension cord suitable for a lamp or radio might well be dangerous used for a heater or power tool.

Electrical Safety

Body tissue is a fairly good electrical conductor because it contains ions in solution. Dry skin has the most resistance and can protect the rest of the body in case of accidental exposure to a high voltage. This protection disappears when the skin is wet.

An electric current in body tissue stimulates nerves and muscles and produces heat. Most people can feel a current as small as 0.0005 A, one of 0.005 A is painful, and one of 0.01 A or more leads to muscle contractions that may prevent a person from letting go of the source of the current. Breathing becomes impossible when the current is greater than about 0.018 A.

Touching a single "live" conductor has no effect if the body is isolated since a complete conducting path is necessary for a current to occur. However, if a person is at the same time grounded by being in contact with a water pipe, by standing on wet soil, or in some other way, a current will pass through his or her body.

The human body's resistance is in the neighborhood of 1000 Ω, so if a potential difference of 120 V is applied via wet skin, the resulting current will be somewhere near $I = V/R = 120 \text{ V}/1000 \text{ }\Omega = 0.12$ A. Such a current is exceedingly dangerous because it causes the heart muscles to contract rapidly and irregularly, which is fatal if allowed to continue.

Electrical devices in bathrooms and kitchens are potential sources of danger because the moisture on a wet finger may be enough to provide a conducting path to the interior of the devices. If a person is in a bathtub and thus is grounded through the tub's water to its drainpipe, or the person has one hand on a faucet, even touching a switch with a wet finger is risky.

Today new electrical installations in bathrooms, kitchens, garages, and outdoors always include **ground fault circuit interruptors** that trip when the current is different in the two nongrounded wires leading to an appliance from an outlet. The difference means that some current is leaking to ground, perhaps through a person's body. Such devices are sensitive to leaks of 0.005 A or more and can break the circuit in 0.025 s.

An important quantity in any discussion of electric current is the rate at which a current is doing work—in other words, the **power** of the current. From Eq. 6-3 we know that $V = W/Q$, where W is the work done in transferring the charge Q through a potential difference of V. Since $W = Pt$ and $Q = It$, we have

$$V = \frac{W}{Q} = \frac{Pt}{It} = \frac{P}{I}$$

Thus we have the useful result that electric power is given by the product of the current and the voltage of the circuit:

$$P = IV \qquad \textit{Electric power} \qquad 6\text{-}5$$

$$\text{Power} = \text{(current)(voltage)}$$

The Watt   Now we can see why electrical appliances are rated in watts; as we learned in Sec. 3.2, the watt is the unit of power. A 60-W lightbulb uses twice the power of a 30-W bulb, and one-tenth the power of a 600-W electric drill (Table 6-1).

A fuse or circuit breaker interrupts a power line if the current exceeds a safe limit. Many of the fuses normally used in homes are rated at 15 A. Since the power-line voltage is 120 V, the greatest power a 15-A line can provide without blowing the fuse is

$$P = IV = (15 \text{ A})(120 \text{ V}) = 1800 \text{ W} = 1.8 \text{ kW}$$

Because $P = IV$, it is easy to find how much current is needed by an appliance rated in watts when connected to a power line of given voltage. For instance, a 60-W bulb connected to a 120-V line needs a current of

$$I = \frac{P}{V} = \frac{60 \text{ W}}{120 \text{ V}} = 0.5 \text{ A}$$

The Kilowatthour   Users of electricity pay for the amount of energy they consume. The usual commercial unit of electric energy is the **kilowatthour**

Table 6-1	Typical Power Ratings of Various Appliances
Appliance	**Power, W**
Charger for electric toothbrush	1
Clothes dryer	5,000
Coffeemaker	700
Dishwasher	1,600
Fan	150
Fax transmitter/ receiver	65
Heater	2,000
Iron	1,000
Personal computer	150
Portable sander	200
Refrigerator	400
Stove	12,000
TV receiver	120
Vacuum cleaner	750

The Grid

The United States, like other developed countries, has an extensive network of electric transmission lines—the **grid**—that connects and interconnects producers and consumers of electric energy. The grid's nationwide scale should allow it to accommodate local and regional variations in electricity demand and supply, but today's grid does this imperfectly. In particular, new sources of sustainable energy often lack adequate transmission lines to take their output to the grid. Thus North Dakota is the windiest state in the United States, but mainly because there is not enough transmission capacity, it is only eleventh in wind energy production.

Extending and improving the grid is expensive and can be difficult to carry out. In a not-unusual case, 8 years were needed to obtain permits for a new 354-km line between Duluth, Minnesota, and Wausau, Wisconsin; only 2 years were needed to build it. Ownership of the 300,000 or so kilometers of existing power lines in the United States is divided among hundreds of companies, all with different ideas about expansion and how costs should be split. State and local governments are reluctant to approve projects that would benefit other regions, and nobody wants to look at huge pylons striding across the landscape in front of their homes. As a result, although electricity use in the United States has climbed by over 50 percent in the recent past, transmission capacity has grown by only 12 percent; half the grid is over 40 years old. Fortunately, this imbalance is on the way to being remedied, which will allow sustainable energy to move closer to its potential and reduce the need for backup generating capacity.

Laying power lines underwater, although more expensive than stringing them overland, has fewer environmental objections and is attractive when rivers and lakes are in the right places. Among a number of proposed submarine lines is one that would carry hydroelectric power from Canada under Lake Champlain and then under the Hudson River to New York City, and from there under Long Island Sound to Connecticut.

Besides being useful in itself, enlarging the grid has another benefit, the opportunity to make it "smarter." A smart grid could increase reliability by automatically detecting and responding to transmission problems as they arise, not after they have disrupted service. Slow responses led to cascading grid failures that blacked out 45 million homes in the eastern United States in 2003.

Example 6.8

Can the energy of lightning strokes be harnessed for human needs? A lightning stroke might be driven by a potential difference of 2 million volts, involve a current of 5000 A, and last for 1 ms (0.001 s). How much energy is released in this stroke?

Solution

The power of the lightning stroke is

$$P = IV = (5 \times 10^3 \text{ A})(2 \times 10^6 \text{ V}) = 1 \times 10^{10} \text{ W}$$

This is 10 billion watts! However, although this is a lot of *power*, the *energy* released is modest:

$$E = Pt = (1 \times 10^{10} \text{ W})(1 \times 10^{-3} \text{ s}) = 1 \times 10^7 \text{ J} = 10 \text{ MJ}$$

Burning a cup of gasoline liberates more energy than this. Hence the response to the question of how to utilize the energy of lightning is, why bother? The reason lightning strokes are so destructive despite their relatively minor energy content is that the release of this energy takes place very quickly in a fairly small volume, which produces an explosive effect.

(kWh), which is the energy supplied per hour when the power level is 1 kilowatt (Fig. 6-22). If electricity is sold at $0.12 per kilowatt-hour, the cost of operating a 1.5-kW electric heater for 7 h would be

$$\text{Cost} = (\text{price per unit of energy})(\text{energy used})$$
$$= (\text{price per unit of energy})(\text{power})(\text{time})$$
$$= (\$0.12/\text{kWh})(1.5 \text{ kW})(7 \text{ h}) = \$1.26$$

Table 6-2 summarizes the various electrical quantities we have been discussing.

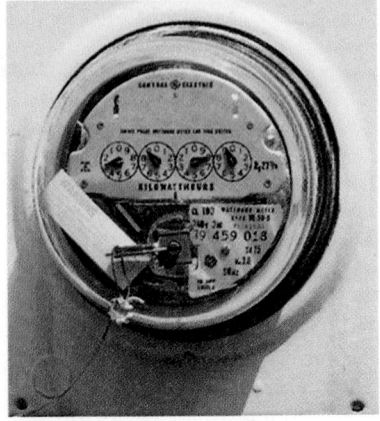

Figure 6-22   A kilowatthour meter registers the electric energy that has been supplied to a house or other user of electricity.

Table 6-2		**Electrical Quantities**		
Quantity	**Symbol**	**Unit**	**Meaning**	**Formula**
Charge	Q	Coulomb (C)	A basic property of most elementary particles. The electron has a charge of -1.6×10^{-19} C.	
Current	I	Ampere (A) (1 A = 1 C/s)	Rate of flow of charge.	$I = \dfrac{Q}{t} = \dfrac{P}{V}$
Potential difference (voltage)	V	Volt (V) (1 V = 1 J/C)	Potential energy difference per coulomb of charge between two points; corresponds to pressure in water flow.	$V = \dfrac{W}{Q} = IR = \dfrac{P}{I}$
Resistance	R	Ohm (Ω) (1Ω = 1 V/A)	A measure of the opposition to the flow of charge in a particular circuit. For a given voltage, the higher the resistance, the lower the current.	$R = \dfrac{V}{I}$
Power	P	Watt (W) (1 W = 1 V · A)	Rate of energy flow.	$P = \dfrac{W}{t} = IV$

Magnetism

Electricity and magnetism were once considered as completely separate phenomena. One of the great achievements of nineteenth-century science was the realization that they are really very closely related, a realization that led to the discovery of the electromagnetic nature of light. And one of the great achievements of nineteenth-century technology was the invention of electric motors and generators, whose operation depends upon the connection between electricity and magnetism.

6.12 Magnets

Attraction and Repulsion

Ordinary magnets are familiar to everybody. The simplest is a bar of iron that has been magnetized in one way or another, say, by having been stroked by another magnet. A magnetized iron bar is recognized, of course, by its ability to attract and hold other pieces of iron to itself. Most of the force a magnet exerts comes from its ends, as we can see by testing the attraction of different parts of a bar magnet for iron nails.

If we pivot a magnet at its center so that it can swing freely, we will find that it turns so that one end points north and the other south. The north-pointing end is called the **north pole** of the magnet, and the south-pointing end is called its **south pole.** The tendency of a magnet to line up with the earth's axis is the basis of the compass, whose needle is a small magnet (Fig. 6-24). (In Chap. 15 we shall find that the reason for this behavior is that the earth itself is a giant magnet.)

If the north poles of two magnets are brought near each other, the magnets repel. If the north pole of one magnet is brought near the south pole of

Series and Parallel

There are two basic ways to connect circuit elements. The resistors in Fig. 6-23a are joined end-to-end in **series** with the same current flowing through all of them. In (b) the resistors are in **parallel** and the total current is split up among them. This is the arrangement used in household wiring, so that each lamp or other appliance has the same voltage (usually 120 V) across it. If the appliances were in series, all would have to be switched on for any of them to work, and each would have a smaller voltage than 120 V.

When batteries are connected in series, as in Fig. 6-23c, their voltages add: three 12-V batteries in series gives 36 V for the set. In parallel, as in (d), the voltage of the set is still 12 V but the set can provide three times as much current as each battery alone. When a car's battery is too weak to start the car, the remedy is another battery connected in parallel to it (+ terminal to +, − terminal to −) using jumper cables.

Figure 6-23 Series and parallel connections. Household electric outlets are always connected in parallel so each one has the same applied voltage of 120 V.

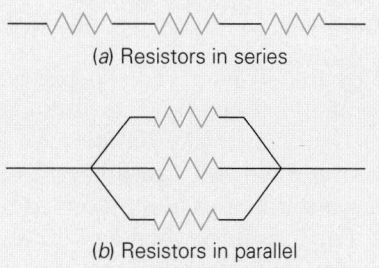

(a) Resistors in series

(b) Resistors in parallel

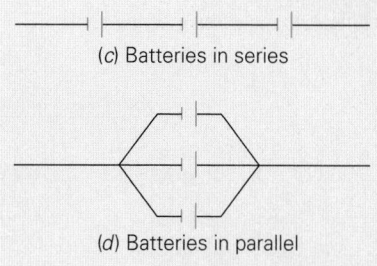

(c) Batteries in series

(d) Batteries in parallel

the other, the magnets attract (Fig. 6-25). This gives us a simple rule like that for electric charges:

> Like magnetic poles repel one another, unlike poles attract one another.

Poles Always Come in Pairs   Positive and negative charges in neutral matter can be separated from each other. Can the north and south poles of a magnet also be separated? It would seem that all we have to do is to saw the magnet in half. But if we do this, as in Fig. 6-26, we find that the resulting pieces each have an N pole and an S pole. We may cut the resulting magnets in two again and continue as long as we like, but each piece, however small, will still have both an N pole and an S pole. There is no such thing as a single free magnetic pole.

Since a magnet can be cut into smaller and smaller pieces indefinitely with each piece a small magnet in itself, we conclude that magnetism is a property of the iron atoms themselves. Each atom of iron behaves as if it has an N pole and an S pole. In ordinary iron the atoms have their poles randomly arranged, and nearby N and S poles cancel out each other's effect. When a bar of iron is magnetized, many or all of the atoms are aligned with the N poles in the same direction, so that the strengths of all the tiny magnets are added together (Fig. 6-27).

A "permanent" magnet can be demagnetized by heating it strongly or by hammering it. Both of these processes agitate the atoms and restore them to their normal random orientations.

All Substances Are Affected by Magnetism   Iron is not the only material from which permanent magnets can be made. Nickel, cobalt, and certain combinations of other elements can also be magnetized. Nor is iron the only material affected by magnetism—*all* substances are, though generally only to a very slight extent. Some are attracted to a magnet, but most are repelled. In the case of mercury the repulsion, though weak, is still enough to be easily observed.

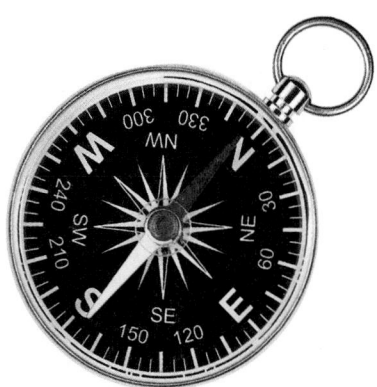

Figure 6-24   A magnetic compass uses the earth's magnetic field to establish direction. The magnetic axis of the earth is not quite aligned with its axis of rotation, so the needle of a magnetic compass does not point exactly to true north.

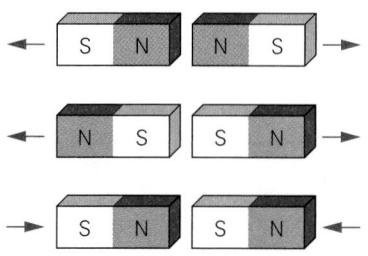

Figure 6-25   Like magnetic poles repel each other; unlike magnetic poles attract.

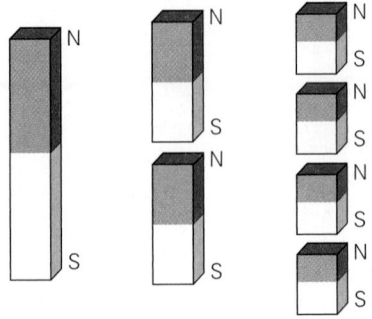

Figure 6-26 Cutting a magnet in half produces two other magnets. There is no such thing as a single free magnetic pole.

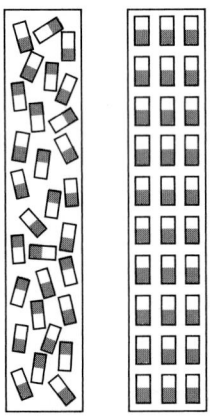

Figure 6-27 The iron atoms in an unmagnetized iron bar are randomly oriented, whereas in a magnetized bar they are aligned with their north poles pointing in the same direction. The ability of iron atoms to remain aligned in this way is responsible for the magnetic properties of iron.

6.13 Magnetic Field

How Magnetic Forces Act

We are so familiar with gravitational, electric, and magnetic forces that we take them for granted. However, if we think about them, it is clear that something remarkable is going on: these forces act without the objects involved touching each other. We cannot move a book from a table by just waving our hand at it, and a golf ball will not fly off until a golf club actually strikes it. An iron nail, however, does not wait until a magnet touches it, but is pulled to the magnet when the two are some distance apart. The properties of space near the magnet are somehow altered by the magnet's presence, just as a mass or an electric charge alters the space around itself, in each case in a different way.

Force Fields The altered space around a mass, an electric charge, or a magnet is called a **force field.** A physicist describes a force field in terms of what it does, which is to exert a force on appropriate objects. Although we cannot see a force field, we can detect its presence by its effects. In fact, even the forces we think of as being exerted by direct contact turn out to involve force fields. For instance, when a golf club strikes a ball, it is the action of electric forces on the molecular level that leads to the observed transfer of energy and momentum to the ball. There is actually no such thing as "direct contact" since the atoms involved never touch each other.

When iron filings are scattered on a card held over a magnet, they form a pattern that suggests the form of the magnet's field. At each point on the card, the filings line up in the direction in which a piece of iron would move if put there, and the filings gather most thickly where the force on the iron would be greatest. Figure 6-28 shows the patterns of iron filings near three bar magnets.

Field Lines It is traditional, and convenient, to think of a **magnetic field** in terms of imaginary **field lines** that correspond to the patterns formed by iron filings. A magnetic field line traces the path that would be taken by a small iron object if placed in the field, with the lines close together where the field is strong and far apart where the field is weak.

Although the notion of field lines is helpful in illustrating a number of magnetic effects, we must keep in mind that they are imaginary—a force field is a continuous property of the region of space where it is present, not a collection of strings. Figure 15-35 shows the field lines of the earth's magnetic field.

6.14 Oersted's Experiment

Magnetic Fields Originate in Moving Electric Charges

Electric currents may not be familiar to us as sources of magnetic fields, yet every current has such a field around it. To repeat a famous experiment first performed in 1820 by the Danish physicist Hans Christian Oersted (Fig. 6-29), we can connect a horizontal wire to a battery and hold under

Figure 6-28 Patterns formed by iron filings sprinkled on a card held over three bar magnets. The filings align themselves in the direction of the magnetic field. It is convenient to think of the pattern in terms of "field lines," but such lines do not actually exist since the field is a continuous property of the region of space it occupies.

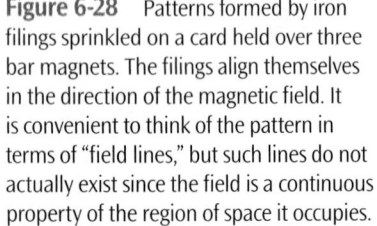

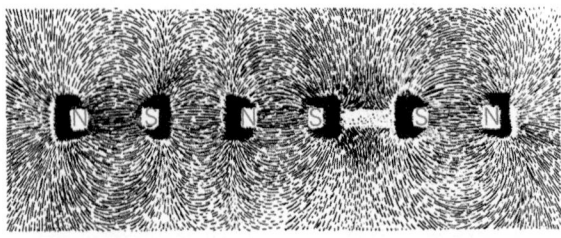

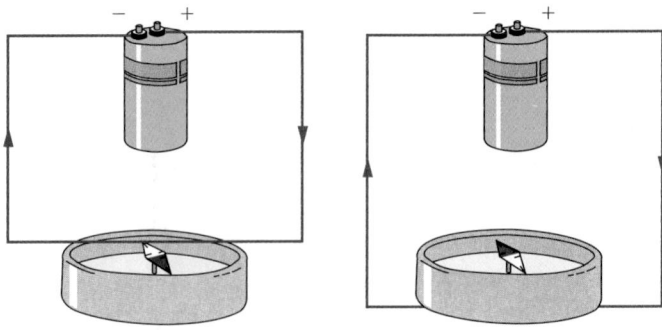

Figure 6-30 Oersted's experiment showed that a magnetic field surrounds every electric current. The field direction above the wire is opposite to that below the wire.

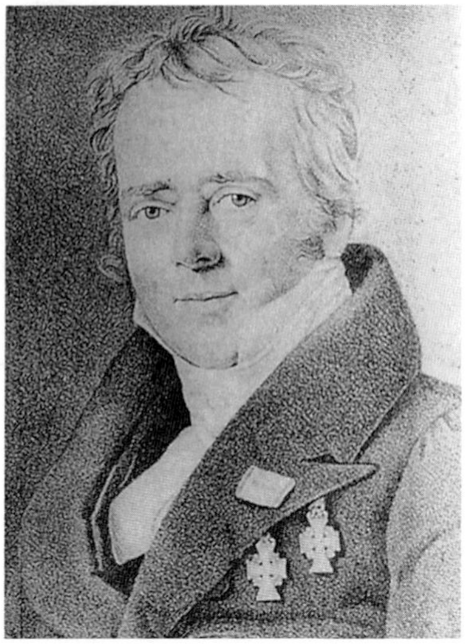

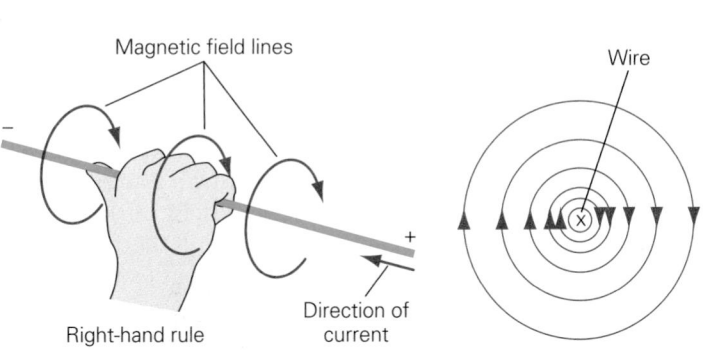

the wire a small compass needle (Fig. 6-30). The needle at once swings into a position at right angles to the wire. When the compass is placed just above the wire, the needle swings around until it is again perpendicular to the wire but pointing in the opposite direction.

We can use iron filings to study the magnetic field pattern around a wire carrying a current. When we do this, we find that the field lines near the wire consist of circles, as in Fig. 6-31. The direction of the field lines (that is, the direction in which the N pole of the compass points) depends on the direction of flow of electrons through the wire. When one is reversed, the other reverses also.

Right-Hand Rule In general, the direction of the magnetic field around a wire can be found by encircling the wire with the fingers of the right hand so that the extended thumb points along the wire in the direction of the current. According to this **right-hand rule,** the current and the field are perpendicular to each other.

Oersted's discovery showed for the first time that a connection exists between electricity and magnetism. It was also the first demonstration of the principle on which the electric motor is based. Magnetism and electricity are related, but only through moving charges. An electric charge *at rest* has no magnetic properties. A magnet is not influenced by a stationary electric charge near it, and vice versa.

When a current passes through a wire bent into a circle, the resulting magnetic field, shown in Fig. 6-32, is the same as that produced by a bar magnet. One side of the loop acts as a north pole, the other as a south pole. If free to turn, the loop swings to a north-south position. A current loop attracts pieces of iron just as a bar magnet does.

The results of Oersted's experiment and of many others allow us to say that

> All moving electric charges give rise to magnetic fields.

Figure 6-29 Hans Christian Oersted (1777–1851).

Figure 6-31 Magnetic field lines around a wire carrying an electric current. The direction of the lines may be found by placing the thumb of the right hand in the direction of the current; the curled fingers then point in the direction of the field lines. In the right-hand diagram the current flows into the paper. (The × represents the tail feathers of an arrow.)

| André Marie Ampère (1775–1836)

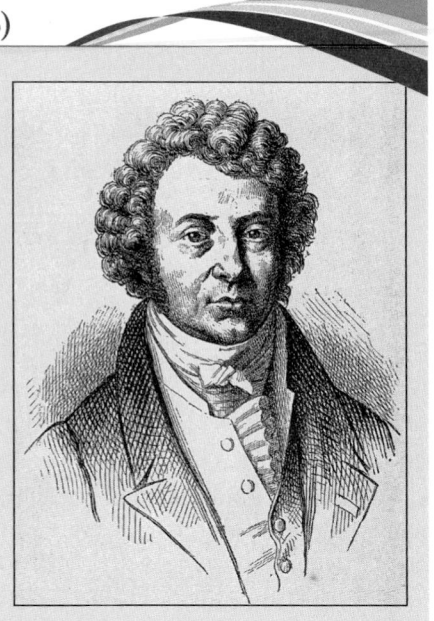

Ampère was largely self-taught and had mastered advanced mathematics by his early teens. Starting as a teacher in local schools near Lyon, he went on to a series of professorships in Paris and was appointed by Napoleon as inspector-general of the French university system. Ampère's personal life was one misfortune after another: the execution of his father during the French Revolution, the early death of his much-loved first wife, a disastrous second marriage, financial problems.

In contrast were the successes of his scientific career. Upon learning of Oersted's discovery that a magnetic field surrounds every electric current, Ampère carried out experiments of his own that resulted in "a great theory of these phenomena and of all others known for magnets," as he wrote to his son only two weeks later. Ampère's results included the law that describes the magnetic force between two currents and the observation that the magnetic field around a current loop is the same as the field around a bar magnet.

Ampère went on to speculate that the magnetism of a material such as iron is due to loops of electric current in its atoms, a concept very much ahead of his time. The unit of electric current is called the ampere because he was the first to distinguish clearly between current and potential difference.

Figure 6-32   The magnetic field of a loop of electric current is the same as that of a bar magnet.

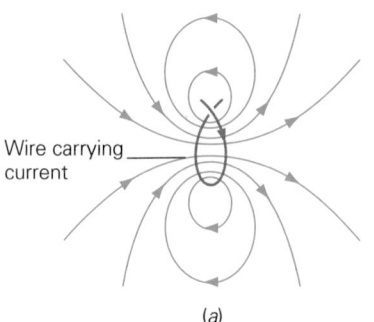

Wire carrying current

(a)

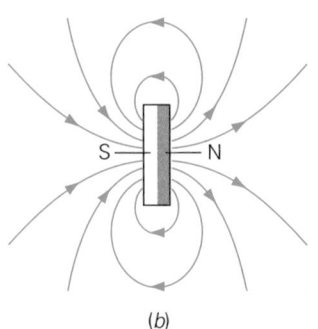

S ⎯ N

(b)

The Electromagnetic Field   An electric charge at rest is surrounded only by an electric field, and when the charge is moving it is surrounded by a magnetic field as well. Suppose we travel alongside a moving charge, in the same direction and at the same speed. All we find now is an electric field—the magnetic field has disappeared. But if we move past a stationary charge with our instruments, we find both an electric and a magnetic field! Clearly the *relative motion* between charge and observer is needed to produce a magnetic field: no relative motion, no magnetic field.

According to the theory of relativity, whatever it is in nature that shows itself as an electric force between charges at rest *must* also show itself as a magnetic force between moving charges. One effect is not possible without the other. Thus the proper way to regard what we think of as separate electric and magnetic fields is that they are both aspects of a single electromagnetic field that surrounds every electric charge. The electric field is always there, but the magnetic field appears only when relative motion is present.

In the case of a wire that carries an electric current, there is only a magnetic field because the wire itself is electrically neutral. The electric field of the electrons is canceled out by the opposite electric field of the positive ions in the wire. However, the positive ions are stationary and therefore have no magnetic field to cancel the magnetic field of the moving electrons. If we simply move a wire that has no current in it, the electric and magnetic fields of the electrons are canceled by the electric and magnetic fields of the positive ions.

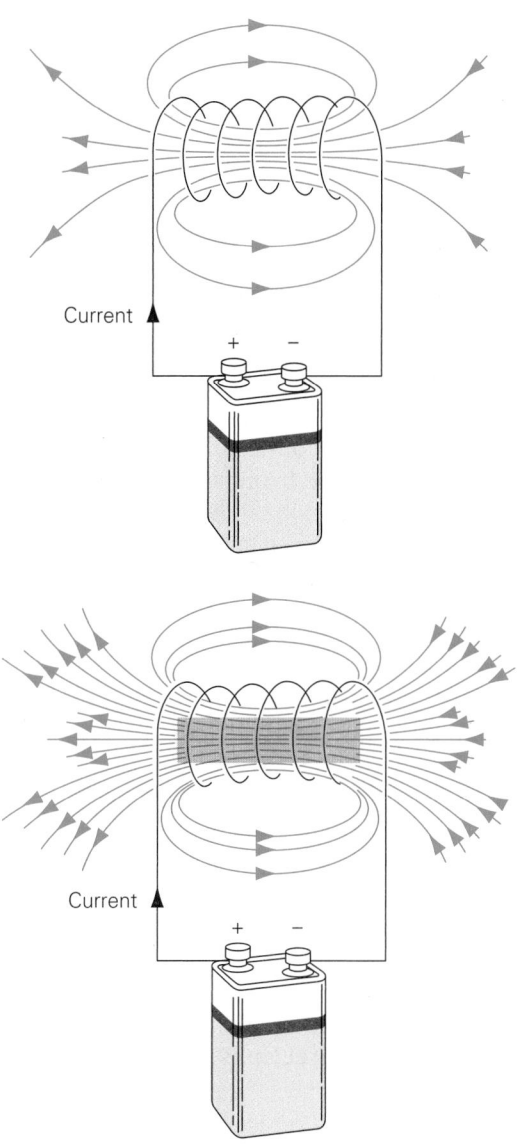

Figure 6-33 The magnetic field of a coil is like that of a single loop but is stronger.

Figure 6-34 An electromagnet consists of a coil with an iron core, which considerably enhances the magnetic field produced.

6.15 Electromagnets

How to Create a Strong Magnetic Field

When several wires that carry currents in the same direction are side by side, their magnetic fields add together to give a stronger total magnetic field. This effect is often used to increase the magnetic field of a current loop. Instead of one loop, many loops of wire are wound into a coil, as in Fig. 6-33, and the resulting magnetic field is as many times stronger than the field of one turn as there are turns in the coil. A coil with 50 turns produces a field 50 times greater than a coil with just one turn.

The magnetic field of the coil is enormously increased if a rod of iron is placed inside it (Fig. 6-34). This combination of coil and iron core is called an **electromagnet.** An electromagnet exerts magnetic force only when current flows through its turns, and so its action can be turned on and off. Also, by using many turns and enough current, an electromagnet can be made far more powerful than a permanent magnet. Electromagnets are widely used and range in size from the tiny coils in telephone receivers to the huge ones that load and unload scrap iron (Fig. 6-35).

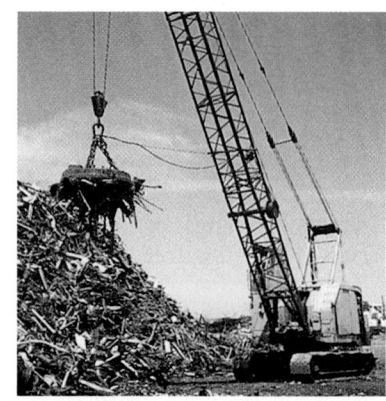

Figure 6-35 Electromagnet loading scrap iron and steel.

Using Magnetism

An electric motor uses magnetic fields to turn electric energy into mechanical energy, and a generator uses magnetic fields to turn mechanical energy into electric energy. As we shall find, magnetic fields also play essential roles in television picture tubes, in sound and video recording, and in the transformers used to distribute electric power over large areas.

6.16 Magnetic Force on a Current

A Sidewise Push

Suppose that a horizontal wire connected to a battery is suspended as in Fig. 6-36, so that it is free to move from side to side, and the N pole of a bar magnet is then placed directly under it. This arrangement is the reverse of Oersted's experiment. Oersted placed a movable magnet near a wire fixed in position, whereas here we have a movable wire near a fixed magnet. We might predict, from Oersted's results and Newton's third law of motion, that in this case the wire will move. It does indeed, swinging out to one side as soon as the current is on. The direction of the wire's motion is perpendicular to the bar magnet's field. Whether the wire swings to one side or the other depends on the direction of flow of electrons in the wire and on which pole of the magnet is used.

Thus the force a magnetic field exerts on an electric current is not a simple attraction or repulsion but a *sidewise push*. The maximum sidewise push occurs when the current is perpendicular to the magnetic field, as in Fig. 6-36. At other angles the push is less, and it disappears when the current is parallel to the magnetic field.

Every current has a magnetic field around it, and as a result nearby currents exert magnetic forces on each other. When parallel currents are in the same direction, as in Fig. 6-37*a*, the forces are attractive; when the currents are in opposite directions, as in Fig. 6-37*b*, the forces are repulsive.

Figure 6-36   A magnetic field exerts a sidewise push on an electric current. In this arrangement, the wire moves to the side in a direction perpendicular to both the magnetic field and the current. A handy way to figure out the direction of the force is to open your right hand so that the fingers are together and the thumb sticks out. When your thumb is in the direction of the current and your fingers are in the direction of the magnetic field, your palm faces in the direction of the force. To remember this rule, think of your thumb in terms of hitchhiking and so as the current, of your parallel fingers as magnetic field lines, and of your palm as pushing on something. The same rule holds for the force on a moving positive charge. The force on a moving negative charge is in the opposite direction.

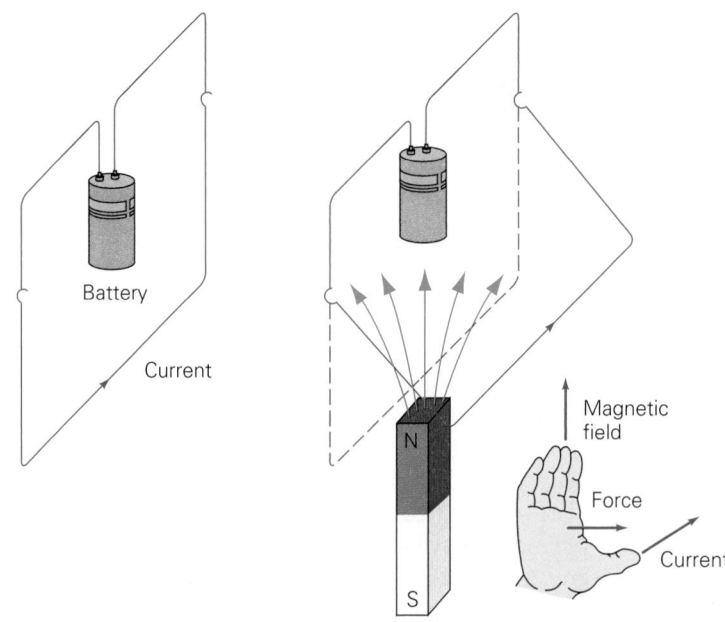

Maglev Trains

Electromagnets can provide enough force to support—"levitate"—trains and so eliminate friction (although air resistance remains). Magnetic forces also propel such **maglev** trains very efficiently. Experimental maglev trains based on pioneering work done in the United States 40 years ago were first built in Germany and Japan. In Germany, attractive forces are developed by conventional electromagnets that curl under a T-shaped guideway. A maglev system of this kind was built in China that connects Shanghai with its new airport 30 km away. The trains carry 600 passengers at 430 km/h (267 mi/h). A proposed 175-km maglev link between Shanghai and Hangzhou that would have cut the journey time between these cities to 30 min from the 140 min that conventional trains take was canceled because of its expected cost of over $5 billion.

In Japan, where an 8.9-km maglev system with nine stations came into service near Nagoya in 2005, the upward force is provided by magnetic repulsion using superconducting coils for the magnetic fields (Fig. 6-38). The Japanese system holds the speed record of 581 km/h (361 mi/h). In both systems the magnetic field of an alternating current passed through electromagnets along the guideway creates attractive forces that pull the train's own magnets forward and repulsive forces that push them from behind. The higher the frequency of the alternating current, the higher the train's speed. Such a **linear motor** is like an ordinary electric motor cut open and unrolled.

A third type of maglev train, called Inductrak, would use powerful permanent magnets in the train cars; a small-scale working model suggests important advantages of efficiency and safety over the German and Japanese approaches.

When perfected, maglev trains are expected to use less than half the energy per person per kilometer than jet aircraft do and ought to be competitive in total trip times for distances of up to perhaps 1000 km, as well as being more convenient. At present, construction costs—

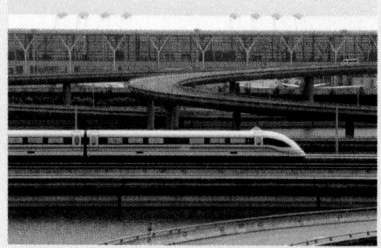

Figure 6-38 This Japanese train uses magnetic forces for both support and propulsion. Such maglev trains are faster and use less energy than conventional trains but are more expensive.

$1.25 billion for the Shanghai airport link—are the chief obstacle to wider use of maglev trains. Even so, a number of maglev systems are being considered around the world. In the United States high-speed maglev links have been proposed to connect Pittsburgh with its airport, Las Vegas with Los Angeles, and Baltimore with Washington, DC. In Japan maglev trains may someday speed at 500 km/h between Tokyo and both Nagoya and Osaka.

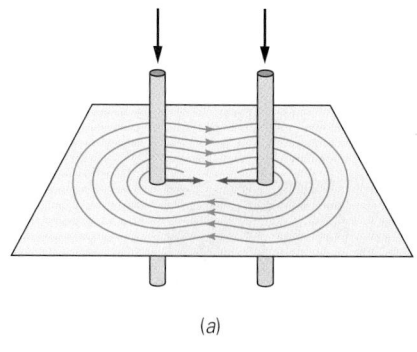

(a)

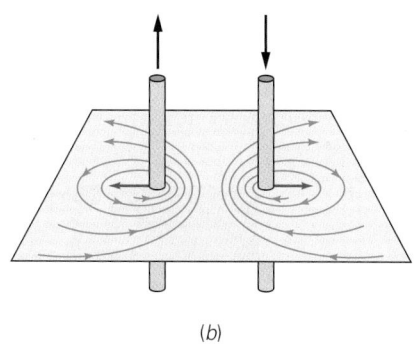

(b)

Figure 6-37 Equal and opposite forces are exerted by parallel currents on each other. (*a*) The forces are attractive when the currents are in the same direction, (*b*) repulsive when they are in opposite directions.

6.17 Electric Motors

Mechanical Energy from Electric Energy

The sidewise push of a magnetic field on a current-carrying wire can be used to produce continuous motion in an arrangement like that shown in Fig. 6-39. A magnet gives rise to a magnetic field inside which a wire loop is free to turn. When the plane of the loop is parallel to the magnetic field, there is no force on the two sides of the loop that lie along the magnetic field. The side of the loop at left in the diagram, however, receives a downward push, and the side at right receives an upward one. Thus the loop is turned counterclockwise.

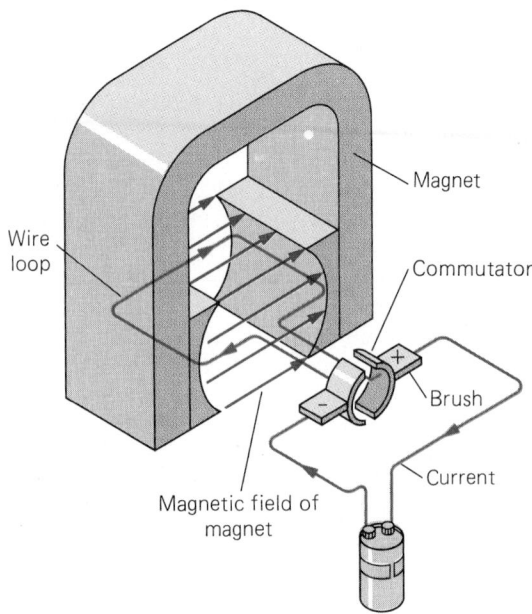

To produce a continuous movement, the direction of the current in the loop must be reversed when the loop is vertical. The reversed current then interacts with the magnetic field to continue to rotate the loop through 180°. Now the current must have its direction reversed once more, whereupon the loop will again swing around through a half-turn. The device used to automatically change the current direction is called a **commutator;** it is visible on the shaft of a direct-current motor as a copper sleeve divided into segments. Normally more than two loops and commutator segments are used in order to yield the maximum turning force.

Actual direct-current motors, such as the starter motor of a car, are more complicated than the one shown in Fig. 6-39, but their basic operating principle is the same. Usually electromagnets are employed rather than permanent ones to create the field (Fig. 6-40), and in some motors the coil is fixed in place and the magnet or magnets rotate inside it. Motors built for alternating rather than direct current do not need commutators because the current direction changes back and forth many times per second.

Figure 6-40   The stationary windings of a large electric motor. Magnetic forces underlie the operation of such motors.

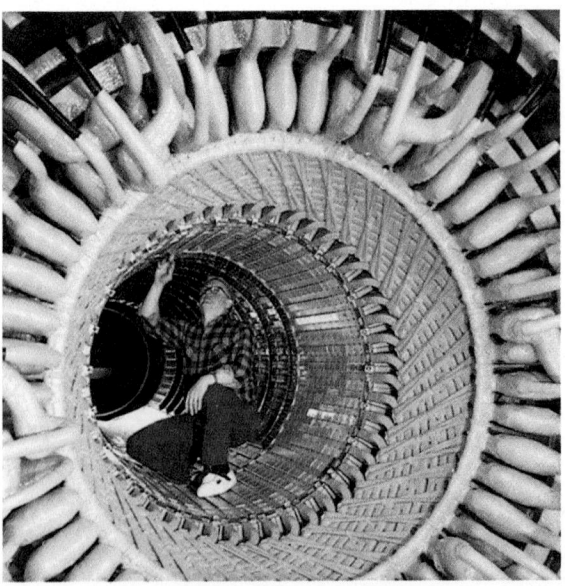

| Michael Faraday (1791–1867)

The son of a blacksmith, Faraday was apprenticed to a bookbinder at 13 and taught himself chemistry and physics from the books he was learning to bind. At 21 he became bottle washer for Humphrey Davy at that noted chemist's laboratory in the Royal Institution in London.

Within 20 years Faraday succeeded Davy as head of the Institution. During that period Faraday had, among other things, liquefied a number of gases for the first time and formulated what are today called Faraday's laws of electrolysis. In the later years of his life came the remarkable work in electricity and magnetism whose results include building the first electric motor and the discovery of electromagnetic induction.

Faraday realized at once the implications of electromagnetic induction and soon had generators and transformers working in his laboratory. Asked by a politician what use these devices were, Faraday replied, "At present I do not know, but one day you will be able to tax them."

To make sense of the electric and magnetic fields he could not see or feel or represent mathematically (he was poor at math), Faraday invented field lines—lines that do not exist but help us to picture what is going on. At his death he left behind notebooks with over 16,000 entries that testify to his originality, intuition, skill, and diligence.

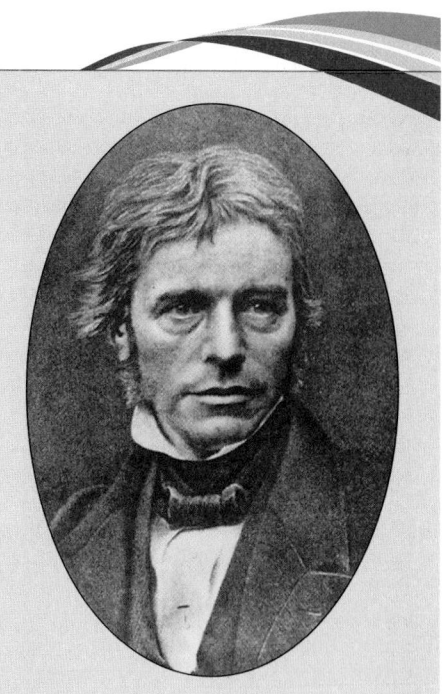

6.18   Electromagnetic Induction

Electric Energy from Mechanical Energy

The electric energy that our homes and industries use in such quantity comes from generators driven by turbines powered by running water or, more often, by steam. In the latter case, as we saw in Fig. 5-49, the boilers that supply the steam obtain heat from coal, oil, or natural gas, or from nuclear reactors. Ships and isolated farms have smaller generators operated by gasoline or diesel engines. In all cases the energy that is turned into electricity is the kinetic energy of moving machinery.

The principle of the generator was discovered by the nineteenth-century English physicist Michael Faraday. Faraday's curiosity was aroused by the research of Ampère and Oersted on the magnetic fields around electric currents. He reasoned that, if a current can produce a magnetic field, then somehow a magnet should be able to generate an electric current.

Induced Current   A wire placed in a magnetic field and connected to a meter shows no sign of a current. What Faraday found instead is that

> A current is produced in a wire when there is relative motion between the wire and a magnetic field.

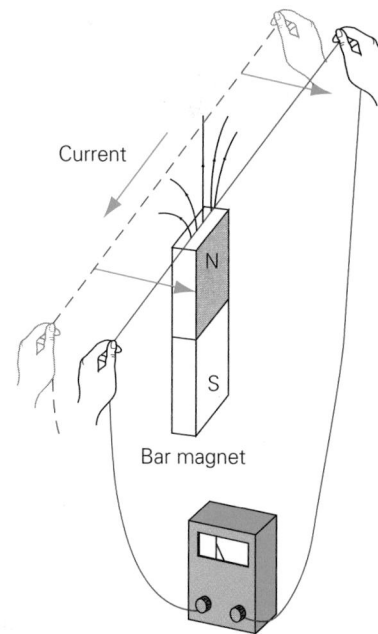

As long as the wire continues to move across magnetic field lines, the current continues. When the motion stops, the current stops. Because it is produced by motion through a magnetic field, this sort of current is called an **induced current.** The entire effect is known as **electromagnetic induction.**

Let us repeat Faraday's experiment. Suppose that the wire of Fig. 6-41 is moved back and forth across the field lines of force of the bar magnet. The meter will indicate a current first in one direction, then in the other. The direction of the induced current through the wire depends on the relative

Figure 6-41   Electromagnetic induction. The direction of the induced current is perpendicular both to the magnetic lines of force and to the direction in which the wire is moving. No current is induced when the wire is at rest.

Current

N

S

Bar magnet

Magnetic Navigation by Animals

A number of animals—notably certain birds, turtles, fish, lobsters, and insects—use the earth's magnetic field to help them find their way on journeys that may cover thousands of kilometers.

Sharks detect the field by means of sense organs in their snouts that respond to tiny electric currents induced by their motion through the field (Fig. 6-42). The amount of current depends on the angle between the field and the direction in which the shark is swimming.

Other animals have bits of magnetite, a mineral that contains iron and is affected by magnetic fields, in their brains. Exactly how animals employ magnetite to sense direction is not known, but experiments leave no doubt that they do. Some bacteria that contain magnetite even use the earth's field to distinguish between up and down when floating in a pond, which enables them to find their preferred habitat in the ooze at the bottom. The human brain also contains magnetite: does that mean we have built-in compasses? Nobody knows for sure.

A third sensing mechanism is based on the presence of certain pigments in the eyes of some animals,

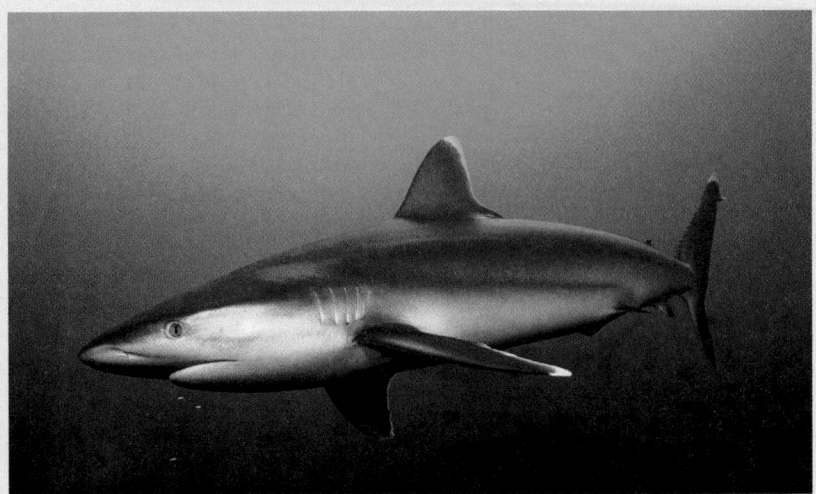

Figure 6-42   Sharks navigate with the help of the earth's magnetic field. They detect the field using electromagnetic induction. Each year 50–100 shark attacks on people are reported worldwide, sometimes as many as 10 of them fatal. Shark fin soup is popular in Asia, and an estimated 70 million sharks are caught each year for making this soup.

for instance, birds, that become weakly magnetic when light falls on them. The signals such eyes send to the brain seem to be affected by a magnetic field.

Magnetic sensing is not the only way that migratory birds navigate on their voyages—as far as 19,000 km for the Arctic tern, which goes from Canada to Antarctica and then back as the seasons change. Such birds also depend for direction on the sun, which traces an east-west arc in the sky with true north (or south in the southern hemisphere) at its highest point, and on the stars, which appear to circle a point in the sky that is always true north (or south). Apparently birds use clues from the sun and stars to calibrate their magnetic compasses as well as directly for navigation.

directions of the wire's motion and of the field lines. Reverse the motion, or use the opposite magnetic pole, and the current is reversed. The strength of the current depends on the strength of the magnetic field and on how rapid the wire's motion is.

Electromagnetic induction is related to the sidewise force a magnetic field exerts on electrons flowing along a wire (Fig. 6-36). In Faraday's experiment electrons are again moved through a field, but now by moving the wire as a whole. The electrons are pushed sidewise as before and, in response to the push, move along the wire as an electric current.

Alternating and Direct Currents   In order to obtain a large induced current, an actual generator uses several coils rather than a single wire and several electromagnets instead of a bar magnet. Turned rapidly between the electromagnets, wires of the coil cut lines of force first one way, then the other. How a generator works is shown in Fig. 6-43, where a coil is shown turning between two magnets. During one part of each turn, each side of the coil cuts the field in one direction. Then, during the other part of the turn, each side of the coil cuts the field in the opposite direction. Hence the induced current flows first one way and then the other. Such a back-and-forth current is an **alternating current.**

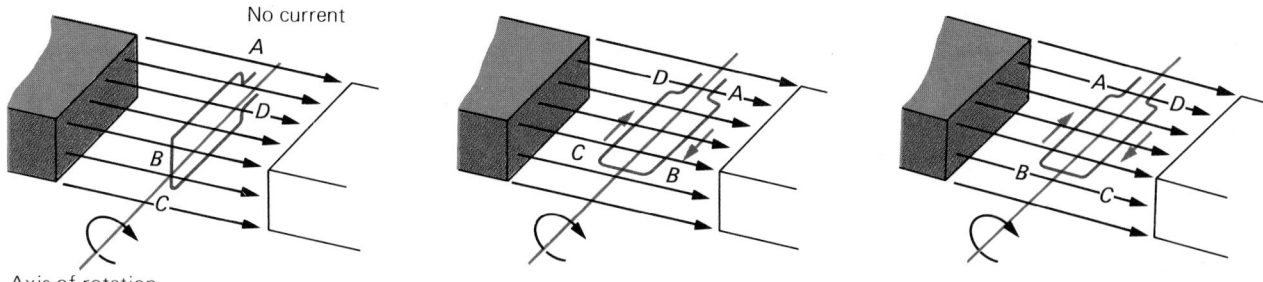

Figure 6-43 An alternating-current generator. As the loop rotates, current is induced in it first in one direction (*ABCD*) and then in the other (*DCBA*). No current flows at those times when the loop is moving parallel to the magnetic field.

The pressure variations of a sound wave (described in detail in Chap. 7) are changed into an alternating current by a microphone, of which there are several kinds. One of them, shown in Fig. 6-44, makes use of electromagnetic induction. A loudspeaker, which changes an alternating current into sound waves, resembles this type of microphone. Its operation is based on the force exerted on a current-carrying wire in a magnetic field.

The Hertz The electric currents that come from such sources as batteries and photoelectric cells are always one-way **direct currents** that can be reversed only by changing the connections. In the 60-Hz (1 **Hz** = 1 **hertz** = 1 cycle/second) alternating current that we ordinarily use in our homes, electrons change their direction 120 times each second (Fig. 6-45). The usual abbreviation for alternating current is ac and that for direct current is dc.

Rectifiers By using commutators like those used on dc motors, generators can be built that produce direct current. Another way to obtain direct current is from an ac generator (or **alternator**) that uses a **rectifier,** a device that permits current to pass through it in only one direction. Because alternators are simpler to make and more reliable than dc generators, they are often used together with rectifiers to give the direct current needed to charge the batteries of cars and trucks.

6.19 Transformers

Stepping Voltage Up or Down

To induce a current requires that magnetic field lines move across a conductor. As in Fig. 6-41, one way to do this is to move a wire past a magnet. Another way is to hold the wire stationary while the magnet is moved. We come now to a third, less obvious, method, which involves no visible motion at all.

Let us connect coil *A* in Fig. 6-46 to a switch and a battery and connect the separate coil *B* to a meter. When the switch is closed, a current flows through *A*, building up a magnetic field around it. The current and field do not reach their full strengths at once. A fraction of a second is needed for the current to increase from zero to its final value, and the magnetic field increases along with the current. As this happens, the field lines from coil *A* spread outward across the wires of coil *B*. This motion of the lines across coil *B* produces in it a momentary current. Once the current in *A* reaches its normal, steady value, the magnetic field becomes stationary and the induced current in *B* stops.

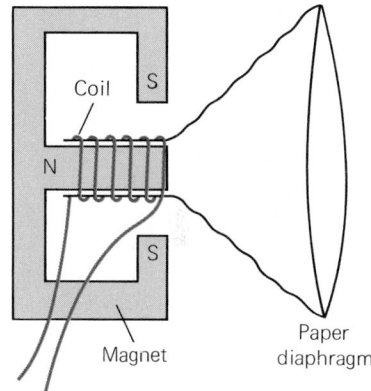

Figure 6-44 A moving-coil microphone. When sound waves reach the diaphragm, it vibrates accordingly. The motion of the coil through the magnetic field of the magnet induces an alternating current in the coil that corresponds to the original sound. A loudspeaker is similar in construction except that an alternating current in its coil causes the diaphragm to vibrate and thereby produce sound waves.

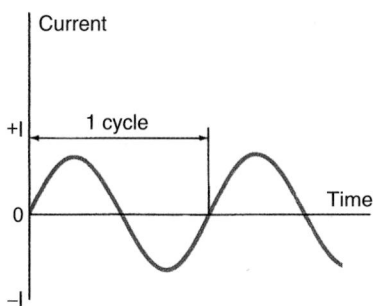

Figure 6-45 How a 60-Hz (60 cycles/s) alternating current varies with time. The frequency of the current is the number of cycles that occur per second. Here each complete cycle takes $\frac{1}{60}$ s. If a current in one direction in a circuit is considered +, a current in the opposite direction is considered −.

Figure 6-46 A simple transformer. Momentary currents are detected by the meter when the current in coil *A* is started or stopped.

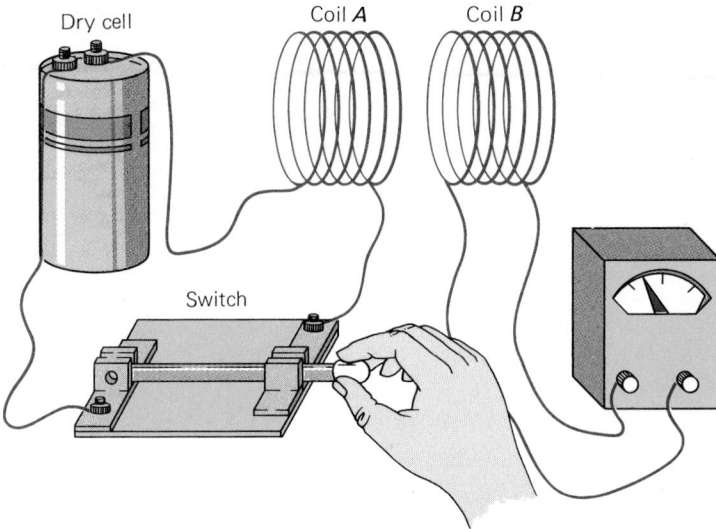

Dry cell   Coil *A*   Coil *B*

Switch

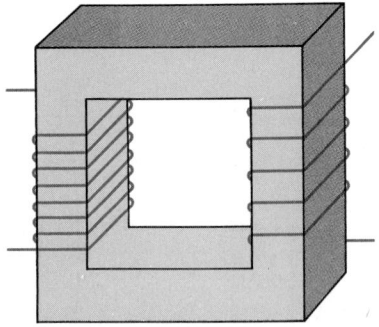

Figure 6-47 Actual transformers usually have iron cores. The winding with the greater number of turns has the higher voltage across it and carries the lower current. The power in both windings is the same.

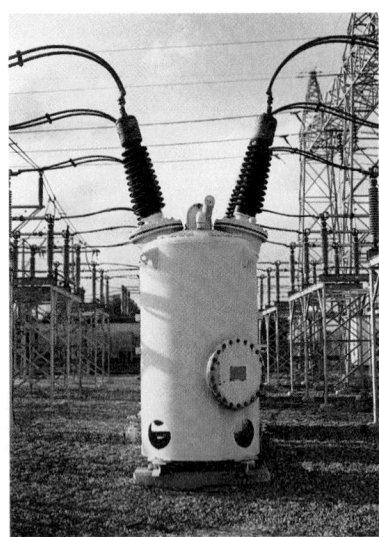

Figure 6-48 Transformers such as this at a power station step up the voltage of the electric power generated there for transmission over long distances. The higher the voltage *V*, the lower the current *I* for the same power *P*, since *P = IV*. The advantage of a low current is that less energy is lost as heat in the transmission lines. Other transformers step down the voltage for the consumer to the usual 220–240 V or 110–120 V.

Next let us open the switch to break the circuit. In a fraction of a second the current in *A* drops to zero, and its magnetic field collapses. Once more field lines cut across *B* to induce a current, this time in the opposite direction since the field lines are now moving the other way past *B*. Thus starting and stopping the current in *A* has the same effect as moving a magnet in and out of *B*. An induced current is generated whenever the switch is opened or closed.

Suppose *A* is connected not to a battery but to a 60-Hz alternating current. Now we need no switch. Automatically, 120 times each second, the current comes to a complete stop and starts off again in the other direction. Its magnetic field expands and contracts at the same rate, and the field lines cutting *B*, first in one direction and then in the other, induce an alternating current similar to that in *A*. An ordinary meter will not respond to these rapid alternations, but an instrument meant for ac will show the induced current.

Thus an alternating current in one coil produces an alternating current in a nearby (but unconnected) coil. Such a combination of two coils and an iron core is a **transformer**. To generate an induced current most efficiently, the two coils should be close together and wound on a core of soft iron (Fig. 6-47). The coil into which electricity is fed from an outside source is the primary coil, and the coil in which an induced current is generated is the secondary coil.

Why Transformers are Useful Transformers are useful because the voltage of the induced current can be raised or lowered by suitable windings of the coils. If the secondary coil has the same number of turns as the primary, the induced voltage will be the same as the primary voltage. If the secondary has twice as many turns, its voltage is twice that of the primary; if it has one-third as many turns, its voltage is one-third that of the primary; and so on. By using a suitable transformer, we can obtain any voltage we like, high or low, from a given alternating current.

When the secondary coil of a transformer has a higher voltage than the primary coil, its current is lower than that in the primary (and vice versa), so that the power *P = IV* is the same in both coils. Thus

$$\frac{N_1}{N_2} = \frac{V_1}{V_2} = \frac{I_2}{I_1} \qquad \textit{Transformer} \qquad 6\text{-}6$$

$$\frac{\text{Primary turns}}{\text{Secondary turns}} = \frac{\text{primary voltage}}{\text{secondary voltage}} = \frac{\text{secondary current}}{\text{primary current}}$$

[For an example, see Sec. 6.19 at www.mhhe.com/krauskopf.]

For many purposes in homes, factories, and laboratories it is desirable to change the voltage of alternating currents. But most valuable of all, transformers permit the efficient long-distance transmission of power. Currents in long-distance transmission must be as small as possible, since large currents mean energy lost in heating the transmission wires. Hence at a power plant electricity from the generator is led into a "step-up" transformer, which increases the voltage and decreases the current, each by several hundred times (Fig. 6-48). On high-voltage lines (sometimes carrying currents at voltages exceeding 1 million V) this current is carried to local substations, where other transformers "step down" its voltage to make it safe for local transmission and use.

Dc Transmission

The advantage of ac over dc in distributing electric power comes from the ability of transformers to easily change the voltage at which the power is sent. This makes it possible to use high voltages and thereby low currents, which reduces the energy lost to heat due to resistance in the transmission lines.

Because there are losses in ac lines that are absent from dc lines, the highest efficiency comes from converting high-voltage ac to high-voltage dc at the production end of a power line and then back to ac at the consumption end. Unfortunately this is expensive: converters at the ends of a 3-GW line might cost $200 million each. Until recently, with fossil-fuel plants located relatively near their markets, ac transmission was almost universal. Alternative energy sources are nowadays often far from their markets, and dc transmission, cheaper than ac over distances longer than about 800 km, is coming into wider use. Over 100 high-voltage dc links already exist: one of them, in China, carries 6.4 GW from an inland dam 2000 km to Shanghai on the coast. In the United States, dc transmission seems ideal to carry wind power from central states and solar power from southwestern states to the rest of the country. Almost all the new underwater transmission lines mentioned in Sec. 6.11 will use direct current.

Important Terms and Ideas

Electric charge is a fundamental property of certain elementary particles of which all matter is composed. The two kinds of charge are called **positive** and **negative.** Charges of the same sign repel each other; charges of opposite sign attract each other. The unit of charge is the **coulomb** (C). All charges, of either sign, occur in multiples of $e = 1.6 \times 10^{-19}$ C.

Atoms are composed of **electrons** whose charge is $-e$; **protons,** whose charge is $+e$; and **neutrons** which have no charge. Protons and neutrons have almost equal masses, which are nearly 2000 times greater than the electron mass. Every atom has a small, central **nucleus** of protons and neutrons with its electrons moving about the nucleus some distance away. The number of protons and electrons is equal in a normal atom, which is therefore electrically neutral. An atom that has lost one or more electrons is a **positive ion,** and an atom that has picked up one or more electrons in excess of its usual number is a **negative ion.**

A flow of charge from one place to another is an **electric current.** The unit of electric current is the **ampere** (A), which is equal to a flow of 1 coulomb/second. Charge flows easily through a **conductor,** with some difficulty through a **semiconductor,** and only with great difficulty through an **insulator.** A **superconductor** offers no resistance at all to the flow of charge.

The **potential difference** (or **voltage**) between two points is the work needed to take a charge of 1 C from one of the points to the other. The unit of potential difference is the **volt** (V), which is equal to 1 joule/coulomb.

According to **Ohm's law,** the current in a metal conductor is proportional to the potential difference between its ends and inversely proportional to its **resistance.** The unit of resistance is the ohm (Ω), which is equal to 1 volt/ampere.

The **power** of an electric current is the rate at which it does work.

Every electric current (and moving charge) has a **magnetic field** around it that exerts a sidewise force on any other electric current (or moving charge) in its presence. All atoms contain moving electrons, and **permanent magnets** are made from substances, notably iron, whose atomic magnetic fields can be lined up instead of being randomly oriented.

Electromagnetic induction refers to the production of a current in a wire when there is relative motion between the wire and a magnetic field.

The direction of an **alternating current** reverses itself at regular intervals. In a **transformer** an alternating current in one coil of wire induces an alternating current in another nearby coil. Depending on the ratio of turns of the coils, the induced current can have a voltage that is larger, smaller, or the same as that of the primary current.

Important Formulas

Columb's law: $F = \dfrac{KQ_1Q_2}{R^2}$

Electric current $= \dfrac{Q}{t}$

Potential difference $= \dfrac{W}{Q}$

Ohm's law: $I = \dfrac{V}{R}$

Electric power: $P = IV$

Transformer: $\dfrac{N_1}{N_2} = \dfrac{V_1}{V_2} = \dfrac{I_2}{I_1}$

Multiple Choice

1. The charge on an electron
   a. is 1 C
   b. depends on the electron's mass
   c. depends on the electron's size
   d. is always the same

2. A positive electric charge
   a. attracts other positive charges
   b. repels other positive charges
   c. does not interact with other positive charges but only with negative ones
   d. consists of an excess of electrons

3. A positively charged rod is brought near an isolated metal ball. Which of the sketches in Fig. 6-49 best illustrates the arrangement of charges on the ball?
   a. *a*
   b. *b*
   c. *c*
   d. *d*

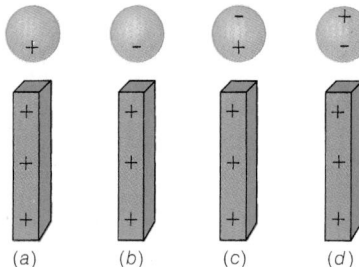

Figure 6-49

4. Protons and electrons have different masses. When they are the same distance apart, the electric force between two electrons
   a. is less than the force between two protons
   b. is the same as the magnitude of the force between two protons
   c. is greater than the force between two protons
   d. Any of these choices could be correct, depending on the distance between each pair of particles.

5. Coulomb's law for the force between electric charges belongs in the same general category as
   a. the law of conservation of energy
   b. Newton's second law of motion

   c. Newton's law of gravitation
   d. the second law of thermodynamics

6. The electric force between a proton and an electron
   a. is weaker than the gravitational force between them
   b. is equal in strength to the gravitational force between them
   c. is stronger than the gravitational force between them
   d. is any of these, depending on the distance between the proton and the electron

7. An atom consists of a
   a. uniform distribution of positive charge in which electrons are embedded
   b. uniform distribution of negative charge in which electrons are embedded
   c. small negative nucleus surrounded at a distance by protons
   d. small positive nucleus surrounded at a distance by electrons

8. The particle easiest to remove from an atom is a(an)
   a. electron
   b. proton
   c. neutron
   d. nucleus

9. An object has a positive electric charge whenever
   a. it has an excess of electrons
   b. it has a deficiency of electrons
   c. the nuclei of its atoms are positively charged
   d. the electrons of its atoms are positively charged

10. A solid conductor is one
    a. whose electrons are firmly bound in place
    b. whose electrons are free to move about
    c. that has no electrons
    d. that has too many electrons

11. Superconductors
    a. have no electrical resistance
    b. have very little electrical resistance
    c. are used in making transistors
    d. have no practical applications

12. Match each of the electrical qualities listed below with the appropriate unit from the list on the right:
   a. resistance   volt
   b. current   ampere
   c. potential difference   ohm
   d. power   watt

13. Electric power is equal to
   a. (current)(voltage)
   b. current/voltage
   c. voltage/current
   d. (resistance)(voltage)

14. The electric energy lost when a current passes through a resistance
   a. becomes magnetic energy
   b. becomes potential energy
   c. becomes heat
   d. disappears completely

15. When a magnetized bar of iron is strongly heated, its magnetization
   a. becomes weaker
   b. becomes stronger
   c. reverses its direction
   d. is unchanged

16. All magnetic fields originate in
   a. iron atoms
   b. permanent magnets
   c. stationary electric charges
   d. moving electric charges

17. The force on an electron that moves in a curved path must be
   a. gravitational
   b. electrical
   c. magnetic
   d. one or more of these

18. Magnetic field lines provide a convenient way to visualize a magnetic field. Which of the following statements is not true?
   a. The path followed by an iron particle released near a magnet corresponds to a field line.
   b. The path followed by an electric charge released near a magnet corresponds to a field line.
   c. A compass needle in a magnetic field turns until it is parallel to the field lines around it.
   d. Magnetic field lines do not actually exist.

19. In a drawing of magnetic field lines, the weaker the field is, the
   a. closer together the field lines are
   b. farther apart the field lines are
   c. more nearly parallel the field lines are
   d. more divergent the field lines are

20. A moving electric charge produces
   a. only an electric field
   b. only a magnetic field
   c. both an electric and a magnetic field
   d. any of these, depending on its speed

21. The magnetic field of a bar magnet resembles most closely the magnetic field of
   a. a straight wire carrying a direct current
   b. a straight wire carrying an alternating current
   c. a wire loop carrying a direct current
   d. a wire loop carrying an alternating current

22. The magnetic field shown in Fig. 6-50 is produced by
   a. two north poles
   b. two south poles
   c. a north pole and a south pole
   d. a south pole and an unmagnetized iron bar

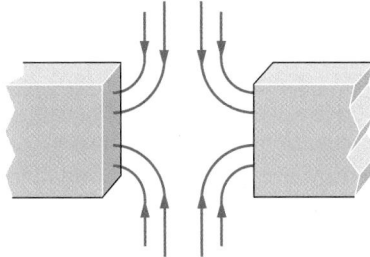

Figure 6-50

23. The magnetic field lines around a long, straight current are
   a. straight lines parallel to the current
   b. straight lines that radiate from the current like spokes of a wheel
   c. concentric circles around the current
   d. concentric helixes around the current

24. A magnetic field does not interact with a
   a. stationary electric charge
   b. moving electric charge
   c. stationary magnet
   d. moving magnet

25. A current-carrying wire is in a magnetic field with the direction of the current the same as that of the field.
   a. The wire tends to move parallel to the field.
   b. The wire tends to move perpendicular to the field.
   c. The wire tends to turn until it is perpendicular to the field.
   d. The wire has no tendency to move or to turn.

26. An electromagnet
   a. uses an electric current to produce a magnetic field
   b. uses a magnetic field to produce an electric current
   c. is a magnet that has an electric charge
   d. operates only on alternating current

27. The nature of the force that is responsible for the operation of an electric motor is
   a. electric
   b. magnetic
   c. a combination of electric and magnetic
   d. either electric or magnetic, depending on the design of the motor

28. A generator is said to "generate electricity." What it actually does is act as a source of
    a. electric charge
    b. electrons
    c. magnetism
    d. electric energy

29. The alternating current in the secondary coil of a transformer is induced by
    a. the varying electric field of the primary coil
    b. the varying magnetic field of the primary coil
    c. the varying magnetic field of the secondary coil
    d. the iron core of the transformer

30. A transformer can change
    a. the voltage of an alternating current
    b. the power of an alternating current
    c. alternating current to direct current
    d. direct current to alternating current

31. If 10^5 electrons are added to a neutral object, its charge will be
    a. -1.6×10^{-24} C
    b. -1.6×10^{-14} C
    c. $+1.6 \times 10^{-24}$ C
    d. $+1.6 \times 10^{-14}$ C

32. A positive and a negative charge are initially 4 cm apart. When they are moved closer together so that they are now only 1 cm apart, the force between them is
    a. 4 times smaller than before
    b. 4 times larger than before
    c. 8 times larger than before
    d. 16 times larger than before

33. The force between two charges of -3×10^{-9} C that are 5 cm apart is
    a. 1.8×10^{-16} N
    b. 3.6×10^{-15} N
    c. 1.6×10^{-6} N
    d. 3.2×10^{-5} N

34. Five joules of work are needed to shift 10 C of charge from one place to another. The potential difference between the places is
    a. 0.5 V
    b. 2 V
    c. 5 V
    d. 10 V

35. When the voltage across a certain resistance is V, the power delivered is P. If the voltage is doubled to $2V$, the power delivered becomes
    a. $2P$
    b. $4P$

    c. P^2
    d. $4P^2$

36. The voltage needed to produce a current of 5 A in a resistance of 40 Ω is
    a. 0.125 V
    b. 5 V
    c. 8 V
    d. 200 V

37. The resistance of a lightbulb that draws a current of 2 A when connected to a 12-V battery is
    a. 1.67 Ω
    b. 2 Ω
    c. 6 Ω
    d. 24 Ω

38. The current in a 40-W, 120-V electric lightbulb is
    a. $\frac{1}{3}$ A
    b. 3 A
    c. 80 A
    d. 4800 A

39. A car's storage battery is being charged at a rate of 75 W. If the potential difference across the battery's terminals is 13.6 V, charge is being transferred between its plates at
    a. 0.18 C/s
    b. 2.8 C/s
    c. 5.5 C/s
    d. 1020 C/s

40. A 120-V, 1-kW electric heater is mistakenly connected to a 240-V power line that has a 15-A fuse. The heater will
    a. give off less than 1 kW of heat
    b. give off 1 kW of heat
    c. give off more than 1 kW of heat
    d. blow the fuse

41. A 240-V, 1-kW electric heater is mistakenly connected to a 120-V power line that has a 15-A fuse. The heater will
    a. give off less than 1 kW of heat
    b. give off 1 kW of heat
    c. give off more than 1 kW of heat
    d. blow the fuse

42. A transformer whose primary winding has twice as many turns as its secondary winding is used to convert 240-V ac to 120-V ac. If the current in the secondary circuit is 4 A, the primary current is
    a. 1 A
    b. 2 A
    c. 4 A
    d. 8 A

Exercises

6.1   Positive and Negative Charge

6.2   What Is Charge?

1. What reasons might there be for the universal belief among scientists that there are only two kinds of electric charge?

2. Electricity was once thought to be a weightless fluid, an excess of which was "positive" and a deficiency of which was "negative." What phenomena can this hypothesis still explain? What phenomena can it not explain?

3. A plastic ball has a charge of $+10^{-12}$ C. (a) Does the ball have more electrons or fewer electrons than when it is electrically neutral? (b) How many such electrons?

4. Why does the production of electricity by friction always yield equal amounts of positive and negative charge?

5. Nearly all the mass of an atom is concentrated in its nucleus. Where is its charge located?

6. Compare the basic characters of electric and gravitational forces.

7. Find the total charge of 1 g of protons.

6.3   Coulomb's Law
6.4   Force on an Uncharged Object
6.5   Matter in Bulk

8. Is there any distance at which the gravitational force between two electrons is greater than the electric force between them?

9. When two objects attract each other electrically, must both of them be charged? When two objects repel each other electrically, must both of them be charged?

10. How do we know that the force holding the earth in its orbit about the sun is not an electric force, since both gravitational and electric forces vary inversely with the square of the distance between centers of force?

11. A hydrogen molecule consists of two hydrogen atoms whose nuclei are single protons. Find the force between the two protons in a hydrogen molecule whose distance apart is 7.42×10^{-11} m. (The two electrons in the molecule spend more time between the protons than outside them, which leads to attractive forces that balance the repulsion of the protons and permit a stable molecule; see Chap. 10.)

12. A charge of $+2 \times 10^{-7}$ C is 10 cm from a charge of -6×10^{-6} C. Find the magnitude and direction of the force on each charge.

13. A charge of $+3 \times 10^{-9}$ C is 50 cm from a charge of -5×10^{-9} C. Find the magnitude and direction of the force on each charge.

14. Two charges repel each other with a force of 0.1 N when they are 5 cm apart. Find the forces between the same charges when they are 2 cm and 8 cm apart.

15. Two charges originally 80 mm apart are brought together until the force between them is 16 times greater. How far apart are they now?

16. Two small spheres are given identical positive charges. When they are 1 cm apart, the repulsive force on each of them is 0.002 N. What would the force be if (a) the distance is increased to 3 cm? (b) one charge is doubled? (c) both charges are tripled? (d) one charge is doubled and the distance is increased to 2 cm?

17. (a) A metal sphere with a charge of $+1 \times 10^{-5}$ C is 10 cm from another metal sphere with a charge of -2×10^{-5} C. Find the magnitude of the attractive force on each sphere. (b) The two spheres are brought in contact and again separated by 10 cm. Find the magnitude of the new force on each sphere.

18. Suppose the force between the earth and the moon were electric rather than gravitational, with the earth having a charge of $+Q$ and the moon a charge of $-Q$. What is the value of Q? (The mass of the earth is 6.0×10^{24} kg and that of the moon is 7.3×10^{22} kg.)

19. How far apart are two charges of $+1 \times 10^{-8}$ C that repel each other with a force of 0.1 N?

6.6   Conductors and Insulators
6.7   Superconductivity

20. How is the movement of electricity through air different from its movement through a copper wire?

21. One terminal of a battery is connected to a lightbulb. What, if anything, happens?

22. Why do you think bending a wire does not affect its electrical resistance, even though a bent pipe offers more resistance to the flow of water than a straight one?

23. What basic aspect of superconductivity has prevented its large-scale application thus far?

6.8   The Ampere
6.9   Potential Difference

24. Sensitive instruments can detect the passage of as few as 60 electrons/s. To what current does this correspond?

25. (a) The capacity of a battery is usually quoted in ampere · hours. Of what is this quantity a unit? (b) How much energy is stored in a 6-V battery rated at 20 A · h?

26. The energy stored in a certain 12-V battery is 3 MJ. (a) How much charge was transferred from one of its terminals to the other when it was charged? (b) How long would a 50-A charger take to charge the battery, assuming a constant current? (Actually, the current decreases as a battery nears a full charge.)

27. The potential difference between a cloud and the ground is 4 MV. A charge of 200 C is transferred in a lightning stroke between the cloud and the ground. How much energy is dissipated?

6.10   Ohm's Law

28. (a) A person can be electrocuted while taking a bath if he or she touches a poorly insulated light switch. Why is the electric shock received under these conditions so much more dangerous than usual? (b) Why does a bird perched on a high-voltage power line remain unharmed?

29. How much current is drawn by a 240-V water heater whose resistance is 24 Ω?

30. A 120-V electric coffeepot draws a current of 0.6 A. What is the resistance of its heating element?

31. What potential difference must be applied across a 1500-Ω resistance in order that the resulting current be 50 mA? (1 mA = 1 milliampere = 0.001 A)

32. A fuse prevents more than a certain amount of current from flowing in a particular circuit. What might happen if too much current were to flow? What determines how much is too much?

33. Should a fuse be connected in series or in parallel with the circuit it is meant to protect? Why?

6.11   Electric Power

34. Heavy users of electric power, such as large electric stoves and clothes dryers, are sometimes designed to operate on 240 V rather than 120 V. What advantage do you think the higher voltage has in these applications?

35. How are the terminals of a set of batteries connected when the batteries are in series? In parallel? What is the advantage of each combination?

36. Wire *A* has a potential difference of 50 V across it and carries a current of 2 A. Wire *B* has a potential difference of 100 V across it and also carries a current of 2 A. Compare the resistances, rates of flow of charge, and rates of flow of energy in the two wires.

37. (a) If a 75-W lightbulb is connected to a 120-V power line, how much current flows through it? (b) What is the resistance of the bulb?

38. A solar cell whose area is 80 cm² produces a current of 2.1 A at 0.5 V in bright sunlight whose intensity is 0.1 W/cm². Find the efficiency with which the cell turns solar energy into electric energy.

39. An electric drill rated at 400 W is connected to a 240-V power line. How much current does it draw?

40. A power of 1 horsepower (hp) is equivalent to 746 W. What is the power output in hp of an electric motor that draws a current of 2.8 A at 120 V and is 75 percent efficient?

41. If your home has a 120-V power line, how much power in watts can you draw from the line before a 30-A fuse will burn out? How many 100-W lightbulbs can you put in the circuit before the fuse will burn out?

42. A 120-V electric motor draws 2.5 A. (a) How many coulombs of charge pass through it in 15 min? (b) How many joules of energy does it use in 15 min?

43. A 240-V clothes dryer draws a current of 15 A. How much energy, in kilowatthours and in joules, does it use in 45 min of operation?

44. When a certain 1.5-V battery is used to power a 3-W flashlight bulb, it is dead after an hour's use. If the battery costs $0.50, what is the cost of a kilowatthour of electric energy obtained in this way? How does this compare with the cost of electric energy supplied to your home?

45. A 1.35-V mercury cell with a capacity of 1.5 A · h is used to power a cardiac pacemaker. (a) If the power required is 0.1 mW (1 mW = 1 milliwatt = 0.001 W), what is the average current? (b) How long will the cell last?

46. A trolley bus whose mass is 10⁴ kg takes 10 s to reach a speed of 8 m/s starting from rest. It operates from a 5-kV overhead power line and is 50 percent

efficient. What is the average current drawn by the bus during the acceleration? (Hint: First calculate the final KE of the bus.)

6.12   Magnets
6.13   Magnetic Field

47. Why is a piece of iron attracted to either pole of a magnet?

48. The magnetic poles of the earth are called geomagnetic poles. Is the north geomagnetic pole a north magnetic pole or a south magnetic pole?

49. Explain why lines of force can never cross one another.

6.14   Oersted's Experiment

50. A current flows west through a power line. Find the directions of the magnetic field above and below the power line; ignore the earth's magnetic field.

51. Figure 6-51 shows a current-carrying wire and a compass. In which direction will the compass needle point?

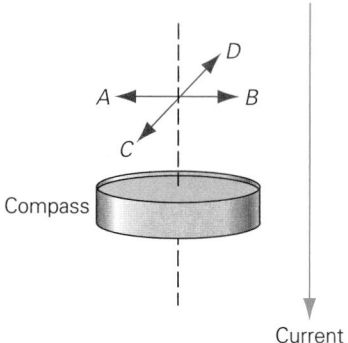

Figure 6-51

52. In an older type of TV picture tube, a beam of electrons perpendicular to a fluorescent screen scans across the screen, which glows where the electrons strike it. When you face the screen, in what direction is the magnetic field of the electron beam?

6.15   Electromagnets
6.16   Magnetic Force on a Current
6.17   Electric Motors

53. Two parallel wires carry currents in the same direction. Do they attract each other, repel each other, or not affect each other? What happens when the currents are in opposite directions?

54. A physicist is equipped to measure electric, magnetic, and gravitational fields. Which will she detect when a proton moves past her? When she moves past a proton?

55. A current-carrying wire is in a magnetic field. What angle should the wire make with the direction of the field for the force on it to be zero? What should the angle be for the force to be a maximum?

56. A current is passed through a helical (corkscrew-shaped) spring. What, if anything, do you think happens to the length of the spring?

57. A length of copper wire *AB* rests across a pair of parallel copper wires that are connected to a battery through a switch, as in Fig. 6-52. The arrangement is placed between the poles of a magnet and the switch is closed. In what direction does the wire *AB* move?

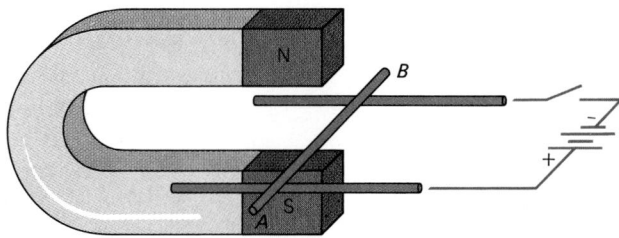

Figure 6-52

58. A beam of protons, at first moving slowly, is accelerated to higher and higher speeds. When the protons are moving slowly, the beam spreads out, but when they are moving fast, the beam diameter decreases. What do you think is the reason for this behavior?

59. When a wire loop is rotated in a magnetic field, the direction of the current induced in the loop reverses itself twice per rotation. Why?

6.18 Electromagnetic Induction

60. Would you expect to find direct or alternating current in (a) the filament of a lightbulb in your home? (b) the filament of a lightbulb in a car? (c) the secondary coil of a transformer? (d) the output of a battery charger?

61. The shaft of a generator is much easier to turn when the generator is not connected to an outside circuit than when such a connection is made. Why?

62. A generator driven by a diesel engine that develops 12 hp delivers 28 A at 240 V. What is the efficiency of the generator?

6.19 Transformers

63. What acts on the secondary winding of a transformer to cause an alternating voltage to occur across its ends even though the primary and secondary windings are not connected?

64. Given a coil of wire and a small lightbulb, how can you tell whether the current in another coil is direct or alternating without touching the second coil or its connecting wires?

65. What would happen if the primary winding of a transformer were connected to a battery?

66. The primary coil of a transformer has 100 turns and its secondary coil has 400 turns. Ignoring the resistance of the coils, compare the input power to the primary coil with the output power from the secondary coil.

67. A transformer rated at a maximum power of 10 kW is used to couple a 5000-V transmission line to a 240-V circuit. What is the maximum current in the 240-V circuit?

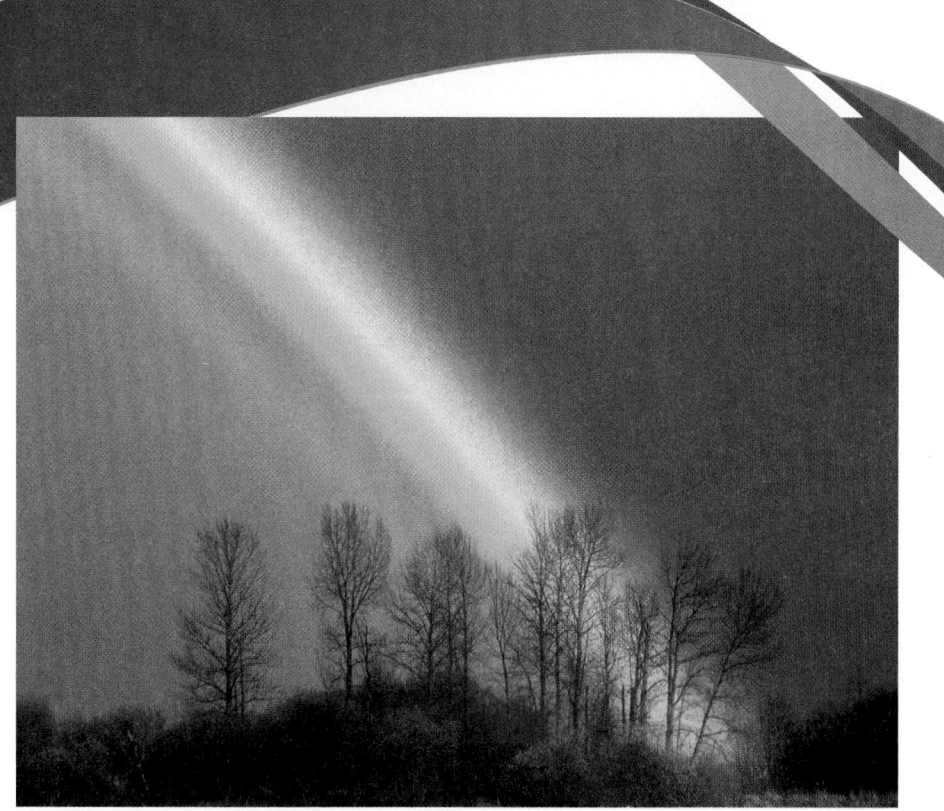

The dispersion of sunlight by water droplets produces rainbows.

GOALS

When you have finished this chapter you should be able to complete the goals
• given for each section below:

Wave Motion

7.1 Water Waves
Crests and Troughs

7.2 Transverse and Longitudinal Waves
Across and Back; Toward and Away
• State what a wave is and give examples of different kinds of waves.
• Distinguish between transverse and longitudinal waves.

7.3 Describing Waves
Wavelength, Frequency, and Speed Are Related
• Use the formula $v = \lambda f$ to relate the frequency and wavelength of a wave to its speed.

7.4 Standing Waves
They Generate Most Musical Sounds
• Describe what a standing wave is and how musical instruments make use of them.

Sound Waves

7.5 Sound
Pressure Waves in a Solid, Liquid, or Gas
• Discuss the nature of sound.

7.6 Doppler Effect
Higher Pitch When Approaching; Lower Pitch When Receding
• State what the doppler effect is and explain its origin.

7.7 Musical Sounds
Fundamentals and Overtones

Electromagnetic Waves

7.8 Electromagnetic Waves
Waves without Matter
• Discuss the nature of electromagnetic waves and describe the difference between polarized and unpolarized light.

7.9 Types of EM Waves
They Carry Information as Well as Energy
• Distinguish between amplitude and frequency modulation of radio signals.
• Explain how a radar works.

7.10 Light "Rays"
The Paths Light Takes
• Describe what is meant by a light ray.

Wave Behavior

7.11 Reflection
Mirror, Mirror on the Wall
• Explain how a mirror produces an image.

7.12 Refraction
A Change in Direction Caused by a Change in Speed
• Describe how refraction occurs.
• Explain how refraction makes a body of water seem shallower than it actually is.
• Explain what is meant by internal reflection and how a glass fiber transmits light.

7.13 Lenses
Bending Light to Form an Image
• Define lens and distinguish between converging and diverging lenses.
• Use ray tracing to find the properties of the image a converging lens produces of an object.

7.14 The Eye
A Remarkable Optical Instrument
• Describe the differences between farsightedness, nearsightedness, and astigmatism.

7.15 Color
Each Frequency of Light Produces the Sensation of a Different Color
• Account for the dispersion of white light into a spectrum when it is refracted.
• Discuss the origin of rainbows and why the sky is blue.

7.16 Interference
Waves in Step and out of Step
• Distinguish between constructive and destructive interference.
• Explain why thin films of soap or oil are brightly colored.

7.17 Diffraction
Why Shadows Are Never Completely Dark
• Describe the diffraction of waves at the edge of an obstacle.
• Discuss the factors that determine the sharpness of the image produced by an optical instrument.

A **wave** is a periodic disturbance—a back-and-forth change of some kind that is repeated regularly as time goes on—that spreads out from a source and carries energy with it. Throw a stone into a lake: water waves move out from the splash. Clap your hands: sound waves carry the noise around you. Switch on a lamp: light waves flood the room. Water waves, sound waves, and light waves are very different from one another in various ways, but all have in common some basic properties that are explored in this chapter.

Wave Motion

Two important categories of waves are **mechanical waves** and **electromagnetic waves.** Mechanical waves, such as water waves and sound waves, travel only through matter and involve the motion of particles of the matter they pass through. Electromagnetic waves, such as light waves and radio waves, consist of varying electric and magnetic fields and can travel through a vacuum as well as through matter. Because mechanical waves are the easier of the two kinds to understand, we shall begin by looking at what they are, how they are described, and how they behave.

7.1 Water Waves

Crests and Troughs

If we stand on an ocean beach and watch the waves roll in and break one after the other, we might guess that water is moving bodily toward the shore (Fig. 7-1). After a few minutes, though, we see that this cannot be true. Between the breakers, water rushes back out to sea, and there is no piling up of water on the beach. The overall motion is really an endless movement of water to and fro.

We can see what is happening better by moving out beyond the breakers, say to the end of a pier. If we study a piece of seaweed floating on the water, we find little change in its position. As the crest of a wave passes, the seaweed rises and moves shoreward. In the trough that follows the crest, the seaweed falls and moves the same distance seaward. On the whole the seaweed moves in a roughly circular path perpendicular to the water surface.

Figure 7-1   Water molecules in deep water move in circular orbits as waves pass by (see Fig. 7-2). When the waves reach shallow water, the molecules in the lower parts of their orbits touch the bottom, which slows them down. The wave crests, however, continue to move forward as before, which causes the fronts of the waves to become steeper and steeper as the water gets shallower. Finally the wave crests topple over, or "break," in a shower of foam that spills down the wave front. At this stage the water depth is about 1.3 times the wave height, and the wave crests may be moving toward the shore twice as fast as the waves themselves.

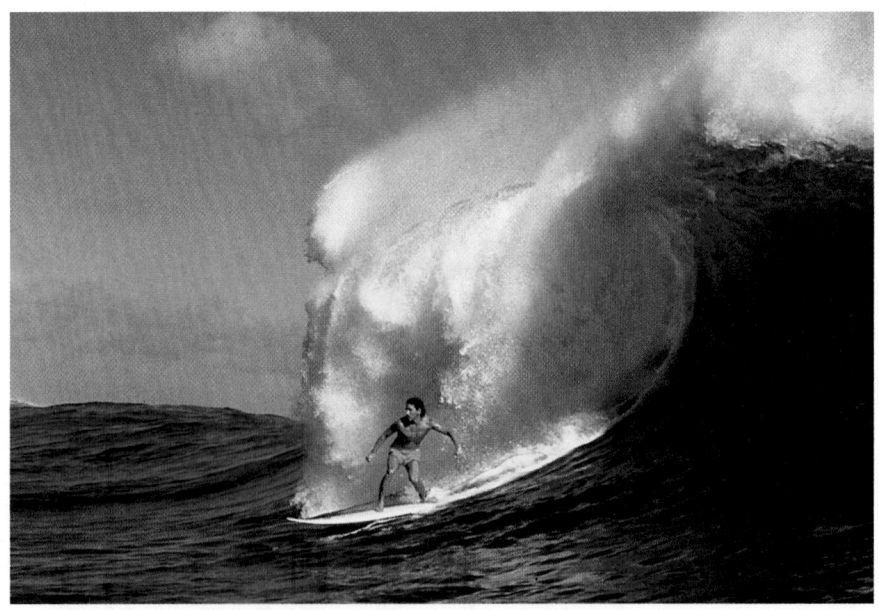

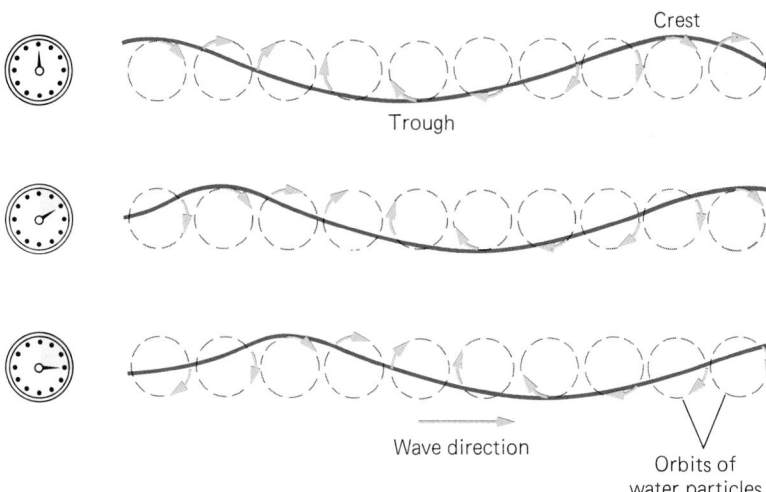

Figure 7-2 Nature of a water wave in deep water. Each water molecule performs a periodic motion in a small circle. Because successive molecules reach the tops of their circles at slightly later times, their combination appears as a series of crests and troughs moving along the surface of the water. There is no net transfer of water by the wave.

The illusion of overall movement toward the shore comes about because each molecule of water undergoes its circular motion a moment later than the molecule behind it (Fig. 7-2). At the crest of a wave the molecules move in the direction of the wave, while in a trough the molecules move in the backward direction.

Waves Carry Energy   What *does* move shoreward is not water but energy. Ocean waves are produced by wind, and it is the energy from the wind out at sea that is carried by means of wave motion to the shore. All mechanical waves behave the same way: they transfer energy from place to place by a series of periodic motions of individual particles but cause no permanent shift in the position of matter.

7.2   Transverse and Longitudinal Waves

Across and Back; Toward and Away

Water waves are familiar but complicated. Simpler are the waves set up when we shake one end of a rope whose other end is fixed in place (Fig. 7-3*a*). Here the rope particles move perpendicular to the direction in which the wave moves. Such waves are said to be **transverse.**

Another type of wave can occur in a long coil spring (Fig. 7-3*b*). If the left-hand end of the spring is moved back and forth, a series of **compressions** and **rarefactions** move along the spring. The compressions are places where the loops of the spring are pressed together; the rarefactions are places where the loops are stretched apart. Any one loop simply moves back and forth, transmitting its motion to the next in line, and the regular series of back-and-forth movements gives rise to the compressions and rarefactions. Waves of this kind, in which the motion of individual units is along the same line that the wave travels, are called **longitudinal waves.**

Water Waves   Water waves are a combination of transverse and longitudinal waves, as Fig. 7-2 shows. Pure transverse mechanical waves can occur only in solids, whereas longitudinal waves can travel in any medium, solid or fluid. Transverse motion requires that each particle, as it moves, drag with it adjacent particles to which it is tightly bound. This is impossible in a fluid, where molecules easily slide past their neighbors. Longitudinal motion, on the other hand, merely requires that each particle push on its neighbors, which can happen as easily in a gas or liquid as in a solid. (Surface waves on

Figure 7-3   Transverse and longitudinal waves. (*a*) Transverse waves travel along the rope in the direction of the black arrow. The individual particles of the rope move back and forth (red arrows) perpendicular to the direction of the waves. (*b*) In longitudinal waves, successive regions of compression and rarefaction move along the spring. The particles of the spring move back and forth parallel to the spring.

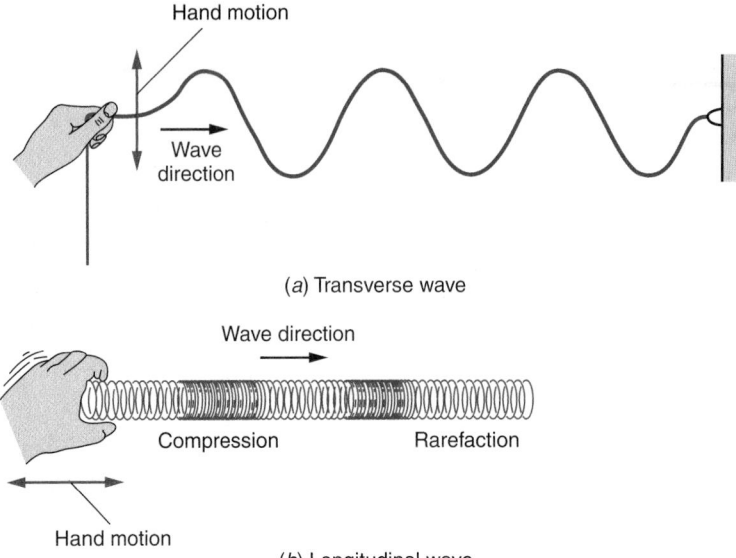

water—in fact any waves at the boundary between two fluids—are an exception to this rule, for in part they involve transverse motion.) The fact that longitudinal waves that originate in earthquakes pass through the center of the earth while transverse earthquake waves cannot is one of the reasons the earth is thought to have a liquid core (Chap. 15).

7.3   Describing Waves

Wavelength, Frequency, and Speed Are Related

All waves can be represented by a curve like that in Fig. 7-4. The resemblance to transverse wave motion is easiest to see; in fact the curve is an idealized picture of continuous waves in a rope like that of Fig. 7-3*a*. As the wave moves to the right, each point on the curve can be thought of as moving up or down just as any point on the rope would move. In the case of a longitudinal wave, the high points of the curve represent the maximum shifts of particles in one direction and the low points represent their maximum shifts in the other direction.

With the help of Fig. 7-4 we can assign numbers to certain key properties of a wave, so that different waves can be compared. The distance from crest to crest (or trough to trough) is called the **wavelength,** usually symbolized by the Greek letter λ (lambda). The **speed** v of the waves is the rate at which each crest moves, and the **frequency** f is the number of crests that pass a given point each second. The **period** T is the time needed for a complete wave (crest + trough) to pass a given point (Table 7-1).

The **amplitude** A of a wave is the height of the crests above the undisturbed level (or the depth of the troughs below this level). Not surprisingly, the energy carried by waves depends on amplitude and frequency, that is, on the violence of the waves and the number of them per second. It turns out that the energy is proportional to the square of each of these quantities.

The unit of frequency is the cycle per second (c/s). As mentioned in Chap. 6, this unit is usually called the **hertz** (Hz), after Heinrich Hertz, a pioneer in the study of electromagnetic waves.

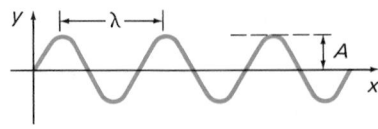

Figure 7-4   A transverse wave moving in the *x* direction whose displacements are in the *y* direction. The wavelength is λ and the amplitude is *A*.

Basic Wave Formula   The number of waves that pass a point per second multiplied by the length of each wave gives the speed with which the waves travel

Quantity	Symbol	Formula	Meaning
Speed	v	$v = f\lambda$	Distance through which each wave moves per second
Wavelength	λ	$\lambda = v/f$	Distance between adjacent crests or troughs
Frequency	f	$f = v/\lambda$	Number of waves that pass a given point per second
Period	T	$T = 1/f$	Time needed for a wave to pass a given point
Amplitude	A		Maximum displacement of oscillating particle from its normal position

Table 7-1 **Wave Quantities**

(Fig. 7-5). Thus frequency f times wavelength λ gives speed v: If 10 waves, each 2 m long, pass in a second, then each wave must travel 20 m during that second to give a speed of 20 m/s. This formula applies to waves of all kinds.

$$v = f\lambda \qquad \textit{Wave speed} \qquad \textit{7-1}$$

Wave speed = (frequency)(wavelength)

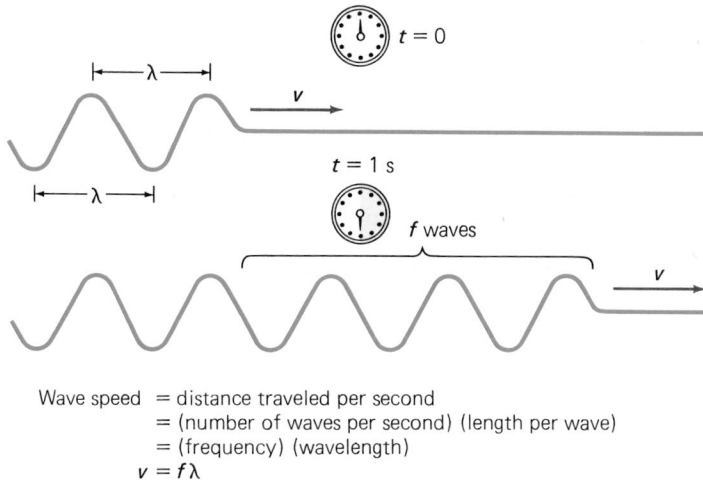

Wave speed = distance traveled per second
= (number of waves per second) (length per wave)
= (frequency) (wavelength)
$v = f\lambda$

Figure 7-5 Wave speed equals frequency times wavelength.

Example 7.1

Waves in the open sea whose wavelength is 50 m travel at about 8.5 m/s (Fig. 7-6). Find their frequency and period.

Solution

The frequency of these waves is

$$f = \frac{v}{\lambda} = \frac{8.5 \text{ m/s}}{50 \text{ m}} = 0.17 \text{ Hz}$$

The period of the waves is

$$T = \frac{1}{f} = \frac{1}{0.17 \text{ Hz}} = 5.9 \text{ s}$$

so a wave passes a given point every 5.9 s. [For another example, see Sec. 7.3 at www.mhhe.com/krauskopf.]

Figure 7-6 Waves whose speed is 8.5 m/s and whose wavelength is 50 m have a frequency of 0.17 Hz. This means that such waves pass an anchored boat once every 5.9 s.

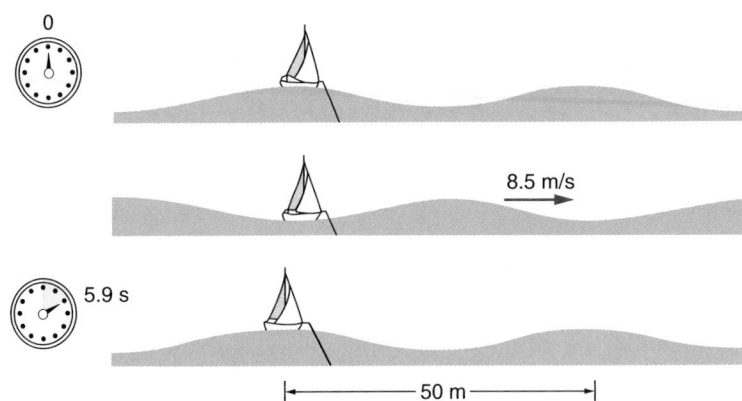

7.4 Standing Waves

They Generate Most Musical Sounds

When a single wave sent down a stretched rope by a shake of the free end meets the attached end, it re-forms itself and travels back along the rope (Fig. 7-7). When a series of waves is sent along the rope, the reflected waves will meet the forward-moving waves head on. Each point on the rope must then respond to two different impulses at the same time. The two impulses add together. If the point on the rope is being pushed in the same direction by both waves, it will move in that direction with an amplitude equal to the sum of the amplitudes of the two waves. If the wave impulses at a point on the rope are in opposite directions, that point will have an amplitude equal to the difference of the two wave amplitudes.

With the timing just right, the two motions may cancel out completely for some points of the rope while other points move with twice the normal amplitude. In this situation the waves appear not to travel at all. Some parts of the rope simply move up and down, and other parts remain at rest (Fig. 7-8). Waves of this sort are called **standing waves.**

Figure 7-7 A wave in a stretched rope is reflected when it reaches a fixed end. The reflected wave is inverted.

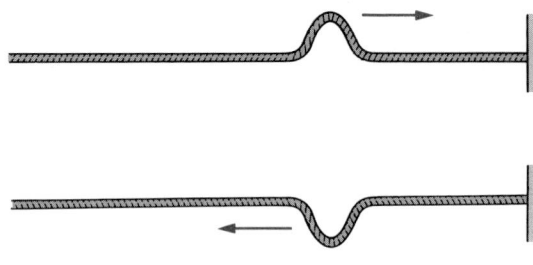

Figure 7-8 Standing waves in a stretched rope.

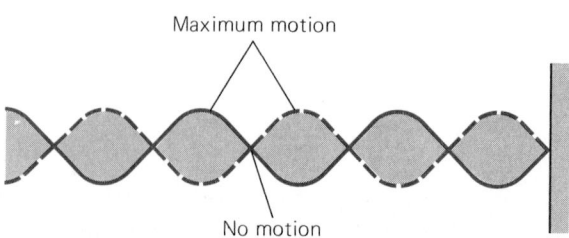

Vibrating strings in musical instruments are the most familiar examples of standing waves (Fig. 7-9). Longitudinal waves traveling in opposite directions over the same path may also set up standing waves, as in the vibrating air columns of whistles, organ pipes, flutes, and clarinets (Fig. 7-10). Standing waves set up in structures, for instance bridges (Fig. 7-11), sometimes lead to severe damage.

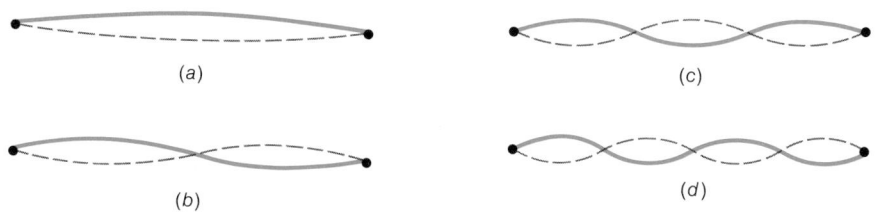

Figure 7-9 A few of the possible standing waves in a stretched string, such as a violin string.

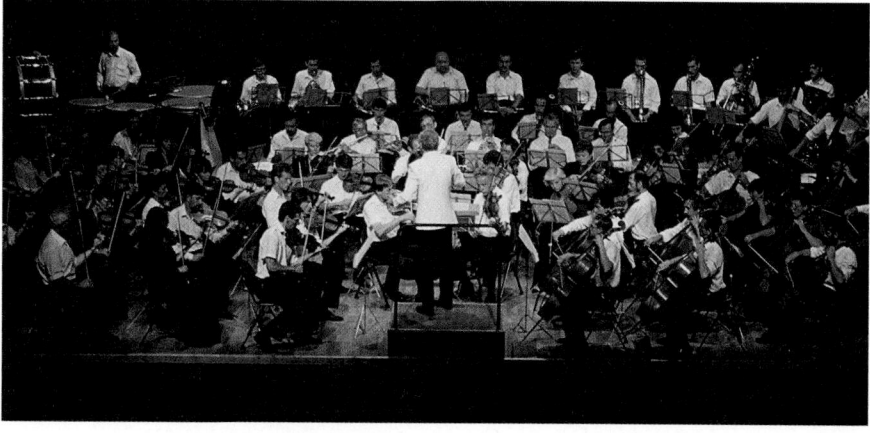

Figure 7-10 Sound waves can be generated in various ways, as by the vibrating strings of a violin, the vibrating air column of a clarinet, and the vibrating membrane of a drum.

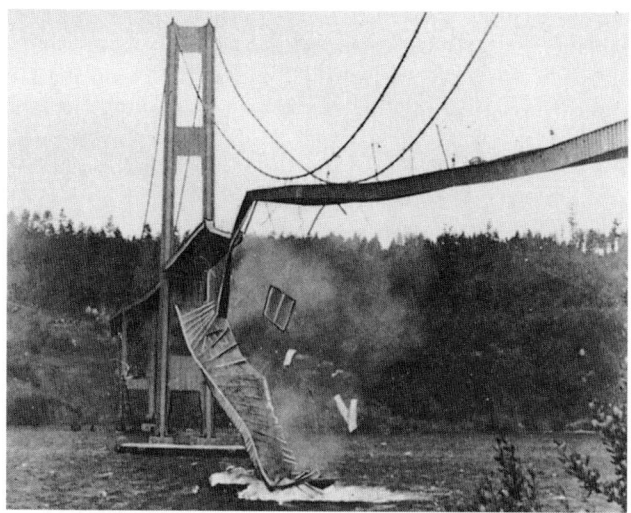

Figure 7-11 Strong winds set up standing waves in the Tacoma Narrows Bridge in Washington State soon after its completion in 1940. The bridge collapsed as a result. Today bridges are stiffened to prevent such disasters.

Sound Waves

7.5 Sound

Pressure Waves in a Solid, Liquid, or Gas

Most sounds are produced by a vibrating object, such as the cone of a loudspeaker (Fig. 7-12). When it moves outward, the cone pushes the air molecules

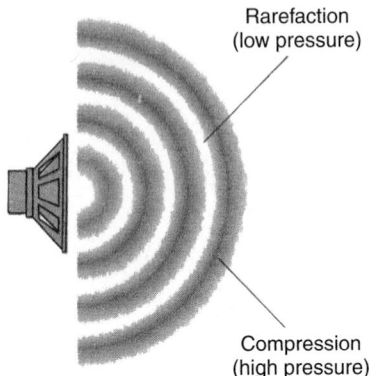

Figure 7-12 Sound waves produced by a loudspeaker. Alternate regions of compression and rarefaction move outward from the vibrating cone of the loudspeaker.

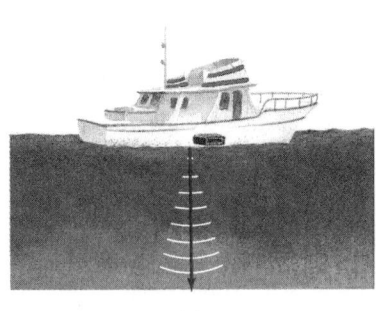

(a)

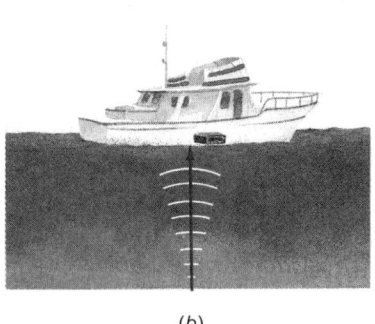

(b)

Figure 7-13 The principle of echo sounding. (*a*) A pulse of high-frequency sound waves is sent out by a suitable device on a ship. (*b*) The time at which the pulse returns to the ship is a measure of the sea depth.

in front of it together to form a region of high pressure that spreads outward. The cone then moves backward, which expands the space available to nearby air molecules. Some of these molecules now flow toward the cone, leaving a region of low pressure that spreads outward behind the high-pressure region. The repeated vibrations of the loudspeaker cone thus send out a series of compressions and rarefactions that constitute sound waves.

Sound waves are longitudinal, because the molecules in their paths move back and forth in the same direction as that of the waves. The air (or other material) in the path of a sound wave becomes alternately denser and rarer, and the resulting pressure changes cause our eardrums to vibrate, which produces the sensation of sound.

The great majority of sounds consist of waves of this type, but a few—the crack of a rifle, the first sharp sound of a thunderclap—are single, sudden compressions of the air rather than periodic phenomena.

The speed of sound is about 343 m/s (767 mi/h) in sea-level air at ordinary temperatures. Since the particles in liquids and solids are closer together than those in gases and therefore respond more quickly to one another's motions, sound travels faster in liquids and solids than in gases: about 1500 m/s in water and 5000 m/s in iron.

Inaudible Sounds Our ears are most sensitive to sounds whose frequencies are between 3000 and 4000 Hz. Almost nobody can hear sounds with frequencies below about 20 Hz (**infrasound**) and above about 20,000 Hz (**ultrasound**), although for many animals the upper limit is higher. Dogs, for instance, respond to sound frequencies up to about 45,000 Hz. Hearing deteriorates with age, most noticeably at the higher frequencies.

Ultrasound has a number of applications, notably in medical imaging and in determining water depths (Fig. 7-13). The latter technique, called **sonar,** is also used to detect submarines and, by bats in air, to detect prey.

The Decibel The more energy a sound wave carries, the louder it sounds. However, our ears respond to sound waves in a peculiar way. Doubling the rate of energy flow of a particular sound gives the sensation of an only slightly louder sound, not nearly twice as loud. This is why a solo instrument can be heard in a concerto even though a full orchestra is playing at the same time, and why you can carry on a conversation at a party even though many others are talking at the same time.

A special scale, whose unit is the **decibel** (dB), is therefore used to describe how powerful a sound is (Fig. 7-15). A sound that can barely be heard by a normal person is given the value 0 dB. Each 10-dB change corresponds to a 10-fold change in sound energy. Thus a 50-dB sound is 10 times stronger than a 40-dB sound and 100 times stronger than a 30-dB sound. The sound of ordinary conversation is usually about 60 dB, which is 10^6—a million—times more intense than the faintest sound that can be heard.

Exposure to sounds of 85 dB or more can lead to permanent hearing damage. Rock concerts (as much as 125 dB) have left many attendees with significant hearing loss, and millions of young people in the United States have damaged hearing due to daily doses of overamplified music. Three-quarters of the hearing loss of a typical older person in the United States is due to exposure to loud sounds.

7.6 Doppler Effect

Higher Pitch When Approaching; Lower Pitch When Receding

We all know that sounds produced by vehicles moving toward us seem higher pitched than usual, whereas sounds produced by vehicles moving away from

Ultrasound Imaging

Ultrasound is used in medicine to produce images of internal parts of the body, including unborn babies. Ultrasound is better able than x-rays to distinguish between soft tissues and liquids, and is far less harmful. What is done is to send a pulse of ultrasound waves in a narrow beam into a patient's body through the skin; the reflections of the pulse from interfaces between different materials return to a detector at different times. A picture of the internal structure of the body can be built up by moving the ultrasound beam in a scanning pattern (Fig. 7-14).

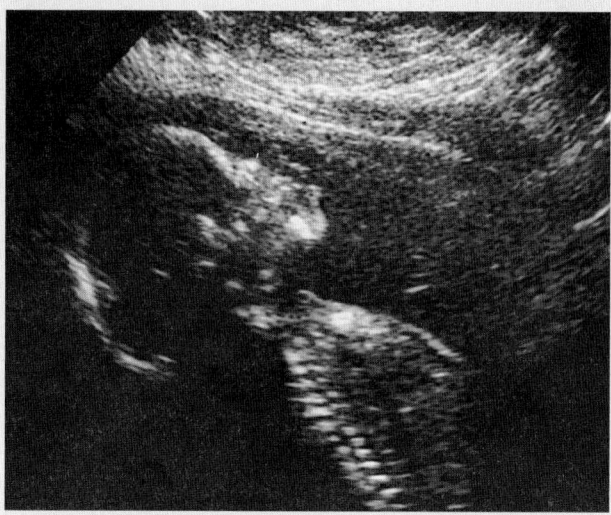

Figure 7-14 Ultrasound image of a fetus 20 weeks old.

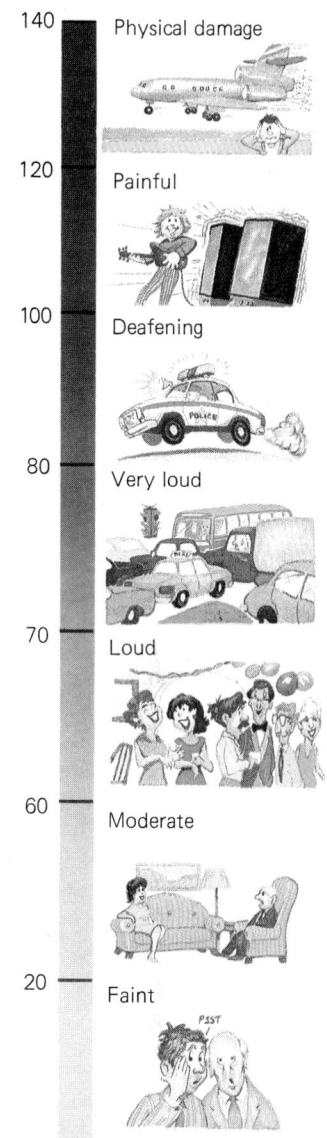

Figure 7-15 Decibel scale for sounds.

us seem lower pitched than usual. Anybody who has listened to the siren of a police car as it passes by at high speed is aware of these changes in frequency, called the **doppler effect.**

The doppler effect arises from the relative motion of the listener and the source of the sound. Either or both may be moving. When the motion reduces the distance between source and listener, as in Fig. 7-16*b*, the wavelength decreases to make the frequency higher. When the motion takes source and listener farther away from each other, as in Fig. 7-16*c*, the wavelength increases to make the frequency lower.

To get an idea of the magnitude of such frequency shifts, the frequency of the sound heard by someone when a fire engine with a 500-Hz siren approaches at 60 km/h (37 mi/h) will be 526 Hz, and it will be 477 Hz when the fire engine has passed and is moving away. The ear can easily pick up frequency changes like these.

A simple way to visualize the doppler effect is to imagine traveling in a boat on a windy day. If we head into the wind, waves strike the boat more often than when the boat is at rest, and the ride may be very choppy. On the other hand, if we head away from the wind, waves catch up with us more slowly than when the boat is at rest, so their apparent frequency is lower.

Using the Doppler Effect An interesting use of the doppler effect is to measure the speed of blood in an artery. When an ultrasound beam is directed

Figure 7-16   The doppler effect. At (*a*) the police car is standing still, and sound waves from its siren reach you at their normal frequency. At (*b*) the car approaches you, moving a distance *x* between two successive waves. To you, the wavelength is shorter by *x* than before and the frequency higher. At (*c*) the car moves away from you, again moving a distance *x* between successive sound waves. Here you find that the wavelength is longer by *x* and the frequency lower.

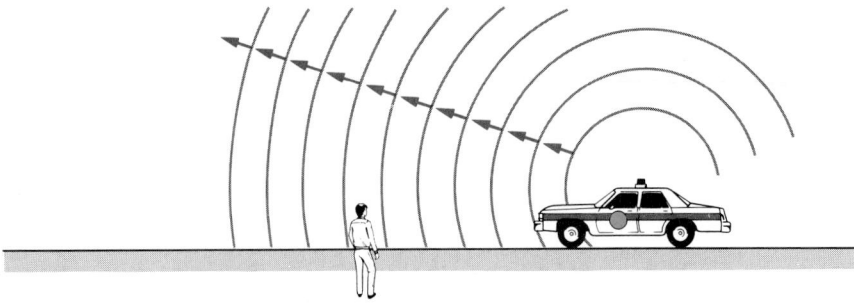

(*a*) Normal frequency is heard

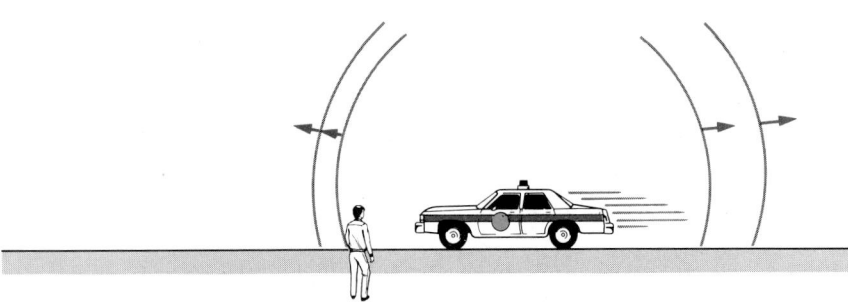

(*b*) Higher frequency (shorter wavelength) is heard

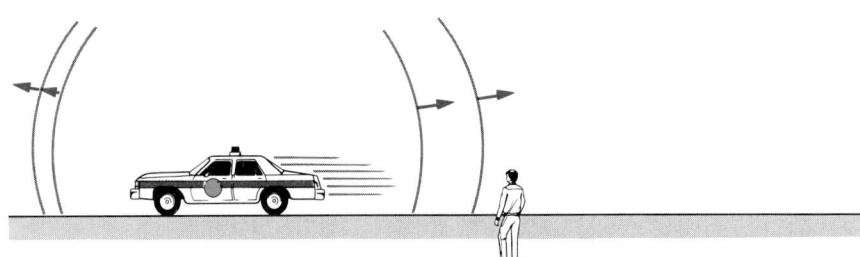

(*c*) Lower frequency (longer wavelength) is heard

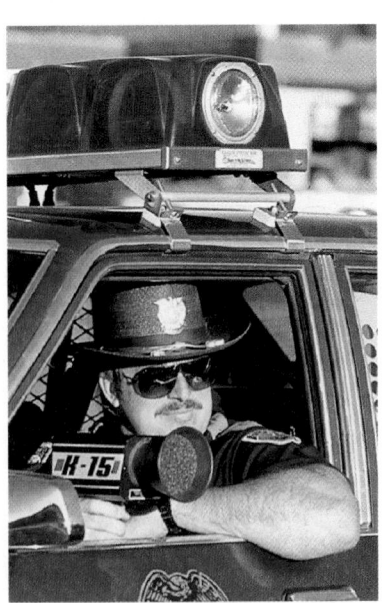

Figure 7-17   Doppler shifts in radar waves are widely used by police to determine vehicle speeds.

at an artery, the waves reflected from the moving blood cells show a doppler shift in frequency because the cells then act as moving wave sources. From this shift the speed of the blood can be calculated. It is a few centimeters per second in the main arteries, less in the smaller ones.

The doppler effect occurs in light waves and is one of the ways by which astronomers detect and measure motions of the stars. Stars emit light that has only certain characteristic wavelengths. When a star moves either toward or away from the earth, these wavelengths appear, respectively, shorter or longer than usual. From the amount of the shift, it is possible to calculate the speed with which the star is approaching or receding. As we shall learn in Chap. 19, this is how the expansion of the universe was discovered. There are still other applications of the doppler effect (Fig. 7-17).

7.7   Musical Sounds

Fundamentals and Overtones

Musical sounds are produced by vibrating objects—stretched gut or wire in stringed instruments, vocal cords in the throat, membranes in drums, air columns in wind instruments. The simplest vibration of a stretched string is one in which a single standing wave takes up the entire length of the string, as in Fig. 7-9a. The frequency may be varied by changing the tension on the string, as a violinist does when tuning the instrument. The tighter the string, the higher the frequency. For a given tension, the frequency can be varied by changing the length of the string, as the violinist does with the pressure of a finger on the string.

Depending on where the string is plucked, bowed, or struck, more complex vibrations may be set up: standing waves may form with two, three, or even more crests (Fig. 7-9b, c, d). Sound waves set up by these shorter standing waves have higher frequencies, and the frequencies are related to the frequency of the longest wave by simple ratios—2:1, 3:1, and so on. The tone produced by the string vibrating as in Fig. 7-9a is called the **fundamental,** and the higher frequencies produced when it vibrates in segments are called **overtones.** [For more, see Sec. 77 at www.mhhe.com/krauskopf.]

Resonance In practice, the strings of a musical instrument give not just the fundamental or a single overtone but a combination of the fundamental plus several overtones. The motion of the string, and so the form of the sound wave, may be very complex (Fig. 7-18). To the ear a fundamental tone by itself seems flat and uninteresting. As overtones are added the tone becomes richer, with the quality, or timbre, of the tone depending on which particular overtones are emphasized. The emphasis largely depends on the shape of the instrument, which enables it to **resonate** at particular frequencies. The sounding part of the instrument—the belly of the violin or the soundboard of the piano—has certain natural frequencies of vibration, and it is more readily set vibrating at these frequencies than at others. The resulting sounds may include a large number of overtones, but the greater emphasis on certain overtones provides the musical quality characteristic of the instrument (Fig. 7-19).

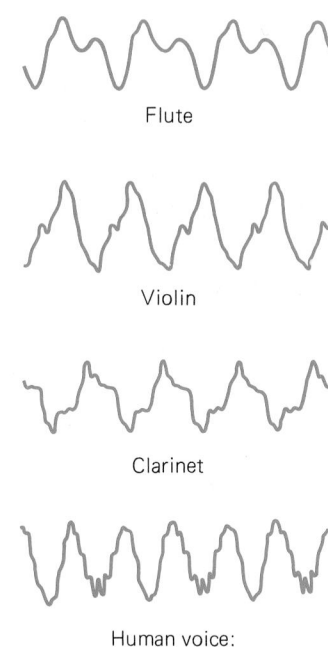

Flute

Violin

Clarinet

Human voice:
vowel sound "e"

Figure 7-18 The waveforms of sounds can be analyzed electronically with the help of an oscilloscope, a device that displays electric signals on a screen like that of a television set. A microphone is used to convert sound waves into electric signals, and these in turn can be displayed on the oscilloscope screen. "Pure" tones, like those produced by a tuning fork, have simple waveforms like that of Fig. 7-4, while musical instruments and the human voice produce complex waveforms. Ordinary nonmusical noises consist of waves with complex and rapidly changing forms.

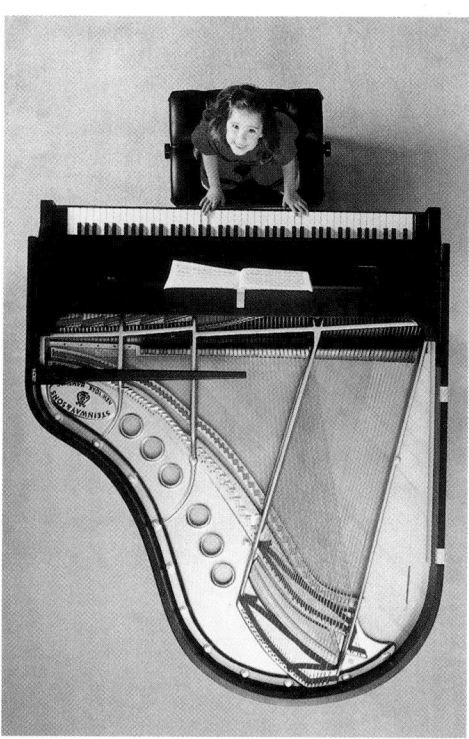

Figure 7-19 The 88 notes of a piano are produced by 220 metal wires (two or three per note to give louder sounds) whose fundamental frequencies range from 27 Hz for the lowest bass note to 4186 Hz for the highest treble note. The total tension of all the wires is about 18 tons and is borne by a heavy cast iron frame.

Earthquake Damage

Earthquakes send out waves that cause the earth's surface to vibrate. A Mexican earthquake in 1985 was especially destructive in Mexico City because the frequency of the waves happened to match the natural frequencies of many buildings there, particularly narrow ones 8 to 15 stories high. The acceleration of the ground due to the waves was about 0.2g, but resonance amplified the building vibrations to produce accelerations of over 1g. This was more than the buildings could withstand, and they collapsed as a result.

Wind instruments produce sounds by means of vibrating air columns. In an organ, there is a separate pipe for each note. The shorter the pipe, the higher the pitch. Woodwinds, such as flutes and clarinets, use a single tube with holes whose opening and closing controls the effective length of the air column. (The oldest known musical instrument is a bone flute 22 cm long with five finger holes. It was found in a German cave and dates back at least 35,000 years.) Most brass instruments have valves connected to loops of tubing. Opening a valve adds to the length of the air column and thus produces a note of lower pitch. In a slide trombone, the length of the air column is varied by sliding in or out a telescoping U tube. A bugle has neither holes nor valves, and a bugler obtains different notes with the lips alone.

The Human Voice   The fundamental frequencies of the speaking voice average about 145 Hz in men and about 230 Hz in women. Even considering the overtones present, the frequencies in ordinary speech are mostly below 1000 Hz. In singing, the first and second overtones may be louder than their fundamentals, and even higher overtones add to the beauty of the sound (Fig. 7-20). Because our ears are more sensitive to higher sound frequencies, the presence of these overtones also helps a singer to be heard over the typically lower sound frequencies of an instrumental background.

Figure 7-20   The human voice is produced when the vocal cords in a person's throat set in vibration an air column that extends from the throat to the mouth and the nasal cavity above it. The shape of this column, which we adjust while speaking or singing by manipulating the mouth and tongue, determines the different vowel sounds by emphasizing some overtones and suppressing others. This shape also gives rise to the subtle differences in sound quality that enable us to tell one person's voice from another's. Vocal power is typically less than 1 W.

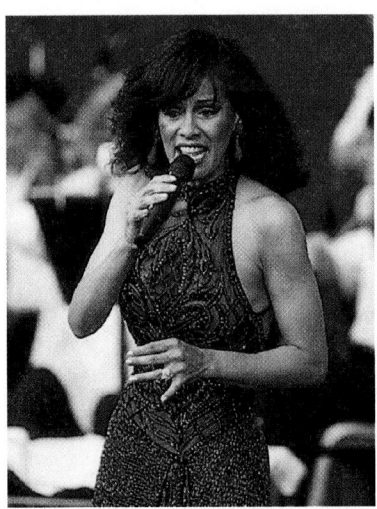

Electromagnetic Waves

In 1864 the British physicist James Clerk Maxwell suggested that an accelerated electric charge generates combined electrical and magnetic disturbances able to travel indefinitely through empty space. These disturbances are called **electromagnetic waves.** Such waves are hard to visualize because they represent fluctuations in fields that are themselves difficult to form mental images of. But they certainly exist—light, radio waves, and x-rays are examples of electromagnetic waves, and like all types of waves, they carry energy from one place to another.

7.8   Electromagnetic Waves

Waves without Matter

We learned in Chap. 6 that a changing magnetic field gives rise by electromagnetic induction to an electric current in a nearby wire. We can reasonably conclude that a changing magnetic field has an electric field associated with it.

James Clerk Maxwell (1831–1879)

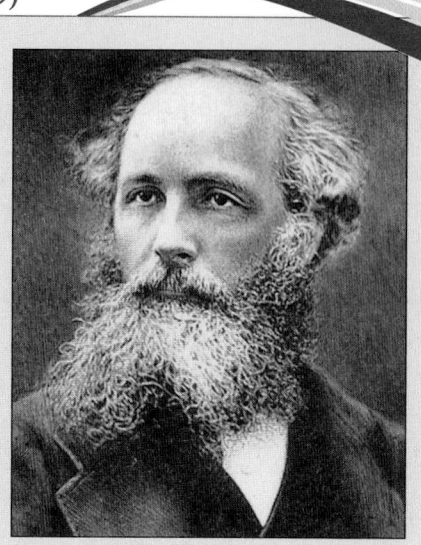

Maxwell was born in Scotland shortly before Michael Faraday discovered electromagnetic induction. While still a student, he used his ideas on color vision to make the first color photograph. At 24 he showed that the rings of Saturn could not be solid or liquid but must consist of separate small bodies. At about this time Maxwell became interested in electricity and magnetism and soon was convinced that these were not separate phenomena but had an underlying unity of some kind.

Starting from the results of Faraday and others, Maxwell created a single comprehensive theory of electricity and magnetism that remains the foundation of the subject today. From his equations Maxwell predicted that electromagnetic waves should exist that travel with the speed of light and surmised that light consisted of such waves.

Sadly, Maxwell did not live to see his work confirmed in the experiments of Heinrich Hertz. He died of cancer at 48 in 1879, the year in which Albert Einstein was born. Maxwell had been the greatest theoretical physicist of the nineteenth century; Einstein was to be the greatest theoretical physicist of the twentieth century. (By a similar coincidence, Newton was born in the year of Galileo's death.)

Maxwell proposed that the opposite effect also exists, so that a changing electric field has an associated magnetic field. The electric fields produced by electromagnetic induction are easy to measure because metals offer little resistance to the flow of electrons. There is no such thing as a magnetic current, however, and it was impossible in Maxwell's time to detect the weak magnetic fields he had predicted. But there is another way to check Maxwell's idea.

If Maxwell was right, then electromagnetic (em) waves must occur in which changing electric and magnetic fields are coupled together by both electromagnetic induction and the mechanism he proposed. The linked fields spread out in space much as ripples spread out when a stone is dropped into a body of water. The energy carried by an em wave is constantly being exchanged between its fluctuating electric and magnetic fields. Calculations show that the wave speed in empty space should have the same value as the speed of light, which is 3×10^8 m/s (186,000 mi/s), regardless of frequency or amplitude. The symbol for the speed of light in empty space is c, so that

$$\textbf{Speed of light} = c = 3 \times 10^8 \text{ m/s}$$

Figure 7-21 shows the relationship between the electric and magnetic fields in an electromagnetic wave. Here the fields are represented by a series of vectors (not field lines) that indicate the magnitude and direction of the fields in the path of the wave. The fields are perpendicular to each other and to the direction of the wave, and they remain in step as they periodically reverse their directions.

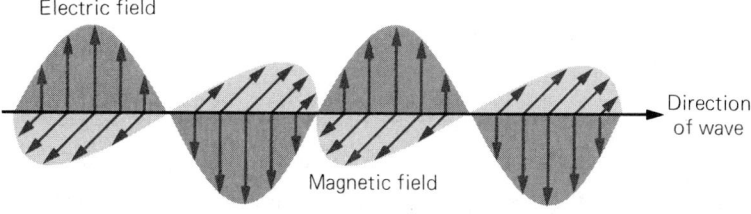

Figure 7-21 The magnitudes of the electric and magnetic fields in an electromagnetic wave vary together. The fields are perpendicular to each other and to the direction of the wave.

Solar Sails

Em waves carry momentum as well as energy, and their impact on a surface gives it a tiny push called **radiation pressure.** A spacecraft could use sunlight from the sun striking a suitable sail to propel it far out into the solar system. Anything bouncing off a surface exerts twice as much force as it would if it were simply absorbed, hence a solar sail should have a reflective surface.

The sail should also be large: for a thrust of only 1 N (0.225 lb) an area of about 10^5 m^2 (nearly 25 acres!) would be needed at the distance of the earth's orbit. But there is no air resistance in space, so even a very small thrust would eventually lead to speeds well beyond those possible for a conventional spacecraft with a fixed fuel supply.

Solar sails are a serious possibility for the future. Unfortunately, trials in 2001, 2005, and 2008 were inconclusive because in each case the launch vehicle failed.

Polarized Light

A polarized beam of light is one in which the electric fields of the waves are all in the same direction. (For simplicity, only the electric fields are considered here; the magnetic fields are perpendicular to them, as in Fig. 7-21.) If the electric fields are in random directions (though, of course, always in a plane perpendicular to the direction of the light beam), the beam is unpolarized. Figure 7-22a corresponds to a polarized beam and b corresponds to an unpolarized beam.

Materials can be made that permit only light polarized in a certain direction to pass through them. Polaroid is a material of this kind. Because skylight is partly polarized, sunglasses with correctly oriented Polaroid lenses reduce glare from the sky while affecting unpolarized light from elsewhere to a lesser extent. Among other applications of polarized light are the liquid-crystal displays used for digital readouts, for instance in watches and some TV screens. These displays are based on the response of certain substances to polarized light when subjected to electric fields.

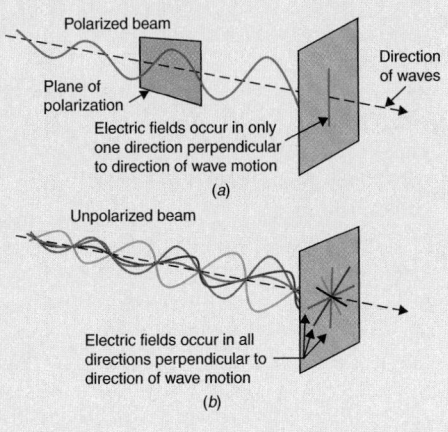

Figure 7-22   (a) A polarized and (b) an unpolarized beam of electromagnetic waves.

7.9   Types of EM Waves

They Carry Information as Well as Energy

During Maxwell's lifetime em waves remained an unproven idea. Finally, in 1887, the German physicist Heinrich Hertz (Fig. 7-23) showed experimentally that em waves indeed exist and behave exactly as Maxwell expected them to.

Radio   Hertz was not concerned with the commercial possibilities of em waves, and other scientists and engineers developed what we now call **radio.** A radio signal is sent by means of em waves produced by electrons that move back and forth hundreds of thousands to millions of times per second in the antenna of the sending station. The signal resides either in variations in the strength of the waves (**amplitude modulation,** or AM) or in variations in the frequency of the waves (**frequency modulation,** or FM), as in Fig. 7-24. Frequency modulation is less subject to random disturbances ("static").

When the waves reach the antenna of a receiver, the electrons there vibrate in step with the waves. The receiver can be tuned to respond only to a narrow frequency band. Since transmitters operate on different frequencies, a receiver can pick up the signals sent out by whatever station we wish. The currents set up in the receiving antenna are very weak, but they are strong enough for electronic circuits in the receiver to extract the signal from them and turn it into sounds from a loudspeaker.

The frequencies of ordinary radio waves extend up to about 2 MHz (1 MHz = 1 megahertz = 10^6 Hz) and those of waves used in long-range short-wave communication extend up to about 30 MHz. Still higher frequencies have found widespread use in television and radar. Such extremely short waves are not reflected by the ionosphere (see opposite page), so direct reception of television is limited by the horizon unless rebroadcast by a satellite station.

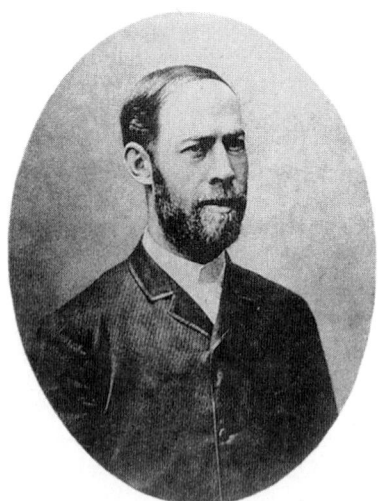

Figure 7-23   Heinrich Hertz (1857–1894).

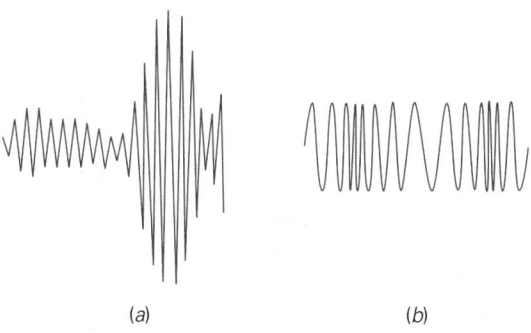

(a) (b)

Figure 7-24 (*a*) In amplitude modulation (AM), variations in the amplitude of a constant-frequency radio wave constitute the signal being sent out. (*b*) In frequency modulation (FM), variations in the frequency of a constant-amplitude wave constitute the signal.

Radar Waves whose frequencies are around 10 GHz (1 GHz = 1 gigahertz = 10^9 Hz), corresponding to wavelengths of a few centimeters, can readily be formed into narrow beams. Such beams are reflected by solid objects such as ships and airplanes, which is the basis of **radar** (from *ra*dio *d*etection *a*nd *r*anging) (Fig. 7-27). A rotating antenna is used to send out a pulsed beam, and the distance of a particular target is found from the time needed for the echo to return to the antenna. The direction of the target is the direction in which the antenna is then pointing. [For an example, see Sec. 7.9 at www.mhhe.com/krauskopf.]

The Ionosphere

Not long after Hertz's experiments with em waves, the Italian engineer Guglielmo Marconi (Fig. 7-25) thought of using them for communication. In Hertz's work the transmitter and receiver were only a few meters apart. Marconi was able to extend the range to many kilometers, and in 1899 he sent a radio message across the English Channel. Two years later he sent signals across the Atlantic Ocean from England to Newfoundland, using kites to raise his antennas.

Radio waves, like light waves, tend to travel in straight lines, and the curvature of the earth should therefore prevent radio communication over long distances. For this reason Marconi's achievements came as a surprise.

The mystery was solved with the discovery of a region of ionized gas called the **ionosphere** that extends from about 70 km to several hundred km above the earth's surface (Fig. 7-26). The ions are produced by the action of high-energy ultraviolet rays and x-rays from the sun. The ionosphere behaves like a mirror to high-frequency radio waves, which can bounce one or more times between the ionosphere and the earth's surface (Fig. 7-26). Low-frequency radio waves are absorbed by the ionosphere, and very-high frequency (VHF) and ultrahigh frequency (UHF) waves pass through it and so can be used to communicate with satellites and spacecraft.

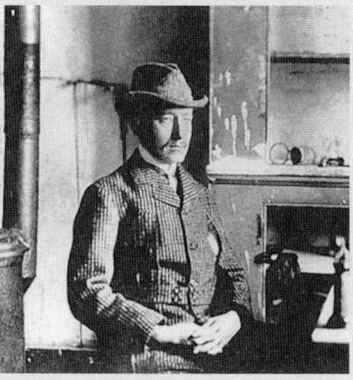

Figure 7-25 Guglielmo Marconi at his laboratory in Newfoundland with the instruments that detected the first radio transmission across the Atlantic Ocean. The radio waves were reflected by the ionosphere.

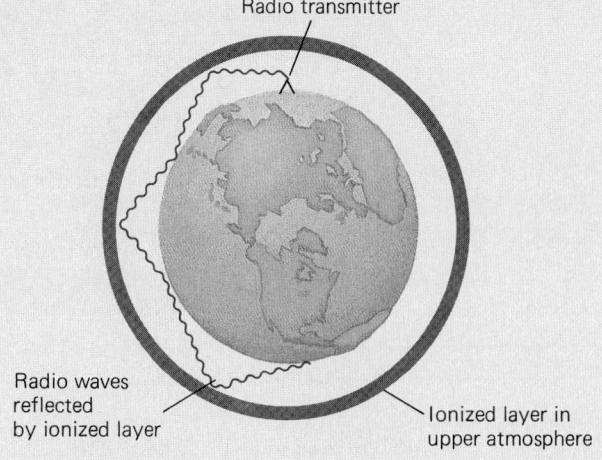

Radio transmitter

Radio waves reflected by ionized layer

Ionized layer in upper atmosphere

Figure 7-26 The ionosphere is a region in the upper atmosphere whose ionized layers make possible long-range radio communication by their ability to reflect short-wavelength radio waves.

Ultraviolet and the Skin

Solar radiation at the longer-wavelength (320–400 nm) end of the ultraviolet part of the spectrum is called UVA and acts on the skin to produce a protective tan. Shorter-wavelength (290–320 nm) ultraviolet radiation is called UVB and causes sunburn. Repeated exposure to both kinds of solar UV ages the skin and, in the case of UVB especially, may lead to skin cancer and cataracts.

Sunscreen products usually block UVB while permitting some UVA to get through, which allows tanning. The sun protection factor (SPF) of a sunscreen is a measure of its effectiveness against UVB. An SPF of 10, for instance, means that 10 hours in the sun with the sunscreen on is equivalent to 1 hour with bare skin. In practice, to achieve its stated SPF value a sunscreen must be applied thickly and fairly often, say every few hours.

There is another consideration here. The action of UVB on skin produces vitamin D, which has turned out to be important in many aspects of health as well as its long-known role in bone formation. Vitamin D is involved in helping the body combat cancers of various kinds, infectious diseases, autoimmune conditions such as multiple sclerosis, heart ailments, diabetes, and possibly dementia. Babies born in late summer or early fall are found to be taller with stronger bones than those born in winter or spring, which is attributed to higher vitamin D levels in their mothers during summer months.

Many people do not receive enough vitamin D in their food. It is now believed that one of the reasons for the general increase in sickness in winter is the reduced exposure of people's skin to strong sunlight then. Evidently, although too much UVB is bad, so is not enough. For most people in North America, 15 to 20 minutes daily of unprotected exposure of the hands, arms, and face to sunlight when the sun is high is sufficient and will not harm the skin. In winter, supplementary vitamin D would be a good idea to accompany diets low in that vitamin.

Sunbeds use UVA and so do not lead to vitamin D production in the skin; they also carry a risk of skin cancer.

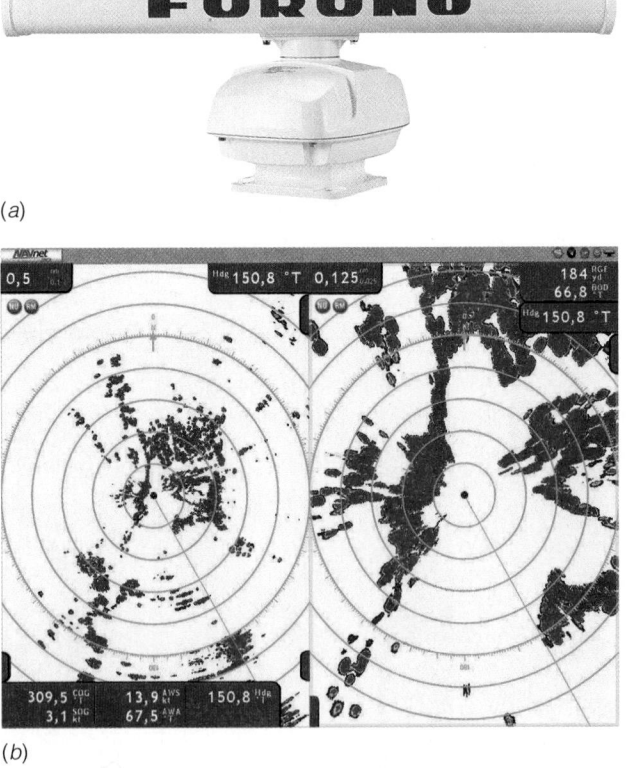

Figure 7-27 *(a)* As a radar scanner rotates, it sends out pulses of high-frequency radio waves in a narrow beam and receives reflections of them from objects around it. The reflections are displayed on a screen. The wider the antenna, the narrower the beam and the more detail in the image. *(b)* Long- and short-range radar images of the surroundings of a ship whose location corresponds in each case to the center of the circles that indicate distance from the antenna. The heading of the ship corresponds to upward in these images.

Figure 7-28 shows the range (or **spectrum**) of em waves. The human eye can detect only light waves in a very short frequency band, from about 4.3×10^{14} Hz for red light to about 7.5×10^{14} Hz for violet light. **Infrared light** has lower frequencies than those in visible light, and **ultraviolet light** has higher frequencies. Still higher are the frequencies of x-rays and of the gamma radiation from atomic nuclei.

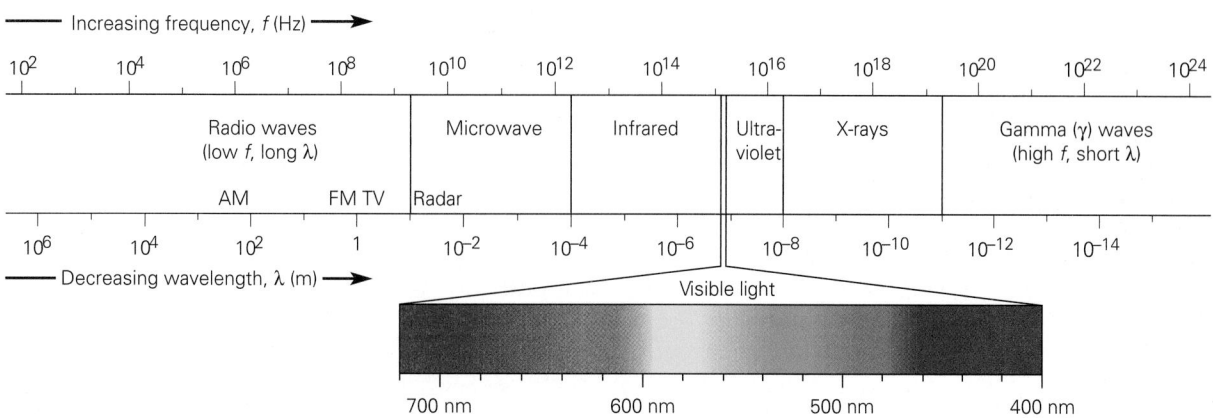

Figure 7-28   The electromagnetic spectrum. All em waves have the same fundamental character and the same speed in a vacuum, but how they interact with matter depends on their frequency (1 nm = 1 nanometer = 10^{-9} m = 1 billionth of a meter).

7.10   Light "Rays"

The Paths Light Takes

Many aspects of the behavior of light waves can be understood without reference to their electromagnetic nature. In fact, we can even use a yet simpler model in many (but far from all) situations by thinking of light in terms of "rays" rather than waves.

Early in life we become aware that light travels in straight lines. A simple piece of evidence is the beam of a flashlight on a foggy night. Actually, our entire orientation to the world about us, our sense of the location of things in space, depends on *assuming* that light follows straight-line paths.

Reflection and Refraction   Just as familiar, however, is the fact that light does not always follow straight lines. We see most objects by reflected light, light that has been turned sharply on striking a surface. The distorted appearance of things seen in water or through the heated air rising above a flame further testifies to the ability of light to be bent from a straight path. In these latter cases the light is said to be **refracted,** and we note that this occurs when light moves from one transparent material to another.

Although the conscious part of our minds recognizes that light can be reflected and refracted, it is easy to be deceived about the true positions of things. When we look in a mirror, for example, we are seeing light that travels to the mirror and then from the mirror to our eyes, but our eyes seem to tell us that the light comes from an image behind the mirror. When we look at the legs of someone standing in shallow water, they appear shorter than they do in air because light going from water into air is bent. Our eyes and brains have no way to take this into account and so we register the illusion rather than the reality.

Much can be learned about the behavior of light by studying the paths that light follows under various circumstances. Since light appears to travel in a straight path in a uniform medium, we can represent its motion by straight lines called **rays.** Rays are a convenient abstraction, and we can visualize what we mean by thinking of a narrow pencil of light in a darkened room.

Wave Behavior

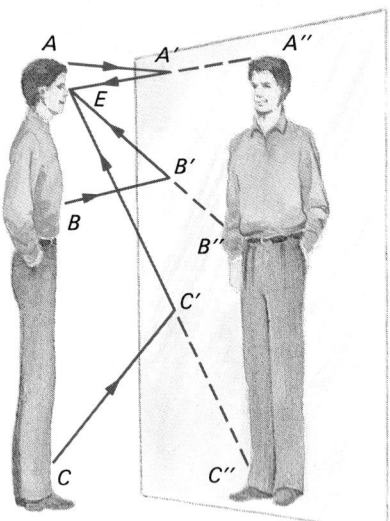

Figure 7-29 Formation of an image in a mirror. The image appears to be behind the mirror because we instinctively respond to light as though it travels in straight lines.

7.11 Reflection

Mirror, Mirror on the Wall

When we look at ourselves in a mirror, light from all parts of the body (this is reflected light, of course, but we may treat it as if it originated in the body) is reflected from the mirror back to our eyes, as in Fig. 7-29. Light from the foot, for example, follows the path $CC'E$. Our eyes, which see the ray $C'E$ and automatically project it in a straight line, register the foot at the proper distance but apparently behind the mirror at C''. A ray from the top of the head is reflected at A', and our eyes see the point A as if it were behind the mirror at A''. Rays from other points of the body are similarly reflected, and in this manner a complete **image** is formed that appears to be behind the mirror.

Left and right are interchanged in a mirror image because front and back have been reversed by the reflection. Thus a printed page appears backward in a mirror, and what seems to be one's left hand is really one's right hand.

Why do we not see images of ourselves in walls and furniture as well as in mirrors? This is simply a question of the relative roughness of surfaces. Rays of light are reflected from walls just as they are from mirrors, but the reflected rays are scattered in all directions by the many surface irregularities (Fig. 7-30). We see the wall by the scattered light reflected from it.

7.12 Refraction

A Change in Direction Caused by a Change in Speed

No matter from where the wind is blowing, waves always approach a sloping beach very nearly at right angles to the shore (Fig. 7-31). Farther out in open water, the wave direction may be oblique (that is, at a slanting angle) to the shore, but the waves swing around as they move in so that their crests become roughly parallel to the shoreline. This is an example of refraction.

The explanation is straightforward. As a wave moves obliquely shoreward, its near-shore end encounters shallow water before its outer end does, and friction between the near-shore end and the sea bottom slows down that part of the wave. More and more of the wave is slowed as it continues to move toward the shore, and the slowing becomes more pronounced as the water gets shallower. As a result the whole wave turns until it is moving almost directly shoreward. The wave has turned because part of it was forced to move more slowly than the rest. Thus refraction is caused by differences in speed across the wave. Figure 7-32 shows an analogy to refraction in the motion of a tracked vehicle.

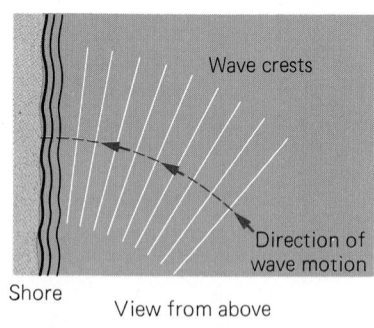

Shore View from above

View from side

Figure 7-31 Refraction of water waves. Waves approaching shore obliquely are turned because they move more slowly in shallow water near shore.

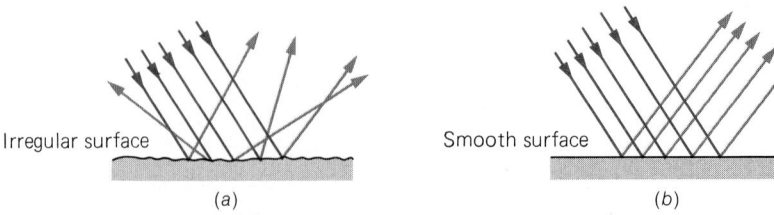

Irregular surface (a)

Smooth surface (b)

Figure 7-30 (a) Light that strikes an irregular surface is scattered randomly and cannot form an image. (b) Light that strikes a smooth, flat surface is reflected at an angle equal to the angle of incidence. Such a surface acts as a mirror.

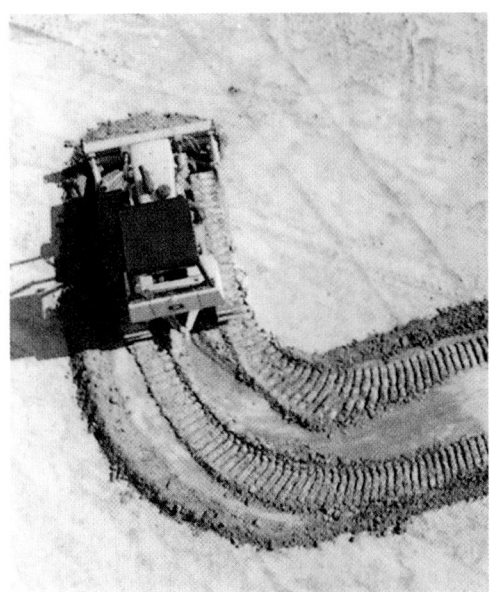

Figure 7-32 Something similar to refraction occurs when a tracked vehicle such as a bulldozer makes a turn. The right-hand track of this bulldozer was slowed down, and the greater speed of its left-hand track then swung the bulldozer around to the right.

The bending will be at a sharp angle if the waves cross a definite boundary between regions in which they move at different speeds. Figure 7-33 shows this effect in ripples that move obliquely from deep water to shallow water in a tank. If the waves approach the boundary at right angles, no refraction occurs because the change in wave speed takes place across each wave at the same time.

Bending Light We all know that the water in a bathtub, a swimming pool, and even a puddle is always deeper than it seems to be. The reason is that light is refracted—changes direction—when it goes from one medium into another medium in which the speed of light is different (Fig. 7-34). The effect is similar to the refraction of water waves. A ray of light from the stone in Fig. 7-35 follows the bent path *ABE* to our eyes, but our brain registers that the segment *BE* is part of the straight-line path starting at *A'*.

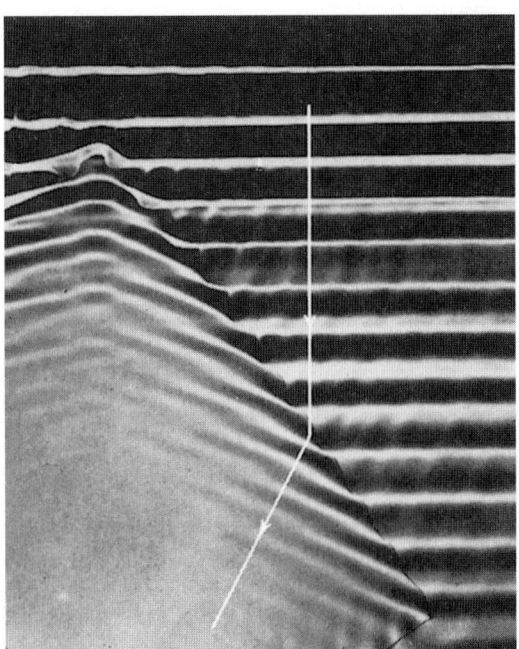

Figure 7-33 The refraction of water waves in a tank. In the left side of the tank is a glass plate over which the water is shallower than elsewhere. Waves move more slowly in shallow water than in deeper water, and hence refraction occurs at the edge of the plate. The arrows show the direction of movement of the waves.

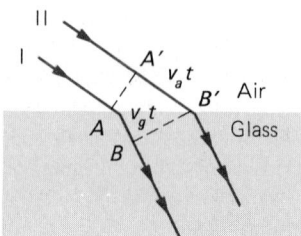

Figure 7-34 Refraction occurs whenever light passes from one medium to another in which its speed is different. Here two rays of light, I and II, pass from air, in which their speed is v_a, to glass, in which their speed is v_g. Because v_g is less than v_a, $A'B'$ is longer than AB, and the beam of which I and II are part changes direction when it enters the glass.

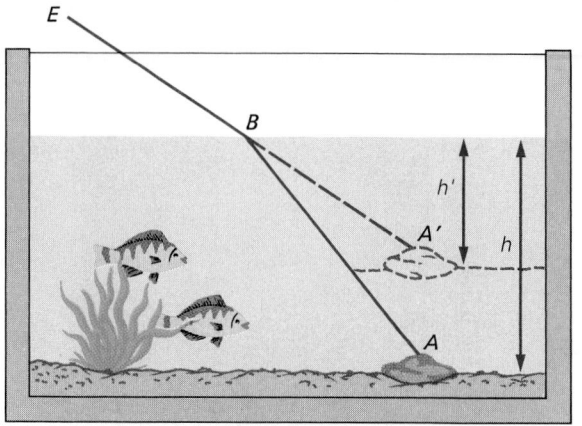

Figure 7-35 Light is refracted when it travels obliquely from one medium to another. Here the effect of refraction is to make the water appear shallower than it actually is.

Index of Refraction The ratio between the speed of light c in free space and its speed v in a medium is called the **index of refraction** of the medium:

$$n = \frac{c}{v} \quad \textit{Index of refraction} \qquad 7\text{-}2$$

$$\text{Index of refraction} = \frac{\text{speed of light in free space}}{\text{speed of light in medium}}$$

The greater the value of n, the more a light ray is deflected when it enters a medium from air at an oblique angle. Here are some examples of indexes of refraction:

Water	1.33
Ordinary glass and clear plastics	1.52
Diamond	2.42

Because the speed of light in air is so close to c, for most purposes we can assume that they are the same with $n = 1$ for air.

The apparent depth h' of the submerged stone in Fig. 7-35 is related to its actual depth h and the index of refraction of the water (or other medium in the tank) by the formula

$$h' = \frac{h}{n} \quad \textit{Apparent depth} \qquad 7\text{-}3$$

$$\text{Apparent depth} = \frac{\text{actual depth}}{\text{index of refraction}}$$

Example 7.2

The water in a swimming pool is 2.0 m deep. How deep does it appear to someone looking into it from its rim?

Solution
For water, $n = 1.33$, so from Eq. 7-3

$$h' = \frac{h}{n} = \frac{2.0 \text{ m}}{1.33} = 1.5 \text{ m}$$

The pool seems only three-quarters as deep as it really is.

In general, light rays that go obliquely from one medium to another are bent toward a perpendicular to the surface between them if light in the second medium travels more slowly than in the first (Fig. 7-36). If light in the second medium travels faster there, the rays are bent *away from* the

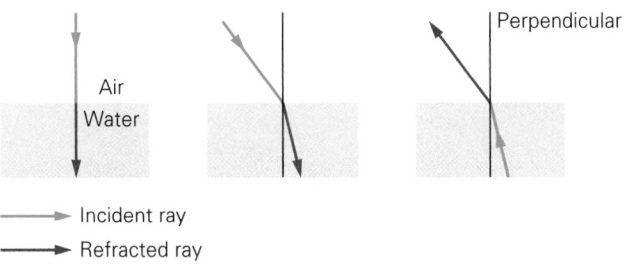

→ Incident ray

→ Refracted ray

Figure 7-36 Light rays are bent toward the perpendicular when they enter an optically denser medium, away from the perpendicular when they enter an optically less dense medium. A ray moving along the perpendicular is not bent. The paths taken by light rays are always reversible.

perpendicular. Light that enters another medium perpendicular to the surface between them does not change direction.

Internal Reflection Since light travels more slowly in glass than in air, light that goes from glass to air at a slanting angle is refracted away from the perpendicular to the glass surface. If the angle is shallow enough, the light will be bent back into the glass (Fig. 7-39). This phenomenon is called **internal reflection** (Fig. 7-40).

Fiber Optics

Internal reflection makes it possible to "pipe" light by means of a series of reflections from the wall of a glass rod, as in Fig. 7-37. If a cluster of thin glass fibers is used instead of a single rod, an image can be transferred from one end to the other with each fiber carrying a part of the image. Because a fiber cluster is flexible, it can be used for such purposes as examining a person's stomach by being passed in through the mouth. Some of the fibers provide light for illumination, and the rest carry the reflected light back outside for viewing.

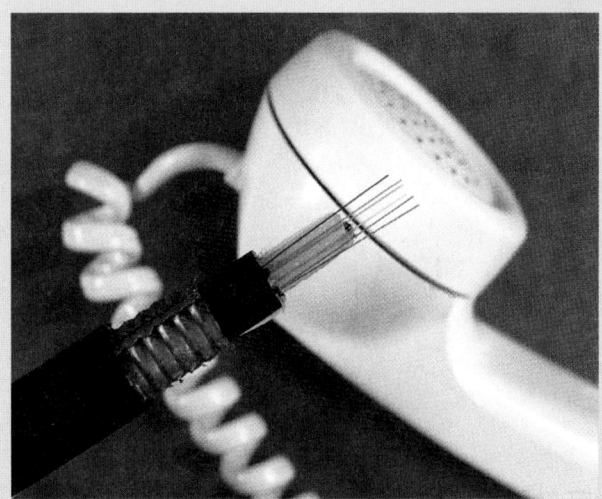

Figure 7-38 Each of the thin fibers in this cable can carry millions of telephone conversations in the form of coded flashes of light distributed among 100 or so different frequencies.

Glass fibers have been used in telephone systems since 1977. The electric signals that would otherwise be sent along copper wires are converted to a series of pulses according to a standard code and then sent as flashes of infrared light down a hair-thin glass fiber. At the other end the flashes are converted back to electric signals (Fig. 7-38). Modern electronic methods allow at most 32 telephone conversations to be carried at the same time by a pair of copper wires, but over a million can be carried by a single fiber with no problems of electrical interference. Telephone fiberoptic systems today link many cities and exchanges within cities everywhere, and fiberoptic cables span the world's seas and oceans.

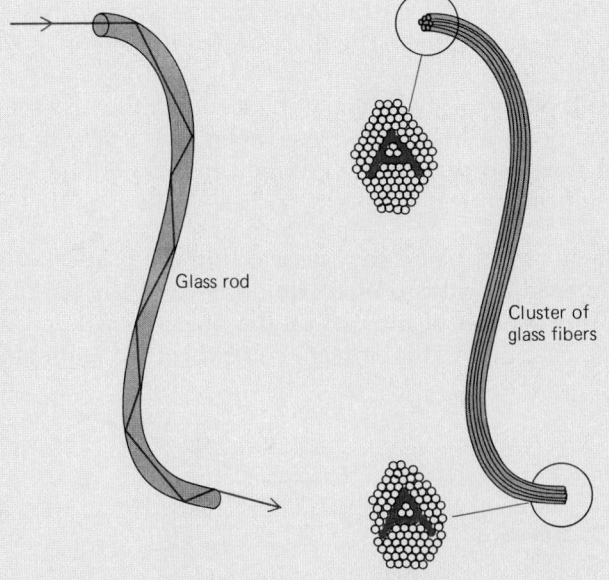

Figure 7-37 Light can be "piped" from one place to another by means of internal reflections in a glass rod. Using a cluster of glass fibers permits an image to be carried in this way.

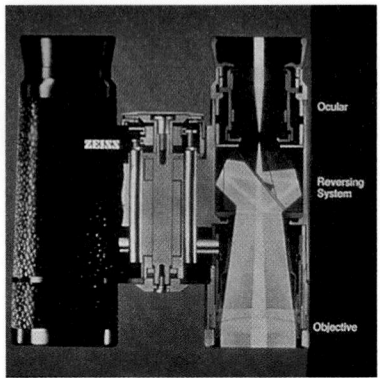

Figure 7-40 The sharpness and brightness of a light beam are better preserved by internal reflection than by reflection from an ordinary mirror. Because of this, optical devices such as binoculars use prisms instead of mirrors when light is to have its direction changed. The prisms used in binoculars have two purposes: they invert the magnified image so that it is right-side-up, and by reversing the optical path twice, they shorten the length of the instrument.

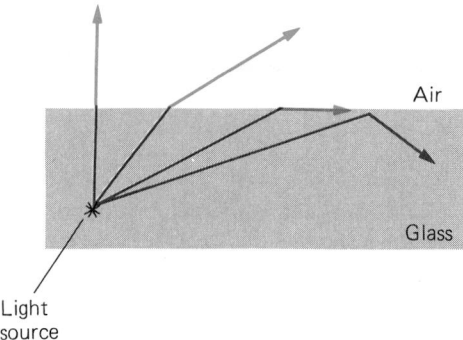

Figure 7-39 Total internal reflection occurs when the angle of refraction for a light ray going from one medium to a less optically dense medium would be more than 90° from the perpendicular to the surface between the media.

What does an underwater fish (or diver) see when looking upward? The paths taken by light rays are always reversible. By reversing the rays of light in Fig. 7-39 we can see that light from above the water's surface can reach the fish's eyes only through a circle on the surface. The rays from above are all brought together in a cone whose angular width turns out to be 98° (Fig. 7-41). Outside the cone is a reflection of the underwater scene.

7.13 Lenses

Bending Light to Form an Image

A **lens** is a piece of glass or other transparent material shaped so that it can produce an image by refracting light that comes from an object. Lenses are used for many purposes: in eyeglasses to improve vision, in cameras to record scenes, in projectors to show images on a screen, in microscopes to enable small things to be seen, in telescopes to enable distant things to be seen, and so forth.

Lenses are of two kinds, **converging** and **diverging.** A converging lens is thicker in the middle than at its rim; a diverging lens is thinner in the middle. As in Fig. 7-42a, a converging lens brings a parallel beam of light to a single focal point F. Here F is called a **real focal point** because the light rays pass through it. If sunlight is used, the concentration of radiant energy may be enough to burn a hole in a piece of paper. The distance from the lens to F is called the **focal length** of the lens.

A diverging lens spreads out a parallel beam of light so that the rays seem to have come from a focal point F behind the lens, as in Fig. 7-42b. In this case F is called a **virtual focal point** because the light rays do not actually pass through it but only appear to.

Ray Tracing A scale drawing gives us an easy way to find the properties of the image of an object formed by a lens. What we do is trace the paths of two different light rays from a point of interest on the object to where they (or their extensions, in the case of a virtual image) come together again after

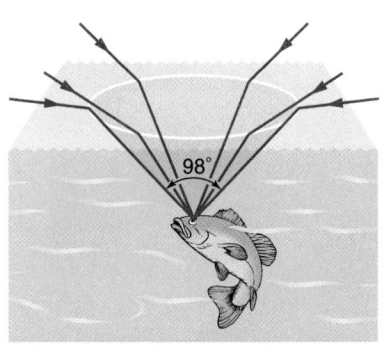

Figure 7-41 All the light reaching an underwater observer from above the surface is concentrated in a cone 98° wide, so that the observer sees a circle of light at the surface when looking upward.

Figure 7-42 (a) A converging lens brings parallel rays of light together to a focal point F. (b) A diverging lens spreads out parallel rays of light so that they seem to originate at a focal point F. In both cases the distance between F and the lens is the focal length f of the lens.

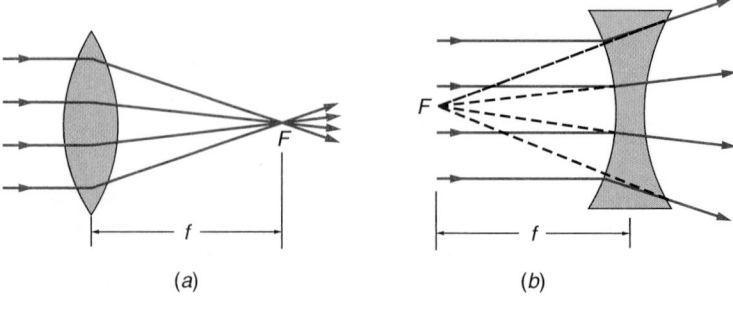

(a)   (b)

passing through the lens. We should note that a lens has two focal points, one on each side, the same distance *f* from its center.

The three simplest rays to trace are shown in Fig. 7-43 for a converging lens:

1. A ray that leaves the object parallel to the lens axis. The lens deviates this ray so that it passes through the focal point of the lens on the far side;
2. A ray that passes through the center of the lens. This ray is not deviated;
3. A ray that passes through the nearest focal point of the lens. The lens deviates the ray so that it continues parallel to the lens axis.

In Fig. 7-43 the object is the distance 2*f* from the lens, and we can see that the image is 2*f* on the other side of the lens. The image is real (the rays actually pass through it), is the same size as the object, and is inverted. This corresponds to the optical system of a photocopier that produces a copy the same size as an original.

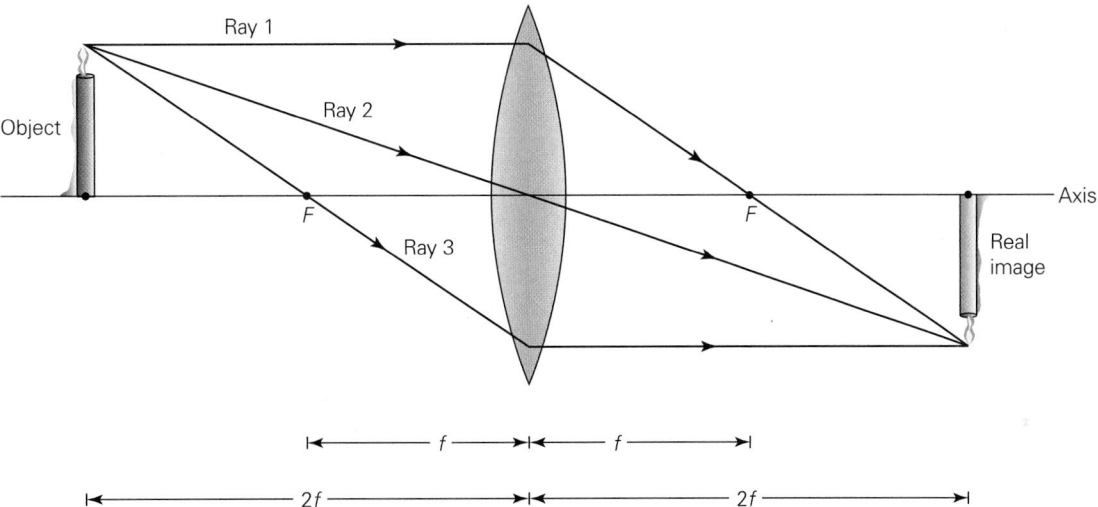

Figure 7-43   Tracing any two of the rays shown will indicate the position and size of the image formed by a converging lens and whether it is erect (right-side-up) or inverted (upside down). The image will be found where the rays come together after being refracted by the lens.

Example 7.3

A slide or movie projector uses a converging lens to produce an enlarged image of a transparent slide on a screen. Use a ray diagram to find the properties of the image when the slide is between *f* and 2*f* from the lens.

Solution
As we see in Fig. 7-44 by tracing rays 1 and 2, the image is real, farther than 2*f* from the lens, larger than the object on the slide, and inverted. This is why slides have to be put upside down in a projector.

Example 7.4

A camera uses a converging lens to produce a reduced image on the sensitive surface (film or electronic sensor). Use a ray diagram to find the properties of the image when the object being photographed is more than 2*f* from the lens.

Solution
As we see in Fig. 7-45, again by tracing rays 1 and 2, the image is real, between *f* and 2*f* from the lens, smaller than the object, and inverted.

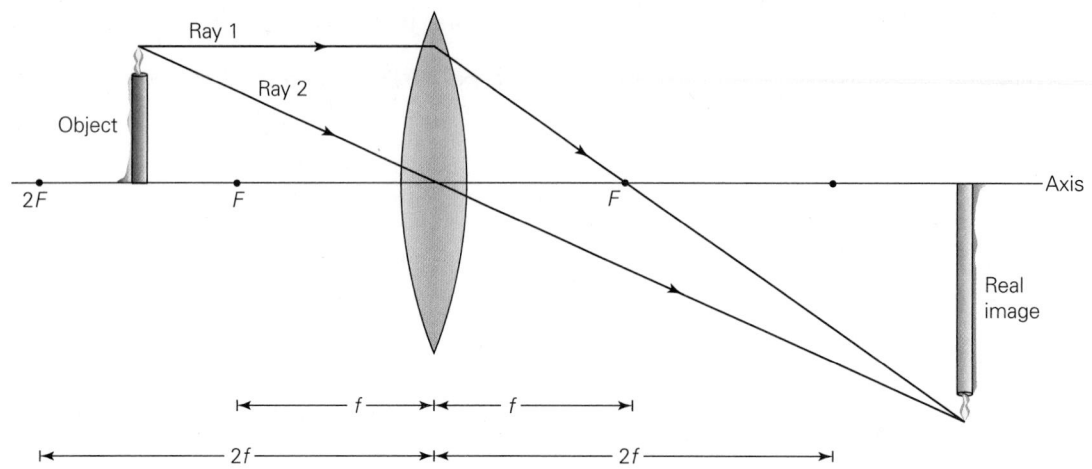

Figure 7-44   Ray diagram for an object a distance between f and $2f$ from a converging lens. This corresponds to the optical system of a projector where a slide or movie film is the object and the image appears on a screen.

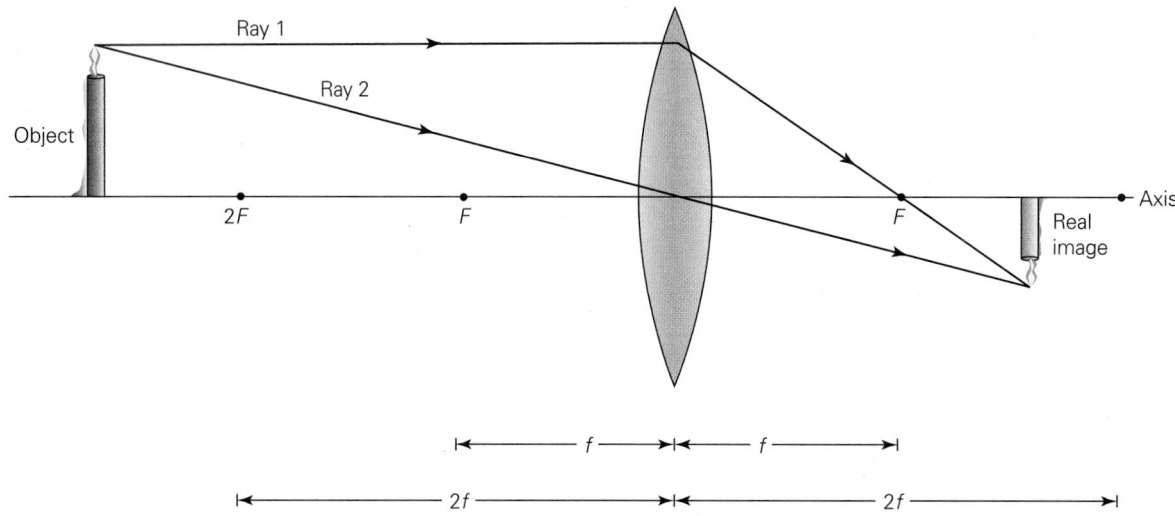

Figure 7-45   Ray diagram for an object farther than $2f$ from a converging lens. This corresponds to the optical system of a camera. The closer the object is to the lens, the farther the sensor screen or film must be from the lens. The appropriate focal length of a camera lens depends upon the desired angle of view. A "normal" lens gives an angle of view of about 45°. A lens of shorter focal length is a wide-angle lens that captures more of a given scene, though at the expense of reducing the sizes of details in the scene. A telephoto lens has a long focal length to give larger images of distant objects, though less of the scene is included. Adjustable "zoom" lenses can cover a wide range of focal lengths.

Example 7.5

A "magnifying glass" uses a converging lens to produce an enlarged image of an object closer than f from the lens. Use a ray diagram to find the properties of the image.

Solution

As we see in Fig. 7-46, the image here seems to be behind the lens because the refracted rays diverge as though coming from a point behind it. This is a **virtual image**: although it can be seen by the eye, it cannot appear on a screen because no rays actually pass through it. The image is farther from the lens than the object, is larger than the object, and is erect.

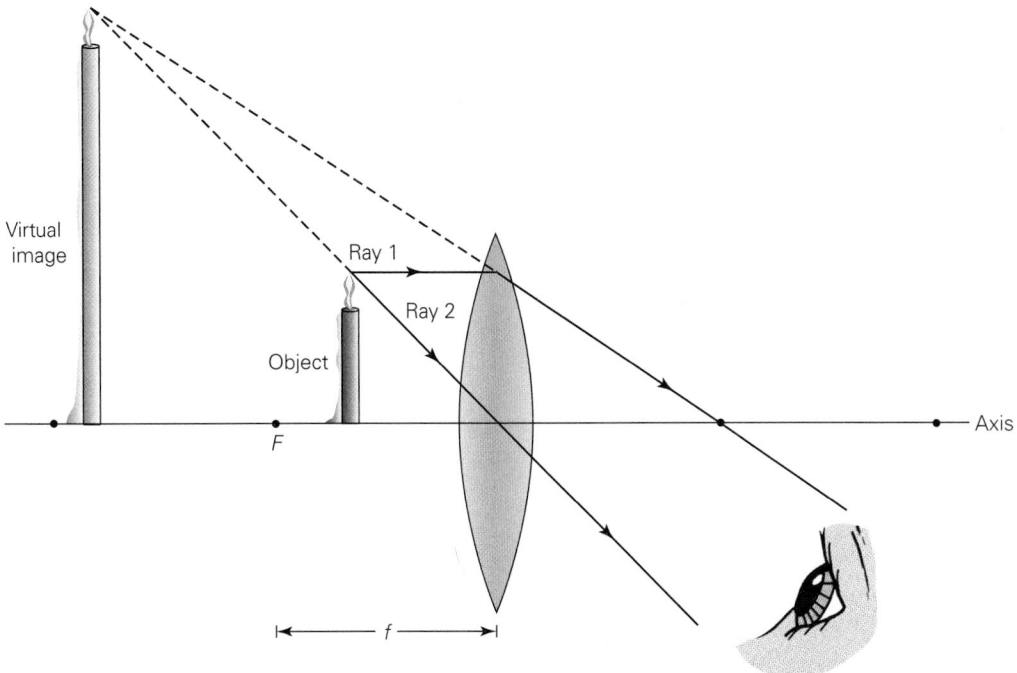

Figure 7-46   Ray diagram for an object closer than f from a converging lens. The image is erect and virtual and larger than the object. This is how a "magnifying glass" works.

Diverging Lens   A diverging lens deviates rays that enter parallel to the axis away from the axis, as we saw in Fig. 7-42b, instead of toward the axis as a converging lens does, as in Fig. 7-42a. As a result, the image of a real object produced by a diverging lens is always virtual, erect, smaller than the object, and closer to the lens than the object is (Fig. 7-47).

7.14   The Eye

A Remarkable Optical Instrument

The structure of the human eye is shown in Fig. 7-48. The **cornea,** the transparent outer membrane, and the jellylike **lens** together focus incoming light on the sensitive **retina,** which converts what is seen into nerve impulses that are carried to the brain by the **optic nerve** (Fig. 7-49). Focusing on objects different distances away is done when the **ciliary muscle** changes the shape and hence the focal length of the lens. The colored **iris** acts like the diaphragm of a camera to control the amount of light entering the **pupil,** which is the opening of the iris. In bright light the pupil is small, in dim light it is

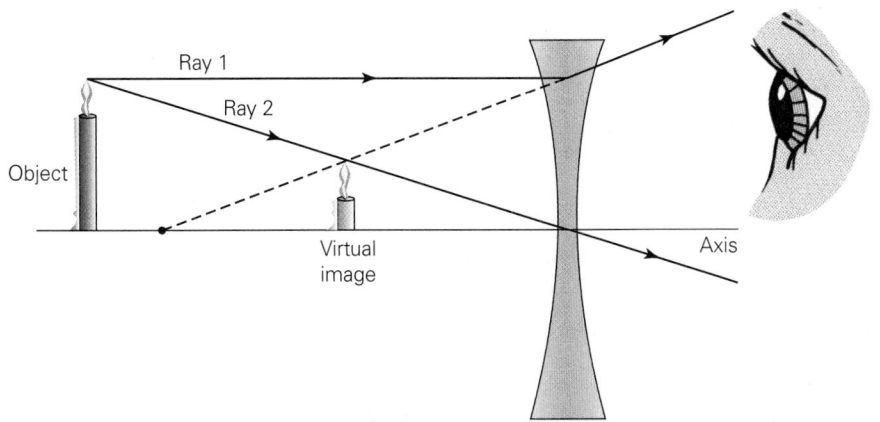

Figure 7-47   A diverging lens produces a virtual image of a real object that is always erect and smaller than the object.

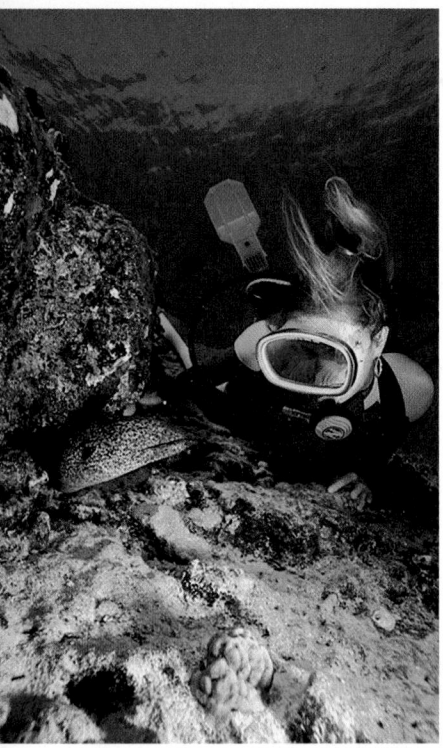

Figure 7-49 Refraction at the cornea gives rise to most of the focusing power of the human eye. When the eye is immersed in water rather than air, the amount of refraction is much less. As a result, underwater objects cannot be brought to a sharp focus unless goggles or a face mask are used to keep water away from the cornea. Beavers cope with this problem by having transparent eyelids that adjust the optical systems of their eyes for underwater vision. Fish avoid the problem by having eyes in which most of the focusing is done by very thick lenses, with the cornea playing only a minor part.

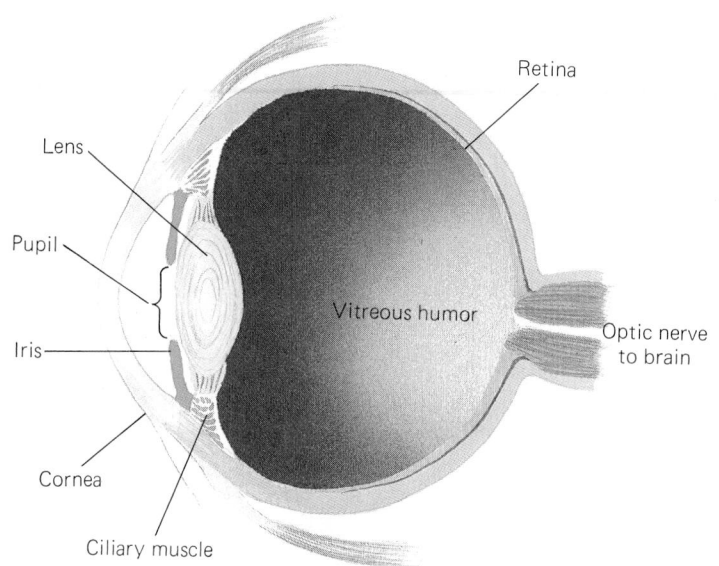

Figure 7-48   The human eye, shown larger than life size. In dim light the iris opens wide to let enough light enter through the pupil for good vision.

large. A fully opened pupil lets in about 16 times as much light as a fully contracted one. The retina itself can also cope with a wide range of brightnesses.

The Retina   The retina has millions of tiny structures called **cones** and **rods** that are sensitive to light. The cones are specialized for color vision and occur in three types that respond respectively to red, green, and blue light. (Mammals other than primates have only two types of cone, so they have poorer color vision than we have; birds have four types, which gives them better color vision, including part of the ultraviolet.) Rods need much less light to be activated than cones do, but rods do not distinguish colors.

In poor illumination, then, what we see is in shades of gray, like a black-and-white photograph. Because the central region of the retina contains only cones, it is easier to see something in a dim light by looking a bit to one side instead of directly at it. This central sensitive region, called the *fovea*, covers a region of the visual field only about the size of the sun or moon in the sky. Because the fovea is so small, each eye constantly darts about a few times a second, stopping each time for a brief moment to register what is in view and then moving on. The brain knits these flashes of information into a seamless picture.

Defects of Vision   Two common defects of vision are **farsightedness** and **nearsightedness** (Fig. 7-50). In farsightedness the eyeball is too short, and light from nearby objects comes to a focus behind the retina. (Distant objects can be seen clearly, however.) A converging eyeglass lens corrects farsightedness. In nearsightedness the eyeball is too long, and light from distant objects comes to a focus in front of the retina. (Nearby objects can be seen clearly, however.) Here the correction is a diverging eyeglass lens.

Sometimes the cornea or lens of an eye has different curvatures in different planes. When light rays that lie in one plane are in focus on the retina of such an eye, rays in other planes are in focus either in front of or behind the retina. This means that only one of the bars of a cross can be in focus at any time (Fig. 7-52), a condition called **astigmatism.** Astigmatism causes eyestrain because the eye continually varies the focus of the lens as it tries to produce a completely sharp image of what it sees. A cylindrical corrective lens (Fig. 7-53) is the remedy for astigmatism.

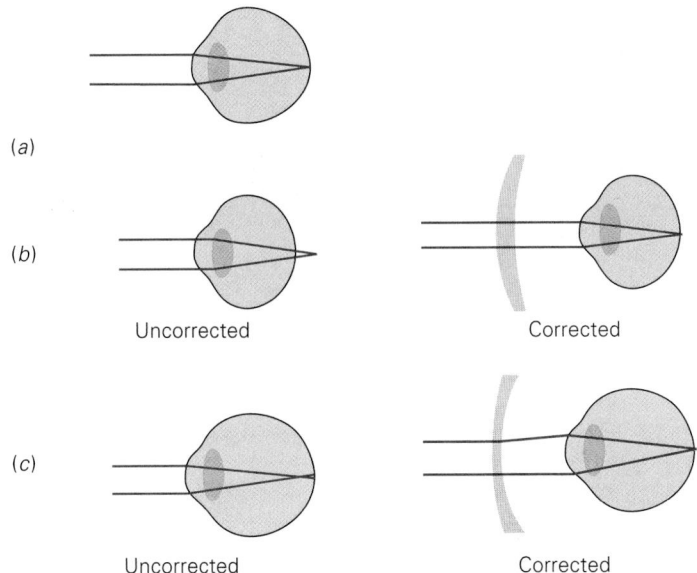

(a)

(b)

Uncorrected   Corrected

(c)

Uncorrected   Corrected

Figure 7-50 *(a)* A normal eye. *(b)* Farsightedness can be corrected with a converging lens. *(c)* Nearsightedness can be corrected with a diverging lens.

7.15 Color

Each Frequency of Light Produces the Sensation of a Different Color

White light is a mixture of light waves of different frequencies, each of which produces the visual sensation of a particular color. To show this, we can direct a narrow beam of white light at a glass prism (Fig. 7-54). Because the speed of light in glass varies slightly with frequency, light of each color is refracted to a different extent. The effect is called **dispersion.** The result is that the original beam is separated by the prism into beams of various colors, with red light bent the least and violet light bent the most.

Dispersion is especially marked in diamond, which is the reason for the vivid play of color when white light shines on a cut diamond. The sparkle of a cut diamond is partly due to its strong refractive power and partly to the way it is cut (Fig. 7-55).

Rainbows The dispersion of sunlight by water droplets is responsible for rainbows, which are seen when we face falling rain with the sun behind us (Fig. 7-56). When a ray of sunlight enters a raindrop, as in Fig. 7-57, the sunlight is first refracted, then reflected at the back of the drop, and finally

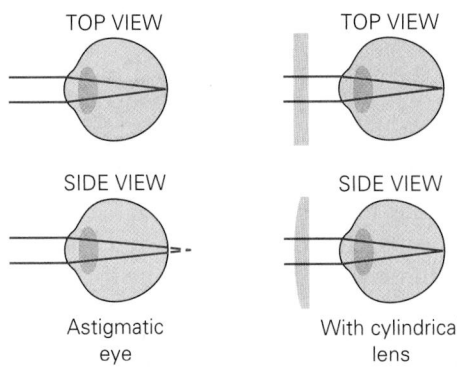

TOP VIEW   TOP VIEW

SIDE VIEW   SIDE VIEW

Astigmatic   With cylindrical
eye   lens

Figure 7-53 A cylindrical lens can improve the image formed by an astigmatic eye.

Two Vision Experiments

The retinas of vertebrate animals, like us, are inside-out (not a very intelligent design, but the result of the unplanned way evolution proceeded): the light-sensitive cells are on the outside, behind the nerves and blood vessels connected to them. A **blind spot** occurs where the nerves and blood vessels pass through the retina.

To experience the blind spot, close your left eye and look directly at the cross in Fig. 7-51 with your right eye. When the cross is about 20 cm from your eye, the dot should disappear.

We are not usually aware of the blind spot for two reasons: the blind spots of the two eyes obscure different fields of vision, and the eyes are in constant scanning motion.

Figure 7-51 Locating the blind spot.

To verify that cones, which are responsible for color vision, are concentrated near the center of the retina, hold something with a bright color off to one side and slowly move it around until it is in front of you. As you do this, you will find the sensation of its color going from weak to strong.

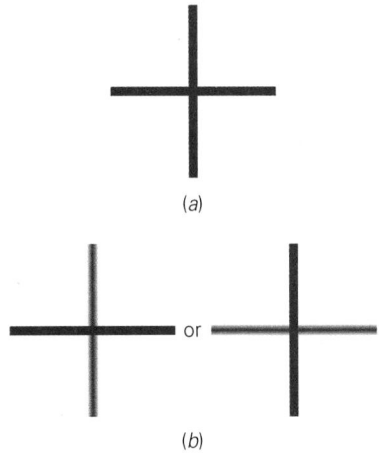

(a)

or

(b)

Figure 7-52 How a cross is seen *(a)* by a normal eye and *(b)* by an astigmatic eye.

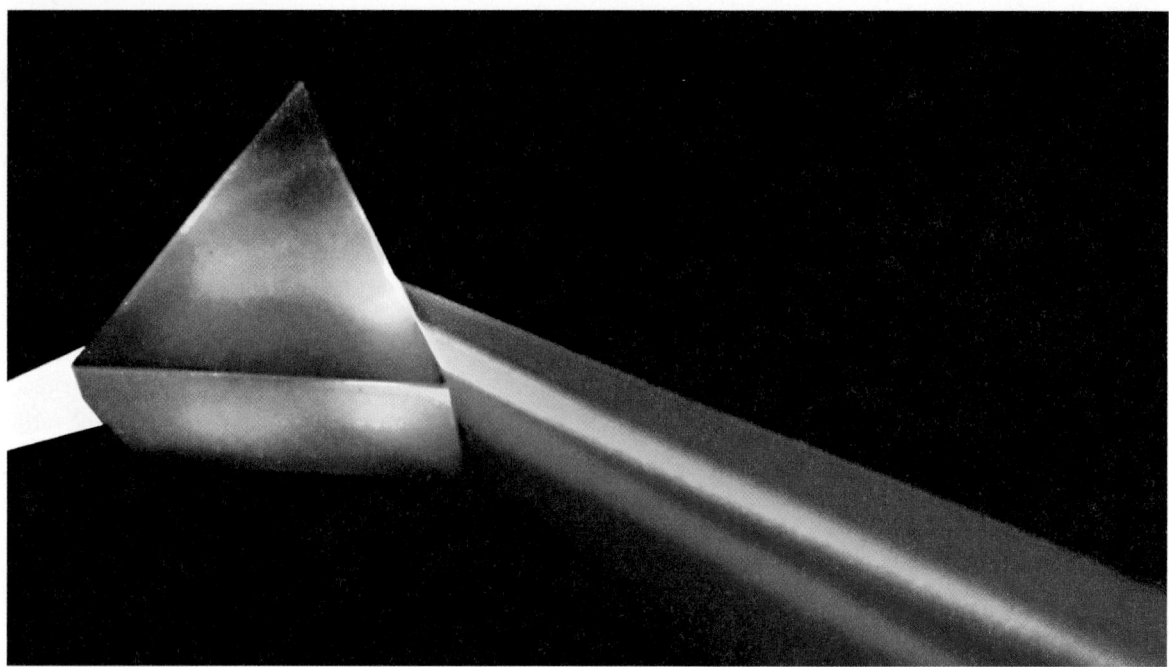

Figure 7-54   A beam of white light is separated into its component wavelengths, each of which appears to the eye as a different color, by dispersion in a glass prism.

Figure 7-55   (*a*) A diamond cut in the "brilliant" style has 33 facets in its upper part and 25 in its lower part. The proportions of the facets are critical in giving the maximum of sparkle.
(*b*) Dispersion gives a cut diamond its fire.

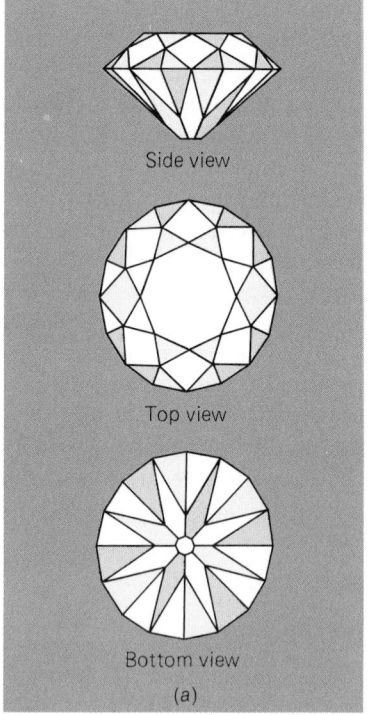

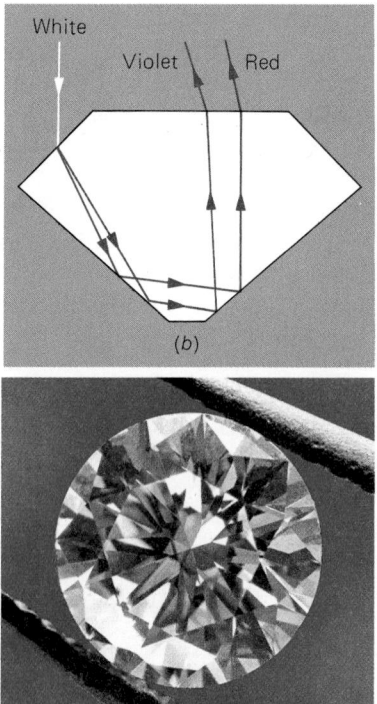

refracted again when it goes back out. Dispersion occurs at each refraction. With the sky full of raindrops, the result is a colored arc that has red light on the outside and violet light on the inside. Someone in an airplane can see the entire ring of color, but from the ground only the upper part is visible.

Color of Reflected Light   The color of an object depends on the kind of light that falls on the object and on the nature of its surface. If a surface

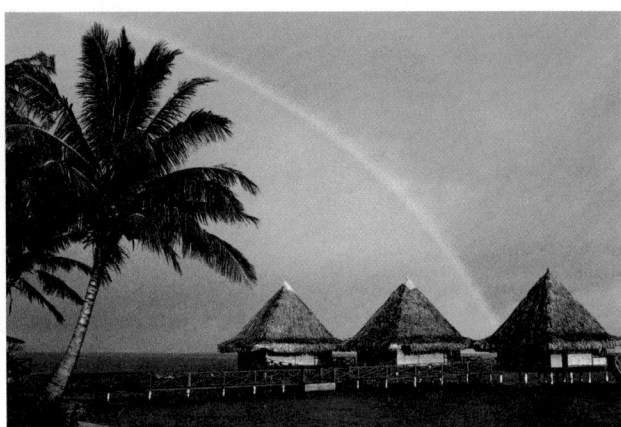

Figure 7-56 A rainbow is caused by the dispersion of sunlight into its component colors when refracted by water droplets in the atmosphere.

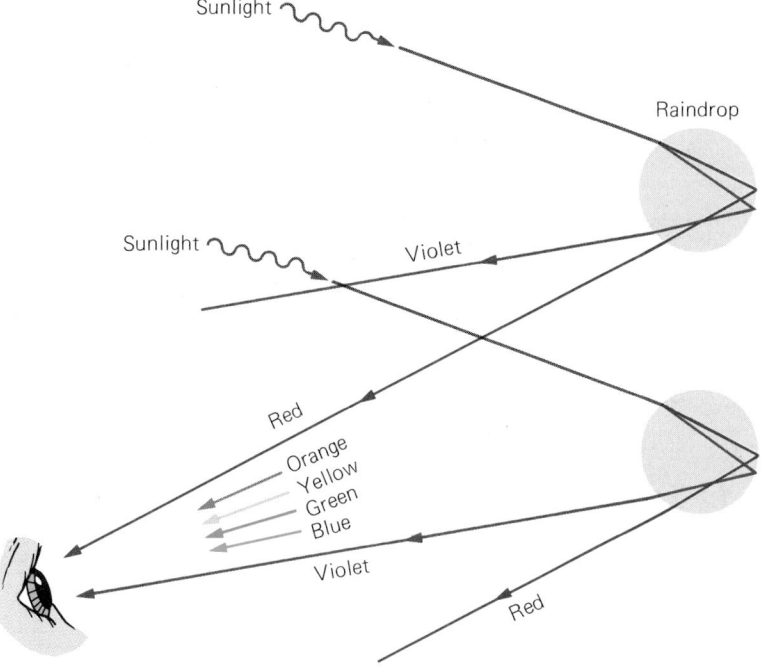

Figure 7-57 Rainbows are created by the dispersion of sunlight by raindrops. Red light arrives at the eye of the observer from the upper drop shown here, violet light from the lower drop. Other raindrops yield the other colors and produce a continuous arc in the sky.

reflects all light that falls on it, the color of the surface will be white when white light illuminates it (Fig. 7-58), red when red light illuminates it, and so on. A surface that reflects only, say, green light will appear green only when the light illuminating it contains green; otherwise it will appear black. A surface that absorbs all light that falls on it appears black.

Blue Sky   The blue color of the sky is due to scattering of the sun's light by molecules and dust particles in the atmosphere. Blue light is scattered more effectively than red light. When we look at the sky, what we see is light from the sun that has been scattered out of the direct beam and hence appears blue (Fig. 7-59). The sun itself is therefore a little more yellowish or reddish than it would appear if there were no atmosphere. At sunrise or sunset, when the sun's light must make a long passage through the atmosphere, much of its blue light is scattered out. The sun may be a brilliant red as a result. Above the atmosphere the sky is black, and the moon, stars, and planets are visible to astronauts in the daytime.

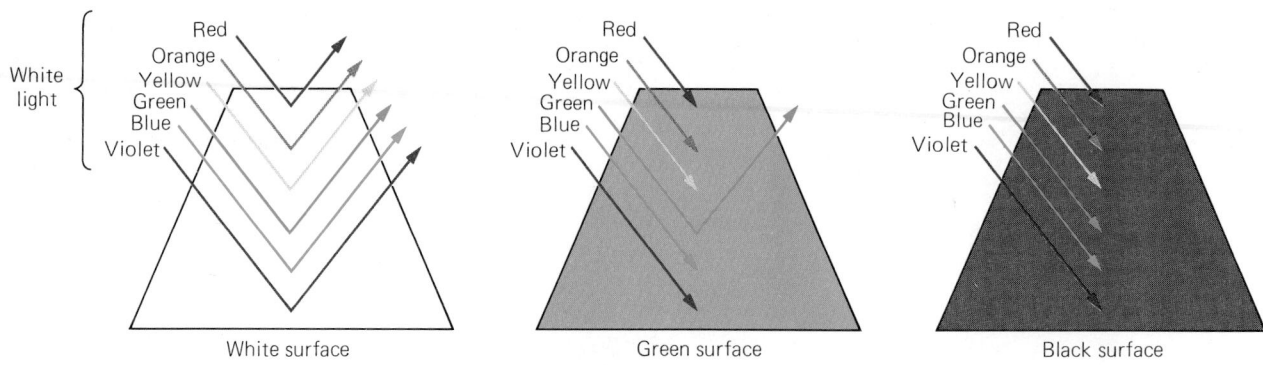

Figure 7-58   A white surface reflects all light that falls on it. A green surface reflects only green light and absorbs the rest. A black surface absorbs all light that falls on it.

Figure 7-59   (*a*) The preferential scattering of blue light in the atmosphere is responsible for the blue color of the sky. (*b*) The remaining direct sunlight is reddish, which is the reason for the red color of the sun at sunrise and sunset.

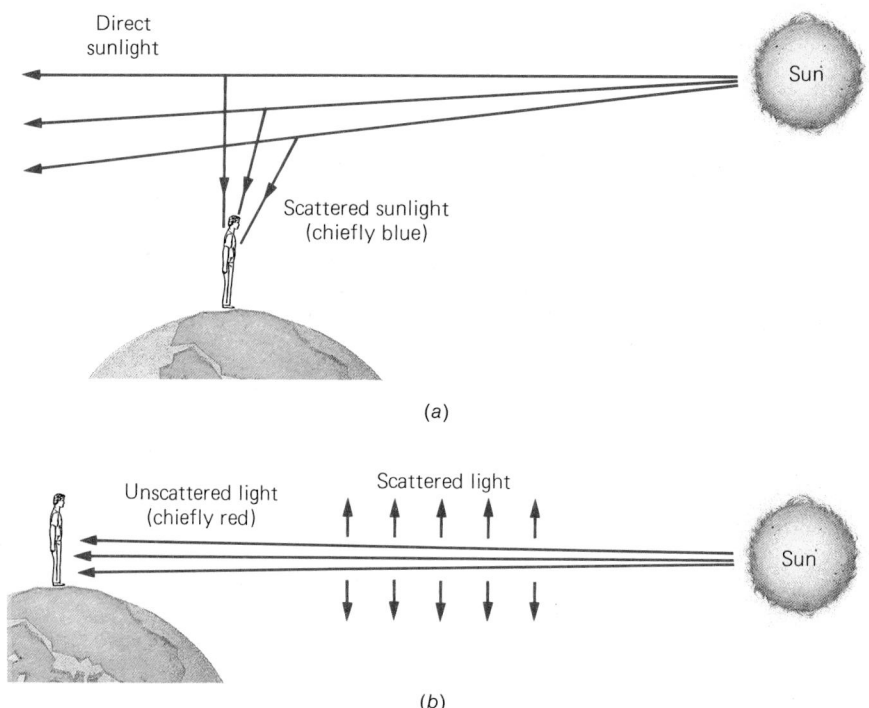

7.16 Interference

Waves in Step and out of Step

Interference refers to the adding together of two or more waves of the same kind that pass by the same point at the same time. The formation of standing waves is an example of interference.

How interference works is shown in Fig. 7-60. Let us shake the stretched strings *AC* and *BC* at the ends *A* and *B*. The single string *CD* is then affected by *both* sets of waves. Each portion of *CD* must respond to two impulses at the same time, and its motion is therefore the total of the effects of the two original waves. Suppose we shake *A* and *B* in step with each other so that, at *C*, crest meets crest and trough meets trough. Then the crests in *CD* are twice as high and the troughs twice as deep as those in *AB* and *BC*. This situation is called **constructive interference.**

On the other hand, if we shake *A* and *B* exactly out of step with each other, wave crests in *AC* will arrive at *C* just when troughs get there from *BC*. As a result, crest matches trough, the wave impulses cancel each other out,

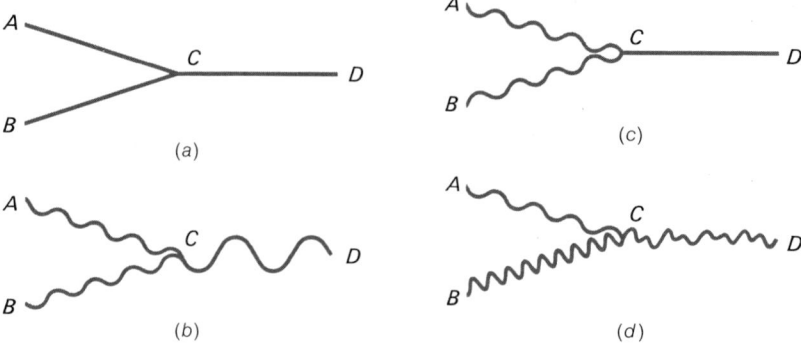

if their amplitudes are the same, and *CD* remains at rest. This situation is called **destructive interference** (Fig. 7-61).

As another possibility, if *A* is shaken through a smaller range than and half as rapidly as *B*, the two waves add together to give the complex waveform of Fig. 7-60*d*. The variations are endless, and the resulting waveforms depend upon the amplitudes, wavelengths, and timing of the incoming waves.

The interference of water waves is shown by ripples in Fig. 7-62. Ripples that spread out from the two vibrating rods affect the same water molecules. In some directions, crests from one source arrive at the same time as crests from the other source and the ripples are reinforced. Between these regions of vigorous motion are narrow lanes where the water is quiet. These lanes represent directions in which crests from one source arrive together with troughs from the other so that the wave motions cancel.

Why Thin Films Are Brightly Colored All of us have seen the brilliant colors that appear in soap bubbles and thin oil films. This effect can be traced to a combination of reflection and interference.

Let us consider what happens when light of only one color, and hence only one wavelength, strikes an oil film. As in Fig. 7-63, part of the light passes right through the film, but some is reflected from the upper surface of the film and some is reflected from the lower surface. The two reflected waves interfere with each other. At some places in the film its thickness is just right for the reflected waves to be exactly out of step (crest-to-trough), as in Fig. 7-63*a*. This is the same effect as the destructive interference shown in Fig. 7-60*c*. Little or no reflection can take place in this part of the oil film, and nearly all the incoming light simply passes right through it. The oil film accordingly seems black in this region.

Where the film is slightly thicker or thinner than in Fig. 7-63*a*, the reflected waves may be exactly in step and therefore reinforce each other, as in *b*. This corresponds to the constructive interference shown in Fig. 7-60*b*. Here the film is a good reflector and appears bright. Shining light of one color on a thin oil film gives rise in this way to areas of light and dark whose pattern depends on the varying thickness of the film.

When white light is used, the reflected waves of only one color will be in step at a particular place while waves of other colors will not. The result is a series of brilliant colors. This is the reason for the rainbow effects we see in soap bubbles and in oil films (Fig. 7-64).

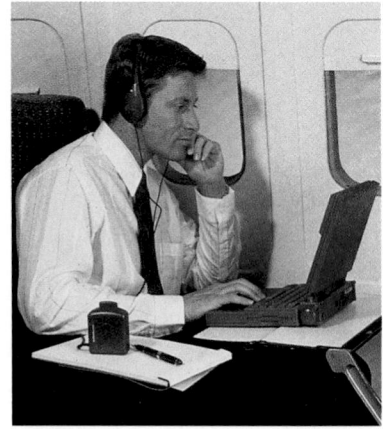

Figure 7-61 Destructive interference provides a way to reduce or eliminate noise. The procedure is to use an electronic device to analyze a particular noise and then produce mirror-image sound waves that cancel it out. If the device is appropriately programmed, wanted sounds such as conversation or music come through clearly. Powerful antinoise systems are already in use to counter the noise of suction grain unloaders, which are as loud as jet engines, and other systems are being developed to make the cabins of turboprop aircraft noise-free. On a smaller scale, the Noise Buster shown here feeds a pair of headphones with antinoise for personal use.

7.17 Diffraction

Why Shadows Are Never Completely Dark

An important property of all waves is their ability to bend around the edge of an obstacle in their path. This property is called **diffraction.**

Figure 7-62   The interference of water waves. Ripples spread out across the surface of a shallow tank of water from the two sources at the top. In some directions (for instance *AB*) the ripples reinforce each other and the waves are more prominent. In other directions (for instance *CD*) the ripples are out of step and cancel each other, so that the waves are small or absent.

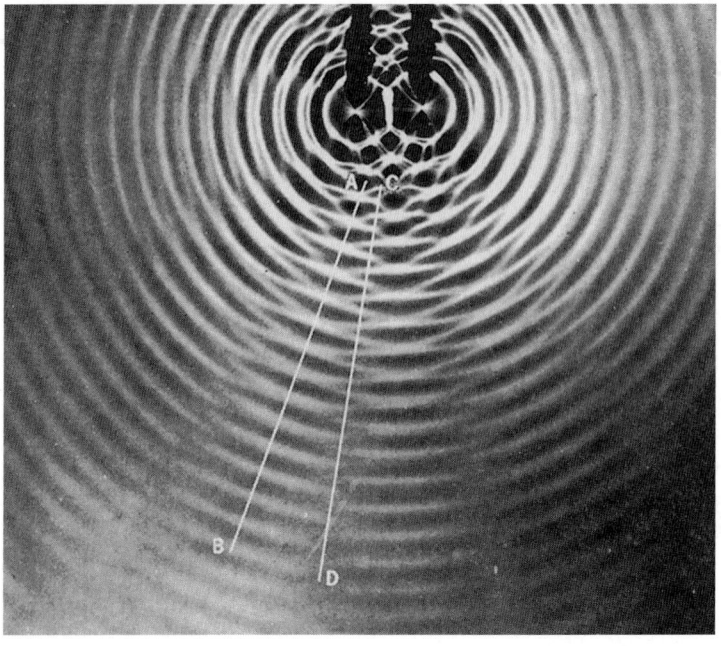

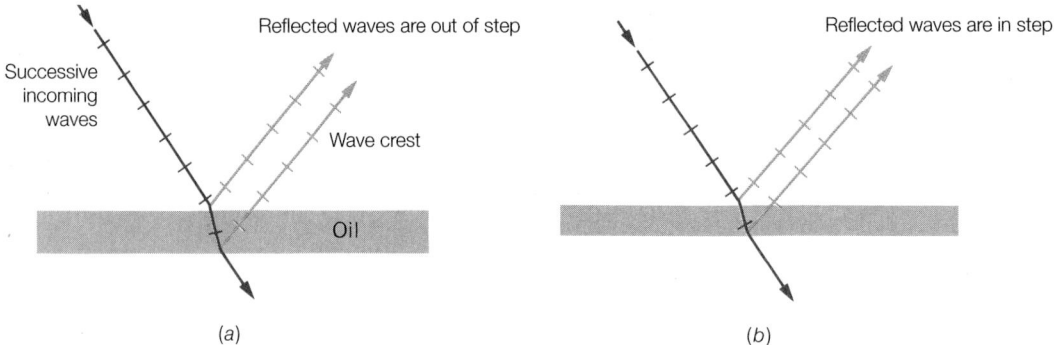

Figure 7-63   (*a*) Destructive and (*b*) constructive interference in a thin film for light of a particular wavelength. When the film has the thickness in (*a*), it appears dark; when it has the thickness in (*b*), it appears bright. Light of other wavelengths undergoes destructive and constructive interference at different film thicknesses.

Coated Lenses

A portion of the light that strikes an air-glass or glass-air interface is reflected, just as in the case of the oil film of Fig. 7-63. Because there are many such interfaces in most optical instruments (10 in the case of each half of a pair of binoculars), the total amount of light lost may be considerable, and the reflections also blur the image.

To reduce reflection at an interface, the glass can be coated with a thin layer of a transparent substance whose thickness is just right for the reflected rays from the top and bottom of the layer to interfere destructively, as in Fig. 7-63a. Of course, the cancellation is exact only for a particular wavelength. What is done is to choose a wavelength in the middle of the visible spectrum, which corresponds to green light, so that partial cancellation occurs over a wide range of colors. The red and violet ends of the spectrum are accordingly least affected, and the light reflected from a coated lens is a mixture of these colors, a purplish hue. Good-quality optical instruments always use coated lenses.

| Thomas Young (1773–1829)

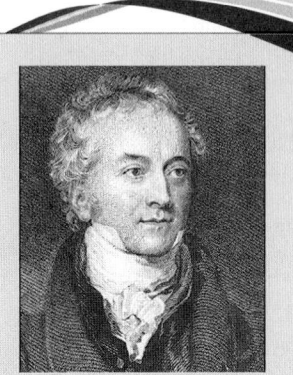

While still a medical student in London, Young discovered that the eye focuses on objects at different distances by changing the shape of its lens, and that astigmatism (from which he suffered) is due to an irregularly shaped cornea. Although a practicing physician all his life, an inherited fortune allowed Young the time to make important discoveries in a number of areas of physics. He was the first to use the word energy in its modern sense and to relate the work done on a body to the change in its kinetic energy.

Young's most notable achievement was to demonstrate the wave nature of light, which until then had been uncertain: many contemporaries still held to Newton's view that light consisted of a stream of particles. What Young did was to show that light from two adjacent narrow slits interferes to produce alternate bright and dark fringes on a screen, the optical equivalent of the interference of water waves shown in Fig. 7-62. From this experiment Young could determine the wavelengths found in light.

Physics and medicine were not all that interested Young: he was a pioneer in deciphering the hieroglyphics of ancient Egypt.

A simple example of diffraction occurs when we hear the noise of a car horn around the corner of a building. The noise could not have reached us through the building, and refraction is not involved since the speed of sound does not change between the source of noise and our ears. What happens is that the sound waves spread out from the corner of the building into the "shadow" as though they come from the corner (Fig. 7-65). The diffracted waves are not as loud as those that proceed directly to a listener, but they go around the corner in a way that a stream of particles, for example, cannot.

The Larger the Lens Diameter, the Sharper the Image   Diffraction, too, occurs in light waves. As mentioned, diffraction refers to the "bending" of waves around the edges of an obstacle in their path. Because of diffraction, a shadow is never completely dark, although the wavelengths of light waves are so short that the effects of diffraction are largely limited to the border of the shadow region.

Diffraction limits the useful magnifications of microscopes and telescopes. The larger the diameter of a lens (or of a curved mirror that acts like a lens), the less significant is diffraction. For this reason a small telescope cannot be used at a high magnification, since the result would be a blurred image instead of a sharp one. The huge Hale telescope at Mt. Palomar in California has a mirror 5 m in diameter, but even so it can resolve objects only 50 m or more across on the moon's surface.

The **resolving power** of a telescope depends upon the wavelength of the light that enters it divided by the diameter of the lens or mirror; the smaller the resolving power, the sharper the image (Fig. 7-66). This relationship poses a severe problem for radio telescopes, which are antennas designed to receive radio waves from space (Chap. 19). Because such waves might have wavelengths as much as a million times greater than those in visible light, an antenna would have to be tens or hundreds of kilometers across to be able to separate sources as close together in the sky as optical telescopes can. In fact, modern electronics permits sufficient resolution to be achieved by combining the signals received by a series of widely spaced antennas. Radio astronomers have established such an antenna array extending from the Virgin Islands across the United States to Hawaii, a span of about 8000 km—nearly the diameter of the earth (Fig. 7-67). This array provides better resolution than even the largest optical telescope.

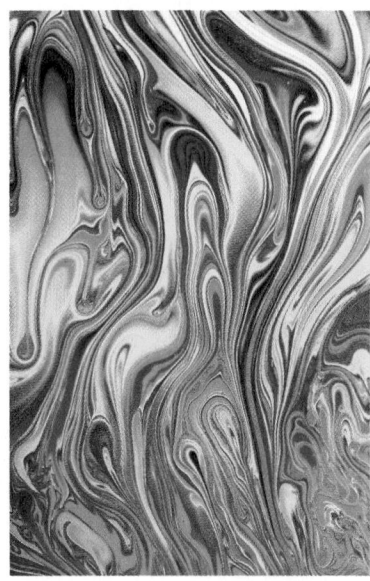

Figure 7-64   A colored pattern occurs when an uneven thin film of oil floats on water, because light of each wavelength undergoes constructive interference at a different oil thickness.

Figure 7-65 Diffraction causes waves to bend around the corner of an obstacle into the "shadow" region. The diffracted waves spread out as though they originated at the corner of the obstacle and are weaker than the direct waves. The waves shown here could be of any kind, for instance, water waves, sound waves, or light waves.

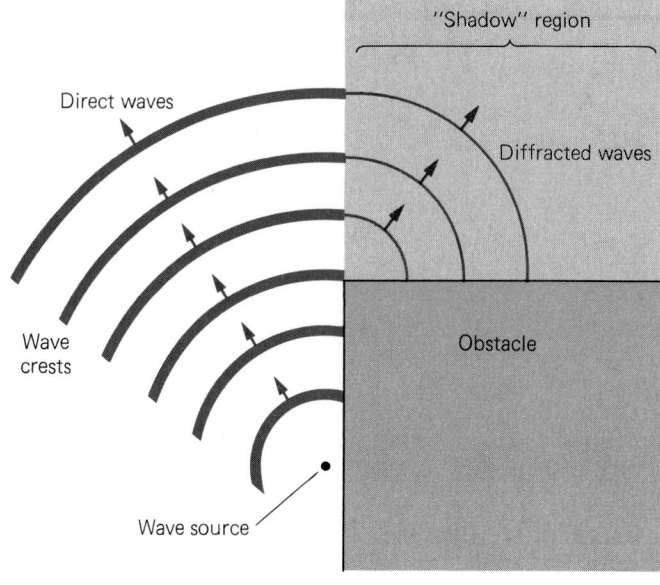

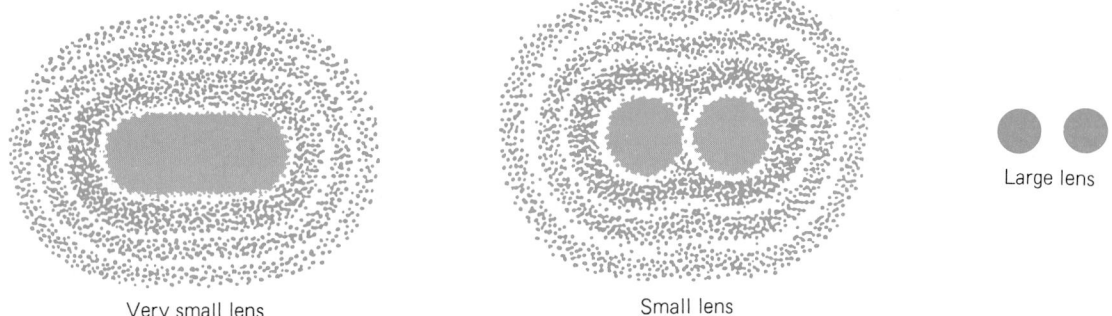

Figure 7-66   A large lens or mirror is better able to resolve nearby objects than a small one.

Figure 7-67   The ten radio telescopes whose locations are shown here operate together to give an angular resolving power of less than a millionth of a degree.

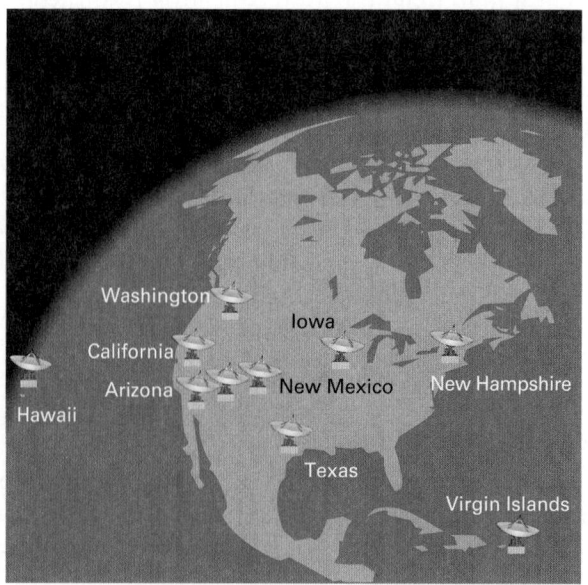

Resolving Power

No matter how perfect an optical system is, the image of a point source of light it produces is always a tiny disk of light with bright and dark interference fringes around it. If we are looking at two objects a distance d apart through an optical system whose diameter is D using light of wavelength λ and we are L away from the objects, we will see a single blob rather than separate objects if their separation is less than

$$d_0 = 1.22 \frac{\lambda L}{D}$$

This minimum distance, its **resolving power,** is a measure of the ability of the optical system to keep distinct the images of two objects that are close together.

The pupils of a person's eyes under ordinary conditions of illumination are about 3 mm in diameter, and for most people the distance of most distinct vision is 25 cm. Let us use $\lambda = 550$ nm, which is in the middle of the visible spectrum of light, to find the resolving power d_0 of the eye. The above formula gives

$$d_0 = 1.22 \frac{\lambda L}{D} = \frac{(1.22)(5.5 \times 10^{-7} \text{ m})(0.25 \text{ m})}{3 \times 10^{-3} \text{ m}}$$
$$= 6 \times 10^{-5} \text{ m} = 0.06 \text{ mm}$$

In fact, the photoreceptors in the retina are not quite close enough together to permit such sharp vision, and 0.1 mm is a more realistic resolving power.

The original generation of DVDs are "read" with lasers that emit red light. Since resolving power is proportional to wavelength, the invention of lasers that emit blue light, whose wavelength is much shorter (see Fig. 7-28), means that DVDs that squeeze more information on each disc can be manufactured and read. Using blue lasers together with improved software enables the second generation of DVDs ("Blu-ray") to each store as much as 13 h of normal video or 2 h of high-definition video.

Important Terms and Ideas

Waves carry energy from one place to another by a series of periodic motions of the individual particles of the medium in which the waves occur. (Electromagnetic waves are an exception.) There is no net transfer of matter in wave motion.

In a **longitudinal wave** the particles of the medium vibrate back and forth in the direction in which the waves travel. In a **transverse wave** the particles vibrate from side to side perpendicular to the wave direction. Sound waves are longitudinal; waves in a stretched string are transverse; water waves are a combination of both since water molecules move in circular orbits when a wave passes.

The **frequency** of waves is the number of wave crests that pass a particular point per second. The **period** is the time needed for a complete wave to pass a given point. **Wavelength** is the distance between adjacent crests or troughs. The **amplitude** of a wave is the maximum displacement of a particle of the medium on either side of its normal position when the wave passes.

The **doppler effect** refers to the change in frequency of a wave when there is relative motion between its source and an observer.

Resonance occurs when an object (such as a musical instrument) vibrates at a frequency equal to one of its natural frequencies of vibration.

Electromagnetic waves consist of coupled electric and magnetic field oscillations. Radio waves, light waves, and x-rays are all electromagnetic waves that differ only in their frequency.

In **amplitude modulation** (AM), information is contained in variations in the amplitude of a constant-frequency wave. In **frequency modulation** (FM), information is contained in variations in the frequency of the wave.

The change in direction of waves when they enter a region in which their speed changes is called **refraction.** In **reflection,** waves strike an obstacle and rebound from it.

The **index of refraction** of a medium is the ratio between the speed of light in free space and its speed in the medium. In **internal reflection,** light that arrives at a medium of lower index of refraction (for instance, glass to air) at a large enough angle is reflected back.

A **lens** is a piece of glass or other transparent material shaped to produce an image by refracting light that comes from an object. A **converging lens** brings parallel light to a single point at a distance called the **focal length** of the lens. A **diverging lens** spreads out parallel light so that it seems to come from a point behind the lens.

A **real image** of an object is formed by light rays that pass through it; the image would therefore appear on a screen. A **virtual image** can only be seen by the eye because the light rays that seem to come from the image do not actually pass through it.

White light is a mixture of different frequencies, each of which produces the visual sensation of a particular color. Because the speed of light in a medium is slightly different for different frequencies, white light is **dispersed** into its separate colors when refracted in a glass prism or a water droplet.

Interference refers to the adding together of two or more waves of the same kind that pass by the same point at the same time. In **constructive interference** the new wave has a greater amplitude than any of the original ones; in **destructive interference** the new wave has a smaller amplitude.

The ability of waves to bend around the edge of an obstacle in their path is called **diffraction.** The **resolving power** of an optical system is a measure of its ability to produce sharp images, which is limited by diffraction.

Important Formulas

Wave speed: $v = f\lambda$

Wave Period: $T = \dfrac{1}{f}$

Index of refraction: $n = \dfrac{c}{v}$

Apparent depth: $h' = \dfrac{h}{n}$

Multiple Choice

1. The distance from crest to crest of any wave is called its
   a. frequency
   b. wavelength
   c. speed
   d. amplitude

2. Of the following properties of a wave, the one that is independent of the others is its
   a. frequency
   b. wavelength
   c. speed
   d. amplitude

3. Energy is carried by which one or more of the following waves?
   a. sound waves
   b. light waves
   c. water waves
   d. waves in a stretched string

4. Water waves are
   a. longitudinal
   b. transverse
   c. a mixture of longitudinal and transverse
   d. sometimes longitudinal and sometimes transverse

5. Sound waves are
   a. longitudinal
   b. transverse
   c. a mixture of longitudinal and transverse
   d. sometimes longitudinal and sometimes transverse

6. Sound cannot travel through
   a. a solid
   b. a liquid
   c. a gas
   d. a vacuum

7. Sound travels slowest in
   a. air
   b. water
   c. iron
   d. a vacuum

8. The greater the amplitude of a wave, the greater its
   a. frequency
   b. wavelength
   c. speed
   d. energy

9. The lower the frequency of a sound wave, the
   a. higher its speed
   b. higher its pitch
   c. louder it is
   d. longer its wavelength

10. Six flutes playing together produce a 60-dB sound. The number of flutes needed to produce a 70-dB sound is
    a. 7
    b. 60
    c. 70
    d. 120

11. The doppler effect occurs
    a. only in sound waves
    b. only in longitudinal waves
    c. only in transverse waves
    d. in all types of waves

12. A spacecraft is approaching the earth. Relative to the radio signals it sends out, the signals received on the earth have
    a. a lower frequency
    b. a shorter wavelength
    c. a higher speed
    d. all of the above

13. Maxwell based his theory of electromagnetic waves on the hypothesis that a changing electric field gives rise to
    a. an electric current
    b. a stream of electrons
    c. a magnetic field
    d. longitudinal waves

14. In a vacuum, the speed of an electromagnetic wave
    a. depends upon its frequency
    b. depends upon its wavelength
    c. depends upon the strength of its electric and magnetic fields
    d. is a universal constant

15. Electromagnetic waves transport
    a. frequency
    b. wavelength
    c. charge
    d. energy

16. Which of the following do(es) not consist of electromagnetic waves?
    a. x-rays
    b. radar waves
    c. sound waves
    d. infrared waves

17. The energy of an electromagnetic wave resides in its
    a. frequency
    b. wavelength
    c. speed
    d. electric and magnetic fields

18. Light waves
    a. require air or another gas to travel through
    b. require some kind of matter to travel through
    c. require electric and magnetic fields to travel through
    d. can travel through a perfect vacuum

19. A beam of transverse waves whose variations occur in all directions perpendicular to their direction of motion is
    a. resolved
    b. diffracted
    c. polarized
    d. unpolarized

20. The ionosphere is a region of ionized gas in the upper atmosphere. The ionosphere is responsible for
    a. the blue color of the sky
    b. rainbows
    c. long-distance radio communication
    d. the ability of satellites to orbit the earth

21. A pencil in a glass of water appears bent. This is an example of
    a. reflection   **c.** diffraction
    b. refraction   **d.** interference

22. A fish that you are looking at from a boat seems to be 60 cm below the water surface. The actual depth of the fish
    a. is less than 60 cm
    b. is 60 cm
    c. is more than 60 cm
    d. may be any of these, depending on the angle of view

23. The index of refraction of a transparent substance is always
    a. less than 1
    b. 1
    c. greater than 1
    d. any of the above

24. A real image formed by any lens is always which one or more of the following?
    a. smaller than the object
    b. larger than the object
    c. erect
    d. inverted

25. The image of a real object farther from a converging lens than f is always which one or more of the following?
    a. smaller than the object
    b. the same size as the object
    c. virtual
    d. inverted

26. The image of a real object closer to a converging lens than f is always which one or more of the following?
    a. smaller than the object
    b. the same size as the object
    c. virtual
    d. inverted

27. The image formed by a diverging lens of a real object is never which one or more of the following?
    a. real   **c.** erect
    b. virtual   **d.** smaller than the object

28. A converging lens of focal length f is being used as a magnifying glass. The distance of an object from the lens must be
    a. less than f **c.** between f and $2f$
    b. f **d.** more than f

29. The quality in sound that corresponds to color in light is
    a. amplitude   **c.** waveform
    b. resonance   **d.** pitch

30. Light of which color has the lowest frequency?
    a. red   **c.** yellow
    b. blue   **d.** green

31. Light of which color has the shortest wavelength?
    a. red   **c.** yellow
    b. blue   **d.** green

32. The Spanish flag is yellow and red. When viewed with yellow light it appears
    a. all yellow   **c.** yellow and black
    b. yellow and red   **d.** white and red

33. The Danish flag is red and white. When viewed with red light it appears
    a. all red   **c.** red and white
    b. all white   **d.** red and black

34. Thin films of oil and soapy water owe their brilliant colors to a combination of reflection, refraction, and
    a. scattering   **c.** diffraction
    b. interference   **d.** doppler effect

35. The sky is blue because
    a. air molecules are blue
    b. the lens of the eye is blue
    c. the scattering of light is more efficient the shorter its wavelength
    d. the scattering of light is more efficient the longer its wavelength

36. Diffraction refers to
    a. the splitting of a beam of white light into its component colors
    b. the interference of light that produces bright colors in thin oil films
    c. the bending of waves around the edge of an obstacle in their path
    d. the increase in frequency due to motion of a wave source toward an observer

37. The useful magnification of a telescope is limited by
    a. the speed of light   **c.** interference
    b. the doppler effect   **d.** diffraction

38. Which one or more of the following will improve the resolving power of a lens?
    a. Increase the wavelength of the light used
    b. Increase the frequency of the light used
    c. Decrease the diameter of the lens used
    d. Increase the diameter of the lens used

39. The speed of sound waves having a frequency of 256 Hz compared with the speed of sound waves having a frequency of 512 Hz is
    a. half as great   **c.** twice as great
    b. the same   **d.** 4 times as great

40. The wavelength of sound waves having a frequency of 256 Hz compared with the wavelength of sound waves having a frequency of 512 Hz is
    a. half as great   **c.** twice as great
    b. the same   **d.** 4 times as great

41. Waves in a lake are observed to be 5 m in length and to pass an anchored boat 1.25 s apart. The speed of the waves is
    a. 0.25 m/s
    b. 4 m/s
    c. 6.25 m/s
    d. impossible to find from the information given

42. A boat at anchor is rocked by waves whose crests are 20 m apart and whose speed is 5 m/s. These waves reach the boat with a frequency of
   a. 0.25 Hz   **c.** 20 Hz
   b. 4 Hz   **d.** 100 Hz

43. One kHz (kilohertz) is equal to 10^3 Hz. What is the wavelength of the electromagnetic waves sent out by a radio station whose frequency is 660 kHz? The speed of light is 3×10^8 m/s.
   a. 2.2×10^{-3} m   **c.** 4.55×10^3 m
   b. 4.55×10^2 m   **d.** 1.98×10^{14} m

44. The speed of light in diamond is 1.24×10^8 m/s. The index of refraction of diamond is
   a. 1.24   **c.** 2.42
   b. 2.31   **d.** 3.72

45. A medal in a plastic cube appears to be 12 mm below the top of the cube. If $n = 1.5$ for the plastic, the depth of the medal is actually
   a. 6 mm   **c.** 18 mm
   b. 8 mm   **d.** 24 mm

Exercises

7.1   Water Waves
7.2   Transverse and Longitudinal Waves
7.3   Describing Waves

1. (a) Distinguish between longitudinal and transverse waves. (b) Do all waves fall into one or the other of these categories? If not, give an example of one that does not.

2. Does increasing the frequency of a wave also increase its wavelength? If not, how are these quantities related?

3. Water waves whose crests are 6 m apart reach the shore every 1.2 s. Find the frequency and speed of the waves.

4. Water waves are approaching a lighthouse at a rate of 1 wave every 1.2 s. The distance between adjacent crests is 7 m. What is the speed of the waves?

5. At one end of a ripple tank 90 cm across, a 6-Hz vibrator produces waves whose wavelength is 50 mm. Find the time the waves need to cross the tank.

6. A 1.2-MHz ultrasonic beam is used to scan body tissue. If the speed of sound in a certain tissue is 1540 m/s and the limit of resolution is one wavelength, what size is the smallest detail that can be resolved?

7.5   Sound

7. Why does sound travel fastest in solids and slowest in gases?

8. The speed of sound in a gas depends upon the average speed of the gas molecules. Why is such a relationship reasonable?

9. Even if astronauts on the moon's surface did not need to be enclosed in space suits, they could not speak directly to each other but would have to communicate by radio. Can you think of the reason?

10. What eventually becomes of the energy of sound waves?

11. A person is watching as spikes are being driven to hold a steel rail in place. The sound of each sledgehammer blow arrives 0.14 s through the rail and 2 s through the air after the person sees the hammer strike the spike. Find the speed of sound in the rail.

12. An airplane is flying at 500 km/h at an altitude of 4.0 km. When the sound of the airplane's engines seems to somebody on the ground to be coming from directly overhead, how far away is she from being directly below the airplane?

13. Find the frequency of sound waves in air whose wavelength is 25 cm.

14. A person determines the direction from which a sound comes by means of two mechanisms. One compares the loudness of the sound in one ear with that in the other ear, which is most effective at low frequencies. The other compares the phases of the waves that arrive at the two ears, which is most effective at high frequencies. (The phase of a wave is the part of its cycle it is in at a particular time and place.) The crossover point of equal effectiveness occurs at about 1200 Hz, and as a result, sound with frequencies in the vicinity of 1200 Hz are difficult to locate. How does the wavelength of a 1200-Hz sound compare with the distance between your ears?

15. How many times stronger than the 60-dB sound of a person talking loudly is the 100-dB sound of a power lawn mower?

16. A violin string vibrates 1044 times per second. How many vibrations does it make while its sound travels 20 m?

7.6   Doppler Effect

17. In what kinds of waves can the doppler effect occur?

18. A "double star" consists of two nearby stars that revolve around their center of mass (see Sec. 18.11). How can an astronomer recognize a double star from the characteristic frequencies of the light that reaches him from its member stars?

19. The characteristic wavelengths of light emitted by a distant star are observed to be shifted toward the red end of the spectrum. What does this suggest about the motion of the star relative to the earth?

7.8   Electromagnetic Waves
7.9   Types of EM Waves

20. Why are light waves able to travel through a vacuum whereas sound waves cannot?

21. How could you show that light carries energy?

22. Why was electromagnetic induction discovered much earlier than its converse, the production of a magnetic field by a changing electric field?

23. Light is said to be a transverse wave. What is it that varies at right angles to the direction in which a light wave travels?

24. Which of the following waves cannot be polarized? X-rays, radio waves, light waves, sound waves.

25. Light waves carry both energy and momentum. Why doesn't the momentum of the sun diminish with time as its energy content does?

26. Give as many similarities and differences as you can between sound and light waves.

27. Visible light of which color has the lowest frequency? The highest frequency? The shortest wavelength? The longest wavelength?

28. A radar signal took 2.7 s to go to the moon and return. How far away was the moon at that time?

29. An opera performance is being broadcast by radio. Who will hear a certain sound first, a member of the audience 30 m from the stage or a listener to a radio receiver 5000 km away?

30. Radio waves of very long wavelength can penetrate farther into seawater than those of shorter wavelength. The U.S. Navy communicates with submerged submarines using 76-Hz radio waves. What is their wavelength in air?

31. A nanosecond is 10^{-9} s. (a) What is the frequency of an em wave whose period is 1 ns? (b) What is its wavelength? (c) To what class of em waves does it belong?

32. A radar sends out $0.05-\mu s$ pulses of microwaves whose wavelength is 24 mm. What is the frequency of these microwaves? How many waves does each pulse contain?

7.10 Light "Rays"

7.11 Reflection

7.12 Refraction

33. When a light ray is reflected, which of the following quantities, if any, is always unchanged? The direction of the ray; its speed; its frequency; its wavelength.

34. When a light ray goes from one medium to another, which of the following quantities, if any, is always unchanged? The direction of the ray; its speed; its frequency; its wavelength.

35. What is the height of the smallest mirror in which you could see yourself at full length? Use a diagram to explain your answer. Does it matter how far away you are?

36. What types of waves can be refracted? Under what circumstances does refraction occur?

37. Can the index of refraction of a substance be less than 1? If not, why not?

38. (a) You are standing on a pier and want to spear a fish that swims by. Should you aim above, below, or exactly where the fish seems to be? (b) What if you are swimming underwater and want to spear a fish?

39. When a fish looks up through the water surface at an object in the air, will the object appear to be its normal size and distance above the water? Use a diagram to explain your answer, and assume that the fish's eye and brain, like the human eye and brain, are accustomed to interpreting light rays as straight lines.

40. A flashlight at the bottom of a swimming pool shines upward at an angle with the surface, as in Fig. 7-68. Which path does the light follow?

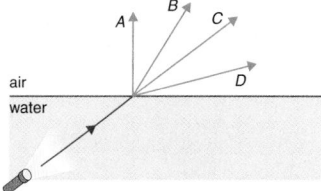

Figure 7-68

41. Which of the paths shown in Fig. 7-69 could represent a ray of light passing through a glass block in air?

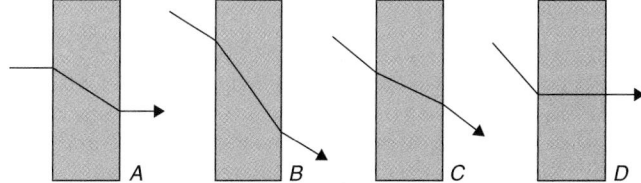

Figure 7-69

42. The olive in a cocktail ($n = 1.35$) seems to be 30 mm below the surface. What is the actual depth of the olive?

43. A leaf frozen into a pond in winter is 40 mm below the surface of the ice. How far down does the leaf seem to be? ($n_{ice} = 1.31$)

7.13 Lenses

44. Does a spherical bubble in a pane of glass act to converge or diverge light passing through it?

45. What is the difference between a real image and a virtual image?

46. A coin is placed at a focal point of a converging lens. Is an image formed? If yes, is it real or virtual, erect or inverted, larger or smaller than the object?

47. Under what circumstances, if any, will a light ray that passes through a converging lens not be deviated? Under what circumstances, if any, will a light ray that passes through a diverging lens not be deviated?

48. Under what circumstances, if any, will a converging lens form an inverted image of a real object? Under what circumstances, if any, will a diverging lens form an erect image of a real object?

49. Is the mercury column in a thermometer wider or narrower than it seems to be?

50. Is there any way in which a converging lens, by itself, can form a virtual image of a real object? Is there any way in which a diverging lens, by itself, can form a real image of a real object?

51. When it leaves the lens, which path will the incoming ray in Fig. 7-70 follow?

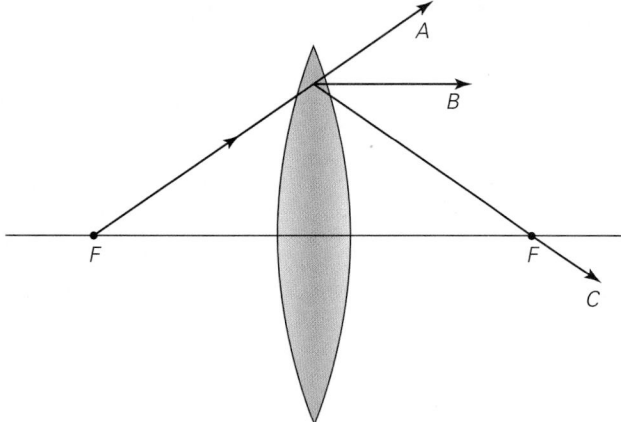

Figure 7-70

52. If the screen is moved farther from a slide projector, how should the projector's lens be moved to restore the image to a sharp focus?

53. A birthday candle 4 cm high is 10 cm from a converging lens whose focal length is 15 cm. Use a ray diagram on a suitable scale (say, $\frac{1}{3}$ full size) to find the location of the image, its height, and whether it is erect or inverted, real or virtual.

54. The candle of Exercise 53 is 15 cm from the lens. Answer the same questions for this situation.

55. The candle of Exercise 53 is 25 cm from the lens. Answer the same questions for this situation.

56. The candle of Exercise 53 is 30 cm from the lens. Answer the same questions for this situation.

57. The candle of Exercise 53 is 50 cm from the lens. Answer the same questions for this situation.

7.14   The Eye

58. Describe the image the lens of the eye forms on the retina.

59. (a) What is the name of the defect of vision in which an eye can see nearby objects clearly but not distant ones? (b) What is the name of the defect of vision in which either bar of a cross can be seen clearly but not both at the same time?

7.15   Color

60. When a beam of white light passes perpendicularly through a flat pane of glass, it is not dispersed into a spectrum. Why not?

61. When white light is dispersed by a glass prism, red light is bent least and violet light is bent most. What does this tell you about the relative speeds of red and violet light in glass?

62. What color would red cloth appear if it were illuminated by (a) white light? (b) red light? (c) green light?

63. (a) What would the American flag look like when viewed with red light? (b) With blue light?

64. If the earth had no atmosphere, what would the color of the sky be during the day?

65. Light of what color is scattered most in the atmosphere? Least?

7.16   Interference

66. How can constructive and destructive interference be reconciled with the principle of conservation of energy?

7.17   Diffraction

67. Which of the following can occur in (a) transverse waves and (b) longitudinal waves? Reflection, interference, diffraction, polarization.

68. Give two advantages that a telescope lens or mirror of large diameter has over one of small diameter.

69. Radio waves are able to diffract readily around buildings, as anybody with a portable radio receiver can verify. However, light waves, which are also electromagnetic waves, undergo no discernible diffraction around buildings. Why not?

70. A radar operating at a wavelength of 3 cm is to have a resolving power of 30 m at a range of 1 km. Find the minimum width its antenna must have.

71. Suppose you are an astronaut orbiting the earth at an altitude of 200 km. The pupils of your eyes are 3 mm in diameter and the average wavelength of the light reaching you from the earth is 500 nm. What is the length of the smallest structure you could make out on the earth with your naked eye, assuming that turbulence in the earth's atmosphere does not smear out the image?

72. At night, the pupils of a certain woman's eyes are 8 mm in diameter. (a) How many km away from a car facing her will the woman be able to distinguish its headlights from each other? (b) What would the distance be if her pupils were 4 mm in diameter (say at twilight)? Assume that the headlights are 1.5 m apart, that the average wavelength of their light is 600 nm, and that her eyes attain half their theoretical resolving power.

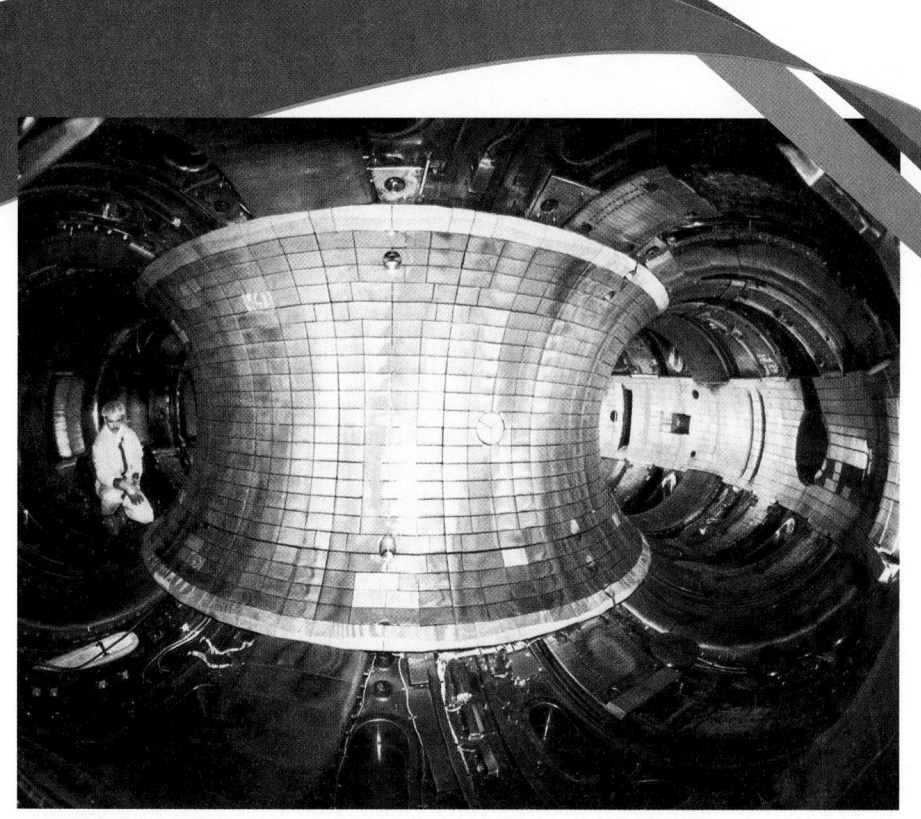

Interior of the Tokamak nuclear fusion test reactor at Princeton.

The Nucleus

GOALS

When you have finished this chapter you should be able to complete the goals
• given for each section below:

Atom and Nucleus

8.1 Rutherford Model of the Atom
An Atom Is Mostly Empty Space
• Discuss how the Rutherford experiment led to the modern picture of atomic structure.

8.2 Nuclear Structure
Protons and Neutrons
• Distinguish between nucleon and nuclide and between atomic number and mass number.
• State in what ways the isotopes of an element are similar and in what ways they are different.

Radioactivity

8.3 Radioactive Decay
How Unstable Nuclei Change into Stable Ones
• Describe the various kinds of radioactive decay and explain why each occurs.

8.4 Half-Life
Less and Less, but Always Some Left
• Define half-life.

8.5 Radiation Hazards
Invisible but Dangerous

• Discuss the sources and hazards of the ionizing radiation we are exposed to in daily life.

Nuclear Energy

8.6 Units of Mass and Energy
The Atomic Mass Unit and the Electronvolt
• Define atomic mass unit and electronvolt and use them in calculations.

8.7 Binding Energy
The Missing Energy That Keeps a Nucleus Together
• Explain the significance of the binding energy of a nucleus.

8.8 Binding Energy per Nucleon
Why Fission and Fusion Liberate Energy
• Sketch a graph of binding energy per nucleon versus mass number and indicate on it the location of the most stable nucleus and the range of mass numbers in which fusion and fission can occur.

Fission and Fusion

8.9 Nuclear Fission
Divide and Conquer
• Discuss nuclear fission and the conditions needed for a chain reaction to occur.

8.10 How a Reactor Works
From Uranium to Heat to Electricity

• Describe how a nuclear reactor works.

8.11 Plutonium
Another Fissionable Material
• Discuss what plutonium is, how it is made, and why it is important.

8.12 Nuclear Fusion
The Energy Source of the Future?
• Describe nuclear fusion and identify the conditions needed for a successful fusion reactor.

Elementary Particles

8.13 Antiparticles
The Same but Different
• Compare a particle with its antiparticle.
• Describe the processes of annihilation and pair production.

8.14 Fundamental Interactions
Only Four Give Rise to All Physical Processes
• List the four fundamental interactions and identify the aspects of the universe that each governs.

8.15 Leptons and Hadrons
Ultimate Matter
• Distinguish between leptons and hadrons and discuss the quark model of hadrons.
• Identify neutrinos and state their properties.

Atoms are the smallest particles of ordinary matter. Every atom has a central core, or **nucleus,** of protons and neutrons that provide nearly all the atom's mass. Outside the nucleus are the much lighter electrons, the same in number as the number of protons in the nucleus so that the atom as a whole is electrically neutral.

The chief properties (except mass) of atoms, molecules, solids, and liquids can be traced to the behavior of atomic electrons. But the atomic nucleus is also significant in the grand scheme of things. The continuing evolution of the universe is powered by energy that comes from nuclear reactions and transformations. Like other stars, the sun obtains its energy in this way. In turn, the coal, oil, and natural gas of the earth, as well as its winds and falling water, owe their energy contents to the sun's rays. Nuclear processes are responsible for the heat of the earth's interior and for the energy produced by nuclear reactors. Thus *all* the energy at our command has a nuclear origin, except for the energy of the tides, which are the result of the gravitational pull of the moon and sun on the waters of the world.

Atom and Nucleus

Until 1911 little was known about atoms except that they exist and contain electrons. Since electrons carry negative charges but atoms are neutral, scientists agreed that positively charged matter of some kind must be present in atoms. But what kind? And arranged in what way?

One suggestion, made by the British physicist J. J. Thomson in 1898, was that atoms are simply positively charged lumps of matter with electrons embedded in them, like raisins in a fruitcake (Fig. 8-1). Because Thomson had played an important part in discovering the electron, his idea was taken seriously. But atomic structure turned out to be very different.

8.1 Rutherford Model of the Atom

An Atom Is Mostly Empty Space

The most direct way to find out what is inside a fruitcake is to poke a finger into it. A similar method was used in 1911 in an experiment suggested by the British physicist Ernest Rutherford to find out what is inside an atom. Alpha particles were used as probes. (As discussed later in this chapter, alpha particles are emitted by certain substances. For now, all we need to know about these particles is that they are almost 8000 times heavier than electrons and each one has a charge of $+2e$.) A sample of an alpha-emitting substance was placed behind a lead screen with a small hole in it, as in Fig. 8-2, so that a narrow beam of alpha particles was produced. This beam was aimed at a thin gold foil. A zinc sulfide screen, which gives off a visible flash of light when struck by an alpha particle, was set on the other side of the foil.

Rutherford expected the alpha particles to go right through the foil with hardly any deflection. This follows from the Thomson model, in which the electric charge inside an atom is assumed to be uniformly spread through its volume. With only weak electric forces exerted on them, alpha particles that pass through a thin foil ought to be deflected only slightly, 1° or less.

What was found instead was that, although most of the alpha particles indeed were not deviated by much, a few were scattered through very large angles. Some were even scattered in the backward direction. As Rutherford remarked, "It was as incredible as if you fired a 15-inch shell at a piece of tissue paper and it came back and hit you."

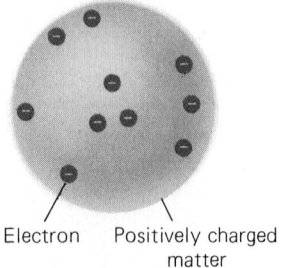

Electron   Positively charged
                      matter

Figure 8-1   The Thomson model of the atom. Experiment shows it to be incorrect.

| Ernest Rutherford (1871–1937)

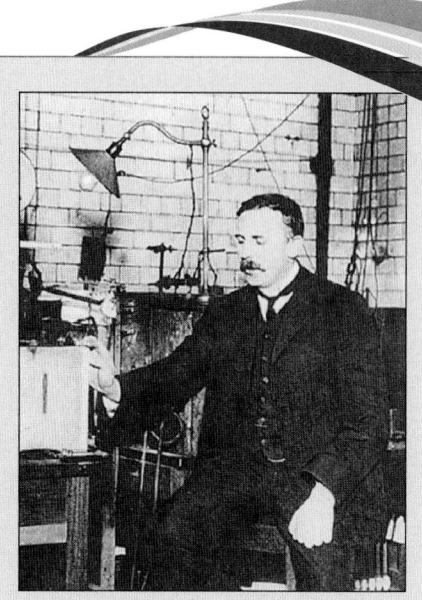

He was digging potatoes on his family's farm in New Zealand when Rutherford learned that he had won a scholarship for graduate study at Cambridge University in England. "This is the last potato I will ever dig," he said, throwing down his spade. Thirteen years later he received the Nobel Prize for his work on radioactivity, which included discovering that alpha particles are the nuclei of helium atoms and that the radioactive decay of an element can give rise to a different element.

In 1911 Rutherford showed that the nuclear model of the atom was the only one that could explain the observed scattering of alpha particles by thin metal foils. Using alpha particles to bombard nitrogen nuclei, Rutherford was the first to artificially transmute one element into another. Notable achievements made in his laboratory by his associates include the discovery of the neutron in 1932 and the construction of the first high-energy particle accelerator for nuclear research.

But Rutherford was not infallible: only a few years before the first nuclear reactor was built, he dismissed the idea of practical uses for nuclear energy as "moonshine." Rutherford is buried near Newton in Westminster Abbey.

Why the Nucleus Must Be Small Since alpha particles are relatively heavy and since those used in this experiment had high speeds, it was clear that strong forces had to be exerted upon them to cause such marked deflections. The only way to explain the results, Rutherford found, was to picture an atom as having a tiny nucleus in which the positive charge and nearly all the mass of the atom are concentrated. The electrons are some distance away, as in Fig. 8-3.

With an atom that is largely empty space, it is easy to see why most alpha particles go right through a thin foil. However, when an alpha particle happens to come near a nucleus, the strong electric field there causes the particle to be deflected through a large angle. The atomic electrons, being so light, have little effect on the alpha particles.

Suppose, as an analogy, that a star approaches the solar system from space at great speed. The chances are good that the star will not be deflected. Even a collision with a planet would not change the star's path to any great extent. Only if the star came near the great mass of the sun would the star's direction change by much. Similarly, said Rutherford, an alpha particle plows straight through an atom, unaffected by striking an electron now and then. Only a close approach to the heavy central nucleus of an atom can turn the alpha particle aside.

Ordinary matter, then, is mostly empty space. The solid wood of a table, the steel that supports a bridge, the hard rock underfoot, all are just collections of electric charges, comparatively farther away from one another than the planets are from the sun. If all the electrons and nuclei in our bodies could somehow be packed closely together, we would be no larger than specks just visible with a microscope.

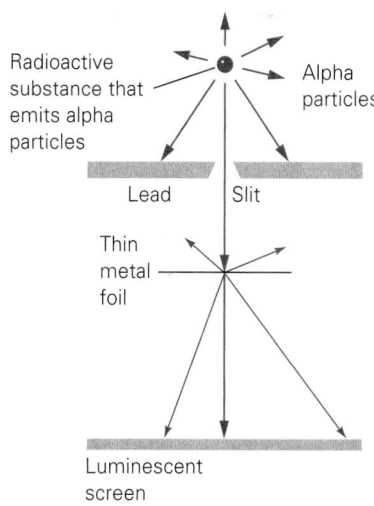

Figure 8-2 Principle of the Rutherford experiment. Nearly all the alpha particles pass through the foil with little or no deflection, but a few of the particles are scattered through large angles, even in the backward direction. This result means that strong electric fields must act on the particles, and such fields can arise only if atoms have very small nuclei in which their positive charge is concentrated.

8.2 Nuclear Structure

Protons and Neutrons

What gives a nucleus its mass and charge? The simplest nucleus, that of the hydrogen atom, usually consists of a single **proton.** As mentioned in Chap. 6, the proton is a particle whose charge is $+e$ and whose mass is 1836 times the electron mass. Nuclei more complex than that of hydrogen contain **neutrons** as well as protons. The neutron has no charge, and its mass, 1839 times that of the electron, is slightly more than that of the proton. The compositions of several atoms are illustrated in Fig. 8-4.

Figure 8-3   In the Rutherford model of the atom, the positive charge is concentrated in a central nucleus with the electrons some distance away. This model correctly predicts that some alpha particles striking a thin metal foil will be scattered through large angles by the strong electric fields of the nuclei.

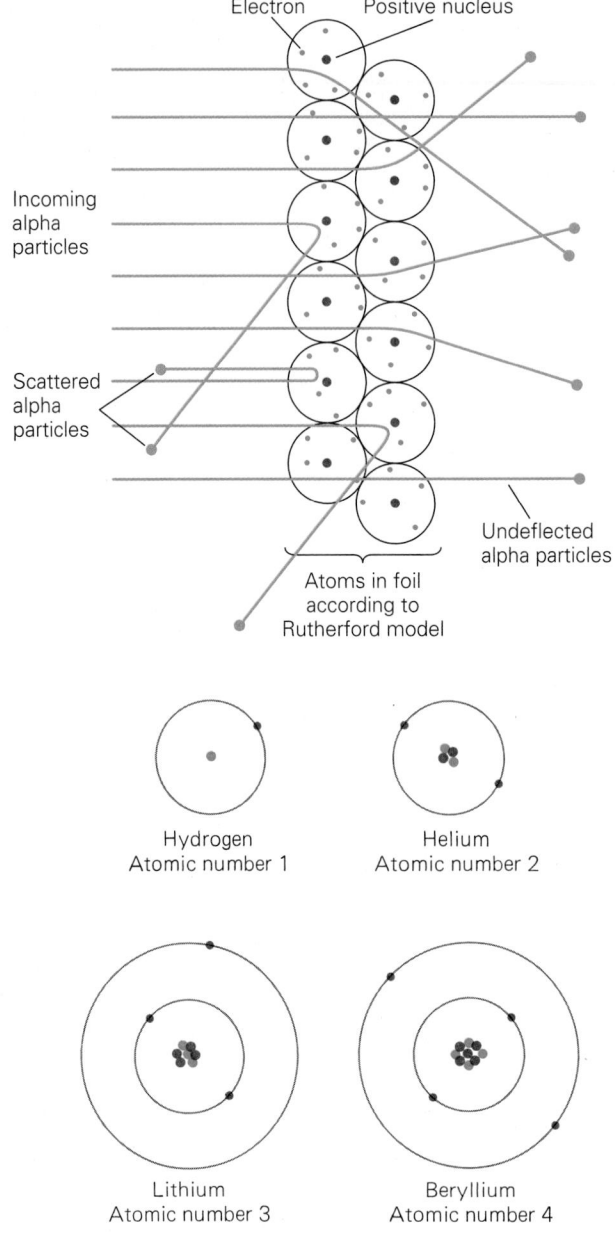

Electron   Positive nucleus

Incoming alpha particles

Scattered alpha particles

Undeflected alpha particles

Atoms in foil according to Rutherford model

Hydrogen
Atomic number 1

Helium
Atomic number 2

Lithium
Atomic number 3

Beryllium
Atomic number 4

● Proton   ● Neutron   ● Electron

Figure 8-4   The elements that correspond to the atomic numbers 1, 2, 3, and 4 are hydrogen, helium, lithium, and beryllium. The particles their atoms consist of are actually far too small to be seen even on this scale, and the structures of the atoms, which are discussed in Chap. 9, are not as simple as those shown here.

Elements   **Elements** are the simplest substances in the bulk matter around us. Over 100 elements are known, of which 11 are gases, 2 are liquids, and the rest are solids at room temperature and atmospheric pressure. Hydrogen, helium, oxygen, chlorine, and neon are gaseous elements, and bromine and mercury are the two liquids. Most of the solid elements are metals. Elements are discussed in more detail in Chap. 10.

In a neutral atom of any element, the number of protons equals the number of electrons. This number is called the **atomic number** of the element. Thus the atomic number of hydrogen is 1, of helium 2, of lithium 3, and of beryllium 4. The atomic number of an element is its most basic property since this determines how many electrons its atoms have and how they are arranged, which in turn govern the physical and chemical behavior of the element.

Atomic numbers and symbols of all the elements are given in Table 10-6, which is reproduced inside the back cover of the book.

Isotopes   All atoms of a given element have nuclei with the same number of protons but not necessarily the same number of neutrons. For instance, even though more than 99.9 percent of hydrogen nuclei are just single protons, a few also contain a neutron as well, and a very few contain two neutrons along with the single proton (Fig. 8-5). The different kinds of hydrogen atom are called **isotopes.** All elements have isotopes.

A nucleus with a particular composition is called a **nuclide.** Symbols for nuclides follow the pattern

$$_Z^A X \qquad Nuclide\ symbol$$

where X = chemical symbol of element
Z = atomic number of element
 = number of protons in nucleus
A = **mass number** of nucleus
 = number of protons and neutrons in nucleus

Thus the nucleus of the chlorine isotope that contains 17 protons and 18 neutrons has the atomic number $Z = 17$ and the mass number $A = 17 + 18 = 35$. Its symbol is accordingly

$$_{17}^{35}\text{Cl}$$

The symbol of this nuclide is sometimes shortened to ^{35}Cl or Cl-35. The symbols of the nuclides of Fig. 8-4 are $_1^1$H, $_2^4$He, $_3^7$Li, and $_4^9$Be.

The term **nucleon** refers to both protons and neutrons, so that the mass number A is the number of nucleons in a particular nucleus.

Radioactivity

In 1896 Henri Becquerel accidentally discovered in his Paris laboratory that the element uranium can expose covered photographic film, can ionize gases, and can cause certain materials (such as the zinc sulfide used in the Rutherford experiment) to glow in the dark. Becquerel concluded that uranium gives off some kind of invisible but penetrating radiation, a property soon called **radioactivity.**

Not long afterward, Pierre and Marie Curie, in the course of extracting uranium from the ore pitchblende at the same laboratory, found two other elements that are also radioactive. They named one polonium, after Marie Curie's native Poland. The other, which turned out to be thousands of times more radioactive than uranium, was called radium.

Chemical reactions do not change the ability of a radioactive material to emit radiation, nor does heating it in an electric arc or cooling it in liquid air. Radioactivity must therefore be associated with atomic nuclei because these are the only parts of atoms not affected by such treatment.

The radioactivity of an element is due to the radioactivity of one or more of its isotopes. Most elements in nature have no radioactive isotopes, though such isotopes can be prepared artificially and are useful in biological and medical research as "tracers." The procedure is to incorporate a radionuclide in a chemical compound and follow what happens to the compound in a living organism by monitoring the radiation from the isotope (Fig. 8-6). Other elements, such as potassium, have some stable isotopes and some radioactive ones. A few, such as uranium, have only radioactive isotopes.

Of the 7000 or so nuclides that might possibly exist, about 2000 have either been found in nature or created in the laboratory, and of those only 256 are stable and do not undergo radioactive decay.

Deuterium and Tritium

About one in every 7000 hydrogen atoms is a deuterium ($_1^2$H) atom (Fig. 8-5). The proportion of tritium ($_1^3$H) atoms is even smaller—only about 2 kg of tritium of natural origin is present on the earth, nearly all of it in the oceans. Tritium is radioactive and decays to a helium isotope. Nuclear reactions in the atmosphere caused by cosmic rays from space (see Sec. 19.5) continually replenish the earth's tritium.

Heavy water is water in which deuterium atoms instead of ordinary hydrogen ($_1^1$H) atoms are combined with oxygen atoms to form H_2O. Because $_1^2$H atoms have about twice the mass of $_1^1$H atoms, heavy water is 10 percent denser than ordinary water. Deuterium does not combine with neutrons as readily as ordinary hydrogen and for this reason heavy water is used in certain types of nuclear reactors.

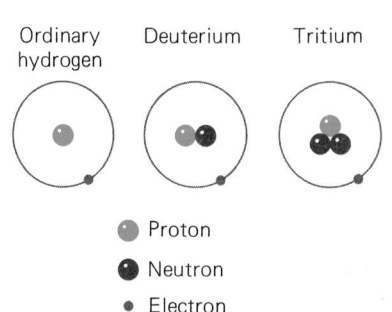

Ordinary hydrogen   Deuterium   Tritium

● Proton
● Neutron
• Electron

Figure 8-5   The isotopes of hydrogen.

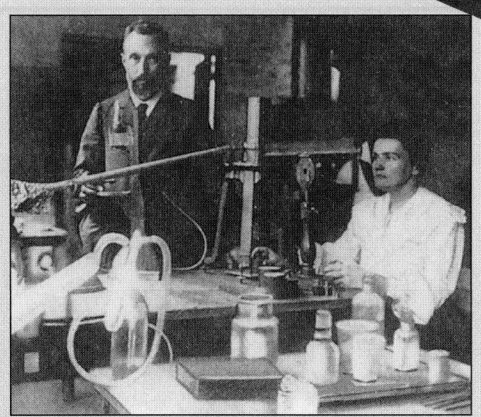

After high school in her native Poland, Marie Sklodowska worked as a governess until she was 24 so that she could study science in Paris, where she had barely enough money to survive. In 1894 Marie married Pierre Curie, who was 8 years older than she and already a noted physicist. In 1897, just after the birth of her daughter Irene (who, like her mother, was to win a Nobel Prize in physics), Marie began to investigate the newly discovered phenomenon of radioactivity—her word—for her doctoral thesis.

After a search of all the known elements, Marie learned that thorium as well as uranium was radioactive. She then examined various minerals for radioactivity and found that the uranium ore pitchblende was far more radioactive than its uranium content would suggest. Marie and Pierre together went on to identify first polonium, named for her native Poland, and

then radium as the sources of the additional activity. With the primitive facilities that were all they could afford (they had to use their own money), they had succeeded by 1902 in purifying a tenth of a gram of radium from several tons of ore, a task that involved immense physical as well as intellectual labor.

Together with Becquerel, the Curies shared the 1903 Nobel Prize in physics. Pierre ended his acceptance speech with these words: "One may also imagine that in criminal hands radium might become very dangerous, and here one may ask if humanity has anything to gain by learning the secrets of nature, if it is ready to profit from them, or if this knowledge is not harmful. . . . I am among those who think . . . that humanity will obtain more good than evil from the new discoveries."

In 1906 Pierre was struck and killed by a horse-drawn carriage in a Paris street. Marie continued work on radioactivity and became world-famous. Even before Pierre's death both Curies had suffered from ill health because of their exposure to radiation, and much of Marie's later life was marred by radiation-induced ailments, including the leukemia from which she died.

Figure 8-6   Substances that contain a radionuclide can be traced in living tissue by the radiation they emit. In this image, different levels of radiation intensity are shown in different colors. The gamma-emitting radionuclide used here is absorbed more readily by cancerous bone than by normal bone. The white area in the spine corresponds to a high rate of gamma emission and indicates a tumor there.

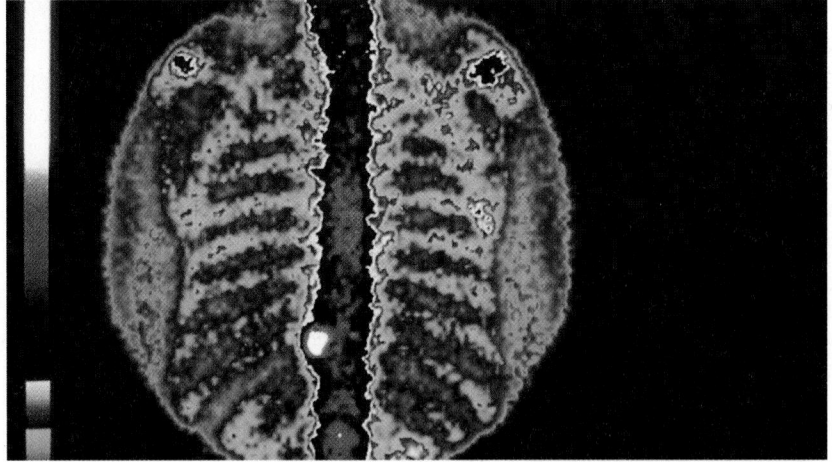

8.3   Radioactive Decay

How Unstable Nuclei Change into Stable Ones

Early experimenters found that a magnetic field splits the radiation from a radioactive material such as radium into three parts (Fig. 8-7). One part is deflected as though it consists of positively charged particles. Called **alpha particles,** these turned out to be the nuclei of helium atoms. Such nuclei contain two protons and two neutrons, so their symbol is $_2^4$He. (These were the probes used in Rutherford's discovery of the nucleus.)

Another part of the radiation is deflected as though it consists of negatively charged particles. Called **beta particles,** these are electrons.

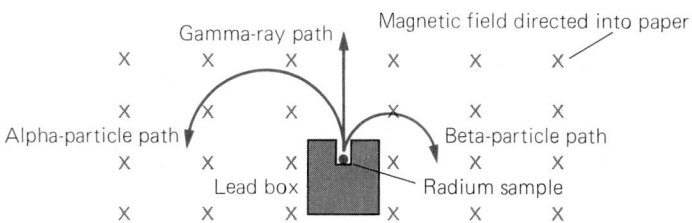

The rest of the radiation, which is not affected by a magnetic field, consists of **gamma rays.** Today these are known to be electromagnetic waves whose frequencies are higher than those of x-rays. A gamma ray is emitted by a nucleus that, for one reason or another, has more than its normal amount of energy. The composition of the nucleus does not change in gamma decay, unlike the cases of alpha and beta decay. Gamma rays are the most penetrating of the three kinds of radiation, alpha particles the least (Fig. 8-8).

Why Decays Occur A nucleus is said to **decay** when it emits an alpha or beta particle or a gamma ray. **Alpha decay** occurs in nuclei too large to be stable (Fig. 8-9). The forces that hold protons and neutrons together in a nucleus act only over short distances. As a result these particles interact strongly only with their nearest neighbors in a nucleus. Because the electrical repulsion of the protons is strong throughout the entire nucleus, there is a limit to the ability of neutrons to hold together a large nucleus. This limit is represented by the bismuth isotope $^{209}_{83}$Bi, which is the heaviest stable (that is, nonradioactive) nucleus. All larger nuclei become smaller ones by alpha decay.

Another cause of radioactive decay is a ratio of neutrons to protons that is too large or too small. A small nucleus is stable with equal numbers of neutrons and protons. However, larger nuclei need more neutrons than protons in order to overcome the electrical repulsion of the protons. In **beta decay,** one of the neutrons in a nucleus with too many of them spontaneously turns into a proton with the emission of an electron, as in Fig. 8-9.

In a nucleus with too few neutrons for stability, one of the protons may become a neutron with the emission of a **positron,** which is an electron that has a positive charge rather than a negative one. Alternatively one of the electrons in the atom may be absorbed by one of the protons to form a neutron. This process, which rarely occurs, is called **electron capture.** (An uncharged particle called a **neutrino,** whose mass is extremely small, is also emitted during beta decay, positron emission, and electron capture. See Sec. 8.15.)

Sometimes a certain nuclide requires a number of radioactive decays before it reaches a stable form. The uranium isotope $^{238}_{92}$U, for instance, undergoes eight alpha decays and six beta decays before it eventually becomes the lead isotope $^{206}_{82}$Pb, which is not radioactive.

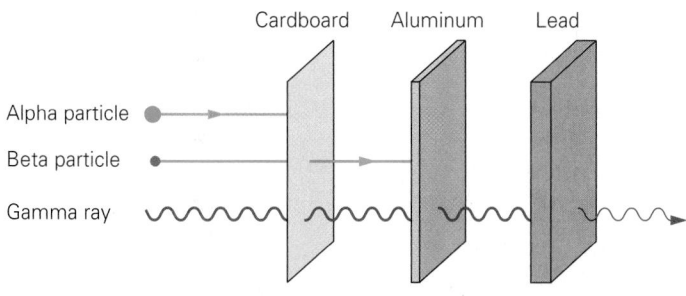

Figure 8-8 Alpha particles from radioactive materials are stopped by a piece of cardboard. Beta particles penetrate the cardboard but are stopped by a sheet of aluminum. Even a thick slab of lead may not stop all the gamma rays.

Figure 8-9   Five kinds of radioactive decay. In all of these processes electric charge is conserved (Sec. 6.1). The neutrinos emitted during beta decay, electron capture, and positron emission are not shown; they are uncharged and have very little mass.

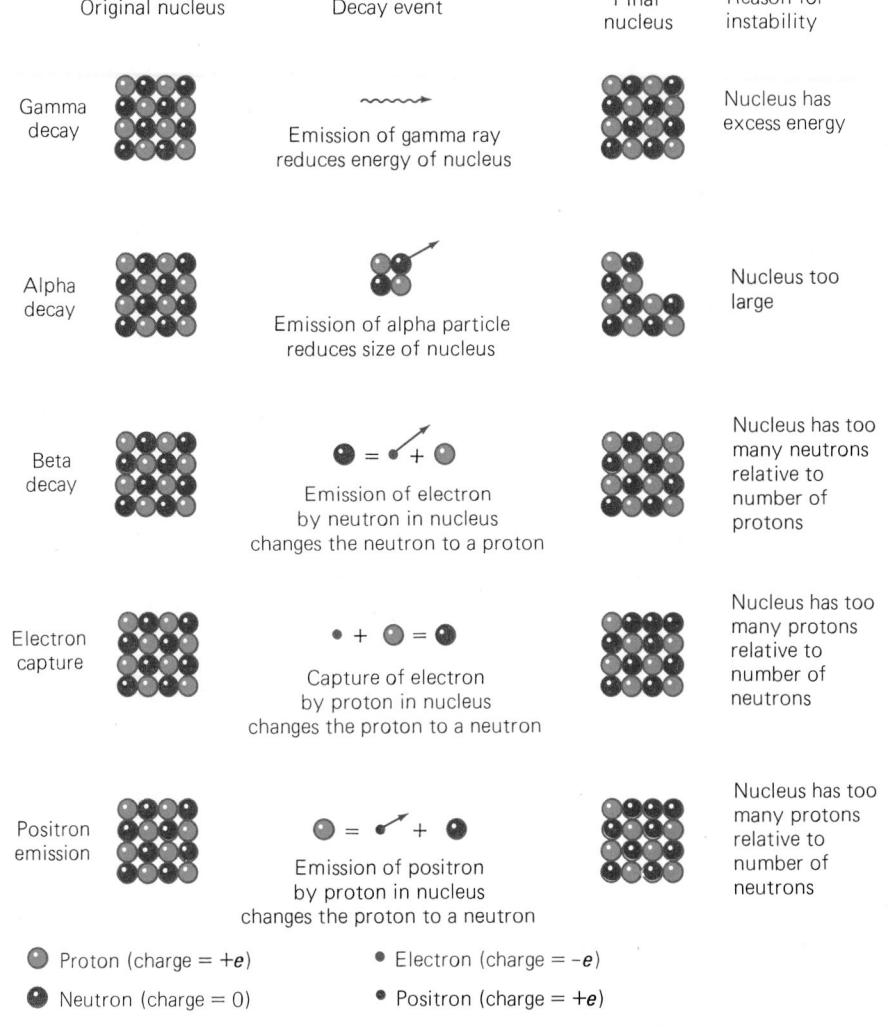

Original nucleus	Decay event	Final nucleus	Reason for instability
Gamma decay	Emission of gamma ray reduces energy of nucleus		Nucleus has excess energy
Alpha decay	Emission of alpha particle reduces size of nucleus		Nucleus too large
Beta decay	Emission of electron by neutron in nucleus changes the neutron to a proton		Nucleus has too many neutrons relative to number of protons
Electron capture	Capture of electron by proton in nucleus changes the proton to a neutron		Nucleus has too many protons relative to number of neutrons
Positron emission	Emission of positron by proton in nucleus changes the proton to a neutron		Nucleus has too many protons relative to number of neutrons

Proton (charge = +e)   Electron (charge = −e)
Neutron (charge = 0)   Positron (charge = +e)

Neutron Decay   Free neutrons outside of nuclei are unstable and undergo radioactive decay into a proton and an electron. The average lifetime of a free neutron is about 15 min before it decays. Nevertheless it is not correct to think of a neutron as a combination of a proton and an electron: a neutron is a separate particle with unique properties. If we were to try to create a neutron by bringing together a proton and an electron, we would merely get a hydrogen atom as the result, not a neutron. Protons outside a nucleus are apparently stable.

Example 8.1

Find the symbol of the nuclide into which the uranium isotope $^{232}_{92}U$ is transformed when it undergoes alpha decay.

Solution

An alpha particle is the ^4_2He nucleus, so when a nucleus undergoes alpha decay its atomic number decreases by 2 (corresponding to a loss of 2 protons) and its mass number decreases by 4 (corresponding to a loss of 4 nucleons). Hence the product of the alpha decay of $^{232}_{92}U$ has the atomic number 90 and the mass number 228. From Table 10-6 (see the inside back cover), thorium, Th, has the atomic number 90, so the result of the decay is $^{228}_{90}Th$.

Example 8.2

The bromine isotope $^{80}_{35}$Br can decay by emitting an electron or a positron or by capturing an electron. What is the equation of the process in each case?

Solution

(a) When a nucleus emits an electron, its charge increases by $+e$ (corresponding to a loss of $-e$), which means that its atomic number increases by 1. Thus the new nucleus has an atomic number of $Z = 35 + 1 = 36$. There is no change in mass number since the number of nucleons (protons + neutrons) stays the same. According to Table 10-6 the element with $Z = 36$ is krypton, Kr, so the equation of the process is

$$^{80}_{35}\text{Br} \rightarrow {}^{80}_{36}\text{Kr} + e^-$$

(b) When a nucleus emits a positron, its charge decreases by $-e$ (corresponding to a loss of $+e$), which means that Z decreases by 1. The new value of Z is therefore $35 - 1 = 34$, which is the atomic number of selenium, Se. Hence

$$^{80}_{35}\text{Br} \rightarrow {}^{80}_{34}\text{Se} + e^+$$

(c) When a nucleus captures an electron, its charge also decreases by $-e$, so the result is again $Z = 34$. In this case

$$^{80}_{35}\text{Br} + e^- \rightarrow {}^{80}_{34}\text{Se}$$

In each case we can see that the net electric charge does not change in the decay, so charge is conserved (as it must be).

8.4   Half-Life

Less and Less, But Always Some Left

The **half-life** of a radionuclide is the period of time needed for half of an initial amount of the nuclide to decay. As time goes on, the undecayed amount becomes smaller, but there is some left for many half-lives.

Suppose we start with 1 milligram (mg) of the radium isotope $^{226}_{88}$Ra, which alpha decays to the radon isotope $^{222}_{86}$Rn, with a half-life of about 1600 years. After 1600 years, 0.5 mg of radium will remain, with the rest having turned into radon (which, by the way, is a gas; radium is a metal). During the next 1600 years, half the 0.5 mg of radium that is left will decay, to leave 0.25 mg of radium (Fig. 8-10). After a further 1600 years, which means a total of 4800 years or 3 half-lives, 0.125 mg of radium will be left—still a fair amount. Even after 6 half-lives, more than 1 percent of an original sample will remain undecayed.

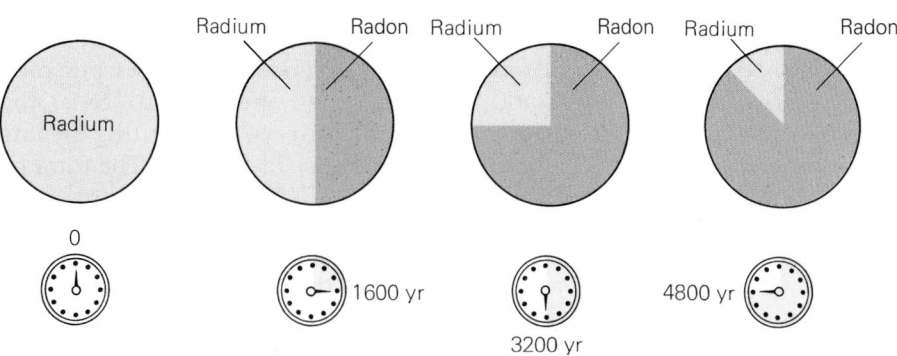

Figure 8-10   The decay of the radium isotope $^{226}_{88}$Ra. The number of undecayed radium atoms in a sample decreases by one-half in each 1600-year period. This time span is accordingly known as the "half-life" of radium. The radium alpha decays into the radon isotope $^{222}_{86}$Rn, whose own half-life is 3.8 days.

Every radionuclide has a characteristic and unchanging half-life. Some half-lives are only a millionth of a second; others are billions of years. Radon, for example, is an alpha emitter like its parent radium, but the half-life of radon is only 3.8 days instead of 1600 years. One of the biggest problems faced by nuclear power plants is the safe disposal of radioactive wastes since some of the isotopes present have long half-lives. The beta decay of neutrons when they are outside nuclei has a half-life of 14.5 min.

The dating of archaeological specimens and rock samples (including those brought back from the moon) by methods based on radioactive decay is described in Chap. 16.

Example 8.3

Potassium contains a small proportion of the radioactive isotope $_{19}^{40}\text{K}$, which decays into the isotope $_{18}^{40}\text{Ar}$ of the gas argon with a half-life of 1.3 billion years. When a rock whose minerals contain potassium is formed, no $_{18}^{40}\text{Ar}$ is present. As time goes on, the $_{19}^{40}\text{K}$ gradually decays into $_{18}^{40}\text{Ar}$, which is trapped in the rock. Comparing the amounts of $_{19}^{40}\text{K}$ and $_{18}^{40}\text{Ar}$ in a rock therefore lets us calculate how long ago the rock was formed. How old is a rock that is found to contain 3 times as much $_{18}^{40}\text{Ar}$ as $_{19}^{40}\text{K}$?

Solution
One-quarter of the original $_{19}^{40}\text{K}$ is left. Since $\frac{1}{4} = \frac{1}{2} \times \frac{1}{2}$, the rock is 2 half-lives old, which is 2.6 billion years.

8.5   Radiation Hazards

Invisible but Dangerous

The various radiations from radionuclides ionize matter through which they pass. X-rays ionize matter, too. All ionizing radiation is harmful to living tissue, although if the damage is slight, the tissue can often repair itself with no permanent effect. Radiation hazards are easy to underestimate because there is usually a delay, sometimes of many years, between an exposure and some of its possible consequences. These consequences include cancer, leukemia, and changes in reproductive cells that lead to children with physical deformities and mental handicaps. The relatively low-frequency em radiation emitted by power lines, cell phones, and the various electronic devices in the home does not ionize matter.

Radiation dosage is measured in **sieverts** (Sv), where 1 Sv is the amount of any radiation that has the same biological effects as those produced when 1 kg of body tissue absorbs 1 joule of x-rays or gamma rays. (A related unit sometimes used is the rem, equal to 0.01 Sv.) Although radiobiologists disagree about the exact relationship between radiation exposure and the likelihood of developing cancer or leukemia, there is no question that such a link exists. Natural sources of radiation lead to a dosage rate per person of about 3 mSv/y averaged over the U.S. population (1 mSv = 0.001 Sv). Other sources of radiation add 0.6 mSv/y, with medical x-rays contributing the largest amount; a typical mammogram involves a dose of 0.7 mSv. The total per person thus averages about 3.6 mSv/y.

Natural Sources   Figure 8-11 shows the relative contributions to the radiation dosage received by an average person in the United States. The most important single source is the radioactive gas radon, a decay product of radium whose own origin traces back to the decay of uranium. Uranium is found in many common rocks, notably granite. Hence radon, colorless and

---

Dose Limits

Many useful processes involve ionizing radiation. Some employ such radiation directly, as in the x-rays and gamma rays used in medicine and industry. In other cases the radiation is an unwanted but inescapable by-product, notably in the operation of nuclear reactors and in the disposal of their wastes.

An estimated 9 million people around the world are exposed to radiation at work. The radiation dosage limit for such people in the United States is 50 mSv per year. The maximum dose to the general public (who have no choice in the matter) from artificial sources has been set internationally at 1 mSv per year. By comparison, smoking 10 cigarettes a day gives a cancer death risk 100 times greater.

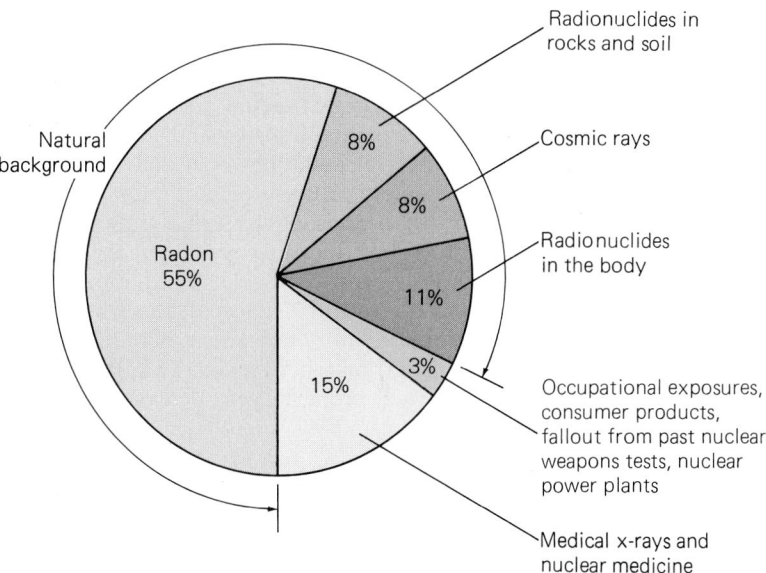

Natural background
Radon 55%

Radionuclides in rocks and soil — 8%

Cosmic rays — 8%

Radionuclides in the body — 11%

3%

15%

Occupational exposures, consumer products, fallout from past nuclear weapons tests, nuclear power plants

Medical x-rays and nuclear medicine

Figure 8-11 Sources of radiation dosage for an average person in the United States. Actual dosages vary widely. For instance, radon concentrations are not the same everywhere, some people receive more medical x-rays than others; cosmic rays are more intense at high altitudes; and so on. Nuclear power stations are responsible for 0.08 percent of the total, although accidents can raise the amount in affected areas to dangerous levels.

odorless, is present nearly everywhere, though usually in amounts too small to endanger health.

Problems arise when houses are built in uranium-rich regions, since it is impossible to prevent radon from entering such houses from the ground under them. Surveys show that millions of American homes have radon concentrations high enough to pose a small but definite cancer risk. As a cause of lung cancer, radon is second only to cigarette smoking. The most effective method of reducing radon levels in an existing house in a hazardous region seems to be to extract air from underneath the ground floor and disperse it into the atmosphere before it can enter the house.

Other natural sources of radiation dosage include cosmic rays from space (see Sec. 19.5) and radionuclides present in rocks and soil. The human body itself contains tiny amounts of radioisotopes of such elements as potassium and carbon. The cosmic-ray dosage depends on altitude because they are gradually absorbed by the atmosphere. Near sea level the dosage is around 0.3 mSv per year, more than that for aircrews and frequent fliers, 2 mSv per year in La Paz, Bolivia, 3700 m above sea level, and as much as 1 mSv per day for astronauts in orbit.

X-Rays   It is not always easy to find an appropriate balance between risk and benefit for medical x-ray exposures, many of which are made for no strong reason and may do more harm than good. In this category are many "routine" x-rays. Particularly dangerous is the x-raying of pregnant women, until not long ago another "routine" procedure, which dramatically increases the chance of cancer in their children. Children themselves are extremely susceptible to harm from x-rays.

Of course, x-rays have many valuable applications in medicine. The point is that every x-ray exposure should have a definite justification that outweighs the risk involved, and patients should never hesitate to question the strength of such justification. Unfortunately not all doctors appreciate the very real hazards of x-rays. This is especially true of CT scans (Fig. 9-11); a typical abdominal CT scan delivers an x-ray dosage 400 times that of an ordinary chest x-ray. Overdoses occur regularly. In one case, for 18 months a major Los Angeles hospital exposed hundreds of patients to as much as eight

MRI Scans

Magnetic resonance imaging (MRI) is a scanning method that does not involve ionizing radiation and so is completely safe (see Fig. 9-39). MRI and CT scans do not respond to body tissues in the same way and one or the other may be superior for a given medical condition; sometimes both are needed. Like CT scans, many MRI scans are unnecessary as well as very expensive, and many of both are of too low quality to show up important details. The best imaging centers are accredited by the American College of Radiology and use certified technicians.

Radiation Therapy

High-energy x-rays are regularly used to treat malignant tumors. In the United States, over half of all cancer patients receive such therapy. Unfortunatly, the radiation beams must pass through healthy tissue before and after attacking cancerous cells, which increases the risk of new cancers later in life. Even worse are inexcusable mistakes made by careless or inadequately trained technicians or therapists (17 states do not require them to be licensed). The usual errors involve incorrect radiation dosages—too little is ineffective, too much may do great harm—and missing the tumor entirely through poor aiming. Sometimes the wrong body part, or even the wrong patient, is irradiated.

An investigation by the *New York Times* in reported all too many dreadful injuries and agonizing deaths caused by powerful machines operated without attention to basic safety procedures. Radiation therapy has saved many thousands of lives that otherwise would have been lost, but that does not mean the associated risks can be disregarded. Because radiation accidents do not always have to be reported, there are no accurate statistics available, but one expert thinks it possible that 1 in 20 patients receiving radiation therapy does not receive a properly aimed correct dose in each exposure.

times the normal (already large) amount of radiation in CT scans before the errors were detected. The overdoses came to light only when the patients complained of hair loss.

In the United States, 70 million CT scans are made every year, and the need for so many has not been established. A recent study estimated that eventually 14,000 people per year in this country will die as a result of the radiation they received from CT scans. Worst of all are CT scans of symptomless people to look for possible hidden abnormalities, which almost all authorities feel seldom justify the very real risks involved. The Food and Drug Administration, which has jurisdiction over medical devices, "has done little to assess whether the rapid proliferation of scans is in the best interests of patients, and whether the machines themselves properly protect patients or are beneficial for all their now-routine uses," according to a report in the *New York Times* in March 2010. The strong public reaction to the report led the FDA, which had until then ignored the concerns of many doctors and members of its own staff, to contemplate steps to promote radiation safety.

Nuclear Energy

The atomic nucleus is the energy source of the reactors that produce more and more of the world's electricity. It is also the energy source of the most destructive weapons ever invented. But there is more to nuclear energy than these applications: nearly all the energy that keeps the sun and stars shining comes from the nucleus as well. Before considering what nuclear energy does, let us look into exactly what it is.

8.6 Units of Mass and Energy

The Atomic Mass Unit and the Electronvolt

Until now we have been using the kilogram as the unit of mass and the joule as the unit of energy. These units are far too large in the atomic world, and physicists find it more convenient to use smaller units for mass and energy in this world.

The **atomic mass unit** (u) has the value

$$1 \text{ atomic mass unit} = 1 \text{ u} = 1.66 \times 10^{-27} \text{ kg}$$

This mass is approximately equal to the mass of the hydrogen atom, whose actual mass is 1.008 u.

The energy unit used in atomic physics is the **electronvolt** (eV), which is the energy gained by an electron accelerated by a potential difference of 1 volt. The joule equivalent of the electronvolt is

$$1 \text{ electronvolt} = 1 \text{ eV} = 1.60 \times 10^{-19} \text{ J}$$

A typical quantity expressed in electronvolts is the energy needed to remove an electron from an atom. In the case of a nitrogen atom this energy is 14.5 eV, for example.

In nuclear physics the electronvolt is too small, and its multiple the **megaelectronvolt** (MeV) is more suitable:

$$1 \text{ megaelectronvolt} = 1 \text{ MeV} = 10^6 \text{ eV} = 1.60 \times 10^{-13} \text{ J}$$

(*Mega* is the prefix for million.) A typical quantity expressed in megaelectronvolts is the energy of the radiation emitted by a radionuclide. The alpha particle emitted by a nucleus of the radium isotope $^{226}_{88}$Ra has an energy of 4.9 MeV, for example.

The energy equivalent ($E_0 = mc^2$) of a rest mass of 1 u is 931 MeV.

8.7   Binding Energy

The Missing Energy That Keeps a Nucleus Together

An ordinary hydrogen atom has a nucleus that consists of a single proton, as its symbol $^1_1$H indicates. The isotope of hydrogen called deuterium, $^2_1$H, has a neutron as well as a proton in its nucleus. Thus we expect the mass of the deuterium atom to equal the mass of a $^1_1$H hydrogen atom plus the mass of a neutron:

Mass of $^1_1$H atom	1.0078 u
+Mass of neutron	+1.0087 u
Expected mass of $^2_1$H atom	2.0165 u

However, the measured mass of the $^2_1$H atom is only 2.0141 u, which is 0.0024 u *less* than the combined masses of a $^1_1$H atom and a neutron (Fig. 8-12).

Deuterium atoms are not the only ones that have less mass than the combined masses of the particles they are composed of—*all* atoms (except $^1_1$H) are like that. We conclude that nuclei are stable because they lack enough mass to break up into separate nucleons.

Where the Mass Goes   What happens when a nucleus is formed is that a certain amount of energy is given off due to the action of the forces that hold the neutrons and protons together. Energy is similarly given off due to the action of gravity when a stone strikes the ground or due to the action of

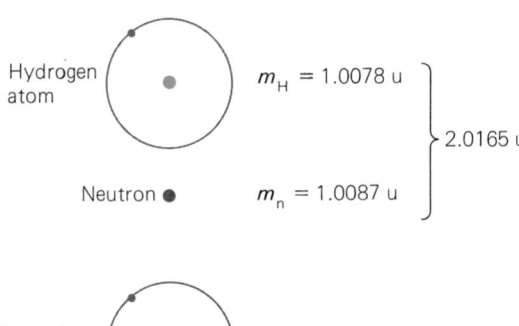

Figure 8-12   The mass of a deuterium atom ($^2_1$H) is less than the sum of the masses of a hydrogen atom ($^1_1$H) and a neutron. The energy equivalent of the missing mass is called the binding energy of the nucleus.

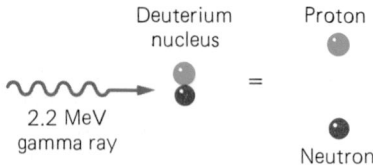

Figure 8-13   The binding energy of the deuterium nucleus is 2.2 MeV. A gamma ray whose energy is 2.2 MeV or more can split a deuterium nucleus into a proton and neutron. A gamma ray whose energy is less than 2.2 MeV cannot do this.

intermolecular forces when water freezes into ice. In the case of a nucleus, the energy comes from the mass of the particles that join together. The resulting nucleus therefore has less mass than the total mass of the particles before they interact.

Since the energy equivalent of 1 u of mass is 931 MeV, the energy that corresponds to the missing deuterium mass of 0.0024 u is

$$\text{Missing energy} = (0.0024 \text{ u})(931 \text{ MeV/u}) = 2.2 \text{ MeV}$$

To test the above interpretation of the missing mass, we can perform experiments to see how much energy is needed to break apart a deuterium nucleus into a separate neutron and proton. The required energy turns out to be 2.2 MeV, as we expect (Fig. 8-13). When less energy than 2.2 MeV is given to a $_1^2$H nucleus, the nucleus stays together. When the added energy is more than 2.2 MeV, the extra energy goes into kinetic energy of the neutron and proton as they fly apart.

> The energy equivalent of the missing mass of a nucleus is called the **binding energy** of the nucleus. The greater its binding energy, the more the energy that must be supplied to break up the nucleus.

Nuclear binding energies are strikingly high. The range for stable nuclei is from 2.2 MeV for $_1^2$H (deuterium) to 1640 MeV for $_{83}^{209}$Bi (an isotope of the metal bismuth). Larger nuclei are all unstable and decay radioactively. To appreciate how high binding energies are, we can compare them with more familiar energies in terms of kilojoules of energy per kilogram of mass. In these units, a typical binding energy is 8×10^{11} kJ/kg—800 billion kJ/kg. By contrast, to boil water involves a heat of vaporization of a mere 2260 kJ/kg, and even the heat given off by burning gasoline is only 4.7×10^4 kJ/kg, 17 million times smaller.

8.8   Binding Energy per Nucleon

Why Fission and Fusion Liberate Energy

For a given nucleus, the **binding energy per nucleon** is found by dividing the total binding energy of the nucleus by the number of nucleons (protons and neutrons) it contains. Thus the binding energy per nucleon for $_1^2$H is 2.2 MeV/2 = 1.1 MeV/nucleon, and for $_{83}^{209}$Bi it is 1640 MeV/209 = 7.8 MeV/nucleon.

Figure 8-14 shows binding energy per nucleon plotted against mass number (number of nucleons). The greater the binding energy per nucleon, the

---

Example 8.4

The binding energy of the neon isotope $_{10}^{20}$Ne is 161 MeV. Find its atomic mass.

Solution

The $_{10}^{20}$Ne atom contains 10 protons and 10 neutrons. The total mass m_0 of 10 H atoms and 10 neutrons is

$$m_0 = 10m_{\text{H}} + 10m_{\text{n}} = 10 \ (1.0078 \text{ u}) + 10 \ (1.0087 \text{ u}) = 20.165 \text{ u}$$

The mass equivalent Δm of 161 MeV is

$$\Delta m = \frac{161 \text{ MeV}}{931 \text{ MeV/u}} = 0.173 \text{ u}$$

and so the atomic mass of $_{10}^{20}$Ne is

$$m = m_0 - \Delta m = 20.165 \text{ u} - 0.173 \text{ u} = 19.992 \text{ u}$$

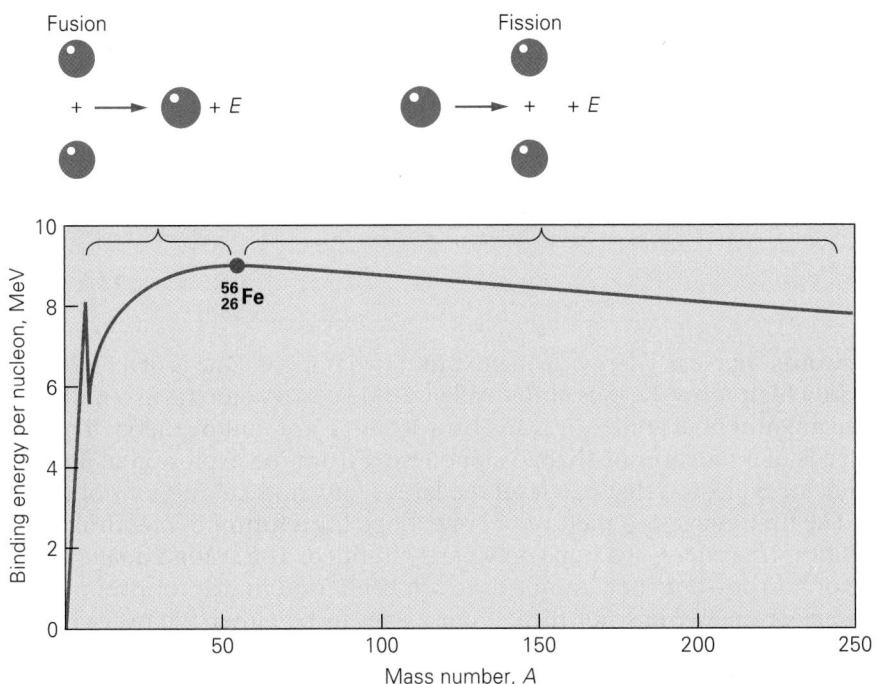

Figure 8-14 The binding energy per nucleon is a maximum for nuclei of mass number $A = 56$. Such nuclei are the most stable. When two light nuclei join to form a heavier one, a process called *fusion*, the greater binding energy of the product nucleus causes energy to be given off. When a heavy nucleus is split into two lighter ones, a process called *fission*, the greater binding energy of the product nuclei also causes energy to be given off. The peak at $A = 4$ corresponds to the $^4_2$He nucleus whose stability enables it to remain intact when emitted in alpha decay (Fig. 8-9).

more stable the nucleus. The graph has its maximum of 8.8 MeV/nucleon when the number of nucleons is 56. The nucleus that has 56 protons and neutrons is $^{56}_{26}$Fe, an iron isotope. This is the most stable nucleus of them all, since the most energy is needed to pull a nucleon away from it. Larger and smaller nuclei are less stable.

Fission Two remarkable conclusions can be drawn from the curve of Fig. 8-14. The first is that, if we somehow split a heavy nucleus into two medium-size ones, each of the new nuclei will have *more* binding energy per nucleon (and hence less mass per nucleon) than the original nucleus did. The extra energy will be given off, and it can be a lot.

As an example, if the uranium nucleus $^{235}_{92}$U is broken into two smaller nuclei, the difference in binding energy per nucleon is about 0.8 MeV. Since $^{235}_{92}$U contains 235 nucleons, the total energy given off is

$$\left(0.8 \, \frac{\text{MeV}}{\text{nucleon}}\right)(235 \text{ nucleons}) = 188 \text{ MeV}$$

This is a truly enormous amount of energy to come from a single atomic event. For comparison, ordinary chemical reactions involve only a few eV per atom. Splitting a large nucleus, which is called **nuclear fission,** thus involves a hundred million times more energy per atom than, say, burning coal or oil.

Fusion The other notable conclusion from Fig. 8-14 is that joining two light nuclei together to give a single nucleus of medium size also means more binding energy per nucleon in the new nucleus. For instance, if two $^2_1$H deuterium nuclei combine to form a $^4_2$He helium nucleus, over 23 MeV is released. Such a process, called **nuclear fusion,** is also a very effective way to obtain energy. In fact, nuclear fusion is the main energy source of the sun and other stars, as described in Chap. 18.

The graph of Fig. 8-14 is extremely significant because it is the key to understanding energy production in the universe. The fact that binding energy exists at all means that nuclei more complex than the single proton of hydrogen can be stable. This stability in turn accounts for the existence of the various elements and consequently for the existence of the many and diverse forms of matter we see around us.

Because the curve peaks in the middle, we have the explanation for the energy that powers, directly or indirectly, the evolution of much of the universe: this energy comes from the fusion of protons and light nuclei to form heavier nuclei. And the harnessing of nuclear fission in reactors and weapons has irreversibly changed modern civilization.

Fission and Fusion

The words "nuclear energy" bring to mind two images. One is of a huge building in which a mysterious thing called a nuclear reactor turns an absurdly small amount of uranium into an absurdly large amount of energy. The other image is of a mushroom-shaped cloud rising from the explosion of a nuclear bomb, an explosion that can level the largest city and kill millions of people.

The first image is a picture of hope, hope for a future of plentiful, cheap, pollution-free energy—a hope only partly fulfilled. The second image is a picture of horror—but such bombs have not been used in war for over 60 years. So nuclear energy has not turned out as yet to be either the overwhelming blessing or the overwhelming curse it might have been.

8.9   Nuclear Fission

Divide and Conquer

As we have seen, a lot of energy will be released if we can break a large nucleus into smaller ones. But nuclei are ordinarily not at all easy to break up. What we need is a way to split a heavy nucleus without using more energy than we get back from the process.

The answer came in 1939 with the discovery that a nucleus of the uranium isotope $^{235}_{92}U$ undergoes fission when struck by a neutron. It is not the impact of the neutron that has this effect. Instead, the $^{235}_{92}U$ nucleus absorbs the neutron to become $^{236}_{92}U$, and the new nucleus is so unstable that almost at once it splits into two pieces (Fig. 8-15). Isotopes of several elements besides uranium were later found to be fissionable by neutrons in similar processes.

Most of the energy set free in fission goes into kinetic energy of the new nuclei. These nuclei are usually radioactive, some with long half-lives. Hence the products of fission, which are found in reactor fuel rods and in the fallout

Figure 8-15   In nuclear fission an absorbed neutron causes a heavy nucleus to split into two parts. Several neutrons and gamma rays are emitted in the process. The smaller nuclei shown here are typical of those produced in the fission of $^{235}_{92}U$.

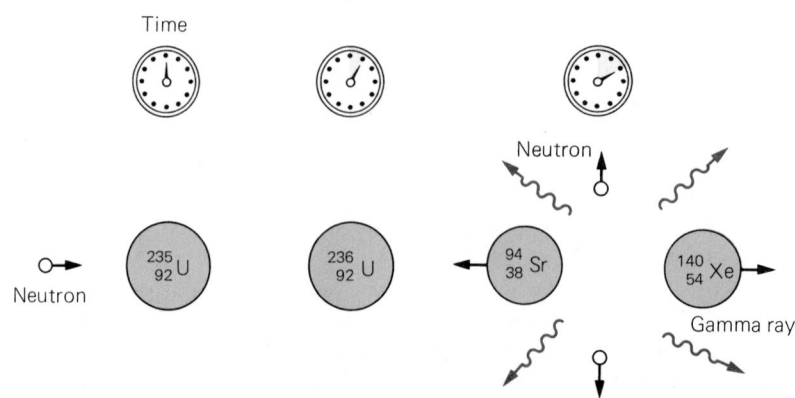

BIOGRAPHY | Lise Meitner (1878–1968)

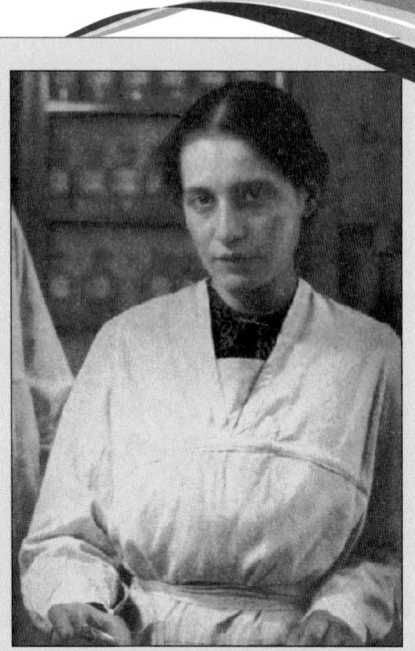

The daughter of a Viennese lawyer, Meitner became interested in science when she read about the Curies and radium. She earned her Ph.D. in physics in 1905 at the University of Vienna, only the second woman to obtain a doctorate there. She then went to Berlin where she began research on radioactivity with the chemist Otto Hahn. Their supervisor refused to have a woman in his laboratory, so they started their work in a carpentry shop. Ten years later she was a professor, a department head, and, with Hahn, the discoverer of a new element, protactinium.

In the 1930s the Italian physicist Enrico Fermi found that bombarding heavy elements with neutrons led to the production of other elements. What happened in the case of uranium was puzzling, and Meitner and Hahn tried to find the answer. At the time the German persecution of Jews had begun, but Meitner, who was Jewish, was protected by her Austrian citizenship. In 1938 Germany annexed Austria, and Meitner fled to Sweden but kept in touch with Hahn and their younger colleague Fritz Strassmann.

Hahn and Strassmann finally concluded that neutrons interact with uranium to produce radium, but Meitner's calculations showed that this was impossible and she urged them to persist in their experiments. They did, and found to their surprise that the lighter element barium in fact had been created. Meitner surmised that the neutrons had caused the uranium nuclei to split apart and, with her nephew Otto Frisch, developed the theoretical picture of what they called fission.

In January 1939, Hahn and Strassmann published the discovery of fission in a German journal; because Meitner was Jewish, they thought it safer to ignore her contribution. Meitner and Frisch later published their own paper on fission in an English journal, but it was too late: Hahn disgracefully claimed full credit, and not once in the years that followed acknowledged her role. Hahn alone received the Nobel Prize in physics for discovering fission. Unfortunately Meitner did not live to see a measure of justice: the element of atomic number 109 is called meitnerium in her honor, while the tentative name of hahnium for element 105 was changed in 1997 to dubnium, after the Russian nuclear research center in Dubna.

from a nuclear weapon explosion, are extremely dangerous and remain so for many generations.

Chain Reaction   When a nucleus breaks apart, two or three neutrons are set free at the same time. This suggests a remarkable possibility. Perhaps, under the right conditions, the neutrons emitted by one uranium nucleus as it undergoes fission can cause other uranium nuclei to split; the neutrons from these other fissions might then go on to split still more uranium nuclei; and so on, with a series of fission reactions spreading through a mass of uranium. A **chain reaction** of this kind was first demonstrated in Chicago in 1942 under the direction of Enrico Fermi, an Italian physicist who had not long before taken refuge in the United States (Fig. 8-16). Figure 8-17 is a sketch of the events that occur in a chain reaction.

For a chain reaction to occur, at least one neutron produced by each fission must, on the average, lead to another fission and not either escape or be absorbed without producing fission. If too few neutrons cause fissions, the reaction slows down and stops. If precisely one neutron per fission causes another fission, energy is released at a steady rate. This is the case in a nuclear reactor, which is an arrangement for producing controlled power from nuclear fission.

Nuclear Weapons   What happens if more than one neutron from each fission causes other fissions? Then the chain reaction speeds up and the energy release is so fast that an explosion results. An "atomic" bomb makes use of

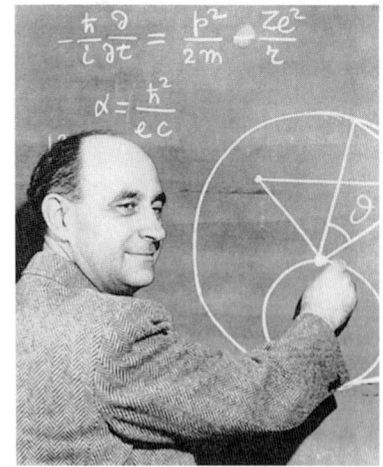

Figure 8-16   Enrico Fermi (1901–1954).

Figure 8-17 Sketch of a chain reaction. The reaction continues if at least one neutron from each fission event on the average induces another fission event. If more than one neutron per fission on the average induces another fission, the reaction is explosive.

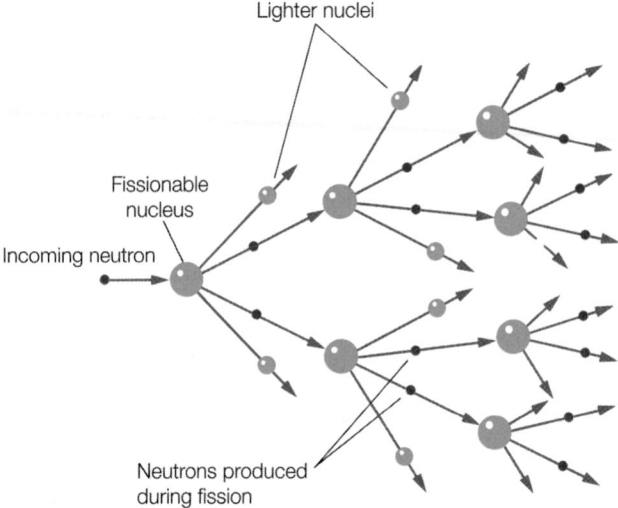

this effect. The destructive power of nuclear weapons does not stop with their detonation but continues long afterward through the radioactive debris that is produced and widely dispersed. A single modern nuclear bomb set off above New York City would leave about 4 million people dead by the next day with millions more fatalities later from radiation exposure.

The discovery of fission became known in the United States in 1939, just before the start of World War II. Its military possibilities were immediately recognized. Expecting that German physicists would come to the same conclusion and would start work on a nuclear bomb, the United States began such a program in earnest. By the time it had succeeded, in 1945, Germany had been defeated, and two nuclear bombs exploded over Hiroshima and Nagasaki then ended the war with Japan. It was later learned that the German effort had amounted to very little.

Not long afterward the Soviet Union, Great Britain, and France also developed nuclear weapons, and later China, Israel, South Africa, India, Pakistan, and North Korea did so as well. South Africa voluntarily abandoned its nuclear weapons program, the only country to do so. The present nuclear powers have among themselves about 23,000 weapons (Table 8-1), many times more than enough to destroy all human life. It is impossible to ascribe a rational purpose to the existence of so many of these weapons.

Table 8-1	**Estimated Stockpiles of Nuclear Weapons**
Country	**Nuclear Warheads**
Russia	13,000
United States	9400
France	300
China	240
Great Britain	185
Israel	80
Pakistan	60
India	60
North Korea	<10

Note: Accurate figures are not available. Not all of the nuclear weapons of Russia and the United States are operational, and both countries have agreed to reduce their stocks of "operationally deployed" weapons in the years to come. In 2010, the nuclear arsenal of the United States contained 5113 operational weapons, down from its peak of 31,255 in 1967. An estimated $8 trillion has been spent on nuclear weapons in the world thus far.

Unfortunately it is not a giant step from a nuclear reactor program for energy generation to a nuclear weapons program. At least 20 countries besides those listed above already have the skills and materials to develop nuclear weapons, and a few may have begun the process. Minimizing the nuclear threat is a continuing task.

8.10   How a Reactor Works

From Uranium to Heat to Electricity

For every gram of uranium that undergoes fission in a reactor, 2.6 tons of coal must be burned in an ordinary power plant of the same rating. The energy given off in a nuclear reactor becomes heat, which is removed by a liquid or gas coolant. The hot coolant is then used to boil water, and the resulting steam is fed to a turbine that can power an electric generator, a ship, or a submarine.

In order for a chain reaction to occur at a steady rate, one neutron from each fission must cause another fission to take place. Since each fission in ^{235}U liberates an average of 2.5 neutrons, no more than 1.5 neutrons per fission can be lost on the average. However, natural uranium contains only 0.7 percent of the fissionable isotope ^{235}U. The rest is ^{238}U, an isotope that captures the rapidly moving neutrons emitted during the fission of ^{235}U but usually does not undergo fission afterward. The neutrons absorbed by ^{238}U are therefore wasted, and since 99.3 percent of natural uranium is ^{238}U, too many disappear for a chain reaction to occur in a solid lump of natural uranium.

Fast and Slow Neutrons   There is an ingenious way around this problem. As it happens, ^{238}U tends to pick up only fast neutrons, not slow ones. In addition, slow neutrons are more apt to induce fission in ^{235}U than fast ones. If the fast neutrons from fission are slowed down, then many more will produce further fissions despite the small proportion of ^{235}U present.

To slow down fission neutrons, the uranium fuel in a reactor is mixed with a **moderator,** a substance whose nuclei absorb energy from fast neutrons that collide with them. In general, the more nearly equal in mass colliding particles are, the more energy is transferred. A ball bounces off a wall with little loss of energy, but it can lose all its energy when it strikes another ball (Fig. 3-24). Since hydrogen nuclei are protons with nearly the same mass as neutrons, hydrogen is widely used as a moderator in the form of water, H_2O, each of whose molecules contains two hydrogen atoms along with an oxygen atom.

Unfortunately a neutron striking a proton has a certain tendency to stick to it to form a deuterium nucleus, ^2_1H. As a result, a reactor whose moderator is water cannot use ordinary uranium as fuel but must instead use **enriched** uranium whose ^{235}U content has been increased to 3 to 5 percent. Uranium enriched to about 90 percent of ^{235}U is used in one type of nuclear weapon.

In a welcome program, both Russia and the United States have begun to dismantle some of their nuclear weapons and convert their cores to reactor fuel by diluting their enriched uranium content. Today about half the reactor fuel in the United States is produced in this way and is used to generate 10 percent of the country's electricity.

8.11   Plutonium

Another Fissionable Material

Some nonfissionable nuclides can be changed into fissionable ones by absorbing neutrons. A notable example is ^{238}U, which becomes ^{239}U when it

---

A Natural Reactor

Because ^{235}U has a shorter half-life than ^{238}U, in the past the ^{235}U/^{238}U ratio in uranium was higher than the 0.7 percent of today. This raises the possibility that, in former times when the ^{235}U/^{238}U ratio was 3 percent or more, a uranium deposit with nearby water to act as moderator could have sustained a chain reaction.

In fact, such a natural reactor seems to have existed 2 billion years ago in West Africa in what is today Gabon, which developed about 100 kW. Studies of rock samples from the area indicate that the reactor operated until the heat it produced boiled away water in the rocks around the uranium deposit, which typically took 30 min. Then the lack of water stopped the chain reaction for typically 2.5 h until enough water had seeped back to restart it. This cycle continued for perhaps 150,000 years. There once may well have been other natural reactors in addition to the one in Gabon.

Nuclear Power Plants

The fuel for a nuclear reactor consists of uranium oxide pellets sealed in long, thin tubes (Fig. 8-18). Control rods of cadmium or boron, which are good absorbers of slow neutrons, can be slid in and out of the reactor core to adjust the rate of the chain reaction.

In the most common type of reactor, water under pressure (to prevent boiling) circulates around the fuel in the core where it acts as both moderator and coolant. As in Fig. 8-19, the pressurized water transfers heat from the chain reaction in the fuel rods to a steam generator. The resulting steam then passes out of the containment shell, which serves as a barrier to protect the outside world from accidents to the reactor, and is piped to a turbine that drives an electric generator. Various aspects of nuclear reactors as commercial energy sources were discussed in Sec. 4.8.

In a typical plant, the steel reactor vessel is 13.5 m high and 4.4 m in diameter and weighs 385 tons. It contains 90 tons of uranium oxide in the form of 50,952 fuel rods, each 3.85 m long and 9.5 mm in diameter. Four steam generators are used, instead of the single one shown in Fig. 8-19, as well as a number of turbine-generators. The reactor operates at 3400 MW and yields 1100 MW of electric power, enough for the needs of over a million people. The fuel must be replaced every few years as the concentration of neutron-absorbing fission products builds up.

New designs for nuclear reactors incorporate what are hoped to be major improvements in efficiency and reliability. Some of the proposed reactors would have higher power outputs than existing ones; others would have much smaller outputs. If all goes well, the

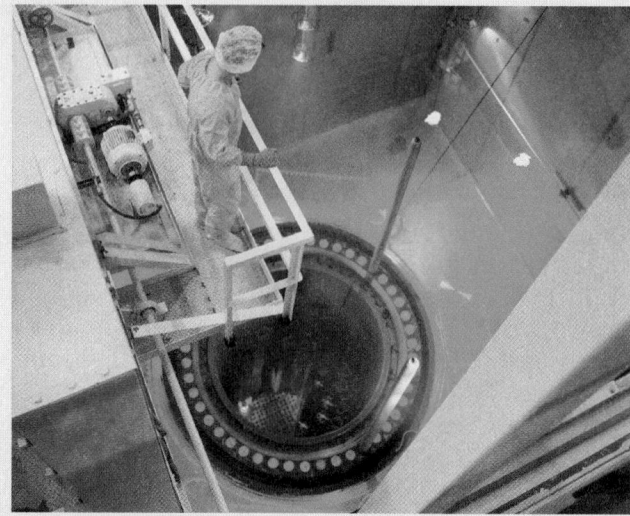

Figure 8-18   Loading fuel rods into a reactor at the Comanche Peak power station in Texas. The rods are metal tubes filled with pellets of uranium oxide. Water circulated through the reactor vessel is both the moderator that slows the fast neutrons liberated in fission events and also the coolant that removes the energy released. The working life of a power reactor is usually assumed to be 40–60 years, after which comes the problem of what to do with it.

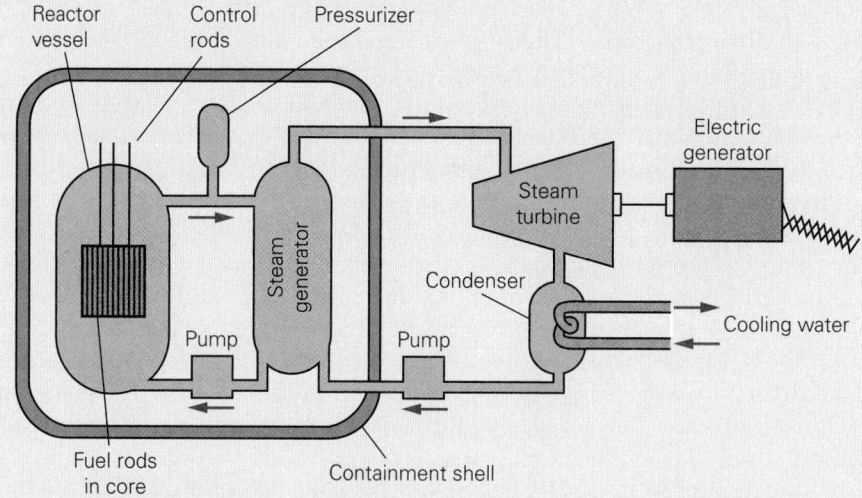

Figure 8-19   Basic design of a typical nuclear power plant.

latter reactors would not only provide cheaper electricity than existing ones but also might be able to act as heat sources to replace the furnaces in plants that now burn coal. The smaller reactors could be built in factories at less cost and in half the time than if built on site. The International Atomic Energy Agency estimates global demand for small reactors to be 500–1000 by 2040.

captures a fast neutron. The latter uranium isotope beta-decays soon after its creation into the neptunium isotope $^{239}_{93}$Np. In turn $^{239}_{93}$Np beta-decays into the plutonium isotope $^{239}_{94}$Pu (Fig. 8-20). Like ^{235}U, ^{239}Pu undergoes fission when it absorbs a neutron and can support a chain reaction.

Both neptunium and plutonium are called **transuranium elements** because their atomic numbers are greater than the 92 of uranium. Other transuranium elements have been created in the laboratory up to atomic number 118 in high-energy collisions of lighter nuclei. Element 110, to give an example, was first produced in 1994 by bombarding lead nuclei with nickel nuclei. No transuranium elements of natural origin are found on the earth because all of them decay too fast to have survived even if they had been present when the earth came into being 4.6 billion years ago.

A certain amount of plutonium is produced in the normal operation of a uranium-fueled reactor, and its fission adds to the energy produced by the reactor. Plutonium separated from the uranium that remains in a used fuel rod can serve as a reactor fuel itself and also, like highly enriched uranium, as the active ingredient in nuclear weapons. Roughly 25 kg of highly enriched uranium or 4 kg of plutonium is the minimum needed for a bomb.

Breeder Reactors   A **breeder reactor** is one especially designed to produce more plutonium than the ^{235}U it consumes. Because the otherwise useless ^{238}U is 140 times more abundant than the fissionable ^{235}U, using breeder reactors would allow reserves of uranium to last much longer. In the past, breeder reactors were expensive and unreliable and few were built. However, new technologies have been proposed that could extract energy from spent reactor fuel while minimizing radioactive waste. If they succeed, uranium reserves would last for many centuries to come, but serious problems remain to be overcome and economic solutions to them may not be possible.

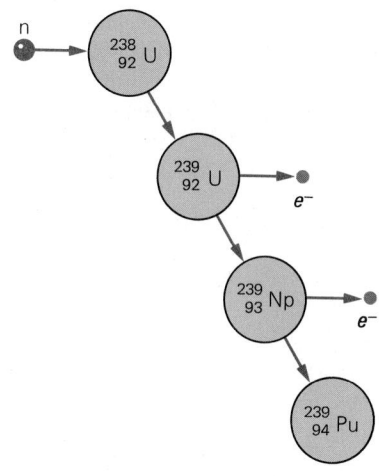

Figure 8-20   The nonfissionable uranium isotope ^{238}U, which makes up 99.3 percent of natural uranium, becomes the fissionable plutonium isotope ^{239}Pu by absorbing a neutron and beta-decaying twice. This transformation is the basis of the breeder reactor, which produces many times more nuclear fuel in the form of plutonium than it uses up in the form of ^{235}U.

8.12   Nuclear Fusion

The Energy Source of the Future?

For all the energy produced by fission, the fusion of small nuclei to form larger ones can yield even more energy per kilogram of starting materials. Nuclear fusion is the energy source of the sun and stars, as discussed in Chap. 18. On the earth, it is possible that fusion will become the ultimate source of energy: safe, almost nonpolluting, and with the oceans supplying limitless fuel.

Three conditions must be met by a successful fusion reactor:

1. A high temperature—100 million °C or more—so that the nuclei are moving fast enough to collide despite the repulsion of their positive electric charges.
2. A high concentration of the nuclei to ensure that such collisions are frequent.
3. The reacting nuclei must remain together for a long enough time to give off more energy than the reactor's operation uses.

The last two conditions are related, since the more nuclei there are in a given volume, the shorter the minimum confinement time for a net energy output.

The fusion reaction that is the basis of current research involves the combination of a deuterium nucleus and a tritium nucleus to form a helium nucleus (Fig. 8-21):

$$\underset{\text{deuterium}}{^{2}_{1}\text{H}} \ + \ \underset{\text{tritium}}{^{3}_{1}\text{H}} \ \rightarrow \ \underset{\text{helium}}{^{4}_{2}\text{He}} \ + \ \underset{\text{neutron}}{^{1}_{0}n} \ + \ \underset{\text{energy}}{17.6 \text{ MeV}} \qquad \textit{Fusion reaction}$$

Most of the energy given off is carried by the neutron that is emitted. To recover this energy, one proposal is to surround the reactor chamber with lithium to absorb the neutrons. The resulting hot lithium would then act as the heat source for a conventional electric generating system.

Figure 8-21 The deuterium-tritium fusion reaction liberates a great deal of energy, most of which is carried off by the neutron as kinetic energy.

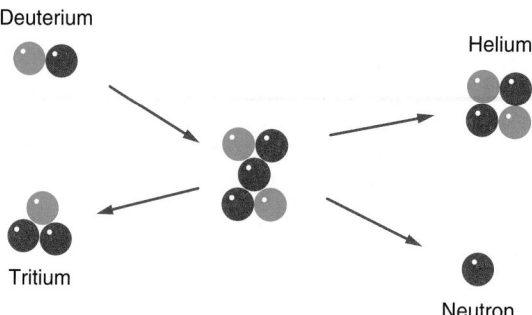

Deuterium

Helium

Tritium

Neutron

About 0.015 percent of the waters of the world is deuterium, which adds up to a total of over 10^{15} tons of ^2_1H—no scarcity there. A gallon of seawater has the potential for fusion energy equivalent to the chemical energy in 600 gallons of gasoline. Seawater contains too little tritium for economic recovery, but as it happens, neutrons react with lithium nuclei to yield tritium and helium. Thus, once a fusion reactor is given an initial charge of tritium, it will make enough additional tritium from the surrounding lithium for its further operation. (Lithium is plentiful in the earth and its oceans.)

Several Approaches   The big problem in making fusion energy practical is to achieve the necessary combination of temperature, density, and confinement time. Two main approaches are being explored. In one, strong magnetic fields are used to keep the reacting nuclei close together. Five decades of research have led to larger and larger experimental magnetic fusion reactors that have brought to light no reasons why eventual success should not be possible.

The larger the reactor, the better its contents can maintain the required high temperature. The current record for size is held by the Joint European Torus (a torus has the shape of a doughnut) in England, which is 15 m across and 20 m high. In 1997 it produced fusion power at a record 16 MW for a brief period and 5 MW for 5 s. An international effort to build a similar reactor, called ITER, with a volume almost six times greater is in progress. If all goes well, commercial fusion reactors could be operating by 2050.

The other chief approach to practical fusion energy uses energetic beams to both heat and compress tiny fuel pellets. Laser beams (see Chap. 9) are being tried for this purpose at the $3.5 billion National Ignition Facility of the Lawrence Livermore National Laboratory in California. An initial laser beam is split into 192 separate beams that are each amplified 3×10^{15} times to give pulses whose total energy is 1.8 MJ. The corresponding power is 500 times the output of all the power stations in the United States, but only for

ITER

The International Thermonuclear Experimental Reactor (ITER) now under construction in Cadarache, France, represents what is hoped to be the final step before practical fusion power by magnetic confinement becomes a reality. ITER is sponsored by the United States, Japan, China, Russia, South Korea, India, and the European Union, which together represent over half the world's population.

ITER is expected to generate 500 MW (10 times the input power) from deuterium-tritium reactions, to weigh 23,000 tons, to cost at least $14 billion (including operation for 20 years), and to be running by 2020 (Fig. 8-22). Superconducting magnets will keep the reacting ions in a doughnut-shaped region whose volume is that of a large house. About 80 percent of the energy released will be carried off by the

neutrons that are produced, and these neutrons will be absorbed by lithium pellets in tubes that surround the reaction chamber. Circulating water will carry away the resulting heat; this is the heat that could be used in a working reactor to power turbines connected to electric generators.

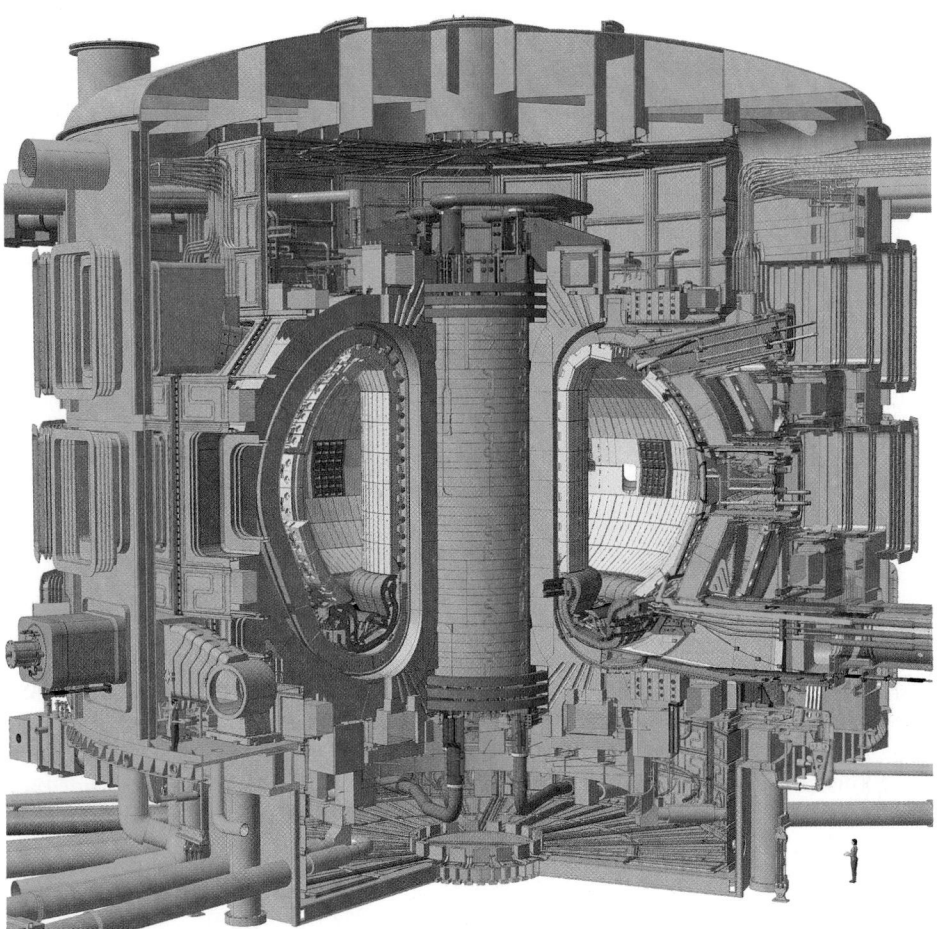

Figure 8-22   Cutaway rendering of the International Thermonuclear Experimental Reactor (ITER) being built in France with international sponsorship. ITER is designed to produce 500 MW of power with an input power of 50 MW when completed in 2020. A successful ITER would be followed in the 2030s by a larger reactor meant to supply electricity to the European grid and thereby start the long-awaited Age of Fusion. In Latin, "iter" means "the way."

3×10^{-9} s—3 billionths of a second. These beams strike a deuterium-tritium fuel pellet 2 mm across from all sides to keep it in place as the conditions inside a star are created. If 10 such pellets are ignited every second, the energy output would be enough to provide electric power to a city of 175,000 people. Other laser fusion projects are under way in France and Japan.

There is a big gap between laboratory experiments, however encouraging, and large-scale production at an economic cost. For all the promise of fusion energy, it is by no means sure that the gap will eventually be bridged and fusion will end up as the ultimate solution to the world's energy needs. An old joke has it that unlimited fusion energy is just 40 years away—and always will be. Still, if fusion energy does prove a success, it could provide possibly a third of global energy needs by 2100 with no fuel supply problems or greenhouse gas emissions.

Elementary Particles

The electrons, protons, and neutrons of which atoms are composed are **elementary particles** in the sense that they cannot be broken down into anything else. Electrons are simply bits of electrically charged matter, but experiments show that nucleons (protons and neutrons) consist of still

Figure 8-23   The search for truly elementary particles has led to the discovery of particles within particles. Today all ordinary matter seems to be made up of electrons and quarks. Shown are the various levels of organization of a lithium $^7_3$Li atom.

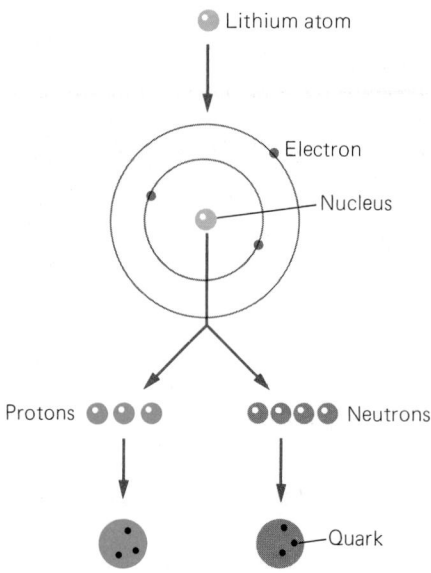

smaller particles called **quarks** (Fig. 8-23). The quarks in a nucleon stick together too tightly to permit the nucleon to be split apart, so nucleons are regarded as elementary particles despite their inner structures.

A great many other elementary particles besides electrons and nucleons are known, some composed of quarks and some not. Few of these other particles seem to have anything to do with ordinary matter, although their discovery has helped physicists in their study of how nature works.

8.13   Antiparticles

The Same but Different

Nearly all elementary particles have **antiparticles.** The antiparticle of a given particle has the same mass as the particle and behaves similarly in most respects, but its electric charge is opposite in sign. Thus the **positron** e^+ is the antiparticle of the electron e^-, and the negatively charged **antiproton** p^-

Antimatter

There seems to be no reason why atoms could not be composed of antiprotons, antineutrons, and positrons. Indeed, hydrogenlike atoms that consist of antiprotons and positrons have already been created in the laboratory. Such **antimatter** ought to behave like ordinary matter.

Of course, if antimatter comes in contact with ordinary matter, the same amount of both will disappear in a burst of energy. A postage stamp of antimatter reacting with a similar stamp of matter would release enough energy to send the space shuttle into orbit.

We might imagine that, when the universe was formed, equal quantities of matter and antimatter came into being that became separate galaxies of stars. If this were true, elsewhere in the universe would be stars, planets, and living things made entirely of antimatter.

The idea that the universe consists of both matter and antimatter is an attractive one, but unfortunately it does not seem to be the case. Although galaxies are far apart on the average, now and then two of them collide. A collision between a matter galaxy and an antimatter galaxy would be a violent explosion

giving rise to a flood of gamma rays with characteristic energies. Very few such gamma rays are observed, from which astronomers conclude that there cannot be much antimatter in the universe.

Current theories of elementary particles suggest that matter and antimatter are not exactly mirror images of each other, and as a result slightly more matter than antimatter was created when the universe came into being in the big bang described in Chap. 19. After all the antimatter had been annihilated, the excess of matter remained to become today's universe.

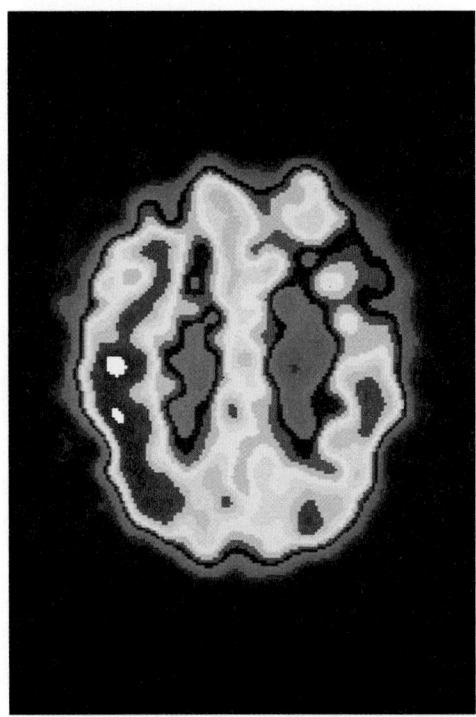

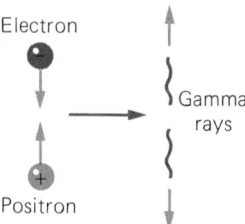

Figure 8-24 The mutual annihilation of an electron and a positron results in a pair of gamma rays whose total energy is equal to mc^2, where m is the total mass of the electron and positron.

Figure 8-25 A positron emission tomography (PET) scan of the brain of a patient with Alzheimer's disease. Different colors correspond to different rates of metabolic activity. In PET, a positron-emitting isotope of an element appropriate to the condition being studied (here an oxygen isotope) is injected and allowed to circulate in a patient's body. When an emitted positron encounters an electron, which it does almost immediately, both are annihilated and a pair of gamma rays is created. Tracing back the directions of the gamma rays gives the location of the annihilation, which is very close to that of the emitting nucleus. In this way, a map of the concentration of the radionuclide can be built up. In a normal brain, metabolic activity produces a similar PET pattern in each side. Here the irregular appearance of the scan indicates that brain tissue has degenerated.

is the antiparticle of the proton p^+. Certain uncharged elementary particles, such as the neutron, have antiparticles because they have properties other than charge that are different in the particle and its antiparticle.

Annihilation   Antiparticles are not easy to find for a very basic reason. When a particle and its antiparticle happen to come together, they destroy each other in a process called **annihilation.** The lost mass reappears as energy in the form of gamma rays when electrons and positrons are annihilated (Figs. 8-24 and 8-25). Unstable particles of various kinds may be produced instead of gamma rays when protons and antiprotons (or neutrons and antineutrons) are annihilated.

Pair Production   The reverse of annihilation can also take place, with energy becoming matter and electric charge being created where none existed before. In the remarkable process of **pair production,** a particle and its antiparticle materialize when a high-energy gamma ray passes near an atomic nucleus (Figs. 8-26 and 8-27). According to Einstein's formula $E_0 = mc^2$, the energy equivalent of the electron mass is 0.51 MeV. To produce an electron-positron pair therefore requires a gamma ray whose energy is at least 1.02 MeV. If the gamma ray has more energy than 1.02 MeV, the excess goes into the kinetic energies of the electron and positron. The minimum energy needed for a proton-antiproton or neutron-antineutron pair is nearly 2 GeV. The antiparticles formed in pair production exist for only a short time before they meet up with their particle counterparts in ordinary matter and are annihilated.

| ## Paul A. M. Dirac (1902–1984)

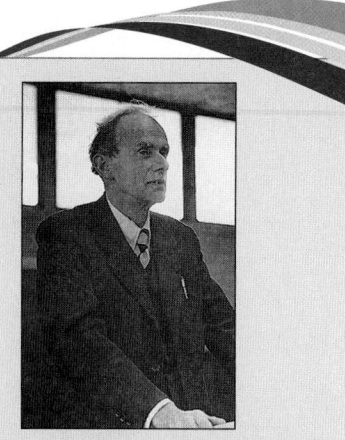

Born in Bristol, England, Dirac originally studied electrical engineering. He then switched to physics and obtained his Ph.D. from Cambridge University in 1926. A new and revolutionary theory of the atom called quantum mechanics (see Sec. 9.12) was just then coming into being, and Dirac made a number of major contributions to it. Soon Dirac had joined special relativity to quantum mechanics to give a theory of the electron that predicted the existence of positively charged electrons, or positrons, which were then unknown.

At first Dirac thought that protons were the positive antiparticles of electrons despite their much greater mass and the fact that they are not annihilated by electrons. Then, in 1932, the American physicist Carl Anderson found that positrons do exist and have the same mass as electrons. In the same year Dirac became Lucasian Professor of Mathematics at Cambridge, the post Newton had held two-and-a-half centuries earlier. Dirac remained active in physics for the rest of his life, after 1969 in the warmer climate of Florida,

but as is often the case in science he will be remembered for the brilliant achievements of his youth.

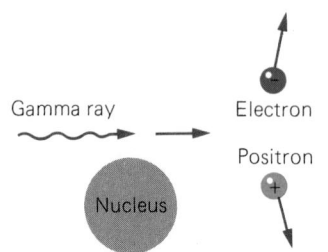

Figure 8-26   Pair production. (The presence of a nucleus is required in order that both momentum and energy be conserved.) Proton-antiproton and neutron-antineutron pairs can also be produced if the gamma ray has enough energy.

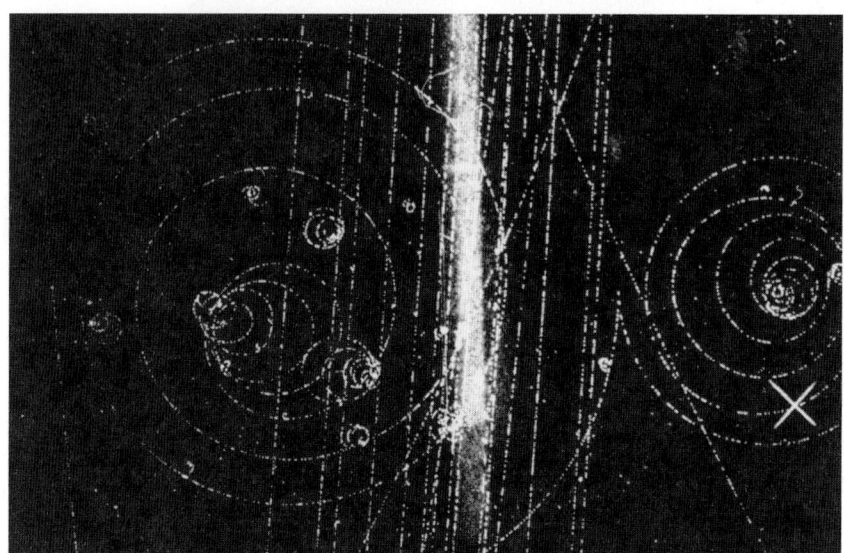

Figure 8-27   A bubble chamber contains liquid hydrogen under high pressure. When the pressure is suddenly released, tiny bubbles form along tracks of fast electrically charged particles. This photograph shows an electron-positron pair that formed in a bubble chamber in which there was a magnetic field perpendicular to the page. The field deflected the electron and positron into oppositely curved paths. These paths are spirals because the particles lost energy as they moved through the hydrogen in the chamber and so were deflected more and more by the field.

8.14   Fundamental Interactions

Only Four Give Rise to All Physical Processes

Elementary particles interact with each other in only four ways. These fundamental interactions seem able to account for all the physical processes and structures in the universe on all scales of size from atomic nuclei to galaxies of stars (Fig. 8-28). In order of decreasing strength these interactions are

1. The **strong interaction,** which holds protons and neutrons together to form atomic nuclei despite the mutual repulsion of the protons. The forces produced by this interaction have short ranges, only about 10^{-15} m, which is why nuclei are limited in size. Because the strong interaction is what its name suggests, nuclear binding energies are high. Electrons are not affected by the strong interaction.

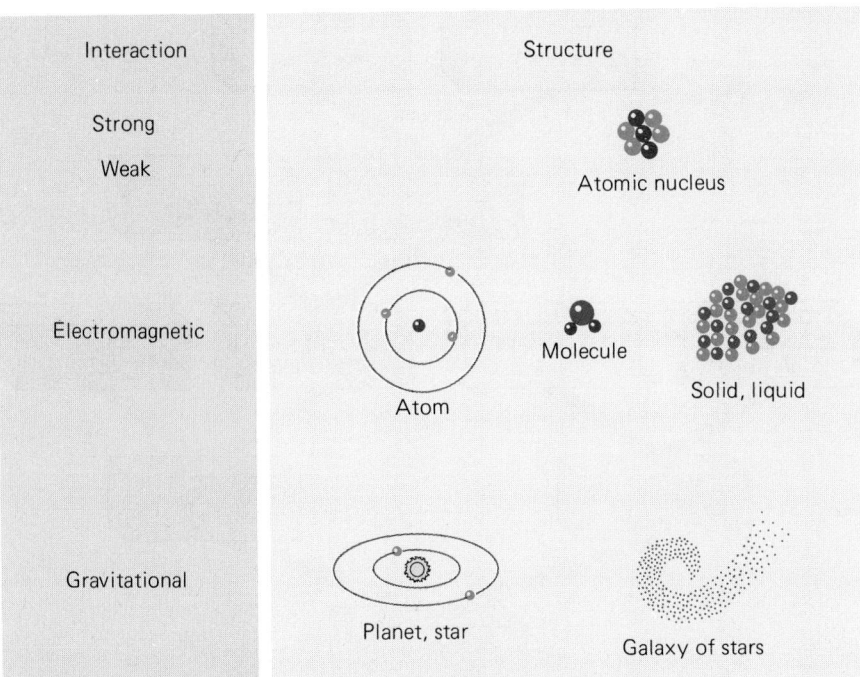

Figure 8-28   The four fundamental interactions determine how matter comes together to form the characteristic structures of the universe.

2. The **electromagnetic interaction,** which gives rise to electric and magnetic forces between charged particles. This interaction is responsible for the structures of atoms, molecules, liquids, and solids. The force exerted when a bat hits a ball is electromagnetic. Although the electromagnetic interaction is about 100 times weaker than the strong interaction at short distances, electromagnetic forces are unlimited in range and, unlike strong forces, act on electrons.

3. The **weak interaction,** which affects all particles. By causing beta decay this interaction helps determine the compositions of atomic nuclei. The range of the weak interaction is even shorter than that of the strong interaction, and 10 trillion times less powerful.

4. The **gravitational interaction,** which is responsible for the attractive force one mass exerts on another. Because the strong and weak forces are severely limited in range and because matter in bulk is electrically neutral, the gravitational interaction dominates on a large scale. Gravitation is what pulls matter together into the planets, stars, and galaxies that populate space. This interaction is nevertheless extremely feeble on a small scale; the gravitational pull of one electron on another is 10^{43} times weaker than their electric repulsion.

Before Newton, it was not clear that the gravity that pulls things down to the earth—which we might call terrestrial gravity—is the same as the gravity that holds the planets in their orbits around the sun. One of Newton's great accomplishments was to show that both terrestrial and astronomical gravity have the same nature. Another notable unification was made by Maxwell when he demonstrated that electric and magnetic forces can both be traced to a single interaction between charged particles.

Unifying the Interactions   What about the four fundamental interactions listed above? Are they all truly fundamental or are any of them, too, related in some way?

Studies made independently by Steven Weinberg and Abdus Salam in the 1960s indicated that the weak and electromagnetic interactions are really

Figure 8-29 One of the goals of physics is a single theoretical picture that unites all the ways in which particles of matter interact with each other. Much progress has been made, but the task is not finished.

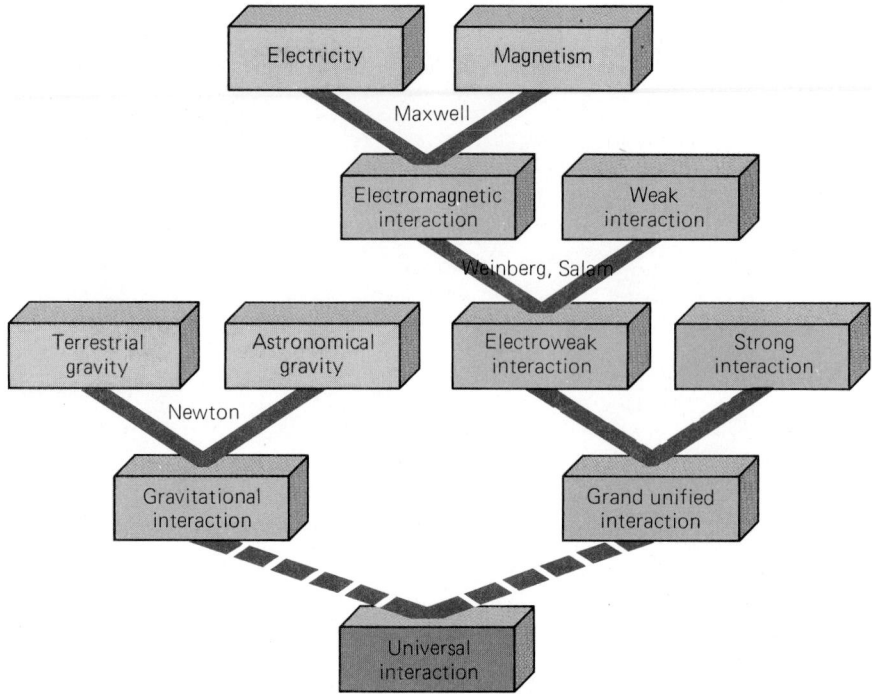

different aspects of the same basic phenomenon, a conclusion supported by experiment (Fig. 8-29). Later work has linked the electroweak and strong interactions as part of the current, very successful Standard Model of elementary particles. One of the merits of this model is that it can explain why the proton and the electron, which are very different kinds of particle (as discussed in the next section), have electric charges of exactly the same size.

What about gravitation? The final step in understanding how nature works would be a single theory that ties together all the particles and interactions that are known—a "theory of everything." What such a theory might illuminate is described in Sec. 19.9.

8.15 Leptons and Hadrons

Ultimate Matter

All elementary particles fall into two broad categories that depend on their response to the strong interaction. **Leptons** (Greek for "light" or "swift") are not affected by this interaction and seem to be point particles with no size or internal structure. The electron is a lepton. **Hadrons** (Greek for "heavy" or "strong") are subject to the strong interaction and have definite sizes—they are about 10^{-15} m across—and internal structures. The proton and neutron are hadrons.

Neutrinos   A very interesting lepton is the **neutrino,** which has no charge and very little mass (a millionth of the electron's mass, so little that until recently it was thought to have no mass at all). The neutrino is associated with the weak interaction. Whenever a nucleus undergoes beta decay, a neutrino as well as an electron (or positron) is emitted. A neutrino can pass through vast amounts of matter—over 100 *light-years* of solid iron on the average—before interacting. (A light-year is the distance light travels in empty space in a year.)

A vast number of neutrinos are produced in the sun in the course of the nuclear reactions that occur within it, and these neutrinos carry into space

New Accelerators

The recently completed Large Hadron Collider (LHC) at the CERN laboratory on the border between France and Switzerland is the most powerful particle accelerator in the world (Fig. 8-30); it uses 120 MW in its operation, as much as a small city.

One of the particles the LHC was designed to produce is the long-sought Higgs boson, which current theories suggest is the key to understanding the nature of mass. Hitherto unknown particles and perhaps new physical laws that apply only at high energies, such as those found in the early universe, may be found as well. No new particles have been discovered since 1995—an unusually long gap in this branch of physics.

Other topics being studied using the LHC include why gravity is so weak compared with the other fundamental interactions and the nature of the mysterious "dark matter" that makes up most of the mass of the universe (see Sec. 19.4). The LHC may also be able to create tiny black holes, miniature versions of the black holes that are the remnants of collapsed stars (Sec. 18.16)

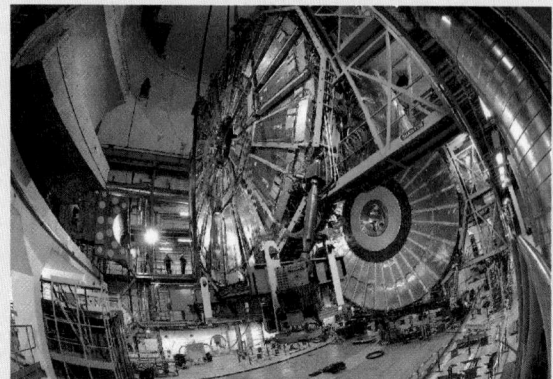

Figure 8-30   One of the four particle detectors, shown under construction, of the Large Hadron Collider at CERN, which is pushing back the frontier of knowledge. Seven thousand magnets, their superconducting windings cooled by liquid helium, guide and focus two beams of 7 TeV protons (the most energetic yet accelerated on the earth) around the 27-km circumference of the collider. At four points on the ring the beams cross to give over 600 million collisions per second. The elementary particles produced in these events are tracked and measured by the detectors. The raw data would fill hundreds of thousands of CDs every second, but only the information about the 100 most interesting events each second is kept for analysis.

and of the immense black holes believed to be at the heart of every galaxy of stars in the universe (Sec. 19.1).

Planning has already begun on the next major accelerator, the International Linear Collider, which would be 35 km long and smash together beams of high-energy electrons and positrons. Collaborating on the design of the projected machine, which is expected to cost $8 billion and be completed in the 2020s, are about 1000 scientists and engineers from 100 countries.

6 to 8 percent of all the energy the sun generates. About 65 billion neutrinos, mostly from the sun, pass through each square centimeter (the area of a fingernail) of your body per second. The energy the neutrinos from the sun and other stars carry is apparently lost forever in the sense that it cannot be changed into any other form. Neutrinos outnumber protons in the universe by about a billion to one, but they represent less than 1 percent of the total energy of the universe.

Besides the proton and the neutron, the hadron family includes several hundred particles with extremely short lifetimes, less than a billionth of a second for some. These particles seem to play no role in the behavior of ordinary matter. They decay in various ways, often in a series of steps, and usually end up as protons, neutrons, or electrons; a few become gamma rays. Some of these decays involve the emission of neutrinos that are different in certain respects from those emitted in the beta decays of atomic nuclei.

Quarks   The discovery that hadrons have internal structures was made with the help of experiments in which fast electrons were scattered by collisions with protons and neutrons. (We recall that the internal structure of the atom was revealed by the similar Rutherford experiment that used alpha particles as probes.) The particles that make up hadrons are the **quarks** mentioned earlier.

Only six kinds of quark are needed to account for all known hadrons. Those hadrons that are lighter than the proton consist of a quark and an

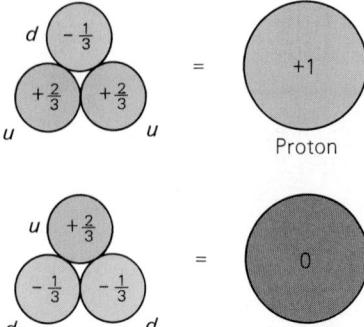

Figure 8-31 Quark models of the proton and neutron. Electric charges are given in units of *e*.

antiquark. The proton, neutron, and heavier hadrons consist of three quarks. This is a welcome simplification, but quarks turn out to have two unprecedented properties. The first is that, unlike any other particle known, their electric charge is less than $\pm e$. Some quarks have a charge of $\pm \frac{1}{3}e$; others have a charge of $\pm \frac{2}{3}e$.

The second unusual aspect of quarks is that they do not seem able to exist outside of hadrons. No quark has ever been found by itself, even in experiments that ought to have been able to set them free. Thus there is no direct way to confirm that quarks have fractional charges, or even that they really exist.

Nevertheless there is a great deal of indirect evidence strongly in favor of quarks. For instance, every known hadron matches up with a particular arrangement of quarks, and predictions of hitherto unknown hadrons made on the basis of the quark model have turned out correct. Furthermore, a theory of the strong interaction based on quarks has been quite successful. This is the theory mentioned in the previous section that has been linked to the theory of the electromagnetic-weak interaction to make a unified picture that accounts for all aspects of the behavior of matter except—thus far—gravitation.

The two quarks that make up the proton and neutron are called *u* (charge $+\frac{2}{3}e$) and *d* (charge $-\frac{1}{3}e$). As shown in Fig. 8-31, a proton consists of one *d* quark and two *u* quarks, and a neutron consists of one *u* quark and two *d* quarks. Thus all the properties of ordinary matter can be understood on the basis of just two leptons, the electron and the neutrino, and two quarks, *u* and *d*. Considering how diverse these properties are, this is an astonishing achievement. The other leptons and quarks are connected only with unstable particles created in high-energy collisions and seem to have nothing to do with ordinary matter. Sensitive experiments, backed up by otherwise successful theories, suggest that leptons and quarks represent the limit of simplification and are not themselves composed of still other, more fundamental particles.

Important Terms and Ideas

An **element** is a substance all of whose atoms have the same number of protons in their nuclei. This number is the **atomic number** of the element and equals the number of electrons that surround each nucleus of the element's atoms. The **isotopes** of an element have different numbers of neutrons in their nuclei. A **nucleon** is a neutron or proton; the **mass number** of a nucleus is the number of nucleons it contains. A **nuclide** is an atom whose nucleus has particular atomic and mass numbers.

In **radioactive decay**, certain atomic nuclei spontaneously emit **alpha particles** (helium nuclei), **beta particles** (electrons), or **gamma rays** (high-frequency electromagnetic waves). A **positron** is a positively charged electron emitted in some beta decays.

The **half-life** of a radionuclide is the time needed for half of an original sample to decay.

The mass of every nucleus is slightly less than the total mass of the same number of free neutrons and protons. The **binding energy** of a nucleus is the energy equivalent of the missing mass and must be supplied to the nucleus to break it up. Nuclei of intermediate size have the highest **binding energies per nucleon**. Hence the **fusion** of

light nuclei to form heavier ones and the **fission** of heavy nuclei into lighter ones are both processes that liberate energy.

An **elementary particle** cannot be separated into other particles. The **antiparticle** of an elementary particle has the same mass and general behavior, but it has a charge of opposite sign and differs in certain other respects. A particle and its antiparticle can **annihilate** each other, with their masses turning entirely into energy. In the opposite process of **pair production**, a particle-antiparticle pair materializes from energy.

The four **fundamental interactions** are, in order of decreasing strength, the strong, electromagnetic, weak, and gravitational.

A **lepton** is an elementary particle that is not affected by the strong interaction and has no internal structure; the electron is a lepton. The **neutrino** is a lepton with no charge and little mass that is emitted during beta decay. A **hadron** is an elementary particle that is affected by the strong interaction and is composed of **quarks**, particles with electric charges of $\pm \frac{1}{3}e$ or $\pm \frac{2}{3}e$ that have not been found outside hadrons as yet. Protons and neutrons are hadrons.

Multiple Choice

1. The basic idea of the Rutherford atomic model is that the positive charge in an atom is
   a. spread uniformly throughout its volume
   b. concentrated at its center
   c. readily deflected by an incoming alpha particle
   d. the same for all atoms

2. Nearly all the volume occupied by matter consists of
   a. electrons   c. neutrons
   b. protons   d. nothing

3. The atomic number of an element is the number of
   a. protons in its nucleus
   b. neutrons in its nucleus
   c. electrons in its nucleus
   d. protons and neutrons in its nucleus

4. The atoms of the isotopes of an element are different in which one or more of the following?
   a. number of electrons
   b. number of protons
   c. number of neutrons
   d. atomic mass

5. Which of the following is not an isotope of hydrogen?
   a. $_0^1$H
   b. $_1^1$H
   c. $_1^2$H
   d. $_1^3$H

6. The atomic number of an element determines its
   a. mass   c. number of neutrons
   b. binding energy   d. chemical behavior

7. The number of protons in a stable nucleus is always
   a. less than the number of neutrons
   b. less than or equal to the number of neutrons
   c. equal to or more than the number of neutrons
   d. more than the number of neutrons

8. An electron is emitted by an atomic nucleus in the process of
   a. alpha decay   c. gamma decay
   b. beta decay   d. nuclear fission

9. Gamma rays have the same basic nature as
   a. alpha particles   c. x-rays
   b. beta particles   d. sound waves

10. Radioactive materials do not emit
    a. electrons   c. alpha particles
    b. protons   d. gamma rays

11. Which of these types of radiation has the least ability to penetrate matter?
    a. alpha particles   c. gamma rays
    b. beta particles   d. x-rays

12. Which of these types of radiation has the greatest ability to penetrate matter?
    a. alpha particles   c. gamma rays
    b. beta particles   d. x-rays

13. When a nucleus undergoes radioactive decay, the number of nucleons it contains afterward is
    a. always less than the original number
    b. always more than the original number
    c. never less than the original number
    d. never more than the original number

14. Which of these particles is radioactive?
    a. electron   c. neutron
    b. proton   d. alpha particle

15. The largest amount of radiation received by an average person in the United States comes from
    a. medical x-rays
    b. nuclear reactors
    c. fallout from past weapons tests
    d. natural sources

16. The half-life of a radionuclide is
    a. half the time needed for a sample to decay entirely
    b. half the time a sample can be kept before it begins to decay
    c. the time needed for half a sample to decay
    d. the time needed for the remainder of a sample to decay after half of it has already decayed

17. As a sample of a radionuclide decays, its half-life
    a. decreases
    b. remains the same
    c. increases
    d. any of these, depending upon the nuclide

18. In a stable nucleus other than $_1^1$H the number of neutrons is always
    a. less than the number of protons
    b. less than or equal to the number of protons
    c. equal to or more than the number of protons
    d. more than the number of protons

19. The electronvolt is a unit of
    a. charge   c. energy
    b. potential difference d. momentum

20. Relative to the sum of the masses of its constituent particles, the mass of an atom is
    a. greater
    b. the same
    c. smaller
    d. any of these, depending on the element

21. The binding energy per nucleon is
    a. the same for all nuclei
    b. greater for very small nuclei
    c. greatest for nuclei of intermediate size
    d. greatest for very large nuclei

22. The splitting of an atomic nucleus, such as that of ^{235}U, into two or more fragments is called
    a. fusion   c. a chain reaction
    b. fission   d. beta decay

23. In a chain reaction
    a. protons and neutrons join to form atomic nuclei
    b. light nuclei join to form heavy ones
    c. neutrons emitted during the fission of heavy nuclei induce fissions in other nuclei
    d. uranium is burned in a type of furnace called a reactor

24. Enriched uranium is a better fuel for nuclear reactors than natural uranium because enriched uranium has a greater proportion of
    a. slow neutrons
    b. deuterium
    c. plutonium
    d. ^{235}U

25. In a nuclear power plant the nuclear reactor itself is used as a source of
    a. neutrons
    b. heat
    c. radioactivity
    d. electricity

26. Fusion reactions on the earth are likely to use as fuel
    a. ordinary hydrogen
    b. deuterium
    c. plutonium
    d. uranium

27. Of the following particles, the one that is not an elementary particle is the
    a. alpha particle
    b. beta particle
    c. neutron
    d. neutrino

28. An example of a particle-antiparticle pair is the
    a. proton and positron
    b. proton and neutron
    c. neutron and neutrino
    d. electron and positron

29. The interaction responsible for the structures of molecules, liquids, and solids is the
    a. gravitational interaction
    b. strong interaction
    c. weak interaction
    d. electromagnetic interaction

30. The weakest of the four fundamental interactions is the
    a. gravitational interaction
    b. electromagnetic interaction
    c. strong interaction
    d. weak interaction

31. The mass of the neutrino is
    a. equal to that of the neutron
    b. equal to that of the electron
    c. equal to that of a quark
    d. very small

32. Quarks are particles that
    a. have no mass
    b. have charges whose magnitudes are less than e
    c. decay into protons
    d. decay into neutrinos

33. A particle that is believed to consist of quarks is the
    a. electron
    b. positron
    c. neutron
    d. neutrino

34. The number of protons in a nucleus of the boron isotope $^{11}_{5}B$ is
    a. 5
    b. 6
    c. 11
    d. 16

35. The number of neutrons in a nucleus of the potassium nucleus $^{40}_{19}K$ is
    a. 19
    b. 21
    c. 40
    d. 59

36. When the nitrogen isotope $^{13}_{7}N$ decays into the carbon isotope $^{13}_{6}C$, it emits
    a. a gamma ray
    b. an electron
    c. a positron
    d. an alpha particle

37. The product of the alpha decay of the bismuth isotope $^{214}_{83}Bi$ is
    a. $^{210}_{79}Au$
    b. $^{210}_{81}Tl$
    c. $^{210}_{83}Bi$
    d. $^{218}_{85}At$

38. The product of the gamma decay of the aluminum isotope $^{27}_{13}Al$ is
    a. $^{27}_{12}Mg$
    b. $^{26}_{13}Al$
    c. $^{27}_{13}Al$
    d. $^{27}_{14}Si$

39. The half-life of a certain radioactive isotope is 6 h. If we start out with 10 g of the isotope, after 1 day there will be
    a. none left
    b. 0.625 g left
    c. 1.6 g left
    d. 2.5 g left

40. After 10 years, 75 g of an original sample of 100 g of a certain radioactive isotope has decayed. The half-life of the isotope is
    a. 5 years
    b. 7.5 years
    c. 20 years
    d. 40 years

Exercises

8.1 Rutherford Model of the Atom
8.2 Nuclear Structure

1. How do the ways in which the mass and the charge of an atom are distributed differ?

2. Alpha particle tracks through gases and thin metal foils show few deflections. What does this tell us about the atom?

3. What are the similarities and differences among the isotopes of an element?

4. Find the number of neutrons and protons in each of the following nuclei: $^{6}_{3}Li$; $^{13}_{6}C$; $^{31}_{15}C$; $^{94}_{40}Zr$.

5. Find the number of neutrons and protons in each of the following nuclei: $^{18}_{8}O$; $^{26}_{12}Mg$; $^{57}_{26}Fe$; $^{109}_{47}Ag$.

8.3 Radioactive Decay

6. The following statements were thought to be correct in the nineteenth century. Which of them are now known to be incorrect? For those that are incorrect, indicate why the statement is wrong and modify it to be in accordance with modern views. (a) Energy can be neither created nor destroyed. (b) The acceleration of an object is proportional to the force applied to it and inversely proportional to its mass. (c) Atoms are indivisible and indestructible. (d) All atoms of a particular element are identical.

7. What limits the size of a nucleus?

8. How does the number of neutrons in a stable nucleus compare with the number of protons? Why is this?

9. (a) What is an alpha particle? A beta particle? A gamma ray? (b) How do they compare in general in ability to penetrate matter?

10. Radium spontaneously decays into helium and radon. Why do you think radium is regarded as an element rather than as a chemical compound of helium and radon in the way that water, for example, is considered a chemical compound of hydrogen and oxygen?

11. What happens to the atomic number and mass number of a nucleus when it emits an alpha particle?

12. What happens to the atomic number and mass number of a nucleus when it emits (a) an electron? (b) a positron? (c) a gamma ray?

13. (a) Under what circumstances does a nucleus emit an electron? A positron? (b) The oxygen nuclei $^{14}_{8}O$ and $^{19}_{8}O$ both undergo beta decay to become stable nuclei. Which would you expect to emit a positron and which an electron?

14. The boron isotope $^{12}_{5}B$ decays into the carbon isotope $^{12}_{6}C$. What kind of particle is emitted in the decay?

15. The polonium isotope $^{210}_{84}Po$ undergoes alpha decay to become an isotope of lead. Find the atomic number and mass number of this isotope.

16. The helium isotope $^{6}_{2}He$ is unstable. What kind of decay would you expect it to undergo? What would the resulting nuclide be?

17. The thorium nucleus $^{233}_{90}Th$ undergoes two successive negative beta decays. Find the atomic number, mass number, and chemical name of the resulting nucleus.

18. A $^{64}_{29}Cu$ nucleus can decay by emitting an electron or a positron and also by capturing an electron. What is the final nucleus in each case?

19. The uranium isotope $^{235}_{92}U$ decays into a lead isotope by emitting seven alpha particles and four electrons. What is the symbol of the lead isotope?

20. A reaction often used to detect neutrons occurs when a neutron is absorbed by a $^{10}_{5}B$ boron nucleus, which then emits an alpha particle. What are the atomic number, mass number, and chemical name of the remaining nucleus?

8.4 Half-Life

21. What happens to the half-life of a radionuclide as it decays?

22. If the half-life of a radionuclide is 1 month, is a sample of it completely decayed after 2 months?

23. After 10 years, 75 g of an original sample of 100 g of a certain radionuclide has decayed. What is the half-life of the nuclide?

24. One-eighth of a sample of $^{227}_{90}Th$ remains undecayed after 54 days. What is the half-life of this thorium isotope?

25. If 1 kg of radium (half-life = 1600 years) is sealed into a container, how much of it will remain as radium after 1600 years? after 4800 years? If the container is opened after a period of time, what gases would you expect to find inside it?

8.6 Units of Mass and Energy

26. When the radium isotope $^{226}_{88}Ra$ undergoes alpha decay, the energy liberated is 4.87 MeV. (a) Identify the resulting nuclide. (b) The alpha particle has a KE of 4.78 MeV. Where do you think the other 0.09 MeV goes?

27. Find the kinetic energy (in eV) of an electron whose speed is 10^6 m/s.

28. Find the kinetic energy (in keV) of a $^{12}_{6}C$ atom of mass 12.0 u whose speed is 2×10^6 m/s.

29. Find the speed of an electron whose kinetic energy is 26 eV.

30. Find the speed of a neutron whose kinetic energy is 60 eV.

8.7 Binding Energy

8.8 Binding Energy per Nucleon

31. How does the energy needed to remove an electron from an atom compare with the energy needed to remove a proton from its nucleus?

32. Why is the $^{56}_{26}Fe$ nucleus the most stable (that is, the most difficult to break apart) nucleus?

33. What property of atomic nuclei makes it possible for nuclear fission and fusion to give off energy?

34. Atomic mass always refers to the mass of a neutral atom, not the mass of its bare nucleus. With this definition in mind, determine by how many electron masses the mass of a parent atom changes when its nucleus emits (a) an electron and (b) a positron. Ignore the kinetic energy of the emitted particle.

35. The binding energy per nucleon in the iron nucleus $^{56}_{26}Fe$ is 8.8 MeV. Find its atomic mass.

36. The binding energy of $^{20}_{10}Ne$ is 161 MeV. Find its atomic mass.

37. The mass of $^{4}_{2}He$ is 4.0026 u. Find its binding energy and binding energy per nucleon.

38. The binding energy per nucleon in the chlorine isotope $^{35}_{17}Cl$ is 8.5 MeV. What is its atomic mass?

39. The neutron decays in free space into a proton and an electron after an average lifetime of

15 min. What must be the minimum binding energy contributed by a neutron to a nucleus in order that the neutron not decay inside the nucleus? How does this figure compare with the observed binding energies per nucleon in stable nuclei?

8.9   Nuclear Fission

8.10   How a Reactor Works

8.11   Plutonium

40. Why can ordinary uranium not be used to fuel a reactor cooled by ordinary water?

41. What is the function of the moderator in a uranium-fueled nuclear reactor?

42. What fuel other than uranium can be used in a nuclear reactor?

43. (a) How much mass is lost per day by a nuclear reactor operated at a 1.0-GW power level? (b) If each fission releases 200 MeV, how many fissions occur per second to give this power level?

44. $^{235}_{92}$U loses loses about 0.1 percent of its mass when it undergoes fission. (a) How much energy is released when 1 kg of $^{235}_{92}$U undergoes fission? (b) A ton of TNT releases about 9×10^9 J when it explodes. How many tons of TNT are equivalent in destructive power to a bomb that contains 1 kg of $^{235}_{92}$U?

8.12   Nuclear Fusion

45. What are the differences and similarities between fusion and fission?

46. Old stars obtain part of their energy by the fusion of three alpha particles to form a $^{12}_{6}$C nucleus, whose mass is 12.0000 u. How much energy is given off in each such reaction?

8.13   Antiparticles

8.14   Fundamental Interactions

8.15   Leptons and Hadrons

47. What distinguishes a charged particle from its antiparticle? What happens when they come together?

48. (a) Could a gamma ray just energetic enough to materialize into a proton-antiproton pair alternatively materialize into a neutron-antineutron pair? (b) Could a gamma ray energetic enough to materialize into a neutron-antineutron pair alternatively materialize into a proton-antiproton pair? Explain.

49. Suppose the strong interaction did not exist, so there were no nuclear binding energies. If the early universe contained protons, neutrons, and electrons, what kind or kinds of matter would eventually fill the universe?

50. Of the following elementary particles, which has the least mass? The most? Proton, neutron, electron, neutrino.

51. List the fundamental interactions in order of decreasing strength. Which, if any, are limited in the distances over which they act?

52. The gravitational interaction alone governs the motions of the planets around the sun. Why are the other fundamental interactions not significant in planetary motion?

53. Discuss the similarities and differences between the neutron and the neutrino.

54. Why can neutrinos travel immense distances through matter whereas other elementary particles cannot?

55. Leptons and hadrons are the two classes of basic particle. How do they differ?

56. Which constituents of an atom consist of quarks and which do not?

57. No particle of fractional charge has yet been observed. If none is found in the future either, does this necessarily mean that the quark hypothesis is wrong?

58. Would you expect the gravitational attractive force between two protons in a nucleus to counterbalance their electrical repulsion? Calculate the ratio between the electric and gravitational forces acting between two protons. Does this ratio depend upon how far apart the protons are?

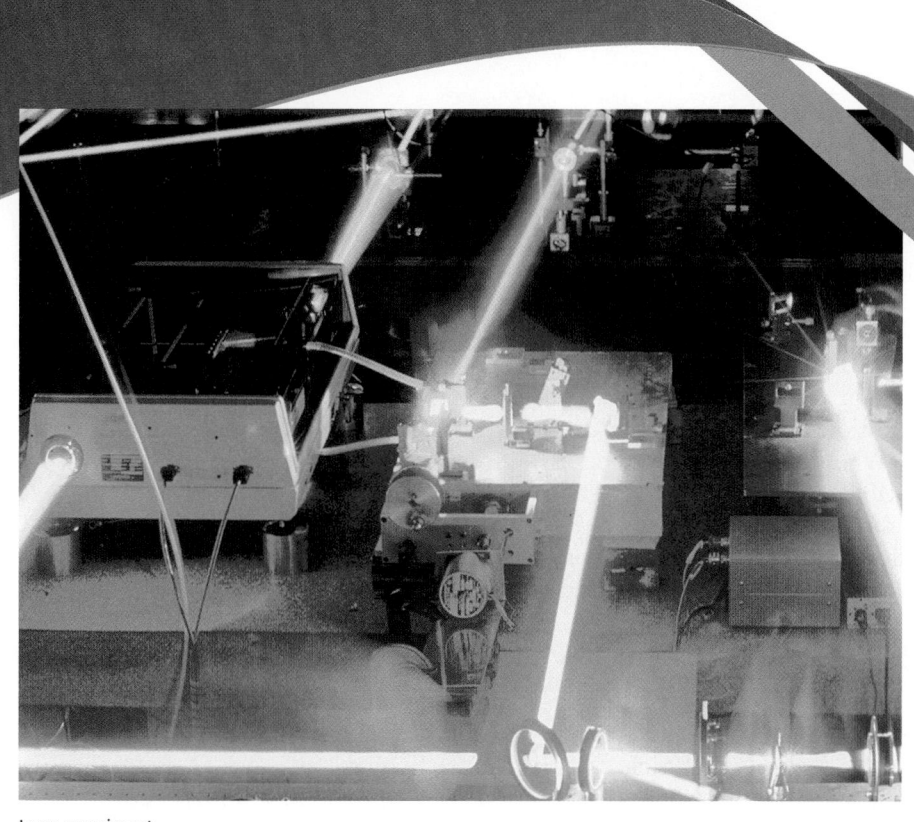

Laser experiment.

9

The Atom

GOALS

When you have finished this chapter you should be able to complete the goals
• given for each section below:

Quantum Theory of Light

9.1 Photoelectric Effect
How Can Electrons Be Set Free from Atoms by Light?
• Describe the photoelectric effect and discuss why the wave theory of light cannot account for it.

9.2 Photons
Particles of Light
• Explain how the quantum theory of light accounts for the photoelectric effect in terms of photons.

9.3 What Is Light?
Both Wave and Particle
• Compare the quantum and wave theories of light and discuss why both are needed.

9.4 X-Rays
High-Energy Photons
• Describe x-rays and interpret their production in terms of the quantum theory of light.

Matter Waves

9.5 De Broglie Waves
Matter Waves Are Significant Only in the Atomic World

9.6 Waves of What?
Waves of Probability
• Discuss what is meant by the matter wave of a moving particle.

9.7 Uncertainty Principle
We Cannot Know the Future Because We Cannot Know the Present
• State the uncertainty principle and interpret it in terms of matter waves.

The Hydrogen Atom

9.8 Atomic Spectra
Each Element Has a Characteristic Spectrum
• Distinguish between emission and absorption spectra and describe what is meant by a spectral series.

9.9 The Bohr Model
Only Certain Electron Energies Are Possible in an Atom

9.10 Electron Waves and Orbits
Standing Waves in the Atom
• Give the basic ideas of the Bohr model of the atom and show how they follow from the wave nature of moving electrons.
• Define quantum number, energy level, ground state, and excited state.
• Explain the origins of emission and absorption spectra and of spectral series.

9.11 The Laser
An Amplifier of Light That Produces Waves All in Step
• Explain how a laser works.
• List the three characteristic properties of laser light.

Quantum Theory of the Atom

9.12 Quantum Mechanics
Probabilities, not Certainties
• Compare quantum mechanics and newtonian mechanics.

9.13 Quantum Numbers
An Atomic Electron Has Four in All
• Describe what is meant by the orbital of an atomic electron.
• List the four quantum numbers of an atomic electron according to quantum mechanics together with the quantity each governs.

9.14 Exclusion Principle
A Different Set of Quantum Numbers for Each Electron in an Atom
• State the exclusion principle and describe how it affects atomic structures.

Every atom consists of a tiny, positively charged nucleus with negatively charged electrons some distance away. What keeps the electrons out there?

By analogy with the planets of the solar system, we might suppose that atomic electrons avoid being sucked into the nucleus by circling around it at just the right speed. This is not a bad idea, but it raises a serious problem. According to Maxwell's theory (see Chap. 6), a circling electron should lose energy all the time by giving off electromagnetic waves. Thus the electron's orbit should become smaller and smaller, and soon it should spiral into the nucleus. However, atomic electrons do not behave like this. Under ordinary conditions atoms emit no radiation, and needless to say, they never collapse.

Whenever they have been tested outside the atomic domain, the laws of motion and of electromagnetism have always agreed with experiment—yet atoms are stable. In this chapter we shall see how the strange and radical concepts of the quantum theory of light and the wave theory of moving particles are needed to understand the world of the atom.

Quantum Theory of Light

The concepts of "particle" and "wave" are clear enough to everybody. We regard a stone as a particle and the ripples in a lake as waves. A stone thrown into a lake and the ripples that spread out from where it lands seem to have in common only that both carry energy from one place to another. **Classical physics,** which refers to the physics covered in Chaps. 1 through 7, treats particles and waves as separate aspects of the reality we find in everyday life.

But the physical reality around us arises from the small-scale world of atoms and molecules, electrons and nuclei. In this world there are neither particles nor waves in our sense of these terms.

We think of electrons as particles because they have charge and mass and behave according to the laws of particle mechanics in such familiar devices as television picture tubes. However, there is plenty of evidence that makes sense only if a moving electron is a type of wave. We think of electromagnetic (em) waves as waves because they can exhibit such characteristic wave behavior as diffraction and interference. However, em waves also behave as though they consist of streams of particles. The wave-particle duality is central to an understanding of **modern physics,** which is the physics of the atomic world.

9.1 Photoelectric Effect

How Can Electrons Be Set Free from Atoms by Light?

A century ago experiments showed that electrons are given off by a metal surface when light is directed onto it (Fig. 9-1). For most metals ultraviolet light is needed for this **photoelectric effect** to occur, but some metals, such as potassium and cesium, and certain other substances as well, also respond to visible light. The photosensitive screen in a digital camera, the solar cell that produces electric current when sunlight falls on it, and the television camera tube that converts the image of a scene into an electric signal are all based upon the photoelectric effect.

Since light is electromagnetic in nature and carries energy, there seems to be nothing unusual about the photoelectric effect—it should be like water waves dislodging pebbles from a beach. But three experimental findings show that no such simple explanation is possible.

1. The electrons are always emitted at once, even when a faint light is used. However, because the energy in an em wave is spread out across the wave, a certain period of time should be needed for an individual electron to

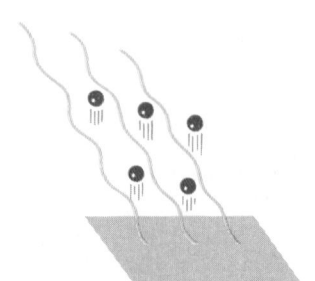

Figure 9-1   In the photoelectric effect, electrons are emitted from a metal surface when a light beam is directed on it.

gather enough energy to leave the metal. Several months ought to be needed for a really weak light beam.

2. A bright light causes more electrons to be emitted than a faint light, but the average kinetic energy of the electrons is the same. The electromagnetic theory of light, on the contrary, predicts that the stronger the light, the greater the KE of the electrons.

3. The higher the frequency of the light, the more KE the electrons have. Blue light yields faster electrons than red light (Fig. 9-2). According to the electromagnetic theory of light, the frequency should not matter.

Until the discovery of the photoelectric effect, the electromagnetic theory of light had been completely successful in explaining the behavior of light. But no amount of ingenuity could bring experiment and theory together in this case. The result was the creation of the entirely new **quantum theory of light** in 1905 by Albert Einstein. The same year saw the birth of his equally revolutionary theory of relativity. All of modern physics has its roots in these two theories.

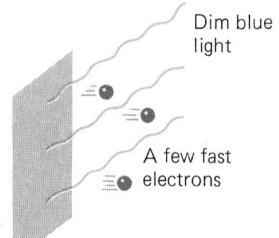
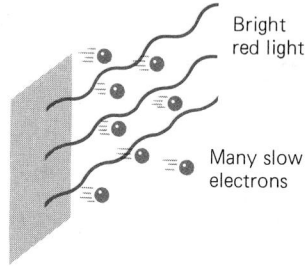

Figure 9-2 The higher the frequency of the light, the more KE the photoelectrons have. The brighter the light, the more photoelectrons are emitted. Blue light has a higher frequency than red light.

9.2 Photons

Particles of Light

Einstein proposed that light consists of tiny bursts of energy called **photons.** He began with a hypothesis suggested 5 years earlier by the German physicist Max Planck (Fig. 9-3) to account for the spectrum of the light given off by hot objects. Figure 9-4 shows how the brightness of this light varies with wavelength for objects at four different temperatures.

Actually, something need not be so hot that it glows for it to radiate em waves—*all* objects radiate such waves whatever their temperatures, though which wavelength appears strongest depends on the temperature. The higher the temperature, the shorter the predominant wavelength (or, equivalently, the higher the predominant frequency); a bar of iron that glows yellow is hotter than one that glows red (Fig. 5-5). For an object at room temperature, or a person, most of the radiation is in the infrared and hence is invisible (Fig. 9-5).

In order to explain the spectrum of emitted radiation, Planck found it necessary to assume that hot objects contribute energy in separate units, or **quanta,** to the light they give off. (Quanta is the plural of quantum, Latin for "how much.") The higher the frequency of the light, the more the energy per quantum. All the quanta associated with a particular frequency f of light have the same energy

$$E = hf \qquad \textit{Quantum energy} \qquad 9\text{-}1$$

Quantum energy = (Planck's constant)(frequency)

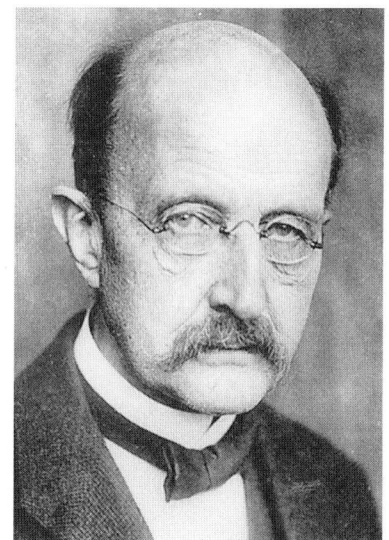

Figure 9-3 Max Planck (1858–1947).

Blackbody Radiation

The ability of a body to emit electromagnetic radiation is closely related to its ability to absorb such radiation: a good absorber is a good emitter. This is to be expected, since a body at the same temperature as its surroundings must be emitting and absorbing radiation at exactly the same rates. When the body is hotter than its surroundings, it emits more radiation than it absorbs, and it is this difference that is pictured in Fig. 9-4.

A perfect absorber is one that absorbs all em radiation that falls on it, regardless of wavelength. Such an absorber, called a **blackbody** (even though real objects painted black actually reflect a little radiation), is therefore also the best possible radiator at any temperature. It is convenient to discuss the thermal radiation of an ideal blackbody so we can disregard the precise nature of whatever is radiating, since all blackbodies at a given temperature behave the same. The graphs of Fig. 9-4 are for blackbodies at the temperatures shown. These are the graphs that Planck needed the quantum theory of light in order to explain.

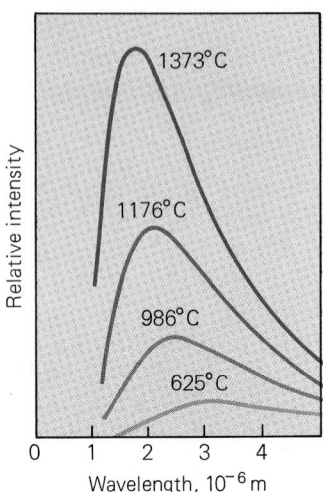

Figure 9-4 Every object gives off electromagnetic radiation. These curves show how the intensity of the radiation varies with wavelength for idealized objects called blackbodies at the temperatures indicated. More energy is given off, and the predominant wavelength decreases, as temperature increases. The greater the surface area of the emitting object, the more radiation is given off.

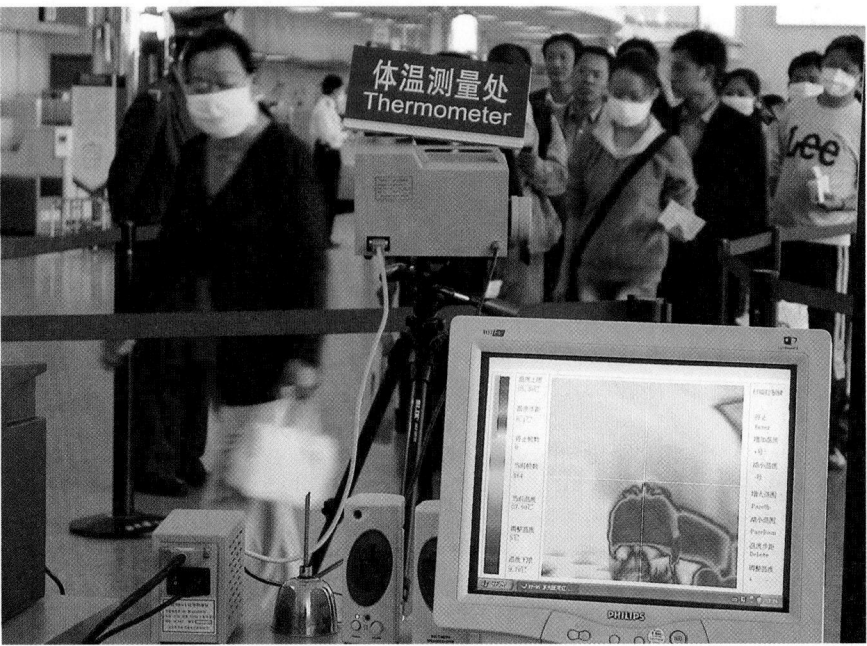

Figure 9-5 The spectrum of the electromagnetic radiation from a surface depends on the temperature of the surface. The system shown here detects people with fevers on the basis of their infrared emissions, with red indicating skin temperatures above normal. In this way people with illnesses that may be infectious can be easily identified in airports, hotels, hospitals, and other public places.

In this formula the quantity *h,* today known as **Planck's constant,** has the value

$$\text{Planck's constant} = h = 6.63 \times 10^{-34} \text{ joule} \cdot \text{second}$$

Planck was not happy about this assumption, which made no sense in terms of the physical theories known at that time. He took the position that, although energy apparently had to be given to the light emitted by a glowing object in small bursts, the light nevertheless traveled with its energy spread out in waves exactly as everybody thought.

Einstein's Hypothesis   Einstein, however, felt that, if light is emitted in little packets, it should also travel through space and finally be absorbed in the same little packets. His idea fit the experiments on the photoelectric effect perfectly (Fig. 9-6). Einstein supposed that some minimum energy *w* is needed to pull an electron away from a metal surface. If the frequency of the light is too low—so that *E*, the quantum energy, is less than *w*—no electrons can come out. When *E* is greater than *w*, a photon of light striking an electron can give the electron enough energy for it to leave the metal with a certain amount of kinetic energy (Fig. 9-7).

Einstein's formula for the photoelectric effect is very simple:

$$hf = \text{KE} + w \qquad \textit{Photoelectric effect} \qquad 9\text{-}2$$

where hf = energy of a photon of light whose frequency is f

KE = kinetic energy of the emitted electron

w = energy needed to pull the electron from the metal

Although the photon has no mass and always moves with the speed of light, it has most of the other properties of particles—it is localized in a small region of space, it has energy and momentum, and it interacts with other particles in more or less the same way as a billiard ball interacts with other billiard balls.

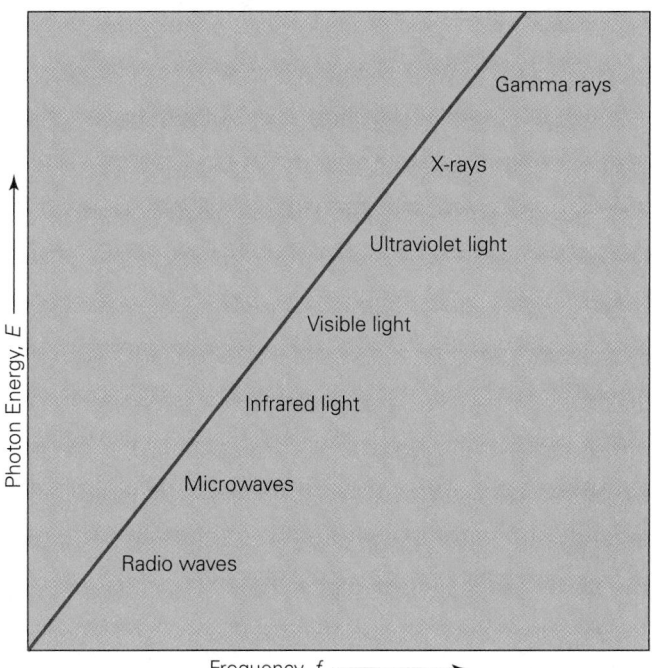

Figure 9-6 The higher the frequency of an electromagnetic wave, the greater the energy of its photons, since $E = hf$. Radio waves have the lowest frequencies, hence their photons have the least energy; gamma rays have the highest frequencies, hence their photons have the most energy. (The spacing of the categories here is not to scale.)

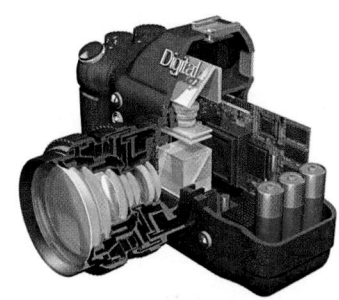

Figure 9-7 All light-sensitive detectors, including the eye and the one used in this digital camera, are based on the absorption of energy from photons of light by electrons in the atoms the light falls on.

Example 9.1

The average frequency of the light emitted by a 100-W lightbulb is 5.5×10^{14} Hz. How many photons per second does the lightbulb emit?

Solution

The energy of each photon is, from Eq. 9-1,

$$E = hf = (6.63 \times 10^{-34} \text{ J} \cdot \text{s})(5.5 \times 10^{14} \text{ Hz}) = 3.6 \times 10^{-19} \text{ J}$$

Since 100 W = 100 J/s, the number of photons emitted per second is

$$\frac{\text{Energy/second}}{\text{energy/photon}} = \frac{100 \text{ J/s}}{3.6 \times 10^{-19} \text{ J/photon}} = 2.8 \times 10^{20} \text{ photons/s}$$

Such an enormous number of photons makes it impossible for us to experience light as a stream of individual particles.

9.3 What Is Light?

Both Wave and Particle

The idea that light travels as a series of little packets of energy is directly opposed to the wave theory of light. And the latter, which provides the only way to explain such optical effects as diffraction and interference, is one of the best established of physical theories. Planck's suggestion that a hot object gives energy to light in separate quanta led to no more than raised eyebrows among physicists in 1900 since it did not apparently conflict with the picture of light as a wave. Einstein's suggestion in 1905 that light travels through space in the form of distinct photons, on the other hand, astonished most of his colleagues.

According to wave theory, light waves spread out from a source in the way ripples spread out on the surface of a lake when a stone falls into it. The energy carried by the light in this picture is spread out through the wave pattern (Fig. 9-8). According to the quantum theory, however, light travels from a source as a series of tiny bursts of energy, each burst so small that it can be

Figure 9-8   (*a*) The wave theory of light accounts for the diffraction of light into the shadow region when it passes through a narrow slit. (*b*) The quantum theory of light accounts for the photoelectric effect. Neither theory by itself can account for all aspects of the behavior of light. The two theories therefore complement each other.

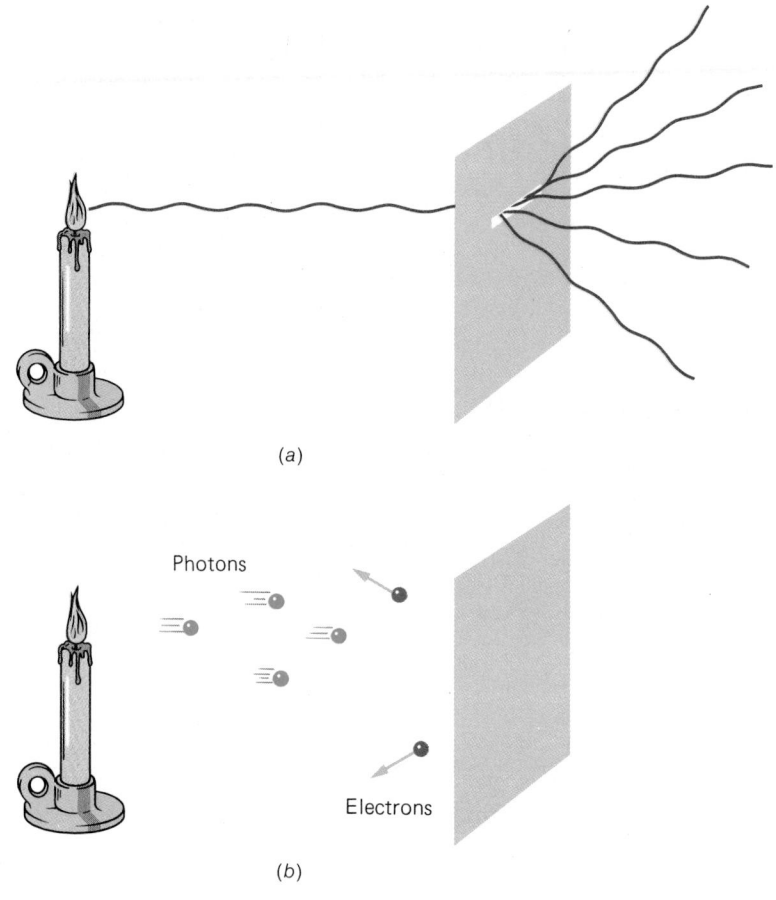

(*a*)

Photons

Electrons

(*b*)

Photons and Gravity

In Sec. 3.13 we saw that light is affected by gravity, which was predicted by Einstein's general theory of relativity and confirmed by measurements on starlight that passes close to the sun. This suggests that photons must be subject to gravity, which is indeed the case.

If we drop a stone, the gravitational pull of the earth accelerates the stone so that it falls faster and thus gains kinetic energy on the way to the ground. All photons travel with the speed of light and so cannot go any faster. However, a photon can manifest a gain in energy by an increase in frequency. This increase, which has been observed, is proportional to the original frequency of the photon and to the height through which it falls. For visible light the frequency change is a few hertz for a fall through 20 m.

taken up by a single electron. Curiously, the quantum theory of light, which treats light as a particle phenomenon, incorporates the light frequency *f*, a wave concept.

Which theory are we to believe? A great many scientific ideas have had to be changed or discarded when they were found to disagree with experiment. Here, for the first time, two entirely different theories are needed to account for a single physical phenomenon.

In any particular event light exhibits *either* a wave nature or a particle nature, never both at the same time. This is an important point. The light beam that shows diffraction in passing the edge of an obstacle can also cause photoelectrons to be emitted from a metal surface, but these processes occur independently:

> The wave theory of light and the quantum theory of light complement each other.

Electromagnetic waves provide the only explanation for some experiments involving light, and photons provide the only explanation for all other experiments involving light. Light incorporates both wave and particle characters even though there is nothing in everyday life like that to help us form a mental picture of it.

9.4   X-Rays

High-Energy Photons

The photoelectric effect shows that photons of light can give energy to electrons. Is the reverse process also possible? That is, can part or all of the kinetic energy of an electron be turned into a photon? As it happens, the inverse photoelectric effect not only does occur but also had been discovered (though not understood) before the work of Planck and Einstein.

In 1895, in his laboratory in Germany, Wilhelm Roentgen (Fig. 9-9) accidentally found that a screen coated with a fluorescent salt glowed every time he switched on a nearby cathode-ray tube. (A cathode-ray tube is a tube with the air pumped out in which electrons are accelerated by an electric field. A TV picture tube is a type of cathode-ray tube.) Roentgen knew that the electrons themselves could not get through the glass walls of his tube, but it was clear that some sort of invisible radiation was falling on the screen.

The radiation was very penetrating. Thick pieces of wood, glass, and even metal could be placed between tube and screen, and still the screen glowed. Soon Roentgen found that his mysterious rays would penetrate flesh and produce shadows of the bones inside. He gave them the name **x-rays** after the algebraic symbol for an unknown quantity. Roentgen refused to benefit financially from his work and died in poverty in the German inflation that followed World War I.

X-rays are given off whenever fast electrons are stopped suddenly. Figure 9-10 shows a cathode-ray tube especially designed to produce x-rays. X-rays are widely used today in medicine (Figs. 9-11 and 9-12) and industry.

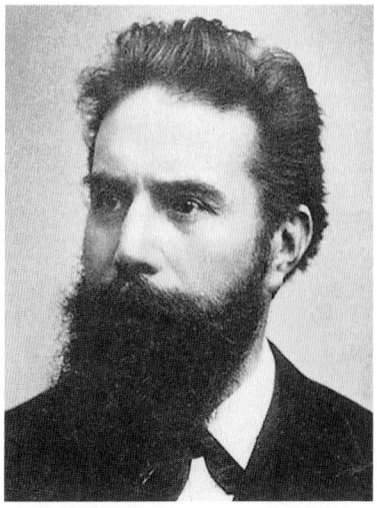

Figure 9-9 Wilhelm Roentgen (1845–1923).

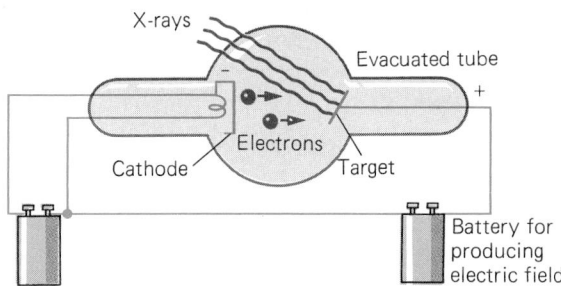

Figure 9-10 A simple x-ray tube. High-frequency electromagnetic waves called x-rays are emitted by a metal target when it is struck by fast-moving electrons. The cathode (negative electrode) is heated to around 1000°C by a filament and emits electrons that are accelerated by an electric field between it and the positively charged target.

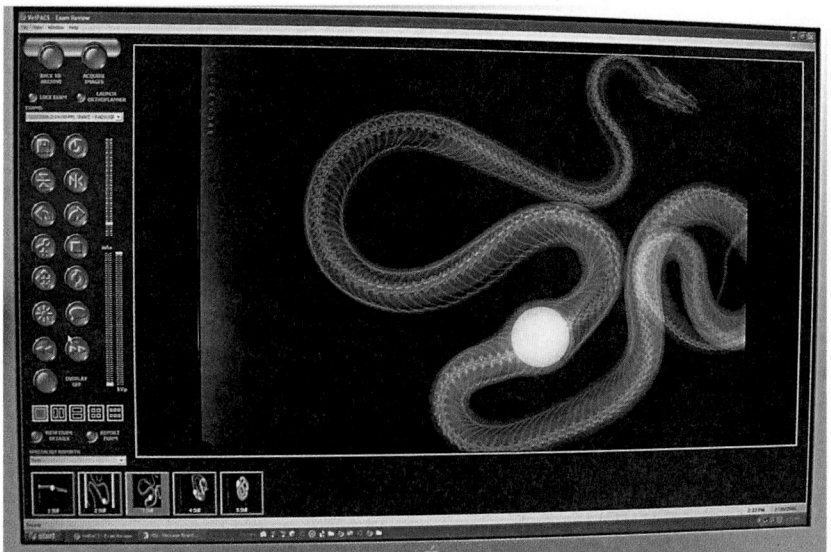

Figure 9-12 X-ray image of a yellow rat snake that had swallowed a golf ball, presumably under the impression it was an egg. The golf ball was later removed by a veterinarian.

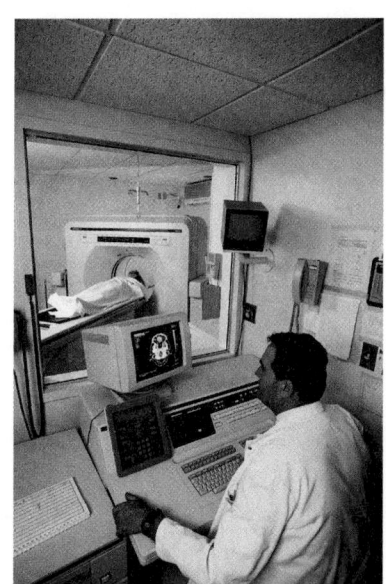

Figure 9-11 In a CT (computerized tomography) scanner, a series of x-ray exposures of a patient taken from different directions are combined by a computer to give cross-sectional images of the part of the body being examined. In effect, the tissue is sliced up by the computer on the basis of the x-ray exposures, and any desired slice can be displayed. This technique enables an abnormality to be detected and its exact location established, which might be impossible to do from an ordinary x-ray picture. The patient's head is being examined here.

What Are X-Rays?   After many attempts had been made to determine their nature, in 1912 Max von Laue was able to show by means of an interference experiment that they are electromagnetic waves of extremely high frequency. X-ray frequencies are much higher than those of ultraviolet light, but somewhat lower than those of the gamma rays produced by radioactive atomic nuclei.

The early workers with x-rays noted that increasing the voltage applied to the tube, which means faster electrons, gave rise to x-rays of greater penetrating power. The greater the penetrating ability, the higher the x-ray frequency turned out to be. Hence high-energy electrons produce high-frequency x-rays. The more electrons in the beam, the more x-rays were produced, but their energy depended only on the electron energy.

The quantum theory of light is in complete accord with these observations. Instead of photon energy being transformed into electron KE, electron KE is transformed into photon energy. The energy of an x-ray photon of frequency f is hf, and therefore the minimum KE of the electron that produced the x-ray should be equal to hf. This prediction agrees with experimental data.

Matter Waves

As we have seen, light has both wave and particle aspects. In the topsy-turvy world of the very small, is it possible that what we normally think of as particles—electrons, for instance—have wave properties as well? So extraordinary is this question that it was not asked for two decades after Einstein's work. Soon after the question was raised came the even more extraordinary answer: yes.

9.5   De Broglie Waves

Matter Waves Are Significant Only in the Atomic World

In 1924 the French physicist Louis de Broglie proposed that moving objects act in some respects like waves. Reasoning by analogy with the properties of photons, he suggested that a particle of mass m and speed v behaves as though it is a wave whose wavelength is

$$\lambda = \frac{h}{mv} \qquad \textit{de Broglie waves} \qquad 9\text{-}3$$

$$\text{de Broglie wavelength} = \frac{\text{Planck's constant}}{\text{momentum}}$$

The more momentum mv a particle has, the shorter its **de Broglie wavelength** λ.

How can de Broglie's hypothesis be tested? Only waves can be diffracted and can reinforce and cancel each other by interference. A few years after de Broglie's work, experiments were performed in the United States and in England in which streams of electrons were shown to exhibit both diffraction and interference. The wavelengths of the electrons could be found from the data, and they agreed exactly with the formula $\lambda = h/mv$. (G. P. Thomson, the English physicist who shared a Nobel Prize for helping establish the wave properties of moving electrons, was the son of J. J. Thomson, who had won an earlier Nobel Prize for establishing the particle properties of electrons.)

There is nothing imaginary about these **matter waves.** They are perfectly real, just as light and sound waves are. Not only electrons but also all other moving objects behave like waves. However, these waves are not necessarily evident in every situation, as Example 9.2 indicates. Only on an atomic scale

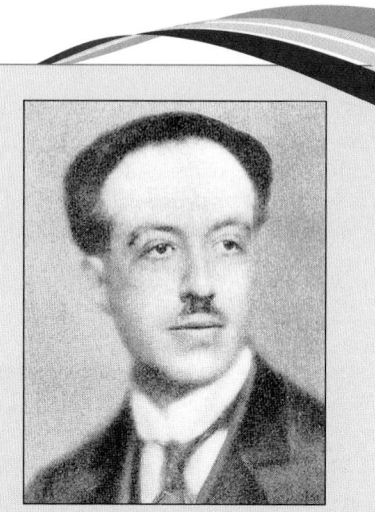

De Broglie originally pursued a career in history but later turned to physics. In his University of Paris doctoral thesis of 1924 de Broglie proposed that moving objects have wave properties that complement their particle properties: these "seemingly incompatible conceptions can each represent an aspect of the truth. . . . They may serve in turn to represent the facts without ever entering into direct conflict."

Looking back, it may seem odd that two decades passed between Einstein's 1905 discovery of the particle behavior of light waves and de Broglie's speculation. It is one thing, however, to suggest a revolutionary concept to explain otherwise mysterious data and quite another to suggest an equally revolutionary concept without such data in hand.

Experiments soon showed that de Broglie's idea was correct, and it was developed by Erwin Schrödinger and others into a detailed theory, called *quantum mechanics*, that explained a wide variety of atomic phenomena. In 1929 de Broglie received the Nobel Prize.

are matter waves significant, and there they turn out to be the key to understanding atomic structure and behavior.

As with electromagnetic waves, the wave and particle aspects of moving bodies can never be observed at the same time. It therefore makes no sense to ask which is the "correct" description. All we can say is that in certain situations a moving body exhibits wave properties and in other situations it exhibits particle properties.

Example 9.2

Find the de Broglie wavelengths of (a) a 46-g golf ball whose speed is 30 m/s, and (b) an electron whose speed is 10^7 m/s.

Solution

(a) From Eq. 9-3, with $m = 46$ g $= 0.046$ kg,

$$\lambda = \frac{h}{mv} = \frac{6.63 \times 10^{-34}\,\text{J} \cdot \text{s}}{(0.046\,\text{kg})(30\,\text{m/s})} = 4.8 \times 10^{-34}\,\text{m}$$

The wavelength of the golf ball is so small compared with its dimensions that we would not expect to find any wave aspects in its behavior.

(b) The electron mass is 9.1×10^{-31} kg, so

$$\lambda = \frac{h}{mv} = \frac{6.63 \times 10^{-34}\,\text{J} \cdot \text{s}}{(9.1 \times 10^{-31}\,\text{kg})(10^7\,\text{m/s})} = 7.3 \times 10^{-11}\,\text{m}$$

The dimensions of atoms are comparable with this wavelength—the radius of the hydrogen atom is 5.3×10^{-11} m, for example. It is therefore not surprising that the wave character of moving electrons is so important in the world of the atom.

9.6 Waves of What?

Waves of Probability

In water waves, the quantity that varies periodically is the height of the water surface. In sound waves, it is air pressure. In light waves, electric and magnetic fields vary. What is it that varies in the case of matter waves?

The quantity whose variations make up matter waves is called the **wave function,** symbol ψ (the Greek letter *psi*). The value of ψ^2 at a given place and time for a given particle determines the probability of finding the particle

Electron Microscopes

The wave nature of moving electrons is the basis of the electron microscope. The resolving power of any optical instrument depends on the wavelength of whatever is used to illuminate the specimen being studied. In the case of a microscope that uses visible light, the highest useful magnification is about 500×. Higher magnifications give larger images but do not show more detail.

Fast electrons, however, have wavelengths much shorter than those of visible light, and electron microscopes can produce useful magnifications of over 1,000,000×. X-rays also have short wavelengths, but it is not (yet?) possible to focus them adequately. In an electron microscope, an electron beam is directed at a thin specimen. Magnetic fields that act as lenses to focus the beam then produce an enlarged image of the specimen on a fluorescent screen or photographic film (Figs. 9-13 and 9-14).

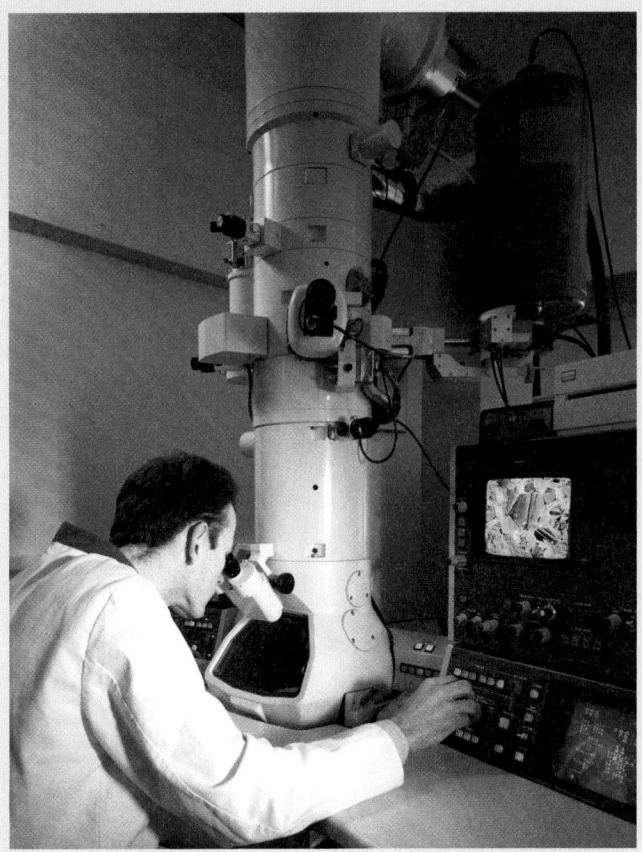

Figure 9-13   An electron microscope.

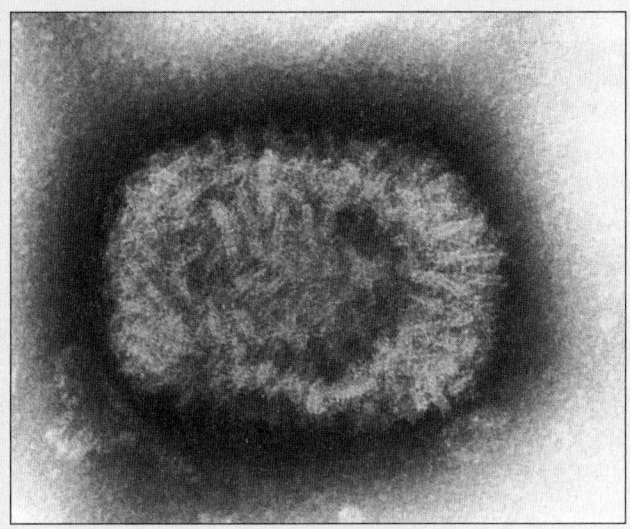

Figure 9-14   Electron micrograph of a smallpox virus particle at a magnification of 310,000×.

there at that time. For this reason ψ^2 is called the **probability density** of the particle. A large value of ψ^2 means the strong possibility of the particle's presence; a small value of ψ^2 means its presence is unlikely.

The de Broglie waves associated with a moving particle are in the form of a group, or packet, of waves, as in Fig. 9-15. This wave packet travels with the same speed v as the particle does. Even though we cannot visualize what is meant by ψ and so cannot form a mental image of matter waves, the agreement between theory and experiment means that we must take them seriously.

9.7   Uncertainty Principle

We Cannot Know the Future Because We Cannot Know the Present

To regard a moving particle as a wave packet suggests that there are limits to the accuracy with which we can measure such "particle" properties as position and speed. The particle whose wave packet is shown in Fig. 9-15 may

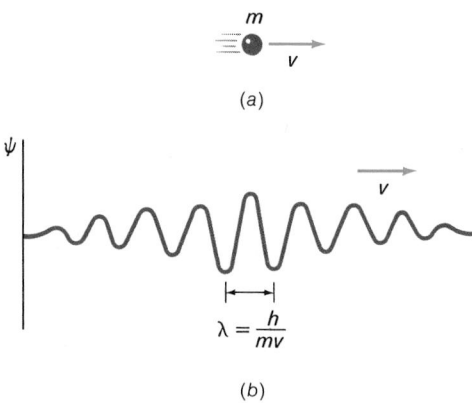

(a)

(b)

$$\lambda = \frac{h}{mv}$$

Figure 9-15 (*a*) Particle description of a moving object. (*b*) Wave description of the same moving object. The packet of matter waves that corresponds to a certain object moves with the same speed *v* as the object does. The waves are waves of probability.

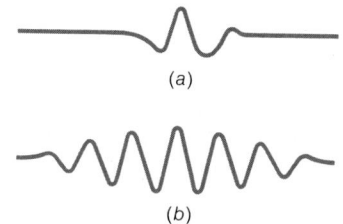

(a)

(b)

Figure 9-16 (*a*) A narrow wave packet. The position of the particle can be precisely determined, but the wavelength (and hence the particle's momentum) cannot be established because there are not enough waves to measure λ accurately. (*b*) A wide wave packet. Now the wavelength can be accurately determined, but not the position of the particle.

be located anywhere within the packet at a given time. Of course, the probability density ψ^2 is a maximum in the middle of the packet, so the particle is most likely to be found there. But we may still find the particle anywhere that ψ^2 is not 0.

The narrower its wave packet, the more precisely a particle's position can be specified (Fig. 9-16*a*). However, the wavelength of the waves in a narrow packet is not well defined. There are just not enough waves to measure λ accurately. This means that, since $\lambda = h/mv$, the particle's momentum *mv* and hence speed *v* are not precise quantities. If we make a series of momentum measurements, we will find a broad range of values.

On the other hand, a wide wave packet such as that in Fig. 9-16*b* has a clearly defined wavelength. The momentum that corresponds to this wavelength is therefore a precise quantity, and a series of measurements will give a narrow range of values. But where is the particle located? The width of the packet is now too great for us to be able to say just where the particle is at a given time.

Thus we have the **uncertainty principle:**

> It is impossible to know both the exact position and the exact momentum of a particle at the same time.

This principle, which was discovered by Werner Heisenberg, is one of the most significant of physical laws.

Since we cannot know exactly both where a particle is right now and what its speed is, we cannot say anything definite about where it will be 2 s from now and how fast it will be moving then. *We cannot know the future for sure because we cannot know the present for sure.* But our ignorance is not total. We can still say that the particle is more likely to be in one place than another and that its speed is more likely to have a certain value than another.

All objects, of whatever size, are governed by the uncertainty principle, which means that their positions and motions likewise can be expressed only as probabilities. There is a chance that this book will someday defy the law of gravity and rise up in the air by itself. But for objects this large—in fact, even for objects the size of molecules—such probabilities are so small as to be practically zero. The likelihood that this book will continue to obey the law of gravity is so great that we can be quite sure it will stay where it is if left alone. Only in the behavior of electrons and other atomic particles do matter waves play an important part. [For more, see Sec. 9.7 at www.mhhe.com/krauskopf.]

B I O G R A P H Y | Werner Heisenberg (1901–1976)

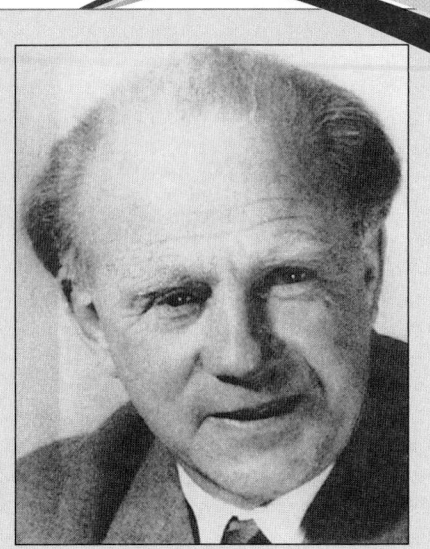

Heisenberg studied theoretical physics in Munich, Germany, where he also became an enthusiastic skier and mountaineer. In 1927 he showed that $\Delta x\Delta(mv)$, the product of the uncertainties in a simultaneous measurement of a particle's position and momentum, can never be less than $h/4\pi$, where h is Planck's constant. This conclusion is an inescapable consequence of the wave nature of moving particles.

Because h is so small, the uncertainty principle is an important factor only in the atomic world, where it tells us what we might be able to know about events in this world and what we cannot ever know. Heisenberg distrusted mechanical models of the atom: "Any picture of the atom that our imagination is able to invent is for that very reason defective," he remarked.

Heisenberg was one of the very few distinguished scientists to remain in Germany during the Nazi period. In World War II he led research there on nuclear weapons, but little progress had been made by the war's end. Poor experimental data seems to have been the reason—there is no evidence that Heisenberg, as he later claimed, had moral qualms about creating such weapons for Hitler and deliberately dragged his feet.

Alarmed by the news that Heisenberg was working on a nuclear bomb, the U.S. government sent the former Boston Red Sox catcher Moe Berg to shoot Heisenberg during a lecture in neutral Switzerland in 1944. Berg, sitting in the second row, found himself uncertain from Heisenberg's remarks about how advanced the German program was, and kept his gun in his pocket. A lawyer who spoke five languages as well as being an athlete, Berg carried out other secret missions in Europe during and after the war.

The Hydrogen Atom

We now have what we need to make sense of atomic structures: the Rutherford model of the atom, the quantum theory of light, and the wave theory of moving particles. When linked together, these concepts give rise to a theory of the atom that agrees with experiment. Our starting point will be the hydrogen atom—the simplest of all—with its single electron outside a nucleus that consists of a single proton.

9.8 Atomic Spectra

Each Element Has a Characteristic Spectrum

When an electric current is passed through a gas, electrons in the gas atoms absorb energy from the current. The gas is said to be **excited.** An excited neon gas gives off a bright orange-red light; other excited gases give off light of other colors. We have all seen signs based on this effect (Fig. 9-17), but not all of us are aware of how closely related the color of the light is to the way the electrons in the gas atoms are arranged.

Figure 9-18 shows an instrument called a **spectroscope** that disperses (spreads out) the light emitted by an excited gas into the different frequencies the light contains. Each frequency appears on the screen as a bright line, and the resulting series of bright lines is called an **emission spectrum** (Fig. 9-19a). Because some of the lines are more intense than the rest, the original undispersed light usually gives the impression of being a specific color, orange-red in the case of neon, even though other colors are present as well.

An emission spectrum is different from a **continuous spectrum,** which is the rainbow band produced when light from a hot object passes through a spectroscope (see Fig. 7-55). A continuous spectrum contains all frequencies, not just a few.

Absorption Spectra   Spectra of a different kind, **absorption spectra,** occur when light from a hot source passes through a cool gas before entering the spectroscope. The light source alone would give a continuous spectrum, but atoms of the gas absorb certain frequencies from the light that goes through it. Hence the original continuous spectrum is now crossed by dark lines, each line corresponding to one of the absorbed frequencies (Fig. 9-19*b*).

If the emission spectrum of an element is compared with the absorption spectrum of the same element, the dark lines in the latter spectrum have the same frequencies as a number of the bright lines in the former spectrum. Thus a cool gas absorbs some of the frequencies of the light that it emits when excited. The spectrum of sunlight has dark lines in it because the luminous part of the sun, which radiates much like an object heated to 6000 K, has around it an envelope of cooler gas (Chap. 18).

Because the line spectrum of each element (either emission or absorption) contains frequencies that are characteristic of that element only, the spectrometer is a valuable tool in chemical analysis (Fig. 9-20). Even the smallest traces of an element can be identified by the lines in a spectrum of an unknown substance. Helium was discovered in the sun through its spectrum 17 years before it was identified on the earth in 1895 (*helios* is Greek for "sun").

Spectral Series   A century ago it was discovered that the frequencies in the spectrum of an element fall into sets called **spectral series** (Fig. 9-21). A simple formula relates the frequencies in each series. When the foundations of the modern picture of the atom had been laid, these spectral series provided the final clues for working out the details of atomic structure.

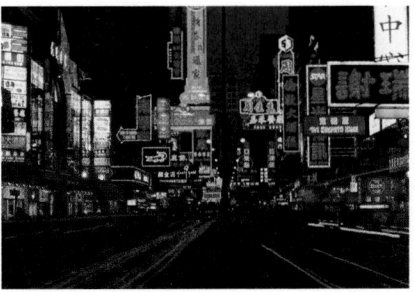

Figure 9-17   Hong Kong at night. Gas atoms excited by electric currents in the tubes of these signs radiate light of wavelengths characteristic of the gas used.

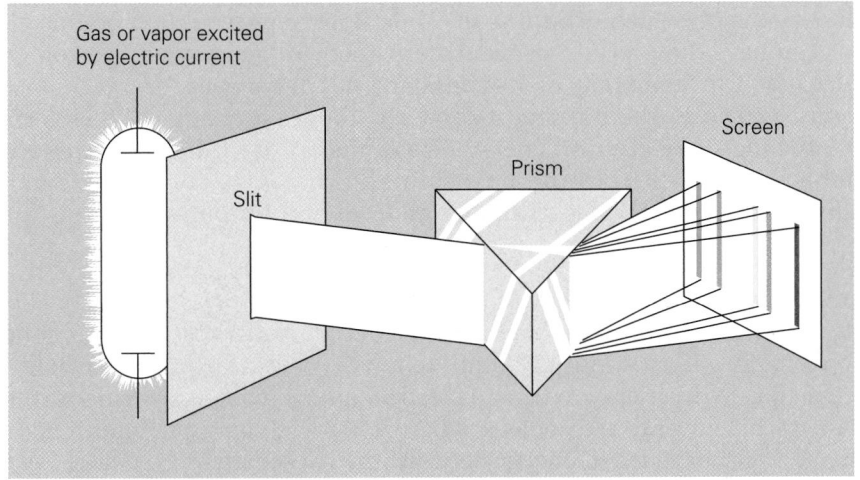

Figure 9-18   An idealized spectroscope. Dispersion in the prism separates light of different frequencies.

Figure 9-19   (*a*) Part of the emission spectrum of sodium. Each bright line represents a specific frequency in the light given off when sodium vapor is excited in an arrangement such as that shown in Figure 9-17. Every element emits a set of frequencies that is characteristic of that element. (*b*) Part of the absorption spectrum of sodium. Each dark line represents a specific frequency in the light absorbed by sodium vapor when white light passes through the vapor. Every dark absorption line corresponds to one of the bright lines in the emission spectrum of the same element.

Figure 9-20 Some of the principal lines in the emission spectra of hydrogen, helium, and mercury. These were produced by passing electric currents through gaseous hydrogen and helium and through mercury vapor, which caused them to radiate light whose frequencies are characteristic of the atoms involved. One of the great triumphs of the modern theory of the atom has been its explanation of why such particular frequencies occur, and from such frequencies a great deal can be learned about the electron structures of the atoms of the elements.

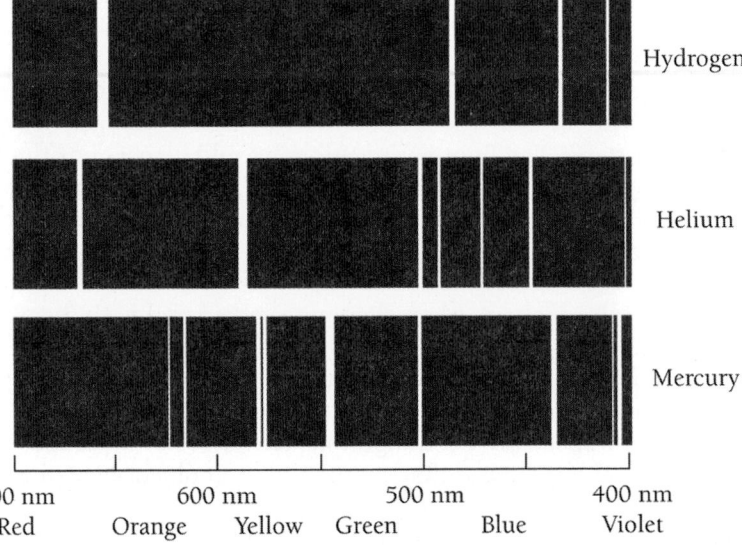

Hydrogen

Helium

Mercury

700 nm　　　　600 nm　　　　500 nm　　　　400 nm
Red　　Orange　Yellow　Green　　Blue　　Violet

Wavelength, nm

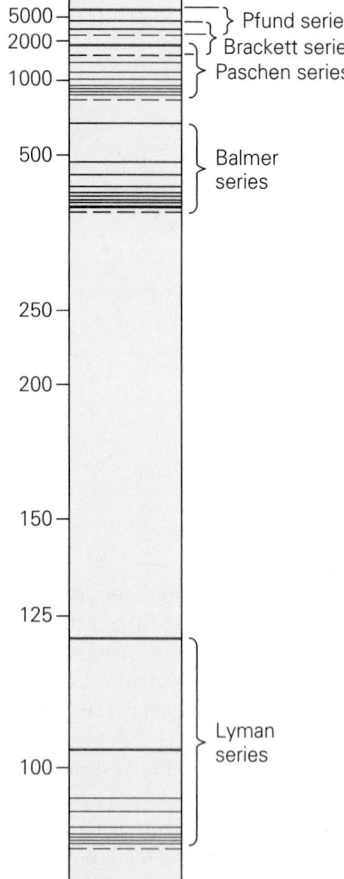

5000 — Pfund series
2000 — Brackett series
1000 — Paschen series

500 — Balmer series

250 —

200 —

150 —

125 —

100 — Lyman series

Figure 9-21 The spectral series of hydrogen. The wavelengths (and hence frequencies) in each series can be related by simple formulas (1 nm = 1 nanometer = 10^{-9} m).

9.9　The Bohr Model

Only Certain Electron Energies Are Possible in an Atom

Niels Bohr, a Dane, put forward in 1913 a theory of the hydrogen atom that could account both for its stability and for the frequencies of the spectral lines of hydrogen. Bohr applied the then-new quantum ideas to atomic structure to come up with a model that, even though later replaced by a more complex picture of greater accuracy and usefulness, is still the mental image many scientists have of the atom.

Bohr began by proposing that an electron in an atom can circle the nucleus without losing energy only in certain specific orbits. Because these orbits are each a different distance from the nucleus, the energy of the electron depends on which orbit it is in. Thus Bohr suggested that atomic electrons can have only certain particular energies. An analogy is a person on a ladder, who can stand only on its rungs and not in between.

An electron in the innermost orbit has the least energy. The larger the orbit, the more the electron energy. The orbits are identified by a **quantum number,** n, which is $n = 1$ for the innermost orbit, $n = 2$ for the next, and so on. Each orbit corresponds to an **energy level** of the atom.

Explaining Spectral Lines　That atoms emit and absorb only light of certain frequencies, which we observe as spectral lines, fits Bohr's atomic model perfectly. An electron in a particular orbit can absorb only those photons of light whose energy will permit it to "jump" to another orbit farther out, where the electron has more energy. When an electron jumps from a particular orbit to another orbit closer to the nucleus, where it has less energy, it emits a photon of light. The difference in energy between the two orbits is hf, where f is the frequency of the absorbed or emitted light.

Figure 9-22 shows the possible orbits of the electron in a hydrogen atom. The circle nearest the nucleus represents the electron orbit under ordinary conditions, when the atom has the lowest possible energy. Such an atom is said to be in its **ground state.** The other circles represent orbits in which the electron would have more energy, since it would then be farther from the nucleus. (Similarly a stone on the roof of a building has more potential energy than it has on the ground, since it is farther from the earth's center when it is on the roof.)

The Bohrs were a distinguished Danish family: Niels's father was a professor of physiology, his brother Harald was a noted mathematician, and his son Aage, like Niels himself, would win a Nobel Prize in physics. After receiving his doctorate in 1911, Bohr visited Rutherford's laboratory in England where he was introduced to the just-discovered nuclear model of the atom.

To understand how atomic spectra are produced by such atomic structures, Bohr began with two revolutionary ideas. The first was that an atomic electron can circle its nucleus only in certain orbits, and the other was that an atom emits or absorbs a photon of light when an electron jumps from one orbit to another. Bohr was able to develop these ideas into a

theory that accounted for the spectral series of hydrogen.

Einstein, who was impressed by Bohr's theory, commented on its bold mix of classical and quantum concepts: "One ought to be ashamed for the successes [of the theory] because they have been earned according to the Jesuit maxim, 'Let not thy left hand know what the other doeth.' "

A decade later de Broglie clarified the basis of Bohr's theory by showing how the restriction of atomic electrons to certain orbits arises from the wave nature of the electrons. Bohr did other important work, including the explanation in 1939 of why nuclear fission, which had just been discovered, occurs in some nuclides but not in others.

Legend has it that, when asked if he really thought the horseshoe

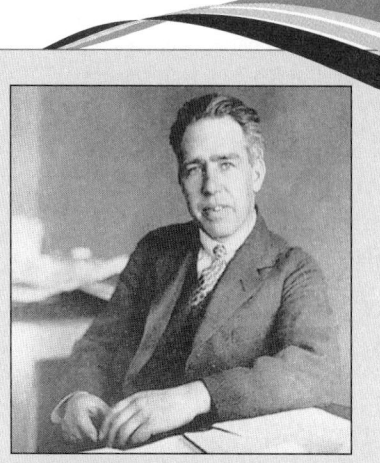

nailed above the door to his summer house brought good luck, Bohr replied, "Of course I don't believe such superstitious nonsense, but I'm told it works even if you don't believe it."

Suppose an atom is in its ground state. If the atom is given energy—by strong heating, by an electric discharge, or by radiation—the electron may jump to a larger orbit (Fig. 9-23). This jump means that the atom has absorbed energy. The atom keeps the added energy as long as it is in the **excited state,** that is, as long as the electron stays in the larger orbit. Because excited states are unstable, in a fraction of a second (usually about 10^{-8} s) the electron drops to a smaller orbit, emitting a photon of light as it does so.

The energy (and hence the frequency) of the photon emitted from a hydrogen atom depends on the particular jump that its electron makes. If the electron jumps from orbit $n = 4$ to orbit $n = 1$ (Fig. 9-24), the energy of the photon will be greater than if the electron jumps from 3 to 1 or 2 to 1. Starting from orbit 4, the electron may return to 1 not only by a single leap but also by stopping at 3 and 2 on the way. Corresponding to these jumps are photons with energies determined by the energy differences between 4 and 3, 3 and 2, 2 and 1.

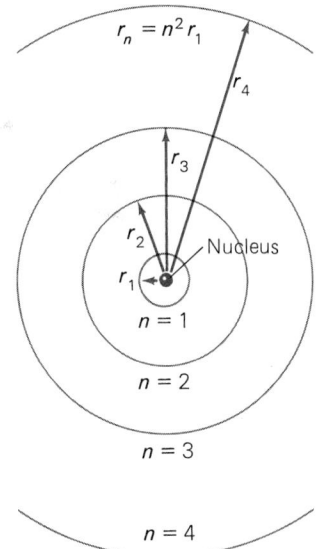

Figure 9-22 Electron orbits in the Bohr model of the hydrogen atom (not to scale). The radius of each orbit is proportional to n^2, the square of the orbit's quantum number. The inner orbit is the electron's normal path, and the outer orbits represent states of higher energy. If the electron absorbs enough energy to jump to an outer orbit, it will return to the $n = 1$ orbit by a single jump or combination of jumps. Each inward jump is accompanied by the emission of a photon.

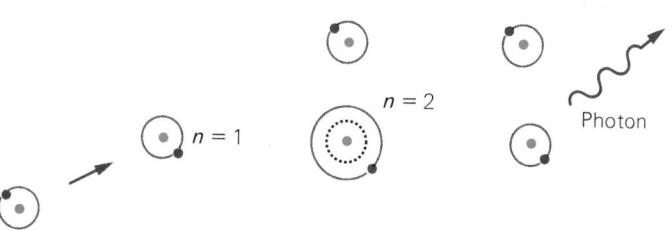

Figure 9-23 Excitation by collision. When two atoms collide, some of the available energy is absorbed by one of the atoms, which goes into an excited energy state. The atom then emits a photon in returning to its ground (normal) state.

Figure 9-24   Spectral lines are the result of jumps between energy levels. The spectral series of hydrogen are shown in Figure 9-21. When $n = \infty$, the electron is free.

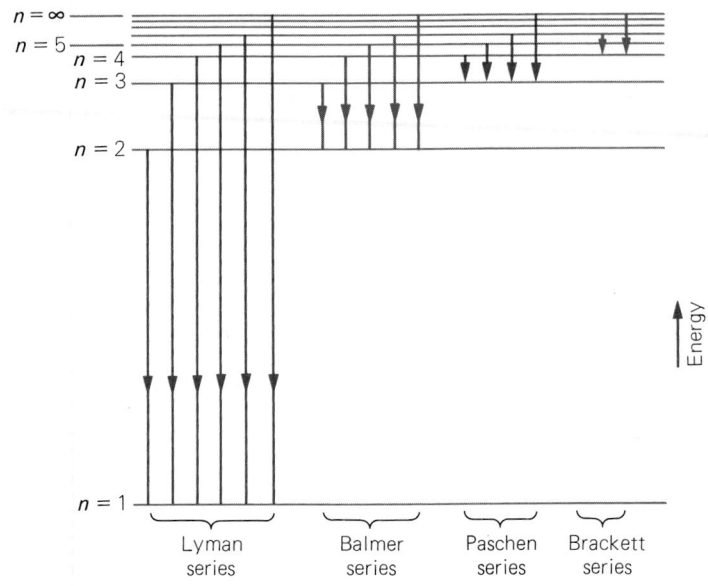

Origin of Absorption Spectra

Figure 9-25 shows how emission and absorption spectra arise. In (a) the jump of an electron from a certain excited state to the ground state of an atom involves the emission of a photon of wavelength λ. This is how an emission (bright) spectrum line originates.

If a photon with the same wavelength λ is absorbed by the atom when it is in its ground state, as in (b), an electron in this state will jump to the same excited state as in (a). This is how an absorption (dark) spectrum line originates.

When white light, which contains all wavelengths, is passed through a gas or vapor, as in Fig. 9-26, photons of those wavelengths that correspond to electron jumps to higher energy levels are absorbed. The resulting excited atoms reradiate their extra energy almost at once, but these photons come off in random directions. Because a few of the reradiated photons are in the direction of the original beam, the dark lines in an absorption spectrum are never completely black.

The lines in an absorption spectrum have the same wavelengths as those of the emission lines that correspond to jumps to the ground state. Hence not all of the emission lines of an element are present in its absorption spectrum, as we saw in Fig. 9-19.

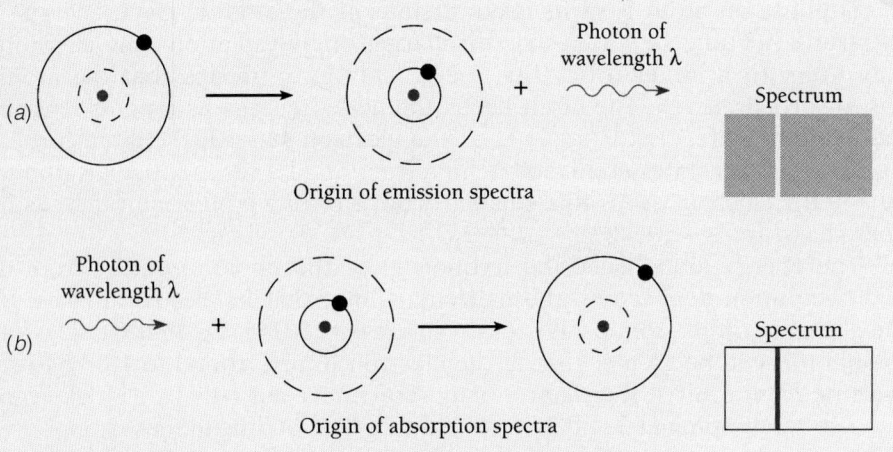

Figure 9-25   How emission and absorption spectra originate.

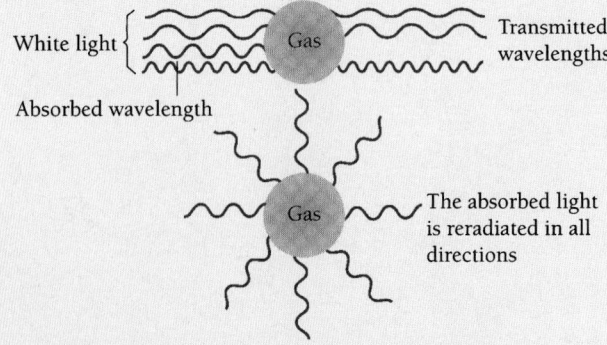

Figure 9-26   The dark lines in an absorption spectrum are never totally dark.

Each electron jump gives a photon of a characteristic frequency and therefore appears in the hydrogen spectrum as a single bright line. The frequencies of the different lines are related since they correspond to different jumps in the same set of orbits. And the relations among the lines that Bohr predicted by this mechanism precisely matched the observed relations among the lines in the hydrogen spectrum. [For an example, see Sec. 9.9 at www.mhhe.com/krauskopf.]

9.10 Electron Waves and Orbits

Standing Waves in the Atom

Why does an atomic electron follow certain orbits only? The answer comes from an analysis of the wave properties of an electron that circles a hydrogen nucleus. It turns out that the de Broglie wavelength of the electron is exactly equal to the circumference of its ground-state (that is, innermost) orbit. Thus the $n = 1$ orbit of the electron in a hydrogen atom corresponds to one complete electron wave joined on itself (Fig. 9-27).

This fact provides us with the final clue we need for a theory of the atom. If we consider the vibrations of a wire loop (Fig. 9-28), we find that their wavelengths always fit a whole number of times into the loop's circumference, so that each wave joins smoothly with the next. These are the only vibrations possible. Regarding electron waves in an atom as analogous to standing waves in a wire loop leads to an interesting concept:

> An electron can circle a nucleus only in orbits that contain a whole number of de Broglie wavelengths.

This idea is the decisive one for understanding the atom. It combines both the particle and the wave characters of the electron into a single statement,

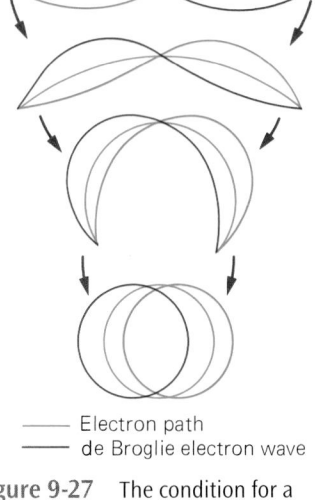

——— Electron path
——— de Broglie electron wave

Figure 9-27 The condition for a stable electron orbit. The orbit of the electron in a hydrogen atom corresponds to a complete de Broglie electron wave joined on itself.

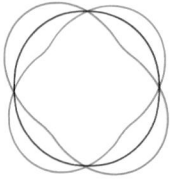 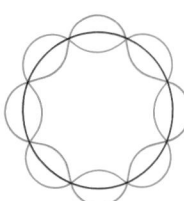 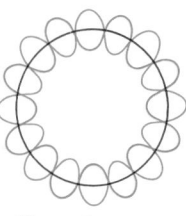

Circumference = 2 wavelengths

Circumference = 4 wavelengths

Circumference = 8 wavelengths

Figure 9-28 Vibrations of a wire loop. In each case a whole number of wavelengths fit into the circumference of the loop.

Quantization in the Atomic World

The presence of energy levels in an atom—which is true for all atoms, not just the hydrogen atom—is a further example of the basic graininess of physical quantities. In the world of our daily lives, matter, electric charge, energy, and so forth seem to be continuous and able to be cut up (so to speak) into chunks of any size at all. But in the world of the atom matter consists of elementary particles with definite masses; charge always comes in multiples of +e and -e; em waves of frequency f appear as streams of photons each with the energy hf; and stable systems of particles, such as atoms, can have only certain energies.

Other quantities in nature are also grainy, or *quantized*. This quantization enters into every aspect of how electrons, protons, and neutrons interact to give the matter around us (and of which we are made) its familiar properties. In the case of an atom, the quantization of energy follows from the wave nature of moving bodies: the electron waves must be standing waves, hence the electrons can have only certain energies.

since the electron wavelength depends upon the orbital speed needed to balance the electrical attraction of the nucleus. These contradictory characters are basic aspects of the atomic world.

Now we see what the quantum number *n* of an orbit means—it is the number of electron waves that fit into the orbit (Fig. 9-29).

9.11   The Laser

An Amplifier of Light That Produces Waves All in Step

A **laser** is a device that produces an intense beam of single-frequency, **coherent** light from the cooperative radiation of excited atoms. The light waves in a coherent beam are all in step with one another, as shown in Fig. 9-30. Ordinary light is incoherent since the atoms in light sources such as lamps and the sun emit light waves randomly.

A laser beam hardly spreads out at all (Fig. 9-31). One sent from the earth to a mirror left on the moon by the Apollo 11 expedition remained narrow enough to be detected on its return to earth, a round-trip distance of over three-quarters of a million km. A light beam produced by any other means would have spread out too much to have been detected. The word *laser* comes from *l*ight *a*mplification by *s*timulated *e*mission of *r*adiation. [For the history of the laser, see Sec. 9.9 at www.mhhe.com/krauskopf.]

Figure 9-29   Energy levels of the hydrogen atom. The energies are negative, which signifies that the electron is bound to its nucleus.

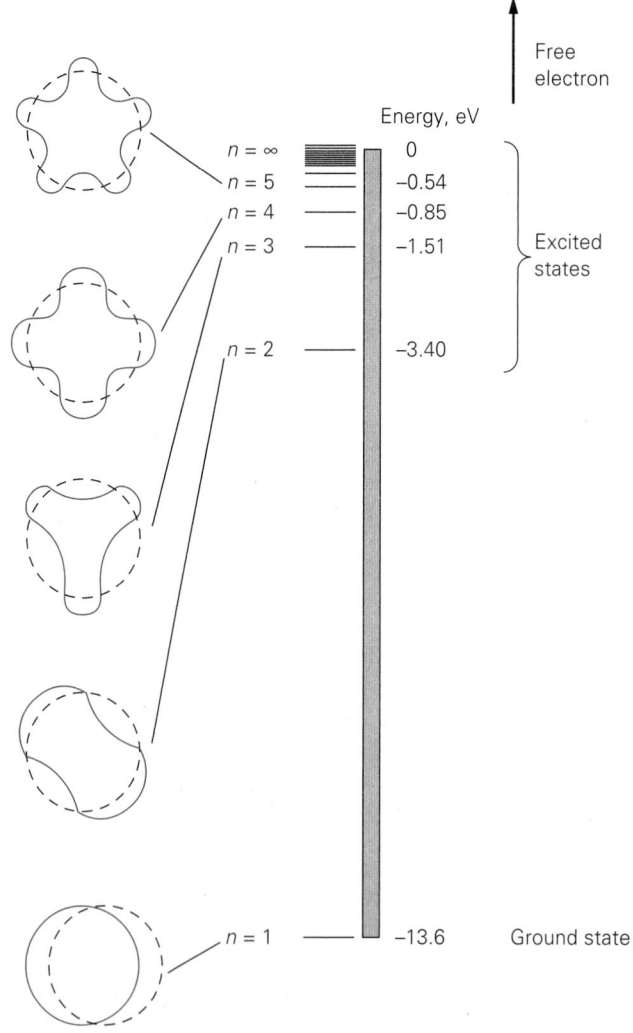

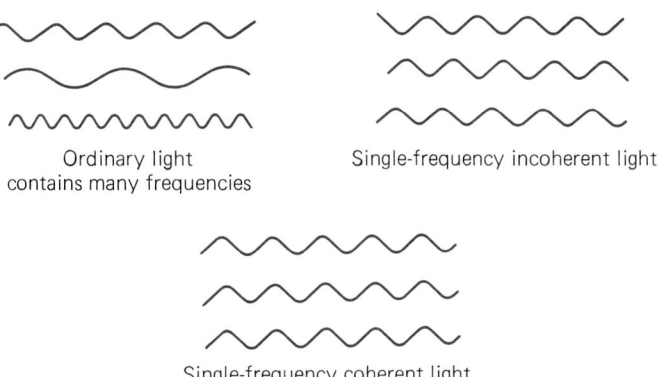

Ordinary light
contains many frequencies

Single-frequency incoherent light

Single-frequency coherent light

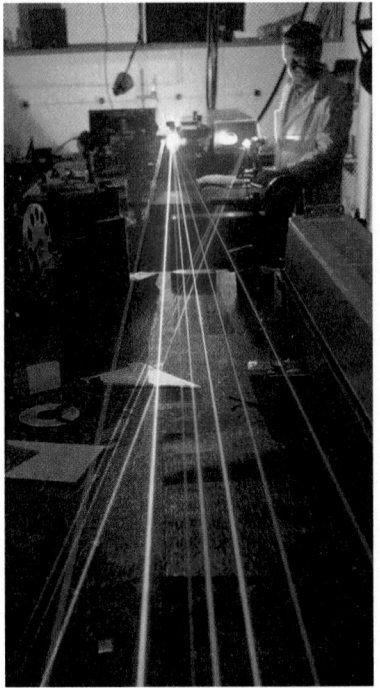

Figure 9-30   A laser produces a beam of light whose waves all have the same frequency and are in step with one another (coherent). The beam is also very narrow and spreads out very little even over long distances.

Figure 9-31   Laser beams at a laboratory in Madrid, Spain.

Metastable States   The key to the laser is that many atoms have one or more excited energy levels whose lifetimes are as much as 0.001 s instead of the usual 10^{-8} s. Such relatively long lived states are called **metastable.**

A laser uses atoms whose metastable states have some excitation energy E_1 (Fig. 9-32). The first step in laser operation is to bring as many of these atoms as possible to this metastable level. Often it is necessary to raise the atoms to a still higher state E_2, from which a number of them fall to the metastable level by emitting a photon of energy $E_2 - E_1$. Several ways exist to do this. In one of them, an external light source provides photons with the right energy. This method was used in the first lasers, in which xenon-filled flash lamps excited chromium ions in ruby rods to the required level E_2 (Fig. 9-33).

Another method is used in the helium-neon laser. Here an electric discharge in the gas mixture produces fast electrons whose impact on the gas

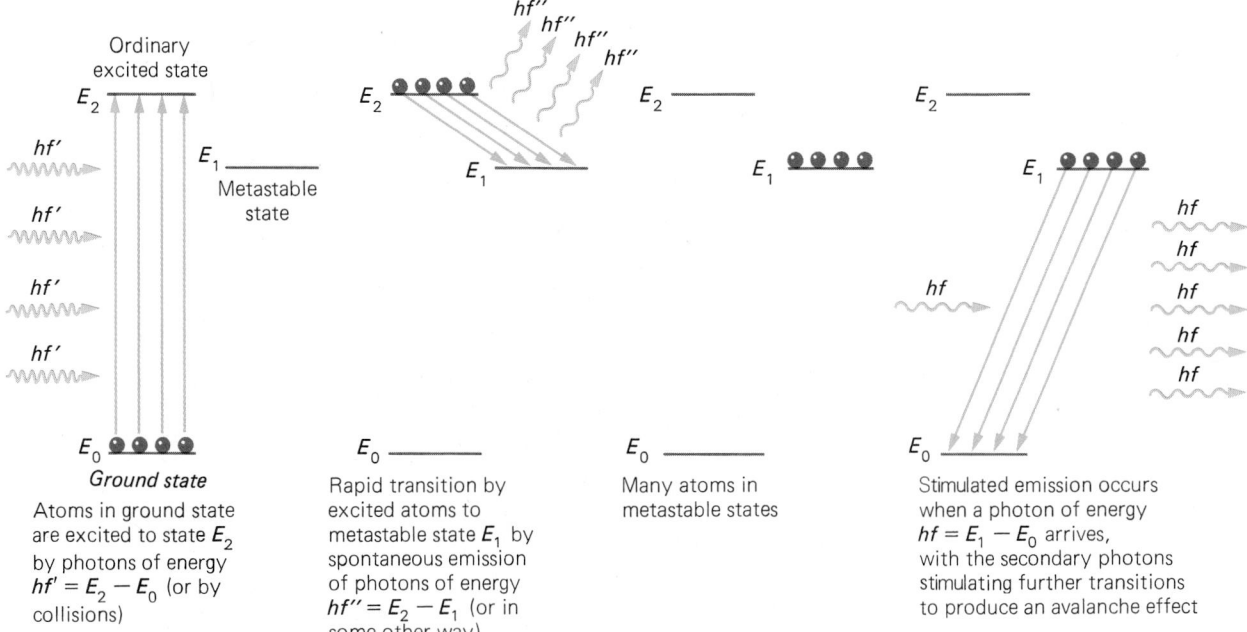

Atoms in ground state are excited to state E_2 by photons of energy $hf' = E_2 - E_0$ (or by collisions)

Rapid transition by excited atoms to metastable state E_1 by spontaneous emission of photons of energy $hf'' = E_2 - E_1$ (or in some other way)

Many atoms in metastable states

Stimulated emission occurs when a photon of energy $hf = E_1 - E_0$ arrives, with the secondary photons stimulating further transitions to produce an avalanche effect

Figure 9-32   The principle of the laser. A metastable atomic state is one that lasts a much longer time than usual before a photon is emitted that brings the atom to a state of lower energy.

Figure 9-33   A ruby laser. A ruby is a crystal that contains Cr^{3+} ions, which are chromium atoms that have lost three electrons each. A Cr^{3+} ion has a metastable level whose lifetime is about 0.003 s. The xenon flash lamp excites the Cr^{3+} ions to a level of higher energy from which they fall to the metastable level by losing energy to other ions in the crystal. Photons from the spontaneous decay of some Cr^{3+} ions cause other excited Cr^{3+} ions to radiate. The result is a large pulse of single-frequency, coherent red light from the partly silvered end of the rod.

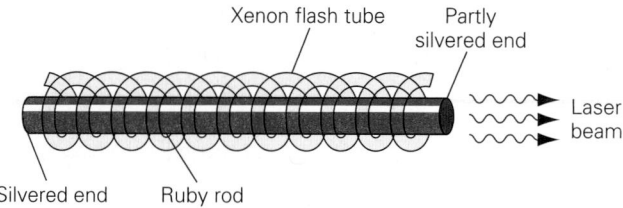

Xenon flash tube   Partly silvered end

Laser beam

Silvered end   Ruby rod

atoms brings them to the required energy level. The advantage is that such a laser can operate continuously, whereas a ruby laser produces separate flashes of light.

Stimulated Emission   With many atoms in the metastable state E_1, a few of them are likely to spontaneously emit photons of energy $hf = E_1 - E_0$ before the others, thereby falling to the ground state E_0. A laser can be a transparent solid (such as a ruby rod) or a gas-filled tube with mirrors at both ends, one of them only partly silvered to allow some of the light inside to get out. The distance between the mirrors is made equal to a whole number of half-wavelengths of light of frequency f, so that the trapped light forms an optical standing wave (Fig. 7-8). This standing wave stimulates the other atoms in metastable states to radiate before they would normally do so. The result is an avalanche of photons, all of the same frequency f and all of whose waves are exactly in step, which greatly increases the power they can deliver.

Practical Lasers

Soon after its invention, the laser was spoken of as "a solution looking for a problem" because few applications were then imagined for it. Today, of course, lasers are widely employed for a variety of purposes.

In a compact disk (CD) or digital video disk (DVD) player, the beam of a tiny solid-state semiconductor laser is focused to a spot a micrometer (a millionth of a meter) across to read data coded as pits that appear as dark spots on a reflective disk 12 cm in diameter. (See sidebar *Resolving Power* in Sec. 7.17.) Similar lasers are used in transmission systems that carry telephone and television signals as flashes of infrared light along thin glass fibers.

Helium-neon gas lasers produce the narrow red beams that read bar codes in shops. More powerful carbon dioxide gas lasers are used in surgery, where a laser beam has the advantage of sealing small blood vessels it cuts through (Fig. 9-34). Lasers find numerous applications in industry, from cutting fabric for clothing and making holes in nipples for babies' bottles to welding pipelines and heat-treating the surfaces of

engine crankshafts to harden them. Lasers have been built for research that deliver pulses of around a joule that last only 10^{-13} s, which means a power of 10^{13} W—more than the

total output of all the power plants of the world, though only for an instant. Lasers are being developed for military use that can deliver over 100 kW for minutes at a time.

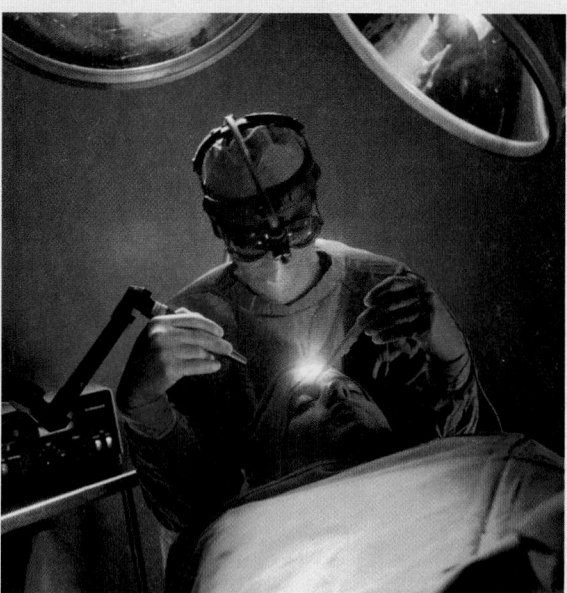

Figure 9-34   A laser produces an intense beam of single-frequency coherent light from the cooperative radiation of excited atoms or molecules. The light waves in a coherent beam are all in step, which greatly increases their effectiveness. A laser beam is here being used in plastic surgery.

Quantum Theory of the Atom

The preceding theory of the hydrogen atom is basically that developed by Bohr in 1913 (although he did not have de Broglie's idea of electron waves to guide his thinking). It can account for much experimental data in a convincing manner. However, it has some severe limitations. For instance, although the Bohr theory correctly predicts the spectral series of hydrogen, it cannot do the same for the spectra of atoms that have two or more electrons each. Perhaps most important of all, it does not give what a really successful theory of the atom ought to: an understanding of how individual atoms interact with one another to form molecules, solids, and liquids.

These objections to the Bohr theory are not meant to be unfriendly, for it was one of those historic achievements that transform scientific thought, but rather to emphasize that a more general approach to the atom is required. Such an approach was developed in 1925–1926 by Erwin Schrödinger, Werner Heisenberg, and others, under the apt name of **quantum mechanics.** By the early 1930s the application of quantum mechanics to problems involving nuclei, atoms, molecules, and matter in the solid state made it possible to understand a vast body of otherwise puzzling data and—vital for any theory—led to predictions of remarkable accuracy.

9.12 Quantum Mechanics

Probabilities, not Certainties

The real difference between newtonian mechanics and quantum mechanics lies in what they describe. The newtonian mechanics of Chap. 2 deals with the motion of an object under the influence of applied forces, and it takes for granted that such quantities as the object's position, mass, velocity, and acceleration can be measured. This assumption agrees completely with our everyday experience. Newtonian mechanics provides the "correct" explanation for the behavior of moving objects in the sense that the values it predicts for observable quantities agree with the measured values of those quantities.

Quantum mechanics, too, consists of relationships between observable quantities, but the uncertainty principle radically alters the meaning of "observable quantity" in the atomic realm. According to the uncertainty principle, the position and momentum of a particle cannot both be accurately known at the same time. (In newtonian physics, of course, such quantities are assumed to always have definite, measurable values.) What quantum mechanics explores are *probabilities*. Instead of saying, for example, that the electron in a normal hydrogen atom is always exactly 5.3×10^{-11} m from the nucleus, quantum mechanics holds that this is the *most probable* distance. In a suitable experiment, many trials would yield different values, but the one most likely to be found would be 5.3×10^{-11} m.

Quantum mechanics does not try to invent a mechanical model based on ideas from everyday life to represent the atom. Instead it deals only with quantities that can actually be measured. We can measure the mass of the electron and its electric charge, we can measure the frequencies of spectral lines emitted by excited atoms, and so on, and the theory must be able to relate them all. But we *cannot* measure the precise diameter of an electron's orbit or watch it jump from one orbit to another, and these notions therefore are not part of the theory.

Two Views of Quantum Physics

According to Eugene Wigner, one of the early workers in the field, "The discovery of quantum mechanics was nearly a total surprise. It described the physical world in a way that was fundamentally new. It seemed to many of us a miracle."

Richard Feynman, one of the most notable of the next generation of quantum physicists, brushed aside the strangeness of the ideas involved: "It is not philosophy we are after, but the behavior of real things," he remarked, and compared the agreement between theory and experiment to finding the distance between New York and Los Angeles to within the thickness of a single hair.

Erwin Schrödinger (1887–1961)

Schrödinger was born in Vienna, Austria, and studied at the university there. Late in 1925, when he was a professor of physics in Zurich, Switzerland, Schrödinger wrote to a friend that he was "struggling with a new atomic theory. If only I knew more mathematics! I am very optimistic about this thing and expect that if I can only . . . solve it, it will be *very* beautiful." The struggle was successful, and early in 1926 Schrödinger published four papers on quantum mechanics that revolutionized physics and were indeed beautiful.

Later, while at Dublin's Institute for Advanced Study, Schrödinger became interested in biology, in particular the mechanism of heredity. He seems to have been the first to make definite the idea of a genetic code and to identify genes as long molecules that carry the code in the form of variations in how their atoms are arranged. Schrödinger's 1944 book *What Is Life?* was enormously influential and started James Watson and Francis Crick on their search for "the secret of the gene," which they discovered in 1953 to be the structure of the DNA molecule (see Sec. 13.16).

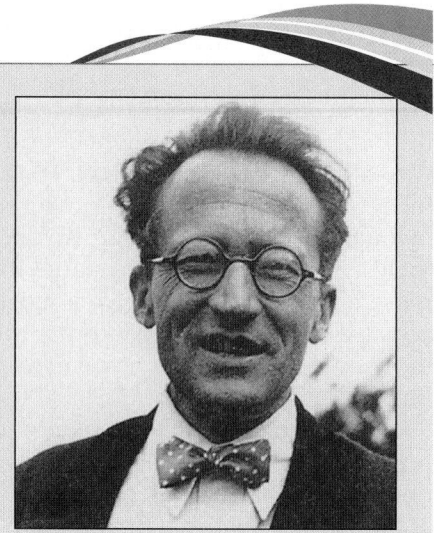

Newtonian and Quantum Mechanics   Quantum mechanics abandons the traditional approach to physics in which models we can visualize are the starting points of theories. But although quantum mechanics does not give us a look into the inner world of the atom, it does tell us everything we need to know about the measurable properties of atoms. And there is something more: *quantum mechanics includes newtonian mechanics as a special case.* The certainties of Newton do not hold on all scales of size. Their agreement with experiment is due to the fact that ordinary objects contain so many atoms that deviations from the most probable behavior are unnoticeable. Instead of two sets of physical principles, one for the world of the large and one for the world of the small, there is only a single set, and quantum mechanics represents our best effort to date at formulating it.

9.13   Quantum Numbers

An Atomic Electron Has Four in All

In the Bohr model of the hydrogen atom, the electron moves around the nucleus in a circular orbit. The only quantity that changes as the electron moves is its position on the circle. The single quantum number n is enough to specify the physical state of such an electron.

In the quantum theory of the atom, an electron has no fixed orbit but is free to move about in three dimensions. We can think of the electron as circulating in a probability cloud or **orbital** that forms a certain pattern in space. Where the orbital is most dense (that is, where ψ^2 has a high value), the electron is most likely to be found. Where the orbital is least dense (ψ^2 has a low value), the electron is least likely to be found (see Sec. 9.6). Figure 9-35a shows a cross section of the orbital of the ground (lowest-energy) state of the hydrogen atom.

Orbital shapes are important in chemistry where, for convenience, an orbital is usually represented not as a probability cloud but instead as a region in which the total probability of finding the electron has some definite value, say 90 percent. Thus, the probability cloud of Fig. 9-35a would be replaced by the **boundary surface diagram** shown in Fig. 9-35b, which is often referred to simply as the orbital of the electron.

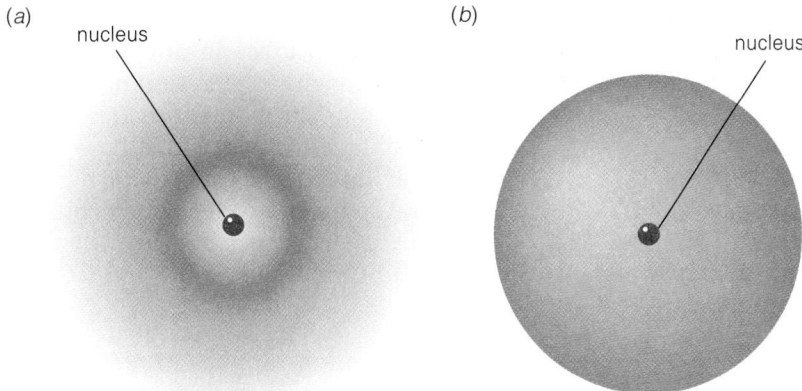

(a) nucleus

(b) nucleus

Figure 9-35 (*a*) The orbital of the electron in the ground state of a hydrogen atom is a probability cloud, which is densest where the electron is most likely to be found. (*b*) Boundary surface diagram of the same orbital shows the region in which the total probability of finding the electron is 90 percent.

Principal Quantum Number Three quantum numbers determine the size and shape of the orbital of an atomic electron as well as the electron's energy. The **principal quantum number,** designated n as in the Bohr theory, is the chief factor that governs the electron's energy: the larger n is, the greater the energy, as shown in Fig. 9-29. The average distance of the electron from the atom's nucleus, and hence the size of its orbital, also increases with increasing n.

Angular Momentum Quantum Number Angular momentum, as we learned in Chap. 3, is the rotational analog of linear momentum. According to quantum mechanics, the angular momentum of an atomic electron, as well as its energy, is quantized—restricted to certain particular values—as the electron moves about the nucleus. These values are determined by l, the **angular momentum quantum number.** Angular momentum states are customarily denoted by a letter according to this scheme:

$$l = 0 \quad 1 \quad 2 \quad 3 \quad 4 \quad 5...$$
$$\quad\; s \quad p \quad d \quad f \quad g \quad h...$$

An electron whose principal quantum number is n can have an angular momentum quantum number of 0 or any whole number up to $n - 1$. For instance, if $n = 3$, the values l can have are 0, 1, or 2. The corresponding atomic states would be called $3s$, $3p$, and $3d$.

Magnetic Quantum Number The angular momentum quantum number l determines the *magnitude* of the electron's angular momentum. However, angular momentum, like linear momentum, is a vector quantity (see Sec. 2.2), and so to describe it completely requires that its *direction* be specified as well as its magnitude (Fig. 9-36). This is the role of the **magnetic quantum number** m_l.

What meaning can a direction in space have for an atom? The answer becomes clear when we reflect that an electron revolving about a nucleus is a current loop and has a magnetic field like that of a tiny bar magnet. In a magnetic field the potential energy of a bar magnet depends both upon how strong the magnet is and upon its orientation with respect to the field. It is the direction of the angular-momentum vector (that is, the direction of the axis about which the electron may be thought to revolve) with respect to a magnetic field that is determined by m_l.

An electron whose orbital quantum number is l can have a magnetic quantum number that is 0 or any whole number between $-l$ and $+l$. The total number of possible m_l values for a given l is $2l + 1$. For instance, if $l = 2$, the five values m_l can have are -2, -1, 0, $+1$, and $+2$.

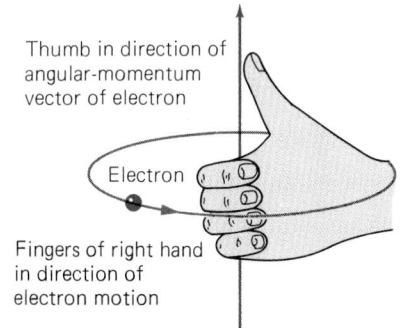

Thumb in direction of angular-momentum vector of electron

Electron

Fingers of right hand in direction of electron motion

Figure 9-36 The right-hand rule for direction of angular-momentum vector.

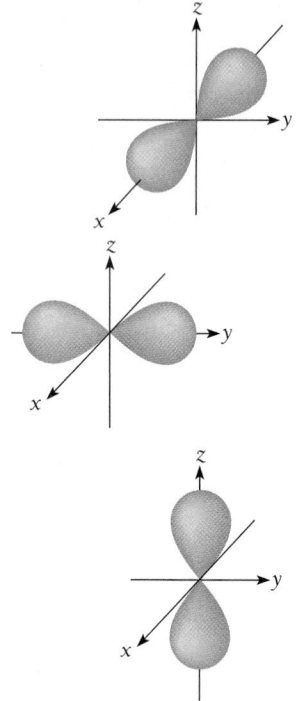

Figure 9-37   The possible *p* orbitals of an atomic electron.

Although all *s* orbitals are spherical in shape, as in Fig. 9-35, those of higher angular momentum have pronounced lobes in different directions. The forms of such orbitals depend on the magnetic quantum numbers of the electrons they contain as well as on their angular momentum quantum numbers. Figure 9-37 shows the three possible *p* orbitals, which have two lobes each that lie along three prependicular directions. Orbitals of higher *l* values are more complicated. Because the shape of an electron's orbital affects the average distance of the electron from the atom's nucleus, the electron's energy depends somewhat on its *l* and m_l values as well as on its principal quantum number *n*.

Electron Spin   There is still another quantum number needed to describe completely an atomic electron. This is the electron **spin magnetic quantum number** m_s.

Electrons behave as though they were, in themselves, little bar magnets, which we can visualize as arising from electrons spinning on their axes. If we picture an electron as a charged sphere, such spinning means a circular electric current and hence magnetic behavior. (This is only a way to help us get a mental handle on what is going on. In reality, an electron has no measurable size; its angular momentum and magnetic properties are built into it, so to speak.) Protons and neutrons also exhibit spin.

An electron can align itself so that its spin is either along a magnetic field, in which case m_s has the value $+\frac{1}{2}$, or opposite to the field, in which case $m_s = -\frac{1}{2}$ (Fig. 9-38). The concept of electron spin is essential for understanding many atomic phenomena such as permanent magnetism. Proton spin underlies the operation of MRI scanners (Fig. 9-39).

Table 9-1 lists the quantum numbers of an atomic electron, their possible values, and their significance.

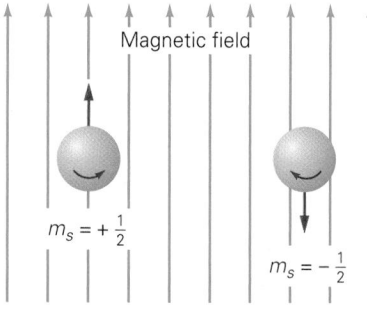

Figure 9-38   The spin magnetic quantum number m_s of an atomic electron has two possible values, $+\frac{1}{2}$ and $-\frac{1}{2}$, depending upon how the electron aligns itself with a magnetic field.

9.14   Exclusion Principle

A Different Set of Quantum Numbers for Each Electron in an Atom

In an unexcited hydrogen atom, the electron is in its quantum state of lowest energy. What about more complex atoms? Are all 92 electrons of a uranium atom in the same quantum state, jammed into a single probability cloud? Many lines of evidence make this idea unlikely.

An example is the great difference in chemical behavior shown by certain elements whose atomic structures differ by just one electron. Thus the elements that have the atomic numbers 9, 10, and 11 are respectively the chemically active gas fluorine, the inert gas neon, and the metal sodium. Since the electron structure of an atom controls how the atom interacts with other atoms, it makes no sense that the chemical properties of the elements should change so sharply with a small change in atomic number if all the electrons in an atom were in the same quantum state.

Table 9-1	**Quantum Numbers of an Atomic Electron**		
Name	**Symbol**	**Possible Values**	**Quantity Determined**
Principal	n	$1, 2, 3, \ldots$	Electron energy; orbital size
Angular momentum	l	$0, 1, 2, \ldots, n-1$	Magnitude of angular momentum; orbital shape
Magnetic	m_l	$-l, \ldots, 0, \ldots, +l$	Direction of angular momentum
Spin magnetic	m_s	$-\frac{1}{2}, +\frac{1}{2}$	Direction of electron spin

Note: Electron energy depends to a lesser extent on *l* and orbital shape to a lesser extent on m_l.

In 1925 Wolfgang Pauli solved the problem of the electron arrangement in an atom that has more than one electron. His **exclusion principle** states that

> Only one electron in an atom can exist in a given quantum state.

Each electron in an atom must have a different set of quantum numbers n, l, m_l, m_s. This means that each orbital can contain at most two electrons, one of each spin direction. Table 9-2 shows the maximum number of electrons that can share the same principal quantum number for $n = 1$ to $n = 4$. In Chap. 10, we will see how the chemical behavior of the elements is connected to Table 9-2.

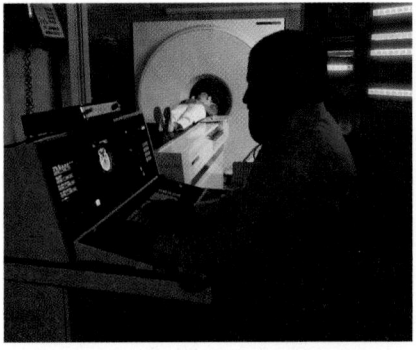

Figure 9-39 Magnetic resonance imaging (MRI) is a method for producing a series of maps of tissue density in the body that reveals details of soft tissues better than x-ray scans do with no radiation hazard (see Sec. 8.5). MRI is based on the magnetic behavior of proton spin. In an MRI scanner, a strong magnetic field aligns the spins of the proton nuclei of hydrogen atoms present in a tissue. A pulse of radio waves with a span of frequencies then bombards the tissue, which causes some of the proton spins to absorb the amount of energy hf needed to flip to the opposite direction. When the pulse stops, the proton spins realign with the magnetic field and in doing so reemit radio waves of frequency f. The exact value of f depends on the environment of the protons and can be interpreted in terms of tissue density. This photograph shows the head of a patient being scanned using MRI.

Table 9-2	Atomic Electron States Permitted by the Exclusion Principle for $n = 1$ to $n = 4$			
Principal quantum number n	Angular momentum state	Possible orbitals per state	Maximum electrons per state	Maximum electrons with given n
1	s	1	2	2
2	s	1	2	
	p	3	6	8
3	s	1	2	
	p	3	6	
	d	5	10	18
4	s	1	2	
	p	3	6	
	d	5	10	
	f	7	14	32

Important Terms and Ideas

The **photoelectric effect** is the emission of electrons from a metal surface when light shines on it. The **quantum theory of light** states that light travels in tiny bursts (or **quanta**) of energy called **photons.** The photoelectric effect can be explained only by the quantum theory of light, whereas the wave theory of light is needed to account for such other phenomena as interference; the two theories complement each other.

X-rays are high-frequency electromagnetic waves given off when matter is struck by fast electrons.

Moving objects have wave as well as particle properties; the smaller the object, the more conspicuous its wave behavior. The **matter waves** that correspond to a moving object have a **de Broglie wavelength** inversely proportional to its momentum. The quantity that varies in a matter wave is called the **wave function,** and its square is the object's **probability density.** The greater the probability density at a certain time and place, the greater the likelihood of finding the object there at that time. The **uncertainty principle** expresses the limit set by the wave nature of matter on finding both the position and the state of motion of a moving object at the same time.

An **emission spectrum** consists of the various frequencies of light given off by an excited substance. An **absorption spectrum** consists of the various frequencies absorbed by a substance when white light is passed through it.

According to the **Bohr model of the atom,** an electron can circle an atomic nucleus only if the electron's orbit is a whole number of de Broglie wavelengths in circumference. The number of wavelengths is the **quantum number** n of the orbit. Each orbit corresponds to a specific energy, and spectral lines originate in electron shifts from one orbit, and hence **energy level,** to another. An atom in its **ground state** has the lowest possible energy; **excited states** correspond to higher energy levels.

A **laser** is a device that produces an intense beam of single-frequency light whose waves are all in step with one another, which greatly increases their effectiveness. Such light is said to be **coherent.**

Quantum mechanics is based on the wave nature of moving things; newtonian mechanics turns out to be a special case of quantum mechanics valid only on large scales of size. Quantum mechanics shows that four quantum numbers are needed to specify the physical state of each atomic electron. One of these quantum numbers governs the direction of the **spin** of the electron. According to the **exclusion principle,** no two electrons in an atom can have the same set of quantum numbers.

In quantum mechanics, an atomic electron does not have a fixed orbit but moves about the nucleus in what can be thought of as a **probability cloud,** called an **orbital,** that is most dense where the electron is most likely to be found. The size and shape of its orbital and its energy depend on three of the electron's quantum numbers. An orbital is usually pictured by a boundary surface diagram that shows the region in which the total chance of finding the electron is, say, 90 percent. Each orbital in an atom can be occupied by, at most, two electrons, one of each spin direction.

Important Formulas

Quantum energy of photon: $E = hf$

Photoelectric effect: $hf = \text{KE} + w$

de Broglie wavelength: $\lambda = \dfrac{h}{mv}$

Multiple Choice

1. When light is directed at a metal surface, the energies of the emitted electrons
   a. vary with the intensity of the light
   b. vary with the frequency of the light
   c. vary with the speed of the light
   d. are random

2. The photoelectric effect can be understood on the basis of
   a. the electromagnetic theory of light
   b. the interference of light waves
   c. the special theory of relativity
   d. none of these

3. In a vacuum, all photons have the same
   a. frequency   c. energy
   b. wavelength   d. speed

4. The mass of a photon
   a. is 0
   b. is the same as that of an electron
   c. depends on its frequency
   d. is the size of the x-rays emitted

5. The rate at which an object emits electromagnetic energy does not depend on its
   a. surface area
   b. mass
   c. temperature
   d. ability to absorb radiation

6. When the speed of the electrons that strike a metal surface is increased, the result is an increase in
   a. the number of x-rays emitted
   b. the frequency of the x-rays emitted
   c. the speed of the x-rays emitted
   d. the size of the x-rays emitted

7. A phenomenon that cannot be understood with the help of the quantum theory of light is
   a. the photoelectric effect
   b. x-ray production
   c. the spectrum of an element
   d. interference of light

8. According to the theories of modern physics, light
   a. is exclusively a wave phenomenon
   b. is exclusively a particle phenomenon
   c. combines wave and particle properties
   d. has neither wave nor particle properties

9. According to the theories of modern physics,
   a. only stationary particles exhibit wave behavior
   b. only moving particles exhibit wave behavior
   c. only charged particles exhibit wave behavior
   d. all particles exhibit wave behavior

10. The speed of the wave packet that corresponds to a moving particle is
    a. less than the particle's speed
    b. equal to the particle's speed
    c. more than the particle's speed
    d. any of these, depending on the circumstances

11. de Broglie waves can be regarded as waves of
    a. pressure   c. electric charge
    b. probability   d. momentum

12. The description of a moving body in terms of matter waves is legitimate because
    a. it is based upon common sense
    b. matter waves have actually been seen
    c. the analogy with electromagnetic waves is plausible
    d. theory and experiment agree

13. The narrower the wave packet of a particle is,
    a. the shorter its wavelength
    b. the more precisely its position can be established
    c. the more precisely its momentum can be established
    d. the more precisely its energy can be established

14. According to the uncertainty principle, it is impossible to precisely determine at the same time a particle's
    a. position and charge
    b. position and momentum
    c. momentum and energy
    d. charge and mass

15. If Planck's constant were larger than it is,
   a. moving bodies would have shorter wavelengths
   b. moving bodies would have higher energies
   c. moving bodies would have greater charges
   d. the uncertainty principle would be significant on a larger scale of size

16. The emission spectrum produced by the excited atoms of an element contains frequencies that are
   a. the same for all elements
   b. characteristic of the particular element
   c. evenly distributed throughout the entire visible spectrum
   d. different from the frequencies in its absorption spectrum

17. A neon sign does not produce
   a. a line spectrum
   b. an emission spectrum
   c. an absorption spectrum
   d. photons

18. Most stars are hot objects surrounded by cooler atmospheres. The spectrum of such a star is a
   a. continuous band of light
   b. band of light crossed by brighter lines
   c. band of light crossed by dark lines
   d. series of bright lines

19. The classical model of the hydrogen atom fails because
   a. an accelerated electron radiates electromagnetic waves
   b. a moving electron has more mass than an electron at rest
   c. a moving electron has more charge than an electron at rest
   d. the attractive force of the nucleus is not enough to keep an electron in orbit around it

20. An electron can revolve in an orbit around an atomic nucleus without radiating energy provided that the orbit
   a. is far enough away from the nucleus
   b. is less than a de Broglie wavelength in circumference
   c. is a whole number of de Broglie wavelengths in circumference
   d. is a perfect circle

21. According to the Bohr model of the atom, an electron in the ground state
   a. radiates electromagnetic energy continuously
   b. emits only spectral lines
   c. remains there forever
   d. can jump to another orbit if given enough energy

22. In the Bohr model of the atom, the electrons revolve around the nucleus of an atom so as to
   a. emit spectral lines
   b. produce x-rays
   c. form energy levels that depend upon their speeds only
   d. keep from falling into the nucleus

23. A hydrogen atom is said to be in its ground state when its electron
   a. is at rest
   b. is inside the nucleus
   c. is in its lowest energy level
   d. has escaped from the atom

24. An atom emits a photon when one of its orbital electrons
   a. jumps from a higher to a lower energy level
   b. jumps from a lower to a higher energy level
   c. is removed by the photoelectric effect
   d. is struck by an x-ray

25. The energy difference between adjacent energy levels in the hydrogen atom
   a. is smaller for small quantum numbers
   b. is the same for all quantum numbers
   c. is larger for small quantum numbers
   d. has no regularity

26. When an atom absorbs a photon of light, which one or more of the following can happen?
   a. An electron shifts to a state of smaller quantum number
   b. An electron shifts to a state of higher quantum number
   c. An electron leaves the atom
   d. An x-ray photon is emitted

27. Which of the following types of radiation is not emitted by the electronic structures of atoms?
   a. ultraviolet light
   b. visible light
   c. x-rays
   d. gamma rays

28. The operation of the laser is based upon
   a. the uncertainty principle
   b. the interference of de Broglie waves
   c. stimulated emission of radiation
   d. stimulated absorption of radiation

29. Which of the following properties is not characteristic of the light waves from a laser?
   a. The waves all have the same frequency
   b. The waves are all in step with one another
   c. The waves form a narrow beam
   d. The waves have higher photon energies than light waves of the same frequency from an ordinary source

30. The quantum-mechanical theory of the atom is
   a. based upon a mechanical model of the atom
   b. a theory that restricts itself to physical quantities that can be measured directly
   c. less accurate than the Bohr theory of the atom
   d. impossible to reconcile with Newton's laws of motion

31. The orbital of an atomic electron is
   a. its orbit around the atom's nucleus
   b. its de Broglie wave
   c. its probability cloud
   d. one of its quantum numbers

32. How many quantum numbers are needed to determine the size and shape of an atomic orbital?
    a. 1   **c.** 3
    b. 2   **d.** 4

33. An electron in a p state of an atom has an angular momentum quantum number l of
    a. 0   **c.** 2
    b. 1   **d.** 3

34. An s orbital
    a. is spherical in shape
    b. is shaped like a doughnut
    c. has two lobes
    d. has six lobes

35. A quantum number is not associated with an atomic electron's
    a. mass
    b. energy
    c. spin
    d. orbital angular momentum

36. Electrons behave like
    a. pure charges with no magnetic properties
    b. tiny bar magnets with different strengths that never change
    c. tiny bar magnets with strengths that may change
    d. tiny bar magnets with the same strength that never changes

37. The electrons in an atom all have the same
    a. speed   **c.** orbit
    b. spin magnitude   **d.** principal quantum number

38. According to the exclusion principle, no two electrons in an atom can have the same
    a. spin direction
    b. speed
    c. orbit
    d. set of quantum numbers

39. The energy of a photon of light whose frequency is 3×10^{14} Hz is
    a. 2.2×10^{-48} J   **c.** 1.98×10^{-19} J
    b. 1.98×10^{-47} J   **d.** 4.5×10^{19} J

40. A lamp emits light of frequency 5×10^{15} Hz at a power of 25 W. The number of photons given off per second is
    a. 1.3×10^{-19} **c.** 7.6×10^{18}
    b. 8.3×10^{-17} **d.** 1.9×10^{50}

41. An x-ray photon has an energy of 3.3×10^{15} J. The frequency that corresponds to this energy is
    a. 3.3×10^{-50} Hz   **c.** 3.3×10^{18} Hz
    b. 3×10^{-19} Hz   **d.** 3.3×10^{20} Hz

42. The de Broglie wavelength of an electron whose speed is 2.0×10^7 m/s is
    a. 3.6×10^{-11} m   **c.** 3.6×10^{-10} m
    b. 2.8×10^{-10} m   **d.** 2.8×10^{10} m

Exercises

9.1 Photoelectric Effect

9.2 Photons

9.3 What Is Light?

1. What differences can you think of between the photon and the electron?

2. The photon and the neutrino are both uncharged. What are the differences between them?

3. Compare the evidence for the wave nature of light with the evidence for its particle nature.

4. If a red star and a white star radiate energy at the same rate, can they be the same size? If not, which must be the larger? why?

5. A bare copper pipe carries hot water to a faucet. What effect, if any, will polishing the pipe have on the rate of heat flow from the pipe to the room?

6. A certain metal surface emits electrons when light is shone on it. (a) How can the number of electrons per second be increased? (b) How can the energies of the electrons be increased?

7. Energy is carried in light by means of separate photons, yet even the faintest light we can see does not appear as a series of flashes. Explain.

8. How does the speed of a photon compare with the speed of an em wave?

9. When the speed of the electrons that strike a metal surface is increased, what happens to the speed, energy, and number per second of the x-ray photons that are emitted?

10. Why do you think the wave aspect of light was discovered earlier than its particle aspect?

11. Find the energy of a photon of ultraviolet light whose frequency is 2×10^{16} Hz. Do the same for a photon of radio waves whose frequency is 2×10^5 Hz.

12. Find the frequency and wavelength of a 50-MeV gamma-ray photon.

13. The eye can detect as little as 10^{-18} J of energy in the form of light. How many photons of frequency 5×10^{14} Hz does this amount of energy represent?

14. A 1.2-kW radio transmitter operates at a frequency of 750 kHz. How many photons per second does it emit?

15. The radiant energy reaching the earth from the sun is about 1400 W/m². If this energy is all green light of wavelength 5.5×10^{-7} m, how many photons strike each square meter per second?

16. A microwave oven operating at 2.4 GHz has a power output of 650 W. (a) What is the wavelength of the microwaves? (b) What is the energy of each photon? (c) How many photons per second does the oven produce?

17. A detached retina is being "welded" back by using 20-ms pulses from a 0.50-W laser operating at a wavelength of 643 nm. How many photons are in each pulse?

18. An electron needs an energy of 2.2 eV to escape from a potassium surface. If ultraviolet light of wavelength 350 nm falls on a potassium surface, what is the maximum KE of the emitted electrons?

19. An energy of 4×10^{-19} J is required to remove an electron from the surface of a particular metal. (a) What is the frequency of the light that will just dislodge electrons from the surface? (b) What is the maximum energy of electrons emitted through the action of light of wavelength 2×10^{-7} m?

9.4 X-Rays

20. What is the shortest wavelength present in the radiation from an x-ray machine whose operating potential difference is 40 kV?

21. In a television picture tube, electrons are accelerated through voltages of about 10 kV. Find the highest frequencies of the em waves emitted when these electrons strike the screen of the tube. What type of waves are they (see Fig. 7-28)?

22. What voltage must be applied to an x-ray tube for it to emit x-rays with a maximum frequency of 2×10^{19} Hz?

9.5 De Broglie Waves
9.6 Waves of What

23. Must a particle have an electric charge in order for matter waves to be associated with its motion?

24. What kind of experiment might you use to distinguish between a gamma ray of wavelength 10^{-11} m and an electron whose de Broglie wavelength is also 10^{-11} m?

25. A photon and a proton have the same wavelength. How does the photon's energy compare with the proton's kinetic energy?

26. A proton and an electron have the same de Broglie wavelength. How do their speeds compare?

27. How does the speed of the wave packet that corresponds to a moving object compare with (a) the object's speed and (b) the speed of light?

28. An electron microscope has a much greater useful magnification than an optical microscope because it can resolve smaller details. What makes the higher resolving power possible?

29. Find the de Broglie wavelength of an electron whose speed is 2×10^7 m/s. How significant are the wave properties of such an electron likely to be?

30. Find the de Broglie wavelength of a 1500-kg car when its speed is 80 km/h. How significant are the wave properties of this car likely to be?

31. An oxygen molecule has a mass of 5.3×10^{-26} kg and an average speed in air at room temperature of about 480 m/s. How does the de Broglie wavelength of such a molecule compare with its diameter of about 4×10^{-10} m? Would you expect such a molecule to exhibit wave behavior?

32. The de Broglie wavelength of a 2-mg grain of sand being blown by the wind is 3.5×10^{-29} m. What is the speed of the grain of sand? How significant are its wave properties likely to be?

33. An electron microscope uses 40-keV (4×10^4 eV) electrons. Find its ultimate resolving power on the assumption that this is equal to the wavelength of the electrons.

9.7 Uncertainty Principle

34. What aspect of nature has the uncertainty principle as a consequence?

35. The uncertainty principle applies to *all* bodies, yet its consequences are significant only for such extremely small particles as electrons, protons, and neutrons. Explain.

9.8 Atomic Spectra

36. Most stars are hot objects surrounded by cooler atmospheres. What kind of spectrum does such a star give rise to?

37. What kind of spectrum is observed in (a) light from the hot filament of a lightbulb; (b) light from a sodium-vapor highway lamp; (c) light from a lightbulb surrounded by cool sodium vapor?

38. Why does the hydrogen spectrum contain many lines, even though the hydrogen atom has only a single electron?

9.9 The Bohr Model
9.10 Electron Waves and Orbits

39. In the Bohr model of the atom, the electron is in constant motion. How can such an electron have a negative amount of energy?

40. Why is the Bohr theory incompatible with the uncertainty principle?

41. (a) What is meant by the ground state of an atom? (b) What is the quantum number of the ground state of a hydrogen atom in the Bohr model?

42. (a) What is an excited atom? (b) How do most excited atoms return to their ground states? (c) What is the usual duration of an excited state: 10^{-8} s, 10^{-2} s, 1 s, 1 min?

43. The atoms of an excited gas are in rapid random motion. What effect do you think this has on the frequencies of the spectral lines in the emission spectrum of the gas?

44. Of the following transitions in a hydrogen atom (a) which emits the photon of highest frequency, (b) which emits the photon of lowest frequency, and (c) which absorbs the photon of highest frequency? $n = 1$ to $n = 2$, $n = 2$ to $n = 1$, $n = 2$ to $n = 6$, $n = 6$ to $n = 2$.

45. Calculate the speed of the electron in the innermost ($n = 1$) Bohr orbit of a hydrogen atom. The radius of

this orbit in 5.3×10^{-11} m. (Hint: Begin by setting the centripetal force on the electron equal to the electrical attraction of the proton it circles around.)

46. With the help of Fig. 9-29 find the frequency of the photon emitted when an electron in the $n = 3$ state of hydrogen falls to the ground state.

47. The earth's mass is 6×10^{24} kg, the circumference of its orbit around the sun is 9.4×10^{11} m, and its orbital speed is 3×10^4 m/s. (a) Find the de Broglie wavelength of the earth. (b) Find the quantum number of the earth's orbit. (c) Do you think quantum considerations play an important part in the earth's orbital motion?

9.11   The Laser

48. What is coherent light? Is the light from a lightbulb coherent? The light from the sun?

49. In what way does light from a laser differ from light from other sources?

50. Why is the optical length of a laser so important?

51. What is a metastable atomic state?

52. For laser action to occur, the medium used must have at least three energy levels. What must the nature of each of these levels be?

9.12   Quantum Mechanics
9.13   Quantum Numbers
9.14   Exclusion Principle

53. How is quantum mechanics related to newtonian mechanics?

54. If Planck's constant were smaller than it is, would quantum phenomena be more or less conspicuous than they are now?

55. The Bohr theory permits us to visualize the structure of the atom, whereas quantum mechanics is very complex and concerned with such ideas as wave functions and probabilities. What reasons would lead to the replacement of the Bohr theory by quantum mechanics?

56. In the Bohr model of the hydrogen atom, the radius of the electron's orbit in the ground state is 5.3×10^{-11} m. What aspect of the quantum mechanical model of this atom would you expect to correspond to this figure?

57. What is the significance of a high value of the probability density ψ^2 of a particle at a certain time and place? Of a low value of ψ^2?

58. What physical quantities are governed by the quantum numbers of an atomic electron?

59. Why is an s orbital spherically symmetric, that is, have its probability density vary in the same way in all directions?

60. Why does the energy of an atomic electron depend on its angular momentum and magnetic quantum numbers as well as on its principal quantum number?

61. What is the angular momentum quantum number of an electron in a p state? How many orbitals are available to such an electron?

62. Can more than one electron occupy an atomic orbital? Is there a limit to how many?

63. Under what circumstances do electrons exhibit spin?

The Periodic Law

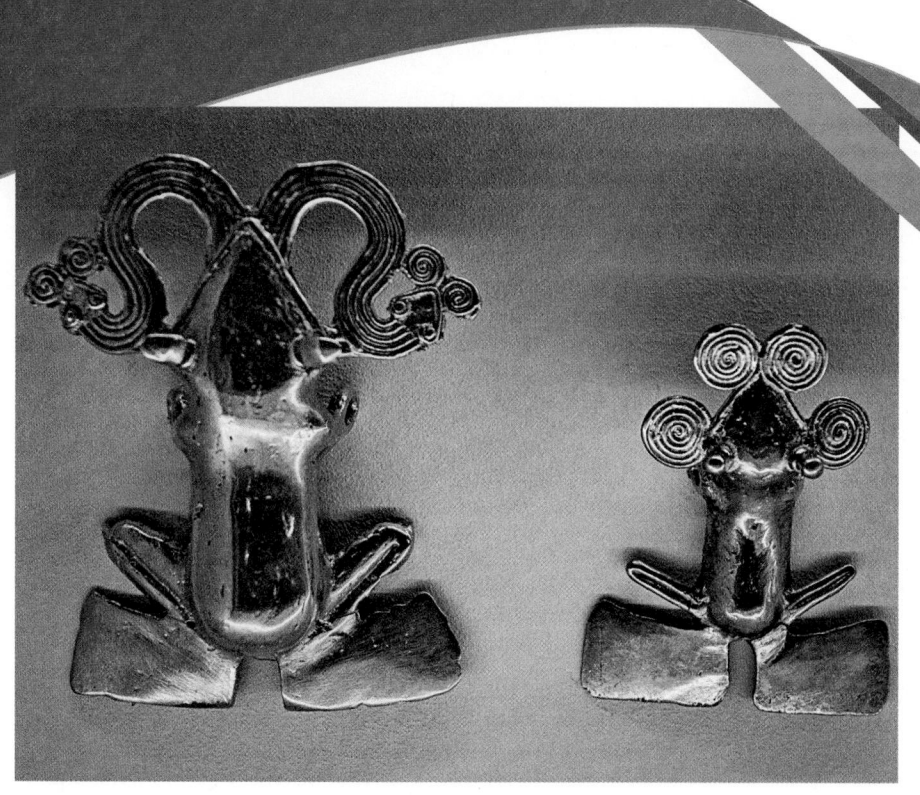

These precolumbian ornaments do not show their age because gold is a relatively inactive element.

GOALS

When you have finished this chapter you should be able to complete the goals
• given for each section below:

Elements and Compounds

10.1 Chemical Change
A Chemical Reaction Alters the Substances Involved

10.2 Three Classes of Matter
Elements, Compounds, and Mixtures
• Distinguish among the three classes of matter—elements, compounds, and mixtures—and describe how they can be told apart.
• State the law of definite proportions.

10.3 The Atomic Theory
The Building Blocks of Matter
• Explain the meanings of the letters, numbers, and parentheses in the chemical formula of a compound, for instance, $Al_2(SO_4)_3$.

The Periodic Law

10.4 Metals and Nonmetals
A Basic Distinction
• Compare the properties of metals and nonmetals.

10.5 Chemical Activity
The More Active an Element, the More Stable Its Compounds
• Discuss the relationship between the chemical activity of an element and the stability of its compounds.

10.6 Families of Elements
Members of Each Family Have a Lot in Common
• List some of the characteristic properties of the halogens, the alkali metals, and the inert gases.

10.7 The Periodic Table
A Pattern of Recurring Similarities among the Elements
• State the periodic law and describe how the periodic table is drawn up.

10.8 Groups and Periods
Elements in a Group Have Similar Properties; Elements in a Period Have Different Ones
• Distinguish between the groups and periods of the periodic table.

Atomic Structure

10.9 Shells and Subshells
They Contain Electrons with Similar Energies
• State what is meant by atomic shells and subshells.

10.10 Explaining the Periodic Table
How an Atom's Electron Structure Determines Its Chemical Behavior
• Distinguish between metal and nonmetal atoms in terms of their electron structures.
• Explain the origin of the periodic law in terms of the electron structures of atoms.

Chemical Bonds

10.11 Types of Bond
Electric Forces Hold Atoms to One Another

10.12 Covalent Bonding
Sharing Electron Pairs Produces an Attractive Force

10.13 Ionic Bonding
Electron Transfer Creates Ions That Attract Each Other
• Compare covalent and ionic bonds.
• State what is meant by a polar covalent molecule.

10.14 Ionic Compounds
Matching Up Ions
• Explain how the formula of an ionic compound can be predicted from the charges on the ions it contains.

10.15 Atom Groups
They Act as Units in Chemical Reactions
• Discuss the nature of an atom group.

10.16 Naming Compounds
The Vocabulary of Chemistry
• Establish the formula of a simple compound from its chemical name.

10.17 Chemical Equations
The Atoms on Each Side Must Balance
• Explain what a chemical equation represents and does not represent.
• Recognize whether a chemical equation is balanced or unbalanced.
• Balance an unbalanced chemical equation.

Although the line between physics and chemistry is hazy, with this chapter we are definitely across it. Chemistry began with a search for a way to change ordinary metals into gold. This fruitless task, called **alchemy** by the Arabs, was not abandoned until the seventeenth century. At that time John Mayow and Robert Boyle in England, Jean Rey in France, and Georg Stahl in Germany, among others, started to look systematically into the properties of matter and how they change in chemical reactions.

After a look at what is meant by chemical change, we go on to consider the periodic law, a natural classification of the elements into groups with similar characteristics. As we shall find, the periodic law has its roots in atomic structure. This is not surprising, since the way in which electrons are arranged in an atom is what determines how that atom interacts with other atoms—in other words, how it behaves chemically.

Elements and Compounds

The properties of matter are altered in a number of processes. When a solid melts into a liquid or a liquid vaporizes into a gas, the cause is a change in the motions and separations of the molecules of the material. In other processes, however, the changes are in the molecules themselves. Examples are the rusting of iron, the burning of wood, and the souring of milk. Such processes are called **chemical reactions.**

10.1   Chemical Change

A Chemical Reaction Alters the Substances Involved

To begin our study of chemistry, let us examine a specific chemical reaction. Suppose we mix some powdered zinc metal with a somewhat larger volume of powdered sulfur on a ceramic surface and then ignite the mixture, say with a gas flame. The result is a small explosion with light and heat given off. When the fireworks have died down, we are left with a brittle white substance that resembles neither the original zinc nor the original sulfur (Fig. 10-1). What has happened?

Further experiments would show (1) that neither zinc nor sulfur alone gives such a reaction when heated; (2) that the explosion takes place just as well in a vacuum as in air; and (3) that the ceramic surface may be replaced by a metal or asbestos one without affecting the reaction. Clearly the process involves both zinc and sulfur, but nothing else. We conclude that zinc and sulfur have joined chemically to form the new material, which is called zinc sulfide.

From Fig. 10-1 we can see that the properties of zinc, sulfur, and zinc sulfide are quite different from one another. Each material is a pure

Figure 10-1   Zinc and sulfur react chemically to give zinc sulfide, a substance whose properties are different from those of zinc and sulfur.

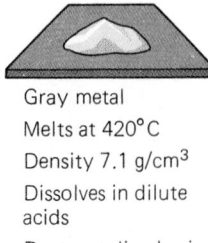

Zinc

Gray metal
Melts at 420°C
Density 7.1 g/cm³
Dissolves in dilute acids
Does not dissolve in carbon disulfide

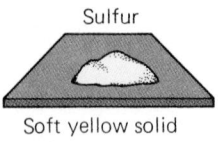

Sulfur

Soft yellow solid
Melts at 113°C
Density 2.0 g/cm³
Does not dissolve in acids
Dissolves in carbon disulfide

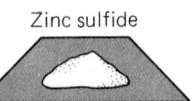

Zinc sulfide

Brittle white solid
Does not melt but decomposes into zinc and sulfur at 600°C
Density 3.5 g/cm³
Does not dissolve in either dilute acids or carbon disulfide

substance. Every particle of sulfur in the sulfur pile is like every other particle of sulfur, and the same is true for zinc and for zinc sulfide. However, if we simply mix zinc and sulfur together without heating them, the result is a **heterogeneous substance** whose properties vary from one particle to the next. With a microscope and tweezers we can separate particles of zinc from those of sulfur, which we cannot do in the case of zinc sulfide. There has been no change at all in the ingredients of the mixture of zinc and sulfur.

10.2 Three Classes of Matter

Elements, Compounds, and Mixtures

Although the alchemists never reached their goal of turning ordinary metals into gold, their work did have an important result. What the alchemists discovered was that certain substances—such as zinc, sulfur, and gold—could be neither broken down nor changed into one another. Slowly the belief grew that only a limited number of such **elements** exist and that all other substances are combinations of them. A new material can be formed from other materials by chemical change only if the elements of the new material are present in the original ones. This observation, little more than two centuries old, marks the beginning of the science of chemistry.

Today more than 100 elements are known, most of them solids at room temperature and atmospheric pressure. About 75 percent (by mass) of the matter in the universe is a single element, hydrogen, and nearly all the rest consists of one other element, helium. The other elements amount to less than 1 percent of the total. As for our planet, the four elements iron, oxygen, silicon, and magnesium make up 96 percent of the earth's mass. In the human body, oxygen is the most abundant element, followed by carbon, hydrogen, nitrogen, calcium, and phosphorus; no other element amounts to more than a fraction of a percent.

The matter around us contains elements by themselves and in a variety of combinations. Some materials consist of two or more elements joined together in chemical **compounds,** as in the case of zinc sulfide. Other materials are mixtures of elements or compounds or both. A mixture may be heterogeneous, with its components obvious to the eye and easy to separate.

Naming the Elements

The names of the elements have a variety of origins. A few elements are identified by their properties: hydrogen, a constituent of water, gets its name from the Greek word for "water maker" and chlorine, a green gas, from the Greek word for green.

Helium, revealed in the sun's atmosphere by its spectral lines before being found on the earth, gets its name from *helios*, Greek for the sun. Mercury, uranium, neptunium, and plutonium are named after planets; europium and americium after continents; francium after France; rhenium after the Rhine River; copper after the island of Cyprus where, according to legend, it was first discovered; and californium and berkelium after the University of California at Berkeley where they were created. Yttrium, ytterbium, terbium, and erbium were identified in ores mined near the Swedish town of Ytterby and were named accordingly. The names of several elements honor notable scientists: curium, einsteinium, fermium, and, appropriately, mendelevium.

The scarcity and inactivity of certain gases kept them from being discovered until only a century ago. Some of their names reflect these properties: neon (from the Greek for "new"); argon ("inert"); krypton ("hidden"); and xenon ("stranger").

The symbol of an element is often an abbreviation of its name. For many elements the first letter is used: O for oxygen, H for hydrogen, C for carbon. When the names of two or more elements begin with the same letter, two letters may be used: Cl for chlorine, He for helium, Zn for zinc. For some elements abbreviations of Latin names are used: Cu for copper (cuprum), Fe for iron (ferrum), Hg for mercury (hydragyrum).

Wood is one example; our mixture of zinc powder and sulfur powder is another. When the components are so thoroughly mixed that the result is uniform, we have a **homogeneous mixture,** or **solution.** Thus seawater is a solution of various solids and gases dissolved in water. Figure 10-2 shows how matter is classified into its different forms.

Compound or Solution?   How can we tell whether two elements have joined to make a compound or are just mixed to make a solution? A number of tests are available. Here are two:

1. See whether the new material can be separated into different substances by boiling or freezing. The changes of state we studied in Chap. 5 occur at specific temperatures for elements and compounds but not for mixtures. Air, for example, is a solution of several gases, mainly nitrogen and oxygen. Nitrogen boils at −196°C and oxygen boils at −183°C. If we heat liquid air to −196°C, most of the gas given off is nitrogen. The liquid left behind is richer in oxygen than the original sample. On the other hand, nitric oxide is a compound of nitrogen and oxygen that has a boiling point of −152°C. If we heat liquid nitric oxide to −152°C, all of it will boil away at this temperature, with no change in composition (Fig. 10-3).

2. Compare the relative masses of the elements in different samples of the material. The elements in a given compound are always present in exactly the same proportions. However, the ingredients of a solution may be present in a range of proportions. At sea level, the mass ratio of

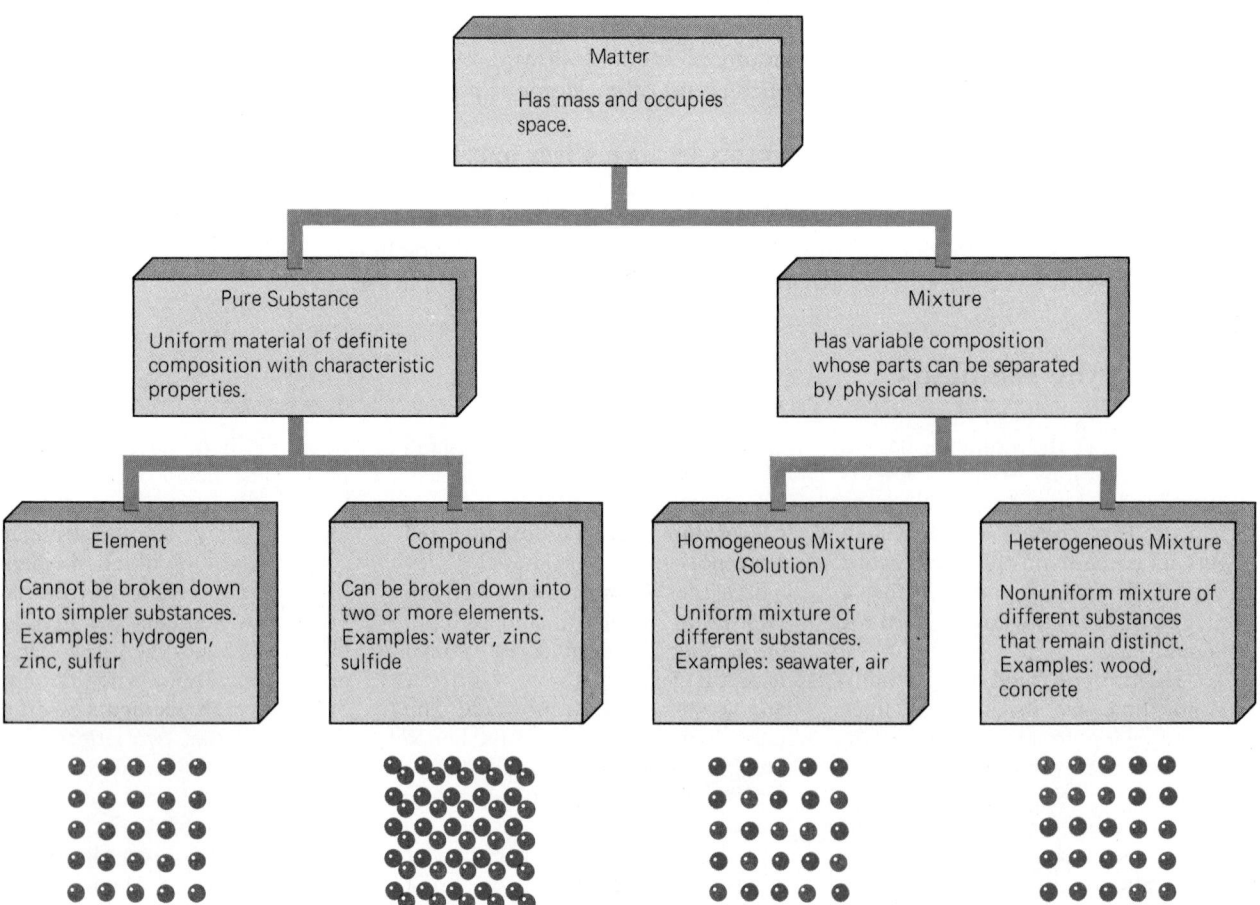

Figure 10-2   Classification of matter.

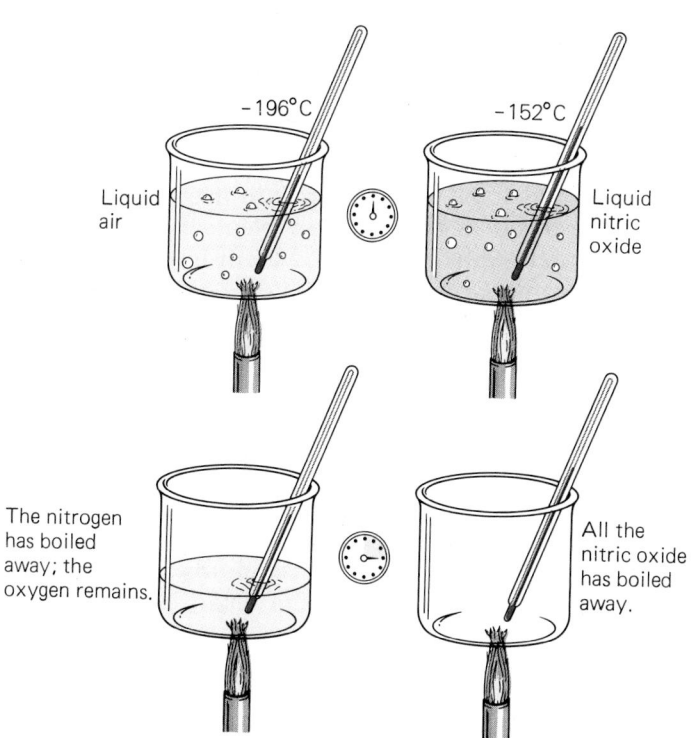

Figure 10-3 Elements and compounds have specific boiling and freezing points. A solution, here air, can therefore be separated into the elements or compounds it contains by boiling or freezing at an appropriate temperature, but a compound, here nitric oxide, cannot. Nitrogen boils at −196°C, oxygen boils at the higher temperature of −183°C, and nitric oxide boils at the still higher temperature of −152°C.

the nitrogen and oxygen in air has an average value of 3.2:1, but there is more nitrogen than this at high altitudes. On the other hand, the mass ratio of these elements in nitric oxide is exactly 0.88:1 everywhere. If there is too much of either nitrogen or oxygen when nitric oxide is being made, the extra amount will not combine but will be left over and can easily be separated (Fig. 10-4). The **law of definite proportions** is as basic to chemistry as the law of conservation of momentum is to physics:

> The elements that make up a compound are always combined in the same proportions by mass.

10.3 The Atomic Theory

The Building Blocks of Matter

Two hundred years ago the structure of matter was still largely a mystery. Nobody knew what really happens when elements combine to form

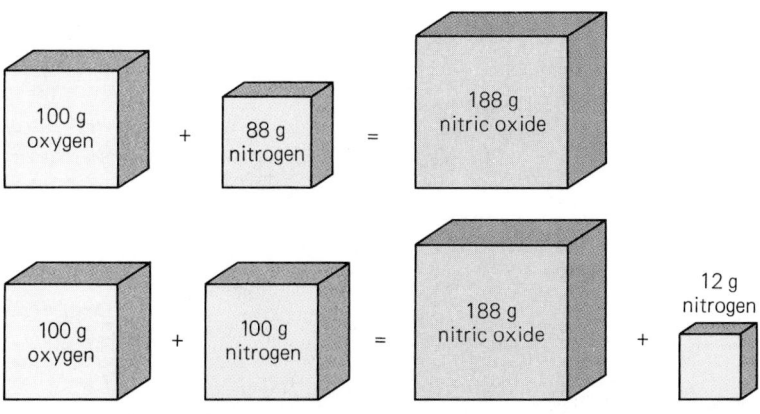

Figure 10-4 An example of the law of definite proportions. Elements combine in a specific mass ratio when they form a compound. The mass ratio between the oxygen and nitrogen in nitric oxide is always 100:88.

compounds. The explanation finally came from an English schoolteacher named John Dalton. Dalton began with the ancient Greek notion that all matter is built from basic particles called **atoms,** but he went much further.

Dalton proposed that all the atoms of each element were the same but were different from the atoms of other elements. He was the first to establish the relative masses of atoms of the known elements, thus taking his ideas from the realm of philosophy and putting them into the realm of science. In Dalton's picture, compounds consist of atoms of different elements, with each compound having fixed ratios of the kinds of atoms present. Chemical reactions represent rearrangements of atoms, not changes in the atoms or the creation or destruction of atoms.

Molecules   Our modern picture of matter grew from Dalton's work. In the case of gases, the ultimate particles of a gaseous compound are its **molecules,** which in turn are made up of atoms of the elements in the compound. Some elemental gases, such as helium and neon, consist of individual atoms. Other elemental gases consist of molecules whose atoms are all the same. Thus each molecule of gaseous oxygen consists of a pair of oxygen atoms bound together.

Atoms and most molecules are very small, and even a tiny bit of matter contains huge numbers of them. If each atom in a penny were worth 1 cent, all the money in the world would not be enough to pay for it.

The molecules of a compound have fixed compositions, as Fig. 10-5 shows. This is the reason for the law of definite proportions. Each water molecule contains two hydrogen atoms and one oxygen atom, for example, and each ammonia molecule contains three hydrogen atoms and a nitrogen atom.

Chemical Formulas   Two or more atoms linked into a molecule are represented by writing the symbols for their elements side by side. Thus a carbon monoxide molecule is CO and a zinc sulfide molecule is ZnS. When a molecule contains two or more atoms of the same kind, a subscript shows the number present. The familiar H_2O means that a molecule of water contains two H atoms and one O atom. A molecule of oxygen, with two O atoms, is written O_2; a molecule of nitrogen pentoxide, with two N atoms and five O atoms, is written N_2O_5. Each subscript number applies only

Figure 10-5   Structures of several common molecules. Ethyl alcohol is also called ethanol.

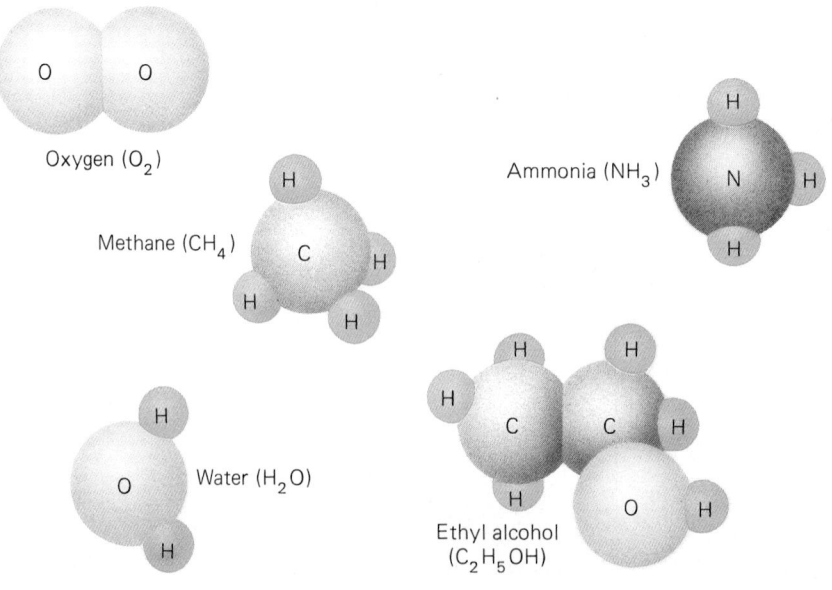

Oxygen (O_2)

Methane (CH_4)

Ammonia (NH_3)

Water (H_2O)

Ethyl alcohol (C_2H_5OH)

John Dalton (1766–1844)

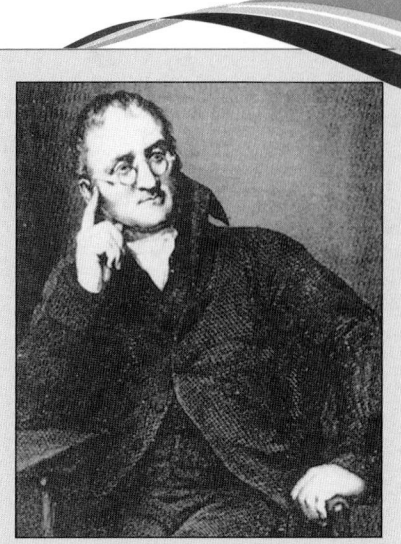

The son of a Quaker weaver in England, Dalton began teaching at the age of 12, a year after his own formal education had ended. Besides having had no instruction in science, Dalton was an inept experimenter, a plodding, literal thinker, and poor at expressing his ideas. But these handicaps did not stop Dalton from placing the atomic theory of matter on a firm foundation. Indeed, by leading him to seek simple explanations for complex phenomena, they gave him an advantage over contemporaries whose minds were full of the misconceptions of the day.

Dalton's initial scientific interest was meteorology: he wrote a book on the subject and recorded weather data every day of his adult life. Studying the atmosphere started Dalton reflecting on the nature of gases and then on the nature of matter in general. He developed the concepts of atom and molecule, element and compound in detail, with numerical values derived from experiment.

For instance, Dalton observed that in what is now called carbon monoxide gas the carbon:oxygen ratio by mass is 3:4 whereas in carbon dioxide it is 3:8. This led him to suggest that carbon monoxide molecules consist of one atom of carbon and one of oxygen (in symbols: CO), and that carbon dioxide molecules consist of one atom of carbon and two of oxygen (CO_2). Ratios such as these enabled Dalton to work out the relative atomic masses of many elements.

Sometimes Dalton's figures were wrong (he assumed that water molecules contain one hydrogen atom for each oxygen atom, so the observed mass ratio of 1:8 means that the atomic mass of oxygen is 8 times that of hydrogen; in fact, of course, there are two H atoms per O atom in water, H_2O, so the O mass is 16 times the H mass), but on the whole he did very well. Soon after his book on this work appeared in 1808, most chemists accepted Dalton's ideas, and he became famous.

The atomic theory was not all that occupied Dalton, who always said he was too busy to marry. Among his other achievements were the first description of color blindness, from which he suffered, and the discovery that the warmer air is, the more water vapor it can hold.

to the symbol just in front of it. These expressions are called **chemical formulas.**

Not All Compounds Consist of Molecules Elements in liquid and solid form are usually assemblies of individual atoms. Some liquid and solid compounds are also assemblies of individual molecules; others are assemblies of ions. For example, crystals of table salt, which is a compound of sodium and chlorine, consist of sodium and chlorine ions rather than of neutral atoms or molecules. The sodium ions are positively charged and the chlorine ions are negatively charged, as in Fig. 10-6. For every sodium ion Na^+, there is a chlorine ion Cl^-, so that the ratio between them is fixed, and the ions are firmly held together in a definite pattern. Sodium chloride is as much a compound as water, even though it is not composed of separate molecules, and its formula is NaCl.

When a compound of any kind is formed from its constituent elements, energy is given off. To break up the compound, the same amount of energy must be provided. This is why compounds are stable; the more the energy needed to break up a compound, the more stable it is.

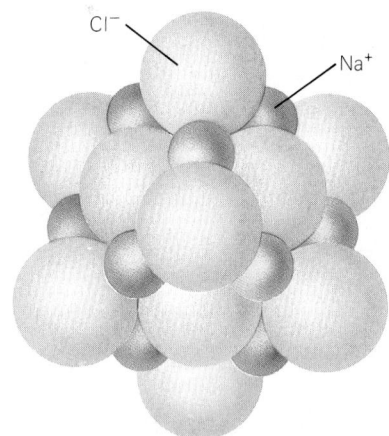

Figure 10-6 Sodium chloride crystals consist of Na^+ and Cl^- ions rather than of neutral Na and Cl atoms or individual NaCl molecules.

The Periodic Law

The periodic law, now over a century old, was a giant step for chemists along the path toward understanding the nature and behavior of the elements. There cannot be many chemistry laboratories in the world that do not have a copy of the periodic table hanging on a wall. Before we examine the periodic law, we shall look at some of the ideas behind its discovery.

10.4   Metals and Nonmetals

A Basic Distinction

The division between metals and nonmetals is a familiar one. All metals except mercury are solid at room temperature. Iron, copper, aluminum, tin, silver, and gold are examples. Nonmetals may be solid (carbon, sulfur), liquid (bromine), or gaseous (chlorine, oxygen, nitrogen) at room temperature. Metals outnumber nonmetals by more than 5:1.

A number of physical properties distinguish metals from nonmetals (Table 10-1). An obvious one is **metallic luster,** the characteristic sheen of a clean metal surface. Related to this sheen is the fact that all metals are opaque—light cannot pass through even the thinnest sheet of a metal. Solid nonmetals do not show metallic luster and nearly all are transparent in thin sheets.

Another typical property of metals is their ability to be shaped by bending or hammering. One gram of gold can be beaten into a square meter of foil (Fig. 10-7), and a copper rod can be pulled through a tiny hole in a steel plate to make a hair-thin wire. Solid nonmetals, though, are brittle and break instead of being deformed when enough force is applied. Metals are all good conductors of heat and electricity; nonmetals are insulators.

Carbon is one of a few elements whose properties put it on the borderline between metals and nonmetals. Carbon conducts heat and electricity better than other nonmetals do, and one form of it, graphite (familiar as the "lead" in pencils), is somewhat lustrous. However, all forms of carbon are brittle. Other elements intermediate between metals and nonmetals are boron, silicon, germanium, arsenic, antimony, and tellurium, which are called **semimetals** or **metalloids.** Modern electronics is largely based on the electrical properties of silicon and germanium.

10.5   Chemical Activity

The More Active an Element, the More Stable Its Compounds

Metals and nonmetals also differ in their chemical properties, but these differences are less clear-cut than the differences in physical properties because the elements in each category vary a great deal among themselves. In particular, some metals and nonmetals are very **active,** which means that they readily combine to form compounds. At the other extreme, **inactive** elements have little tendency to react chemically.

Sodium is an example of an active metal and gold is an example of an inactive one. A few seconds in the open air and sodium has lost its luster through chemical reactions, but a gold ring remains bright after a lifetime of exposure to perspiration as well as air. Sodium combines spectacularly with chlorine, giving off much heat and light. Gold combines with chlorine only sluggishly, with little energy set free. Sodium reacts with dilute acids and even with water. Gold is affected only by a mixture of concentrated hydrochloric and nitric acids.

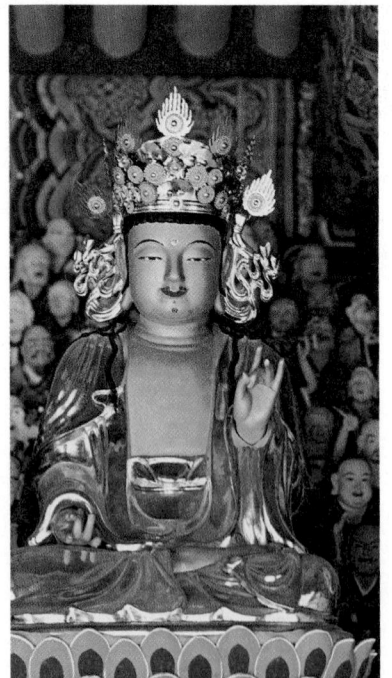

Figure 10-7   Gold leaf thinner than this page was glued to this statue of Buddha. Metals differ from other solids in their ability to be rolled into thin sheets or be otherwise deformed without breaking.

Table 10-1	Some Physical Properties of Metals and Nonmetals	
Property	**Metals**	**Nonmetals**
Metallic luster	Yes	No
Opaque to light	Yes	Only a few
Can be deformed without breaking	Yes	No
Conducts heat and electricity	Yes	No

Determining Activities The relative activities of different elements can be established by measuring the amounts of heat given off in similar chemical reactions. Suppose we combine a given mass of chlorine with sodium and then the same mass of chlorine with gold. We would find that forming sodium chloride gives off more than 15 times as much heat as forming gold chloride. The conclusion is that sodium is much more active than gold (Fig. 10-8).

Or we might start with similar compounds and ask how easily they can be separated into their component elements. In the case of gold chloride and sodium chloride, the results are that gold chloride breaks up when it is heated to about 300°C, but sodium chloride must be heated to well over 1000°C for this to happen. Gold chloride is accordingly considered to be a relatively unstable compound and sodium chloride to be a relatively stable compound. In general, the more active an element is, the more difficulty we have in decomposing its compounds.

Both metals and nonmetals can be arranged in order of their activities. In the partial listing of Table 10-2 the most active elements are at the top of each series and the least active are at the bottom.

The more active a metal is, the harder it is to extract from its ores, which are the minerals that contain compounds of the metal. Lead is more active than copper. If we heat the copper sulfide Cu_2S in air, the result is metallic copper and sulfur dioxide gas, SO_2. But if we heat lead sulfide, PbS, in air, we get lead oxide, PbO, and sulfur dioxide. Refining lead is evidently more difficult than refining copper.

10.6 Families of Elements

Members of Each Family Have a Lot in Common

Some elements resemble one another so much that they seem to be members of the same natural family. Three examples of such families are a group of active nonmetals called the *halogens,* a group of active metals called the *alkali metals,* and a group of gases that undergo almost no chemical reactions, the *inert gases.*

Halogens The **halogens** (Table 10-3) are all highly active elements. In fact, fluorine is the most active element of all and can even corrode platinum, one of the most stable metals. The halogens are responsible for some of the worst odors (*bromos* is Greek for "stink") and most brilliant colors (*chloros* is Greek for "green") to be found in the laboratory. The name halogen means "salt former," a token of the fact that these elements combine with many metals to give white solids that resemble table salt (which is NaCl, sodium chloride).

At room temperature fluorine is a pale-yellow gas, chlorine is a greenish-yellow gas, bromine is a reddish-brown liquid, iodine is a steel-gray solid, and astatine is a radioactive solid.

What are the similarities among the halogens? For one thing, their molecules contain two atoms at ordinary temperatures: F_2, Cl_2, Br_2, I_2. (The half-life of astatine is too short for its chemical properties to be known.) Also, the compounds they form with metals have similar formulas. Here are three examples:

NaF	ZnF_2	AlF_3
NaCl	$ZnCl_2$	$AlCl_3$
NaBr	$ZnBr_2$	$AlBr_3$
NaI	ZnI_2	AlI_3

All the halogens react with hydrogen to form HF, HCl, HBr, and so on. These compounds can be dissolved in water to form acids, of which hydrochloric acid is a familiar example. The halogens dissolve readily in a

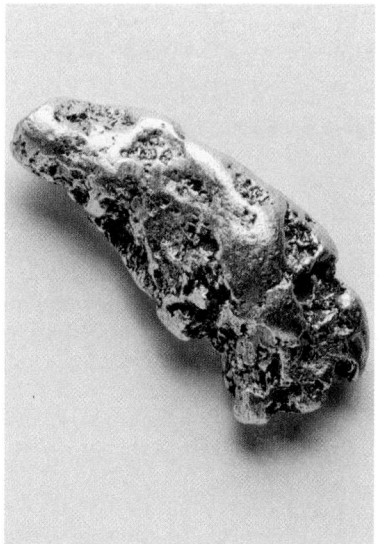

Figure 10-8 Gold occurs as the free metal because it is very inactive chemically, which is why gold objects such as rings and this nugget do not tarnish or corrode.

Table 10-2	Relative Activities of Metals and Nonmetals

Metals	Nonmetals
Potassium	Fluorine
Sodium	Chlorine
Lithium	Bromine
Calcium	Oxygen
Magnesium	Iodine
Aluminum	Sulfur
Zinc	
Iron	
Tin	
Lead	
Copper	
Mercury	
Silver	
Gold	
Platinum	

(arrows indicate: More active ↑ / Less active ↓)

Table 10-3	The Halogens

Element	Symbol	Atomic Number
Fluorine	F	9
Chlorine	Cl	17
Bromine	Br	35
Iodine	I	53
Astatine	At	85

Uses of the Halogens

Fluorine is a constituent of the non-stick plastic Teflon and is added in small quantities to water to help prevent tooth decay by making tooth enamel more resistant to acid attack. About one part of chlorine per million parts of water is enough to kill any bacteria present, which is why chlorine is added to water supplies and to swimming pools; it is also widely used as a bleach. Silver bromide, a compound of bromine and silver, is the light-sensitive material in photographic film and paper.

Because the thyroid hormone thyroxine contains iodine, this halogen is essential in the diet, and accordingly table salt in the United States and elsewhere is usually "iodized" with a small percentage of KI or NaI. Iodine is the active ingredient in various antiseptics.

In an ordinary incandescent lightbulb a tungsten filament glows when it is heated by the passage of an electric current. As the bulb is used, the tungsten gradually evaporates and condenses on the glass envelope until the bulb eventually "burns out." To achieve a brighter light, the filament would have to be hotter and its lifetime would then be correspondingly shorter.

A way around this problem is to fill the bulb with an appropriate vapor; usually the halogen element iodine is chosen. The evaporated tungsten cools after it leaves the filament and reacts with the iodine to form tungsten iodide vapor instead of being deposited on the glass. When tungsten iodide vapor comes in contact with the hot filament, it breaks up, and the tungsten returns to the filament to leave the iodine vapor free once more. This cycle allows a halogen bulb to be operated at much higher temperatures than an ordinary bulb, and hence to be much brighter, without reducing its lifetime.

Table 10-4	The Alkali Metals	
Element	**Symbol**	**Atomic Number**
Lithium	Li	3
Sodium	Na	11
Potassium	K	19
Rubidium	Rb	37
Cesium	Cs	55
Francium	Fr	87

liquid called carbon tetrachloride to give solutions colored in the same way as their vapors, but the halogens are only slightly soluble in water.

Alkali Metals   The **alkali metals** (Table 10-4) are all soft and very active chemically. They lose their lusters quickly in air, liberate hydrogen from water and dilute acids, and combine with active nonmetals to form very stable compounds. Formulas for their compounds follow similar patterns, for instance,

Bromides:	LiBr	NaBr	KBr	RbBr	CsBr	FrBr
Sulfides:	Li_2S	Na_2S	K_2S	Rb_2S	Cs_2S	Fr_2S
Hydroxides:	LiOH	NaOH	KOH	RbOH	CsOH	FrOH

Sodium is quite abundant, making up about 2.5 percent of the earth's crust, but its activity prevents it from occurring free in nature. Its compounds are widely distributed in rocks, soil, and, in solution, in bodies of water.

All the alkali metals have rather low melting points for metals: cesium melts on a really hot day, and even lithium, with the highest melting point of the group, melts at only 186°C. Because the isotopes of francium are radioactive with very short half-lives, little is known about its properties. If enough of it could be gathered together, francium would probably join bromine and mercury as the only elements that are liquid at room temperature.

Inert Gases   The **inert gases** (Table 10-5), in contrast with the active halogens and alkali metals, are so inactive that they form only a handful of compounds with other elements. In fact, these elements are so inactive that their atoms do not even join together into molecules as the atoms of other gaseous elements do. All the inert gases are found in small amounts in the atmosphere, with argon making up about 1 percent of the air and the others much less.

A volume of helium weighs much less than the same volume of air. Because it also cannot burn or explode, helium is ideal for lighter-than-air craft such as balloons and blimps (Fig. 10-9). We have already met radon, a radioactive product of radium decay, in Chap. 8. The other inert gases glow in various colors when excited by an electric current and are widely used in signs. Argon is often used in welding as a shield to prevent the hot metal from reacting with atmospheric oxygen.

Table 10-5	The Inert Gases	
Element	**Symbol**	**Atomic Number**
Helium	He	2
Neon	Ne	10
Argon	Ar	18
Krypton	Kr	36
Xenon	Xe	54
Radon	Rn	86

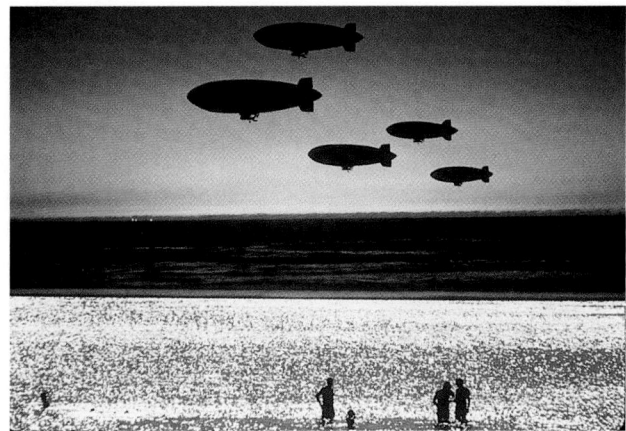

Figure 10-9   The inert gas helium is used in these blimps because helium cannot burn or explode, besides being less dense than air. Helium is found in small amounts in natural gas. To separate it out, the raw gas is cooled to a temperature at which the other gases present (mainly methane) have become liquid, leaving gaseous helium behind.

10.7   The Periodic Table

A Pattern of Recurring Similarities among the Elements

A curious feature of the elements listed in Tables 10-3, 10-4, and 10-5 is that each halogen is followed in atomic number by an inert gas and then by an alkali metal. Thus fluorine, neon, and sodium have the atomic numbers $Z = 9$, $Z = 10$, and $Z = 11$, a sequence that continues through astatine (85), radon (86), and francium (87). When the properties of all the elements are checked to see what other regularities occur, the result is the **periodic law:**

> When the elements are listed in order of atomic number, elements with similar chemical and physical properties appear at regular intervals.

The periodic law was first formulated in detail by the Russian chemist Dmitri Mendeleev about 1869, although the general idea was not new. While the modern quantum theory of the atom was many years in the future, Mendeleev was fully aware of the significance of his work. As he remarked, "The periodic law, together with the revelations of spectrum analysis, have contributed to again revive an old but remarkably long-lived hope—that of discovering, if not by experiment then at least by mental effort, the *primary matter.*"

A **periodic table** is a listing of the elements according to atomic number in a series of rows such that elements with similar properties form vertical columns. Table 10-6 is a simple form of the periodic table. Let us see how it organizes our knowledge of the elements.

Building the Periodic Table   The first element in the table is hydrogen, which behaves chemically much like an active metal although physically it is a nonmetal. Next comes the inert gas helium, the alkali metal lithium, and the less active metal beryllium. Then follows a series of nonmetals of increasing nonmetallic activity: boron, carbon, nitrogen, oxygen, and finally the halogen fluorine. Thus from lithium to fluorine we have a complete sequence that goes from a highly active metal to a highly active nonmetal.

Following fluorine is neon, an inert gas like helium, and after neon is sodium, an alkali metal like lithium. Clearly it makes sense to break off the rows at helium and neon and start new rows with lithium and sodium under hydrogen. In the seven elements beyond neon, we find again a transition from active metals to active nonmetals.

After calcium, in the fourth row, complications appear. Scandium, the next element, is similar to aluminum in some properties but different in

Atomic Mass

As we recall from Chap. 8, nearly all elements have isotopes whose nuclei have different numbers of neutrons and hence whose atomic masses are different. The atomic mass of an element that chemists use is the *average* mass of the atoms of its various isotopes in the proportion in which they occur in nature. For instance, chlorine consists of 76 percent of the $^{35}_{17}Cl$ isotope, whose atomic mass is 34.97 u, and 24 percent of the $^{37}_{17}Cl$ isotope, whose atomic mass is 36.97 u. The average atomic mass of chlorine is 35.45 u, and this is the value given in Table 10-6.

Table 10-6 The Periodic Table of the Elements

The number above the symbol of each element is its atomic number, and the number below its name is its average atomic mass. The elements whose atomic masses are given in parentheses do not occur in nature but have been created in nuclear reactions. The atomic mass in such a case is the mass number of the most long-lived radioisotope of the element. The elements with atomic numbers 113–118 have also been created in the laboratory.

Period	Group 1	Group 2	Group 3	Group 4	Group 5	Group 6	Group 7	Group 8
1	1 **H** Hydrogen 1.008							2 **He** Helium 4.003
2	3 **Li** Lithium 6.941	4 **Be** Beryllium 9.012	5 **B** Boron 10.81	6 **C** Carbon 12.01	7 **N** Nitrogen 14.01	8 **O** Oxygen 16.00	9 **F** Fluorine 19.00	10 **Ne** Neon 20.18
3	11 **Na** Sodium 22.99	12 **Mg** Magnesium 24.31	13 **Al** Aluminum 26.98	14 **Si** Silicon 28.09	15 **P** Phosphorus 30.97	16 **S** Sulfur 32.07	17 **Cl** Chlorine 35.45	18 **Ar** Argon 39.95
4	19 **K** Potassium 39.10	20 **Ca** Calcium 40.08	31 **Ga** Gallium 69.72	32 **Ge** Germanium 72.59	33 **As** Arsenic 74.92	34 **Se** Selenium 78.96	35 **Br** Bromine 79.90	36 **Kr** Krypton 83.80
5	37 **Rb** Rubidium 85.47	38 **Sr** Strontium 87.62	49 **In** Indium 114.8	50 **Sn** Tin 118.7	51 **Sb** Antimony 121.8	52 **Te** Tellurium 127.6	53 **I** Iodine 126.9	54 **Xe** Xenon 131.8
6	55 **Cs** Cesium 132.9	56 **Ba** Barium 137.3	81 **Tl** Thallium 204.4	82 **Pb** Lead 207.2	83 **Bi** Bismuth 209.0	84 **Po** Polonium (209)	85 **At** Astatine (210)	86 **Rn** Radon (222)
7	87 **Fr** Francium (223)	88 **Ra** Radium 226.0						

Alkali metals (Group 1) — Inert gases (Group 8) — Halogens (Group 7)

Transition metals

Period	Group 3	4	5	6	7	8				1	2
4	21 **Sc** Scandium 44.96	22 **Ti** Titanium 47.88	23 **V** Vanadium 50.94	24 **Cr** Chromium 52.00	25 **Mn** Manganese 54.94	26 **Fe** Iron 55.8	27 **Co** Cobalt 58.93	28 **Ni** Nickel 58.69	29 **Cu** Copper 63.55	30 **Zn** Zinc 65.39	
5	39 **Y** Yttrium 88.91	40 **Zr** Zirconium 91.22	41 **Nb** Niobium 92.91	42 **Mo** Molybdenum 95.94	43 **Tc** Technetium (98)	44 **Ru** Ruthenium 101.1	45 **Rh** Rhodium 102.9	46 **Pd** Palladium 106.4	47 **Ag** Silver 107.9	48 **Cd** Cadmium 112.4	
6	57 **La** Lanthanum 138.9	72 **Hf** Hafnium 178.5	73 **Ta** Tantalum 180.9	74 **W** Tungsten 183.9	75 **Re** Rhenium 186.2	76 **Os** Osmium 190.2	77 **Ir** Iridium 192.2	78 **Pt** Platinum 195.1	79 **Au** Gold 197.0	80 **Hg** Mercury 200.6	
7	89 **Ac** Actinium (227)	104 **Rf** Rutherfordium (261)	105 **Db** Dubnium (262)	106 **Sg** Seaborgium (263)	107 **Bh** Bohrium (262)	108 **Hs** Hassium (265)	109 **Mt** Meitnerium (266)	110 **Ds** Darmstadtium (271)	111 **Rg** Roentgenium (272)	112 **Cn** Copernicium (285)	

Lanthanides (rare earths)

57 **La** Lanthanum 138.9	58 **Ce** Cerium 140.1	59 **Pr** Praseodymium 140.9	60 **Nd** Neodymium 144.2	61 **Pm** Promethium (145)	62 **Sm** Samarium 150.4	63 **Eu** Europium 152.0	64 **Gd** Gadolinium 157.3	65 **Tb** Terbium 158.9	66 **Dy** Dysprosium 162.5	67 **Ho** Holmium 164.9	68 **Er** Erbium 167.3	69 **Tm** Thulium 168.9	70 **Yb** Ytterbium 173.0	71 **Lu** Lutetium 175.0

Actinides

89 **Ac** Actinium (227)	90 **Th** Thorium 232.0	91 **Pa** Protactinium 231.0	92 **U** Uranium 238.0	93 **Np** Neptunium (237)	94 **Pu** Plutonium (244)	95 **Am** Americium (243)	96 **Cm** Curium (247)	97 **Bk** Berkelium (247)	98 **Cf** Californium (251)	99 **Es** Einsteinium (252)	100 **Fm** Fermium (257)	101 **Md** Mendelevium (260)	102 **No** Nobelium (259)	103 **Lw** Lawrencium (262)

| **Dmitri Mendeleev (1834 –1907)**

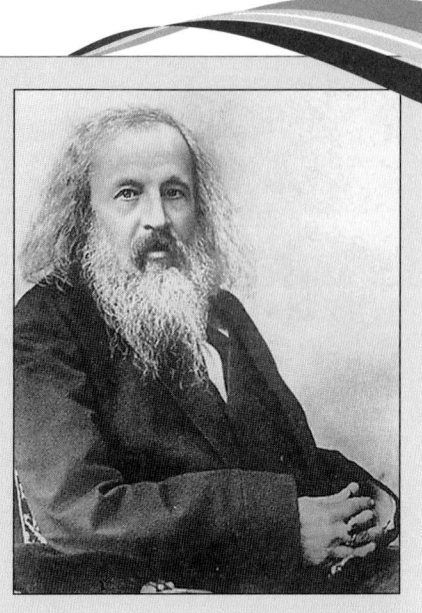

Mendeleev was born in Siberia and grew up there, going on to Moscow and later France and Germany to study chemistry. In 1866 he became professor of chemistry at the University of St. Petersburg and 3 years later he published the first version of the periodic table.

The notion of atomic number was then unknown and Mendeleev had to deviate from the strict sequence of atomic masses for some elements and to leave gaps in the table in order that the known elements (only 63 at that time) occupy places appropriate to their properties. Other chemists of the time were thinking along the same lines, but Mendeleev went further in 1871 by proposing that the gaps correspond to then-unknown elements. When his detailed predictions of the properties of these elements were fulfilled upon their discovery, Mendeleev became world-famous.

A further triumph for the periodic table came at the end of the nineteenth century when the inert gases were discovered. Here were six elements of whose existence Mendeleev (and everybody else) had been unaware, but they fit perfectly as a new group in the table. The element of atomic number 101 is called mendelevium in his honor.

others. Titanium (Ti) is even less like carbon and silicon. Then come 10 metals (including iron, copper, and zinc) that are quite similar among themselves but conspicuously different from the nonmetals at the end of the first three rows. Only after the 10 metals do three relatives of these nonmetals appear, arsenic (As), selenium (Se), and bromine (Br).

Between the gases helium and neon is a sequence of eight elements, and between neon and argon is another sequence of eight. However, between argon and krypton the sequence includes 18 elements. Beyond krypton is a second sequence of 18, including again a dozen metals with many properties in common. From xenon to the last inert gas, radon, is an even more complex sequence of 32 elements.

10.8   Groups and Periods

Elements in a Group Have Similar Properties; Elements in a Period Have Different Ones

The periodic table arranges families of similar elements in vertical columns called **groups.** The horizontal rows, called **periods,** contain elements with widely different properties (Fig. 10-10). Across each period is a steady change from an active metal through less active metals and weakly active nonmetals to highly active nonmetals and finally to an inert gas (Fig. 10-11). Within each column there is also a steady change in properties. Thus activity increases in

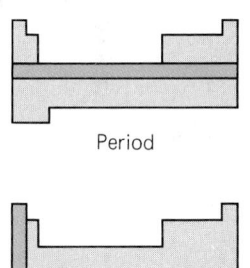

Figure 10-10   The elements in a group of the periodic table have similar properties whereas those in a period have different properties.

Figure 10-11   How chemical activity varies in the periodic table.

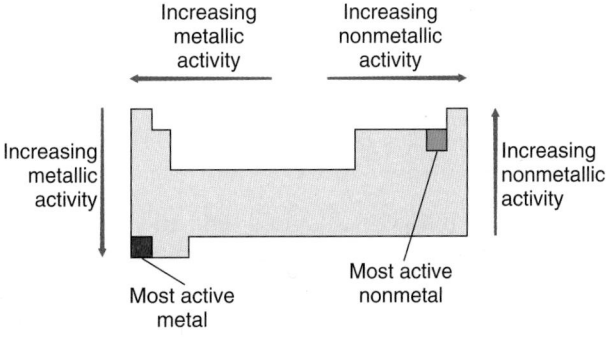

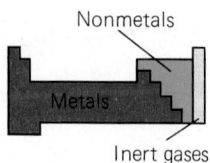

Figure 10-12   The majority of the elements are metals. The semimetals lie just to the right of the division between metals and nonmetals.

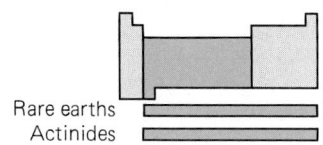

Figure 10-13   The transition elements are metals.

the alkali metal family as we go from top to bottom down the group 1 column, and activity decreases in the halogen family as we go down the group 7 column.

Eight of the groups in Table 10-6 are numbered. The inert gases of group 8 are placed at the right since this puts them with the other nonmetals (Fig. 10-12). Each of the eight-element periods (periods 2 and 3) is broken after the second element in order to keep the members of the period in line with the most closely related elements of the long periods, which are 4 to 7.

Transition Metals   The **transition metals** in periods 4 and 5 are metals that resemble one another in chemical behavior but do not much resemble elements in the numbered groups (Fig. 10-13). They are what we usually think of as typical metals. Iron, nickel, copper, and gold are transition metals, all of which are less reactive than the metals in groups 1 and 2. Period 6 contains 32 elements, but 15 of them are brought out to a separate box. These **rare-earth** metals, which are so much alike that they are hard to separate chemically, are all placed together in the spot just to the right of barium, $Z = 56$. A similar group of closely related elements, the **actinides,** appears in the same position in period 7, and these elements are also shown in a separate box.

The relationships brought out by the periodic table are a little vague in places, but on the whole the table brings together similar elements with considerable accuracy. Mendeleev's achievement is all the more remarkable when we recall that in 1869, when the periodic law was developed, the notion of atomic number had not been discovered and only 63 elements were known. Mendeleev used average atomic mass, not atomic number, to arrange the elements in the periodic table, and he and later chemists found it necessary to deviate from the strict sequence of atomic masses for certain elements. When atomic numbers were later determined for the elements, the values of Z were found to fit the sequence in the periodic table perfectly.

Mendeleev's Predictions   Because so few elements were known in his time, Mendeleev had to leave gaps in his table in order to have similar elements fall in line. Sure of the correctness of his classification, he proposed that these gaps represented undiscovered elements. From the position of each gap, from the properties of the elements around it, and from the variation of these properties across the periods and down the columns, he went on to predict the properties of the unknown elements. His predictions included not only general chemical activity but also numerical values for boiling points, melting points, and so on.

As the unknown elements were discovered one by one and as their properties were found to agree with Mendeleev's predictions, the validity and usefulness of the periodic table became firmly established. Perhaps its greatest triumph came at the end of the nineteenth century, when the inert gases were discovered. Here were six new elements whose existence Mendeleev was not aware of, but they fitted perfectly as one more family of similar elements into the periodic table. The history of the periodic table is a beautiful example of the scientific method in action.

Atomic Structure

Now we return to the atomic theory of Chap. 9 to seek the basis of the periodic law. Two basic principles determine the structure of an atom that contains more than one electron:

1. The exclusion principle, which states that only one electron can exist in each quantum state of an atom. Thus each electron in a complex atom must have a different set of the four quantum numbers n, l, m_l, and m_s (see Table 9-1).

2. An atom, like any other system, is stable when its total energy is a minimum. This means that the various electrons in a normal atom are in the quantum states of lowest energy permitted by the exclusion principle.

10.9   Shells and Subshells

They Contain Electrons with Similar Energies

Let us look into how electron energy varies with quantum state. In any atom, all the electrons with the same quantum number n are, on the average, about the same distance from the nucleus. These electrons therefore move around in nearly the same electric field and have similar energies. Such electrons are said to occupy the same atomic **shell.** The higher the value of n, the larger the shell.

The energy of an electron in a particular shell also depends to some extent on the electron's angular momentum quantum number l, because l influences the shape of the electron's orbital and hence its average distance from the nucleus. The higher the value of l, the higher the energy. Electrons that share a certain value of l in a shell are said to occupy the same **subshell.** All the electrons in a subshell have very nearly the same energy.

The subshells in a shell of given n can have any value of l from 0 to $n - 1$. Thus the $n = 1$ shell has only the s ($l = 0$) subshell; the $n = 2$ shell has s and p ($l = 1$) subshells; the $n = 3$ shell has s, p, and d ($l = 2$) subshells; and so on.

Closed Shells and Subshells   The exclusion principle limits the number of electrons that can occupy a given shell or subshell. A shell or subshell that contains its full quota of electrons is said to be **closed.**

The larger the orbital quantum number l, the more electrons the corresponding subshell can hold (see Table 9-2). Adding up the electrons in its closed subshells gives the maximum number of electrons in a closed shell.

How Subshells Are Filled

Subshells are filled in order of increasing energy, and the energies of atomic electrons depend on the shapes of their orbitals. Hence, with l as well as with n, all the available subshells in a given shell may not be filled before subshells of low l in the next shell begin to be occupied. This can be seen in Fig. 10-14. It is customary to identify a subshell by its quantum number n followed by a letter corresponding to its quantum number l, so that 3p refers to the p subshell of shell $n = 3$. In this notation, the sequence in which atomic subshells are filled is as follows:

1s 2s 2p 3s 3p 4s 3d 4p
5s 4d 5p 6s 4f 5d 6p 7s 6d 5f

The transition elements in any period have similar properties because their outer electron shells are the same and they add electrons successively to inner shells.

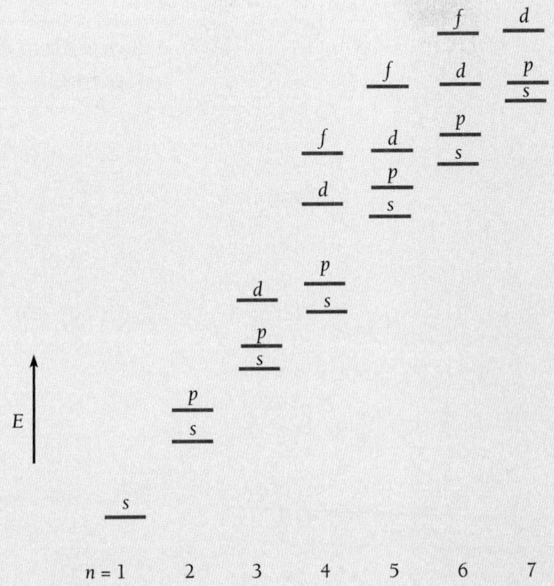

Figure 10-14   The sequence of quantum states in an atom. Not to scale.

Thus a closed $n = 1$ shell holds 2 s electrons; a closed $n = 2$ shell holds 2 s electrons plus 6 p electrons for a total of 8 electrons; a closed $n = 3$ shell holds these 8 electrons plus 10 more d electrons for a total of 18 electrons; and so on.

The concept of electron shells and subshells fits perfectly into the pattern of the periodic table, which turns out to mirror the atomic structures of the elements. Let us see how this pattern arises.

10.10   Explaining the Periodic Table

How an Atom's Electron Structure Determines Its Chemical Behavior

Table 10-7, which is illustrated in Fig. 10-15, shows the number of electrons in the shells of a number of elements. The table is arranged in the same manner as the periodic table to emphasize the relationship between the two tables.

Inert Gas Atoms   In order to interpret Table 10-7 we note that the electrons in a closed shell are all tightly bound to the atom, since the positive nuclear charge that attracts them is large relative to the negative charge of any electrons in inner shells. An atom that contains only closed shells or subshells has its electric charge uniformly distributed, so it does not attract other electrons and its electrons cannot be easily removed. We would expect such atoms to be passive chemically, like the inert gases—and the inert gases all turn out to have closed-subshell electron structures!

Hydrogen and Alkali Metal Atoms   Hydrogen and the alkali metals have single outer electrons. In the case of the hydrogen atom, the attractive force on the electron is due to a nuclear charge of only $+e$ and is not very great. In the case of the sodium atom, the total nuclear charge of $+11e$ acts on the two inner electrons, which are held very tightly. These two electrons shield part of the nuclear charge from the 8 electrons in the second shell, which are therefore attracted by a net charge of $+9e$. All 10 electrons in the first and second shells act to shield the outermost electron. This electron "sees" a net nuclear charge of only $+e$ and is held much less securely to the atom than any of the other electrons (Fig. 10-16a).

Table 10-7	Simplified Table of Electron Structures of Some Atoms (Subshells Are Filled When a Shell Has 2, 8, or 18 Electrons)							
Electrons in	H							He
1st shell	1							2
Electrons in	Li	Be	B	C	N	O	F	Ne
1st shell	2	2	2	2	2	2	2	2
2nd shell	1	2	3	4	5	6	7	8
Electrons in	Na	Mg	Al	Si	P	S	Cl	Ar
1st shell	2	2	2	2	2	2	2	2
2nd shell	8	8	8	8	8	8	8	8
3rd shell	1	2	3	4	5	6	7	8
Electrons in	K	Ca					Br	Kr
1st shell	2	2	. . . .				2	2
2nd shell	8	8					8	8
3rd shell	8	8					18	18
4th shell	1	2					7	8
Electrons in	Rb	Sr					I	Xe
1st shell	2	2	. . . .				2	2
2nd shell	8	8					8	8
3rd shell	18	18					18	18
4th shell	8	8					18	18
5th shell	1	2					7	8

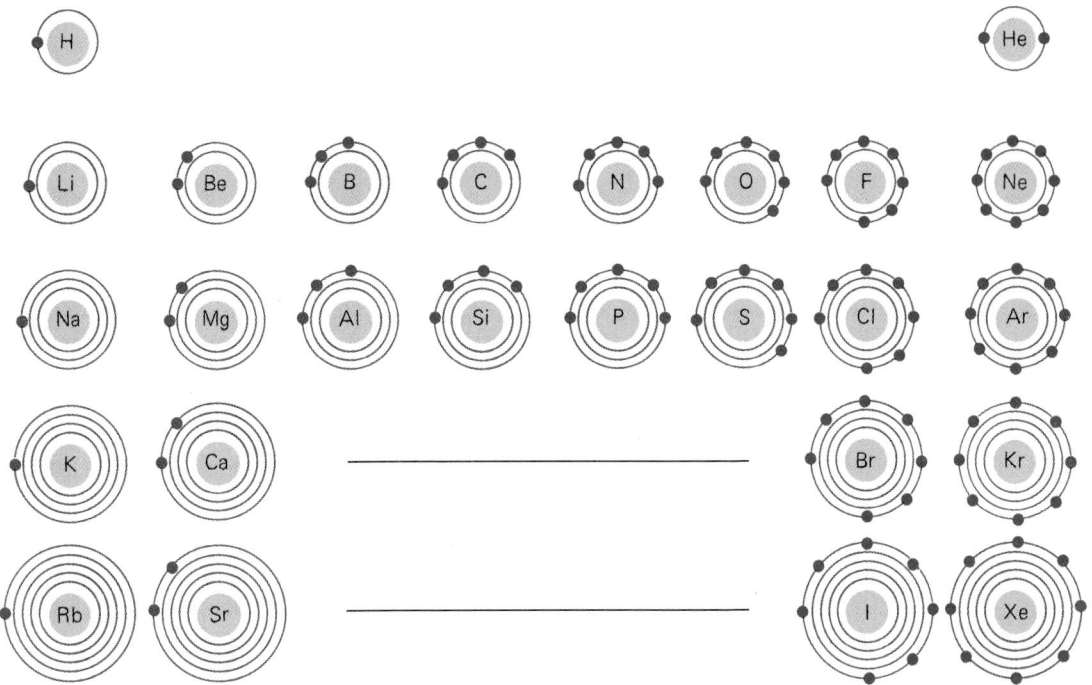

Figure 10-15 Electron structures of some atoms. In this schematic illustration of Table 10-7 the circles without dots represent closed (that is, completely filled) inner shells.

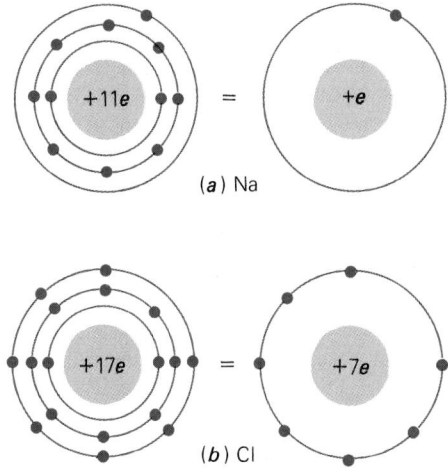

Figure 10-16 Electron shielding in sodium (*a*) and chlorine (*b*). Each outer electron in a Cl atom is acted upon by an effective nuclear charge 7 times greater than that acting upon the outer electron in a Na atom, even though the outer electrons in both cases are in the same shell.

An analysis of this kind also holds for the other alkali metals. As a result, atoms of hydrogen and of the alkali metals all tend to lose their outermost electrons in chemical reactions and therefore have similar chemical behavior.

As noted in Fig. 10-11, the alkali metals become more active going down group 1. This is because atoms become larger with increasing atomic number in group 1. As a result, their outer electrons are farther and farther from the nucleus, so the electric force on them is progressively weaker. Therefore these electrons are held less tightly and are more easily given up in a reaction.

Halogen Atoms An atom whose outer shell lacks one electron from being closed tends to pick up such an electron through the strong attraction of the poorly shielded nuclear charge. The chemical behavior of the halogens is the result. In the chlorine atom, for instance, there are 10 electrons in the inner two shells, just as in the sodium atom. However, the nuclear charge of chlorine is +17e as compared with only +11e for sodium (Fig. 10-16b). Hence the net charge "felt" by each of the 7 outer electrons in chlorine is +7e, not the +e in the case of the single outer electron of sodium, and the attractive force on an outer electron in chlorine is 7 times greater.

In contrast to the alkali metals, the halogens become *less* reactive going down group 7. The reason again is the increase in atomic size with increasing atomic number. The halogens react by picking up electrons, and the larger the atom, the weaker the attractive electric force on the electrons in the outer shell. Thus the smaller the halogen atom, the more strongly it attracts an electron from elsewhere to fill its outer shell and the more reactive it is, as shown in Fig. 10-11.

Metals and Nonmetals   These considerations lead us to general descriptions of metal and nonmetal atoms:

> A metal atom has one or several electrons outside closed shells or subshells. Such an atom combines chemically by losing these electrons to nonmetal atoms.

> A nonmetal atom needs one or several electrons to achieve closed shells or subshells. Such an atom combines chemically by picking up electrons from metal atoms or by sharing electrons with other nonmetal atoms.

The inert gases are exceptions to these statements, of course, since their atomic structures make it hard for them to gain or lose electrons. As a result, they have almost no ability to react chemically.

The steady change in chemical properties as we go across a period from an alkali metal on the left to a halogen on the right is easy to account for. An atom of an element in group 2, for instance magnesium (Mg), has two electrons outside closed inner shells, as we see in Fig. 10-15. These electrons "feel" an effective nuclear charge of +2e and so are more tightly held than the single outer electron in sodium, which "feels" an effective nuclear charge of only +e.

Not surprisingly, the outer electrons in an Mg atom are harder to pull away than the outer electron in Na. Hence Mg is less active as a metal than Na. Aluminum (Al), with three outer electrons, holds them still more securely, which is why Al is less active than Mg.

In a nonmetal atom, the more the gaps in its outer shell, the weaker the electric field that attracts additional electrons to complete the shell. Sulfur (S), with two electrons missing from its outer shell, is therefore less active a nonmetal than chlorine, which is missing just one electron. Phosphorus (P), with three electrons missing, is even less active. We can now see why, in any period, metallic activity (losing electrons) decreases going to the right, while nonmetallic activity (gaining electrons) increases going to the right (Fig. 10-11).

[For a sidebar on atomic sizes, see Sec. 10.10 at www.mhhe.com/krauskopf.]

Chemical Bonds

What is the nature of the forces that bond atoms together when compounds are formed? This question is of basic importance to the chemist. It is also important to the physicist because the quantum theory of the atom cannot be complete unless it provides a satisfactory answer. The ability of the quantum theory to explain chemical bonding is further testimony to the power of this approach.

10.11 Types of Bond

Electric Forces Hold Atoms to One Another

Let us consider what happens when two atoms are brought closer and closer together. Three extreme situations may occur:

1. A **covalent bond** is formed. The outermost orbitals of the atoms overlap and one or more pairs of electrons are shared by them. The shared electrons spend more time between the atoms than on their far sides, which produces an attractive force. An example is H_2, the hydrogen molecule, whose two electrons belong jointly to the two protons (Fig. 10-17).
2. An **ionic bond** is formed. One or more electrons from one atom shift to another atom, and the resulting positive and negative ions attract each other. An example is NaCl, where the bond exists between Na^+ and Cl^- ions and not between Na and Cl atoms (Fig. 10-18).
3. No bond is formed. The atoms do not interact to produce an attractive force.

In H_2 the bond is purely covalent and in NaCl it is purely ionic, but in many other molecules an intermediate type of bond occurs in which the atoms share electrons to an unequal extent. An example is the HCl molecule, where the Cl atom attracts the shared electrons more strongly than the H atom.

Ionic bonds usually do not result in the formation of molecules. Strictly speaking, a molecule is an electrically neutral group of atoms that is held together strongly enough to be experimentally observable as a particle. Thus the individual units that constitute gaseous hydrogen each consist of two hydrogen atoms, and we are entitled to regard them as molecules.

Crystals   Crystals of table salt (NaCl), on the other hand, are aggregates of sodium and chlorine ions (Fig. 10-19). Although arranged in a certain definite way, as we saw in Fig. 10-6, the ions do not pair off into individual molecules consisting of one Na^+ ion and one Cl^- ion. Salt crystals may in fact be of almost any size. There are always equal numbers of Na^+ and Cl^- ions in salt, so that the formula NaCl correctly represents its composition. Despite the absence of individual NaCl molecules in solid NaCl, the electric force between adjacent Na^+ and Cl^- ions makes NaCl as characteristic an example of chemical bonding as H_2.

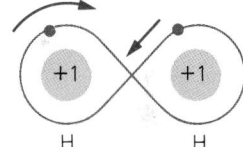

Figure 10-17 A simplified model of covalent bonding in hydrogen. The shared electrons spend more time on the average between their parent nuclei than on the far sides of the nuclei and therefore lead to an attractive internuclear force.

Figure 10-18 A simplified model of ionic bonding. Sodium and chlorine combine chemically by the transfer of electrons from sodium atoms to chlorine atoms. The resulting ions attract electrically.

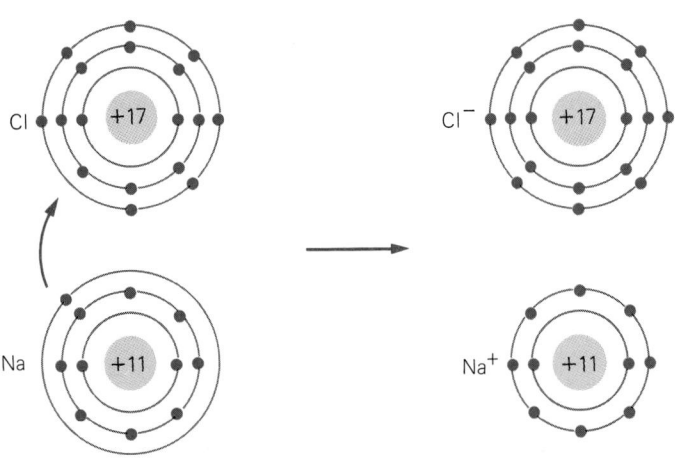

| **Linus Pauling (1901–1994)**

A native of Oregon, Pauling received his Ph.D. from the California Institute of Technology and remained there for his entire scientific career except for a period in the middle 1920s when he was in Germany to study the new quantum mechanics. A pioneer in applying quantum theory to chemistry, Pauling provided many of the key insights that led to an understanding of the details of chemical bonding.

Pauling also did important work in molecular biology, in particular protein structure: with the help of x-ray diffraction, he discovered the helical and pleated sheet forms that protein molecules can have. It was Pauling who realized that sickle cell anemia is a "molecular disease"

due to hemoglobin with one wrong amino acid resulting from a genetic fault. He received the Nobel Prize in chemistry in 1954.

In 1923 Pauling met Ava Helen Miller in a chemistry class and she married him despite his admission that, "if I had to choose between you and science, I'm not sure that I would choose you." She introduced him to the world outside the laboratory, and in his later years he became more and more politically active. Pauling fought to stop the atmospheric testing of nuclear weapons with its attendant radioactive fallout, a crusade that led to a 2500-page FBI file, the nuclear test ban treaty, and the Nobel Peace Prize in 1965.

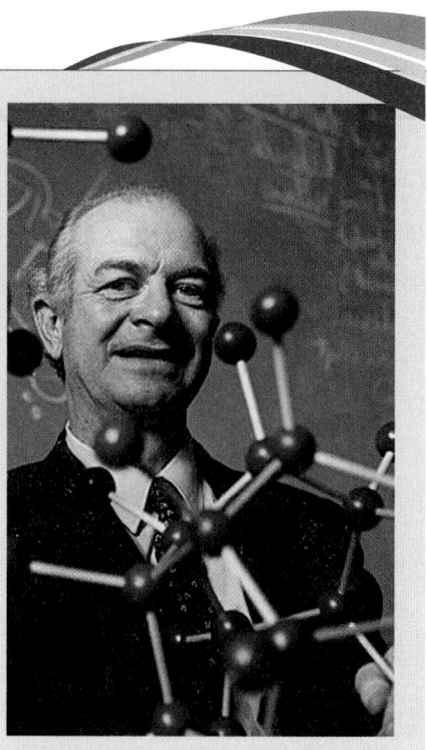

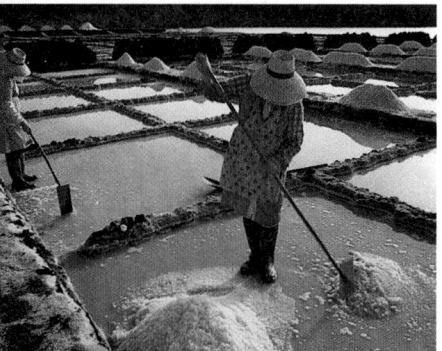

Figure 10-19   Much of the world's salt was once produced by evaporating seawater, as is still done in the Canary Islands.

10.12   Covalent Bonding

Sharing Electron Pairs Produces an Attractive Force

We saw in Fig. 10-17 how two identical atoms, in this case hydrogen atoms, can bond together by sharing a pair of electrons. In some molecules more than one pair of electrons is shared. Examples are O_2, which has two shared electron pairs, and N_2, which has three. If we use a pair of dots to stand for a shared pair of electrons, the H_2, O_2, and N_2 molecules can be represented as follows:

$$H : H \qquad\qquad O : : O \qquad\qquad N : : : N$$

hydrogen   oxygen   nitrogen
molecule   molecule   molecule

Substances whose atoms are joined by shared electron pairs are called **covalent.** In general, they are either nonmetallic elements or else compounds of one nonmetal with another, although some compounds that contain metals belong to this class. The shared pair or pairs of electrons between two atoms constitute a **bond.** In general, double or triple bonds are stronger than single ones. The triple bonds in nitrogen molecules are among the strongest known. As a result, nitrogen molecules are extremely stable and do not react readily; what this means for living things, which need nitrogen for their proteins, is discussed in Sec. 13.15.

Polar Covalent Compounds   In some covalent compounds the shared electron pairs are closer to one atom than to the other. Two examples are HCl (hydrochloric acid) and H_2O:

$$H : Cl \qquad\qquad H \quad : \overset{..}{O}$$

$$H$$

These substances are called **polar covalent compounds,** because one part of the molecule is relatively negative and another part is relatively positive.

All gradations can be found between uniformly covalent molecules at one extreme, through polar covalent molecules, to ionic compounds at the other extreme. For example,

Covalent	Cl	:	Cl
Polar covalent	H	:	Cl
Ionic	Na	: Cl	

Organic Compounds   The carbon atom has four outer electrons to share with each other and with other atoms in covalent bonds. Covalent compounds that contain carbon are called **organic compounds.** Organic compounds are so important that all of Chap. 13 is devoted to them.

10.13   Ionic Bonding

Electron Transfer Creates Ions That Attract Each Other

The simplest example of a chemical reaction that involves electron transfer is the combination of a metal and a nonmetal. For a specific case, let us consider the burning of sodium in chlorine to give sodium chloride. From Fig. 10-15 it is clear that Na and Cl are perfect mates—one has an electron to lose, the other an electron to gain. In the process of combination, an electron goes from Na to Cl, as shown in Fig. 10-18.

The stability of the resulting closed electron shells in both ions is shown by the large amount of energy given off in the form of heat and light when this reaction takes place. The compound NaCl is quite unreactive because each of its ions has a stable electron structure. To break NaCl apart, which means to return the electron from Cl^- to Na^+, requires the same considerable energy that was set free when the compound was formed.

As we know, metal atoms tend to lose their outer electrons, like sodium in NaCl. Nonmetal atoms, on the other hand, tend to gain electrons so as to fill in gaps in their outer shells. In most reactions of this sort the metal loses all its outer electrons, and the nonmetal fills all the gaps in its structure.

When sodium combines with sulfur, for instance, each S atom has two spaces to fill for a closed outer shell (Fig. 10-20), but each Na atom has only one electron to give. Hence two Na atoms are needed for each S atom, and the resulting compound is Na_2S. When calcium combines with oxygen, each Ca atom contributes two electrons to each O atom, and the formula of the compound is CaO.

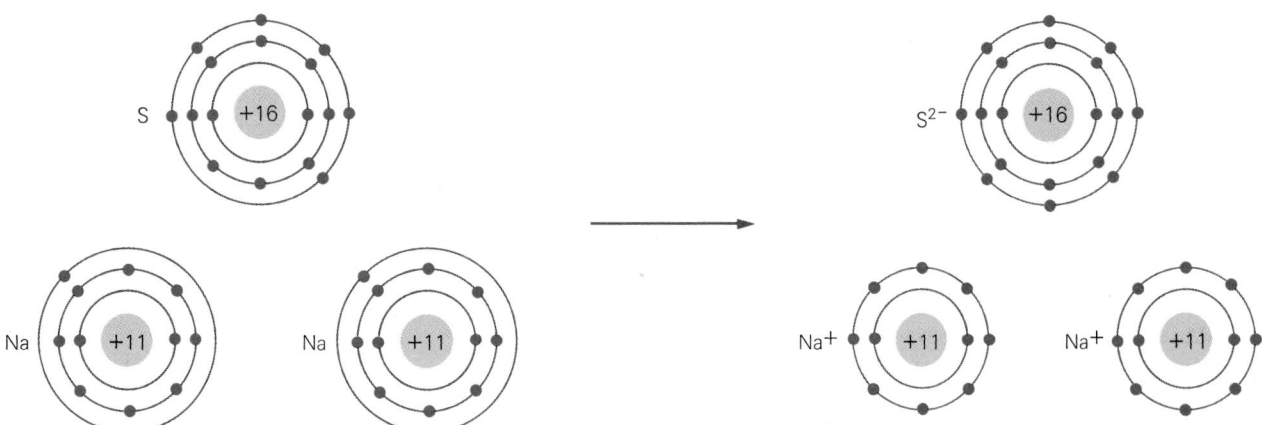

Figure 10-20   Ionic bonding in Na_2S. Each sodium atom contributes one electron to the sulfur atom, and the resulting S^{2-} ion attracts the two Na^+ atoms.

Table 10-8	Ions of Some Common Elements
Element	**Ion**
Hydrogen	H^+
Lithium	Li^+
Sodium	Na^+
Potassium	K^+
Silver	Ag^+
Copper	Cu^+, Cu^{2+}
Mercury	Hg^+, Hg^{2+}
Magnesium	Mg^{2+}
Calcium	Ca^{2+}
Barium	Ba^{2+}
Zinc	Zn^{2+}
Iron	Fe^{2+}, Fe^{3+}
Aluminum	Al^{3+}
Tin	Sn^{2+}, Sn^{4+}
Lead	Pb^{2+}, Pb^{4+}
Fluorine	F^-
Chlorine	Cl^-
Bromine	Br^-
Iodine	I^-
Oxygen	O^{2-}
Sulfur	S^{2-}
Nitrogen	N^{3-}
Phosphorus	P^{3-}

Compounds formed by electron transfer are called **ionic compounds.** Some are simple compounds like NaCl, Na_2S, and CaO. Others have more complex formulas, such as Na_2SO_4, KNO_3, and $CaCO_3$. In these latter compounds electrons from the metal atoms have been transferred to nonmetal **atom groups** (SO_4, NO_3, CO_3) instead of to single nonmetal atoms.

Ionic compounds in general contain a metal and one or more nonmetals, and their crystal structures have alternate positive and negative ions. Most of them are crystalline solids with high melting points. We expect this, since melting involves separating the ions.

Example 10.1

Why do only the outermost electrons of an atom usually participate in bonding?

Solution

Inner electrons are much more tightly held to a nucleus both because they are closer to it and because they are shielded by fewer intervening electrons. Hence the inner electrons are unable either to transfer to another atom in an ionic bond or to be shared with another atom in a covalent bond.

10.14   Ionic Compounds

Matching Up Ions

When a metal and a nonmetal combine to form an ionic compound, the atoms of the metal give up one or more electrons to atoms of the nonmetal. We can figure out the formula of the compound by knowing how many electrons the metal atoms tend to lose and how many electrons the nonmetal atoms tend to gain.

As we have already seen, Na tends to lose one electron to become Na^+ and Cl tends to gain one electron to become Cl^-. Hence the formula of sodium chloride is NaCl. Similarly sulfur tends to gain two electrons to become S^{2-}, so sodium sulfide must have the formula Na_2S in order that two electrons be available for each S atom. Calcium forms Ca^{2+} ions, hence calcium sulfide must have the formula CaS with two electrons shifting from each Ca atom to each S atom.

Ions of Different Charge   Table 10-8 shows the ions formed by some common elements when they enter into compounds. A few elements form different ions under different circumstances, for example copper (Cu^+, Cu^{2+}) and iron (Fe^{2+}, Fe^{3+}). In such cases the name of the element in its compound is followed by a Roman numeral to indicate the ionic charge. Thus $FeCl_2$ is called iron(II) chloride (in speech, "iron-two chloride") because it contains Fe^{2+} ions, and $FeCl_3$ is called iron(III) chloride because it contains Fe^{3+} ions.

With the help of Table 10-8 we can see what happens when a given metal combines with a given nonmetal. The positive and negative charges on the ions must always balance out, and a little thought may be needed to find the right combination.

Figure 10-21   The charges in each unit of an ionic compound, such as Al_2O_3, must be in balance. Here the 6 positive charges of $2Al^{3+}$ are balanced by the 6 negative charges of $3O^{2-}$.

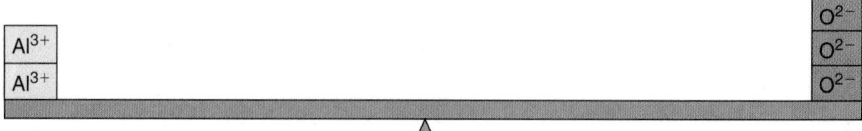

Example 10.2

Find the formula of aluminum oxide, which consists of aluminum and oxygen ions.

Solution

From Table 10-8 we see that aluminum forms Al^{3+} ions, and oxygen forms O^{2-} ions. Because the ion charges are different in magnitude, the formula cannot be simply AlO. A straightforward way to arrive at the correct formula is to first write down the symbols for each ion in parentheses:

$$(Al^{3+}) \quad (O^{2-})$$

Now we put a subscript after each parentheses equal to the magnitude of the charge on the *other* ion (that is, the amount of charge regardless of sign):

$$(Al^{3+})_2(O^{2-})_3$$

Finally we delete the ionic charges and, where possible, the parentheses:

$$Al_2O_3$$

This is the formula of aluminum oxide (Fig. 10-21).

10.15   Atom Groups

They Act as Units in Chemical Reactions

Certain groups of atoms appear as units in many compounds and remain together during chemical reactions. An example is the group SO_4, which consists of a sulfur atom joined to four oxygen atoms. This **sulfate group,** whose ion has a charge of -2, is found in a number of compounds:

Sodium sulfate	Na_2SO_4
Potassium sulfate	K_2SO_4
Copper(II) sulfate	$CuSO_4$
Magnesium sulfate	$MgSO_4$

How can we be sure that the sulfate group enters into chemical reactions as a unit? One way is to mix solutions of magnesium sulfate and barium chloride, $BaCl_2$. What happens is that a precipitate is formed, which analysis shows consists of barium sulfate, $BaSO_4$. (A **precipitate** is an insoluble solid that results from a chemical reaction in solution.) The solution left behind contains magnesium ions and chlorine ions (Fig. 10-22). The sulfate group has changed partners.

When two or more groups of a single kind are present in each molecule of a compound, the formula is written with parentheses around the group. An example is

Calcium nitrate $Ca(NO_3)_2$

The Ca^{2+} ion needs two NO_3^- ions to combine with in order that the charges balance out. Table 10-9 is a list of common atom groups and the charges their ions have.

10.16   Naming Compounds

The Vocabulary of Chemistry

Here are some of the rules chemists use to name compounds:

1. The ending *-ide* usually indicates a compound having only two elements:

Sodium chloride	NaCl
Calcium oxide	CaO

Figure 10-22   When magnesium sulfate ($MgSO_4$) and barium chloride ($BaCl_2$) are dissolved in water, a precipitate of the insoluble compound barium sulfate is produced. The magnesium and chlorine ions remain in solution.

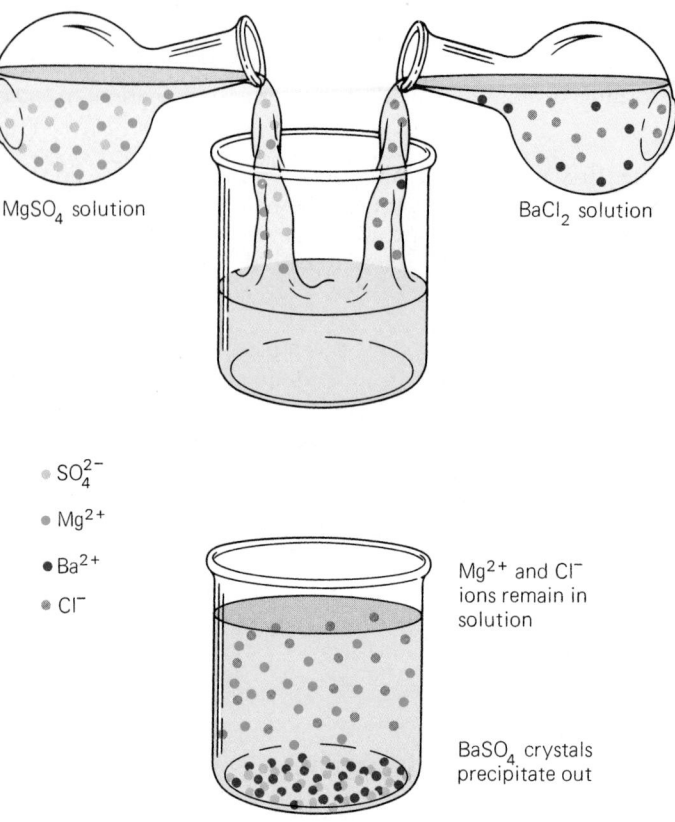

MgSO₄ solution

BaCl₂ solution

• SO_4^{2-}

• Mg^{2+}

• Ba^{2+}

• Cl^-

Mg^{2+} and Cl^- ions remain in solution

BaSO₄ crystals precipitate out

Table 10-9	Ions of Some Common Atom Groups
Atom Group	**Ion**
Ammonium	NH_4^+
Nitrate	NO_3^-
Permanganate	MnO_4^-
Chlorate	ClO_3^-
Hydroxide	OH^-
Cyanide	CN^-
Sulfate	SO_4^{2-}
Carbonate	CO_3^{2-}
Chromate	CrO_4^{2-}
Silicate	SiO_4^{2-}
Phosphate	PO_4^{3-}

The hydroxides, which contain the OH^- ion, are the most common exceptions to this rule:

Barium hydroxide $Ba(OH)_2$

2. The ending *-ate* indicates a compound that contains oxygen and two or more other elements:

Sodium sulfate Na_2SO_4
Potassium nitrate KNO_3

3. When the same pair of elements occurs in two or more compounds, a prefix (*mono-* = 1, *di-* = 2, *tri-* = 3, *tetra-* = 4, *penta-* = 5, *hexa-* = 6, and so on) may be used to indicate the number of one or both kinds of atom in the molecule:

Carbon monoxide   CO
Carbon dioxide CO_2

4. When one of the elements in a compound is a metal that can form different ions, the scheme mentioned in Sec. 10.14 is used. In this scheme the ionic charge of the metal is given by a roman numeral:

Iron(II) chloride $FeCl_2$
Iron(III) chloride $FeCl_3$

The names of molecular compounds that contain hydrogen often follow tradition instead of a definite system. Thus

Methane CH_4
Water H_2O
Ammonia NH_3

10.17 Chemical Equations

The Atoms on Each Side Must Balance

A **chemical equation** is a shorthand way to express the results of a chemical change. In a chemical equation the formulas of the **reactants** (reacting substances) appear on the left-hand side and the formulas of the products appear on the right-hand side. When charcoal (which is almost pure carbon) burns in air, for instance, what is happening is that carbon atoms are reacting with oxygen molecules in the air to form carbon dioxide molecules. The corresponding equation is therefore

$$C \quad + \quad O_2 \quad \rightarrow \quad CO_2$$

$$\underset{\text{atom}}{\text{carbon}} + \underset{\text{molecule}}{\text{oxygen}} \rightarrow \underset{\text{molecule}}{\text{carbon dioxide}}$$

Electrolysis   In order to correctly represent a chemical reaction, a chemical equation must be **balanced:** the number of atoms of each kind must be the same on both sides of the equation. Let us consider the decomposition (breaking down) of water that occurs when an electric current is passed through a water sample (Fig. 10-23). The process is called **electrolysis** and is written in words as

$$\text{Water} \rightarrow \text{hydrogen} + \text{oxygen}$$

Using the formulas for these substances, we might write

$$H_2O \rightarrow H_2 + O_2 \qquad \textit{Unbalanced equation}$$

Here two atoms of oxygen are shown on the right-hand side but only one atom of oxygen on the left. The equation is therefore **unbalanced.** We cannot just write O instead of O_2 on the right because gaseous oxygen has the formula O_2. Nor can we write a subscript "2" after the O in H_2O because H_2O_2 is the formula for hydrogen peroxide, not water.

Balancing an Equation   The first step toward balancing the equation is to show two molecules of H_2O on the left:

$$2H_2O \rightarrow H_2 + O_2 \qquad \textit{Oxygen atoms balanced}$$

Now we have two O atoms on both sides of the equation, which means that these atoms are balanced. However, there are four H atoms on the left but

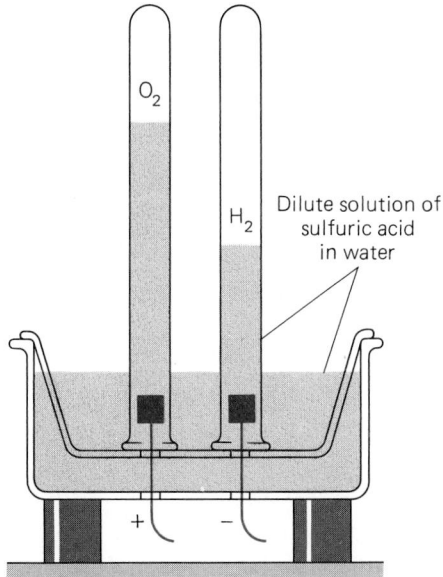

Figure 10-23   Electrolysis of water. An electric current decomposes water into gaseous hydrogen and oxygen. The volume of the hydrogen evolved is twice that of the oxygen, since water contains twice as many hydrogen atoms as oxygen atoms. A trace of sulfuric acid is used to enable the water to conduct electricity.

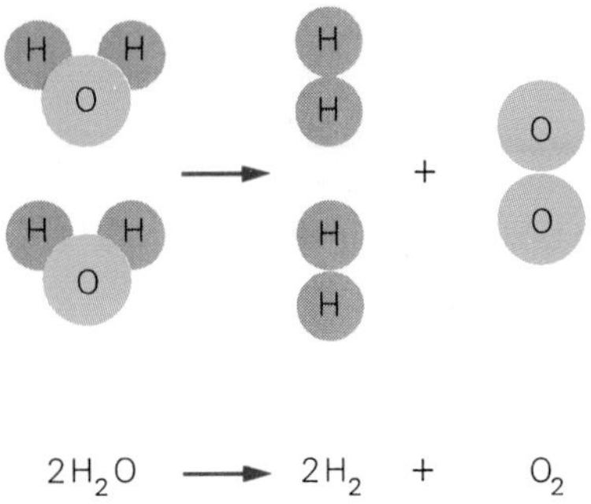

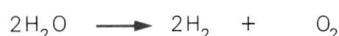

$$2H_2O \longrightarrow 2H_2 + O_2$$

Figure 10-24   Schematic diagram of the electrolysis of water.

only two H atoms on the right. The remedy is to put two H_2 molecules on the right:

$$2H_2O \rightarrow 2H_2 + O_2 \qquad \textit{Balanced equation}$$

2 water molecules → 2 hydrogen molecules + 1 oxygen molecule

Since two O atoms and four H atoms appear on each side, the equation is balanced (Fig. 10-24). [For another example, see Sec. 10.17 at www.mhhe.com/krauskopf.]

An important point is that a number in front of a formula multiplies everything in the formula, whereas a subscript applies only to the symbol before it. Thus $2H_2O$ refers to two complete H_2O molecules, each one of which has two H atoms and one O atom.

It is worth noting that being able to balance the chemical equation for a certain reaction does not necessarily mean that the reaction can occur. And even if a reaction can take place, the balanced equation for the reaction does not tell us the particular conditions (of temperature and pressure, for instance) that might be needed.

Important Terms and Ideas

Elements are the simplest substances present in bulk matter. An element cannot be decomposed or changed into other elements by chemical means. Two or more elements may combine chemically to form a **compound**, a new substance whose properties are different from those of the elements it contains. According to the **law of definite proportions**, the elements that make up a compound are always combined in the same proportions by mass.

Other materials are **mixtures** of elements or compounds or both. The constituents of a mixture keep their characteristic properties. A **solution** is a uniform (or **homogeneous**) mixture.

The ultimate particles of any element are called **atoms.** The ultimate particles of gaseous compounds consist of atoms of the elements they contain joined together in separate **molecules.** Some compounds in the liquid and solid state also consist of molecules, but in many others the atoms are linked in larger arrays. In a given compound, however, the ratios between its various atoms are fixed.

The **periodic law** states that if the elements are listed in order of atomic number, elements with similar chemical and physical properties appear at regular intervals. Such similar elements form **groups.** The halogens, the alkali metals, and the inert gases are examples.

The electrons in an atom that have the same principal quantum number n are said to occupy the same **shell.**

Electrons in a given shell that have the same orbital quantum number l are said to occupy the same **subshell.** Shells and subshells are **closed** when they contain the maximum number of electrons permitted by the exclusion principle. Atoms that contain only closed shells and subshells are extremely stable. The concept of shells and subshells is able to account for the periodic law.

A **metal** atom has one or several electrons outside closed shells or subshells. It combines chemically by losing these electrons to nonmetal atoms. A **nonmetal** atom lacks having closed shells or subshells by one or several electrons. It combines chemically by picking up electrons from metal atoms or by sharing electrons with other nonmetal atoms. **Semimetals,** or **metalloids,** are elements whose properties are intermediate between metals and nonmetals.

In a **covalent bond** between atoms, the atoms share one or more electron pairs. In an **ionic bond,** electrons are transferred from one atom to another and the resulting ions then attract each other. Many bonds in liquids and solids are intermediate between covalent and ionic.

Atom groups, such as SO_4^{2-} (the sulfate group), appear as units in many compounds and remain together during chemical reactions.

A **chemical equation** expresses the result of a chemical change. When the equation is **balanced,** the number of each kind of atom is the same on both sides of the equation.

Multiple Choice

1. A pure substance that cannot be decomposed by chemical means is
   a. an element
   b. a compound
   c. a solid
   d. a solution

2. Elements can be distinguished unambiguously by their
   a. hardnesses
   b. colors
   c. atomic numbers
   d. electrical properties

3. The number of known elements is approximately
   a. 50
   c. 200
   b. 100
   d. 500

4. At room temperature and atmospheric pressure, most elements are
   a. gases
   c. metallic solids
   b. liquids
   d. nonmetallic solids

5. Which of the following substances is a homogeneous mixture?
   a. iron
   c. salt
   b. seawater
   d. paper

6. Which of the following substances is a compound?
   a. iron
   c. salt
   b. seawater
   d. paper

7. The nonmetal whose chemical behavior is most like that of typical metals is
   a. hydrogen
   c. chlorine
   b. helium
   d. carbon

8. Which one or more of the following properties are characteristic of all metals?
   a. Conducts electricity well
   b. Conducts heat well
   c. Is a solid at room temperature
   d. Is transparent to light

9. Iodine is an example of
   a. an inert gas
   c. a halogen
   b. an alkali metal
   d. a compound

10. Which of the following is (are) true for active elements?
    a. They form compounds readily
    b. They form stable compounds
    c. They never occur as gases at room temperature
    d. They liberate more heat when they react than inactive elements do

11. Of the following metals, the most active chemically is
    a. gold
    c. iron
    b. aluminum
    d. sodium

12. Of the following metals, the least active chemically is
    a. gold
    c. iron
    b. aluminum
    d. sodium

13. Of the following nonmetals, the most active chemically is
    a. helium
    c. oxygen
    b. fluorine
    d. sulfur

14. At room temperature, chlorine is
    a. a colorless gas
    b. a greenish-yellow gas
    c. a reddish-brown liquid
    d. a steel-gray solid

15. Of the following nonmetals, the one not a halogen is
    a. fluorine
    c. sulfur
    b. bromine
    d. iodine

16. The place of an element in the periodic table is determined by its
    a. atomic number
    c. density
    b. atomic mass
    d. chemical activity

17. Each vertical column of the periodic table includes elements with chemical characteristics that are, in general,
    a. identical
    b. similar
    c. different
    d. sometimes similar and sometimes different

18. The periodic table of the elements does not
    a. permit us to make accurate guesses of the properties of undiscovered elements
    b. reveal regularities in the occurrence of elements with similar properties
    c. include the inert gases
    d. tell us the arrangement of the atoms in a molecule

19. The elements in group 1 of the periodic table (except for hydrogen) are
    a. all metals
    b. all nonmetals
    c. both metals and nonmetals
    d. neither metals nor nonmetals

20. Of the elements in group 8 of the periodic table, at room temperature and atmospheric pressure
    a. all are gases
    b. all are liquids
    c. some are gases and the others liquids
    d. some are liquids and the others solids

21. In each period of the periodic table, metallic activity
    a. increases to the right
    b. remains constant
    c. decreases to the right
    d. varies with no regular pattern

22. An alkali metal atom
    a. has one electron in its outer shell
    b. has two electrons in its outer shell
    c. has a filled outer shell
    d. lacks one electron of having a filled outer shell

23. A halogen atom
    a. has one electron in its outer shell
    b. has two electrons in its outer shell
    c. has a filled outer shell
    d. lacks one electron of having a filled outer shell

24. An inert gas atom
    a. has one electron in its outer shell
    b. has two electrons in its outer shell
    c. has a filled outer shell
    d. lacks one electron of having a filled outer shell

25. The most important factor in determining the chemical behavior of an atom is its
    a. nuclear structure
    c. atomic mass
    b. electron structure
    d. solubility

26. An atom that loses its outer electron or electrons readily is
    a. an active metal
    b. an active nonmetal
    c. an inactive metal
    d. an inactive nonmetal

27. When they combine chemically with metal atoms, nonmetal atoms tend to
    a. gain electrons to become negative ions
    b. lose electrons to become positive ions
    c. remain electrically neutral
    d. any of these, depending upon the circumstances

28. When a molecule breaks up into its constituent atoms,
    a. energy is absorbed
    b. energy is given off
    c. there is no energy change
    d. any of these choices could be correct, depending on the molecule

29. Relative to the number of electrons in the atoms that join to form a molecule, the number of electrons in the molecule is
    a. smaller
    b. the same
    c. larger
    d. any of the above, depending on the molecule

30. In a covalent molecule,
    a. at least one metal atom is always present
    b. one or more electrons are transferred from one atom to another
    c. adjacent atoms share one or more electrons
    d. adjacent atoms share one or more pairs of electrons

31. An element that can form an ionic compound with chlorine is
    a. carbon   c. sulfur
    b. copper   d. neon

32. Sodium chloride crystals consist of
    a. NaCl molecules
    b. Na and Cl atoms
    c. Na^+ and Cl^- ions
    d. Na^- and Cl^+ ions

33. A compound whose name ends in -ate always contains
    a. hydrogen   c. hydrogen and oxygen
    b. oxygen   d. carbon

34. The number of atoms in a molecule of $Ca_3(PO_4)_2$ is
    a. 8   c. 13
    b. 12   d. 16

35. The number of hydrogen atoms in a molecule of $C_3H_5(OH)_3$ is
    a. 2   c. 8
    b. 6   d. 18

36. Chlorine forms Cl^- ions. The compound $FeCl_3$ is called
    a. iron(I) chloride
    b. iron(III) chloride
    c. iron(I) chlorate
    d. iron(III) chlorate

37. Which one or more of the following equations is (are) balanced?
    a. $PCl_2 + 4H_2O \rightarrow H_3PO_4 + 5HCl$
    b. $6H_2O + 6CO_2 \rightarrow C_6H_{12}O_6 + 6O_2$
    c. $C_7H_{16} + 11O_2 \rightarrow 7CO_2 + 8H_2O$
    d. $Fe_3O_4 + 4H_2 \rightarrow 3Fe + 4H_2O$

38. Which of the following chemical equations is unbalanced?
    a. $2Hg + O_2 \rightarrow 2HgO$
    b. $2H_2S + 3O_2 \rightarrow 2H_2O + 2SO_2$
    c. $Na_2O + H_2O \rightarrow 2NaOH$
    d. $SO_2 + H_2O \rightarrow H_2SO_4$

39. The missing number in the equation
    $(\ )C_4H_{10} + 13O_2 \rightarrow 8CO_2 + 10H_2O$ is
    a. 1   c. 3
    b. 2   d. 4

40. The missing number in the equation
    $2HNO_3 + Ca(OH)_2 \rightarrow Ca(NO_3)_2 + (\ )H_2O$ is
    a. 1   c. 3
    b. 2   d. 4

Exercises

10.1   Chemical Change
10.2   Three Classes of Matter
10.3   The Atomic Theory

1. The conversion of water to ice is considered a physical change, whereas the conversion of iron to rust is considered a chemical change. Why?

2. How can you show that water is a compound rather than a homogeneous mixture of hydrogen and oxygen?

3. Heating is a physical process. When mercuric oxide is heated, it becomes mercury and oxygen. Does this mean that mercuric oxide is a mixture rather than a compound?

4. Which of the following substances are homogeneous and which are heterogeneous? Blood, carbon dioxide gas, solid carbon dioxide, rock, steak, iron, rust, concrete, air, oxygen, salt, milk.

5. Which of the following homogeneous liquids are elements, which are compounds, and which are solutions? Alcohol, mercury, liquid hydrogen, pure water, seawater, beer.

6. How does the law of definite proportions help to distinguish between a compound of certain elements and a mixture of the same elements?

7. What is the most abundant element in the universe? In the human body?

8. What kind(s) of particles make up (a) gaseous compounds, (b) liquid compounds, and (c) solid compounds?

9. The formula for liquid water is H_2O, for solid zinc sulfide ZnS, and for gaseous nitrogen dioxide NO_2. Precisely what information do these formulas convey? What information do they *not* convey?

10. What is the difference in meaning between C_4 and 4C?

10.4 Metals and Nonmetals

11. From what physical and chemical characteristics of iron do we conclude that it is a metal? From what physical and chemical characteristics of sulfur do we conclude that it is a nonmetal?

10.5 Chemical Activity

12. The Bronze Age got its name from the ability of people in that stage of human development to refine tin and copper from their ores; bronze is an alloy (mixture) of tin and copper and is stronger than either of these metals by itself. In the later Iron Age, the still stronger iron could be won from its ores. Nowadays metals such as aluminum and magnesium are refined electrically. Relate this sequence of metallurgical skill to the sequence of metal activity in Table 10-2.

13. Sodium never occurs in nature as the free element, and platinum seldom occurs in combination. How are these observations related to the chemical activities of the two metals?

14. What energy change would you expect when a molecule breaks up into its constituent atoms?

10.6 Families of Elements
10.7 The Perodic Table
10.8 Groups and Periods

15. Are the chemical properties of the elements in a vertical column or in a horizontal row of the periodic table similar to one another?

16. The element astatine (At), which appears at the bottom of the halogen column in the periodic table, has been prepared artificially in minute amounts but has not been found in nature. Using the periodic law and your knowledge of the halogens, predict the properties of this element, as follows:

   a. At room temperature, is it solid, liquid, or gaseous?

   b. How many atoms does a molecule of its vapor contain?

   c. Is it very soluble, moderately soluble, or slightly soluble in water?

   d. What is the formula for its compound with hydrogen?

   e. What are the formulas for its compounds with potassium and calcium?

   f. Is its compound with potassium more or less stable than potassium iodide?

17. The following metals are listed in order of decreasing chemical activity: potassium, sodium, calcium, magnesium. How does this order agree with their positions in the periodic table? Where would you place cesium in the above list?

10.9 Shells and Subshells
10.10 Explaining the Periodic Table

18. A century ago an entirely new group of elements, the inert gases, was discovered. Is it possible that, in the future, another as yet unknown group of the periodic table might be found?

19. (a) What is characteristic about the outer electron shells of the alkali metals? (b) Of the halogens? (c) Of the inert gases?

20. Group 2 of the periodic table contains the family of elements called the **alkaline earths.** How active chemically would you expect an alkaline earth element to be compared with the alkali metal next to it? Why?

21. Why do fluorine and chlorine exhibit similar chemical behavior?

22. Why do lithium and sodium exhibit similar chemical behavior?

23. Electrons are much more readily liberated from metals than from nonmetals when irradiated with visible or ultraviolet light. Can you explain why this is true? From metals of what group would you expect electrons to be liberated most easily?

24. Would you expect magnesium or calcium to be the more active metal? Explain your answer in terms of atomic structure.

25. Why are chlorine atoms more chemically active than chlorine ions?

26. What is the difference in atomic structure between the two isotopes of chlorine? How would you account for the great chemical similarity of the two isotopes?

27. The transition elements in any period have the same or nearly the same outer electron shells and add electrons successively to inner shells. How does this bear upon their chemical similarity?

28. (a) Would you expect N or Br to differ most in its chemical properties from F? (b) B or Si from C? (c) P or O from N?

29. The rare element selenium has the following arrangement of electrons: 2 in the first shell, 8 in the second, 18 in the third, and 6 in the fourth. Would you expect selenium to be a metal or a nonmetal?

30. What is the effective nuclear charge that acts on each electron in the outer shell of the sulfur ($Z = 16$) atom? Would you think that such an electron is relatively easy or relatively hard to detach from the atom?

31. What is the effective nuclear charge that acts on each electron in the outer shell of the calcium ($Z = 20$) atom? Would you think that such an electron is relatively easy or relatively hard to detach from the atom?

32. The energy needed to remove an outer electron from an atom is called the atom's ionization energy. (a) Use Fig. 9-29 to find the ionization energy in eV of lithium (atomic number 3) on

the basis that its two inner electrons completely shield $2e$ of the nuclear charge from the outer electron. (Hint: Begin by establishing the principal quantum number n of the outer electron.) (b) The observed value of this energy is 5.4 eV. If this is not the same as the answer to (a), account for the difference.

33. The ionization energies of the elements of atomic numbers 20 through 29 are very nearly equal. Why should this be so when considerable variations exist in the ionization energies of other consecutive sequences of elements?

34. The ionization energies of Li, Na, K, Rb, and Cs are respectively 5.4, 5.1, 4.3, 4.2, and 3.9 eV. All are in Group 1 of the periodic table. Explain the decrease in ionization energy with increasing atomic number in this group.

35. In each of the following pairs of atoms, which would you expect to be larger in size: Li and F, Li and Na, F and Cl, Na and Si? Why?

10.11   Types of Bond

10.12   Covalent Bonding

10.13   Ionic Bonding

36. Illustrate with electronic diagrams (a) the reaction between a lithium atom and a fluorine atom, and (b) the reaction between a magnesium atom and a sulfur atom. Would you expect lithium fluoride and magnesium sulfide to be ionic or covalent compounds?

37. More energy is needed to remove an electron from a hydrogen molecule than from a hydrogen atom. Why do you think this is so?

38. Which of the following compounds do you expect to be ionic and which covalent? IBr, NO_2, SiF_4, Na_2S, CCl_4, RbCl, Ca_3N_2.

39. Why do the inert gas atoms almost never participate in covalent bonds?

40. Under what circumstances would you expect the shared electron pair to be equal distances on the average from each of the atoms participating in a covalent bond?

10.14   Ionic Compounds

41. What is the charge on alkali metal ions? On halogen ions? On oxygen ions?

42. With the help of Tables 10-8 and 10-9 find the formulas of the following compounds: silicon carbide; lead(II) oxide; manganese(IV) oxide; sodium nitride.

43. With the help of Tables 10-8 and 10-9 find the formulas of the following compounds: barium iodide; ammonium chlorate; tin(II) chromate; lithium phosphate.

10.15   Atom Groups

44. How many atoms of which elements are present in a molecule of $CH_3(CH_2)_2Cl$?

45. How many atoms are present in a molecule of $C_3H_5(OH)_3$? How many of them are hydrogen atoms?

10.16   Naming Compounds

46. Name these compounds: $CaMnO_2$, $CaWO_4$, $Ca_3(AsO_4)_2$.

47. Name these compounds: BaH_2, Li_3PO_4, PbO, $CuBr_2$, KOH.

48. Write the formulas of these compounds: sulfur trioxide; phosphorus pentachloride; dinitrogen tetroxide.

10.17   Chemical Equations

49. Which of the following equations are balanced?

    a. $Zn + H_2SO_4 \rightarrow H_2 + ZnSO_4$

    b. $Al + 3O_2 \rightarrow Al_2O_3$

    c. $H_2CO_3 \rightarrow H_2O + CO_2$

    d. $3CO + Fe_2O_3 \rightarrow 3CO_2 + 2Fe$

50. Which of the following equations are balanced?

    a. $6Na + Fe_2O_3 \rightarrow 2Fe + 3Na_2O$

    b. $MnO + 4HCl \rightarrow MnCl_2 + 2H_2O + Cl_2$

    c. $C_4H_{10} + 9O_2 \rightarrow 4CO_2 + 5H_2O$

    d. $3H_2S + 2HNO_3 \rightarrow 3S + 2NO + 4H_2O$

51. Insert the missing numbers in the following equations:

    a. $Ca + [\ ]H_2O \rightarrow Ca(OH)_2 + H_2$

    b. $2Al + [\ ]H_2SO_4 \rightarrow Al_2(SO_4)_3 + 3H_2$

    c. $C_7H_{16} \rightarrow 11O_2 \rightarrow 7CO_2 + [\ ]H_2O$

    d. $6H_3BO_3 \rightarrow H_4B_6O_{11} + [\ ]H_2O$

52. Insert the missing numbers in the following equations:

    a. $4NH_3 + 3O_2 \rightarrow 2N_2 + [\ ]H_2O$

    b. $4NH_3 + 5O_2 \rightarrow 4NO + [\ ]H_2O$

    c. $4FeS_2 + 11O_2 \rightarrow 2Fe_2O_3 + [\ ]SO_2$

    d. $2HNO_3 + 3H_2S \rightarrow 2NO + [\ ]H_2 + 3S$

53. When nitroglycerin [$C_3H_5(NO_3)_3$] explodes, carbon dioxide, water vapor, nitrogen, and another substance are produced. What is the other substance? Give the equation of the process. (Hint: Start with four nitroglycerin molecules.)

54. When chlorine gas is bubbled through a solution of sodium hydroxide (NaOH), sodium hypochlorite (NaOCl), sodium chloride, and another substance are produced. What is the other substance? Give the equation of the process.

Write balanced equations for the following reactions:

55. Sodium reacts with water to give sodium hydroxide and gaseous hydrogen.

56. Calcium hydride reacts with water to give gaseous hydrogen and calcium hydroxide.

57. Aluminum reacts with gaseous chlorine to give aluminum chloride.

58. Sulfur dioxide and carbon react to give carbon disulfide and carbon monoxide.

59. Ethane (C_2H_6) burns in air—that is, reacts with oxygen—to give carbon dioxide and water.

60. Heating magnesium nitrate gives magnesium oxide, nitrogen dioxide, and oxygen.

61. Butane (C_4H_{10}) burns in air to give carbon dioxide and water.

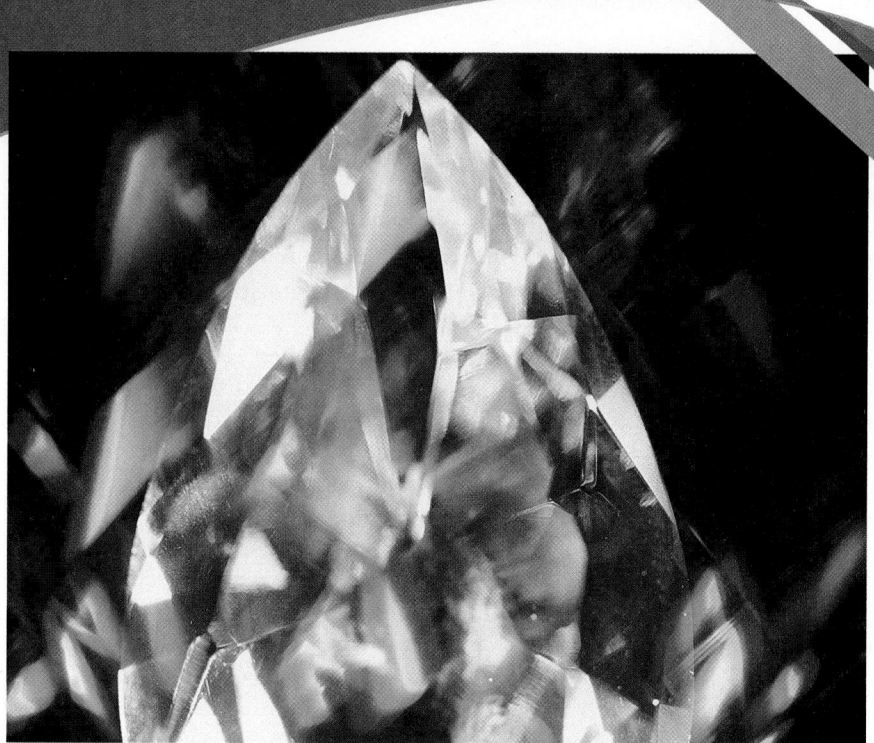

Diamond is one of the crystalline forms of carbon.

Crystals, Ions, and Solutions

GOALS

When you have finished this chapter you should be able to complete the goals
• given for each section below:

Solids

11.1 Ionic and Covalent Crystals
Electron Transfer and Electron Sharing in Solids

11.2 The Metallic Bond
The Electron "Sea" That Bonds Metals Makes Them Good Conductors

11.3 Molecular Crystals
Van der Waals Forces Can Hold Molecules Together
• Distinguish between crystalline and amorphous solids.
• List the four classes of crystalline solids and identify the nature of the bonds in each class.
• Explain the origin of van der Waals forces.

Solutions

11.4 Solubility
Solvent and Solute
• Distinguish between solvent and solute.

• Define the solubility of a substance.
• Describe what is meant by unsaturated, saturated, and supersaturated solutions.
• Discuss how the solubilities of gases and solids in water vary with temperature and, in the case of gases, with pressure.

11.5 Polar and Nonpolar Liquids
Like Dissolves Like
• Compare polar and nonpolar liquids as solvents.

11.6 Ions in Solution
Ions Have Characteristic Properties of Their Own

11.7 Evidence for Dissociation
A Daring Idea a Century Ago
• Give some of the reasons why an ionic crystal is believed to dissociate into ions when it dissolves.
• Explain how dissociation occurs.

11.8 Water
The Most Important Liquid

11.9 Water Pollution
A Menace Hard to Eliminate
• Discuss some of the chief causes of water pollution.

Acids and Bases

11.10 Acids
Hydrogen Ions Give Acidic Solutions Their Characteristic Properties

11.11 Strong and Weak Acids
The More It Dissociates, the Stronger the Acid
• Define acid and distinguish between strong and weak acids.

11.12 Bases
Hydroxide Ions Give Basic Solutions Their Characteristic Properties
• Define base and distinguish between strong and weak bases.

11.13 The pH Scale
Less Than 7 Is Acidic; More Than 7 Is Basic
• Describe the pH scale.

11.14 Salts
An Acid Plus a Base Gives Water and a Salt
• Explain what happens when an acid and a base neutralize each other.
• Describe how to prepare a salt.
• Give some examples of acids, bases, and salts.

Solids

The modern theory of the atom provides deep insights into many properties of matter. Exactly how are atoms held together in a solid? Why do metals conduct electricity but other solids do not? Why do some substances dissolve only in water and others dissolve only in liquids like alcohol or gasoline? In this chapter we shall look into the answers to these questions and others like them.

A solid consists of atoms, ions, or molecules packed closely together and held in place by electric forces. Most solids are **crystalline,** which means that the particles they are made of are arranged in regular, repeated patterns. Every crystal of a given kind, whether large or small, has the same geometric form. The word *crystal* suggests salt and sugar grains, mineral samples, sparkling gemstones. But metals and snowflakes are crystalline, too, as are the fibers of asbestos and the clear, flat plates of mica. Clay is composed of tiny crystals that can trap water between them to give an easily shaped material.

Solids whose particles are irregularly arranged with no definite pattern are called **amorphous** (Greek for "without form"). Examples of amorphous solids are glass, pitch, and various plastics. One way to distinguish between the two kinds of solid is to see what happens when samples of each kind are heated. A crystalline solid melts at a specific temperature when the thermal energy of its particles is enough to break the bonds between them. An amor-

Glass

Glass is a transparent, amorphous solid that consists of silica (silicon dioxide, SiO_2, the chief constituent of most sands) combined with other oxides (Fig. 11-1). Some glasses slowly crystallize with time and crack easily when that happens. Silica alone forms an excellent temperature-resistant glass ("quartz glass") that is transparent to ultraviolet light, unlike other glasses, but is too difficult to make for everyday use. Ordinary glass consists of about 75 percent SiO_2, 15 percent Na_2O, and 10 percent CaO.

Pyrex glass, more resistant to temperature changes, is largely silica and B_2O_3 with small amounts of other oxides. Lead glass, a soft, highly refractive glass used in optical instruments and expensive glassware, is made up of SiO_2, PbO, and K_2O.

Traces of certain metal oxides are responsible for most colored glass. The green glass of cheap bottles contains a little of the iron oxide FeO that was originally present as an impurity in its ingredients. Cobalt oxide gives glass a blue color, manganese oxide a violet color, and uranium oxide a yellow color. Red glass

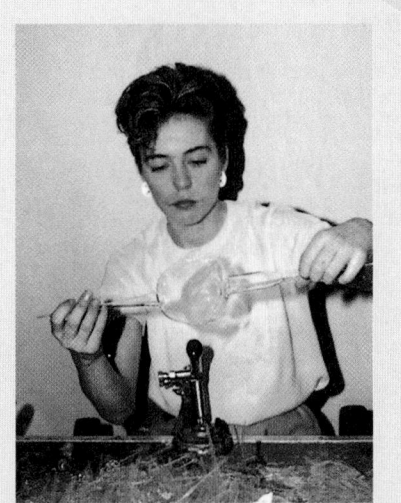

Figure 11-1   Glass is an amorphous solid that softens gradually when heated instead of melting at a specific temperature as crystalline solids do. For this reason hot glass is easily shaped.

gets its hue from tiny particles of gold and copper.

Glass has been made for a long time; the Egyptians used glass containers 5000 years ago. The energy saved by recycling a glass bottle could power a 100-W lightbulb for nearly an hour.

phous solid is really a very stiff liquid and softens gradually when heated because of the random nature of the bonds between its particles.

Crystalline solids fall into four classes, depending on how their particles are bonded together: **ionic, covalent, metallic,** and **molecular.** Let us look into how each type of bond arises.

11.1   Ionic and Covalent Crystals

Electron Transfer and Electron Sharing in Solids

As we know, ionic bonds occur when metal atoms, which tend to lose electrons, interact with nonmetal atoms, which tend to pick up electrons. The result is a stable assembly of positive and negative ions. Ionic bonds are usually fairly strong and result in hard crystals with high melting points.

X-rays are often used to study the structure of a solid. The basic particles—atoms, ions, or molecules—in a solid diffract a beam of x-rays at angles that vary with the wavelength of the x-rays, the spacing of the particles, and their arrangement. From the pattern of diffracted x-rays, the corresponding pattern of particles in the solid can be found (Fig. 11-2).

Figure 11-4 shows the arrangement of Na⁺ and Cl⁻ ions in a sodium chloride crystal. The ions of each kind may be thought of as located at the corners and centers of the faces of a series of cubes, with the Na⁺ and Cl⁻ cubes overlapping. Each ion thus has six nearest neighbors of the other kind.

A different structure is found in cesium chloride crystals, where each ion is located at the center of a cube at whose corners are ions of the other kind (Fig. 11-5). Here each ion has eight nearest neighbors of the other kind. Still other types of structures are found in ionic crystals.

The forces that hold covalent crystals together can be traced to electrons between adjacent atoms. Each atom involved in a covalent bond donates an electron to the bond, and these electrons are shared by both atoms. Few purely covalent crystals are known; some examples are diamond, silicon, germanium, and silicon carbide ("Carborundum"). They are not soluble in water and do not conduct electricity.

As in the case of molecules, it is not always possible to classify a given crystal as being wholly ionic or wholly covalent. Silicon dioxide (quartz) and tungsten carbide, for instance, contain bonds of mixed character.

Diamond and Graphite   Figure 11-6 shows the structure of a diamond crystal. This is the most symmetrical crystal structure possible. In diamond, each carbon atom has four nearest neighbors and shares an electron pair with each of them. Since all the electrons in the outer shells of the carbon atoms participate in the bonding, it is not surprising that diamonds are extremely hard and must be heated to over 3500°C before they melt. (The name comes from the Greek *adamas,* which means "unconquerable.")

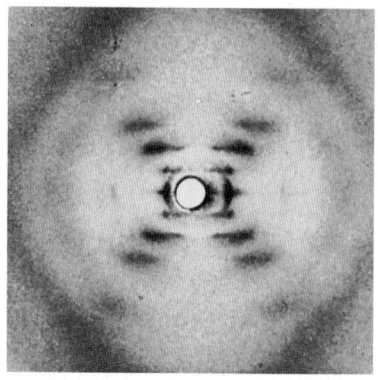

Figure 11-2   An x-ray diffraction photograph of a DNA fiber obtained in 1952 by the English crystallographer Rosalind Franklin (Fig. 11-3). From this photograph and others like it, the helical structure of DNA and its dimensions can be inferred. Franklin's work was essential to Watson and Crick in their analysis of DNA (see Sec. 13.16).

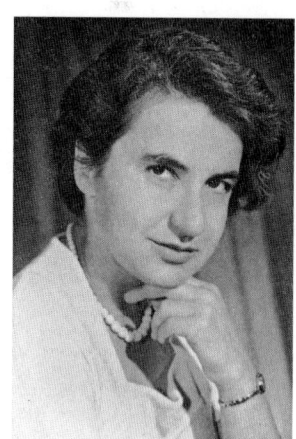

Figure 11-3   Rosalind Franklin (1921–1958).

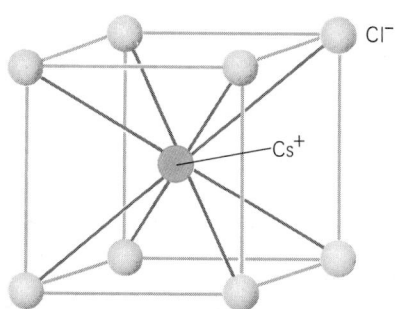

Figure 11-5   The crystal structure of cesium chloride.

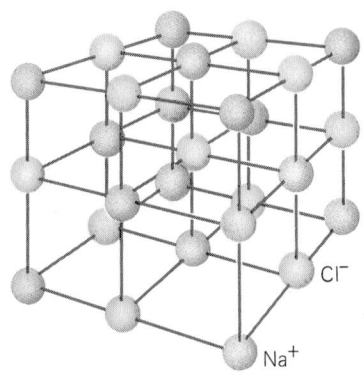

Figure 11-4   The crystal structure of sodium chloride.

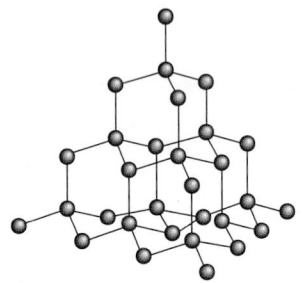

Figure 11-6   The crystal lattice of diamond. The carbon atoms are held together by covalent bonds, which are shared electron pairs.

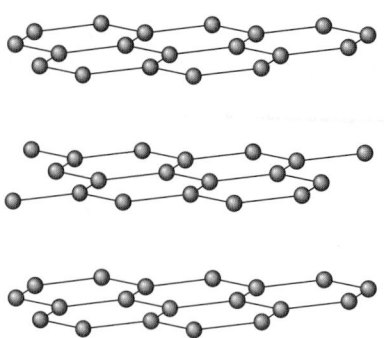

Figure 11-7   Graphite is a form of carbon that consists of layers of carbon atoms in hexagonal arrays. The layers are held together by the weak van der Waals forces described in Sec. 11.3.

Carbon can occur in other forms besides diamond. One is the familiar **graphite,** a soft, black, lustrous solid that is a fair conductor of electricity—all properties very different from those of diamond. Coke, charcoal, and soot are composed mainly of small graphite crystals. Figure 11-7 shows the structure of graphite, which consists of sheets of carbon atoms in hexagonal arrays in which each atom is linked to three others. Weak van der Waals forces (see Sec. 11.3) bond the layers together. The layers can slide past each other readily and are easily flaked apart, which is why graphite is so useful as a lubricant and in pencils, where it is mixed with a clay binder. Graphite does not melt but becomes a gas directly from its solid form when heated above 3000°C.

Under ordinary conditions graphite is more stable than diamond, so crystallizing carbon produces only graphite. Because graphite is less dense than diamond, high pressures favor the formation of diamond. Natural diamond originates deep in the earth where pressures are enormous. To synthesize diamonds, graphite is dissolved in molten cobalt or nickel and the mixture is compressed at 1400°C or more to about 60,000 atmospheres. The diamonds that form are less than 1 mm across and are widely used for grinding and cutting tools; a small number are of gem quality (Fig. 11-8). About 100 tons of synthetic diamonds are produced each year, 10 times the amount of natural diamonds mined.

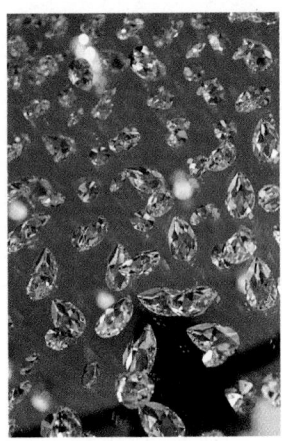

Figure 11-8   Extremely high temperatures and pressures are needed to change graphite, the ordinary form of carbon, into diamond. Only relatively small diamonds, such as these, have been produced artificially.

11.2   The Metallic Bond

The Electron "Sea" That Bonds Metals Makes Them Good Conductors

A metal atom has only one or a few electrons in its outer shell, and these electrons are loosely attached. When metal atoms come together to form a solid, their outer electrons are given up to a common "sea" of electrons that move relatively freely through the assembly of metal ions. This negatively charged electron sea acts to hold together the positively charged metal ions.

The electron-sea picture of the **metallic bond** accounts nicely for the properties of metals. Metals conduct heat and electricity well because the free electrons can move about easily. In nonmetallic solids, all the electrons are bound firmly to particular atoms or pairs of atoms, which is why nonmetals are poor conductors (in other words, good insulators). Free electrons in metals respond readily to electromagnetic waves, which is why metals are opaque to light and have shiny surfaces (Fig. 11-10). Since neighboring atoms in a metal are not linked to each other by specific bonds, most alloys—mixtures of different metals—do not obey the law of definite proportions discussed in Sec. 10.2. The copper and zinc in brass, for instance, need not be present in any exact ratio.

[For a sidebar on metallic hydrogen, see Sec. 11.2 at www.mhhe.com/krauskopf.]

Buckyballs, Nanotubes, and Graphene

A form of carbon other than diamond or graphite was accidentally discovered in 1985 at Rice University in Texas. The commonest version consists of 60 carbon atoms arranged in a cage structure of 12 pentagons and 20 hexagons whose geometry is the same as that of a soccer ball (Fig. 11-9). This extraordinary molecule was called "buckminsterfullerene" in honor of the American architect R. Buckminster Fuller, whose geodesic domes it resembles; the name is usually shortened to **buckyball.**

Buckyballs can be made in the laboratory from graphite, and are present in small quantities in ordinary soot and in a carbon-rich rock found in Russia. The original C_{60} buckyball is not the only form of fullerene known: C_{28}, C_{32}, C_{50}, C_{70} (also present in the Russian rock), C_{76}, C_{78}, and still larger ones have been made.

Fullerene molecules are held together to form solids by weak van der Waals forces (like those that hold together the layers of C atoms in graphite); solid C_{60} is yellowish-brown, and C_{70} is reddish-brown. Since their discovery, the fullerenes and their offshoots have shown some remarkable properties. For instance, solid C_{60} with potassium atoms in the spaces between the buckyballs ("potassium buckide") is a superconductor.

Carbon nanotubes, relatives of buckyballs, consist of tiny cylinders of carbon atoms arranged in hexagons, like rolled-up chicken wire. They were first made over a century

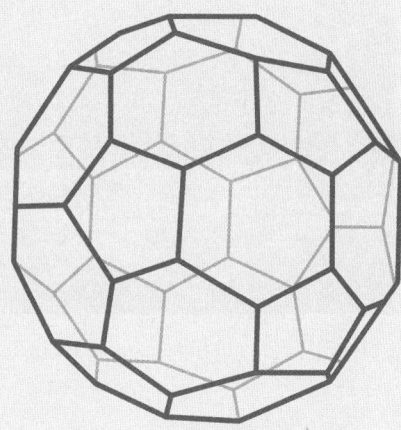

Figure 11-9   In a buckyball, carbon atoms form a closed cagelike structure in which each atom is bonded to three others. Shown here is the C_{60} buckyball that contains 60 carbon atoms. The lines represent carbon-carbon bonds; their pattern of hexagons and pentagons closely resembles the pattern made by the seams of a soccer ball. Other buckyballs have different numbers of carbon atoms.

ago for use as filaments in early lightbulbs, although their structures are a much more recent discovery. Their name comes from nanometer, a billionth of a meter, which is about the diameter of the thinnest nanotubes.

Depending on whether their rows of hexagons are straight or wind around in a helix, carbon nanotubes act either as electrical conductors or as semiconductors and various possible applications in electronics are under active study. Most of today's cars have carbon nanotubes embedded in their nylon

fuel lines to carry away any electronic charge that may build up during fuel flow and cause dangerous sparks.

Carbon nanotubes form exceedingly strong fibers, 50 times stronger than steel wires of the same size although a quarter as dense, that are highly flexible as well. They have a remarkable ability to repair themselves when tears occur in their structures. If carbon nanotubes can be made long enough cheaply, fibers like this would be ideal in composite materials, a big improvement on the glass and graphite fibers currently used to reinforce polyester and epoxy resins in aircraft components, boat hulls, wind turbine blades, and so forth. Virtually crashproof cars? Perhaps.

Nanotubes also have promise for use in water desalination membranes and for storing the hydrogen needed for the fuel cells of future electric cars without the use of heavy steel containers.

Imagine unrolling a nanotube. The result, called **graphene,** is a one-atom-thick sheet of carbon atoms linked by bonds arranged in hexagons, like one layer of the carbon atoms in graphite (Fig. 11-7). (Graphene is not actually made this way.) Graphene is the strongest material known. It can be embedded in a plastic matrix to form stiff, tough composites that could be used in lightweight structures and as protective coatings. Experimental eleronic devices of great promise have been made with graphene.

Example 11.1

(a) The freely-moving electrons in the electron "sea" of a metal come from the outer shells of the metal's atoms. Why is it relatively easy for these electrons to be detached from metal but not from nonmetal atoms? (b) Like those of alkali metals, hydrogen atoms have single outer-shell electrons. Why is hydrogen not a metal?

Solution

(a) Electrons in the inner shells of metal atoms shield the outer electrons from most of the nuclear charge. The outer electrons are therefore not held as securely as the less-shielded outer electrons of nonmetal atoms. (b) A hydrogen atom has only one vacancy in its outer shell and so cannot bond to more than one other H atom. A metal atom has many such vacancies.

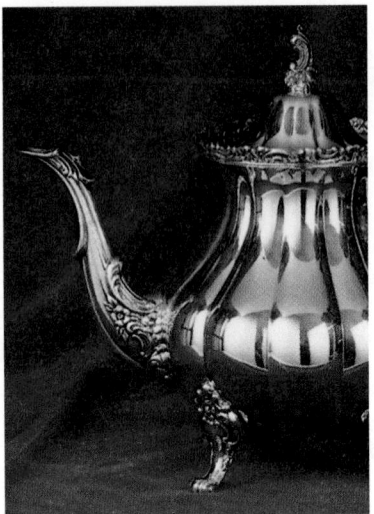

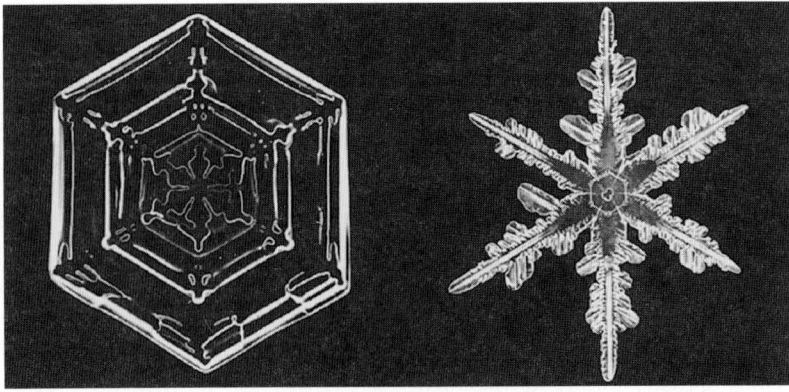

Figure 11-11   The water molecules in a snowflake are held together by van der Waals bonds.

Figure 11-10   The electron "sea" in a metal is responsible for the shiny surfaces of metal objects such as this silver teapot.

11.3   Molecular Crystals

Van der Waals Forces Can Hold Molecules Together

Many molecules are so stable that they have no tendency to join together by transferring or sharing electrons. However, even these stable molecules can form liquids and solids through the action of what are called **van der Waals forces** (Fig. 11-11). These forces are named after the Dutch physicist Johannes van der Waals, who suggested their existence nearly a century ago to account for the small but definite departures of actual gases from the ideal gas law. The explanation of how the forces come into being is more recent, of course, since it is based on the quantum theory of the atom.

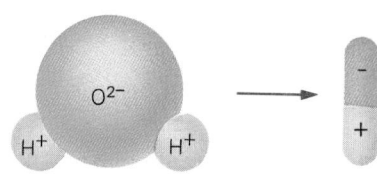

Figure 11-12   The electron distribution in a water molecule is such that the end where the H atoms are attached behaves as if positively charged and the opposite end behaves as if negatively charged. The water molecule is therefore polar.

Polar Molecules   We recall from Sec. 10.12 that molecules held together by polar covalent bonds behave as though they are negatively charged at one end and positively charged at the other end. An example is the H_2O molecule. In this molecule, the tendency for the shared electrons to favor the O atom makes the oxygen end of the molecule more negative than the end where the hydrogen atoms are (Fig. 11-12). Such **polar molecules** line up with the ends that have opposite charges adjacent, as in Fig. 11-13. This is a **polar-polar** interaction.

A polar molecule can also attract nonpolar molecules through a **polar-nonpolar** interaction. Figure 11-14 shows a polar molecule approaching a nonpolar molecule. When the two molecules are close enough, the electric field of the polar molecule causes charges in the nonpolar molecule to separate. The two molecules now have charges of opposite sign facing each other, which produces an attractive force.

The thin plastic sheets that stick so readily to whatever they touch do so because of polar molecules on their surfaces (Fig. 11-15). The polar molecules cause molecules in the other material (the glass of the bowl you cover with cling film, for instance) that were originally nonpolar to become polar, and as a result, the plastic sheet is held firmly in place.

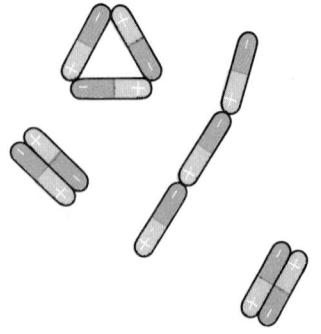

Figure 11-13   Polar molecules attract each other by means of a polar-polar interaction.

Nonpolar-Nonpolar Attraction   More remarkably, two nonpolar molecules can attract each other electrically. The electrons in a **nonpolar molecule** are distributed evenly *on the average*. However, the electrons are in constant motion, and so *at any moment* one part of the molecule has more than the usual number of electrons and the rest of the molecule has less. When two nonpolar molecules happen to get close together, their changing charge distributions tend to shift together, with adjacent ends always having opposite signs (Fig. 11-16). The result of this **nonpolar-nonpolar**

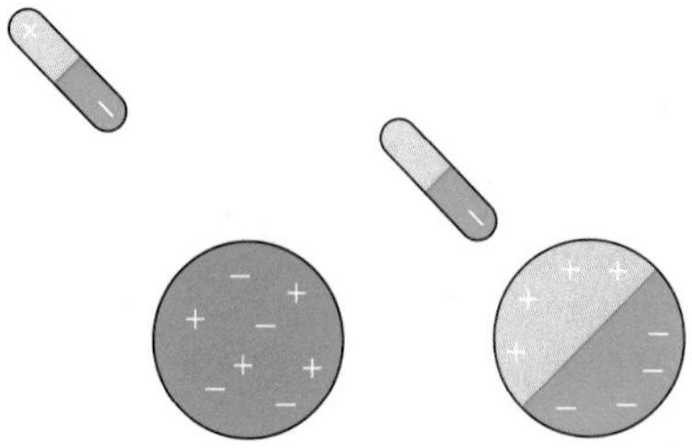

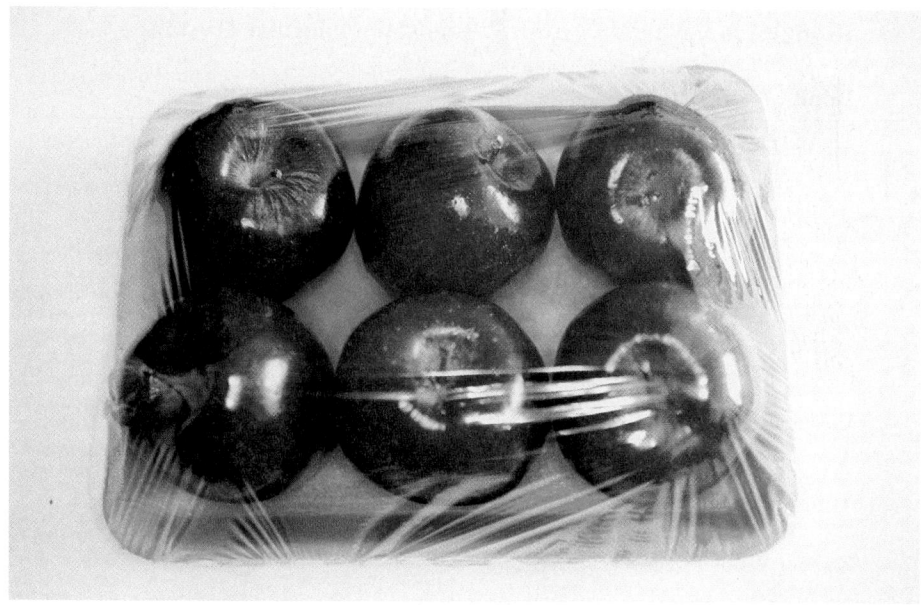

Figure 11-15   Cling film owes its properties to polar molecules on its surface.

Figure 11-14   Polar molecules attract normally nonpolar molecules by means of a polar-nonpolar interaction.

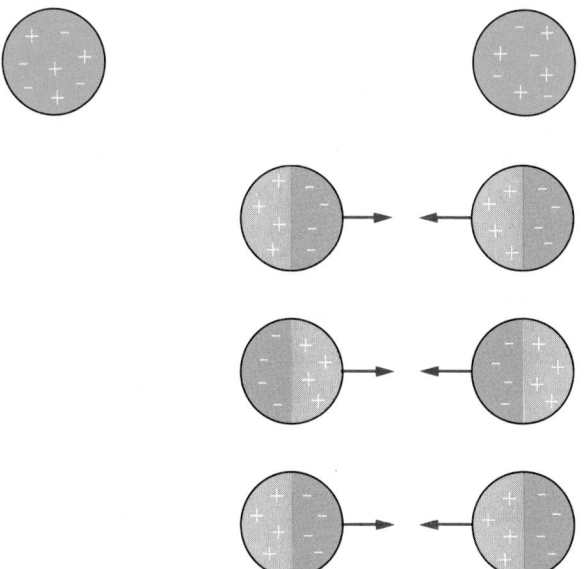

Figure 11-16   Nonpolar molecules normally have, on the average, uniform distributions of charge, but at any one moment the distributions may be uneven. When two nonpolar molecules are close together, the fluctuations in their charge distributions keep in step, which leads to an attractive force between them. This is a nonpolar-nonpolar interaction.

Geckos

Geckos are small lizards famous for their ability to scamper up walls and across ceilings (Fig. 11-17). Insects do this by means of sticky secretions, but geckos use van der Waals forces. The bottom of each of their toes is covered with several hundred thousand tiny hairs, with each hair ending in a number of minute pads. These pads are so small that they come in intimate contact with any surface they touch, which enables the short-range van der Waals forces to act.

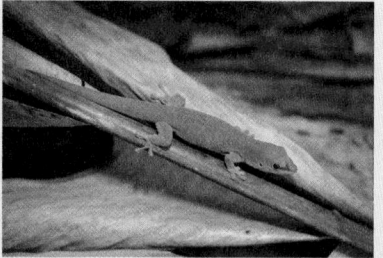

Figure 11-17   A gecko.

The total of 6.5 million hairs on a gecko's feet could altogether support about 130 kg—a gecko could hang from a ceiling suspended from just one toe. This raises the question of how a gecko manages to lift its feet to walk. The answer is that a toe hair can act as a lever to help peel its pads away from a surface; a change in angle of only about 30° is enough to release the grip, and only a few hairs need be detached at a time.

Synthetic gecko hairs have been made with promising results, but there is a long way to go before wearing a pair of the right gloves will enable us to walk across a ceiling.

Table 11-1	**Crystal Types (Bonds Are Strongest in Covalent Crystals, Weakest in Molecular Crystals)**			
Type		**Bond**	**Example**	**Properties**
Covalent	Shared electrons	Shared electrons	Diamond C	Very hard; high melting point
Ionic	Negative ion Positive ion	Electrical attraction	Sodium chloride NaCl	Hard; high melting point
Metallic	Electron sea Metal ion	Electron sea	Copper Cu	Can be deformed; metallic luster; high electrical and thermal conductivity
Molecular	Instantaneous charge separation in molecule	Van der Waals forces	Ice H_2O	Soft; low melting point

interaction is an attractive force. Although individual van der Waals bonds are relatively weak, they can add up to substantial forces in some situations.

Van der Waals forces occur not only between all molecules but also between all atoms, including those of the inert gases that do not otherwise interact. Van der Waals bonds are much weaker than ionic, covalent, and metallic bonds. As a result, molecular crystals generally have low melting and boiling points and little mechanical strength. Ordinary ice and dry ice (solid CO_2) are examples of molecular solids.

Table 11-1 summarizes the characteristics of the four kinds of crystalline solids.

Solutions

A solution is an intimate mixture of two or more substances. Solutions can be formed of any of the three states of matter. Thus air is a solution of several gases, seawater is a solution of various solids and gases in a liquid, and many alloys, such as brass, are "solid solutions" of two or more metals. Here our concern will be with solutions in liquids.

11.4 Solubility

Solvent and Solute

In a solution that contains two substances, the substance present in the larger amount is called the **solvent** and the other substance is called the **solute.** When solids or gases dissolve in liquids, the liquid is always considered the solvent. When sugar is stirred into water, the sugar is the solute and the water is the solvent. Water is by far the most common and most effective of all solvents.

Concentration   The **concentration** of a solution is the amount of solute in a given amount of solvent. Solutions, like compounds, are homogeneous, but

Ice

The molecular solid ice deserves an additional word. The crystal structure of ice is very open (Fig. 11-18) because an H_2O molecule can form bonds with only four other H_2O molecules. In other solids, each atom or molecule may have as many as 12 neighbors, which gives crystals that are much more compact than ice crystals.

The molecules in liquid water are closer together on the average than those in ice. Water therefore expands when it freezes, which is why water pipes may burst on a cold winter's day. The expansion also means that a given volume of ice weighs less than the same volume of water, which is why ice cubes float in a glass of water (Fig. 11-19).

Since ice floats, a body of water outdoors freezes from the top down. Ice is a fair insulator of heat, and so a layer of it on the surface of a body of water helps prevent further freezing. As a result, many lakes, rivers, and arms of the sea do not freeze solid in winter, which allows their plant and animal life to survive until the following spring.

When seawater freezes, its salt content is not incorporated in the ice crystals that form but ends up as brine (concentrated salt solution) in tiny pockets and channels around the crystals. As time goes on, the brine gradually drains away into the seawater below the ice. After a few months the upper layers of sea ice contain very little brine, and when melted, yield water that is fresh enough to drink. This was known by nineteenth century whalers and explorers, who replenished their water supplies in the Arctic by melting sea ice.

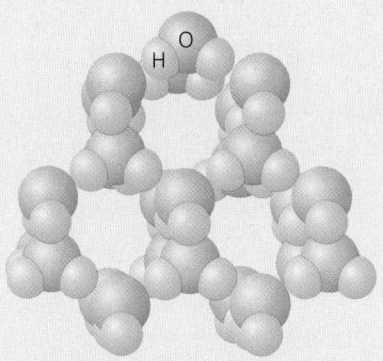

Figure 11-18 Top view of an ice crystal, showing the open hexagonal arrangement of the H_2O molecules. The molecules in liquid water are randomly arranged; hence water is denser and ice floats.

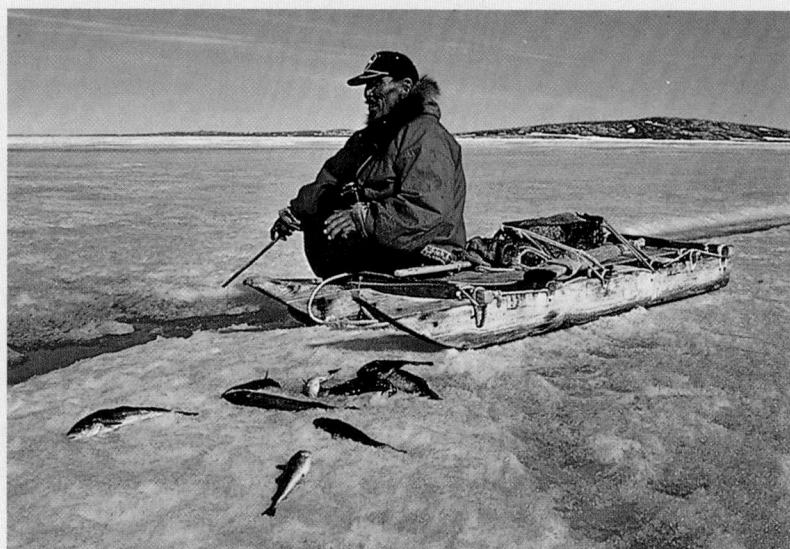

Figure 11-19 Fishing through floating ice in the Arctic.

unlike compounds, solutions do not have fixed compositions. To a sodium chloride solution whose concentration is 10 g of NaCl in 100 g of water, for example, we can add somewhat more NaCl or as much more water as we like. The concentration of the solution is altered, but it remains uniform.

Some pairs of liquids form solutions in all proportions. Any amount of alcohol may be mixed with any amount of water to form a homogeneous liquid, for instance. In general, however, a given liquid will dissolve only a limited amount of another substance. Sodium chloride can be stirred into water at 20°C until the solution contains 36 g of the salt for every 100 g of water. More salt will not dissolve, no matter how much we stir (Fig. 11-20). This figure, 36 g per 100 g of water, is called the **solubility** of NaCl in water at 20°C:

> The solubility of a substance is the maximum amount that can be dissolved in a given quantity of a particular solvent at a given temperature and pressure.

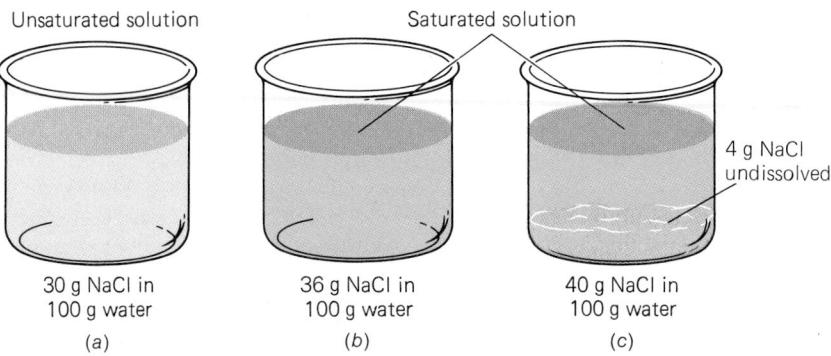

Unsaturated solution

Saturated solution

4 g NaCl
undissolved

30 g NaCl in
100 g water

(a)

36 g NaCl in
100 g water

(b)

40 g NaCl in
100 g water

(c)

Figure 11-20   The solubility of NaCl is 36 g per 100 g of water at 20°C. (*a*) 30 g of NaCl in 100 g of water produces an unsaturated solution. (*b*) 36 g of NaCl is the maximum amount that can dissolve, and it produces a saturated solution. (*c*) If 40 g of NaCl is added to 100 g of water, 4 g will remain undissolved.

Saturated Solutions   A solution that contains the maximum amount of solute possible is said to be **saturated.** The solubilities of most solids increase with increasing temperature (Fig. 11-21). We all know that hot water is a better solvent than cold water; for example, hot tea can dissolve about twice as much sugar as iced tea. When a solution that is saturated at a high temperature is allowed to cool, some of the solute usually crystallizes out (Fig. 11-22).

Sometimes, if the cooling of a saturated solution is allowed to take place slowly and without disturbance, a solute may remain in solution even though its solubility is exceeded. The result is a **supersaturated** solution. Supersaturated solutions are often unstable, with the solute crystallizing out suddenly when the solution is jarred or otherwise disturbed.

In contrast to the case of solids, the solubilities of gases in liquids *decrease* with increasing temperature. We all know that warming a glass of soda water, which is a solution of carbon dioxide gas in water, causes some of the gas to escape as bubbles. The solubility of a gas in a liquid depends on the pressure as well, increasing with increasing pressure. Soda water is bottled under high pressure (over twice that of the atmosphere), and when a bottle of it is opened, the drop in pressure causes some of the gas to leave the solution and form bubbles (Fig. 11-23).

Boiling and Freezing Points   The boiling point of a solution is usually higher than that of the pure solvent, and its freezing point is lower. Thus

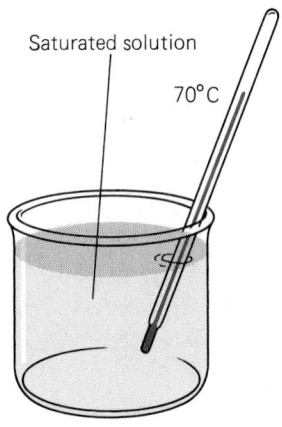

Saturated solution

70°C

136 g KNO₃ dissolved in
100 g water

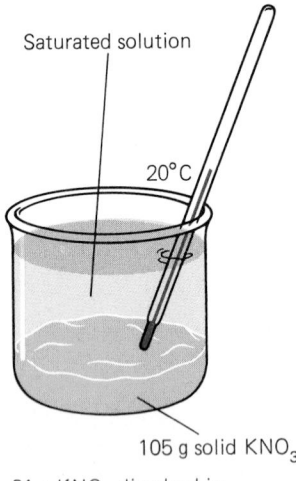

Saturated solution

20°C

105 g solid KNO₃

31 g KNO₃ dissolved in
100 g water

Figure 11-22   The solubility of potassium nitrate, KNO_3, is 136 g per 100 g of water at 70°C and 31 g at 20°C. Cooling a saturated solution of KNO_3 from 70°C to 20°C causes 136 g − 31 g = 105 g of the salt per 100 g of water to crystallize out.

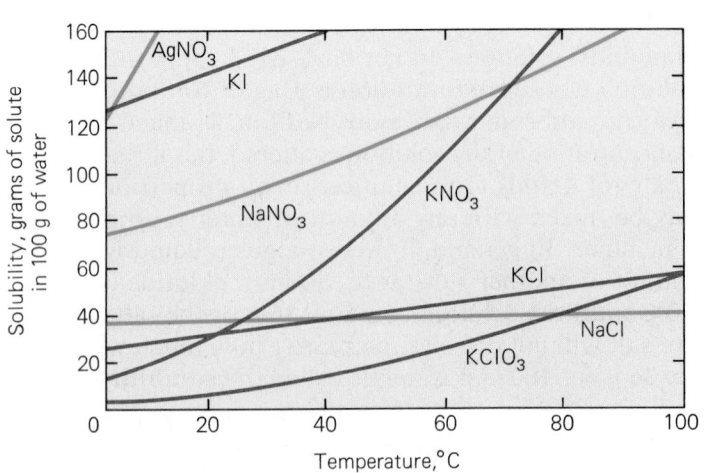

Figure 11-21   How the solubilities of various compounds in water vary with temperature. The higher the temperature, the greater the solubility.

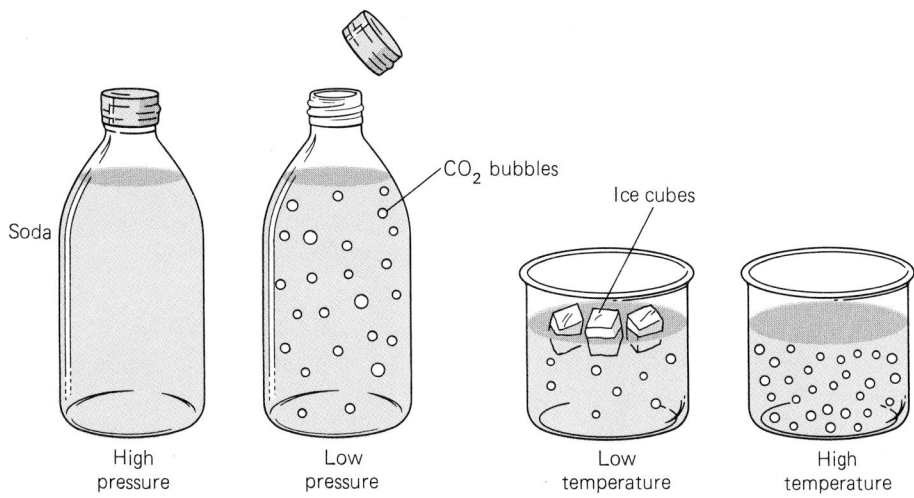

Figure 11-23   The higher the pressure and the lower the temperature, the greater the solubility of a gas in water.

seawater, which contains about 3.5 percent of various salts (chiefly NaCl), boils at 100.3°C and freezes at −1.2°C. The more concentrated the solution, the greater the changes in boiling and freezing points. Ethylene glycol, $C_2H_4(OH)_2$, is often added to the water in the cooling system of a car to prevent the water from freezing in cold weather. A solution of 83 g of ethylene glycol per 100 g of water will not freeze until −25°C.

11.5   Polar And Nonpolar Liquids

Like Dissolves Like

Some liquids are better solvents for some substances than for others. Water readily dissolves salt and sugar but not fats or oil. Gasoline, on the other hand, dissolves fats and oils but not salt or sugar.

The explanation for this behavior depends upon the electrical characters of the solvent and solute. Water is a **polar liquid** since its molecules behave as if negatively charged at one end and positively charged at the other (Fig. 11-12). Gasoline is a **nonpolar liquid** since the charges in its molecules are evenly distributed. Let us see what difference this makes.

The Bends

As a diver goes down to greater and greater depths, the pressure of the air being breathed increases as the water pressure increases. Because of the higher pressure, more oxygen and nitrogen are dissolved in the blood and tissues of the diver than usual. The extra oxygen is mostly used up in the normal metabolism of the diver's body, but the inert nitrogen can build up to a high concentration.

If the diver returns to the surface slowly, the added nitrogen comes out of solution gradually and is simply breathed out. However, if the diver ascends rapidly, nitrogen bubbles form in his or her body. Nitrogen bubbles in the joints cause great pain—"the bends." More dangerous are bubbles in the blood, which can block arteries and lead to nervous system damage and even death. Apparently sperm whales also suffer from the bends from time to time when they ascend too rapidly, and this may be true for other whales as well.

The only remedy for the bends is to put the diver into a decompression chamber at a high enough pressure to redissolve the nitrogen and then to gradually reduce the pressure. Among the first things student divers are taught is the proper way to ascend after a deep dive. Professional divers often use a mixture of helium and oxygen instead of air because helium is less soluble than nitrogen and so less likely to cause trouble.

Divers evidently have to be careful people. As the saying goes, "There are old divers and bold divers, but there are no old bold divers."

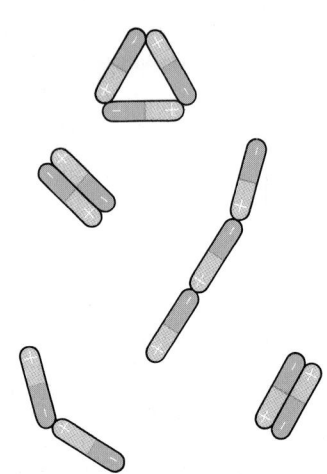

Figure 11-24 Water molecules cluster together because of electric forces that arise from their polar character.

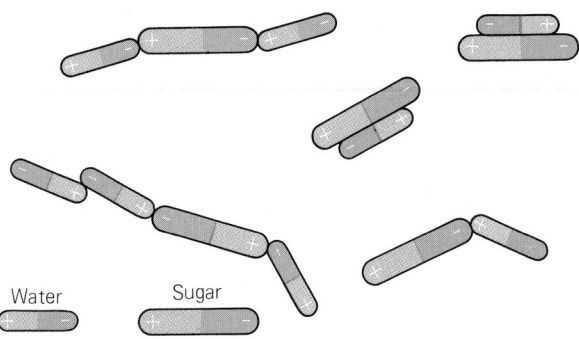

Figure 11-25 Sugar dissolved in water. Polar compounds readily dissolve in water because their molecules can link up with water molecules.

Water and other polar liquids consist of groups of molecules rather than single, freely moving molecules. The molecules join together in clumps, positive charges near negative charges, as in Fig. 11-24. Water molecules can join together in a similar way with polar molecules of other substances, such as sugar (Fig. 11-25), so water dissolves these substances with ease.

Molecules of fats and oils are nonpolar and so do not interact with water molecules. If oil is shaken with water, the strong attraction of water molecules for one another squeezes out the nonpolar oil molecules from between them and the oil and water separate into layers. Oil or fat molecules mix readily, however, with the similarly nonpolar molecules of gasoline (Fig. 11-26).

A covalent substance, then, dissolves only in liquids whose molecules have similar electrical structures. In general, "like dissolves like."

Soaps and Detergents Some dirt is water soluble, but much is greasy and thus nonpolar, so plain water will not wash it away. Soap molecules are negatively charged at one end and nonpolar at the other, and in water they clump together to form clusters called **micelles** with the nonpolar ends of the molecules inside (Fig. 11-27). Nonpolar dirt particles are absorbed inside micelles, which, unlike the particles themselves, move freely through water because their outsides are polar. In this manner dirt on skin, clothing, and other surfaces is loosened by soapy water and can then be rinsed away.

Soap is not effective in "hard" water (see Sec. 11.8) because the minerals dissolved in it interfere with micelle formation. Synthetic **detergents** act in the same way as soaps even in hard water.

Dissociation Ionic compounds consist of positive and negative ions and therefore dissolve only in highly polar liquids. Figure 11-28 shows how

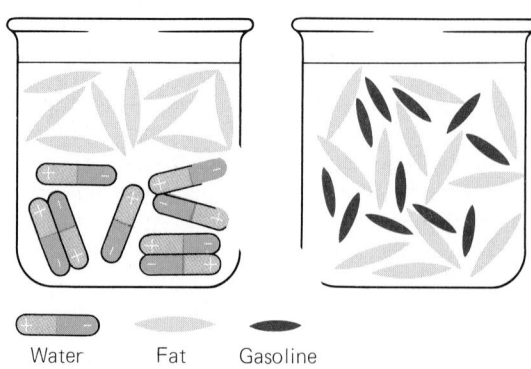

Figure 11-26 Gasoline dissolves fat; water does not. Nonpolar compounds dissolve only in nonpolar liquids.

Microwave Ovens

In a **microwave oven,** the alternating electric fields of the microwaves cause water molecules (and any other polar molecules present) in the food to flip back and forth several billion times a second as they try to become aligned with the changing directions of the fields. As the molecules turn, they collide with other molecules present, which increases the average kinetic energy of all the food molecules and thereby the temperature of the food. Microwave cooking is faster because the microwaves penetrate the food and generate heat in its interior instead of having heat added through its surface as in ordinary cooking. (Microwaves cannot escape through an oven window because a fine-mesh metal screen is embedded in the glass that reflects microwaves back inside.)

NaCl dissolves in water. At the surface of a salt crystal, water molecules are attracted to the ions, positive ends toward negative ions and negative ends toward positive ions. The pull of several water molecules is enough to overcome the electric forces that hold an ion to the crystal. The ion then moves off into the solution with its cluster of water molecules. As each layer of ions is removed, the next is attacked, until either the salt is completely dissolved or the solution becomes saturated. The separation of a compound into ions when it dissolves is called **dissociation.**

The ions released when an ionic compound dissolves are the same as those in its crystal structure. This is true not only for such simple compounds as NaCl, which dissociates into Na^+ and Cl^- ions, but also for more complex compounds that involve atom groups. An example is potassium nitrate, KNO_3, which dissociates into K^+ and NO_3^- ions.

Electrolytes   Substances that separate into ions when dissolved in water are called **electrolytes.** Electrolytes include all ionic compounds soluble in water and some covalent compounds containing hydrogen (for example, hydrochloric acid, HCl) that form ions by reaction with water. Soluble covalent compounds, such as sugar and alcohol, that do not dissociate in solution are **nonelectrolytes.**

Electrolytes can be recognized by the ability of their solutions to conduct electric current. Hence their name. Conduction is possible because the ions are free to move, with positive ions migrating through the solution toward the negative terminal, negative ions migrating toward the positive terminal (Fig. 11-29). The electric currents in nerves are carried by ions.

11.6   Ions in Solution

Ions Have Characteristic Properties of Their Own

One of the early objections to the theory of ionic solutions was that sodium chloride was supposed to break down into separate particles of sodium and chlorine, yet the solution remains colorless. Why, if chlorine is present as free

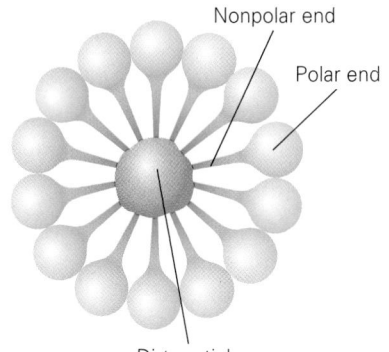

Figure 11-27   Soap and detergent molecules are polar at one end and nonpolar at the other. In water they form spherical cages, called micelles, of several dozen molecules with the nonpolar ends of the molecules on the inside. Micelles trap nonpolar dirt particles as shown. Because the outside of a micelle is polar, it moves freely in water, whereas the dirt particle inside cannot. Micelles that have picked up dirt from a surface can then be rinsed away, taking the dirt with them.

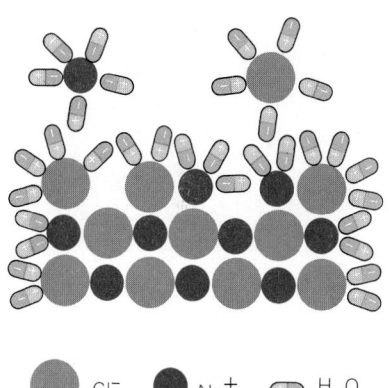

Figure 11-28   Solution of sodium chloride crystal in water. Water molecules exert electric forces on the Na^+ and Cl^- ions that are strong enough to remove them from the crystal lattice.

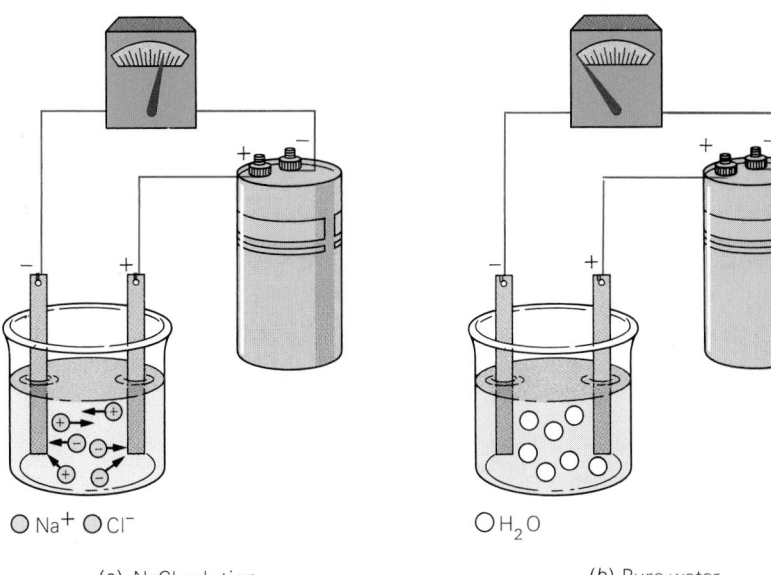

(a) NaCl solution   (b) Pure water

Figure 11-29   (a) An electrolyte such as NaCl in solution conducts electric current through the motion of its ions. (b) Pure water is a nonelectrolyte, as are solutions of compounds that do not dissociate.

Breath Analyzer

The difference in color between the chromic ion (Cr^{3+}), which is green, and the dichromate ($Cr_2O_7^{2-}$) ion, which is yellow-orange, is used by police to determine the level of ethanol—ethyl alcohol—in the breath of a person suspected of drunken driving (Fig. 11-31). A sample of the breath is mixed with a solution of potassium dichromate in sulfuric acid, and any ethanol present reacts with the solution to give chromic ions. The amount of ethanol can be found from the extent of the color change, which is measured in a device called a breath analyzer. Because ethanol in the bloodstream passes into air in the lungs, the proportion of ethanol vapor in a breath sample indicates the percentage of ethanol in the person's blood.

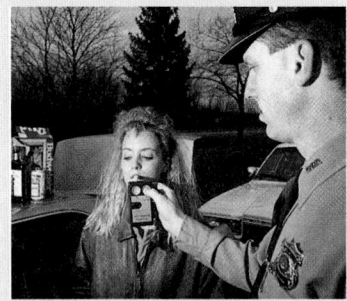

Figure 11-31 This device uses the color difference between chromic and dichromate ions to measure the alcohol concentration in a person's breath.

ions, should we not find the greenish-yellow color of chlorine in the solution? The answer is that chloride ion Cl^- has altogether different properties from gaseous chlorine—a different color, a different taste, different chemical reactions.

We must regard a solution of sodium chloride not as a solution of NaCl or of Na and Cl atoms but as a solution of the two ions Na^+ and Cl^-. Each of these ions in solution has its own set of properties, properties quite different from those of NaCl crystals or of the active metal Na and the poisonous gas Cl_2. Each ion in an electrolytic solution is a new and separate substance.

Properties of an Ion   The "properties of an ion" are really the properties of solutions in which the ion occurs. A solution of a single kind of ion, all by itself, cannot be prepared; positive ions and negative ions must always be present together, so that the total number of charges of each sign will be the same. But each ion gives its own characteristic properties to all solutions containing it, and these properties can be recognized whenever they are not masked by other ions.

Let us look at some examples. A property of the copper ion Cu^{2+} is its blue color, and all solutions of this ion are blue (unless some other ion that has a stronger color is present). A characteristic of the hydrogen ion H^+ is its sour taste, and all solutions containing this ion (namely acids) are sour. The silver ion Ag^+ forms an insoluble white precipitate of AgCl when mixed with solutions of the chloride ion Cl^-. (As we recall from Chap. 10, a precipitate is an insoluble solid that results from a chemical reaction.) Any solution of an electrolyte that contains silver will give this precipitate when mixed with a solution of any chloride (Fig. 11-30).

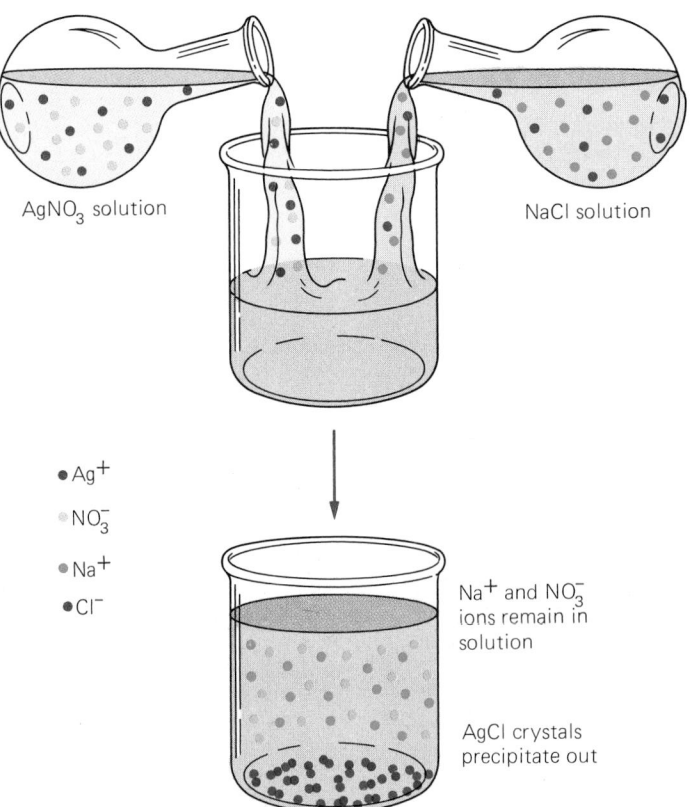

Figure 11-30   When silver nitrate (AgNO₃) and sodium chloride (NaCl) are dissolved in water, a precipitate of the insoluble compound silver chloride is produced. The sodium and nitrate ions remain in solution.

Table 11-2	The Properties of Molecular Chlorine and Chloride Ion in Solution

Cl_2	Cl^-
Greenish-yellow color	Colorless
Strong, irritating taste and odor	Mild, pleasant taste
Combines with all metals	Does not react with metals
Combines readily with hydrogen	Does not react with hydrogen
Does not react with Ag^+	Forms AgCl with Ag^+

To emphasize the differences between the properties of an ion and those of the corresponding neutral substance, Table 11-2 compares the chloride ion, Cl^-, and molecular chlorine, Cl_2. In general, Cl_2 is much more active chemically. This is to be expected, since Cl atoms have only seven outer electrons whereas Cl^- ions have closed outer shells with eight electrons.

For any ion we can list the properties common to all its solutions. In general, the properties of a solution of an electrolyte are the sum of the properties of the ions that the solution contains. The properties of a sodium chloride solution are the properties of Na^+ plus those of Cl^-; the properties of a copper sulfate solution are the properties of Cu^{2+} plus those of SO_4^{2-}. Instead of learning the individual properties of hundreds of different electrolytes, we need only learn the properties of a few ions to be able to predict the behavior of any electrolytic solution that contains them.

11.7 Evidence for Dissociation

A Daring Idea a Century Ago

The hypothesis that many substances exist as ions in solution was proposed in 1887 by a young Swedish chemist, Svante Arrhenius. Today the idea of ions in solution follows naturally from our knowledge of the electrical structure of matter. We know that some compounds are formed by the shift of electrons from one kind of atom to another, so that some of the atoms become positive ions and the others negative ions. It is not hard for us to imagine that a polar liquid like water can separate these ions from a crystal. But in 1887 the modern picture of the atom was not even a dream. Without this knowledge Arrhenius's fellow chemists were hard to convince that neutral substances can break up into electrically charged fragments in solution.

Until the work of Arrhenius, Faraday's explanation for the ability of certain solutions to conduct electricity was generally accepted. Faraday held that the passage of a current caused the substance in solution to break up into ions. Arrhenius instead felt that ions are set free whenever an electrolyte dissolves, and he gave a number of reasons to support this notion.

Reaction Speed One of the points Arrhenius made was that reactions between electrolytes take place almost instantaneously in solution, but occur very slowly or not at all if the electrolytes are dry. An example is the reaction between the silver nitrate and sodium chloride solutions shown in Fig. 11-30, which is very rapid. The speed with which the insoluble AgCl is formed suggests that its silver and chlorine components are already free in the original solutions and so are ready to combine at once. However, if dry $AgNO_3$ is mixed with dry NaCl, nothing happens because the components of each salt are held firmly in their respective crystals.

Freezing and Boiling Points Another piece of evidence cited by Arrhenius was the unexpectedly low freezing points of electrolyte solutions. The

| Svante Arrhenius (1859–1927)

Born near Uppsala, Sweden, Arrhenius attended the university there. As a graduate student, he developed his theory that electrolytes dissociate into ions in solution and presented this as part of his Ph.D. thesis in 1884. His examiners found the ideas difficult to swallow—not only was atomic structure then unknown, but the electron itself was unknown as well—and gave him the lowest passing grade.

In the years that followed a few other chemists agreed with Arrhenius, but most, Mendeleev among them, did not. Once the electron had been discovered (by the English physicist J. J. Thomson in 1897), though, it became clear that atoms were not indivisible particles,

and in 1903 Arrhenius received the Nobel Prize in chemistry.

Arrhenius did other notable work, for instance, in proposing the concept of activation energy in chemical reactions (see Sec. 12.7). The connection between the greenhouse effect and climate was another of his contributions. He pointed out that carbon dioxide in the atmosphere absorbs infrared radiation emitted by the sunwarmed earth, just as the windows of a greenhouse absorb the infrared emitted by its interior. As a result, said Arrhenius, changes in the CO_2 content of the atmosphere would be followed by changes in its temperature and so might be responsible for such variations in climate as the ice ages.

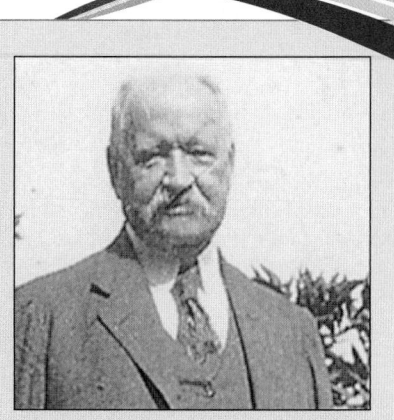

Arrhenius recognized that industrialization would lead to an increase in atmospheric CO_2 but, not foreseeing its eventual extent, thought the result would be beneficial rather than the potential catastrophe it has turned out to be.

amount by which the freezing point of a solution is reduced (or its boiling point increased) depends upon the concentration of solute particles present, not upon their nature. Equal numbers of sugar and of alcohol molecules dissolved in the same amount of water lower its freezing point by almost exactly the same amount. But the same number of NaCl units lowers the freezing point nearly *twice as much*. This suggests that there are no NaCl molecules as such and that solid NaCl breaks up into Na^+ and Cl^- ions when it dissolves. Similarly calcium chloride, $CaCl_2$, lowers the freezing point of water by nearly three times as much as sugar or alcohol, because each $CaCl_2$ unit dissociates in solution into three particles, one Ca^{2+} ion and two Cl^- ions.

11.8   Water

The Most Important Liquid

Although a minor constituent of the earth as a whole, water covers three-quarters of its surface. Most of the earth's water was once part of the rock of its interior and was freed as a result of geological processes. As evidence, water is present in meteorites, which are leftovers from the youth of the solar system, and water vapor is common in the gases that present-day volcanoes emit (see Chap. 15). Some water has also been brought to the earth's surface by comets, whose impacts were frequent in the earth's early history. Life may have begun in or near the early oceans, and water is essential to all living things.

Seawater has a salt content (or **salinity**) that averages 3.5 percent. The composition of seawater is shown in Fig. 11-32. The ions Na^+ and Cl^- account for over 85 percent of the total salinity. Figure 11-33 shows where the ions found in seawater come from.

Waste Not, Want Not   Only 3 percent of the world's water is fresh, and of that 3 percent, two-thirds is trapped as ice in the Arctic and Antarctic. Half of the rest is already being employed for various human purposes: roughly

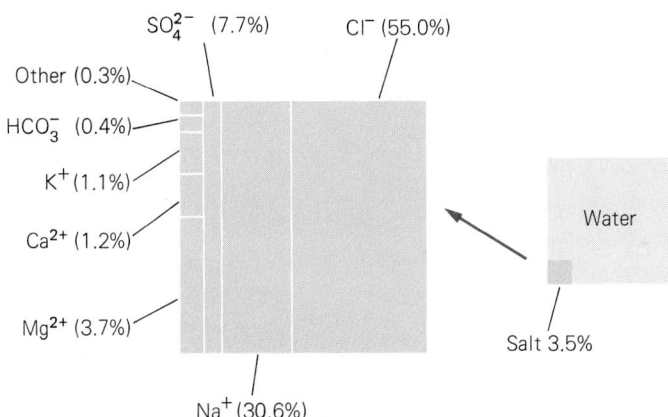

Figure 11-32 The composition of seawater. In the open ocean the total salt content varies about an average of 3.5 percent, but the relative proportions of the various ions are quite constant. (Percentages given are by mass.)

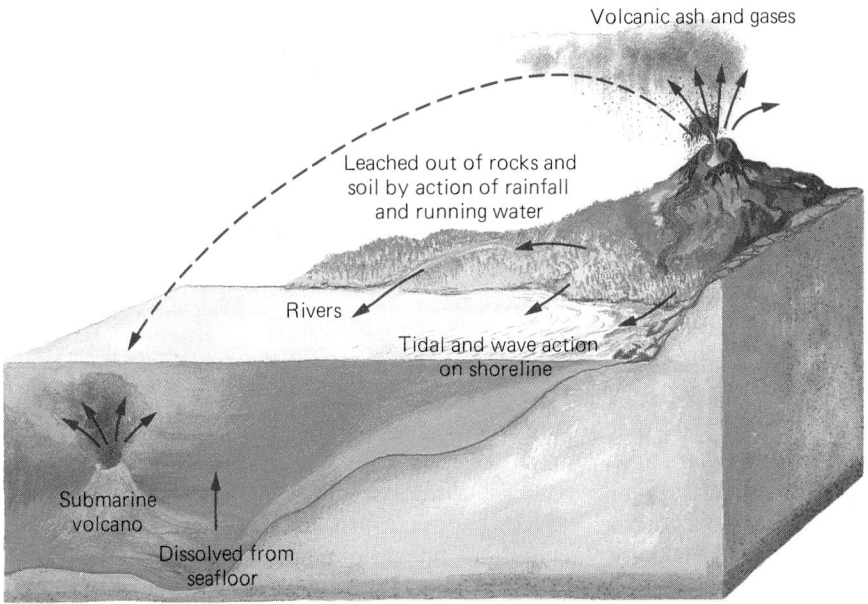

Figure 11-33 Origins of seawater salts.

70 percent by farms and ranches (about 1000 liters of water per kilogram of wheat, up to 15,000 liters/kg of beef); 20 percent by industry; and 10 percent for drinking, washing, and other domestic uses. In North America, water consumption for all uses averages about 4500 liters per day per person, twice the world average. Biofuel production gulps water: over 9000 liters per liter of biodiesel (34 tons/gallon!), for instance. World water demand is increasing even faster than population (Fig. 11-34).

Some aquifers (underground water sources; see Sec. 15.13) store ancient water deposits that are not renewable and are being steadily emptied. The water in many other aquifers is being pumped out faster than rainfall can replenish it. As a result of all these factors, readily available freshwater is well on the way to becoming a scarce commodity: over a billion people today lack reliable access to safe drinking water, and a United Nations estimate has water shortages affecting two-thirds of the world's people by 2025. China is already in a serious situation with 20 percent of the world's population but only 7 percent of the world's water resources (and most of them in its south, whereas demand is mainly in its north).

Although freshwater can be made by desalinating seawater, the process is costly in both money and energy and is practical only in a limited number of

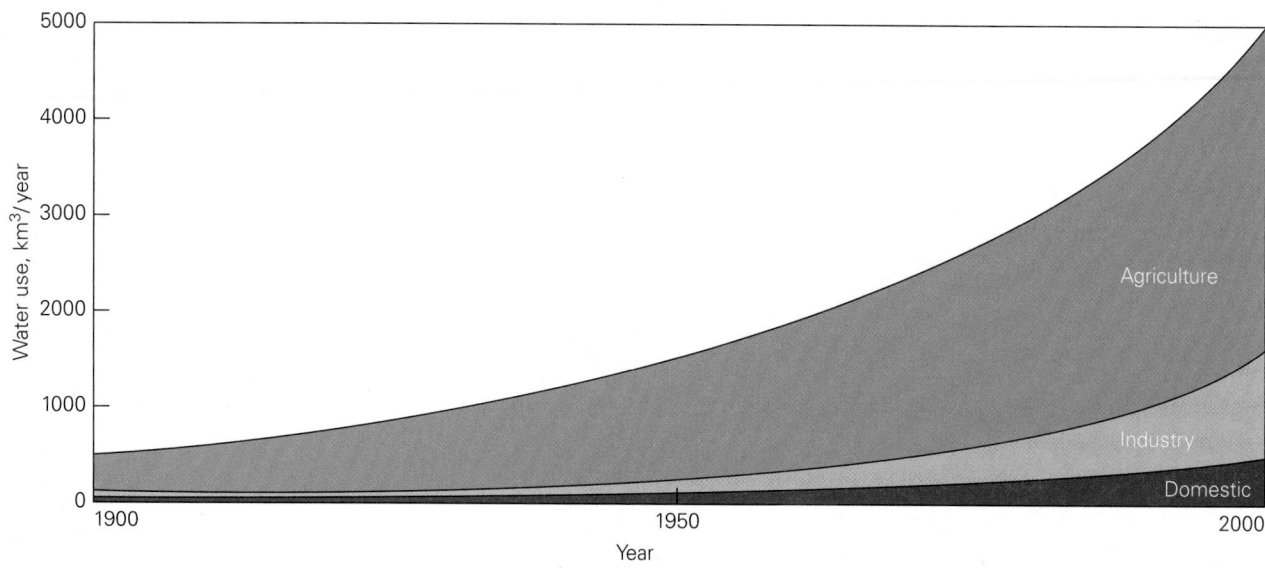

Figure 11-34 Worldwide use of freshwater in cubic kilometers per year. The rate of increase is somewhat greater than the rate of population increase. Without effective conservation, serious water shortages are sure to become widespread in years to come.

locations. The only real way to prevent large-scale water shortages is conservation. Simply charging appropriate prices for water has reduced water wastage wherever it has been tried. Repairing leaky water delivery systems and recycling industrial water are other practical strategies. As much as 100 tons of water once had to be supplied to make a ton of steel, but today less than 6 tons of new water is needed; the remainder is water that was formerly discarded. And in agriculture, by far the biggest user (and waster) of water, new irrigation techniques are being adopted. Merely burying perforated pipes in the soil to deliver water directly to plant roots minimizes water losses by evaporation and runoff, which can be substantial in traditional agriculture. Another approach is to replace, where possible, water-hungry crops such as rice with others, such as wheat, that need less. So there is hope, but much remains to be done.

Desalination

Modern desalinators use special semipermeable membranes that allow water molecules to pass through while holding back salt ions. If pure water is on one side of such a membrane with salt water on the other side and both are under the same pressure, more water molecules will migrate through the membrane from the pure side to the salt side than the other way. This process is called **osmosis.**

However, if the salt water is under higher pressure than the pure water, more water molecules will migrate from the salt side to the pure side. This is **reverse osmosis.** An extremely high pressure is needed for a reasonable output of pure water, which means expensive pumps that consume a great deal of energy. As a result reverse osmosis desalinators are currently in use only in places where water is really scarce.

The largest desalination plant built thus far, at Ashkelon on Israel's Mediterranean coast, produces over 300,000 tons of pure water per day, 6 percent of the country's water consumption. The plant is extremely efficient because it generates much of its input energy from the high-pressure salt water left over from the reverse osmosis process. Desalination plants worldwide currently provide less than 0.5 percent of human water needs.

Improved membranes are being developed, some using the carbon nanotubes mentioned in Sec. 11.2, that could reduce the energy required considerably and make desalination realistic anywhere that freshwater is in short supply and salt water is available, which is a lot of the world.

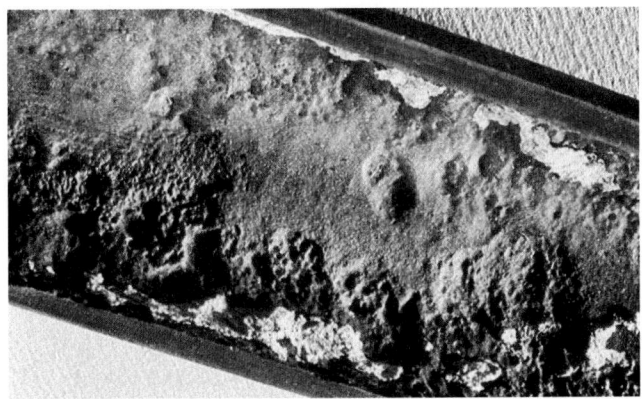

Figure 11-35   Hard water left a deposit of scale in this pipe.

"Hard" Water   Even freshwater is rarely free of ions in solution. "Hard" water contains dissolved minerals that prevent soap from forming suds and react with soap to produce a precipitate. When heated, hard water forms deposits called scale in boilers, water heaters, and tea kettles that decrease their efficiency by acting as heat insulators (Fig. 11-35). Hot water pipes often become partly or even completely blocked by scale. These deposits are insoluble in water but not in acids, which provides a way to remove them. Calcium and magnesium ions are usually responsible for hard water.

Groundwater commonly becomes hard by flowing past limestone deposits on or near the earth's surface. Although calcium carbonate ($CaCO_3$), the main constituent of limestone, is insoluble in pure water, water with dissolved carbon dioxide (which is present in air) can react with $CaCO_3$ as follows:

$$CaCO_3 + CO_2 + H_2O \longrightarrow Ca^{2+} + 2HCO_3^-$$

The HCO_3^- ion is the *hydrogen carbonate ion*, also known as the *bicarbonate ion*. When water that contains Ca^{2+} and HCO_3^- ions is heated, this reaction occurs in reverse to precipitate solid $CaCO_3$ as scale.

11.9   Water Pollution

A Menace Hard to Eliminate

Water can be polluted—that is, rendered unsuitable for a particular purpose, not necessarily human consumption only—in a variety of ways. Now that the dangers of water pollution are widely recognized, a great deal of effort is going into minimizing it. But so widespread are the existing sources of pollution, together with new ones appearing as patterns of industry and agriculture evolve, that this is a problem that will never go away.

Industry   Common sources of pollution are industry and mining. Some pollutants are especially dangerous because they are concentrated in the food chain of living things. A notorious example is mercury, which is widely used in the production of sodium hydroxide (NaOH) and chlorine gas from solutions of NaCl by electrolysis, as well as in other processes. Mercury-containing wastes have traditionally been dumped into the nearest body of water on the assumption that, since most mercury compounds are insoluble in water, no harm would result. Unfortunately some bacteria are able to convert mercury into the soluble compound dimethyl mercury, $(CH_3)_2Hg$, which is highly toxic. As lower forms of life are eaten by higher ones, the concentration of dimethyl mercury in the organisms increases. A number of years ago in Japan, thousands of people who regularly ate fish caught in Minamata Bay were afflicted with mercury poisoning due to wastes dumped by a nearby factory: brain

Water Softeners

Hard water can be softened by removing the Ca^{2+} and Mg^{2+} ions it contains, which can be done in several ways. In one common method, hard water is passed through a column filled with either a synthetic ion-exchange resin or a natural material called zeolite (Fig. 11-36). Both absorb Ca^{2+} and Mg^{2+} ions into their structures while releasing an equivalent number of Na^+ ions. Since Na^+ ions do not affect soap or form compounds that precipitate out from hot water, the water is now "soft." When the ion-exchange column has reached its capacity of Ca^{2+} and Mg^{2+} ions, it can be flushed with a concentrated solution of NaCl to reverse the process and replace the accumulated Ca^{2+} and Mg^{2+} ions with Na^{2+} ions.

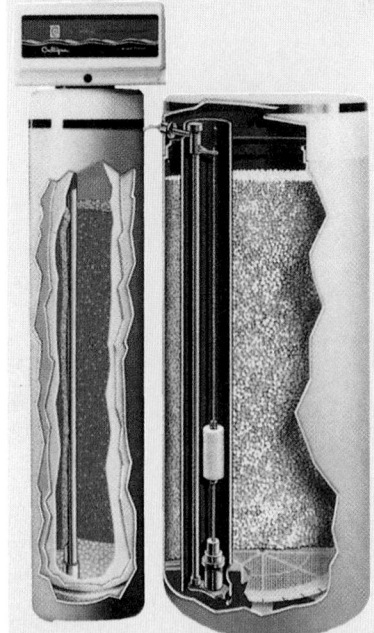

Figure 11-36   These household water softeners use ion-exchange resins.

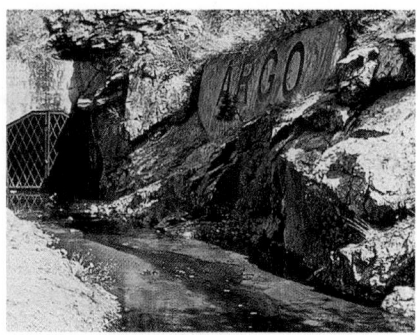

Figure 11-37 Water pollution from a mine. Public anger has forced governments to act against such abuse of the environment.

damage, paralysis, blindness, and deformed children were the result, and hundreds died. "Minamata disease" is only one of many occurrences of poisoning due to industrial pollution.

For four decades, the United States has had federal and state laws to control water pollution. However, these laws have been largely ignored; a survey by the New York Times showed less than 3 percent of reported violations resulted in any government action. As a result, according to a top official of the Environmental Protection Agency, the country's water "does not meet public health goals." Cancer and birth defects in affected populations are among the possible consequences of toxic materials that lax enforcement has allowed to enter water supplies.

Today nearly half of all toxic releases in the United States are from metal mines and refineries in Nevada, Utah, Arizona, and Alaska (Fig. 11-37). About 500,000 abandoned mines continue to pollute streams in the West. In China, whose industrialization has led to severe environmental damage, 70 percent of the lakes and rivers are polluted, with resulting harm to the health of people and crops. At least half a million Chinese die every year as a result of water and air pollution.

Agriculture The fertilizers and pesticides used in agriculture are another major source of water pollution. Unlike the case of industry, where proper procedures can control the dispersion of harmful wastes, there is no way to keep chemicals deposited on the soil from spreading further. What can happen is illustrated by the potent and long-lasting insecticide DDT, now banned in the United States and elsewhere. Washed from farmland into a body of water such as a lake, DDT enters the chain of life through tiny plant and animal organisms called plankton. With less than 0.1 part per million (ppm) of DDT in the lake water, the plankton may contain several ppm of DDT. The DDT concentration increases rapidly in the fish that eat plankton because DDT is retained in their fat and can reach over 1000 ppm in birds that eat the fish. One way that DDT affects birds is by weakening the shells of their eggs, which tend to break before the chicks hatch. This can wipe out whole species of birds in a DDT-polluted region.

Because pesticides are of great benefit to agriculture and, in many parts of the world, to disease control, it is not satisfactory merely to stop using them. The remedy is to develop pesticides that decompose rapidly, and much has already been done in this respect. But unfortunately no really effective alternative to DDT has yet been found for preventing the spread of malaria, whose parasites are carried by mosquitoes. More people may have died from malaria over history than from any other disease. Because its drawbacks led to a major decline in the use of DDT, malarial regions were left with the disastrous consequence that this disease, once on the way out, flourished once more and now kills or contributes to the deaths of perhaps 3 million people, mainly in Africa, each year. As a result, DDT has been reintroduced for malarial control as an indoor spray and as a coating for bed nets, both of which use much less of the pesticide than its former agricultural employment and so affects the environment to only a minor extent.

Dissolved Oxygen Fertilizers contain the plant nutrients nitrogen, phosphorus, and potassium. (Nitrogen goes into the proteins in plant tissues; phosphorus promotes root growth and fruit ripening; potassium helps plants to cope with disease and frost and promotes seed growth.) When a body of water becomes rich in these elements as a result of pollution by fertilizers, tiny organisms called algae cover its surface (Fig. 11-38). As the algae die, aerobic bacteria (which need oxygen to live) use oxygen dissolved in the water to break down the algae into simple compounds, largely water and

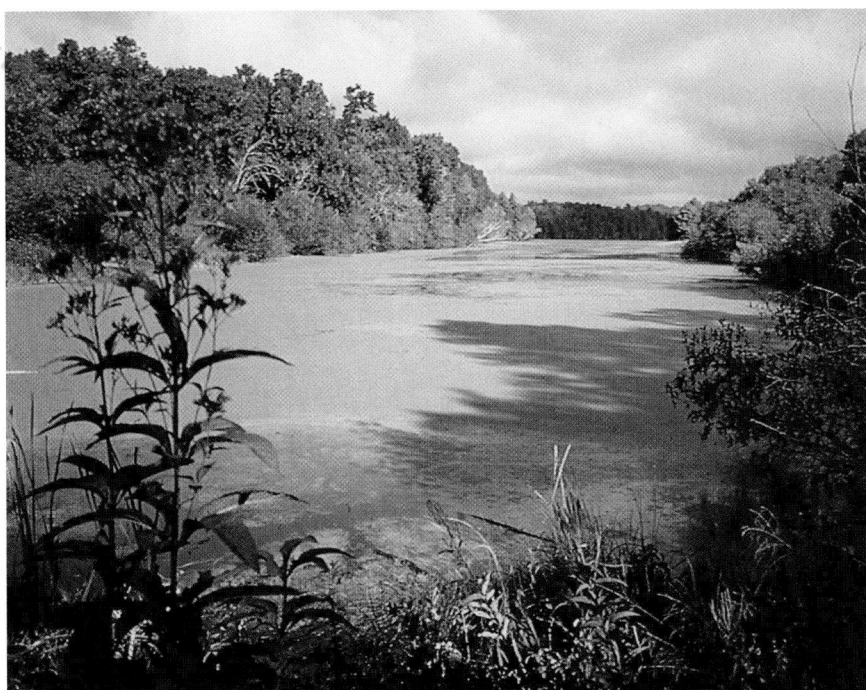

Figure 11-38 Water pollution by fertilizers caused this algal bloom on the surface of a lake in Wisconsin.

CO_2. Sewage and other organic wastes (such as those from food-processing plants and paper mills) are similarly attacked by these bacteria.

The oxygen needed to completely oxidize the organic debris in a given sample of water is called the **biochemical oxygen demand,** or BOD, of the water. BOD is a useful index of pollution because, when it is too great, the oxygen content of the water falls to the point where fish and other creatures in the water die out. A huge (sometimes over 8000 square miles) dead zone of this kind forms each summer in the Gulf of Mexico south of Louisiana and has significantly harmed the fishing industry there. The Mississippi River and the rivers that flow into it drain 40 percent of the continental United States, and since 1960 the amount of nitrogen in the water the Mississippi delivers to the Gulf has tripled and the amount of phosphorus doubled. Fertilizer runoff from farms in the Middle West is largely responsible and the dead zone is widening as more and more corn is being grown for conversion into ethanol.

More than half the other river mouths of the United States have also been degraded by nutrient pollution, though not to the same extent as in the dead zone of the Gulf. In Europe's Black Sea, a dead zone the size of Switzerland occurs off the mouth of the Danube River. In all, over 400 dead zones lie off the world's coasts.

A sufficiently high BOD can lower the oxygen content of water so far that aerobic bacteria are unable to break down organic wastes. Anaerobic bacteria (which do not need oxygen) then take over to produce such gases as methane (CH_4), which is flammable, and hydrogen sulfide (H_2S), whose unpleasant odor is that of rotten eggs.

Another way in which the oxygen content of a body of water can be lowered is by heating, since the solubility of a gas in water decreases with increasing temperature. Because the heat output of an electric power plant is two or more times its electric output, such a plant has plenty of heat to get rid of. Using water from a nearby river or lake for cooling is the most common method, but the resulting thermal pollution does not benefit the local fish population.

Acids and Bases

We continue our study of ions in solution by considering the three important classes of electrolytes: acids, bases, and salts. All are familiar in everyday life.

11.10 Acids

Hydrogen Ions Give Acidic Solutions Their Characteristic Properties

Acids are hydrogen-containing substances whose water solutions taste sour and change the color of the dye litmus from blue to red. In concentrated form such strong acids as the sulfuric acid used in storage batteries are poisonous, cause painful burns if allowed to remain on skin, and damage many materials. Hydrochloric acid, another strong acid, helps to digest food in our stomachs. Weak acids—such as the acetic acid of vinegar, the citric acid of lemons, and the lactic acid of yogurt—are far from being harmful and add a pleasant sour taste to foods and drinks.

What is it that underlies the behavior of acids? We have two clues:

1. All acids consist of hydrogen in combination with one or more nonmetals.
2. Solutions of acids conduct electricity and hence must contain ions.

It is therefore tempting to think that acids such as hydrochloric acid, HCl, and sulfuric acid, H_2SO_4, dissociate into hydrogen and nonmetal ions as follows:

$$HCl \longrightarrow H^+ + Cl^- \qquad \textit{Dissociation of}$$
$$\textit{hydrochloric acid}$$

$$H_2SO_4 \longrightarrow H^+ + HSO_4^- \quad \textit{Dissociation of}$$
$$\textit{sulfuric acid}$$

From this it is natural to conclude that the characteristic properties of acid solutions are the properties of the hydrogen ion H^+.

This simple picture presents difficulties, however. For one thing, pure acids in liquid form do not conduct electric current, so a pure acid cannot be made up of ions. Because acids are covalent rather than ionic substances, they form ions not by the separation of ions already present but by reacting with water.

Hydronium   A second problem with the above simple picture of acids is that the ion H^+ is just a single proton—the nucleus of a hydrogen atom without its electron. All other ions are particles of the same general size as atoms, particles that consist of nuclei and electron clouds. The H^+ ion would be entirely different, a naked proton a million billion times smaller than other ions. Such a particle cannot exist by itself in a liquid but must become attached immediately to some other atom or molecule.

To avoid these difficulties, we could think in terms of reactions like this:

$$HCl + H_2O \longrightarrow H_3O^+ + Cl^-$$

Here the acid HCl is shown reacting with water instead of simply splitting up into ions, and the proton (the H^+ ion) is shown attached to a water molecule rather than free in solution. The ion H_3O^+ is a combination of H^+ with H_2O and is called the **hydronium ion** (Fig. 11-39). The characteristic properties of acids are described more correctly as properties of the hydronium ion than as properties of the simple hydrogen ion.

Nevertheless, chemists customarily write H^+ for the characteristic ion of acids rather than H_3O^+ because it is more convenient to do so. For most purposes, then, we can say that

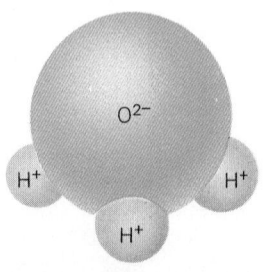

Figure 11-39   A model of the hydronium ion, H_3O^+.

> An acid is a substance that contains hydrogen and whose solution in water increases the number of H^+ ions present.

Although not strictly true, it is still legitimate to think of free hydrogen ions as being present in all acid solutions and giving these solutions their common properties. When we say that acid solutions taste sour, turn litmus pink, and liberate hydrogen gas by reaction with metals, we mean that the hydrogen ion does these things.

11.11   Strong and Weak Acids

The More It Dissociates, the Stronger the Acid

Acids differ greatly in how much they dissociate. Some acids, called **strong acids,** dissociate completely. The three most common strong acids are HCl (hydrochloric), H_2SO_4 (sulfuric), and HNO_3 (nitric). Other acids, called **weak acids,** dissociate only slightly.

The stronger an acid, the weaker the attachment of hydrogen in its molecules. In a strong acid like HCl the link is so weak that all the H^+ and Cl^- ions split apart and go their separate ways in solution. In a weak acid like acetic acid, $HC_2H_3O_2$, on the other hand, the link is strong enough so that most of the molecules remain undissociated—in the case of acetic acid, 98 out of 100.

The greater dissociation of strong acids means that, in solutions of the same total concentration, a strong acid has a much larger proportion of hydrogen ions than a weak acid. It has a more sour taste, it is a better conductor of electricity, and if the two acids are poured on zinc, hydrogen gas is given off much faster from the reaction with strong acid.

Why Carbon Dioxide Solutions Are Acidic   Certain substances that do not contain hydrogen still yield acidic solutions by reacting with water to liberate H^+ from H_2O. An interesting example is the gas CO_2, which when dissolved in water produces H^+ and HCO_3^- (hydrogen carbonate) ions:

$$CO_2 + H_2O \longrightarrow H^+ + HCO_3^-$$

Some HCO_3^- ions further dissociate into H^+ and CO_3^{2-} (carbonate) ions:

$$HCO_3^- \longrightarrow H^+ + CO_3^{2-}$$

It is customary to consider a solution of CO_2 in water (which is what soda water is) as containing "carbonic acid," although H_2CO_3 rarely exists as such. "Carbonic acid" is weak because relatively little of the dissolved CO_2 reacts with water to give H^+ ions. Rain and snow are slightly acidic because of the dissolved CO_2 they contain.

11.12   Bases

Hydroxide Ions Give Basic Solutions Their Characteristic Properties

Bases are familiar as substances whose solutions in water have a bitter taste, a slippery or soapy feel, and an ability to turn red litmus to blue. Their formulas, such as $NaOH$ for sodium hydroxide and $Ba(OH)_2$ for barium hydroxide, show that bases consist of a metal together with one or more hydroxide (OH) groups. On dissolving in water, bases dissociate into ions according to reactions such as

$$NaOH \longrightarrow Na^+ + OH^- \qquad \textit{Dissociation of sodium hydroxide}$$

Alkali

The name **alkali** is sometimes used for a substance that dissolves in water to give a basic solution. Alkali is an old Arabic word that referred originally to a bitter extract obtained from the ashes of a desert plant. Because $NaOH$ and KOH are strong alkalis, sodium and potassium are known as alkali metals. An alkaline solution is one that contains OH^- ions; the terms alkaline and basic mean the same thing.

$$Ba(OH)_2 \longrightarrow Ba^{2+} + 2OH^- \quad \textit{Dissociation of barium hydroxide}$$

Just as H^+ is the characteristic ion of acidic solutions, so OH^- is the characteristic ion in water solutions of bases. The properties of bases are properties of the OH^- ion. We may therefore say that

> A base is a substance that contains hydroxide groups and whose solution in water increases the number of OH^- ions present.

The last part of the definition is needed because not all compounds that contain OH groups release them as OH^- ions in solution. An example is methanol (methyl alcohol), CH_3OH.

Like acids, bases may be classed as strong and weak according to how they dissociate in solution. Thus potassium hydroxide, KOH, is a strong base because it breaks up completely into K^+ and OH^- ions when it dissolves. The most common strong bases are KOH (caustic potash), NaOH (lye or caustic soda, used in oven cleaners), and $Ca(OH)_2$ (slaked lime, used in the mortar that holds the bricks of a building together). Widely employed in industry, these bases are all poisonous and just as destructive to flesh and clothing as the strong acids.

Why Ammonia Solutions Are Basic   Bases differ from acids in that soluble weak bases are rare. However, many substances that do not contain OH in their formulas give basic solutions because they react with water to release OH^- ions from H_2O molecules. An example is the gas ammonia, NH_3, which reacts with water as follows:

$$NH_3 + H_2O \longrightarrow NH_4^+ + OH^- \quad \textit{Solution of ammonia}$$

The process is analogous to that by which CO_2 reacts with water to give an acidic solution. Ammonia solutions are often used in household cleansers. Two other compounds that are not bases but that give basic solutions are sodium carbonate (washing soda), Na_2CO_3, and sodium tetraborate (borax), $Na_2B_4O_7$, both also used as cleansing agents. [For another example, see Sec. 11.12 at www.mhhe.com/krauskopf.]

11.13   The pH Scale

Less Than 7 Is Acidic; More Than 7 Is Basic

Even pure water dissociates to a small extent. The reaction can be written

$$H_2O \longrightarrow H^+ + OH^- \quad \textit{Dissociation of water}$$

The hydroxide ion OH^- attracts protons much more strongly than the neutral water molecule H_2O, and the reverse reaction

$$H^+ + OH^- \longrightarrow H_2O \quad \textit{Recombination of water}$$

occurs readily. Thus we can write

$$H_2O \rightleftharpoons H^+ + OH^-$$

where the double arrow means that both reactions take place all the time in water.

The dissociation of water means that there are always some H^+ and OH^- ions in pure water, and the tendency for these ions to recombine keeps their concentration low. Only 0.0000002 percent of pure water is dissociated into ions on the average: 2 molecules out of every billion. In an acidic solution the

Gastric Fluid

Gastric fluid, produced by glands in the stomach lining, acts upon food in the stomach. This fluid contains pepsin, an enzyme that helps break down proteins in food, and hydrochloric acid, which creates the acid environment needed for pepsin to act. (Most digestion occurs in the small intestine, not the stomach.)

Gastric fluid normally has a pH of about 1.0, acidic enough to dissolve some metals. If the acid concentration is too high, the stomach lining can become inflamed (gastritis), which causes pain and sometimes bleeding. To reduce excess acidity, an antacid can be taken to neutralize some of the HCl. A number of antacids are widely used, one of which is magnesium hydroxide, $Mg(OH)_2$, commonly known as milk of magnesia. It reacts with HCl as follows:

$$Mg(OH)_2 + 2HCl \longrightarrow MgCl_2 + 2H_2O$$

Some antacids are not bases like $Mg(OH)_2$ but nevertheless can neutralize HCl; see the discussion at the end of Sec. 11.12. An example is sodium bicarbonate, $NaHCO_3$:

$$NaHCO_3 + HCl \longrightarrow NaCl + H_2O + CO_2$$

The carbon dioxide gas that is produced may cause discomfort and belching.

concentration of H^+ is greater than in pure water, and the concentration of OH^- is lower. In a basic solution, the concentration of OH^- is greater than in pure water, and that of H^+ is lower.

The **pH scale** is a method for expressing the exact degree of acidity or basicity of a solution in terms of its H^+ ion concentration (Fig. 11-40). This scale is so widely used that an acquaintance with it is worth having, but we need not concern ourselves here with its mathematical basis.

What pH Values Mean   A solution that, like pure water, is neither acidic nor basic is said to be **neutral** and has, by definition, a pH of 7. Acidic solutions have pH values of less than 7; the more strongly acidic they are, the lower the pH. Basic solutions have pH values of more than 7; the more strongly basic they are, the higher the pH. A change in pH of 1 means a change in H^+ concentration by a factor of 10. Thus a solution of pH 4 is 10 times more acidic than a solution of pH 5 and 100 times more acidic than a solution of pH 6. Figure 11-41 illustrates the pH scale and Fig. 11-42 shows typical pH values of some familiar solutions.

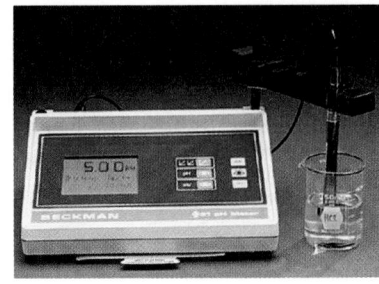

Figure 11-40   This device determines the pH of a solution electrically. Its pH is a measure of how strongly acidic or basic the solution is.

11.14   Salts

An Acid Plus a Base Gives Water and a Salt

When a sodium hydroxide solution is added slowly to hydrochloric acid, there is no visible sign that anything is happening. Both original solutions are colorless, and the resulting solution is also colorless. That a reaction does indeed occur can be shown in several ways, however. One sign is that the mixture becomes warm, which means that chemical energy is being liberated. In addition, if we measure the pH of the mixture as we add the NaOH, we would find that it gets closer and closer to 7 as the base is added—the concentration of H^+ ions is decreasing.

Evidently a base destroys, or **neutralizes,** the characteristic properties of an acid, and the reaction is accordingly called **neutralization.** In the same way the characteristic properties of a base can be neutralized by adding a strong acid.

Neutralization   What is the chemical change in the neutralization of HCl by NaOH? We could write simply

$$HCl + NaOH \longrightarrow H_2O + NaCl$$

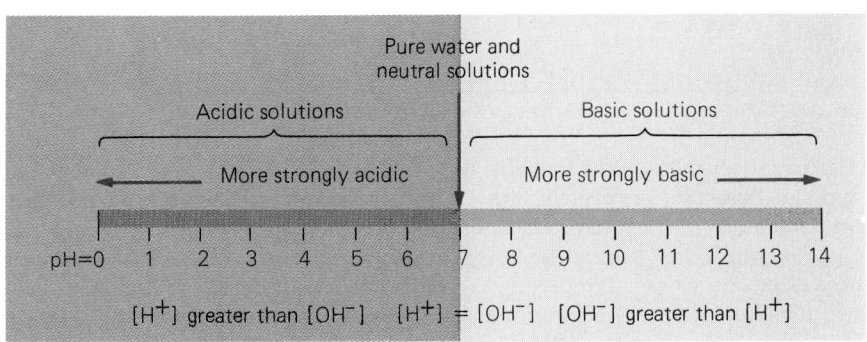

Figure 11-41   The pH scale. The concentration of hydrogen ion is symbolized by [H^+] and that of the hydroxide ion by [OH^-]. A neutral solution has a pH of 7. Litmus paper is red in an acidic solution, blue in a basic solution. An increase of 1 in pH corresponds to a decrease of a factor of 10 in H^+ concentration.

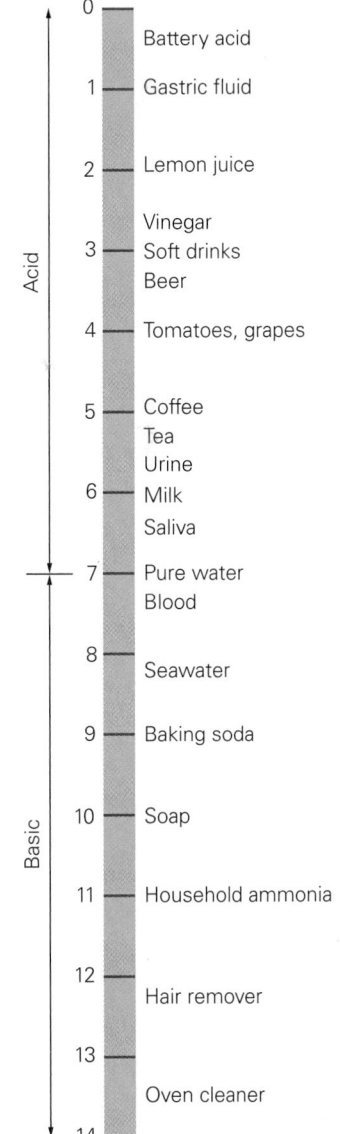

Figure 11-42   Typical pH values.

However, we gain more insight into the process by considering the ions involved. HCl, a strong acid, dissociates completely in water to give H^+ and Cl^-; NaOH, a strong base, dissociates into Na^+ and OH^-; the product NaCl, also a soluble electrolyte, remains dissociated in solution. Of the four substances shown, only water is a nonelectrolyte, so it alone should appear intact in the equation. Hence we have

$$H^+ + Cl^- + Na^+ + OH^- \longrightarrow H_2O + Na^+ + Cl^-$$

Since Na^+ and Cl^- appear on both sides, we can omit them, leaving

$$H^+ + OH^- \longrightarrow H_2O \qquad \textit{Neutralization}$$

This is the chemical change stripped of all nonessentials. The neutralization of a strong acid by a strong base in water solution is really a reaction between hydrogen ions and hydroxide ions to form water.

When an NaOH solution is neutralized with HCl, the resulting solution contains only the ions Na^+ and Cl^-. If the solution is evaporated to dryness, the ions combine to form the white solid NaCl. This substance, ordinary table salt, gives its name to an important class of compounds. Most **salts** are crystalline solids at ordinary temperatures and consist of a metal combined with one or more nonmetals.

How to Prepare a Salt   Any salt can be made by mixing the appropriate acid and base and evaporating the solution to dryness. Thus potassium nitrate, KNO_3, is formed when solutions of potassium hydroxide, KOH, and nitric acid, HNO_3, are mixed and evaporated; copper sulfate, $CuSO_4$, is formed when sulfuric acid, H_2SO_4, is poured on insoluble copper hydroxide, $Cu(OH)_2$, and the resulting solution is evaporated. In general, then, neutralization reactions give water and a solution of salt.

It is important to remember that a salt itself is not produced directly by a neutralization. Neutralization is a reaction between hydrogen ions and hydroxide ions. As a result of neutralization, ions may be left in solution that combine to form a salt when the solution is evaporated.

Table salt, NaCl, is not the only salt familiar to us in everyday life. Washing soda, Na_2CO_3, and borax, $Na_2B_4O_7$, have already been mentioned. Here are a few other examples. Baking soda, $NaHCO_3$, is used in baking powder, as a deodorizer, and in medicine as an antacid; it is also known as bicarbonate of soda and, to chemists, as sodium hydrogen carbonate. Epsom salt, $MgSO_4 \cdot 7H_2O$ (this formula means that seven water molecules are associated with each $MgSO_4$ unit in its crystals), has various medical uses. Saltpeter, KNO_3, is used to preserve meat and in gunpowder. Gypsum, $CaSO_4 \cdot 2H_2O$, is an ingredient of plaster. Many other salts can be added to this list.

Important Terms and Ideas

Solids that consist of particles arranged in repeated patterns are called **crystalline**. If the particles are irregularly arranged, the solid is called **amorphous**. The four types of bonds in crystals are **ionic, covalent, metallic,** and **molecular.**

The **metallic bond** arises from a "sea" of electrons that can move freely through a solid metal. These electrons are also responsible for the ability of metals to conduct heat and electricity well.

Van der Waals forces arise from the electric attraction between nonuniform charge distributions in atoms and molecules. They enable atoms and molecules to form solids without sharing or transferring electrons.

In a solution, the substance present in larger amount is the **solvent;** the other is the **solute.** When a solid or gas is dissolved in a liquid, the liquid is always considered the solvent. The **solubility** of a substance is the maximum amount that can be dissolved in a given quantity of solvent at a given temperature. A **saturated** solution is one that contains the maximum amount of solute possible.

Polar molecules behave as if negatively charged at one end and positively charged at the other; in **nonpolar molecules,** electric charge is uniformly distributed on the average. **Polar liquids** dissolve only ionic and polar covalent compounds, whereas **nonpolar liquids** dissolve only nonpolar covalent compounds. Water is a highly polar liquid, which is why it is so good a solvent.

Ionic compounds **dissociate** into free ions when dissolved in water; ions of a given kind in solution have properties that differ from those of the corresponding neutral substance. An **electrolyte** is any substance that separates into ions when dissolved in water.

Solutions of **acids** in water contain H^+ ions; solutions of **bases** in water contain OH^- ions. **Strong** acids and bases dissociate completely in solution; **weak** acids and bases only partially. The **pH** of a solution is a measure of its degree of acidity or basicity. Acid solutions have pH values of less than 7; basic solutions have pH values of more than 7. A **neutral** solution is neither acidic nor basic and has a pH of 7.

In acid-base **neutralization,** H^+ and OH^- ions join to form H_2O molecules.

Salts are usually crystalline solids that consist of positive metal ions and negative nonmetal ions. A salt can be formed by neutralizing the acid that contains the appropriate nonmetal ion with the base that contains the appropriate metal ion and then evaporating the solution to dryness.

Multiple Choice

1. A solid whose particles are irregularly arranged is said to be
   a. a van der Waals solid
   b. nonpolar
   c. amorphous
   d. unsaturated

2. An amorphous solid is closest in structure to
   a. a covalent crystal
   b. an ionic crystal
   c. a van der Waals crystal
   d. a liquid

3. Ionic crystals
   a. consist of positive ions only
   b. consist of negative ions only
   c. dissolve only in polar liquids
   d. are soft and melt at low temperatures

4. A "sea" of freely moving electrons is present in
   a. ionic crystals
   b. covalent crystals
   c. molecular crystals
   d. metal crystals

5. A polar molecule can attract
   a. only ions
   b. only other polar molecules
   c. only nonpolar molecules
   d. all of these

6. Van der Waals forces between atoms and between molecules arise from
   a. uniform charge distributions
   b. nonuniform charge distributions
   c. electron transfer
   d. electron sharing

7. Which solids have the lowest melting points in general?
   a. covalent   c. van der Waals
   b. ionic   d. metallic

8. Ice is an example of
   a. a covalent solid   c. a metallic solid
   b. an ionic solid   d. a van der Waals solid

9. Diamond is an example of
   a. a covalent solid   c. a metallic solid
   b. an ionic solid   d. a van der Waals solid

10. A property of metals that is not due to the electron "sea" in them is their ability to
    a. conduct electricity
    b. conduct heat
    c. reflect light
    d. form oxides

11. Diamond and graphite are forms of solid carbon. They both
    a. conduct electricity well
    b. can be used as lubricants
    c. are very hard
    d. form CO_2 when burned in air

12. Suppose there were molecules that had no attraction whatever for one another. A collection of such molecules would form a (an)
    a. gas   c. amorphous solid
    b. liquid   d. crystalline solid

13. A saturated solution is a solution that
    a. contains the maximum amount of solute
    b. contains the maximum amount of solvent
    c. is in the process of crystallizing
    d. contains polar molecules

14. A gas is dissolved in a liquid. When the temperature of the solution is increased, the solubility of the gas
    a. increases
    b. decreases
    c. remains the same
    d. any of these, depending upon the nature of the solution

15. A solid is dissolved in a liquid. When the temperature of the solution is increased, the solubility of the solid
    a. increases
    b. decreases
    c. remains the same
    d. any of these, depending upon the nature of the solution

16. Dissolving a solute in a liquid
    a. decreases the liquid's freezing point
    b. increases the liquid's freezing point
    c. does not change the liquid's freezing point
    d. any of these, depending on the substances involved

17. A molecule that behaves as though positively charged at one end and negatively charged at the other is called a (an)
   a. hydronium ion
   b. acid molecule
   c. polar molecule
   d. nonpolar molecule

18. The most strongly polar liquid of the following is
   a. water
   b. alcohol
   c. a detergent
   d. gasoline

19. In general, ionic compounds
   a. are insoluble in all liquids
   b. dissolve best in polar liquids
   c. dissolve best in nonpolar liquids
   d. dissolve equally well in polar and nonpolar liquids

20. Nonpolar substances usually dissolve most readily in
   a. polar liquids
   b. nonpolar liquids
   c. acids
   d. bases

21. A substance that separates into free ions when dissolved in water is said to be
   a. polar
   b. saturated
   c. an electrolyte
   d. covalent

22. Which of the following would you expect to be a strong electrolyte in solution?
   a. H_2O
   b. HCl
   c. sugar
   d. alcohol

23. Which of the following has the least ability to conduct electric current?
   a. an acid solution
   b. a basic solution
   c. a salt solution
   d. a nonpolar liquid

24. The ions and atoms (or molecules) of an element
   a. have very nearly the same properties except that the ions are electrically charged
   b. may have strikingly different properties
   c. always exhibit different colors
   d. differ in that the ions are always more active chemically than the atoms or molecules

25. Dissociation refers to
   a. the formation of a precipitate
   b. the separation of a mixture of polar and nonpolar liquids (such as oil and water) into separate layers
   c. the separation of a solution containing ions into separate layers of + and − ions
   d. the separation of a substance into free ions

26. When an electrolyte is dissolved in water,
   a. the freezing point of the water is raised
   b. the solution is acidic
   c. the solution contains free ions
   d. the solution contains free electrons

27. The average salinity of seawater is about
   a. 0.1 percent
   b. 1.5 percent
   c. 3.5 percent
   d. 10 percent

28. The ions usually responsible for "hard" water are
   a. H^+ and OH^-
   b. Na^+ and Cl^-
   c. Ca^{2+} and Mg^{2+}
   d. SO_4^{2-} and NO_3^-

29. Acids invariably contain
   a. hydrogen
   b. oxygen
   c. chlorine
   d. water

30. The reason pure acids in the liquid state are not dissociated is that their chemical bonds are
   a. ionic
   b. covalent
   c. metallic
   d. van der Waals

31. While it is convenient to regard acidic solutions as containing H^+ ions, it is more realistic to describe them as containing
   a. hydronium ions
   b. hydroxide ions
   c. polar molecules
   d. hydrogen atoms

32. A common strong acid is
   a. acetic acid
   b. boric acid
   c. nitric acid
   d. citric acid

33. A base dissolved in water liberates
   a. H^-
   b. OH
   c. OH^+
   d. OH^-

34. A substance whose formula does not contain OH yet yields a basic solution when dissolved in water is
   a. NH_3
   b. CO_2
   c. HCl
   d. NaCl

35. The symbol of the ammonium ion is
   a. NH_3^-
   b. NH_3^+
   c. NH_4^-
   d. NH_4^+

36. The net reaction between a strong acid and a strong base is
   a. $H_2O \rightarrow H^+ + OH^-$
   b. $H^+ + OH^- \rightarrow H_2O$
   c. $H_2O + H_2O \rightarrow H_3O^+ + OH^-$
   d. $H^+ + H_2O \rightarrow H_3O^+$

37. The formula for iron(III) hydroxide is
   a. FeOH
   b. Fe_3OH
   c. $Fe(OH)_3$
   d. $Fe_3(OH)_3$

38. A strong acid or base in solution is completely
   a. dissociated
   b. neutralized
   c. hydrolyzed
   d. precipitated

39. Pure water contains
   a. only H^+ ions
   b. only OH^- ions
   c. both H^+ and OH^- ions
   d. neither H^+ nor OH^- ions

40. A pH of 7 signifies a (an)
   a. acid solution
   b. basic solution
   c. neutral solution
   d. solution of polar molecules

41. A concentrated solution of which of the following has the lowest pH?
   a. hydrochloric acid
   b. acetic acid
   c. sodium hydroxide
   d. ammonia

42. A concentrated solution of which of the following has the highest pH?
   a. hydrochloric acid
   b. acetic acid
   c. sodium hydroxide
   d. ammonia

Exercises

11.1   Ionic and Covalent Crystals

11.2   The Metallic Bond

11.3   Molecular Crystals

1. (a) State the four principal types of bonding in crystalline solids and give an example of each. (b) What is the fundamental physical origin of all of them? (c) What kind of particle is present in the crystal structure of each of them?

2. What kind of solid is ice? Why does ice float when nearly all other solids sink when they freeze?

3. Are ionic or covalent crystals more common?

4. You are given two solids that look nearly alike, one of which is held together by ionic bonds and the other by van der Waals bonds. How could you tell them apart?

5. How could you tell experimentally whether a fragment of a clear, colorless material is glass or a crystalline solid?

6. From which class of solids would you expect electrons to be liberated most readily by the photoelectric effect when light is shined on a sample?

7. What kind of solid contains a "sea" of freely moving electrons? Does this sea include all the electrons present?

8. Lithium atoms, like hydrogen atoms, have only a single electron in their outer shells, yet lithium atoms do not join together to form Li_2 molecules the way hydrogen atoms form H_2 molecules. Instead, lithium is a metal with each atom part of a crystal structure. Can you think of the reason for this difference?

9. Van der Waals forces are strong enough to hold inert gas atoms together to form liquids at low temperatures, but these forces do not lead to inert gas molecules at higher temperatures. Why not?

10. What ions would you expect to find in the crystal structures of MgO and K_2S?

11. What ions would you expect to find in the crystal structures of CaF_2 and KI?

11.4   Solubility

11.5   Polar and Nonpolar Liquids

12. Why is the solubility of one gas in another unlimited?

13. Why do bubbles of gas form in a glass of soda water when it warms up?

14. Ordinary tap water tastes different after it has been boiled. Can you think of the reason why?

15. How do unsaturated, saturated, and supersaturated solutions differ?

16. How can an unsaturated solution of a solid in a liquid become saturated? How can a saturated solution of a solid in a liquid become supersaturated (if this is possible in a particular case)?

17. Give two ways to tell whether a sugar solution is saturated or not.

18. At 10°C, which is more concentrated, a saturated solution of potassium nitrate or a saturated solution of potassium chloride? At 60°C?

19. You have saturated solutions of silver nitrate ($NaNO_3$) and potassium nitrate (KNO_3) at 60°C. What is an easy way to tell which is which?

20. What is the difference between a molecular ion and a polar molecule?

11.6   Ions in Solution

11.7   Evidence for Dissociation

21. How could you distinguish experimentally between an electrolyte and a nonelectrolyte?

22. The ions of potassium (K) and calcium (Ca) both contain 18 electrons. Would you expect the chemical behaviors of these elements to be similar?

23. You have a solution that contains Cl^- ions and another that contains NO_3^- ions. How would adding a solution that contains Ag^+ ions to these solutions enable you to tell which is which?

24. You have a solution that contains Ca^{2+} ions and another that contains Na^+ ions. How would adding a solution that contains CO_3^{2-} ions enable you to tell which is which?

25. You have a solution that contains Ag^+ ions and another that contains Na^+ ions. How would adding a solution that contains Cl^- ions to these solutions enable you to tell which is which?

26. What is the easiest way to distinguish between a solution that contains Cu^{2+} ions from one that contains Ca^{2+} ions?

27. How does the reactivity of the chloride ion Cl^- compare with the reactivity of the chlorine molecule Cl_2? Does the answer depend on temperature?

28. Seawater freezes at a lower temperature than pure water because of the salts dissolved in it. How does the boiling point of seawater compare with that of pure water?

11.8   Water

11.9   Water Pollution

29. When water that contains Ca^{++} and HCO_3^- ions is heated, calcium carbonate precipitates out. Carbon dioxide and something else are also produced. What is the something else? Give the equation of the process, which is the cause of the scale found in boilers, water heaters, and tea kettles.

30. What are the two chief ions found in seawater?

31. (a) Is the percentage of the world's water that is freshwater 1 percent? 3 percent? 10 percent? 50 percent? (b) Is the proportion of freshwater in the form of ice in the polar regions about one-third? One-half? Two-thirds?

32. The pesticide DDT concentrates in the fat of animals and tends to remain in the soil despite heavy rain that washes away other contaminants. What do these observations tell you about the nature of the DDT molecule?

11.10 Acids

11.11 Strong and Weak Acids

33. Do pure acids in the liquid state contain H^+ ions? If not, what do such acids consist of?

34. Which of the following are weak acids? Hydrochloric acid, nitric acid, acetic acid, sulfuric acid, citric acid.

35. Would you expect HBr to be a weak or strong acid? Why?

11.12 Bases

36. Even though ammonia is not a base because its molecules do not contain OH groups, its solution in water is basic. Why?

37. What is the difference, if any, between a basic solution and an alkaline solution?

11.13 The pH Scale

38. Is it correct to say that the only ions an acidic solution contains are H^+ ions and that the only ions a basic solution contains are OH^- ions? If not, what would correct descriptions of such solutions be?

39. Which is more strongly acidic, a solution of pH 3 or one of pH 5? Which is more strongly basic, a solution of pH 8 or one of pH 10?

40. In an acidic solution, why is the OH^- concentration lower than it is in pure water?

41. Justify the statement that water is both a weak acid and a weak base.

11.14 Salts

42. When a salt that contains the negative ion of a weak acid is dissolved in water, the solution is basic. For example, a solution of sodium acetate (the corresponding acid is acetic acid) is basic. Why?

43. Give the ionic equation for the neutralization of potassium hydroxide by nitric acid. What chemical changes does this equation show?

44. What salt is formed when a solution of calcium hydroxide is neutralized by phosphoric acid, H_3PO_4? Give the equation of the process.

45. What salt is formed when a solution of calcium hydroxide is neutralized by hydrochloric acid? Give the equation of the process.

46. What salt is formed when a solution of sodium hydroxide is neutralized by sulfuric acid? Give the equation of the process.

47. What salt is formed when a solution of potassium hydroxide is neutralized by acetic acid, $HC_2H_3O_2$? Give the equation of the process.

48. Give the equation of the reaction described below:

Johnny, finding life a bore,
Drank some H_2SO_4.
Johnny's father, an MD,
Gave him $CaCO_3$.
Now he's neutralized, it's true,
But he's full of CO_2.

49. The fertilizer ammonium sulfate can be made by using sulfuric acid to neutralize a solution of ammonia in water. Give the overall equation of the process.

50. Boric acid (H_3BO_3) is a very weak acid. What would happen if solutions of Na_3BO_3 (sodium borate) and HCl were mixed?

51. The Al^{3+} ion tends to form $AlOH^{2+}$ ions in water solution. Would you expect a solution of $AlCl_3$ to be acidic, basic, or neutral? Why?

52. From the fact that H_2S is a weak acid, would you predict that a solution of Na_2S would be acidic, basic, or neutral? Why?

53. How could you prepare the weak acid H_2S from the salt Na_2S (sodium sulfide)?

Chemical Reactions

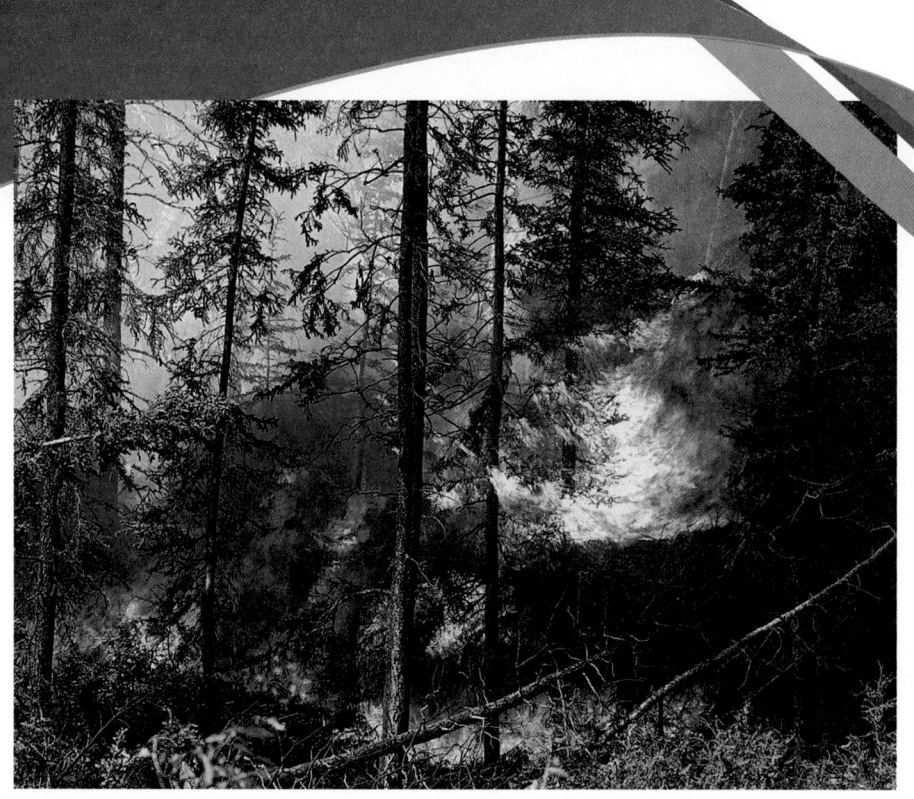

A fire is an exothermic chemical reaction.

GOALS

When you have finished this chapter you should be able to complete the goals
• given for each section below:

Quantitative Chemistry

12.1 Phlogiston
Now It's There, Now It Isn't
• Discuss the phlogiston hypothesis and explain how Lavoisier's experiments showed it to be incorrect.

12.2 Oxygen
Combustion Is Rapid Oxidation
• Define oxide and oxidation.

12.3 The Mole
The Chemist's Unit of Quantity

12.4 Formula Units
A Mole of Anything Contains Avogadro's Number of Formula Units
• Define mole, Avogadro's number, and formula mass.
• Explain why the mole is so valuable as a unit in chemistry.

Chemical Energy

12.5 Exothermic and Endothermic Reactions
Some Reactions Liberate Energy; Others Absorb It

• Distinguish between exothermic and endothermic reactions.

12.6 Chemical Energy and Stability
The Less PE Its Electrons Have, the More Stable the Compound
• Identify the nature of chemical energy.
• Describe the relationship between the chemical energy absorbed or given off in a chemical change and the stabilities of the substances involved.

12.7 Activation Energy
The Initial Energy Needed to Start an Exothermic Reaction
• Explain what is meant by activation energy.

Reaction Rates

12.8 Temperature and Reaction Rates
Hotter Means Faster
• Explain why reaction rates depend strongly on temperature.

12.9 Other Factors
Concentration, Surface Area, and Catalysts
• List the four factors that affect the speed of a chemical reaction.

12.10 Chemical Equilibrium
One Step Forward; One Step Back
• Describe what is meant by a chemical equilibrium.

12.11 Altering an Equilibrium
How to Get Farther Up the Down Escalator
• List the three main ways in which a chemical equilibrium can be altered to favor one direction over the other.

Oxidation and Reduction

12.12 Oxidation-Reduction Reactions
They Always Go Together
• Distinguish between oxidation and reduction in terms of the electrons transferred in each case.
• Describe electrolysis.

12.13 Electrochemical Cells
Turning Chemical Energy into Electric Energy
• Explain the basic principle behind the operation of electrochemical cells.
• Compare batteries and fuel cells.

Chemical reactions have significant aspects quite apart from the changes that occur when the reactants combine to form the products. An important one concerns the quantities involved, for instance, how much of *A* must be added to how much of *B* to give a certain amount of *C?* Energy considerations are also relevant. After all, the energy given off in chemical reactions powers our cars, airplanes, and ships, heats our homes, cooks most of our food, and is the energy source of the generating plants that produce most of our electricity. Our own bodies obtain the energy they need from chemical reactions in which the food we eat combines with oxygen from the air we breathe.

Not all chemical reactions liberate energy—some reactions must be supplied with energy in order to occur. Even those reactions that liberate energy may not take place unless some initial energy is furnished to start the process. Another aspect of chemical reactions is that they take time to be completed: a fraction of a second to many years, depending on a number of factors. Not all reactions even go to completion. Instead, an intermediate equilibrium situation often occurs with the products undergoing reverse reactions to form the starting substances just as fast as the primary reaction proceeds. These are some of the topics considered in this chapter.

Quantitative Chemistry

The most spectacular chemical change our ancestors were familiar with was **combustion,** the process of burning. Early explanations of how wood turns into smoke and ashes amid dancing flames were based on demons and spirits. The fire god has a respected place in many religions.

The ancient Greeks made the first attempt at a nonsupernatural explanation, as recorded by Aristotle. Every flammable material was supposed to consist of "earth" and "fire." When the material burned, the fire escaped, leaving the earth behind as ashes. This idea persisted in various forms until the time of the French Revolution two centuries ago when Antoine Lavoisier gave combustion its modern explanation.

Lavoisier's discovery was made possible by his use of the balance and by his insistence on the importance of mass in studying chemical reactions. This emphasis on mass marked a profound change in viewpoint and is one of Lavoisier's great contributions to chemistry. From his day to ours the balance has remained the chemist's most valuable tool.

12.1 Phlogiston

Now It's There, Now It Isn't

The notion of fire as a basic substance was developed by two Germans, Johann Becher (1635–1682) and his student Georg Stahl (1660–1734), into the **phlogiston** hypothesis. The starting point was the same as Aristotle's, but Becher and Stahl showed how it could be extended to reactions other than burning. They used the word phlogiston (from the Greek word for "flame") for the substance that supposedly escaped during combustion. The story of the downfall of the phlogiston hypothesis and the growth of the modern picture of chemical change is a notable chapter in the history of ideas.

Today we never hear the word phlogiston, but once there was no more respected concept in chemistry. All substances that can be burned were supposed to contain phlogiston, which escapes as the burning takes place. Combustion requires air, but this is explained by assuming that phlogiston can leave a substance only when air is present to absorb it. When heated in air, many metals change slowly to soft powders: zinc and tin give white powders, mercury a reddish powder, iron a black scaly material. These changes, like the changes in ordinary burning, were ascribed to the escape of phlogiston.

A metal was assumed to be a compound of the corresponding powder plus phlogiston, and heating the metal simply caused the compound to decompose. Now, many of these powders can be changed back into metal by heating with charcoal. This observation was interpreted to mean that charcoal must be a form of phlogiston that simply reunited with the powder to form the compound (the metal). When hydrogen was discovered in 1766, its ability to burn without leaving any ash suggested that it was another form of phlogiston. One could predict, then, that heating one of these powders with hydrogen would form a metal, and this prediction was confirmed by experiment.

So far so good, but soon the phlogiston hypothesis ran into serious trouble. When wood burns, its ashes weigh less than the original wood, and the decrease in mass can reasonably be explained as due to the escape of phlogiston. But when a metal is heated until it turns into a powder, the powder weighs *more* than the original metal! The believers in phlogiston were forced to assume that it sometimes could have negative mass, so that if phlogiston left a substance, the remaining material could weigh more than before. To us this notion of negative mass is nonsense, but in the eighteenth century it was taken quite seriously.

The Downfall of Phlogiston The French chemist Antoine Lavoisier carried out a series of experiments in the latter part of the eighteenth century that overthrew the phlogiston hypothesis. Lavoisier knew that tin changed into a white powder when heated and that the powder weighed more than the original metal. To study the process in detail, he placed a piece of tin on a wooden block floating in water, as in Fig. 12-1. He covered the block with a glass jar and heated the tin by focusing sunlight on it with a magnifying glass—a common method of heating before gas burners and electric heaters were invented. The tin was partly changed into a white powder and the water level rose in the jar until only four-fifths as much air was left in the jar as there had been at the start. Further heating caused nothing more to happen.

In another experiment, Lavoisier heated tin in a sealed flask until as much as possible was turned into powder. The flask was weighed before and after heating, and the two masses were the same. Then the flask was opened, and air rushed in. With the additional air, the mass of the flask was more than it had been at the start. The increase in mass was equal to the increase in mass of the tin.

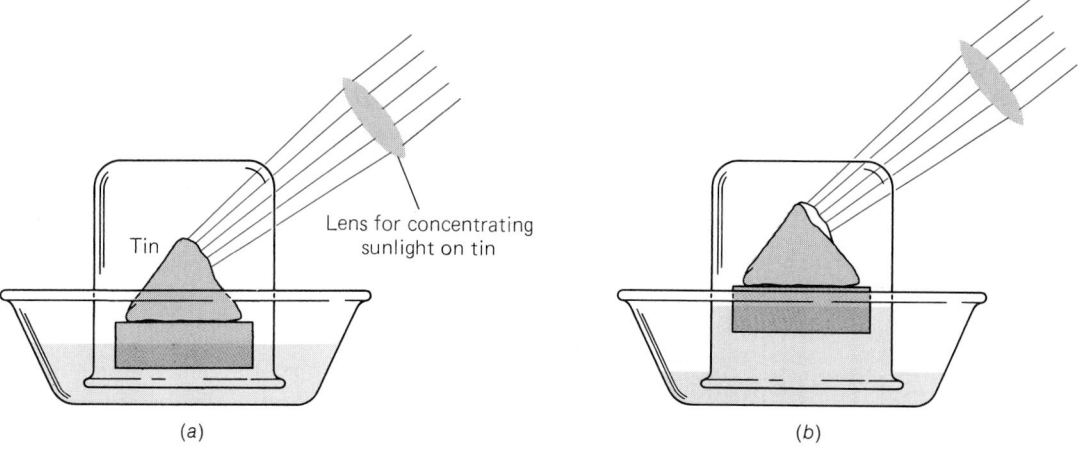

Figure 12-1 Lavoisier's experiment showed that tin, upon heating, combines with a gas from the air. (*a*) Before heating; (*b*) after heating. The tin is partly changed to a white powder, and the water level rises until only four-fifths as much air is left as there was at the start. Further heating causes no additional change.

Tin

Lens for concentrating sunlight on tin

(a)

(b)

| Antoine Lavoisier (1743–1794)

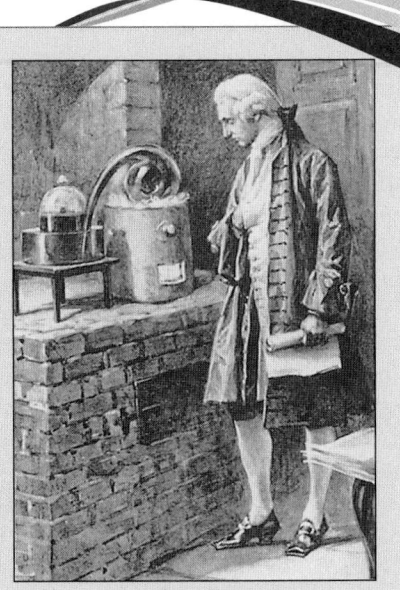

The son of a wealthy French lawyer, Lavoisier studied law at first but soon became fascinated by chemistry and published his first paper, on the mineral gypsum, when he was 22. In that paper, as in his later work, Lavoisier stressed the importance of accurate measurements of mass in chemistry. This emphasis on reliable data marked the start of the modern era of chemistry.

Lavoisier's influence on chemistry was much like that of Galileo on physics. With the help of a sensitive balance and a large magnifying glass for focusing sunlight, Lavoisier carried out a series of experiments that, among other achievements, demolished the notion of phlogiston and made clear the role of oxygen in combustion and other processes.

In his research Lavoisier was greatly aided by his wife, Marie-Anne, who was 14 to his 28 when they were married. Besides work in the laboratory, Marie-Anne made engravings of the apparatus for publication and translated scientific books and papers from English to French. Benjamin Franklin and Thomas Jefferson were among the visitors to the Lavoisier laboratory.

In 1787 Lavoisier and several colleagues systematized the language of chemistry in the book *Methode de Nomenclature Chimique*. They listed 55 substances they could not decompose, most of which (but not caloric or light, which were included) indeed proved to be elements, and named compounds after their constituents according to a standard scheme. Such familiar terms as oxide, nitrate, and sulfate were thereby introduced for the first time. Two years later Lavoisier published the first modern textbook on chemistry, an influential book in which the central place of the law of conservation of mass was made clear.

In order to support his research, while still a young man Lavoisier had invested in the Ferme Générale, a private company that collected taxes for the French government, and he became an official of the company, as was his father-in-law. Brutal and corrupt, the Ferme Générale was the most hated institution in the country. In 1793, after the French Revolution, Lavoisier was arrested because of his association with the Ferme

Générale; when he protested that he was a scientist, he was told that "the Republic has no need of scientists." In 1794 he and his father-in-law were guillotined. Lavoisier's widow later married Count Rumford, who proved that caloric did not exist 25 years after Lavoisier had done the same for phlogiston, but it was an unhappy union.

To Lavoisier these results suggested that the tin had combined with a gas from the air. Since four-fifths of the original air was left after the reaction, he reasoned that one-fifth of air consisted of a gas that can combine with tin. Then the powder was a compound formed from this gas and tin, and the increase in mass of the powder over the tin was the mass of the gas. Water rose in the jar of Fig. 12-1 to take the place of the gas that had combined with the tin. When the sealed flask was opened in the second experiment, air rushed in to take the place of the gas that had combined with the tin. These explanations are simple and direct and involved substances that, unlike phlogiston, had definite masses.

12.2   Oxygen

Combustion Is Rapid Oxidation

At about the time he was making these experiments, Lavoisier learned that Joseph Priestley (Fig. 12-2) had prepared a new gas with remarkable properties. Priestley was the poverty-striken minister of a small church in England, with only limited time and equipment, yet his scientific talents led him to a number of significant discoveries. The gas he had found caused lighted candles to flare up brightly and glowing charcoal to burst into flames. A mouse kept in a closed jar of the gas lived longer than one kept in a closed jar of air.

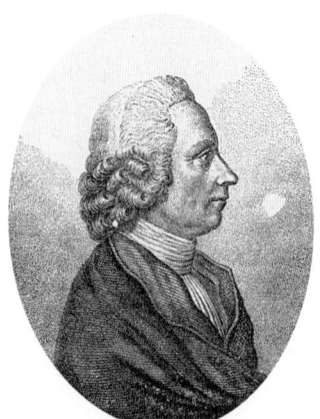

Figure 12-2   Joseph Priestley (1733–1804).

Lavoisier gave Priestley's new gas its modern name, **oxygen,** and found it to be involved not only in the changes that occur in metals when heated but in the process of combustion as well. The burning of candles, wood, and coal, according to Lavoisier, involves combining their materials with oxygen. When they burn, these materials seem to lose mass only because some of the products of the reactions are gases. Actually, as experiment shows, the total mass of the products in each case is more than the original mass of the solid material.

Under ordinary conditions, oxygen is a colorless, odorless, tasteless gas. Air owes its ability to support combustion to its oxygen content. Air cannot support combustion as well as pure oxygen because air consists of only about one-fifth oxygen (Fig. 12-3). The other four-fifths is mainly nitrogen, together with small amounts of other inactive gases.

Priestley discovered a number of other gases—for instance, ammonia, sulfur dioxide, hydrogen sulfide, and carbon monoxide. His political opinions—one of his books provided ideas to Thomas Jefferson—and religious beliefs—he opposed the Church of England—were unpopular, and after his house and laboratory were burnt down by a mob he left England and spent the last 10 years of his life in Pennsylvania.

Oxidation   When oxygen combines chemically with another substance, the process is called **oxidation,** and the other substance is said to be **oxidized.** In the experiments of Lavoisier, the tin reacted with oxygen in the air to become oxidized to a white powder. Rapid oxidation in which a lot of heat and light are given off is the process of combustion (Fig. 12-4). As Priestley found, a lighted candle oxidizes rapidly in air, even more rapidly in pure oxygen.

Slow oxidation is involved in many familiar processes. One of them is the rusting of iron, in which iron is oxidized into the reddish-brown material we call rust (Fig. 12-5). The energy to maintain life comes from the steady oxidation of food by oxygen taken in through our lungs and carried to all parts of our bodies by blood.

Oxide   A substance formed by the union of another element with oxygen is called an **oxide.** The white powder that Lavoisier obtained by heating tin is tin oxide. Rust is largely iron oxide. In general, oxides of metals are solids. Oxides of other elements may be solid, liquid, or gaseous. Thus one of the oxides of sulfur is the foul-smelling gas sulfur dioxide (SO_2). Carbon forms two gaseous oxides, carbon monoxide (CO) and carbon dioxide (CO_2). The oxide of silicon SiO_2 is found in nature as the solid called quartz, the chief constituent of ordinary sand and abundant in rocks (see Figs. 15-2 and 15-6). The oxide of hydrogen is water, H_2O.

Ozone

The molecules of ordinary oxygen consist of two oxygen atoms: O_2. A less stable form of oxygen is **ozone,** whose molecules consist of three oxygen atoms: O_3. The pungent odor of ozone is familiar near electrical discharges, such as sparks and lightning, which can produce O_3 from atmospheric O_2. Ozone is used industrially as a bleach and to purify water; it is toxic to living things and damages various materials, notably rubber.

Two important processes in the atmosphere, one bad and one good, involve the small amount of ozone it contains. At low altitudes ozone damages our lungs and contributes to the formation of smog, which is also harmful to our health. At high altitudes, however, ozone provides a vital service by absorbing dangerous ultraviolet radiation from the sun (see Sec. 14.1).

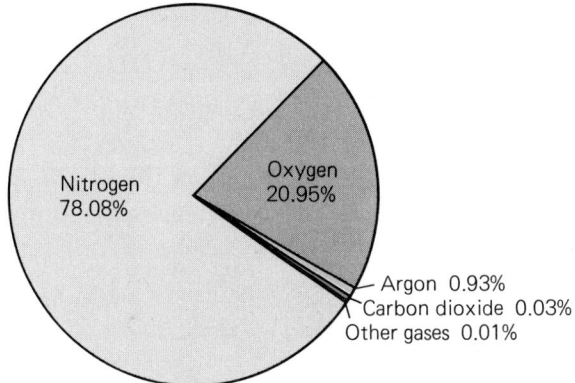

Figure 12-3   Composition of dry air near ground level. A variable amount of water vapor is usually present also.

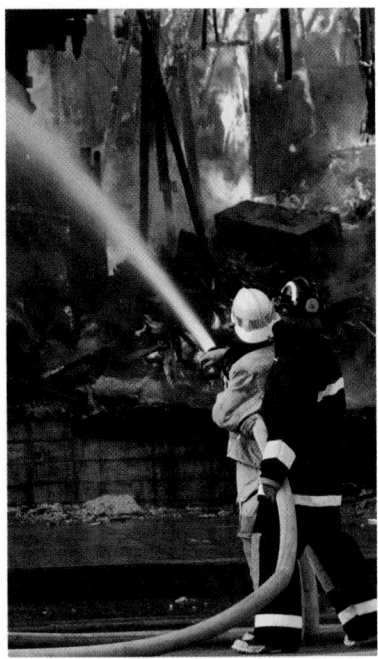

Figure 12-4 A fire can be put out in three ways. (1) Water can be sprayed on to cool the burning material below its ignition temperature. (2) The fire can be smothered by a heavier-than-air agent (such as carbon dioxide or a foam that contains carbon dioxide bubbles) that does not support combustion and keeps out air and hence oxygen. (3) A chemical that interferes with the oxidation process can be sprayed on the fire.

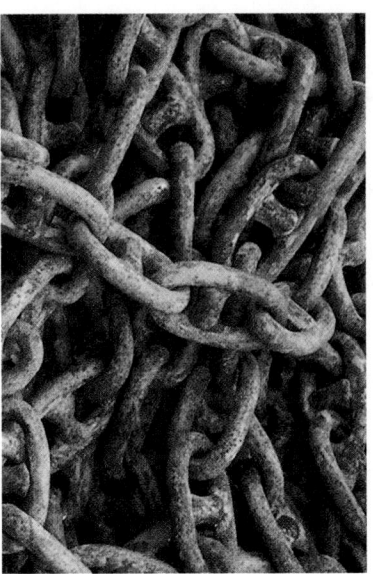

Figure 12-5 Rust forms when iron or steel reacts with oxygen and water. The formula for rust is often written $2Fe_2O_3 \cdot xH_2O$, which means that a variable number of water molecules are associated with every two iron(III) oxide units. Because rust is porous, oxygen and water vapor can penetrate it and continue to react with the metal underneath. A rusty object may therefore have very little strength left. On the other hand, the oxidation of aluminum to Al_2O_3, which occurs naturally in air, produces a hard, durable coating that prevents further corrosion. This is why steel cans are plated with tin to protect them, whereas aluminum cans need no treatment. For even greater protection of aluminum, an electrical process called anodization produces a much thicker layer of Al_2O_3.

Oxides of nearly all the elements can be prepared, most of them simply by heating the elements with oxygen. A few oxides (mercury oxide, lead oxide, barium peroxide) are easily decomposed by heating, which provides a convenient laboratory method for preparing oxygen. Other oxides, such as lime (calcium oxide), are not decomposed even at the temperature of an electric arc, 3000°C.

Example 12.1

The most common building material is concrete, which is often reinforced by embedded steel rods. Iron is the chief ingredient of steel, and if the iron in the steel rods rusts, the concrete may crack. Why?

Solution
Rust is a compound of iron and oxygen and so occupies more volume than the same amount of iron by itself. As their iron content rusts, the rods expand and thus may crack the concrete.

Stainless Steel

Chromium reacts with atmospheric oxygen to produce a thin airtight oxide coating on a chromium surface, which prevents further oxidation. If the oxide layer is scratched, new oxide rapidly covers the exposed metal. For this reason chromium surfaces are always shiny, which is why many metal objects are chrome plated.

When iron and ordinary steel are oxidized, on the other hand, the resulting rust does not seal the surface and oxidation can continue underneath. With enough chromium alloyed (mixed) with steel, the chromium is able to form an oxide coating that protects the entire surface. Such an alloy is called **stainless steel.** To be sure, some "stainless" steels do not have enough expensive chromium to be completely stainless and corrode in certain environments.

12.3   The Mole

The Chemist's Unit of Quantity

Regardless of how small may be the samples of matter involved in a chemical process in industry or the laboratory, so many atoms are present that counting them is out of the question. To measure the mass of a sample, however, is easy. What the chemist therefore needs is a way to relate the number of atoms in a chemical formula or equation to the corresponding masses of the substances.

To make clear the train of thought used to set up such a method, let us consider atoms of carbon and of oxygen. Since the mass of a carbon atom is 12 u and the mass of an oxygen atom is 16 u, the ratio of their masses is exactly 12:16. (We recall from Chap. 8 that u is the abbreviation of the atomic mass unit, which is equal to 1.66×10^{-27} kg.)

Now suppose we have samples of carbon and of oxygen that contain many atoms. However, no matter how many atoms the samples contain, if the ratio between the carbon and oxygen masses is the same 12 : 16 as the ratio between their atomic masses, the samples contain the same numbers of each kind of atom.

This reasoning can be extended to the atoms of any element. For convenience a quantity called the **mole** is defined in this way:

> A mole of any element is that amount of it whose mass in grams is equal to its atomic mass expressed in u.

The abbreviation of the mole is just mol. Thus the molar mass of carbon is 12 g and the molar mass of oxygen is 16 g (Fig. 12-6).

Avogadro's Number   The definition of the mole means that *a mole of any element contains the same number of atoms as a mole of any other element.* This number is a constant of nature called **Avogadro's number** (Fig. 12-7):

$$N_0 = 6.02 \times 10^{23} \text{ atoms/mol} \quad \textit{Avogadro's number}$$

Avogadro's number = number of atoms per mole of any element

The number of atoms in a sample of any element is just the number of moles in the sample multiplied by N_0.

Atom of carbon   Atom of oxygen

$m = 12$ u $m = 16$ u

Mole of carbon   Mole of oxygen

$m = 12$ g $m = 16$ g

Figure 12-6   The molar mass of any element is equal to its atomic mass expressed in grams.

Example 12.2

How many atoms are present in 100 g of iron?

Solution

Since the atomic mass of iron is 55.85 u, the mass of 1 mole of iron is 55.85 g. The number of moles in 100 g of iron is

$$\text{Moles of iron} = \frac{\text{mass of Fe}}{\text{molar mass of Fe}}$$

$$= \frac{100 \text{ g}}{55.85 \text{ g/mol}} = 1.79 \text{ mol}$$

The number of iron atoms is therefore (Fig. 12-8)

$$\text{Atoms of iron} = (\text{moles of iron})(\text{atoms/mol})$$

$$= (1.79 \text{ mol})(6.02 \times 10^{23} \text{ atoms/mol})$$

$$= 1.08 \times 10^{24} \text{ atoms}$$

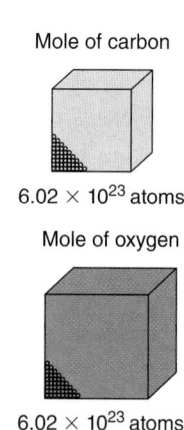

Mole of carbon

6.02×10^{23} atoms

Mole of oxygen

6.02×10^{23} atoms

Figure 12-7   A mole of any element contains 6.02×10^{23} atoms, which is Avogadro's number.

Figure 12-8   How the number of atoms in 100 g of iron can be calculated. (*a*) First the number of moles is found. (*b*) Then the total number of atoms is determined.

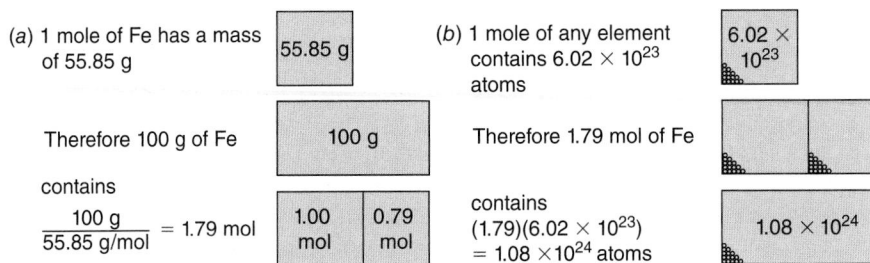

12.4   Formula Units

A Mole of Anything Contains Avogadro's Number of Formula Units

The concept of the mole is not limited to the elements. For instance, the gas carbon monoxide, CO, is a compound of carbon and oxygen whose molecules contain one atom of each kind. A molecule of CO therefore has a mass of $12 \text{ u} + 16 \text{ u} = 28 \text{ u}$, and a mole of CO has a mass of 28 g. There are N_0 molecules of CO in each mole of it.

Because many compounds, such as sodium chloride, $NaCl$, do not consist of individual molecules, it is more appropriate to deal with **formula units** rather than molecules in generalizing the definition of the mole. A formula unit of a substance is just the set of atoms given by its formula. In the case of CO, a formula unit is the same combination of one C atom and one O atom each molecule contains. For $NaCl$, a formula unit consists of one Na atom and one Cl atom. For the more complex compound sodium sulfate, Na_2SO_4, a formula unit consists of two Na atoms, one S atom, and four O atoms.

> The **formula mass** of a substance is the sum of the atomic masses of the elements it contains, each multiplied by the number of times it appears in the formula of the substance.

Evidently the formula mass of carbon monoxide is the same as its molecular mass of 28 u. Here is how the formula masses of sodium chloride and sodium sulfate, which do not exist in molecular form in the solid state, are found:

$$\begin{array}{ll}
\text{NaCl: 1 Na} = 22.99 \text{ u} & \text{Na}_2\text{SO}_4\text{: 2Na} = 2 \times 22.99 = 45.98 \text{ u} \\
\phantom{\text{NaCl: }} 1 \text{ Cl} = \underline{35.45 \text{ u}} & \phantom{\text{Na}_2\text{SO}_4\text{: }} 1\text{S} = 1 \times 32.06 = 32.06 \text{ u} \\
\text{Formula mass} = 58.44 \text{ u} & \phantom{\text{Na}_2\text{SO}_4\text{: }} 4\text{O} = 4 \times 16.00 = \underline{64.00 \text{ u}} \\
& \phantom{\text{Na}_2\text{SO}_4\text{: }} \text{Formula mass} = \overline{142.04 \text{ u}}
\end{array}$$

Now we can give a general definition of Avogadro's number:

$$N_0 = 6.02 \times 10^{23} \text{ formula units/mol} \qquad \textit{Avogadro's number}$$

Avogadro's number = number of formula units per mole of any substance

For a grocer, the normal unit of quantity for eggs is the dozen, equal to 12. For a paper manufacturer, the normal unit of quantity for his product is the ream, equal to 500 sheets. For a chemist, the normal unit of quantity of any substance is the mole, equal to N_0 formula units:

> A mole of any substance is that amount of it whose mass in grams is equal to its formula mass expressed in u.

Molarity of a Solution

The *molarity* of a solution is the number of moles of solute per liter of solution. A solution that contains 2 mol of sulfuric acid per liter is designated $2M$ H_2SO_4.

When a certain number of moles of a compound is needed for a particular reaction, it is convenient to be able just to pour out the corresponding volume of a solution of known molarity. Suppose we need 0.082 mol of sulfuric acid and have a bottle of $2M$ H_2SO_4. Since molarity = moles/liter,

$$\text{Volume needed} = \frac{\text{moles needed}}{\text{molarity}}$$

$$= \frac{0.082 \text{ mol}}{2 \text{ mol/liter}}$$

$$= 0.041 \text{ liter}$$

$$= 41 \text{ ml}$$

A mole of NaCl has a mass of 58.44 g, and a mole of Na_2SO_4 has a mass of 142.04 g.

The number of formula units in a mole is Avogadro's number.

Mass Relationships in Reactions   Owing to the way the mole is defined, a chemical equation can be interpreted in terms of moles as well as in terms of molecules or formula units.

As an example, let us consider the burning of propane, a gas that is widely used as a fuel for cooking and heating. When it burns, propane combines with oxygen from the air to form carbon dioxide and water vapor (Fig. 12-9). The process obeys the equation

$$C_3H_8 + 5O_2 \longrightarrow 3CO_2 + 4H_2O$$

which means that 1 molecule of C_3H_8 combines with 5 molecules of O_2 to yield 3 molecules of CO_2 and 4 molecules of H_2O. The equation equally correctly states that 1 mole of C_3H_8 combines with 5 moles of O_2 to yield 3 moles of CO_2 and 4 moles of H_2O:

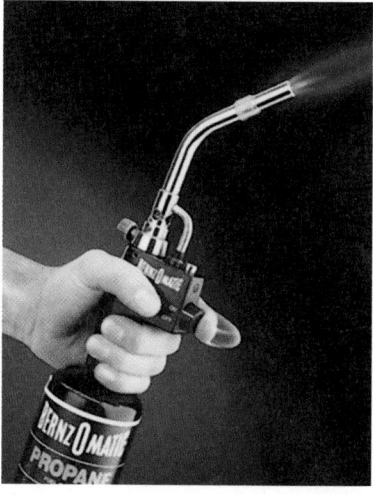

Figure 12-9   The combustion of propane produces carbon dioxide and water vapor and releases a great deal of energy.

$$\underset{\substack{\text{1 mole of}\\\text{propane}}}{C_3H_8} + \underset{\substack{\text{5 moles of}\\\text{oxygen}}}{5O_2} \longrightarrow \underset{\substack{\text{3 moles of}\\\text{carbon}\\\text{dioxide}}}{3CO_2} + \underset{\substack{\text{4 moles of}\\\text{water}}}{4H_2O}$$

Example 12.3

How many grams of oxygen are needed to burn 100 g of propane?

Solution

We start by finding the formula masses of oxygen and propane:

$$O_2: 2O = 2 \times 16.00 = 32.00 \text{ u} \qquad \begin{aligned} C_3H_8: 3C &= 3 \times 12.00 = 36.00 \text{ u}\\ 8H &= 8 \times 1.008 = \underline{8.06 \text{ u}}\\ & 44.06 \text{ u} \end{aligned}$$

Therefore the molar masses of oxygen and propane are, respectively, 32.00 g and 44.06 g. The number of moles in 100 g of propane is

$$\text{Moles of propane} = \frac{\text{mass of } C_3H_8}{\text{molar mass of } C_3H_8} = \frac{100 \text{ g}}{44.06 \text{ g/mol}} = 2.27 \text{ mol}$$

From the equation of the reaction, 5 moles of O_2 are needed for every mole of C_3H_8, so the number of moles of oxygen we need is

$$\text{Moles of oxygen} = \left(\frac{\text{moles of } O_2}{\text{mole of } C_3H_8}\right)(\text{moles of } C_3H_8)$$
$$= (5)(2.27 \text{ mol}) = 11.35 \text{ mol}$$

The mass of oxygen needed is

$$\text{Mass of oxygen} = (\text{moles of } O_2)(\text{molar mass of } O_2)$$
$$= (11.35 \text{ mol})(32.00 \text{ g/mol}) = 363 \text{ g}$$

A total of 363 g of oxygen is needed for the complete combustion of 100 g of propane (Fig. 12-10). Propane and other hydrocarbon gases, such as butane and methane (natural gas), need surprisingly large amounts of oxygen to burn completely.

Figure 12-10 How the mass of oxygen needed to burn 100 g of propane is calculated. (*a*) First the number of moles of propane is found. (*b*) Then the number of moles of oxygen is found. (*c*) Finally the mass of oxygen is determined. The formula for the process is $C_3H_8 + 5O_2 \longrightarrow 3CO_2 + 4H_2O$.

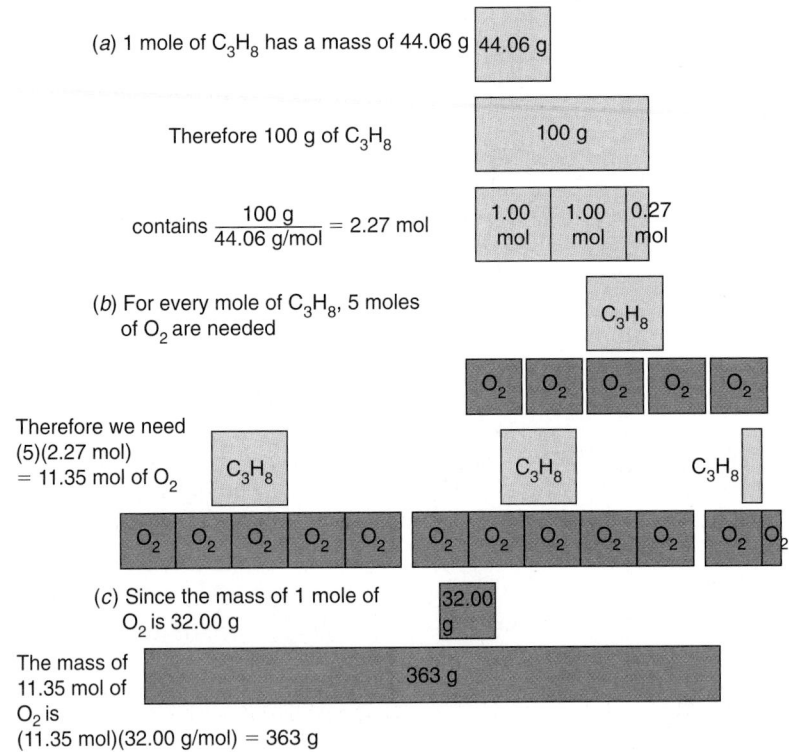

Chemical Energy

Ever since our ancestors learned to control fire, people have been putting chemical energy to practical use. Today we transform it not only into heat and light but into mechanical energy and electric energy as well. Locked up in matter, chemical energy long remained a mystery. The modern picture of the atom and of the chemical bond, however, is able to explain the nature of this energy.

12.5 Exothermic and Endothermic Reactions

Some Reactions Liberate Energy; Others Absorb It

Chemical changes that *give off* energy are called **exothermic reactions.** (In Greek, *exo* means "outside.") The burning of coal, which is largely carbon, and of hydrogen are both exothermic:

$$C + O_2 \longrightarrow CO_2 + E \qquad E = 9 \text{ kJ/g of } CO_2 \qquad \textit{Formation of carbon dioxide}$$

$$2H_2 + O_2 \longrightarrow 2H_2O + E \qquad E = 13.6 \text{ kJ/g of } H_2O \qquad \textit{Formation of water}$$

Chemical changes that take place only when heat or some other kind of energy is *absorbed* are called **endothermic reactions.** (In Greek, *endo* means "inside.") The decomposition of water into hydrogen and oxygen requires heating to very high temperatures or the supply of electric energy during electrolysis (see Fig. 10-23), so it is endothermic:

$$2H_2O + E \longrightarrow 2H_2 + O_2 \qquad E = 13.6 \text{ kJ/g of } H_2O \qquad \textit{Decomposition of water}$$

The *Hindenburg* Fire

The German airship *Hindenburg* was filled with hydrogen. In 1937, after crossing the Atlantic, it caught fire while landing at Lakehurst, New Jersey (Fig. 12-11). The combustion of hydrogen is an exothermic reaction whose product is water. Today's airships use the inert gas helium, which is denser than hydrogen and so less buoyant but is completely safe.

Because the *Hindenburg* fire was bright whereas flames from a hydrogen fire are almost invisible, it has been proposed that the *Hindenburg* fire occurred primarily in the paint on its envelope.

However, experiments on surviving pieces and replica samples of the airship's envelope show that they burn far too slowly to account for the event; instead of the observed 34 seconds, the fire would have lasted 40 hours. Of course, if the hydrogen had been ignited first, as seems probable from the available evidence, the envelope would then burn brightly and other materials in the airship would glow in the way the mantle of a gas lantern does. Both effects would have contributed to the spectacle shown in the photograph.

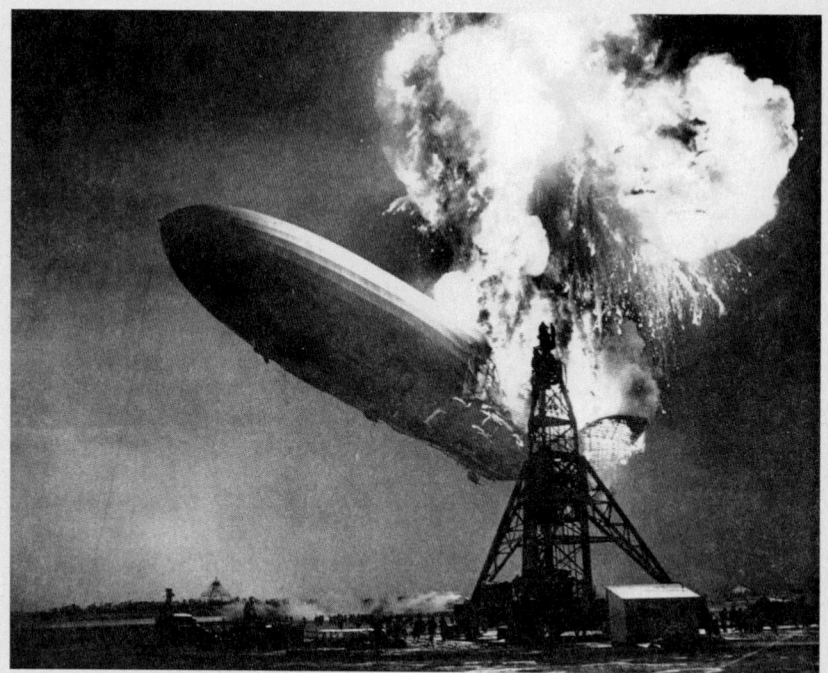

Figure 12-11   The hydrogen-filled airship *Hindenburg* took only 34 seconds to burn up.

The formation of nitric oxide (NO) from the elements N_2 and O_2 is an endothermic reaction that takes place only at high temperatures (Fig. 12-12):

$$N_2 + O_2 + E \longrightarrow 2NO \qquad E = 3 \text{ kJ/g of NO}$$

Formation of nitric oxide

Direct and Reverse Reactions   From the law of conservation of energy we can predict that, if a given reaction is exothermic, the reverse reaction will be endothermic. Furthermore, the amount of heat liberated by the exothermic reaction must be the same as the amount of heat absorbed by the endothermic reaction. This prediction is borne out in the case of water, as we just saw, and is also verified in all other reactions where it can be tested. An example is sodium reacting with chlorine:

$$2Na + Cl_2 \longrightarrow 2NaCl + E \quad E = 7 \text{ kJ/g of NaCl}$$

Formation of sodium chloride (Exothermic)

To break up NaCl takes the same amount of energy:

$$2NaCl + E \longrightarrow 2Na + Cl_2 \qquad E = 7 \text{ kJ/g of NaCl}$$

Decomposition of sodium chloride (Endothermic)

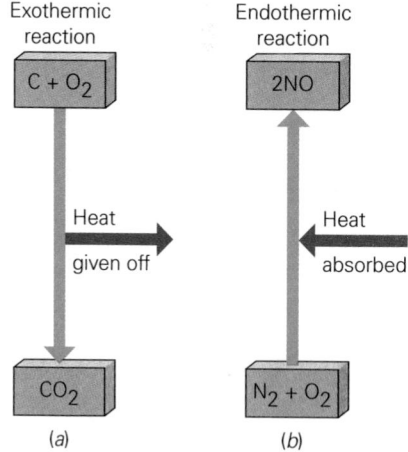

Figure 12-12   Examples of exothermic and endothermic reactions. (*a*) The burning of coal to form carbon dioxide gas gives off 9 kJ of heat per gram of CO_2. (*b*) The formation of nitric oxide requires 3 kJ of heat to be absorbed per gram of NO.

Dissociation and Neutralization   The dissociation of most salts is an endothermic process. For example, when KNO_3 is dissolved in water,

Hot and Cold Packs

Although most salts absorb heat when they dissolve in water, some give off heat in this process. These effects are used in the hot and cold packs that are sometimes applied as first aid for minor injuries. A hot pack contains a plastic bag of water and a salt whose solution is exothermic, for example calcium chloride. In a cold pack the salt is one whose solution is endothermic, for example ammonium nitrate. Squeezing the pack breaks the water bag and, as the salt dissolves, the pack becomes hot or cold depending on what kind of salt is present.

the container becomes cold, since the dissociation of the salt requires energy:

$$KNO_3 + E \longrightarrow K^+ + NO_3^- \quad E = 0.36 \text{ kJ/g of } KNO_3 \qquad \textit{Dissociation of potassium nitrate}$$

Neutralization, on the other hand, is an exothermic process. If concentrated solutions of NaOH and HCl are mixed, for instance, the mixture quickly becomes too hot to touch:

$$H^+ + OH^- \longrightarrow H_2O + E \quad E = 3.2 \text{ kJ/g of } H_2O \qquad \textit{Neutralization}$$

The Na^+ and Cl^- ions are omitted here because the principal chemical change in all neutralizations is simply the joining together of hydrogen ions and hydroxide ions. For the same reason the neutralization of any other strong acid by any other strong base liberates almost precisely the same amount of heat for each gram of water produced.

12.6 Chemical Energy and Stability

The Less PE Its Electrons Have, the More Stable the Compound

The heat given off or absorbed in a chemical change is a measure of the stabilities of the substances (or mixtures of substances) involved. If a great deal of energy is needed to decompose a substance, the substance is (with rare exceptions) relatively stable. If the decomposition is either exothermic or weakly endothermic, the substance is normally unstable.

From the reactions given in Sec. 12.5 we can see at a glance that CO_2, H_2O, and NaCl are stable compounds, since the formation of each is strongly exothermic and its decomposition is endothermic. NO, on the other hand, is unstable, since its decomposition liberates heat. The combinations H_2 and O_2, Na and Cl_2, H^+ and OH^- are relatively unstable, since they react to give off energy. On the other hand, N_2 and O_2 form a stable mixture since energy must be supplied for them to react.

Bond Energies and Reaction Energy We can interpret chemical-energy changes in terms of atomic structure (Fig. 12-13). When sodium reacts with chlorine, for example, the outer electron of each Na atom is transferred to

Explosives

An explosive is a material in which a violent reaction can occur whose products are rapidly expanding gases. Most explosives contain nitrogen compounds because N_2 molecules, which have triple covalent bonds between their N atoms (see Sec. 10.12), are very stable and so their formation in an explosion is strongly exothermic.

The earliest explosive in wide use was gunpowder, a mixture of potassium nitrate (KNO_3), charcoal, and sulfur. The Chinese invention of gunpowder over a thousand years ago, together with their later inventions of

printing and the magnetic compass, began the modern era of human history. Until the fifteenth century, China was the most technologically advanced country in the world.

When gunpowder is ignited, oxygen from the KNO_3 combines with carbon in the charcoal to give CO_2 and with sulfur to give SO_2, and the nitrogen in the KNO_3 becomes N_2. The temperature of the explosion is thought to be about 2700°C.

More recent explosives, such as nitroglycerin and trinitrotoluene (TNT), consist of molecules that each contain carbon, hydrogen,

oxygen, and nitrogen whose recombination yields gaseous products. For instance, when nitroglycerin explodes,

$$4C_3H_5(NO_3)_3 \longrightarrow 12CO_2 + 10H_2O + 6N_2 + O_2$$

Nitroglycerin is dangerous to handle because it blows up at the slightest shock. Dynamite is a mixture of nitroglycerin and other explosives with inert ingredients that make the combination safe to work with. Dynamite is set off by a small explosive detonator that is activated electrically (see Fig. 13-11).

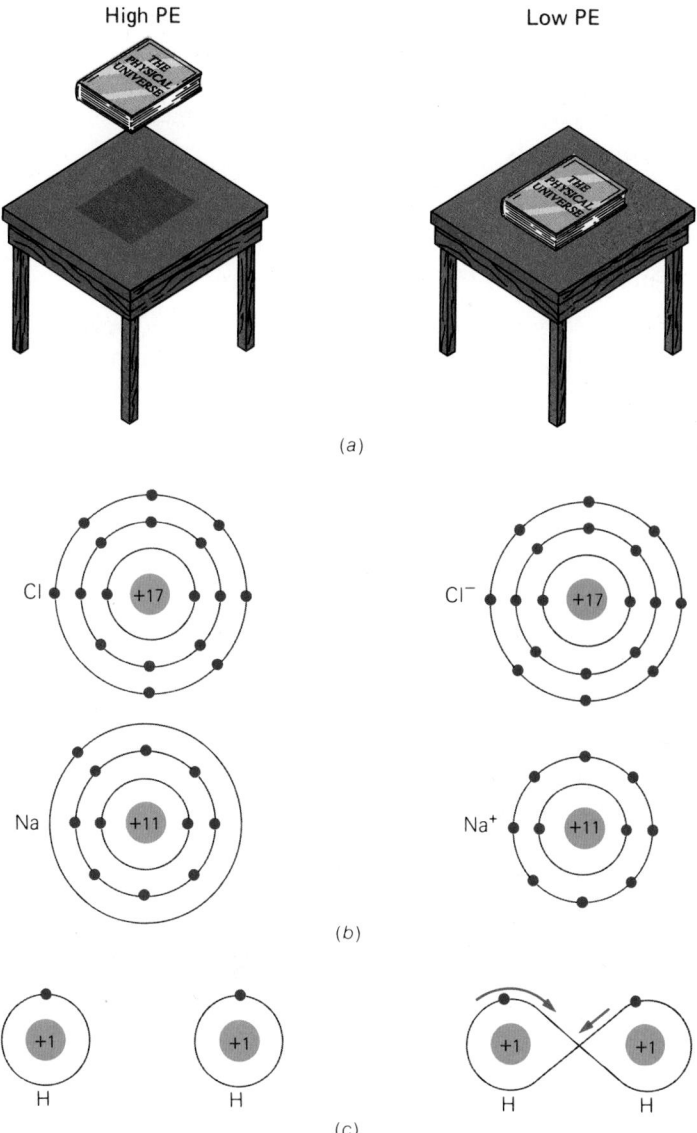

High PE   Low PE

(a)

(b)

(c)

Figure 12-13 (a) A book raised above a table has more PE than the same book lying on the table because the attractive force the earth exerts on the book is greater when the book is closer to the earth. (b) The outer electron in an Na atom has more PE than the same electron has when it is attached to a Cl atom to form a Cl⁻ ion because the electron is more strongly attracted to the nucleus of the Cl⁻ ion (see Fig. 10-16). (c) The electron in an H atom has more PE than the same electron has when it is part of an H molecule because in the H molecule the electron is attracted by two protons rather than one proton.

the outer shell of a Cl atom. In its new position the electron has less potential energy with respect to the atomic nuclei because it is held more firmly to the chlorine nucleus than it was to the sodium nucleus. The same is true for other ionic bonds.

When two hydrogen atoms react to form a hydrogen molecule, the atoms are joined by shared electrons. Such a covalent bond involves a decrease in the PE of the electrons because each is now attracted by two nuclei instead of a single nucleus. The same is true for other covalent bonds.

When electrons move to new locations during an exothermic reaction, some of their original PE is liberated. This released energy may show itself in faster atomic or molecular motions that correspond to a higher temperature. Or the freed energy may excite outer electrons into higher energy levels from which they return to lower levels by giving off photons of light. In endothermic reactions, energy must be supplied to the atoms involved to enable some of their electrons to form bonds in which their PEs are greater than before.

Whether a reaction is endothermic or exothermic thus depends on the difference between the energy needed to break the chemical bonds in the reacting substances—by separating atoms in the molecules of covalent compounds or the ions in ionic compounds—and the energy released in the formation of new bonds in the reaction products. If the energy needed to break the initial bonds is greater than the energy released as the final bonds are made, the reaction is endothermic. If the reverse is true, the reaction is exothermic. Bond energies vary, so the energy changes in different reactions are correspondingly different.

12.7 Activation Energy

The Initial Energy Needed to Start an Exothermic Reaction

Wood burns in air to give off great quantities of heat. However, we can store a pile of firewood indefinitely without its catching fire. A mixture of hydrogen and oxygen can explode violently. However, hydrogen does not explode when mixed with air unless a flame or spark sets off the reaction. Why do not all exothermic reactions take place at once of their own accord?

Clearly, in order to begin, many exothermic processes must first be supplied with energy. The preceding discussion gives the reason. A mixture of hydrogen and oxygen is like the car of Fig. 12-14, whose potential energy may be converted to kinetic energy if it moves down into the valley. However, the car cannot begin to go downward unless it is first given enough energy to climb to the top of the hill. Similarly the chemical energy of a mixture of hydrogen and oxygen can be freed only if the molecules have enough energy, or are sufficiently **activated,** to make the reaction start. The energy needed for activation, corresponding to the energy required to move the car up the hill, is called the **activation energy** of the reaction.

The electron picture of chemical combination suggests the reason for activation energy. The reaction of oxygen and hydrogen involves the formation of bonds between O and H atoms, a process that gives out energy. However, before these bonds can be formed, the covalent bonds between the hydrogen atoms in H_2 molecules and the oxygen atoms in O_2 molecules must be broken. To break these bonds takes energy. Once the reaction starts, the energy already liberated can supply the needed energy, but in the beginning some activation energy must be supplied from outside. Thus a mixture of hydrogen and oxygen need only be touched with a flame for the reaction to spread so rapidly that an explosion results. When a bed of coal is set on fire it continues to burn, since the heat liberated in one place is sufficient to ignite the coal around it.

Activated Molecules   A molecule with enough energy to react is called an **activated molecule.** In reactions that take place spontaneously at room temperature (for example, the reaction between hydrogen and fluorine), enough of the initial molecules have the required KE of thermal motion for their bonds to break during collisions without further activation. Ions in solution are, so to speak, already activated and react almost instantaneously. But a large number of exothermic reactions must have the preliminary activation of some molecules before the reactions can take place in a self-sustaining way.

Figure 12-14   Activation energy. The potential energy of the car will be converted into kinetic energy if it moves down into the valley. However, the car requires initial kinetic energy in order to climb the hill between it and the valley, analogous to the activation energy required in many exothermic reactions.

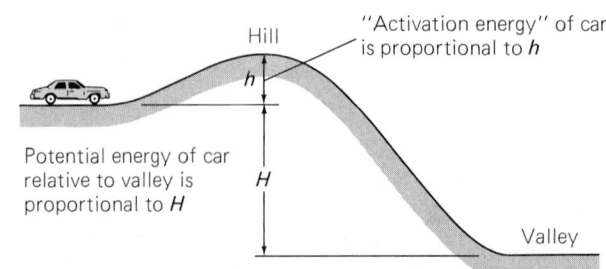

Reaction Rates

Some chemical changes are practically instantaneous. Thus in neutralization the acid and base react as soon as they are stirred together. Silver chloride is precipitated immediately when solutions that contain silver ions and chloride ions are mixed. The reaction involved in a dynamite explosion takes a fraction of a second. In contrast, other chemical changes, like the rusting of iron, take place slowly.

Reaction rates depend first of all on the nature of the reacting substances: iron corrodes faster than copper, for example. In any particular reaction the rate is influenced by four principal factors (Table 12-1). These are temperature, concentrations of the reacting substances, the exposed surface area in the case of reactions that involve solids, and the presence of an appropriate catalyst.

12.8   Temperature and Reaction Rates

Hotter Means Faster

Reaction rates are always increased by a rise in temperature. This is why we use hot water rather than cold for washing. Reaction rates for many common processes that occur at or near room temperature are approximately doubled for every 10°C increase in temperature.

The kinetic theory of matter suggests one obvious reason for the increase of reaction rates with temperature. Most reactions depend on collisions between particles, and the number of collisions increases with rising temperature because molecular speeds are increased. But a 10°C rise is nowhere near enough to double the number of collisions in a particular sample. To find the principal explanation, we must go back to the idea of activation energy.

Why Reaction Rates Vary with Temperature   If molecules must be activated before they can react, reaction rates should depend not on the total number of collisions per second but on the number of collisions between *activated* molecules (see Sec. 12.5). Activated molecules in a fluid (liquid or gas) are produced by ordinary molecular motion as a result of exceptionally energetic collisions. Such molecules remain activated only a short time before losing energy in further collisions (unless they react in the meantime).

In any fluid, then, a certain fraction of the molecules is activated at any time. The fraction may be very small at ordinary temperatures, but it increases rapidly as the temperature rises and molecular motion speeds up. Reaction rates increase with temperature chiefly because the number of activated molecules increases, to a smaller extent because collisions are more frequent.

At room temperature, for instance, a mixture of hydrogen and oxygen contains very few molecules with sufficient energy to react. The reaction is so slow that the gases may remain mixed for years without anything happening.

Table 12-1	Factors That Affect Reaction Rates

Factor	Effect
Temperature	The higher the temperature, the faster the reaction
Concentration	The higher the concentration of the reactants, the faster the reaction
Surface area	The greater the surface area of a solid reactant, the faster the reaction
Catalyst	Increases the reaction rate

Even at 400°C the rate is small, but at 600° enough of the molecules are activated to make the reaction fast, and at 700° so many are activated that the mixture explodes.

This kind of behavior is typical of many reactions between molecules. At low temperatures the chemical changes are so slow that for all practical purposes they do not occur; in a range of intermediate temperatures the reactions are moderately rapid; and at high temperatures they become practically instantaneous. Reactions between ions, on the other hand, occur immediately even at room temperature, since the ionic state itself is a form of activation.

12.9   Other Factors

Concentration, Surface Area, and Catalysts

The effect of concentration on reaction speed is illustrated by rates of burning in air and in pure oxygen. The pure gas has almost 5 times as many oxygen molecules per cubic centimeter as air, and combustion in pure oxygen is correspondingly faster.

As a general rule, the rate of a simple chemical reaction is proportional to the concentration of each reacting substance. The number of collisions between activated molecules, which determines the reaction speed, depends on the total number of collisions and this, in turn, depends on how many molecules each cubic centimeter contains.

Surface Area   When a reaction takes place between two solids or between a fluid and a solid, the reaction speed depends markedly on the amount of solid surface exposed. A finely powdered solid presents vastly more surface than a few large chunks (Fig. 12-15), and reactions of powders are accordingly much faster. Granulated sugar dissolves more rapidly in water than lump sugar; finely divided zinc is attacked by acid quickly, larger pieces are attacked slowly; ordinary iron rusts slowly, but the oxidation of iron powder is fast enough to produce a flame.

The explanation is obvious: the greater the surface, the more quickly atoms and molecules can get together to react. For a similar reason, efficient stirring speeds up reactions between fluids.

Catalysts   A **catalyst** is a substance that speeds up a reaction without being permanently changed itself. As an example of catalytic action, let us consider the decomposition of hydrogen peroxide, H_2O_2. At ordinary temperatures solutions of hydrogen peroxide are unstable and slowly turn into water and oxygen:

$$2H_2O_2 \longrightarrow 2H_2O + O_2$$

Figure 12-15   Cutting a cube into 8 smaller cubes doubles its original surface area. Cutting the smaller cubes further gives a still larger total surface area, and grinding them into a fine powder increases the area by a huge amount. When a solid undergoes a chemical reaction, the greater its surface area, the faster the reaction.

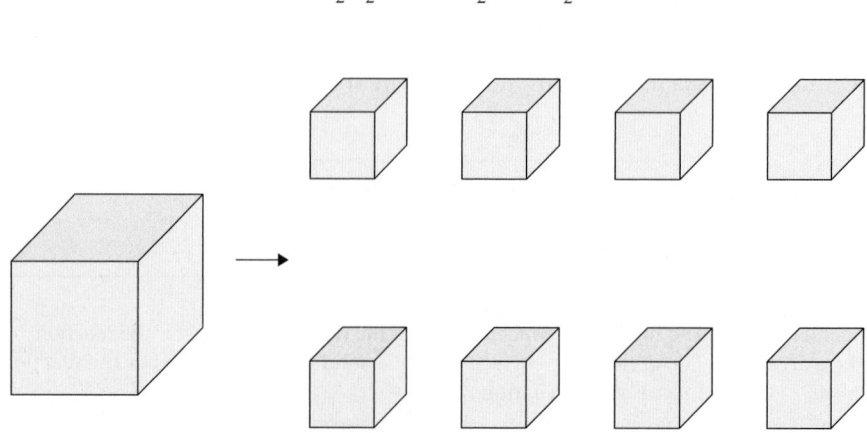

If a little powdered manganese dioxide is added to the solution, the decomposition goes much faster, with oxygen bubbling up violently. At the end of the reaction the manganese dioxide remains unchanged. Commercial solutions of hydrogen peroxide usually contain a trace of the compound acetanilid, which acts to retard their decomposition.

Catalysts accelerate reactions in different ways. In some cases the catalyst forms an unstable intermediate compound with one of the reacting substances, and this compound decomposes later in the reaction. Most catalysts, notably certain metals such as platinum, increase reaction rates by producing activated molecules at their surfaces. No adequate explanation is known for the action of some catalysts. A given reaction is usually influenced only by a few catalysts, and these may or may not affect other reactions. Catalysts are essential in many industrial processes, for instance, oil refining (Sec. 13.3).

Enzymes   The many chemical processes that take place in living things, for instance the digestion of food, are controlled by catalysts called **enzymes.** An enzyme is a protein molecule whose physical structure is such that it attracts specific molecules to its surface, promotes their reaction, and then releases the products. Each enzyme catalyzes a particular reaction, and thousands of different ones are present in the human body. The reacting molecules fit into the outside of the enzyme for a process much as a key fits into a lock: if their shapes do not match, nothing will happen. Enzymes in yeast promote the fermentation of sugars into ethanol (ethyl alcohol) described in Sec. 13.9.

12.10 Chemical Equilibrium

One Step Forward; One Step Back

Most chemical reactions are reversible. That is, under suitable conditions the products of a chemical change can usually be made to react "backward" to give the original substances. We have seen many examples in other connections. Hydrogen burns in oxygen to form water, and water decomposes into these elements during electrolysis. Mercury and oxygen combine when heated moderately, and the oxide decomposes when heated more strongly. Carbon dioxide reacts with water to give hydrogen and hydrogen carbonate (HCO_3^-) ions, and these ions recombine all the time to form the original CO_2 and H_2O.

There is no reason why, under the right conditions, the forward and backward processes of a chemical change cannot take place at the same time. In a bottle of soda water (Fig. 12-16), some of the CO_2 reacts with the water. But a number of the resulting H^+ and HCO_3^- ions then join together to give CO_2 and H_2O. The recombination rate increases with the ion concentration until, finally, as many ions recombine each second as are being formed. At this point the rates of the forward and backward reactions are the same, and the amounts of the various substances do not change. The situation can be represented by the single equation

$$H_2O + CO_2 \rightleftharpoons H^+ + HCO_3^-$$

The double arrow indicates that reactions in both directions occur together.

A State of Balance   Such a situation is called **chemical equilibrium.** It is a state of balance determined by two opposing processes. The two processes do not reach equilibrium and stop, but instead continue indefinitely because each process constantly undoes what the other accomplishes.

As an analogy, we might imagine a person walking up an escalator while the escalator is moving down. If the person walks as fast in one direction as the escalator is moving in the other, the two motions will be in equilibrium and the person will remain in the same place indefinitely.

Catalytic Converters

Ideally, the engine of a car should burn its fuel completely and emit only carbon dioxide and water vapor in its exhaust. Actual engines and fuels, however, also produce carbon monoxide and various hydrocarbons, which are toxic, and nitrogen oxides, which contribute to acid rain through the nitric acid they form. One way to reduce the amount of such pollutants is to use a catalytic converter in which exhaust gases pass through an assembly of small tubes lined with a porous ceramic that contains particles of platinum and rhodium. The platinum is a catalyst for the oxidation of carbon monoxide and the hydrocarbons to CO_2 and H_2O, and the rhodium is a catalyst for the decomposition of the nitrogen oxides to N_2 and O_2. Most of the polluting gases are eliminated in this way. [For more on carbon monoxide, see Sec. 12.9 at www.mhhe.com/krauskopf.]

Self-cleaning Windows

The compound titanium dioxide, which is what makes most white paint white, is also an efficient photocatalyst that promotes the dissociation of water molecules by ultraviolet light. The resulting OH^- ions disrupt organic molecules of all kinds.

Because water vapor is always present in the atmosphere and sunlight contains ultraviolet light, titanium dioxide coatings thin enough to be transparent are being used on window glass to make them self-cleaning. The breakdown products of dirt on the windows are easily washed away by rain. Titanium dioxide is also used in a similar way to treat polluted water and to sterilize hospital surfaces using artificial sources of ultraviolet light.

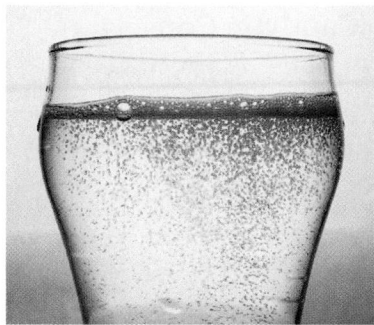

Figure 12-16   In soda water, dissolved carbon dioxide reacts with water to give hydrogen and hydrogen carbonate ions. At the same time, hydrogen and hydrogen carbonate ions are recombining to form carbon dioxide and water. The forward and reverse reactions occur at the same rate, which is an example of chemical equilibrium.

A great many chemical changes reach a state of equilibrium instead of going to completion. Equilibrium may be established when a reaction is nearly complete, or when it is only just starting, or when both products and reacting substances are present in comparable amounts.

The point at which equilibrium occurs depends on the rates of the opposing reactions. The initial reaction always dominates until the products are abundant enough for the reverse reaction to go at the same rate. Thus the extent to which an acid is dissociated depends on how fast its molecules break down into ions compared with how fast the ions recombine. HCl dissociates so rapidly in solution into H^+ and Cl^- that the reverse reaction has no chance to maintain a measurable amount of HCl. On the other hand, acetic acid dissociates slowly, and when only a small concentration of ions has been built up, the recombination occurs at the same rate as the dissociation.

Example 12.4

Under what circumstances will a liquid-phase reaction go to completion instead of an equilibrium being established?

Solution

When one of the products of a reaction leaves the system, the reaction must go to completion since the reverse reaction then cannot occur. A reaction in a liquid will go to completion if one of the products is (a) a gas that escapes; (b) an insoluble precipitate; or (c) composed of molecules that do not dissociate when the reaction involves ions.

12.11   Altering an Equilibrium

How to Get Farther Up the Down Escalator

Often a chemist wishing to prepare a compound finds that the reaction reaches equilibrium before very much of the compound has been formed. Once this happens, waiting for more of the product to form is useless, for its amount does not change after that. How can equilibrium conditions be altered to increase the yield of the product?

Since equilibrium represents a balance between two rates, what is needed to increase the yield is a way to change the speed of one reaction or the other. Speeding up or slowing down one of the reactions in an equilibrium is not as simple as changing the rate of a single reaction, but the same factors that affect reaction rates also influence equilibrium. The chemist has three chief methods available for shifting an equilibrium to favor one direction or the other. These are:

1. Change the concentration of one or more substances. For example, removing the gaseous product of a reaction will retard the reverse reaction. Thus opening a soda bottle allows CO_2 to escape, which decreases the rate of formation of H^+ and HCO_3^- and so lowers the acidity of the solution.
2. Change the temperature. If one reaction in an equilibrium is exothermic (gives off energy), the other is necessarily endothermic (absorbs energy). A rise in temperature, although it makes both reactions go faster, will favor the endothermic one.
3. Change the pressure. This is most effective in gas reactions where the number of product molecules differs from the number of initial molecules. Increasing the pressure favors the reaction that gives the

The Haber Process

Fritz Haber (1868–1934) was the German chemist who perfected the synthesis of ammonia from nitrogen and hydrogen. Carl Bosch adapted the process for the commercial production of ammonia, which began in 1913, just in time to provide Germany with the nitrogen compounds it needed to manufacture explosives for World War I. Without the Haber-Bosch process, German guns would have run out of ammunition in 6 months.

After the war, the same process was used to "fix" nitrogen for use in fertilizers; nitrogen is an essential constituent of all proteins (see Sec. 13.14). Much of the world's agriculture today depends on fertilizers based on synthetic ammonia, for whose development Haber received the Nobel Prize in chemistry in 1919. The

breakthrough was hailed as *Brot aus Luft*, bread from the air.

In what he saw as a humanitarian effort to minimize overall casualties by bringing about a quick German victory in World War I, Haber pioneered the use of poison gas as a battlefield weapon. Horrified, his wife committed suicide, and the Allies labeled Haber a war criminal for the immense suffering gas warfare caused.

Despite his contributions to the war effort, Haber, who was Jewish, had to flee Germany in 1933 to escape the increasing persecution of Jews there. The insecticide Zyklon B, whose development Haber had worked on in the 1920s, was later used in modified form by the Nazis to kill millions of people, mainly Jews, among whom were members of Haber's family.

fewest molecules. An example is the synthesis of ammonia from nitrogen and hydrogen in the reaction

$$N_2 + 3H_2 \rightleftharpoons 2NH_3 \qquad \textit{Ammonia synthesis}$$

A rise in pressure increases the yield of ammonia because the ammonia occupies only half the volume of the gases that react to form it. Pressures of 150 to 350 atm are used in modern ammonia production plants.

Example 12.5

Hydrogen sulfide gas dissolves in water and ionizes very slightly:

$$H_2S \rightleftharpoons 2H^+ + S^{2-}$$

How would the acidity of the solution (that is, the concentration of H^+) be affected by (a) increasing the pressure of H_2S? (b) Raising the temperature? (c) Adding a solution of silver nitrate? (Silver sulfide, Ag_2S, is insoluble.)

Solution

(a) The acidity would increase because the greater the gas pressure, the more of it dissolves. (b) The acidity would decrease because the solubility of gases decreases with increasing temperature. (c) The acidity would increase because removing S^{2-} ions reduces the rate at which H_2S leaves the solution without affecting the rate at which H_2S enters it.

Oxidation and Reduction

Until now we have used the term **oxidation** to mean the chemical combination of a substance with oxygen. A related term is **reduction,** which refers to the removal of oxygen from a compound. When oxygen reacts with another substance (except fluorine), the oxygen atoms pick up electrons donated by the atoms of that substance. When the resulting compound is reduced, the atoms of the substances that had been oxidized regain the electrons initially lost to the oxygen atoms.

12.12   Oxidation-Reduction Reactions

They Always Go Together

It is convenient to generalize oxidation and reduction to refer to *any* chemical process in which electrons are transferred from one element to another, regardless of whether or not oxygen is involved. Hence

> Oxidation refers to the loss of electrons by the atoms of an element, and reduction refers to the gain of electrons.

The oxidation of one element is always accompanied by the reduction of another. The two processes must take place together. For example, when zinc combines with chlorine, electrons are given up by the zinc atoms to the chlorine atoms. Thus the zinc is oxidized and the chlorine is reduced in the reaction:

$$Zn \longrightarrow Zn^{2+} + 2e^- \qquad \textit{Oxidation}$$
$$Cl_2 + 2e^- \longrightarrow 2Cl^- \qquad \textit{Reduction}$$

Reactions that involve electron transfer are called **oxidation-reduction reactions,** and they make up a large and important category of chemical reactions.

Example 12.6

Chlorine is a powerful oxidizing agent, which is the reason it is used as a bleach. Do you think a chlorine solution would remove a rust stain on a piece of clothing?

Solution

Because the iron in rust is already oxidized, the chlorine solution will have no effect.

Electrolysis   Electrolysis is an oxidation-reduction process. Let us consider the electrolysis of molten sodium chloride, which consists of the ions Na^+ and Cl^-. An **electrode** is a conductor through which electric current enters or leaves a solution. When electrodes in the molten NaCl are connected to the terminals of a battery, Na^+ ions are attracted to the negative electrode and Cl^- ions to the positive electrode, as in Fig. 12-17. At the positive electrode each Cl^- is neutralized by giving up its extra electron and becomes a chlorine atom:

$$Cl^- \longrightarrow Cl + e^- \qquad \textit{Oxidation}$$

The Cl atoms pair off to form molecules of chlorine gas, Cl_2. At the negative electrode each Na^+ is neutralized by gaining an electron and becomes a sodium atom:

$$Na^+ + e^- \longrightarrow Na \qquad \textit{Reduction}$$

The net result of sending a current through molten salt, then, is to break up the compound NaCl into its constituent elements:

$$2NaCl \longrightarrow 2Na + Cl_2 \qquad \textit{Electrolysis of sodium chloride}$$

The sodium, a liquid at the temperature of molten salt, collects around the negative electrode, and chlorine gas bubbles up around the positive electrode. This procedure is commonly used to prepare metallic sodium.

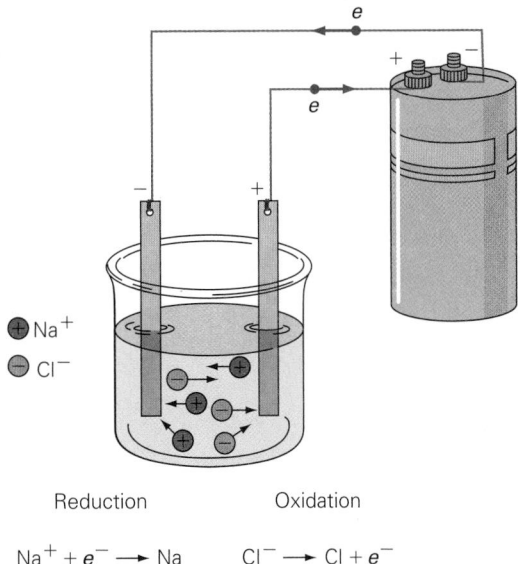

Figure 12-17 The electrolysis of molten sodium chloride. The current in the liquid consists of moving Na^+ and Cl^- ions; the current in the wires consists of moving electrons.

Reduction   Oxidation

$$Na^+ + e^- \longrightarrow Na \qquad Cl^- \longrightarrow Cl + e^-$$

Electroplating Electrolysis is used in the process of **electroplating** in which a thin layer of one metal is deposited on an object made of another metal. Sometimes this is done because the plating metal is expensive, for instance gold or silver. In other cases the object is to protect the base metal from corrosion, as in the tin or chromium plating of steel (Fig. 12-18). Nonmetallic items can be plated by first coating them with a conducting material such as graphite.

Figure 12-19 shows how a spoon can be silver-plated. The procedure uses a solution of silver nitrate, which dissociates into Ag^+ and NO_3^- ions. Silver atoms lose electrons (which flow to the battery) at the positive electrode and enter the solution as Ag^+ ions. These ions are attracted to the spoon, which acts as a negative electrode, from which they pick up electrons (supplied by the battery) to become silver atoms again. In this way silver atoms are transferred from the positive electrode to the spoon. Because an Ag atom loses an electron to become Ag^+ more readily than an NO_3^- ion loses its extra electron, the NO_3^- ions stay in solution and do not participate in the plating process.

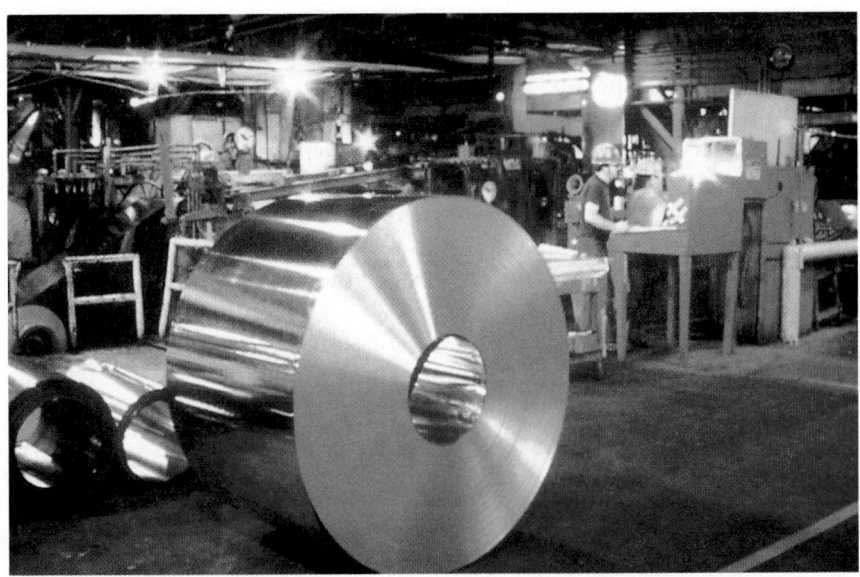

Figure 12-18 Steel plated with tin to prevent corrosion is widely used for food and beverage containers.

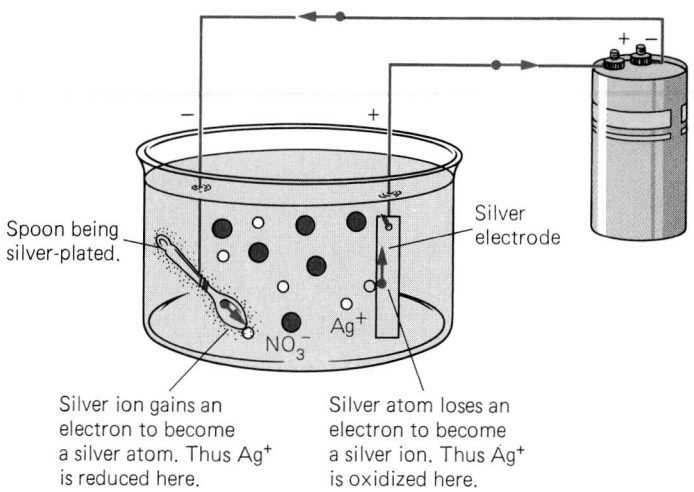

Figure 12-19 Silver plating. The bath is a solution of silver nitrate, $AgNO_3$. The nitrate ions remain in solution because Ag atoms lose electrons at the positive electrode more readily than NO_3^- ions do.

Spoon being silver-plated.

Silver electrode

Silver ion gains an electron to become a silver atom. Thus Ag^+ is reduced here.

Silver atom loses an electron to become a silver ion. Thus Ag^+ is oxidized here.

Aluminum

Although aluminum is the third most abundant element in the earth's outer layer and the most abundant metal there, it was not discovered until 1827. Chemical methods for preparing aluminum were so expensive then that for some time its main use was in jewelry, and attempts to refine aluminum by electrolysis were balked by the difficulty of melting or dissolving aluminum ores.

Finally, in 1886, a 22-year-old American, Charles Martin Hall, found that cryolite, a mineral abundant in Greenland, when melted would dissolve the chief aluminum ore, Al_2O_3. Passing an electric current through a solution of Al_2O_3 in molten cryolite liberates aluminum at the negative electrode and oxygen at the positive one: this is the process used today to refine aluminum.

About 11 kJ of electric energy is needed to produce each gram of aluminum metal, which is a lot of energy: 2 percent of all the world's energy is used to refine aluminum. To recycle aluminum, notably the aluminum cans discarded by the billion every year, basically involves heating it to its melting point and then melting it, which takes less than 1 kJ/g. Hence recycling aluminum uses less than 9 percent as much energy as refining it from its ores, a vast saving on the scale at which aluminum cans are used. About 20 percent of all the aluminum produced in the world is used for beverage cans in the United States alone.

12.13 Electrochemical Cells

Turning Chemical Energy into Electric Energy

Oxidation-reduction reactions can produce electric currents. What we must do is arrange to have the electrons transferred in such a reaction pass through an external wire as they go from one reactant to the other. All batteries and fuel cells are based on oxidation-reduction reactions. They are known as **electrochemical cells.**

In some types of batteries, the oxidation-reduction reactions cannot be reversed; when the reactants are used up, the battery is "dead." Examples are the familiar zinc-carbon and alkaline "dry cell" batteries that power flashlights and small electrical and electronic devices. In a rechargeable battery, the reactions can be reversed by passing a current through it in the opposite direction. The electrode reactions then proceed backwards to restore the battery to its original state.

Rechargeable Batteries   An example of a rechargeable battery is the storage battery of a car in which plates of lead and of lead dioxide, PbO_2, are in a solution of sulfuric acid which is dissociated into H^+ and SO_4^{2-} ions. The reactions that take place at each electrode when the battery is providing current are shown in Fig. 12-20. As the battery provides current, insoluble lead sulfate, $PbSO_4$, builds up on its plates. When the reactants have been used up, the battery cannot supply any more current. Recharging the battery brings the plates and the acid bath back to their initial compositions.

The potential difference across a storage battery cell is 2.1 V; a "12-V" battery contains six cells connected together. The lower the temperature of the acid in a storage battery, the slower its ions move and the less current the battery can provide. In freezing weather, the current available for the starting motor of a car may be less than half that available on a warm day, and it may be difficult or impossible to start the car's engine.

Other types of rechargeable batteries are also common. Nickel cadmium (NiCd) and nickel metal hydride (NiMH) batteries are widely used instead of dry cells. NiMH batteries have higher energy densities (that is, they store more energy per kilogram) than NiCd batteries but are less durable. Lithium ion (Li-ion) batteries have the highest energy densities by far, about three times those of NiMH batteries, which is why the latest electric cars and such power-hungry portable devices as cell phones and laptop computers have them. Li-ion batteries have other advantages also, for instance they keep their charge for a relatively long time and they can provide many hundreds

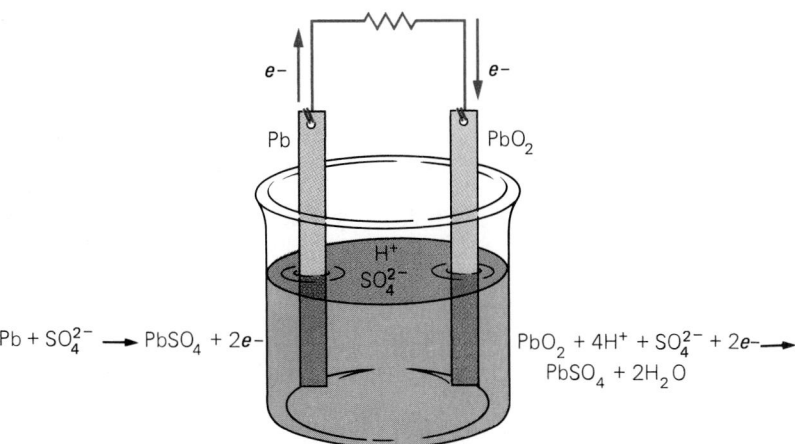

Figure 12-20 The lead-acid storage battery. The reactions shown are those that occur at each electrode when the battery provides current. These reactions are reversed when the battery is being charged.

of charge-discharge cycles. Disadvantages include expense, a lifetime of only a few years from manufacture regardless of how much they are used, and the possibility of catching fire if mistreated in various ways or even, on rare occasions, spontaneously.

Fuel Cells In a **fuel cell,** the reacting substances are fed in continuously. As a result the cell can provide current indefinitely without having to be replaced or recharged. Fuel cells are used in spacecraft since they are very light in proportion to the electric power they can supply. In the future it is possible that fuel cells will be perfected to the point where they are economical sources of power for individual homes, electric cars, and large-scale electric plants.

Combining 1 kg of hydrogen and 8 kg of oxygen in a hydrogen-oxygen fuel cell produces over 2×10^8 J of electric energy, enough to power a 100-W lightbulb for 4 weeks. The overall reaction in such a cell is simply

$$2H_2 + O_2 \longrightarrow 2H_2O$$

and involves the flow of 4 electrons each time the reaction occurs (Fig. 12-21). If a mixture of two volumes of hydrogen gas and one volume of oxygen gas is ignited, the result is a violent explosion with water as the product. In a hydrogen-oxygen fuel cell the same chemical combination takes place, but the liberated energy is released in the form of electric current.

Several types of fuel cells have been developed. The fuel cells used in spacecraft are very light in weight but are extremely expensive and rely on pure oxygen, rather than the oxygen in air, because their potassium hydroxide electrolyte reacts with the CO_2 in air. More practical on earth is a cell with a phosphoric acid electrolyte that can be fed with methane or hydrogen and air. Thousands of phosphoric-acid fuel cells, some quite large, today supply uninterruptible electricity to hospitals, banks, and computer centers. The reliability of these cells compensates for their cost, which is declining but still higher than that of conventional generators.

Using fuel cells in remote locations can be cheaper and more convenient than running power lines to distant electric grids. Thus a police station in New York's Central Park was equipped with a 200-kW fuel cell because it was less expensive than digging up the park for cables. In Japan, phosphoric-acid cells totalling 2000 MW have been installed in a number of small power stations to supply local needs.

PEM Fuel Cells A hydrogen fuel-cell design that employs a solid proton-exchange membrane (PEM) instead of a liquid electrolyte is better suited for vehicles. Their operation is shown in Fig. 12-21. Such cells are relatively light in weight and small in size but need very pure fuel. The membrane is

Fuel Cell Efficiency

A fuel cell does not function in the way a heat engine does and therefore is not subject to the thermodynamic limits on efficiency of heat engines (Sec. 5.14). A hydrogen fuel cell is about twice as efficient as a gasoline or diesel engine. Because there are hundreds of millions of cars and trucks in the world, the saving in energy could be large if the energy used to produce and distribute the hydrogen is not excessive.

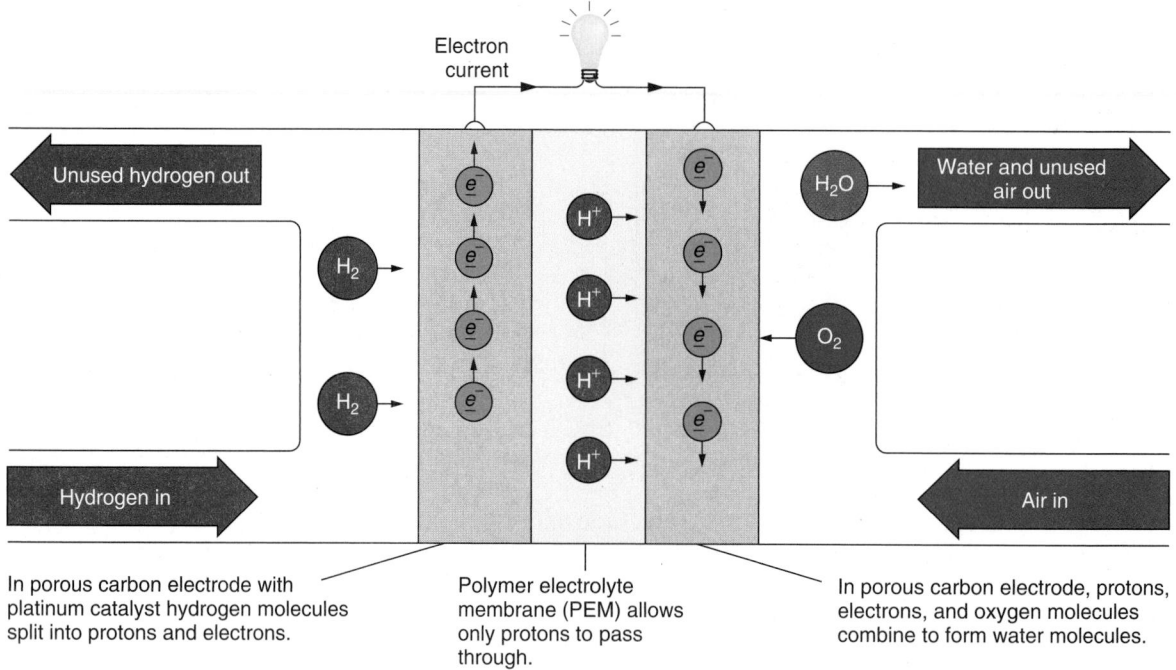

Electron current

Unused hydrogen out

H_2

H_2

e^-
e^-
e^-
e^-

H^+
H^+
H^+
H^+
H^+

e^-
e^-
e^-
e^-

H_2O

O_2

Water and unused air out

Hydrogen in

Air in

In porous carbon electrode with platinum catalyst hydrogen molecules split into protons and electrons.

Polymer electrolyte membrane (PEM) allows only protons to pass through.

In porous carbon electrode, protons, electrons, and oxygen molecules combine to form water molecules.

Figure 12-21   How a hydrogen PEM fuel cell operates. The overall reaction is $2H_2 + O_2 \longrightarrow 2H_2O$.

made of Teflon treated to permit protons but not electrons to pass through it. The membrane acts as the electrolyte and is sandwiched between two electrodes coated with platinum particles that act as catalysts. Hydrogen is fed to one electrode, where it breaks up into protons and electrons. The protons migrate through the membrane to the other electrode where their positive charge attracts the electrons through an external circuit. (These electrons carry the energy the cell generates to the outside world.) Air is fed to this electrode, where its oxygen reacts with the protons and electrons to form water, which passes out of the cell and is the only by-product.

A single PEM cell has a voltage of only about 0.7 V, so stacks of them must be connected in series (Fig. 6-24) to provide the higher voltages needed in practical applications; car motors, for instance, need about 300 V (Fig. 12-22). A number of cars and buses use PEM cells to power electric motors (Fig. 4-34).

Figure 12-22   The power densities of PEM fuel cell stacks used in cars have improved from 0.1 kW/liter (at left) to 1.1 kW/liter (at right). The stack at right can deliver 50 kW to a car's motors.

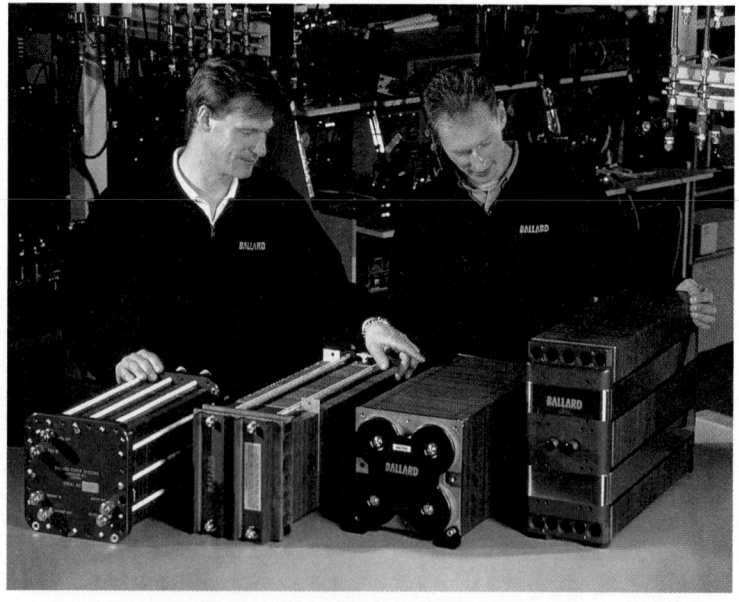

Important Terms and Ideas

Combustion is the rapid combination of oxygen with another substance during which heat and light are given off.

The **formula mass** of a substance is the sum of the atomic masses of the elements it contains, each multiplied by the number of times it appears in the formula of the substance. A **mole** of a substance is that amount of it whose mass in grams is equal to its formula mass expressed in atomic mass units (u). A mole of anything contains the same number of formula units as a mole of anything else; this number is called **Avogadro's number.** Because of the way the mole is defined, a chemical equation can be interpreted in terms of moles as well as in terms of formula units such as atoms, molecules, or ions.

Endothermic reactions absorb energy and **exothermic reactions** liberate energy. Many exothermic reactions require initial **activation energy** in order to take place.

A **catalyst** is a substance that can change the rate of a chemical reaction without itself being permanently changed.

In a **chemical equilibrium,** forward and reverse reactions occur at the same rate, so the concentrations of the reactants and products remain constant.

Oxidation involves the loss of electrons by the atoms of an element in a chemical reaction, and **reduction** involves the gain of electrons. An example of an oxidation-reduction reaction is **electrolysis,** in which free elements are liberated from a liquid by the passage of an electric current. **Batteries** and **fuel cells** produce electric current by means of oxidation-reduction reactions.

Multiple Choice

1. When something burns,
   a. it combines with phlogiston
   b. it gives off phlogiston
   c. it combines with oxygen
   d. it gives off oxygen

2. The chief constituent of dry air is
   a. oxygen   c. carbon dioxide
   b. nitrogen   d. argon

3. A substance of unknown composition is heated in an open container. As a result,
   a. its mass decreases
   b. its mass remains the same
   c. its mass increases
   d. any of these, depending on the nature of the substance and the temperature reached

4. When 1 g of a metal is oxidized, the resulting oxide has a mass that is
   a. less than 1 g
   b. equal to 1 g
   c. more than 1 g
   d. any of these, depending on the metal

5. A chemical reaction that absorbs energy is called
   a. endothermic   c. activated
   b. exothermic   d. oxidation-reduction

6. An example of an endothermic reaction is
   a. the dissociation of a salt in water
   b. the neutralization of an acid by a base
   c. the freezing of water
   d. combustion

7. If a given reaction is exothermic, the reverse reaction
   a. is exothermic
   b. is endothermic
   c. may involve no energy change
   d. any of these, depending on the reaction

8. The energy change in a chemical reaction depends on
   a. the bond energies of the reactants
   b. the bond energies of the products
   c. both of the above
   d. neither of the above

9. When a catalyst promotes a chemical reaction, it usually does so by
   a. providing energy
   b. providing electrons
   c. producing activated molecules
   d. becoming permanently altered

10. The neutralization of a strong acid by a strong base
    a. absorbs energy
    b. liberates energy
    c. involves no energy change
    d. requires a catalyst to occur

11. Reaction rates increase with temperature primarily because
    a. dissociation into ions is more complete
    b. more collisions occur between the molecules involved
    c. more activated molecules are formed
    d. equilibrium does not occur at high temperatures

12. For a reaction that occurs near room temperature, an increase of 10°C
    a. has little effect on the reaction speed
    b. increases the reaction speed by about 10 percent
    c. increases the reaction speed by about 50 percent
    d. approximately doubles the reaction speed

13. The speeds of reactions between ions in solution
    a. depend critically upon temperature
    b. are essentially independent of temperature
    c. depend upon which catalyst is used
    d. are slow in general

14. When the temperature at which a certain reversible reaction occurs is increased, the final amount of the reaction product or products
    a. increases
    b. remains the same
    c. decreases
    d. any of the above, depending on the reaction

15. At equilibrium,
    a. both forward and reverse reactions have ceased
    b. the forward and reverse reactions are proceeding at the same rate
    c. the forward reaction has come to a stop, and the reverse reaction is just about to begin
    d. the mass of reactants equals the mass of products

16. The yield of the product C in the reversible reaction A + B + energy $\rightleftharpoons$ C can be increased by
    a. decreasing the temperature
    b. increasing the temperature
    c. increasing the surface area of the reactants
    d. changing the catalyst

17. When a gas reaction involves a decrease in the total number of molecules, the equilibrium can be shifted in the direction of higher yield by
    a. increasing the pressure
    b. decreasing the pressure
    c. increasing the temperature
    d. decreasing the temperature

18. When a substance gains electrons in a chemical reaction, the substance is said to be
    a. reduced   c. electrolysed
    b. oxidized   d. activated

19. A catalyst affects which one or more of the following?
    a. The energy needed for a chemical reaction to occur
    b. The energy a chemical reaction gives off
    c. The speed of a chemical reaction
    d. Whether a substance is oxidized or reduced in a chemical reaction

20. When an electric current is passed through molten sodium chloride,
    a. sodium metal is deposited at the positive electrode
    b. sodium ions are deposited at the positive electrode
    c. chlorine gas is liberated at the positive electrode
    d. chlorine ions are liberated at the positive electrode

21. The quantity actually stored in a "storage battery" is
    a. electric charge   c. voltage
    b. electric current   d. energy

22. Batteries and fuel cells employ
    a. oxidation reactions only
    b. reduction reactions only
    c. both oxidation and reduction reactions
    d. acid-base neutralization reactions

23. A fuel cell does not require
    a. a positive electrode
    b. a negative electrode
    c. oxidation-reduction reactions
    d. recharging

24. One mole of an element has a mass equal to
    a. Avogadro's number
    b. its atomic number expressed in grams
    c. its mass number expressed in grams
    d. its atomic mass expressed in grams

25. A mole of any compound contains Avogadro's number of
    a. atoms   c. molecules
    b. ions   d. formula units

26. The formula mass of gaseous carbon dioxide, CO_2,
    a. is 28 u
    b. is 44 u
    c. is 56 u
    d. depends on the mass of the sample

27. An oxygen atom has a mass of 16.0 u. The number of moles of molecular oxygen, O_2, in 64 g of oxygen gas is
    a. 2   c. 32
    b. 4   d. 64

28. How many moles of H atoms are present in 1 mole of H_2O?
    a. $\frac{2}{3}$ c. 2
    b. 1   d. 3

29. The number of moles of carbon present in 3 mol of glucose, $C_6H_{12}O_6$, is
    a. 2   c. 6
    b. 3   d. 18

30. The atomic mass of helium is 4.0 u and that of carbon is 12.0 u.
    a. The mass of 1 mole of carbon is $\frac{1}{3}$ the mass of 1 mole of helium
    b. The mass of 1 mole of carbon is 3 times the mass of 1 mole of helium
    c. One mole of carbon contains $\frac{1}{3}$ as many atoms as 1 mole of helium
    d. One mole of carbon contains 3 times as many atoms as 1 mole of helium

31. One mole of which of the following compounds contains the greatest mass of bromine?
    a. HBr   c. $AlBr_3$
    b. Br_2 d. $SiBr_4$

32. In round numbers, the atomic mass of nitrogen is 14 u and Avogadro's number is $N_0 = 6 \times 10^{23}$ formula units/mole. One mole of molecular nitrogen, N_2, contains
    a. 6×10^{23} molecules   c. 84×10^{23} molecules
    b. 12×10^{23} molecules   d. 168×10^{23} molecules

33. The mass of 1 mole of molecular nitrogen is
    a. 14 g   c. 84×10^{23} g
    b. 28 g   d. 168×10^{23} g

34. The mass of 6×10^{23} molecules of N_2 is
    a. 14 g   c. 84×10^{23} g
    b. 28 g   d. 168×10^{23} g

35. Six moles of O_2 are consumed in a certain run of the reaction $2H_2S + 3O_2 \longrightarrow 2H_2O + 2SO_2$. The number of moles of water produced in the run is
    a. 1   c. 4
    b. 2   d. 6

Exercises

12.1 Phlogiston
12.2 Oxygen

1. What aspect of Lavoisier's work marked the beginning of chemistry as a science?

2. (a) What is the formula of ozone? (b) Ozone in the atmosphere is both harmful to and essential for our health. Explain.

3. What role does air play in combustion?

4. For a given amount of energy to be used for its propulsion, a spacecraft must have much larger tanks than an airplane. Why?

12.3 The Mole
12.4 Formula Units

5. Which of the following quantities are the same for both a mole of hydrogen molecules and a mole of oxygen molecules at the same temperature? (a) The mass of each sample; (b) the number of molecules present; (c) the average molecular energies.

6. When hydrogen is burned in oxygen, water is formed according to the reaction $2H_2 + O_2 \longrightarrow 2H_2O$. How many moles of H_2 and how many of O_2 are needed to produce 3 mol of H_2O?

7. How many moles of aluminum are present in 5 mol of $MgAl_2O_4$?

8. How many moles of atomic oxygen are present in 1 mol of $Ca_3(PO_4)_2$?

9. How many moles of propane, C_3H_8, can be prepared from 1 mol of carbon? From 1 mol of hydrogen?

10. How many moles of Al are needed to react with each mole of $CuSO_4$ in the reaction $2Al + 3CuSO_4 \longrightarrow 3Cu + Al_2(SO_4)_3$?

11. Ammonia is produced by the reaction $N_2 + 3H_2 \longrightarrow 2NH_3$. How many moles of N_2 and how many of H_2 are needed to produce 1 mol of ammonia?

12. Find the mass of 1.6 mol of magnesium, Mg. How many atoms are present in such a sample?

13. Find the mass of 10 mol of uranium, U. How many atoms are present in such a sample?

14. Find the mass of 5 mol of ethylene, C_2H_4. How many carbon atoms are present in the sample?

15. Find the mass of 2 mol of iron(III) oxide, Fe_2O_3.

16. Find the mass of 30 mol of sulfuric acid, H_2SO_4.

17. How many moles of glucose are present in 500 kg of glucose, $C_6H_{12}O_6$?

18. How many moles of lead nitrate are present in 100 g of lead nitrate, $Pb(NO_3)_2$?

19. Three compounds used as fertilizers are urea, $CO(NH_2)_2$; ammonium nitrate, NH_4NO_3; and ammonium sulfate, $(NH_4)_2SO_4$. What is the percentage of nitrogen by mass in each compound? (Hint: Divide the formula mass of the nitrogen in each compound by the formula mass of the compound and then express the result as a percentage.)

20. When potassium chlorate, $KClO_3$, is heated, it decomposes into potassium chloride and oxygen in the reaction $2KClO_3 \longrightarrow 2KCl + 3O_2$. How much oxygen is liberated when 50 g of potassium chlorate is heated?

21. How much chlorine is needed to react with 50 g of sodium to form sodium chloride, NaCl? How much sodium chloride is produced?

22. How much CO_2 is produced when 100 g of butane (C_4H_{10}) is burned in the reaction $2C_4H_{10} + 13O_2 \longrightarrow 8CO_2 + 10H_2O$?

23. How much sulfur is needed to react with 200 g of potassium to form potassium sulfide, K_2S?

12.5 Exothermic and Endothermic Reactions
12.6 Chemical Energy and Stability
12.7 Activation Energy

24. What is the origin of the energy liberated in an exothermic reaction?

25. In what fundamental way is the explosion of an atomic bomb different from the explosion of dynamite?

26. From the observation that the slaking of lime [addition of water to CaO to form $Ca(OH)_2$] gives out heat, would you conclude that the following reaction is endothermic or exothermic?

$$Ca(OH)_2 \longrightarrow CaO + H_2O$$

27. Which of the following are exothermic reactions and which are endothermic?

   a. The explosion of dynamite

   b. The burning of methane

   c. The decomposition of water into its elements

   d. The dissociation of water into ions

   e. The burning of iron in chlorine

   f. The combination of zinc and sulfur to form zinc sulfide

28. When carbon in the form of diamond is burned to produce CO_2, more heat is given off than when carbon in the form of graphite is burned. What form of carbon is more stable under ordinary conditions? What bearing does this conclusion have on the origin of diamonds?

29. What is the fundamental role of activation energy in starting an exothermic reaction?

30. Do ions in solution need activation energy to react with one another? If not, why not?

12.8 Temperature and Reaction Rates
12.9 Other Factors

31. What is the chief reason that reaction rates increase with temperature?

32. Why does an increase in temperature increase the rate of exothermic as well as endothermic reactions?

33. Suggest three ways to increase the rate at which coarse salt dissolves in a pan of water.

34. Suggest three ways to increase the rate at which zinc dissolves in sulfuric acid.

35. Give an example of a reaction that is (a) practically instantaneous at room temperatures, (b) fairly slow at room temperatures.

36. Under ordinary circumstances coal burns slowly, but the fine coal dust in mines sometimes burns so rapidly as to cause an explosion. Explain the difference in rates. Would you expect the danger from spontaneous combustion to be greater in a coal pile containing principally large chunks or in one containing finely pulverized coal? Why?

37. Why is a reaction with a high activation energy slow at room temperature?

38. To what extent does the time needed for a strong acid to neutralize a strong base in solution depend on temperature?

12.10 Chemical Equilibrium

12.11 Altering an Equilibrium

39. How common are reversible chemical reactions?

40. The solubility of a gas in a liquid decreases with increasing temperature. From this observation and what you know of how a change in temperature can affect an equilibrium, would you expect that dissolving a gas in a liquid is an exothermic or an endothermic process?

41. Changing the pressure has no effect on the equilibrium

$$CO + H_2O \rightleftharpoons CO_2 + H_2$$

in which all the substances involved are gases. Why not?

42. The reaction $2SO_2 + O_2 \longrightarrow 2SO_3$ is exothermic. (a) How will a rise in temperature affect the yield of SO_3 in an equilibrium mixture of the three gases? (b) Will an increase in pressure raise or lower the yield? (c) In what possible way can the speed of the reaction be increased at moderate temperatures?

43. The reaction $2SO_2 + O_2 \longrightarrow 2SO_3$ is exothermic. How will a rise in temperature affect the yield of SO_3 in an equilibrium mixture of the three gases? Will an increase in pressure raise or lower this yield? In what possible way can the speed of the reaction be increased at moderate temperatures?

44. Hydrogen sulfide gas dissolves in water and dissociates very slightly: $H_2S \rightleftharpoons 2H^+ + S^{2-}$. How would the acidity of the solution be affected by

   a. increasing the pressure of H_2S?

   b. raising the temperature?

   c. adding a solution of KOH?

   d. adding a solution of silver nitrate? (Silver sulfide, Ag_2S, is insoluble.)

45. The three gases N_2, O_2, and NO are in equilibrium. The formation of NO is exothermic. Write the equation for the equilibrium. How would a decrease in temperature affect the equilibrium? A decrease in pressure? A lower concentration of N_2? A lower concentration of NO? The presence of a catalyst?

12.12 Oxidation-Reduction Reactions

46. A displacement reaction is an oxidation-reduction reaction in which one element displaces another from solution. In each of the following displacement reactions identify the element that is oxidized and the element that is reduced:

$$Zn + Cu^{2+} \longrightarrow Zn^{2+} + Cu$$
$$Fe + 2H^+ \longrightarrow Fe^{2+} + H_2$$
$$Cl_2 + 2Br^- \longrightarrow 2Cl^- + Br_2$$

47. Which loses electrons more easily, Na or Fe? Al or Ag? I^- or Cl^-? Which gains electrons more easily, Cl or Br? Hg^{2+} or Mg^{2+}? (Hint: Reread Sec. 10.10.)

48. When magnesium is placed in an acid solution, hydrogen gas is given off. Is magnesium or hydrogen the better reducing agent?

49. Lithium reacts with water to produce lithium hydroxide. What else is produced? Write the equation of the process. Which element is reduced and which is oxidized?

50. In the refining of iron, the iron(III) oxide, Fe_2O_3, in iron ore is reduced by carbon (in the form of coke) to yield metallic iron and carbon dioxide. Write the balanced equation of the process.

51. When an electric current is passed through a solution of hydrochloric acid, what substance is liberated at the positive electrode? At the negative electrode?

52. When an electric current is passed through a solution of copper chloride, what substance is liberated at the positive electrode? At the negative electrode?

53. Which of the following metals will be deposited in the greatest mass when 1 C of charge is passed through appropriate electrolytic cells? Aluminum, nickel, silver. The ions of these metals in solution are respectively Al^{3+}, Ni^{2+}, Ag^+.

12.13 Electrochemical Cells

54. What becomes of the electric energy provided in electrolysis? In what device is this energy transformation reversed?

55. What do you think happens when a charging current is passed through a fully charged storage battery?

56. In what basic way is a fuel cell different from a dry cell or a storage battery?

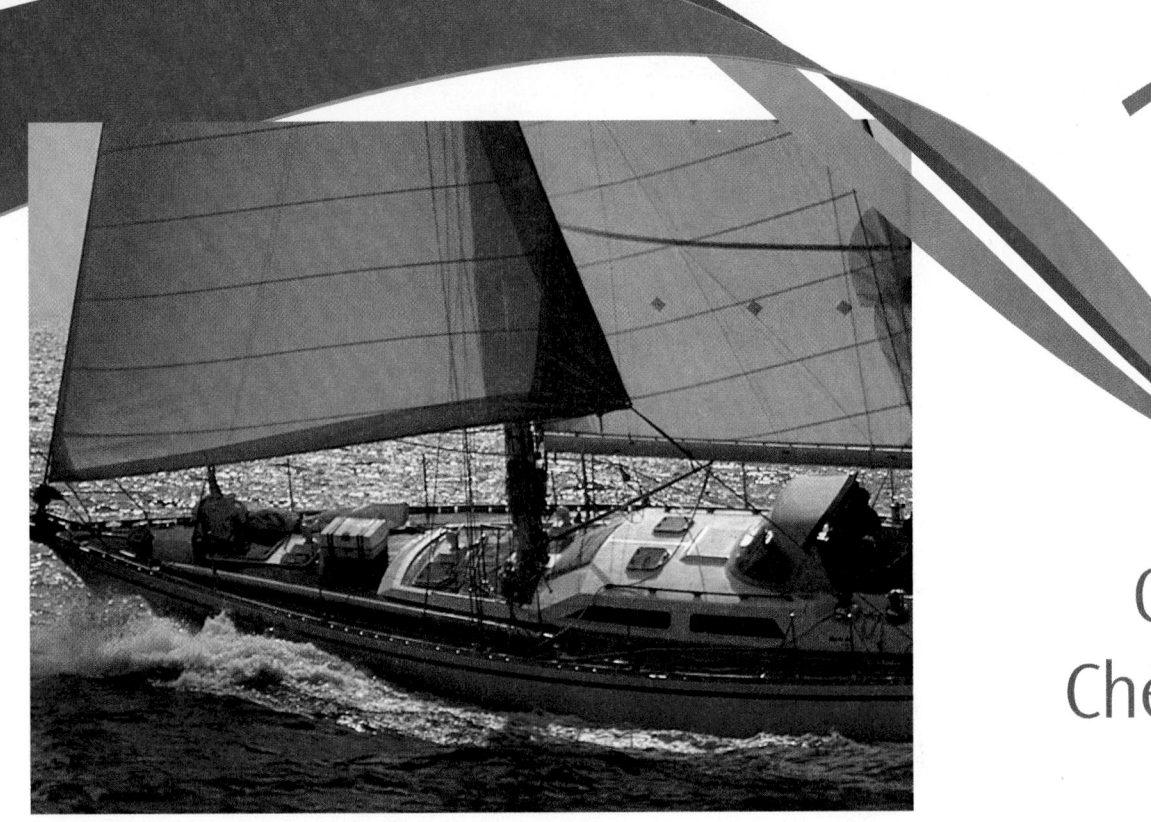

Organic Chemistry

Synthetic polyester resins are used in the hull and sails of this yacht.

GOALS

When you have finished this chapter you should be able to complete the goals
• given for each section below:

In many ways carbon is the most remarkable element. Hundreds of thousands of carbon compounds are known, far more than the number of compounds that do not contain carbon. Furthermore, carbon compounds are the chief constituents of all living things—hence the name **organic chemistry** to describe the chemistry of carbon and the name **inorganic chemistry** to describe the chemistry of all the other elements.

Carbon Compounds

At one time it was thought that carbon compounds—with the exception of the carbon oxides, the carbonates, and a few others—could be produced only by plants and animals (or indirectly from other compounds produced by them). Carbon was supposed to unite with other elements only under the influence of a mysterious "life force" possessed by living things.

This ancient idea was disproved in 1828 by the German chemist Friedrich Wöhler, who prepared the organic compound urea by reacting the inorganic compounds lead cyanate and ammonia. Since Wöhler's time a great number of organic compounds have been made in the laboratory from inorganic materials, but the general distinction between the chemistry of carbon compounds and inorganic chemistry nevertheless remains useful.

13.1 Carbon Bonds

Carbon Atoms Can Form Covalent Bonds with Each Other

Let us see what the periodic table can tell us about carbon. Carbon is in period 2 at the top of group 4, which means it is halfway between the active metal lithium and the active nonmetal fluorine. Active metals tend to lose their outer electrons when they react chemically, and active nonmetals tend to gain electrons. Carbon, in the middle, does neither. Instead, it forms covalent bonds in which it shares four electron pairs.

As we saw in Table 10-7 and Fig. 10-15, the carbon atom has four electrons in its outer shell. For a carbon atom to achieve a closed outer shell, it can lose these four electrons, pick up four more for a total of eight, or share its four electrons with other atoms that contribute four electrons so that eight electrons—four pairs—are shared.

The effective nuclear charge on the outer electrons in a carbon atom is $+4e$ (Fig. 13-1). The resulting force on the outer electrons is sufficient to keep them from being detached to leave a C^{4+} ion. However, the effective nuclear charge is not enough for a carbon atom to attract and hold four more electrons to give a C^{4-} ion. (See Fig. 10-16 for the reason why Na readily becomes Na^+ and Cl readily becomes Cl^-.) The result is that carbon atoms participate in four covalent bonds each when they form molecules with other atoms.

Why Carbon Forms Many Compounds   A carbon atom can bond strongly not only with many metallic and nonmetallic atoms but with *other carbon atoms* as well. This is the reason for the immense number and variety of carbon

Figure 13-1   Electron shielding in carbon. Each outer electron is acted on by an effective nuclear force of $+4e$ because the inner electrons shield part of the actual nuclear charge of $+6e$.

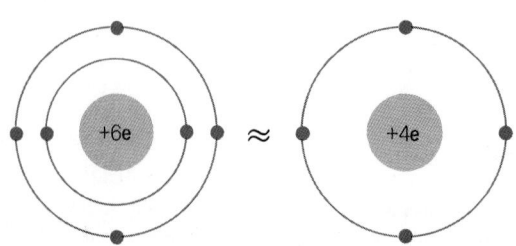

compounds, whose molecules have skeletons of linked carbon atoms. The strength of the bonds between carbon atoms is shown by the hardness of diamond, a crystalline form of carbon in which each atom is joined to four others by electron pairs (see Fig. 11-6). Atoms of a few elements near carbon in the periodic table, notably boron and silicon, are also able to bond with each other, but the range of their compounds is far more limited.

Because the bonds formed by carbon atoms are covalent, carbon compounds are mostly nonelectrolytes, and their reaction rates are usually slow. The affinity of carbon and hydrogen for oxygen makes many organic compounds subject to slow oxidation in air and to rapid oxidation if heated. Even in the absence of air most organic compounds are unstable at high temperatures; very few of them resist decomposition at temperatures over a few hundred degrees celsius.

Organic molecules are either nonpolar or nearly so, hence the van der Waals forces between them are weak and as a class, organic compounds have low melting and boiling points. Some polymers (large molecules that consist of a great many subunits joined together) are exceptions; a notable example is Teflon.

13.2 Alkanes

The Hydrocarbons in Petroleum and Natural Gas

The simplest organic compounds are the **hydrocarbons** that contain only carbon and hydrogen. A group of hydrocarbons called the **alkanes** includes the familiar gases methane (CH_4), propane (C_3H_8), and butane (C_4H_{10}), all widely used as fuels in stoves and furnaces. Alkane molecules have single covalent bonds between their carbon atoms. The freezing points and boiling points of the alkanes all increase regularly as the molecular size increases (Table 13-1). Other series of organic compounds show similar regular changes in properties as the number of carbon atoms per molecule increases.

Table 13-1	The Alkane Series of Hydrocarbon			
Formula	**Name**	**Freezing Point, °C**	**Boiling Point, °C**	**Commercial Name**
CH_4	Methane	−183	−160	Fuel gases
C_2H_6	Ethane	−184	−89	Fuel gases
C_3H_8	Propane	−188	−42	Fuel gases
C_4H_{10}	Butane	−139	−1	
C_5H_{12}	Pentane	−130	36	Naphtha
C_6H_{14}	Hexane	−95	69	
C_7H_{16}	Heptane	−91	98	
C_8H_{18}	Octane	−57	126	Gasoline
C_9H_{20}	Nonane	−54	151	
$C_{10}H_{22}$	Decane	−30	174	Kerosene,
$C_{11}H_{24}$	Undecane	−27	197	jet fuel
$C_{16}H_{34}$	Hexadecane	18	287	
$C_{14}H_{30}$ to $C_{18}H_{38}$				Diesel fuel, heating oil
$C_{16}H_{34}$ to $C_{18}H_{38}$				Lubricating oil
$C_{16}H_{34}$ to $C_{32}H_{68}$				Petroleum jelly
$C_{20}H_{42}$ and up				Paraffin wax
$C_{36}H_{74}$ and up				Asphalt

Note: The data refer to the straight-chain compounds. Isomers of these hydrocarbons (see Sec. 13.5) have somewhat different properties.

Natural gas (see Sec. 4.6) and petroleum (see Sec. 4.5) consist mainly of alkanes. About 80 percent of natural gas is methane, 10 percent ethane, and the rest mostly propane and butane. Alkanes with five or more carbon atoms are the main ingredients of petroleum ("crude oil"), whose exact composition varies from source to source. Methane is also one of the emissions from active volcanoes and a product of the bacterial decay of plant matter in the absence of oxygen. The "marsh gas" that bubbles up from the black ooze at the bottom of stagnant pools is largely methane, as is the "fire damp" that sometimes causes explosions in coal mines.

13.3   Petroleum Products

Fractional Distillation, Catalytic Cracking, and Polymerization

The separation of petroleum into its different alkanes is difficult because their properties are so similar. Suppose we want to separate pentane and hexane. Because pentane boils at 36°C and hexane at 69°C, it would seem that if we heated a mixture of the two, all the pentane would boil away first to leave pure hexane. The trouble is that hexane evaporates readily at 36°C, so the vapor produced by heating the mixture to that temperature would contain a certain amount of hexane as well as pentane. This procedure would thus give a vapor rich in pentane and a remaining liquid rich in hexane, but would not separate the two compounds completely.

Usually a complete separation of the alkanes in petroleum is not necessary, however. The basic process in petroleum refining is **fractional distillation,** in which crude oil is heated and its vapors are led off and condensed at progressively higher temperatures. A diagram of a distillation tower together with some of the possible fractions is given in Fig. 13-3. The cracking process mentioned in the figure is described below. Grease is not one of the fractions because it consists of oil to which a thickening agent has been added to prevent the mixture from running out from between the surfaces being lubricated.

Gasoline   Of all these products the most valuable, of course, is gasoline, needed to fuel many of the world's hundreds of millions of cars. The United States alone uses over 100 billion gallons of gasoline each year. Unfortunately the constituents of gasoline are present only to a minor extent in most petroleums. Two methods have been developed to increase the yield of gasoline. In one of them, the heavier hydrocarbons are **cracked** into smaller molecules by heating them under pressure in the presence of catalysts (Fig. 13-2). A typical cracking reaction is

$$C_{16}H_{34} \longrightarrow C_8H_{18} + C_8H_{16} \qquad \textit{Cracking reaction}$$

Here hexadecane, one of the heavier alkanes in kerosene and diesel fuel, is broken down into lighter hydrocarbons that vaporize and burn more readily.

The second procedure is to **polymerize** lighter hydrocarbons, which means to join small molecules into larger ones under the influence of heat, pressure, and appropriate catalysts. An example is

$$C_3H_8 + C_4H_8 \longrightarrow C_7H_{16} \qquad \textit{Polymerization reaction}$$

in which heptane, a liquid, is formed by the polymerization of two gases. Figure 13-5 shows what a barrel of crude oil typically yields.

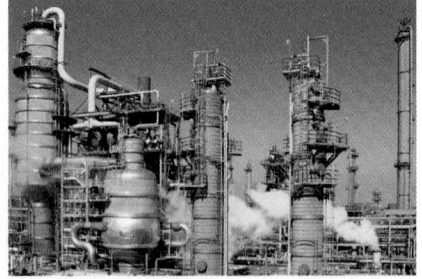

Figure 13-2   Catalytic cracking units at an oil refinery break down complex hydrocarbons into simpler ones. There have been no new oil refineries in the United States for 30 years, mainly because of environmental concerns. Many refineries have been built recently or are under construction abroad.

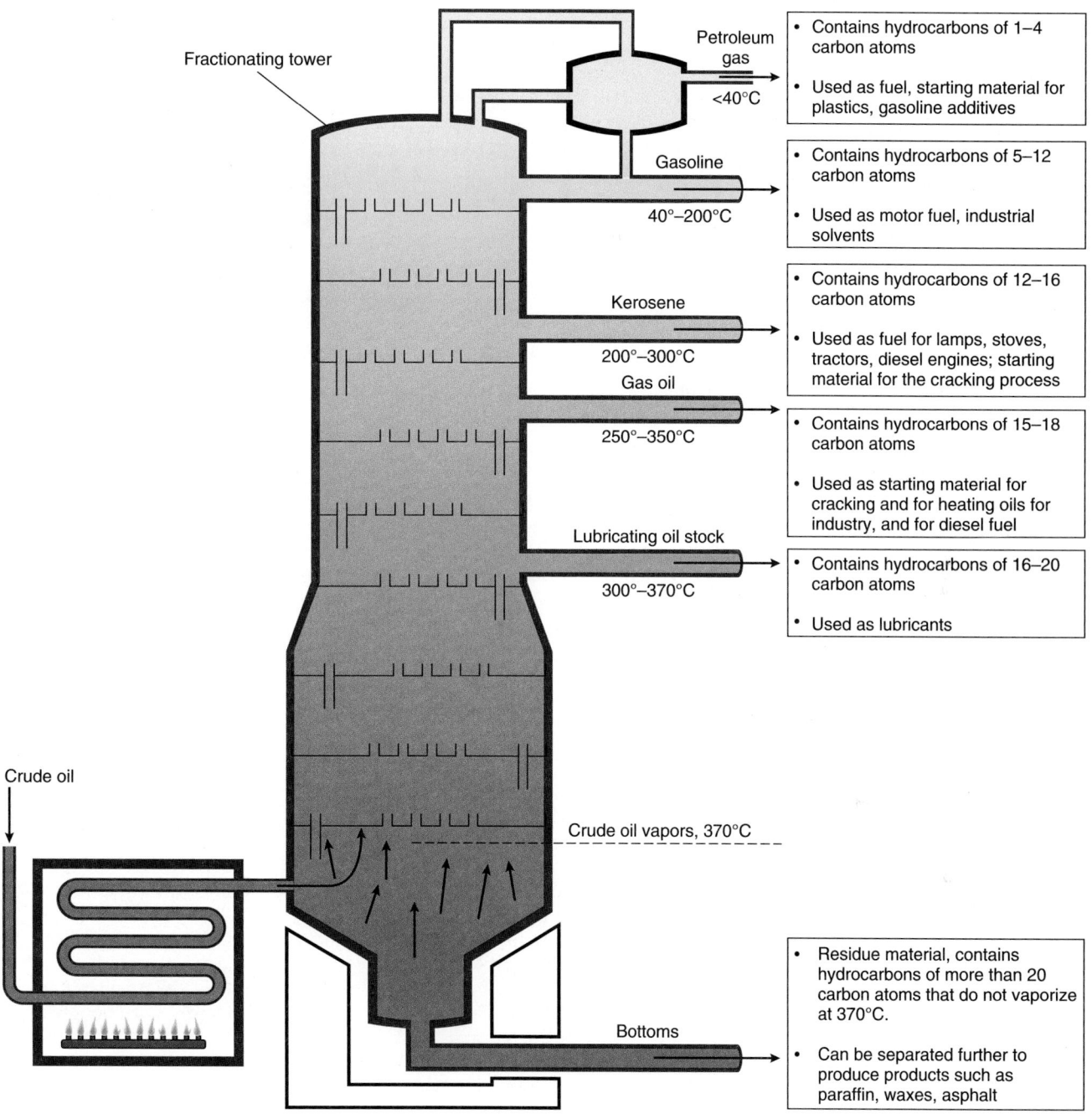

Figure 13-3 A distillation tower like the simplified one shown here separates crude oil into fractions according to their boiling points.

Alkane molecules have chains of carbon atoms linked together in line, as we shall see in Sec. 13.4. Such molecules, as we might expect, are nonpolar, with neither end much more positive or negative than the other. Because of this nonpolar character, the alkane hydrocarbons are insoluble in water. Chemically they are rather unreactive, and neither concentrated acids and bases nor most oxidizing agents affect them at moderate temperatures. Nor do biological agents such as bacteria attack them to any great extent. The combination of insolubility, relative inertness, and toxicity to living things is what makes the discharge of petroleum and its products into the sea such a serious matter.

Octane Rating

When a car's gasoline engine is under stress, for instance when climbing a hill in high gear, the gasoline-air mixture in its cylinders may ignite early, while being compressed instead of when the spark plugs fire (Fig. 5-47). The result is a rattle called "knocking." The octane rating of a gasoline (Fig. 13-4) is a measure of its ability to prevent knocking: the higher the octane rating, the less likely knocking is to occur. On the octane scale, heptane (a straight-chain hydrocarbon) is rated as 0, and isooctane (a branched-chain hydrocarbon) is rated as 100; branched-chain hydrocarbons are the more effective in reducing knocking.

A compound called tetraethyl lead was once widely used to increase the octane rating of gasoline. Because the exhausts of engines

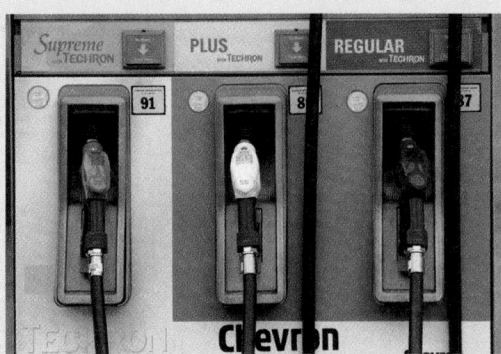

Figure 13-4   Gasoline with the correct octane rating is needed for optimum performance from a car engine.

using leaded gasoline discharge lead, which is toxic, into the atmosphere and the catalytic converters that reduce other pollutants are inactivated by lead, unleaded gasoline is now standard in the United States (but not everywhere else in the world, unfortunately). To obtain a high octane rating for "super" or "premium" fuel, branched-chain hydrocarbons of various kinds are incorporated in unleaded gasoline.

The Deepwater Horizon Disaster

Oil spills are common. Some are accidental, the result of shipwreck or a malfunction at an offshore oil well, but others are deliberate, the result of tankers illegally flushing out waste oil. Although the lighter hydrocarbons soon evaporate, the heavier ones remain floating on the surface or are washed ashore on adjacent coastlines. Of every thousand tons of oil shipped around the world, one is spilled at sea.

Depending on the nature of the residues and the region, the effects of the residues on marine life may be drastic and immediate—dead plankton, dead fish, dead animals, dead birds—or they may be gradual, taking the form of an altered balance of nature with declining populations. The lumps of tar that are one result of oil spills are a prominent feature on the surface of much of the world's oceans and are familiar sights on many beaches.

The worst environmental disaster in United States history was an oil spill that began in April 2010

when the drilling rig Deepwater Horizon, under charter to the oil company BP, exploded and sank in the Gulf of Mexico. Eleven workers on the rig died and tens of thousands of barrels of crude oil gushed out every day for 5 months afterward. The well penetrated 4 km into the seabed, itself 1.5 km below the surface of the Gulf, and its drilling was behind schedule and over budget. To save time and money, BP and its contractors took dangerous shortcuts that deviated from standard procedures. Signs of trouble were ignored for days before the explosion.

In its application for a drilling permit, BP claimed to have "proven equipment and technology" to respond to such a blowout, but in fact had neither. In the absence of effective action oil spread through the Gulf to damage fisheries (the Gulf region usually produces a third of the country's seafood) and other ecosystems and to wash up on adjacent coasts.

Even before the Gulf event, BP was notorious for putting profit ahead of responsible management: in 2005, a BP refinery in Texas exploded, killing 15 workers, and a year later badly-maintained BP pipelines in Alaska ruptured to flood the countryside with oil. BP was fined for criminal violations in both cases, but evidently not enough to change its attitude to risk. U.S. government agencies then ignored BP's history and waived inconvenient safety regulations at its request.

BP is the leading producer of oil and gas in the United States, the largest deepwater operator in the Gulf of Mexico, and the second most profitable oil company in the world.

Almost no oil deposits can still be found that are easy and safe to exploit, and the result is a possibility of further catastrophes as more and more difficult wells are drilled, even when this is done carefully.

For more, see Sec. 13.3 at www.mhhe.com/krauskopf.

Barrel of Crude Oil

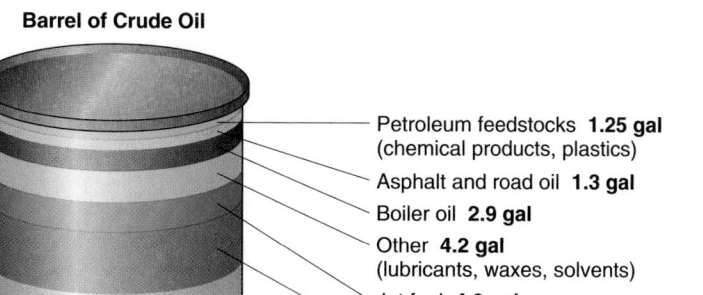

Petroleum feedstocks **1.25 gal**
(chemical products, plastics)

Asphalt and road oil **1.3 gal**

Boiler oil **2.9 gal**

Other **4.2 gal**
(lubricants, waxes, solvents)

Jet fuel **4.2 gal**

Diesel and home heating oil **8.4 gal**

Gasoline **19.7 gal**

Figure 13-5 End products from the refining of a barrel (42 gallons) of crude oil. Over 80 percent is merely burnt, mostly in vehicle engines. The proportion that becomes feedstocks for plastics, fibers, pharmaceuticals, and other synthetic products, which is increasing, will be hardest to replace when crude oil becomes rare. The United States, with less than 5 percent of the world's population, consumes a quarter of the world's oil production. Two-thirds of the oil used in the United States is imported.

Structures of Organic Molecules

13.4   Structural Formulas

They Show How Atoms Are Linked Together

Instead of a molecular formula such as CH_4 and C_2H_6, an organic compound is often represented by a **structural formula** in which the covalent bonds between the atoms in each molecule are shown by dashes. Each dash stands for a shared pair of electrons. Thus the structural formulas of the alkanes methane, ethane, and propane are

$$
\begin{array}{ccccc}
 & H & & H\ \ H & & H\ \ H\ \ H \\
 & | & & |\ \ \ | & & |\ \ \ |\ \ \ | \\
H- & C & -H & H-C-C-H & & H-C-C-C-H \\
 & | & & |\ \ \ | & & |\ \ \ |\ \ \ | \\
 & H & & H\ \ H & & H\ \ H\ \ H \\
 & \text{methane} & & \text{ethane} & & \text{propane}
\end{array}
$$

A molecular formula tells us only how many atoms of each kind are present in each molecule of a compound. A structural formula tells us more. For instance, in the above three molecules we can see that each hydrogen atom is attached to a carbon atom and that in ethane and propane the carbon atoms are linked together. Figure 13-6 shows a three-dimensional model of the methane molecule.

The number of bonds an atom forms in an organic compound is the same as the number of electrons it has to gain or lose to achieve a closed outer shell. A carbon atom always participates in four bonds, as we have learned. A hydrogen atom always participates in a single bond, as does a chlorine atom; an oxygen atom participates in two bonds. Here are some examples:

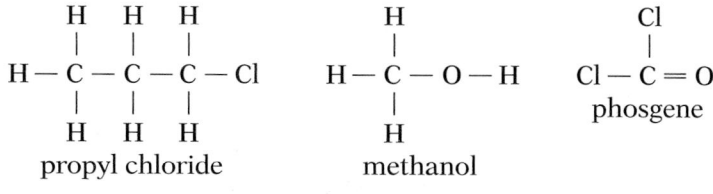

propyl chloride

methanol

phosgene

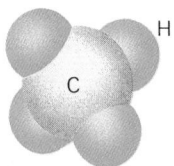

Figure 13-6 Model of the methane molecule, CH_4.

13.5   Isomers

The Same Atoms but Arranged Differently

For methane, ethane, and propane the structural formulas given earlier are the only possible arrangements of carbon and hydrogen atoms that will satisfy the combination rules. Butane, on the other hand, may have its 4 C atoms and 10 H atoms arranged in two ways:

$$
\begin{array}{cccc}
\text{H} & \text{H} & \text{H} & \text{H} \\
| & | & | & | \\
\text{H}-\text{C}-\text{C}-\text{C}-\text{C}-\text{H} \\
| & | & | & | \\
\text{H} & \text{H} & \text{H} & \text{H}
\end{array}
\qquad\qquad
\begin{array}{ccc}
\text{H} & \text{H} & \text{H} \\
| & | & | \\
\text{H}-\text{C}-\text{C}-\text{C}-\text{H} \\
| & | & | \\
\text{H} & \text{C} & \text{H} \\
& /\,|\,\backslash & \\
\text{H} & \text{H} & \text{H}
\end{array}
$$

normal butane   isobutane

These formulas show that there are two different compounds with the molecular formula C_4H_{10}. They differ in that one of the carbon atoms in isobutane is linked to three other carbon atoms, while in normal butane the carbon atoms are linked to only one or two others.

The physical properties of isobutane are different from those of normal butane because of this difference in molecular structure. The boiling point of isobutane, for instance, is $-12°C$, whereas that of normal butane, as listed in Table 13-1, is $-1°C$. Another difference is their densities (masses per unit volume): that of isobutane is 0.622 g/cm^3 whereas that of normal butane is 0.604 g/cm^3. Figure 13-7 shows three-dimensional models of the two kinds of butane.

Compounds that have the same molecular formulas but different structural formulas are called **isomers.** The number of possible isomers increases rapidly with the number of carbon atoms in the molecule; $C_{13}H_{28}$ has 813 theoretically possible isomers and $C_{20}H_{42}$ has 366,319. Only a few of the possible isomers have actually been prepared.

Merely flipping a structural formula end-for-end does not give the formula of an isomer. For instance, we can show the structure of methanol (methyl alcohol) in two ways:

$$
\begin{array}{c}
\text{H} \\
| \\
\text{H}-\text{C}-\text{OH} \\
| \\
\text{H}
\end{array}
\qquad\qquad
\begin{array}{c}
\text{H} \\
| \\
\text{OH}-\text{C}-\text{H} \\
| \\
\text{H}
\end{array}
$$

However, the molecule is exactly the same in both cases.

13.6   Unsaturated Hydrocarbons

Double and Triple Carbon-Carbon Bonds

Hydrocarbons are not limited to the alkanes. A simple example of a nonalkane hydrocarbon is **ethene,** also called **ethylene,** whose formula is C_2H_4. The alkane with two C atoms is ethane, C_2H_6, whose structural formula is

$$
\begin{array}{cc}
\text{H} & \text{H} \\
| & | \\
\text{H}-\text{C}-\text{C}-\text{H} \\
| & | \\
\text{H} & \text{H}
\end{array}
$$

ethane

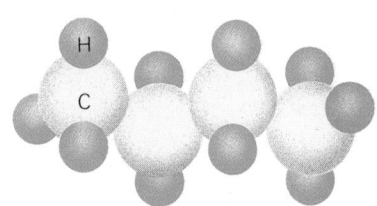

Normal butane

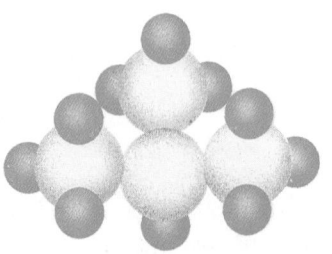

Isobutane

Figure 13-7   The two isomers of butane, C_4H_{10}. Their physical properties are different.

How can ethene, with two fewer H atoms, still have each C atom share four electron pairs? The answer is that there are *two* covalent bonds between the C atoms in ethene:

$$H\diagdown \diagup H$$
$$C = C$$
$$H\diagup \diagdown H$$

ethene

Such a link between carbon atoms is called a **double bond** and involves the sharing of two electron pairs.

Triple bonds, with carbon atoms sharing three electron pairs, are also possible. The simplest case is that of acetylene, C_2H_2, a gas widely used in welding and metal-cutting torches (Fig. 13-8). The structural formula of acetylene is

$$H - C \equiv C - H$$
acetylene

Multiple Bonds and Reactivity   Compounds with double and triple bonds are much more reactive than the alkanes, which have only single bonds. Both HCl and Cl_2 combine readily with ethene, for instance:

$$\begin{array}{ccc} H\diagdown \diagup H & & HH \\ C = C & + \ HCl \longrightarrow & H - C - C - H \\ H\diagup \diagdown H & & HCl \end{array}$$

$$\begin{array}{ccc} H\diagdown \diagup H & & HH \\ C = C & + \ Cl_2 \longrightarrow & H - C - C - H \\ H\diagup \diagdown H & & ClCl \end{array}$$

The other halogens and many other acids give similar reactions. Since compounds with multiple bonds are able to add other atoms to their

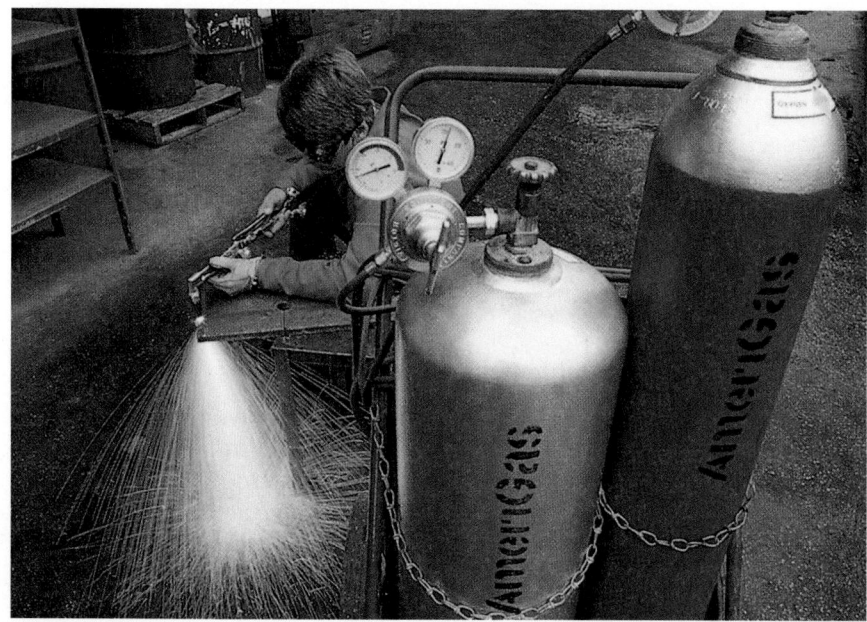

Figure 13-8   Oxyacetylene cutting torch. The short cylinder contains acetylene and the tall one contains oxygen. The flame temperature can reach 3000°C. The reaction is extremely exothermic because the acetylene molecule contains a triple carbon-carbon bond.

Example 13.1

The compound pentene has the molecular formula C_5H_{10}. Draw the structural formula(s) of pentene and its isomers, if any. Is it a saturated or unsaturated compound?

Solution

Each C atom must participate in four bonds. We begin by drawing the C atoms with single bonds between them and lines to represent the remaining bonds they can form:

$$-\overset{|}{\underset{|}{C}}-\overset{|}{\underset{|}{C}}-\overset{|}{\underset{|}{C}}-\overset{|}{\underset{|}{C}}-\overset{|}{\underset{|}{C}}-$$

Now we distribute the ten H atoms among these bonds:

$$H-\overset{\overset{\displaystyle H}{|}}{\underset{\underset{\displaystyle H}{|}}{C}}-\overset{\overset{\displaystyle H}{|}}{\underset{\underset{\displaystyle H}{|}}{C}}-\overset{\overset{\displaystyle H}{|}}{\underset{\underset{\displaystyle H}{|}}{C}}-\overset{\overset{\displaystyle H}{|}}{\underset{\underset{\displaystyle H}{|}}{C}}-\overset{\overset{\displaystyle H}{|}}{\underset{|}{C}}-$$

Two bonds are left over, which means that one of the carbon-carbon bonds is a double bond. Thus the structural formulas of the two possible isomers of pentene are

$$H-\overset{\overset{\displaystyle H}{|}}{\underset{\underset{\displaystyle H}{|}}{C}}-\overset{\overset{\displaystyle H}{|}}{\underset{\underset{\displaystyle H}{|}}{C}}-\overset{\overset{\displaystyle H}{|}}{\underset{\underset{\displaystyle H}{|}}{C}}-\overset{\overset{\displaystyle H}{|}}{C}=C\overset{\diagup H}{\diagdown H}$$

$$H-\overset{\overset{\displaystyle H}{|}}{\underset{\underset{\displaystyle H}{|}}{C}}-\overset{\overset{\displaystyle H}{|}}{\underset{\underset{\displaystyle H}{|}}{C}}-\overset{||}{\underset{\underset{\displaystyle C}{}}{C}}-\overset{\overset{\displaystyle H}{|}}{\underset{\underset{\displaystyle H}{|}}{C}}-H$$
$$\underset{H \quad H}{\diagup \diagdown}$$

(If we put the double bond between either of the other pairs of C atoms the result will not be a new isomer because it would just be a flipped version of one of the above formulas.) Pentene is evidently an unsaturated compound.

---

molecules, they are called **unsaturated compounds.** The alkanes and similar compounds whose molecules have only single carbon-carbon bonds are called **saturated compounds** because they cannot add other atoms to their molecules.

13.7 Benzene

Its Molecule Contains a Stable Ring of Six Carbon Atoms

Benzene, C_6H_6, is a clear liquid that does not mix with water and has a strong odor. Benzene is widely used as a solvent and in the manufacture of more complex organic compounds.

The six C atoms in benzene are arranged in a flat hexagonal ring, as shown in Fig. 13-9. What is especially interesting about this molecule is the manner in which its C atoms are attached to one another. In addition to single bonds between these atoms, six electrons are shared by the entire

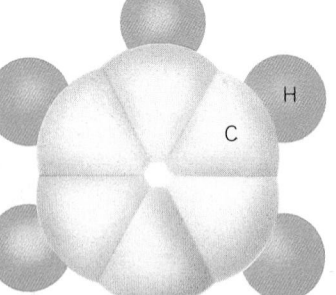

Figure 13-9 Model of the benzene molecule, C_6H_6. Over 5 million tons of benzene are produced in the United States each year.

BIOGRAPHY | August Kekulé (1829–1896)

A native of Germany, Kekulé studied architecture before he became a chemist, and in fact his most notable work was on the architecture of molecules. He introduced the idea of structural formulas, proposed that a carbon atom forms four bonds when it combines, and suggested that carbon atoms could join with each other to form chains. All this came before the nature of chemical bonds was understood; indeed, even the electron was unknown until after Kekulé's death.

Kekulé's greatest achievement was to establish the structure of benzene, C_6H_6, a compound which had been discovered by Michael Faraday in 1826. Exactly how benzene's atoms were arranged was a mystery for the next 40 years until Kekulé (so he said) had a dream in which dancing snakes swallowed their tails. This led him to the concept of a flat ring of carbon atoms linked by alternate single and double bonds, with a hydrogen atom attached to each carbon atom:

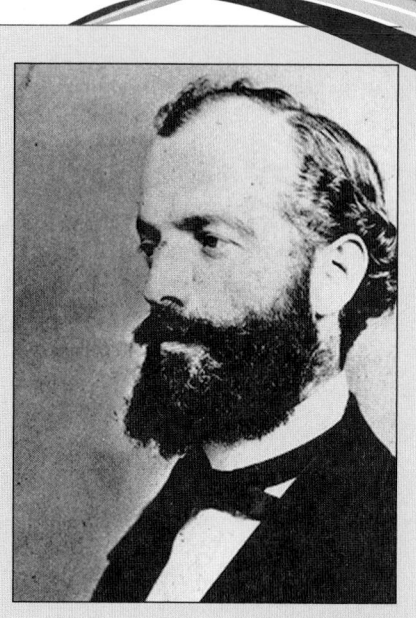

Although this picture accounted for most of the properties of benzene and was the key to many of the extraordinary successes of organic chemistry, it had a flaw: experiments show that all of the carbon-carbon bonds in benzene are exactly the same, not alternate single and double ones. Not until quantum theory was applied to molecular structure in the next century did it become clear that six of the bonding electrons could be shared equally by the entire ring.

ring. The latter electrons belong to the molecule as a whole and not to any particular pair of atoms; these electrons are **delocalized.** (We recall from Chap. 11 that the outer-shell electrons in a metal are similarly delocalized.) The six delocalized electrons in benzene can be represented by an inner circle in its structural formula:

benzene

Aromatic Compounds   An **aromatic** compound is defined as one that contains a ring of six carbon atoms like that in benzene. The name arose because many of these compounds have strong odors. An example is toluene, which is a common solvent and paint thinner:

toluene

The C and H atoms that are part of a benzene ring are often omitted in representing the structures of aromatic molecules, as shown above.

Some aromatic compounds contain two or more benzene rings fused together, as in the case of naphthalene:

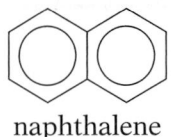

naphthalene

Naphthalene is familiar as the active ingredient in mothballs.

Organic compounds whose molecules do not contain ring structures are said to be **aliphatic.**

Organic Compounds

The remarkable range of organic compounds is hinted at in the hydrocarbons, which contain only carbon and hydrogen. Add just oxygen and the possibilities are multiplied many times over, giving compounds as diverse as they are numerous. Add still other elements and the result is staggering in variety and complexity. Fortunately, regularities exist that permit the orderly classification of organic compounds and lead to an understanding of how their molecular structures govern their behavior. Given this understanding, the organic chemist can create compounds tailored to exhibit specific properties. Evidence of the success of this endeavor is found in the synthetic materials, from textile fibers to drugs, so widely used today.

13.8   Hydrocarbon Groups

A Handy Classification Scheme

In the classification system used for organic compounds that contain other elements besides carbon and hydrogen, the compounds are often regarded as **derivatives** of hydrocarbons—that is, as compounds obtained by substituting other atoms or atom groups for one or more of the H atoms in hydrocarbon molecules. Ordinarily such compounds are *not* prepared in this way, but their structural formulas suggest that they might be. For example, ethanol can be regarded as a derivative of ethane, with an OH group replacing an H atom:

$$
\begin{array}{ccc}
\text{H} & \text{H} \\
| & | \\
\text{H} - \text{C} - \text{C} - \text{H} \\
| & | \\
\text{H} & \text{H}
\end{array}
\qquad
\begin{array}{ccc}
\text{H} & \text{H} \\
| & | \\
\text{H} - \text{C} - \text{C} - \text{OH} \\
| & | \\
\text{H} & \text{H}
\end{array}
$$

ethane   ethanol

Similarly acetic acid can be regarded as a derivative of methane, with a COOH group replacing an H atom:

methane   acetic acid

Hydrocarbon Groups   The carbon-hydrogen atom groups that appear in hydrocarbon derivatives are named from the hydrocarbons. Groups corresponding to the hydrocarbons methane, ethane, and propane are methyl group   ethyl group   propyl group

Thus the compound CH_3Cl is methyl chloride, C_3H_7I is propyl iodide, and $CH_3C_2H_5SO_4$ is methyl ethyl sulfate.

13.9 Functional Groups

Atom Groups with Characteristic Behaviors

Inorganic compounds that contain a particular atom group, such as OH or SO_4, have important aspects of their chemical behavior in common, as we know. The chemical behavior of many organic compounds is also determined to a large extent by the presence of certain atom groups, called **functional groups.** Table 13-2 shows some of the main functional groups found in organic molecules.

| Example 13.2

The following compound can be called either bromoethane or ethyl bromide. Why?

Solution

Since CH_3CH_3 is ethane, substituting a Br (bromine) atom for one of the H atoms leads to the name bromoethane. Since CH_3CH_2 is the ethyl group, the compound can also be called ethyl bromide.

Alcohols The hydroxyl (OH) group they contain makes many alcohol molecules somewhat polar, and the simpler alcohols are soluble in water. The polarity is not enough, however, to prevent them from mixing with many compounds less polar than water, which makes the alcohols useful as solvents. Ethanol (ethyl alcohol) is, of course, the active ingredient in wine, beer, and spirits. Ethanol is a poison that is removed from a person's blood by the liver; one of the hazards of regularly drinking too much ethanol is permanent liver damage.

The ethanol in beverages is produced by fermentation. In this process sugar is converted to ethanol and carbon dioxide, with yeast enzymes acting as catalysts. For example,

$$C_6H_{12}O_6 \xrightarrow[\text{enzymes}]{\text{yeast}} 2C_2H_5OH + 2CO_2 \qquad \textit{Fermentation}$$

glucose (a sugar)   ethanol   carbon dioxide

Wine is made by fermenting fruit juice, usually grape juice; traces of wine have been found in jars dating back to 5400 B.C. Beer is made by fermenting grain, usually barley, and then adding a bitter extract of a plant called hop for flavor. Since yeast cells die before the alcohol concentration reaches about

Animals and Alcohol

In nature, it is possible for the sugar in the fruit, sap, and nectar of various plants to ferment. The resulting alcohol may find its way into the diets of a number of animals, from bees to elephants, whose behavior afterward suggests the behavior of people who have overindulged in alcohol, including later hangovers.

Table 13-2	Common Functional Groups

Name of Group	Structural Formula	Class of Compound	Example	Formula	Comments
Hydroxyl	—OH	Alcohol	Ethanol	$CH_3—CH_2—OH$	Used as a solvent and in beverages; prepared by fermenting sugar solution and synthetically from ethene and water.
Ether	—O—	Ether	Diethyl ether	$CH_3—CH_2—O—CH_2—CH_3$	Once widely used as an anesthetic, its side effects and flammability led to its replacement by safer compounds.
Aldehyde	$—C(=O)H$	Aldehyde	Formaldehyde	$H—C(=O)H$	A gas used to preserve biological specimens and as an embalming fluid when dissolved in water ("formalin").
Carbonyl	$—C(=O)—$	Ketone	Acetone	$CH_3—C(=O)—CH_3$	A common solvent with a toxic vapor used in paints and as nail polish remover.
Carboxyl	$—C(=O)OH$	Acid	Acetic acid	$CH_3—C(=O)OH$	Responsible for characteristic taste of vinegar; a weak acid like other organic acids.
Ester	$—C(=O)O—$	Ester	Methyl acetate	$CH_3—C(=O)O—CH_3$	A solvent formed in the reaction of methyl alcohol and acetic acid with water as the other product; used in fast-drying paints, in perfumes, and in dye manufacturing.

15 percent, wine and beer cannot be stronger than this. In fact, fermentation generally stops somewhat earlier because the sugar runs out.

Distillation can produce stronger liquors. The fermented liquid is heated and the alcohol-rich vapor is then led off and condensed to give brandy (starting from fruit), whiskey (grain), rum (sugar cane), vodka (traditionally potatoes), and so on. The proof of an alcoholic beverage is twice its percentage content of ethanol. Thus 80 proof whiskey contains 40 percent ethanol, and pure ethanol is 200 proof.

Ethanol for industrial purposes is usually made by reacting ethene, a by-product of petroleum refining, with steam under high pressure. As mentioned in Sec. 4.12, ethanol for fuel is made today by fermenting the sugar in sugarcane or corn. Probably suitable catalysts will eventually be developed to enable cellulose from plant material—which is cheap, plentiful, and does not compete with food supply—to be processed efficiently into ethanol.

When an H atom is replaced by an OH group in an aromatic hydrocarbon, the result is a compound whose properties are different from those of ordinary alcohols. The simplest example is phenol ("carbolic acid"), C_6H_5OH, which was the first antiseptic and today is one of the raw materials for the plastic Bakelite and for the phenolic glues used in plywood:

phenol

Familiar alcohols with more than one OH group are ethylene glycol and glycerol:

ethylene glycol   glycerol

Ethylene glycol is used as an antifreeze in car engines. Glycerol, also known as glycerin, is a sweetish, viscous liquid used in many skin lotions and to prevent tobacco from drying out.

Ethers   An ether has an oxygen atom bonded between two carbon atoms. Relatively inert chemically, ethers are widely used as solvents in organic processes since there is little or no danger they will interfere with the reactions.

Aldehydes and Ketones   These compounds have similar chemical behavior because both contain the carbonyl atom group $\diagdown C = O$. In aldehydes the carbonyl group is at the end of a molecule with a hydrogen atom attached to the carbon atom, while in ketones the group is inside a molecule between two other carbon atoms. The double bond between C and O is highly polar, and as a result aldehydes and ketones are soluble in water.

Ethanol is oxidized in the liver into acetaldehyde:

ethanol   oxygen   acetaldehyde   water

Most of the acetaldehyde is oxidized further in the liver to acetic acid, which is then oxidized in the muscles to CO_2 and H_2O. The acetaldehyde that survives enters the bloodstream and is responsible for many of the ill effects of drinking too much, which include damage to most of the body's organs as well as nausea and hangovers. Acetaldehyde is also present in tobacco smoke and contributes to the harm it causes. Methanol (methyl alcohol) is oxidized in the liver to the poisonous formaldehyde, which is believed to be the reason why methanol is so toxic.

The solvent acetone is the most familiar ketone.

Organic Acids   Compounds that contain the carboxyl group, —COOH, are acids because the H atom is loosely held and can detach itself as H^+. A C–H bond is stronger. Most organic acids are very weak. Familiar examples are the formic acid that causes insect bites to sting, the acetic acid of vinegar, the butyric acid of rancid butter and some cheeses, the citric acid of citrus fruits, the lactic acid of sour milk, and the acetylsalicylic acid of aspirin.

When an opened bottle of wine is stored for some time, the ethanol it contains gradually turns into acetic acid and the eventual result is vinegar.

The conversion of ethanol to acetic acid is promoted by enzymes produced by bacteria in the wine:

$$H-\overset{\overset{\displaystyle H}{|}}{\underset{\underset{\displaystyle H}{|}}{C}}-\overset{\overset{\displaystyle H}{|}}{\underset{\underset{\displaystyle H}{|}}{C}}-OH + O_2 \longrightarrow H-\overset{\overset{\displaystyle H}{|}}{\underset{\underset{\displaystyle H}{|}}{C}}-C\overset{\displaystyle O}{\underset{\displaystyle O-H}{\diagup}} + H_2O$$

ethanol   oxygen   acetic acid   water

Esters   Alcohols are, so to speak, organic hydroxides, but unlike their inorganic cousins they do not dissociate appreciably in water. They react slowly with acids to form compounds called esters, which are analogous to the salts of inorganic chemistry but are not electrolytes. An example is ethyl acetate, which is made by reacting ethanol with acetic acid:

$$H-\overset{\overset{\displaystyle H}{|}}{\underset{\underset{\displaystyle H}{|}}{C}}-\overset{\overset{\displaystyle H}{|}}{\underset{\underset{\displaystyle H}{|}}{C}}-O-\overset{\overset{\displaystyle O}{\|}}{C}-\overset{\overset{\displaystyle H}{|}}{\underset{\underset{\displaystyle H}{|}}{C}}-H$$

ethyl acetate

This ester is an important commercial solvent. Several hundred thousand tons of it are used each year in the United States in manufacturing coatings of various kinds, from paint to nail polish.

Many esters have pleasant fruity or flowerlike odors and find extensive use in perfumes and flavors. Propyl acetate is responsible for the fragrance and taste of pears, octyl acetate for those of oranges, ethyl butyrate for those of apricots, and butyl butyrate for those of pineapples. When wine is aged, some of its alcohol content reacts with organic acids also present to produce a variety of esters that improves its flavor and aroma. Some wines need little aging but many, especially red wines, benefit from several years of storage. The explosive nitroglycerin is an ester formed by the reaction of nitric acid with the alcohol glycerol (Fig. 13-10). Animal and vegetable fats are all esters of glycerol as well.

13.10   Polymers

Molecules Linked into Giant Chains

Polymers are giant molecules that consist of hundreds or thousands of identical (or almost identical) subunits. Proteins, starch, cellulose, and rubber are natural polymers. Polythene, polyvinyl chloride (PVC), Styrofoam, Teflon, nylon, and Dacron are synthetic polymers; the solid ones are usually called just plastics.

For a long time polymers were thought to be merely assemblies of small molecules held together by van der Waals forces. Finally, in work that began in 1926, the German chemist Hermann Staudinger (Fig. 13-11) showed that polymers are true molecules of huge size held together with covalent bonds. Nearly 60 million tons of polymers are made every year in the United States, about 0.25 percent ("bioplastics") from plant material and the rest from oil and natural gas feedstocks.

Polythene   We are already acquainted with the unsaturated hydrocarbon ethene:

$$\overset{\displaystyle H}{\diagdown}\underset{\displaystyle H}{\diagup}C=C\overset{\displaystyle H}{\diagdown}\underset{\displaystyle H}{}$$

ethene

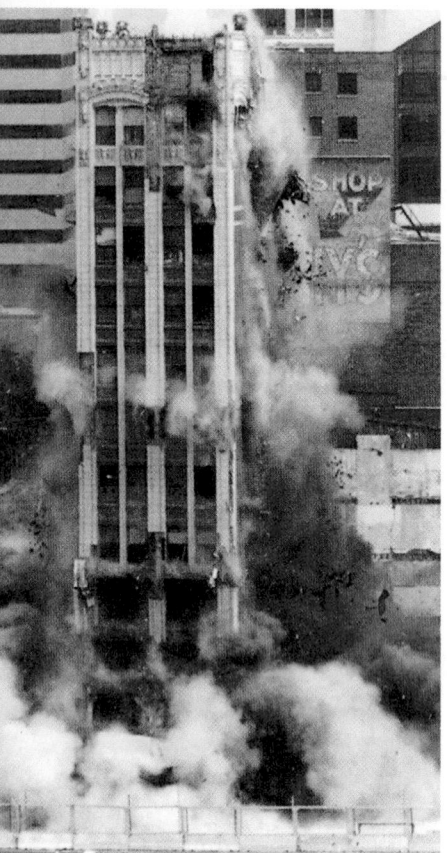

Figure 13-10   The ester nitroglycerin is the active ingredient in the explosive dynamite. Dynamite was used to demolish this building in Indianapolis.

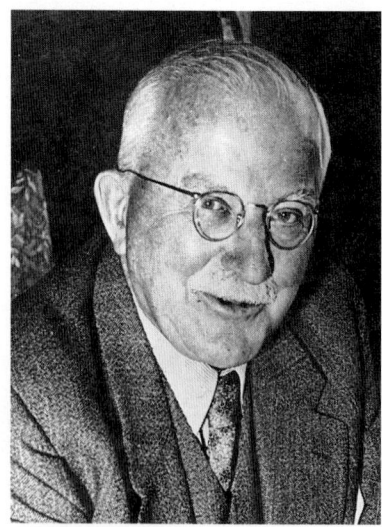

Figure 13-11   Hermann Staudinger (1881–1965).

Plastic Waste

Modern civilization produces huge amounts of plastic waste that are a problem to dispose of because ordinary polymers, unlike traditional materials such as wood, paper, and natural fibers, do not readily decompose. Dumped in landfills, where most rubbish ends up, plastic waste remains intact for a very long time. Burning plastic waste reduces its volume and provides useful heat—more than the same mass of coal or oil—but it must be carried out in expensive special incinerators because toxic gases, such as sulfur dioxide, hydrogen chloride, and hydrogen cyanide, may be given off.

Another approach is to create plastics that degrade naturally. An example is the plastic collars used to hold beer cans together, which contain polymer chains with atom groups that split the chains when

exposed to light; the fragments that result decompose more readily than intact chains. Biodegradable plastics are available that incorporate starch, which bacteria consume and thereby break down the polymer chains. Still other ways to produce degradable plastics are being explored, including the use of bacteria to convert sugar or starch to a biodegradable compound called polyactic acid (PLA).

The best thing to do with plastic waste, of course, is to recycle it into new products. But not all polymers can be reused, and the needed careful sorting is often more expensive than starting from new materials. One successful recycling process starts with beverage bottles made of polyethylene terephthalate(PET). The PET is melted down and turned into fibers that are used in such items as blankets, fleece garments,

and insulation. In India, discarded plastic bags are processed and added to the asphalt used to pave roads, which makes the roads more durable. Overall, though, relatively little plastic waste is recycled today.

Of course, the problem of plastic waste can be reduced just by wasting less plastic. For instance, durable shopping bags could replace the usual plastic bags provided by stores, 100 billion or so of which are thrown away in the United States every year. To encourage such good sense, a growing number of cities and countries now tax plastic bags, which in the case of Ireland has led to a 90 percent drop in their use. San Francisco has simply banned its larger groceries and pharmacies from providing nonbiodegradable plastic bags at all. The city's goal is for all waste to be biodegradable or recyclable by 2020.

Because of the double bond, ethene molecules can, under the proper conditions of heat and pressure, polymerize to form chains thousands of units long whose formula we might write as

$$\cdots - \underset{\underset{H}{|}}{\overset{\overset{H}{|}}{C}} - \underset{\underset{H}{|}}{\overset{\overset{H}{|}}{C}} - \underset{\underset{H}{|}}{\overset{\overset{H}{|}}{C}} - \underset{\underset{H}{|}}{\overset{\overset{H}{|}}{C}} - \underset{\underset{H}{|}}{\overset{\overset{H}{|}}{C}} - \underset{\underset{H}{|}}{\overset{\overset{H}{|}}{C}} - \cdots$$

polythene

This material is polythene (or polyethylene), which is widely used as a packaging material because of its inertness and pliability. The ethene is called the **monomer** in the process, and polythene the polymer. (In Greek, *mono* means "alone" or "single," and *poly* means "many.") A train can be thought of as a polymer, with each of its cars as a monomer. Because of the large size of their molecules, polymers are usually solids.

Vinyls   One of the H atoms in ethene can be replaced by another atom or atom group to form the monomer for a polymer whose properties differ from those of polythene. Because the group

$$\overset{\displaystyle H}{\underset{\displaystyle H}{\diagdown}} C = C \overset{\displaystyle H}{\diagdown}$$

vinyl group

is called the **vinyl group,** such polymers are classed as vinyls. Some familiar examples are shown in Table 13-3 with Fig. 13-12 illustrating the corresponding monomers.

Table 13-3   **Some Common Vinyl Polymers**

Monomer	Polymer	Uses
vinyl chloride	polyvinylchloride	Tubing, insulation, imitation leather, rainwear (PVC, Geon, Koroseal)
acrylonitrile	polyacrylonitrile	Textiles, carpets (Acrilon, Orlon)
propene	polypropylene	Carpets, ropes, molded objects, thermal underwear
styrene	polystyrene	Molded objects, insulation, packing material (Styrofoam)

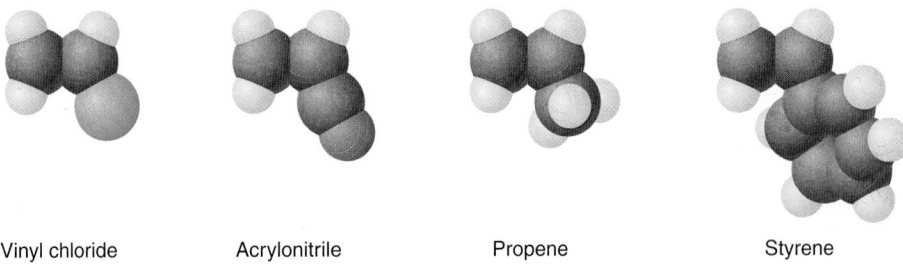

Figure 13-12 Models of the monomers listed in Table 13-3.

Vinyl chloride   Acrylonitrile   Propene   Styrene

The benzene rings attached to alternate C atoms in polystyrene are relatively large and project like knobs from the polymer chain. This prevents adjacent chains from sliding past one another, and as a result polystyrene is relatively stiff. If a substance that gives off a gas is added to the liquid monomer mixture, gas bubbles will form throughout the liquid as it polymerizes. The result is the familiar lightweight, rigid Styrofoam.

Lucite and Plexiglas   In some monomers, such as methyl methacrylate, two of the H atoms in ethene are replaced by atom groups. Methyl methacrylate polymerizes to form the transparent plastics whose trade names are Lucite and Plexiglas. A feature of this material is that it is **thermoplastic,** which means that it softens and can be shaped when heated but becomes rigid again upon cooling.

The Cup and the Environment

Styrofoam cups have nonrenewable petroleum as their ultimate raw material, their manufacture involves the carcinogen styrene, they cannot be recycled, and they are not biodegradable. Surely paper cups, with trees as their raw material and disposable in various ways, are more friendly to the environment? And are not china cups really the greenest of all, since they can be used over and over again?

Well, it all depends (Fig. 13-13). Paper cups need more energy and are more polluting to produce than Styrofoam cups. Since paper cups weigh more than Styrofoam cups, their transportation uses more energy, too. China cups have to be washed, which involves energy, detergents, and water. Whether Styrofoam, paper, or china cups are best varies according to whether the criterion is energy use, nature and amount of raw materials, air pollution, water pollution, or volume of solid wastes. Overall, china cups win only if they are washed with the least water and detergent possible and are used several thousand times before breaking. (Dishwashing a full load by machine uses less water and less electricity for heating it than dishwashing by hand.) Between the throwaway cups, Styrofoam seems less harmful than paper, although this is not entirely certain.

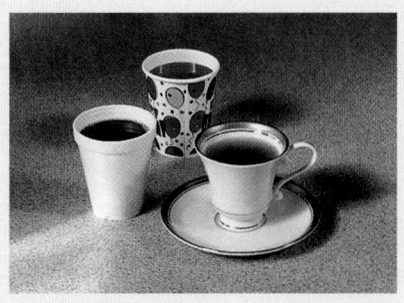

Figure 13-13   Life-cycle studies of the environmental impacts of Styrofoam, paper, and china cups give no firm answer as to which is best on an overall basis.

Teflon   The monomer for Teflon is tetrafluorethene, which is ethene with all the H atoms replaced by fluorine atoms:

F   F
 \   /
  C = C
 /   \
F   F

tetrafluorethene

           F   F
           | |
••• — C — C — •••
           | |
           F   F
        Teflon

The bond between fluorine and carbon is extremely strong, which makes Teflon tough and inert and able to withstand much higher temperatures than other polymers. Teflon has a very slippery surface, too. These properties make Teflon useful industrially for seals and bearings as well as for nonstick coatings for cooking utensils (Fig. 13-14).

Copolymers   Some polymers consist of two different monomers. An example of such a **copolymer** is Dynel, used among other things to make fibers for wigs, whose monomers are vinyl chloride and vinyl acetate. The kitchen wrap Saran is another copolymer.

Elastomers   Certain monomers that contain two double bonds in each molecule form flexible, elastic polymers called **elastomers.** Rubber is a natural elastomer (Fig. 13-15). A widely used synthetic elastomer is neoprene, which has the valuable property that liquid hydrocarbons such as gasoline affect it less than they do natural rubber. Another elastomer, nitrile rubber, is still more resistant to hydrocarbons and is used to line gasoline hoses.

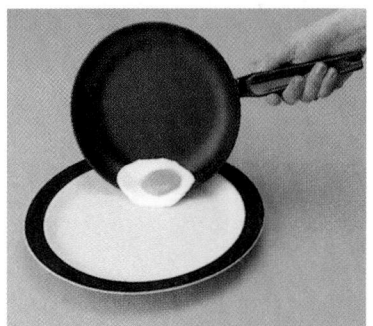

Figure 13-14   The strong bond between carbon and fluorine accounts for the durability and inertness of Teflon, which was used to coat this frying pan.

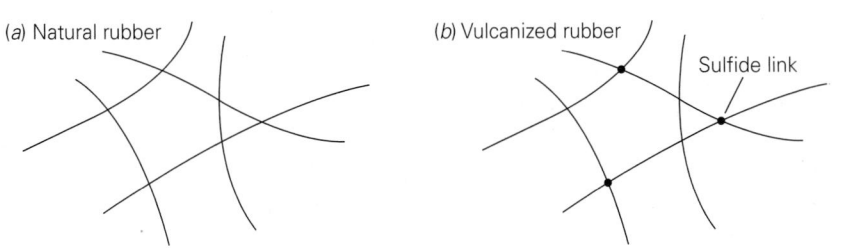

(a) Natural rubber

(b) Vulcanized rubber

Sulfide link

Figure 13-15   (a) Natural rubber is a sticky liquid whose polymer chains can slide past one another easily. (b) In the process of vulcanization, natural rubber is heated with sulfur, which produces links between polymer chains. The result is a material that is locally flexible but solid overall. The greater the number of sulfide links, the stiffer the result.

Silicones

Silicon is just below carbon in the periodic table and, like carbon, its atoms each participate in four covalent bonds. Polymers can be made in which silicon atoms replace some of the carbon atoms in their structures. Such polymers are called **silicones.** Some silicones are liquids, others are gels or elastomers, and some are solids with varying degrees of rigidity. Silicone surgical implants are widely used.

Fibers   Of the various kinds of synthetic fibers that have been developed, nylon and Dacron are the most familiar. Both are composed of chains of structural elements, just like polymers, but they are produced by chemical reactions rather than by the polymerization of monomer molecules. In the case of nylon, the result is a chain whose elements can be written

$$-\text{N}-\text{C}-\text{C}-\text{C}-\text{C}-\text{C}-\text{C}-\text{N}-\text{C}-\text{C}-\text{C}-\text{C}-\text{C}-\text{C}-$$

The atom group

$$\begin{array}{c} \text{H} \quad \text{O} \\ | \quad \parallel \\ -\text{N}-\text{C}- \end{array} \qquad \textit{Amide linkage}$$

is known as an amide linkage, so nylon is called a **polyamide.** The N—H and C $=$ O groups in nylon are polar, and their mutual attraction is what holds adjacent chains of molecules firmly together (Fig. 13-16).

Dacron, whose structural elements are different from those of nylon, is a **polyester** because its elements are linked together by groups of the form

$$\begin{array}{c} \text{O} \\ \parallel \\ -\text{C}-\text{O}- \end{array} \qquad \textit{Ester linkage}$$

(see Table 13-2). Polyester resins reinforced with glass fibers are often used in boat hulls, truck bodies, and other large structures (Fig. 13-17).

The strongest synthetic fiber yet developed—10 times as strong as steel for the same weight—is a form of polythene called Spectra. The molecules in Spectra are as much as 100 times as long as those in ordinary polythene, and great care is taken when they are formed into fibers to keep them aligned in the fiber direction.

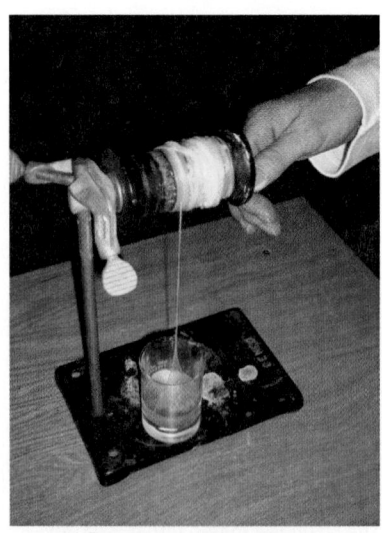

Figure 13-16   Winding a nylon filament from liquid polyamide in the laboratory.

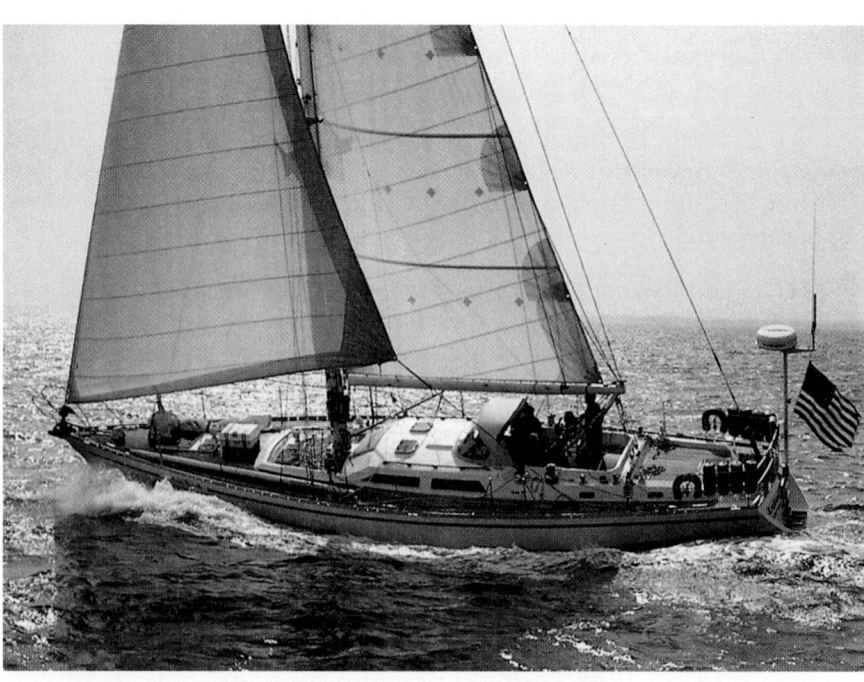

Figure 13-17   The hull of the yacht *Ardent Spirit* consists of fiberglass-reinforced polyester resin, and polyester fibers were woven to make the cloth for its sails.

Chemistry of Life

At one time the physical and biological worlds seemed two separate realms. They interacted with each other to be sure, but nevertheless they were thought to be distinct in that an intangible "life force" was thought to be present in living things but absent everywhere else.

Nowadays it is clear there is no life force. Instead there is a continuous chain of development from simple chemical compounds through more elaborate ones through viruses (which are neither "alive" nor "dead" by conventional definitions) through primitive one-celled organisms to complex plants and animals. Given the right chemical and physical conditions and plenty of time, there is every reason to believe that life will inevitably come into being from inorganic matter, as it has on our planet.

The four chief classes of organic compounds found in living matter are carbohydrates, lipids, proteins, and nucleic acids, which we shall examine in turn.

13.11 Carbohydrates

The First Link in the Food Chain

Carbohydrates are compounds of carbon, hydrogen, and oxygen whose molecules generally contain two atoms of hydrogen for every one of oxygen. They are manufactured in the leaves of green plants from carbon dioxide and water in the process of **photosynthesis,** with energy for the reaction being provided by sunlight. Sugars, starches, and cellulose are all carbohydrates.

An important group of sugars consists of isomers that have the same molecular formula, $C_6H_{12}O_6$. These sugars exist both as straight chains of C atoms and as ring structures. The ring forms are more stable and so occur in nature most often, but a sugar molecule of this kind can shift back and forth between the two forms. Here are the straight-chain and ring forms of glucose, which is the sugar circulated by the blood to provide the body with energy:

glucose
(straight-chain form)

glucose
(ring form)

The isomers of glucose—among them fructose (the sweetest-tasting of all), galactose, and mannose—have somewhat different structures and properties.

Simple sugars like those above are called **monosaccharides.** Two monosaccharide rings can link together to form a **disaccharide.** Thus sucrose (ordinary table sugar) consists of one ring of glucose and one of fructose; lactose (milk sugar) consists of one ring of glucose and one of galactose; and maltose (malt sugar) consists of two rings of glucose. The molecular formula of all three of these disaccharides is $C_{12}H_{22}O_{11}$, but of course their structures are different.

Polysaccharides   **Polysaccharides** are complex sugars that consist of chains of more than two simple sugars. They are naturally occurring polymers. In living things the polysaccharides serve both as structural components and as a medium of energy storage. In plants **cellulose,** which consists of a chain of about 1500 glucose rings, is the chief constituent of cell walls. Wood is mostly cellulose, as is cotton (Fig. 13-18). In fact, cellulose is the most abundant organic compound on earth.

Starch, whose 300 to 1000 glucose units are joined together in a slightly different way from those in cellulose, is a polysaccharide that plants use to store energy for later use. Starch occurs in grains that have an insoluble outer layer, and so remains in the cell in which it is formed until, when needed as fuel, it is broken down into soluble glucose molecules. (Chew a mouthful of white bread without swallowing. After a while the bread will begin to taste sweet as its starch molecules are broken up into glucose molecules by the action of enzymes in your saliva.)

A polysaccharide found in animals is **chitin,** which forms the outer shells of insects and crustaceans such as lobsters and crabs. Chitin is much like cellulose in structure and is also very abundant. Another polysaccharide is **glycogen,** which is present in the liver and muscles of animals and is released when energy is required. Glycogen, the animal equivalent of starch, is soluble, but its molecules are so large that they cannot pass readily through cell walls. When glucose is needed by an animal, its stored glycogen is split into the much smaller glucose molecules. When the stored glycogen of an endurance athlete such as a distance runner is used up, he or she "hits the wall" as extreme fatigue sets in.

Plant and Animal Energy   Living things obtain the energy they need by the oxidation of nutrient molecules. Generally the nutrient molecule most directly involved is glucose, and its oxidation is an exothermic reaction that yields carbon dioxide and water as products:

$$C_6H_{12}O_6 \;+\; 6O_2 \;\longrightarrow\; 6CO_2 \;+6H_2O \;+ \text{energy} \qquad \textit{Oxidation of}$$

glucose   oxygen   carbon   water   *glucose*
                               dioxide

This reaction takes place not all at once, as this equation would indicate, but in a complex series of steps that involve a number of other substances.

Figure 13-18   The cellulose in wood is extracted and made into paper at this mill in Maine.

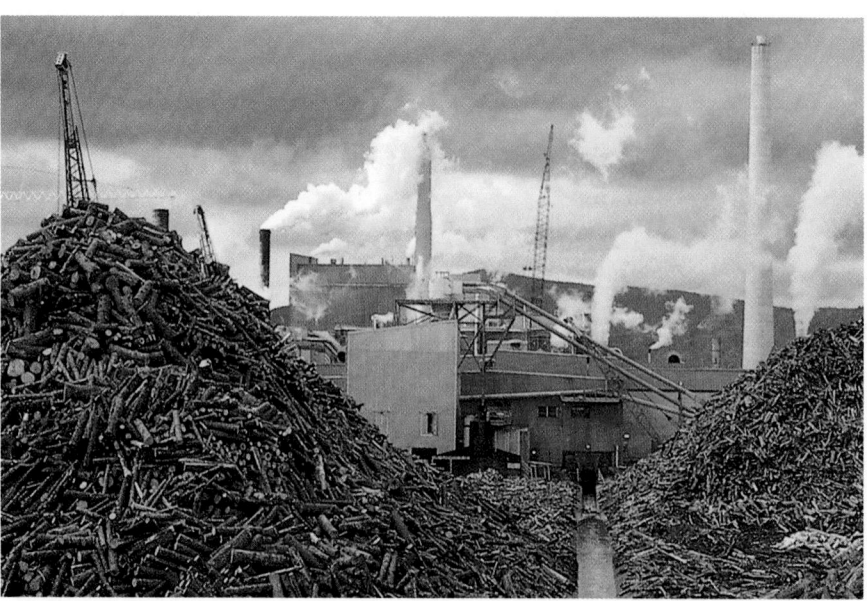

However, the net effect is the oxidation of glucose. The oxidation of glucose is evidently the reverse of photosynthesis and is the final process by which the energy in sunlight is turned into the energy used by living things.

Usually the carbohydrates in the food we eat are in the form of disaccharides and polysaccharides. In digestion these are **hydrolyzed** with the help of water to monosaccharides. Hydrolysis is promoted by enzymes, which are the specialized protein molecules that act as catalysts in most biochemical processes.

Although many animals can hydrolyze starch to glucose, very few can hydrolyze cellulose. Some plant-eating animals, for instance cattle, have microorganisms such as yeasts, protozoa, and bacteria in their digestive tracts, and enzymes from these microorganisms hydrolyze cellulose in the plants that are eaten. The resulting glucose can then be used by the animal (Fig. 13-19).

After digestion, glucose passes into the bloodstream to be circulated throughout the body. Glucose not immediately needed by the cells is converted into glycogen in the liver and elsewhere. If there is too much glucose to be stored as glycogen, the excess is synthesized into fats.

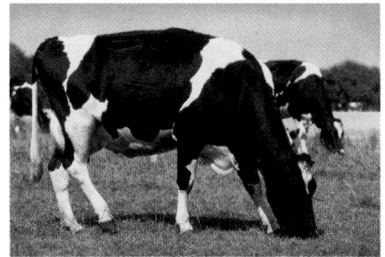

Figure 13-19   Microorganisms in their digestive systems enable cattle to convert the cellulose in plants to glucose. A great deal of methane, a greenhouse gas, is produced in the process and ends up in the atmosphere. The methane emitted by the world's meat and dairy cattle is an important contributor to global warming (see Sec. 4.4).

13.12   Photosynthesis

How the Sun Powers the Living World

As just mentioned, plants combine carbon dioxide from the air with water absorbed through their roots to form carbohydrates in photosynthesis (Fig. 13-20). Photosynthesis is highly endothermic, with the necessary energy coming from sunlight:

$$6CO_2 + 6H_2O + energy \longrightarrow C_6H_{12}O_6 + 6O_2 \quad \textit{Photosynthesis}$$

The energy is absorbed not directly by the CO_2 and H_2O but instead by a substance called **chlorophyll,** which is part of the green coloring matter of leaves. Chlorophyll acts as a catalyst that passes solar energy to the reacting molecules in a complicated way.

Perhaps 70 billion tons of carbon dioxide is cycled each year, about half by land plants and the rest by free-floating plantlike organisms (algae and certain bacteria) in the upper part of the oceans (Fig. 13-21). Photosynthesis is only about 1 percent efficient on the average in utilizing the sunlight that reaches plants. A few plants have much higher efficiencies—as much as 11 percent for sugarcane, which is why the cheapest ethanol sometimes used to replace or supplement gasoline is made from this source of sugar.

Origin of Atmospheric Oxygen   Photosynthesis not only maintains the oxygen content of the atmosphere but seems to have been responsible for it in the first place. The early atmosphere of the earth, which is thought to have consisted of gases emitted during volcanic action, contained oxygen only in combination with other elements in compounds such as water (H_2O), carbon dioxide (CO_2), and sulfur dioxide (SO_2). Primitive organisms, which probably obtained their own energy originally from such sources as sulfur, iron, and methane, eventually began to produce free oxygen by photosynthesis. There is evidence that photosynthesis has been going on for at least 3.5 billion years.

In time the oxygen content of the atmosphere increased to the point where more complex organisms could evolve (see Fig. 16-37). Besides the oxygen now in the atmosphere, photosynthesis is believed to account for much of the oxygen that is combined with other elements in the oxides, carbonates, and sulfates found in sediments and sedimentary rocks.

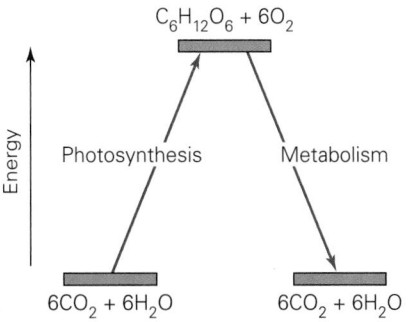

Figure 13-20   The energy needed for the photosynthesis of carbohydrates (shown is glucose) in plants comes from sunlight. The energy stored in carbohydrates is released during their metabolism by plants and animals.

Figure 13-21 The oxygen-carbon dioxide cycle in the atmosphere.

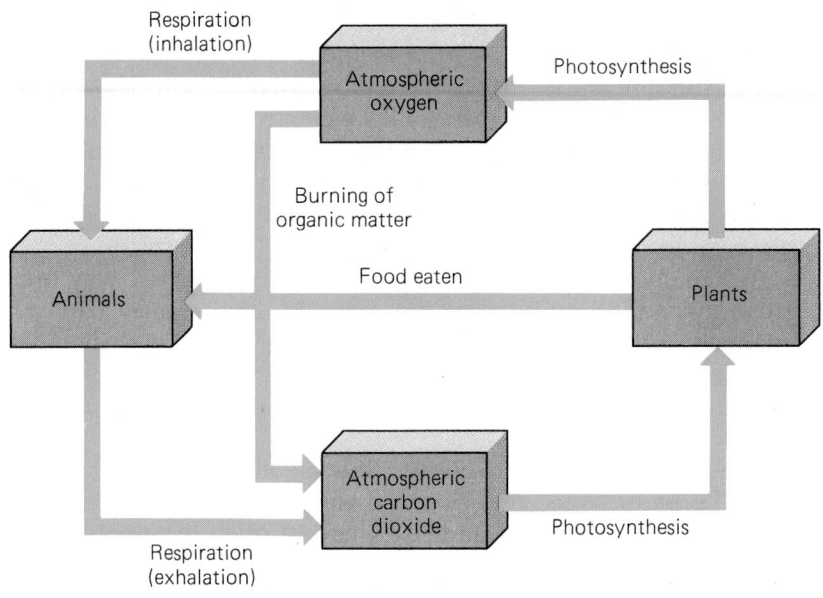

13.13 Lipids

Where the Calories Are

Fats and such fatlike substances as oils, waxes, and sterols are collectively known as **lipids.** Like carbohydrates, lipids contain only the elements C, H, and O. This is natural since lipids are synthesized in plants and animals from carbohydrates. The proportions and arrangements of these elements are different in lipids, though.

Fat Molecules A fat molecule consists of a glycerol molecule with three **fatty acid** molecules attached to it. The hydrocarbon chains in solid fats have only single bonds between their carbon atoms; hence they are saturated. Most animal fats are saturated. Liquid fats, such as vegetable oils, are unsaturated, with double bonds linking one or more carbon atoms. Polyunsaturated fats have more than one double bond per molecule. The double bonds introduce bends in such molecules, which prevents them from being closely packed together. As a result the interactions between nearby molecules are weaker than in the case of saturated fat molecules, and unsaturated fats are liquid at room temperature whereas saturated fats are solid.

Adding hydrogen atoms to the double-bonded carbon atoms in a liquid fat saturates the chains and gives a solid fat. Margarine is produced by such a **hydrogenation** process, with vegetable oils such as soybean and cottonseed oils being heated with hydrogen in the presence of a catalyst.

Fats are used for energy storage and other purposes, such as waterproofing, insulation against cold, and mechanical protection, in most living things. The digestion of a fat molecule involves the breaking of the ester links between its glycerol and fatty acid parts. The oxidation of the glycerol and fatty acids then proceeds in a fairly complicated way and releases nearly twice as much energy as in the case of the same mass of carbohydrate.

Cholesterol and Health **Cholesterol** is a lipid found in the bloodstream. Some comes from food of animal origin that we eat, and some is synthesized by the body itself from other lipids. **Atherosclerosis** ("hardening of the arteries") is a serious condition caused by deposits, largely of cholesterol, that restrict the flow of blood. Heart attacks occur when partly blocked arteries prevent

Plants and People

Suppose you are in a sealed room (perhaps in a space station) with plenty of light, either from the sun or from artificial sources. What area of plant life would there have to be to provide you with the oxygen you need and to absorb the carbon dioxide you exhale?

If you spend all your time resting, your body will require around 1750 kcal of energy per day. To obtain this much energy by metabolizing food will take a little less than 500 g of oxygen, which can be produced by plants that cover an area between 2.5 and 18 m², depending on the plants used and assuming optimum illumination. The same vegetation will absorb the CO_2 you breathe out.

In Russian experiments using algae to recycle air in this way, an area of 8 m² per person did the trick with artificial light powering the photosynthesis. A square plot of this area would be 9.3 ft on a side.

enough blood from reaching its muscles for the heart to function properly. These attacks are a leading cause of death. Eating unsaturated rather than saturated fats has been found to keep the cholesterol level in the blood low and so helps prevent atherosclerosis.

13.14 Proteins

The Building Blocks of Living Matter

Proteins are the principal constituent of living cells. They are compounds of carbon, hydrogen, oxygen, nitrogen, and often sulfur and phosphorus; some proteins contain still other elements.

Amino Acids   The basic chemical units of which protein molecules are composed are 20 **amino acids.** The simplest amino acid is glycine,

in which we recognize the characteristic carboxyl group —COOH of organic acids. Typical protein molecules consist of several hundred amino acids joined together in chains, and their structures are accordingly quite complex. The formula of one of the proteins found in milk is $C_{1864}H_{3012}O_{576}N_{468}S_{21}$, which gives an idea of the size of some protein molecules.

Plant and animal tissues contain proteins both in solution, as part of the fluid present in cells and in other fluids such as blood, and in insoluble form, such as the skin, muscles, hair, nails, horns, and so forth of animals. Silk is an almost pure protein. The human body contains thousands of different proteins, all of which it must make from the 20 amino acids it obtains from the digestion of the food proteins it takes in. One of the great successes of modern biochemistry was the discovery of how living cells build the complex arrangements of amino acids in their proteins.

Polypeptide Chains   In a protein molecule, the links between the amino acids consist of **peptide bonds** that are like the amide bonds in nylon. These chains of amino acids, called **polypeptide chains,** are usually coiled or folded in intricate patterns (Fig. 13-23). An important aspect of the patterns is the cross-linking that occurs between different chains and between different parts of the same chain.

The sequence of amino acids in a protein is just as important as which ones they are. The amino acid units in even a small protein molecule, such as insulin with 51 units, can be arranged in a great many different ways. However, only one arrangement has the biological effects associated with insulin. A parallel is with the formation of a word from the 26 letters of the alphabet. *Run* and *urn* have the same letters but mean different things because the order of the letters is different.

The alphabet of the proteins has only 20 letters, corresponding to the various amino acids, but the words may contain hundreds of letters whose relative positions in three dimensions are significant. The extraordinary number of different proteins, each serving a specific biological need in an organism, is not surprising in view of this picture of protein structure.

Every protein has a specific shape it must assume in order to carry out its function in the body. A number of serious diseases—for instance, Alzheimer's, Parkinson's, Huntington's, and several kinds of cancer—seem to be the result of incorrect protein folding.

Tissue Matching

The carbohydrates and the lipids do not share the specificity of the proteins. Glucose, for instance, is a carbohydrate found in all plants and animals, but no protein is similarly widespread. Even individuals of the same species have some proteins that are not quite identical, so that tissues cannot ordinarily be transplanted because of the danger of "rejection" of the graft. The matching of blood types before a transfusion is to ensure that the proteins in the blood of the donor are the same as those in the blood of the recipient (Fig. 13-22).

Drugs have been developed that can prevent transplanted organs such as kidneys and hearts from being rejected. Unfortunately such drugs also weaken the body's ability to defend itself from infection since both responses of the body to foreign proteins involve the same mechanisms.

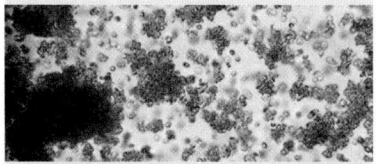

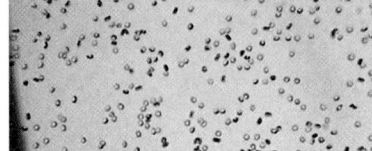

Figure 13-24   Matching blood types before a transfusion. *Top:* The blood types of donor and recipient are incompatible, which causes the red cells to clump together. *Bottom:* When the blood types are compatible, no clumping occurs.

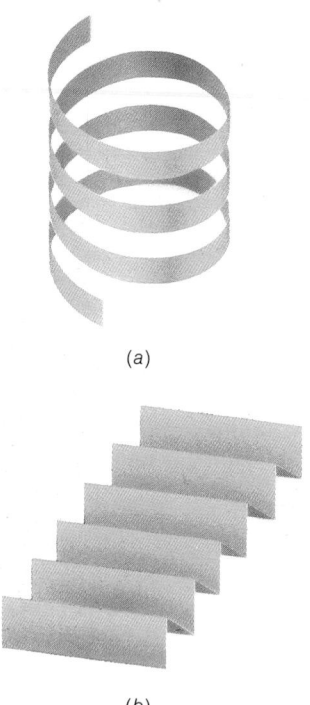

(a)

(b)

Figure 13-23   (a) The alpha helix form of a protein molecule. Each amino acid unit in the helix is linked by hydrogen bonds (a type of van der Waals bond) to other units above and below it. Most proteins have molecules like this. (b) The pleated sheet form of a protein molecule. Two or more chains of amino acid units are linked side-to-side along the sheet by hydrogen bonds. Fibrous proteins—such as those in hair, silk, cartilage, and horn—are of this kind. Some proteins have still other forms.

Spider Silk

A strand of spider silk is about five times as strong as a steel wire of the same size and is more elastic. Such strands consist chiefly of a protein polymer called fibroin that is similar to keratin, the protein found in hair and horns.

When a spider squeezes liquid fibroin out through a tiny orifice, some of the amino acid chains in the fibroin align into highly ordered crystals whose peptide bonds are exceptionally strong. The rest of the fibroin is in the less-ordered form of helices, as in Fig. 13-24a. The result is a composite material in which the crystals provide strength and the helices provide elasticity.

The diameter of a typical strand is 1 micrometer, a thousandth of a millimeter. Spider silk is used in medicine to make mats and sponges that serve as scaffolds on which human cells of various kinds are grown.

Dietary Protein   The human body can synthesize only some of the 20 amino acids it requires. The others must be present in our diets or else our bodies will not be able to manufacture the various proteins essential to life. A proper diet must therefore include not just an adequate total amount of proteins but also the right ones.

Most proteins of animal origin—such as those in meat, fish, eggs, and milk—contain all the needed amino acids, but plant proteins do not. The important amino acid lysine is missing in corn, wheat, and rice; isoleucine and valine are missing in wheat; threonine is missing in rice; and so on. Although it is certainly possible to live without eating meat or other animal products, a vegetarian diet not only must be sufficiently varied to include all the required amino acids but must provide all of these acids every day since they are not stored in the body and are needed together to manufacture proteins.

13.15   Soil Nitrogen

A Vital Component

The amino acids of which proteins are composed all contain nitrogen. The ultimate source of all our protein is plants, although much of it comes to us secondhand in such animal proteins as those in meat, eggs, and milk. Plants manufacture their proteins from simpler nitrogen compounds that enter their roots from the soil in which they grow.

Green plants cannot draw upon the stable molecules of free nitrogen in the air around them. All their nitrogen, and therefore all the nitrogen that goes into animal bodies as well, comes from nitrogen compounds in the soil. The nitrogen molecules we breathe can do us no good either, for the atoms in these molecules are held together by strong triple bonds that our body processes are unable to break. Like a shipwrecked sailor surrounded by seawater but dying of thirst, we are surrounded by an ocean of nitrogen but would perish except for the combined nitrogen that plants can absorb through their roots.

The formation of plant proteins steadily removes nitrogen compounds from the soil. Just as steadily, nitrogen compounds are returned to the soil by the decay of animal wastes and of dead plants and animals. The nitrogen of proteins is converted by decay into ammonia and ammonium salts, which are then oxidized to nitrates by soil bacteria. But the replenishment is never complete. Some nitrogen is lost permanently from the soil when nitrates and ammonium salts dissolve in streams and rainwash, and when bacteria decompose nitrates into free nitrogen.

Cooking

Two of the ways in which the heat of cooking affects raw food are to break up starch molecules and to "denature" protein molecules so that their amino-acid chains unfold. In both cases, the transformations make it easier for digestive enzymes to act.

Dorothy Crowfoot was fascinated at the age of 10 by the growth of crystals in alum and copper sulfate solutions as their solvent water evaporated. This fascination with crystals never left her. She studied chemistry at Oxford University despite the difficulties women students of science had to face in those days, and as an undergraduate had mastered x-ray crystallography well enough to have a research paper published. In this technique a narrow beam of x-rays is directed at a crystal from various angles and the resulting interference patterns are analyzed to yield the arrangement of the atoms in the crystal.

Dorothy Crowfoot went next to Cambridge University to work with J. D. Bernal, who had just begun to use x-rays to investigate biological molecules. Under the right conditions many such molecules form crystals from whose structures the structures of the molecules themselves can be inferred. In particular,

the structures of protein molecules are important because they are closely related to their biological functions. She and Bernal were the first to map the arrangement of the atoms in a protein, the digestive enzyme pepsin.

After two intense years at Cambridge, Dorothy Crowfoot returned to Oxford where she married Thomas Hodgkin and had three children while continuing active research. Her most notable work was on penicillin (then the most complex molecule to be successfully analyzed), vitamin B_{12}, and insulin (it took 35 years of on-and-off effort to finish the job). She was a pioneer in using computers to interpret x-ray data, an arduous task for all but the simplest molecules.

For all her achievements and their recognition in the scientific world, Hodgkin was for many years shabbily treated at Oxford: poor laboratory facilities, the lowest possible official status, half the pay of her

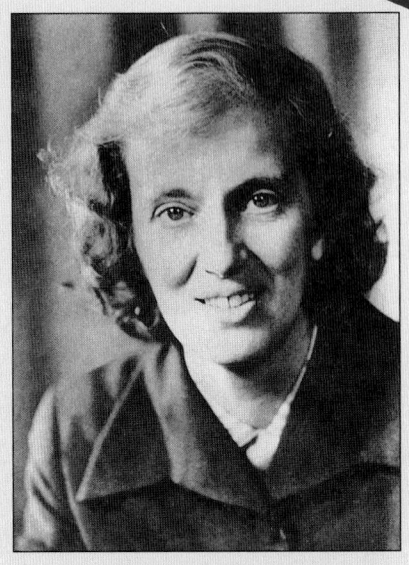

male colleagues with continual worries about making ends meet until outside support (much of it from the Rockefeller Foundation of the United States) became available. She received the Nobel Prize in chemistry in 1964, the third woman to do so.

Replacing Soil Nitrogen   Nature makes good these losses in two ways. Another kind of soil bacteria, the "nitrogen-fixing" bacteria, have the ability to break down the stable nitrogen molecules of the air and to manufacture nitrates from the atoms. Also, lightning causes atmospheric nitrogen and oxygen to combine into nitrogen oxides, which are brought down to the earth in rainwater. So in nature nitrogen goes through a continuous cycle (Fig. 13-24) that keeps the amount of fixed nitrogen in the soil approximately constant.

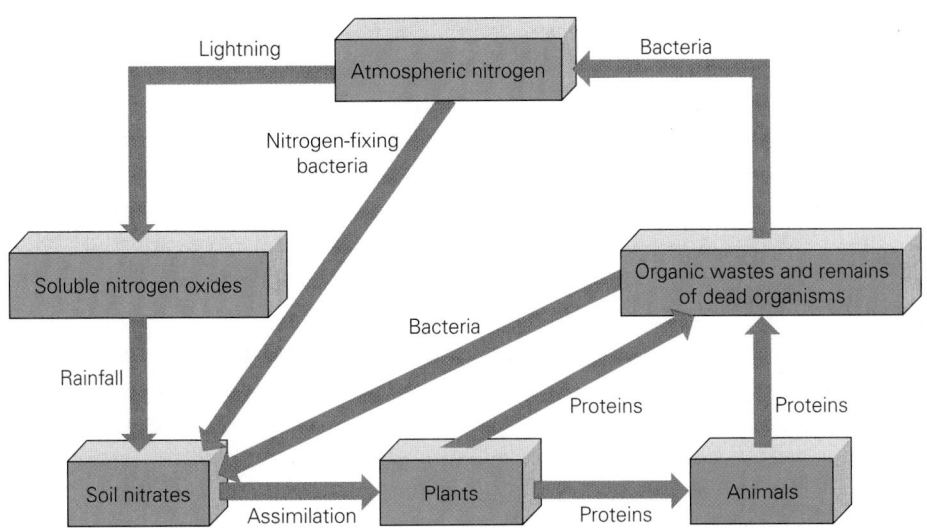

Figure 13-24   The nitrogen cycle on land.

Figure 13-25   Pure ammonia (NH$_3$) is sometimes applied directly to soil to supply it with the nitrogen that plants (here soybeans) need to manufacture proteins.

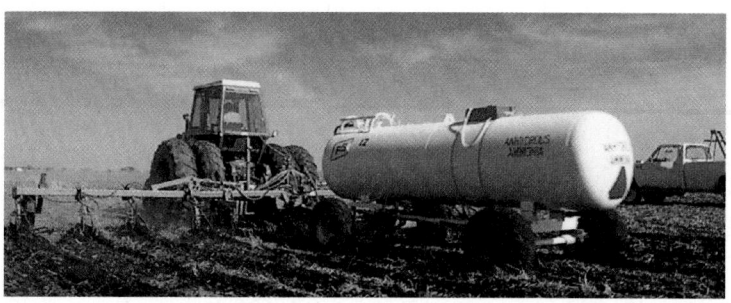

We have drastically disturbed this natural cycle. Much of the protein that enters our bodies is not returned to the soil but instead is dumped as sewage into various bodies of water. The use of plant material and manure for cooking fires in primitive areas further adds to the conversion of fixed nitrogen to free nitrogen. To be sure, manure is still used as fertilizer in some regions, and legumes, which are plants (such as peas and beans) on which nitrogen-fixing bacteria grow, are widely cultivated, but artificial fertilizers have become essential as sources of nitrogen for a large part of the world's agriculture (Fig. 13-25). Fertilizer manufacture uses about 1 percent of the world's energy supply.

On a global basis, a third of the protein in the human diet contains nitrogen derived from artificial fertilizers. Eighty million tons of nitrogen contained in such fertilizers is used each year, much of it ending up in groundwater, lakes, and rivers. Some of the consequences of this pollution were described in Sec. 11.9; nitrates in drinking water are also a health hazard.

13.16   Nucleic Acids

The Genetic Code

The **nucleic acids** are very minor constituents of living matter from the point of view of quantity. However, because they control the processes by which cells and organisms manufacture their proteins and reproduce themselves, these acids are extremely important. If anything may be said to be the key to the distinction between living and nonliving matter, it is the nucleic acids.

Nucleic acid molecules consist of long chains of units called **nucleotides.** As in the case of the amino acids in a polypeptide chain, both the kinds of nucleotide present and their arrangement govern the biological behavior of a nucleic acid.

Each nucleotide has three parts, a **phosphate group** (PO$_4$), **pentose sugar,** and a **nitrogen base.** A pentose sugar is one that contains five carbon atoms. In **ribonucleic acid** (RNA) the sugar is **ribose,** C$_5$H$_{10}$O$_5$, and in **deoxyribonucleic acid** (DNA) the sugar is **deoxyribose,** C$_5$H$_{10}$O$_4$, which has one O atom fewer than ribose. Nitrogen bases have characteristic ring structures of nitrogen and carbon atoms. Four nitrogen bases are found in DNA: adenine, guanine, cytosine, and thymine. The nitrogen bases in RNA are the same except that uracil replaces thymine.

DNA Structure   The structure of a DNA molecule is shown in Fig. 13-26. Pairs of nitrogen bases form the links between a double chain of alternate phosphate and deoxyribose groups. Adenine and thymine are always coupled together, as are cytosine and guanine. The chains are not flat but spiral around each other in a double helix, as in Fig. 13-26*b*. The double helix structure of DNA was discovered in 1953 by the American biologist

James D. Watson and the English physicist Francis H. C. Crick, who were working together at Cambridge University (Fig. 13-27).

Figure 13-26c shows the four "letters" of the genetic code. There may be hundreds of millions of such letters in a DNA molecule, and their precise sequence governs the properties of the cell in which the molecule is located. DNA molecules thus represent the biological blueprints that are translated into the processes of life.

The complexity of living things is mirrored in the complexity of DNA molecules, which are the largest known to science (Fig. 13-28). DNA molecules are normally folded and coiled into microscopic packages called **chromosomes.** If the 23 human chromosomes were stretched out, they would total about a meter in length. If DNA were as thick as a strand of spaghetti, a chromosome would be over 10 km long.

What DNA and RNA Do   DNA controls the development and functioning of a cell by determining the proteins the cell makes. This is only one aspect of the role of DNA in the life process. Another follows from the ability of DNA molecules to reproduce themselves, so that when a cell divides, all the new cells have the same characteristics (that is, the same **heredity**) as the original cell (Fig. 13-29). Finally, changes in the sequence of bases in a DNA molecule can occur under certain circumstances, for example, during exposure to x-rays. These changes will be reflected in alterations in the cell containing the DNA molecule. If such a **mutation** occurs in the DNA of a reproductive cell of an organism, the result may be that the descendants of the original organism will be different in some way from their ancestor.

Thus four fundamental attributes of life can be traced to DNA: the structure of every organism, how it functions, its ability to reproduce, and its ability to evolve into different forms in later generations.

The other type of nucleic acid, RNA, differs from DNA in a number of respects. RNA molecules are much smaller than DNA molecules, for example, and usually consist of only single strands of nucleotides. One type of RNA carries instructions for the synthesis of specific proteins from the DNA in a cell's nucleus to the place where the synthesis occurs. The instructions are in the form of a code in which each successive group of three nucleotides determines the particular amino acid to be added next to the protein polypeptide chain being formed. For example, the group GCA (guanine-cytosine-adenine) corresponds to the amino acid alanine, and GGA corresponds to glycine.

The Human Genome   Every cell in a plant or animal contains in its DNA coded instructions for making all the proteins the organism needs. The set of instructions for each protein is called a **gene;** human genes are 1000 to 1500 base pairs long. Genes make up only 2 percent of the human **genome,** the 3 billion or so base pairs present in our chromosomes. The rest of the genome (once dismissed as "junk DNA") contains a number of base-pair sequences that regulate the action of various genes. Some sequences that do not code for genes, amounting to 3.8 percent of the genome, are also found in other mammals, which suggests they are not random but either have an unknown function or once did. Perhaps raw material for new genes is part of the genome.

The human genome seems to contain about 23,000 genes. Preparing a detailed map that shows not only each gene but also its sequence of base pairs was an immense task that was started in 1988 and is now largely complete—an extraordinary accomplishment. The result is nothing less than a blueprint for human life. It is remarkable that such a linear code is able to produce enormously complex three-dimensional living things (such as us).

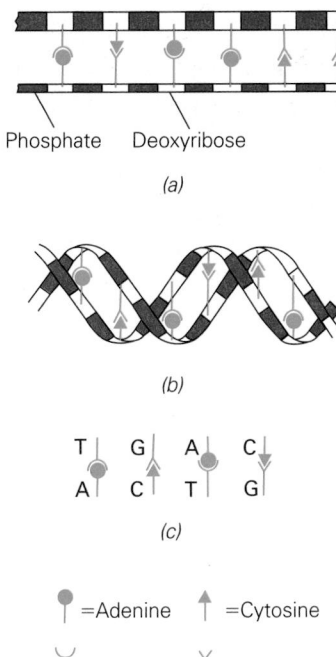

Phosphate   Deoxyribose

(a)

(b)

T | G   A | C
●   ▲   ▲   ●
A | C   T | G

(c)

● =Adenine   ▲ =Cytosine
Y =Thymine   Y =Guanine

Figure 13-26   The structure of DNA. (a) The nitrogen bases link a double chain of alternate phosphate and deoxyribose groups. Adenine and thymine are always paired, and cytosine and guanine are always paired. (b) The chains are not flat but form a double helix, like a twisted ladder. (c) The four "letters" of the genetic code.

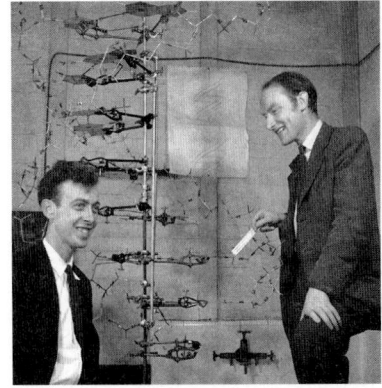

Figure 13-27   James D. Watson (1928–) *at left* and Francis H. C. Crick (1916–2004).

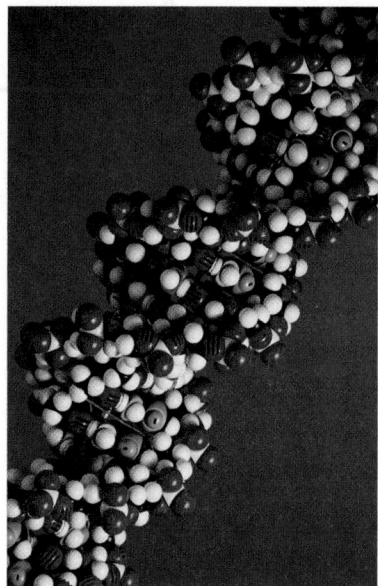

Figure 13-28   Model of a small part of a DNA molecule, which has the form of a double helix. The development and functioning of every living organism are ultimately controlled by the DNA in its cells. When the organism reproduces, copies of its DNA are passed on to the new generation. One cubic centimeter of DNA can hold more information than a trillion CDs.

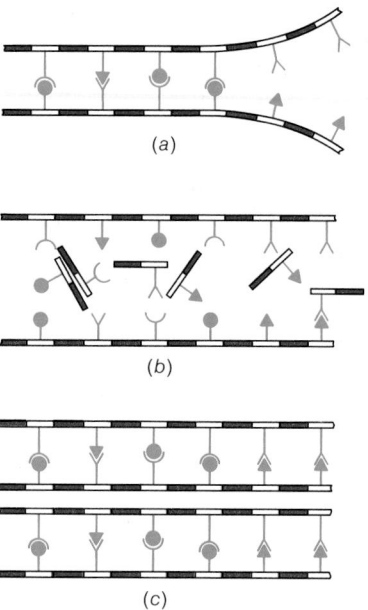

Figure 13-29   Simplified model of DNA replication. (*a*) When a cell reproduces, each double DNA chain it contains breaks into two single ones, much like a zipper opening. (*b*) The single chains then pick up from the cell material the nucleotides needed to complete their structures. (*c*) The result is two identical DNA chains.

The genomes of over a thousand species have either been or are being decoded today, with more to come. About 500 genes seem to be universal: every known genome contains them. The human genome, with 3 billion base pairs, is not unusual in size: the range in animals is from 350 million (the pufferfish) to 130 billion (the marbled lungfish). Plants may have surprisingly large genomes. That of the mere onion, with 17 billion base pairs, is over five times the size of ours. Why? Nobody knows.

A knowledge of the genome has practical importance apart from its intrinsic interest. Many diseases have a specifically genetic basis (for instance, cystic fibrosis and muscular dystrophy), and most, if not all, others have some genetic linkage. An example of a genetic linkage is the increased tendency members of some families have to contract a particular disease, such as cancer or Alzheimer's. The human genetic map is a guide toward better health for everybody.

13.17   Origin of Life

An Inevitable Result of Natural Processes

Whatever the earth's beginnings may have been, it is safe to assume that, at some time in the remote past, the surface was considerably warmer than it is at present. The atmosphere of the young earth almost certainly contained compounds of hydrogen, oxygen, carbon, and nitrogen; the most likely were water, methane, ammonia, and carbon dioxide (Fig. 13-30).

When an electric discharge simulating lightning is passed through a mixture of water vapor, hydrogen, methane, and ammonia, amino acids and other compounds of biological importance are formed (Fig. 13-31). This result seems to suggest that the raw materials for living things could have come into being in the early atmosphere of the earth. However, it is uncertain whether the young earth's atmosphere contained enough hydrogen and hydrogen-rich compounds, notably methane (CH_4) and ammonia (NH_3), to

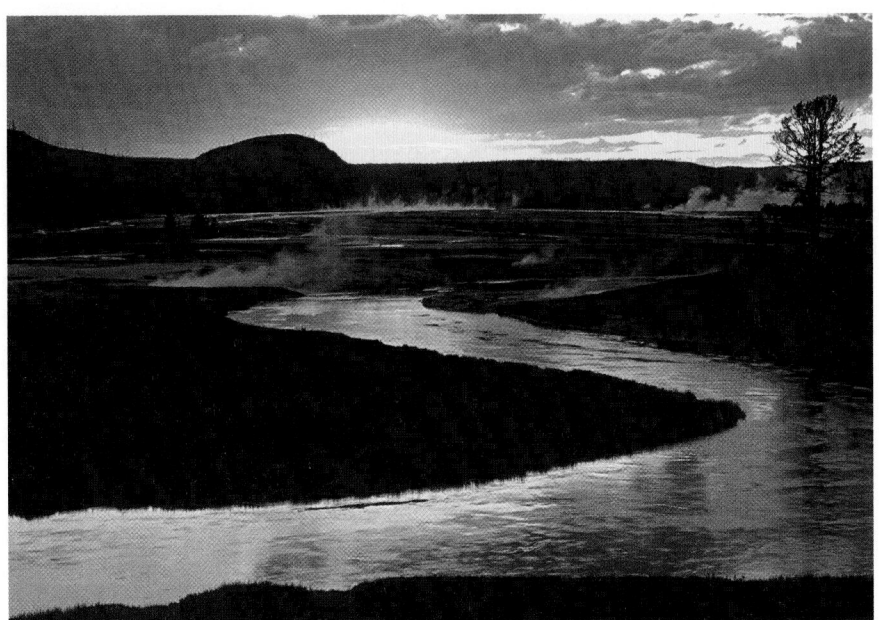

Figure 13-30 **Fumaroles** are vents in the earth's surface associated with volcanic activity that give out a mixture of gases, mainly water vapor, carbon dioxide, and nitrogen and sulfur compounds. The earth's oceans and atmosphere are believed to be the result of similar outgassing on a large scale early in the earth's history. These fumaroles are in Yellowstone National Park.

get very far on the journey to life. An atmosphere dominated by carbon dioxide, such as those of Venus and Mars, seems more probable.

Another hypothesis is that the ingredients of life came from space, where molecules of many compounds, including amino acids, have been identified both in clouds of matter from which stars and planetary systems condense (see Sec. 19.10) and in comets, which peppered the earth long ago. But, among other objections, the number of these compounds with biological significance is too few to fill in the blanks in any plausible picture of how life began.

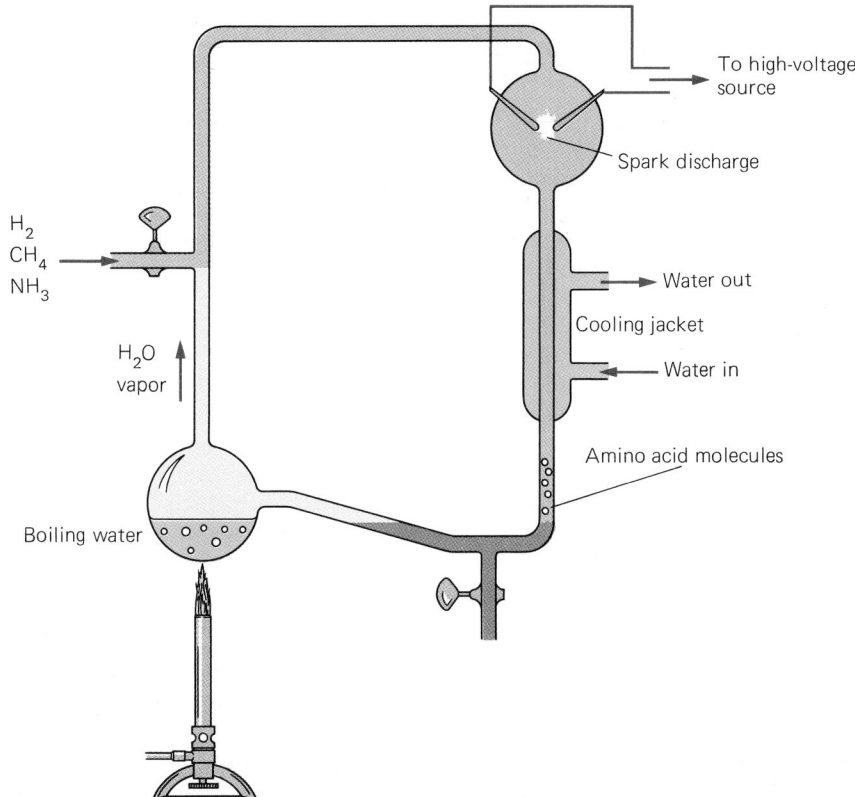

Figure 13-31 In this experiment, first performed in 1952 by Stanley Miller under the direction of Harold Urey, a number of the amino acids that constitute proteins were created by passing sparks that simulate lightning through a mixture of water vapor, hydrogen, methane, and ammonia.

Shadow Life

However the life we see around us originated, we know that it happened at least once. Could it have happened more than once, with "shadow" life forms coming into being independent of the life forms familiar to us? Although there are unlikely to be any undiscovered large-scale shadow plants or animals, fewer than 1 percent of single-celled microbe species have been thoroughly investigated. It seems entirely possible that shadow microbes exist somewhere, perhaps everywhere, and various studies are under way to look for them.

A more promising line of thought proposes that at least some of the building blocks of life were formed near hydrothermal vents, like those on the floors of modern oceans, from which scalding hot, chemical-laden water gushes out. Chemical reactions occur most readily in liquids, water is the best solvent, and there is ample energy here to power such reactions. And, indeed, not only individual amino acids but also short chains of them—miniature proteins—are created around today's vents. The nitrogen bases of RNA and DNA could perhaps also have such vents in their ancestry.

Good arguments put RNA rather than DNA as the first genetic molecule. For one thing, RNA molecules are both simpler and more stable than those of DNA. For another, RNA plays many more roles in life than just being a messenger for instructions from DNA, such as acting as a catalyst in various biochemical reactions.

Where could RNA have come from? One idea is that certain clays acted as templates for selecting the starting molecules for RNA and as scaffolds for assembling them. In experiments, RNA molecules up to 50 letters long developed on the surface of a variety of clay called montmorillonite. Another proposal details how RNA and proteins could have appeared together, each acting as a catalyst for the production of the other. Or, since recent work shows that the nucleotides of which RNA is composed seem able to link themselves together to form RNA chains without a catalyst, perhaps RNA came first and the amino acids in the primordial soup then became associated with it. Given proteins and RNA, all that remains to make a living cell able to function and reproduce is a fatty membrane to act as a container, and it is known that such membranes can spontaneously form in certain circumstances.

Living organisms certainly did not come into existence with the neatness and dispatch with which, say, a baker combines certain ingredients, puts the mixture in an oven, and takes out a cake an hour later. Although there is no agreement on which, if any, of the proposed pathways from individual molecules to the first cells was actually followed, nothing is known that conflicts with such a transformation. And plenty of time—hundreds of millions of years—was available between the origin of the earth 4.6 billion years ago and the existence of well-established life, probably primitive bacteria, that left traces in ancient rocks (see Sec. 16.13).

Important Terms and Ideas

Organic chemistry concerns the chemistry of carbon compounds. The number and variety of organic compounds result from the ability of carbon atoms to form covalent bonds with each other as well as with other atoms.

Structural formulas show not only the numbers of each kind of atom in a molecule but also how the atoms are joined together. **Isomers** are compounds with the same molecular formulas but different structural formulas, corresponding to different arrangements of the same atoms.

Double bonds and **triple bonds** are possible between carbon atoms in addition to single ones. The molecules of a **saturated** organic compound contain only single carbon-carbon bonds; those of an **unsaturated** compound contain one or more double or triple bonds. Unsaturated compounds react more readily than saturated ones.

A **functional group** is a group of atoms whose presence in an organic molecule determines its chemical behavior to a large extent. Thus the hydroxyl (OH) group characterizes the alcohols, the carboxyl (COOH) group characterizes the organic acids, and so on.

A **polymer** is a long chain of simple molecules (**monomers**) linked together. Plastics, synthetic fibers, and synthetic elastomers are polymers.

Carbohydrates are compounds of carbon, hydrogen, and oxygen manufactured in green plants from carbon dioxide and water by **photosynthesis** with sunlight providing the needed energy. Sugars, starches, and cellulose are carbohydrates. **Lipids** are fats and fatlike substances such as oils and waxes synthesized from carbohydrates by plants and animals. **Proteins,** the principal constituents of living matter, consist of long chains of **amino acid** molecules. The sequence of amino acids in a protein molecule together with the shape of the molecule determines its biological role.

The **nucleic acid** molecules DNA and RNA consist of long chains of **nucleotides,** atom groups whose precise sequence governs the structure and function of cells and organisms. DNA has the form of a double helix and carries the genetic code; one type of RNA has the form of a single helix and acts as a messenger in protein synthesis.

Multiple Choice

1. The science of organic chemistry has as its subject
   a. compounds produced by plants and animals
   b. carbon compounds
   c. compounds with complex molecules
   d. the determination of structural formulas

2. In comparison with organic compounds in general, most inorganic compounds
   a. are less soluble in water
   b. are more stable when heated
   c. are more likely to contain carbon
   d. react more slowly

3. The number of covalent bonds each carbon atom has in organic compounds is usually
   a. one   c. four
   b. two   d. six

4. The number of covalent bonds possible between two carbon atoms in organic molecules is
   a. one
   b. one or two
   c. one, two, or three
   d. one, two, three, or four

5. As a class, the alkanes are
   a. highly reactive
   b. soluble in water
   c. unaffected by acids and bases
   d. harmless to living things

6. In general, in the alkane series of hydrocarbons, a high molecular mass implies a (an)
   a. low boiling point
   b. high boiling point
   c. low freezing point
   d. artificial origin

7. Gasoline is a mixture of
   a. alkanes
   b. isomers of octane
   c. hydrocarbon derivatives
   d. unsaturated hydrocarbons

8. Compounds that have the same molecular formulas but different structural formulas are called
   a. hydrocarbons   c. polymers
   b. isomers   d. derivatives

9. Unsaturated hydrocarbon molecules are characterized by
   a. double or triple bonds between carbon atoms, so that additional atoms can be added readily
   b. the ability to absorb water
   c. the ability to dissolve in water
   d. benzene rings in their structural formulas

10. Hydrocarbon molecules with only single bonds between carbon atoms are
    a. fairly reactive   c. extremely dense
    b. fairly unreactive   d. unsaturated

11. In comparison with hydrocarbon molecules that have double or triple bonds between carbon atoms, hydrocarbon molecules with only single bonds are in general
    a. less reactive
    b. about the same in reactivity
    c. more reactive
    d. no generalization is possible

12. A molecule in which three bonds occur between carbon atoms is
    a. C_2H c. C_2H_4
    b. C_2H_2 d. C_2H_6

13. Which one or more of the following compounds cannot exist?
    a. C_2H_2 c. C_2H_4
    b. C_2H_3 d. C_4H_8

14. The number of electrons shared among all the carbon atoms in a benzene ring is
    a. 1   c. 6
    b. 2   d. 12

15. Hydrocarbon derivatives in general are
    a. formed by burning hydrocarbons in air
    b. alcohols
    c. hydrocarbons that have had H atoms replaced by other atoms or atom groups
    d. hydrocarbons that have more than one bond between carbon atoms

16. The alcohols are organic equivalents of inorganic
    a. acids   c. salts
    b. bases   d. oxides

17. The conversion of sugar to ethanol and carbon dioxide with enzymes acting as catalysts is called
    a. fermentation
    b. polymerization
    c. photosynthesis
    d. digestion

18. An organic acid molecule contains one or more carboxyl group whose molecular formula is
    a. CO   c. COH
    b. OH   d. COOH

19. Organic acids are
    a. strong and highly corrosive
    b. rather weak
    c. not found in nature but must be artificially made
    d. characterized by simple molecules

20. The reaction of ethanol with acetic acid produces ethyl acetate, which is a (an)
    a. aldehyde   c. aromatic compound
    b. ester   d. polymer

21. The structural elements of a polymer are called
    a. isomers   c. monomers
    b. elastomers   d. esters

22. Dacron is an example of a
  a. monomer   **c.** isomer
  b. polymer   **d.** elastomer

23. Living cells consist mainly of
  a. carbohydrates   **c.** proteins
  b. lipids   **d.** nucleic acids

24. Living things differ most from one another in their constituent
  a. carbohydrates   **c.** amino acids
  b. lipids   **d.** proteins

25. The most abundant organic compound on earth is
  a. methane   **c.** glucose
  b. benzene   **d.** cellulose

26. Photosynthesis produces
  a. carbohydrates
  b. proteins
  c. lipids
  d. all of these choices are correct

27. Animals store energy in the form of
  a. starch   **c.** chitin
  b. cellulose   **d.** glycogen

28. Plants store energy in the form of
  a. starch   **c.** chitin
  b. cellulose   **d.** glycogen

29. Fermentation can convert sugars to carbon dioxide and
  a. ethanol   **c.** starch
  b. acetic and   **d.** proteins

30. Cellulose is not
  a. a carbohydrate
  b. the chief constituent of wood
  c. present in all plants
  d. easily digested by most animals

31. Fats and oils are
  a. proteins   **c.** nucleic acids
  b. carbohydrates   **d.** lipids

32. Lipids are synthesized in plants and animals from
  a. proteins   **c.** enzymes
  b. carbohydrates   **d.** nucleic acids

33. A given mass of fat compared with the same mass of carbohydrate can provide the body with about
  a. half as much energy
  b. the same amount of energy
  c. twice as much energy
  d. 10 times as much energy

34. It is healthier to eat unsaturated rather than saturated fats because unsaturated fats
  a. are easier to digest
  b. contain more energy
  c. keep the cholesterol content of the blood low
  d. keep the glucose content of the blood low

35. Proteins consist of combinations of
  a. amino acids
  b. nucleic acids
  c. esters of glycerin with organic acids
  d. DNA and RNA molecules

36. The number of amino acids important to life is
  a. 2   **c.** 20
  b. 8   **d.** 69

37. Which of the following statements is correct?
  a. The human body can synthesize all the amino acids it requires.
  b. The human body can synthesize some of the amino acids it requires.
  c. The human body can synthesize none of the amino acids it requires.
  d. Different people require different groups of amino acids.

38. A transplanted body tissue or organ is "rejected" by the recipient's body when the donor and recipient have different
  a. carbohydrates
  b. proteins
  c. lipids
  d. all of these choices are correct

39. Most biochemical processes in living matter are catalyzed by
  a. enzymes   **c.** lipids
  b. glycogen   **d.** DNA

40. The structure of a DNA molecule resembles a
  a. single helix   **c.** pleated ribbon
  b. double helix   **d.** straight chain

41. Each three-nucleotide group in a DNA molecule corresponds to a particular
  a. amino acid   **c.** enzyme
  b. nucleic acid   **d.** protein

42. DNA is involved in which one or more of the following attributes of every living organism?
  a. Its structure.
  b. How it functions.
  c. Its ability to transmit its characteristics to its descendants.
  d. The ability of these characteristics to evolve, that is, to change in succeeding generations.

Exercises

13.1   Carbon Bonds

1. Why are there more carbon compounds than compounds of any other element?

2. In what ways do organic compounds, as a class, differ from inorganic compounds?

3. What is the principal bonding mechanism in organic molecules?

13.2   Alkanes
13.3   Petroleum Products

4. How can the different alkanes in petroleum be separated? What property of the alkanes makes this procedure possible?

5. Is gasoline a compound? If not, what is it?

13.4   Structural Formulas
13.5   Isomers
13.6   Unsaturated Hydrocarbons

6. Why are structural formulas more important in organic chemistry than in inorganic chemistry?

7. The isomers of a compound have the same chemical formula. In what way do they differ from one another?

8. Distinguish between unsaturated and saturated hydrocarbons, giving examples of each.

9. How many electrons are shared in a double bond between two carbon atoms?

10. What kind of carbon-carbon bonds are found in alkane molecules?

11. How many covalent bonds are present between the carbon atom and each oxygen atom in carbon dioxide, CO_2?

12. In general, how do the reactivities of hydrocarbon molecules that contain only single bonds compare with the reactivities of hydrocarbon molecules that contain double or triple bonds as well?

13. Why are substances whose molecules contain triple carbon-carbon bonds relatively rare?

14. The alkanes of Sec. 13.2 are saturated hydrocarbons with the general formula C_nH_{2n+2}. Another group of hydrocarbons called **alkenes** have molecules with two fewer H atoms than the corresponding alkane molecules, so their general formula is C_nH_{2n}. (a) Would you expect the alkenes to be saturated or unsaturated? (b) Would you expect more, less, or about the same reactivity in the alkenes as in the alkanes?

15. The structural formula of propane is given in Sec. 13.4. In bromopropane, one of the H atoms is replaced by a Br (bromine) atom. How many isomers does bromopropane have? What are their structural formulas?

16. Why does this structural formula not represent an actual molecule?

$$
\begin{array}{cc}
\text{H} & \text{H} \\
| & | \\
\text{H} - \text{C} - \text{C} \\
| & | \\
\text{H} & \text{H}
\end{array}
$$

17. Why does this structural formula not represent an actual molecule?

$$
\begin{array}{ccc}
\text{H} & \text{H} & \quad \text{H} \\
| & | & \diagup \\
\text{H} - \text{C} - \text{C} = \text{C} \\
| & | & \diagdown \\
\text{H} & \text{H} & \quad \text{H}
\end{array}
$$

18. In which of the compounds C_2H_2, C_2H_4, and C_4H_{10} are the carbon-carbon bonds single, in which are they double, and in which are they triple?

19. Is it possible for a molecule with the formula C_4H_2 to exist? If not, why not?

20. Is it possible for a molecule with the formula C_2H_3 to exist? If not, why not?

21. Is it possible for a molecule with the formula C_2H_6 to exist? If not, why not?

22. Each molecule of butyne, C_4H_6, has a triple bond between two of its carbon atoms. What is the structural formula of the butyne isomer in which the triple bond is in the middle of the molecule?

23. Each molecule of butene, C_4H_8, has a double bond between two of its carbon atoms. (a) Give the structural formulas for the isomers of butene in which the carbon atoms form a straight chain. (b) Another isomer is possible in which the carbon atoms form a branched chain. What is its structural formula?

24. Each molecule of propene, C_3H_6, has a double bond between two of its carbon atoms. Give the structural formula(s) for propene and its isomers, if any.

13.7   Benzene

25. What is the difference between aromatic and aliphatic compounds?

26. Why are all aromatic compounds unsaturated?

27. The carbon atoms in normal hexane, C_6H_{14}, form a straight chain. All the bonds are single. In cyclohexane the six carbon atoms are arranged in a ring. Give the structural formula of cyclohexane. Are all the bonds single?

13.8   Hydrocarbon Groups
13.9   Functional Groups

28. Ethanol can be used as an automotive fuel either by itself or added to gasoline. Give the equation for the combustion of ethanol.

29. When sugar undergoes fermentation to produce ethanol, what other compound is also formed?

30. To what class of organic compounds does the compound belong whose structure is shown below?

$$
\begin{array}{ccccc}
 & & \text{H} & & \\
\text{O} & & | & & \text{O} \\
\diagdown & & | & & \diagup \\
 \text{C} - &\text{C} - &\text{C} - &\text{C} \\
\diagup & & | & & \diagdown \\
\text{HO} & & \text{OH} & & \text{OH}
\end{array}
$$

31. To what class of organic compounds does the compound belong whose structure is shown below?

$$
\begin{array}{cccc}
\text{H} & \text{H} & & \\
| & | & & \text{O} \\
\text{H} - \text{C} - \text{C} - \text{C} & & \diagup\!\diagup \\
| & | & & \diagdown \\
\text{H} & \text{H} & & \text{H}
\end{array}
$$

32. What have the compounds in each of these pairs in common? How could you distinguish one from the other? (a) CH_3COOH and CH_3OH? (b) C_2H_5OH and H_2O?

33. What have the compounds in each of these pairs in common? How could you distinguish one from the other? (a) CH_4 and C_2H_4? (b) CH_4 and O_2?

34. Which of the following (a) dissolve in water, (b) are acids, (c) react with ethyl alcohol to give esters, (d) react with acetic acid to give esters?

C_2H_5COOH	C_3H_8
C_2H_4	C_2H_5OH
HCl	$C_3H_5(OH)_3$

35. Compare the properties of a simple ester, for instance, methyl acetate, with those of a salt, for instance, sodium chloride.

36. Why do you think the compound whose structure is shown below is called dimethyl ether?

$$
\begin{array}{ccc}
H & & H \\
| & & | \\
H-C-O-C-H \\
| & & | \\
H & & H
\end{array}
$$

37. Why do you think the compound whose structure is shown below is called trichloroethene?

$$
\begin{array}{ccc}
Cl & & H \\
\diagdown & & \diagup \\
 & C=C & \\
\diagup & & \diagdown \\
Cl & & Cl
\end{array}
$$

38. Use structural formulas to show the reaction between methyl alcohol and acetic acid to produce methyl acetate.

39. Give structural formulas for the two isomeric propyl alcohols that share the molecular formula C_3H_7OH.

40. What is the structural formula of methyl ethyl ketone?

41. (a) Give structural formulas for the three isomers of pentane, C_5H_{12}. (b) One of these isomers is also known as methylbutane. Which is it? (c) Another of these isomers is also known as dimethyl propane. Which is it?

13.10 Polymers

42. Teflon is inert, tough, and can tolerate high temperatures because the bonds between carbon and fluorine in its structure are extremely strong. What does this suggest about the chemical activity of fluorine?

13.11 Carbohydrates

13.12 Photosynthesis

13.13 Lipids

43. How does a plant obtain its carbohydrates and fats? An animal?

44. What are the products of the oxidation of glucose? Is the process endothermic or exothermic?

45. What is believed to be the origin of atmospheric oxygen?

46. The ultimate source of the energy in food is the energy liberated when hydrogen is converted to helium in thermonuclear reactions in the sun. Trace this energy from the sun to the food you eat.

47. Can you think of any function other than energy storage that body fat might have?

13.14 Proteins

13.15 Soil Nitrogen

48. Why do plants need nitrogen? Why can they not use nitrogen from the air? Where do nitrogen compounds in the soil come from?

49. What are the basic structural units of proteins? How does the human body obtain them?

13.16 Nucleic Acids

50. How many letters are there in the genetic code by which DNA governs protein synthesis? How many letters are used to specify a particular amino acid?

51. What change in a gene is involved in a mutation? What is the significance of mutations in reproduction?

52. To which class of organic compounds do most of the constituents of living cells belong?

Atmosphere and Hydrosphere

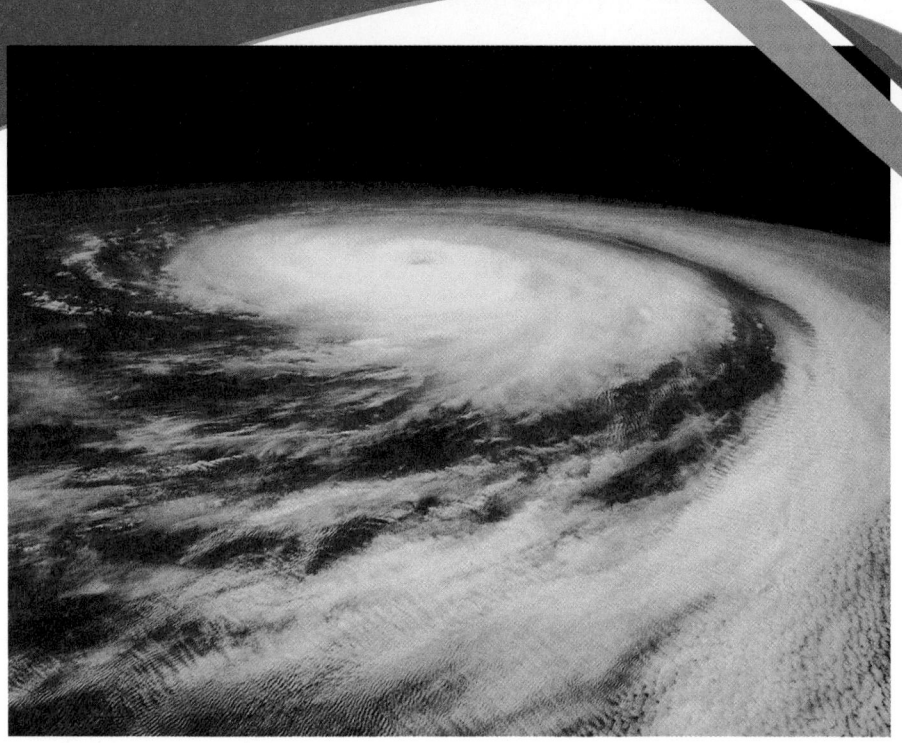

Hurricane Fefa east of Taiwan in 1991.

GOALS

When you have finished this chapter you should be able to complete the goals
• given for each section below:

The Atmosphere

14.1 Regions of the Atmosphere
Four Layers
• List in order of abundance the four chief ingredients of dry air near ground level.
• Distinguish among the troposphere, stratosphere, mesosphere, and thermosphere.
• Define ozone and explain why the ozone layer in the upper atmosphere is so important.

14.2 Atmospheric Moisture
Another Vital Cycle
• State what is meant by saturated air and by the relative humidity of a volume of air.

14.3 Clouds
Some Are Water Droplets, Others Are Ice Crystals
• List the three principal ways in which clouds form.
• Describe what causes rain and snow to fall from a cloud.

Weather

14.4 Atmospheric Energy
A Giant Greenhouse in the Sky
• Define insolation and describe the greenhouse effect.

• Discuss why temperatures vary around the earth.

14.5 The Seasons
They Are Due to the Tilt of the Earth's Axis
• Explain how the seasons of the year originate.

14.6 Winds
Currents of Air Driven by Temperature Differences
• Describe what is meant by a convection current.
• State the influence of the coriolis effect on wind direction in the northern and southern hemispheres.

14.7 General Circulation of the Atmosphere
Alternate Belts of Wind and Calm
• Sketch on a map the main surface wind systems of the world and name them and the belts of relative calm that separate them.
• Describe what a jet stream is.
• Describe what an El Niño is.

14.8 Middle-Latitude Weather Systems
Why Our Weather Is So Fickle
• Compare cyclones and anticyclones and describe the motion of air in each of them.
• Compare warm and cold fronts and describe what happens when a cold front overtakes a warm front.

Climate

14.9 Tropical Climates
Hot and Wet or Hot and Dry
• Explain how tropical cyclones originate and where they usually occur.

14.10 Middle- and High-Latitude Climates
Variety Is the Rule
• Account for the differences in climates in the United States.
• Give the reason why relatively little snow falls in the polar regions.

14.11 Climate Change
An Icy Past, a Warm Future
• Describe the ice ages and the variations in the earth's motions that may be responsible for them.

The Hydrosphere

14.12 Ocean Basins
Water, Water Everywhere
• Describe what a tsunami is and how it is caused.

14.13 Ocean Currents
Four Great Whirlpools
• List the ways in which the oceans affect climates.
• Describe how the Gulf Stream affects European climate and why it has little influence on climate in the United States.

The earth's **atmosphere** is an invisible envelope of gas we hardly notice except when the wind blows or when rain or snow falls. The atmosphere is also responsible for the blue of the sky, for the colors of sunrise and sunset, and for the rainbow, as we learned in Chap. 7. Less obvious but more important is the role of the atmosphere in the living world. Its oxygen, nitrogen, and carbon dioxide are essential for life. It screens out deadly ultraviolet and x-rays from the sun. It carries energy and water over the face of the earth. And, by weathering away rocks, it helps form the soil in which plants grow.

All the water of the earth's surface is included in the **hydrosphere.** Oceans, seas, rivers, and lakes cover about three-quarters of the surface area of our planet. The oceans, of course, make up by far the greatest part of the hydrosphere, and they are a major factor in shaping the environment of life on earth.

The Atmosphere

14.1   Regions of the Atmosphere

Four Layers

The chief gases of the atmosphere and their average abundances are given in Table 14-1. Water vapor is also present but to a variable extent, from nearly none to about 4 percent. In addition, the lower atmosphere contains a great many small particles of different kinds, such as soot, bits of rock and soil, salt grains from the evaporation of seawater droplets, and spores, pollen, and bacteria.

Those of us who have been among mountains know that the higher up we go, the thinner and colder the air becomes. In the lower atmosphere, air temperature falls an average of 6.5°C per km of altitude. At an elevation of only 5 km (about 16,400 ft) the pressure is down to half what it is at sea level (Fig. 14-1) and the temperature is about −20°C. At about 11 km (36,000 ft) the pressure is only one-fourth its sea-level value, which means that 75 percent of the atmosphere lies below. The temperature at 11 km is about −55°C, which is cold but no colder than it sometimes is at ground level in Siberia and northern Canada. The atmosphere stays that cold for 14 km more.

Table 14-1	The Composition of Dry Air Near Ground Level

Gas	Average Percentage by Volume
Nitrogen	78.08
Oxygen	20.95
Argon	0.93
Carbon dioxide	0.03
Neon	0.0018
Helium	0.00052
Methane	0.00015
Krypton	0.00011
Hydrogen, carbon monoxide, xenon, ozone	<0.0001

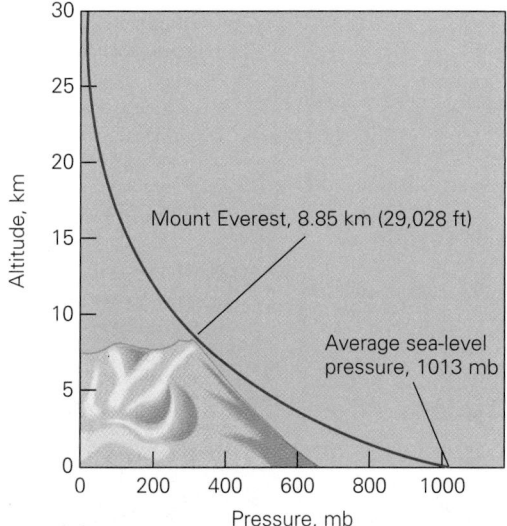

Figure 14-1   The variation of atmospheric pressure with altitude. The **millibar** (mb) is the pressure unit used in meteorology, where 1 mb = 100 Pa = 1 hPa. The average sea-level pressure of 1013 mb corresponds to 14.7 lb/in.^{2}. The lowest and highest surface pressures ever recorded are respectively 870 mb (in a Pacific typhoon) and 1084 mb (in a Siberian winter).

BIOGRAPHY   Evangelista Torricelli (1608–1647)

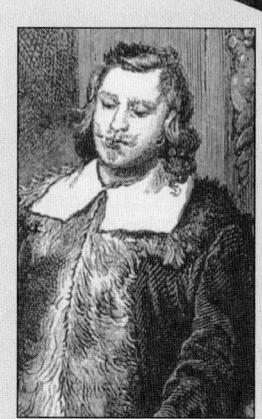

Born near Ravenna, Italy, Torricelli studied mathematics in Rome. He revered Galileo and was his secretary in Florence for the last few months of Galileo's life. Torricelli then became court mathematician to the Grand Duke of Tuscany, Galileo's old position. Galileo had found it odd that, on the upstroke of its piston, a suction pump could lift water no more than about 10 m, and he suggested that Torricelli investigate the matter. As others did in those days, Galileo thought that pumps were able to lift water because "nature abhors a vacuum," so there seemed no reason for the observed limit of 10 m.

Torricelli concluded that the behavior of a lift pump made sense if air has mass, so that the atmosphere presses on the water feeding the pump and thereby pushes it upward in the cylinder as the piston is raised. The limit of 10 m meant that the atmosphere was finite in extent and did not fill the entire universe, despite the belief of many scientists then.

To test his ideas, in 1643 Torricelli filled a glass tube, closed at one end, with mercury, whose density is nearly 14 times that of water. Holding his thumb over the open end of the tube, Torricelli turned it upside down and placed the open end in a dish of mercury. When he removed his thumb, the mercury level dropped in the tube but stopped when its height was about 760 mm above the mercury in the dish, $\frac{1}{14}$ of the maximum height that water could be lifted by a pump. This was

the first barometer, with the mercury height directly proportional to the pressure of the atmosphere. (Fig. 14-2).

Torricelli observed that the mercury height varied slightly from day to day and interpreted this to mean that atmospheric pressure varied similarly. Three years later the French mathematician and physicist Blaise Pascal realized that, if atmospheric pressure is due to the weight of the atmosphere, then it should decrease with altitude. Himself not very robust, Pascal gave his brother-in-law two barometers to take up a mountain. The mercury columns dropped by several centimeters, which verified Torricelli's insights.

A pressure unit equal to the pressure exerted by a mercury column 1 mm high is called the **torr** in honor of Torricelli; blood pressures in medicine are conventionally expressed in torr (Sec. 5.5).

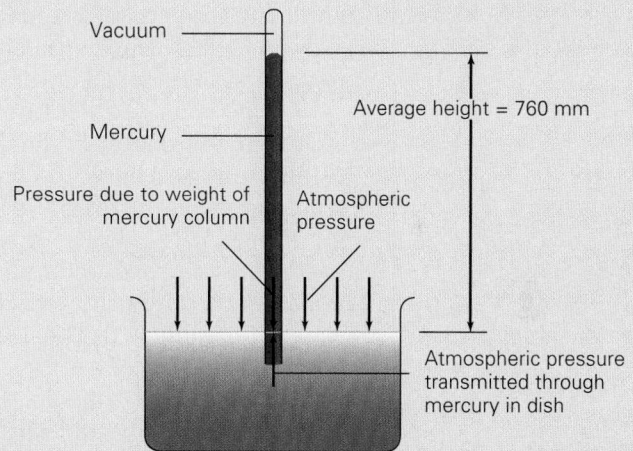

Figure 14-2   In a mercury barometer, the pressure due to the weight of a column of mercury is balanced by atmospheric pressure due to the weight of the air above the mercury in a dish. Atmospheric pressure varies with weather conditions over a range of about 20 percent of its average value of 1013 mb (see Fig. 14-1), which corresponds to a mercury height of 760 mm. Another type of barometer is shown in Fig. 5-16.

A passenger in an airplane climbing past 11 km would notice a marked change in the atmosphere. Above that level there are almost no clouds, no storms, not even dust. Since the character of the atmosphere changes so abruptly at the 11-km level, this is taken as the boundary between the two lowest layers of the atmosphere. The dense part near the ground is called the **troposphere,** and the clear layer above it is called the **stratosphere.** Such features of the weather as clouds and storms, fog and haze, belong to the troposphere. Figure 14-3 shows how the atmosphere is divided into regions based on temperature behavior.

Ozone   An important aspect of the stratosphere is the presence of ozone, O_3, which was described in Sec. 12.2. Ozone is produced in the stratosphere

Figure 14-3   The variation of temperature with altitude. The altitudes of the boundaries between regions of the atmosphere are averages.

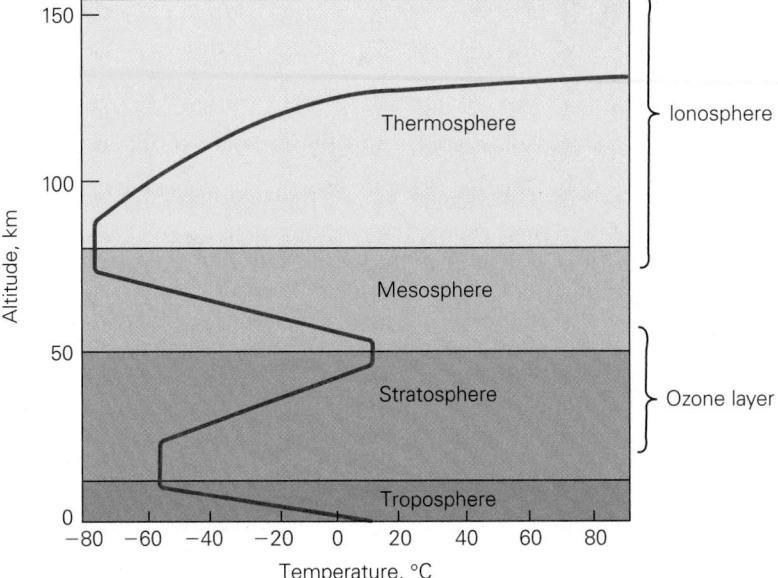

when solar radiation breaks up O_2 molecules into O atoms. Some O atoms then join O_2 molecules to give ozone molecules: $O + O_2 \rightarrow O_3$. As O_3 molecules are being formed, others are combining with O atoms to give O_2 molecules: $O + O_3 \rightarrow 2O_2$. Hence the situation is one of equilibrium, with ozone being formed and destroyed at the same rates.

Ozone is an excellent absorber of ultraviolet radiation. It is so good, in fact, that the relatively small amount of ozone in the stratosphere is able to filter out nearly all the dangerous short-wavelength ultraviolet radiation reaching the earth from the sun. Because this radiation is so harmful to living things, it is believed that life did not leave the protection of the sea to become established on land until the ozone layer had come into being. The maximum concentration of ozone occurs at 22 km, where less than one molecule in 4 million is O_3—hardly an impressive amount for so efficient an absorber.

Because the ozone in the stratosphere is so valuable, pollutants that attack it are highly undesirable. Among the worst such pollutants are artificially made gases called chlorofluorocarbons (CFCs) and hydrochlorofluorocarbons (HCFCs). An example is $CHClF_2$, usually referred to as HCFC-22, R-22, or Freon 22. These gases are widely used in refrigerators and air conditioners, as cleaning solvents, as the propellants in spray cans, and in making foam-plastic objects. In each application some CFCs or HCFCs escape into the atmosphere. The chlorine in them catalyzes the breakdown of O_3 molecules, and once in the stratosphere, the chlorine can remain there for a very long time. One chlorine molecule can destroy around 100,000 ozone molecules during its stay in the stratosphere.

The Ozone Hole   By now the CFCs and HCFCs have measurably weakened the ozone shield. This is a serious matter since the additional ultraviolet radiation that reaches the earth as a result increases skin cancer and cataract rates, depresses immune systems, and reduces crop yields, among other effects. Over Antarctica, weather patterns have enabled the CFCs and HCFCs to punch a huge seasonal "hole" of low O_3 concentration in the ozone layer larger in size than North America, and something similar seems to be happening in the Arctic.

By international agreement production of CFCs and HCFCs (and similarly destructive gases that contain bromine) is being phased out and other gases,

Smog in Los Angeles and Elsewhere

On an average day 9000 tons of carbon monoxide, various hydrocarbons, nitrogen and sulfur oxides, and small particles such as soot are emitted in the Los Angeles basin, mainly by vehicles and industry. (On some days, 25 percent of the particulate matter has been blown over from China, where 400,000 people die prematurely every year from diseases linked to air pollution.) Sunlight acting on this already nasty mixture adds toxic ozone to it. The result of breathing such polluted air is a high rate of respiratory diseases such as bronchitis and asthma and an increased risk of cancer. The air in Los Angeles is unhealthful on half the days each year (Fig. 14-4).

Los Angeles is not alone in having dirty air: all 20 of the world's largest cities exceed World Health Organization limits in at least one pollutant (Fig. 14-5). According to the Environmental Protection Agency, 95 percent of the U.S. population has an increased likelihood of developing cancer due to breathing toxic substances in the air. The EPA believes that as many as 12,000 premature deaths per year could be avoided with stricter limits on ground-level ozone. The American Petroleum Institute, which represents most oil companies, opposes such limits.

The situation in the Los Angeles basin is made worse by the frequent **temperature inversions** that occur there; Mexico City is another victim of this phenomenon. Ordinarily air temperature falls steadily with increasing altitude in the lower atmosphere. Sometimes, however, a temporary situation arises in which a layer of air aloft is warmer than the air below it. This is called a temperature inversion. Polluted air cannot rise past an inversion because

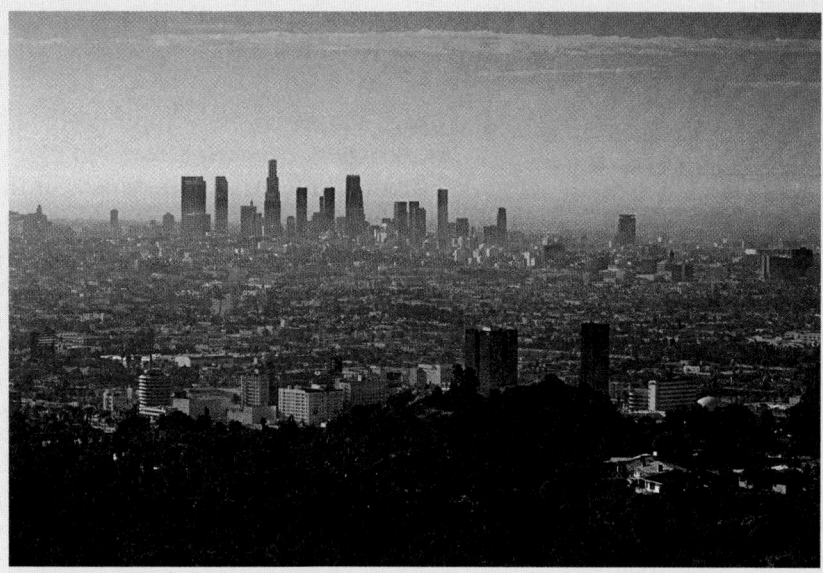

Figure 14-4 Smog in Los Angeles. When cool air from the Pacific blows into the Los Angeles basin, it forms a dense layer under warm air above it that stops polluted air from rising upward. The result of such a temperature inversion is heavy smog, made worse by nearby mountains that prevent the smog from escaping inland.

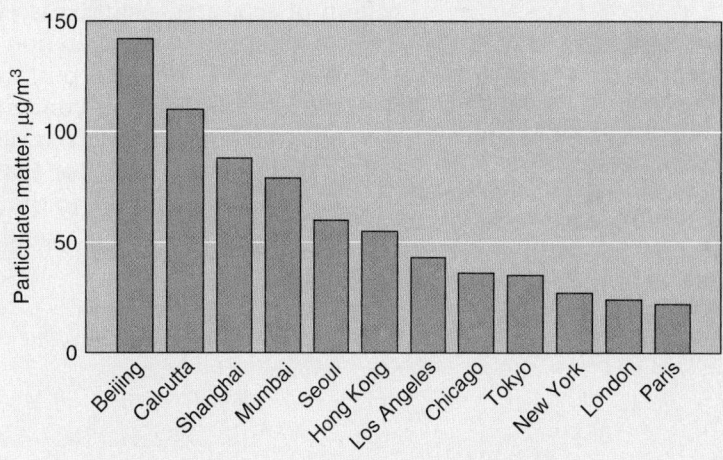

Figure 14-5 Average densities of particulate matter, mainly soot and dust, in the air of various cities. In the United States, densities of over 50 μg/m^3 (micrograms per cubic meter) are considered unhealthy; the European Union figure is 40 μg/m^3. The World Health Organization has found that deaths due to cardiopulmonary diseases and lung cancer increase above a density of 10 μg/m^3.

when it reaches the inversion, the density of the polluted air is greater than that of the warm air layer on top. Hence the inversion acts to trap the polluted air, which results in a persistent smog.

less harmful to the ozone layer, are replacing them. In the United States, production and import of some CFCs and HCFCs are becoming increasingly restricted, with a complete ban on all of them to come in 2030. But because the changeover is taking place gradually, because air conditioners are being installed at rapid rates in China and India with their huge populations, and because these gases in the atmosphere take an average of 75 years to release their chlorine, the ozone layer will not fully recover for a long time to come.

Mesosphere and Thermosphere   The ozone of the stratosphere causes a rise in temperature to 10°C or so in the vicinity of 50 km. At this altitude the atmosphere is $\frac{1}{1000}$ of its density at sea level. The temperature then falls once more to another minimum of about −75°C at 80 km. The portion of the atmosphere between 50 and 80 km is known as the **mesosphere.**

Above 80 km the properties of the atmosphere change radically, for now ions become abundant. The **thermosphere** extends from 80 km to about 600 km, with the temperature increasing to about 2000°C. (We must keep in mind that the density of the thermosphere is extremely low, so that despite the high temperatures a slowly moving object there would not get hot if shielded from direct sunlight.) The thermosphere is the home of the ionosphere, which was described in Sec. 7.9; it is where auroras—"northern lights"—occur (Sec. 18.5) and also where most small meteoroids burn up when they approach the earth (Sec. 17.3).

14.2 Atmospheric Moisture

Another Vital Cycle

Water vapor consists of water molecules that have escaped, or **evaporated,** from a body of water at a temperature below the boiling point of water. The moisture content, or **humidity,** of air refers to the amount of water vapor that it contains. Most of the atmosphere's water vapor comes from the evaporation of seawater. A little also comes from evaporation of water in lakes, rivers, moist soil, and vegetation (Fig. 14-6).

Since water vapor is continually being added to air by evaporation and periodically removed by condensation as clouds, fog, rain, and snow, the humidity of the atmosphere varies a lot from day to day and from one region to another. If it were not for the ability of water to evaporate, to be carried by winds, and later to fall to the ground, all the earth's water would be in its oceans and the continents would be lifeless deserts.

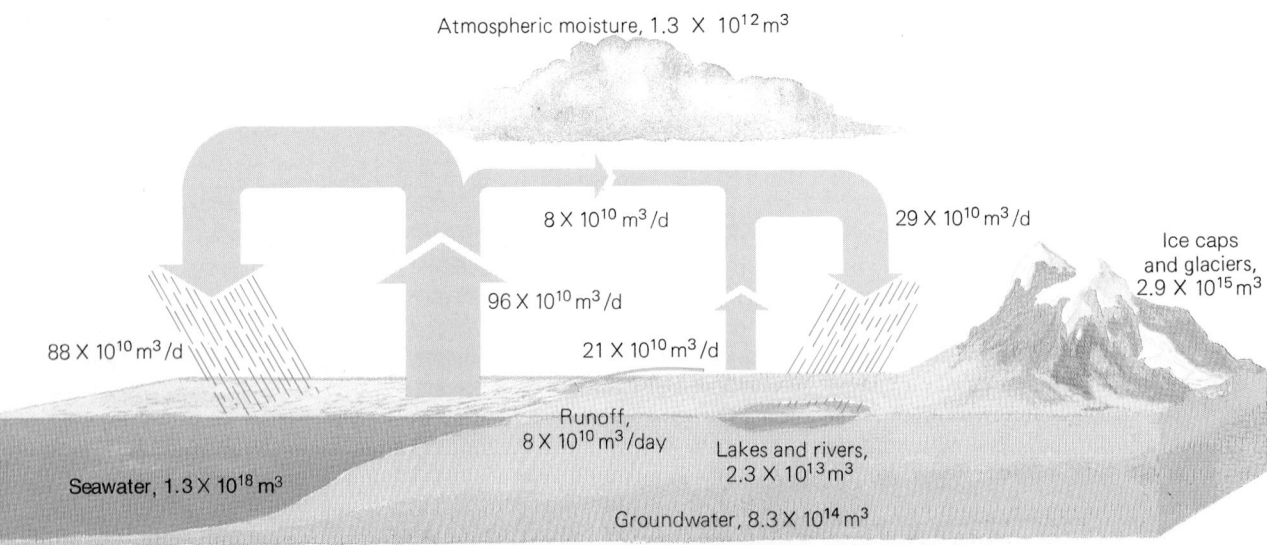

Atmospheric moisture, $1.3 \times 10^{12}\,m^3$

$8 \times 10^{10}\,m^3/d$ $29 \times 10^{10}\,m^3/d$

Ice caps and glaciers, $2.9 \times 10^{15}\,m^3$

$96 \times 10^{10}\,m^3/d$

$88 \times 10^{10}\,m^3/d$ $21 \times 10^{10}\,m^3/d$

Runoff, $8 \times 10^{10}\,m^3/day$

Lakes and rivers, $2.3 \times 10^{13}\,m^3$

Seawater, $1.3 \times 10^{18}\,m^3$

Groundwater, $8.3 \times 10^{14}\,m^3$

Figure 14-6 The world's water content and its daily cycle. Upward arrows indicate evaporation; downward arrows indicate precipitation. If all the water vapor in the atmosphere were condensed, it would form a liquid layer only about 2.5 cm thick. Rainfall in the United States varies from region to region; the average is about 76 cm per year.

We can regard air as a sort of sponge for water vapor, and like an ordinary sponge, air at a given temperature can absorb only so much water and no more. Air is said to be **saturated** when it holds this maximum amount of water vapor. (To be accurate, air has nothing to do with evaporation. Even if there were no air, vapor would still escape from bodies of water. But, since moving air carries water vapor from one region to another and since air is the medium in which water vapor condenses as clouds, fog, rain, or snow, it is convenient to think of the air as "taking up" and "holding" different amounts of vapor.)

We usually describe air as humid if it is saturated or nearly saturated, and as dry if it is highly unsaturated. Humid weather is uncomfortable because little moisture can evaporate from the skin into saturated air, and so perspiration does not produce its usual cooling effect. Very dry air is harmful to the skin and mucous membranes because their moisture evaporates too rapidly to be replaced.

14.3 Clouds

Some Are Water Droplets, Others Are Ice Crystals

When air that contains water vapor is cooled past its saturation point, some of the vapor condenses to a liquid. Dew forms because the temperature of the

---

Relative Humidity and Dew Point

Meteorologists express the moisture content of air in terms of **relative humidity,** a percentage that indicates the extent to which air is saturated with water vapor. (The **absolute humidity** is the actual density of water vapor.) A relative humidity of 100 percent means that the air is completely saturated with water vapor, 50 percent means that the air contains half of the maximum it could hold, and 0 percent means perfectly dry air.

The amount of moisture that air can hold increases with temperature (Fig. 14-7). As a result, a sample of air becomes less saturated when it is heated (its relative humidity goes down) and more saturated when it is cooled (its relative humidity goes up).

Suppose outside air at, say, 10°C and 70 percent relative humidity is taken inside a house and heated to 20°C. The relative humidity indoors will then drop to only about 35 percent, even though the actual vapor density stays the same. Such a low relative humidity is not desirable, so a way to add more moisture to heated air in winter should be provided.

On the other hand, if summer air at, say, 30°C and 70 percent relative humidity is cooled, it will reach saturation (100 percent relative humidity) at only 24°C. Further cooling will cause water to condense out. An air-conditioning system should therefore include a way to remove water vapor from the air being cooled to keep the relative humidity at a comfortable level.

The **dew point** of air with a certain water vapor content is the temperature at which the air would be saturated. Suppose the air somewhere contains 9.4 g/m³ of water vapor. According to Fig. 14-7, air with this vapor content is saturated at 10°C, so the dew point of this air is 10°C. At temperatures above 10°C, the relative humidity

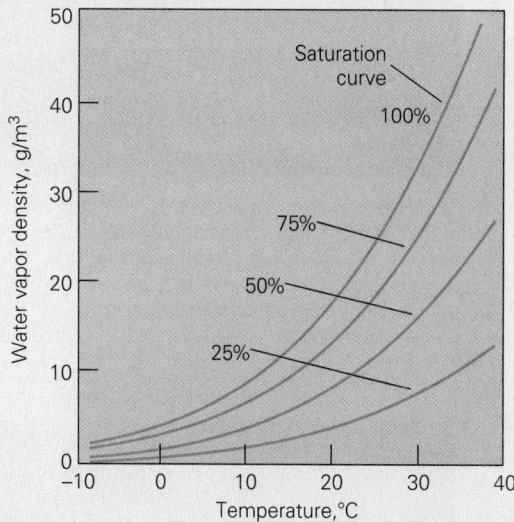

Figure 14-7 How the density of water vapor varies with temperature for various relative humidities. Each curve corresponds to a different relative humidity. The curve for 100% relative humidity represents saturation, when the air can hold no more water vapor.

of the air is below 100 percent; at 20°C, for instance, it would be 54 percent. If the temperature of the air drops to 10°C or less, however, some moisture will condense out. Dew point can be used as a guide to the possibility of fog. When the air temperature is well above the dew point, the relative humidity is low, and there is no danger of fog. When the air temperature is near the dew point and is decreasing, though, fog is likely.

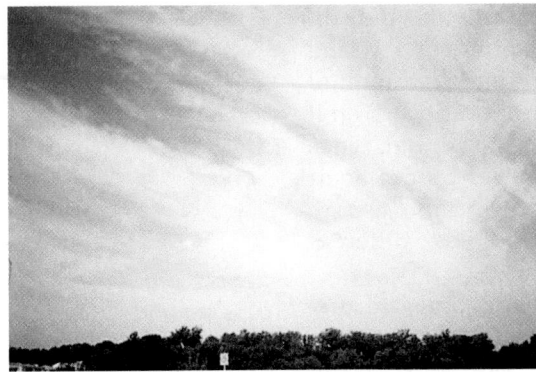

Cirrus clouds consist of ice crystals and occur at high altitudes. They are wispy or featherlike. *Stratus* clouds occur in broad, flat layers. The *cirrostratus* clouds shown combine features of both types. If such clouds grow thicker and darker, a storm is approaching.

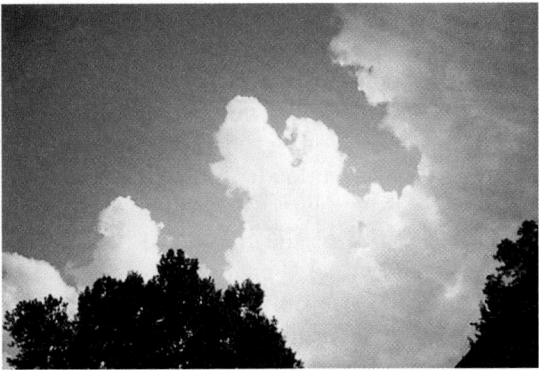

Cumulus clouds, such as these, are dense and heaped upwards with flat bottoms and puffy tops. They are common features of fair weather and usually dissipate at night.

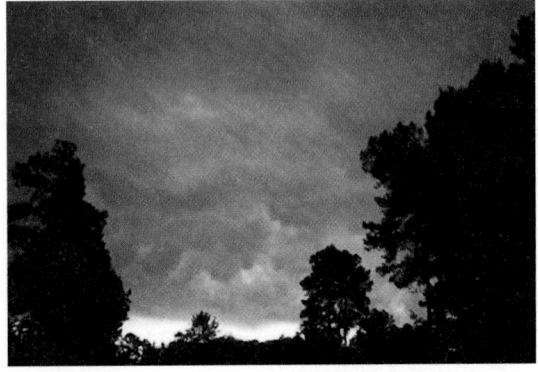

Clouds from which rain or snow fall have the word *nimbus* in their names. Shown are *cumulonimbus* clouds, which are dark and heavy with mountainous tops that constantly change shape. Strong winds, rain (sometimes hail), and thunderstorms are associated with them.

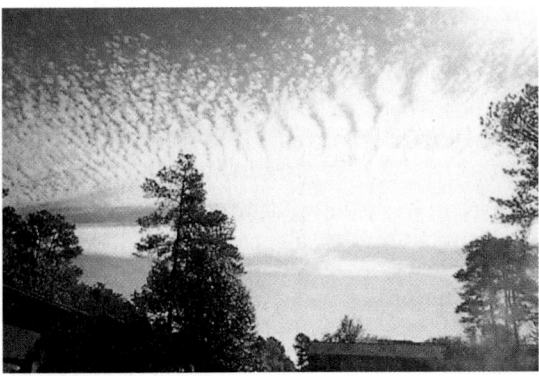

A "mackerel sky" like this contains small, round, high-altitude *cirrocumulus* clouds that happen to form patterns that suggest the scales of this fish. Such clouds indicate a change in weather with winds that fluctuate in speed and direction.

A cloud that occurs at a higher altitude than usual for its type is given the prefix *alto*, as in the case of the *altocumulus* clouds shown. Altocumulus clouds look lumpy, like cotton balls, and, if white against a blue sky, indicate fair weather. If they are dark and tightly packed, squalls may follow.

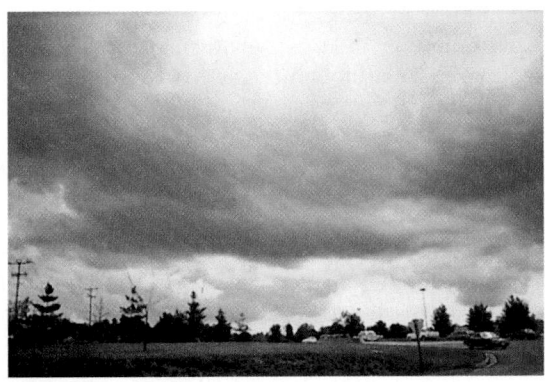

Nimbostratus clouds are low, thick, and relatively shapeless. Their presence is usually accompanied by steady rain or snow.

Figure 14-8   Six common cloud types.

ground falls at night, which cools the nearby air. Fogs result when large volumes of air come in contact with cold land or water. Clouds come into being when air is cooled by expansion when it rises. Clouds cover about half the earth's surface at any time.

Compressing a gas causes it to heat up, as anyone who has used a tire pump knows. The opposite effect is the cooling of a gas when it expands. When a warm, moist air mass moves upward, it expands because the pressure decreases, and it becomes cooler. A cooling rate of about 0.65°C for each 100 m of rise is normal. If the temperature drop is large enough, the air becomes saturated and some of its water vapor condenses on dust specks or other microscopic particles into clouds of tiny water droplets or ice crystals, depending on the temperature, that are small enough to remain suspended aloft indefinitely. High clouds consist of ice crystals, low clouds of water droplets (Fig. 14-8).

The three chief processes in the atmosphere that can cause clouds to form are these.

1. A warm air mass moving horizontally meets a land barrier such as a mountain and rises (Figs. 14-9 and 14-10). Coastal mountains that lie in the paths of moisture-laden ocean winds may have permanent cloud caps over them.
2. An air mass is heated by contact with a warm part of the earth's surface. The air mass expands, and its buoyancy causes it to rise. This process, called **convection,** is discussed in Sec. 14.6 (see Fig. 14-17).
3. A warm air mass meets a cooler air mass and, being less dense, is forced upward over the cooler mass. This process is discussed in Sec. 14.8 (see Fig. 14-29).

Other sources of clouds include water vapor emitted by volcanoes and water vapor in the exhaust gases of aircraft engines. The latter condenses into ice crystals at high altitudes to form streaks of cirrus clouds ("contrails") that may persist for several hours.

Rain, Snow, Sleet, and Hail   Rain falls when a cloud (or part of one) is cooled suddenly, usually by a rapid updraft, so that condensation is quick. Some of the water droplets in the cloud become larger than others and because air resistance affects them less, they move within the cloud faster than the smaller droplets. The smaller droplets tend to stick to the larger ones when they come in contact, and the result is larger and larger droplets. Finally the droplets become drops usually 1 to 2 mm in diameter (about the size of the letter "o" in this typeface), 100 times larger than typical cloud droplets. These drops are too heavy to stay aloft and the result is rain. Drops less than 0.5 mm in diameter fall as drizzle.

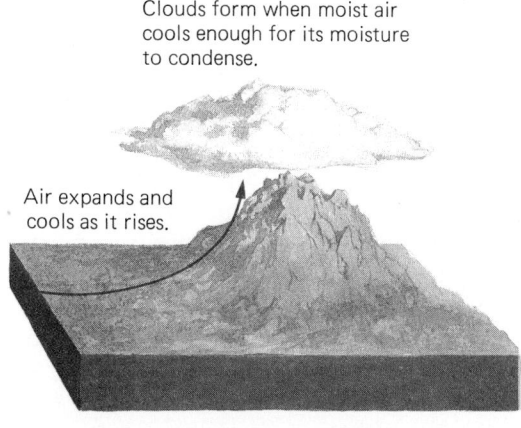

Clouds form when moist air cools enough for its moisture to condense.

Air expands and cools as it rises.

Figure 14-9   Why mountains often have cloud caps over them.

Figure 14-10   Cloud cap over the mountainous island of Saba in the West Indies.

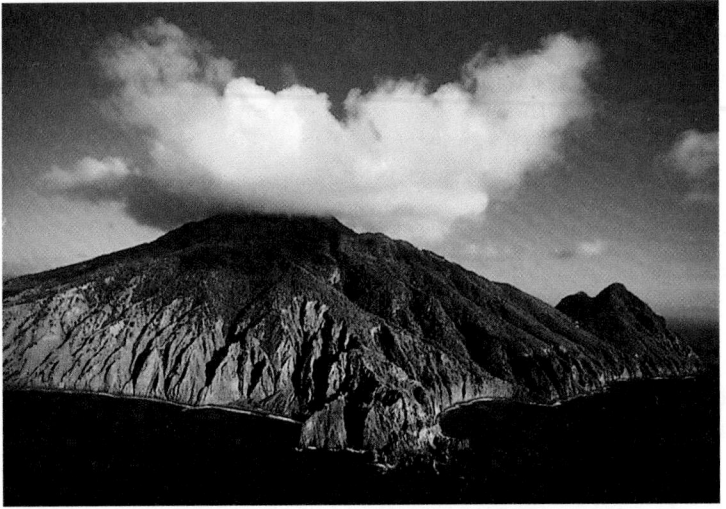

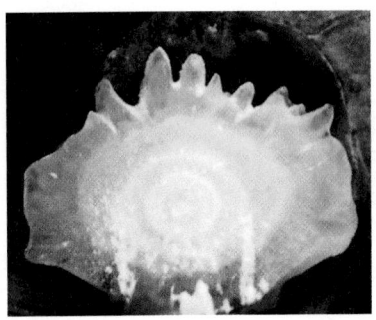

Figure 14-11   Cross section of a hailstone the size of a grapefruit that fell in Kansas in 1970.

If a cloud is cold enough, it consists of ice crystals rather than water droplets, and these crystals can grow into snowflakes. As the photographs in Fig. 11-11 show, snowflakes have very open structures. As a result, 7 cm of snow is typically equivalent to only about 1 cm of rain.

Sleet consists of raindrops that have frozen on the way to the ground. **Hail** is associated with the violent up- and downdrafts in thunderclouds. When a raindrop rises high enough, it freezes; then when it falls it picks up more water, which freezes as the drop rises again; and so on. The result is a rocklike lump of ice layered like an onion that may be larger than a golfball (Fig. 14-11).

Clouds are sometimes **seeded** with silver iodide to induce rain to fall from them. The crystal structure of silver iodide resembles that of ice; hence water molecules and droplets in a cloud can readily become attached to a silver iodide crystal. Such crystals are thus efficient condensation nuclei and so promote rain from a cloud. "Dry ice" (solid carbon dioxide) can also be used to seed clouds. However, the usual reason for not enough rain is not enough clouds of the right kind in the first place, so cloud seeding is seldom of much help in a drought.

Weather

Meteorology, the study of weather and weather patterns, is concerned with what we can think of as a vast air-conditioning system. Our spinning planet is heated strongly at the equator and weakly at the poles, and its water content is concentrated in the great ocean basins. From our point of view, it is the task of the atmosphere to redistribute this heat and moisture so that large areas of the land surface are habitable.

But air-conditioning by the atmosphere is far from perfect. It fails miserably in deserts, on mountaintops, in the polar regions. On sultry midsummer nights or on bitter January mornings we may question its efficiency even in our favored part of the world. Still, the atmosphere does succeed in making a surprisingly large part of the globe fit for people to live in.

Besides regulating air temperature and humidity, we expect the atmosphere to provide us with water in the form of rain or snow. The weather and climate of a region describe how effectively these things are done. **Weather** refers to the temperature, humidity, air pressure, cloudiness, and rainfall (or snowfall) at any given time. **Climate** is a summary of weather conditions over a period of years, including how temperature and rainfall vary with the seasons. For instance, a notable feature of the climate of North Dakota is its extreme warmth in summer and extreme cold in winter, whereas comfortable year-round temperatures with rainfall concentrated in the winter months characterize the climate of southern California. The speeds and directions of winds are often significant in describing weather and climate.

14.4 Atmospheric Energy

A Giant Greenhouse in the Sky

The energy that warms the air, evaporates water, and drives the winds comes to us from the sun. Solar energy arriving at the upper atmosphere is called **insolation** (for *in*coming *sol*ar radi*ation*). Bright sunlight can bring energy at a rate of as much as 1.4 kW to each square meter on which it falls perpendicularly. However, because the earth is round, sunlight arrives at a glancing angle almost everywhere (see Fig. 14-13), and this angle changes with the time of day and with the seasons (see Fig. 14-15). As a result, the average intensity of sunlight at the top of the atmosphere at a given location is less than 1.4 kW/m^2; the average at noon is around 1 kW/m^2 for the continental United States.

Every object gives off electromagnetic waves whose intensity and predominant wavelength depend on the temperature of the object (Fig. 9-4). The hotter the object, the more energy it emits and the shorter the predominant wavelength. The sun, whose surface temperature is about 5700°C, gives off a great deal of energy and its radiation is mainly visible light. The earth, whose surface temperature averages about 15°C, is a feebler source of energy, and its radiation is mainly in the long-wavelength infrared part of the spectrum to which the eye is not sensitive.

About 30 percent of the insolation is reflected directly back into space, chiefly by clouds (Fig. 14-12). The atmosphere absorbs perhaps 19 percent of the insolation, with ozone, water vapor, and water droplets in clouds taking up most of this amount. Slightly over half of the total insolation therefore reaches the earth's surface, where it is absorbed and becomes heat. A little of this heat is given to the atmosphere through contact with the warm surface, somewhat more by means of water evaporated from the oceans.

The warm earth also radiates energy back into the atmosphere, but the energy now is in the form of long-wavelength infrared radiation. These long waves are readily absorbed by atmospheric carbon dioxide and water vapor, whose molecules then transfer energy to the rest of the atmosphere. Thus a

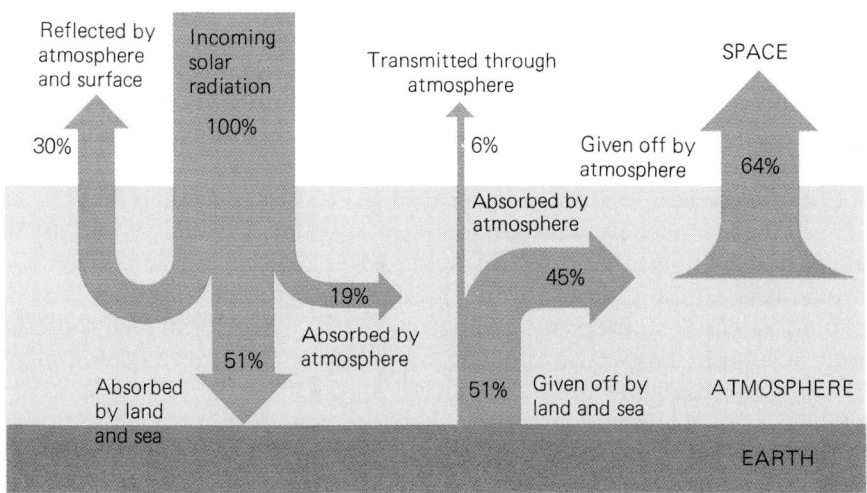

Figure 14-12 The greenhouse effect. Much of the energy in the short-wavelength visible light from the sun that is absorbed by the earth's surface is in turn radiated by the earth as long-wavelength infrared light that is absorbed by CO_2, H_2O, and other gases in the atmosphere. Some energy also reaches the atmosphere by contact with the earth and by means of water evaporated from the sea. Thus the atmosphere is heated mainly from below by the earth rather than from above by the sun. Without the greenhouse effect the earth would average −18°C instead of its present average of 15°C.

major source of atmospheric energy is radiation from the earth, not direct sunlight.

Greenhouse Effect   The way in which the atmosphere is heated from below rather than from above is often called the **greenhouse effect.** The interior of a greenhouse is warmer than the outside air because sunlight can enter through its windows, but the infrared radiation that the warm interior gives off cannot go through glass. As a result much of the incoming energy is trapped inside before being reemitted by the warm windows themselves. The atmosphere thus behaves like a giant greenhouse, with atmospheric gases that absorb infrared radiation acting like the windows of a greenhouse.

Normally, incoming and outgoing energy flows are in balance, but an increasingly more efficient atmospheric greenhouse leads to more energy arriving than leaving. As a result the earth is warming up (see Sec. 4.3), but the enormous mass involved means that the earth's surface temperature responds only slowly to changes in energy supply. Eventually the two flows will be in balance again, though at a higher surface temperature.

Example 14.1

Air temperatures in the troposphere decrease with altitude whereas those in the stratosphere increase with altitude. Why do these variations occur?

Solution

The troposphere is heated largely through the absorption by carbon dioxide and water molecules of infrared radiation emitted by the earth's surface. Because it is heated from below, the temperature of the troposphere decreases with altitude.

The stratosphere is heated largely through the absorption by ozone molecules of ultraviolet radiation from the sun. Because it is heated from above, the temperature of the stratosphere increases with altitude.

Factors That Govern Air Temperatures   If the earth had no atmosphere, it would grow intensely hot during the day and unbearably cold at night, as the airless moon does. The earth's atmosphere prevents these extremes. The constant movement of air around the world keeps daytime temperatures in any one place from climbing very high, and the ability of moist air to absorb the earth's infrared radiation prevents the rapid escape of heat by night.

How hot the atmosphere becomes over any particular region depends on a number of factors. Air near the equator is on the average much warmer than air near the poles because the sun's rays are more effective in heating the surface when they come from overhead than when they come at a slanting angle (Fig. 14-13). Air over a mountaintop may become warm at midday but cools quickly because it is thinner and contains less carbon dioxide and water vapor than air lower down. Clouds reflect sunlight, so a region with clouds overhead usually has lower air temperatures than a nearby region whose sky is clear.

Because the temperature of water changes more slowly than that of rocks and soil, the atmosphere near large bodies of water is usually cooler by day and warmer by night than the atmosphere over regions far from water. Desert regions commonly show abrupt changes in air temperature between day and night because so little water vapor is there to absorb infrared radiation. The atmospheric temperatures of some regions are influenced profoundly by winds and by ocean currents.

The earth's average temperature does not change very much with time, even with today's global warming, hence there must be an approximate balance between incoming and outgoing energy. This can be seen with the help

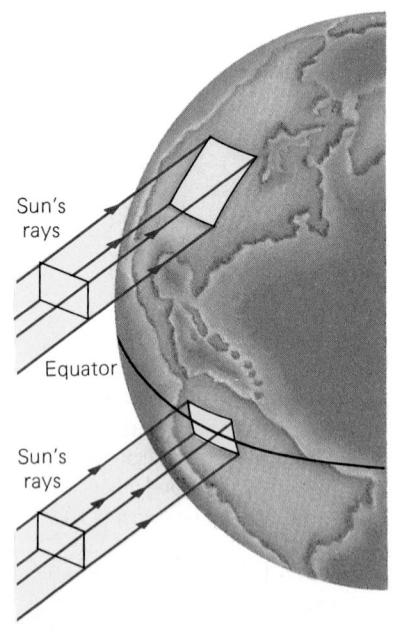

Figure 14-13   The equatorial regions of the earth are on the average warmer than the polar regions because at the equator the sun's rays are spread over a smaller surface.

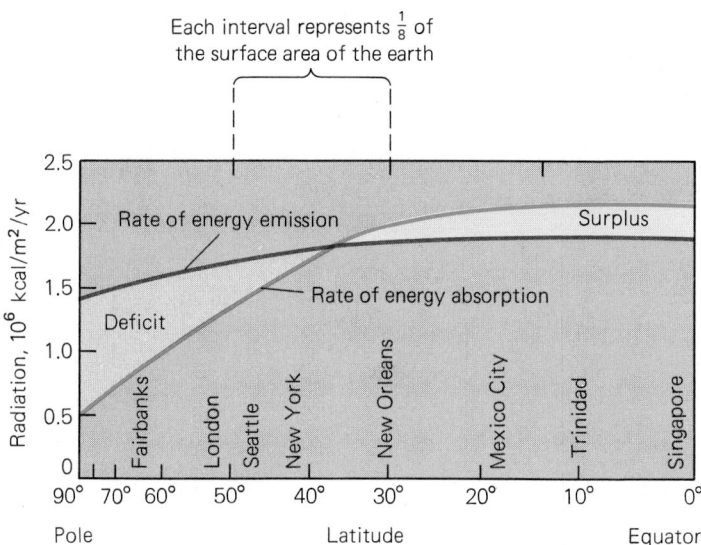

Each interval represents $\frac{1}{8}$ of the surface area of the earth

Figure 14-14 The annual balance between incoming solar radiation and outgoing radiation from the earth. More energy is gained than lost in the tropical regions, and more energy is lost than gained in the polar regions. The latitude scale is spaced so that equal horizontal distances on the graph correspond to equal areas of the earth's surface. [For the meaning of latitude, see Sec. 14.4 at www.mhhe.com/krauskopf.]

of Fig. 14-14, which shows how the rates at which radiant energy enters and leaves the earth vary with latitude.

Heat Transfer   More energy arrives at the tropical regions than is lost there, and the opposite is true at the polar regions. Why then do not the tropics grow warmer and warmer while the poles grow colder and colder? The answer is to be found in the motions of air and water that shift energy from the regions of surplus to the regions of deficit. About 80 percent of the energy transport around the earth is carried by winds in the atmosphere, and the remainder is carried by ocean currents. We shall look at both of these mechanisms in the rest of this chapter.

14.5   The Seasons

They Are Due to the Tilt of the Earth's Axis

The average distance between the earth and the sun is about 150 million km. Because the earth's orbit is an ellipse rather than a circle, the earth-sun distance varies during the year from about 2.4 million km closer than the average to the same amount farther away. The earth is nearest the sun early in January and farthest from the sun early in July.

We might be tempted to attribute the seasons to the shape of the earth's orbit, especially if we happen to live in the southern hemisphere where January is a summer month and July a winter month. But this cannot be the reason, if only because the seasons are reversed in the northern hemisphere. In fact, the sunlight that reaches the earth varies in intensity by too little between the orbital extremes to give rise to the difference between summer and winter. After all, the earth's orbit differs from a perfect circle by only ±1.6 percent.

The 23.5° tilt of the earth's axis, not the shape of its orbit, is what causes the seasons. As a result of this tilt, for half of each year one hemisphere receives more direct sunlight than the other hemisphere, and in the other half of the year it receives less (Fig. 14-15). A beam of light that arrives at an angle to a surface delivers less energy per m² than does a similar beam that arrives perpendicularly, as we can see in Fig. 14-13.

Solstices and Equinoxes   The noon sun is at its highest in the sky in the northern hemisphere on about June 22 when the North Pole is tilted most toward the sun. The period of daylight in the northern hemisphere is longest on this

Figure 14-15 The seasons are caused by the tilt of the earth's axis together with its annual orbit around the sun. As a result, the daylight side of the northern hemisphere is tilted away from the sun in January, which means that sunlight strikes this hemisphere at a glancing angle and delivers less energy to a given area than in June. The seasons are reversed in the southern hemisphere.

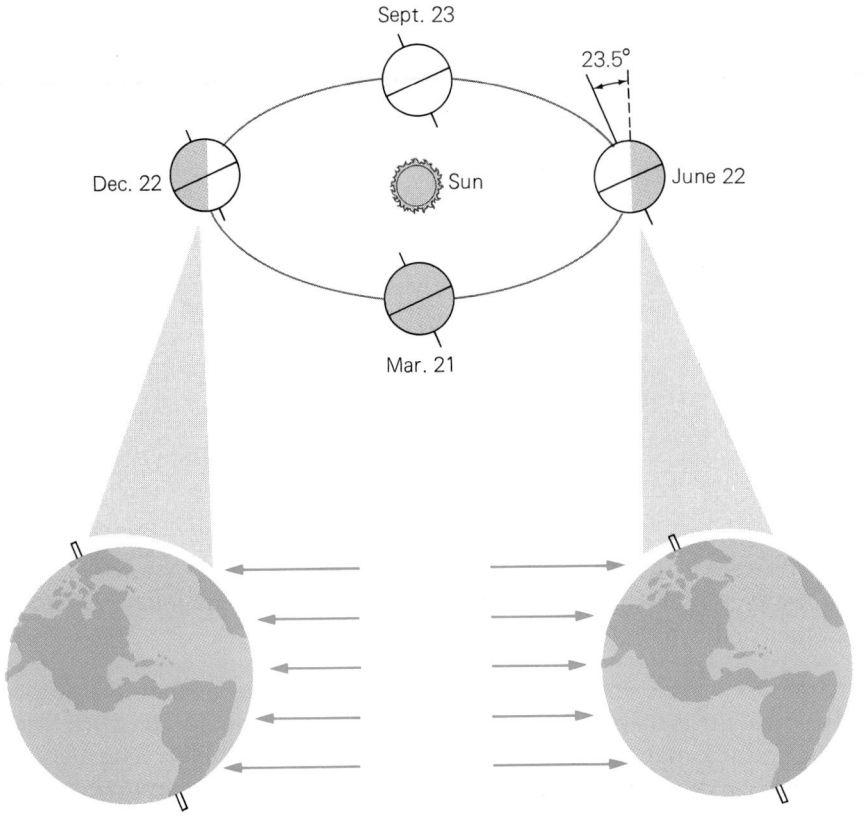

Arctic and Antarctic Circles

On December 22, the shortest day of the year in the northern hemisphere, the 23.5° tilt of the earth's axis (see Fig. 14-15) means that no sunlight reaches any point within 23.5° of the North Pole. The Arctic Circle is the boundary of this region of unbroken darkness. It is thus the northernmost latitude at which the sun is above the horizon every day of the year.

December 22 is also the longest day of the year in the southern hemisphere. On this day there are 24 hours of daylight at all points within 23.5° of the South Pole, and the Antarctic Circle is the boundary of this region of unbroken daylight. On June 22 the situations in the two hemispheres are reversed.

The latitude of the North Pole is 90°N, hence that of the Arctic Circle is 90°N − 23.5° = 66.5°N. The circle passes through northern Canada, Alaska, Siberia, Scandinavia, and southern Greenland. The latitude of the Antarctic Circle is similarly 66.5°S; it lies south of South America and Africa.

Example 14.2

If the earth's axis were not tilted, would there still be seasons?

Solution
There would be seasons because the earth's orbit is an ellipse rather than a circle. As a result, the earth's distance from the sun varies during the year, but because the earth's orbit differs from a circle by very little, the seasons would be much less pronounced than the current seasons.

date. The noon sun is at its lowest 6 months later, on or about December 22, when the North Pole is tilted most away from the sun. The period of daylight is then at its shortest; these times are called **solstices.** In the southern hemisphere the situation is, of course, reversed.

On about March 21 and September 23, the sun is directly overhead at noon at the equator. The periods of daylight and darkness are then equal everywhere on the earth; these times are called **equinoxes.**

14.6 Winds

Currents of Air Driven by Temperature Differences

Winds are horizontal movements of air caused by pressure differences in the atmosphere. The greater the pressure difference between two regions, the faster the air between them moves. All pressure differences between places on the earth's surface can be traced to temperature differences.

When a region is warmer than its surroundings, the air above it is heated and expands (Fig. 14-16). The hot air rises, leaving behind a low-pressure zone into which cool air from the high-pressure neighborhood flows. The

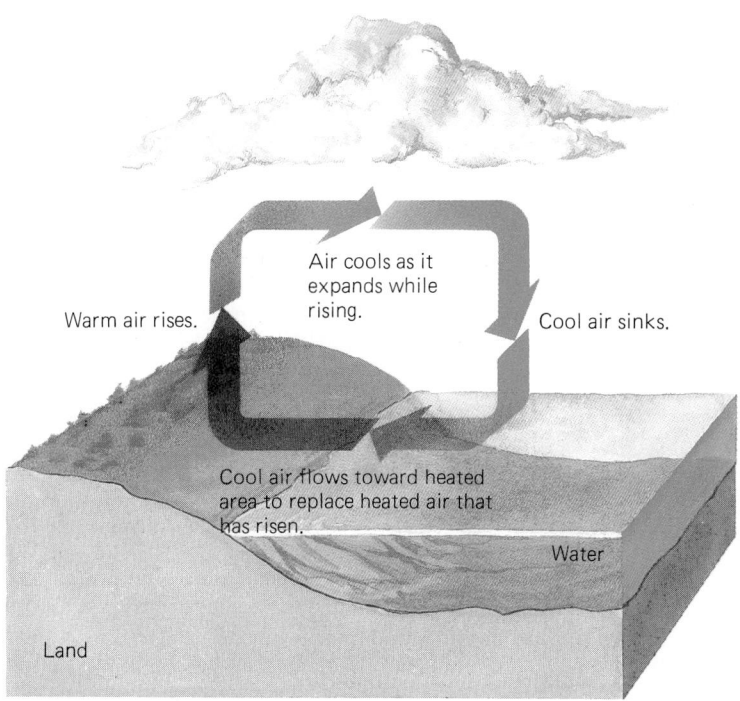

Figure 14-16 Convection currents are produced by unequal heating. The temperature of a land surface rises more rapidly in sunlight than the temperature of a water surface. The resulting convection produces the **sea breeze** found on sunny days near the shores of a body of water. At night, the land cools more than the sea, and the convection current is reversed to give a **land breeze** that blows offshore.

flow toward the heated region at low altitudes is balanced by an outward flow of the air that has risen. This air then cools and sinks to replace the air that has moved inward. Air movements of this kind, produced as the result of unequal heating of the earth's surface, are called **convection currents.**

Coriolis Effect   The rotation of the earth affects the path of something that moves above its surface as this path is seen from the surface. This phenomenon is called the **coriolis effect,** and it has these results:

> In the northern hemisphere, a path that would be a straight line over a stationary earth instead is curved to the right. In the southern hemisphere the curvature is to the left.

Only motion along the equator is not affected by the coriolis effect.

Because of the coriolis effect, winds are deflected from straight paths into curved ones. Thus the air rushing into a low-pressure region does not move directly inward but instead follows a spiral path that is counterclockwise in the northern hemisphere and clockwise in the southern (Fig. 14-17). Examples of such spiral motion are, in order of decreasing size (but increasing violence), middle-latitude weather systems, hurricanes and other tropical storms, and tornados.

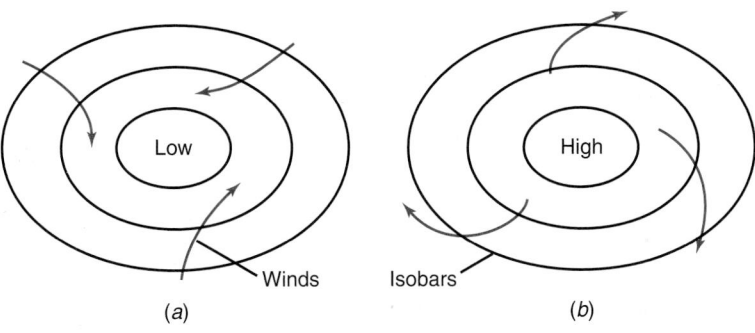

(a) (b)

Figure 14-17 (a) Because of the coriolis effect, which is a consequence of the earth's rotation, winds in the northern hemisphere are deflected to the right. As a result, air does not flow directly toward the center of a low-pressure region but spirals inward in a counterclockwise direction. (b) Similarly, air flows away from the center of a high-pressure region in a clockwise spiral. In the southern hemisphere these directions are reversed. An **isobar** is a line of constant pressure on a weather map; it corresponds to a contour line of constant altitude on an ordinary map.

Monsoons

The seasonal winds called **monsoons** are large-scale sea and land breezes modified by the coriolis effect. During the summer, a continent is warmer than the oceans around it. The rising air over the continent creates a low-pressure region that pulls in moisture-laden sea breezes that bring rain. In winter the situation is reversed, with dry air moving seaward.

Monsoons are most pronounced in certain parts of Africa and Asia. Figure 14-18 shows how the summer and winter monsoons of India and southeast Asia arise. In summer, the motion of air around the low-pressure center on land is counterclockwise, and it is clockwise around the high-pressure center in the Indian Ocean. The result is a wet southwest monsoon that blows from May to September as in Fig. 14-18a. Every few years this monsoon is weaker than usual, less rain falls, crops suffer, and there may be widespread famine.

From October to April dry winds blow from the northeast, as in Fig. 14-18b. The shifts in wind patterns usually take a few weeks but sometimes only a few days. About half the world's population depends on summer monsoons to provide the rain needed for agriculture. One of the reasons global warming is so serious is that, if it continues unabated, the Asian monsoons may no longer occur.

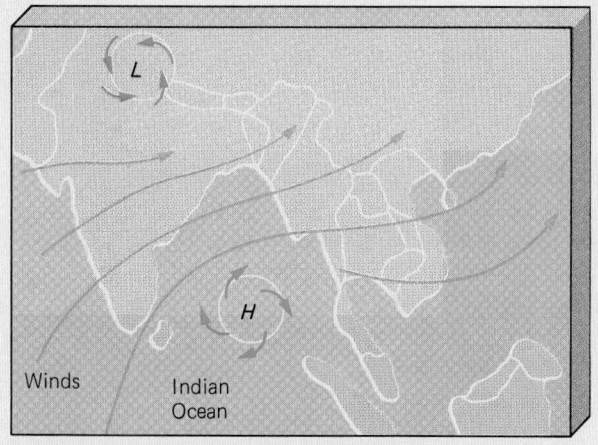

(a) Summer monsoon

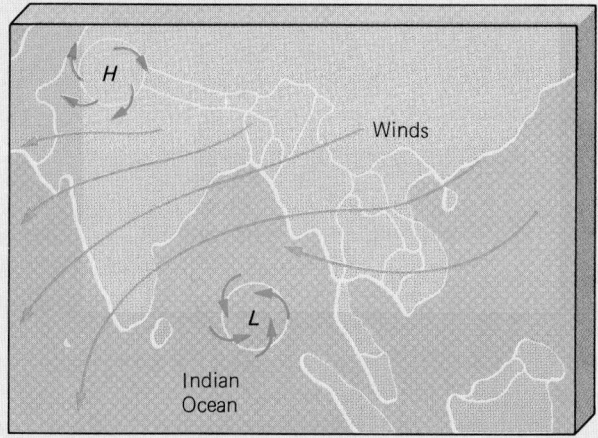

(b) Winter monsoon

Figure 14-18   (a) The summer monsoon of India and south Asia. Heating of the land produces a low-pressure region (L) centered inland and a high-pressure region (H) centered in the Indian Ocean that together cause southwest winds to occur. Rice cultivation in this part of the world depends on the warm, moist air brought by the summer monsoon. (b) The winter monsoon. Now the land is cooler than the ocean, so the low- and high-pressure regions are reversed to give dry northeast winds.

14.7   General Circulation of the Atmosphere

Alternate Belts of Wind and Calm

The earth is heated most at the equator and least at the poles. We therefore expect to find convection currents as part of the general atmospheric circulation.

Suppose for the moment that our planet did not rotate and that its surface was made up entirely of either land or water. On such an earth, air circulation would depend only on the difference in temperature between equator and poles. Air would rise along the heated equator, flow at high altitudes toward the poles, and at low altitudes return from the poles toward the equator (Fig. 14-19). We in the northern hemisphere would experience a steady north wind. (Winds are named for the direction they come from, so a north wind blows from the north.) Around the equator would be a belt of relatively low pressure, and near each pole a region of high pressure.

Because the earth does rotate, however, the north and south winds coming from the poles are deflected by the coriolis effect into large-scale eddies that lead to a generally eastward drift in the middle of each hemisphere and a westward drift in the tropics. The main features of the general circulation of the atmosphere are shown in Fig. 14-20.

The various wind zones were important to shipping in the days of sail, as their names indicate. Thus the steady easterlies on each side of the equator became known as the **trade winds** because they could be relied upon by sailing ships. The region of light, erratic wind along the equator, where the principal movement of air is upward, constitutes the **doldrums.** The **horse latitudes** that separate the trade winds in both hemispheres from the **prevailing westerlies** poleward of them are also regions of calm and light winds. Their name is supposed to have come from the practice of throwing overboard horses from sailing ships when the ships were becalmed and ran short of drinking water.

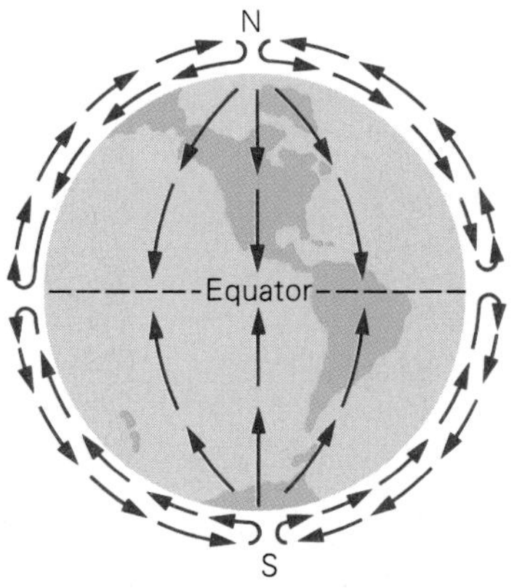

Jet Streams   With increasing altitude the belts of westerly winds broaden until almost the entire flow of air is west to east at the top of the troposphere. The westerly flow aloft is not uniform but contains narrow cores of high-speed winds called **jet streams,** usually only a few hundred kilometers wide but with winds of up to 500 km/h. The jet streams form zigzag patterns around the earth that change continuously and affect the

Figure 14-19   The convectional circulation that would occur if the earth did not rotate. The arrows in the center of the diagram indicate surface winds.

Example 14.3

The crew of a yacht is planning to sail from the east coast of the United States to England and later to sail home. What routes should the crew follow across the Atlantic on the passages out and back to have the courses more or less downwind as much of the time as possible?

Solution

To England, the crew should first sail northeast to reach the prevailing westerlies and then head eastward. Back to the United States, the crew should first sail south to the trade winds, then west, and finally north.

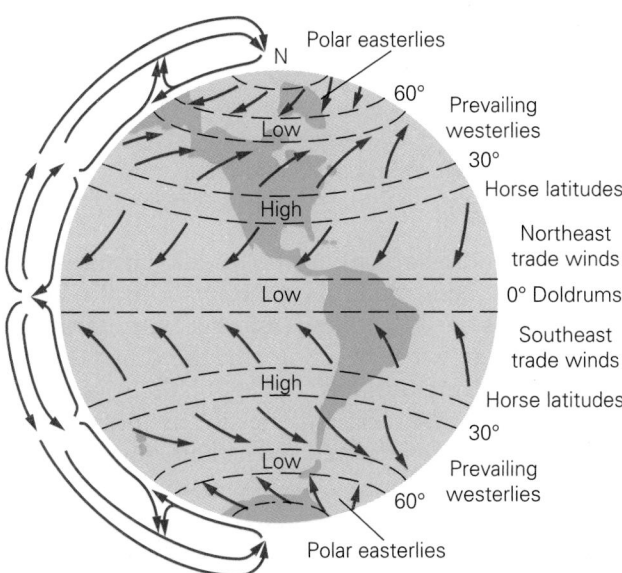

Figure 14-20   Simplified pattern of horizontal and vertical circulation in the actual atmosphere. Regions of high and low pressure are indicated. In general, the trade winds consist of warm, dry air; the westerlies of warm, damp air; and the polar easterlies of cold, dry air.

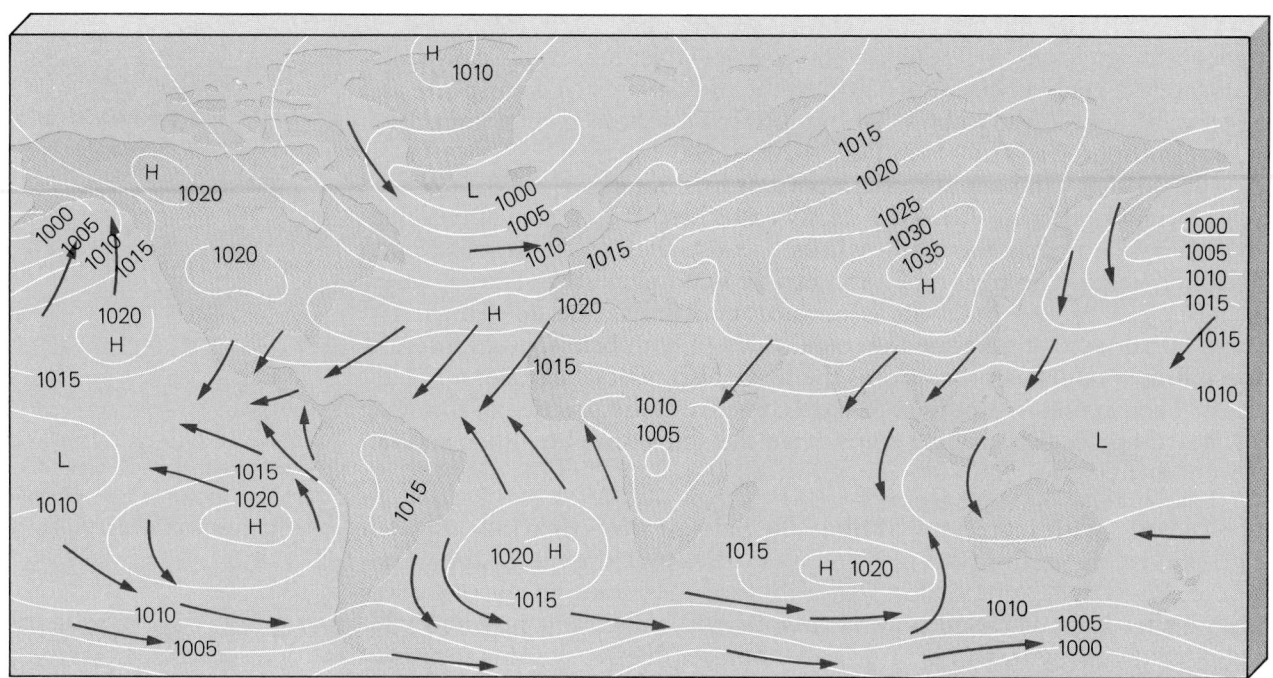

Figure 14-21 Average January sea-level pressures (in millibars) and wind patterns (red arrows). High- and low-pressure systems are indicated. Isobars connecting points of equal pressure are shown in white.

variable weather of the middle latitudes by their influence on the paths of air masses closer to the surface. They are important to aircraft—an hour or more can be saved on a long west-east flight by using a route with a jet stream as a tail wind, and a corresponding addition to the flight time can be prevented in the other direction by avoiding a jet stream as much as possible.

At any given time the circulation near the earth's surface is more complicated than the pattern given in Fig. 14-20. An important factor is the presence of large seasonal low- and high-pressure regions caused by unequal heating due to the irregular distribution of landmasses and sea areas (Fig. 14-21). Smaller, short-lived cells also occur and profoundly affect local weather conditions, as we shall see next.

14.8   Middle-Latitude Weather Systems

Why Our Weather Is So Fickle

Day-to-day weather is more variable in the middle latitudes than anywhere else on earth. If we visit central Mexico or Hawaii, in the belt of the northeast trades, we find that one day follows another with hardly any change in temperature, humidity, or wind direction. On the other hand, in nearly all parts of the continental United States, drastic changes in weather are commonplace. The reason for this variability lies in the movement of warm and cold air masses and of storms derived from them through the belts of the westerlies.

Air Masses   In the northern part of the westerly belt an irregular boundary separates air moving generally northward from the horse latitudes and air moving southward from the polar regions. Great bodies of cold air at times sweep down over North America, and at other times warm air from the tropics extends far northward. The cold air is ultimately warmed and the warm

El Niño and La Niña

The surface winds of the tropical Pacific often blow westward from the Americas, as in the top part of Fig. 14-22. These are the easterly trade winds shown in Fig. 14-20. Together with the ocean currents they drive, the trade winds create a huge pool of warm water in the western side of the Pacific basin. The heated moist air above this pool rises to give an area of low pressure and brings abundant rain to Indonesia and northern Australia.

Every few years, however, a different pattern takes over. For reasons that are not completely understood, the trade winds weaken and the warm water pool shifts eastward. Now there is high pressure over the western Pacific and droughts parch Australia and East Asia. Low pressure over the eastern Pacific brings storms that lash California and torrential rains that soak Chile, Peru, and Ecuador on South America's west coast (Fig. 14-22).

The upwelling of nutrient-rich cold water along this coast when the surface waters were blown westward then stops and the coastal water becomes warm. As a result the fish population drops sharply in the eastern Pacific and the economies of Peru and Ecuador suffer accordingly. The entire phenomenon is called **El Niño,** Spanish for "the little boy," a reference to the infant Jesus, because the warm water appears around Christmas. The other pattern is called **La Niña,** "the little girl."

The influence of an El Niño can extend well beyond the Pacific, in part by disrupting the jet streams. The severe El Niño of 1982–1983 brought droughts that devastated agriculture in India, southern Africa, and Brazil, and abnormally heavy rains gave rise to floods in California. All the continents were affected in some way. In North America milder winters coincide with El Niños, and there are fewer tropical storms and hurricanes in the Atlantic.

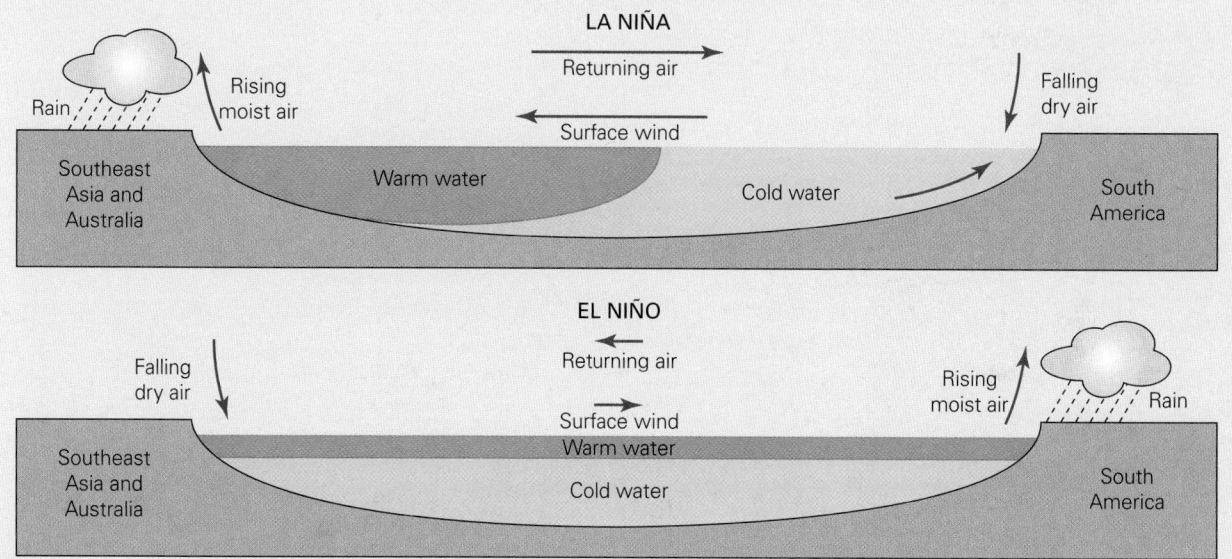

Figure 14-22   Simplified pictures of La Niña and El Niño conditions in the Pacific Ocean. In a La Niña year, the easterly trade winds push warm surface water away from South America and cold, nutrient-laden water from below rises to feed an abundant fish population. About 10 percent of all the fish caught in the world come from Peruvian waters. Descending dry air produces droughts along the coast, much of which is desert. In an El Niño year, the winds weaken and may vary in direction, or even reverse as shown. As a result, the surface water is warm everywhere, there is no upwelling, and the fish population declines. Now there are storms and heavy rain on the South American coast with droughts on the western side of the Pacific.

air cooled, but a large volume of air can maintain nearly its original temperature and humidity for days or weeks.

These huge tongues of air, or isolated bodies of air detached from them, are the **air masses** of meteorology. The kind of air in an air mass depends on its source (Fig. 14-23). A mass formed over northern Canada is cold and dry, one from the North Atlantic or North Pacific is cold and humid, one from the Gulf of Mexico warm and humid, and so on. Weather prediction in the United States depends largely on following the movements of air masses from these various source areas.

Cyclones and Anticyclones   Weather systems associated with air masses are usually several hundred to a thousand or more km across and move from west to east. A **cyclone** is an air mass in which the pressure is low at the center. As air rushes in toward the center of a cyclone, the moving air is deflected toward the right in the northern hemisphere and toward the left in the southern because of the coriolis effect (Fig. 14-18). As a result cyclonic winds blow in a counterclockwise spiral in the northern hemisphere and in a clockwise spiral in the southern hemisphere (Fig. 14-24).

An **anticyclone** is centered on a high-pressure region from which air moves outward. The coriolis effect therefore causes anticyclonic winds to blow

Figure 14-23   The air masses that affect weather in North America. The importance of the various air masses depends upon the season. In winter, for instance, the continental tropical air mass disappears and the continental polar air mass exerts its greatest influence.

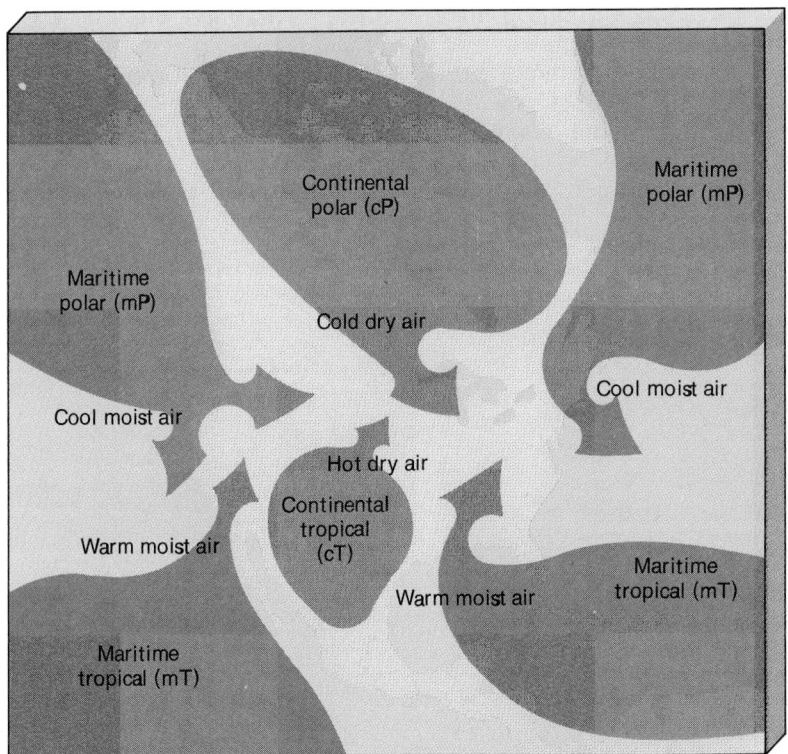

Figure 14-24   Cyclonic weather systems are responsible for the variable weather of the middle latitudes. A typical system is 1500 km in diameter and moves eastward at 40 km/h; its characteristic winds usually do not exceed 65 km/h. The system here was centered about 2000 km north of Hawaii when it was photographed from a spacecraft.

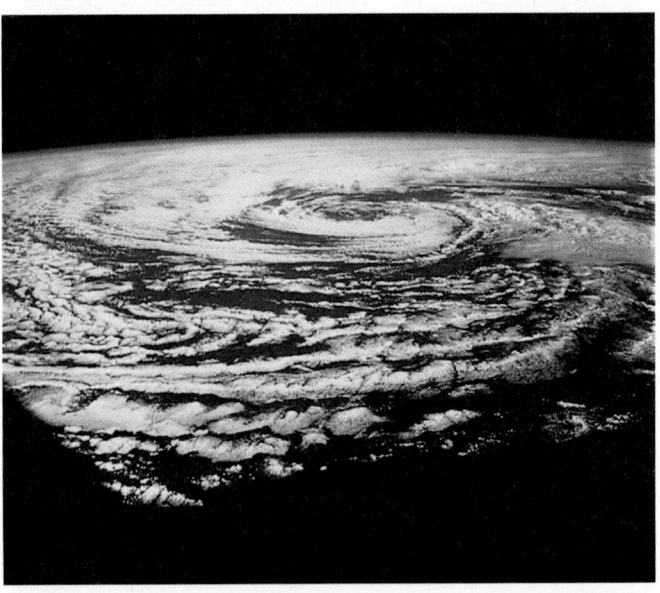

in a clockwise spiral in the northern hemisphere and in a counterclockwise spiral in the southern hemisphere. These spirals are conspicuous in cloud formations photographed from earth satellites.

A cyclone is a region of low pressure, and air flowing into one rises in an upward spiral (Fig. 14-25). The rising air cools and its moisture

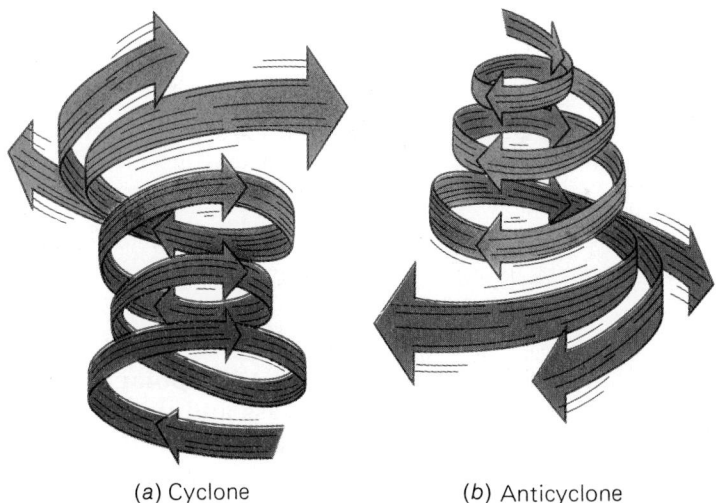

(a) Cyclone   (b) Anticyclone

Figure 14-25 (*a*) In a cyclone in the northern hemisphere, the coriolis effect causes surface air to spiral counterclockwise as it moves toward the low-pressure center and rises. The air cools as it moves upward, which causes its moisture to condense out as clouds and rain. (*b*) In an anticyclone, cold air from above spirals outward from the high-pressure center as it sinks. The falling air warms, which decreases its relative humidity to give a clear sky. In the southern hemisphere the directions of spin are reversed.

Tornados

A tornado is a narrow but extremely violent cyclonic storm (Fig. 14-26). In the central United States, particularly in Kansas, Oklahoma, and Texas, about a thousand of them occur every year.

Tornados typically form in the spring when warm, moist air moving north from the Gulf of Mexico collides with cold, dry air moving south from Canada (see Fig. 14-23). The warm air rises through the cold air to create a strong updraft that can power a severe thunderstorm. If the rising air in the thundercloud is swirling rapidly, the result may be a tornado. Waterspouts are weak tornados that form over open water.

Most tornados are about 50 m across, travel at about 50 km/h, and last for only a few minutes. Severe tornados may be over a kilometer across, travel at 100 km/h, and last for over an hour. Wind speeds up to 512 km/h (318 mi/h) have been recorded in especially violent tornados, and debris is sometimes found over 100 km from where the twister struck. In fact, much of the damage

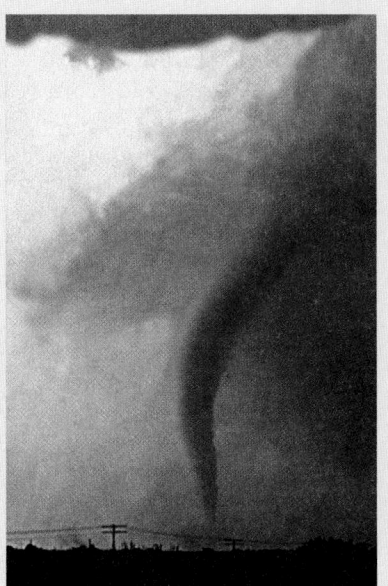

Figure 14-26 A tornado in Oklahoma. The spinning column of air spreads out as it rises because air pressure decreases with altitude.

tornados cause is due to churned-up debris shredding whatever it encounters.

content condenses into clouds. As a rule, cyclones bring unstable weather conditions with clouds, rain, strong shifting winds, and abrupt temperature changes. An anticyclone is a region of high pressure, and air flows out of it in a downward spiral. The descent warms the air and its relative humidity accordingly drops, hence condensation does not occur. The weather associated with anticyclones is usually settled and pleasant with clear skies and mild winds.

Example 14.4

Why are most of the world's deserts found in the horse latitudes, which separate the trade winds from the prevailing westerlies in both hemispheres?

Solution

As shown in Fig. 14-20, airflow in the horse latitudes is anticyclonic, which means that little rain falls there.

Fronts   Middle-latitude cyclones originate at the **polar front,** which is the boundary between the cold polar air mass and the warmed air mass next to it. It is common for a kink to develop in this front with a wedge of warm air protruding into the cold air mass. This produces a low-pressure region that moves eastward as a cyclone. The eastern side of the warm-air wedge is a **warm front** since warm air moves in to replace cold air in its path; the western side is a **cold front** since cold air replaces warm air (Fig. 14-27).

As warm air rises along an inclined front, it is cooled and part of its moisture condenses out. Clouds and rain are therefore associated with both kinds of fronts (Fig. 14-28). A cold front is generally steeper, since cold air is actively burrowing under warm air. The temperature difference is greater as well, so rainfall on a cold front is heavier and of shorter duration than on a

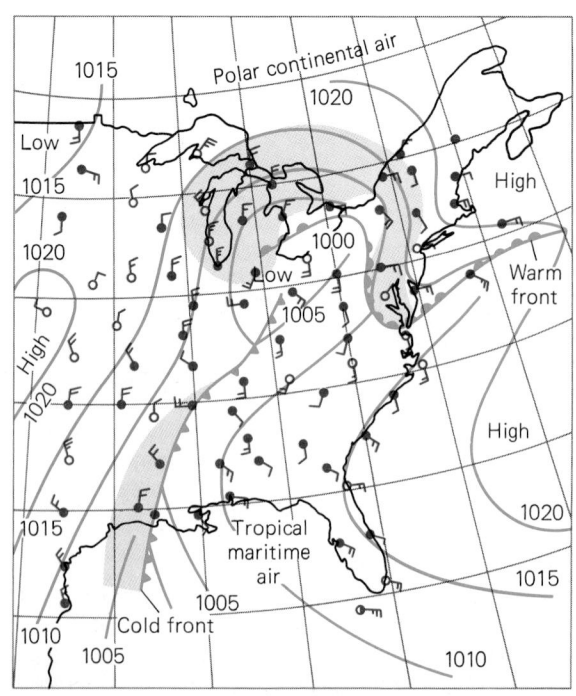

Figure 14-27   Weather maps show pressure patterns, winds, rain, and snow. This is a weather map of the eastern United States one April morning. A cold air mass on the west and north (polar continental air) is separated from a warm air mass (tropical maritime air) by a cold front extending from Louisiana to Michigan and by a warm front from Michigan to Virginia. Where the north end of the warm air mass lies between the two fronts a cyclone has formed, bringing rain (colored area) to the Great Lakes region. The unit of pressure in this map is the millibar. The small circles indicate clear skies; solid dots indicate cloudy skies. The small lines show wind direction, which is toward the circle or dot, and wind strength; the greater the number of tails, the faster the wind.

Jacob A. B. Bjerknes (1897–1975)

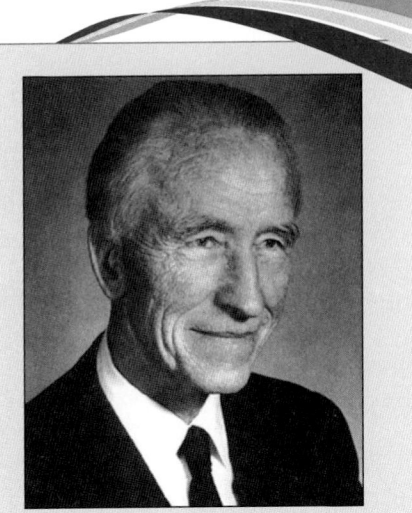

The son and grandson of physics professors at Norway's University of Christiania (later Oslo, renamed after Norway became independent of Sweden in 1905), Bjerknes began his work in meteorology in collaboration with his father, Vilhelm. They established a network of observing stations all over Norway during World War I, and from the data they developed the concept of air masses that keep their identities for relatively long periods of time. They called the boundaries between air masses "fronts."

Bjerknes studied how fronts evolve and applied his findings to weather forecasting. In 1940 he joined the University of California at Los Angeles, where he extended his analysis of weather phenomena to include heat exchange between the atmosphere and the oceans. An especial interest was the phenomenon of El Niño. In 1952 Bjerknes pioneered the use of cloud photographs taken from rockets as an aid in forecasting. Today, of course, satellite-borne cameras are a routine tool of the meteorologist.

warm front. A cold front with a large temperature difference is often marked by violent thundersqualls.

A warm front typically moves eastward at about 150 km/day. The cold front behind it moves faster, up to twice as fast, and eventually it overtakes the warm front to force the wedge of warm air upward (Fig. 14-29). The resulting **occluded front** is the last stage in the evolution of a cyclone, which soon afterward disappears. The total life span of a middle-latitude cyclone may be as little as a few hours or as much as a week, though the usual range is 3 to 5 days.

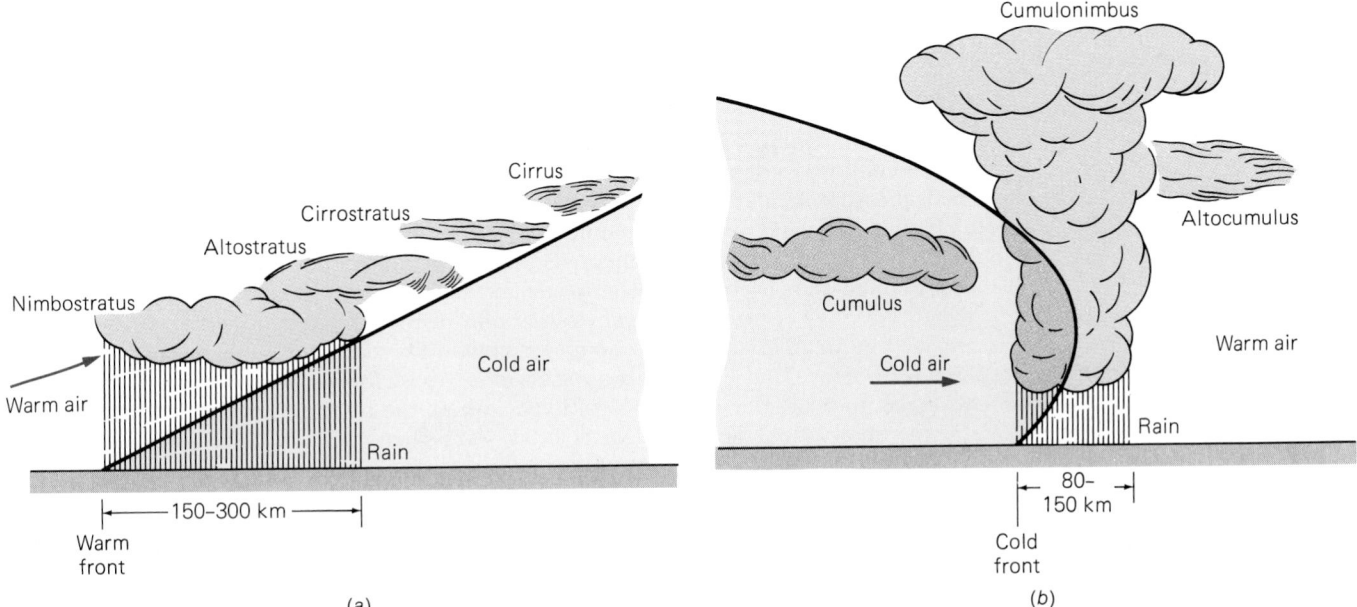

Figure 14-28   Cross-section diagrams of (a) a warm front and (b) a cold front. In each case the front is moving to the right. Photographs of the various cloud forms appear in Fig. 14-8. A warm front is the boundary between a warm, moist air mass that has moved (usually eastward) up and over a cool air mass ahead of it. The rising air cools, and its water vapor condenses into clouds and rain. A cold front is the boundary between a cool, relatively dry air mass that pushes warm, moist air ahead of it upward and out of its (usually eastward) path; it is steeper than a warm front. Again the rising warm air cools to produce clouds and rain, but now the weather change is more rapid and dramatic with stronger winds.

Figure 14-29 Life cycle of a middle-latitude cyclone in the northern hemisphere. Conventional weather-map symbols are used for cold, warm, and occluded fronts.

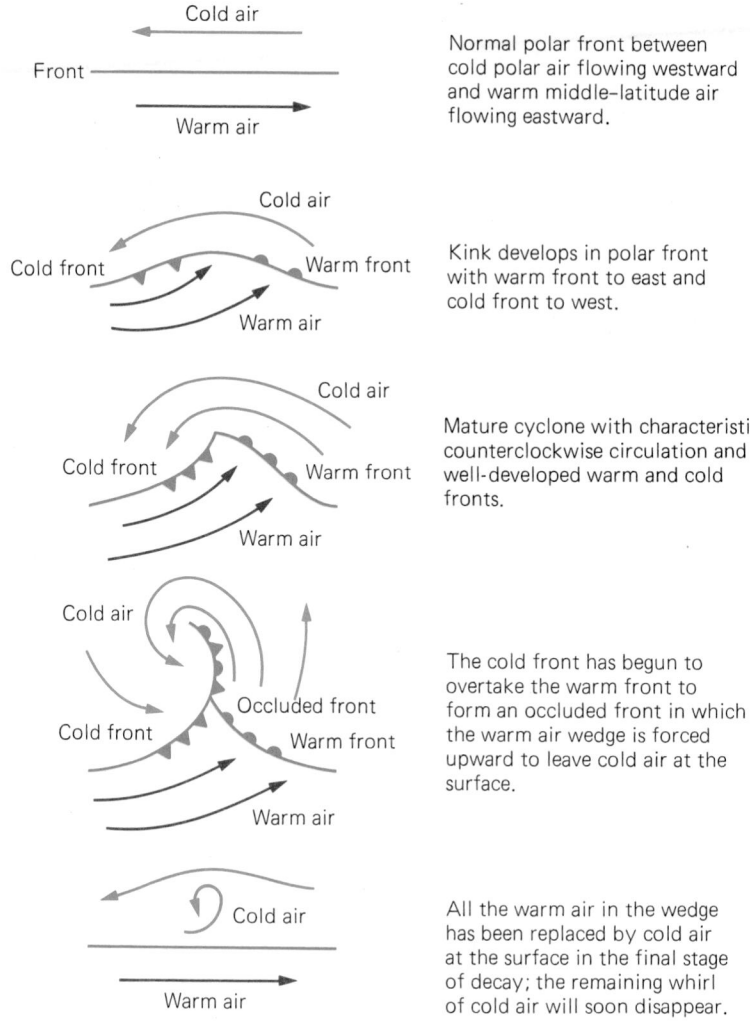

Normal polar front between cold polar air flowing westward and warm middle–latitude air flowing eastward.

Kink develops in polar front with warm front to east and cold front to west.

Mature cyclone with characteristic counterclockwise circulation and well-developed warm and cold fronts.

The cold front has begun to overtake the warm front to form an occluded front in which the warm air wedge is forced upward to leave cold air at the surface.

All the warm air in the wedge has been replaced by cold air at the surface in the final stage of decay; the remaining whirl of cold air will soon disappear.

Weather Forecasting

In order to predict the weather for a certain region, it is necessary to know present and past conditions in detail over a much larger area. Data on air pressure, temperature, humidity, cloud cover, precipitation, and winds are collected every 3 hours at about 10,000 weather stations around the world and are available to forecasters everywhere in a standard code.

Additional information is provided by weather satellites that look at the atmosphere from above and by balloon-borne instruments that make measurements at various altitudes. In both cases the observations are radioed to ground stations.

The first step in preparing a forecast is to draw a weather map, called a **synoptic** map, that shows the current situation. By comparing this map with the synoptic maps for the past day or two, a meteorologist can see how the various weather systems are developing and moving and may be able to spot new ones in their early stages. Then a **prognostic** map is prepared that shows for a future time the weather pattern the meteorologist thinks will have evolved from the current situation.

The prognostic map indicates the weather that can be expected at that time.

Nowadays computers are used to digest the vast amounts of data that go into synoptic maps and also to help predict what will happen next. People are still essential, though: an educated guess by someone familiar with local weather may be more reliable than the calculations of a supercomputer. Forecasts for a day ahead are usually quite accurate, those for longer periods in the future less so. Even with all the resources available to meteorologists today, some phenomena, such as hurricanes, do not always behave as expected.

Are more accurate long-range forecasts a realistic prospect? The trouble is that the atmosphere is a very complex system and it interacts with land and sea in complicated ways. Although weather exhibits many regularities, even small differences in initial conditions may lead to entirely different outcomes. Because, to give a famous example, a tornado in Texas could, in principle, be triggered by the fluttering of a butterfly's wings in Brazil, some element of uncertainty will always exist in weather prediction.

Tropical Cyclones

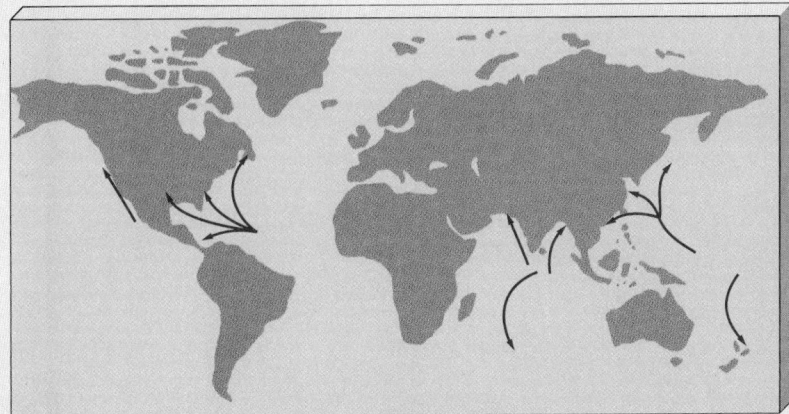

Figure 14-30   Typical storm tracks of tropical cyclones.

Compared with the cyclonic weather systems of the middle latitudes, tropical cyclones are less common—only 80 or 90 occur worldwide in an average year—but are much more violent with half of them having winds that exceed 120 km/h (75 mi/h). The hurricanes that several times a year batter the West Indies and the eastern coast of the United States are tropical cyclones, as are the typhoons of the western Pacific Ocean and the cyclones of the Indian Ocean (Fig. 14-30).

A mature hurricane, one of the most powerful events on earth, has as much energy as all the electric energy used in the United States in 3 or 4 years.

A tropical cyclone begins as a small area of low pressure over warm (above 26.5°C) ocean water near the equator in late summer or early fall. Moist air flows into the depression and cools as it spirals upward (see Fig. 14-25*a*). The water vapor in this air condenses into cloud and rain droplets, a process that liberates heat; this is the

reverse of the vaporization process described in Sec. 5.11, and it is what powers the cyclone. The heat given off causes the air pressure to drop further, which leads to more moisture from the ocean surface being sucked into the rising, spinning air column.

The above self-reinforcing sequence produces an increasingly intense storm that may end up as much as 2000 km across whose raging winds whirl around a calm "eye" of low pressure that is usually 20 to 100 km across (Fig. 14-31). The lowest surface pressure ever measured, 870 mb, occurred in the eye of a Pacific typhoon in 1979. Outside the eye rain falls in torrents. The most vigorous phase of these storms lasts for a few days to a week or so.

A typical North Atlantic hurricane originates near the bulge of Africa and gathers strength as it is swept westward by the trade winds. Then it turns north to swing around the permanent high-pressure region of the mid-Atlantic, and finally is blown eastward by the westerlies of the higher latitudes until it weakens and dies out without warm seawater to feed it energy.

Hurricanes usually move at 15 to 50 km/h but may remain stationary for a day or two. Some of them, instead of staying at sea, curve across the eastern or southern United States, where their winds may do immense damage inland. Seawater surging ashore to batter low-lying coastal areas is even more destructive. This was the case when Hurricane Katrina struck New Orleans in August 2005. The storm drove flood waters past inadequate earthen levees and concrete walls to devastate much of the low-lying city, killing 1500 people, leaving tens of thousands homeless, and doing at least $80 billion worth of damage (Fig. 14-32).

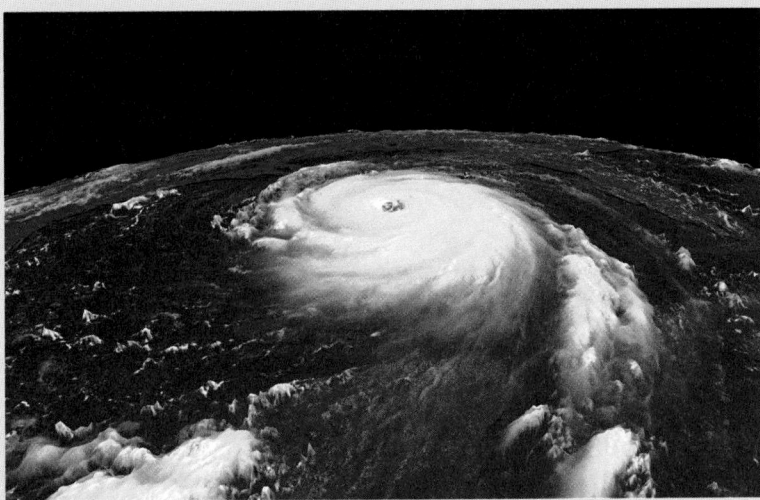

Figure 14-31   This satellite photograph of Hurricane Katrina in the Gulf of Mexico was taken on August 28, 2005, when it had grown to category five with sustained winds of 260 km/h (160 mi/h), over twice the wind speeds of category one hurricanes.

(Continued)

Tropical Cyclones   (continued)

Over the past twenty years, tropical storms around the world have been increasing in strength. There has always been a natural variation in the violence of such storms. However, the consensus among atmospheric scientists is that the current upswing can be traced to global warming (Sec. 4.3): rising ocean temperatures mean more energy being fed into the storms that form over them—bad news for coastal dwellers.

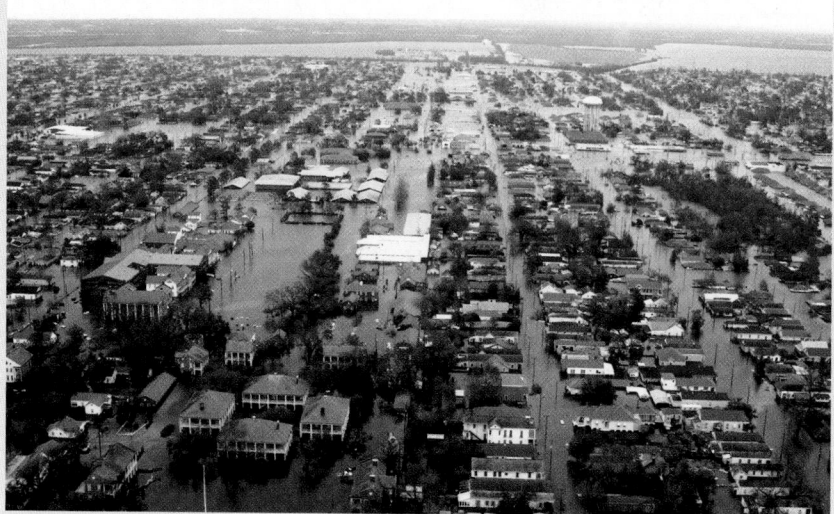

Figure 14-32   New Orleans after Hurricane Katrina in 2005. The flood defenses were known not to be robust enough for such an assault; the savings were a fraction of the cost of the disaster, which had been predicted. And, of course, there is the question of how wise it was in the first place to develop so important a city nearly 10 m below sea level in a vulnerable location almost surrounded by water.

Climate

The climate of a region refers both to its average weather over a period of years and to the typical variations in its weather elements during each day and during each year. The most significant weather elements in determining climate are temperature and precipitation. Climates differ considerably around the world, ranging from the tropics, where there is no winter, to the polar regions, where summer is brief.

14.9   Tropical Climates

Hot and Wet or Hot and Dry

The equatorial belt of the doldrums, with its rapid evaporation and strong rising air currents, provides an ideal situation for abundant rain. Throughout the year the weather is hot with almost daily rains and light, changeable winds. The steaming rain forests of Africa, South America, and the East Indies occur where this belt crosses land (Fig. 14-33).

The horse latitudes, roughly 30° north and south of the equator, are also belts of little wind, but their climate is anything but humid. Air in these belts moves downward to become warmer and hence less saturated with water vapor. Thus the climate is dry, with clouds and rain only at long intervals. In a few areas, however, such as the Gulf Coast of the United States, the prevailing dryness is modified by moisture-laden winds of local origin.

Air returning to the warm equatorial belt from the horse latitudes tends to keep the little moisture it contains, except where a mountain range or strong convection currents force the air upward. Hence the trade-wind belts are for the most part dry regions. Seasonal shifts of the trade-wind belts give rainfall during part of the year to the equatorial margins of these belts. The poleward portions of the trade-wind belts, together with the adjacent horse latitudes, are the regions of the world's great deserts—the Sahara, the deserts of South Africa, the dry districts of Mexico and northern Chile, the dry interior of Australia.

14.10 Middle- and High-Latitude Climates

Variety Is the Rule

The belts of prevailing westerlies generally have moderate average temperatures, although continental interiors show great variations with the seasons. On the other hand, oceanic islands and the western coasts of continents in these belts have even temperatures throughout the year.

In the northern hemisphere the huge landmasses of North America and Eurasia bring complications that are well illustrated by climates in the United States. Damp winds from the Pacific Ocean are forced upward by mountain ranges along the West Coast, and the western sides of the mountains therefore receive abundant rainfall. Once across the mountain barriers the westerlies have little remaining moisture, so that the region from the mountains east to the Great Plains is largely dry.

If the westerlies kept their direction as steadily as do the trade winds, dry conditions would continue across the continent to the East Coast. Instead, the cyclonic storms characteristic of this belt often bring moisture-laden air from the Gulf of Mexico and the Atlantic Ocean into the Mississippi Valley and the eastern states. Rainfall increases eastward across the country, becoming very abundant along the Gulf of Mexico.

Temperatures on the West Coast are conditioned by the prevailing wind from the ocean and change relatively little from season to season. In most other parts of the country, however, the difference between summer and winter is very marked. The fine climates of Florida and southern California owe their mildness to nearby warm oceans and to their locations near the junction of the belt of the westerlies and the horse latitudes.

In the bleak arctic and antarctic regions, summer warmth is a brief respite from the deep cold of the rest of the year. Moderate winds are the rule, although violent gales occur at times. The total amount of snow during the year is small simply because the low temperatures prevent the accumulation of much water vapor in the air.

14.11 Climate Change

An Icy Past, a Warm Future

Weather we expect to vary, both from day to day and from season to season. Nor are we surprised when one year has a colder winter or a drier summer than the one before. Less familiar are changes in climate. Even though climate represents averages in weather conditions over periods of, say, 20 or 30 years, there is plenty of evidence that it, too, is not constant but instead fluctuates markedly over long spans of time. The most dramatic fluctuations were the **ice ages** of the distant past.

The last ice age reached its peak about 20,000 years ago when huge ice sheets as much as 4 km thick covered much of Europe and North America (see Chap. 16). The vast amount of water locked up as ice lowered sea level nearly 100 m below what it is today. Then the ice began to melt and climates became progressively less severe; in a period of 12,000 years the average annual temperature of central Europe rose from −4°C to +9°C. By about 4000 B.C. average temperatures were a few degrees higher than those of today.

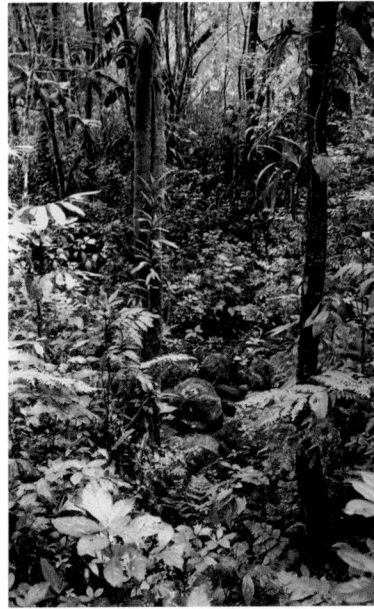

Figure 14-33 Year-round high temperatures and abundant rainfall are characteristic of the equatorial regions and encourage plant growth. This rain forest is in Costa Rica.

Why Is the South Pole Colder Than the North Pole?

The main reason is the altitude difference between the North Pole region (a winter average of −30°C), which consists of sea ice floating on the Arctic Ocean, and the South Pole region (−60°C), which is over 2 km high on the world's loftiest continent. The water of the Arctic Ocean is also a more effective heat reservoir than the rock and ice of Antarctica. A third factor is the presence of tall mountain ranges in Antarctica that prevent warm air from the middle latitudes from reaching its interior.

A time of declining temperatures then set in, reaching a minimum in Europe between 900 and 500 B.C.

A gradual warming-up followed and came to a peak between A.D. 800 and 1200. So generally fine were climatic conditions then that the Vikings established flourishing colonies in Iceland and Greenland from which they went on to visit North America (Fig. 14-34). But then came cooler summers and exceptionally cold winters with extensive freezing of the Arctic Sea. The extreme weather from the fifteenth to the nineteenth centuries in Europe led it to be called the "Little Ice Age." Greenland became a less attractive place than formerly and the colony there disappeared; the coast of Iceland was surrounded by ice for several months per year (in contrast to a few weeks per year today); and glaciers advanced farther across mountain landscapes than ever before or since in recorded history. The average temperature in Europe then was around 1°C less than it is these days. This does not seem like much, but it made a considerable difference in climates.

Late in the nineteenth century a trend toward higher temperatures led to a marked shrinkage of the world's glaciers. In the first half of the twentieth century especially pronounced temperature increases took place whose most noticeable consequences were milder winters in the higher latitudes. These balmy conditions peaked about 1940, after which average worldwide temperatures did not change by much for 40 years. Then temperatures again started upward (see Sec. 4.3 and especially Fig. 4–7). The increase in average temperature has been 0.83°C since 1880.

Why Do Climates Change?   A number of factors can influence climate, and it is not always clear which one is responsible for which change.

The most obvious factor is the sun's energy output. This is not constant but increases and decreases during the 11-year sunspot cycle (Sec. 18.6). Variations in a number of weather phenomena (for instance, in the paths of winter storms across the North Atlantic Ocean) parallel the sunspot cycle. Although the connections with the sunspot cycle seem to be real, nobody yet knows exactly how they come about. Longer-term rises and falls in solar radiation occur as well; the Little Ice Age may have been caused by one of them.

The most promising explanation for the large-scale climatic changes, however, relates them to periodic changes that occur in the tilt of the earth's axis, the shape of its orbit, and the time of year when the earth is closest to

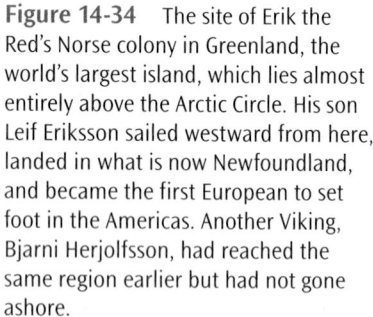

Figure 14-34   The site of Erik the Red's Norse colony in Greenland, the world's largest island, which lies almost entirely above the Arctic Circle. His son Leif Eriksson sailed westward from here, landed in what is now Newfoundland, and became the first European to set foot in the Americas. Another Viking, Bjarni Herjolfsson, had reached the same region earlier but had not gone ashore.

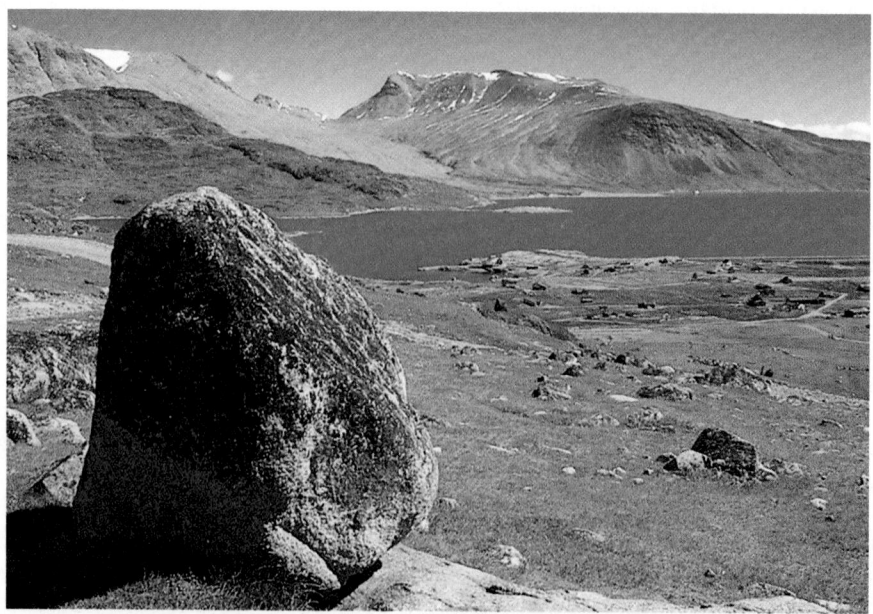

Climate and Collapse

The Viking Erik the Red established a colony in Greenland in the tenth century, which was a time of warm climate (Fig. 14-34). The colony, a few thousand strong, lasted for nearly 5 centuries until the Arctic climate deteriorated in the Little Ice Age.

The colonists contributed to their fate: they cut down trees for fuel and construction until none were left, they used nonsustainable farming methods that led to soil erosion and a consequent shortage of food, and when starvation loomed, cultural taboos kept them from eating the abundant fish or learning from their Inuit ("Eskimo") neighbors how to hunt effectively. The

Greenland Norse, already near the edge, could not survive the changing climate, unlike the more adaptable Inuit.

In his book *Collapse*, Jared Diamond examines the Greenland colony and other failed societies and then considers the "nagging thought: might such a fate eventually befall our own wealthy society?" His themes are "human environmental impact and climate change intersecting, environmental and population problems spilling over into warfare, the strengths but also the dangers of complex non-self-sufficient societies dependent on imports and exports, and societies collapsing swiftly after attain-

ing peak population numbers and power."

Elizabeth Kolbert, another worried observer, has this to say about a worldwide peril in her book *Field Notes from a Catastrophe:* "As the effects of global warming become more and more difficult to ignore, will we react by finally fashioning a global response? Or will we retreat into ever narrower and more destructive forms of self-interest? It may seem impossible to imagine that a technologically advanced society could choose, in essence, to destroy itself, but that is what we are now in the process of doing."

the sun (Fig. 14-35). Seventy years ago Milutin Milankovitch (1879–1958), a Yugoslav mathematician and physicist, worked out how these changes might affect climate by altering the amount of sunlight (that is, insolation) received by the earth.

The differences in insolation on a global basis are small, 0.3 percent at most, but Milankovitch argued that what really counts is not the total insolation but the insolation in the polar regions in summer, which varies by up to 20 percent. Too little summer sunshine would not melt all the snow that fell during the winter before, and in time the accumulated snow would turn into great sheets of ice. In the southern hemisphere the ice would melt when it left the Antarctic continent and fell into the sea, but in the northern hemisphere the ice would move down across North America and Eurasia to produce an ice age.

Major ice ages have occurred every 100,000 years or so, with smaller cycles of cold and warm at closer intervals. The strongest evidence in favor of Milankovitch's hypothesis is that the periods of advance and retreat of the ice sheets are in accord with the various periods of the earth's orbital variations. Additional support comes from current theoretical models of the earth's climate, which respond to the known insolation changes with a prediction of regular ice ages.

Global Warming What about the warming trend of recent years? A few degrees more (which seem on the way) and we will be living in the warmest environment since humans evolved millions of years ago. It is clear today that the steady rise in CO_2 levels is increasing global temperatures (Sec. 4.4). Exactly how life on earth will ultimately be affected can only be guessed at, but it is sure to mean profound changes. We are in the midst of a gigantic experiment in climate modification, one that our descendants will surely regret. It is too late to stop the experiment because the persistence of greenhouse gases in the atmosphere means that global warming will continue for decades to come no matter what is done now. But a drastic cut in their emissions on a worldwide scale, though not easy to accomplish, may allow us to moderate the experiment before we go the way of the Greenland Vikings.

Figure 14-35 Three variations in the earth's motion that may be responsible for causing ice ages. (*a*) The time of year when the earth is nearest the sun varies with a period of about 23,000 years. (*b*) The angle of tilt of the earth's axis of rotation varies with a period of about 41,000 years. (*c*) The shape of the earth's elliptical orbit varies with a period of about 100,000 years. These variations have relatively little effect on the total sunlight reaching the earth but a considerable effect on the sunlight reaching the polar regions in summer. The ellipticity of the earth's orbit is vastly exaggerated here; the orbit is actually less than 2 percent away from a perfect circle.

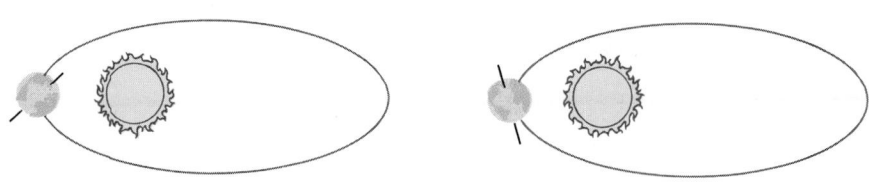

(*a*) Time of the year when earth is nearest the sun

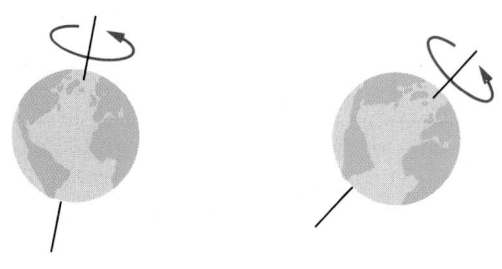

(*b*) Angle of tilt of earth's axis

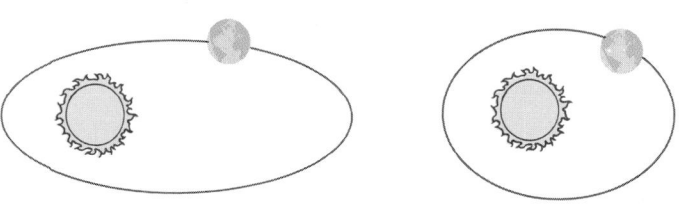

(*c*) Shape of earth's orbit

How long do we have? For an even chance of keeping global warming to no more than 2°C by 2100 (as we saw earlier in this chapter probably the maximum rise if catastrophe is to be avoided), greenhouse gas emissions would have to be cut to below half of today's figure by 2050. Such a goal seems barely possible, and even that would require intensive international efforts on a scale that has yet to come into being.

The Hydrosphere

Over 70 percent of the earth's surface is covered by the oceans and the seas that join with them. These waters are filled with plant and animal life—indeed, the early oceans were home to living things for more than a billion years before they began to move ashore. In addition, the oceans influence continental life in a variety of indirect ways. The oceans provide the reservoir from which water is evaporated into the atmosphere, later to fall as rain and snow on land. The oceans participate in the oxygen–carbon dioxide cycle both through the life they support and through the vast quantities of these gases dissolved in them. And the oceans help determine climates by their ability to absorb solar energy and transport it around the world.

14.12 Ocean Basins

Water, Water Everywhere

Each of the world's oceans lies in a vast basin bounded by continental landmasses. Typically an ocean bottom slopes gradually downward from the shore to a depth of 130 m or so before starting to drop more rapidly (Fig. 14-36).

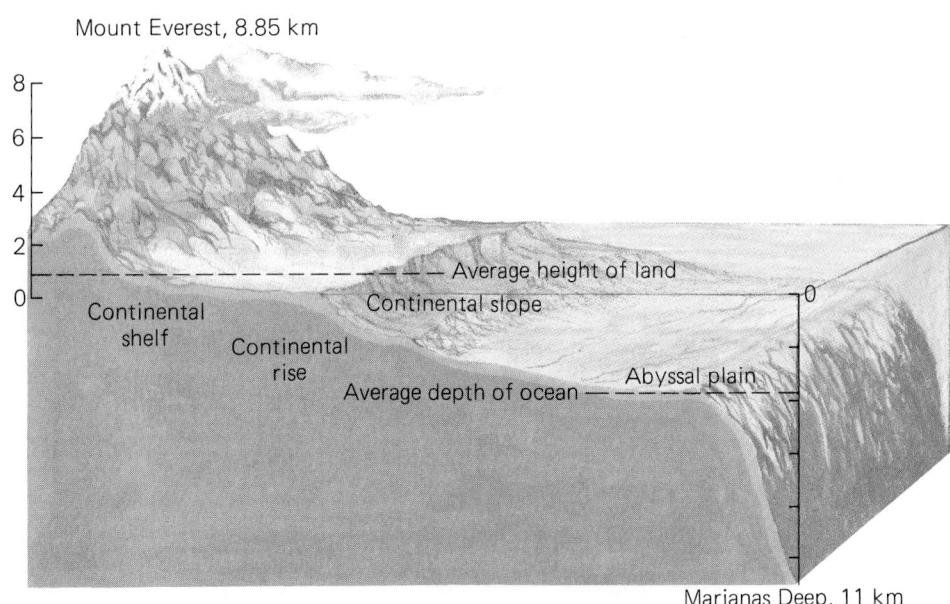

Figure 14-36   Profile of the earth's surface with heights above sea level and depths below it in km. In general, ocean depths are greater than land heights—the Marianas Deep can swallow Mt. Everest with over 2 km to spare. The vertical scale is greatly exaggerated here: the earth is actually quite smooth. Although the earth's circumference is about 40,000 km, the vertical distance from the deepest point in the oceans to the top of the highest mountain is less than 20 km. A car on a level road can easily go this far in 15 min.

The average width of this **continental shelf** is 65 km, but it ranges from less than a kilometer (off the mountainous western coast of South America) to over 1000 km (off the low arctic coasts of the Eurasian landmass). The North, Irish, and Baltic Seas are part of the European continental shelf, while the Grand Banks off Newfoundland are part of the North American shelf. A sharp change in steepness marks the change from the continental shelf to the steeper **continental slope,** which after a fall of perhaps 2 km joins the **abyssal plain** of the ocean floor via the gentle **continental rise.**

The ocean basins average 3.7 km in depth, while the continents average only about 0.8 km in height above sea level. If the earth were smooth, it would be covered with a layer of water perhaps 2.4 km thick, but it seems likely that the oceans have always been confined to more or less distinct basins and presumably will continue to be. The waves that ruffle ocean surfaces are caused by winds that blow across them (Fig. 14-37).

The Ocean Floor   The ocean floor, like the continents, has mountain ranges and valleys, volcanoes, and vast plains, many of them rivaling or exceeding in size their counterparts on land. The Hawaiian Islands, for instance, are volcanoes that rise as much as 9000 m above the ocean floor, about half of their altitude being above sea level. Less conspicuous from the surface is the Mid-Atlantic Ridge, an immense submarine mountain range that extends from Iceland past the tip of South America before swinging into the Indian Ocean. Such islands as the Azores, Ascension Island, and Tristan da Cunha are all that protrude from the ocean of this ridge.

Much remains to be learned about the ocean floor—only 10 percent of its area has been surveyed well enough to reveal details smaller than 300 m. By contrast, 90 percent of the surface of Venus has been mapped to that extent by instruments carried on spacecraft.

Seawater and Freshwater   By far the greatest part of the earth's surface water is in the form of seawater, as Fig. 14-6 shows. Much of the freshwater is stored as ice in the form of the glaciers and ice caps that cover one-tenth

Figure 14-37 Winds that blow over the surface of a body of water churn up waves that range from the ripples produced by a gentle breeze to the towering seas produced by a hurricane. The stronger the wind, the longer it blows, and the greater the distance over which the wind has been in contact with the water, the greater the average height of the waves that result. These three factors govern the amount of energy transferred to the water and thus govern how violent the resulting disturbance will be. At a given time and place in the ocean, wave heights vary considerably about their average. A third of the waves are normally higher than average, a tenth of them twice as high, and a very few three times as high. The record is held by a wave 29 m (95 ft!) high measured off the coast of Scotland by an oceanographic vessel in 2000. How such waves are formed is not fully understood.

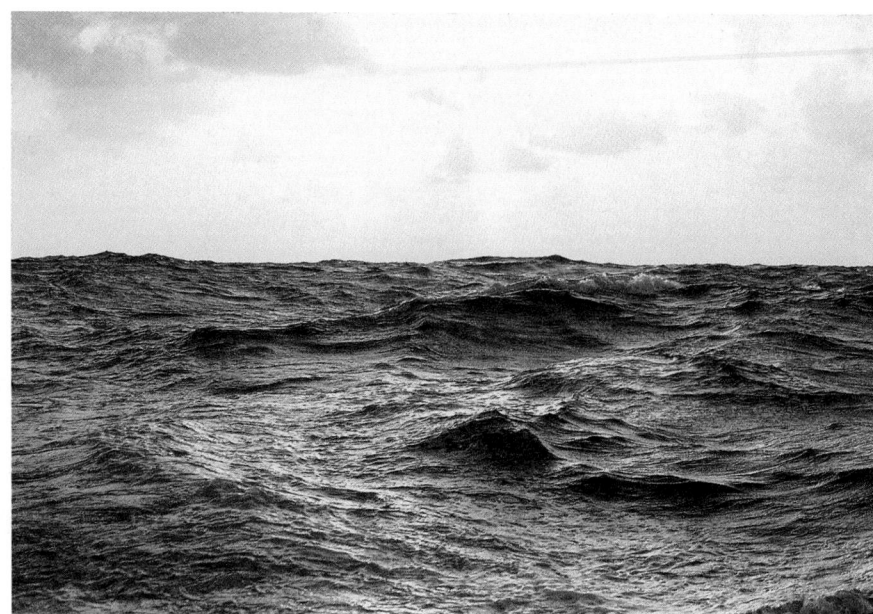

Tsunamis

A **tsunami** consists of ocean waves usually caused by an earthquake on the seabed. In the open ocean tsunamis may be less than a meter high and, since their crests are many kilometers apart, ships at sea do not notice them and they lose little energy as they go. In deep water, tsunami speeds can exceed 700 km/h, as fast as a jet airliner. When the waves reach shallow water, they slow down, steepen to heights of as much as 30 m, and can go on to do immense damage on land (Fig. 14-38).

Because the location and magnitude of a major earthquake can be established soon after it occurs, even in midocean, warnings of a possible tsunami can usually be given a few hours before the first wave arrives. Tsunamis used to be called "tidal waves," but since they have nothing to do with tides, scientists now use the Japanese word for them, which means "harbor wave." Over 800 tsunamis have occurred since 1900, most of them in the Pacific Ocean and a few of which caused serious damage on shore. Reports of tsunamis go back to ancient Greece and Rome; one recorded in 365 A.D. killed thousands in the Egyptian port of Alexandria.

There is evidence that some tsunamis in the past were induced by large-scale landslides into the ocean. Of concern today is the instability of a volcano on La Palma, one of the Canary Islands in the Atlantic near Africa. It seems possible that its huge (half a trillion tons) western flank may someday split off and tumble into the ocean. The resulting tsunami might be 20 m high when it reaches the eastern coast of North America 8 h later where it would surge inland, devastating everything in its path.

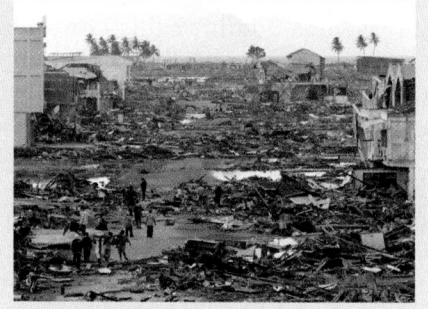

Figure 14-38 During a severe earthquake—the most violent in 40 years—on December 26, 2004, off the northwestern corner of the Indonesian island of Sumatra, a massive section of the earth's crust was abruptly thrust upward along a rupture hundreds of kilometers long. The result was a huge tsunami that spread across the Indian Ocean and smashed into the coasts of Indonesia, Sri Lanka, India, and Thailand. It reached East Africa 7 hours later. In all, at least 280,000 people, mainly in Indonesia and Sri Lanka, lost their lives and perhaps 2 million others were left homeless by waves up to 10 m high that surged ashore.

the land area of the earth. About 90 percent of this ice is located in the Antarctic ice cap, about 9 percent in the Greenland ice cap, and the remaining 1 percent in the various glaciers of the world. If suddenly melted, the ice would raise the sea level by perhaps 70 m. (By comparison, if all the water vapor in the atmosphere were condensed, the sea level would go up by only about 2.5 cm.)

Most of the earth's surface water probably appeared about 4 billion years ago when the young earth assumed its present internal structure. The water came from the rocks of the interior and took with it the same ions found in seawater today: the oceans have always been salty.

Additional salts have been added to the oceans in the various ways illustrated in Fig. 11-33. However, seawater salinity has not changed very much because of various mechanisms that remove salt from the oceans. One of these mechanisms is quite direct: the loss of salt to the atmosphere when wind blows spray off wave tops. The resulting salt particles serve as nuclei for water molecules to stick to, and a substantial amount falls on land in rain and snow. Another mechanism that reduces salinity is the incorporation of various compounds in the shells of marine organisms, which end up in the sediments that coat the ocean floors.

14.13 Ocean Currents

Four Great Whirlpools

The oceans affect climate in two ways. First, they act as heat reservoirs that moderate seasonal temperature extremes; more heat is stored in the upper few meters of the oceans than in the entire atmosphere. In spring and summer the oceans are cooler than the regions they border, since the insolation they receive is absorbed in a greater volume than on solid, opaque land. The heat stored in the ocean depths means that in fall and winter the oceans are warmer than nearby land areas. Heat flows readily between moving air and water. With enough of a temperature difference, the rate of energy transfer from warm water to cold air (or from warm air to cold water) can exceed the rate at which solar energy arrives at the earth.

Lacking such an adjacent heat reservoir, continental interiors experience lower winter temperatures and higher summer temperatures than those of coastal districts. In Canada, for instance, temperatures in the city of Victoria on the Pacific coast range from an average January minimum of 9°C to an average July maximum of 20°C, whereas in Winnipeg, in the interior, the corresponding figures are −13°C and 27°C.

The second way oceans influence climate is through surface currents, which are produced by the friction of wind on water. Such currents are much slower than movements in the atmosphere, with the fastest normal surface currents having speeds of about 10 km/h.

The wind-driven surface currents parallel to a large extent the major wind systems (Fig. 14-39). The northeast and southeast trade winds drive water before them westward along the equator, forming the **equatorial current.** In the Atlantic Ocean this current runs into South America and in the Pacific the current runs into the East Indies. At each of these contacts the current divides into two parts, one flowing south and the other north. Moving away from the equator along the continental edges, these currents then come under the influence of the westerlies, which drive them eastward across the oceans. Thus gigantic whirlpools are set up in both the Atlantic and the Pacific on either side of the equator. Many complexities are produced in the four great whirls by islands, continental projections, and undersea mountains and valleys.

The Gulf Stream   The western side of the North Atlantic whirl—a warm current moving partly into the Gulf of Mexico, partly straight north along our southeastern coast—is the famous **Gulf Stream.** Forced away from the coast in the latitude of New Jersey by the westerlies, this current moves northeastward

Sea Ice

Even in the intense cold of the polar regions, sea ice is seldom more than a few meters deep. (Icebergs are huge masses of ice that have broken off from ice caps or glaciers that formed from accumulated snow on a land base.)

There are several reasons why sea ice is so relatively thin. The chief one is that, as water under a surface layer of ice cools, it becomes denser and sinks, to be replaced by warmer water from underneath. Another reason is that ice itself acts as an insulator. Also, as seawater freezes, its salt content is not incorporated in the ice crystals but stays behind to increase the salinity of the remaining water, whose freezing point is accordingly lowered (see Sec. 11.4).

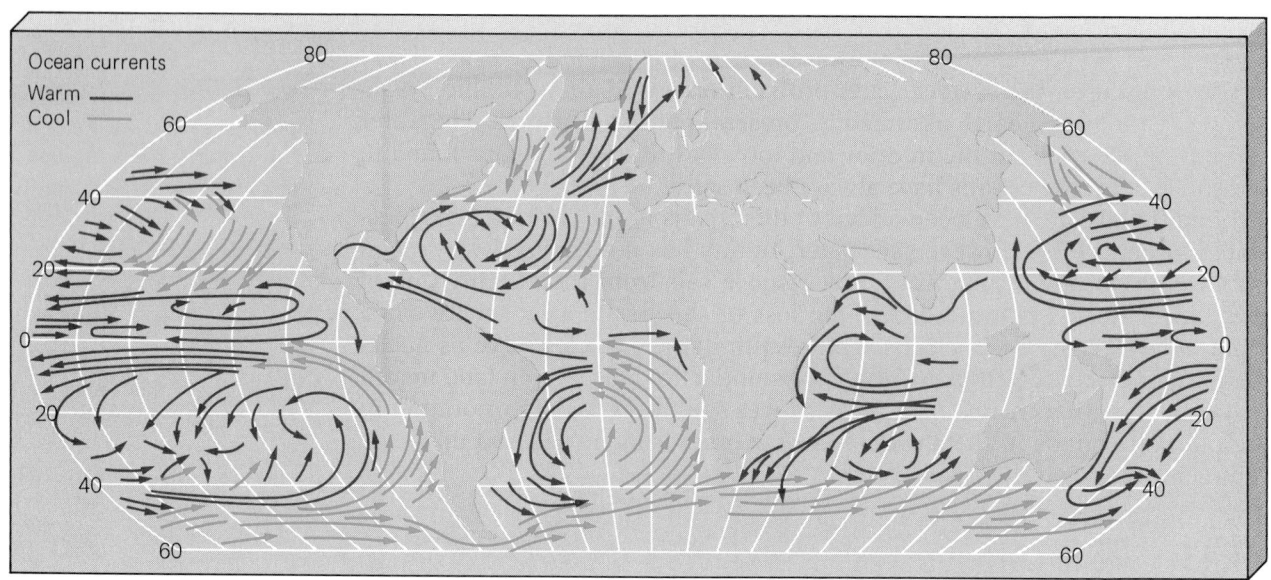

Figure 14-39 Principal ocean currents of the world. The swirling currents of the Pacific Ocean contain an estimated 100 million tons of rubbish, mainly plastic bags and bottles, that floats just below the surface and covers a total area twice that of the continental United States. The plastic debris will take hundreds of years to disintegrate.

Figure 14-40 Surface temperatures of the North Atlantic Ocean are shown in this computer simulation. Temperatures range from about 28°C (dark red) in the tropics to 0°C (dark blue) near Greenland. The ribbon of dark red off the southern part of the American coast is the Gulf Stream, whose continuation across the Atlantic is responsible for the relatively warm water shown in yellow and green. Global warming is reducing the rate of flow of the Gulf Stream, a process that will eventually have the paradoxical effect of chilling the climate of northern Europe, perhaps by as much as 5°C.

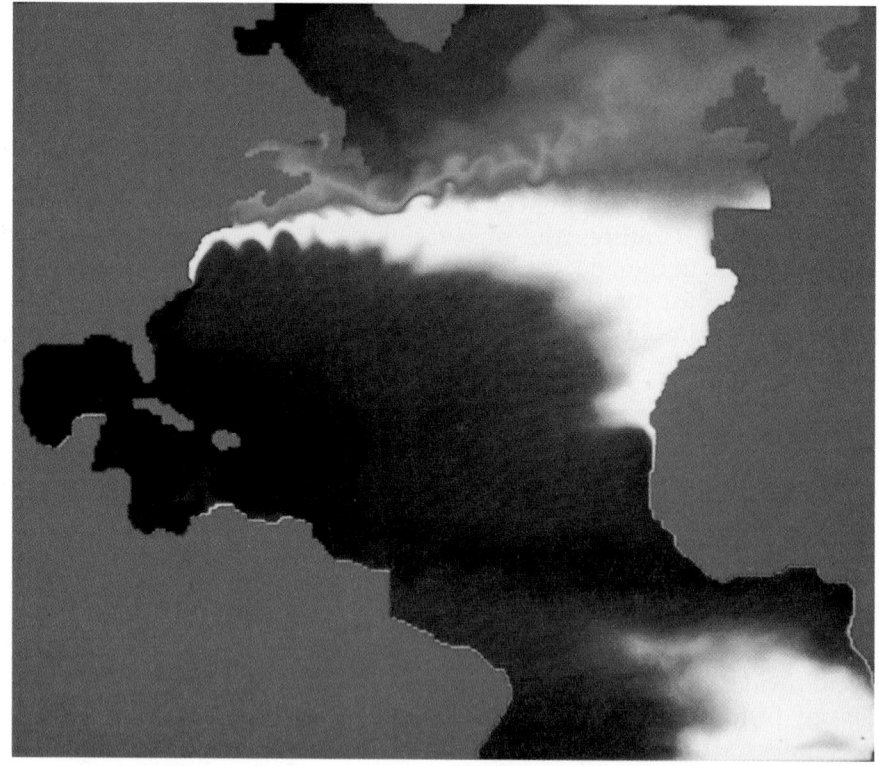

across the Atlantic (Fig. 14-40). The current splits on the European side into one part that moves south to complete the whirl and another part that continues northeastward past Great Britain and Norway into the Arctic Ocean. To compensate for the addition of water into the polar sea, the cold **Labrador Current** moves southward along the east coast of North America as far as New York. Down the west coast of North America moves the **California Current,** the southward-flowing eastern part of the North Pacific whirl.

Since ocean currents retain the temperatures of the latitudes from which they come for a long time, they exert a direct influence on the temperatures of neighboring lands. The influence is greatest, of course, where prevailing winds blow shoreward from the sea. The warm Gulf Stream has a far greater effect in tempering the climate of northwestern Europe than that of eastern United States, since prevailing winds in these latitudes are from the west. Cyclonic storms bring east winds to the Atlantic seaboard often enough, however, for the Gulf Stream to help raise temperatures in the South Atlantic states, and for the same reason the Labrador Current is in part responsible for the rigorous climate of New England and eastern Canada.

Thus the oceans, besides acting as water reservoirs for the earth's atmosphere, play a direct part in temperature control—both by preventing abrupt temperature changes in lands along their borders and by aiding the winds, through the motion of ocean currents, in their distribution of heat and cold over the surface of the earth.

Important Terms and Ideas

The earth's **atmosphere** is its envelope of air, which consists mainly of nitrogen and oxygen. The lowest part of the atmosphere is the **troposphere,** in which such weather phenomena as clouds and storms occur. Next comes the **stratosphere,** whose content of **ozone** (O_3) absorbs most of the ultraviolet radiation from the sun. Above the stratosphere is the **mesosphere** and still higher is the **thermosphere,** which contains most of the ions that make up the **ionosphere.** The ionosphere reflects radio waves.

Air at a given temperature is said to be **saturated** when it contains the maximum amount of water vapor possible without liquid water condensing out. The **relative humidity** of a volume of air is the ratio between the water vapor it contains and the amount that would be present at saturation. Low-altitude **clouds** consist of tiny water droplets; high-altitude clouds consist of ice crystals.

The energy that powers weather phenomena is **insolation,** which is **in**coming **sol**ar radi**ation.** Most of the insolation passes through the atmosphere and is absorbed by the earth's surface. The warm earth then radiates energy back into the atmosphere which absorbs some of it. This indirect heating of the atmosphere is called the **greenhouse effect.**

The **seasons** occur because the earth's axis is tilted, so that in half of each year one hemisphere receives more direct sunlight than the other hemisphere.

Convection currents are due to the uneven heating of a fluid: the warmer parts of the fluid expand and rise while the cooler parts sink. Such currents occur where air in the equatorial regions is heated strongly, expands and rises, and moves toward the poles. In the polar regions the air cools and sinks and then flows back on the surface toward the equator. In this way energy is shifted from the tropics to the higher latitudes.

The **coriolis effect** is the deflection of winds to the right in the northern hemisphere, to the left in the southern, as a consequence of the earth's rotation. Because of the coriolis effect, the convection currents in the atmosphere follow curved paths. A **cyclone** is a weather system centered on a low-pressure region. In the northern hemisphere the coriolis effect deflects winds moving inward in a cyclone into a counterclockwise spiral, in the southern hemisphere into a clockwise spiral. An **anticyclone** is a weather system centered on a high-pressure region; winds blowing outward from an anticyclone spiral clockwise in the northern hemisphere and counterclockwise in the southern hemisphere.

A **front** is the boundary between a mass of warm air and a mass of cold air; clouds and rain usually occur at a front.

Climate refers to averages in weather conditions over a period of years. The **ice ages** were times of severe cold in which ice sheets covered much of Europe and North America. Such long-term climatic changes are probably caused by changes in the earth's motions around the sun.

A **tsunami** consists of ocean waves caused by earthquakes on the seabed or by gigantic landslides into the ocean.

The **Gulf Stream** is a warm current that flows northeastward in the Atlantic Ocean. Westerly winds that blow across the Gulf Stream carry heat that moderates the climate of northwestern Europe.

Multiple Choice

1. Arrange the following gases in the order of their abundance in the earth's atmosphere:

   a. oxygen   **c.** nitrogen

   b. carbon dioxide   **d.** argon

2. Much of Tibet lies in altitudes above 5.5 km (18,000 ft). At such altitudes the Tibetans are above approximately

   a. 10 percent of the atmosphere

   b. 50 percent of the atmosphere

   c. 90 percent of the atmosphere
   d. 99 percent of the atmosphere

3. Weather phenomena such as clouds and storms are found in the
   a. thermosphere   **c.** troposphere
   b. stratosphere   **d.** ionosphere

4. Temperatures in the stratosphere increase with altitude because of the presence there of
   a. water vapor   **c.** pollutants
   b. ozone   **d.** CFCs

5. The ozone in the stratosphere
   a. reflects radio waves
   b. reflects solar ultraviolet radiation
   c. absorbs solar ultraviolet radiation
   d. is responsible for the blue color of the sky

6. The breakdown of the ozone layer is promoted by the emission into the atmosphere of
   a. carbon dioxide from the burning of fossil fuels
   b. sulfuric acid from the burning of fossil fuels
   c. unburned hydrocarbons in the exhausts of gasoline engines
   d. chlorofluorocarbon (CFC) gases used in refrigeration

7. Saturated air has a relative humidity of
   a. 0   **c.** 50 percent
   b. 1 percent   **d.** 100 percent

8. The higher the temperature of a volume of air, the
   a. more water vapor it can hold
   b. less water vapor it can hold
   c. greater its possible relative humidity
   d. lower its possible relative humidity

9. When saturated air is cooled,
   a. it becomes able to take up more water vapor
   b. some of its water content condenses out
   c. the relative humidity goes down
   d. convection currents result

10. Clouds consist of
   a. water droplets at all altitudes
   b. ice crystals at all altitudes
   c. water droplets at low altitudes and ice crystals at high altitudes
   d. ice crystals at low altitudes and water droplets at high altitudes

11. If the atmosphere contained fewer salt crystals and dust particles than it now does,
   a. clouds would form less readily
   b. clouds would form more readily
   c. the formation of clouds would be unaffected
   d. snow would never fall

12. When an air mass moves upward, it cools because
   a. it contracts
   b. it expands
   c. its ozone content increases
   d. it comes in contact with clouds

13. Insolation is
   a. the insulating effect of the atmosphere
   b. another name for the greenhouse effect
   c. incoming solar radiation
   d. incoming heat from the equator

14. The chief source of atmospheric heat is
   a. incoming solar radiation
   b. infrared radiation from the earth itself
   c. ultraviolet radiation absorbed by ozone
   d. ultraviolet radiation absorbed by clouds

15. Energy is transported from the tropics to the polar regions chiefly by
   a. winds   **c.** carbon dioxide
   b. ocean currents   **d.** ozone

16. The seasons occur as a result of
   a. variations in the sun's energy output
   b. variations in the distance between the earth and the sun
   c. variations in the orbital speed of the earth
   d. the tilt of the earth's axis

17. Because of the coriolis effect, a wind in the northern hemisphere is deflected
   a. upward   **c.** toward the right
   b. downward   **d.** toward the left

18. Because of the coriolis effect, a wind in the southern hemisphere is deflected
   a. upward   **c.** toward the right
   b. downward   **d.** toward the left

19. On a summer day sunlight warms coastal land until its temperature is higher than that of the adjacent sea. The result is a "sea breeze" that blows
   a. from sea to land
   b. from land to sea
   c. parallel to the shore
   d. any of these, depending on the part of the world

20. The flow of air in the upper atmosphere is largely from
   a. east to west   **c.** north to south
   b. west to east   **d.** south to north

21. The middle latitudes usually experience winds from the
   a. north   **c.** east
   b. south   **d.** west

22. The generally easterly winds that blow on both sides of the equator are called
   a. trade winds   **c.** cyclones
   b. monsoons   **d.** doldrums

23. An airplane flies at the same speed relative to the air at a high altitude from New York to Paris and back.
   a. The New York to Paris flight takes less time.
   b. The Paris to New York flight takes less time.
   c. The two flights take the same time on the average.
   d. Any of these, depending on the season.

24. The trade-wind belts are regions of generally
   a. little rainfall   **c.** low temperatures
   b. much rainfall   **d.** westerly winds

25. A cyclone is a weather system centered about a
   a. region of low pressure
   b. region of high pressure
   c. hurricane
   d. cold front

26. The winds in an anticyclone
   a. blow directly toward its center
   b. spiral toward its center
   c. blow directly away from its center
   d. spiral away from its center

27. Unstable weather is associated with
   a. cyclones   **c.** trade winds
   b. anticyclones   **d.** the greenhouse effect

28. Tornados
   a. are narrow cyclonic storms
   b. are narrow anticyclonic storms
   c. are the central parts of hurricanes
   d. occur mainly in the winter

29. The chief reason why the equatorial regions are warmer than the polar regions is that
   a. the equator is closer to the sun
   b. sunlight falls more nearly vertically on the equatorial regions
   c. sunlight is reflected by ice and snow in the polar regions
   d. there is more CO_2 in the air over the equatorial regions

30. The greatest seasonal variations in temperature occur in
   a. the west coasts of the continents
   b. the east coasts of the continents
   c. continental interiors
   d. isolated islands

31. Rain is most abundant in the
   a. prevailing westerlies of the middle latitudes
   b. horse latitudes between the middle latitudes and the trade-wind belts
   c. trade-wind belts
   d. doldrums of the equatorial regions

32. Ice ages
   a. cover the entire earth with a sheet of ice
   b. freeze all the oceans

   c. occurred seldom in the past
   d. occurred frequently in the past

33. The approximate percentage of the earth's surface covered by water is
   a. 10 percent   **c.** 70 percent
   b. 50 percent   **d.** 90 percent

34. Compared with the average height of the continents above sea level, the average depth of the ocean basins below sea level is
   a. smaller
   b. greater
   c. about the same
   d. sometimes smaller and sometimes greater, depending upon the tides

35. The deepest known point of the oceans is found in the
   a. Atlantic Ocean   **c.** North Sea
   b. Pacific Ocean   **d.** Panama Canal

36. The Hawaiian Islands are
   a. part of a sunken continent
   b. floating on the surface of the ocean
   c. located in shallow water
   d. volcanic peaks

37. Tsunamis are caused by
   a. monsoons
   b. typhoons
   c. icebergs
   d. undersea earthquakes

38. Most surface ocean currents are due to
   a. melting glaciers
   b. rivers
   c. winds
   d. differences in the altitude of the ocean surface

39. The Gulf Stream is a
   a. warm current in the North Atlantic
   b. cool current in the North Atlantic
   c. river that flows into the Gulf of Mexico
   d. warm wind blowing over the North Atlantic

40. The climate of northwestern Europe is greatly affected by the
   a. Gulf Stream   **c.** Labrador Current
   b. abyssal zone   **d.** trade winds

Exercises

14.1   Regions of the Atmosphere

1. What causes ionization to occur in the upper atmosphere?

2. Suppose you are climbing in an airplane that has no altimeter. How could you tell when you are approaching the top of the troposphere?

3. The tropopause, stratopause, and mesopause are respectively the upper boundaries of the troposphere,

stratosphere, and mesosphere. What is characteristic of the air temperature at each of these boundaries?

4. What would happen if ozone were to disappear from the upper atmosphere? From the lower atmosphere?

5. Why are chlorofluorocarbon (CFC) gases, which are widely used in refrigeration and in foam plastics, harmful when released into the atmosphere?

14.2 Atmospheric Moisture

6. What does it mean to say that a certain volume of air has a relative humidity of 50 percent? Of 100 percent?

7. Under what circumstances, if any, can saturated air take up more water? Under what circumstances, if any, can some of the water content of saturated air condense out?

8. Why does the air in a heated room tend to be dry?

9. The air in a closed container is saturated with water vapor at 20°C. (a) What is the relative humidity? (b) What happens to the relative humidity if the temperature is reduced to 10°C? (c) If the temperature is increased to 30°C?

10. (a) Why does dew form on the ground during clear, calm summer nights? (b) What is the dew point of a body of air?

11. What does Fig. 14-5 tell us about the relative amounts of freshwater present on or near the earth's surface as groundwater, in lakes and rivers, in ice caps and glaciers, and as moisture in the atmosphere? How does the total amount of freshwater compare with the amount of seawater?

14.3 Clouds

12. What do high-altitude clouds consist of? Low-altitude clouds?

13. What initiates the fall of rain from a cloud? The fall of snow?

14. (a) The three basic cloud types are cirrus, stratus, and cumulus. What is characteristic of each type? (b) What is the origin of the streaks of cirrus cloud produced by high-altitude aircraft?

14.4 Atmospheric Energy

15. What is insolation? How does it affect the atmosphere?

16. (a) On a clear day, solar radiation is most intense at noon. Why? (b) The highest air temperatures occur a few hours later. Why?

17. What is the greenhouse effect and how is it related to the absorption of solar energy by the earth's atmosphere?

18. Compare the ways in which the troposphere and the stratosphere are heated.

19. If the earth's atmosphere were to disappear, what would happen to the rate at which the earth would radiate energy back into space?

20. Why does the average air temperature decrease going from the equator to the poles?

21. What are the two mechanisms by which energy of solar origin is transported around the earth? Which is more important?

22. Account for the abrupt changes in temperature between day and night in desert regions.

14.5 The Seasons

23. In the northern hemisphere, the longest day is in June and the shortest day is in December, but the warmest weather occurs in July and August and the

coldest weather in January and February. What is the reason for these time lags?

24. If the earth's axis were tilted more than its present 23.5°, in what way, if any, would the seasons be affected?

25. The *Tropic of Cancer* is the most northerly latitude in the northern hemisphere at which the sun is ever directly overhead at noon. The *Tropic of Capricorn* is the corresponding latitude in the southern hemisphere. What are the latitudes of these tropics?

26. (a) At what times of year are the periods of daylight and darkness the same everywhere on the earth? What are these times called? (b) Where is the noon sun directly overhead at these times?

27. What is a solstice?

14.6 Winds

28. What is the basic cause of winds?

29. Distinguish between an isobar and a millibar.

30. A wind in the northern hemisphere starts to blow toward the equator. Toward what direction is the wind deflected by the coriolis effect? What about a wind in the southern hemisphere also starting to blow toward the equator?

31. On a summer night coastal land cools below the temperature of the adjacent sea. Does the resulting "land breeze" blow offshore or onshore? Does the coriolis effect influence the land breeze? If so, how?

14.7 General Circulation of the Atmosphere

32. Where in the atmosphere do the jet streams occur? What is their general direction?

33. An airplane flies at the same speed relative to the air at a high altitude from Chicago to London and then back to Chicago. How do the flight times for each leg compare?

34. The prevailing westerly winds of the middle latitudes of the northern hemisphere are generally weaker than those of the southern hemisphere. Can you think of why this is so?

14.8 Middle-Latitude Weather Systems

35. (a) What is the name of weather systems centered about regions of high pressure? (b) In what direction do winds in the northern hemisphere spiral around such a region? (c) In the southern hemisphere?

36. (a) What is the name of weather systems centered about regions of low pressure? (b) In what direction do winds in the northern hemisphere spiral around such a region? (c) In the southern hemisphere?

37. How does the weather associated with a cyclone differ from that associated with an anticyclone?

38. Why are clouds and rain more likely to be associated with a cyclone than with an anticyclone?

39. When you face a wind associated with a cyclone in the northern hemisphere, in what approximate direction will the center of low pressure be? In what direction will the center of low pressure be if you do this in the southern hemisphere?

40. What is the approximate sequence of wind directions when the center of a cyclone passes north of an observer in the northern hemisphere?

41. What is the approximate sequence of wind directions when the center of an anticyclone passes south of an observer in the northern hemisphere?

42. What is the difference between the rainfall that accompanies the passage of a warm front and that which accompanies the passage of a cold front?

43. Cumulus clouds form when warm air rises vertically by convection, and stratus clouds form when a warm air mass moving horizontally encounters a cooler mass and is forced upward on top of the cooler mass. Which kind of clouds would you expect to be characteristic of a warm front?

44. Why can a hurricane be regarded as a heat engine?

14.9   Tropical Climates

45. The northeast and southeast trade winds meet in a belt called the doldrums. What is the characteristic climate of the doldrums and why does it occur?

46. A feature of most autumns in the northeastern United States is a period of mild, sunny weather called Indian summer, which occurs when an anticyclone happens to stall for a few days off the East Coast. Explain the connection.

47. Most of the world's deserts occur in the horse latitudes between the trade winds and the prevailing westerlies in each hemisphere. Why?

14.11   Climate Change

48. Water vapor is an important "greenhouse gas" in the atmosphere, yet much more attention is paid in this respect to carbon dioxide. Why do you think this is so?

49. The Milankovitch theory of ice ages relates them to variations in the tilt of the earth's axis, the shape of its orbit, and the time of year when the earth is closest to the sun. However, these variations affect the total amount of solar energy reaching the earth by no more than 0.3 percent. How did Milankovitch account for this apparent contradiction?

50. From time to time a gigantic volcanic explosion sends a large amount of dust into the atmosphere, where it may remain for some years. How many consequences of such an event can you think of?

51. When did the Little Ice Age occur: several hundred years ago, several thousand years ago, several million years ago? By roughly how much did average European temperatures fall in the Little Ice Age?

14.12   Ocean Basins

52. How does the average depth of the ocean basins below sea level compare with the average height of the continents above sea level?

53. A wind begins to blow over the surface of a calm body of deep water. What factors govern the height of the waves that are produced?

54. Why is it believed that seawater has always been salty?

14.13   Ocean Currents

55. The salinity of seawater varies with location, but the relative proportions of the various ions in solution are almost exactly the same everywhere regardless of local circumstances. What is the significance of the latter observation?

56. The giant whirls of the oceans involve clockwise flows in the northern hemisphere and counter-clockwise flows in the southern. Why?

57. In what two ways do the oceans influence climates on land?

58. England and Labrador are at about the same latitude on either side of the North Atlantic Ocean, but England is considerably warmer than Labrador on the average. Why?

59. The California Current along the California coast is cooler than the ocean to the west. How does this fact explain the numerous fogs on this coast?

60. The island of Oahu (one of the Hawaiian Islands) is at latitude 21°N and is crossed by a mountain range trending roughly northwest to southeast. Account for the more abundant rainfall on the northeastern side of the range.

61. Why does the equatorial current flow westward?

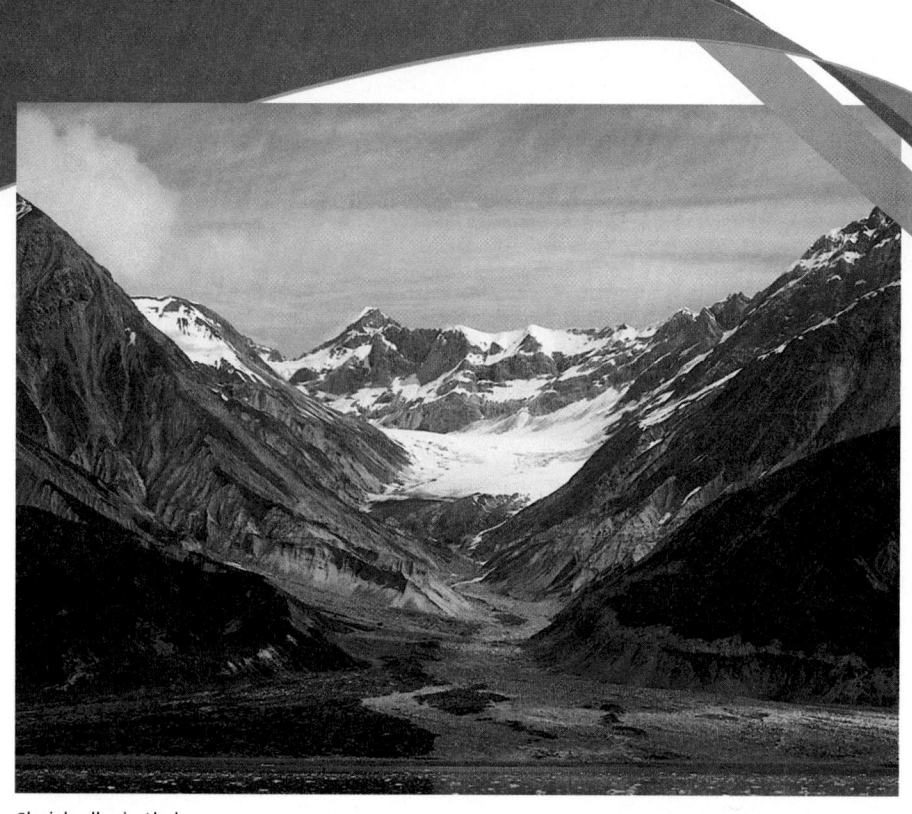

Glacial valley in Alaska.

The Rock Cycle

GOALS

When you have finished this chapter you should be able to complete the goals
• given for each section below:

Rocks

15.1 Composition of the Crust
Oxygen and Silicon Are the Most Abundant Elements
• List in order of abundance the four chief elements in the earth's crust.
• Explain why the silicates can vary so much in composition and crystal structure.

15.2 Minerals
What Rocks Are Made Of
• Distinguish between rocks and minerals.
• Briefly describe quartz, feldspar, mica, the ferromagnesian minerals, the clay minerals, and calcite.

15.3 Igneous Rocks
Once Molten, Now Solid
• Distinguish among igneous, sedimentary, and metamorphic rocks.
• Compare the origins of the fine-grained and coarse-grained igneous rocks and give several examples of each type.

15.4 Sedimentary Rocks
Compacted Sediments or Precipitates from Solution
• Describe several fragmental sedimentary rocks.
• State the main characteristics of limestone and describe how it is formed.

15.5 Metamorphic Rocks
Formed from Other Rocks by Heat and/or Pressure
• Describe several metamorphic rocks and give their origins.

Within the Earth

15.6 Earthquakes
When Our Planet Trembles
• Distinguish among the four kinds of earthquake waves.

15.7 Structure of the Earth
Core, Mantle, and Crust
• Explain the evidence that suggests the division of the earth into core, mantle, and crust.

15.8 The Earth's Interior
A Mantle of Rock, a Core of Molten Iron
• Give several reasons for the belief that earth's core is largely molten iron.
• Identify the main source of heat that flows out of the earth's interior.

15.9 Geomagnetism
Electric Currents in the Core Seem to Be Responsible
• Compare the earth's magnetic field with the magnetic field of a bar magnet, and explain why no actual permanent magnet can give rise to the earth's field.

Erosion

15.10 Weathering
How Exposed Rocks Decay
• Describe the chemical and mechanical weathering of rocks.

15.11 Stream Erosion
Running Water Is the Chief Agent of Erosion
• Discuss the development of a valley carved by a river.

15.12 Glaciers
Rivers and Seas of Ice
• Discuss the development of a valley carved by a glacier.

15.13 Groundwater
Water, Water Everywhere (Almost)
• Define groundwater, saturated zone, water table, spring, and aquifer.

15.14 Sedimentation
What Becomes of the Debris of Erosion
• Discuss the deposition of stream and glacier sediments.
• Describe the processes by which sediments become rock.

Vulcanism

15.15 Volcanoes
Rivers of Lava, Clouds of Gas and Dust
• Describe the events that occur in a typical volcanic eruption.
• Identify the parts of the world where most volcanoes occur.

15.16 Intrusive Rocks
They Have Hardened Underground from Magma
• Describe the different kinds of intrusive bodies of igneous rock.

15.17 The Rock Cycle
Rocks Are Not Necessarily Forever
• Draw the rock cycle.

Soil, vegetation, and rock fragments form a thin surface layer on most land areas, but solid rock is always underneath. Rock underlies the sediments on the ocean floors as well. The deepest oil wells, which go down over 8 km, are drilled through rock similar to that at the surface. Some of the rock now out in the open was once buried several km inside the earth, and the material that makes up some volcanic rock probably rose in molten form from still greater depths, perhaps as much as 100 km down. These samples of rock from well below the earth's surface also turn out to be very much like rock that formed close to the surface.

Such direct observation tells us that the outer part of the earth, called its **crust,** is composed almost entirely of rock. However, the thickness of the crust is only 0.5 percent of the earth's 6400-km radius. There is no firsthand information about the rest of our planet, but its interior can be probed by indirect methods. After we have learned something about the structure of our planet and about the rocks that clothe it, we shall turn to the processes whose action has produced the landscapes around us.

Rocks

15.1 Composition of the Crust

Oxygen and Silicon Are the Most Abundant Elements

The average composition of the earth's crust is shown in Fig. 15-1. Only a few elements are abundant in the crust, while others are present in quite small amounts. Oxygen makes up nearly half the mass of the crust, most of it combined with silicon. Silicon and the two metals iron and aluminum account for three-fourths of the rest of the crust's mass. Lumped together in the 1.4 percent of "all others" are the carbon, hydrogen, and nitrogen present in all living things and such familiar metals as copper, lead, and silver.

Silicon never occurs by itself on the earth, but its compounds make up about 87 percent of the rock and soil of the earth's crust. In the chemistry of the earth, silicon has the same sort of central role that carbon has in the chemistry of living things.

Nearly all the earth's silicon is combined either with oxygen in silicon dioxide (SiO_2), sometimes called **silica,** or with oxygen and one or more metals in the **silicates.** The differences in composition and structures of the silicates are reflected in a variety of colors, hardnesses, and crystal forms. The softness of talc and the hardness of zircon and beryl, the transparency of

Figure 15-1 Average chemical composition of the earth's crust. Percentages are by mass. The total is not 100 percent because of rounding.

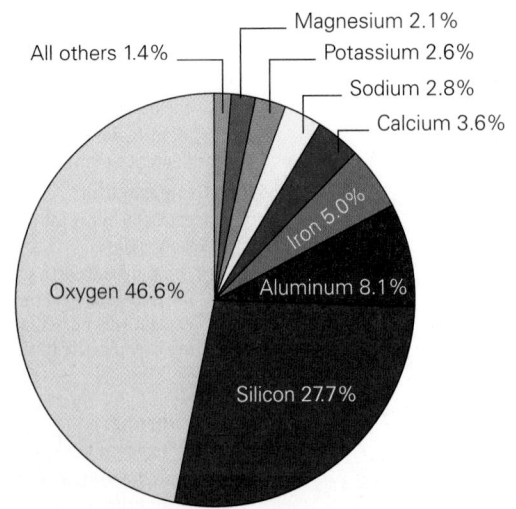

topaz and the deep color of garnet, the platy crystals of mica and the fibrous crystals of asbestos give some idea of the range of silicate properties. Glass consists largely of silicates.

Silicate Structures   The basic structural unit of all silicates is the SiO_4^{4-} tetrahedron (a pyramid with a triangular base) shown in Fig. 15-2. In some silicates these units occur as single ions linked by positive metal ions. In more complex silicates the units form continuous chains, as in asbestos, or sheets, as in mica, with metal ions lying between them. Three-dimensional networks of SiO_4^{4-} units also occur. The number and variety of silicate minerals are due to the many different ways in which the basic SiO_4^{4-} unit can combine with metal ions to form stable crystal structures.

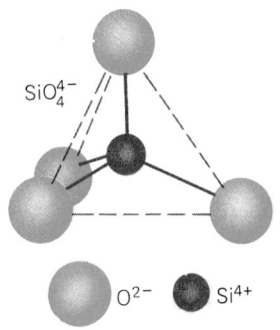

Figure 15-2   The silicon-oxygen tetrahedron is the fundamental unit in all silicate structures. Dashed lines show the tetrahedral form of SiO_4^{4-}; solid lines are bonds between the ions.

15.2   Minerals

What Rocks Are Made Of

Most rocks are heterogeneous solids. The different homogeneous materials, called **minerals,** in a coarse-grained rock like granite are obvious to the eye.

Asbestos

Asbestos is the name given to a group of fibrous minerals whose silicon-oxygen units are arranged in long chains. Because of its fibrous nature, mechanical strength, inertness, and resistance to fire, asbestos was once widely employed as reinforcement for building materials, as insulation in walls and around steam pipes, for fireproof theater curtains, in filters, in brake linings, and so on. The peak year for asbestos was 1973, when almost a million tons were used in the United States alone.

Unfortunately, asbestos fibers can cause serious lung and intestinal diseases such as cancer. For many years after their discovery nearly a century ago, the dangers of asbestos were ignored by both industry and government, sometimes even deliberately hidden by them. Hundreds of thousands of people around the world have died prematurely or will do so as a result of ingesting asbestos fibers at work or in their daily lives. One asbestos-related disease, mesothelioma, may take up to 50 years to show up after an exposure, after which it is usually fatal within 2 years. The eventual bill for compensation will total over $100 billion.

When the perils of asbestos finally became widely known, its use became severely restricted and asbestos already in buildings such as schools was removed. There are two types of asbestos: the amphiboles, whose stiff, hard fibers are mainly responsible for the maladies associated with asbestos, and chrysotile, whose softer fibers are less likely to cause illness (Fig. 15-3).

Chrysotile is still widely used in construction in a number of countries, notably Russia, China, and Brazil, and to a certain extent in the United States in certain applications where there is no adequate substitute. It is banned as a health hazard in the European Union and elsewhere.

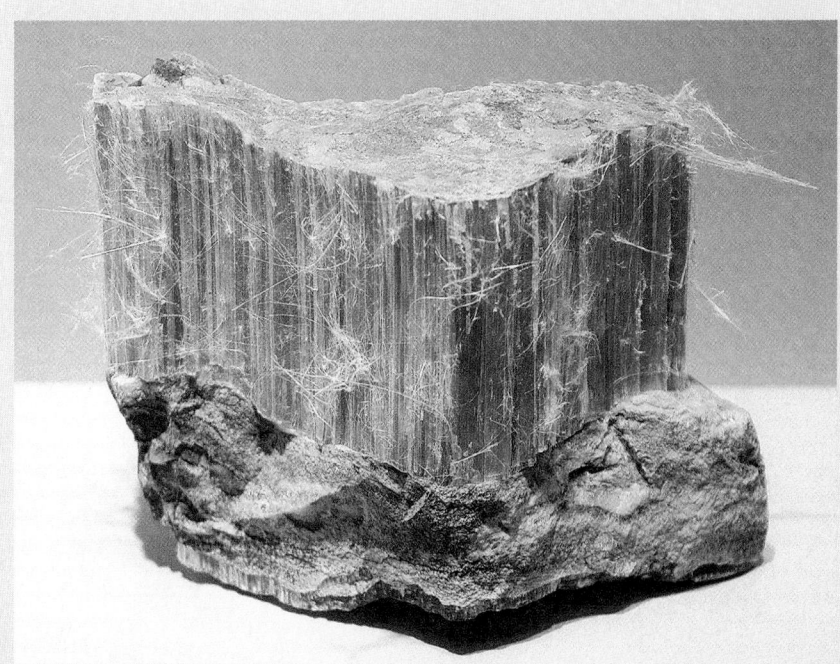

Figure 15-3   Chrysotile asbestos.

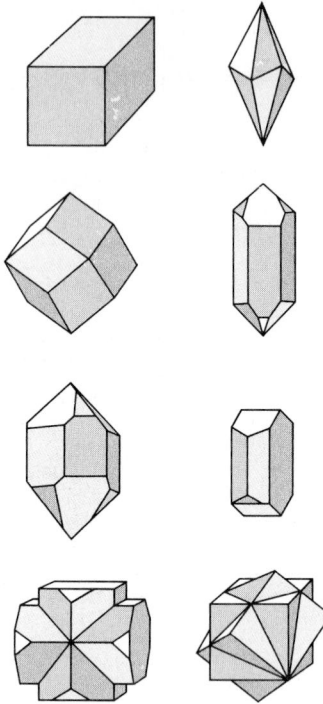

Figure 15-4   Some crystal forms found in minerals.

For a fine-grained rock, a microscope may be needed to distinguish the minerals that compose it.

A mineral is a crystalline inorganic solid found in nature that has a fairly specific chemical composition. Minerals are not usually identified by chemical names for two reasons. First, the same compound may occur in different forms: for instance, the minerals calcite and aragonite are both largely calcium carbonate ($CaCO_3$), but they differ in crystal form, hardness, density, and so on. Second, most minerals vary somewhat in composition from sample to sample, whereas the compositions of chemical compounds are invariable. About 4000 minerals are known, but the great majority are rare. The number of minerals important in ordinary rocks is so small that knowing something about only half a dozen minerals or mineral groups is enough for an introduction to geology.

Crystal Form and Cleavage   In describing minerals, two important properties are **crystal form** and **cleavage.** Minerals are crystalline solids, which means that their atoms are arranged in lattice structures with definite geometric patterns. When a mineral hardens in a location where its crystals can grow freely, as in a cavity, perfect crystals are formed with smooth faces that meet each other at sharp angles. Each mineral has crystals of a distinctive shape, so that well-formed crystals make it easy to recognize a mineral (Fig. 15-4). Unfortunately good mineral crystals are rare, since neighboring crystals usually interfere with one another's growth.

When well-developed crystals are not present, the characteristic crystal structure of a mineral may still reveal itself in the property called cleavage. This is the tendency of a substance to split along certain planes, which are determined by the arrangement of atoms in its lattice. When a mineral sample is struck with a hammer, its cleavage planes are revealed as the preferred directions in which it breaks.

Even in its original state, a mineral may show cleavage by flat, parallel faces and minute parallel cracks. The flat surfaces of mica flakes, for instance, and the ability of mica to be peeled apart in thin sheets show that this mineral has almost perfect cleavage in one direction (Fig. 15-5). Some minerals (for example, quartz) have no cleavage at all. When struck they shatter, like glass, along random curved surfaces.

Example 15.1

Opals are used in jewelry because of the beautiful play of colors that some specimens exhibit. An opal consists of SiO_2 and H_2O in various proportions linked together in microscopic crystals that form an amorphous material. Would you expect opals to exhibit cleavage?

Solution
Because an opal is amorphous, it has no regular structure and therefore cannot exhibit cleavage.

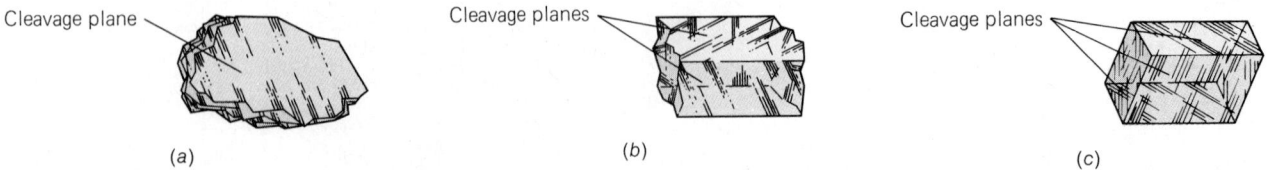

Cleavage plane

(a)

Cleavage planes

(b)

Cleavage planes

(c)

Figure 15-5   (*a*) Mica has one direction of cleavage and fractures irregularly if broken across its cleavage plane. (*b*) Feldspar has two perpendicular cleavage planes and fractures irregularly if broken across them. (*c*) Calcite has three directions of cleavage that are not perpendicular to each other.

Six Common Minerals   Here are details of six common minerals and mineral groups.

Quartz   Well-formed quartz (SiO_2) crystals are six-sided prisms and pyramids that show no cleavage (Fig. 15-6). They are colorless or milky (often gray, pink, or violet because of impurities), have a glassy luster, and are hard enough to scratch glass. They occur in many kinds of rock, sometimes appear as long, narrow deposits called **veins,** and often form assemblies of crystals inside cavities. Clear quartz (rock crystal) is used in jewelry and in optical instruments. Smoky quartz, rose quartz, and amethyst are colored varieties used in jewelry. Quartz sand is the chief raw material for making glass.

Feldspar   This is the name of a group of minerals with very similar properties. The two classes of feldspar are a silicate of K and Al called orthoclase and a series of silicates of Na, Ca, and Al collectively called plagioclase. The crystals are rectangular, with blunt ends; they show good cleavage in two directions approximately at right angles (Fig. 15-7). They are sometimes clear; if not, their color is white or light shades of gray and pink. Feldspar is slightly harder than glass but not as hard as quartz. It is the most abundant single constituent of rocks, making up about 60 percent of the total weight of the earth's crust. Pure feldspar is used in the making of porcelain and as a mild abrasive.

Mica   The two chief varieties of this familiar mineral are white mica—a silicate of H, K, and Al—and black mica—a silicate of H, K, Al, Mg, and Fe. Mica is easily recognized by its perfect and conspicuous cleavage in one plane (Fig. 15-8). It is a very soft mineral, only a trifle harder than a fingernail. Large sheets of white mica free from impurities are used as insulators in electrical equipment.

Ferromagnesian Minerals   This name refers to a large group of minerals with varied properties. All of them are silicates of iron and magnesium, and most of them contain other metallic elements as well (for instance, calcium). Black mica belongs to this group; its composition includes H, K, and Al in addition to Fe and Mg. Nearly all ferromagnesian minerals are dark green to black (Fig. 15-9), but apart from composition and color the members of this group differ greatly from one another. The most abundant dark-colored constituents of common rocks belong to this group.

Clay Minerals   This is a group of closely related minerals that are the chief constituents of clay. All are silicates of aluminum, some with a little Mg, Fe, and K. They consist of microscopic crystals, white or light-colored when pure, often discolored with iron compounds. They have a dull luster and are very soft, forming a smooth powder when rubbed between the fingers. Clay minerals have a low density and absorb water readily. They are distinguished from chalk by softness. Kaolin, one of the clay minerals, is an important ingredient in the manufacture of ceramics, paper, paint, and certain plastics (Fig. 15-10).

Calcite   Calcite (calcium carbonate, $CaCO_3$) crystals are hexagonal, somewhat like those of quartz (Fig. 15-11). Unlike quartz they show perfect cleavage in three directions at angles of about 75°, so that fragments of calcite have a characteristic rhombic shape in which opposite sides are parallel. They are colorless or light in color, with a glassy luster. They are hard enough to scratch mica or a fingernail, but can be scratched by glass or by a knife blade. Like quartz, calcite is a common mineral of veins and crystal aggregates in cavities. It is the chief constituent of the common rocks limestone and marble and commercially serves as a source of lime for glass, mortar, and cement. Eggshells are mainly calcite, incidentally.

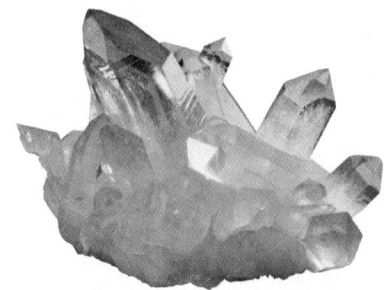

Figure 15-6   Quartz consists of silicon dioxide crystals and is found in many kinds of rock.

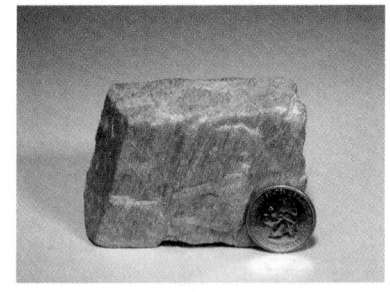

Figure 15-7   Feldspar is the most abundant mineral in the earth's crust. Shown is a sample of orthoclase feldspar. The salmon-pink color is characteristic of this mineral.

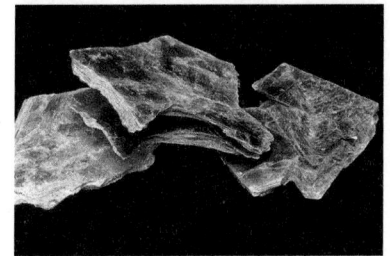

Figure 15-8   The micas are aluminum silicates having a sheet-type cleavage. As fine flakes, mica is the shiny mineral in some metamorphic rocks. Shown is white mica.

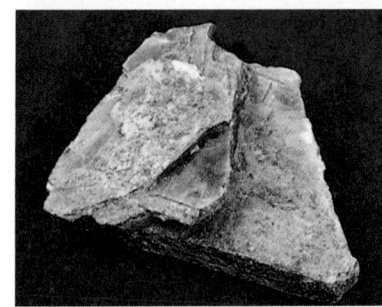

Figure 15-9   Olivine is an olive-green ferromagnesian mineral (a magnesium-iron silicate) that occurs mainly in igneous rocks.

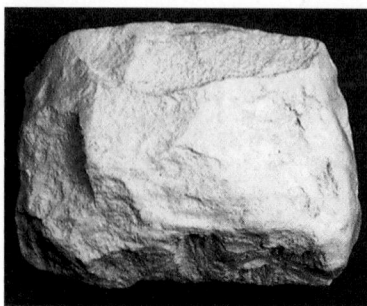

Figure 15-10   Water molecules fit readily into the layered structures of clay minerals such as kaolin, shown here. When baked, wet clay loses its water content and becomes hard due to the formation of silicates that bind together the clay particles. The transformation of clay from a soft, easily shaped material into a rigid one is the basis of such ceramic products as bricks, pottery, and porcelain.

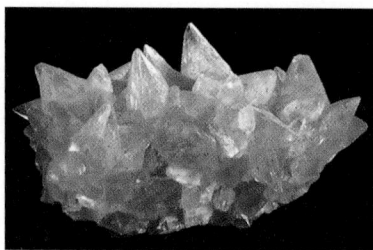

Figure 15-11   Calcite, the chief constituent of limestone and marble, consists of calcium carbonate crystals.

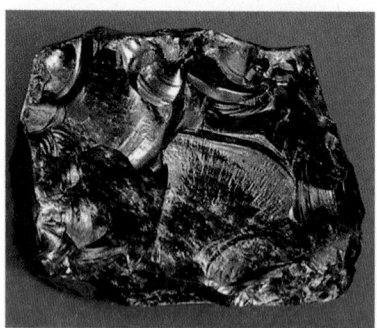

Figure 15-12   Obsidian is a glassy rock of volcanic origin.

15.3   Igneous Rocks

Once Molten, Now Solid

There seems no limit to the variety of rocks on the earth's surface. We find coarse-grained rocks and fine-grained rocks, light rocks and heavy rocks, soft rocks and hard rocks, rocks of all sizes, shapes, and colors. But if we look closely, we will find order in this diversity, and a straightforward scheme for classifying rocks according to their origin has been developed.

1. **Igneous rocks** are rocks that have cooled from a molten state. The formation of some igneous rocks can actually be observed when molten lava cools on the side of a volcano. For others an igneous origin inside the earth is inferred from their composition and structure. Two-thirds of crustal rocks are igneous.
2. **Sedimentary rocks** consist of materials derived from other rocks and deposited by water, wind, or glacial ice. Some consist of separate rock fragments cemented together; others contain material precipitated from solution in water. Although sedimentary rocks make up only about 8 percent of the crust, three-quarters of surface rocks are of this kind.
3. **Metamorphic rocks** are igneous or sedimentary rocks that have been changed, or metamorphosed, by heat and pressure deep under the earth's surface. The changes may involve the formation of new minerals or simply the recrystallization of minerals already present.

Properties of Igneous Rocks   The minerals in igneous rocks usually appear in the form of irregular grains that consist of interlocking crystals. This is to be expected when crystals grow together and interfere with one another's development. The principal minerals of these rocks contain silicon: quartz, feldspar, mica, and the ferromagnesians.

The siliceous liquids from which igneous rocks form are thick and viscous, much like molten glass. Sometimes, in fact, molten lava has the right composition and cools rapidly enough for crystals to have no time to develop. The result is a natural glass—the black, shiny rock called **obsidian** (Fig. 15-12).

More often cooling is slow enough to allow mineral crystals to form. If cooling is fairly rapid and if the molten material is highly viscous, the resulting rock may consist of tiny crystals or partly of crystals and partly of glass (Fig. 15-13). If cooling is very slow, mineral crystals grow large and a coarse-grained rock is formed (Fig. 15-14). Table 15-1 lists some common igneous rocks according to composition and grain size.

Grain size usually tells us not only the rate of cooling but also the environment in which a rock was cooled. Sufficiently fast cooling to give fine-grained rocks is common when molten lava reaches the earth's surface from a volcano and spreads out in a thin flow. Coarse-grained rocks, on the other hand, have cooled slowly, which must have occurred well beneath the surface. Such rocks are now exposed only because erosion has carried away the material that once covered them.

15.4   Sedimentary Rocks

Compacted Sediments or Precipitates from Solution

Sediments laid down by wind, water, or ice can become rock through the pressure of overlying deposits and by the gradual cementing of their grains with material deposited from underground water. The resulting rocks usually have distinct, somewhat rounded grains that have not grown together like the crystals of igneous rocks. A few sedimentary rocks, however, consist of intergrowing mineral grains that precipitated from solution in water.

Since sediments are normally deposited in layers, most sedimentary rocks have a banded appearance owing to slight differences in color or grain size from one layer to the next. Sedimentary rocks may often be recognized at a glance by the presence of fossils—remains of plants or animals buried with the sediments as they were laid down.

Types of Sedimentary Rocks   Sedimentary rocks may be divided into two groups according to the nature of the original sediments, as in Table 15-2. The three **fragmental rocks** are distinguished by their grain size. **Conglomerate** is cemented gravel whose fragments may have any composition and any size, from pebbles to boulders (Fig. 15-15). Conglomerate becomes **sandstone** as fragment size decreases. Sand grains may consist of many different minerals, but quartz is generally the most abundant. The

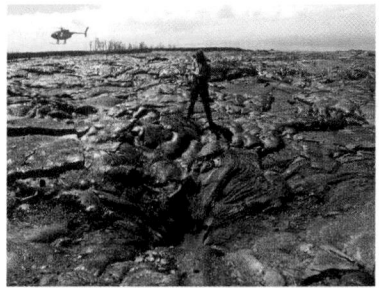

Figure 15-13   Basalt is a dark, fine-grained rock that emerged molten from the earth's interior. The ocean floors, under a thin sedimentary layer, consist of basalt, as do the volcanic islands of Hawaii and Iceland. Shown is pahoehoe basalt whose smooth, ropy surface resulted from the rapid cooling of a very fluid lava that came out of the opening in the foreground.

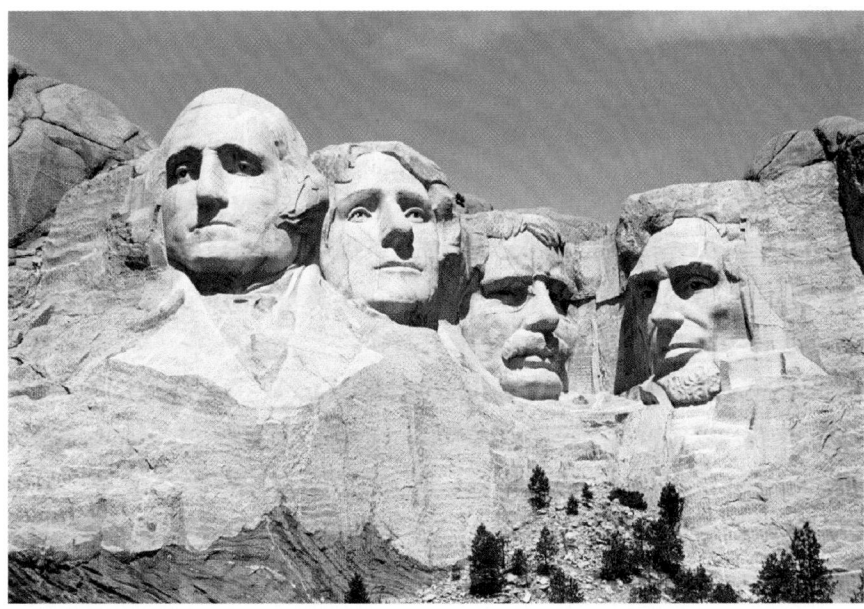

Figure 15-14   The faces of four American presidents (Washington, Jefferson, Theodore Roosevelt, and Lincoln) are carved in the granite of Mt. Rushmore, South Dakota. Granite is a coarse-grained igneous rock, generally light in color, in which quartz and feldspar are abundant. The faces of the feldspar crystals glisten, which gives granite an attractive appearance. Granite and similar rocks underlie the continents.

Table 15-1	Some Igneous Rocks	
Mineral Composition	**Coarse-Grained Rocks**	**Fine-Grained Rocks**
Quartz Feldspar Ferromagnesian minerals	Granite	Rhyolite
No quartz Feldspar predominant Ferromagnesian minerals	Diorite	Andesite
No quartz Feldspar Ferromagnesian minerals predominant	Gabbro	Basalt

Table 15-2	**Some Sedimentary Rocks**	
Group	**Type**	**Constituents**
Fragmental rocks	Conglomerate	Rock fragments
	Sandstone	Quartz usually most abundant
	Shale	Clay minerals
Chemical and biochemical precipitates	Chert	Microcrystalline quartz
	Limestone	Calcite

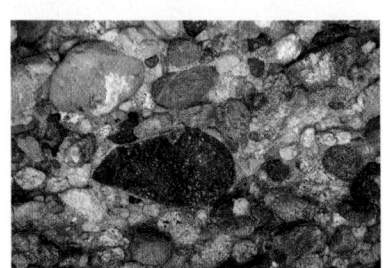

Figure 15-15   This conglomerate incorporates rounded volcanic and granitic rock fragments.

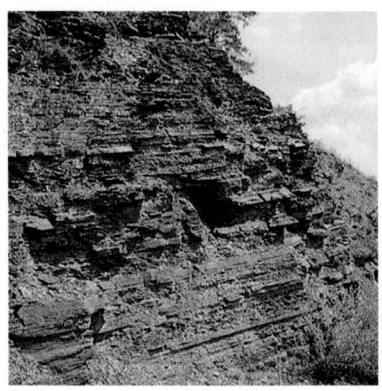

Figure 15-16   Shale is a soft sedimentary rock that has consolidated from mud deposits. These shale layers in the Hudson River Valley of New York were formed over 400 million years ago.

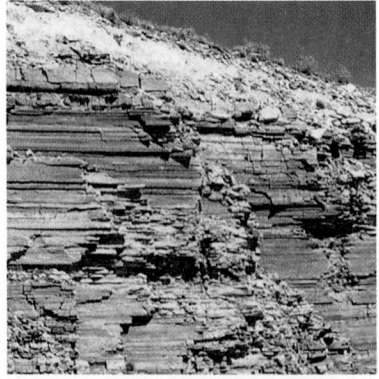

Figure 15-17   Limestone deposit in western Texas. Some limestones originate as precipitates from solution; others have consolidated from the shells of marine organisms.

hardness of sandstone and conglomerate depends largely on how well their grains are cemented together. Some varieties crumble easily. Others, especially those with silica as the cementing material, are among the toughest of rocks. **Shale** is consolidated mud or silt; it is a soft rock usually composed of thin layers (Fig. 15-16).

Limestone is a fine-grained rock that consists chiefly of calcite. It may be formed either as a chemical precipitate or by the consolidation of shell fragments (Fig. 15-17). Small amounts of impurities may give limestone almost any color. **Chalk** is a loosely consolidated variety of limestone, often made up mainly of the shells of tiny one-celled animals.

Many Native American arrowheads are made of either the igneous rock obsidian or the sedimentary rock **chert** (microcrystalline quartz). Both rocks are hard and have sharp edges when broken. Two familiar varieties of chert are **flint** (Fig. 15-18) and **jasper.** Fragments of chert show the same sharp edges and smooth, concave surfaces as broken quartz or obsidian, but the surfaces have a characteristic waxy luster. Chert may have almost any color; often a single specimen shows bands and pockets of several different colors. Not nearly as abundant as the other sedimentary rocks just described, chert is nevertheless common in pebble beds and gravel deposits because its hardness and resistance to chemical decay enable it to survive rough treatment from streams, waves, and glaciers.

15.5   Metamorphic Rocks

Formed from Other Rocks by Heat and/or Pressure

The enormous pressures and high temperatures below the earth's surface can profoundly change sedimentary and igneous rocks that become deeply buried. Minerals stable at the surface are often unstable when crushed and baked and may react to form different substances. Other minerals keep their identities but their crystals increase in size. Hot liquids may add some new materials and dissolve out others. So many kinds of change are possible that no general rules can be set down to tell metamorphic rocks from others.

Many metamorphic rocks are characterized by a property called **foliation,** which refers to the arrangement of flat or elongated mineral grains in parallel layers. This effect is caused by extreme pressure in one direction, with the mineral grains growing out sideward as the rock is squeezed. Foliation gives a rock a banded or layered appearance, and when it is broken, the rock tends to split along the bands. Layering is also characteristic of sedimentary rocks, but in them the layering is caused by slight variations in color or grain size; layering in metamorphic rocks is due to the lining up of mineral grains.

Coral Reefs

A common feature of shallow waters in the tropics is limestone coral reefs (Fig. 15-19). These reefs are produced by tiny creatures called coral polyps, which extract calcium carbonate from seawater to form hard external skeletons. When the polyps die, their skeletons remain behind, with new polyps growing on top. Coral reefs harbor plants and animals of many kinds, a profusion of life comparable with that in a rain forest.

The Great Barrier Reef off Australia's east coast is a series of coral reefs that extends for about 2000 km; it is the only structure of biological origin visible from space. Bermuda, the Bahamas, and the Florida Keys are coral islands and the Pacific Ocean contains many atolls, which are rings or horseshoes of coral reefs that enclose lagoons. Numerous coral reefs have been severely damaged in recent years, mainly by the use of dynamite to kill fish near them, by pollution of various kinds from agriculture on nearby shores, and by rising water temperatures.

In all, coral reefs cover about a million square kilometers of the earth's surface. The fossil record shows that reefbuilding organisms first appeared 225 million years ago. Limestone deposits that were once coral reefs are found in Wisconsin, Illinois, Indiana, and Texas.

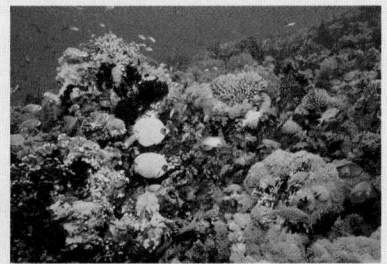

Figure 15-19   A coral reef in Egypt.

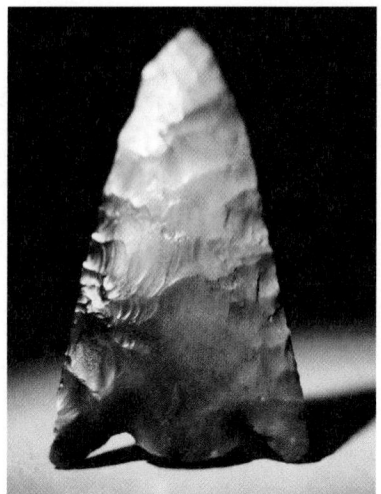

Figure 15-18   Flint, a type of chert, consists largely of microcrystalline quartz and hence is hard and durable. Many Native American arrowheads, like this one, were made from flint.

Table 15-3	Some Metamorphic Rocks		
Group	**Type**	**Constituents**	**Origin**
Foliated rocks	Slate	Mica and usually quartz, both in microscopic grains	Shale
	Schist	Mica and/or a ferromagnesian mineral, usually quartz also	Shale or fine-grained igneous rock
Foliated and banded rocks	Gneiss	Quartz, feldspar, mica	Various
Unfoliated rocks	Marble	Chiefly calcite	Limestone
	Quartzite	Chiefly quartz	Sandstone

Some Common Metamorphic Rocks   The more common metamorphic rocks may be classified according to the presence or absence of foliation, as in Table 15-3.

Slate is produced by the low-temperature metamorphism of the sedimentary rock shale, whose clay minerals form tiny flakes of mica. Although the individual flakes are too small to be seen, mica is responsible for the shiny surfaces seen whenever slate is split along its foliation (Fig. 15-20). Slate is harder than shale, finely foliated, and usually black or dark gray but sometimes light-colored.

Schist is formed from shale at higher temperatures than those that give slate, or from fine-grained igneous rocks. In it the mineral grains responsible for the foliation are large enough to be visible, giving the foliation surfaces a characteristic spangled appearance. Schist does not split as easily along the foliation as slate does, and its surfaces are rougher.

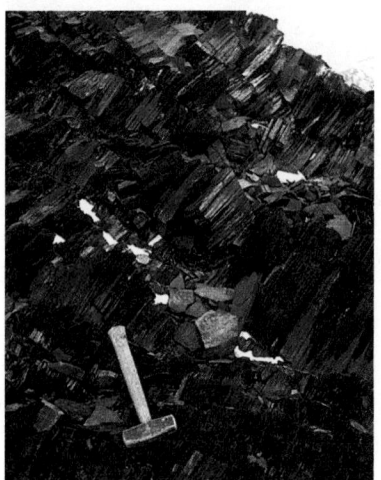

Figure 15-20   Slate results from the metamorphism of shale under pressure. This outcrop is in Antarctica.

Portland Cement

Portland cement, invented in 1824, is made by heating limestone and clay together in a rotating furnace at a high temperature until they partly melt. This produces various combinations of calcium, aluminum, and silicon oxides that are ground up together with additives that prevent the mixture from setting too quickly when water is added. The resulting Portland cement—so called because, when hard, it resembles a rock found near Portland, England—reacts with water to form a strong and durable adhesive that sets in a few hours and continues to harden over a period of weeks.

Most Portland cement is mixed with water, sand, and gravel to form concrete, an artificial rock that is the most widely used building material, often reinforced with embedded steel rods.

Every year 2 billion tons of Portland cement are used worldwide, an average of over a quarter of a ton per person. China is the largest consumer of cement, next is India, then the United States. Cement plants account for 5 percent of all CO_2 emissions. About a ton of CO_2 is given off in making a ton of cement, some from the burning of fossil fuels for the required heat but most from the chemical reactions involved. For this reason improved methods of heating, though helpful, are unable to counterbalance the growing use of cement. Fortunately, stronger types of cement and concrete are coming into use that permit smaller amounts for a given application, and processes are being explored that reduce CO_2 emissions during cement manufacture, in some cases considerably.

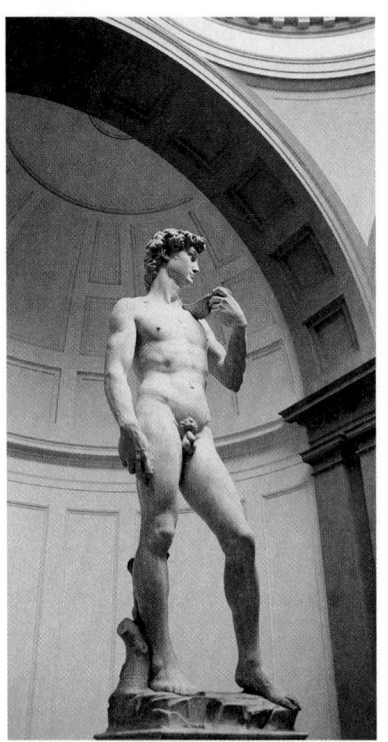

Figure 15-22   The metamorphic rock marble is often used for statues, such as this larger-than-life one of David by Michelangelo in Florence, Italy.

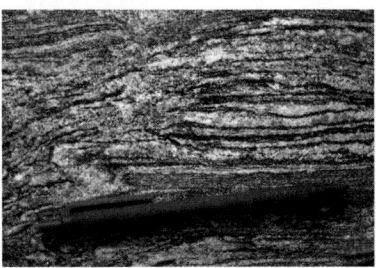

Figure 15-21   The metamorphic rock gneiss is foliated and has bands of different material.

Gneiss is a coarse-grained rock formed under conditions of high temperature and pressure from almost any other rock except pure limestone and pure quartz sandstone. Its composition naturally depends on the nature of the original rock, but quartz, feldspar, and mica are the commonest minerals. In appearance gneiss resembles granite, except for its banding and foliation (Fig. 15-21).

The metamorphism of pure limestone and of pure quartz sandstone are relatively simple processes. Since each consists of a single mineral of simple composition, heat and pressure can produce no new substances but instead cause the growth and interlocking of crystals of calcite and quartz. Thus limestone becomes **marble** (Fig. 15-22), a rock composed of calcite in crystals large enough to be easily visible, and sandstone becomes the hard rock **quartzite.** Quartzite sometimes looks like sandstone, but its grains are so firmly intergrown that it splits across separate grains when broken to give smooth fracture surfaces in contrast to the rough surfaces of sandstone.

Within the Earth

The earth's solid crust together with the atmosphere and oceans above is directly accessible to our instruments, and we may legitimately hope one day to understand their structures and behavior in detail. The interior of the earth, however, is beyond our direct reach. What we need to study it is some kind of indirect probe, and the waves sent out by earthquakes have turned out to be ideal for this purpose. Largely through the analysis of earthquake waves we now know a great deal about the earth's interior, which is hardly less remote than the most distant star, and we are continually learning more.

15.6 Earthquakes

When Our Planet Trembles

An **earthquake** consists of rapid vibrations of rock near the earth's surface. A single shock usually lasts no more than a few seconds, though severe quakes may last for as much as 3 min. Even in such brief times the damage done may be immense. Widespread fires often follow earthquakes in inhabited regions with broken water mains hindering their control, and landslides are common. Usually the first shock is the most severe, with weaker and weaker disturbances following from time to time for days or months afterward. Some aftershocks are severe: 18 of them with magnitudes of over 6.0 followed a 7.1-magnitude earthquake in western China in 2010. A major earthquake may be felt over many thousands of square kilometers, but its destructiveness is limited to a much smaller area.

The Richter Scale

Earthquake magnitudes are often expressed on the **Richter scale.** Each step of 1 on this scale represents an increase in vibration amplitude of a factor of 10 and an increase in energy release of a factor of about 30. Thus an earthquake of magnitude 5 produces vibrations 10 times larger than a quake of magnitude 4 and releases 30 times more energy.

An earthquake of magnitude 0 is barely detectable; if the energy given off by such an earthquake could be concentrated, it would be just about enough to blow up a tree stump. An earthquake of magnitude 3 would be felt by people living near the location of the quake, and some damage to structures would occur when the magnitude is 4 or 5. Significant destruction is likely if the magnitude is 6 or more.

The energy given off in a magnitude 9.5 earthquake, the strongest observed in the past century—it occurred off the Chilean coast (Fig. 15-23) and left 2 million people homeless—is perhaps 20 times the energy content of the world's yearly production of coal and oil. The Indonesian earthquake of 2004 that caused the tsunami described in Sec. 14.12 was nearly this severe; it moved every spot on the earth's surface by at least a centimeter, although so slowly far from the quake itself that the motion could not be felt. A magnitude 8 earthquake occurs somewhere an average of once a year, a magnitude 9 earthquake once every 30 or 40 years.

The 8.8-magnitude Chilean earthquake of 2010 is especially significant because, following previous major quakes, the country put in force strict construction codes to minimize the consequences of such events. However, in 2010 these codes did not prevent extensive damage to many buildings in the affected region, including their collapse. Because construction codes on the U.S. west coast are not as rigorous as those in Chile, future severe quakes there, in the Pacific Northwest as well as in California, may well be even more destructive.

Figure 15-23 Some major earthquakes and their magnitudes on the Richter scale. The San Francisco and Tokyo earthquakes, together with the fires that followed them, led to the almost complete destruction of those cities.

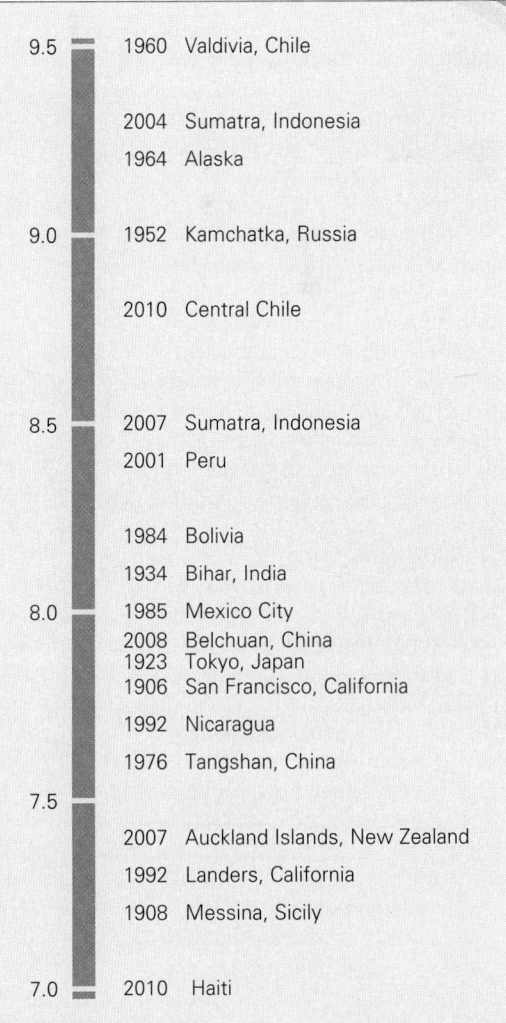

9.5	1960 Valdivia, Chile
	2004 Sumatra, Indonesia
	1964 Alaska
9.0	1952 Kamchatka, Russia
	2010 Central Chile
8.5	2007 Sumatra, Indonesia
	2001 Peru
	1984 Bolivia
	1934 Bihar, India
8.0	1985 Mexico City
	2008 Belchuan, China
	1923 Tokyo, Japan
	1906 San Francisco, California
	1992 Nicaragua
	1976 Tangshan, China
7.5	
	2007 Auckland Islands, New Zealand
	1992 Landers, California
	1908 Messina, Sicily
7.0	2010 Haiti

Figure 15-24 Highway affected by the earthquake that shook Loma Prieta, California, and its vicinity in 1989. Horizontal vibrations of the ground are usually responsible for most of the damage an earthquake causes.

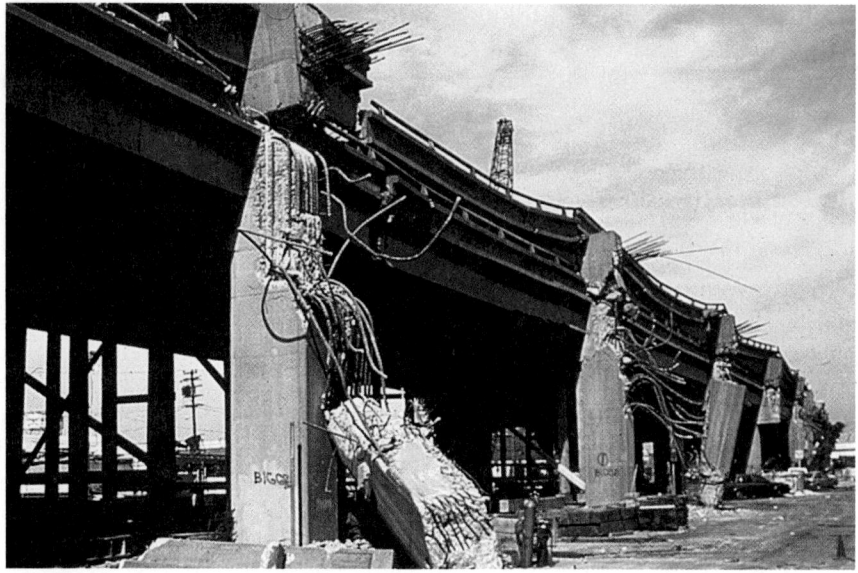

Earthquakes and Clean Energy

The pursuit of clean energy has had the unfortunate side effect of setting off several earthquakes. By far the largest was the 7.9-magnitude tremor that shook Belchuan, China, in 2008 and left 87,000 people dead or missing. Four years earlier, the huge new Zipingpu dam, located near a major fault that passed close to the town, had been filled with 320 million tons of water. U.S. and Chinese seismologists have evidence that the pressure of the water disturbed the fault and thereby triggered the earthquake. In fact, local geologists had warned of the possibility when the dam was being planned.

Smaller earthquakes have occurred as the result of injecting water into hot underground rock formations to bring geothermal energy to the surface (Sec. 4.9). A related source of concern is the proposed large-scale pumping of CO_2 emitted by fossil-fuel power plants into underground reservoirs (Sec. 4.7) to keep it from the atmosphere where it would promote global warming. Might this procedure also be enough to trigger earthquakes in sensitive regions?

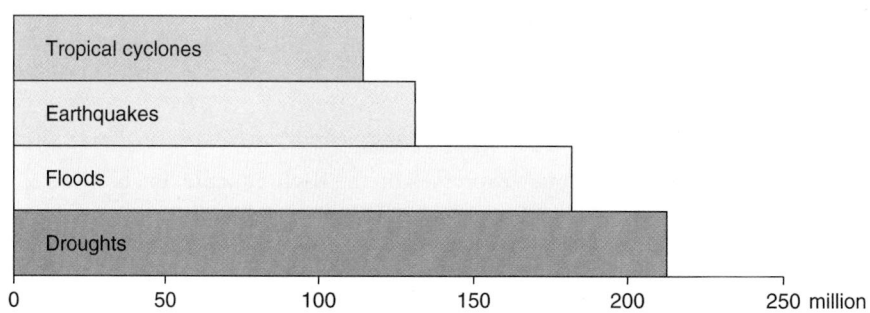

Figure 15-25 The average number of people affected by the 700 or so major natural disasters that occur each year.

Of the million or so earthquakes per year strong enough to be noticed, only a few liberate enough energy to do serious damage (Fig. 15-24). About 15 really violent earthquakes occur each year on the average. When one of them happens to involve a densely populated urban area, the effects can be appalling: more than 250,000 people (possibly many more) died in the 1976 earthquake in Tangshan, China, as buildings collapsed around them (Fig. 15-25).

The great majority of earthquakes are caused by the sudden movement of large blocks of the earth's crust less than 70 km from the surface along fracture lines called **faults.** When the stresses that develop in the crust in a certain region become too great for the rock there to support, one side of a fault slips past the other side (Fig. 15-26). This movement causes vibrations that send out waves that may travel for long distances from their origin.

Most earthquakes are over in a few seconds, but some last longer. For instance, the earthquake that caused the giant tsunami of 2004 continued for almost 10 minutes as the sides of a fault under the seabed off the Indonesian island of Sumatra shifted by 15 m over a distance of hundreds of kilometers.

Where Earthquakes Occur Regions in which severe earthquakes are comparatively frequent include the mountain chains that fringe the Pacific and a broad belt that extends from the Mediterranean basin across southern Asia

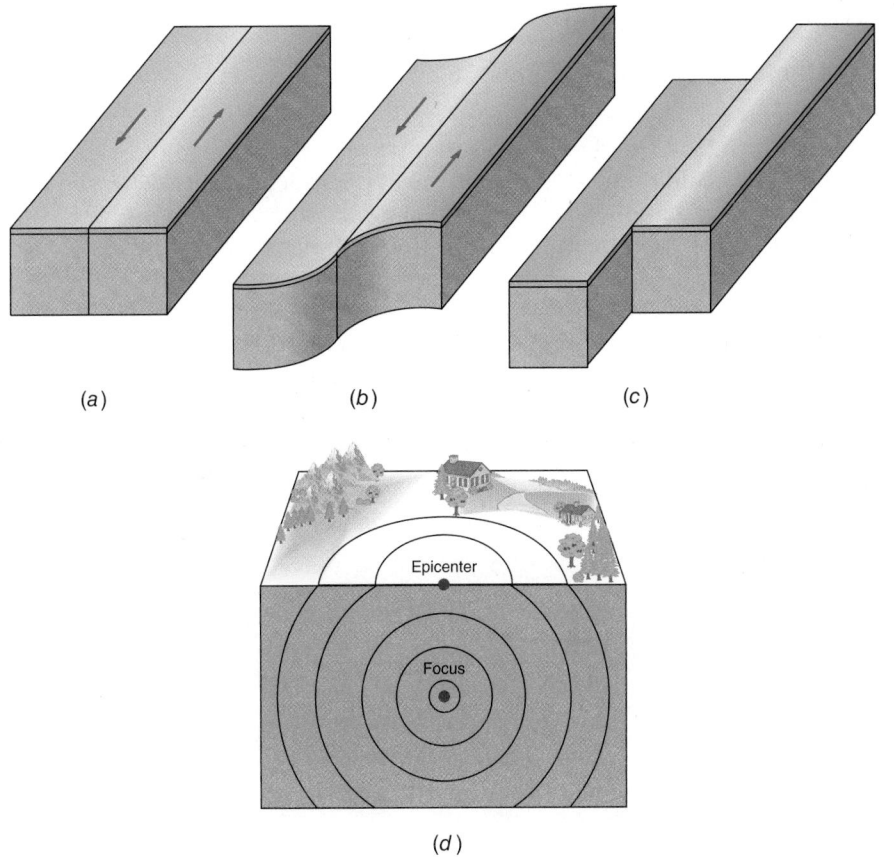

Figure 15-26 How an earthquake occurs. (*a*) The sides of a fault between crustal blocks have stuck together, preventing movement even though the forces (arrows) on them remain active. (*b*) As time goes on, stresses build up in the adjacent blocks, which deform as a result. (*c*) When the locked-in stresses become too great, the blocks suddenly shift to release them. The stored-up elastic energy powers the vibrations that constitute an earthquake. (*d*) The **focus** of an earthquake is the place where the crustal blocks moved; the **epicenter** of the quake is the point on the surface directly over the focus. Most earthquakes have foci less than 100 km below the surface.

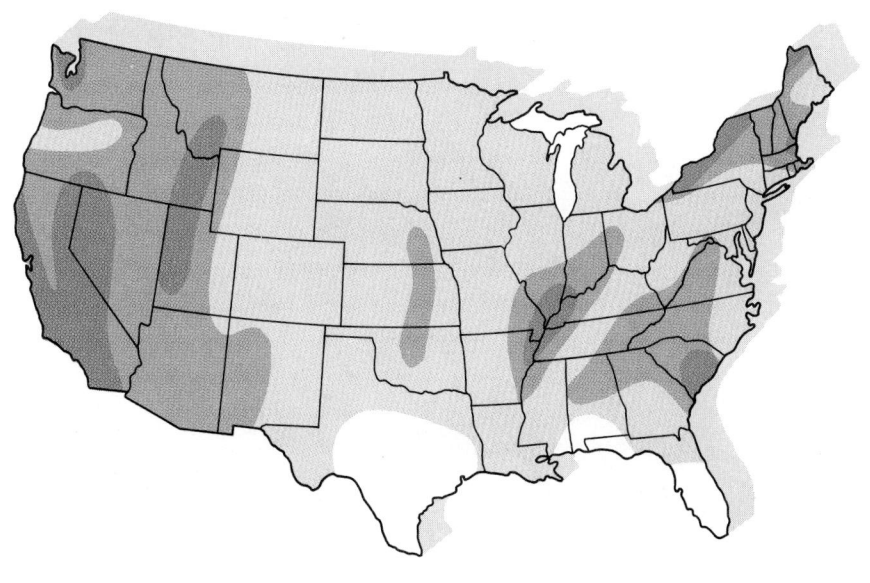

Figure 15-27 Earthquakes are expected during the next 100 years in the parts of the United States shown in color. The darker the color, the greater the likely damage. The earthquake probability is especially high in California because locked-in stresses have built up in many of the thousands of faults that riddle the region. The most severe earthquakes in U.S. history were a trio that occurred in the winter of 1811–1812 at New Madrid in southeastern Missouri, which is in the dark spot south of the Great Lakes in this map. The quakes were felt over most of the country east of the Rockies; the vibrations set church bells ringing as far away as Boston. The map does not show Hawaii or Alaska. In fact, the most earthquake-prone state is Alaska, which experiences a quake of magnitude 7 or so in most years.

to China (see Fig. 15-57). Major earthquakes have occurred now and then elsewhere, but most have been concentrated in these zones. In or near the earthquake belts lie most of the world's active volcanoes— which, as we shall see in Chap. 16, is no coincidence. Figure 15-27 is a map prepared by the U.S. Coast and Geodetic Survey that shows where earthquakes may be expected in the United States in the next 100 years.

Although the regions where earthquakes are likely to occur are fairly well known, their timing is another matter. Earthquakes give no obvious warning other than weak foreshocks that occasionally warn of larger quakes to come. Various subtle effects were at one time or another claimed to precede earthquakes, but none has proved a reliable predictor. For example, various animals, such as dogs, snakes, and cockroaches, have been reported to sometimes behave strangely before earthquakes, but nobody knows exactly what they may be responding to.

Despite intensive monitoring, the severe earthquakes that rocked California in 1989 and 1993 came as surprises. Possibly earthquakes are inherently unpredictable: once crustal stresses have built up somewhere, the situation may be so unstable that even a fairly minor event of some kind may be enough to initiate a quake without giving an unambiguous advance signal.

15.7   Structure of the Earth

Core, Mantle, and Crust

When an earthquake occurs at a fault in the crust, the rocks on both sides of the fault vibrate and send out waves that travel both through the earth's interior—"body waves"—and along its surface—"surface waves." The two kinds of body waves and the two kinds of surface waves are shown in Fig. 15-28.

An easy way to remember the difference between P and S waves is to think of P waves as "push-pull" vibrations and of S waves as "shakes." P waves are the fastest and so arrive first at a distant point when an earthquake occurs somewhere (Fig. 15-29). The S waves, which are slower, come next.

The surface waves, which have to travel along the ground rather than the shorter distance through the earth, appear last. However, the surface waves

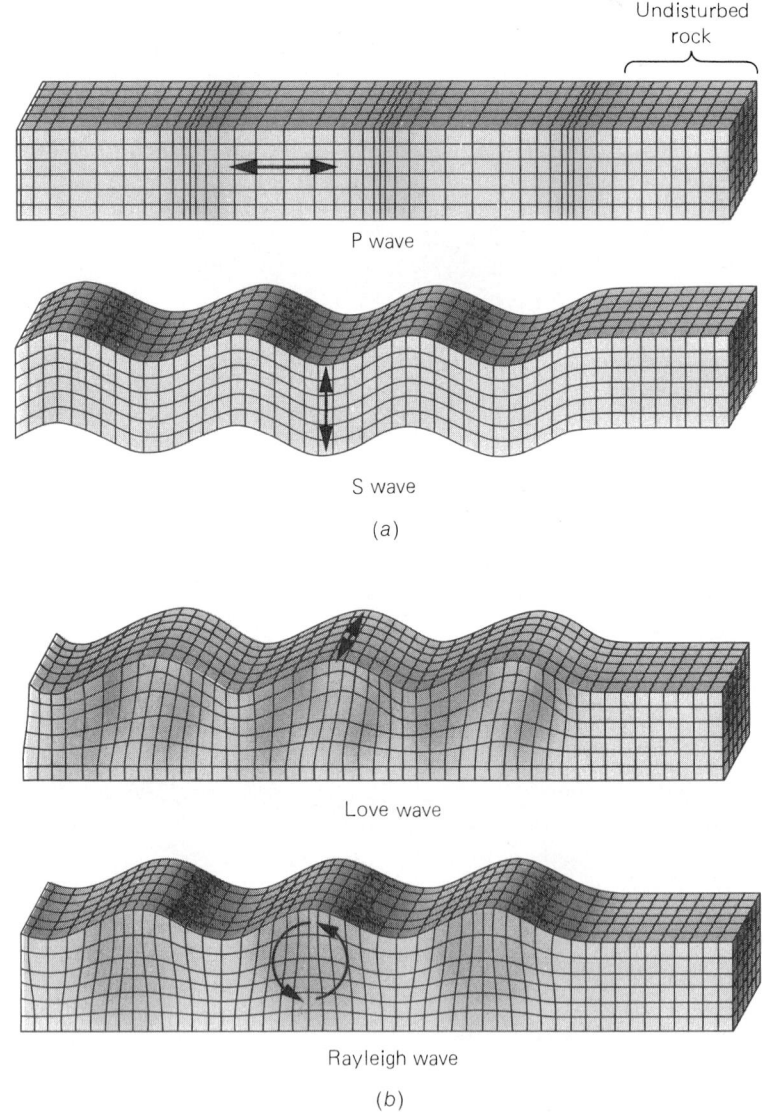

Figure 15-28   (*a*) Earthquake body waves travel through the earth's interior. P waves are longitudinal, like sound waves. S waves are transverse, like waves in a stretched string. P waves can move through a liquid; S waves cannot. (*b*) Earthquake surface waves travel on the earth's surface. Love waves are transverse, with their vibrations parallel to the surface. Rayleigh waves involve rotary motions, like the water waves of Fig. 7-2. All the waves shown here are moving from left to right. The arrows show the directions in which the rock particles move. (Love waves are named after the English mathematician Augustus Love and Rayleigh waves after the English physicist Lord Rayleigh.)

may produce the strongest vibrations, particularly when the distance is no more than a few thousand kilometers. The Love surface waves, which involve horizontal motions, are responsible for most earthquake damage to buildings and other structures. The Rayleigh waves, which resemble water waves, are the slowest of all.

Wave Speeds Change with Depth The internal structure of the earth was discovered with the help of P and S earthquake waves. These waves do not travel in straight lines inside the earth (except directly downward toward the earth's center) because of refraction. As we learned in Chap. 7, refraction refers to the change in direction of a wave when its speed changes. The speeds of P and S waves change with depth in the earth in two ways, which have different effects on these waves due to the increasing pressure.

One change in speed is a gradual increase with depth. This causes the P and S waves to travel in curved paths within the earth, as shown in Fig. 15-30. Figure 7-31 shows a similar effect in ocean waves as they approach the shore.

The other change in speed is more abrupt and occurs because the earth's interior consists of layers of different materials. When an earthquake body wave crosses the boundary between two layers, its speed changes, and the

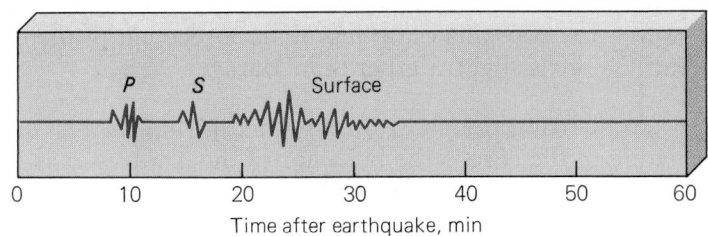

0   10   20   30   40   50   60
Time after earthquake, min

Figure 15-29 Earthquake waves are detected by instruments called **seismographs.** This is a record of waves from an earthquake that occurred about 5000 km from the location of the seismograph.

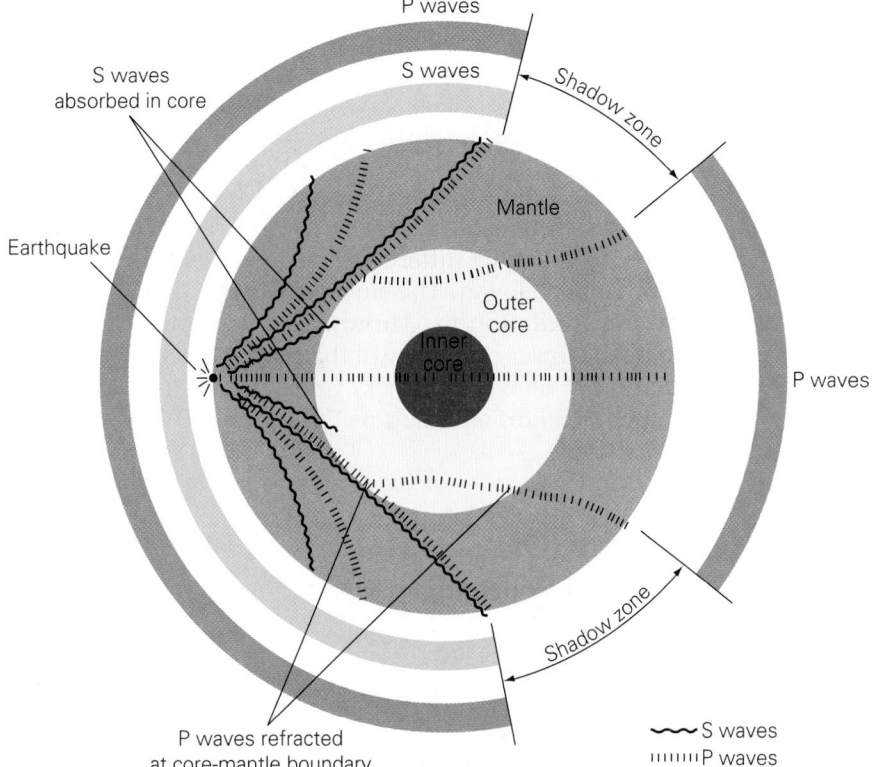

Figure 15-30 How earthquake waves travel through the earth. The existence of a shadow zone where neither P nor S waves arrive is evidence for a core. The inability of S waves to get through the core suggests that at least the outer part of it is liquid. The inner core is believed to consist of iron crystals.

result is a sharp change in direction. Figure 7-34 shows a similar effect in light waves as they go from air into glass. As we see in Fig. 7-36, waves that move perpendicularly through a boundary are not deflected.

Shadow Zones   Let us suppose an earthquake occurs somewhere. We consult various seismograph stations and find that most of them—never all—have detected P waves from this event. Curiously, the stations that P waves did not reach lie along a large band on the side of the earth opposite the quake. We would find, if we looked at the records of other earthquakes, that no matter where they took place, similar **shadow zones** for their P waves existed. This is the chief clue that confirmed an early suspicion that the earth's interior is not uniform.

Figure 15-30 shows why this conclusion is necessary. In the picture, the earth below its thin outer crust is divided into a central **core** and a surrounding **mantle.** P waves from an earthquake that move only through the mantle are refracted so that they reach only a little over half the earth's surface. Those P waves that enter the core are bent sharply toward the center of the earth, and as a result the only part of the earth's surface they reach is a region opposite the quake. The shadow zone separates P waves that have reached the surface through the mantle only from P waves that have also passed through the core.

Analyzing the data shows that the mantle is about 2900 km thick, which means that the core has a radius of about 3470 km, over half the earth's total radius. However, the core makes up less than 20 percent of the earth's volume. The earth's core is slightly larger than Mars.

Liquid Core   Supporting the above finding and giving further information about the nature of the core is the behavior of the S waves. It is found that these cannot get through the core at all (see Fig. 15-30). Because they are transverse, S waves cannot pass through a liquid, so the conclusion is that the earth's core is liquid! A liquid core accounts not only for the behavior of S waves but also for the marked changes in the speed of P waves when they enter and leave the core.

Sensitive seismographs have detected faint traces of P waves in the shadow zones, which suggested to Inge Lehmann (Fig. 15-31), a Danish geologist, that within the liquid core is a smaller, solid inner core. This idea is now well-established; the inner core is believed to have a radius of 1216 km, almost 2/3 that of the moon. Thus the earth's interior has the onionlike structure shown in Fig. 15-32.

The Moho   From observations of the waves from a 1909 earthquake it became clear that there is a distinct difference between the outer shell of the earth and the denser mantle below it. The surface between them is known as the **Mohorovicic discontinuity** (or just **Moho**), after its Croatian discoverer, and is considered to be the lower boundary of the crust. Under the oceans the crust is seldom much more than 5 km thick. Under the continents, though, the crust averages about 35 km, as much as 70 km under some mountain ranges (Fig. 15-33).

15.8   The Earth's Interior

A Mantle of Rock, a Core of Molten Iron

In the absence of a hole over 6000 km deep, anything said about the composition of the earth's interior must be a hypothesis, but a great deal of evidence supports the hypotheses that have been made.

In the case of the upper mantle, most studies point to igneous rocks composed mainly of ferromagnesian minerals. Deep in the mantle enormous

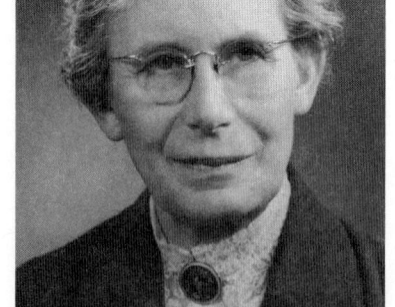

Figure 15-31   Inge Lehmann (1888–1993).

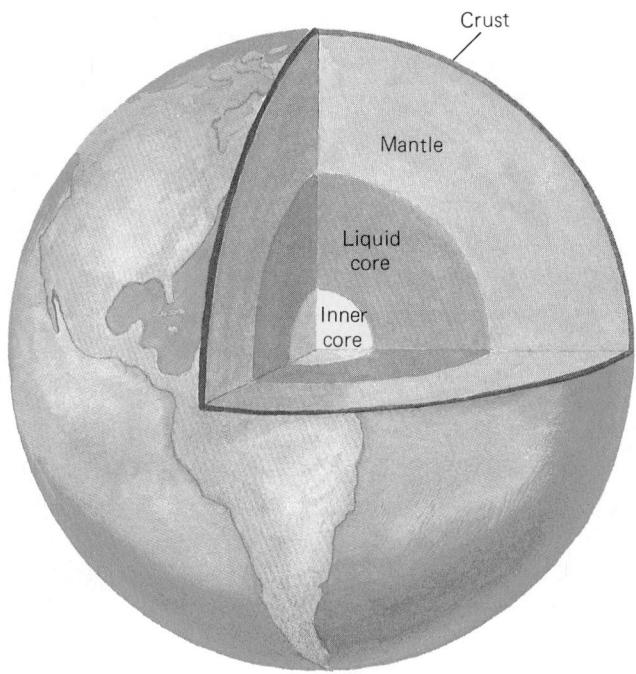

Crust

Mantle

Liquid core

Inner core

Figure 15-32   Structure of the earth. The mantle constitutes 80 percent of the earth's volume and about 67 percent of its mass.

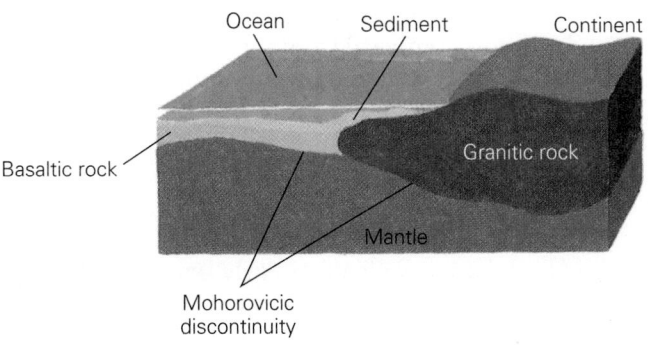

Ocean   Sediment   Continent

Basaltic rock

Granitic rock

Mantle

Mohorovicic discontinuity

Figure 15-33   The Mohorovicic discontinuity separates the earth's crust from the mantle below it. The crust is thicker and has a different composition under the continents than under the oceans.

pressures squeeze minerals into crystal structures that are the most compact possible. Olivine (Fig. 15-9), probably the most abundant mineral in the mantle, is known to occur in two forms, the normal one of the crust and another whose particles are packed together in an especially tight arrangement. In the upper mantle the more open variety is probably the main component with the denser variety predominant lower down. In the innermost part of the mantle, minerals have probably separated into very dense oxides of silicon, iron, and magnesium that occupy even less space.

The Core   Now we come to the liquid outer core. The average density of the earth is about twice the average density of the rocks at the earth's surface. The material of the mantle is only moderately denser than surface rocks, so that the core must be very heavy indeed.

Several clues point to iron as the logical candidate for most (80–85 percent) of the core material. It has almost the right density, it is liquid at the estimated pressure and temperature of the core, and it is abundant in the universe generally. Furthermore, iron is a good conductor of electricity, which is necessary in order to explain the earth's magnetism (Sec. 15.9). Because those meteorites that contain iron also contain some nickel, a reasonable conclusion is that there is nickel in the core also. As for the solid inner core, the kernel of the earth, many geophysicists believe it to be crystalline,

Figure 15-34   Diamond-bearing rock about to be blasted out in a mine several kilometers deep near Pretoria in South Africa. Such rock originates in the mantle where temperatures and pressures are high enough for diamonds to be formed. An average of 5 tons of rock must be mined for each carat of rough diamonds found. The world's deepest mine is a gold mine in South Africa that goes down 3.8 km. Rough diamonds worth about $13 billion are mined every year. Leading producers are Botswana, Russia, South Africa, and Canada in that order.

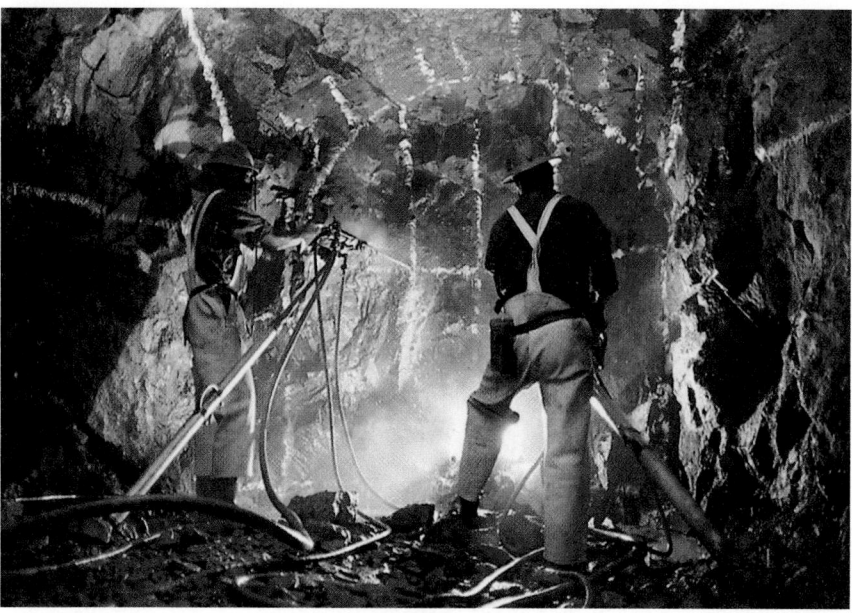

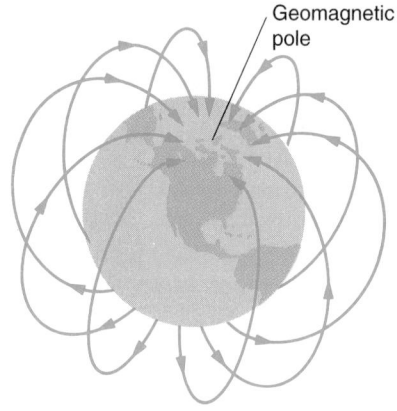

Figure 15-35   The earth's magnetic field originates in electric currents in its core of molten iron. The magnetic axis is tilted by 11° from the axis of rotation, so magnetic compasses do not point to true north.

because of the pressures there, and to consist of iron plus nickel and one or more lighter elements, such as silicon, sulfur, carbon, and oxygen.

The Earth's Heat   Below its surface the earth is extremely hot (Fig. 15-34). The rate at which heat flows outward from the interior is immense, about 100 times greater than the energy involved in such geological events as volcanoes and earthquakes. There is plenty of heat to spare to account for mountain building and other deformations that occur in the crust. In fact, the geological history of the earth is mainly a consequence of the steady heat streaming through its outer layers. Temperatures inside the earth are believed to go from perhaps 375°C at the top of the mantle to perhaps 5000°C in the core.

Part of the earth's heat is a relic of its early history, but most of it comes from radioactive uranium, thorium, and potassium isotopes. These isotopes are present in the minerals of the earth, and their radiations, which were discussed in Sec. 8.3, give up their energy to the minerals as they are absorbed. The earth is believed to have come into being 4.6 billion years ago as a cold clump of smaller bodies of metallic iron and silicate minerals that had been circling the sun. Heat due to radioactivity accumulated in the interior of the infant earth and in time caused partial melting. The influence of gravity then caused the iron to migrate inward to form the core while the lighter silicates rose to form the mantle and crust.

Today most of the earth's radioactivity is concentrated in the crust and upper mantle, where the heat it produces escapes through the surface and cannot collect to remelt the rest of the mantle or the inner core.

15.9   Geomagnetism

Electric Currents in the Core Seem to Be Responsible

Although the earliest known description of the compass and its use in navigation was published by Alexander Neckham in 1180, knowledge of the compass seems to have been widespread even further back in antiquity. Until 1600, however, it was believed that a force exerted by Polaris, the North Star, is what attracted magnetized needles. In that year Sir William Gilbert wrote of experiments he had performed with spherical pieces of lodestone, a naturally magnetized mineral. By comparing the direction of the magnetic force

BIOGRAPHY   William Gilbert (1544 –1603)

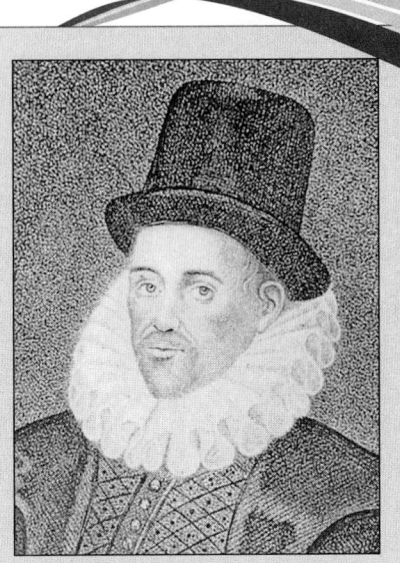

Gilbert practiced medicine in London and became the personal physician to Queen Elizabeth I in 1600. At about that time he published *De Magnete,* a book that described the results of his years of research on magnetism. An early advocate of experiment and observation in science—Galileo admired his work—Gilbert found that iron objects can be magnetized by rubbing them with a lodestone (an iron oxide mineral that is naturally magnetic); that heating an iron magnet causes it to lose its magnetism; that like magnetic poles repel and unlike poles attract (he introduced the word pole for the end of a magnet); and, most significant of all, that the earth itself is a giant magnet.

In addition Gilbert showed that a number of popular beliefs were incorrect, for instance that garlic destroys magnetism and that magnetism cures headaches. Not until two centuries after *De Magnete* were any major additions made to our knowledge of magnetism.

Gilbert also studied static electricity, which the ancient Greeks had discovered by rubbing amber with silk, and found that other substances, too, can be charged by rubbing. Gilbert called all such substances *electrics*, after the Greek for "amber," and clearly distinguished between magnetic and electric attractions.

In astronomy, Gilbert was the first prominent Englishman to support the copernican model of the universe, and he believed that the stars were at different distances from the earth, perhaps circled by habitable planets. The **gilbert** is a magnetic unit named after this remarkable man.

on an iron needle at various positions near a lodestone sphere with similar measurements made in other parts of the world by explorers, Gilbert concluded that the earth behaves like a giant magnet—*"magnus magnes ipse est globus terrestris."*

The earth's magnetic field is much like the field that would come from a giant bar magnet located near the earth's center and tilted by 11° from the direction of the earth's axis of rotation (Fig. 15-35). No such magnet can possibly exist, since iron loses its magnetic properties above about 770°C and most of the earth's interior is much hotter than that. Instead, the magnetic field is believed to arise from electric currents generated in the swirling liquid iron of the core, a hypothesis supported by laboratory experiments. We recall from Fig. 6-33 that an electric current in the form of a loop has around it a magnetic field of the same kind as that of a bar magnet. Less than a billionth of the earth's rotational energy is needed to generate the observed magnetic field. The geomagnetic field is believed to have come into being about 3.5 billion years ago when the earth was a billion or so years old (see Sec. 19.10).

Field Reversals

When deposits of rock that contain magnetizable minerals are dated, specimens of different ages may have opposite magnetic polarities. The only explanation in most cases is that the earth's magnetic field has reversed itself periodically while these rocks were being formed. In the past 76 million years, 171 field reversals have apparently occurred. Such flip-flops fit in with the notion that the field is due to electric currents in the outer core, since changes may well take place in the patterns of flow in the liquid iron there from time to time. As we shall see in Sec. 16.6, these reversals helped to establish that the ocean floors are spreading, an important part of the plate tectonics picture of the earth that includes the drift of the continents.

The most recent field reversal occurred 780,000 years ago, nearly double the average interval between past reversals, so we seem to be overdue for another one. What will happen is that the field strength will decrease over a period of a few thousand years (a blink of the eye, geologically speaking) and then build up again with the field in the opposite direction. In the past hundred years the field has weakened by about 10 percent, which suggests that perhaps a reversal has already begun.

Erosion

It is not obvious that this solid earth under us, made up largely of hard, strong rock, is in a state of constant change. But rocks, hills, and mountains are permanent only by comparison with the brief span of human life, and the long history of the earth goes back not scores of years but billions of years. In this immense stretch of time continents have shifted across the globe, mountain ranges have been thrust upward and then leveled, and broad seas have appeared and disappeared.

All the processes by which rocks are worn down and by which the debris is carried away are included in the general term **erosion.** The underlying cause of erosion is gravity. Such agents of erosion as running water and glaciers derive their destructive energy from gravity, and gravity is responsible for the transport of the removed material.

15.10   Weathering

How Exposed Rocks Decay

We have all seen the rough, pitted surfaces of old stone buildings and monuments (Fig. 15-36). This kind of disintegration, brought about by rainwater and the gases in the air, is called **weathering.** Weathering contributes to erosion by preparing rocks for easy removal by the more active erosional agents, such as running water.

Some of the minerals in igneous and metamorphic rocks are especially susceptible to **chemical weathering,** since they were formed under conditions very different from those at the earth's surface. Ferromagnesian minerals are readily attacked by atmospheric oxygen, aided by carbon dioxide dissolved in water (which gives an acid solution) and by organic acids from decaying vegetation. This results in the formation of iron oxides, which give the red and brown colors that commonly appear as stains on the surface of rocks containing these minerals. Feldspars and other silicates containing aluminum are broken down to clay minerals.

Among common sedimentary rocks limestone is most readily attacked by chemical weathering because calcite dissolves in weak acids (Fig. 15-37). Exposures of limestone can often be identified simply from the pitted surfaces and enlarged cracks that solution produces.

Quartz and white mica resist chemical attack and usually remain as loose grains when the rest of a rock is thoroughly decayed. Rocks consisting wholly of silica, like chert and most quartzites, are practically immune to chemical weathering.

Example 15.2

Both marble and slate are metamorphic rocks. Would you expect a marble tombstone or a slate one to be more resistant to chemical weathering?

Solution

When exposed to the atmosphere marble weathers fairly readily because its calcite content is soluble in rainwater that contains carbon dioxide. Slate consists largely of clay minerals that have metamorphosed to white mica, which is nearly as resistant as quartz to chemical weathering.

Mechanical weathering is often aided by chemical attack. Not only is the structure of a rock weakened by the decomposition of its minerals, but fragments of it are wedged apart because the chemical changes in a mineral grain usually result in an increased volume. The most effective process of mechanical disintegration that does not require chemical action is the freezing of water

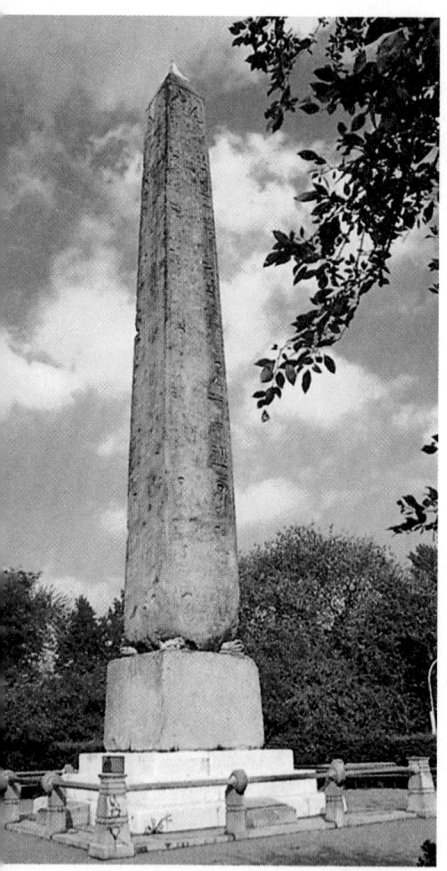

Figure 15-36   After standing in the clean, dry air of Egypt for about 36 centuries, the carvings on Cleopatra's Needle were still sharp and clear. In 1881 the granite obelisk was moved to New York City, where the combination of climate and atmospheric pollution has almost erased the carvings. Acid rain running down the obelisk is the reason the damage increases toward the base.

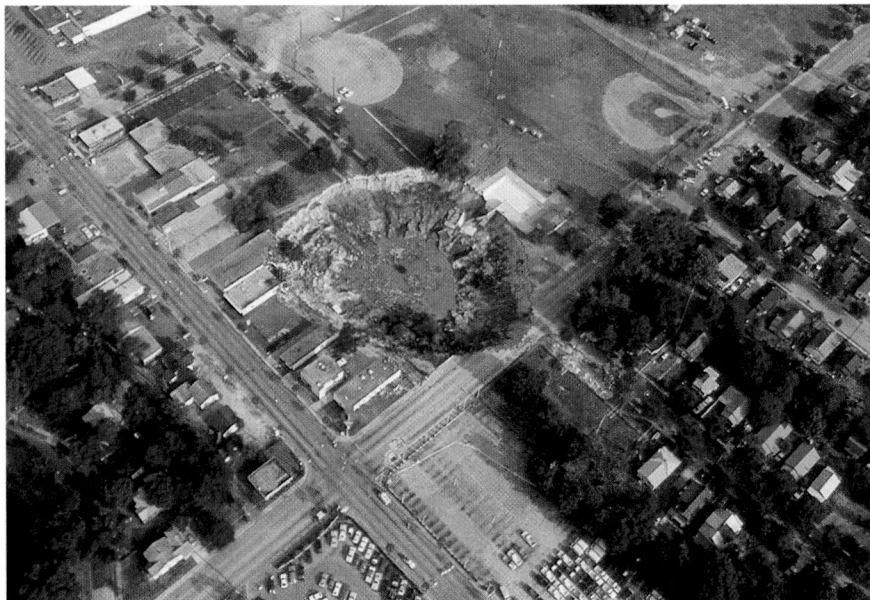

Figure 15-37 Underground limestone gradually dissolves in acid water that seeps through it. When the limestone is near the surface, its disappearance can lead to a collapse of the ground above to leave a **sinkhole.** This sinkhole occurred in Winter Park, Florida. When limestone farther underground is dissolved, the result is a cave. Mammouth Cave in Kentucky is the world's longest; its various passages total 560 km.

Soil

Though the bulk of the earth's crust is solid rock, what we see on that part of the surface not covered by water is mainly soil with only occasional outcrops of bedrock. Soil originates in the weathering of rock, a complex disintegration process whose result is a coat of rock fragments and clay minerals mixed with varying amounts of organic matter.

Any type of rock may form the parent material of a soil. The particles of rock typically vary in size down to microscopic fineness and are intimately mixed with dark, partly decomposed plant debris called humus. The humus content decreases with depth (Fig. 15-38).

A great many factors are involved in the production of soil, including microorganisms such as bacteria and fungi that are responsible for the decay of plant and animal residues and are important in maintaining the nitrogen content of soil. A significant fraction of the organic matter in soil, in fact, consists of the bodies, living and dead, of these microorganisms. Even so lowly a creature as the worm plays a vital role in mixing together the various soil constituents.

Some dust is always present in the lower atmosphere, but at various times and places gigantic dust storms of soil particles occur that can blot out daylight, make it hard to breathe, and damage crops on a large scale. In the 1930s such storms were a feature of the "dust bowl" in the Middle West of the United States. Today, on a much larger scale, they are taking place in northern China where they create dust clouds thousands of miles across that sometimes cross the Pacific to deposit dust on western North America.

The chief factors responsible for dust clouds are the overcultivation of marginal soils, overgrazing of vegetation by sheep and goats, the cutting down of trees that anchor the soil, and the overpumping of groundwater that leaves the soil dry. Strong winds sweep millions of tons of loose soil into the air in late winter and early spring in the affected regions to produce the dust storms, which leave deserts behind. Harvests in China have been declining as a result of such ecological catastrophes, and its worried government is trying various schemes to keep the remaining soil in place.

The problem of soil erosion is not confined to China: erosion by water as well as by wind contributes to the loss of farmland soils in much of the world faster than new soil is formed. Iowa has lost about half its topsoil in the past 150 years.

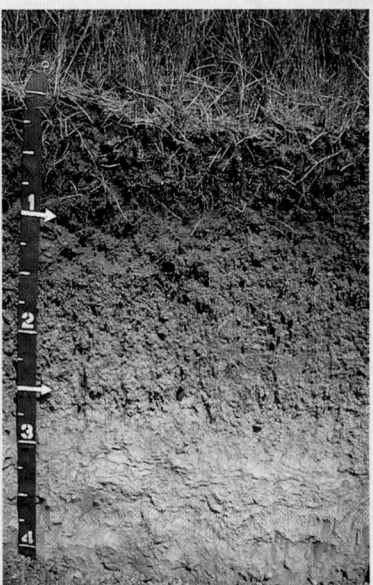

Figure 15-38 Cross section of a typical soil. The darkening toward the top is due to the presence of humus.

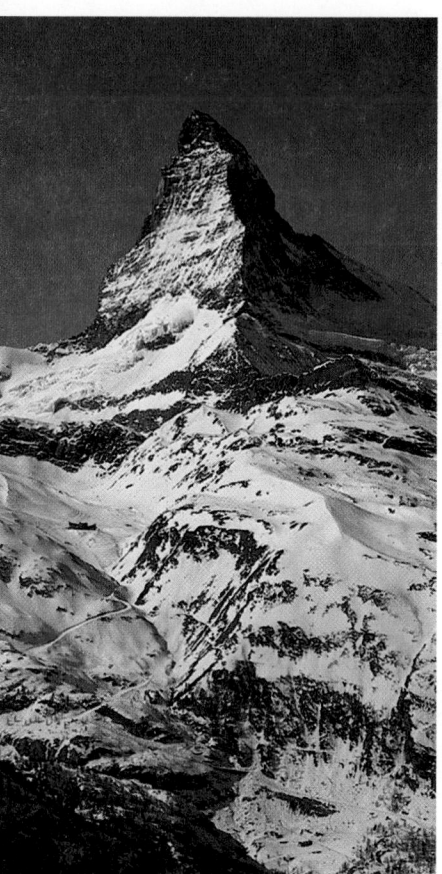

Figure 15-39 The expansion of water as it freezes into ice in cracks in rock has carved the sharp peak of the Matterhorn, a mountain on the border between Switzerland and Italy.

in crevices. Just as water freezing in a car's engine on a cold night may split the engine block, so water freezing in tiny cracks is effective in disrupting rocks (Fig. 15-39). Plant roots help in rock disintegration by growing in cracks.

Weathering processes coat the naked rock of the earth's crust with a layer of debris made up largely of clay mixed with rock and mineral fragments. The upper part of the weathered layer, in which rock debris is mixed with decaying vegetable matter, is the **soil.** The formation of soil is an important result of weathering.

15.11 Stream Erosion

Running Water Is the Chief Agent of Erosion

By far the most important agent of erosion is the running water of streams and rivers. The work of glaciers, wind, and waves is impressive locally, but compared with running water, these other erosion agents play only minor roles in shaping the earth's landscapes. Even in deserts, mountainsides are carved with the unmistakable forms of stream-made valleys.

In a young landscape, streams and rivers are just starting their work and flow downhill swiftly with many rapids and waterfalls (Fig. 15-40). At first a

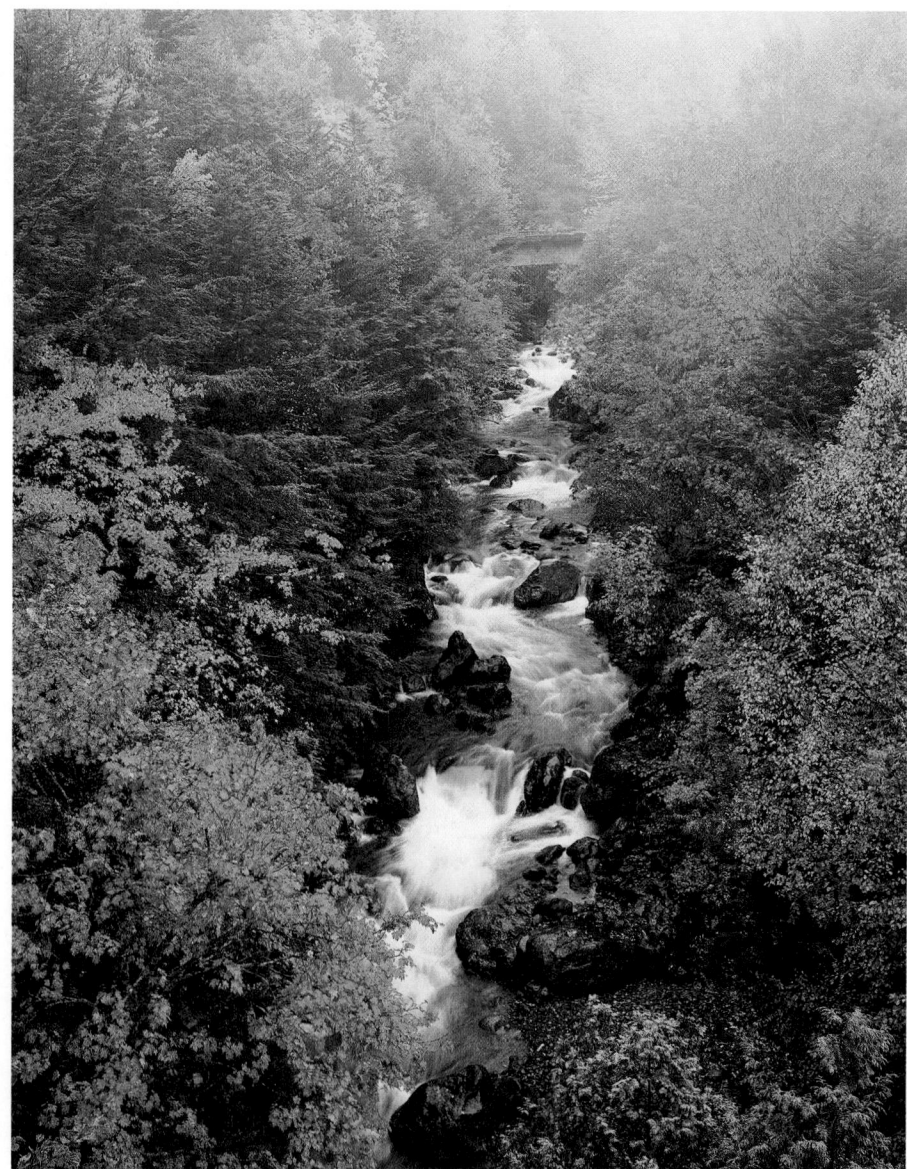

Figure 15-40 The running water of a stream may accomplish more erosion during a few hours of heavy rain than in months or years of normal flow. What does the work is not the moving water itself but the sand and pebbles hurled by the water at the sides and bed of its channel.

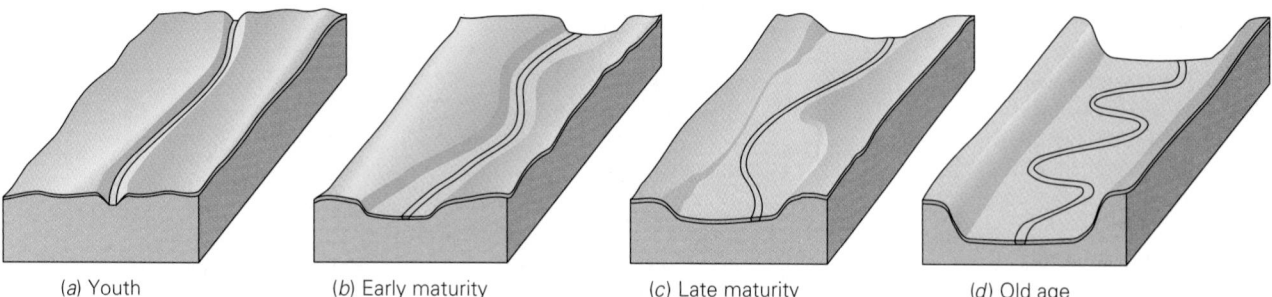

(a) Youth   (b) Early maturity   (c) Late maturity   (d) Old age

Figure 15-41   Successive stages in the development of a river valley.

river carves a narrow V-shaped channel (Fig. 15-41*a*). As time goes on, the channel deepens until the river's lower end is near the level of a nearby valley or perhaps nearly at sea level. As the rest of the channel becomes less steep, its sides begin to be cut away to broaden it (Fig. 15-41*b*). The eventual result is a **floodplain** with a flat floor (Fig. 15-41*c*). In dry weather the river wanders over its plain in a meandering course; in very wet weather it overflows its channel and spreads across the plain. The floodplain grows wider and wider, the river becomes more and more sluggish, and the sides of its valley become lower and lower (Fig. 15-41*d*).

During this development of the major valley, secondary streams extend their smaller valleys on either side. Soon a characteristic treelike pattern develops, separated from the patterns of adjacent rivers by sharp divides of high ground (Fig. 15-42). As floodplains widen along the main streams, divides are lowered by attack from the streams on either side. In the final stages of valley growth, when floodplains are wide and rivers broadly meandering, most of the divides are erased and those remaining are low and rounded (Fig. 15-43).

Actual Landscapes   Actual landscapes seldom conform exactly to the simple valley shapes and patterns just described. One reason is the presence of rocks of different hardness: hard rocks usually remain as cliffs and high ridges, while the more easily eroded soft rocks wear away (Fig. 15-44). Many of the striking landforms produced by erosion are due simply to differences in resistance from one rock layer to the next.

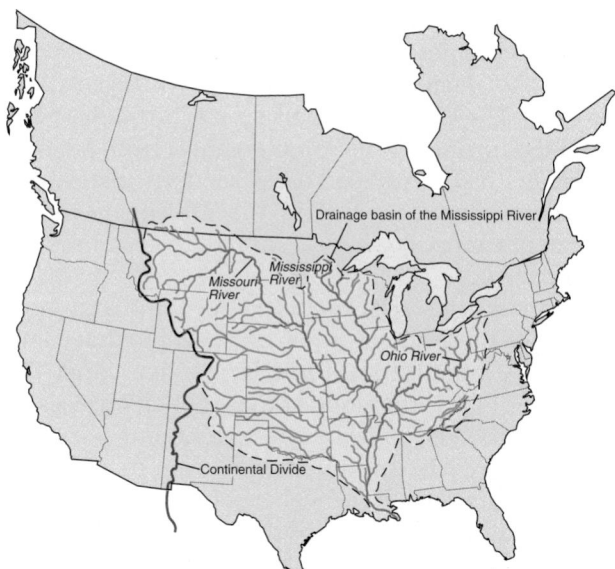

Figure 15-42   The treelike drainage pattern of the Mississippi River covers more than 2.5 million square kilometers. Rivers to the west of the Continental Divide flow into the Pacific, those to its east flow into the Atlantic and the Gulf of Mexico.

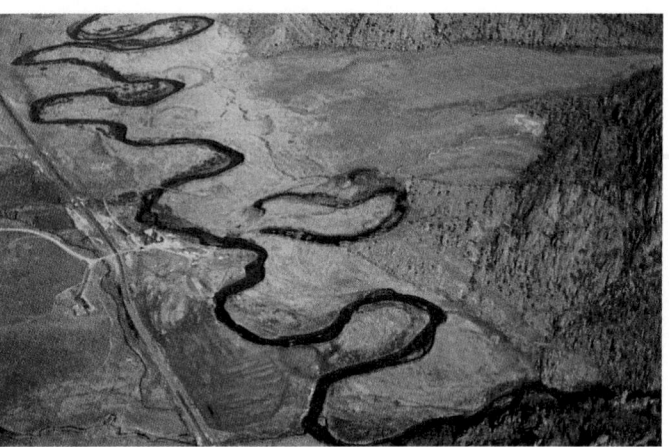

Figure 15-43 The floodplain of the Sweetwater River in Wyoming. The wandering, shifting channel is typical of the old age of a river. The bends grow larger as their outer banks (where the water flows faster) are eroded, while sediments are deposited on the inner banks. Sometimes a bend becomes so extreme that its ends join together at a time of high water, which cuts a straight connection that leaves behind an oxbow lake. Such a lake can be seen to the right of the river in the middle of this photograph.

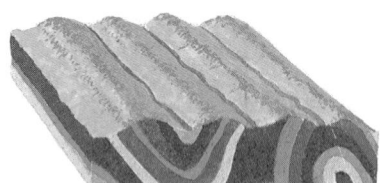

Figure 15-44 Parallel ridges and valleys produced by stream erosion in tilted layers of hard and soft rocks. Soft layers underlie the valleys; hard layers, the ridges. Landscapes and rock structures of this sort are typical of the Appalachian Mountains.

Whatever the valley shapes produced in various stages of landscape development, whatever different kinds of rock may be present, the tendency of stream erosion is to reduce the land surface to a flat plain almost at sea level. However, this outcome is seldom reached because, as we shall learn, other geologic processes continually counteract the effects of running water. There are very few regions in which geologic processes involving uplift do not occur at the same time as stream erosion. Thus most landscapes are the result of a complex of factors and reflect a balance among them rather than the action of stream erosion alone.

15.12 Glaciers

Rivers and Seas of Ice

In a cold climate with abundant snowfall, the snow of winter may not completely melt during the following summer, and a deposit of snow accumulates from year to year. Partial melting and the continual increase in pressure cause the lower part of a snow deposit to change gradually into ice. If the ice is sufficiently thick, its weight forces it slowly downhill. A moving mass of ice formed in this manner is called a **glacier**. About 10 percent of the earth's land area is today covered by glacial ice, which contains three-quarters of its freshwater.

Today's glaciers are of two main kinds:

1. **Valley glaciers**—found, for instance, in the Alps, on the Alaskan coast, in the western United States—are patches and tongues of ice lying in mountain valleys. These glaciers move slowly down their valleys and melt at their lower ends. The combination of downward movement and melting keeps their ends in roughly the same position from year to year. Valleys carved by glaciers have U-shaped cross sections instead of the V shapes produced by stream erosion (Fig. 15-45). Movement in the faster valley glaciers (a meter or more per day) is enough to keep their lower ends well below the timber line.

2. Glaciers of another type cover most of Greenland and Antarctica. These huge masses of ice thousands of square km in area that engulf hills as well as valleys are called **continental glaciers** or **ice caps.** They, too, move downhill, but the "hill" is the slope of their upper surfaces. An ice cap has the shape of a broad dome with its surface sloping outward from a thick central portion of greatest snow accumulation. Its motion is outward in all directions from its center. The icebergs of the polar seas are fragments that have broken off the edges of ice caps (see Fig. 4-7). Similar sheets of ice extended across Canada and northern Eurasia during the ice ages.

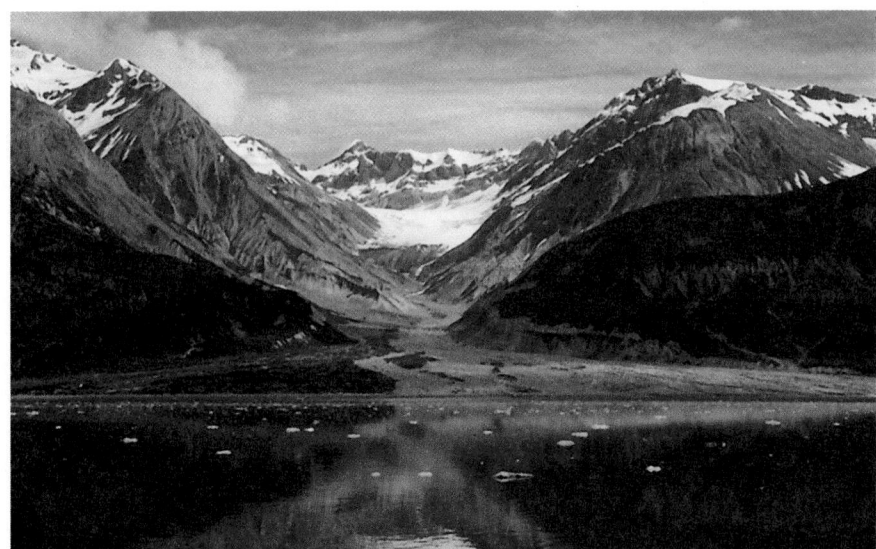

Figure 15-45 The U-shaped cross section of this valley in Alaska suggests that it was cut by the ancestor of today's glacier at a time when the climate there was colder than at present. Today's glaciers range in length up to the 109-km Hubbard Glacier in western Canada; all are smaller than in the past due to global warming.

Glacial Erosion As a glacier moves, rock fragments held firmly by the ice at its bottom are dragged along. These fragments scrape and polish the underlying rock and are themselves ground down. Smooth, grooved rock surfaces and deposits of debris that contain boulders with flattened sides are common where the lower end of a valley glacier has melted back to reveal some of its bed. When such evidence of ice erosion is found far from present-day glaciers, we can infer that glaciers must have been active there in the past.

Glacial erosion is locally very impressive, particularly in high mountains. The amount of debris and the size of the boulders that a glacier can carry or push ahead of itself are often startling. But overall, the erosion accomplished by glaciers is small. Only rarely have they gouged rock surfaces deeply, and the amount of material they carry long distances is little compared with that carried by streams. Most glaciers of today are only feeble descendants of mighty ancestors, but even these ancestors succeeded only in modifying landscapes already shaped by running water.

15.13 Groundwater

Water, Water Everywhere (Almost)

Most of the water that falls as rain does not run off at once in streams but instead soaks into the ground. All water that thus penetrates the surface is called **groundwater.** There is more groundwater than all the freshwater of the world's lakes and rivers, though less than the water locked up in ice caps and glaciers (see Fig. 14-6).

The Water Table The soil, the layer of weathered rock under it, and any porous rocks below act together as a sponge that can absorb huge quantities of water. During and just after a heavy rain all empty spaces in the sponge may be filled, and the ground is then said to be **saturated** with water. When the rain has stopped, water slowly drains away from hills into the adjacent valleys. A few days after a rain porous material in the upper part of a hill contains relatively little moisture, while that in the lower part may still be saturated. Another rain would raise the upper level of the saturated zone, prolonged drought would lower it. The fluctuating upper surface of the saturated zone is called the **water table.**

Beneath valleys the water table is usually closer to the surface than beneath nearby hills (Fig. 15-46). Groundwater in the saturated zone seeps slowly downward and sideward into streams, lakes, and swamps. The motion is rapid through coarse material like sand or gravel, slow through fine material like clay. It is this flow of groundwater that maintains streams when rain is not falling; a stream goes dry only when the water table drops below the level of its bed. A **spring** is formed where groundwater comes to the surface in a more or less definite channel.

Aquifers   An **aquifer** is a body of porous rock through which groundwater moves. Aquifers underlie more than half the area of the continental United States (Fig. 15-47) and supply about half its drinking water and much of the water used by industry and agriculture. Rivers supply most of the rest.

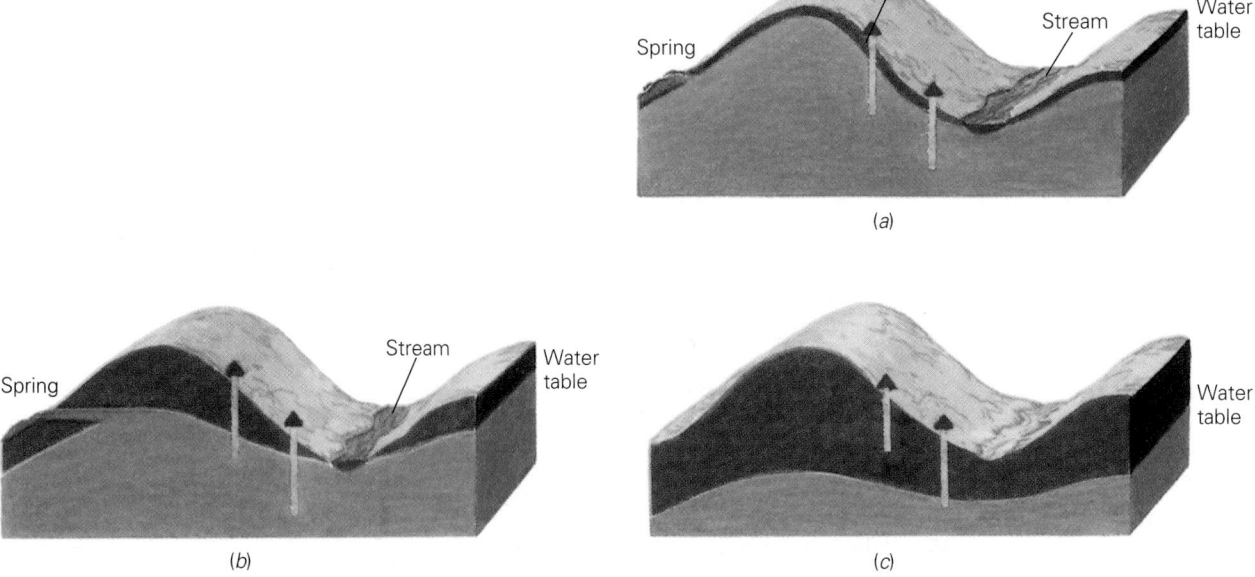

Figure 15-46   Cross sections through a landscape underlain by porous material. The position of the water table is shown (*a*) just after a heavy rain, (*b*) several days later, and (*c*) after a prolonged drought. The spring, the stream, and the upper well would be dry during the drought.

Figure 15-47   The Ogallala aquifer, the largest in the United States, supplies water for agricultural use in a heavily farmed region. It is shrinking and becoming contaminated by fertilizer runoff. Water from other aquifers throughout the world is also being withdrawn faster than natural processes can replenish it.

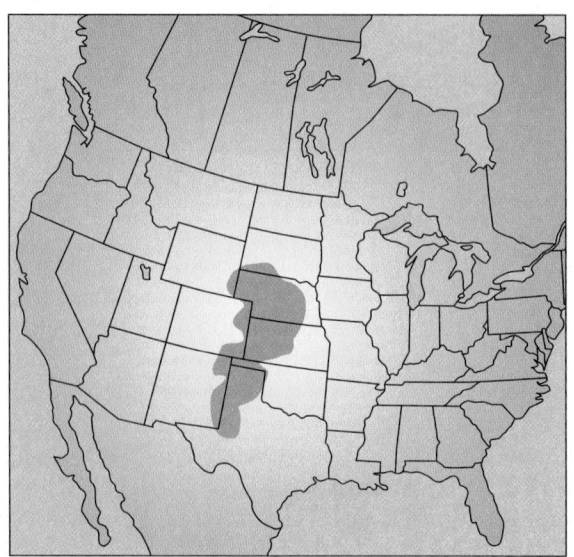

Because groundwater moves slowly, it can accomplish little mechanical wear, but its prolonged contact with rocks and soil allows it to dissolve much soluble material. Some of the dissolved material remains in solution (hence the "hardness" of water from many wells), and some is redeposited elsewhere. In regions underlain by limestone, the most soluble of ordinary rocks, caves are produced when water moving through tiny cracks enlarges the cracks by dissolving and removing the adjacent limestone.

15.14   Sedimentation

What Becomes of the Debris of Erosion

Most of the material transported by the agents of erosion is eventually deposited to form **sediments** of various sorts. The ultimate destination of erosional debris is the ocean, and the most widespread sediments collect in shallow parts of the ocean near continental edges. But much sedimentary material is carried to the sea in stages, deposited first in thick layers elsewhere—in lakes, in desert basins, in stream valleys. Each erosional agent has its own ways of giving up its load, and these ways leave their stamps on the deposits formed.

Stream Deposits   Rivers and streams, the chief agents of erosion, lose some of the abundant debris they carry whenever their speeds drop or their volumes of water decrease. Four sites of deposition are common:

1. Debris carried in time of flood is deposited in gravel banks and sandbars on the streambed when the swiftly flowing waters begin to recede.
2. The floodplain of a meandering river is a site of deposition whenever the river overflows its banks and loses speed as it spreads over the plain. In Egypt, for example, before construction of the Aswan Dam, the fertility of the soil was maintained for centuries by the deposit of black silt left each year when the Nile was in flood.
3. A common site of deposition, especially in the western United States, is the point where a stream emerges from a steep mountain valley and slows down as it flows onto a plain. Such a deposit, usually taking the form of a low cone pointing upstream, is called an **alluvial fan** (Fig. 15-48).
4. A similar deposit is formed when a stream's flow is stopped abruptly as the stream enters a lake or sea. This kind of deposit, built largely underwater and with a surface usually flatter than that of an alluvial fan, is called a **delta.**

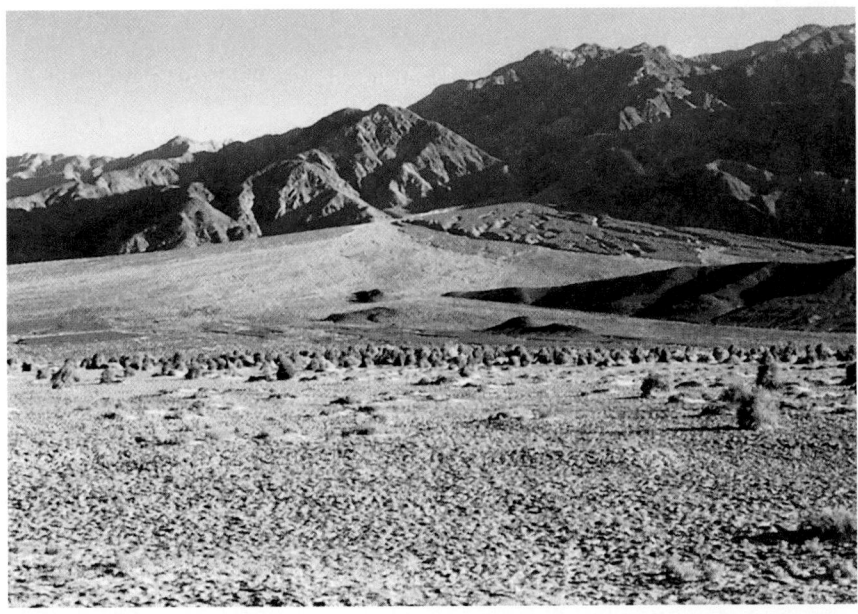

Figure 15-48   An alluvial fan consists of debris deposited by a mountain stream when it slowed down on reaching the plain.

Glacial Deposits   Some of the material a glacier scrapes from its channel is spread as a layer of irregular thickness under the ice, and some is heaped up at the glacier's lower end where the ice melts. The pile of debris around the end and along the sides of the glacier, called a **moraine,** is left as a low ridge when the glacier melts back. Moraines in mountain valleys and in the North Central states are part of the evidence for a former wide extent of glaciation.

All the material deposited directly by ice goes by the name of **till,** an indiscriminate mixture of fine and coarse material. Till includes huge boulders that are often embedded in the fine, claylike material a glacier produces by its polishing action. Typically, most of the boulders are angular, but a few are rounded and show the flat scratched faces produced as they were dragged along the bed of the glacier.

Ocean Currents and Ground Water   Most important of the agents of deposition, because they handle by far the largest amount of sediment, are ocean currents. Currents deposit not only the materials eroded from coastlines by wave action but also the abundant debris brought to the ocean by rivers, wind, and glaciers. Visible deposits of waves and currents include beaches and sandbars, but the great bulk of the sediments brought to the ocean are laid down underwater (Fig. 15-49).

Groundwater deposits material in the pore spaces of sediments, a process that helps to convert the sediments to rock. Much dissolved material precipitates in cracks to form **veins,** which are found in all kinds of rocks. Quartz and calcite are common in veins, and the ores of various metals are also found there. Spectacular examples of groundwater deposition are the **stalactites** that hang from the roofs of limestone caves, the **stalagmites** that rise from their floors (Fig. 15-50), and the colorful deposits often found around hot springs and geysers.

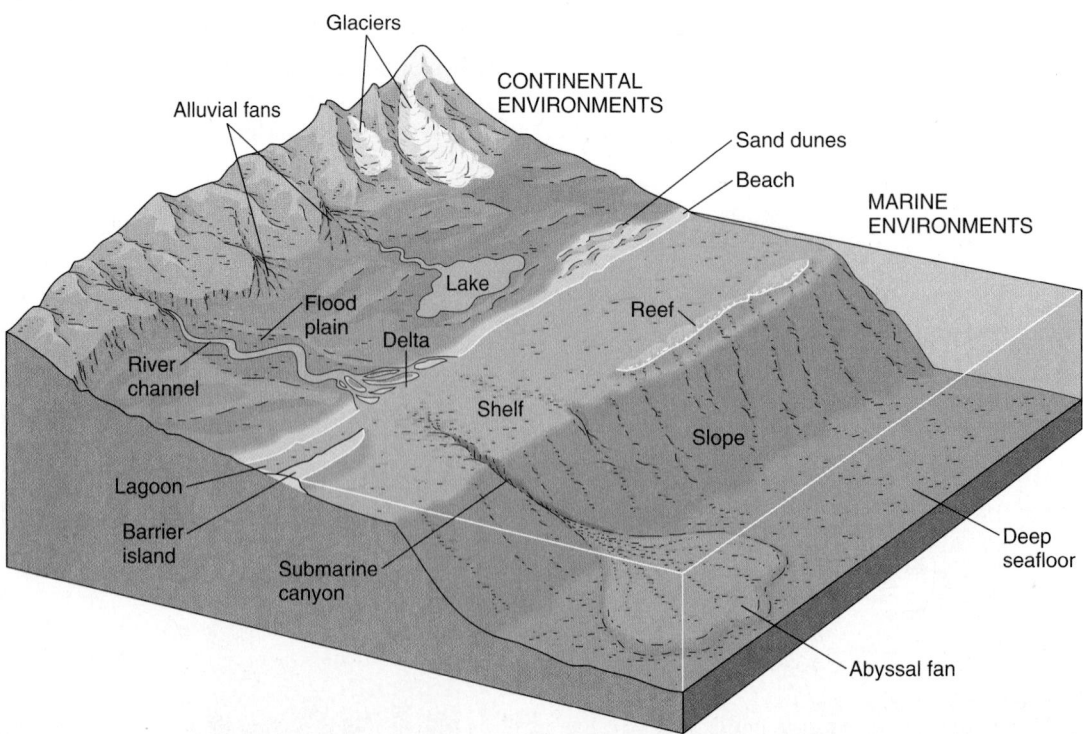

Figure 15-49 Erosion and sedimentation on land and sea.

Example 15.3

Why are mineral deposits around hot springs thicker than those around ordinary springs?

Solution

Minerals are more soluble in hot water than in cold water, hence hot water contains a greater mineral load to deposit.

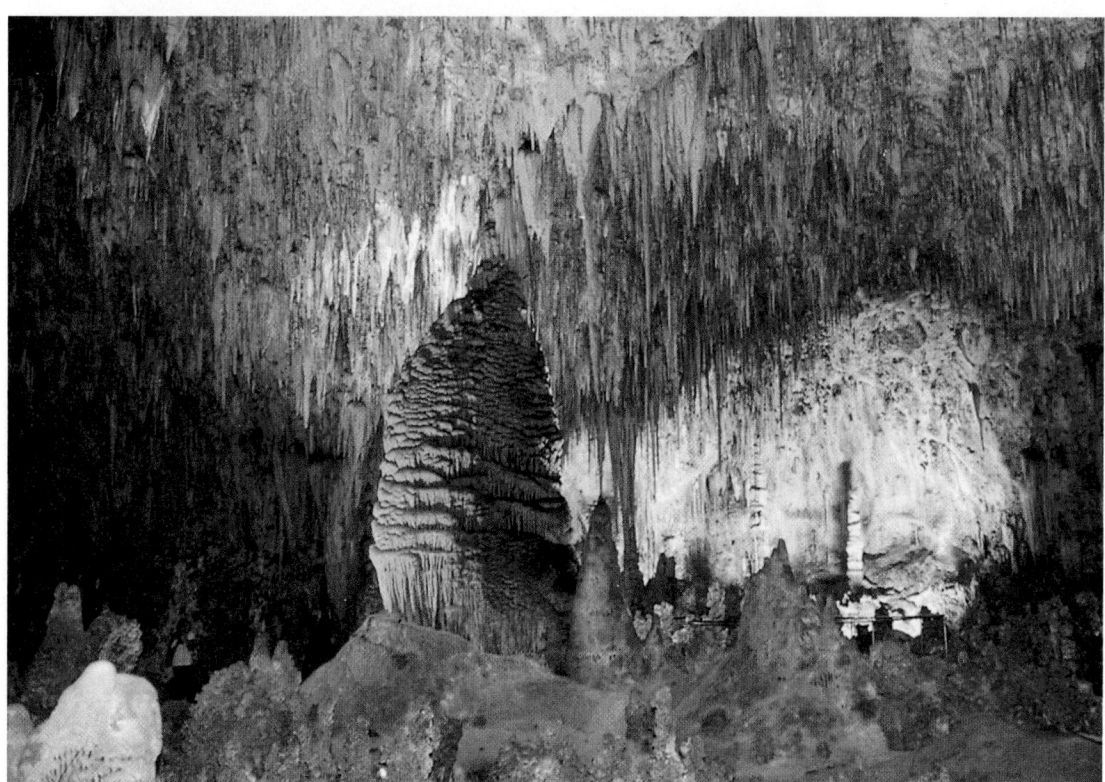

Figure 15-50 Carlsbad Caverns in New Mexico. Caves such as this occur when groundwater dissolves limestone and carries it away. The stalactites that hang like icicles from the roof of the cave and the stalagmite columns that grow from its floor consist of material that has precipitated from solution.

Lithification Sediments buried beneath later deposits are gradually hardened into rock, a process called **lithification.** Lithification can be a complex process, taking thousands or even millions of years. One important change in the sediment is compaction, the squeezing together of its grains under the pressure of overlying deposits. Some recrystallization may accompany compaction. The calcite crystals of limy sediments, in particular, grow larger and interlock with one another.

Chemical changes brought about by circulating groundwater contribute to the hardening of many sediments. The grains of coarse sediments are cemented by material precipitated from solution in groundwater, and some sediments have much of their original material dissolved away and replaced by other substances. In petrified wood the original organic compounds have been removed, molecule by molecule, and replaced by silica. The whole process takes place so gradually that the finest details of the wood structure may be preserved (Fig. 15-51).

Sedimentary rocks are especially important in geology because they contain material that was deposited at or near the earth's surface and so record

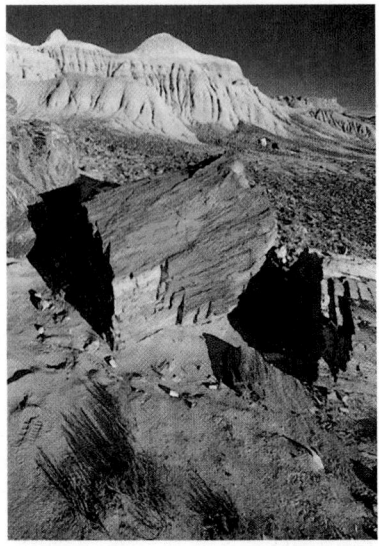

Figure 15-51 Petrified wood (this example is in Arizona) consists mainly of silica. Its beautiful colors come from other minerals deposited with the silica: those that contain iron give the reds and yellows, those that contain chromium give the greens, and those that contain cobalt give the blues.

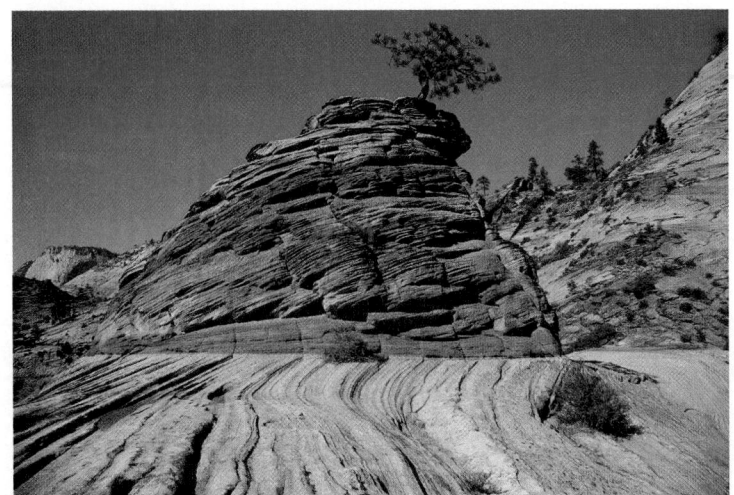

Figure 15-52 These sandstone beds in Zion National Park, Utah, were once sand dunes that had been deposited by winds.

the changing surface conditions of past time. If we read the evidence with sufficient insight and imagination, we find before us a panorama of earth history: seas that once spread widely over the land, the advance and retreat of immense glaciers, the shifting sand dunes of ancient deserts (Fig. 15-52), and much more. Revealed are the living creatures that inhabited lands and seas of the past, for many sedimentary rocks contain fossil remains of plants and animals.

Igneous and metamorphic rocks tell us by their structures something about conditions in the earth's interior; sedimentary rocks tell us about the history of surface landscapes.

Vulcanism

Erosion and sedimentation are leveling processes through which the higher parts of the earth's surface are worn down and the lower parts are filled with the resulting debris. If their work could be completed, the continents would disappear and the earth would become a smooth globe covered with water. The fact that the continents still exist, not to mention mountain ranges on them, testifies to the action of two other processes:

1. Processes of **vulcanism,** which involve movements of molten rock
2. Processes of **diastrophism** (or **tectonism**), which involve movements of the solid materials of the crust

Vulcanism and diastrophism often occur together. The flow of molten rock may cause adjacent rock structures to be distorted, and it is common for major crustal shifts to be accompanied by volcanic eruptions and subsurface migrations of molten rock.

15.15 Volcanoes

Rivers of Lava, Clouds of Gas and Dust

A **volcano** is an opening in the earth's crust through which molten rock, usually called **magma** while underground and **lava** above ground, pours forth. Because lava accumulates near their openings, most volcanoes in the course of time build up mountains with a characteristic conical shape that steepens toward the top, with a small depression, or **crater,** at the summit. Lava escapes almost continuously from a few volcanoes, but the majority are active only at intervals.

A volcanic eruption is one of the most awesome spectacles on earth (Figs. 15-53 and 15-54). Earthquakes may provide warning of an eruption a few hours or a few days beforehand—minor shocks probably caused by the movement of gases and liquids underground. Eruptions follow a variety of patterns. Usually an explosion comes first, sending a great cloud of gases, dust, and rock fragments billowing from the crater. The exceptionally violent Tambora eruption in Indonesia in 1815, which killed 92,000 people, is thought to have blown over 100 km³ of debris into the atmosphere. Enough stayed aloft to markedly reduce the sunlight reaching Europe and North America the following year—the "year without a summer." New England had blizzards in July and in Switzerland the 18-year-old Mary Shelley, kept indoors by constant rain, wrote *Frankenstein*. A number of airplanes have been damaged by flying into volcanic ash aloft. In 2010, clouds of ash from a volcano in Iceland kept aircraft out of European skies for almost a week, stranding millions of travelers as nearly 100,000 flights were canceled.

Most deaths from volcanoes are due not to lava flows but rather to clouds of gas and ash that sweep down from the craters and destroy everything in their paths. Sometimes a heavy rain washes ash and rock fragments down the slopes of a volcano; such a mudflow killed 25,000 people in 1985 in the town of Armero, Columbia.

Example 15.4

An experiment is performed to determine the lowest temperature at which a certain magma can exist within the earth by melting a sample of rock that has hardened from this magma in a furnace. How meaningful are the results of this experiment?

Solution

The results mean little because the effect of the immense pressure within the earth on the melting point of the magma is not being taken into account.

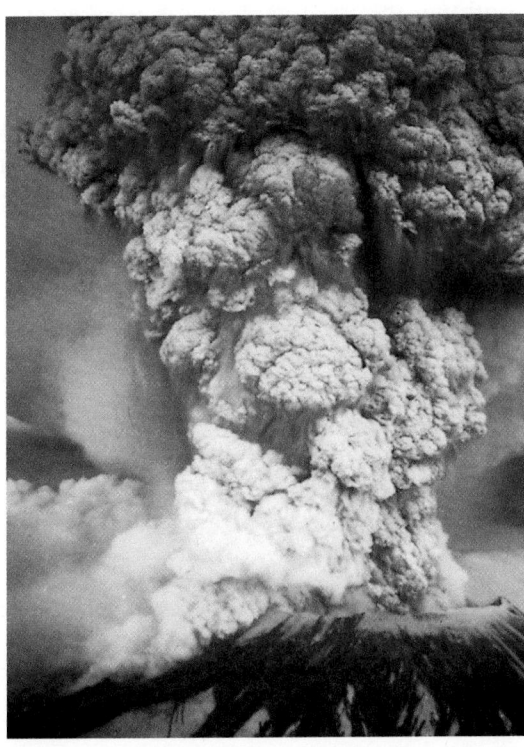

Figure 15-53 The eruption of Mt. St. Helens on May 18, 1980, began with an explosion that devastated an area of over 500 km² in Washington State and sent a column of ash and smoke to a height of 20 km (see Fig. 15.54). Winds carried ash as far as Oklahoma. About 2.7 km³ of volcanic rock, 0.5 km³ of it molten, was expelled. The energy released was about 1.7×10^{18} J, equivalent to 400 million tons of TNT. Mt. St. Helens had also erupted a number of times in the past, leading Native Americans in the region to call it Coowit, the Lady of Fire.

Figure 15-54   What happened at Mt. St. Helens in 1980.
(*a*) A few weeks before the eruption, magma began welling up into the mountain and created a huge bulge (over 100 m outward) in its northern side. Small earthquakes and emissions of gas and ash occurred as the bulge formed.
(*b*) Then the bulge broke loose and the rock that had sealed in the magma slid down the slope.
(*c*) The sudden drop in pressure released the gases dissolved in the magma, and in the resulting explosion a froth of magma and gases poured out of the side of the mountain to devastate a wide area while dense clouds of ash shot upward for more than a day. Since the 1980 eruption magma has been flowing upward to the surface where it is oozing out to produce a lava dome. Because of this another violent eruption like that of 1980 seems unlikely, at least for some time to come.

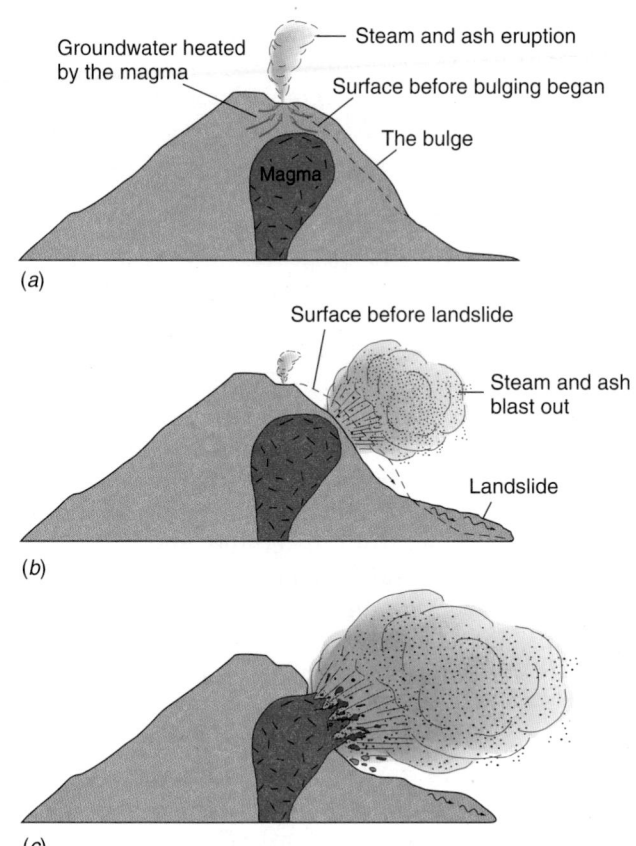

Gas may continue to come out after the first explosion, and further bursts may recur at intervals. The cloud may persist for days or weeks with its lower part glowing red at night. Activity gradually slackens, and soon a tongue of white-hot (1100°C or so) lava spills over the edge of the crater or pours out of a fissure on the mountain slope. Other flows may follow the first, and explosions may continue, though they become weaker and weaker. Slowly the volcano quiets down, with only a small cloud of water vapor above to suggest its activity.

Volcanic Violence   The chief factors that determine whether an eruption will be a quiet lava flow or a furious explosion are the **viscosity** of the magma and the amount of gas it contains. (The greater the viscosity of a liquid, the less freely it flows; honey is more viscous than water.) Magma is a complex mixture of various metal oxides and silica and usually has a lot of gas dissolved in it under pressure. Lavas vary in viscosity but commonly

Predicting an Eruption

Unlike earthquakes, which often occur with little or no warning, volcanoes commonly show signs that an eruption is coming hours or days before. Movements of gases and magma underground give rise to characteristic vibrations that can be heard as creaks, groans, and rumbles; sometimes small earthquakes are felt.

Analyzing these vibrations gives clues as to when the eruption will begin, though not (yet?) how large it will be.

Other signs of an impending eruption are changes in the shape of a volcano (see Fig. 15-54), sudden rises in its surface temperature, and the emission of volcanic gases such as sulfur dioxide. These effects can

be detected by satellite measurements, which is often cheaper and easier than making observations on the volcanoes themselves. However, only a few satellites are suitably equipped, and these satellites survey the entire earth, so they only pass over a particular place every two weeks or so.

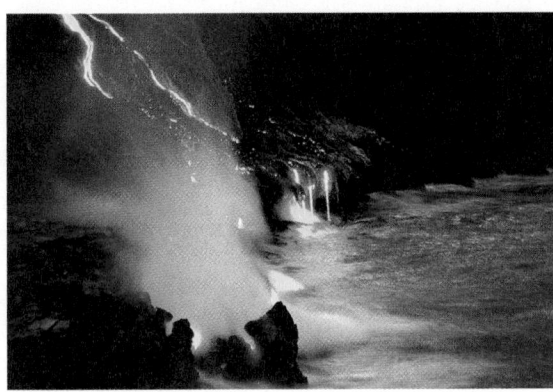

Figure 15-55   Rivers of red-hot lava pour into the Pacific Ocean from a volcano in Hawaii. The magma is relatively poor in silica, so the lava flows freely. Mauna Loa, also in Hawaii, is the largest volcano on earth; it rises over 15 km above the ocean floor. Mauna Loa's weight has depressed the ocean floor under it by about 8 km.

creep downhill slowly, like thick syrup or tar. The viscosity depends largely upon chemical composition: magmas with high percentages of silica are the most viscous.

Gas also affects viscosity: magmas with little gas in them are the most viscous. If the magma feeding a volcano happens to be rich in both gas and silica, the eruption will be explosive. A magma with modest gas and silica contents results in a quiet eruption (Fig. 15-55).

Volcanic gases include water vapor, carbon dioxide, nitrogen, hydrogen, and various sulfur compounds. The most prominent is water vapor. Some of it comes from groundwater heated by magma, some comes from the combination of hydrogen in the magma with atmospheric oxygen, and some was formerly incorporated in rocks deep in the crust and carried upward by the magma. Much of the water vapor condenses when it escapes to give rise to the torrential rains that often accompany eruptions.

Volcanic Rocks   Lava hardens into one or another of the various volcanic rocks (Fig. 15-56), which are all fine-grained because lava cools too rapidly for large mineral crystals to grow. Basalt is by far the most common volcanic rock and, when molten, is fluid enough to spread out over a wide area. The more viscous andesite usually produces steep, conical mountains and generally is associated with more rugged landscapes than basalt. Rhyolite, the most siliceous of ordinary lavas, forms small, thick flows and domes. Rhyolitic lava is sometimes so viscous and cools so rapidly that crystallization does not take place, leaving the natural glass obsidian.

Volcanic rocks of all kinds frequently have rounded holes due to gas bubbles that were trapped during the final stages of solidification. Viscous lavas may harden with so many cavities that the light, porous rock **pumice** results. Pumice is so light that it floats in water; it is sometimes used as a gentle abrasive.

Volcanic Regions   About 530 volcanoes are active today around the borders of the Pacific Ocean (the "Ring of Fire"), on some of the Pacific Islands, in Iceland, in the Mediterranean, and in East Africa. Fifty or so of them erupt in an average year; see Fig. 15-57 and Table 15-4. One in ten of the world's people lives near an active volcano. There are many thousands of undersea volcanoes.

In many other parts of the world volcanoes were active in earlier times. Where volcanoes became extinct in the recent geological past, their former splendor is suggested by isolated conical mountains, by solidified lava flows, and by hot springs, geysers, and steam vents. Some of the great mountains in the western United States are old volcanoes, scarred here and there with lava flows so recent that vegetation has not yet gained a foothold on them.

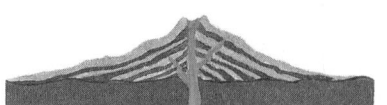

Figure 15-56   Cross section of an idealized volcano. During explosive eruptions much liquid rock flies apart when it emerges from the opening at the top, which becomes a crater afterward. Deposits of the finer material may form the rock **tuff,** and deposits of the coarser material may form a kind of conglomerate called **volcanic breccia** whose fragments are angular rather than rounded. In the volcano shown, lava flows (solid color) alternate with beds of tuff and volcanic breccia.

Figure 15-57 The principal earthquake (light color) and volcanic (dark color) regions of the world.

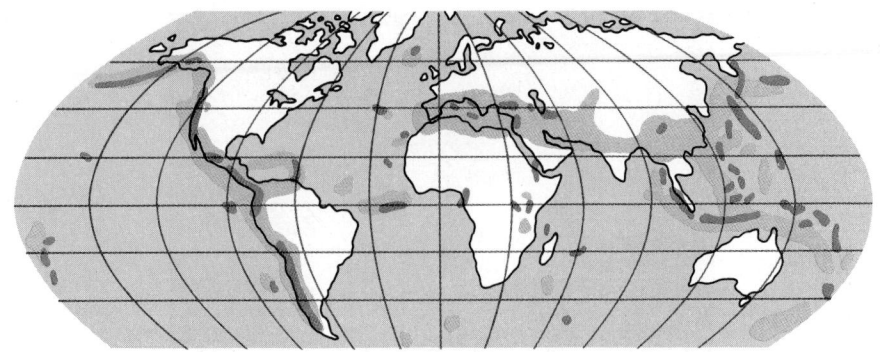

In regions where volcanoes have been inactive for still longer, erosion may have removed all evidence of the original mountains and left only patches of volcanic rocks to indicate former igneous activity.

15.16 Intrusive Rocks

They Have Hardened Underground from Magma

Molten rock that rises through the earth's crust but does not reach the surface solidifies to form intrusive bodies (often called **plutons**) of various kinds. Because these bodies cool slowly, intrusive igneous rocks are coarser-grained than volcanic rocks that cool rapidly on the surface. We find intrusive rocks exposed only where erosion has uncovered them after they hardened.

The igneous origin of volcanic rocks is clear enough, for we can actually watch lava harden to solid rock. But no one has ever seen an intrusive rock like granite in a liquid state in nature. The belief that granite was once molten follows from indirect evidence such as the following:

1. Granite shows the same relations among its minerals that a volcanic rock shows. The separate grains are intergrown, and those with higher melting points show by their better crystal forms that they crystallized a little earlier than the others.
2. Some small intrusive formations show a continuous change between coarse granite and a rock indistinguishable from the volcanic rock rhyolite, whose igneous origin is clear.

Table 15-4	Volcanoes Near Population Centers Around the World That Could Erupt at Any Time	
Region	**Country**	**Volcano**
Western Pacific	Indonesia	Merapi
	Philippines	Taal
	Japan	Unzen
	Japan	Sakurajima
Hawaii	United States	Mauna Loa
Western North America	United States	Rainier
Central America	Mexico	Colima
	Guatemala	Santa Maria/Santiaguito
	Colombia	Galeras
Mediterranean	Italy	Vesuvius
	Italy	Etna
	Greece	Santorini
East Africa	Congo	Niragongo

3. Granite is found in masses that cut across layers of sedimentary rock and from which small irregular branches penetrate into the surrounding rocks. Sometimes blocks of the sedimentary rocks are found completely engulfed by the granite.

4. That granite was at a high enough temperature to be molten is shown by the baking and recrystallization of the rocks that it intrudes.

These four types of evidence apply equally well to the other intrusive rocks.

Plutons   A **dike** is a wall of igneous rock that cuts across existing rock layers (Fig. 15-58). The largest dikes are hundreds of meters thick, but more often their thickness is between a few tenths of a meter and a few meters. The distinction between dikes and veins is that a dike is molten rock that has filled a fissure and solidified, whereas a vein consists of material deposited along a fissure from solution in water (Fig. 15-59).

Any kind of igneous rock may occur in a dike. Rapid cooling in small dikes may produce rocks similar to those of volcanic origin, and slow cooling in larger dikes gives rise to coarse-grained rocks. Dikes may cut any other kind of rock. They are often associated with volcanoes: some of the magma forces its way into cracks instead of moving upward through the central orifice. In regions of intrusive rocks, dikes are often found as offshoots of larger masses, as in Fig. 15-58. Also shown in the figure are **sills** and **laccoliths,** intrusive bodies that lie parallel to the strata in which they are found.

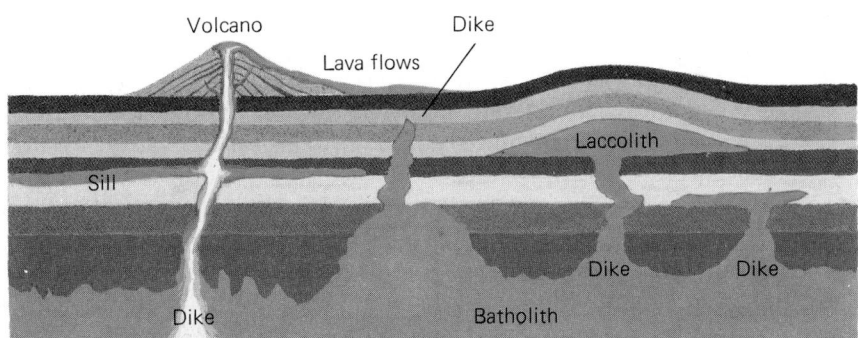

Figure 15-58   A batholith and associated dikes and sills; a laccolith and a volcano are also shown.

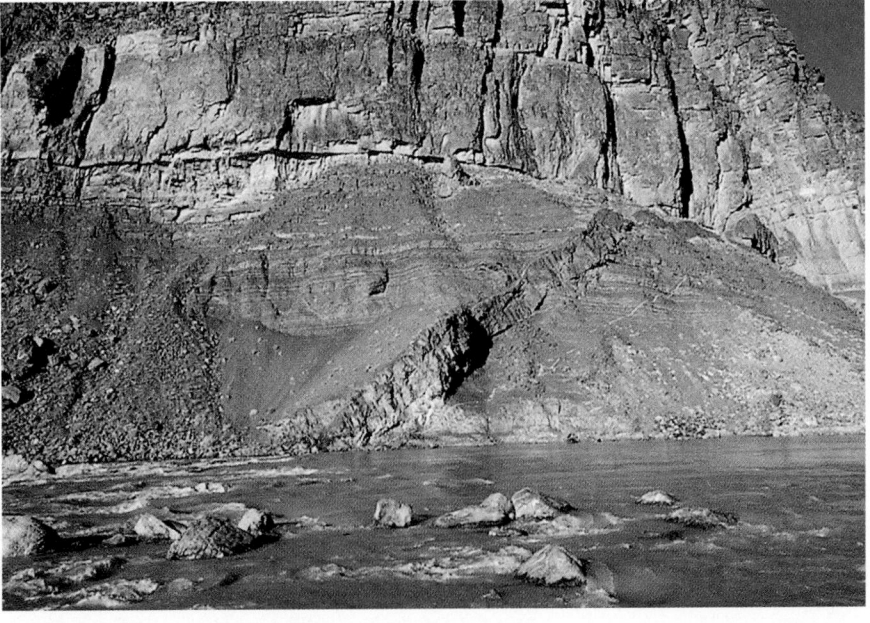

Figure 15-59   A dike of igneous rock intruded in sedimentary beds in Arizona's Grand Canyon. The beds on either side of the dike do not match, which suggests that the dike was intruded along a fault.

Batholiths are very large plutons that extend downward as much as several km. Visible exposures of batholiths cover hundreds of thousands of square km. The great batholith that forms the central part of the Sierra Nevada in California, for example, is about 800 km long and, in places, over 160 km wide. Granite is the principal rock in batholiths, although many have local patches of diorite and gabbro. Batholiths are always associated with mountain ranges, either mountains of the present or regions whose rock structure shows evidence of mountains in the distant past. The intrusion of a batholith is evidently one of the events that occurs in the process of mountain building.

Example 15.5

Suppose you find a nearly vertical contact between granite and sedimentary rocks with the sedimentary beds ending abruptly against the granite. How could you tell whether the granite had intruded into the sedimentary rocks or after solidifying had moved against the sedimentary rocks during a deformation of the crust?

Solution

If the granite had intruded the sedimentary rocks, they would show evidence of thermal metamorphism.

15.17   The Rock Cycle

Rocks Are Not Necessarily Forever

As we have seen, rocks can change from one kind to another in a variety of ways. An igneous rock, for instance, can be broken up by erosion into fragments that eventually end up in a deposit of sediments that in time lithifies into sedimentary rock. Heat and pressure can later transform this rock into a metamorphic counterpart, which may later be melted underground into magma and still later harden into an igneous rock—probably not the same as the one the cycle began with, but perhaps a cousin to it. Other life histories are also possible, as shown in Fig. 15-60.

Figure 15-60   The rock cycle. Depending upon circumstances, different transformations are possible, including the conversion of one kind of metamorphic rock into another.

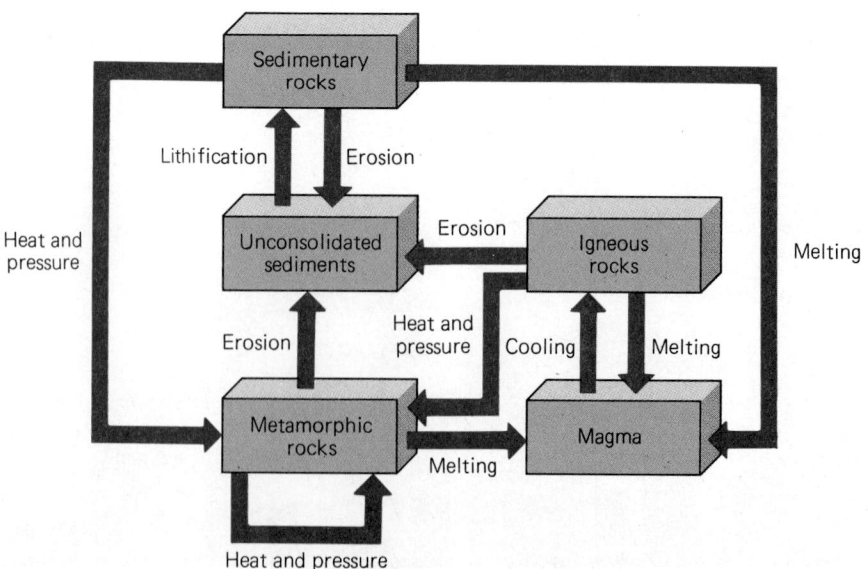

Important Terms and Ideas

The earth's outer shell of rock is called its **crust.** Oxygen and silicon are the most abundant elements in the crust. Crystalline **silicates** consist of continuous structures of oxygen and silicon ions, usually with metal ions as well. **Minerals** are the substances of which rocks are composed. The most abundant minerals are silicates; also common are carbonates and oxides. Quartz, feldspar, mica, calcite, and the ferromagnesian and clay minerals are six important kinds of minerals.

Igneous rocks (such as granite and basalt) have cooled from a molten state. **Sedimentary rocks** (such as sandstone and limestone) have consolidated from materials derived from the disintegration or solution of other rocks and deposited by water, wind, or glaciers. **Metamorphic rocks** (such as slate and marble) have been altered by heat and pressure beneath the earth's surface. **Soil** consists of rock fragments mixed with varying amounts of organic material.

Nearly all **earthquakes** are due to the sudden movement of solid rock along fracture surfaces called **faults** that are near the earth's surface. Earthquakes send out **body waves,** which pass through the earth's interior, and **surface waves,** which travel along the earth's surface. The two kinds of body waves are **P waves,** which are longitudinal, and **S waves,** which are transverse. The two kinds of surface waves are **Love waves,** which are transverse, and **Rayleigh waves,** which are rotary, like water waves.

The analysis of earthquake wave records shows that the earth's interior contains a **core,** probably consisting mainly of molten iron with a small solid inner core, and a solid **mantle** of ferromagnesian silicates. The temperature of the earth's interior increases with depth.

The **earth's magnetic field** resembles the magnetic field that would be produced by a huge bar magnet located near the earth's center. The field is due to electric currents in the molten iron core, and the direction of the field has reversed itself many times in the past.

The processes by which rocks are worn down and the debris carried away are included in the term **erosion.** The chief agent of erosion is running water, although **weathering** (the gradual disintegration of exposed rocks), **glaciers** (rivers and seas of ice formed from accumulated snow), and **groundwater** (subsurface water) also contribute. An **aquifer** is a body of porous rock through which groundwater moves. Most of the eroded material is deposited to form sediments, the bulk of which are laid down on ocean bottoms. **Lithification** refers to the gradual hardening into rock of sediments buried under later deposits.

A **volcano** is an opening in the earth's crust through which molten rock (called **magma** while underground, **lava** above ground) comes out. Intrusive bodies called **plutons** are formed by the solidification of magma under the surface.

Multiple Choice

1. The most abundant element in the earth's crust is
   a. oxygen
   b. nitrogen
   c. silicon
   d. carbon

2. The second most abundant element is
   a. iron
   b. silicon
   c. carbon
   d. aluminum

3. Minerals are
   a. silicon compounds
   b. common types of rock
   c. homogeneous solids of which rocks are composed
   d. always compounds

4. The tendency of certain minerals to split along particular planes is called
   a. foliation
   b. faulting
   c. cleavage
   d. gneiss

5. Feldspar is
   a. relatively rare in the earth's crust
   b. the most abundant mineral in the earth's crust
   c. composed of calcium carbonate
   d. similar to mica

6. Quartz is
   a. a variety of feldspar
   b. a variety of white mica
   c. composed of calcium carbonate
   d. composed of silicon dioxide

7. A mineral that is not a silicate is
   a. quartz
   b. mica
   c. feldspar
   d. calcite

8. The ferromagnesian minerals are usually
   a. transparent
   b. white or pink
   c. bluish
   d. dark green or black

9. Igneous rocks have been formed by
   a. cooling from a molten state
   b. precipitation from solution
   c. the alteration of other rocks by heat
   d. the alteration of other rocks by pressure

10. Rocks that have been altered by heat and pressure beneath the earth's surface are called
    a. igneous rocks
    b. sedimentary rocks
    c. metamorphic rocks
    d. precipitated rocks

11. Most crustal rocks
    a. were formed from compacted sediments
    b. were formed from chemical or biochemical precipitates
    c. solidified from a molten state
    d. were metamorphosed by heat and pressure under the earth's surface

12. A general characteristic of rocks of volcanic origin is
    a. the presence of shale
    b. a light color
    c. coarse-grained structure
    d. fine-grained structure

13. Foliation occurs in
    a. sedimentary rocks
    b. metamorphic rocks
    c. igneous rocks
    d. all of the above

14. An example of a foliated rock is
    a. marble   c. slate
    b. sandstone   d. granite

15. An example of a light-colored, coarse-grained intrusive igneous rock is
    a. granite   c. gneiss
    b. shale   d. basalt

16. Limestone may be metamorphosed into
    a. marble   c. gneiss
    b. quartzite   d. schist

17. Shale may be metamorphosed into
    a. marble   c. slate
    b. sandstone   d. granite

18. Mica is present in
    a. marble   c. basalt
    b. chert   d. gneiss

19. Fossils are most likely to be found in
    a. granite   c. gneiss
    b. shale   d. basalt

20. Most earthquakes are caused by shifts of rocks along faults
    a. on the earth's surface
    b. in the crust
    c. in the mantle
    d. in the core

21. Regions in which earthquakes are frequent are also regions in which
    a. the geomagnetic field is strong
    b. hurricanes are common
    c. volcanoes occur
    d. petroleum is found

22. Relative to an earthquake of magnitude 5 on the Richter scale, an earthquake of magnitude 6 releases
    a. 2 times more energy
    b. 10 times more energy
    c. 30 times more energy
    d. 100 times more energy

23. Which one or more of the following statements apply to earthquake P waves?
    a. They are back-and-forth vibrations like sound waves.
    b. They are transverse vibrations like waves in a taut string.
    c. They travel in straight lines through the earth's interior.
    d. They can pass through the earth's core.

24. The earth's crust
    a. has very nearly the same thickness everywhere
    b. varies irregularly in thickness
    c. is always thinnest under the continents
    d. is always thinnest under the oceans

25. The part of the earth with the greatest volume is the
    a. inner core   c. mantle
    b. outer core   d. crust

26. The radius of the earth's core is roughly
    a. $\frac{1}{10}$ the earth's radius
    b. $\frac{1}{4}$ the earth's radius
    c. $\frac{1}{2}$ the earth's radius
    d. $\frac{3}{4}$ the earth's radius

27. The rocks of the mantle are believed to consist largely of
    a. feldspar   c. clay minerals
    b. quartz   d. ferromagnesian minerals

28. Among the reasons why the earth's core is believed to consist mainly of molten iron is (are)
    a. the density of iron
    b. the electrical conductivity of iron
    c. the relative abundance of iron in the universe
    d. that earthquake S waves do not pass through the core

29. The chief source of the energy that powers geological processes today is
    a. the sun
    b. heat left over from the earth's formation
    c. electric currents in the earth's core
    d. radioactivity in the earth's interior

30. The earth's magnetic field
    a. never changes
    b. has reversed itself many times
    c. is centered exactly at the earth's center
    d. originates in a permanently magnetized iron core

31. If we travel around the earth, we would find that the earth's magnetic field
    a. is the same in direction and strength
    b. is the same in direction but not in strength
    c. is the same in strength but not in direction
    d. varies in both direction and strength

32. A rock readily attacked by chemical weathering is
    a. limestone
    b. obsidian
    c. granite
    d. chert

33. The principal agent of erosion is
 a. groundwater   **c.** ice
 b. running water   **d.** wind

34. Which of the following is not produced by rivers?
 a. flood plains   **c.** alluvial fans
 b. deltas   **d.** moraines

35. Glaciers produce which one or more of the following?
 a. U-shaped valleys   **c.** batholiths
 b. V-shaped valleys   **d.** caves

36. The last stage in the erosion of a river is the production of a (an)
 a. delta   **c.** moraine
 b. alluvial fan   **d.** floodplain

37. The approximate percentage of the earth's land area covered by ice today is
 a. 1 percent   **c.** 10 percent
 b. 2 percent   **d.** 30 percent

38. A fairly fast valley glacier might have a speed of
 a. 1 m/h   **c.** 1 m/month
 b. 1 m/day   **d.** 1 m/year

39. Most of the groundwater present in soil and underlying porous rocks comes from
 a. streams and rivers **c.** springs
 b. melting glaciers   **d.** rain

40. An aquifer is
 a. a river or stream on the surface
 b. an underground stream
 c. a water table
 d. a body of porous rock that contains groundwater

41. The largest amounts of sediment are deposited
 a. by glaciers   **c.** on the ocean floors
 b. on river beds   **d.** by chemical precipitation

42. Minerals deposited by groundwater in rock fissures form
 a. dikes   **c.** sills
 b. veins   **d.** moraines

43. Most caves are produced by the solvent action of groundwater on
 a. limestone   **c.** granite
 b. sandstone   **d.** schist

44. The chief constituent of volcanic gases is
 a. nitrogen   **c.** carbon dioxide
 b. oxygen   **d.** water vapor

45. Molten rock underneath the earth's surface is called
 a. magma   **c.** obsidian
 b. lava   **d.** till

46. The most common volcanic rock is
 a. granite   **c.** limestone
 b. basalt   **d.** shale

47. The holes found in most volcanic rocks are due to
 a. gases trapped in solidifying lava
 b. erosion
 c. marine organisms
 d. rapid cooling

48. Active volcanoes are not found
 a. in the West Indies
 b. in the Mediterranean region
 c. on the rim of the Pacific Ocean
 d. in eastern Canada

49. A batholith is a
 a. fissure from which groundwater emerges
 b. natural rock pillar
 c. large body of intrusive rock
 d. volcanic cone

Exercises

15.1   Composition of the Crust
15.2   Minerals

1. Arrange these elements in decreasing order of their abundance on the earth: silicon, carbon, oxygen, aluminum.

2. Do silicon compounds make up less than a quarter, between a quarter and a half, between half and three-quarters, or more than three-quarters of the mass of the crust?

3. What is the relationship between rocks and minerals?

4. What mineral is most abundant in the earth's crust? Does it make up more or less than half of the mass of the crust?

5. Both cleavage and crystal form are characteristic mineral properties. What is the difference between the two?

6. Graphite consists of layers of carbon atoms in hexagonal arrays (see Fig. 11-7), with each atom covalently bonded to three others. The layers are bonded together by van der Waals forces. Would you expect graphite to exhibit cleavage?

7. In the silicate minerals each Si^{4+} ion is always surrounded by four O^{2-} ions, yet no mineral has the formula SiO_4. Why not?

8. How could you distinguish calcite crystals from quartz crystals?

15.3   Igneous Rocks

9. Are the mineral grains in an igneous rock usually regular in form? What is the usual arrangement of the grains in an igneous rock?

10. Granite and rhyolite have similar compositions, but granite is coarse-grained whereas rhyolite is fine-grained. What does the difference in grain size indicate about the environments in which each rock formed?

11. Diorite is an igneous rock that has hardened slowly underground, and andesite, whose composition is similar, is an igneous rock that has hardened on the earth's surface. How can they be distinguished from one another?

12. Obsidian is a rock that resembles glass, in particular by sharing the property that its structure is closer to that of a liquid than to that of a crystalline solid. What does this observation suggest about the manner in which obsidian is formed?

15.4   Sedimentary Rocks

13. In what way does calcite differ from almost all other minerals? What rocks are largely calcite?

14. Of what rock do coral reefs consist?

15. What is the nature of chert and why is it so resistant to chemical and mechanical attack?

15.5   Metamorphic Rocks

16. What kind of rocks are most abundant in the earth's crust? On the earth's surface?

17. What happens to the density of a rock that undergoes metamorphism?

18. Why is gneiss the most abundant metamorphic rock?

19. The mineral grains of many metamorphic rocks are flat or elongated and occur in parallel layers. (a) What is this property called? (b) How does it originate?

20. Shale is a sedimentary rock that consolidated from mud deposits. What are the various metamorphic rocks that shale can become under progressively increasing temperature and pressure?

21. (a) What is the origin of limestone? (b) What rock is formed by the metamorphism of limestone? (c) What is the difference in structure that the metamorphism produces?

22. Distinguish between the foliation of a metamorphic rock and the stratification of a sedimentary rock.

23. Distinguish between quartz and quartzite.

24. How could you distinguish (a) chert from obsidian? (b) conglomerate from gneiss? (c) quartz from calcite?

25. How could you distinguish (a) granite from gabbro? (b) basalt from limestone? (c) schist from diorite?

26. Name the following rocks: (a) a rock consisting of intergrown crystals of quartz; (b) the rock resulting from the metamorphism of limestone; (c) an intrusive igneous rock with the same composition as andesite.

27. Name the following rocks: (a) a fine-grained, unfoliated rock with intergrowing crystals of quartz, feldspar, and black mica; (b) a finely foliated rock with microscopic crystals of quartz and white mica; (c) a fine-grained rock consisting principally of clay minerals.

15.6   Earthquakes

28. What is the difference between the focus of an earthquake and its epicenter?

29. Each step of 1 on the Richter scale of earthquake magnitude represents an increase in vibration amplitude of a factor of 10. What is the approximate increase in the energy released?

30. What can be said about an earthquake whose magnitude is 0 on the Richter scale? Whose magnitude is 8 or more?

15.7   Structure of the Earth

31. Why is the mantle thought to be solid?

32. (a) Distinguish between earthquake P and S waves. (b) Which of them can pass through the mantle? (c) Through the core?

33. In what part of the earth does the rock motion occur that causes an earthquake?

34. An earthquake occurs far from an observing station and produces P, S, and surface waves. Do all the waves arrive at the same time? If not, which arrives first and which last?

35. How does the radius of the earth's core compare with the total radius of the earth?

36. Where is the earth's crust thinnest? Where is it thickest?

15.8   The Earth's Interior

37. What evidence is there in favor of the idea that the earth's interior is very hot?

38. What is the source of the energy that powers most geological processes other than erosion?

39. (a) Why is it believed that the earth's outer core is a liquid? (b) Why is it believed that the liquid is mainly molten iron?

15.9   Geomagnetism

40. Why does a compass needle in most places not point due north?

41. Why is it unlikely that the earth's magnetic field originates in a huge bar magnet located in its interior?

15.10   Weathering

42. What is the most important mechanism of mechanical weathering?

43. Why are igneous and metamorphic rocks in general more susceptible to chemical weathering than sedimentary rocks?

44. Both marble and slate are metamorphic rocks. Would you expect a marble tombstone or a slate tombstone to be most resistant to weathering?

45. In what way is the weathering of rock important to life on earth?

15.11   Stream Erosion

46. What is the source of energy that makes possible the erosion of landscapes?

47. Is there a limit to the depth to which streams can erode a particular landscape? Is there a limit in the case of glaciers?

48. Why are streams and rivers so effective as agents of erosion on the earth's surface?

15.12 Glaciers

49. Under what circumstances does a glacier form?

50. Which is the more important agent of erosion today, running water or glaciers? Why?

51. What agent of erosion produces valleys with a V-shaped cross section? A U-shaped cross section?

52. How is it possible for glaciers to wear down rocks that are harder than glacial ice?

15.13 Groundwater

53. What is a water table? An aquifer?

54. What is the immediate destination of most of the water that falls as rain on land?

15.14 Sedimentation

55. What is the eventual site of deposition of most sediments?

56. Distinguish between an alluvial fan and a moraine.

57. Why are clay minerals and quartz particles abundant in sediments that have not been chemically deposited?

58. In sand derived from the attack of waves on granite, what mineral would you expect to be most abundant?

59. What is the probable origin of the following sedimentary rocks?

 a. A thick limestone

 b. A conglomerate with well-rounded boulders and numerous thin beds of sandy and clayey material

 c. A sandstone consisting of well-sorted, well-rounded grains of quartz

15.15 Volcanoes

60. What characteristic landscape features do active volcanoes produce? From what features could you conclude that volcanoes were once active in a region where eruptions have long since ceased?

61. What kinds of rocks are likely to be found in lava flows? What is the most common volcanic rock?

62. What factors determine the viscosity of a magma? What kinds of landscapes are produced by volcanoes whose lavas have relatively high and relatively low viscosities?

63. What is the cause of the holes found in many volcanic rocks?

64. What is the main constituent of volcanic gases?

15.16 Intrusive Rocks

65. (a) Why are metamorphic rocks often found near plutons? (b) Where would you expect to find the wider zone of thermal metamorphism, near a dike or near a batholith?

66. Distinguish between a dike and a vein.

16

The Evolving Earth

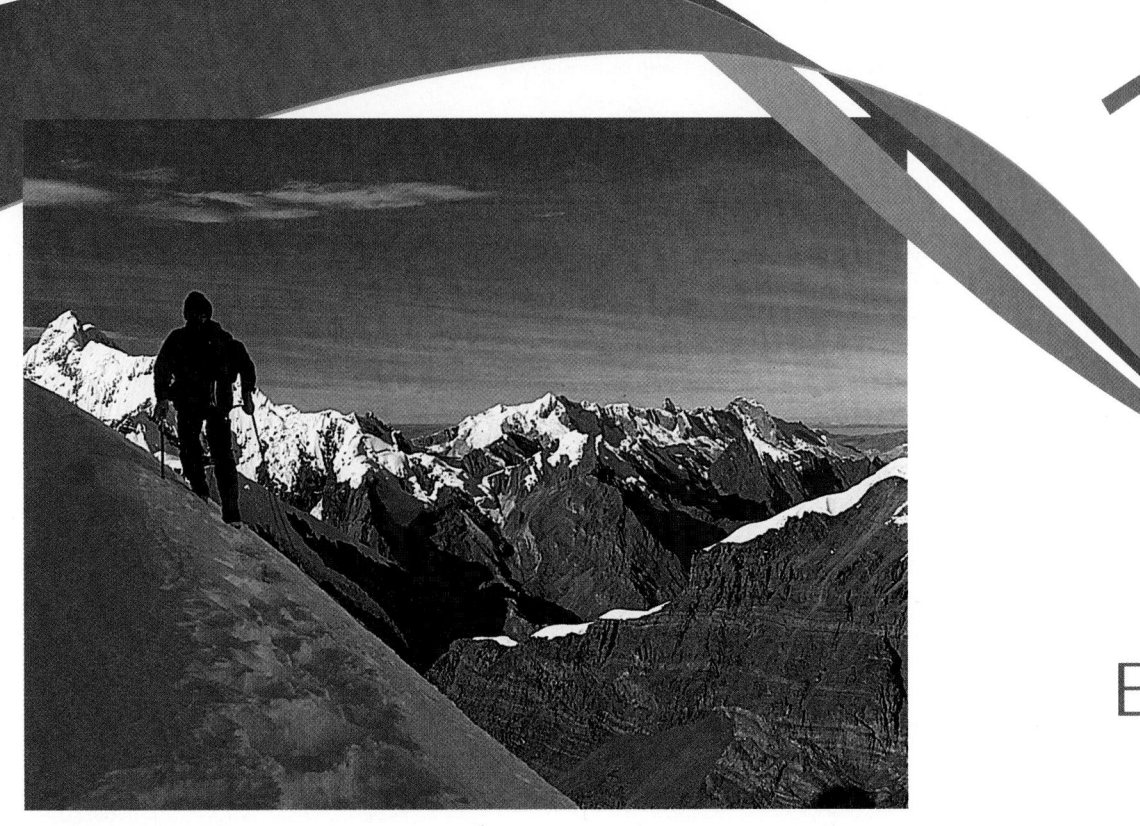

The Andes Mountains of South America are relatively young.

GOALS

When you have finished this chapter you should be able to complete the goals
• given for each section below:

Nothing about the earth is fixed, permanent, unchanging. What is today a great mountain that pierces the sky may in the future be nibbled down into a mere hill, while elsewhere an undersea mass of sediments may be thrust upward into a lofty plateau. How do we know that such things can happen? After all, though plenty of geologic activity is taking place around us, for the most part the pace is exceedingly slow. Only after millions of years can the processes now at work yield large-scale changes in the pattern of the continents and in their landscapes. What justifies the belief that the earth's crust never stops evolving is the record of the past, a record that can be read in the rocks of the present.

During the past few decades a major advance has occurred in our understanding of the large-scale forces that shape and reshape the earth's crust. The notion that the continents are slowly drifting relative to one another—a notion going back three-quarters of a century but largely scorned for most of that period—has turned out to be the only way to explain a variety of striking observations. These same observations also provide clues as to what makes the continents drift. So far-reaching are the implications of the new dynamic picture of the crust, and so suddenly did they come to light, that it is legitimate to speak of a revolution in geologic thought.

Tectonic Movement

Terra firma, the solid earth, is a symbol of stability and strength. On foundations of rock we anchor our buildings, our dams, our bridges. The massive rock of mountain ranges seems strong enough to withstand any force.

Yet even casual observation shows how naive such notions of the earth's stability are. High up on mountainsides we find shells of marine animals, shells that can be there only if rock formed beneath the sea has been lifted far above sea level. Sedimentary rocks, which must have been deposited originally in horizontal layers, are found tilted at steep angles or folded into arches and basins. Other layers have broken along cracks, and the fractured ends have moved apart. Gigantic forces must occur in the crust in order to lift, bend, and break even the strongest rocks. Such forces and the changes they cause are called **tectonic** (from the Greek word for "carpenter").

16.1   Types of Deformation

Faults and Folds, Tilts and Warps, Rises and Falls

Cracks are found in rock formations of all kinds, some due to molten rock contracting as it cools and others due to mechanical stresses in the crust. A fracture surface along which motion has taken place is called a **fault.** In a rock outcrop a fault appears as a fairly straight line against which sedimentary layers and other structures end abruptly (Fig. 16-1). Near the fault, layers may be bent or crumpled, and along the fault streaks of finely powdered material may have developed from friction during movement. Three important kinds of fault are shown in Fig. 16-2.

Movement along faults usually takes place as a series of small, sudden displacements, with intervals of years or centuries between successive jerks. An immediate effect of displacement along a reverse fault or normal fault is a small cliff. Erosion then attacks the cliff and may level it before the next movement. If successive movements follow one another fast enough, erosion may not be able to keep up, with a high cliff as the result. Cliffs of this sort are called **fault scarps.** Good examples of scarps produced by

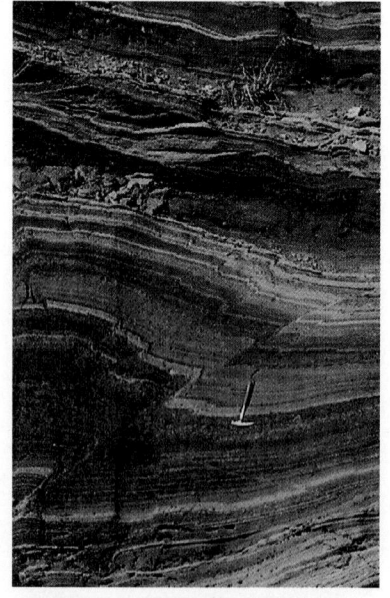

Figure 16-1   Reverse fault in sandstone near Klamath Falls, Oregon. A reverse fault occurs when a rock mass moves upward relative to adjacent rock.

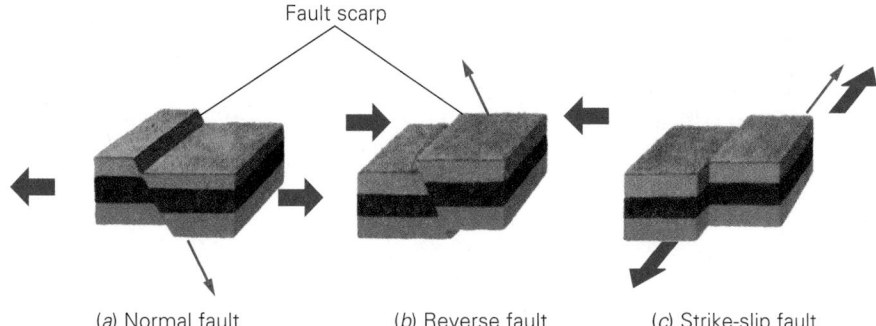

(a) Normal fault   (b) Reverse fault   (c) Strike-slip fault

Figure 16-2   (a) A normal fault is an inclined surface along which a rock mass has slipped downward; it is the result of forces that tend to stretch the earth's crust. (b) A reverse fault is an inclined surface along which a rock mass has moved upward to override the neighboring mass; it is the result of forces that tend to compress the crust. (c) A strike-slip fault is a surface along which one rock has moved horizontally with respect to the other; it is the result of oppositely directed forces in the crust that do not act along the same line. Erosion modifies the fault scarps left by normal and reverse faults.

normal faults are the steep mountain fronts of many of the desert ranges in Utah, Nevada, and eastern California. A more deeply eroded scarp produced by reverse faulting is the eastern front of the Rocky Mountains in Glacier National Park.

Folding takes place by slow, continuous movement, in contrast to the sudden displacements along faults (Figs. 16-3 and 16-4). Sometimes folding produces hills and depressions in the landscape directly, but more often erosion keeps pace with folding. Indirectly folds affect landforms by exposing tilted beds of varying degrees of resistance to the action of streams, so that long, parallel ridges and valleys develop, like those of the Appalachian Mountains (see Fig. 15-44). In these mountains, as in many others, the folding is very ancient. The present ridges are due to deep erosion after successive uplifts of the stumps of the old folds.

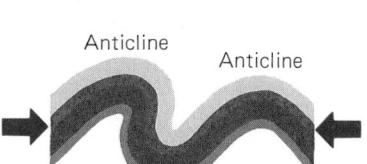

Figure 16-3   Cross section showing effect of folding in horizontal strata. Folds always shorten the crust and hence are produced by compressional forces. An anticline is an arch (a fold convex upward), and a syncline is a trough (a fold convex downward). In regions of intense folding, anticlines and synclines follow one another in long series.

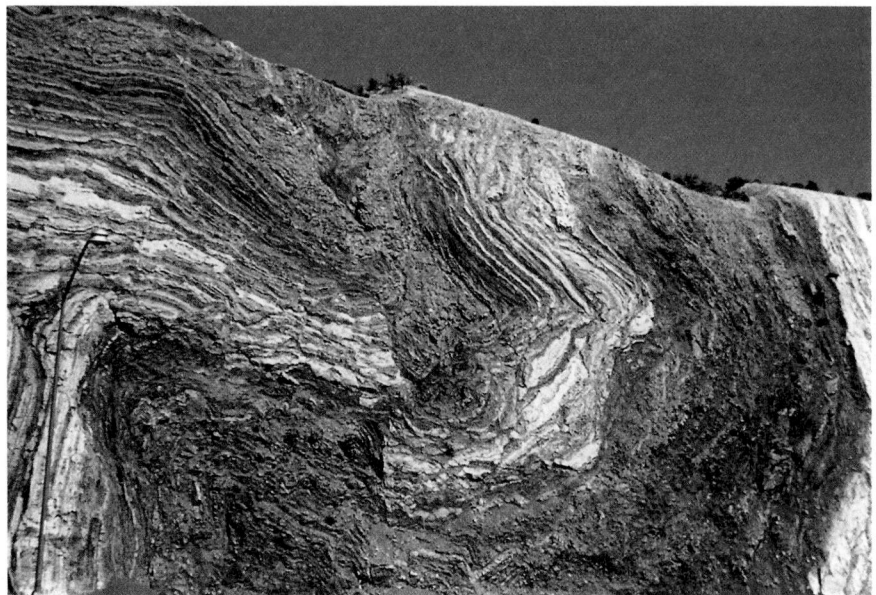

Figure 16-4   Folded shale beds near Palmdale, California.

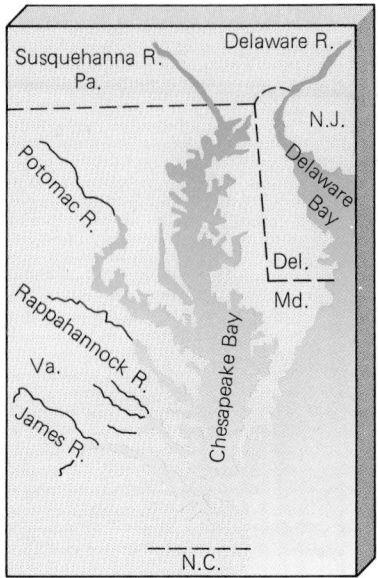

Figure 16-5 Drowned valleys on the Atlantic Coast of the United States.

Large-Scale Movements Large-scale crustal movements may involve whole continents or large parts of them, which may rise or fall, tilt or warp. Such events are occurring today as they have in the past. Coastal features in many parts of the world provide obvious evidence. For instance, a wave-cut cliff and terrace high above the present shore means that the coast there has been raised in fairly recent times, or stream erosion would have eaten these features away.

The sinking of land with respect to sea level is shown by long, narrow bays that fill the mouths of large stream valleys. A body of water like Chesapeake Bay (Fig. 16-5) could not be formed by wave erosion, since wave attack normally straightens a coastline rather than deeply indenting it. Instead, the shape of the bay suggests that it lies in a stream-carved valley whose lower part has been submerged beneath the sea. Elsewhere in the landscapes and sedimentary rocks of the United States a multitude of regional movements are recorded.

16.2 Mountain Building

The Rock Record Tells a Complicated Story

Mountains can form in a number of ways. Some mountains are accumulations of lava and fragmental material ejected by a volcano. Others are small blocks of the earth's crust raised along faults (Fig. 16-6). But the great mountain ranges of the earth, like the Appalachians, the Rockies, the Alps, and the Himalayas (where all 10 of the world's highest mountains are located), have a much longer and more complex history involving sedimentation, folding, faulting, igneous activity, repeated uplifts, and deep erosion. How the forces originate that push together and pull apart, lift and depress parts of the earth's crust is one of the principal themes of this chapter.

The layers of sedimentary rock in a mountain range are usually thicker than layers of similar age found under adjacent plains. Most of the layers in both mountains and plains, as shown by their sedimentary structures and their fossils, were formed from deposits that accumulated in shallow seas or on low-lying parts of the land—that is, on surfaces not far above or below sea level. As deposition continued, the surface must have been slowly sinking at

Figure 16-6 The Teton mountain range in Wyoming came into being when the eastern end of a crustal block was raised along a fault. As a result the Teton range slopes gradually toward the west from a steep eastern front (shown here). The rugged landscape is largely the result of extensive glacial erosion in the past.

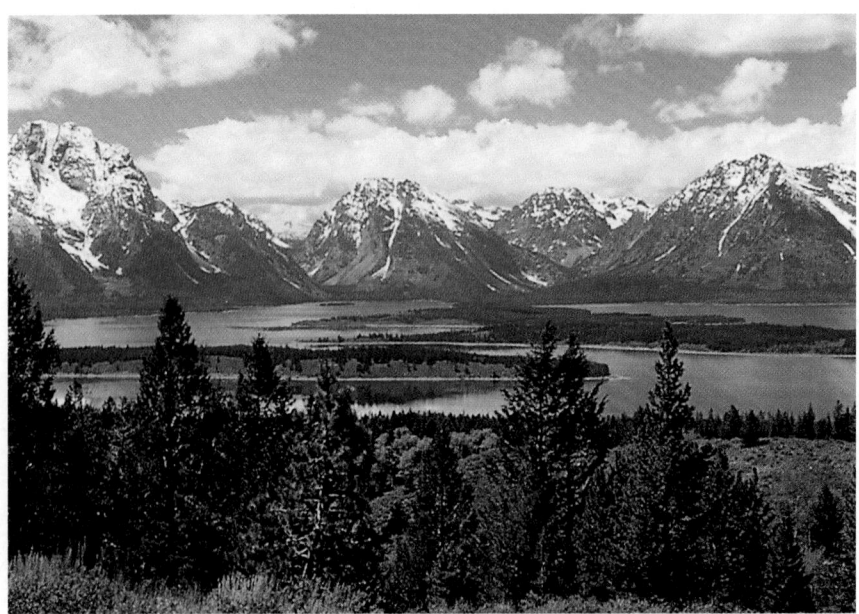

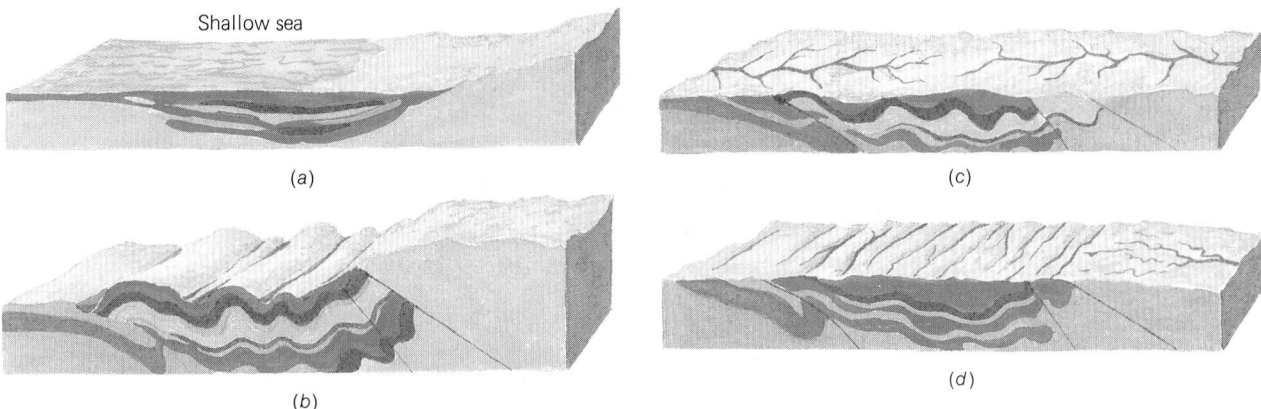

Figure 16-7 Successive stages in the evolution of the Appalachian Mountains. (*a*) Sediments accumulating in the Appalachian basin; (*b*) folding and reverse faulting of rocks in the basin; (*c*) original mountains worn down to a nearly level plain by stream erosion; (*d*) renewed erosion of the folded strata following vertical uplift, producing the parallel ridges and valleys of the present landscape.

the same time. The greater thickness of the strata in the present mountain area means that this part of the earth's surface was sinking more rapidly than nearby areas.

Besides their thickness, another conspicuous feature of the sedimentary rocks in major mountain ranges is their complex structure (Fig. 16-7). They are crumpled by intense folding and locally broken along huge reverse faults and minor normal faults. Thus in the development of a mountain range the next step must be a period in which the piled-up sediments are subjected to intense compressional forces that act horizontally. The compression raises the folded layers high above the sea, and erosion begins to wear down the exposed beds as folding continues. The appearance of most present-day mountain landscapes is not due directly to the compressions that folded and faulted their rocks but instead to erosion between periodic uplifts.

16.3 Continental Drift

An Evolving Jigsaw Puzzle

A glance at a map of the world suggests that at some time in the past the continents may have been joined together in one or two giant supercontinents. If the margins of the continents are taken to be on their continental slopes (see Fig. 14-36) at a depth of 900 m instead of their present sea-level boundaries, the fit between North and South America, Africa, Greenland, and western Europe is remarkably exact, as Fig. 16-8 shows.

But merely matching up outlines of continents is not by itself proof that the continents have migrated around the globe. A detailed hypothesis of continental drift was proposed almost a century ago by Alfred Wegener, building on the work of others before him, who based his argument on biological and geologic evidence.

Wegener was troubled by the parallel evolution of living things. Going back through the ages, the fossil record shows that, until about 200 million years ago, whenever a new species appeared, it did so in many now-distant regions where suitable habitats existed. Evolution, in other words, proceeded at the same rate and in the same way in continents and oceans that today are widely separated. Only in the last 200 million years have plants and animals in the different continents developed in markedly different ways.

Figure 16-8 How some of the continents fit together. The boundary of each continent is taken at a depth of 900 m on its continental slope; the tan regions represent land above sea level at present, and the light orange regions represent submerged land on the continental shelf and slope. Overlaps are shown in dark orange and gaps in blue.

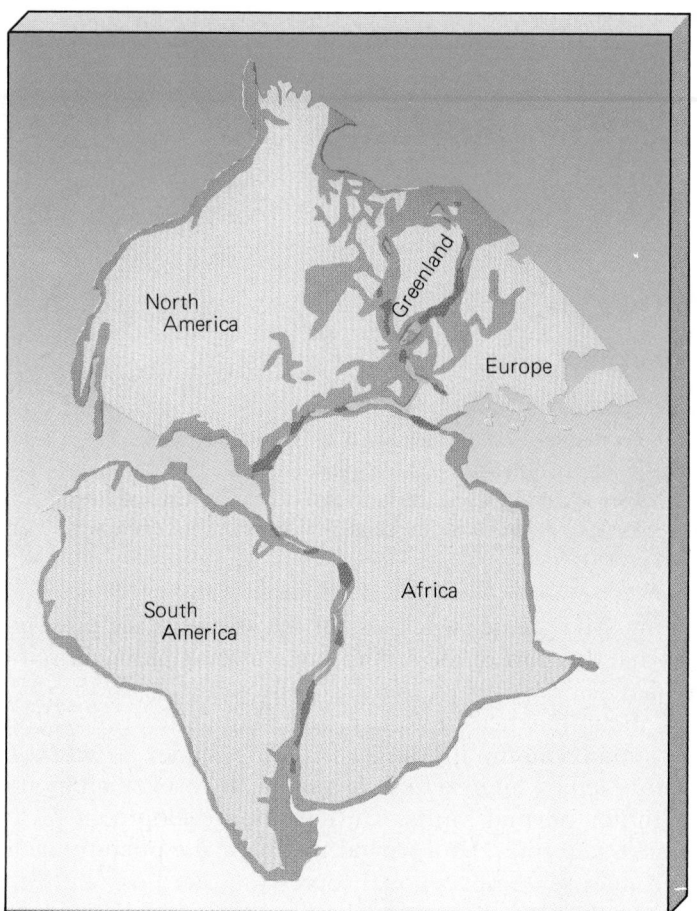

Pangaea   Wegener brought back an earlier idea that the continents were once all part of one huge landmass he called **Pangaea** ("all earth"). Then Pangaea broke up, and the continents slowly drifted to their present locations. This model found additional support in geologic data regarding prehistoric climates. Somewhat over 200 million years ago South Africa, India, Australia, and part of South America were burdened with great ice sheets, while at the same time a tropical rain forest covered North America, Europe, and China. At various other times, there was sufficient vegetation in Alaska and Antarctica for coal deposits to have resulted, and so currently frigid a place as Baffin Bay, which lies between Canada and Greenland, was a desert.

Wegener and his followers examined what was known about the climates of the distant past and tried to arrange the continents in each geologic period so that the glaciers of that period were near the poles and the hot regions were near the equator. Their efforts were, in general, quite successful, and in some cases startlingly so. Deposits of glacial debris and fossil remains of certain distinctive plant species follow each other in the same succession in Argentina, Brazil, South Africa, Antarctica, India, and Australia, for example. A recent discovery of this kind was the identification of a skull of the reptile Lystrosaurus in a sandstone layer in the Alexandra mountain range of Antarctica. This creature, which was about 90 cm long, flourished long ago in Africa.

Laurasia and Gondwana   Today it seems clear that Pangaea did exist. About 200 million years ago it began to break apart into two supercontinents,

BIOGRAPHY | Alfred Wegener (1880–1930)

Wegener was a German meteorologist with a special interest in the Arctic. He participated in four expeditions to Greenland and died on the last of them. Like others before him, going back 3 centuries, Wegener was struck by the apparent fit of the continents shown in Fig. 16-8, but unlike them he went on to develop biological and geological arguments to support the notion that the continents had once been united.

Wegener did not stop with tracing the subsequent movements of the continents but also considered other effects of their motions. He believed that mountain ranges were forced up by pressure on the leading edges of the drifting continents, with the Rockies and Andes as examples. The trailing edges of the drifting continents, in Wegener's view, left behind fragments that ended up as such island arcs as the West Indies.

Wegener first presented his ideas in 1912 and continued to refine them until his death. Some geologists were immediately attracted by the boldness and comprehensiveness of his scheme. Others were strongly opposed, at least partly because Wegener, a meteorologist, seemed to them an outsider heedlessly trying to overthrow established geological concepts. Doubters of Wegener explained the similarity of patterns of early life around the world by postulating a series of land bridges linking the continents. But no traces of such bridges were ever found.

As for the mountains, it was widely believed that the earth was in the process of shrinking, with its surface becoming wrinkled the way a baked apple does as its water content evaporates. But the massive earth cannot contract as a baked apple does: the wrinkles of its continents can only have been produced by horizontal forces.

A more serious objection to continental drift was Wegener's inability to come up with a convincing mechanism for pushing the continents around. Today such a mechanism is known, and even though he got some details seriously wrong, Wegener now can be seen as a brilliant pioneer and not

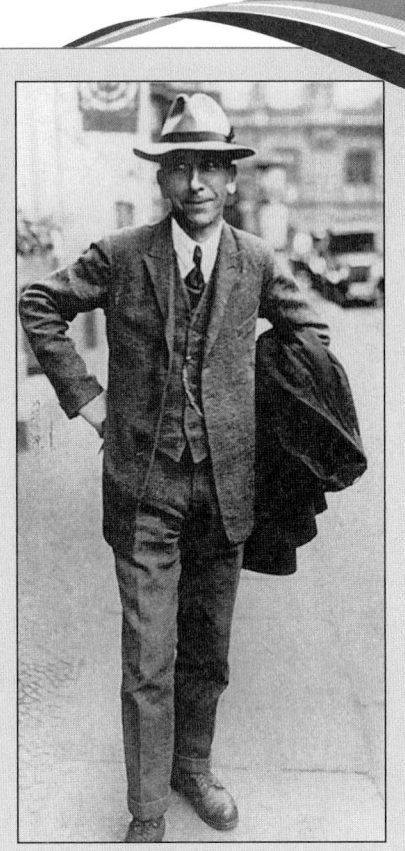

as the "pseudo-scientist" his opponents called him.

Laurasia (which consisted of what is now North America, Greenland, and most of Eurasia) and **Gondwana** (South America, Africa, Antarctica, India, and Australia). Laurasia and Gondwana were almost equal in size (Fig. 16-9). The separation of Pangaea into these supercontinents is supported by detailed geologic and biological evidence, for instance the differences between Laurasian and Gondwana fossils of the same age after the breakup.

Laurasia and Gondwana were separated by a body of water called the **Tethys Sea.** Today a little of the Tethys Sea survives as the Mediterranean, Caspian, and Black Seas. Its original extent can be gauged from the sediments that were subsequently uplifted to form the mountain ranges that stretch from Gibraltar eastward to the Pacific. The Pyrenees, Alps, and Caucasus of Europe, the Atlas Mountains of North Africa, and the Himalayas of Asia all were once part of the Tethys Sea.

Not long after Pangaea divided into Laurasia and Gondwana, the supercontinents themselves started to break up. The North Atlantic and Indian Oceans were the first to open, followed by the South Atlantic. Perhaps 80 million years ago Greenland began to move away from North America; 45 million years ago Australia split off from Antarctica and India finished its journey north to Asia; and 20 million years ago Arabia separated from Africa.

Figure 16-9   The landmasses of the earth as they may have appeared in the past and as they are today. The breakup of Pangaea into Laurasia and Gondwana began about 200 million years ago. There is evidence of even earlier continental drift, possibly as far back as 3.8 billion years ago.

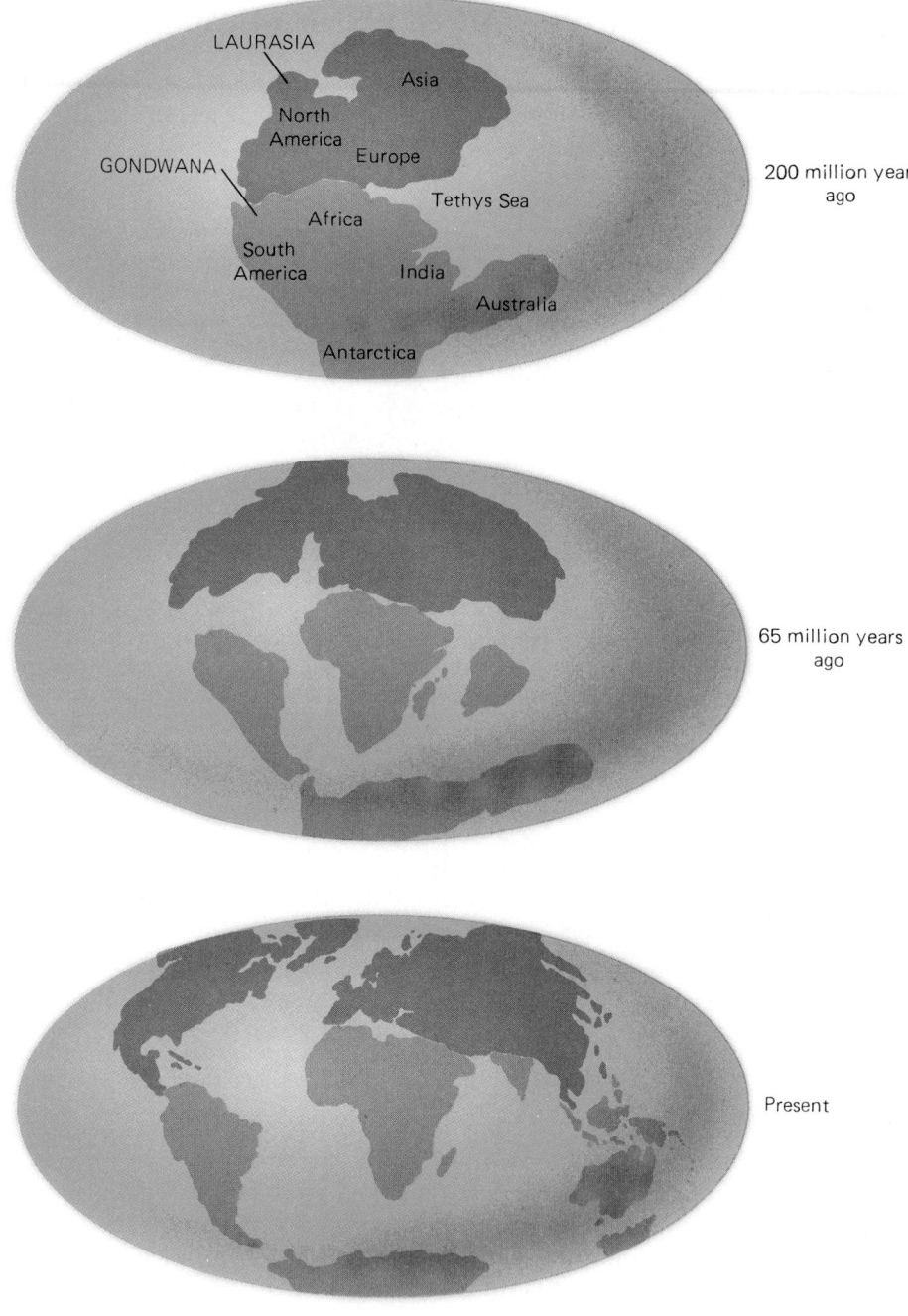

Plate Tectonics

"Continental drift" is not too accurate a description because the continents turn out to be merely passengers on a number of rigid rock plates that are continually moving across the face of the earth. Before we examine how this motion occurs and what its consequences are, we must first see why it is possible in the first place.

16.4   Lithosphere and Asthenosphere

A Hard Layer over a Soft Layer

At the heart of all current explanations for major crustal changes is the idea that the mantle of the earth is not a stiff structure, like the crust, but rather contains a layer near the top that is able to flow.

Why Continents Have Deep Roots

The notion of a relatively soft asthenosphere makes it possible to understand both why the continents are raised above the rest of the crust and why the crust is much thicker beneath them than beneath the oceans (see Fig. 15-33).

Suppose that we place several blocks of wood of different sizes in a pool of water. The larger blocks float higher than the smaller while simultaneously extending down farther into the water (Fig. 16-10). Thus, if the lithosphere with its continents is imagined as floating on a denser asthenosphere, we can refer for guidance to the floating wooden blocks. This analogy suggests that exceptionally high regions—mountain ranges and plateaus—have roots that extend far downward.

Such is actually the case; in fact, its discovery led the British scientist George Airy a century ago to propose the floating of the entire lithosphere.

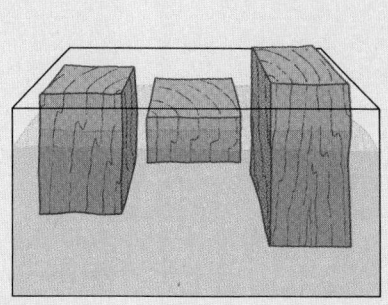

Figure 16-10   Large blocks of wood float higher and extend farther downward than smaller blocks of wood. This is why the thicker continental crust extends lower into the mantle than the oceanic crust, as shown in Fig. 15-33.

The crust and the outermost part of the mantle together make up a shell of hard rock mostly 50 to 100 km thick called the **lithosphere.** The lithosphere has no sharp boundary, as the crust does, but gradually turns into the softer **asthenosphere,** a region 100 to 200 km thick. (*Lithos* means "rock" in Greek and *astheno* means "weak.") The asthenosphere is soft because its material is close to the melting point at the temperature and pressure found at such depths. Above the asthenosphere the temperature is too low and below it the pressure is too high for the material to deform easily.

The speeds of earthquake waves in the crust are different from their speeds in the mantle, which suggests that the two regions differ in their compositions or crystal structures or both. The difference between the lithosphere and the asthenosphere instead lies in their degrees of rigidity. In response to suddenly applied forces, the asthenosphere behaves like a solid and so can transmit the transverse S waves of earthquakes, for example. But when forces act on the asthenosphere over long periods of time, it responds like a thick, viscous fluid.

16.5 The Ocean Floors

The Youngest Part of the Crust

The mountains and valleys, plains and plateaus of the continents were mapped long ago, and few surprises are in store for future explorers. But the continents occupy less than 30 percent of the area of the earth's crust, while the rest lies hidden in darkness thousands of meters under the seas and oceans. Only in the past few decades have the floors of the oceans been studied and their physical characteristics determined. It is largely these findings that have clarified the evolution of the crust.

Methods used to investigate the ocean floors are not particularly subtle—the real problem is the vastness of the area to be covered. These days depths are charted by means of echo sounders. An instrument of this kind sends out a pulse of high-frequency sound waves and the time needed for the pulse to reach the seafloor, be reflected there, and then return to the surface is a measure of how deep the water is (Fig. 7-13). A variant of this method reveals something of the structure of the sea floor itself. What is done is to set off an explosive charge in the water and study the returning echoes—one echo will come from the top of the sediment layer, and a later one from the hard rock underneath.

Samples of the seafloor can be obtained by dropping a hollow tube to the bottom on a long cable and then pulling it up filled with a core of the sediments into which it sank. Longer sediment cores can be obtained by drilling. These sediments can be examined later in the laboratory for their composition, their age, their fossil content, their magnetization, and so forth (Fig. 16-11). Another important technique is to tow a magnetometer behind a survey ship to obtain an idea of the direction and intensity of the magnetization of the rocks of the ocean floor over wide areas.

Four Important Findings   Four findings about ocean floors have proved of crucial importance:

1. The ocean floors are, geologically speaking, very young. The oldest oceanic crust dates back only about 200 million years, in contrast to continental rocks that date back as much as 3800 million years. Many parts of the ocean floor are much younger still, so that about one-third of the earth's surface has come into existence in $1\frac{1}{2}$ percent of the earth's history.

2. A worldwide system of narrow **ridges** and somewhat broader **rises** runs across the oceans (Fig. 16-12). An example is the Mid-Atlantic Ridge, which runs down the Atlantic Ocean from north to south. Iceland, the Azores, Ascension Island, and Tristan da Cunha are some of the higher peaks in this ridge. These ridges are offset at intervals by fracture zones that indicate sideways shifts of the ocean floors.

3. There is also a system of **trenches** several kilometers deep that rims much of the Pacific Ocean. These trenches parallel the belts in which most of today's earthquakes and volcanoes occur. Some of the trenches have **island arcs** on their landward sides that consist largely of volcanic mountains projecting above sea level.

4. The direction in which ocean-floor rocks are magnetized is the same along strips parallel to the midocean ridges, but the direction is reversed from strip to strip going away from a ridge on either side (Fig. 16-13).

Figure 16-11   Samples from a core of sediments extracted from the ocean floor are removed for examination. The record of the past is most complete in marine sediments.

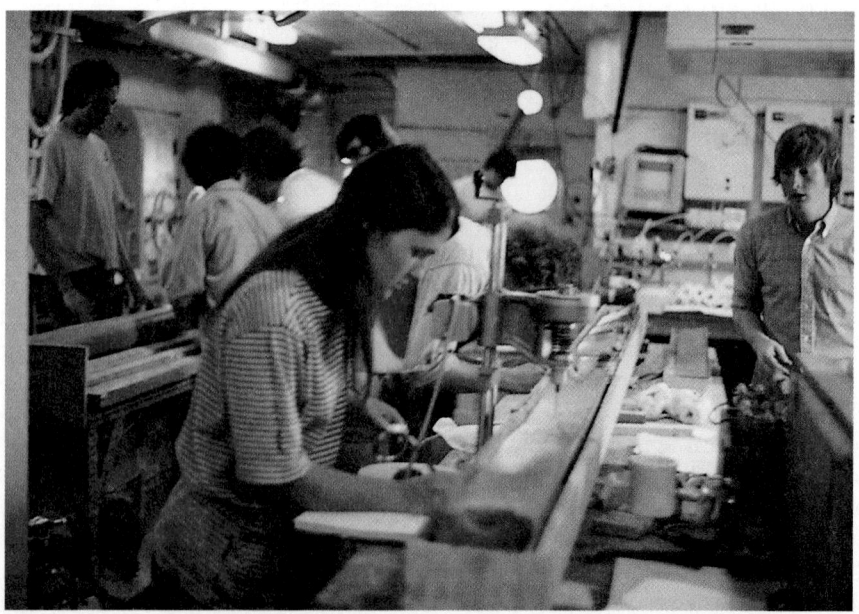

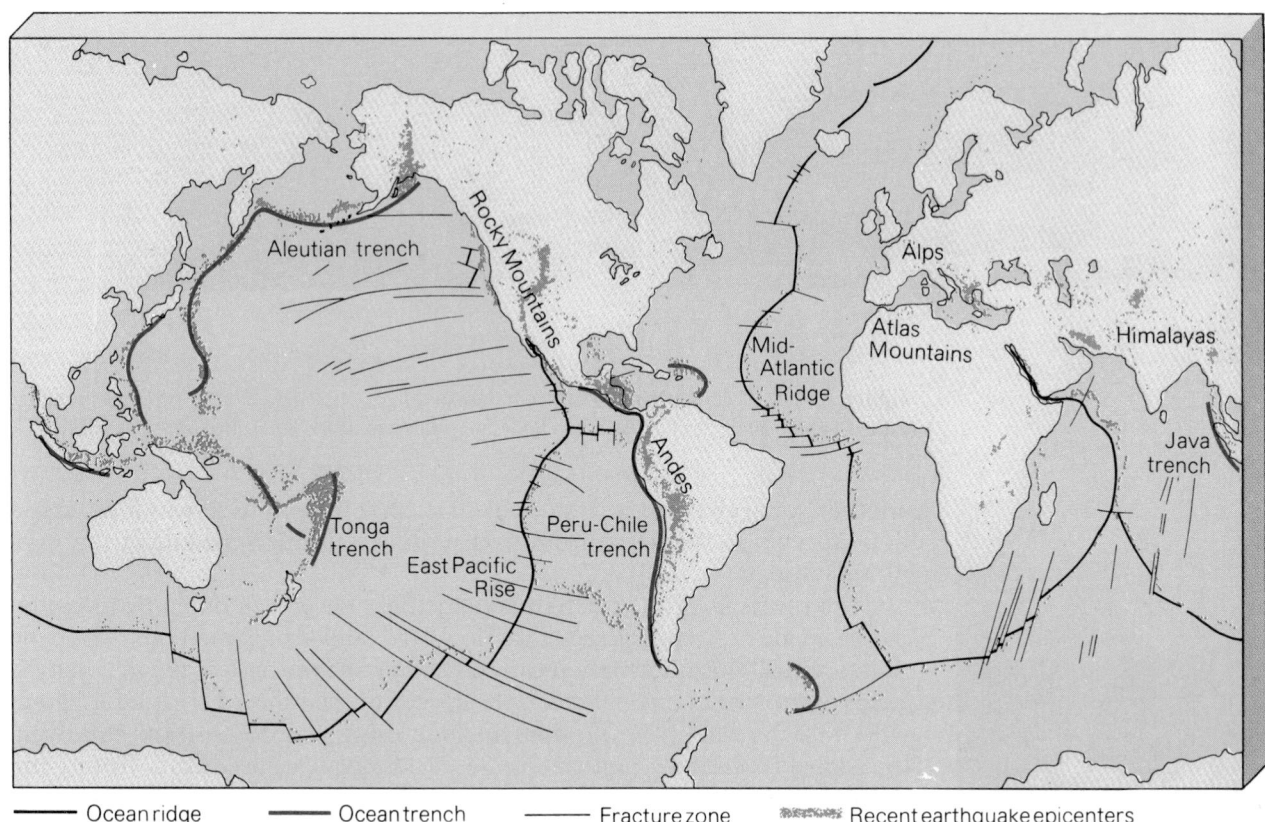

— Ocean ridge   — Ocean trench   — Fracture zone   ▨▨▨ Recent earthquake epicenters

Figure 16-12   The worldwide system of oceanic ridges, rises, and trenches. The ridges and rises are offset by transverse fracture zones. The American oceanographers Marie Tharp and Bruce Heezen were pioneers in identifying these features of the ocean floors.

16.6   Ocean-Floor Spreading

Alternate Magnetization Is the Proof

The first step toward understanding the above observations was taken in the early 1960s by the American geologists Harry H. Hess and Robert S. Dietz, who independently proposed that the ocean floors are spreading. (A similar hypothesis was put forward in 1928 by Arthur Holmes in England, but it remained practically unnoticed because supporting data were lacking.)

The basic idea of ocean-floor spreading is that molten rock is continually rising up along the midocean ridges (Figs. 16-14 and 16-15). The parts of the lithosphere on either side of a ridge move apart at speeds of a few centimeters per year—about as fast as fingernails grow—with the new material filling the gap as it hardens.

The fourth key observation mentioned earlier, which concerns the magnetization of rocks on either side of an ocean ridge, confirms the hypothesis of seafloor spreading in a convincing way. As Fig. 16-13 shows in the case of a portion of the Mid-Atlantic Ridge southwest of Iceland, successive strips of rock lying parallel to the ridge are magnetized in alternate directions.

To interpret this pattern, we draw upon the fact that the earth's magnetic field has periodically reversed itself many times in the past (see Sec. 15.9). What must have been happening is clear. As molten rock, unmagnetized in its liquid state, comes to the surface of the crust at a ridge, it hardens and the iron content of its minerals becomes magnetized in the same direction as that of the geomagnetic field at the time. When the direction of the geomagnetic field reverses, the new molten rock that cools then becomes magnetized in the opposite direction. Thus strips of alternate magnetization follow one

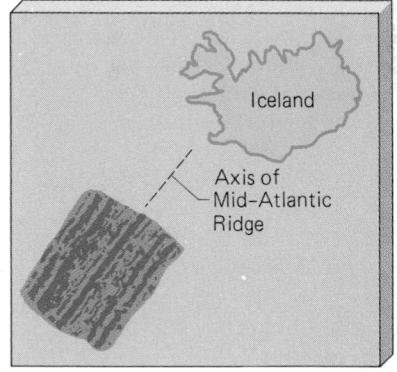

Figure 16-13   Pattern of magnetization along the Mid-Atlantic Ridge southwest of Iceland. Seafloor rocks whose directions of magnetization are the same as that of today's geomagnetic field are shown in dark blue; the intervening spaces represent rocks whose magnetization is in the opposite direction.

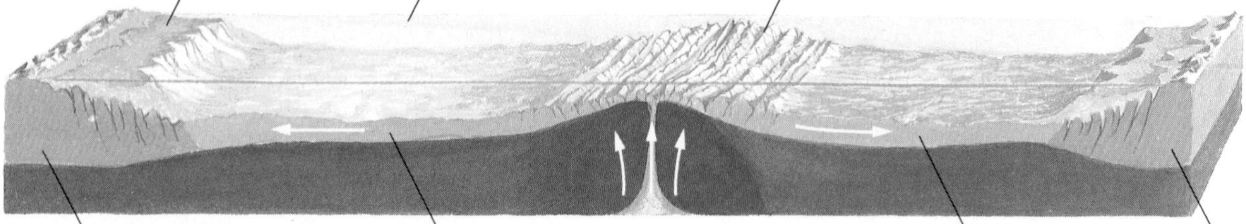

Continental shelf   Ocean   Midocean ridge

Continental crust   Oceanic crust   Oceanic crust   Continental crust

Figure 16-14   Ocean-floor spreading. A midocean ridge forms where molten rock rises from the asthenosphere along a rift in the ocean floor and pushes apart the lithosphere on both sides.

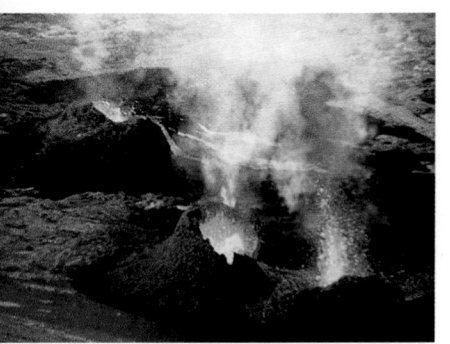

Figure 16-15   The island of Surtsey came into being in 1963 as a volcano that grew from the sea south of Iceland on the Mid-Atlantic Ridge. Molten rock rises to become new oceanic crust along this ridge, which forms the boundary between the North Atlantic and Eurasian plates. These plates are moving apart at about 1 cm per year.

another going away on both sides from a ridge. Iceland itself was formed less than 70 million years ago from magma rising through the rift in the Mid-Altantic Ridge.

The reversals of the earth's magnetic field have been dated by measurements made on magnetized lava flows on land using methods based on radioactivity. This information can be used to find the ages of the magnetized strips of the seafloor, which gives the speeds of the lithospheric plates. Other ways to determine plate motions include using precise position data from the Global Positioning System (see Sec. 2.14). Typical speeds vary from 1 cm/year in the North Atlantic Ocean to 10 cm/year in the Pacific. The record is 15 cm/year near Easter Island—about as fast as the hair on your head grows.

16.7   Plate Tectonics

How the Continents Drift

Although the ocean floors are spreading at the midocean ridges, the earth as a whole does not expand. The spread of the ocean floors must therefore be balanced by other large-scale processes in the lithosphere. The study of these processes, which do not occur on any other planet, and their consequences has come to be known as **plate tectonics.**

The starting point of plate tectonics is the observation that the lithosphere is split not only along the ridges of the ocean floors but also along the trenches and fracture zones of Fig. 16-12. These cracks divide the lithosphere into seven huge **plates** and a number of smaller ones, all of which float on the plastic asthenosphere (Fig. 16-16).

New lithosphere is created where plates move apart at the midocean ridges, as we saw in Fig. 16-14. Where plates come together, on the other hand, lithosphere may be destroyed: the edge of one of the plates may slide under the edge of the other and partially melt upon reaching the hot asthenosphere. Figure 16-17 shows the three possible kinds of collision. To understand what is happening, we must keep in mind that continental crust (largely granitic rock) is less dense than oceanic crust (largely basaltic rock).

1. **Oceanic-continental plate collision.** When a plate whose edge is covered with oceanic crust moves against a plate whose edge is covered with continental crust, the denser oceanic slab slides underneath the continental slab (Fig. 16-17a). The region of contact is called a **subduction zone,** and a trench is formed there. Some of the oceanic slab melts in the asthenosphere, and magma from the lighter materials in the slab is carried upward by its buoyancy. The magma rises through cracks in the

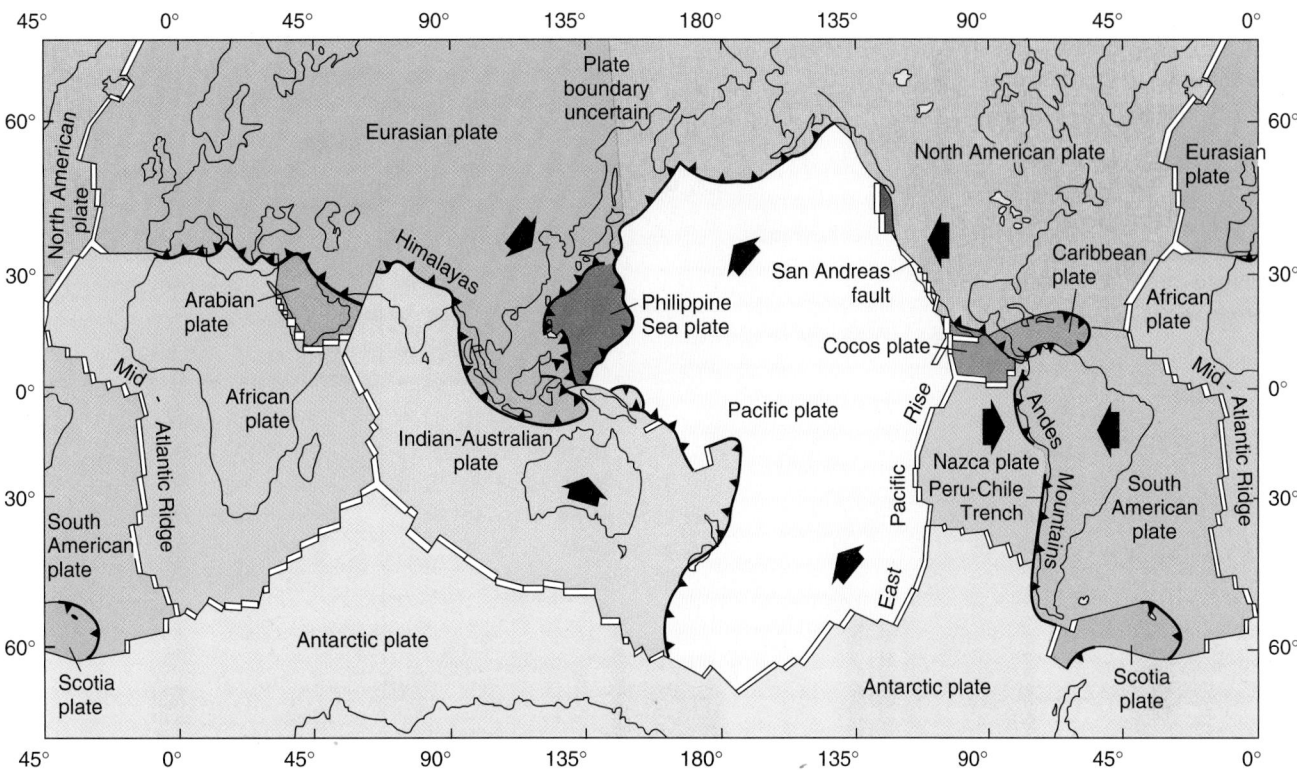

Figure 16-16 The chief lithospheric plates whose motion results in continental drift. The arrows show the directions of plate motions; the African plate is thought to be stationary. Diverging plate boundaries are shown as double lines. Converging boundaries are shown as heavy lines with triangles that point down subduction zones. Transform boundaries are shown as single lines. Because Japan lies on or near the intersections of four plates, one-tenth of the world's earthquakes rock its islands.

continental plate above to produce volcanoes at the surface and bodies of intrusive rock below the surface. An example of such a collision occurs at the western edge of South America, where the oceanic Nazca plate (which is moving eastward) meets the continental South American plate (which is moving westward). The result is a trench along the coasts of Peru and Chile and a range of volcanic mountains, the Andes (Figs. 16-18 and 16-19). Many of the world's 530 or so active volcanoes are found above subduction zones.

2. **Oceanic-oceanic plate collision.** When two plates whose edges are covered with oceanic crust collide, one of them slides underneath the other in a subduction zone (Fig. 16-17*b*). Volcanoes are again formed, this time on the ocean floor. Where these volcanoes are high enough to rise above the ocean, they appear as the chains of islands called **island arcs.** The island arcs that border the Asiatic side of the Pacific—the Aleutians, Japan, the Philippines, Indonesia, the Marianas—are believed to have come into being in this way. The West Indies in the Atlantic form another example of an island arc.

3. **Continental-continental plate collision.** Here both plates are too light relative to the underlying asthenosphere and too thick for either one to be forced under. The result is that the plate edges are pushed together and buckle, forming a mountain range (Fig. 16-17*c*). The massive Himalayas that divide India from the rest of Asia were thrust upward in this manner. The geological evidence for this event is backed up by the fossil record. The oldest mammal fossils in India date back only 45 million years, just when the Indian and Eurasian plates came together, and these

Figure 16-17 Three situations can occur when lithospheric plates come together. (*a*) Oceanic-continental plate collision. The Andes Mountains of South America are the result of such a collision. (*b*) Oceanic-oceanic plate collision. The islands of the West Indies originated in this way. (*c*) Continental-continental plate collision. A collision of this kind thrust up the Himalaya Mountains between India and the rest of Asia.

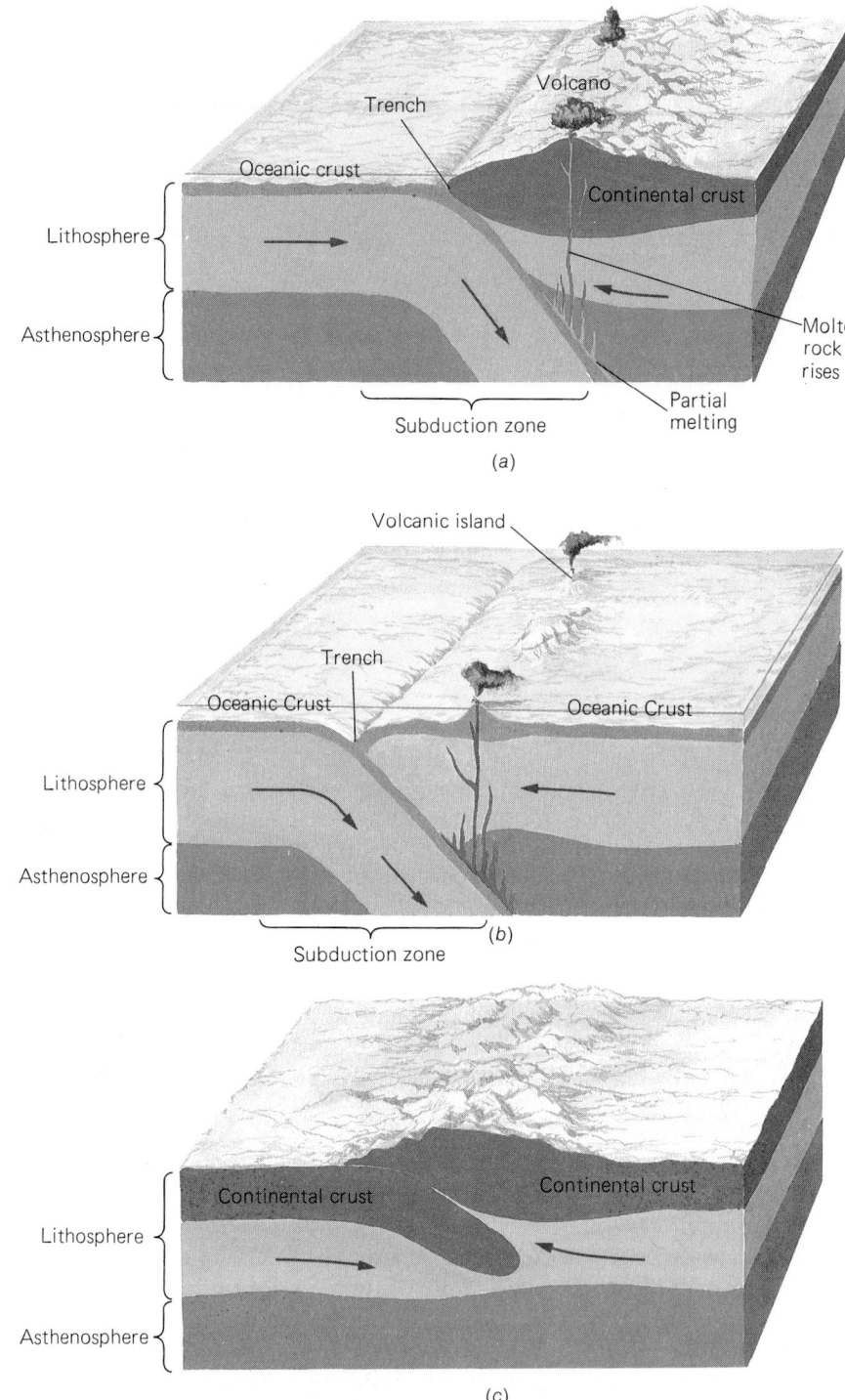

fossils are similar to those found in Mongolia, the part of Asia that India joined. The Ural Mountains between Europe and Asia are a much older range that formed in the same manner.

Crustal Ages Because the earth's crust under the oceans is being continuously created at midocean ridges and destroyed at subduction zones, all of it is relatively young. On the other hand, most continental crust is quite old, as much as 3.8 billion years old as compared with less than 180 million years for oceanic crust. Figure 16-21 on page 547 shows the various geological processes that take place in the vicinity of a convergent plate boundary.

Example 16.1

The Andes are a young, still-growing mountain range on the west coast of South America. Why is there no similar mountain range on the east coast of South America?

Solution

The boundary of the western Atlantic plate is along the western edge of South America, and the Andes are the result of the collision between this plate, which is moving westward, and the eastern Pacific plate, which is moving eastward. The eastern edge of South America is not near a plate boundary so there is nothing to force a mountain range upward there.

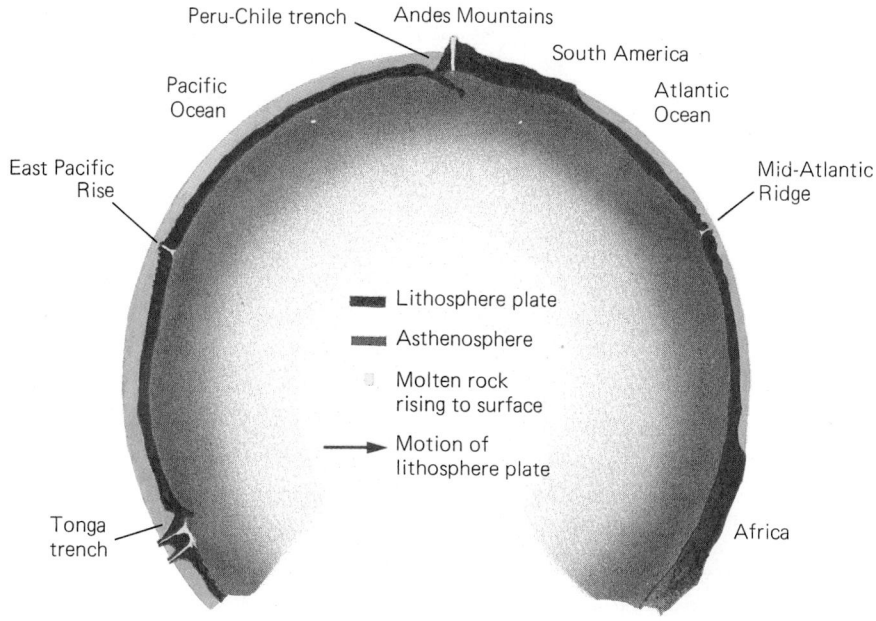

Figure 16-18 The seafloor spreads apart at midocean ridges where molten rock rises to the surface of the lithosphere. At a trench, one lithosphere plate is forced under another into the asthenosphere, where it melts. Mountain ranges, volcanoes, and island arcs are found where plates collide. The vertical scale is greatly exaggerated.

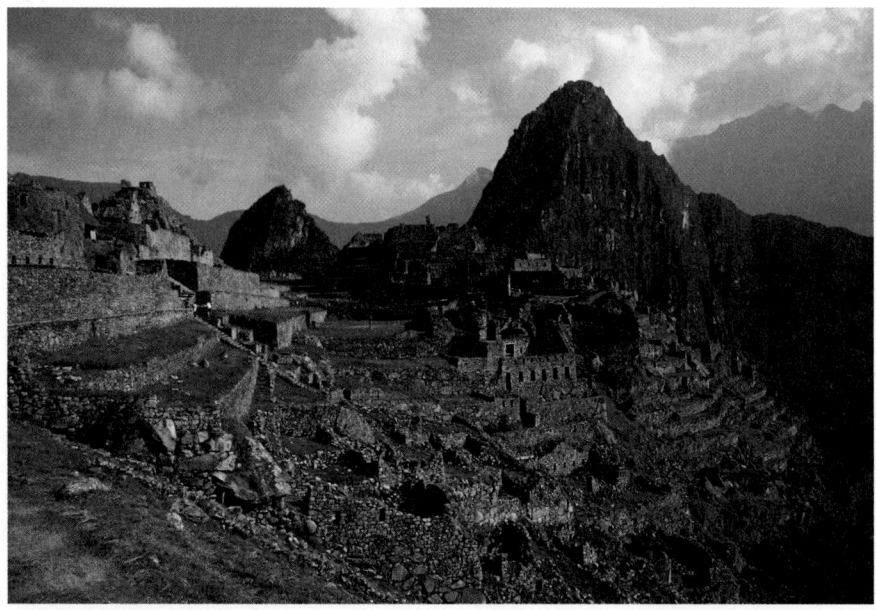

Figure 16-19 The Andes are a young mountain range thrust upward along the western edge of South America where the eastward-moving Nazca plate is forced under the westward-moving Atlantic plate. These ruins in the Peruvian Andes are of the Inca city of Machu Picchu, which was built about 1450 and abandoned a century later at the time of the Spanish conquest of Peru.

Mount Everest

Mt. Everest, the highest mountain above sea level on earth, has an altitude of 8.85 km (29,028 ft) and is part of the Himalaya range in Asia (Fig. 16-20). Its Tibetan name is Chomolungma, "Mother Goddess of the Earth." The mountain was named after Sir George Everest, who supervised the Great Trigonometrical Survey of India, which mapped the subcontinent between 1823 and 1843.

Measured from its base on the ocean floor, the Hawaiian mountain Mauna Kea is actually 1.4 km taller than Everest. Because the earth bulges at the equator as a consequence of its rotation, Mt. Chimborazo in Ecuador, which lies almost on the equator, is 2.2 km farther from the earth's center than Mt. Everest. However, Mt. Chimborazo, only 6.3 km above sea level, is not even the highest peak in the Andes.

The Himalayas were forced upward when the Indian plate plowed into the Eurasian plate about 45 million years ago. Before the collision the northward speed of the Indian plate was 15–20 cm/year. Afterward the plate slowed to around 5 cm/year as it advanced roughly 2000 km into the Eurasian plate. The Indian plate is still moving north, today at 2 cm/year, and the Himalayas are still rising. The world's 10 highest mountains are currently in the Himalayas, but the Andes are going up faster and some of their peaks may well look down on Everest in time.

Most of Mt. Everest consists of granite and metamorphic rocks with a topping of limestone that contains fossils of marine life from the Tethys Sea (see Fig. 16-9).

As we would expect, major earthquakes occur regularly along the still-active fault between the Indian and Eurasian plates. The most recent was the magnitude 7.6 quake of October 2005 that devastated Kashmir and adjacent northern Pakistan. About 87,000 people were

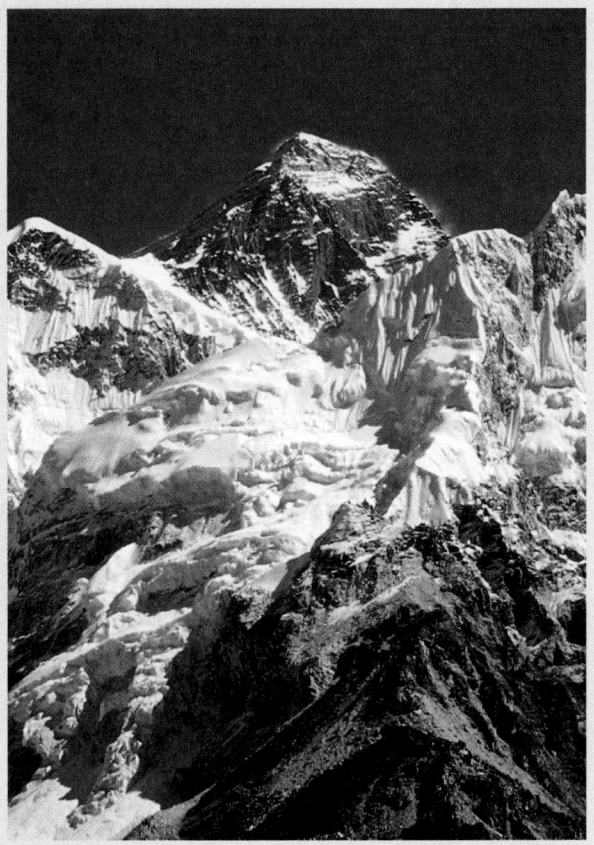

Figure 16-20   Mt. Everest lies on the border between Nepal and Tibet. Its summit was first reached in 1953 after many failed attempts.

killed, at least 130,000 were injured, and 2 million were left homeless as winter approached.

Transform Faults   Another type of plate boundary is a **transform fault,** which occurs where the edges of two plates slide past each other. (A transform fault is a large-scale version of the strike-slip fault shown in Fig. 16-2.) Earthquakes are common along transform faults, as we would expect. Since most transform faults are in ocean basins (see Fig. 16-16), the quakes associated with them usually are unnoticed except by geologists.

A conspicuous exception is the 1200-km-long San Andreas Fault in California, which is one of the faults that lie along the boundary between the Pacific and North American plates (Figs. 16-23 and 16-24). Movement along the fault occurs continuously in some regions but elsewhere in sudden jerks that release accumulated stresses. The San Francisco earthquakes of 1906 and 1989 were caused by such abrupt slippages, and further earthquakes along the fault are sure to happen in the future.

How Tectonic Forces Arise   What drives the lithosphere plates as they shape and reshape the earth's surface? Several plausible mechanisms have been put forward and it is possible that all contribute to some extent to plate motion.

An obvious one is convection in the plastic asthenosphere due to uneven heating from the mantle below. Rock hot enough to flow gradually is

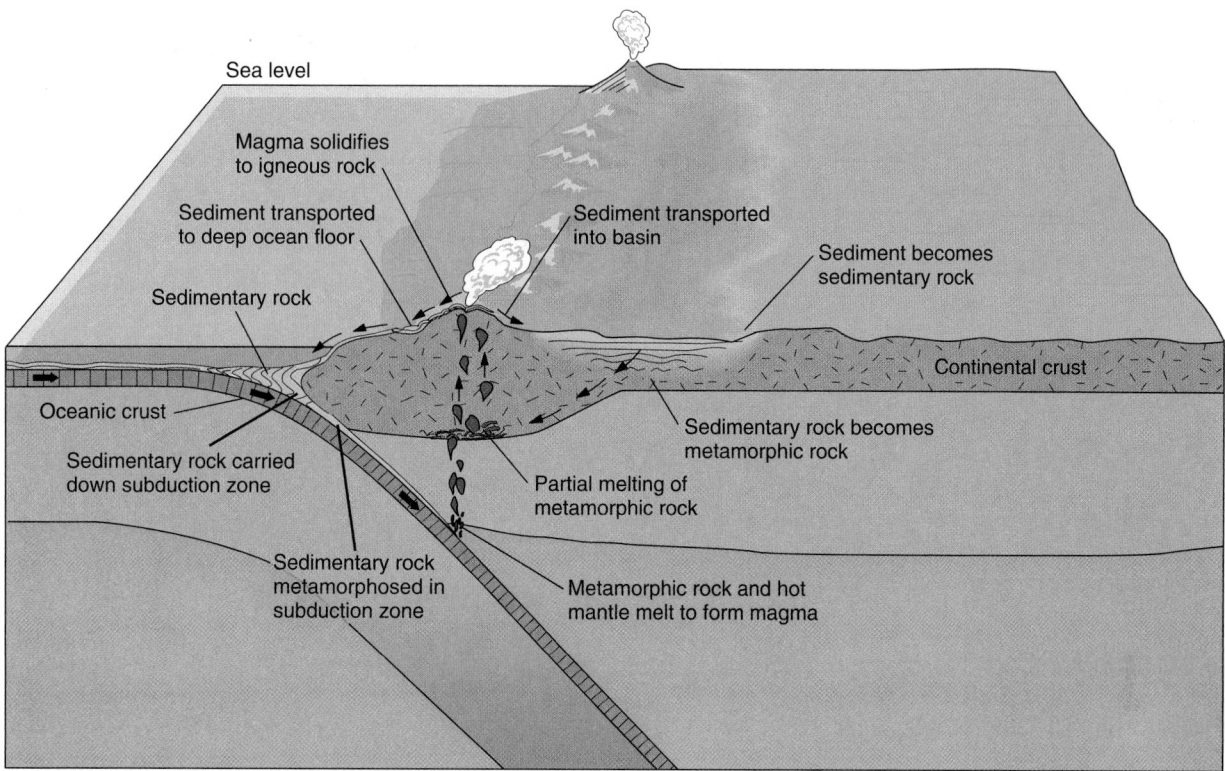

Figure 16-21   How the various transformations of the rock cycle shown in Fig. 15-60 occur where an oceanic plate collides with a continental plate.

supposed to rise at diverging plate edges (where midocean ridges occur) and spread out horizontally while dragging along the plates above. Then, having cooled, the rock sinks at subduction zones. (Convection in the atmosphere is shown in Fig. 14-16.)

Alternatively, the raised material in a midocean ridge pushes the adjacent plates apart by virtue of its weight; an analogy is a person standing with a foot in each of two adjacent canoes that then move apart. A third hypothesis,

The Hawaiian Islands

Many of the world's active volcanoes occur along the rifts between plates that are moving apart; an example is shown in Fig. 16-15. Another common location is above a subduction zone, as in Fig. 16-17a and b.

A third class of volcanoes are those produced by molten rock that comes to the surface above hot spots in the mantle. The Hawaiian Islands were formed as the Pacific plate moved northwestward at about 9 cm/year over such a hot spot (Fig. 16-22). From time to time a plume of molten rock erupted from this hot spot to create a volcano above it that rose above the ocean floor. These volcanoes, now the islands of the Hawaiian chain, became extinct after they passed the hot spot.

The only volcanic activity in that region today is on the island of Hawaii, whose southeastern part is over the hot spot, and on a young undersea volcano called Loihi that is 30 km southeast of Hawaii and feeding off the same plume. Eventually Loihi will grow into the next member of the Hawaiian island chain. There is evidence that the hot spot as well as the Pacific plate have been moving, which is why the islands do not lie along a straight line. About 20 other hot spots are active today around the world.

(Continued)

The Hawaiian Islands   (Continued)

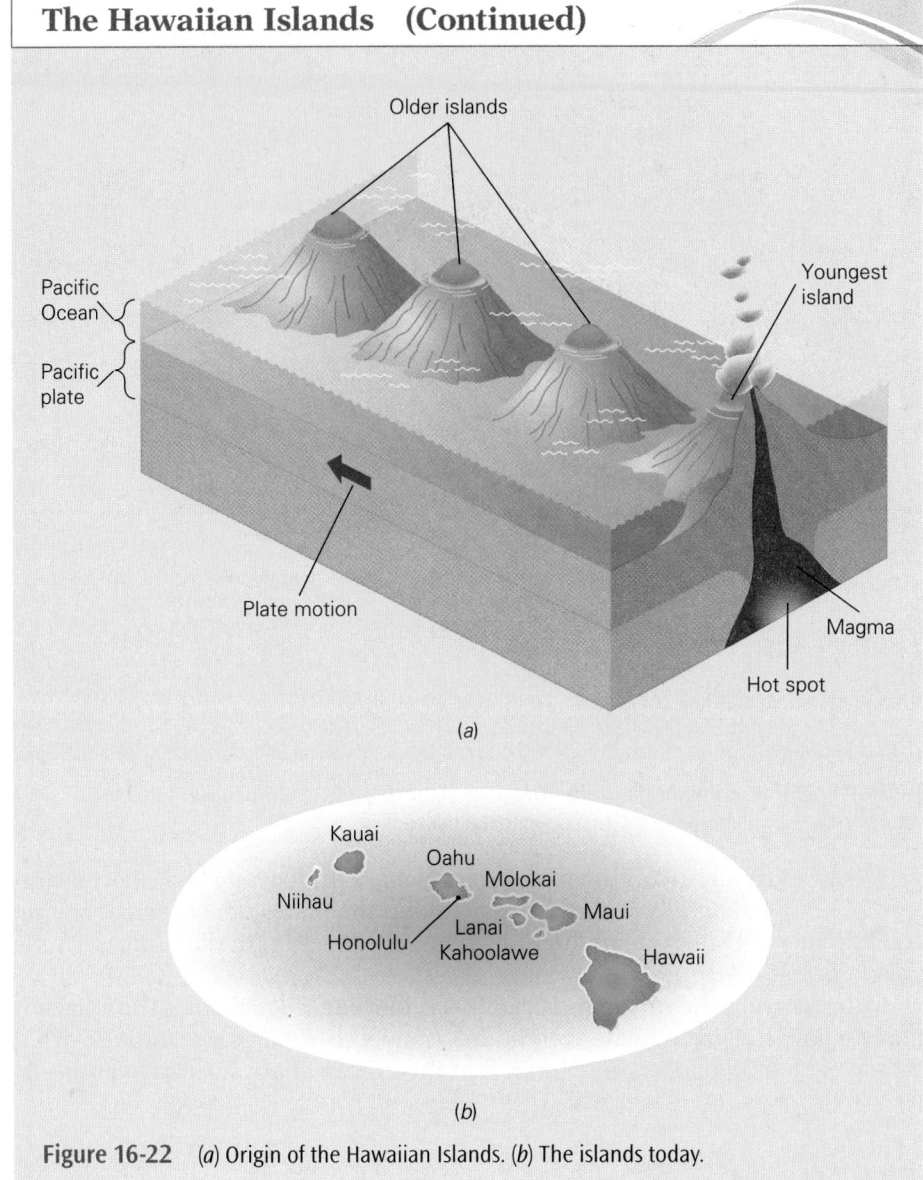

(a)

(b)

Figure 16-22   (a) Origin of the Hawaiian Islands. (b) The islands today.

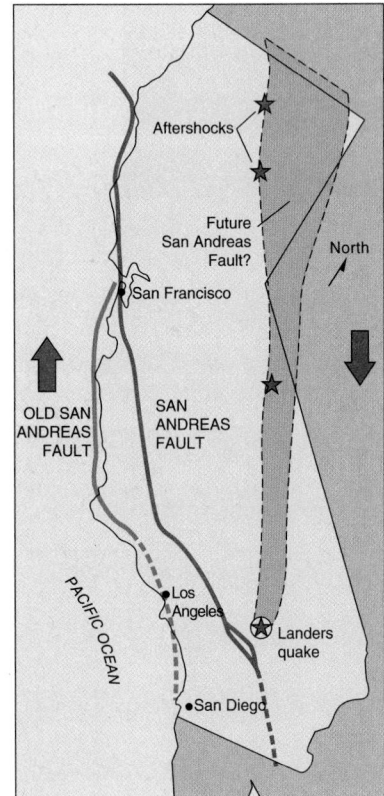

Figure 16-23   Until about 5 million years ago, motion along the transform boundary between the Pacific and North American plates occurred along a fault west of the present San Andreas Fault. Today the motion takes place along the latter fault at about 6 cm per year. The 1992 Landers earthquake had aftershocks along a line extending to the north, which suggests that perhaps in the future more of California will become attached to the Pacific plate and slide northwestward with it past the North American plate.

currently favored, has the oceanic plates pulled apart by the weights of their sinking edges as these edges descend into subduction zones (Fig. 16-17a and b). The ability of the plates to bend is possibly helped by the lubricating effect of water trapped in their rock.

The Future   When present trends in the evolution of the earth's crust are projected 30 million years into the future, the result is a picture like that shown in Fig. 16-25. The Atlantic Ocean has grown wider, the Pacific narrower. Part of California has broken off from the rest of North America, and the Arabian peninsula has been forced around to become an integral part of Asia. The islands of the West Indies have grown into a land bridge between the Americas, and the western Pacific islands have also increased markedly in extent.

And after that? All that can be said is that the face of the earth will probably continue to change in the future, just as it has been changing as far back in the past as we have any evidence. One projection has all the continents merged again into a new Pangaea 250 million or so years from now. And then another breakup? Quite possibly.

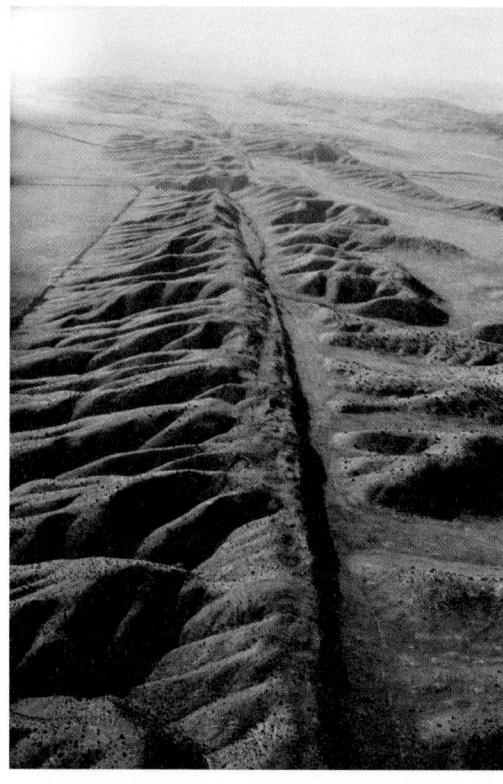
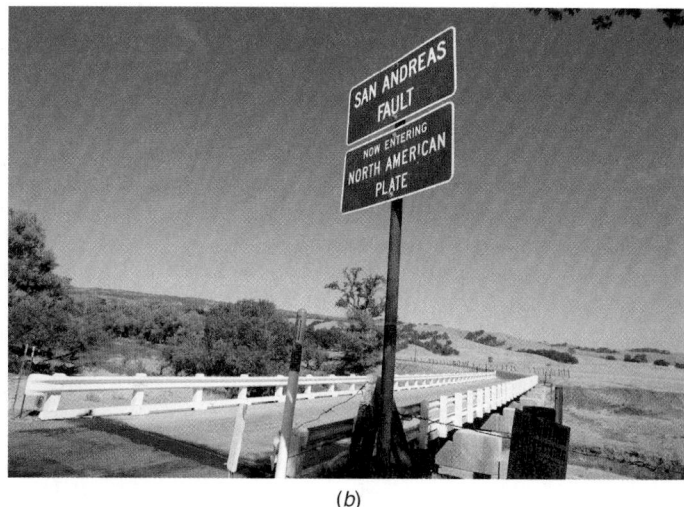

(a) (b)

Figure 16-24 (a) Part of the San Andreas Fault in California. The earthquake of October 17, 1989, that rocked San Francisco originated in a zone of this fault whose sides shifted by about 2 m relative to each other. The slippage occurred underground. (b) Geology is taken seriously in California.

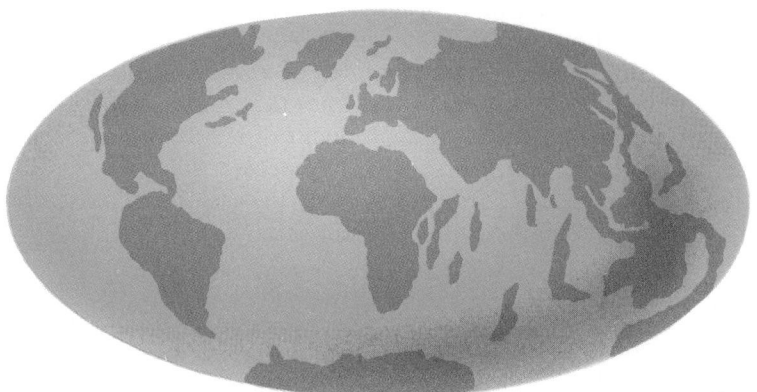

Figure 16-25 How the earth may appear 30 million years from now if present plate motions continue. Figure 16-9 shows the earth's landmasses as they were and as they are today to the same scale.

Methods of Historical Geology

Two kinds of events in the history of the crust are significant. In one category are physical changes such as the drift of the continents, the upthrust and wearing away of mountains, the spread and retreat of glaciers and ice sheets. In the other are changes in the living things that populate the earth, from primitive one-celled organisms to the complex plants and animals of today. Although the rock record is less complete the farther back we go, it is still possible to trace the physical and biological evolution of the crust for billions of years into the past. Let us see how this is done.

16.8   Principle of Uniform Change

"No Vestige of a Beginning, No Prospect of an End"

The modern view of geologic evolution had its start two centuries ago. Before then a major obstacle to scientific thinking about the earth's history was the Bible. The Book of Genesis tells about the earth's beginning with beauty and simplicity. A seventeenth-century theologian, Bishop James Ussher, used the stories in the Bible to pinpoint the moment when our planet was created from a formless void: 9 o'clock in the morning of October 12, 4004 B.C.

However, even the smallest knowledge of geology shows that the events recorded in today's landscapes cannot possibly have occurred in only a few thousand years. Early investigators nevertheless devoted their efforts to trying to fit what they found in the rocks around them into a literal interpretation of Genesis.

Even when freed from biblical shackles, geologists of the past usually went far astray in their arguments. One reason was their habit of generalizing from limited evidence. Another was their readiness to postulate tremendous events to explain particular findings. For instance, a comprehensive theory was formulated by Abraham Gottlob Werner on the basis of the geologic structures he found near his home in Freiberg, Germany. What he saw was granite overlain by folded, somewhat metamorphosed rocks, with these in turn overlain by flat sedimentary beds.

Untraveled and deaf to the reports of others, Werner considered this sequence to be the same worldwide. Each of the three types of rocks, he presumed, was deposited by a universal ocean, with granite precipitating first and the upper beds last. All rocks, in Werner's system, were sedimentary rocks, and the geologic history of the earth consisted of three sudden precipitations from an ancient ocean that were followed by the disappearance of most of the water.

The French biologist Georges Cuvier greatly influenced geology at the beginning of the nineteenth century by studying **fossils,** which are the remains or traces of organisms preserved in rocks. In successive rock layers around Paris, Cuvier found distinct groups of animal fossils, different from one another and from the present animals of that region. He concluded that each group appeared on the earth as a result of a special creation and that each was destroyed by a universal disaster before the next creation. Thus Cuvier also regarded the earth's history as a succession of catastrophes that were separated by intervals of stable conditions.

Hutton, Lyell, and Darwin   James Hutton, a Scot, based his thinking on a much larger body of observational evidence than Werner or Cuvier. By accepting that the earth is very old, Hutton found no need to invoke special mechanisms since he could account for what he saw in terms of processes under way in the present-day world: "In the phenomena of the earth," he concluded, "I see no vestige of a beginning, no prospect of an end."

Hutton's ideas, outlined in his 1785 book *Theory of the Earth,* were soon taken up by others who modified and extended them. Chief among Hutton's followers was Charles Lyell, whose goal was "to explain the former changes of the earth's surface by forces now in operation." This he was largely able to do, and his guiding idea became known as the **principle of uniform change.** Of course, the vigor of geologic processes has varied from time to time and from place to place, so that uniform is not the best word. However, with a few exceptions, such variations are quite different from the catastrophic happenings earlier thinkers were so fond of.

An important link in the chain of ideas that was forming was supplied by Lyell's friend Charles Darwin in 1859 (Fig. 16-26). Darwin's **theory**

Charles Lyell (1797–1875)

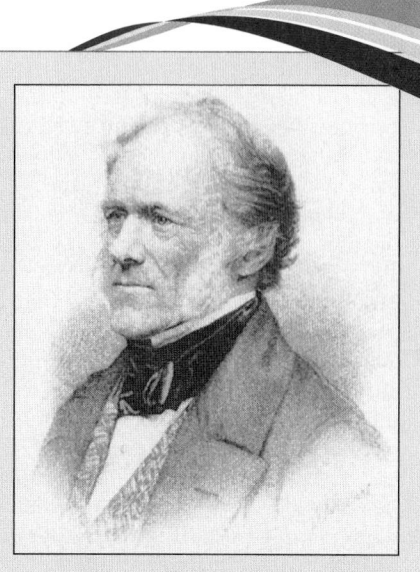

A Scot, Lyell studied law at Oxford. Fascinated by geology, he traveled extensively and observed geologic changes then taking place—the shifting of streams, the building of deltas, the advances and retreats of shorelines, the outpouring of lava and ash from volcanoes. From rocks and landscapes he read the slow accumulation of these changes through the long past—rivers now cutting far below their former channels, coasts with remnants of old beaches high above the present shore, immense lava flows where no volcanoes exist today.

Lyell was the first to distinguish metamorphic rocks as a group, and so to understand clearly the cycle by which rocks are formed, destroyed, and re-formed. He continued the work of Cuvier and his English followers in tracing the succession of animals whose remains are entombed in rocks. Nowhere did he find signs of past changes brought about by agencies other than those in the world around him. Lyell reemphasized his predecessor Hutton's point that processes that seem unable to alter the landscape by very much may nevertheless have large-scale consequences if given enough time. If the earth is only a few thousand years old, catastrophism is indeed the only explanation, but if the earth is millions of years old, the slow pace of geologic change can explain what we see around us.

Lyell's accumulation of evidence was overwhelming, and not long after his *Principles of Geology* was published, most geologists, initially skeptical, accepted his views.

of evolution showed that changes in living things as well as those in the inorganic world of rocks could be explained in terms of processes operating all around us. The fossil groups found by Cuvier near Paris did not come from special creations but were stages in a continuous line of development. Lyell understood at once the significance of Darwin's work and became one of his most active supporters.

How far back does the principle of uniform change hold? It must break down eventually because the earth in its early stages as a planet was certainly different from today's earth. All geology can say for certain is that the oldest rocks now exposed contain a clear record of processes very similar to those of the present. Beyond that lies the realm of hypothesis, and in Chap. 19 we shall see how theories of the origin of the earth connect up with geologic history.

16.9 Rock Formations

History under Our Feet

The crustal events of the past are recorded in the rocks and landscapes of the present. It is usually possible to reconstruct these events in terms of processes still at work reshaping the face of the earth. Thus from moraines, lakes, and U-shaped valleys we learn of the spread and retreat of ancient glaciers. Wave-cut cliffs and terraces above the sea suggest recent elevation of the land. Hot springs and isolated, cone-shaped mountains signify past volcanic activity.

Other past events have left their traces as well. A geologist finds a bed of salt or gypsum buried beneath other strata, and he or she knows that the region must once have had a desert climate in which a lake or an arm of the sea evaporated. A layer of coal implies an ancient swamp in which partly decayed vegetation accumulated. A limestone bed with numerous fossils suggests a clear, shallow sea in which lived clams, snails, and other hard-shelled

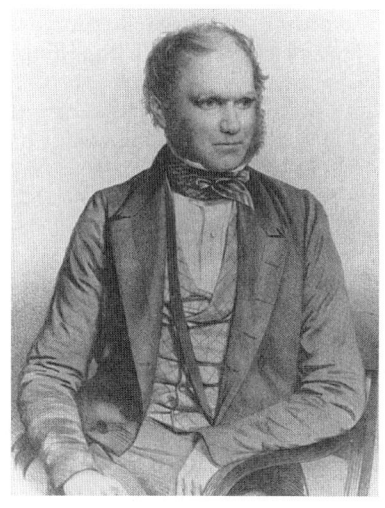

Figure 16-26 Charles Darwin (1809–1882).

Evolution

Evolution is the "view of life" (in Darwin's words) that has turned out to be the only organizing principle from which all the different aspects of biology make sense. "I had two distinct objects in view: firstly to show that species had not been separately created, and secondly, that natural selection has been the chief agent of change." Starting from the simplest organisms, "endless forms most beautiful and most wonderful have been, and are being, evolved."

The ability to evolve can be considered one of the chief distinctions—perhaps the primary one—between life and nonlife.

Evolution operates through two mechanisms. The first is reproduction with variation: the members of each generation are not necessarily the same as each other or as their parents. Darwin did not know how variation comes about, but today we can trace it to changes (called mutations) in the DNA of which the genes of living things are composed.

The second mechanism is natural selection: the individual plants and animals that are best adapted to their environments are most likely to thrive and produce similarly successful offspring. In simple terms, "survival of the fittest."

When living conditions alter drastically, which has happened often in the history of the earth, the pace of evolution is faster than during periods of stability. At such times previously dominant species (such as the dinosaurs) may even disappear entirely, while previously marginal species (such as the mammals) may become favored. Darwin's view was that "it is not the strongest of the species that survive, nor the most intelligent, but the ones most responsive to change."

It is sometimes said that evolution cannot have led to complex life forms because it involves chance events. However, although each individual mutation is indeed a chance event, whether the mutation survives as an element in the genetic makeup of the descendants of an organism does not depend on chance but on how well the descendants meet the challenges of life. Thus evolution is not random overall because it is directed by natural selection.

The descendants of a particular organism may later follow different evolutionary paths, which leads to the diversity of living things, but this branching, too, is shaped by natural selection. In this way immense numbers of random events occurring over immense reaches of time have, under the nonrandom guidance of natural selection, produced a living world of variety and complexity. Only evolution can explain how this world came about in terms of natural processes, and it does this with complete success.

A huge body of evidence drawn from many disciplines supports the basic concepts of evolution. Thus the fossil record shows the development of new forms of life from older ones, with a time scale established by radiometric methods that is long enough (billions of years) for this development to have taken place. Attempts to discredit evolution always point to gaps that remain in the fossil record between some old and new forms of life. But these gaps are being steadily filled in with transitional fossils, confirming Darwin's vision.

A notable example of such gap-filling is the discovery in 2004 in the Canadian Arctic of fossils of a 2.75-m-long, 375-million-year-old creature that seems to be the missing link between fish and land-dwelling animals. Called Tiktaalik roseae, it had anatomical features of both fish and land animals, for instance, lungs as well as gills, fins that contained primitive limbs with shoulders, wrists, and fingers, the scales of a fish, and the flexible neck of a land animal. From the transitional Tiktaalik evolved amphibians, reptiles (such as dinosaurs; birds descended from them), and mammals (such as us).

The theory of evolution is a good example of the scientific method (Sec. 1.1) in action. Darwin formulated a hypothesis based on observations, further observations supported the hypothesis, and it was so successful in explaining a large variety of findings that it was accepted as a theory. And quite a theory it is: according to the National Academy of Sciences, the theory of evolution is no less than "the foundation of modern biology."

The distribution of life forms around the world shows the effects of evolution: Australia was long isolated from the other continents, and many plants and animals there are distinct from those elsewhere. The anatomies of different species often show great similarities (human arms have much in common with whale flippers), which suggests descent from a common ancestor. Certain body parts that today have no function can be traced back to forebears that needed them: an example is the coccyx at the base of the spine, the remnant of a tail. And, of course, even before Darwin farmers speeded up evolution by choosing plant and animal variations to breed that were especially desirable for their purposes.

Even this very brief account shows the power of evolution to account for the history, variety, and relatedness of life on earth.

organisms (Fig. 16-27). As the long history is carried further and further back, the evidence becomes more shadowy and the geologist's reconstruction of the earth's surface similarly imprecise.

In trying to figure out how the earth's crust evolved, geology is faced with two fundamental problems: to arrange in order the events recorded

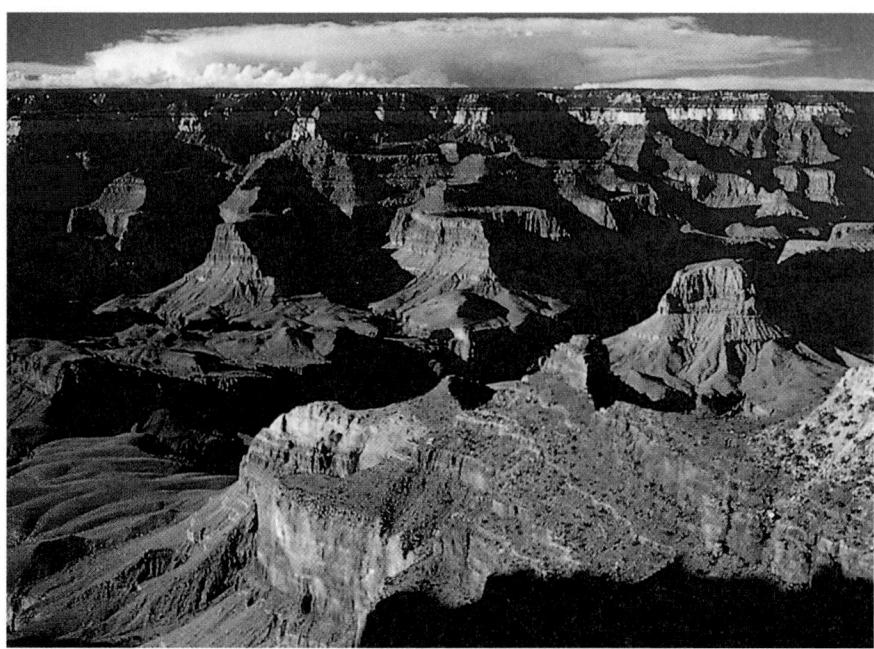

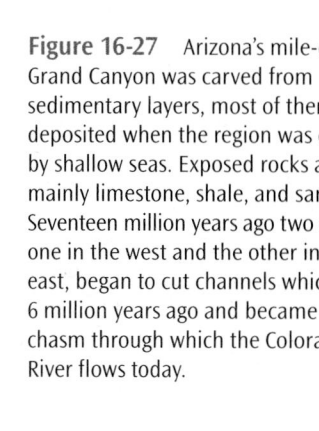

Figure 16-27 Arizona's mile-deep Grand Canyon was carved from sedimentary layers, most of them deposited when the region was covered by shallow seas. Exposed rocks are mainly limestone, shale, and sandstone. Seventeen million years ago two streams, one in the west and the other in the east, began to cut channels which met 6 million years ago and became a single chasm through which the Colorado River flows today.

in the rocks of a single outcrop or small region, and to correlate events in various regions of the world to give a connected history of the earth as a whole.

Reading the Rocks Some of the principles used by geologists to figure out the history of a small area are straightforward:

1. In a sequence of sedimentary rocks, the lowest bed is the oldest and the highest bed is the youngest. In Fig. 16-28 bed *A* must have been deposited before the others and bed *E* last.
2. Sedimentary beds were originally deposited in approximately horizontal layers.
3. Tectonic movement took place after the deposition of the youngest bed affected. Thus the layers of Fig. 16-28 were not folded until after bed *D* was laid down, and the fault must be younger than bed *C*.
4. An igneous rock is younger than the youngest bed it intrudes. The granite pluton shown in Fig. 16-28 is younger than bed *D*. (The age of an igneous rock refers to the time at which it solidified.)

Obvious as these rules are, much ingenuity may be needed to apply them to regions of heavily folded and faulted layers. The problem is especially difficult in regions where much of the rock structure is hidden by later sediments or vegetation.

Unconformity A structure like that shown in Fig. 16-29 requires further attention. Here the lower, tilted beds are cut off by an uneven surface on which rest the upper horizontal beds. An irregular surface of this sort, separating two series of rocks, is called an **unconformity.**

An unconformity is a buried surface of erosion. It always involves at least four geologic events: the deposition of the oldest strata; tectonic movement that raises and perhaps tilts the existing strata; erosion of the elevated strata to produce an irregular surface; and finally a new period of deposition that buries the eroded surface (Fig. 16-30). Usually this last event involves the lowering of the eroded surface either beneath the sea or to a level where stream deposition can occur.

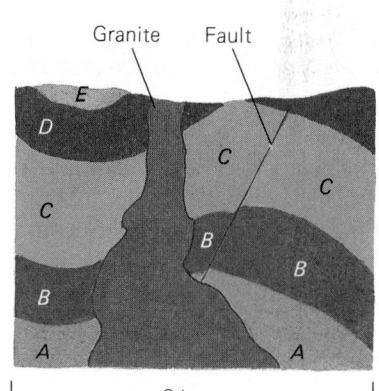

Figure 16-28 Schematic cross section showing folded sedimentary rocks that were displaced along a fault and then intruded by granite.

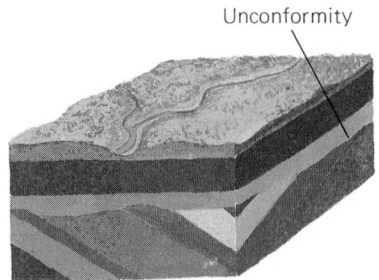

Figure 16-29 An unconformity is an irregular eroded surface that separates one set of rock layers from an earlier set. Shown is an unconformity above tilted lower layers; the layers above and below an unconformity can also be parallel.

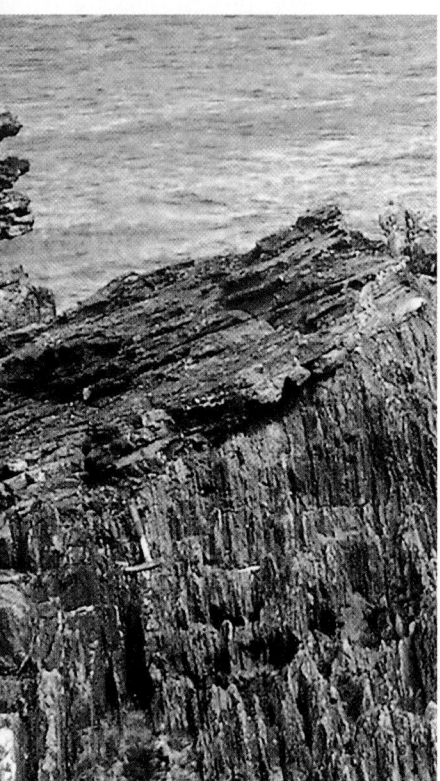

Figure 16-30 This angular unconformity in Scotland consists of sandstone layers from the Devonian Period that overlie layers of Silurian rock that have been tilted almost vertically.

Example 16.2

In parts of Colorado and Wyoming, a long period during which marine sediments were deposited in a sinking basin ended with intense tectonic movement. A mountain range rose there that was later worn down by erosion to a nearly level plain. On parts of this plain stream and lake sediments were deposited. What rocks and rock structures would be expected in this region?

Solution

The original sedimentary deposits will have been converted into such metamorphic rocks as slate, schist, and marble, which will be exposed by the subsequent erosion. The outcrops of metamorphic rocks will be intruded by igneous rocks— granite batholiths and dikes of various kinds. Unconformities will occur where the later stream and lake sediments are deposited. Sandstone, shale, and conglomerate will predominate in the overlying sedimentary rocks.

16.10 Radiometric Dating

A Clock Based on Radioactivity

To trace the sequence of geologic events in various places is not enough. We also need to know which events happened at the same time in different places if we are to understand how the earth's crust evolved. We could get the data we need by following rock layers from one region to another around the globe, but in fact after a shorter or longer distance the layers are always either cut off by erosion or concealed by later deposits.

Two methods can be used to figure out the worldwide sequence of the events that have shaped the earth's surface: radioactive dating and fossil identification. As we shall find, each method has different advantages and disadvantages.

Methods based on radioactive decay make it possible to establish the ages of many rocks on an absolute rather than a relative time scale. Because the decay of any particular radionuclide proceeds at a steady rate, the ratio between the amounts of that nuclide and its eventual stable daughter in a rock sample indicates the age of the rock. (There may be several decays into intermediate daughter radionuclides before a stable daughter is reached.) The more there is of the daughter, the older the rock (Fig. 8-10). Radiometric dating can be accurate to ±2500 years per million years, but only certain rock specimens can be dated in this way.

Table 16-1 lists the radionuclides that have been found most useful in dating rocks. Age measurements of fossil-bearing rocks with the radioactive clock reveal that relatively large-brained humanlike creatures walked erect in Africa about 2 million years ago; that primitive mammals existed about 200 million years ago; that sea animals with hard shells first became abundant about 600 million years ago. The most ancient rocks whose ages have been established are found in northwestern Canada and are 4 billion years old; zircon samples have been discovered in Australia that seem to have crystallized even earlier.

Table 16-1	Radionuclides Used for Dating Rocks	
Parent Nuclide	**Stable Daughter Nuclide**	**Half-Life, Billion Years**
Potassium 40	Argon 40	1.3
Rubidium 87	Strontium 87	49
Thorium 232	Lead 208	14.1
Uranium 235	Lead 207	0.7
Uranium 238	Lead 206	4.5

Example 16.3

What are the chief assumptions made in the radiometric dating of the age of a rock?

Solution

(a) The rates of decay of the parent and any daughter radionuclides are constant, independent of time, temperature, and pressure.

(b) There has been no addition to or loss from the rock of any of the nuclides involved in the decay series from the radioactive parent to the eventual stable daughter.

Radiocarbon   Another radionuclide permits the dating of more recent remains of living things. The carbon isotope ^{14}C, called **radiocarbon,** is beta radioactive with a half-life of 5700 years. Radiocarbon is produced in small quantities in the earth's atmosphere by the action of cosmic rays (discussed in Chap. 19) on nitrogen atoms, and the carbon dioxide of the atmosphere accordingly contains a small proportion of radiocarbon. Green plants take in carbon dioxide in order to live, and so every plant contains radioactive carbon that it absorbs along with intake of ordinary carbon dioxide. Animals eat plants and thus become radioactive themselves; there are about 13 decays of ^{14}C per minute per gram of carbon in living tissue.

Every living thing on earth is therefore slightly radioactive because of the radiocarbon it takes in. The mixing of radiocarbon with ordinary carbon is very efficient and so living plants and animals all have the same proportion of radiocarbon to ordinary carbon (^{12}C).

After death, however, the remains of living things no longer absorb radiocarbon, and the radiocarbon they contain keeps decaying away to nitrogen. After 5700 years, then, they have only half as much radiocarbon left—relative to their total carbon content—as they had as living matter, after 11,400 years only one-fourth as much, and so on. Determining the proportion of radiocarbon to ordinary carbon thus makes it possible to evaluate the ages of ancient objects and remains of organic origin (Figs. 16-31 and 16-32). This elegant method permits the dating of archeological specimens such as mummies, wooden implements, cloth, leather, charcoal from campfires, and similar remains of ancient civilizations that are between 1000 and 40,000 years old.

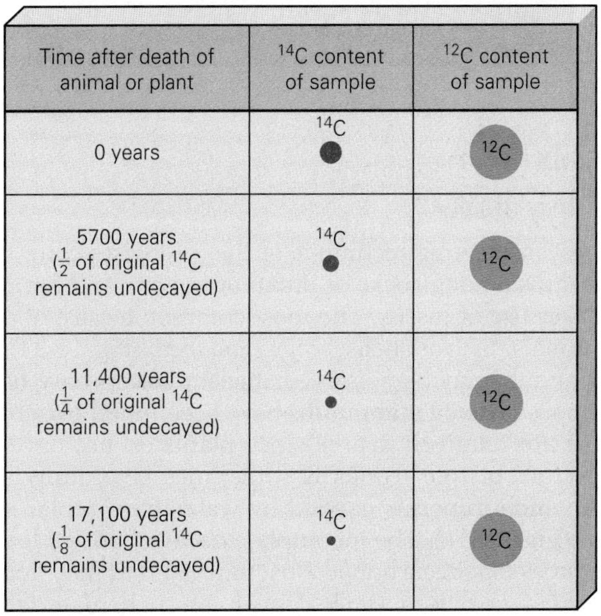

Time after death of animal or plant	^{14}C content of sample	^{12}C content of sample
0 years	^{14}C ●	^{12}C
5700 years ($\frac{1}{2}$ of original ^{14}C remains undecayed)	^{14}C ●	^{12}C
11,400 years ($\frac{1}{4}$ of original ^{14}C remains undecayed)	^{14}C ●	^{12}C
17,100 years ($\frac{1}{8}$ of original ^{14}C remains undecayed)	^{14}C ●	^{12}C

Figure 16-31   The principle of radiocarbon dating. The radioactive ^{14}C content of a sample of dead animal or plant tissue decreases steadily, while its ^{12}C content remains constant. Hence the ratio of ^{14}C to ^{12}C contents indicates the time that has elapsed since the death of an organism. The half-life of ^{14}C is 5700 years. (The relative proportions of ^{14}C and ^{12}C are greatly exaggerated here; there is actually very little ^{14}C in a carbon sample from animal or plant tissue.)

| ## Arthur Holmes (1890–1965)

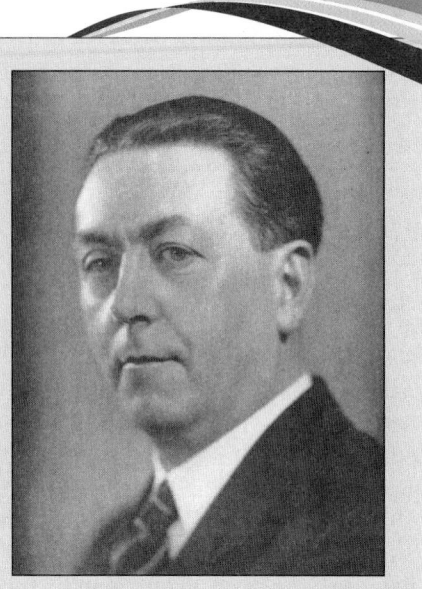

Although Holmes was interested first in physics, he turned to geology because he felt it was more likely to lead to a good job. As it turned out, Holmes's great achievements in geology were largely due to his application of physics and chemistry to a subject that, in his student days, was much less of a science than he helped it to become.

After graduating from the Imperial College of Science in London, Holmes worked for a time in Africa and later for an oil company in what was then Burma. In 1924 he became head of the geology department at Durham University and in 1947 went to Edinburgh University where he remained until just before his death.

Holmes's main interest was petrology, the study of rocks, in particular igneous rocks and their origins, and he worked in this field with his wife Doris Reynolds, herself a distinguished geologist. However, his contributions to geology covered a wide span. He is best known for using radioactive methods to date rocks, which established a timescale for the geological record and provided a figure for the age of the earth based on measurements rather than on speculation: "It is perhaps a little delicate to ask of our Mother Earth her age, but Science admits no shame," he wrote.

Holmes was an early champion of continental drift when it was a heretical idea, and his imaginative insight led him to anticipate some of the concepts of plate tectonics long before this theory became recognized as the key to understanding how the earth's surface evolves.

Figure 16-32   A mass spectrometer such as this one at the University of Minnesota can measure the proportion of ^{14}C atoms in carbon from a sample of plant or animal material. Because ^{14}C is radioactive whereas the more abundant ^{12}C isotope is not, their ratio indicates how long ago a plant or animal died.

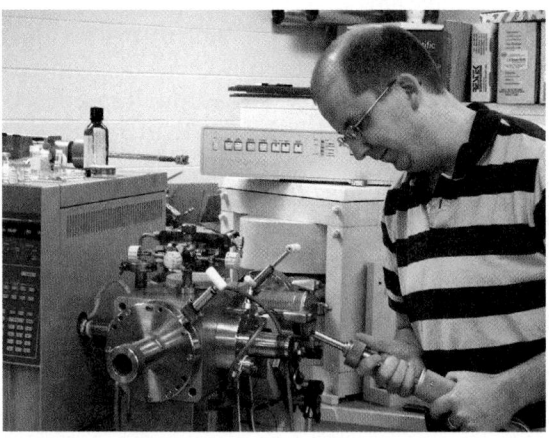

16.11   Fossils

Tracing the History of Life

Perhaps the most fascinating technique at the geologist's command for establishing relationships among rocks of different regions and for arranging beds in sequence makes use of fossils. The most common fossils, of course, are the hard parts of animals, such as shells, bones, and teeth (Fig. 16-33). On rare occasions an entire animal may be preserved: ancient insects have been trapped in amber, and immense woolly mammoths have been found frozen in the Arctic.

Plant fossils are relatively scarce since plants do not have durable hard parts. The structure of tree trunks is sometimes beautifully shown in petrified wood in which minerals carried by water have replaced the original plant tissue (see Fig. 15-51). The incomplete decay of buried leaves and wood fragments produces black, carbonaceous material that may keep the original organic structures—coal is a thick deposit of such material (Fig. 16-34).

Occasionally fine sediments show impressions of delicate structures like leaves, feathers, and skin fragments. Some fossils are merely trails or footprints left in soft mud and covered by later sediments.

Conditions necessary for preservation have been much the same throughout geologic history. Chemical decay, bacteria, and scavengers have quickly disposed of most of the organisms that have lived on the earth, and only special conditions of burial permit the survival of fossil groups. These conditions most often occur on the floor of shallow seas, where life is abundant and sediments are sometimes deposited rapidly. Our picture of marine life in the past is accordingly far more complete than our picture of the organisms that lived on land, but even the marine record is fragmentary.

What Fossils Tell Us An important conclusion from the fossil record is that groups of organisms show a progressive change from those buried in ancient rocks to those of the most recent strata. In general, the degree of complexity increases, from forms very different from those in the present world to creatures much like those around us today. Some older forms may continue to exist with the newer ones. These observations are part of the foundation for Darwin's theory that life has evolved by a steady development from simple organisms to complex ones.

Because plants and animals have changed continuously through the ages, rock layers from different periods can be recognized by the kinds of fossils they contain. This fact makes possible the arrangement of beds in a relative time sequence, even when their relationships are not directly apparent, and also provides a means of correlating the strata of different localities. If, for example, fossil snail shells and clamshells are found in a rock layer in New York that are similar to fossil shells from a layer in the Grand Canyon, the two layers are likely to be approximately the same age.

Fossils are useful not only in tracing the development of life and in correlating strata but in helping us to reconstruct the environment in which the organisms lived. Some creatures, like barnacles and scallops, live only in the sea, and it is likely that their close relatives in the past were similarly restricted to salt water. Other animals can exist only in freshwater. On land some organisms prefer desert climates, others cold climates, others warm and humid climates. Evidently many details about the conditions in which a rock was formed can be revealed by its fossil organisms.

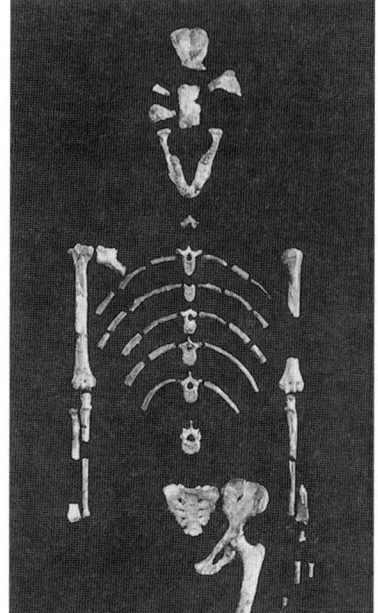

Figure 16-33 Fossil skeleton of "Lucy," a humanlike creature who lived 3 million years ago in what is today Ethiopia. She was between 1 and 1.5 m tall with long arms and curved fingers and toes that suggest she was at home both in trees and upright on the ground.

16.12 Geologic Time

Precambrian, Paleozoic, Mesozoic, Cenozoic

Fossils enable us to arrange in sequence geologic events over the entire earth. Enough of these events can be dated accurately by radioactive methods for good estimates to be made for the dates of the others. The most recent 542 million years of the earth's history have been divided by geologists into three major divisions called **eras** (Table 16-2):

Cenozoic ("recent life") Era; began 66 million years ago
Mesozoic ("intermediate life") Era; began 251 million years ago and lasted 185 million years
Paleozoic ("old life") Era; began 542 million years ago and lasted 291 million years

Geologists have divided the 4 billion years before the Paleozoic Era—a shadowy span that covers over seven-eighths of the history of our planet—into just two major parts, the **Archaean** ("ancient") **Eon** and the later **Proterozoic** ("former life") **Eon,** that together make up **Precambrian time.** The dates of the various divisions of geologic time are changed from time to time as new evidence turns up; those in this book are the most recent ones.

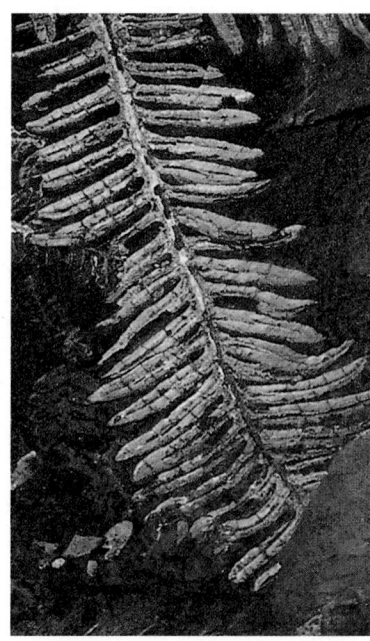

Figure 16-34 Fossil fern found in a coal deposit in Pennsylvania.

Table 16-2   Geologic Time (The Earth Came into Existence About 4600 Million Years Ago).

Millions of Years Ago	Era	Period	Epoch	Duration, Million Years	The Biologic Record	The Geologic Record
66	Cenozoic	Neogene	Holocene	0.01	Humans become dominant	Ice Age
			Pleistocene	1.8	Rise of humans; large mammals abundant	
			Pliocene	3.5	Flowering plants abundant; early humans	Atlantic Ocean widens
			Miocene	18	Grasses abundant; rapid spread of grazing mammals	Alps and Himalayas form; Red Sea opens
		Paleogene	Oligocene	11	Apes and elephants appear	India collides with Asia; Australia separates from Antarctica
			Eocene	22	Primitive horses, camels, rhinoceroses; first grasses	Norwegian Sea and Baffin Bay open
			Paleocene	10	First large mammals and modern plants	
251	Mesozoic	Cretaceous		80	Spread of flowering plants; dinosaurs die out at end	Laurasia and Gondwana begin to break up
		Jurassic		54	First birds; dinosaurs at their peak	Laurasia separates from Gondwana
		Triassic		51	Dinosaurs and first mammals appear	Pangaea complete
542	Paleozoic	Permian		48	Rise of reptiles; insects abundant	Laurasia and Gondwana come together to form Pangaea
		Carboniferous		60	Large nonflowering plants in enormous swamps; extensive forests; large insects and amphibians; sharks abundant	Coal being formed; Africa moves against Europe and North America
		Devonian		57	First forests and amphibians; fish abundant	Greenland and North America join Europe
		Silurian		28	First land plants and large coral reefs	
		Ordovician		44	First vertebrates (fish) appear	
		Cambrian		54	Marine shelled invertebrates (earliest abundant fossils)	Early supercontinent breaks up
	Precambrian time	Ediacaran		88	Various forms of simple multicellular life	
2100		Proterozoic Eon		1958	Before Ediacaran: complex one-celled organisms and algae colonies; atmospheric oxygen appears	Early supercontinent forms; "Snowball Earth" occurs
		Archaean Eon		2100	Primitive bacteria and stromatolites	Continents, oceans, and atmosphere form
4600						

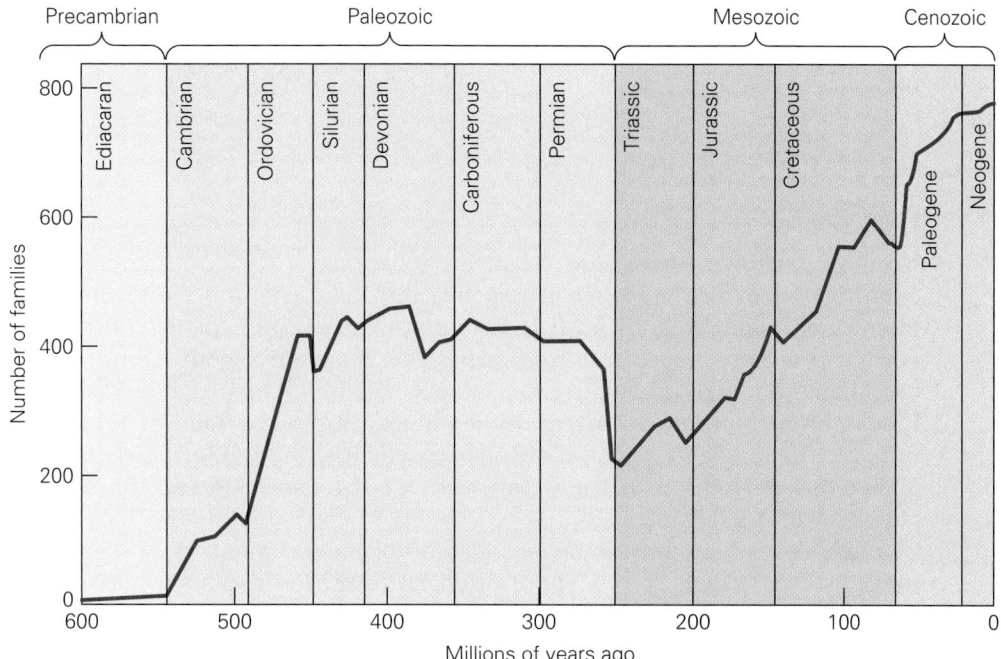

Figure 16-35   How the number of families of living things has varied in the past 600 million years. A family is a group of related species, and the greater the number of families, the greater the diversity of life. Each dip in the curve represents a biological extinction; there have been 20 major ones in all. The most severe extinction marks the end of the Paleozoic Era; the dinosaurs disappeared in the extinction at the end of the Mesozoic Era. Life is at its most diverse today, although human activity has begun to turn the graph downward.

Extinctions   The divisions of geologic time shown in Table 16-2 are based on dramatic changes that occurred from time to time in the earth's history—changes in landscapes, in climates, in types of organisms. In particular, the fossil record reveals a number of occasions, called **extinctions,** when animal and plant life became sharply reduced in both number and variety, to be followed in each case by the evolution of new forms (Fig. 16-35). Although it is hard to be precise, extinctions—with the exception of the one that ended the Mesozoic Era—seem to have taken place over periods of 100,000 years or more of environmental disturbances that involved drastic climate changes—a long time to us, but a relatively brief time in geology.

Extinctions are used to divide geologic history into **periods.** During a typical period an expansion of living things is followed by an interval in which biological change is more gradual; then a time of more sudden change ends the period. Periods are similarly subdivided into shorter **epochs;** only the epochs of the Cenozoic Era are shown in Table 16-2.

The division into eras was based on exceptionally marked worldwide extinctions and subsequent expansions, and correlations were found between large-scale events in the earth's crust and the biological record. Not all these correlations have turned out to be as clear-cut as they once appeared, but the traditional organization of geologic time is still convenient and is universally used by scientists.

Earth History

The earth came into being about 4.6 billion years ago. Current ideas on its origin are discussed in Chap. 19. With the oldest surface rocks the story of the earth leaves the realm of speculation. These rocks, which are found in northern Canada and date back over 4 billion years, consist of sedimentary and metamorphic rocks intruded by igneous rocks. This suggests that the cycle of erosion and renewal of continental crust was already well established as far back as the visible record of the earth's history extends.

Precambrian Time
PROTEROZOIC EON (2500–542)
Ediacaran (630–542)
various forms of simple multicellular life
Before Ediacaran: complex one-celled organisms and algae colonies; atmospheric oxygen appears
ARCHAEAN EON (4600–2500)
primitive bacteria and stromatolites
(dates are millions of years ago)

16.13 Precambrian Time

Long Ago But Not Far Away

Nothing is known for certain about the locations of the continents in Precambrian time. The splitting of Pangaea into Laurasia and Gondwana and their subsequent breakup into today's continents began about 200 million years ago, a mere 4 percent of the earth's age. Plate movement seems to have been going on farther back in the past, perhaps much farther back, with the Precambrian continents differently arranged across the face of the earth. Possibly the long-ago collision of the early earth with another newly formed planet that gave birth to the moon (Sec. 17.16) also triggered the start of plate-tectonic activity.

Although practically unaltered Precambrian sedimentary and igneous rocks are sometimes found, more often Precambrian rocks show considerable metamorphism and in many places have been greatly deformed. Both stream deposits and marine deposits are found in the sedimentary beds (Fig. 16-36). The volcanic rocks include all types, with basalt flows then as now the most common. Intrusive rocks are represented in great abundance and variety.

Evidently geologic processes a billion years ago were not very different from those in the modern world. Precambrian rocks are exposed at the surface over a broad area covering most of eastern Canada and nearby parts of the United States.

Late in Precambrian time declines in the concentration of greenhouse gases in the atmosphere led to a series of at least three global ice ages—"Snowball Earth"—during which glaciers hundreds of meters thick covered land and sea everywhere. These big freezes occurred between 850 and 635 million years ago. Probably each ice age ended when volcanic eruptions released greenhouse gases sufficient for the earth's surface to become warm again. Subsequent ice ages were never as extreme as these earliest ones.

Early Life   Precisely when and where life began on earth nobody knows, because primitive organisms seldom leave traces. Nevertheless, old rocks that *could* show signs of life usually *do* show such signs. Apparently life began not long after the environment of the early earth allowed. In the Archaean Eon, evidence of some sort of primitive single-celled organisms, probably bacteria without nuclei, is found that dates back as far as 3.8 billion years ago.

Figure 16-36 Sample of Precambrian rock from northern Canada that shows ripples and cracks characteristic of fine sediments deposited in shallow water and occasionally dried by exposure to the sun. Similar conditions occur along the shores of present-day lakes and seas.

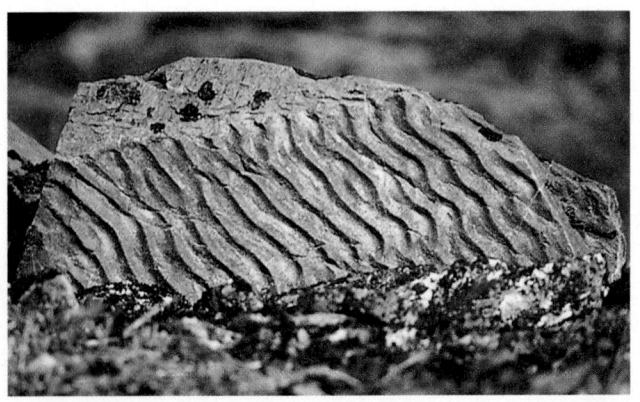

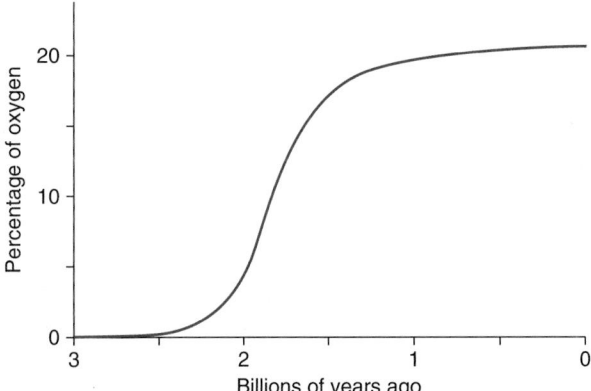

Figure 16-37 Free oxygen began to appear in the atmosphere about 2.5 billion years ago as the result of photosynthesis by primitive bacteria. The exact shape of the curve to today's level of nearly 21 percent is uncertain. The oxygen-carbon dioxide cycle is shown in Fig. 13-22.

By 2.7 billion years ago cyanobacteria ("cyan" comes from the Greek for blue) had developed and began to spread in the oceans. Joined together by sticky mucus into bluish-green mats, these bacteria could survive solar ultraviolet light deadly to most other life, and their photosynthetic activity started to provide the atmosphere with oxygen. (The original atmosphere was rich in CO_2 but lacked free O_2.) Besides producing O_2 the cyanobacteria caused the precipitation of calcium carbonate into characteristic structures of thin sheets of limestone called **stromatolites.** Stromatolites continue to be formed today in a few locations, notably in Australia.

In most of the Proterozoic Eon cyanobacteria were the dominant form of life and contributed to the increase in the oxygen content of the atmosphere (Fig. 16-37). They are still common today. More complex single-celled organisms that contained nuclei arose, including algae that formed colonies in the oceans. When the last Snowball Earth ice age had thawed out, the bacteria that had survived were joined by a variety of simple multicellular organisms that began to develop.

The newcomers did not have hard parts such as shells that could be preserved but did leave impressions in sediments that could be deciphered. The members of one group were apparently similar to modern coral polyps and jellyfish; the members of another had quiltlike structures up to a meter across but less than a centimeter thick that have no counterparts today.

Ediacaran Period Evidence of such life forms in the Ediacara Hills of southern Australia led to the name Ediacaran Period for the time interval that bridged the end of Snowball Earth and the start of the Paleozoic Era with its abundant fossils. Ediacaran mementos have been found in many other parts of the world as well, for instance in Newfoundland where frondlike patterns were discovered in sediments laid down in this period. The Ediacaran Period was not formally recognized until 2004; the more recent geological divisions were finalized in 1891.

16.14 The Paleozoic Era

Plants and Animals in Variety and Abundance

The history of the Paleozoic Era is remarkably complete. No longer are there the doubts and vagueness that characterize Precambrian events, for Paleozoic strata are widely exposed, and their wealth of fossils makes possible correlation of rocks and events from one side of the earth to the other.

The oldest fossils of the Paleozoic Era are those of marine **invertebrates,** creatures without internal skeletons but with external shells of various kinds. All the major groups of the invertebrates are represented. Clams and snails

Paleozoic Era
Permian (299–251)
rise of reptiles, insects abundant
Carboniferous (359–299)
large nonflowering plants in enormous swamps; extensive forests; large insects and amphibians; sharks abundant
Devonian (416–359)
first forests and amphibians; fish abundant
Silurian (444–416)
first land plants and large coral reefs; first insects
Ordovician (488–444)
first vertebrates (fish) appear
Cambrian (542–488)
marine invertebrates with shells (earliest abundant fossils)
(dates are millions of years ago)

Trilobites

Trilobites were abundant in Paleozoic seas and oceans. Their fossils are common because they were among the first animals to have hard shells, which they shed periodically as they grew, like today's lobsters.

Trilobites were the first creatures to have eyes, which appeared about 543 million years ago. These eyes had lenses of crystalline calcite, a feature not found elsewhere. Genetic evidence suggests that trilobite eyes could have been the ancestors of all other eyes, but it also seems possible that eyes evolved independently in as many as 65 different life forms.

Because trilobites evolved rapidly, fossils of their successive species are valuable markers that indicate the ages of rocks in which they are found. Trilobites ranged in length from a few millimeters to 70 cm (Fig. 16-38). Newly evolved predatory fish and squid may have been responsible for the disappearance of the trilobites near the end of the Paleozoic.

Horseshoe crabs are the closest living relatives of trilobites. They are not true crabs but, like trilobites, are distant cousins of spiders and scorpions.

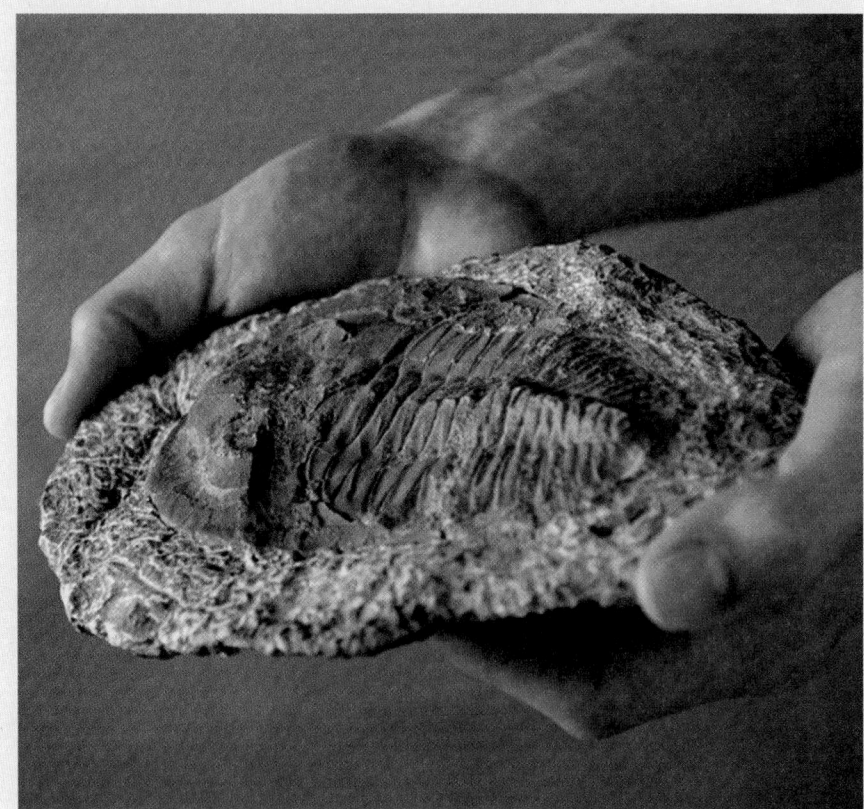

Figure 16-38   Trilobite fossil from the Paleozoic era.

Cambrian Explosion

Living things blossomed in the Paleozoic in an evolutionary riot that began in the Cambrian period—the "Cambrian explosion" of life. The ancestors of most modern life forms arose at this time.

The first life was water-dwelling probably because there was not yet enough ozone in the atmosphere to screen out lethal ultraviolet light from the sun. The early Paleozoic was also a time when the earth's surface was being drastically reshaped; for instance, it was then that North America migrated from near the South Pole to the equator. Shifts such as this stressed living things through changes in climate and thus accelerated their rates of evolution.

increased in number and evolved considerably in the Paleozoic seas. Tiny coral polyps built widespread reefs in the middle Devonian Period. Starfish and sea urchins were not common, but some of their distant relatives that today are rare or extinct were more numerous then. Fishes were many and varied.

In late Paleozoic rocks there is for the first time much evidence of land-dwelling organisms. In the coal swamps of Carboniferous times grew dense forests of primitive plants—huge fernlike trees, enormous horsetails,

The Great Dying

As Fig. 16-35 shows, the most severe mass extinction yet marks the divide between the Paleozoic and Mesozoic Eras. In all, 95 percent of the earth's plant and animal species vanished a quarter of a billion years ago. Not for millions of years was the normal complexity of ecosystems reestablished. What had happened?

Because the Great Dying (as it has been called) took place so long ago, geological processes have inexorably erased most potential evidence. But some clues remain, and they point to a series of immense volcanic eruptions that lasted half a million years and covered much of Siberia with lava. Vast clouds of ash and poisonous gases billowed into the atmosphere.

A huge amount of carbon dioxide was also released, which caused global warming that raised world temperatures by around 6°C. Plant life died off on a large scale, which led oxygen levels to drop as the decay of the remains absorbed oxygen that could not be replaced by photosynthesis. Starved of oxygen, animal life suffered as well.

Further harm was done by toxic hydrogen sulfide (H_2S) gas produced in the oceans by anaerobic bacteria (Sec. 11.9) which do not need oxygen. The H_2S that bubbled into the atmosphere was lethal to both plants and animals and also attacked the protective ozone layer, allowing solar ultraviolet radiation through to do more damage to living things.

Eventually the volcanic activity subsided and conditions more favorable to living things returned. The biological world began to flourish again, now with a different mix of life forms.

The Great Dying set the stage for the rise of the dinosaurs by leaving ecological niches vacant for them, just as the later extinction that ended the Mesozoic saw off the dinosaurs and allowed mammals (such as our ancestors) to thrive afterward.

primitive conifers. A modern person wandering through such a forest would find no bright-colored flowers, no grasses, few plants at all familiar except possibly some of the ferns and mosses.

Animals   In and near the primeval forests lived a great variety of animals, including giant scorpions and the largest insects that ever lived, dragonflies whose wings spanned nearly a meter. The land-living vertebrates of the late Paleozoic are early members of our own family tree. In fact, the basic body plans that appeared in the Paleozoic have served for all animals ever since.

Fossil amphibians, oldest of the land vertebrates, appear first in Devonian rocks. These are relatives of modern frogs and salamanders, sluggish creatures that laid their eggs and spent the early part of their lives in water. Fossils of reptiles begin to appear in late Carboniferous rocks. These animals looked at first much like their amphibian ancestors but had the great advantage of being able to lay their eggs on land. The dry climate at the end of this era was hard on the amphibians, but the reptiles, not needing water to hatch their eggs, multiplied rapidly and developed many different species. During the Permian Period reptiles became the dominant creatures of the land.

The Paleozoic Era ended with a time of intense tectonic activity, which affected many parts of the world including the North American continent. The sediments that had accumulated for more than 300 million years in the Appalachian trough were crumpled, fractured, and uplifted into a mountain chain that must have rivaled any modern range in height and grandeur. It is not hard to connect these dramatic geologic events with the crushing together of the continental masses that formed the supercontinent Pangaea at this time.

16.15   Coal and Petroleum

Both Came from Once-Living Matter

Coal is plentiful in Paleozoic rocks. Coal was formed from plant matter that accumulated under conditions where complete decay was prevented. A bed of coal nearly always implies an ancient swamp. Coal has been formed in swamps from the Devonian to the present day, but seldom have conditions been so favorable as in the Carboniferous Period. (The first part of this period is sometimes called the Pennsylvanian Period and the last part the Mississippian Period.) Apparently there were broad swamps almost at sea level that became periodically submerged so that partly decayed vegetation was covered with thin layers of marine sediments.

The formation of coal begins with the slow bacterial decay of the cellulose content of plants. Taking place underwater and in the absence of air, this decay results in a gradual removal of oxygen and hydrogen from the cellulose to leave a residue that is largely carbon. Also contributing to coal formation was the action of heat and pressure resulting from burial beneath later sediments.

The origin of petroleum is more obscure, for two reasons: fossils are not preserved in a fluid, and petroleum often migrates long distances from where it forms. Because petroleum hydrocarbons can be detected in modern marine sediments, because oils resembling petroleum can be prepared artificially from organic material, and because petroleum is associated with rocks formed from sediments deposited in shallow seas, there seems to be little doubt that marine life such as algae and plankton is the source of petroleum. Most petroleum apparently was formed more recently than coal: over half in the Cenozoic Era, about a quarter in the Mesozoic, and the rest in the Paleozoic.

Petroleum Formation   Three steps seem to have been involved in producing petroleum. The first was bacterial decay in the absence of oxygen, an ideal site being the floor of a shallow sea. Then, as the organic debris was buried under later sediments, it was further modified by low-temperature chemical reactions. The final step was the "cracking" of complex hydrocarbons to straight-chain alkane hydrocarbons (see Chap. 13) under the influence of temperatures of 70°C to 130°C deep underground. If the temperatures became higher, the result was natural gas rather than oil.

Both gas and petroleum, like groundwater, can migrate freely through such porous rocks as loosely cemented sandstones and conglomerates. Wherever formed, they often find their way into porous beds, and it is from these beds that they are obtained by drilling. Since both gas and petroleum are lighter than water, they may be displaced by groundwater and so move upward to the surface to form oil seeps.

Petroleum reservoirs consist of porous sandstones or carbonates capped by layers of impermeable clays or shales. The most common kinds of reservoir are shown in Fig. 16-39. The locations of the world's chief oil and gas deposits are shown in Fig. 4-16.

Figure 16-39 Two common types of structural traps in which petroleum accumulates: (*a*) a trap formed by an anticline (see Fig. 16-3); (*b*) a trap formed by a fault. In both cases petroleum in a porous reservoir rock (such as sandstone) is prevented from migrating upward by an impermeable cap rock (such as shale). A well drilled at A would strike petroleum, one drilled at B would strike gas, and one at C only water. About 80 percent of known petroleum deposits are found in anticline traps. Commercial oil deposits are typically 500–700 m deep; the deepest wells go down about 6 km.

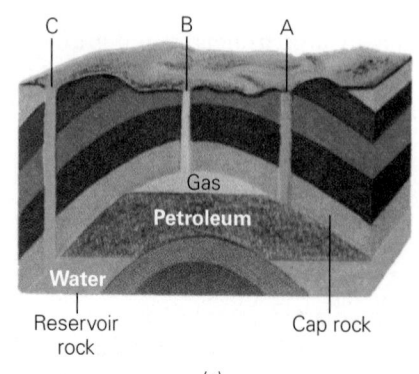

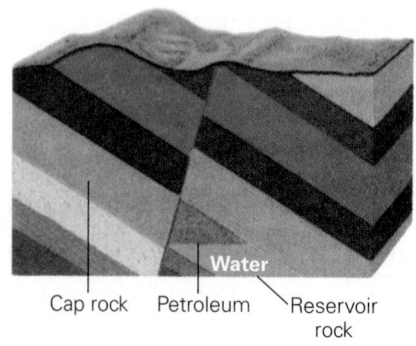

(a)   (b)

16.16   The Mesozoic Era

The Age of Dinosaurs

The earliest Mesozoic sediments were laid down about 251 million years ago, a long time by ordinary reckoning. But the earth was already very old. Some 291 million years had elapsed since the beginning of the Paleozoic and $3\frac{1}{2}$ billion years since the oldest known rocks of the Precambrian. All the time that we include in the Mesozoic and Cenozoic Eras is only one-sixteenth of the history recorded in rocks of the earth's crust.

The Mesozoic Era saw Pangaea split into Laurasia and Gondwana, and this division was followed by their own breakup (see Fig. 16-9). Early in the Mesozoic Era North America began to part from Europe, and somewhat later, perhaps 120 million years ago, South America and Africa began to drift apart. By the end of the era Gondwana no longer existed. Australia, New Zealand, and India had all left Africa, though Arabia still remained attached. Africa itself was in the process of a shift northeastward, thus closing the western end of the Tethys Sea, while India, well on its way toward Asia, was moving into the eastern end. The Mid-Atlantic Ridge was already a prominent feature of the floor of the infant Atlantic Ocean.

The Rise of Dinosaurs   At the end of the Paleozoic Era the world became hot and dry with widespread deserts and less plant life to provide oxygen to the atmosphere by photosynthesis. Reptiles, then the dominant land animals, had evolved when the oxygen level was high, and most of them found it difficult to survive when the level fell. A small class of reptiles, however, happened to have especially efficient respiratory systems, and they took over under the new conditions. These were the **dinosaurs,** some of which developed into the largest land animals the earth has ever seen. (The word *dinosaur* comes from the Greek for "terrible lizard.") Birds are direct descendants of dinosaurs and share their remarkable respiratory systems, which allow geese to fly over the Himalayas at altitudes where the air is too thin for humans to live.

Some dinosaurs were carnivores with bodies designed for pursuing and eating other animals. Some were herbivores with jaws and digestive organs adapted for a vegetarian diet. Active species lived in open plains, more sluggish ones in swamps. Some had bony armor for protection, others depended on speed to escape their enemies. The fastest dinosaurs could outrun today's sprinters, though not today's racehorses. The really large dinosaurs, though, moved sedately at a pace slower than that of a person walking. Not all the dinosaurs by any means were huge, but among the largest were the 80-ton *Futalognkosaurus* ("giant chief lizard"), which were 32 to 34 m (over 100 ft) long from head to tail. They were herbivores that ate a ton or so of vegetation daily, and lived in what is now northern Argentina 80 million years ago. Blue whales, the largest of today's animals and almost extinct due to overhunting, are heavier but a few meters shorter. The smallest known dinosaurs, not much larger than a cat, lived in Colorado late in the Jurassic Period. The largest modern land animal, the African elephant, weighs in at a mere 5–6 tons.

Meanwhile other land organisms were developing. Flowering plants appeared in mid-Mesozoic and with them a host of modern-looking insects suited for helping in the pollination of flowers. The first true birds, with feathered wings rather than membranes, arose from dinosaur ancestors in the Jurassic and were probably four-winged gliders. Birds with two flapping wings and lightweight skeletons, like modern ones, evolved later.

Mammals   Sometime in the Triassic appeared the first **mammals,** creatures that probably descended from a group of small Permian reptiles.

Mesozoic Era
Cretaceous (146–66)
spread of flowering plants; dinosaurs die out at end
Jurassic (200–146)
first birds; dinosaurs at their peak
Triassic (251–200)
dinosaurs and first mammals appear
(*dates are millions of years ago*)

Dinosaurs and Pterosaurs

Dinosaur forms can be inferred by comparing their skeletons with the skeletons of living reptiles. Impressions of dinosaur skins sometimes occur in the rocks in which their bones are found, although the skin colors can only be guessed at. The dinosaurs shown in Fig. 16-40 were all plant-eaters except Tyrannosaurus rex ("king of the tyrant lizards") at upper right, which was about 3 m high at the hips, 11 m long, and had a mass of about 8 tons. The teeth of this creature were 15 cm long and the biting force of its jaws is estimated as at least 13.4 kilonewtons (almost 3 tons!) based on toothmarks found on fossil dinosaur bones discovered in Montana. With a top speed of perhaps 40 km/h, T. Rex could run faster than its herbivorous prey could flee. Thirty T. Rex skeletons have been identified thus far, the first in 1905. The largest modern land predator is the polar bear, whose mass is at most around 700 kg.

Pterosaurs (Greek for "winged lizards") took to the skies in the Mesozoic. The smallest were the size of robins, the largest were over 6 m long with wingspans of 12 m—the size of a small airplane. The toothless beaks of the latter giants were 1.8 m long and tapered to narrow points. What did such a creature eat? Perhaps, like today's storks, it probed for tasty morsels on the bottoms of shallow lakes. Did pterosaurs build up speed to take off by running on the ground or by dropping off a tree or a cliff? In the air, did they soar on thermal updrafts like a glider or did they flap their wings? Nobody is sure about the answers; today's birds are relative pygmies with masses of less than 15 kg, so we can't use them as guides. Dinosaurs, not pterosaurs, were the ancestors of modern birds. Crocodiles are the closest living relatives of birds.

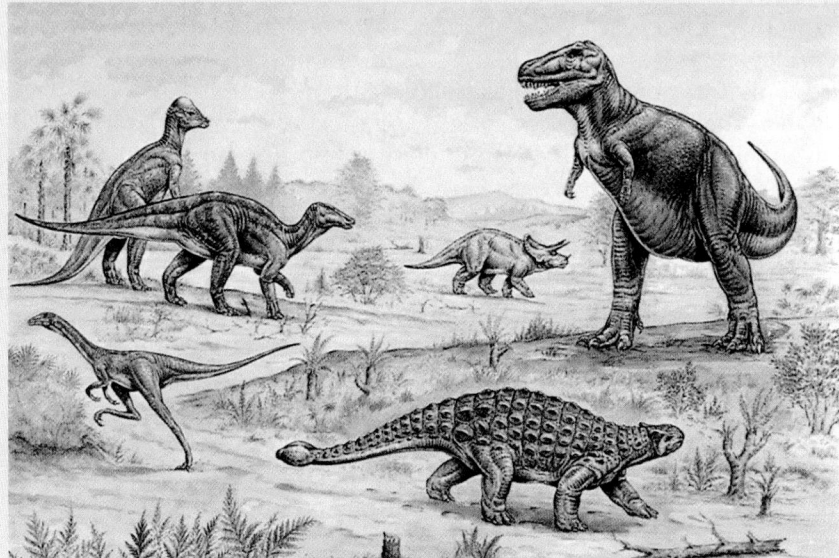

Figure 16-40   A painting of some of the dinosaurs that lived in North America 65 to 70 million years ago at the end of the Mesozoic Era.

All during the Mesozoic mammals remained inconspicuous, seldom much larger than a cat. However, in several respects mammals represented an evolutionary advance over reptiles: they were warm-blooded (constant body temperatures), hence better able to cope with changes of temperature; they had bigger brains relative to their body size; and (except for the egg-laying spiny anteater and duck-billed platypus) they gave birth to well-developed live offspring which they cared for relatively long after birth, so some of the experience of one generation could be passed on to the next.

Although most early mammals filled minor ecological niches, like rodents today, some were predators: the bones of a young dinosaur were found in the belly of a fossil opossum-sized mammal in China. One small mammal had flaps of skin that probably allowed it to glide through the air, like today's flying squirrels; bats arose much later.

Disappearance of the Dinosaurs   For over 100 million years dinosaurs large and small roamed the earth. Then, 66 million years ago, at the height of their diversity and success, all of them disappeared. Not a single dinosaur fossil has ever been found in rocks formed after the end of the Mesozoic Era. The largest animals to survive were crocodiles, close cousins of dinosaurs. Dinosaurs were not the only victims: as many as 70 percent of the plant and animal species of the world were wiped out at about the same time. (Insects were more durable: most of the insect species present at the end of the Mesozoic are still with us. Today there are 200 million insects for each person on the earth.) This mass extinction is what divides the Mesozoic from the Cenozoic.

Throughout geological history extinctions of organisms have been by no means unusual. New species have evolved, flourished, and then died out as far back as the fossil record exists. There is no shortage of past events that could have led to these extinctions. The shifting of the continents and surges in volcanic activity associated with such shifts certainly led to repeated changes in climate, in sea level, in the amount of sunlight reaching the surface (which affects the photosynthesis that is at the base of the chain of life), in the carbon dioxide content of the atmosphere, and so forth. In particular, the end of the Mesozoic was a time of worldwide tectonic and volcanic activity, and it would have been surprising if a large-scale extinction had not occurred then. The late Mesozoic extinction is famous because the dinosaurs disappeared so suddenly and completely, but in fact, as Fig. 16-35 shows, other extinctions, notably the Great Dying that ended the Paleozoic, saw more species disappear.

What Happened?   Until 1979 there seemed no reason to suppose that the fate of the dinosaurs was unusual in any fundamental way. In that year came the discovery of exceptionally large traces of the element iridium in a thin clay layer in Gubbio, Italy, that separated marine limestones of the late Mesozoic from younger limestones. Iridium, a metal similar to platinum, is rare in the earth's crust but relatively abundant in the meteorites that bombard the earth from space. Other late-Mesozoic deposits rich in iridium were soon found elsewhere. The obvious inference was that an asteroid, perhaps 10 or 15 km across, struck the earth 65 million years ago. The impact could have sent up a vast cloud of debris that remained in the stratosphere for months, perhaps years, blocking sunlight and, together with widespread fires that destroyed habitats and spread out everywhere, wiped out much of the life on our planet.

Supporting the impact theory was the discovery in 1991 of the remains of a huge crater about 150 km across (as big as Maryland) that is centered on the edge of Mexico's Yucatán peninsula (Fig. 16-41). The crater's size and age are about right. Furthermore, the clay layer that marks the end of the Mesozoic seems to have originated in both ocean-floor and continental rocks that were pulverized by the impact, which fits in with the crater's location at the rim of an ocean basin.

Volcanic Activity   There is another aspect to the disappearance of the dinosaurs. Intense volcanic activity took place at the end of the Mesozoic, leaving 300,000 km^2 of India covered with several km of lava (Fig. 16-42). Certainly the noxious gases and ash thrown into the atmosphere by the eruptions did life on our planet no good. Furthermore, iridium is abundant in the mantle and could have been brought to the surface in the volcanic magma. Nevertheless, the bulk of the available evidence points strongly to the asteroid impact as the reason for the disappearance of the dinosaurs. Were it not for this impact, dinosaurs might well exist today. Would we? Nobody can say.

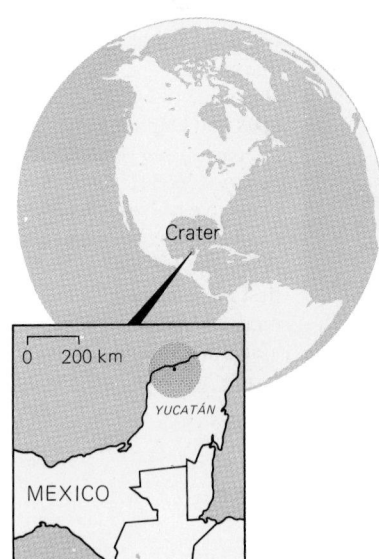

Figure 16-41   A gigantic crater whose traces were found at Chicxulub in Mexico's Yucatán peninsula may have been formed by the impact of the asteroid that led to the extinction of the dinosaurs and many other forms of life at the end of the Mesozoic Era.

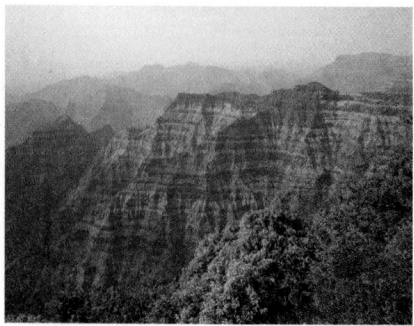

Figure 16-42   Volcanic eruptions at the end of the Mesozoic flooded a huge area of what is now India with basalt to form landscapes like this. Debris flung into the air by the eruptions could have partly blocked sunlight for a long period and thus contributed to the biological extinction at that time.

Cenozoic Era

Neogene {
Holocene (0.01–0) humans are the most complex and successful form of life
Pleistocene (1.8–0.01) rise of humans; large mammals abundant
Pliocene (5.3–1.8) flowering plants abundant; early humans
Miocene (23–5.3) grasses abundant; rapid spread of grazing mammals
}

Paleogene {
Oligocene (34–23) apes and elephants appear
Eocene (56–34) primitive horses, camels, rhinoceroses; first grasses
Paleocene (66–56) first large mammals and modern plants
(dates are millions of years ago)
}

Example 16.4

The widespread biological extinctions of the past, for instance the drastic one in which the dinosaurs disappeared, lead to an interesting question. How can the events that caused them be squared with the principle of uniform change, according to which the earth's geologic history can be explained, in Lyell's words, by "forces now in operation"?

Solution

Certainly the event that caused not only the dinosaurs but a large proportion of the world's other living things to perish is a catastrophe in the usual sense of the word. But the ideas proposed to account for this catastrophe are all in accord with the laws of nature in today's universe. Such is not the case with Werner's idea that all rocks were formed in three precipitations from a universal ocean or with Cuvier's idea of the periodic destruction and re-creation of life by divine edict. Their catastrophes make no sense in terms of physics, chemistry, and biology. On the other hand, volcanoes and asteroids do exist, and even though they may affect the earth on a large scale only rarely, they still fit into the pattern of the principle of uniform change.

16.17   The Cenozoic Era

The Age of Mammals

In many ways the Cenozoic Era of today has been different from preceding eras. During the Cenozoic the continents have stood for the most part well above sea level. No longer do shallow seas spread widely. In North America, beds originating from marine deposits are found only in narrow strips along the Pacific Coast and on the Atlantic Coast from New Jersey south to Yucatán. The thick Paleogene beds east and west of the Rocky Mountains are river, lake, and wind deposits made in continental basins.

Climates during much of the Cenozoic had a diversity like those of the present. The distribution of plants and animals shows that, instead of having widespread moderate climates like those of other eras, Cenozoic continents had zones of distinct hot, cold, humid, and dry climates.

A characteristic of Cenozoic times has been widespread volcanic activity. From the Rockies to the Pacific Coast, lava flows and tuff beds testify to former volcanoes, some of which have only recently become extinct. Immense flows of basalt inundated an area of nearly a half-million km^2 in Oregon, Idaho, and Washington. Some of these flows today form the somber cliffs of the Columbia River Gorge.

Tectonic Activity   The Cenozoic has also been a time of almost continuous tectonic disturbance, in contrast with the long periods of crustal stability in previous eras. Movements associated with the mountain-building episodes that divide the Cenozoic from the Mesozoic lasted well into the Paleogene. In mid-Paleogene the Alps and Carpathians of Europe and the Himalayas of Asia were folded and uplifted. Toward the end of the Paleogene the Cascade range of Washington and Oregon was formed, and other mountain ranges that have been active to the present day began to form around the border of the Pacific. Mountain ranges that had been folded earlier—the Appalachians, the Rockies, the Sierra Nevada—were repeatedly uplifted during the Cenozoic, and erosion following these uplifts has created their present topography.

It is not hard to associate this reshaping of continental landscapes with the spreading of seafloors and the grinding together of lithospheric plates that are still in action today. In the Cenozoic the continents continued their earlier drifts (see Fig. 16-9). In addition Greenland parted from Norway,

Australia parted from Antarctica (New Zealand had done so earlier), and the Bay of Biscay opened up. More recently the Arabian peninsula broke off from Africa, the Gulf of California opened to separate Baja California from mainland Mexico, and Iceland rose above the surface of the Atlantic Ocean.

Mammals   Thanks to their great adaptability, many mammals managed to survive the mass extinction that ended the Mesozoic Era. They continued an evolution and expansion that had begun during the Mesozoic. Carnivores like cats and wolves, armored beasts like rhinoceroses, agile creatures like deer and rabbits—ancestors of all these modern forms roamed the Paleogene landscape. A few mammals, like the whales and porpoises, took to life in the sea; another line, the bats, developed wings.

By the start of the Neogene Period, mammals began to dominate the earth as reptiles had before them. The most numerous of today's mammals are the rodents; a total of 4554 mammalian species are known. Side by side with the mammals developed modern birds and the trees of modern forests. As the Neogene continued, both the physical and the biological worlds assumed more and more closely their present aspects.

Recent Epochs   In the ice ages of the Pleistocene Epoch, great ice caps formed every 100,000 years or so in Canada and northern Europe, and valley glaciers advanced in high mountains elsewhere. (See Sec. 14.11.) Glacial deposits in North America show that ice spread outward from three centers of accumulation in Canada, as shown in Fig. 16-43. The changing climates proved a severe ordeal for living things. Nowadays mammals are still dominant, but in numbers of diversity of species they have declined markedly since the Pliocene.

The current interglacial period, now 10,000 years old, is known as the Holocene Epoch. This length of time is typical of interglacial periods in the past, which suggests another big chill may be about to begin. However, the interglacial period just before the most recent ice age lasted for an unusual 20,000 years, and it seems quite possible that the Holocene may follow

Supersnake

The largest snake known to have existed left fossil remains that date back to the start of the Cenozoic Era. A cousin of boa constrictors, it lived in a rain forest in what is now Colombia, weighed over a ton, and was 13 m long. (Today's snakes max out at around 10 m.) Crocodiles are thought to have been among its prey.

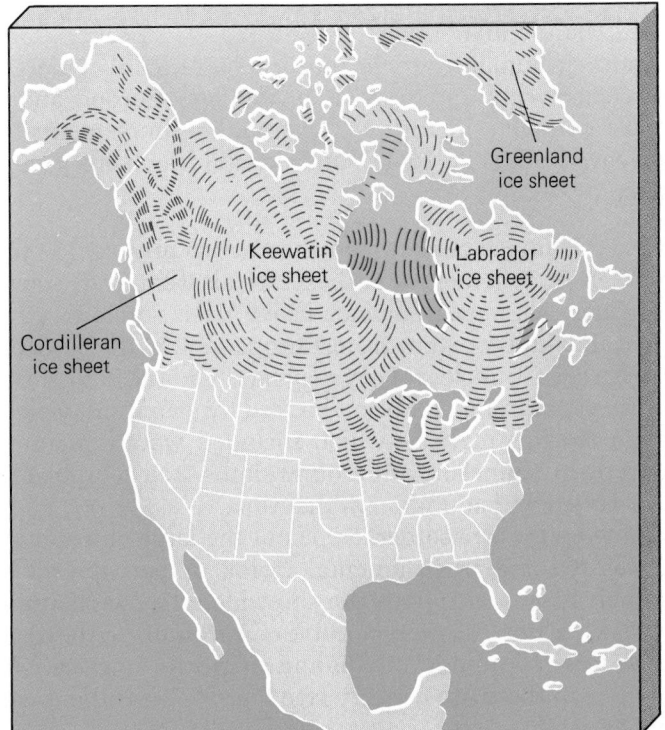

Figure 16-43   The maximum extent of Pleistocene glaciers, some over a kilometer thick, in North America. The major ice advances covered up to 30 percent of the earth's land surface about 20,000 years ago. Today we are in a warm interglacial period with about 10 percent under ice. Average worldwide temperatures when the last ice age was at its peak were 6°C colder than at present and sea level was more than 100 m lower.

Ardi

The oldest hominin fossil known dates back 4.4 million years and is the partial skeleton of an adult female about 1.2 m tall. Her brain was somewhat smaller than that of a chimpanzee and she walked upright. She is called Ardi, short for *Ardipithecus ramidus*, and her ancestors apparently had split away from the lineage that eventually led to modern humans. Ardi's bones were found in Ethiopia together with the remains of 35 other members of the same species.

suit. And there is the global warming discussed in Chap. 4. Although its duration thus far hardly registers on the geological clock, if the warming persists at its current rate, the ice-age cycle may well be disrupted, at least temporarily.

Example 16.5

Suppose the Cenozoic Era follows the patterns of the Paleozoic and Mesozoic Eras. In that case, what will the next phase of the geological story of the earth be like?

Solution

If history repeats itself, the vigorous tectonic and volcanic activities of the Cenozoic thus far (the growth of the Andes and Himalayas, for example) will eventually subside. Mountain building will then lose its major role in shaping landscapes, and erosion will become the chief influence. Today's mountain ranges will be worn down and shallow seas will spread across continental interiors to cover much of their areas.

16.18   Human History

We Are a Recent Species

According to the fossil record, our own species had its infancy in the Great Rift Valley of eastern Africa. Anatomic and genetic evidence indicates that the descendants of a common ancestor split into two branches, about 7 million years ago, one that evolved into some of today's apes and the other into today's humans (Fig. 16-44). The earliest of the **hominins**—humanlike creatures—walked on two legs but still had small brains and eventually died out. There was not a continuous development from then on but rather a succession of closely related species hominin, usually overlapping, with each flourishing for a time and then either disappearing or turning into another. By a little over 2 million years ago some early humans had larger brains than before and were making and using stone tools (hence their species name *Homo habilis*, "handy man"). Farther into the Pleistocene, around 200,000 years ago, modern humans (*Homo sapiens*, "wise man") emerged in Africa and about 65,000 years ago started to populate Europe and Asia. Their record is most complete in Europe, where stone implements, burial sites, drawings on cave walls (Fig. 16-45), and skeletal fragments give a fairly connected history.

North America   Humans came to North America around 15,000 years ago, perhaps even earlier. Whether the earliest arrivals went from Siberia to Alaska over a land bridge that appeared when heavy glaciation lowered sea level (as later ones certainly did) or went from Europe to Canada via Greenland over frozen northern seas is unclear. They may have had the help of boats for part of either journey; Australia had been reached by watercraft well before then. Animal life in North America—which included woolly mammoths, lions, saber-toothed tigers, camels, giant ground sloths, and zebralike horses—was spectacularly varied and abundant at that time.

Did hunting by the newcomers wipe out the large animals about 13,000 years ago, was it some environmental factor, or perhaps the immigrants brought animals that carried pathogens to which they were immune but the native animals were not. All seem possible contributors to the disappearance. There were at least 10 million inhabitants of North America when the first Europeans came in the tenth century (see Fig. 14-34) and more than that in South America.

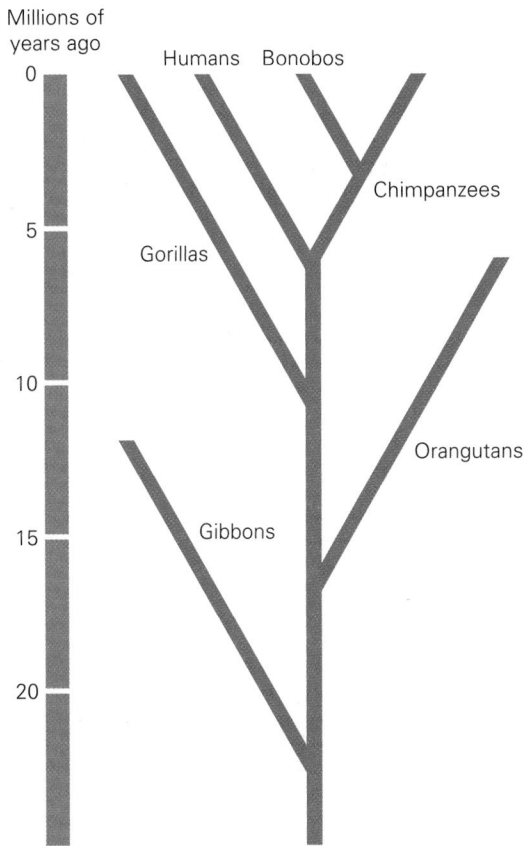

Millions of years ago

Figure 16-44 Evolutionary tree of humans and apes, based on DNA evidence. Monkeys split off earlier. Chimpanzees, bonobos, and humans have nearly all of their genes (and every bone in their bodies) in common; a notable anatomic difference is that the human brain is three times larger than those of the others. All other living things are also our relatives, if more distant. We share around 40 percent of our genes with fish and 25 percent with dandelions.

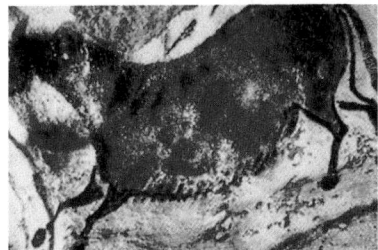

Evolution in humans is still continuing, as it is in other living things. Over 700 genes have been identified that have changed in the past 15,000 years. Most of these genes are involved in bone structure, skin color, digestion, brain function, and the senses of taste and smell. The time period covers the introduction and spread of farming, which changed the characteristics that promoted success in life from what they had been when people were

Figure 16-45 This painting is one of many that were made in a cave at Lascaux, France, during the most recent Ice Age 15,000 years ago.

Recent Cousins

Four hundred thousand years ago the Neanderthals, cousins of ours who were strongly built hunters with large brains (Fig. 16-46), diverged from the lineage that ultimately became modern humans and migrated from their original home in Africa to populate Europe and the Near East. (They are named after the German valley where their remains were first found in 1857.) About 44,000 years ago our direct ancestors began a major expansion north from Africa to Europe where they coexisted with the Neanderthals, the last of whom died out 30,000 years ago. Why they vanished is not known although there are plenty of ideas.

Was there any interbreeding? Apparently Neanderthals and humans were close enough genetically for this to have been possible. Comparing DNA from Neanderthal bones found in a Croatian cave with the DNA of modern humans suggests that many of us indeed have a number of Neanderthal genes in our genomes.

What may have been another cousin species, whose members were less than a meter tall with grapefruit-sized skulls, lived on the Indonesian island of Flores for thousands of years and used relatively advanced tools. They disappeared about 17,000 years ago after a major volcanic eruption on Flores. The leading hypothesis (though not

the only one) is that these little people in several million years of isolation had evolved away from the lineage that led to us.

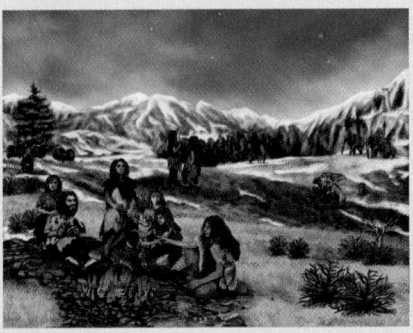

Figure 16-46 What a Neanderthal family might have looked like.

The Next Extinction

Will the next mass extinction be our fault? Thousands of years of hunting for food, skins, and furs have already caused numerous animal species to vanish. The ballooning human population and the accompanying expansion of agriculture have destroyed natural ecosystems everywhere. And global warming is altering the world's climates in ways that stress many life forms. It seems possible that, if these patterns of human behavior continue, their result will be a biological extinction large enough to show up on a graph like that of Fig. 16-35.

Some biologists believe that two-thirds of present bird, mammal, and plant species will be gone by the year 2100. Will we be on the way out in 2100? Humans are extremely adaptable, but there is surely a limit to how much we can abuse our planet and still flourish. How ironic if our mental capacities, which have enabled us to dominate life on earth despite other creatures being larger, stronger, faster, and with superhuman abilities such as flight, should be what brings about our decline.

migratory hunter-gatherers. An example is the emergence of the gene for lactase, the enzyme that permits adults to digest milk; today this gene is most common among people whose ancestors came from northern Europe, where cattle raising became widespread.

People and the Environment   In the past, biological changes were brought about largely by changes in the physical environment, so the biological narrative follows the physical one through the ages. The modern world seems to be witnessing a reversal of this sequence. Not only are we able by virtue of our ingenuity to flourish in the environment that nature has provided, but we are able to alter that environment in a number of ways. These alterations have permitted a vast number of people to live relatively free (by historical standards) of starvation and disease. Today deaths due to ailments brought on by diets of plenty exceed those due to famine.

If continued into the future and swollen in scale by population growth, however, our present patterns of industry and agriculture menace the interplay between people and environment that has been so successful in the past. The indiscriminate use of pesticides and artificial fertilizers has already destroyed the ecological balance in many areas; numerous inland waters have been poisoned by industrial waste; noxious gases fill the air in densely populated regions; acid rain due to power-plant emissions has damaged forests and lakes on a large scale; vast areas of forest have had their trees cut and their soil washed away as a result; global warming due to carbon dioxide emissions is increasing; deposits of radioactive wastes lie waiting for chance catastrophe to disperse them; and so on.

Although a lot has been done in developed countries to limit environmental damage, it is accelerating in the poorer ones as their people climb out of poverty. Most ominous of all is that, whatever we do in the future, a lot more of us will be doing it (see Sec. 4.1).

Important Terms and Ideas

Movements of the solid materials of the earth's crust are called **tectonic.** The principal kinds of tectonic movement are faulting, folding, and regional uplift, sinking and tilting. A **fault** is a fracture surface along which motion has taken place. **Mountain building** begins with the deposition of sediments in a sinking area, followed by tectonic movement and erosion.

The crust and the upper part of the mantle make up a shell of hard rock called the **lithosphere.** Below the lithosphere is a layer of hot, soft rock called the **asthenosphere.**

According to the theory of **plate tectonics,** the lithosphere is divided into seven huge **plates** and a number of smaller ones. The plates can move relative to one another in four ways: two plates can move apart with molten rock rising to form new ocean floor at the gap; one plate can slide under another and melt in a **subduction zone;** two plates can collide and buckle to form a mountain range; and adjacent plates can slide past each other along a **transform fault.**

Continental drift occurs because of plate motion. Today's continents were once part of two supercontinents called **Laurasia** (North America, Greenland, Europe, and most of Asia) and **Gondwana** (South America, Africa, Antarctica, India, and Australia) that were separated by the **Tethys Sea.**

According to the **principle of uniform change,** geologic processes in the past were the same as those in the present. An **unconformity,** which is a buried surface of erosion, indicates that tectonic uplift, erosion, and sedimentation have occurred in that order.

Radionuclides and their decay products in rocks make it possible to date geologic formations. The remains of living things can be dated with the help of **radiocarbon,**

the radioactive carbon isotope ^{14}C. **Fossils,** the remains of organisms preserved in rocks, are useful in correlating strata, in tracing the development of living things, and in reconstructing ancient environments.

Geologic time is divided into **Precambrian time** and the **Paleozoic, Mesozoic,** and **Cenozoic Eras.** Eras are subdivided into periods and the periods into **epochs.** The divisions are marked by mass **extinctions** in which environmental changes cause the disappearance of many species of plants and animals. Dinosaurs were among the victims of the extinction at the end of the Mesozoic Era.

Multiple Choice

1. A crack in the earth's crust along which movement has taken place is called
   - **a.** a fault
   - **b.** a fold
   - **c.** an earthquake
   - **d.** a moraine

2. A long, narrow bay with an irregular outline, such as Chesapeake Bay, was formed by
   - **a.** wave action
   - **b.** stream erosion and later submersion
   - **c.** glacier erosion and later submersion
   - **d.** faulting

3. The rugged character of mountain landscapes is largely the result of
   - **a.** folding
   - **b.** faulting
   - **c.** stream erosion
   - **d.** glacier erosion

4. The ancient supercontinents Laurasia and Gondwana were separated by the
   - **a.** Atlantic Ocean
   - **b.** Pacific Ocean
   - **c.** Tethys Sea
   - **d.** Caribbean Sea

5. A mountain range that was not once part of the Tethys Sea is the
   - **a.** Alps
   - **b.** Pyrenees
   - **c.** Andes
   - **d.** Himalayas

6. North America, Greenland, and most of Eurasia once made up the supercontinent of
   - **a.** Pangaea
   - **b.** Laurasia
   - **c.** Gondwana
   - **d.** Atlantis

7. The shell of rigid rock that makes up the earth's crust and the outer part of the mantle is called the
   - **a.** lithosphere
   - **b.** asthenosphere
   - **c.** thermosphere
   - **d.** subduction zone

8. As compared with the earth's crust under the oceans, under the continents it is
   - **a.** thinner
   - **b.** thicker
   - **c.** about the same in thickness
   - **d.** in some places thinner and in others thicker

9. As compared with the continents, the ocean floors are
   - **a.** much younger
   - **b.** much older
   - **c.** about the same age
   - **d.** in some places older and in others younger

10. The ocean floor near a midocean ridge
    - **a.** has the same constant magnetization on both sides
    - **b.** is magnetized in one direction on one side and in the opposite direction on the other side
    - **c.** has strips of alternate magnetization on both sides
    - **d.** has no consistent pattern of magnetization

11. According to the hypothesis of seafloor spreading, molten rock is rising up along the
    - **a.** trenches that rim the Pacific Ocean
    - **b.** ridges on midocean floors
    - **c.** location of the Tethys Sea
    - **d.** equator

12. The number of large plates into which the lithosphere is divided is
    - **a.** 3
    - **b.** 7
    - **c.** 20
    - **d.** 50

13. In the course of 100 years, a lithosphere plate will typically have moved
    - **a.** 3 mm
    - **b.** 3 m
    - **c.** 3 km
    - **d.** 300 km

14. A region where an edge of a lithospheric plate slides under an edge of another plate is called a
    - **a.** transform fault
    - **b.** fault scarp
    - **c.** moraine
    - **d.** subduction zone

15. Most volcanoes are found
    - **a.** where continental plates collide with each other
    - **b.** in the interior of continents
    - **c.** along subduction zones
    - **d.** along transform faults

16. The Indian subcontinent
    - **a.** was always part of Asia
    - **b.** came into being 45 million years ago as the result of extensive vulcanism
    - **c.** collided with Asia 45 million years ago
    - **d.** began to move away from Asia 45 million years ago

17. Iceland was once
   a. a coral reef
   b. magma that rose from the Mid-Atlantic Ridge
   c. part of Laurasia
   d. part of the Appalachian mountain range

18. The San Andreas Fault in California is the result of the Pacific plate moving
   a. toward the North American plate
   b. away from the North American plate
   c. vertically upward with respect to the North American plate
   d. parallel to the North American plate

19. If the processes of plate tectonics were to stop acting, which of the following would be the last to cease?
   a. earthquakes   **c.** erosion
   b. volcanic eruptions   **d.** tsunamis

20. The theory of evolution is supported by which one or more of the following?
   a. the fossil record of organisms in the past
   b. the distribution of life forms around the world
   c. similarities in the anatomies of different species
   d. the occurrence of mutations

21. An uneven surface on which a horizontal upper bed rests is called a (an)
   a. stratum
   b. fault
   c. dike
   d. unconformity

22. Radiocarbon dating is based upon the fact that
   a. ^{14}C is continually being formed in the remains of living things after their death
   b. ^{14}C is not radioactive
   c. the ^{14}C content of the remains of living things depends upon the time in the past when they came into being
   d. the ^{14}C content of the remains of living things depends upon the time in the past when they died

23. Radiocarbon dating is limited to the remains of plants and animals that died no longer ago than about
   a. 100 years   **c.** 40,000 years
   b. 5700 years   **d.** 1,000,000 years

24. Fossils are least likely to be found in
   a. limestone   **c.** shale
   b. sandstone   **d.** granite

25. Conditions for the preservation of fossils are best fulfilled
   a. in the desert
   b. on the floors of shallow seas
   c. on ocean floors
   d. on river beds

26. The division of geologic time into eras and periods is based upon
   a. the coming of ice ages
   b. the disappearance of continents
   c. biological extinctions
   d. worldwide flooding

27. The earth was formed
   a. in 4004 B.C.
   b. about 2 million years ago
   c. about 4.6 billion years ago
   d. about 10 billion years ago

28. Arrange the following divisions of geologic time in their proper sequence, starting with the oldest:
   a. Paleozoic Era   **c.** Cenozoic Era
   b. Precambrian time   **d.** Mesozoic Era

29. Precambrian rocks are
   a. never found
   b. extremely rare
   c. exposed in a number of regions
   d. the most common rocks

30. Living things have been present on the earth
   a. only in the most recent geological era
   b. only since Pangaea split into Laurasia and Gondwana
   c. for most of its existence
   d. for all of its existence

31. The oxygen in the atmosphere
   a. was present since the earth was formed
   b. was emitted by volcanoes
   c. is the result of sunlight decomposing water vapor
   d. was produced by photosynthesis

32. Ancient geologic processes as revealed in Precambrian strata were
   a. primarily volcanic
   b. primarily glacial
   c. primarily erosion and sedimentation
   d. of the same kinds as those of the present time

33. Coal is composed of
   a. petrified wood
   b. buried plant material that has partially decayed
   c. buried animal material that has partially decayed
   d. a variety of igneous rock

34. A bed of coal usually implies that the region was once a
   a. desert   **c.** swamp
   b. coniferous forest   **d.** river bed

35. The oldest land vertbrates were
   a. reptiles   **c.** mammals
   b. dinosaurs   **d.** amphibians

36. Amphibians, fishes, and marine invertebrates were the dominant form of life in the
   a. Cenozoic   **c.** Paleozoic
   b. Mesozoic   **d.** Precambrian

37. The dinosaurs were which one or more of the following?
   a. reptiles
   b. primitive mammals
   c. all carnivorous
   d. still living when early humans appeared

38. Dinosaurs were abundant in the
   a. Cenozoic   **c.** Paleozoic
   b. Mesozoic   **d.** Precambrian

39. Dinosaurs were the dominant form of animal life for a period of about
   a. 1000 years   **c.** 100 million years
   b. 1 million years   **d.** 1 billion years

40. The leading explanation for the disappearance of the dinosaurs involves
   a. the Little Ice Age
   b. a worldwide flood
   c. an asteroid impact
   d. competition from mammals

41. The ancestors of the birds were
   a. reptiles   **c.** amphibians
   b. mammals   **d.** insects

42. During the Cenozoic Era
   a. Laurasia and Gondwana split into today's continents
   b. lithospheric plates stopped moving
   c. shallow seas covered most of the continents
   d. mammals became the dominant form of animal life

43. Pangaea broke up into Laurasia and Gondwana, which themselves then broke up in the
   a. Cenozoic   **c.** Paleozoic
   b. Mesozoic   **d.** Precambrian

44. The line of descent of humans broke away from that of the apes roughly
   a. 15,000 years ago   **c.** 7 million years ago
   b. 100,000 years ago   **d.** 100 million years ago

45. The Cenozoic Era represents a period
   a. of almost continuous tectonic activity
   b. of relative stability, with erosion and sedimentation the chief geologic processes
   c. of relatively uniform climate around the world
   d. in which the reptile was the most advanced form of life

46. During the Ice Age
   a. there was a single glacial advance
   b. there were several glacial advances and retreats
   c. the entire earth was covered with an ice sheet
   d. all animal life perished and had to start over again afterward

Exercises

16.1 Types of Deformation

1. What landscape features are associated with faults?

2. List all the evidence you can for each of the following statements:
   a. Granite is an igneous rock.
   b. Mica schist is a rock that has been subjected to nonuniform pressure.
   c. Compressional forces exist in the earth's crust.
   d. Tectonic movement is going on at present.

16.2 Mountain Building

3. What geologic process is chiefly responsible for the landscape of a mountain range?

4. Deposits of igneous rocks are found intruded in the folded sedimentary and metamorphic rocks of large mountain ranges. What do you think is the sequence of events that occurred when these ranges were formed?

5. Why is it believed that the region where the Rocky Mountains now stand was once near or below sea level?

16.3 Continental Drift

6. What kind of biological evidence supports the notion that all the continents were once part of a single supercontinent? What kind of climatological evidence supports the concept of continental drift?

7. The eastern coast of South America is a good fit against the western coast of Africa. What sort of evidence would you look for to confirm that the two continents were once part of the same landmass?

8. (a) Where was the Tethys Sea located? (b) Are there any remnants of this body of water in existence today? If so, what are they? (c) What mountain ranges of today were once part of the Tethys Sea? (d) What kind of evidence indicates that the region where these mountains are was once below sea level?

9. Which of today's continents were once part of Laurasia? of Gondwanaland?

16.4 Lithosphere and Asthenosphere

10. Which is denser, the granitic rock of the continents or the basaltic rock of the ocean floors? Which extends deeper into the crust, the continents or the ocean floors?

11. (a) What is the difference between the earth's crust and its lithosphere? (b) How is it possible for a plastic asthenosphere to occur between a rigid lithosphere and a rigid mantle? (c) If the asthenosphere is plastic, how can transverse seismic waves travel through it?

16.5 The Ocean Floors

16.6 Ocean-Floor Spreading

12. North America, Greenland, and Eurasia fit quite well together in reconstructing Laurasia, but there is no space available for Iceland. Why is the omission of Iceland from Laurasia reasonable?

13. How do the ages of the ocean floors compare with the ages of continental rocks? What is the reason for the difference, if any?

16.7 Plate Tectonics

14. When continental drift was proposed almost a century ago, it was assumed that the continents move through soft ocean floors. Why is this hypothesis no longer considered valid? How does continental drift actually occur?

15. The energy source of erosional processes is the sun. Where does the energy involved in tectonic activity come from?

16. Where do subduction zones occur? What happens at them? What becomes of a subducted plate edge?

17. The Himalayas are the highest mountain range on earth. Why are they still rising?

18. How does the origin of the Himalayas differ from that of the oceanic mountains that constitute the Mid-Atlantic Ridge?

19. Which are younger, the Rocky Mountains or the Himalayas?

20. Is the Atlantic Ocean becoming narrower or wider? The Pacific Ocean?

21. The San Andreas Fault in California is a strike-slip fault that lies along the boundary between the Pacific and American plates. What does this indicate about the nature of the boundary?

22. In what geological zones are most volcanoes found?

23. Which plate collisions are responsible for creating island arcs such as the West Indies, the Aleutians, and Indonesia?

24. The distance between the continental shelves of the eastern coast of Greenland and the western coast of Norway is about 1300 km. If Greenland separated from Norway 65 million years ago and their respective plates have been moving apart ever since at the same rate, find the average speed of each plate.

25. The oldest sediments found on the floor of the South Atlantic Ocean, which are 1300 km west of the axis of the Mid-Atlantic Ridge, were deposited about 70 million years ago. What rate of plate movement does this finding suggest?

16.9 Rock Formations

26. In Fig. 16-47, beds *A* to *F* consist of sedimentary rocks formed from marine deposits and rocks *G* and *H* are granite. What sequence of events must have occurred in this region?

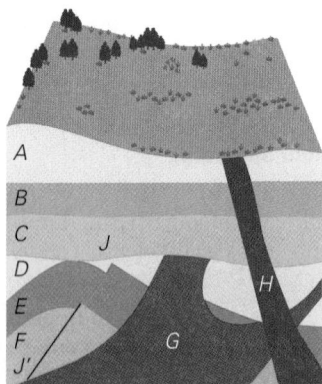

Figure 16-47

27. (a) What is an unconformity? (b) If one is shown in Fig. 16-47, where is it?

28. What is a fault? If one is shown in Fig. 16-47, where is it?

16.10 Radiometric Dating

29. What is the basis of the radiocarbon dating procedure?

30. The half-life of rubidium 87 is 47 billion years, and that of potassium 40 is 1.3 billion years. Would you expect the rubidium-strontium or potassium-argon method of radiometric dating to be more generally useful? Why?

31. The half-life of potassium 40 is 1.3 billion years. If a rock sample contains 0.010 percent of this radionuclide today, what was its percentage in the rock 3.9 billion years ago?

16.11 Fossils

32. Why are fossils still useful in dating rock formations despite the development of radioactive methods?

33. List as many different kinds of fossils as you can.

34. Why are most fossils found in beds that were once the floors of shallow seas?

35. Why are fossils never found in igneous rocks and only rarely in metamorphic rocks?

16.12 Geologic Time

36. What is the basis for the division of geologic time into eras and periods?

37. What is the oldest division of geologic time? In what division are we living today?

38. During what divisions of geologic time have living things existed on the earth?

39. The earth's history is sometimes divided into two **eons,** Cryptozoic ("hidden life") and Phanerozoic ("visible life"), with the first corresponding to Precambrian time and the second extending from the beginning of the Paleozoic Era to the present day. What do you think is the reason for this division?

16.13 Precambrian Time

40. The early atmosphere of the earth probably consisted of carbon dioxide, water vapor, and nitrogen, with little free oxygen. What is believed to be the source of oxygen in the present-day atmosphere? What bearing has this question on the relatively rapid development of varied and complex forms of life that marks the start of the Paleozoic Era?

41. Precambrian rocks include sedimentary, igneous, and metamorphic varieties. What does this suggest about the geologic activity in Precambrian time?

42. Precambrian rocks are exposed over a large part of eastern Canada. What does this suggest about the geologic history of this region since the end of Precambrian time?

43. What conspicuous difference is there between Precambrian sedimentary rocks and those of later eras?

44. What are the chief kinds of organisms that have left traces in Precambrian sedimentary rocks?

16.14   The Paleozoic Era

45. Paleozoic sedimentary rocks derived from marine deposits are widely distributed in all the continents. What does this indicate about the height of the continents relative to sea level in the Paleozoic Era?

46. Which of the following are found in Paleozoic rock formations? Dinosaur fossils; early human fossils; coal deposits; radiocarbon deposits.

47. Why is it believed that large parts of the United States were once covered by shallow seas?

16.15   Coal and Petroleum

48. Under what circumstances is coal formed?

49. What is believed to be the origin of petroleum? Of natural gas?

16.16   The Mesozoic Era

50. What are some of the chief differences between reptiles and mammals?

51. What kind of animals were the dinosaurs? Were they mostly small, mostly large, or were they of all sizes?

52. What is believed to be the reason or reasons for the disappearance of the dinosaurs? What is the evidence for this belief?

53. From what type of animal did birds evolve? Are modern birds closest anatomically to butterflies, bats, flying fish, or crocodiles?

16.17   The Cenozoic Era

54. About 200 million years ago today's continents were all part of the supercontinent Pangaea. During what geologic era did Pangaea break apart into Laurasia and Gondwana? During what era did Laurasia break up into North America, Greenland, and Eurasia?

55. The same reptiles were present on all continents during the Mesozoic Era, but the mammals of the Cenozoic Era are often different on different continents. Why?

56. In rocks of what era or eras would you expect to find fossils of (a) horses; (b) ferns; (c) clams; (d) insects; (e) apes?

57. What were the ice ages? When did they occur?

58. The Scandinavian landmass of Norway and Sweden has been rising since the end of the most recent ice age. Can you think of the reason for this?

59. Minnesota has a great many shallow lakes. How do you think they originated?

The Solar System

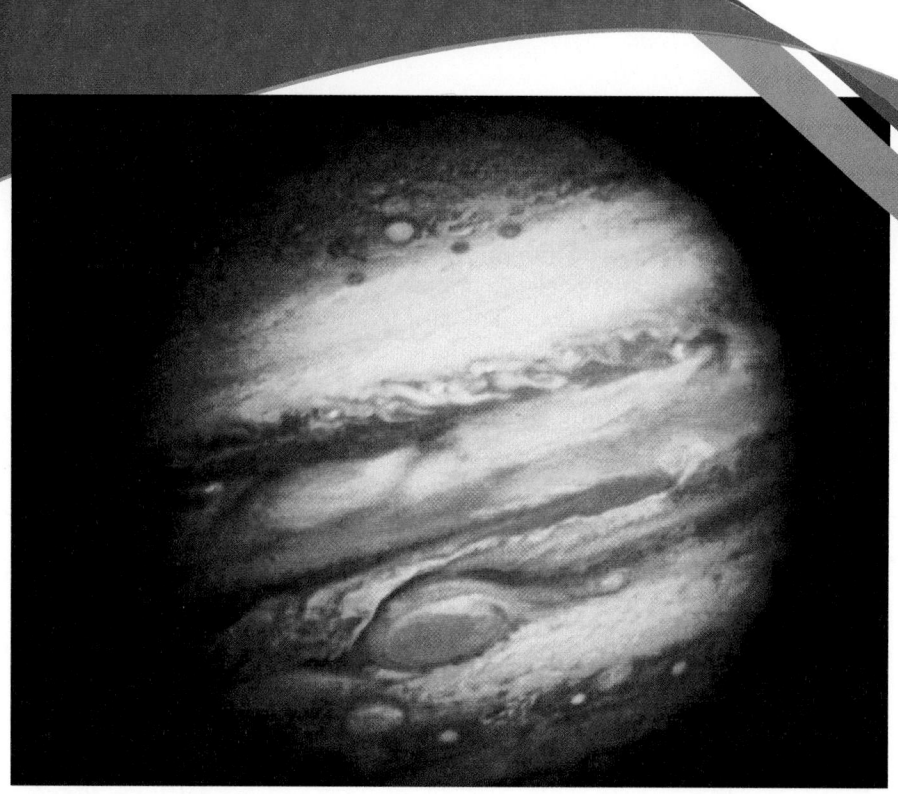

Jupiter is the largest planet.

GOALS

When you have finished this chapter you should be able to complete the goals
• given for each section below:

Whether we look at them with the naked eye or with the help of the largest telescope, the stars are just points of light. On the other hand, most of the planets appear as disks in a telescope of even modest power. This does not mean, of course, that the planets are larger than the stars, only that the planets are much closer to us. The sun, like other stars, glows brightly because it is extremely hot. The planets are too cool to shine by themselves and we see them by the sunlight they reflect. The sun together with its accompanying planets, their satellites, and other smaller bodies make up the **solar system.** The members of the solar system dwell in emptiness and are separated by vast distances from everything else in the universe.

The Family of the Sun

Until the seventeenth century the solar system was thought to consist of only the five planets Mercury, Venus, Mars, Jupiter, and Saturn besides the sun, the earth, and the moon. In 1609, soon after having heard of the invention of the telescope in Holland, Galileo built one of his own. With his telescope, Galileo found four additional members of the solar system: the brighter of the moons (or **satellites**) that circle Jupiter. Since Galileo's time, improved telescopes have led to the discovery of many more members of the sun's family.

The list of planets, in order of average distance from the sun, comprises Mercury, Venus, Earth, Mars, Jupiter, Saturn, Uranus, and Neptune (Fig. 17-1). Pluto, once considered a planet, was reclassified in 2006 as a **dwarf planet** (Secs. 17.8 and 17.11), a new category with other members. All except Mercury and Venus have satellites. Thousands of small objects called **asteroids,** all less than 1000 km in diameter, follow separate orbits about the sun in the region between Mars and Jupiter. Similar objects, one larger than Pluto, are in orbit outside Pluto. Comets and meteors, in Galileo's time thought to be atmospheric phenomena, are now recognized as also belonging to the solar system.

In recent years our knowledge of the solar system has been greatly increased by the voyages of spacecraft, most of them from the United States but with some notable European ones as well. There have been around 200 missions thus far, about two-thirds of them successful, with more in flight or planned. Spacecraft have landed on Venus and Mars, inspected comets and asteroids at close range, and astronauts have walked on the surface of the moon.

So remarkable is modern technology that signals from the tiny 8-W transmitter on Pioneer 10 were still being picked up on the earth in 2003,

Figure 17-1 The solar system. The orbits of Mercury and Venus are too small to be shown on this scale. Diameters of sun and planets are exaggerated.

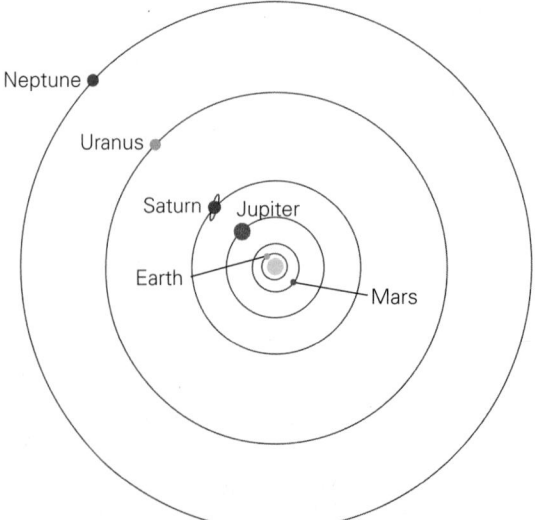

20 years after it left the solar system, over 30 years after it left Florida. The spacecraft was then so far away that its signals took more than 11 hours, traveling at the speed of light, to reach the earth. Effective contact was finally lost in that year.

Over 400 planets have been discovered that orbit stars other than the sun. These exoplanets are the subject of Sec. 19.11.

17.1   The Solar System

Inner Planets Mostly Rock, Outer Planets Mostly Liquified Gas

Not only is the solar system isolated in space, but also each of its principal members is far from the others. From the earth to our nearest neighbor, the moon, is about 384,000 km; from the earth to the sun is about 150 million km. It took the Apollo 11 spacecraft 3 days to reach the moon. Traveling at the same speed, Apollo 11 would take more than 3 years to reach the sun.

If we use a golf ball to represent the sun, a grain of sand 4 m away would represent the earth on the same scale. The moon would be a dust speck about 1 cm from the sand grain. The largest planet, Jupiter, would be a small pebble 18 m from the golf ball, and Neptune would be a still smaller pebble 120 m from the golf ball. The total mass of the planets is only 0.13 percent of the mass of the sun. The relative sizes of the planets are shown in Fig. 17-2.

Planets **revolve** around the sun and **rotate** on their axes. Two aspects of these motions are notable:

1. Nearly all the revolutions and rotations are in the same direction. Only the rotation of Venus and the revolutions of a few minor satellites about their parent planets run contrary to the general motion. (Uranus is an exception of a different kind, since it rotates about an axis only 8° from the plane of its orbit.)
2. All the orbits lie nearly in the same plane (Fig. 17-3).

The principal data about the planets and their orbits are summarized in Table 17-1. The **inner planets** of Mercury, Venus, Earth, and Mars are relatively small, have similar densities, and are composed largely of rocky material. All have cores that probably consist mainly of iron. They rotate fairly slowly on their axes. Among them is only one satellite of any size, the moon; the two satellites of Mars are only a few km across.

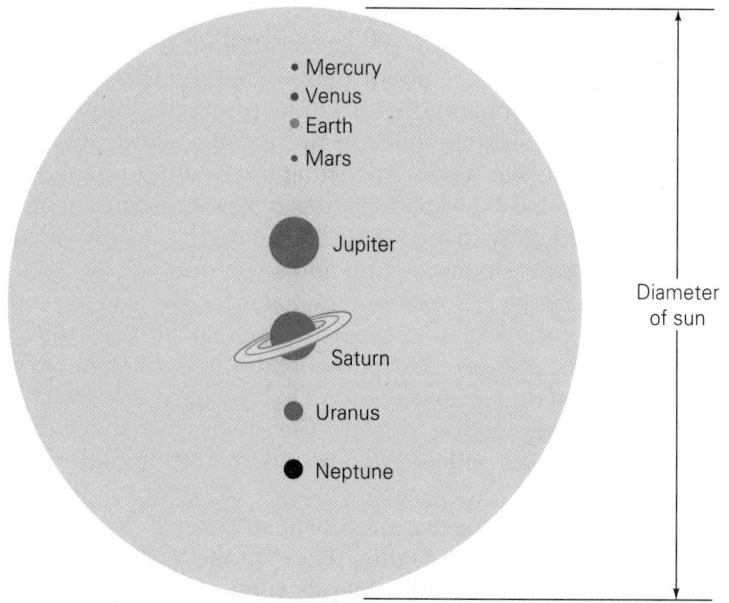

Figure 17-2   Relative sizes of planets and sun.

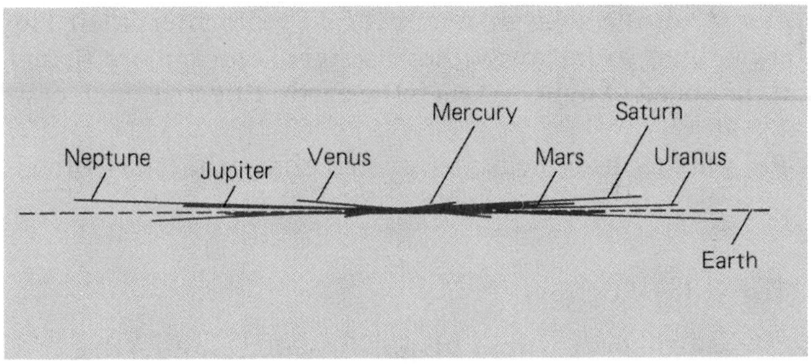

Figure 17-3   The orbits of the planets seen edgewise. The orbits all lie nearly in the same plane.

The **outer planets** of Jupiter, Saturn, Uranus, and Neptune are large, not very dense compared with the earth (Saturn would float if placed in a large enough bathtub), and are composed largely of gases compressed to liquid form without iron cores. They rotate fairly rapidly on their axes. These giant planets have among them a total of over 130 satellites, a few large, most quite small. The inner planets have low escape speeds; the giant ones have high escape speeds. (Escape speed is discussed in Sec. 2.14.)

The dwarf planets are discussed in Secs. 17.8 and 17.11.

17.2   Comets

Regular Visitors from Far Away in the Solar System

Besides the stars, planets, and moon that are its permanent inhabitants, the night sky is occasionally host to transient visitors known as **comets** (Fig. 17-4). Until the work of the Danish astronomer Tycho Brahe, it was not clear whether comets were luminous clouds in the upper atmosphere or were heavenly bodies in space. In 1577 Brahe compared the positions in the sky of a comet as seen from different places in Europe and found them the same within the accuracy of his instruments, which meant that the comet was more distant than the moon.

Comets are thought to be leftover matter from the early history of the solar system that did not become part of larger bodies such as the planets. A comet is composed chiefly of ice and dust—a "dirty snowball"—in some cases mixed with polymerized organic molecules. In addition, smaller amounts of various frozen gases are present, for instance carbon monoxide, carbon dioxide, methane, ammonia, and hydrogen cyanide.

Spacecraft Interception   A number of spacecraft have been sent out to intercept comets and find out more about them. On July 4, 2005, one of these spacecraft, NASA's Deep Impact, fired a 370-kg projectile into the path of the comet Tempel 1. The resulting collision produced a giant plume of debris and left a crater behind (Fig. 17-5). Analyzing the wealth of images and spectroscopic data sent back by the spacecraft as it flew past and by other spacecraft, as well as recorded by instruments on the earth, has provided detailed information on the comet's composition and structure.

Apparently the comet is loosely held together by gravity rather than packed hard, and contains clay and carbonates, substances that need liquid water to form. But comets like Tempel 1 are thought to have originated from smaller bits of matter past Neptune's orbit where any water would be frozen. Unexpected findings like this are the rewards of space exploration, and solving such mysteries will add to our understanding of the universe we live in.

In 2004 another NASA spacecraft, Stardust, passed close enough to the comet Wild 2 to take samples of its dust. The samples, parachuted down near Salt Lake City in 2006, contained minerals such as olivine (Fig. 15-9) that

Where Comets Live

Most of the comets in the solar system, perhaps 10^{13} of them, make up the Oort Cloud, which lies about 50,000 times farther from the sun than the earth, a fifth of the distance to the nearest star. At that distance the sun is only as bright as Venus is in our sky. The cloud is named for the Dutch astronomer Jan Oort, who proposed its existence after studying the orbits of known comets.

Because the Oort Cloud is so far from the sun, the orbits of its members are easily disturbed, for instance by stars that happen to pass not too far away, which occurs from time to time. Some of the changed orbits bring the corresponding comets to the inner solar system, where we are. The Hale-Bopp comet that decorated the sky in 1997 is believed to have leaked from the Oort Cloud.

A smaller number of comets form a swarm outside Neptune called the Kuiper Belt (named for the American astronomer Gerard Kuiper). Many objects in the Kuiper Belt—over 800 of them are known at present—are more like asteroids (see Sec. 17.8). Some of these objects are huge, over 1000 km across. There may be many more like these far out in space and therefore hard to find.

Table 17-1 | The Planets

Planet	Symbol	Mean Distance from Sun, Earth = 1[a]	Diameter, Thousands of km	Mass, Earth = 1[b]	Mean Density, Water = 1[c]	Surface Gravity, Earth = 1[d]	Escape Speed, km/s[e]	Period of Rotation on Axis	Period of Revolution around Sun	Eccentricity of Orbit[h]	Inclination of Orbit to Ecliptic[i]	Known Satellites[j]
Mercury	☿	0.39	4.9	0.055	5.4	0.38	4.3	59 days	88 days	0.21	7°00'	0
Venus	♀	0.72	12.1	0.82	5.25	0.90	10.4	243 days[f]	225 days	0.01	3°34'	0
Earth	⊕	1.00	12.7	1.00	5.52	1.00	11.2	24 h	365 days	0.02		1
Mars	♂	1.52	6.8	0.11	3.93	0.38	5.0	24.5 h	687 days	0.09	1°51'	2
Jupiter	♃	5.20	143	318	1.33	2.6	60	10 h	11.9 yr	0.05	1°18'	63
Saturn	♄	9.54	120	95	0.71	1.2	36	10 h	29.5 yr	0.06	2°29'	60
Uranus	♅	19.2	51	15	1.27	1.1	22	16 h[g]	84 yr	0.05	0°46'	27
Neptune	♆	30.1	50	17	1.70	1.2	24	16 h	165 yr	0.01	1°46'	13

[a]The mean earth-sun distance is called the astronomical unit, where $1 AU = 1.496 \times 10^{11}$ km.
[b]The earth's mass is 5.98×10^{24} kg.
[c]The density of water is $1 g/cm^3 = 10^3 kg/m^3$.
[d]The acceleration of gravity at the earth's surface is $9.8 m/s^2$.
[e]Speed needed for permanent escape from the planet's gravitational field.
[f]Venus rotates in the opposite direction from the other planets.
[g]The axis of rotation of Uranus is only 8° from the plane of its orbit.
[h]The difference between the minimum and maximum distances from the sun divided by the average distance.
[i]The ecliptic is the plane of the earth's orbit.
[j]Probably more small ones around Jupiter, Saturn, and Uranus.

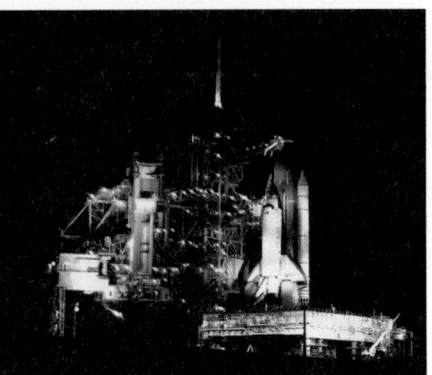

Figure 17-4   The comet Hale-Bopp, one of the largest ever to come near the earth, was a spectacular sight in the night sky for the first few months of 1997. It appears here to the left of the Space Shuttle *Columbia* on its launching platform. Comets are named after their discoverers, here the professional astronomer Alan Hale and the amateur Thomas Bopp, who independently noticed a faintly glowing speck moving across the fields of their telescopes on the same night in July 1995. (About half a dozen comets are spotted every year by amateur astronomers.) The comet was then farther away than Jupiter. When it was closest to the earth, Hale-Bopp's tail stretched across 20° of the sky; for comparison, the apparent diameter of the full moon is 0.5°.

form only at high temperatures. But Wild 2, like Tempel 1, came from the Kuiper Belt beyond Neptune, where it is bitterly cold. This suggests that at least some of the material in both comets came into being closer to the sun before somehow ending up far out in the Kuiper Belt. In addition, organic compounds of various kinds were found, among them two that contain biologically usable nitrogen, which supports the idea (mentioned in Sec. 13.17) that the comets that rained down on the young earth may have had a role in the origin of life.

Comet Orbits   The paths followed by comets that periodically pass near the earth are quite different from the nearly circular planetary orbits. A typical comet approaches the sun from far out in space beyond Pluto, swings around the sun, and then retreats. The orbit is a long, narrow ellipse, and the comet returns at regular intervals.

Although most orbits are so large that their periods range up to millions of years, a few are smaller. Halley's comet, for instance, reappears every 76 years and has returned 28 times since the first sure record of its observation was made in 239 B.C. It was named after the English astronomer Edmund Halley, a contemporary of Newton, who in 1705 predicted that a comet last seen in 1682 would reappear in 1758, as it did. Halley's comet came within 93 million km of the earth in November 1985 on its most recent visit, when it was studied at close range by various spacecraft. The comet's solid nucleus was about 16 km long and 8 km across, with a mass of about 100 billion tons.

Heads and Tails   In the far reaches of the solar system comets are fairly small, only a few km across. Near the sun the frozen gases vaporize and take with them dust to form the huge but thin clouds that make up the comet heads and tails we see. Comets are visible only when close to the sun. This is partly because of sunlight scattered by cometary material but mainly because the gases are excited to luminescence by solar radiation.

Comets appear as small, hazy patches of light, often accompanied by long, filmy tails—hence their name, which comes from the Greek word for "hairy." Most comets are visible only with the help of a telescope, but from time to time one becomes conspicuous enough to be seen with the naked eye. Watched for a few weeks or months, a comet at first grows larger and its tail longer and more brilliant. Then it fades gradually, loses its tail, and eventually disappears.

A comet's tail always points away from the sun regardless of which way the comet is heading (Fig. 17-6). One reason is the **solar wind,** the stream of ions that constantly flows outward from the sun, which tends to sweep the comet's gases with it. Another reason is the pressure of solar radiation on the tail's dust particles.

Comet tails may stretch for millions of km across the sky. Near the sun, a comet loses material to space, and so is fainter each time it returns. Far from the sun, it contracts again into a relatively small body.

17.3   Meteors

"Shooting Stars" Usually Smaller Than a Grain of Sand

Meteoroids are small fragments of matter that the earth meets as it travels through space. Most meteoroids are smaller than grains of sand. The majority are believed to be the result of asteroid collisions; others are the debris of comets.

Moving swiftly through the atmosphere, meteoroids are heated rapidly by friction. Usually they burn up completely about 100 km above the

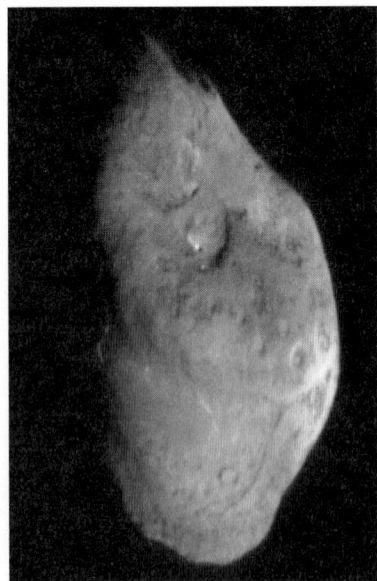

Figure 17-5   The NASA Deep Impact probe collided with the comet Tempel 1 in 2005 and left the crater just above the center of this photograph. The crater is 20 m deep.

earth, appearing as bright streaks in the sky—**meteors,** or "shooting stars" (Fig. 17-7). Sometimes, though, they are so large to begin with that a substantial portion may get through the atmosphere to the earth's surface (Fig. 17-8). The largest known fallen meteoroids, called **meteorites,** weigh many tons. The smallest meteoroids are so light that they float through the atmosphere without burning up. Around a hundred tons of these fine, dust-like micrometeoroids reach our planet daily.

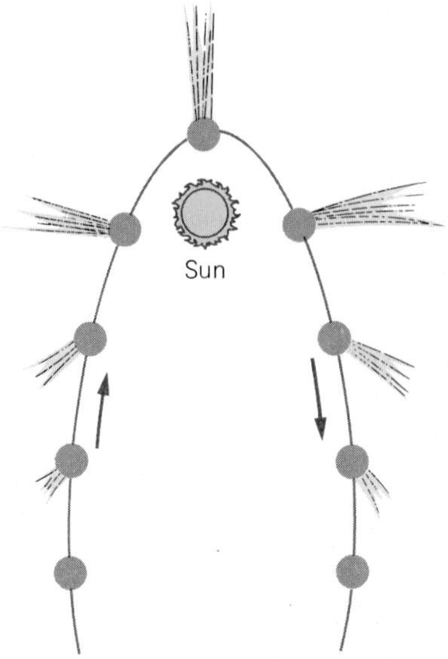

Meteor Showers   A keen observer on an average clear night can spot 5 to 10 meteors an hour. Most of these meteors are random in occurrence and follow no particular pattern either in time or place in the sky. At several specific times of year, however, great meteor showers occur, with 50 or more meteors sometimes visible per hour that appear to come from the same part of the sky. The showers occur when the earth moves through a swarm of meteoroids that follow the same orbit about the sun.

When the meteoroids of a shower are spread out along their common orbit, the number of meteors seen is about the same each year. This is the case with the Perseid showers of mid-August. When the meteoroids are bunched together, the number of meteors seen varies from year to year. The Leonid showers of mid-November are an example, with intense displays every 33 years. Other conspicuous meteor showers are listed in Table 17-2. The Eta Aquarid and Orionid showers are due to dust particles from Halley's comet that are spread out in its orbit. The earth crosses this orbit twice a year with the showers as a result.

Meteoroid speeds range up to 72 km/s. This limit is significant, because a higher speed would imply an object arriving from outside the solar system. The conclusion is that all meteoroids, random as well as shower, are members of the solar system that follow regular orbits around the sun until they collide with the earth or another planet.

Meteorites   Most meteorites that have been examined fall into two classes: stony meteorites, the great majority, which consist of silicate minerals much like those in common rocks of the earth's crust, and iron meteorites, which, like the earth's core, consist largely of iron with a small percentage of nickel (Fig. 17-9). A few meteorites are intermediate in character. All meteorites are sufficiently different from terrestrial rocks to be recognized as such, notably by smooth surface crusts, usually black, that formed when their surfaces melted on entry into the atmosphere and later hardened.

Figure 17-6   The tail of a comet always points away from the sun because of pressure from the sun's radiation and from the solar wind of ions. The tail is longest near the sun, when it is millions of km long, and seems to be absent far away from the sun.

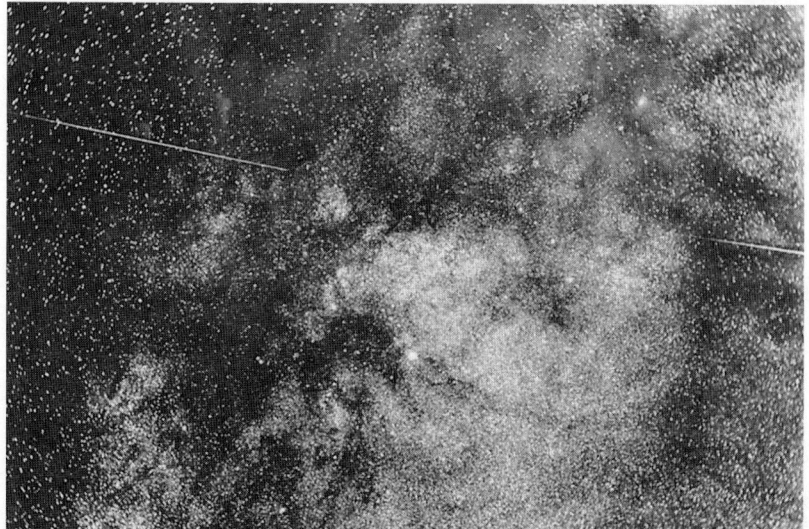

Figure 17-7   Time exposure showing a meteor streak in the night sky. Few meteoroids are larger than a grain of sand, and those that enter the earth's atmosphere usually burn up before they can reach the ground. On a clear dark night, 5 to 10 meteors per hour can be seen.

Figure 17-8   The Barringer Meteor Crater near Winslow, Arizona, 1200 m across and 175 m deep, was formed about 50,000 years ago. Its origin was ascribed to a meteoroid impact by the mining engineer D. M. Barringer in 1906. The meteoroid may have been 50 m across, weighed several hundred thousand tons, and traveled at over 40,000 km/h. It was completely destroyed upon impact.

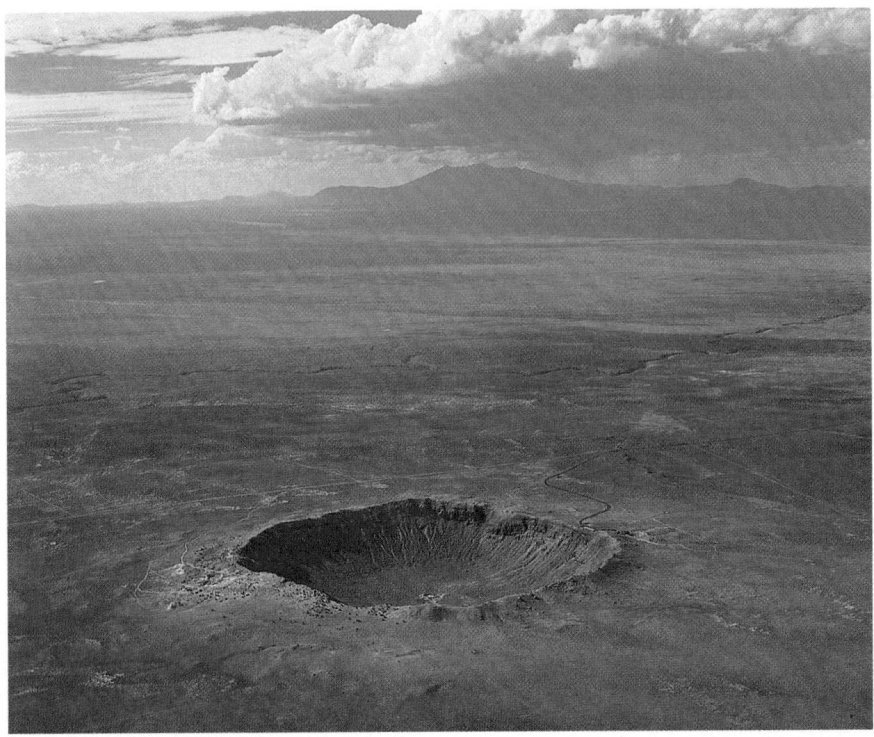

Table 17-2	Some Major Meteor Showers	
Shower	**Maximum Display**	**Average Hourly Rate**
Quadrantid	Jan. 3, 4	40
Eta Aquarid	May 5, 6	10
Delta Aquarid	July 28, 29	20
Perseid	Aug. 12, 13	60
Orionid	Oct. 21, 22	20
Leonid	Nov. 17, 18	40
Geminid	Dec. 13, 14	60

Figure 17-9   Discovered in Greenland in 1894, this iron meteorite is 3.3 m long. The largest known meteorite has a mass of 55,000 kg and was found in Namibia. About 4 percent of meteorites are iron, 94 percent are stony, and the rest are stony-iron.

The best place to seek meteorites is the Antarctic, where conditions for preservation are ideal and on whose ice sheets scattered rocks are conspicuous in various regions. Most such rocks came from nearby mountains, but quite a few fell from the sky. Almost 20,000 meteorites have been collected thus far in the Antarctic in the last two decades, far more than have been found in the rest of the world in all the past. Stony meteorites classed as chondrites are the most common, and are not hard to identify because they are studded with tiny white mineral spheres ("chondrules"). The chondrules solidified from once-liquid rock 4.6 billion years ago when the solar system came into being.

The earth's neighbors in space—the moon, Mercury, Venus, Mars, and the satellites of Mars—are all deeply pitted with many huge meteor craters.

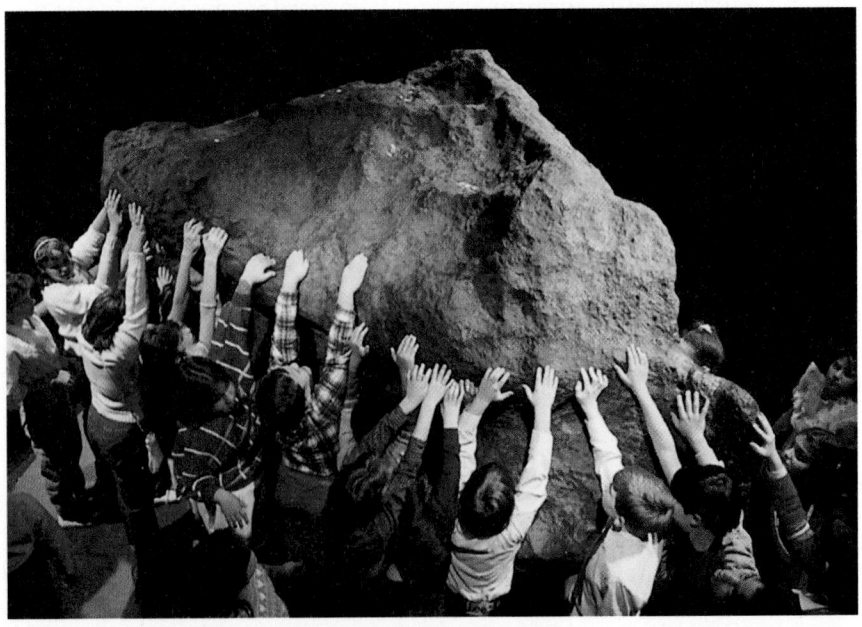

Visitors from the Moon and Mars

Not everything that falls on the earth is a meteoroid from space. In 1982 an unusual greenish brown rock about the size of a golf ball was found in Antarctica. The composition of this rock turned out to be identical with that of rocks brought back from the moon by Apollo 15 astronauts in 1971. A number of other similar moon rocks were found later, in Australia as well as in Antarctica. It seems possible that the impact of large meteoroids on the moon could have hurled the rocks out fast enough to escape the moon's gravitational pull.

Over 30 other rocks found in Antarctica, India, Egypt, and France show signs of having come from Mars—the gas trapped in them has the same composition as the Martian atmosphere, for instance (Fig. 17-10). One such rock, the size and shape of a potato, seems to have been chipped off Mars and flung into space 15 million years ago by an asteroid collision. The rock then drifted through the solar system until it passed near enough to the earth about 13,000 years ago for the earth's gravity to pull it in. This much is well established; the time spans come from measurements of nuclides formed in the rock by cosmic ray bombardment in space and on the earth's surface. (Cosmic rays are the subject of Sec. 19.5.) Less certain are what seem to be traces of past life in the rock but which may have alternative explanations as well. Despite much study the origin of these traces remains a matter of controversy.

Since rocks ejected from the moon and Mars are found on the earth, perhaps rocks from the earth now lie on the surfaces of the moon and Mars. Those reaching Mars long ago would have been slowed down by its dense early atmosphere and got through more or less intact. Finding ancient earth rocks on Mars would help in figuring out how the earth's crust developed and might also provide clues on the origin of earthly life, because the abundance ratios of the isotopes of some elements are affected by life processes.

Indeed, it is not at all impossible that microbes from the earth, protected from solar ultraviolet radiation by being embedded in a lump of ejected matter, could have ended up alive on Mars. After all, live bacteria have been found on the earth inside solid rock. If life is ever found to exist, or have existed, on Mars, one of the first questions is whether it is related to life on earth.

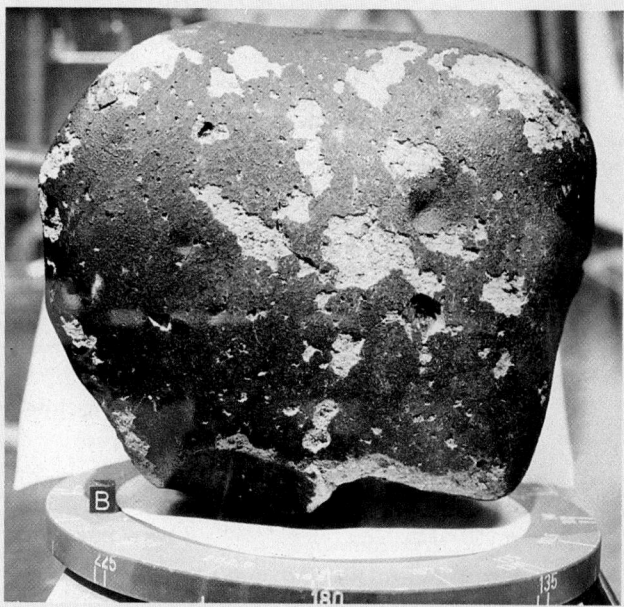

Figure 17-10 This meteorite, found in Antarctica in 1979, is one of a dozen or so believed to have come from Mars. Unlike other meteorites, which solidified about 4.5 billion years ago, these solidified much later, only 1.3 billion years ago, when Mars was still volcanically active. The meteorite here has a mass of 8 kg and is 15 cm long.

Erosion on the earth has left traces of only 100 or so large craters, but there is no reason to think that a similar rain of giant meteoroids many km across did not fall long ago on our planet as well. By about 3 billion years ago the sizes and rate of arrival of the bombarding objects seem to have fallen to their present levels. This suggests that the planets and their satellites had by then finished sweeping up most of the larger debris left over after the solar system was formed.

The Inner Planets

17.4 Mercury

It Always Appears near the Sun

Mercury was named after the fleet-footed messenger of the gods in classical mythology because its position relative to the stars changes rapidly. Its symbol represents a winged helmet.

Messenger

Mariner 10 has thus far been the only spacecraft to visit Mercury, about which we know less than any other planet. In 2004 a spacecraft appropriately called Messenger was sent to Mercury, where it was planned to arrive in March 2011 after a roundabout voyage to prevent the sun's gravity from accelerating it to too great a speed to permit its injection into an orbit around Mercury.

The images radioed back by Mariner 10 only covered 45 percent of Mercury's surface at a resolution of about 1 km. Messenger was equipped to return images of Mercury's entire surface at much higher resolution. It will also make various measurements that should vastly increase our knowledge of the planet and its history. Messenger was meant to orbit Mercury for an earth year and then crash into the planet.

What should the many geological features that Messenger might discover be called? The International Astronomical Union has prescribed that notable writers, musicians, and artists should be so honored; three prominent craters on Mercury are already named Shakespeare, Mozart, and Monet.

The innermost planet, Mercury always appears in the sky as a companion to the sun. Although as brilliant an object as Sirius, the brightest star, it is hard to see during the day because it is so near the sun; the best times for observation are near sunrise and sunset. To an observer on the earth, Mercury shows phases like those of the moon and Venus because its orbit lies within that of the earth. Mercury's apparent diameter is about 3 times greater when it is closest to the earth than when it is farthest away.

Mercury takes 59 of our days to make a complete turn on its axis and 88 of our days to circle the sun. As a result of its slow rotation, a day on Mercury—one sunrise to the next, say—is as long as two of its years (two circuits of the sun). Thus a day on Mercury is 176 of our days.

The long days on Mercury and its closeness to the sun lead to high temperatures on the sunlit side, as much as 450°C (more than enough to melt lead). There is almost no atmosphere to transfer heat from the sunlit side to the dark side or to trap heat radiated by the surface. As a result the night temperature drops to less than −200°C just before sunrise. The only gases found near Mercury are the inert gases helium, argon, neon, and xenon, and only traces of them. Mercury is altogether an inhospitable place.

Surface and Interior In 1974 the Mariner 10 spacecraft passed within a few hundred kilometers of Mercury and radioed back photographs (Fig. 17-11) as well as data of various kinds. Mercury turns out to have a surface pocked by meteoroid craters, much like the surface of the moon. Hills and valleys as well as craters abound in the rugged landscape. The youthful earth must also have suffered its share of assault by large meteoroids. The resulting craters on the earth, however, were later erased by the melting of the crust and by the erosive processes that continue to this day.

There is no evidence that Mercury ever melted, which presents a problem. Mercury seems to have a crust of silicate rocks whose density is much lower than the high average density of the planet; Mercury is the densest planet. Hence the interior probably has an iron-rich core like that of the earth but considerably larger in proportion to Mercury's size. Furthermore, Mercury has a magnetic field, which suggests that at least part of its interior is even now liquid. But if Mercury never completely melted after it had been formed, how did its heavy and light constituents separate, and why is the core molten today? Another puzzle.

Figure 17-11 A mosaic of false color photographs of Mercury radioed back from the Mariner 10 spacecraft. The surface is heavily cratered as a result of meteoroid bombardment, probably several billion years ago when similar craters were formed on the moon.

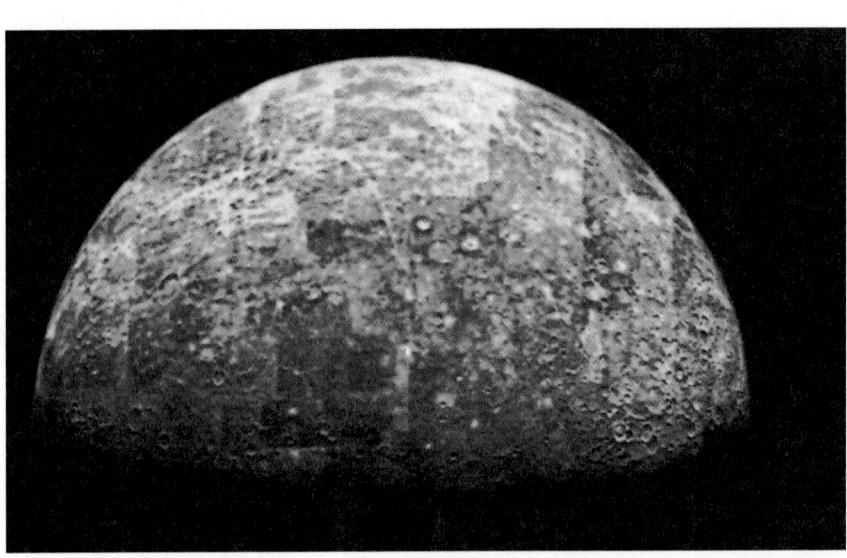

17.5 Venus

Our Sister Planet

Venus is the brightest object in the sky apart from the sun and moon (Fig. 17-12). If we know where to look, we can sometimes see Venus during the day. Because its orbit, like that of Mercury, lies inside the earth's orbit, Venus never gets very far away in the sky from the sun and appears alternately as a "morning star" and an "evening star" (Fig. 17-13). Venus is usually farther from the sun than Mercury, however, and so is visible for longer periods than Mercury. Venus was named after the Roman goddess of love and beauty and is represented by the traditional symbol of a mirror.

Venus has the distinction of spinning "backward" on its axis. That is, looking downward on its north pole, Venus rotates clockwise, whereas the earth and the other planets rotate counterclockwise. As a result the sun rises in the west on Venus, not in the east as on the earth. The rotation of our twisted sister is also extremely slow, so that a day on that planet represents 243 of our days.

The Surface of Venus   In size and mass Venus is more like the earth than any other member of the sun's family. Mountains, craters, and fault-like cracks mar its surface (Fig. 17-14), which has two major highland regions, the larger with about the area of the United States. These "continents" cover only about 5 percent of Venus in contrast to the 30 percent extent of the earth's continents, and no water laps their edges.

Some of the mountains of Venus are quite high, one of them topping Everest (Fig. 17-15). Evidence of volcanism is abundant, including volcanic peaks, extensive lava flows, and a huge volcanic crater about 100 km across. There are about 1600 large volcanoes, perhaps a million smaller ones. The amount of sulfur dioxide in the Venusian atmosphere varies from time to time, which suggests that a few of the volcanoes are still active since this gas is belched out by volcanoes on the earth.

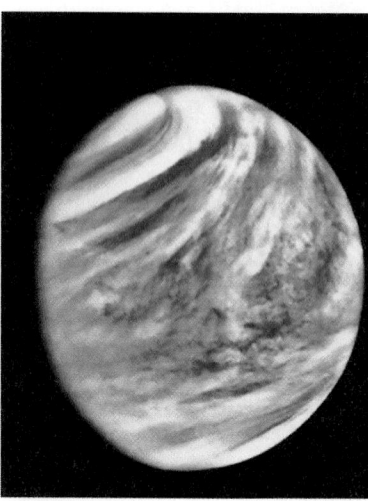

Figure 17-12   The cloudy atmosphere of Venus as photographed by the Mariner 10 spacecraft on its way to Mercury. Like Mercury, Venus has no satellites.

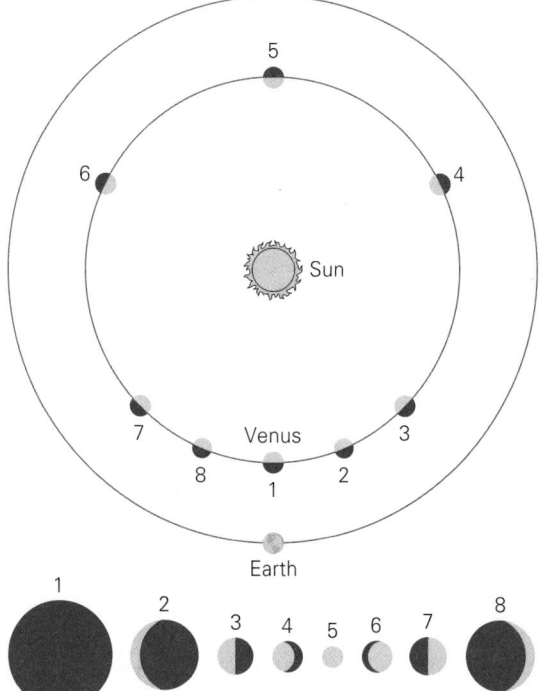

Figure 17-13   The appearance and apparent size of Venus as seen from the earth depend upon the relative positions of the two planets and the sun. The "new Venus" at 1 is 6 times larger than the "full Venus" at 5. Venus appears brightest between 1 and 2 and between 8 and 1. To an observer on the earth, Venus never appears very far from the sun and either rises just before sunrise or sets just after sunset.

The Phases of Venus

Galileo, the first person to study Venus with a telescope, found that it has phases like those of the moon and that its apparent size changes cyclically. He correctly interpreted this evidence as supporting the copernican thesis that Venus revolves around the sun. A good pair of binoculars can reveal the phases of Venus.

Figure 17-13 shows how these effects arise. A year on Venus is only 225 earth days long, so the positions of Venus and the earth relative to each other and to the sun change continually. When Venus is between the sun and the earth, as at 1, it appears dark to an observer on earth. If it could be seen, it would have its largest apparent diameter.

At 2 and 8 Venus appears as a crescent, but because it is still fairly close to the earth, it is quite bright. At 3 and 7 we see half of Venus illuminated, and at 4 and 6 more than half. Although the sun gets in the way of our seeing the full Venus at 5, it is so far from the earth that it would not be especially brilliant even if it were visible.

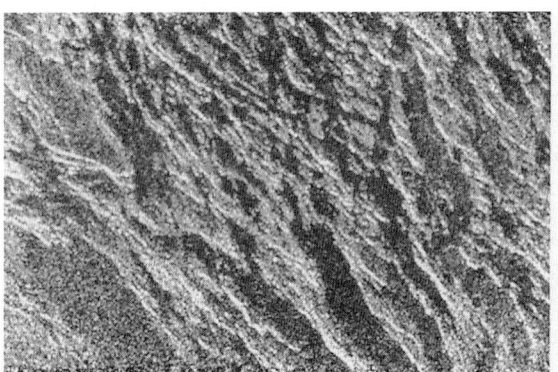 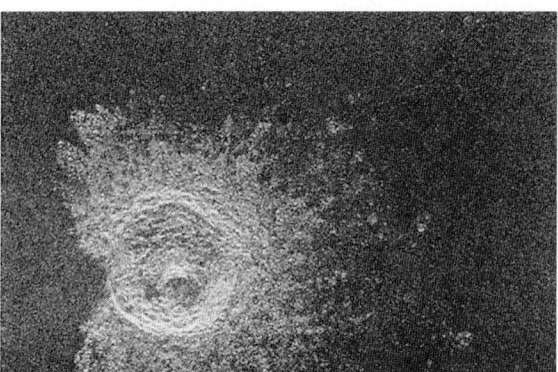

Figure 17-14   In 1990 the United States space probe Magellan began to circle Venus and to radio back radar images of its rugged surface. Features as small as 120 m across could be detected. The picture at left shows a ridge and valley network formed by intersecting faults that resembles the landscape of a region in the western United States. The picture at right shows an impact crater 12.5 km in diameter probably formed by a meteoroid moving at a shallow angle with the surface when it hit. The central peak in the crater consists of material that rebounded after the impact. Volcanic mountains and rivers and plains of hardened lava were also found. Some volcanic activity apparently continues today.

Unanswered Questions   There is no evidence that the crust of Venus, like that of the earth, consists of huge shifting plates, which is odd since the two planets are otherwise so similar. Perhaps the absence of water on Venus is responsible: it is thought that water in the rock of the earth's plates might help the plates to bend and thus be tugged across the surface by the weight of their sinking edges (Sec. 16.7). Another mystery is why Venus, which is thought to have a molten iron core like that of the earth, has no magnetic field.

Meteoroids less than a kilometer or so across cannot make it through the dense atmosphere of Venus without burning up, but larger ones can and should have left far more impact craters on Venus's surface than the mere 968 that spacecraft have found. Without liquid water on Venus (it is too hot) there is no erosion to wear away craters, and the observed craters show little alteration by volcanic or tectonic activity. Something happened a half-billion years ago to blot out the impact craters that then existed, but what?

The best guess is that immense lava flows at that time paved over Venus's surface one or more kilometers deep. Could such a lava inundation flood the earth in the future? Much of the earth's internal heat, which is what drives geologic processes, is spent in shaping and reshaping its lithosphere. This leaves a smaller proportion of the available energy for vulcanism, unlike the case of Venus where there is no plate activity. One less worry.

Life on Venus   Is there life on Venus? Bernard de Fontanelle thought so when he wrote in 1686 that the inhabitants of Venus must "resemble the Moors of

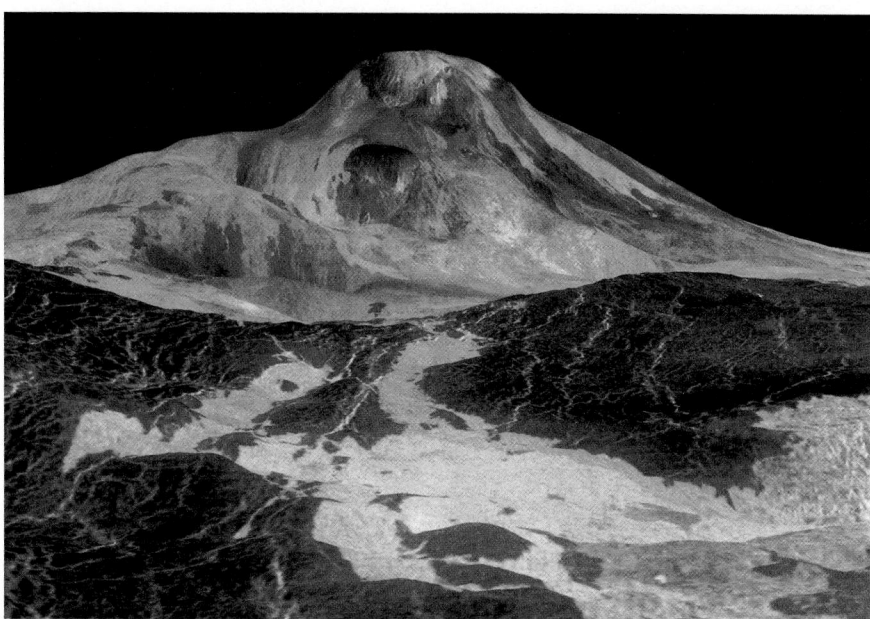

Figure 17-15 Radar images from the Magellan spacecraft were combined to give this false color perspective view of Maat Mons, at 8 km high the second tallest mountain on Venus. Lava flows extend for hundreds of kilometers across the fractured plains in the foreground. The mountains of Venus reflect radar signals much more strongly than ordinary rocks do. Perhaps metallic compounds emitted by its volcanoes were deposited on the mountains and turned into metal coatings, but nobody knows for sure.

Granada; a small, dark people, burned by the sun, full of wit and fire, always in love, writing verse, fond of music, arranging festivals, dances, and tournaments every day."

Alas, the truth is less romantic. American and European spacecraft have passed close to Venus and Soviet ones have parachuted instruments to its surface. The information radioed back shows that the atmosphere of Venus is almost all carbon dioxide with a little nitrogen and traces of other gases. Lightning occurs there fairly often. The thick lemon-yellow clouds that permanently shroud Venus consist mainly of sulfuric acid droplets and are driven around the planet by strong east-to-west winds. Tornadoes whirl near its poles. At the surface, the pressure of the atmosphere is about 90 times the corresponding figure for the earth.

On the earth the small amount of carbon dioxide in the atmosphere absorbs most of the reradiation from the ground—the greenhouse effect (see Fig. 14-12). Venus, blanketed more effectively by far than the earth and closer to the sun, has a surface temperature that averages 470°C, enough to melt lead (as in the case of Mercury's daylit surface). The existence of life on Venus seems impossible.

The surface of Venus is actually hot enough to glow a dull red, which can be seen at times on its night side through its clouds with even a small telescope. This glow was first observed by an Italian monk in 1643 when it was attributed to bonfires used to illuminate cities at night, or alternatively to firework displays set off by joyful inhabitants.

17.6 Mars

Small and Cold with a Varied Landscape

When it is at its closest to us, Mars is second only to Venus in brightness. Reddish orange in color, it has always been associated with violence and disaster (Fig. 17-16). The Romans named it after their god of war. The discoverer of its two satellites, the American astronomer Asaph Hall, continued the tradition by calling them Phobos (fear) and Deimos (terror) after the two sons of the Greek war god Ares. The symbol of Mars is a circle with an arrow, which is also the conventional male symbol.

The Moons of Mars

In what must be among the most bizarre coincidences in astronomy, the existence of two Martian satellites was conjectured in 1600 by Kepler and elaborated upon by Jonathan Swift in 1726 in *Gulliver's Travels*. Neither of them seems to have had the slightest justification for his belief. In the Voyage to Laputa, Swift has Gulliver learn not only that such satellites existed but that their periods of revolution were 10 h and $20\frac{1}{2}$ h, not far from their actual periods.

Figure 17-16   Mars at the beginning of summer in its northern hemisphere as seen from the Hubble Space Telescope. Iron oxides in the Martian soil are responsible for its red color. The ice cap around the north pole of Mars consists of water ice; the ice cap around its south pole consists of water ice and frozen carbon dioxide. Wispy white clouds of water ice cover about 1 percent of Mars on the average. Violent dust storms with winds of up to 150 km/h sometimes lash the entire planet and may last for months.

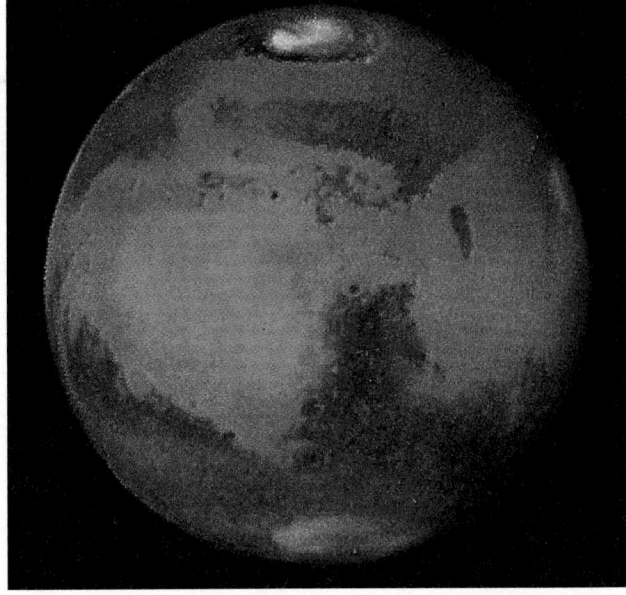

The satellites of Mars were not discovered until 1877 because they are such tiny objects, far too insignificant to deserve the names they were given. Phobos, the inner one, is only 20 km high and 28 km across. It is expected to crash into Mars in about 50 million years. Deimos, the outer one, is even smaller, 12 km high and 16 km across (Fig. 17-17). Shapes like these are possible only for astronomical bodies so small that the rigidity of their material is able to withstand the tendency of gravity to impose a spherical form, as discussed in Sec. 1.9.

Phobos is so close to Mars that its orbital period of 7 h 39 min is shorter than the length of the Martian day, and as a result it rises in the west and sets in the east, speeding across the Martian sky three times each day. The period of Deimos is 30 h 18 min, and it passes from east to west just as the earth's moon does. It seems possible that both satellites were originally asteroids that became trapped in orbits around Mars by its gravitational pull.

The diameter of Mars is slightly over half that of the earth, and its mass is 11 percent of the earth's mass. As a result the surface gravity on Mars is 38 percent of the earth's. An astronaut weighing 150 lb on the earth would weigh 57 lb on Mars. Although the overall density of Mars is 3.97 g/cm^3 as compared with 5.52 g/cm^3 for the earth, the difference is misleading because materials in the interior of the less massive Mars are not compressed as much as those in the earth's interior. Figured on a comparable basis, the two planets have about the same density, which suggests that Mars probably has about the same composition as the earth. Also like the earth, Mars seems to have a liquid core.

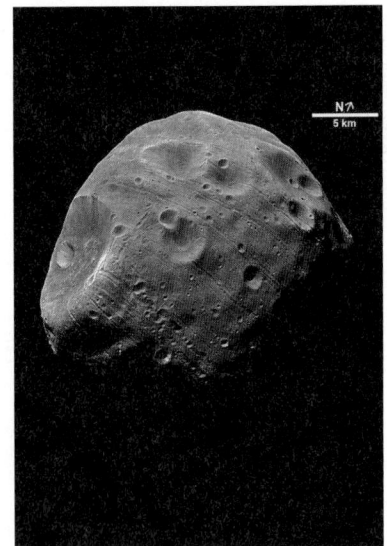

Figure 17-17   The two satellites of Mars may be captured asteroids. Conceivably Phobos and Deimos long ago passed close enough to Mars to be slowed down by its atmosphere, which was denser in the past than it is today, and this allowed them to be trapped in orbits by Martian gravity. Phobos has a huge crater called Stickney visible at the left side of this photograph. The impact that created Stickney must have come close to shattering Phobos.

Example 17.1

If you were living on Mars, where in the sky would you expect to see the earth? When would be the best time to look?

Solution

Because the earth's orbit is inside the orbit of Mars, the earth would always appear near the sun in the sky, just as in the case of Venus as seen from the earth (see Fig. 17-13). The earth would best be seen just before sunrise or just after sunset, depending on the relative positions of Mars and the earth in their orbits. During the day the sky would be too bright to see the earth from Mars.

Geological Activity   Mars today lacks the internal heat to power processes like those that shift and renew the earth's crustal plates or to drive a dynamo in its core to produce a magnetic field. But that may not have always been true: the Mars Global Surveyor, orbiting the planet, found a region where the Martian crust is magnetized in strips of alternating polarity. This also occurs in the earth's oceanic crust where molten rock comes to the surface, spreads out, and hardens while the geomagnetic field reverses itself periodically, thus locking the back-and-forth magnetic directions into the rock. The magnetized strips on Mars are about 200 km wide and up to 2000 km long on its southern highlands.

The first conclusion from the new findings is that, although Mars no longer has a magnetic field, it must once have had a strong one originating in a liquid iron core that reversed itself a number of times. Second, although the Martian surface today consists of an unbroken shell of rock, large-scale tectonic movements must have taken place there in the past. During Mars's first half-billion years, its interior evidently was sufficiently hot to support both a magnetic dynamo and plate-tectonic surface movement. Then, 4 billion years ago, the dynamo seems to have faded away, and not long afterward new crust stopped being formed.

Mars has nevertheless not been geologically dead since those early events. Its surface sports a host of intriguing features, some apparently of recent origin. The Martian landscape is extremely varied, with vast plains pitted with impact craters, regions broken up into irregular short ridges and depressions, a deep canyon as long as the distance from New York City to Los Angeles, deserts of windblown sand, and extinct volcanoes, some not very old and one of them three times the height of Everest (Fig. 17-18).

Water   A lot of evidence points to running water in the past. Spacecraft (of the 38 missions sent thus far, 18 were successful) have sent back pictures of what seem to be dried-up river channels and drainage basins, dried-up lake beds, and structures that look like sedimentary deposits (Fig. 17-19). Seas and oceans were quite possibly parts of the Martian landscape. Eventually the water must have stopped flowing, though, because there are undisturbed meteoroid craters in areas that show signs of earlier carving by running water. The number of these craters suggests that no major erosion has taken place on Mars for a long time, probably billions of years.

Mars should have been cold and dry in the past, as it is now, and it has been a mystery how warm and wet periods occurred in its history. The discovery that the Martian river valleys and the craters made by giant asteroid impacts

Visiting Mars

Astronauts have already set foot on the moon; will Mars be next? After all, motorized vehicles have successfully been landed there and explored its surface. [See Sec. 17.6 at www .mhhe.com/krauskopf.] Of the problems associated with such a venture, the only one that does not seem to have a path to a solution concerns radiation in space. Cosmic rays (Sec. 19.5) are atomic nuclei, mostly protons, that zoom through space at nearly the speed of light and pose a danger to astronauts who leave the protection of the earth's atmosphere and magnetic field. NASA limits the lifetime risk of a fatal cancer from radiation in space to 3 percent. This means that a spacecraft with sufficient shielding for a round trip to Mars taking a year each way would be far too heavy for the mission.

Probably in the future, as at present, robotic explorers would be a better choice. But perhaps astronauts could be found who would accept the radiation risk, perhaps even be willing to make a one-way voyage and spend the rest of their lives on Mars, which would solve other problems as well. Any volunteers?

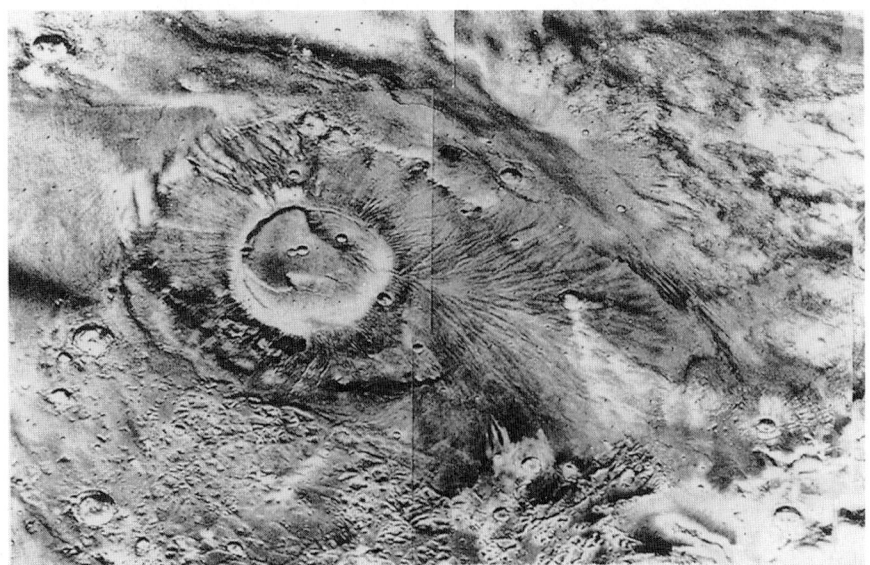

Figure 17-18   The crater of the Martian volcano Apollinaris Patera is 100 km across and has been scarred by running water. The lava flows that extend about 200 km southeast of the crater seem to have originated in a fissure. Although all are inactive today, some Martian volcanoes may just be dormant and may erupt again in the future. Another Martian volcano, Olympus Mons, is the largest in the solar system.

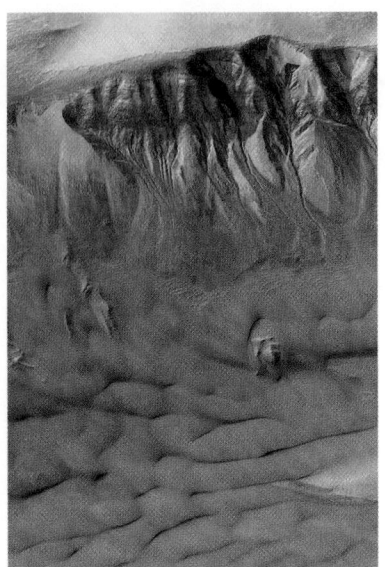

Figure 17-19   Gullies on the wall of a crater on Mars look just like gullies carved by streams of water on the earth.

are about the same age suggests what may have happened. The kinetic energy of an asteroid of rock and ice 100 to 200 km across that smashed into Mars would have heated the planet's surface, and the asteroid's ice content would have become scalding rain that fell for many years, caused flash floods, and fed the streams that carved the valleys seen today. Frozen groundwater would also have melted and come to the surface. After some thousands of years Mars would have cooled down and the water turned to ice although underground water could have remained liquid for much longer. There seem to have been 25 such impacts 3.5 billion years ago, 10 to 20 million years apart.

Today there are caps of water ice around both poles of Mars (Fig. 17-16) and elsewhere water ice mixed with subsurface soil, perhaps like the permafrost of the earth's Arctic regions. As for liquid water, a little may flow even now on the surface once in a while: high-resolution images from the Mars Global Explorer revealed thousands of small gullies that resemble gullies cut by water gushing out of hillsides on earth. A typical Martian gully is 2 m deep and a few hundred meters long. The gullies appear to be fresh, geologically speaking, having come into being "perhaps a million years ago, perhaps 10 thousand, perhaps yesterday," according to one of the researchers involved. After carving a gully, the water would have evaporated or frozen. [For more on Martian water, see Sec. 17.6 at www.mhhe.com/krauskopf.]

17.7   Is There Life on Mars?

Maybe

Mars rotates on its axis in a little over 24 h. Its revolution about the sun requires nearly 2 years, and its axis is inclined to the plane of its orbit at nearly the same angle as the earth's. Thus the Martian day and night have about the same lengths as ours, and the Martian seasons are 6 months long and at least as pronounced as ours. Mars has long fascinated astronomers and laypeople alike because it is in so many ways similar to the earth, which leads to the question of whether life of some kind is present there.

Although the conditions on Mars were once as hospitable to life as those on the earth, if life exists today it is adapted to an environment that would soon destroy most earthly organisms. For a start, Martian climates are severe by our standards. Over half again farther from the sun than the earth, Mars receives much less solar energy per m² than we do. Its atmosphere, largely carbon dioxide, is extremely thin—equivalent to the earth's atmosphere at an altitude of nearly 40 km—so little of the heat from the sun remains after nightfall. Daytime temperatures in summer at the equator rise to over 0°C, but at night drop to a chilly −23°C. The average surface temperature of the entire planet is about −55°C.

The scanty Martian atmosphere is also unable to screen out harmful solar ultraviolet radiation, a function carried out in the earth's atmosphere

Example 17.2

Photographs of Martian gullies taken in 2004 and 2005 show what seem to be fresh light-colored mineral deposits on the sides of two gullies that were absent in photographs taken in 1999 and 2000. Is any explanation possible that does not involve running water?

Solution

The deposits could conceivably be of windblown dust that slid down the gullies. However, this is thought unlikely because such dust elsewhere on Mars is always darker than its surroundings.

by the ozone present at high altitudes (see Sec. 14.1). At times giant dust storms blow for months across the entire planet.

Extreme Life   The fact that most terrestrial life requires a regular supply of liquid water and oxygen plus protection from solar ultraviolet radiation does not necessarily mean that life of some kind could not exist without them. The life processes of certain bacteria on the earth do not require oxygen, so an oxygen-containing atmosphere is not indispensable, at least for primitive forms of life. Conceivably there could have evolved on Mars organisms that can thrive on traces of water gleaned from the minerals in surface rocks. And shells of some sort might protect Martian life from ultraviolet radiation. Or life there could exist underground where water ice or pehaps liquid water is present, the energy source heat from the interior rather than sunlight, as in some places on the earth.

In fact, extra heat may not be needed: bacteria have been found deep in the ice sheets of Greenland and Antarctica that seem to have survived for hundreds of thousands of years at temperatures as low as $-40°C$. One species remained alive at $-196°C$ when immersed in liquid nitrogen. Thin films of water often cling to the surfaces of mineral grains frozen inside ice deposits, and they could take care of the water needs of bacteria inside Mars.

Since conditions there long ago may have been comparable for a long period to those on the earth, life of some kind could have come into being on Mars. The loss of most of the carbon dioxide of its atmosphere, vital for the greenhouse effect, and the disappearance of its surface water, some ending up frozen underground, were gradual, and it is not at all absurd to speculate that living things there could have adapted to the progressively harsher environment and have survived in some form to the present.

Methane on Mars   In 2004 three different studies, made using spectrometers on the earth and on a spacecraft orbiting Mars, found evidence for methane in several regions of the Martian atmosphere above icy ground. Later work confirmed the presence of methane and was able to locate plumes of it in various locations. This was very exciting, because methane molecules are broken down in an average of a few hundred years by sunlight. Hence what was detected must have originated relatively recently.

On the earth, nearly all the methane in the air is produced by plants and by bacteria, for instance those that rot plant matter and those that populate the digestive systems of cows. Nonbiological explanations are also possible, but the most obvious one, that the Martian methane has a volcanic origin, is unlikely because if so it should be accompanied by sulfur dioxide, which is absent. The discovery of Martian methane gives even more immediacy to the search for definitive signs of life, past and present, on our neighbor in space: nobody laughs at the possibility any longer.

17.8   Asteroids

Millions of Tiny Planets between Mars and Jupiter

The asteroids are small, rocky objects, many of which circle the sun in a belt between Mars and Jupiter. A few pass inside the earth's orbit, at least one has an orbit entirely inside that of the earth, and another, Icarus, gets even closer to the sun than Mercury. Similar bodies are also found in the Kuiper Belt outside Neptune; see Sec. 17.11.

The largest asteroid, Ceres, is 950 km across, roughly the extent of Texas. It was the first to be discovered, on January 1, 1801, by the Italian astronomer Giuseppe Piazzi, who named it after the patron goddess of his native Sicily. Ceres is today classified as a dwarf planet.

Dawn

In 2007 NASA launched the spacecraft Dawn on a voyage to the asteroid Vesta and the dwarf planet Ceres. Dawn was expected to reach Vesta in 2011 to begin 6 months of studies from an orbit around it, and then go on to Ceres for 5 months of similar studies.

Unlike previous spacecraft, once Dawn left the earth it was propelled by the reaction force (see Sec. 3.9) of xenon ions accelerated electrically to 34 km/s. The high ion speed means that very little xenon is needed—only 425 kg of xenon for the entire mission, far less than the many tons of chemical fuel needed by a conventional rocket engine.

The reaction force on Dawn is less than the weight of a sheet of paper, but its effect grows steadily over time. In the 4 years of its flight to Vesta, Dawn's speed will have climbed to nearly 11 km/s, about the same as a conventional spacecraft although taking longer to go that fast.

For a long time asteroids were thought to be fragments from the breakup of a planet that was supposed to have once existed between Mars and Jupiter. Nowadays asteroids are considered to be bits of matter from the early solar system that never became part of a larger body because of the gravitational influence of the nearby giant planet Jupiter. Thus their study should tell us something about the raw materials from which the planets were formed 4.6 billion years ago.

The larger asteroids, several thousand in all with relatively few over 100 km across, have been tracked and named. Although there are millions more, the asteroid belt is so vast that they are usually far apart. But not always: most of the meteoroids that reach the earth are believed to be debris from asteroid collisions (the others come from the breakup of comets). Most asteroids are irregular in shape, too small for gravity to have pulled them into spheres (Fig. 17-20). At least one asteroid, Ida, has a satellite. Called Dactyl (after the Dactyli, mythical creatures supposed to live on Mount Ida in Greece), the moonlet is 1.4 km across.

The Asteroid Danger Because some asteroids have paths that intersect the earth's orbit, there is a chance that one of them might someday collide with the earth, which has occurred before. What would happen? Small asteroids would not threaten life on our planet. But a really big asteroid, of which there are plenty, is another story. As we saw in Sec. 16.16, an asteroid about 10 km across struck Mexico 65 million years ago, an event whose consequences may have led to the extinction of the dinosaurs as well as many other forms of life.

How often asteroids of various sizes collide with the earth can be estimated from their numbers in space and the distribution of crater sizes on the moon (where there is no erosion, unlike the earth). Figure 17-22 shows how the probable frequency of arrival varies with asteroid size. An asteroid 2 km across, which can be expected an average of every million years, could create catastrophe on a global scale. Its impact would release energy equivalent to 100,000 megatons of TNT—over 10,000 times the energy of the largest hydrogen bomb ever tested—and leave a crater 30 km in diameter. Hundreds of asteroids of that size or larger have been detected that periodically pass near the earth's orbit, and there are no doubt thousands of smaller ones potentially able to cause serious damage if they fall on inhabited land.

Figure 17-20 The first close-up photograph of an asteroid was taken in 1991 from the Galileo spacecraft. Called Gaspra, the asteroid is 19 km long and 12 km wide and is pocked with craters, some over a kilometer across. It rotates with a period of 7 h. Gaspra seems to have a magnetic field as strong as the earth's. Asteroids can be named after almost anybody except religious, political, or military leaders; one has been called Jerry Garcia after the former singer.

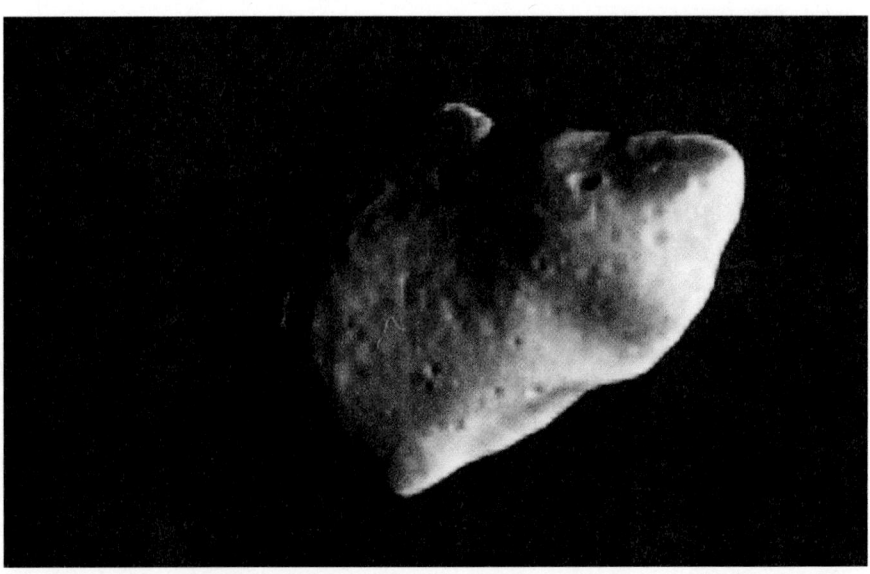

The Tunguska Event

On the morning of June 30, 1908, in the Tunguska River region north of Lake Baikal in Siberia, there was a brilliant flash in the sky and a great blast that devastated over 2000 km^2 of forest (Fig. 17-21). Here is how the event appeared to a Siberian farmer 200 km away: "When I sat down to have my breakfast beside my plow, I heard sudden bangs, as if from gunfire. My horse fell to its knees. From the north side above the forest a flame shot up. Then I saw that the fir forest had been bent over by the wind, as I thought of a hurricane. I seized hold of my plow with both hands so it would not be carried away. The wind was so strong it carried soil from the surface of the ground, and then the hurricane drove a wall of water up the Angora River."

Because no crater was found under the center of the blast, the most likely explanation for the Tunguska event seems to be the violent disintegration of an asteroid about 50 m across in the atmosphere at an altitude of 6 to 8 km. This origin is still a hypothesis because, although the breakup of so large an asteroid should have flung out thousands of tons of cosmic debris, 35 expeditions to Tunguska have turned up only relatively few iron and silicate particles of the expected kinds. Recently a deep lake 8 km from the point on the ground under the blast was found to have features that suggest an impact crater. It remains to be seen whether an asteroid remnant is buried under the lake.

In March 2009, an asteroid of about the same size as the one proposed for the Tunguska event passed 78,000 km from the earth, only twice as far away as some communication satellites.

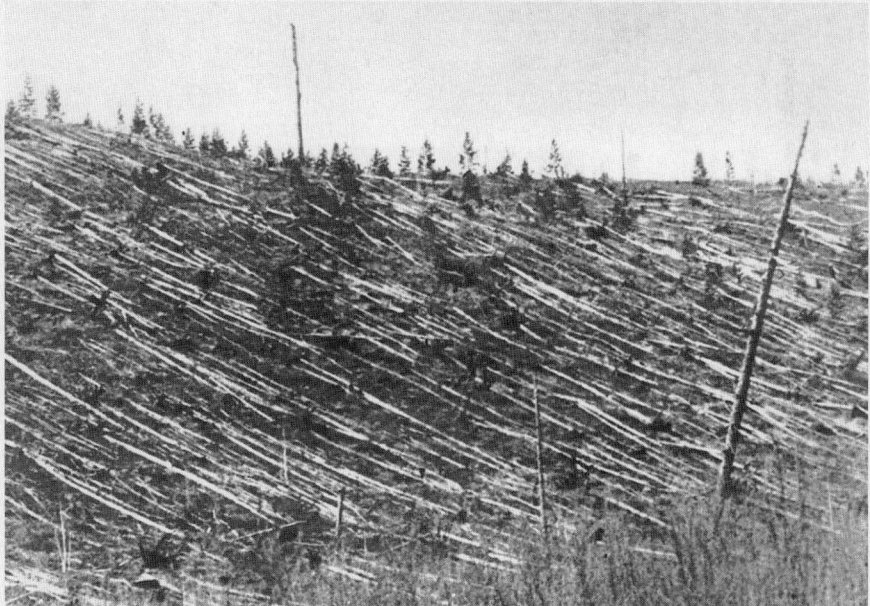

Figure 17-21   The Tunguska event blew down millions of trees over a large area in a radial pattern like the spokes of a wheel. It may have been caused by an asteroid exploding above the ground.

Of the larger asteroids that have been tracked, the first that may pose a risk is expected in the earth's neighborhood in 2029, 2036, and 2068. Called Apophis, it is about 270 m across, big enough to destroy a major city, but is very likely to be, at worst, a near miss. What may be the next to arrive, known as 1999 RQ36, is twice as large and has a greater chance—still only 1 in 1400—of striking the earth when it approaches somewhat over a century later.

If a large asteroid definitely headed for the earth were to be noticed in time, say at least 20 y ahead, a spacecraft could be sent to divert it by impact or explode a nuclear weapon on its surface to either divert it or blow it apart. However, if the asteroid is not a solid chunk of rock but a clump of cosmic rubble loosely held together mainly by gravity, as most asteroids seem to be,

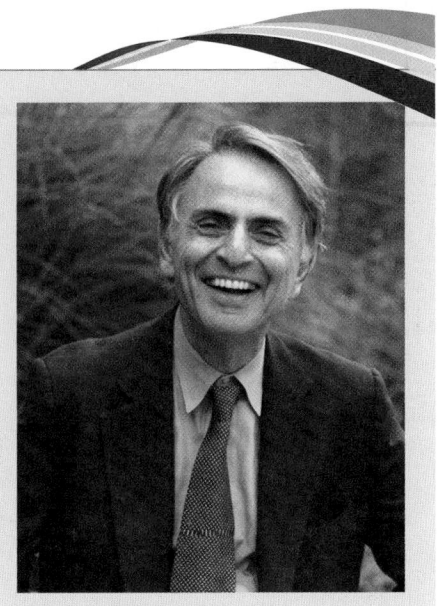
Figure 17-22 Large asteroids are much less likely to collide with the earth than small ones, but those more than about 2 km across would devastate life on earth. (The scales are not linear.)

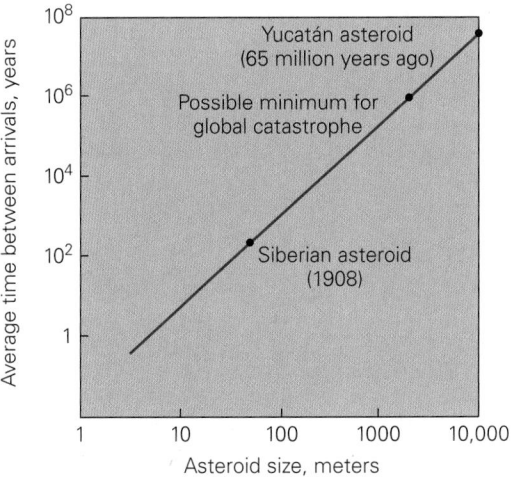

absorbing a shock would give it an unpredictable deflection; an explosion would also have an unpredictable result. So a better idea might be to have a spacecraft spend a few years nearby where it could exert enough of a gravitational tug—very little would be needed—to edge the asteroid into a safer orbit.

The Outer Planets

17.9 Jupiter

Almost a Star

The mammoth planet Jupiter, fittingly named after the most important of the Roman gods, is represented by a stylized lightning bolt because lightning was supposed to come from the god Jupiter. The symbolism has turned out to be appropriate since electric discharges regularly occur in Jupiter's atmosphere that produce bursts of radio waves detectable on the earth.

Jupiter, like Venus, is shrouded in clouds, but those of Jupiter are more spectacular (Fig. 17-23). The clouds are responsible for Jupiter's relatively high reflectivity, which together with its size makes it a bright object in the sky despite its distance from the sun. The clouds occur in alternate light and dark bands whose colors—mostly in the yellow-orange-red family—and markings change slightly from time to time.

One marking is particularly conspicuous, the Great Red Spot that today is about 25,000 km long and 10,000 km high, as large as two earths. Though its size, shape, and color are known to vary, the Spot itself does not seem to be a temporary phenomenon. It was definitely identified as long ago as 1831 and is probably the same marking described in 1660 by the French astronomer Jean Dominique Cassini.

Although the nature and origin of the Great Red Spot remain uncertain, a plausible suggestion is that it is a kind of permanent hurricane into which energy is constantly fed by the Jovian wind system. The red color may be due to phosphorus from the breakup of the phosphorus compounds believed to contribute to the colors of the bands that circle the planet.

Cassini used the spot he found, whatever it was, to determine Jupiter's period of rotation. This is a little less than 10 h, which means that points on Jupiter's equator travel at the enormous speed of 45,000 km/h. (The earth's equatorial speed is only 1670 km/h.) Because of its rapid rotation, Jupiter bulges much more at the equator than the earth does.

Satellites   Of Jupiter's 63 known satellites, the 4 that Galileo discovered in 1610 are easy to see with a pair of binoculars or a small telescope. The innermost, Io, is slightly larger than our moon and is spangled with active volcanoes. Indeed, no other body in the solar system is so volcanically active. Apparently the energy involved comes from the gravitational pulls of Jupiter and two of its other satellites, Ganymede and Europa, which knead Io like a lump of clay. Io flexes by nearly 100 m, which heats its interior and thereby powers over 100 active volcanoes that belch white-hot lava and jets of sulfurous gas. The most vigorous volcano, Loki, pours out more heat than all the earth's active volcanoes together.

The other large Jovian satellites are coated with ice: Europa, smaller than the moon; the giant Ganymede, larger than Mercury; and Callisto, a bit more modest in size (Fig. 17-24). All but Callisto show signs of geological activity.

The rest of Jupiter's satellites are very small, only 2 to 250 km across, and most have large noncircular orbits that do not lie in the plane of Jupiter's orbit. Apparently these satellites were originally asteroids somehow captured by Jupiter as they circulated through the early solar system. A number of the irregular satellites revolve "backward" around Jupiter, from east to west. Jupiter also has a ring, like those of Saturn but so faint that it can be detected only by spacecraft. The ring seems to consist of dust knocked off Jupiter's innermost satellites by micrometeoroid impacts and/or debris from volcanic eruptions on Io.

Structure   Jupiter's volume is about 1300 times that of the earth, but its mass is only 318 times as great. The resulting low density—only a quarter that of the earth—means that Jupiter cannot be composed of rock and iron as is the earth. Like the other large planets—Saturn, Uranus, and Neptune—Jupiter must consist chiefly of hydrogen and helium, the two lightest elements.

Possibly Jupiter has a relatively small rocky inner core, perhaps the size of the earth, surrounded by a large outer core of liquid hydrogen under such enormous pressure that it behaves like a liquid metal. The interior is believed to be very hot, possibly 20,000°C. This is not hot enough for nuclear reactions to occur in its hydrogen content that would turn Jupiter into a star. However,

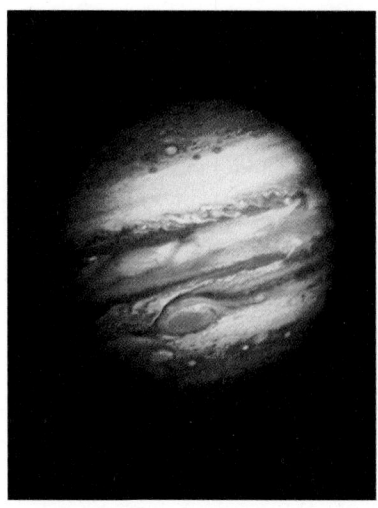

Figure 17-23   Jupiter, the largest planet, has a mass $2\frac{1}{2}$ times that of all the other planets together. The Great Red Spot in its southern hemisphere is larger than the earth; it consists of swirling gases and varies in size and appearance.

Figure 17-24 Jupiter and its four largest satellites, which were first seen and named by Galileo almost 400 years ago. In this composite image, Io, the innermost, is at the top, then in order of distance from Jupiter are Europa, Ganymede, and Callisto.

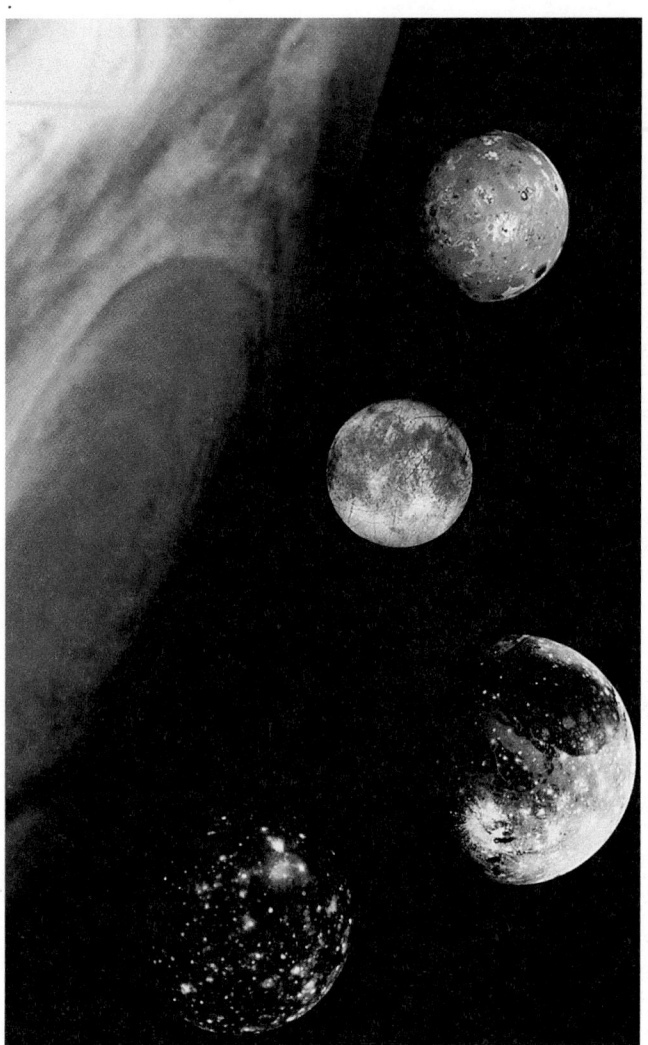

if Jupiter's mass were perhaps 80 times greater than it is, the internal temperatures would be high enough for Jupiter to be a miniature star (see Sec. 18.13). Surrounding the core is a dense layer of liquid hydrogen and helium that gradually turns into a gas with increasing distance. The outer part of Jupiter's atmosphere contains such gases as ammonia, methane, and water vapor as well as hydrogen and helium.

Spacecraft Visits   United States spacecraft passed close to Jupiter after a number of journeys that lasted several years and covered over a billion km. Of the wealth of information radioed back, a few items are especially notable. For example, Jupiter has a magnetic field many times stronger than the earth's. This field traps high-energy protons and electrons from the sun in belts that extend many Jovian radii outward. The earth has such belts too, but they are 10,000 times weaker than those of Jupiter. It is plausible that Jupiter's magnetic field is connected with the metallic nature of part of its volume, with the "metal" being highly compressed liquid hydrogen instead of the molten iron of the earth's core.

Another important finding confirmed that Jupiter radiates over twice as much energy as it receives from the sun. By contrast the atmospheres of Venus, Earth, and Mars are on average in balance, and radiate only as much energy as the sun provides. Apparently Jupiter is still cooling down, so that the extra heat has been left over from the planet's formation.

Europa

The Jovian satellite Europa (Fig. 17-25) is nearly the size of our moon but, unlike the moon, it is covered with a layer of water ice several kilometers thick. The ice is scarred by a network of curved, intersecting fracture lines, like a cracked eggshell (Fig. 17-26). A surface of this kind is to be expected if the ice is floating on a vast ocean of liquid water; currents in the ocean regularly break up the ice, and water wells up into the cracks and freezes there to give the patterns we see.

Where does the heat come from that keeps Europa's subsurface water liquid and powers its currents? Some may be the result of radioactivity in Europa's rocky core, but most arises from the continual squeezing and stretching due to tidal forces caused by the gravitational pulls of Jupiter and its other large satellites, as in the case of Io.

Given liquid water and heat, could life have arisen on Europa? After all, organisms have been discovered on earth that thrive in perpetual darkness with no need for sunlight, and living things have been found beneath Antarctic ice.

Comet impacts on Europa may well have dumped on its surface billions of tons of such elements needed for life as carbon, nitrogen, and sulfur. Many scientists think that Europa, not Mars, is the most likely candidate for extraterrestrial life in the solar system today.

NASA hopes to launch a spacecraft to visit Europa, Callisto, and Ganymede. If liquid water is indeed under Europa's ice coat, a lander may follow that will inspect the cracks and burrow through the ice to look for life.

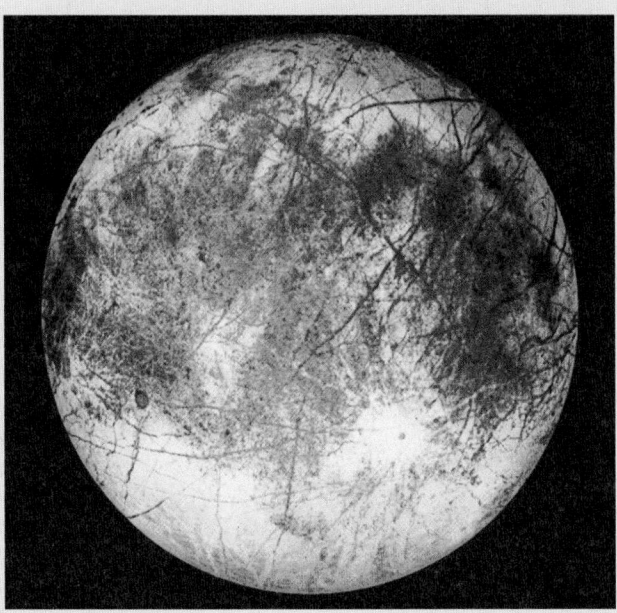

Figure 17-25   Jupiter's satellite Europa.

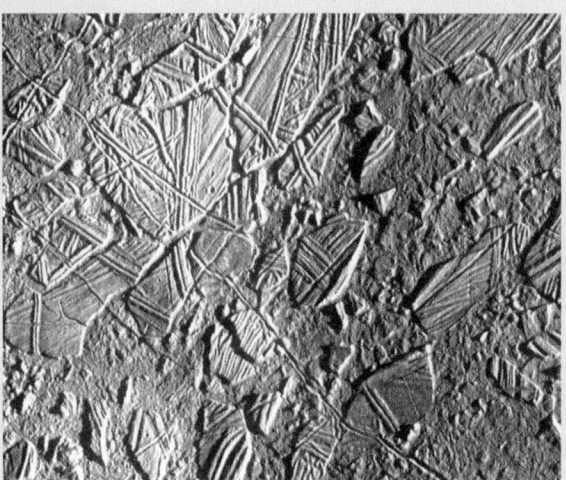

Figure 17-26   Europa's shell of ice is covered with cracks and floats on an ocean of liquid water. This image, which covers an area 5 km wide, was radioed back by the spacecraft Galileo, which went into orbit around Jupiter late in 1995.

17.10   Saturn

Lord of the Rings

In its setting of brilliant rings, Saturn is the most striking and beautiful of the earth's kin (Fig. 17-27). Saturn, the Roman god of sowing seed and the father of Jupiter, was called Kronos in Greek mythology, from which the planet's symbol of a stylized K probably derives. The midwinter festivals of worship to Saturn, the saturnalia, were always splendid occasions of joy and revelry. Saturday is named after him.

Saturn resembles Jupiter in many respects, though smaller and less massive. Like Jupiter it consists largely of hydrogen and helium, radiates more heat than it receives from the sun, is flattened at the poles by rapid rotation, has a strong magnetic field and a dense atmosphere of hydrogen with some helium, and is surrounded by banded clouds in which gigantic lightning

Slingshot Effect

Spacecraft are often helped by the "slingshot effect" when they explore the solar system. When a spacecraft passes behind a planet (in terms of its orbital motion), the planet's gravitational pull accelerates the spacecraft. NASA's New Horizons probe, which was launched in 2006, received such a gravity assist when it passed by Jupiter 13 months later. The slingshot effect boosted the probe's speed by 2 m/s, which will save 3 years on the journey to Pluto, where it should arrive in 2015, and beyond.

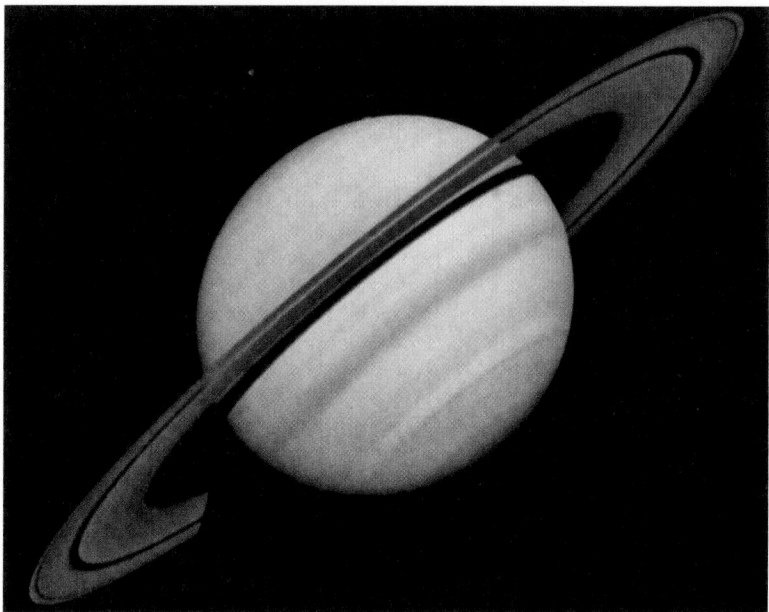

Figure 17-27 The rings of Saturn are not solid or gaseous but consist of small rock and ice fragments that orbit the planet. Galileo called Saturn "the planet with ears," but in 1655 the Dutch astronomer Christian Huygens recognized that the "ears" were actually rings. He also discovered Titan, Saturn's largest satellite.

storms occur. Auroras occur in the atmospheres of both planets. However, Saturn's core seems to have less liquid metallic hydrogen than Jupiter's core, perhaps with a large rocky kernel inside. Farther from the sun than Jupiter, Saturn is considerably colder, only about −180°C at the surface. Winds blow harder on Saturn, over 1800 km/h at its equator.

The satellites of Saturn—at least 60, probably with more small ones—range in size from 6 km across to the giant Titan, whose 5140 km diameter makes it only slightly smaller than Jupiter's Ganymede (Fig. 17-28). An outer moon, Phoebe, orbits in the opposite direction to the others and may be a captured asteroid, as in the cases of many of Jupiter's outer satellites.

Titan Titan is the only satellite in the solar system with an atmosphere, which seems to consist largely of nitrogen with some methane and small amounts of other organic compounds. Titan's atmosphere is more like ours than that of any other body in the solar system. Reddish clouds of organic compounds float in this atmosphere and send showers of methane rain and perhaps snow from time to time to feed the liquid methane rivers and seas on Titan's surface. Methane apparently plays the same geological role on Titan that water does on the earth, although the gaseous methane in its atmosphere seems to come from its interior rather than from the evaporation of liquid methane on its surface. Titan and the earth are the only bodies in the solar system on which rain or snow of some kind falls to the ground.

Could life have developed on Titan? The answer seems to be that it might have had Titan been warmer. Titan's atmosphere, in particular, is similar to that of the earth before life emerged. However, chemical processes are slow at low temperatures. If life took a half billion years to come into being on the earth, a reasonable estimate, then the solar system is not old enough for this process to have occurred on the frigid (−179°C) surface of Titan. But conceivably heat from Titan's interior or from comet impacts produced local pools of liquid water that could persist under crusts of ice for long periods,

Cassini and Huygens

In 2004 the Cassini spacecraft, a $3.3-billion American-European collaboration, reached Saturn after a 7-year journey. Cassini, 6.5 m long with the mass of a small elephant, carried a dozen instruments of various kinds to study Saturn, its rings, and several of its moons from orbit. Originally planned for 4 years of studies, Cassini was so successful that its mission has been extended to 2017 when it will plunge through Saturn's rings into the planet itself.

Six months after its arrival Cassini sent off the smaller Huygens probe to Titan, Saturn's largest moon (Fig. 17-28), where it parachuted through the orange haze that hides its surface to land on soft ground that apparently is soaked with liquid methane. Huygens found a varied terrain with evidence of flowing hydrocarbon liquid (it is too cold there for liquid water) in the form of drainage channels and eroded plains. The presence of smooth, rounded pebbles supports this inference. Dark, featureless areas were seen that resemble lakes and seas with sharp boundaries that could be shorelines. Few craters scar Titan's landscape, unlike the landscapes of Mars and the moon, which confirms that erosion and deposition are continuing on Titan.

Huygens had power enough to operate for only a short time on Titan, but Cassini flew close to it several dozen times. When all the images and data are analyzed, we will know much more about the still-active geology and chemistry of this remote world.

Cassini also inspected other of Saturn's satellites. One of them, the tiny (diameter 505 km) Enceladus, seems to have abundant liquid water below its surface that spews out in geysers of water vapor and ice crystals near its south pole. The vapor plumes show traces of organic compounds. Even though distant from the sun, Enceladus is warm enough for subsurface liquid water to be present, perhaps heated by the same tidal kneading that heats Jupiter's moon Europa. Given warmth, water, and organic compounds, did life of some kind appear? There is a long way to an answer, but right now there is nothing to rule it out.

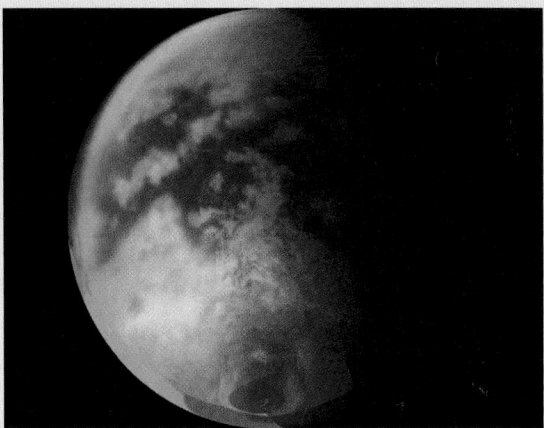

Figure 17-28   Titan, Saturn's largest satellite.

which makes a search for life more reasonable. As far as astronomers can tell at present, conditions on Enceladus, a much smaller satellite of Saturn, may also be able to support life.

Example 17.3

You are in a spacecraft orbiting Saturn. Would you find that Jupiter shows phases like those of Venus? Would you find that Uranus does this?

Solution

Jupiter shows phases to you because its orbit is inside that of Saturn (see Fig. 17-13). Uranus does not show phases because its orbit is outside that of Saturn.

Saturn's Rings   A number of rings surround Saturn at its equator, two of them bright and the others faint. The rings are inclined by 27° with respect to the plane of the earth's orbit, so we see them from different angles as Saturn proceeds in its leisurely 29½-year tour around the sun (Fig. 17-29). Twice in each period of revolution the rings are edgewise to the earth, which happened last in 1996 and will happen again in 2011. In this orientation the rings are practically invisible, suggesting that they are very thin. In fact, they

Figure 17-29   The appearance of Saturn's rings from the earth varies with Saturn's location in its orbit. Saturn's period of revolution is 29.5 years.

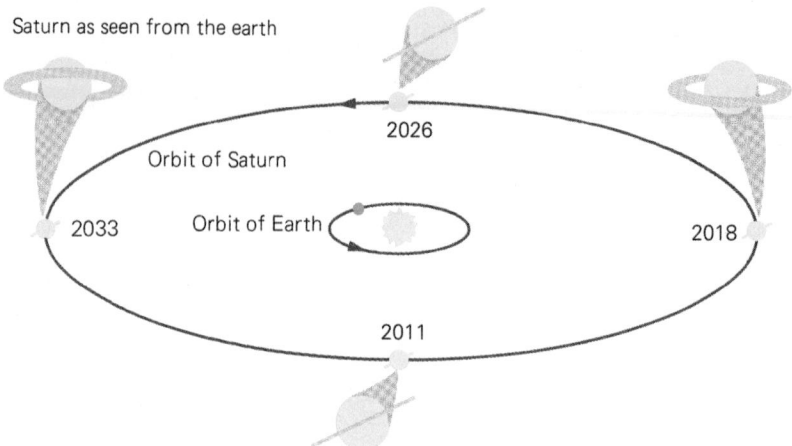

Saturn as seen from the earth

Orbit of Saturn

Orbit of Earth

2026

2033

2018

2011

average only about 50 meters thick. Since the outer bright ring is 270,000 km in diameter, a sheet of paper is fat by comparison. In 2018 we will be able to see Saturn's rings in their fullest glory, tipped by 27° so that their upper (northern) surfaces face us.

The rings are not the solid sheets they appear to be but instead consist of a multitude of small bodies, each of which revolves around Saturn as a miniature satellite. How do we know that Saturn's rings are not solid? One piece of evidence is that we can see stars through them. Another is that doppler-effect measurements show that the inner part of each ring moves faster than the outer part. This is in accord with Kepler's third law, which calls for a decrease in orbital speed with an increase in orbital size. (Thus Mercury's orbital speed is 48 km/s, and Pluto's is only 5 km/s.) If the rings were solid, their outer parts would have the highest speeds, contrary to what is found.

Nor can the rings be gaseous—they reflect sunlight and radar signals far too well. The only question left is the size and nature of the particles of which they consist. In 1980 and 1981 two Voyager spacecraft reached Saturn after 4-year journeys. They radioed back vast amounts of data on the planet, its satellites, and, of course, its rings. The findings about the rings confirmed what astronomers had suspected earlier: the particles are mainly ice with some rock and range in size from small stones to boulders.

The rings we see from the earth are not uniform but are split into thousands of narrow ringlets. Two of the ringlets in one of the outer, faint rings seem to be braided around each other, a peculiarity that may result from the gravitational pulls of two small satellites whose orbits are just inside and just outside the ringlets.

Were Saturn's rings always there? Many—not all—astronomers think they are relatively young, perhaps fragments of a comet torn to shreds by Saturn's gravity or else the debris of a collision between an asteroid and one of Saturn's moons. Probably the rings are migrating inward and, in several hundred million years, will disappear into Saturn itself.

17.11   Uranus, Neptune, Pluto, and More

Far Out

Uranus, Neptune, and the dwarf planet Pluto owe their discovery to the telescope. Uranus was found in 1781 by the great English astronomer William Herschel. In Greek mythology, Uranus personifies the heavens and is the father of Saturn and the grandfather of Jupiter.

Herschel at first suspected Uranus to be a comet because, through his telescope, it appeared as a disk rather than as a point of light like a star.

Observations made over a period of time showed its position to change relative to the stars, and its orbit, found from these data, revealed it to be a planet. Neptune was discovered in 1846 as the result of predictions based on its gravitational effects on the orbit of Uranus (see Chap. 1). Neptune was named after the Roman god of the sea.

Uranus has the distinction of rotating about an axis only 8° from the plane of its orbit, so we can think of it as spinning on its side. The most likely reason is a collision with a large object, perhaps the size of the earth, early in the history of the solar system. Because of this tilt, summer at a particular place on Uranus is a 42-year period of continuous sunshine, and winter is a 42-year period of continuous darkness. Uranus and Neptune are about the same size, smaller than Jupiter and Saturn but much larger than the other planets. Like Jupiter and Saturn they consist chiefly of hydrogen and helium.

The spacecraft Voyager 2 passed near Uranus in 1986 and near Neptune 3 years later (Fig. 17-30). Photographs radioed back to the earth show that both planets have several rings around them. Like the rings of Saturn, these rings consist of small particles but are too narrow to be seen from the earth. Uranus has 27 known satellites and Neptune has 13.

Voyager 2 found that Neptune's atmosphere is in much more violent motion than that of Uranus. Strong, turbulent winds blow across Neptune, and a huge hurricane can be seen that is nearly the width of the earth. From its appearance this storm is called the Great Dark Spot, and it is much like Jupiter's Great Red Spot (Fig. 17-23). A smaller hurricane is near Neptune's south pole. Both hurricanes are accompanied by white cirrus clouds of methane ice. Since Neptune is farther from the sun than Uranus and so receives less solar energy, why Neptune has stormier weather than Uranus is a puzzle.

Pluto Pluto was discovered in 1930 by the American astronomer Clyde Tombaugh, then 24 years old, who spent 10 months meticulously looking for a new planet whose existence was suspected on the basis of irregularities in the orbits of Uranus and Neptune. As it happens, the total mass of Pluto and its satellite is not enough to account for these irregularities, and Tombaugh seems to have found it purely by accident. Pluto was considered as a planet until 2006; it is now regarded as a dwarf planet. Pluto was named after the Greek god of the underworld, the home of the dead.

Pluto is so small, so far away, and so dimly lit that reliable information about it is hard to obtain. It is about two-thirds the size of our moon and seems to consist of rock and water ice with a thin atmosphere of nitrogen,

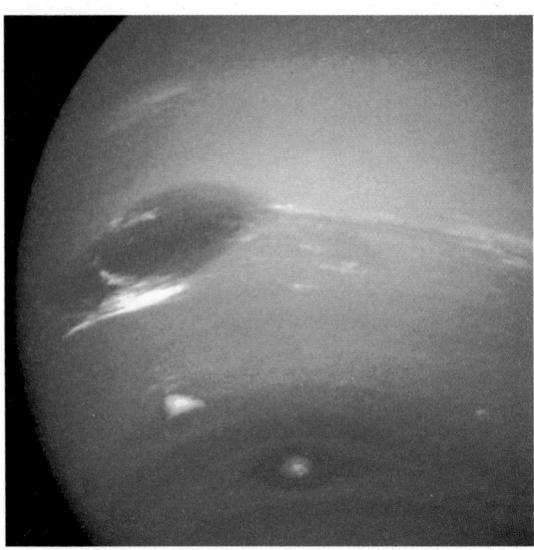

Figure 17-30 The spacecraft Voyager 2 left Florida in 1977 and arrived at Neptune 12 years later. This photograph radioed back by Voyager 2 shows Neptune's Great Dark Spot, which is almost as large as the earth. White patches are clouds that consist of methane ice crystals.

BIOGRAPHY | William Herschel (1738–1822)

Herschel was born in Germany (his name was originally Friedrich Wilhelm) and went to England in 1757 to avoid military service. In England Herschel prospered as an organist and music teacher, and composed 24 symphonies. He also found time for his hobby of astronomy.

Good telescopes were expensive, so Herschel, with the help of his sister Caroline, built his own. By 1774 Herschel had made the finest telescope in the world, a reflector whose mirror he and his sister had ground themselves. With this telescope he systematically searched the sky, a labor rewarded in 1781 by the discovery of a seventh planet, Uranus. This created a great stir everywhere, both because Uranus was the first new planet to be identified for many centuries and because its distance from the sun was twice that of Saturn, thus doubling the size of the solar system.

Six years later Herschel found 2 satellites circling Uranus and called them Titania and Oberon. Today 27 are known, some very small.

Caroline Herschel did important work herself, among other things discovering 8 comets. In her day—she lived from 1750 to 1848—women were unusual in science, but eventually her achievements were recognized with a gold medal from the Royal Astronomical Society in

1828 and another from the king of Prussia on her 96th birthday.

In 1788 Herschel married a rich widow, which enabled him to become a full-time observer of the heavens. The list of his achievements is unparalleled in astronomy. Among his other discoveries were binary (double) stars, and he established that each member of a pair revolved around the other. Using a thermometer to measure the heat produced, he studied the intensity of sunlight in various parts of its spectrum. To his surprise, the heating continued past the red end, which suggested to him that the sun emits invisible (today called infrared) radiation besides visible light.

Most significantly, Herschel's studies of the Milky Way led him to conclude that it is a vast disk-shaped galaxy of stars, one of which is the sun. He speculated—correctly—that a number of fuzzy objects in the sky were other galaxies far away in space.

Herschel's renown became such that King George III provided the money for a huge new telescope with a mirror 1.2 m across. The first time the telescope was used, Herschel discovered two more satellites

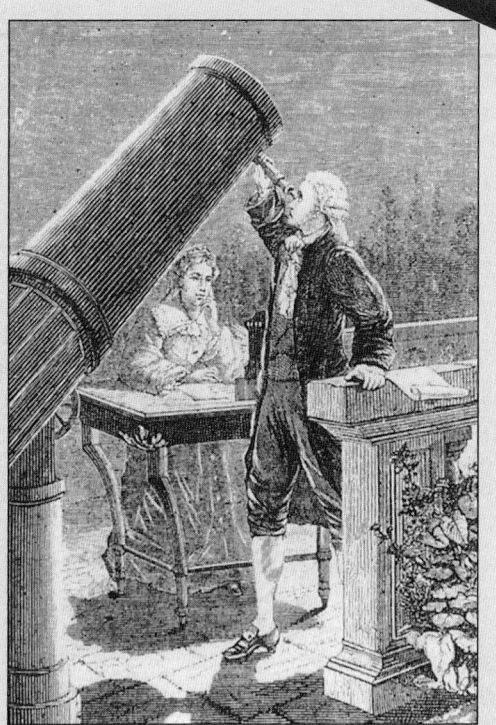

of Saturn to add to the five already known, and he was soon able to show that Saturn's rings are not stationary but revolve about their mother planet. He remained active almost until his death at 84 (the same span as the orbital period of Uranus). Herschel's work was carried on by his son John, who was a pioneer in photography (his word) and its application to astronomy.

---

carbon monoxide, and methane. Six other satellites in the solar system are also larger than Pluto. Pluto's average surface temperature is −230°C and it has prominent polar caps of frozen gas. It takes 248 of our years to orbit the sun. As in the case of Uranus, Pluto's axis is horizontal, that is, it lies near the plane of Pluto's orbit.

Satellites Pluto has a satellite, Charon, named for the ferryman who takes the dead across the river Styx to Pluto's domain (Fig. 17-31). Charon's diameter of 1200 km is a little over half that of Pluto, and it probably consists largely of ice with some rock as well. Charon is relatively close to Pluto and circles it every 6.4 days. Since Pluto also rotates with a 6.4-day period, Pluto and Charon always show the same sides to each other.

There are signs that Charon, like Jupiter's satellite Europa, has an ocean of liquid water under a covering of ice. It is possible, again like Europa, that Charon is heated by tidal forces that knead its interior. Could there be underground life on Charon that draws its energy from this heat rather than from the extremely feeble sunlight? What little we know about Charon does not seem to rule it out.

Dwarf Planets

Because Pluto is much smaller than the eight first-discovered planets (and indeed is smaller than seven of their satellites), is very different from the outer planets nearest it, and has an unusual orbit, many astronomers have never regarded it as a genuine planet. In 2006 the International Astronomical Union agreed that a planet must (1) orbit the sun, (2) have been forced by gravity into a spherical shape (see Sec. 1.9), and (3) be large enough to have cleared other objects from the neighborhood of its orbit.

A new class of dwarf planets was established that need meet only the first two of these criteria. As for the third one, each of the eight "genuine" planets has a mass more than five thousand times the total mass of all the fragmentary bodies in its orbital vicinity; the masses are comparable for dwarf planets.

The first dwarf planets to be nominated were Pluto, the asteroid Ceres, and a Kuiper Belt member called Eris, which is somewhat larger and more massive than Pluto and has a satellite, Dysnomia. (Eris is the Greek goddess of discord; Dysnomia is her daughter.)

As mentioned in Sec. 17.2, the Kuiper Belt beyond Neptune is home to comets and to many asteroids of various sizes. At present, four objects in the Kuiper Belt are officially classed as **plutoids:** Pluto itself, Eris, and the smaller Maumea and Makemake (named respectively for the Hawaiian and Easter Island fertility gods). Maumea has two satellites. Several dozen other Kuiper Belt objects may also qualify as plutoids. Ceres remains the only dwarf planet not a plutoid.

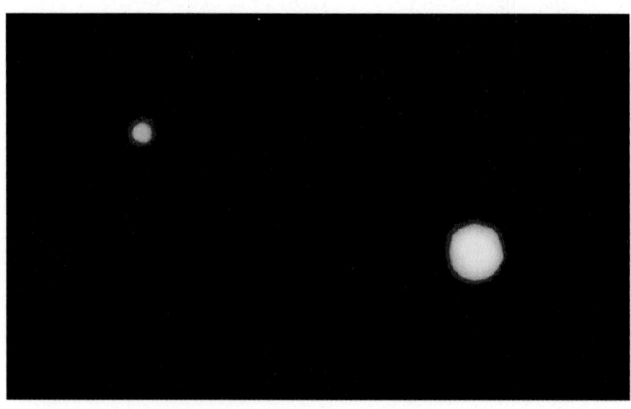

Figure 17-31   Pluto and its satellite Charon as seen by the Hubble Space Telescope. Pluto has two other, smaller satellites that are farther away.

In 2005 the Hubble Space Telescope discovered two more moons that orbit Pluto. Both are over twice as far from Pluto as Charon and are quite small, not much over a tenth of Charon's diameter.

A spacecraft called New Horizons was launched in 2006 to inspect Pluto and its moons, which it should reach in 2015, the first spacecraft to do so. New Horizons will then go on past Pluto to examine Kuiper Belt objects, some comparable in size with Pluto. Clyde Tombaugh, who discovered Pluto, died in 1997 and New Horizons carries some of his ashes.

The Moon

The light that reaches us from the moon is reflected sunlight. Although closer to the earth than any other celestial body, the moon is nevertheless an average of 384,400 km away. Its diameter of 3476 km—a little more than a quarter of the earth's diameter—places it among the largest satellites in the solar system.

The moon circles the earth every $27\frac{1}{3}$ days and, like the earth, turns on its axis as it revolves. In the case of the moon, the rotation keeps pace exactly with the revolution, so the moon turns completely around only once during each circuit of the earth. This means that the same face of our satellite is always turned toward us and that the other side remains hidden from the earth (though not from spacecraft).

The earth-moon synchronization is a consequence of tidal bulges raised in the moon itself by the earth's gravitational pull, as described in Sec. 1.10 for the case of surface water on the earth attracted by the moon. Friction between the water bulges and the ocean bottoms is currently slowing down the earth's rotation on its axis. Friction involved in its tidal flexing similarly slowed the moon's spin in the past to the point where the tidal bulges are locked in place along a line between the moon and the earth. Most of the other large satellites in the solar system have their spin and orbital motions synchronized in the same way.

17.12 Phases of the Moon

A Little Less Than a Month per Cycle

The properties of the moon are given in Table 17-3. The $27\frac{1}{3}$-day period of the moon's orbit quoted previously is the time needed for the moon to go through a complete circuit of the earth. *If* the earth did not move around the sun, we would see the moon in the same place in the sky relative to the stars at the same time of day every $27\frac{1}{3}$ days. But while the moon is circling the earth, the earth is carrying the moon with it in the earth's own motion around the sun. As a result, to us the moon's orbital period is increased to $29\frac{1}{2}$ days. *Relative to the stars,* the moon's period is $27\frac{1}{3}$ days; *relative to the sun,* the moon's period is $29\frac{1}{2}$ days. Since time on earth is figured relative to the sun, we see the moon return to the same place in the sky at the same time of day every $29\frac{1}{2}$ days.

Example 17.4

If the moon circled Jupiter in an orbit the same size as its orbit around the earth, would its period of revolution be different from its period around the earth?

Solution

The period of the orbit around Jupiter would be shorter since the greater gravitational attraction of Jupiter would require a higher orbital speed for a stable orbit.

Table 17-3	The Moon (Percentages Are with Respect to the Same Property of the Earth)
Diameter	3476 km (27%)
Mass	7.35×10^{22} kg (1.2%)
Average density	3.3 g/cm³ (60%)
Acceleration of gravity	1.7 m/s² (17%)
Escape speed	2.4 km/s (21%)
Average distance from the earth	384,400 km
Rotational period	27.3 days
Orbital period:	
Relative to the stars	27.3 days
Relative to the sun	29.5 days

During each $29\frac{1}{2}$-day period the moon goes through its familiar cycle of **phases** (Fig. 17-32). First there is only a thin crescent in the western sky at sunset that soon falls below the horizon (Fig. 17-33). Each night afterward the illuminated part of the moon grows wider and moves eastward relative to the stars. After 2 weeks the moon has become full and rises in the east at sunset to light up the sky all night. Next the illuminated part of the moon grows narrower until, after 2 more weeks, it is a thin crescent that rises just before sunrise. Finally the moon disappears altogether for a few days before we see it again as a crescent at sunset.

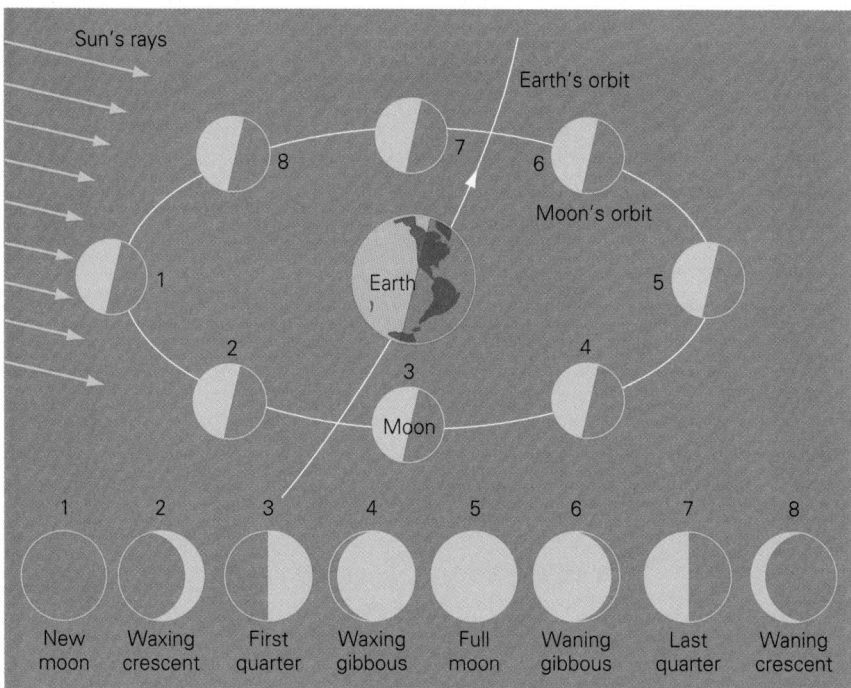

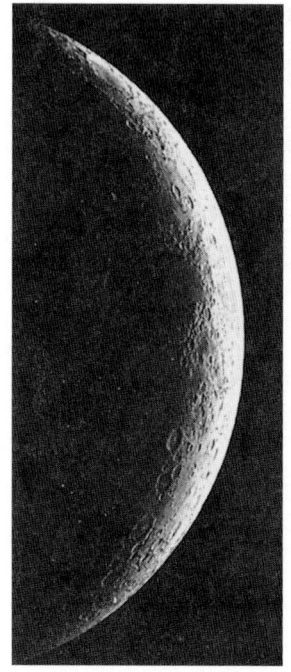

Figure 17-32 The origin of the moon's phases. As the moon revolves around the earth, we see it from different angles. When it is between us and the sun, we see only the dark side (new moon), and when it is on the opposite side of us from the sun, we see only the illuminated side (full moon). At other times we see parts of both sides. When the moon is approaching full moon, it is said to be **waxing;** when it is approaching new moon it is said to be **waning.** A way to remember what the moon looks like when it is waxing and waning is the rule of opposites: when the moon looks like a C, it is really Departing (waning); when it looks like a D, it is really Coming (waxing).

Earthshine These different aspects represent the amounts of the moon's illuminated surface visible to us in different parts of its orbit. When the moon is full, it is on the opposite side of the earth from the sun, so the side facing us is fully illuminated. In the "dark of the moon" (or new moon), the moon is moving approximately between us and the sun, so the side toward the earth is in shadow. But the shadow is not completely dark—there is a ghostly glow because of **earthshine,** sunlight reflected from the earth's surface that reaches the moon. In addition to clouds and surface ice, whitecaps on ocean waves contribute significantly to earthshine.

17.13 Eclipses

Now You See It, Now You Don't

When the earth is between the sun and the moon (that is, at full moon), how can the sun illuminate the moon at all? Why doesn't the earth's shadow hide the moon completely? And when the moon passes between the sun and the earth, why isn't the sun hidden from our view?

The answers to these questions follow from the fact that the moon's orbit is tilted at an angle of 5.2° to the earth's orbit. Ordinarily the moon passes either slightly above or slightly below the direct line between sun and earth (Fig. 17-34). On the rare occasions when the moon does pass more or less directly before or behind the earth, an **eclipse** occurs—an eclipse of the moon when the earth obscures the moon, an eclipse of the sun when the moon's shadow touches the earth. The circular shape of the earth's shadow during a lunar eclipse is evidence for its spherical form, as the ancient Greek astronomers realized.

Figure 17-33 Waxing crescent moon 3 days after new moon.

A Remarkable Coincidence Total eclipses of the sun occur because, though the sun's diameter is about 400 times as great as that of the moon, the sun is also about 400 times as far away from the earth during much of its orbit. At these times the apparent diameters of both sun and moon are the same as seen from the earth, and total eclipses are possible (Fig. 17-35). Partial

Moonrise and Moonset

From Fig. 17-32 we can figure out the times of moonrise and moonset for each phase, keeping in mind that the earth spins counterclockwise when viewed from above the North Pole. Because a number of factors will be ignored, actual times of moonrise and moonset may vary by an hour or more from those we shall find.

Let us start with the new moon. Since the new moon is nearly in line with the sun, the new moon rises when the sun does at about 6 A.M. local time, is at its highest point at noon, and sets at about 6 P.M. The full moon is along the same earth-sun line but on the opposite side of the earth. The full moon therefore rises at 6 P.M. when the sun sets, is at its highest point in the sky at midnight, and sets at 6 A.M. A first-quarter moon is halfway between new moon and full moon; hence it rises at noon and sets at midnight. A last-quarter moon is halfway between full moon and new moon; hence it rises at midnight and sets at noon.

The rises and sets of crescent and gibbous phases can be estimated in the same way (Table 17-4). For instance, a waxing crescent moon, which is at position 2 in Fig. 17-32, is intermediate between new moon and first quarter, and therefore rises at about 9 A.M. and sets at about 9 P.M.

Table 17-4	Approximate Times of Moonrise and Moonset	
Phase	**Rise Time**	**Set Time**
New moon	6 A.M.	6 P.M.
Waxing crescent	9 A.M.	9 P.M.
First quarter	Noon	Midnight
Waxing gibbous	3 P.M.	3 A.M.
Full moon	6 P.M.	6 A.M.
Waning gibbous	9 P.M.	9 A.M.
Last quarter	Midnight	Noon
Waning crescent	3 A.M.	3 P.M.

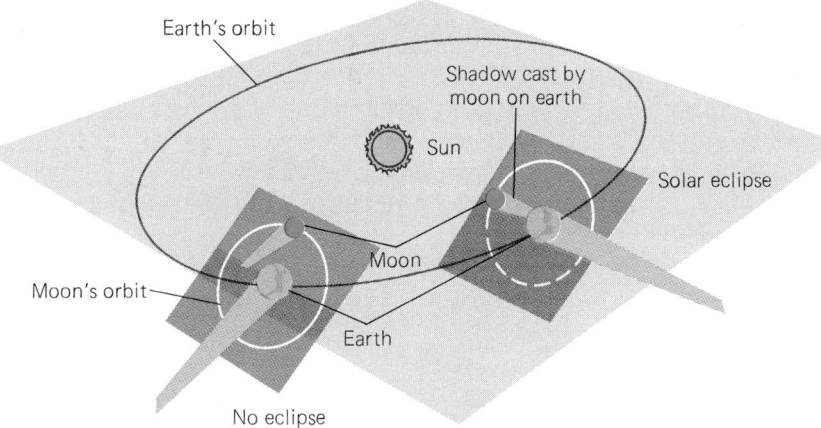

Figure 17-34 The orbit of the moon is tilted with respect to that of the earth. For this reason the moon normally passes above or below the direct line from the sun to the earth. Eclipses occur only on the rare occasions when the moon passes exactly between the earth and the sun (a solar eclipse, with the moon blocking out light from the sun) or exactly behind the earth (a lunar eclipse, with the earth blocking out light from the sun).

eclipses of the sun take place when the moon is not quite aligned with the sun, so that only part of the solar disk is obscured.

When the moon is farthest from the earth, its apparent diameter is less than that of the sun. The moon cannot then block the entire solar disk even when the moon lies directly between the sun and the earth. In this situation the result is an **annular** eclipse of the sun, with a ring of sunlight appearing around the rim of the moon. Table 17-5 lists the eclipses that will occur in the next few years.

17.14   Lunar Surface and Interior

Mountains and Maria, Probably Ice but No Atmosphere

To look at the moon is to wonder (Fig. 17-36). What is it made of? What is its origin? What is the nature of its landscape? What geologic processes occur on its surface and in its interior? Is there life on the moon? What is the ultimate destiny of the earth-moon system?

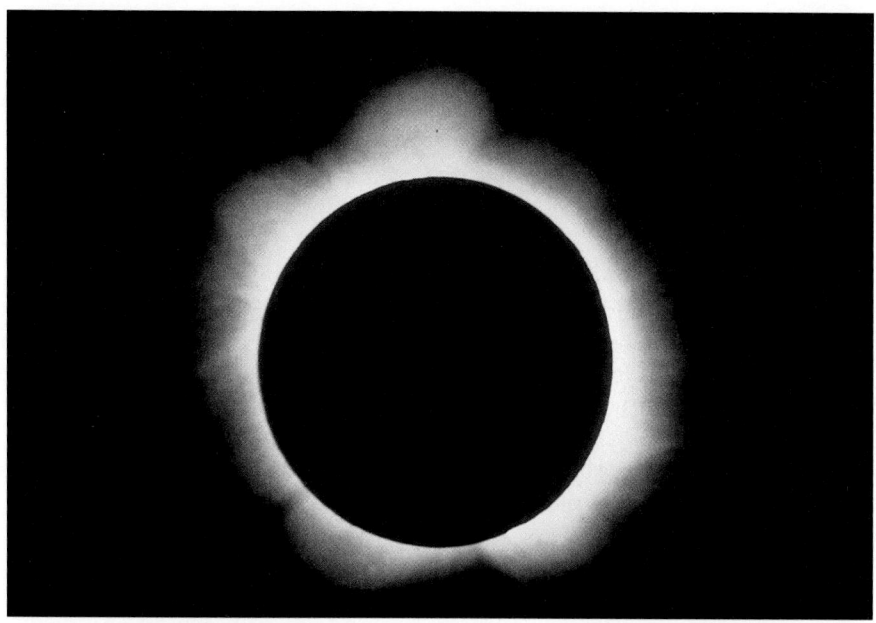

Figure 17-35 In a total solar eclipse, the sun's disk is exactly obscured by the moon. The solar corona, a glowing gas cloud, can be seen during such an eclipse. Most total eclipses last less than 5 min. A total eclipse is visible somewhere on the earth about every year and a half, but there may be hundreds of years between successive eclipses at the same place.

Future Eclipses

The friction of the earth's tidal bulges (see Sec. 1.10) on the ocean floors means that the bulges are always slightly ahead of the direct line between the centers of the earth and moon. The gravitational pull of the bulge nearest the moon is gradually speeding up the moon in its motion around the earth, which means that its orbit is increasing in size all the time.

Radar measurements show that the moon is moving away from the earth at about 4 cm per year. As a result, in the distant future—perhaps 150 million years from now—the apparent size of the moon in the sky will be smaller than that of the sun and total solar eclipses will no longer take place, only annular eclipses.

Table 17-5	Solar and Lunar Eclipses 2009–2013*	
Date	**Type**	**Where Visible**
January 4, 2011	Partial solar	Europe, Africa, Asia
June 1, 2011	Partial solar	Asia, North America
June 15, 2011	Total lunar	South America, Europe, Asia, Australia
July 1, 2011	Partial solar	Indian Ocean
November 25, 2011	Partial solar	Africa, Antarctica, New Zealand
December 10, 2011	Total lunar	Europe, Africa, Asia, Australia
May 20, 2012	Annular solar	Asia, Pacific, North America
June 4, 2012	Partial lunar	Asia, Australia, Pacific, Americas
November 13, 2012	Total solar	Australia, Pacific, South America
November 28, 2012	Partial lunar	Europe, Africa, Asia, Australia, Pacific, North America
April 25, 2013	Partial lunar	Europe, Africa, Asia, Australia
May 10, 2013	Annular solar	Australia, Pacific
May 25, 2013	Partial lunar	Americas, Africa
October 18, 2013	Partial lunar	Americas, Europe, Africa, Asia
November 3, 2013	Partial solar	Americas, Europe, Africa
April 15, 2014	Total lunar	Australia, Pacific, Americas
April 29, 2014	Annular solar	Indian Ocean, Australia, Antarctica
October 8, 2014	Total lunar	Asia, Australia, Pacific, Americas
October 23, 2014	Partial solar	Pacific, North America
March 20, 2015	Total solar	Europe, Africa, Asia
April 4, 2015	Total lunar	Asia, Australia, Pacific, Americas
September 13, 2015	Partial solar	Africa, Indian Ocean, Antarctica
September 28, 2015	Total lunar	Pacific, Americas, Europe, Africa, Asia
March 9, 2016	Total solar	Asia, Australia, Pacific
March 23, 2016	Partial lunar	Asia, Australia, Pacific, Americas
August 18, 2016	Partial lunar	Australia, Pacific, Americas
September 1, 2016	Annular solar	Africa, Indian Ocean
September 16, 2016	Partial lunar	Europe, Africa, Asia, Australia, Pacific

*Predictions by Fred Espenak, NASA/GSFC

Until July 20, 1969, the study of the moon was more notable for the questions asked than for the answers available. On that day Neil Armstrong set foot on the moon, the first person ever to do so, after a 3-day voyage aboard the spacecraft Apollo 11 with two companions. Four days after that they returned to earth, bringing with them samples of the lunar surface. That historic expedition and the others that followed it (Fig. 17-37) answered a great many questions about our companion in space. But others still remain, notably about its interior.

The moon was not entirely a mystery even before the voyages of Apollo 11 and of the other manned spacecraft that followed it there. Even a small telescope reveals the chief features of the lunar landscape: wide plains, jagged mountain ranges, and innumerable craters of all sizes. Each mountain stands out in vivid clarity, with no clouds or haze to hide the smallest detail. Mountain shadows are black and sharp-edged. When the moon passes in front of a star, the star remains bright and clear up to the moon's very edge. From these observations we conclude that the moon has little or no atmosphere.

Figure 17-36 The moon rotates on its axis at the same rate that it orbits the earth. As a result, the moon always presents this face to us. The dark areas are the maria, ancient lava flows that have been broken up by meteoroid bombardment.

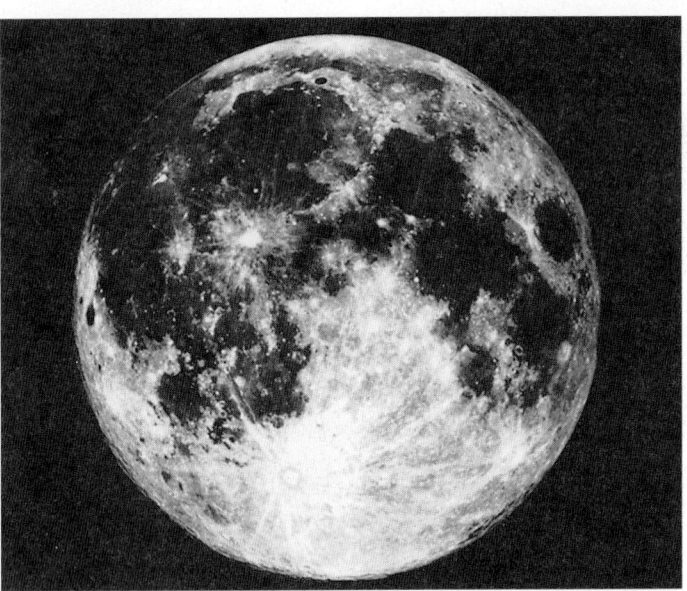

Figure 17-37 Astronaut Charles M. Duke, Jr., collecting lunar samples during the Apollo 16 expedition in 1972. The crater at left is 40 m in diameter and 10 m deep. Behind it is the Lunar Roving Vehicle that permitted Duke and his fellow astronaut John W. Young to explore the lunar surface some distance from the landing craft. Possible projects for future landings include installing an array of radiotelescopes on the dark side of the moon, studying x-rays from space, and accurately measuring the earth-moon distance.

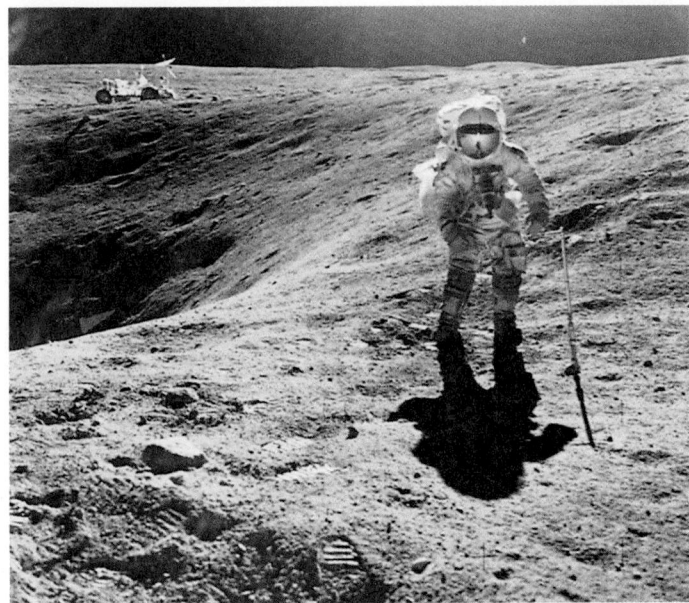

Liquid water is absent from the moon's surface—no lakes, rivers, or seas. However, a lot of ice is there in places permanently in the shadow of nearby mountains and so always cold. With no sunlight shining on it, the ice remained undiscovered until recently. Then, in 2009, NASA aimed a spent rocket stage at a region of constant shadow and detected a significant amount of water in the plume of debris that was thrown up. The water may have been brought to the moon by the comets and asteroids that pelted down upon it long ago. In addition, some may be the result of protons, which are hydrogen nuclei, in the solar wind (Sec. 18.4) binding to oxygen atoms in the lunar soil to form H_2O molecules.

Example 17.5

Why does the moon not have an atmosphere although the earth does?

Solution
The moon's gravitational attraction is not great enough to prevent the escape of the rapidly moving gas molecules in an atmosphere. From Table 17-3 the escape speed of the moon is only 2.4 km/s, about a fifth of the escape speed of the more massive earth.

But there is still no substitute for direct observation and laboratory analysis. Each spacecraft that visited on the moon, whether piloted by human beings or not, has brought back information of the greatest value. The lack of a protective atmosphere and of running water to erode away surface features means there is much to be learned on the moon about our common environment in space, both past and present. And from the composition and internal structure of the moon hints can be gleaned of its history, hints that bear upon the history of the earth as well. Thus the study of the moon is also a part of the study of the earth, doubly justifying the effort of its exploration.

Landscape Features   With the help of no more than binoculars it is easy to distinguish the two main kinds of lunar landscape, the dark, relatively smooth **maria** (the singular is **mare**) and the lighter, ruggedly mountainous highlands. The mountains of the moon are thousands of meters high, which means that the moon's surface is about as irregular as the earth's.

Mare means "sea" in Latin, but the term is still used even though it has been known for a long time that these regions are not covered with water. The largest of the maria is Mare Imbrium, the Sea of Showers, which is over 1000 km across.

The maria are circular depressions covered with dark, loosely packed material—not solid rock. They are not perfectly smooth but are marked by small craters, ridges, and cliffs. The maria consist of lava flows similar to basalt that have been broken up by meteoroid impacts. It is curious that nearly all the maria are on the lunar hemisphere that faces the earth (Fig. 17-38).

The lunar highlands are scarred by innumerable craters, some with mountain peaks at their centers (Fig. 17-39). Certain craters, such as Tycho and Copernicus, have conspicuous streaks of light-colored matter radiating outward. These **rays** may extend for hundreds or thousands of km, and seem to consist of lunar material sprayed outward after the meteoroid impacts that caused the craters. The impacts melted this material, and it cooled quickly in flight into glassy particles that reflect light well.

The **rilles** of the highlands are especially intriguing. These are narrow trenches up to 250 km long that look like dried-up riverbeds. The rilles were probably created by the collapse of subsurface channels through which molten rock once flowed from active volcanoes.

A Base on the Moon

A life-support system that does not rely exclusively on supplies from the earth is necessary for a long-term lunar base. What is exciting about the discovery of water (as ice) on the moon is not only that it might be used in the daily lives of visitors, who would anyway recycle most of their water, but that electrolysis (Sec. 10.17) powered by solar energy could separate it into hydrogen and oxygen for rocket fuel. Then visitors to the moon would not have to carry with them fuel for their return to the earth, an enormous advantage.

The combination of weak lunar gravity and a local fuel supply would make the moon a much better base for exploring the solar system than the earth itself. It remains to be seen how practical it will be to actually collect lunar ice, melt it, and convert it into rocket fuel.

Water is not the only lunar material that could help visitors. A cubic meter of the rock dust on the moon's surface contains, according to one researcher, the equivalent of two cheese sandwiches, two cola drinks, and two plums in such elements important to life as hydrogen, oxygen, carbon, nitrogen, and potassium. How to turn rock dust into lunch efficiently may or may not be worked out eventually, but a better bet for the first menus is something like nutritious and easily grown (though not necessarily very appetizing) blue-green algae.

Figure 17-38   The far side of the moon, which always faces away from the earth, was photographed from the Galileo spacecraft in 1990. The dark markings are basaltic lava flows formed over 3 billion years ago. The dark region at lower left is a huge basin that was probably caused by the impact of a giant meteoroid.

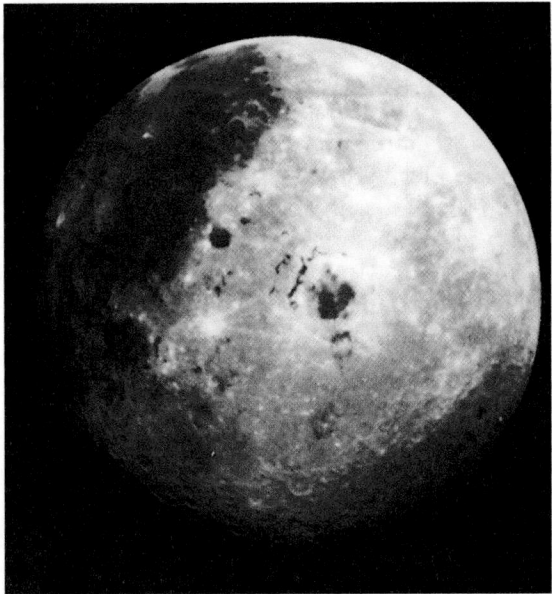

Figure 17-39   Cratered landscapes of the lunar highlands were caused by meteoroid impacts.

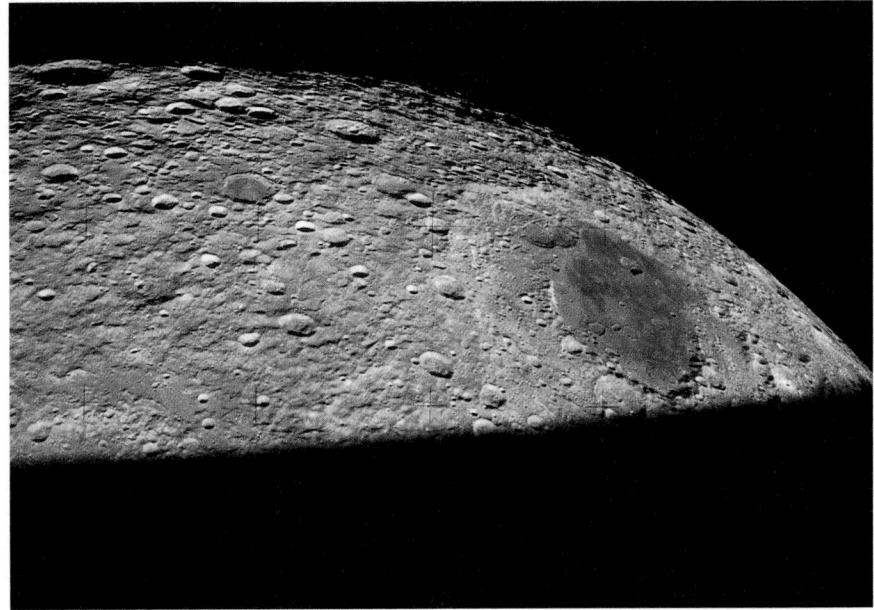

Interior   Four of the Apollo missions planted seismometers that for 9 years radioed measurements of several thousand moonquakes to the earth. As in the case of the earth, the data show the moon to consist of a rigid crust, a thick semisolid mantle, and a small, dense core. Evidence in lunar rocks of a magnetic field in the past suggests that the core then consisted of molten iron, as the earth's core does today. Later the core cooled, which stopped the motions that generated the magnetic field, though it may still be liquid. Because the moon's average density is only 60 percent of the earth's average density, the moon's core must be much smaller, relative to its size, than the earth's core.

17.15   Evolution of the Lunar Landscape

A Violent Past, a Quiet Present

The analysis of lunar rock and soil samples (2200 of them, totalling 382 kg) has led to a number of conclusions about the history of our satellite. On

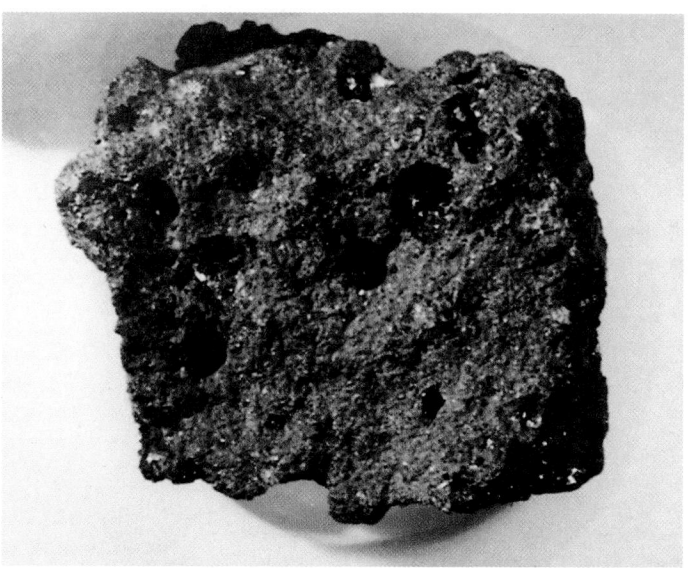

Figure 17-40 This 2-cm rock fragment collected during the Apollo 11 expedition to the moon in 1969 resembles certain volcanic rocks on the earth, although it is different chemically and no weathering has taken place.

the basis of such samples the moon's story can be taken farther back than the earth's because, since the moon lacks an atmosphere, weathering did not occur there (Fig. 17-40). Even particles of pure iron have been found on the moon's surface, whereas only iron compounds occur on the earth's surface.

Rocks have been found on the moon that radioactive dating reveals crystallized earlier than the most ancient terrestrial rocks, which are nearly 4 billion years old. Some lunar samples apparently solidified very soon after the solar system came into being. These rocks are older than any found on the earth.

As the molten outer part of the early moon gradually hardened into a light-colored crust, meteoroids of all sizes rained down. Some, as large as Rhode Island and better described as asteroids, smashed great basins hundreds of km across. About 4 billion years ago, as the bombardment moderated, radioactivity inside the moon produced enough heat to melt rock there. Lava that reached the surface flowed into the impact basins to form the dark maria that today cover about 20 percent of the moon's surface.

The youngest rocks found on the moon are 3 billion years old, so all igneous activity there must have stopped at that time. Meteoroids continued to crater the landscape and to pulverize surface rock into the powdery debris that today coats the moon.

17.16 Origin of the Moon

A Collision was Probably Responsible

Until recently, theories of the origin of the moon fell into three categories (Fig. 17-41):

1. The moon was initially part of the earth and split off to become an independent body.
2. The moon was formed elsewhere in the solar system and was later captured by the earth's gravitational field.
3. The moon and the earth came into being together as a double-planet system.

Each of these approaches once seemed quite attractive, but strong arguments against all of them eventually appeared.

A fourth proposal is today widely accepted. Suppose that early in the history of the solar system (see Sec. 19.10), another planet a little larger than

Figure 17-41 Four theories of the moon's origin: (1) The moon split away from the earth. (2) The moon was captured as it approached the earth from elsewhere. (3) The earth and moon were formed together from different clouds of particles. (4) Another early planet struck the earth and formed a larger earth plus the moon. The last theory seems the most plausible.

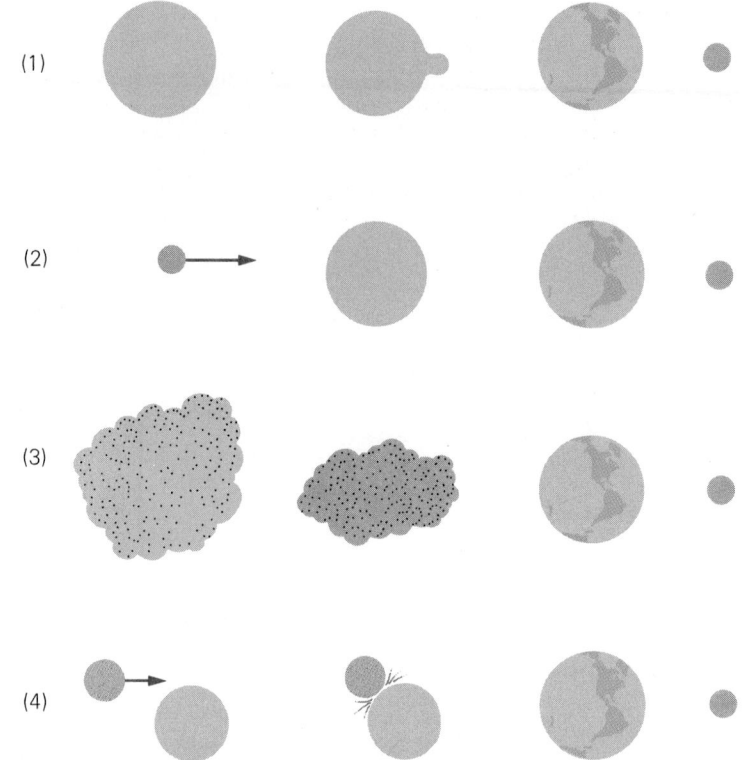

Mars and with a composition slightly different from that of the infant earth had developed nearby, and this planet crashed into the earth sometime during the first 100 million years after it had formed. The mantle of the other planet and some of the earth's would have been thrown off into orbit around the earth by the impact, a year or so later to form the moon. In this picture of the moon's origin, the other planet's iron core was added to the earth's core. The orbital angular momentum that the moon has today can be accounted for if the collision were a glancing one rather than head-on.

Pulling so dramatic an event as a collision between two planets out of a hat always arouses suspicion among scientists. Why should we take this idea any more seriously than the discarded hypotheses mentioned earlier?

The basic answer is that detailed computer simulations of such a collision and its aftermath fit well with what we know about the earth and moon and with what is strongly believed about the early history of the solar system. In addition, if similar collisions also occurred elsewhere in the solar system, then a number of other long-standing oddities can also be understood. For instance, we have already noted that a large-scale collision could have knocked Uranus into its sideways rotation, so it is possible that the moon's origin is just one example of a normal phenomenon.

Important Terms and Ideas

Comets and **meteoroids** are relatively small objects that pursue regular orbits in the solar system. Comets glow partly by the reflection of sunlight but mainly through the excitation of their gases by solar ultraviolet radiation. **Meteors** are the flashes of light that meteoroids produce when they enter the earth's atmosphere. Fallen meteoroids are called **meteorites.**

In order from the sun, the planets are **Mercury, Venus, Earth, Mars, Jupiter, Saturn, Uranus,** and **Neptune.** All but Mercury and Venus have satellites. There are also a number of **dwarf planets,** notably **Pluto.** In addition, thousands of **asteroids** are in orbits that lie between those of Mars and Jupiter and outside Neptune's orbit. All these bodies are visible by virtue of the sunlight they reflect.

The **inner planets** (Mercury, Venus, Earth, and Mars) are considerably smaller, less massive, and denser than the **outer planets,** which apparently consist largely of hydrogen, helium, and hydrogen compounds such as methane, ammonia, and water vapor. Jupiter, Saturn, Uranus, and Neptune are circled by **rings** of particles.

The **moon** shines by virtue of reflected sunlight. The **phases** of the moon occur because the area of its illuminated side visible to us varies with the position of the moon in its orbit. A **lunar eclipse** occurs when the earth's shadow obscures the moon, a **solar eclipse** when the moon obscures the sun.

The moon has neither an atmosphere nor liquid surface water although ice is present. Geologically inactive at present, the lunar surface shows signs of having once melted and of having experienced many volcanic eruptions long ago. Meteoroid bombardment has been a more recent factor in shaping its landscapes.

Multiple Choice

1. Comets
  a. follow orbits around the earth
  b. follow orbits around the sun
  c. move randomly through the solar system
  d. are the tracks left in the atmosphere by meteoroids

2. Comets consist of
  a. leftover matter from the early solar system
  b. the debris of a shattered planet
  c. luminous gases
  d. particles from the solar wind

3. Comet tails always
  a. are longest near the sun
  b. are shortest near the sun
  c. are of constant length
  d. point away from their direction of motion

4. Meteor showers occur
  a. at the same times each year
  b. at random times
  c. in connection with solar eclipses
  d. in connection with lunar eclipses

5. When visibility is good and there are no meteor showers, it is possible to see about 5 to 10 meteors per
  a. minute   **c.** night
  b. hour   **d.** week

6. Meteoroids
  a. come from the sun
  b. come from the moon
  c. come from outside the solar system
  d. are members of the solar system

7. The majority of meteoroids consist of
  a. silicate minerals   **c.** iron
  b. calcite   **d.** nickel

8. The planets are visible because
  a. their atmospheres are excited to luminescence by the solar wind
  b. they are hot enough to radiate light
  c. they reflect sunlight
  d. they reflect starlight

9. The planet nearest the sun is
  a. Mercury   **c.** Saturn
  b. Venus   **d.** Neptune

10. The smallest of the following planets is
  a. Mars   **c.** Saturn
  b. Jupiter   **d.** Uranus

11. The largest of the following planets is
  a. Mars   **c.** Saturn
  b. Jupiter   **d.** Uranus

12. The planet closest to the earth in size and mass is
  a. Mercury   **c.** Mars
  b. Venus   **d.** Uranus

13. The planet with the longest year is
  a. Mercury   **c.** Saturn
  b. Jupiter   **d.** Neptune

14. A planet with virtually no atmosphere is
  a. Mercury   **c.** Jupiter
  b. Mars   **d.** Saturn

15. Of the following planets, the least conspicuous in the sky is
  a. Venus   **c.** Jupiter
  b. Mars   **d.** Neptune

16. The planet whose surface most resembles that of the moon is
  a. Mercury   **c.** Jupiter
  b. Venus   **d.** Saturn

17. An astronaut would weigh least on the surface of
  a. Venus   **c.** Mars
  b. Earth   **d.** Jupiter

18. A dense atmosphere of carbon dioxide is found on
  a. Mercury   **c.** Mars
  b. Venus   **d.** the moon

19. The two planets of the solar system that do not have satellites are
  a. Mercury and Venus
  b. Mars and Saturn
  c. Jupiter and Neptune
  d. Neptune and Uranus

20. The surface of Titan, Saturn's largest moon,
  a. has many active volcanoes
  b. shows signs of erosion by flowing liquid
  c. is covered with liquid water
  d. is covered with water ice

21. The largest of Jupiter's satellites is about the size of
  a. a large ship   **c.** Mercury
  b. the moon   **d.** the earth

22. Of the following members of the solar system, the one that never exhibits phases to us is
    a. the moon
    b. Mercury
    c. Venus
    d. Mars

23. Compared with the earth, Mars has
    a. a denser atmosphere
    b. more surface water
    c. a lower average surface temperature
    d. a shorter year

24. The spacecraft that traveled to Mars did not find
    a. heavily cratered regions
    b. lava flows
    c. dust storms
    d. living things

25. The rings of Saturn
    a. are gas clouds
    b. are sheets of liquid
    c. are sheets of solid rock
    d. consist of separate particles

26. Meteor craters are observed on the surface of which of the following?
    a. Mercury
    b. Venus
    c. Mars
    d. the moon

27. A planet that consists largely of hydrogen and helium is
    a. Mercury
    b. Venus
    c. Mars
    d. Jupiter

28. Asteroids are found
    a. spread evenly throughout the solar system
    b. mainly in a belt between the earth and the moon
    c. mainly in a belt between the earth and Mars
    d. mainly in a belt between Mars and Jupiter

29. Polar ice caps are found on
    a. Mercury
    b. Venus
    c. Mars
    d. Jupiter

30. The dwarf planets have diameters of about
    a. 1 km
    b. 10 km
    c. 1000 km
    d. that of the moon

31. The asteroids probably consist largely of
    a. ice
    b. frozen methane
    c. silicate minerals
    d. metallic iron

32. The largest known asteroid is about as far across as
    a. New York City
    b. Texas
    c. the United States
    d. the moon

33. An asteroid 2 km or more across could cause a worldwide catastrophe. Such an asteroid is thought to collide with the earth an average of roughly every
    a. thousand years
    b. million years
    c. billion years
    d. 10 billion years

34. Relative to the time the moon takes to circle the earth, the period of its rotation on its axis is
    a. shorter
    b. the same
    c. longer
    d. any of these, depending on the time of the year

35. The durations of "day" and "night" at a given place on the moon each correspond to about
    a. 1 day on earth
    b. 1 week on earth
    c. 2 weeks on earth
    d. 4 weeks on earth

36. The moon's diameter is about
    a. $\frac{1}{10}$ that of the earth
    b. $\frac{1}{4}$ that of the earth
    c. $\frac{1}{2}$ that of the earth
    d. $\frac{3}{4}$ that of the earth

37. At new moon, the moon is
    a. between the earth and the sun
    b. on the opposite side of the earth from the sun
    c. on the opposite side of the sun from the earth
    d. to the side of a line between the earth and the sun

38. An eclipse of the sun can occur
    a. only when the moon passes directly between the earth and the sun
    b. only when the sun passes directly between the earth and the moon
    c. only when the earth passes directly between the sun and the moon
    d. at any time

39. Eclipses of the sun occur at
    a. new moon
    b. first or last quarter
    c. full moon
    d. any time

40. Eclipses of the moon occur at
    a. new moon
    b. first or last quarter
    c. full moon
    d. any time

41. The average density of the moon is
    a. lower than that of the earth
    b. about the same as that of the earth
    c. higher than that of the earth
    d. unknown

42. The moon's surface is
    a. perfectly smooth
    b. irregular but relatively smoother than the earth's surface
    c. about as irregular as the earth's surface
    d. much more irregular than the earth's surface

43. The moon's maria are
    a. bodies of water like the earth's oceans
    b. solid lava flows
    c. lava flows pulverized by meteoroid impacts
    d. hardened sediments

44. Most of the craters on the moon are probably the result of
    a. volcanic action
    b. meteoroid bombardment
    c. erosion
    d. collisions with asteroids

45. The moon's surface shows no signs of
   a. volcanic action
   b. meteoroid bombardment
   c. ever having melted
   d. glacier erosion

46. The time needed for the Apollo spacecraft to reach the moon was about
   a. 3 h   **c.** 3 weeks
   b. 3 days   **d.** 3 months

47. Relative to the oldest rocks that have been found on the moon, the oldest rocks found on the earth are
   a. younger
   b. about the same age
   c. somewhat older
   d. very much older

48. The interior of the moon is probably entirely or almost entirely
   a. liquid   **c.** gaseous
   b. solid   **d.** hollow

Exercises

17.1 The Solar System

1. Which planets are visible to the unaided eye?

2. (a) How is it possible to distinguish the planets from the stars by observations with the unaided eye? (b) By observations with a telescope?

3. Which is the largest planet? The smallest? Which planet is nearest the sun?

4. Why do the planets shine?

5. Which planets, if any, have no satellites?

6. Is the mass of the solar system concentrated in the sun or in the planets?

7. On which planets would a person weigh less than on the earth? On which planets would a person weigh more?

8. Suppose you were on Mars and watched the earth with the help of a telescope. What changes would you see in the earth's appearance as it moves around the sun in its orbit?

17.2 Comets

9. How do the orbits of comets compare in shape with the orbits of the planets?

10. Why do comets have tails only in the vicinity of the sun? Why do these tails always point away from the sun, even when the comet is receding from it?

11. When a comet is close enough to the sun to be seen from the earth, stars are visible through both the comet's head and tail. What does this imply about the danger to the earth from a collision with a comet?

17.3 Meteors

12. The Perseid meteor shower appears early every August. Does this mean that the orbits of the meteoroids in the Perseid swarm all have periods of exactly 1 year?

13. Over 90 percent of the meteorites found after a known fall are stony, yet most of the meteorites in museums are iron. Why do you think this is so?

14. If the earth had no atmosphere, would comets still be visible from its surface? Would meteors?

15. Why are most meteorites found in Antarctica?

16. Why are meteoroids believed to come from within the solar system?

17.4 Mercury

17. Why is it very unlikely that there is life on Mercury?

18. Mercury takes 59 of our days to turn completely on its axis, but the period of time between one sunrise and the next on Mercury is 176 of our days. What do you think is the reason for the difference?

17.5 Venus

19. Why are Mercury and Venus always seen either around sunrise or around sunset?

20. Venus is the brightest planet in the sky. How does its brightness compare with that of the brightest stars?

21. Why are Mercury and Venus the only planets that show phases like those of the moon?

22. Venus is brighter when it appears as a crescent than when we can see its full disk. Why?

23. Far fewer meteoroid craters of ancient origin have been observed on Venus than expected. Could running water have eroded the others? If not, what might be the reason?

24. Give two reasons why the surface of Venus is so much hotter than the earth's surface.

17.6 Mars

17.7 Is There Life on Mars?

25. Give three reasons why Venus is a brighter object in the sky than Mars.

26. Compare the likelihood that an astronaut on Mars will be struck by a meteoroid with its likelihood on earth.

27. Mars has surface features that seem to be the result of erosion by running water. Why does the presence of many meteoroid craters in some of these regions suggest that the running water disappeared there long ago?

28. Why do temperatures on the surface of Mars vary between day and night more than they do on the earth's surface?

29. Why does Mars appear red?

30. Are any volcanoes active on Mars today?

31. Why is ultraviolet radiation from the sun more of a hazard to life on Mars than on the earth?

17.8 Asteroids

32. Distinguish between asteroids and meteoroids.

33. What is believed to be the origin of the asteroids?

34. Why are few asteroids spherical, as planets are?

35. Is there any evidence that an asteroid ever collided with the earth? Could such a collision occur in the future?

17.9 Jupiter

36. Why is Jupiter thought not to consist mainly of rock with an iron core, as does the earth? Of what does it mainly consist?

37. What is believed to be the nature of the Great Red Spot on Jupiter?

38. When did conditions on the earth resemble those on Jupiter's satellite Europa today? Was there any life on the earth at that time?

39. The interior of Jupiter's satellite Io is thought to be heated through being flexed by the gravitational pulls of Jupiter and two other satellites. Why is Io's interior believed to be hot?

17.10 Saturn

40. What are the chief similarities between Jupiter and Saturn? The chief differences?

41. Why are Saturn's rings believed to consist of small particles rather than being solid sheets of matter or thin gas clouds?

42. Is it likely that Saturn's rings are permanent features?

43. Saturn's satellite Titan has an atmosphere. Do any of the other planetary satellites also have atmospheres?

17.11 Uranus, Neptune, Pluto, and More

44. Which planet resembles the earth most in size and mass? In surface conditions?

45. Is there any evidence that planets other than the earth today have crusts that consist of huge moving plates?

46. (a) Which planets besides Saturn have rings? (b) What is the nature of these rings?

47. What are thought to be the chief constituents of the giant planets Jupiter, Saturn, Uranus, and Neptune?

48. (a) What is the chief distinction between planets and dwarf planets? (b) What are the chief similarities? (c) What is the chief distinction between dwarf planets and planetary satellites? (d) Do any dwarf planets have satellites?

49. How does Pluto compare in size with the moon? With the satellites of the other planets?

17.12 Phases of the Moon

50. We always see the same hemisphere of the moon. Why?

51. What is wrong with the statement that the moon is more useful to us than the sun because the moon provides illumination at night when it is needed most?

52. The moon rises in the east at midnight on a certain night. Can it appear as a full moon?

53. Approximately how much time elapses between new moon and full moon?

54. Is the moon the largest satellite in the solar system? The smallest?

55. To what approximate length of time on the earth does the length of "day" at a given place on the moon correspond? The length of "night"?

56. Relative to the stars, the moon takes 27.3 days to orbit the earth. As seen from the earth, the moon drifts eastward relative to the stars. Through what angle does the moon move eastward each day relative to the stars?

17.13 Eclipses

57. If the moon were smaller than it is, would total eclipses of the sun still occur? Would total eclipses of the moon still occur?

58. Eclipses of the sun and of the moon do not occur every month. Why not?

59. In what phase must the moon be at the time of a solar eclipse? At the time of a lunar eclipse?

17.14 The Lunar Surface and Interior

17.15 Evolution of the Lunar Surface

60. The moon's surface is about as irregular as that of the earth. What does this imply about temperatures in the moon's interior?

61. The moon's maria are dark, relatively smooth regions conspicuous even to the naked eye. What is their nature?

62. Moonquakes are weaker and occur much less often than earthquakes. What do these facts imply about temperatures in the moon's interior?

63. Why is it believed that the moon's interior is different in composition from the earth's interior?

64. Why is it believed that large-scale igneous activity ceased on the moon about 3 billion years ago?

65. What has been the chief influence that shaped the lunar landscape during the past 3 billion years?

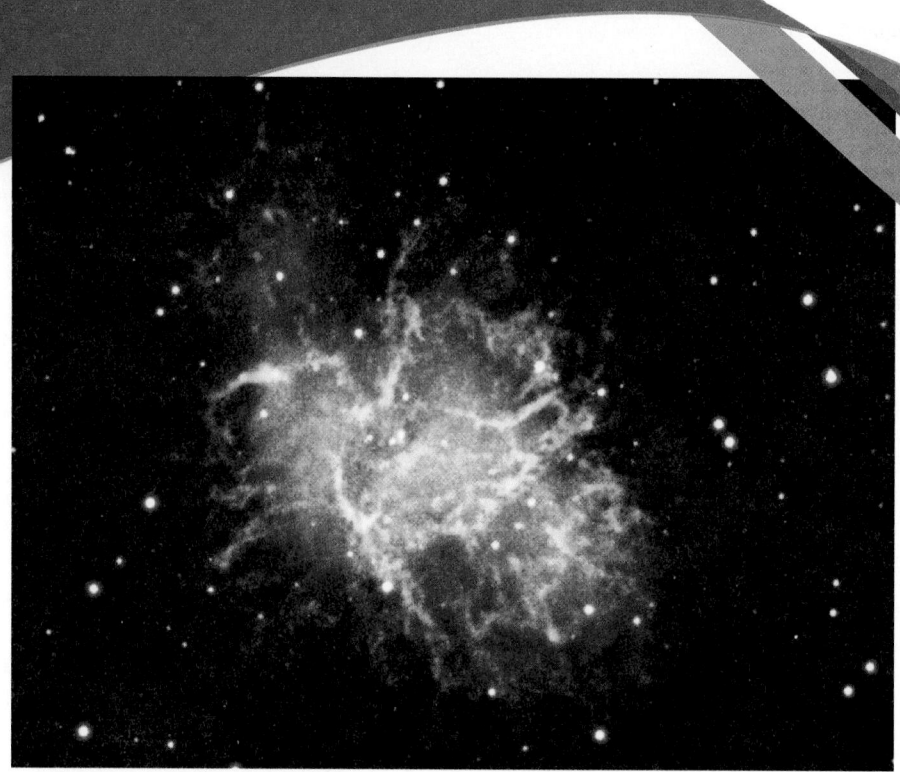

The Crab Nebula has a pulsar at its heart.

GOALS

When you have finished this chapter you should be able to complete the goals
given for each section below:

Tools of Astronomy

18.1 The Telescope
All Modern Ones Are Reflectors
- Give two advantages of large telescopes.

18.2 The Spectrometer
Without It, Little Would Be Known about the Stars
- Describe the operation of a spectrometer.

18.3 Spectrum Analysis
Spectra Can Tell Us a Surprising Amount
- Describe how the spectrum of a star can provide information on the star's structure, temperature, composition, condition of matter, magnetism, and motion.
- Interpret in terms of stellar structure the observation that nearly all stars have absorption (dark line) spectra.

The Sun

18.4 Properties of the Sun
The Nearest Star
- State what is meant by the photosphere of the sun.

18.5 The Aurora
Fire in the Sky
- Describe the appearance in the sky and the origin of auroras.

18.6 Sunspots
They Come and Go in an 11-Year Cycle

- Discuss sunspots, the sunspot cycle, and some effects on the earth that are correlated with sunspot activity.

18.7 Solar Energy
It Comes from the Conversion of Hydrogen to Helium
- Explain why solar energy cannot come from combustion.
- Identify the basic process that gives rise to solar energy.
- Describe how the elements more massive than hydrogen are created and distributed throughout the universe.

The Stars

18.8 Stellar Distances
Not Easy to Measure
- Define light-year.
- Describe the parallax method of finding the distance to a star.
- Describe how the distance to a star can be found by comparing its apparent and intrinsic brightness.

18.9 Variable Stars
Stars Whose Brightness Changes, Usually in Regular Cycles
- Explain how Cepheid variable stars are used to find the distances of star groups.

18.10 Stellar Motions
The Stars Are Not Fixed in Space
- Explain how stellar motions are detected.

18.11 Stellar Properties
Mass, Temperature, and Size

- Describe how the mass and size of a star can be found.
- Account for the relatively small range of stellar masses.

Life Histories of the Stars

18.12 H-R Diagram
Most Stars Belong to the Main Sequence
- State what is plotted on a Hertzsprung-Russell (H-R) diagram.
- Draw an H-R diagram and indicate the positions of main-sequence stars, giants, and white dwarfs.
- Compare the properties of giants and white dwarf stars.

18.13 Stellar Evolution
Life History of a Star
- Outline the life history of an average star like the sun.
- State what a brown dwarf is.

18.14 Supernovas
Exploding Stars
- Outline the life history of a very massive star.
- State what a supernova is.

18.15 Pulsars
Spinning Neutron Stars
- Define neutron star and pulsar and discuss the connection between them.

18.16 Black Holes
Even Light Cannot Escape from Them
- Describe what black holes are and explain how they can be detected.

The study of the stars began in earnest toward the end of the eighteenth century with the work of William Herschel. Herschel sought among the stars some kind of order, something as profound as the regularities Copernicus, Kepler, and Newton had found in the solar system. Like a pioneer in any other branch of science, Herschel began with observation and spent many years cataloging stars and measuring their apparent motions. From this study he was able to verify a structure for the universe that is not far from the one that today's astronomers believe to be correct.

Of the billions of stars in the universe, none (besides the sun) appears as more than a point of light to even the most powerful telescope. Less than a century ago, most scientists despaired of ever knowing the physical nature of the stars. Today, however, thanks to spectroscopic analysis, we not only have a great deal of detailed information on thousands of stars but also are able to trace the evolution of a star from its birth through maturity to its last agonies and eventual fate.

Tools of Astronomy

Light is the messenger that brings us information about the universe. Because the information arrives in code, so to speak, the astronomer must decipher it before being able to assess its significance. The tools of astronomy are devices that collect light and sort it into its component wavelengths, which are the elements of the code.

18.1   The Telescope

All Modern Ones Are Reflectors

In Herschel's time, as in ours, the telescope (invented in Holland in 1608) was the basic astronomical instrument. Much of his success was due to the improvements he introduced in telescope construction. Herschel was the first to build and use a large reflecting telescope, an instrument in which light is reflected from a concave mirror instead of being refracted through a lens (Fig. 18-1). A large lens tends to sag under its own weight, with the change in shape producing a distorted image, whereas even a sizable mirror can be adequately supported from behind. In addition, there is no problem of the dispersion of light of different wavelengths with a mirror (see Sec. 7.15).

Modern astronomical telescopes are reflectors. The 5-m-diameter Hale Telescope on Mt. Palomar, California, was the largest single mirror reflector from 1948 to 1999, when the 8.3-m Subaru reflector was installed on Mauna Kea in Hawaii. All other modern large reflectors do not rely on single mirrors, which are limited in size by practical difficulties. Instead, a number of individual mirrors are linked to produce a single image. In one approach, hexagonal mirror segments are used to give a large collecting surface (Fig. 18-2). In another, separate circular mirrors are used. A telescope of this type with four 8.2-m mirrors has been installed on a Chilean mountain where the air is especially dry, stable, and clear; it should be able to observe an astronaut on the moon.

Future Telescopes   A still larger such telescope will have seven 8.4-m mirrors to give it more collecting area plus 10 times the resolving ability of the Hubble Space Telescope. Called the Giant Magellan Telescope (GMT), it will also be installed in Chile and—it is hoped—will start in 2015 to help solve such deep remaining astronomical mysteries as the natures of dark matter and dark energy, which we shall meet in Chap. 19.

Being considered for even farther in the future is OWL—the name comes both from the keen-eyed bird and from the telescope's *overwhelmingly large* size—whose mirror, 100 m in diameter, would consist of 3048 adjustable hexagonal segments; its total weight would be 15,000 tons.

Twinkling stars, the result of turbulent motions in the atmosphere that create density fluctuations, delight poets but not astronomers. A cure for such flickering images, called adaptive optics, uses light from a bright "guide" star or from a reflected laser beam to detect the distortions, which are continuously corrected by adjusting a deformable mirror in the optical path of the telescope. Such a system can produce images as sharp as those of a telescope in space.

Size Matters   In stellar astronomy the purpose of a big telescope is not magnification, for the stars are too distant to ever appear as more than points of light. One virtue of large mirrors and lenses lies in their light-gathering power, which enables more light from a given object to be collected. Thus faint objects that would otherwise be invisible are revealed by a large telescope, and more light from brighter objects is available for study.

The second advantage of a large telescope is its ability to distinguish, or **resolve,** small details. As mentioned in Sec. 7.17, the diffraction of light waves causes every optical image to be blurred to a certain extent. The larger the lens or mirror, the less the blurring and the sharper the image.

Originally the light collected by a telescope went to an astronomer's eye, but later photographic plates were used and today electronic sensors are preferred. The latter methods have the advantage that they respond to the *total amount* of light that falls on them over the period of time they are exposed. The eye, on the other hand, responds only to the *brightness* of the light that reaches it. A telescope with a camera or sensor attached can be trained on the same area of the sky for hours or, if necessary, for several nights to detect objects too faint for the eye to pick up. Photographic plates (over 2 million in

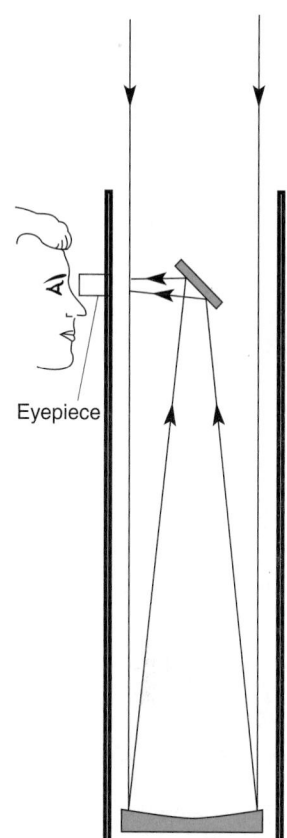

Figure 18-1   Simplified sketch of one type of reflecting telescope. The concave mirror produces a real image (see Chap. 7) of a distant object that is reflected outside the telescope by another mirror, normally for recording electronically or for spectroscopic analysis. When used in this way the telescope does not need additional optics—it acts as a giant telephoto lens. However, for direct viewing, a lens or set of lenses called an eyepiece is needed to give a virtual image whose object is the image produced by the mirror.

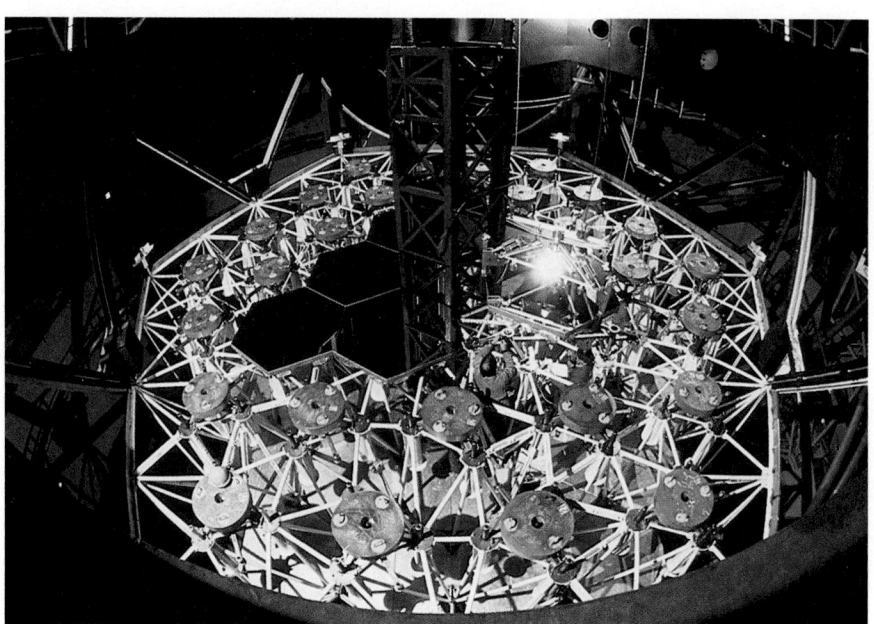

Figure 18-2   Each of the twin Keck telescopes atop Hawaii's Mauna Kea volcano has a mosaic mirror 10 m in diameter that consists of 36 hexagonal segments. The segments can be continuously adjusted to compensate for any distortions that may arise. Because the Keck telescopes are so much larger than the Hubble Space Telescope, they can see much fainter objects, but atmospheric turbulence reduces their resolving ability below that of the Hubble. Only four mirror segments were in place when this photograph was taken. A telescope with a still larger segmented mirror, 10.4 m across, has been installed on a peak on La Palma, one of Spain's Canary Islands.

Telescopes in Space

A telescope orbiting the earth in a satellite has a number of advantages over its earthbound cousins. An important one is that there is no atmosphere in the way to blur images and absorb various wavelengths of incoming radiation. Nor is there background radiation from the earth to swamp faint signals from space.

The first major telescope in orbit operating at visible wavelengths, the Hubble Space Telescope, named for the astronomer Edwin Hubble (biography in Sec. 19.6), has a mirror 2.4 m in diameter and was launched in 1990 (Fig. 18-3); it orbits the earth 5800 times each year. An unceasing stream of marvels has been revealed by the Hubble telescope, from closeups of the planets to views of distant galaxies. It has been repaired and upgraded during four space shuttle missions, the last in 2009, and is expected to continue to expand our knowledge of the heavens at least until 2014. Other telescopes in orbit operate in the x-ray and infrared parts of the spectrum and future ones will extend the range to include microwave, ultraviolet, and gamma radiations.

Future space telescopes will be able to see yet farther into the depths of the universe. One of them, the James Webb Space Telescope (named for a past chief of NASA), is planned for launch in 2013. It will have a mirror 6.5 m in diameter that will give it 7 times the light-gathering ability of the Hubble telescope. To get the mirror into space, it will be made in 18 lightweight beryllium segments folded together that will unfurl when the telescope is in place. Each hexagonal segment will be very thin and have four actuators to control its shape precisely.

Because it orbits the earth, the Hubble telescope cannot make continuous observations of all parts of the sky. To avoid this limitation, the Webb telescope will hover in space at a place called a Lagrange point where the gravitational forces of the earth and sun always balance out exactly. (There are five Lagrange points; this one is four times as far away from the earth as the moon.) The Webb telescope will operate in the infrared because the expansion of the universe (Sec. 19.6) shifts the light from distant objects to this part of the spectrum through the doppler effect—the farther away an object is, the faster it appears to be receding from us, and the greater the shift. It is hoped that the new telescope will be able to study the formation of the earliest stars and galaxies. The telescope should also be able to detect Jupiter-sized planets that may orbit nearby stars.

Finding planets is also the task of several existing space telescopes. The next generation of them will be able to detect signs of water, oxygen, and carbon dioxide, suggestive of the possibility of life, on any planets seen around other stars.

Figure 18-3   The Hubble Space Telescope was put in orbit in 1990 and is still in operation. Its record of discoveries is unsurpassed in variety and importance.

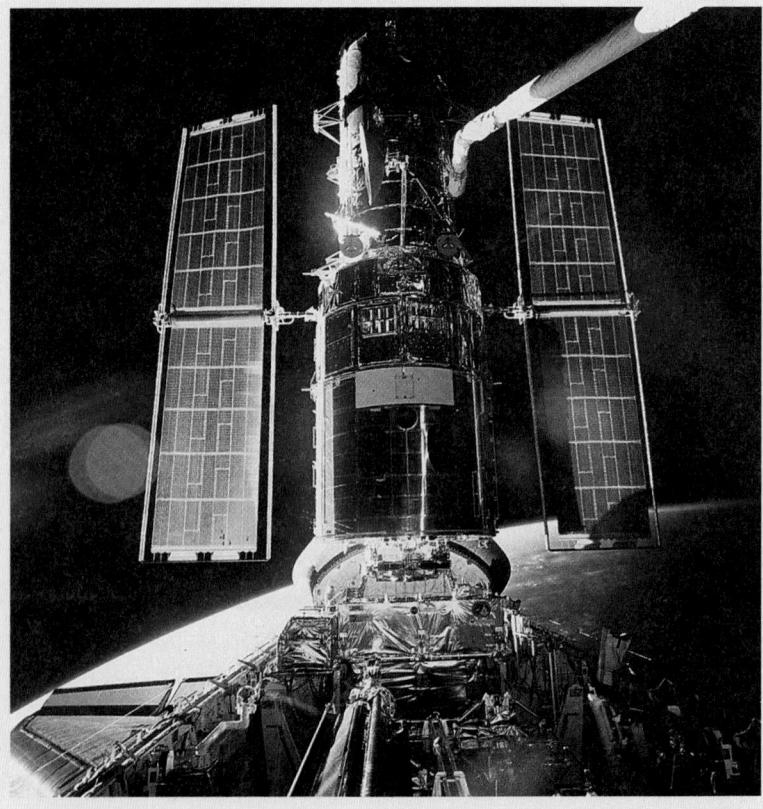

storage, some a century old) and, today, electronic methods of data storage provide permanent records that enable positions and properties of stars as they appear today to be compared with what they were years ago and with what they will be in years to come.

18.2 The Spectrometer

Without It, Little Would Be Known about the Stars

By itself, a telescope is of limited use in studying the stars. What is needed is a combination of a telescope and a spectrometer, the same instrument that contributed so much to our knowledge of atomic structure (see Chap. 9). A spectrometer breaks light up into its separate wavelengths, as shown in Fig. 9-18. The resulting band of colors, with each wavelength separate from the others, is the spectrum that is recorded on a photographic plate or electronic medium.

The spectrum of a star does not seem impressive. If photographed in natural colors, it generally consists of a rainbow band crossed by a multitude of fine dark lines. Ordinarily color film is not used, so the spectrum shows simply black lines on a light gray background.

At first glance it does not seem that a few black lines on a photographic plate can get us very far in understanding the stars. But each of those lines has its own story to tell about how it was produced, and a specialist can piece together data from different lines into a comprehensive picture of a star. Some types of information obtainable from spectra are outlined in the next section.

A serious problem in astronomical spectroscopy is the absorption of light in the earth's atmosphere. Spectrometers mounted in sounding rockets, high-altitude balloons, satellites, and spacecraft are needed to study those parts of solar and stellar spectra that cannot reach the earth's surface.

18.3 Spectrum Analysis

Spectra Can Tell Us a Surprising Amount

Structure A spectrum of dark lines on a continuous colored background is an **absorption spectrum;** it is produced when light from a hot object passes through a cooler gas (see Sec. 9.8). Atoms and molecules of the gas absorb light of certain wavelengths and so leave narrow gaps in the band of color. Thus a star that has this kind of spectrum (and nearly all of them do) reveals at once something of its structure: it must have a hot, glowing interior surrounded by a relatively cool gaseous atmosphere.

Temperature From the continuous background of a star's spectrum, astronomers can find the temperature of its surface. What they need to know is where in the spectrum the star's radiation is brightest. Since the wavelength of maximum intensity decreases as the temperature rises, the point of maximum intensity in the spectrum is a measure of temperature (Figs. 9-4 and 18-4). Thus the hottest stars are blue-white (maximum intensity at the short-wavelength end of the spectrum), stars of intermediate temperature are orange-yellow, and the coolest visible stars are red. This relation holds for materials on the earth as well as for the stars, as we know from experience (see Fig. 5-5).

Composition Each element has a spectrum of lines with characteristic wavelengths. The elements present in a star's atmosphere can therefore be identified from the dark lines in its spectrum. In principle, all we have to do is measure the wavelength of each line in the spectrum and compare these wavelengths with those produced by various elements in the laboratory.

Condition of Matter In practice the identification of lines in a star's spectrum is not quite so easy. The wavelengths and intensities of the lines characteristic

Figure 18-4 Relative intensity of the wavelengths of light emitted by bodies with the temperatures indicated. The wavelength of greatest intensity is shorter for hot bodies than for cooler ones. The red curve represents measurements of the sun's photosphere. (1 nm = 10^{-9} m)

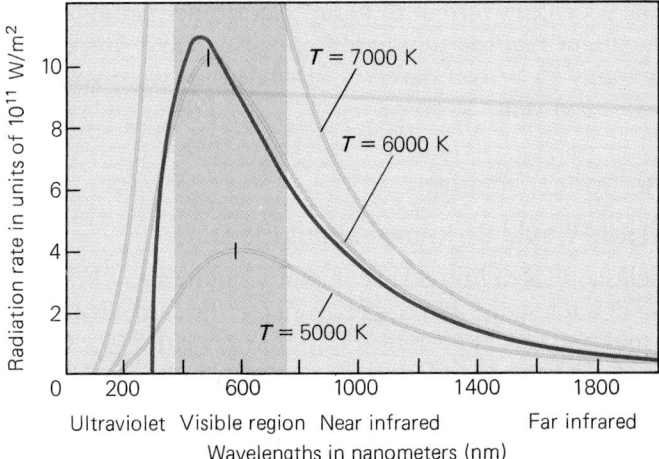

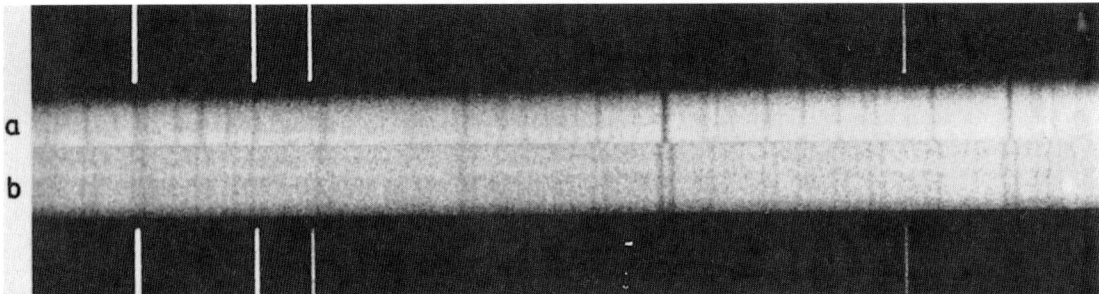

Figure 18-5 Spectra of the double star Mizar, which consists of two stars that circle each other, taken 2 days apart. In (*a*) the stars are in line with no motion toward or away from the earth, so their spectral lines are superimposed. In (*b*) one star is moving toward the earth and the other is moving away from the earth, so the spectral lines of the former are doppler shifted toward the blue end of the spectrum and those of the latter are shifted toward the red end.

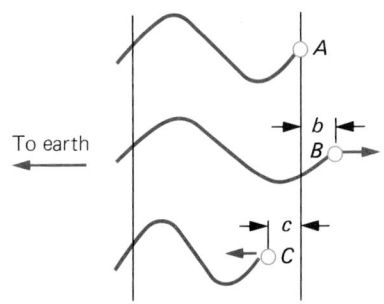

Figure 18-6 The doppler effect in stellar spectra. Star *A* is stationary with respect to the earth. Star *B* is moving away from the earth; it moves the distance *b* during the emission of one light wave, whose wavelength is therefore increased by *b*. Star *C* is approaching the earth; it moves the distance *c* during the emission of one wave, whose wavelength is thus decreased by *c*. Hence stars receding from the earth have spectral lines shifted toward the red (long-wavelength) end, while stars approaching the earth have spectral lines shifted toward the blue (short-wavelength) end.

of a given element depend not only on the element but also on such conditions as temperature, pressure, and degree of ionization. These difficulties prove to be blessings in disguise, however, for once the lines are identified, they tell us not only which elements are present in a star's atmosphere but also something about the physical conditions in which the elements exist.

Chemical compounds also have spectral lines of recognizable wavelengths, so spectra provide a means of determining how much of the matter in a star's atmosphere is in the form of molecules rather than atoms.

Magnetic Fields   The presence of a magnetic field causes individual energy levels within atoms to divide into several sublevels. When such atoms are excited and radiate, their spectral lines are accordingly split, each into a number of lines close to the original one. This phenomenon is called the **Zeeman effect** after its discoverer, the Dutch physicist Pieter Zeeman. With the help of the Zeeman effect the magnetic nature of sunspots has been established, and a large number of stars and clouds of matter in space have been discovered that appear to be strongly magnetized.

Motion   As we learned in Chap. 7, the doppler effect causes sounds produced by vehicles moving toward us to seem higher pitched than usual, whereas sounds produced by vehicles receding from us seem lower pitched than usual. Similarly a star moving toward the earth has a spectrum whose lines are shifted toward the blue (high-frequency) end, and a star moving away from the earth has a spectrum in which each line is shifted toward the red (low-frequency) end, as in Figs. 18-5 and 18-6. From the amount of the shift we can calculate the speed with which the star is approaching or receding.

The Sun

The sun is the glorious orb that dominates the solar system, and the origin and destiny of the earth are closely connected with its life cycle. The astronomer has another reason for studying the sun closely, for it is in many ways a typical star, a rather ordinary member of the assembly of perhaps 10^{20} stars that make up the known universe. Thus the properties of the sun that we can observe by virtue of its relative closeness are interesting not only in themselves but also because they give us information about stars in general that would otherwise be out of reach.

18.4   Properties of the Sun

The Nearest Star

The sun's mass can be found from the characteristics of the earth's orbital motion around it. The result is a mass of 1.99×10^{30} kg, more than 300,000 times the earth's mass. The sun's radius of 6.96×10^8 m can be established by simple geometry from the fact that its angular diameter as seen from the earth is 0.53°. The volume of the sun is such that 1,300,000 earths would fit into it.

The Photosphere   The gases in the sun's interior are very hot, so they emit light copiously, and they are very dense, so the light is reabsorbed almost at once. Because both temperature and density fall off with distance from the sun's center, eventually there is a region in which the gases are still hot enough to radiate a great deal of light but not dense enough to prevent the light from escaping (Fig. 18-7). This region, called the **photosphere,** is what we see as the "surface" of the sun, although it has no sharp boundary. The temperature of the photosphere, 5800 K, is found in two ways: from the shape of its spectrum (see Fig. 18-4) and from the rate at which it gives off energy.

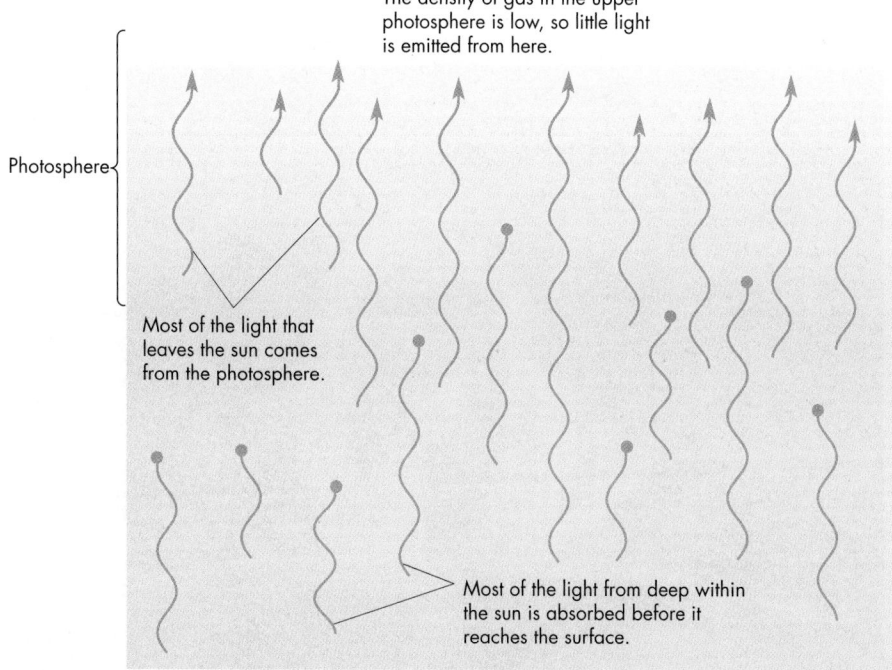

The density of gas in the upper photosphere is low, so little light is emitted from here.

Photosphere

Most of the light that leaves the sun comes from the photosphere.

Most of the light from deep within the sun is absorbed before it reaches the surface.

Figure 18-7   The light the sun emits comes from a thin outer layer called the photosphere. The photosphere is so thin (only 0.03 percent of the sun's radius) that it appears as a sharp surface.

Of the thousands of lines in the sun's spectrum, about half have been traced to specific elements. The others probably come from highly excited energy levels or energy levels in ions rather than atoms. Lines of few compounds are found since the photosphere is hot enough to break up nearly all molecules.

Although conditions on the sun are very different from those on the earth, the basic matter of the two bodies appears to be the same. Even the relative amounts of different elements are similar, except that there is much more of the light elements hydrogen (72 percent by mass) and helium (27 percent) on the sun. At the relatively low temperatures here on the earth, most elements have combined to form compounds; in the sun's interior the elements occur as individual atoms or ions.

Above the Photosphere   A rapidly thinning atmosphere, mainly of hydrogen and helium, extends past the photosphere. From this atmosphere great flamelike **prominences** sometimes project into space, much like sheets of gas standing on their sides (Fig. 18-8). Prominences occur in a variety of forms; a typical example is about 200,000 km long, 10,000 km wide, and 50,000 km high. Prominences are often associated with sunspots and, like sunspots, seem to have magnetic fields associated with them.

During a total eclipse of the sun, when the moon obscures the sun's disk completely (see Fig. 17-37), a wide halo of pearly light can be seen around the dark moon. This halo, or **corona,** may extend out as much as a solar diameter and seems to have a great number of fine lines extending outward from the sun immersed in its general luminosity. The corona consists of ionized atoms, mainly protons, and electrons in extremely rapid motion; its temperature can reach 2 million K.

Solar Wind   Although the corona we see during eclipses is relatively near the sun, it is found in very diffuse form much farther out, well beyond the earth's orbit. The outward flow of ions (mostly protons) and electrons in this extension of the sun's atmosphere is the **solar wind,** which leaves the sun at about 400 km/s. The solar wind has been detected by spacecraft and helps deflect comet tails away from the sun as well as causing auroras in the earth's upper atmosphere.

Figure 18-8   These solar prominences follow magnetic field lines.

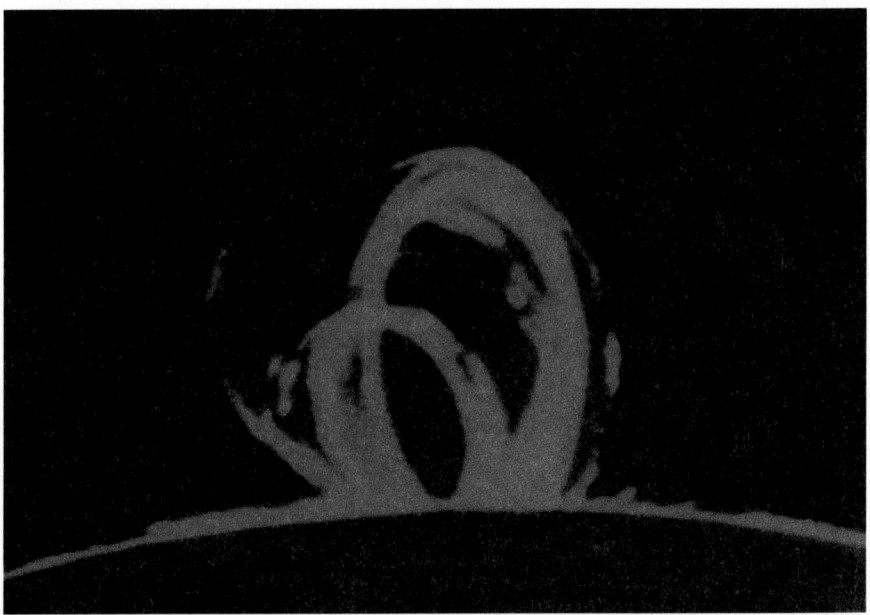

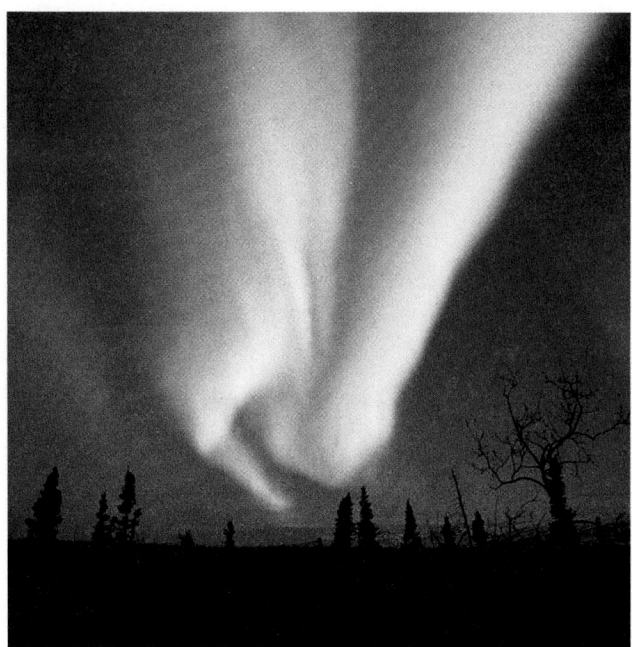

Figure 18-9 Aurora in Alaska. Auroras are caused by streams of fast protons and electrons from the sun that excite gases in the upper atmosphere to emit light.

18.5 The Aurora

Fire in the Sky

The aurora (or "northern lights") is one of nature's most awesome spectacles. In a typical auroral display, colored streamers seem to race across the sky, and glowing curtains of light pulsate as they change their shapes into weird forms and images. In the climax of the display the heavens seem on fire, with silent green and red flames dancing everywhere (Fig. 18-9). Then, after a while, the drama fades away, and only a faint reddish arc remains.

Auroras are most common in the far north and far south. **Aurora borealis** is the name given (by Galileo) to this phenomenon in the northern hemisphere, and **aurora australis** in the southern. (Aurora was the Roman god of the dawn, boreas is Greek for "north wind," and australis is Greek for "of the south.")

Origin of Auroras Auroras are caused by the solar wind. The protons and electrons take about a day to reach the earth. When they enter the upper atmosphere, they interact with the nitrogen and oxygen there so that light is given off. The process is similar to what occurs in a neon-filled glass tube when electricity is passed through it. The gas molecules are excited by charged particles moving near them, and this energy is then radiated as light in the characteristic wavelengths of the particular element. The green hues of an auroral display come from oxygen, the blues from nitrogen, and the reds from both oxygen and nitrogen.

Auroras have also been observed in the atmospheres of Venus, Mars, Jupiter, and Saturn.

The incoming streams of solar protons and electrons are affected by the earth's magnetic field in a complicated way. As a result most auroral displays occur in doughnutlike zones about 2000 km in diameter centered about the geomagnetic North and South Poles. Sometimes, though, the cloud of particles from the sun is so immense that auroras are visible elsewhere as well.

Even when auroras are not obvious as such, there is a faint glow in the night sky due to less concentrated streams of solar particles that interact

An Aurora in Russia

Here is how an aurora that occurred in Russia in 1370 was described at the time: "During the autumn there were many signs in the sky. For many nights, people saw pillars in the sky and the sky itself was red, as if covered with blood. So red was the sky that even on the earth covered with snow all seemed red like blood, and this happened many times."

Figure 18-10   This photograph of an aurora seen from above was taken from the American satellite Spacelab when it was halfway between Australia and Antarctica in 1985. The blue-green band and the tall red rays are the aurora. The brownish band along the earth's rim is the airglow, a faint luminescence of the atmosphere excited by streams of particles from the sun less concentrated than those responsible for the aurora.

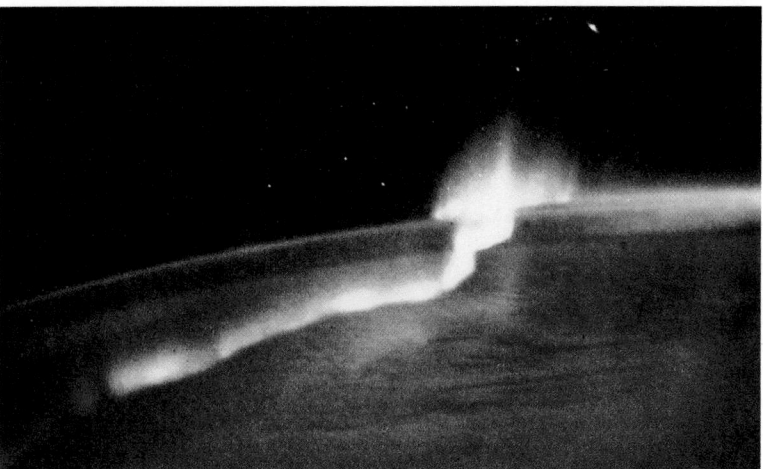

with the upper atmosphere. The brightness of this **airglow** varies with solar activity, but it is always present to some extent (Fig. 18-10). Auroras and the airglow occur during the day as well as the night but are too dim to be visible in the daytime.

18.6   Sunspots

They Come and Go in an 11-Year Cycle

Dark patches called **sunspots** at times mar the intense luminosity of the sun's surface. Sunspots are cooler areas that appear dark only because we see them against a brighter background (Fig. 18-11). A spot whose temperature is 4500 K is hot enough to glow brilliantly but is considerably cooler than the rest of the solar surface, whose temperature is about 5800 K. They were first recorded by Chinese astronomers over 2000 years ago.

Sunspots change continually in form, each one growing rapidly and then shrinking, with lifetimes of from 2 to 3 days to more than a month. The largest sunspots are many thousands of km across, large enough to swallow several earths. Galileo noted in 1610 that they moved across the sun's disk,

Figure 18-11   Sunspots appear dark because they are cooler than the rest of the solar surface, although quite hot themselves. Some sunspots are larger across than the earth. Most sunspots occur in groups.

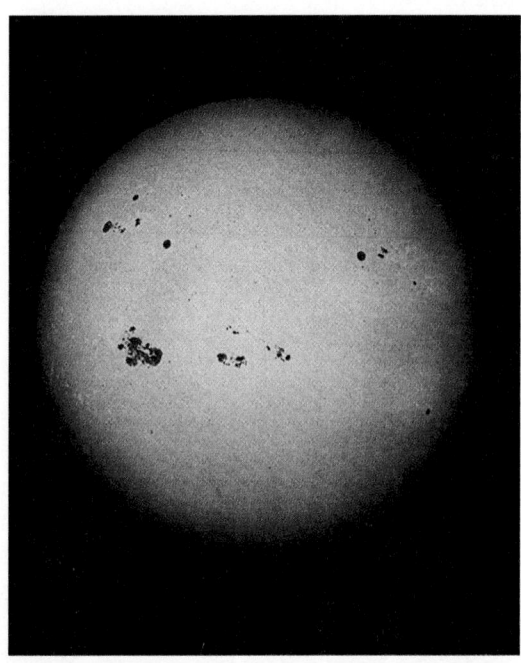

Solar Storms

Solar storms can have serious consequences. The fluctuating magnetic fields of a major storm in 1989 induced currents in electric transmission lines in eastern Canada strong enough to trip protective devices. This triggered power failures over a wide area by a domino effect: as one section of the electric grid became overloaded and shut down, its load was automatically shifted to another section that in turn became overloaded and shut down, and so on. Six million people lost electricity for 9 hours.

Today's larger and higher-voltage grids are even more vulnerable to solar storms than those of two decades ago, and much of our lives depends on reliable electricity supplies. A really severe solar storm could lead to power failures over the developed world that might take a long time, not just hours, to recover from. Damaged transformers (Fig. 6-48) would be a particular problem because there are few spares and new ones take a long time to build. The scale of a disaster of this kind could be reduced, however, by relatively simple modifications to protect transformers.

At present, the ACE spacecraft, which is in a solar orbit that keeps it between the sun and the earth, can give up to an hour's warning of the arrival of a solar storm. This would help power companies prepare for the storm. The spacecraft, launched in 1997, has enough fuel to maintain its position until about 2024.

The particle streams of solar storms can affect spacecraft by damaging the solar cells that provide their energy, by altering control software in their computers, and by producing flashes of light in the glass windows of star tracker navigation systems, which can cause the systems to lose their bearings. A satellite failure due to a solar storm in 1998 silenced most of the pagers in North America and in 2003 a large solar storm knocked two Japanese satellites out of service and affected communication and power grids around the world. A solar storm to come could jeopardize land, sea, and air navigation by GPS (Sec. 2.14).

which he interpreted, as we do today, as a sign that the sun rotates on its axis. Solar rotation is confirmed by doppler shifts in the spectral lines of radiation from the edges of the sun's disk. The sun rotates faster at its equator, where a complete turn takes 27 days, than near its poles, where a complete turn takes about 31 days.

Sunspots generally appear in groups, each with a single large spot together with a number of smaller ones. Some groups contain as many as 80 separate spots. They tend to occur in two zones on either side of the solar equator and are rarely seen either near the equator or at latitudes on the sun higher than 35°. Strong magnetic fields are associated with sunspots, and there is little doubt these fields are involved in sunspot formation.

The number of spots on the sun increases and decreases with time in a regular cycle that covers about 11 years (Fig. 18-12). There is evidence that other stars also have cool spots, some of which come and go periodically like those on the sun. Many of these starspots are much larger than sunspots.

Sunspots and the Earth   The sunspot cycle has aroused much interest because a number of effects observable on the earth—such as disturbances in its magnetic field, shortwave radio fadeouts, changes in cosmic-ray intensity, and unusual auroral activity—follow this cycle. It seems likely that the ionosphere changes that affect radio transmissions are due to intense bursts of ultraviolet and x-radiation that are more frequent during sunspot maximum. The magnetic, cosmic-ray, and auroral effects are due to vast streams of energetic protons and electrons that shoot out of the sun from the vicinity of sunspot groups to produce **solar storms** at the earth about 30 hours later.

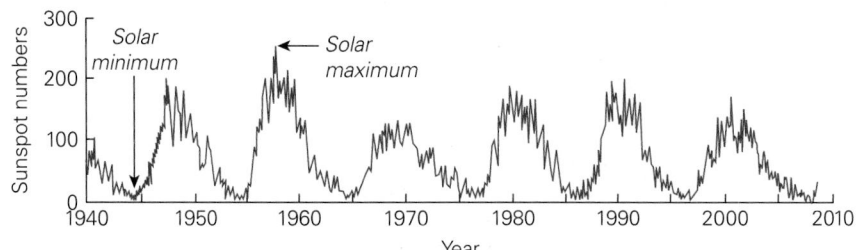

Figure 18-12   Sunspot numbers since 1940. Each cycle averages 11 years. The current cycle is one of the weakest on record with an average of 90 or even fewer sunspots expected at its maximum in 2013.

Some aspects of weather and climate seem to be synchronized with sunspot activity. For instance, very few sunspots appeared between 1645 and 1715, a period during which temperatures worldwide were lower than usual—the "Little Ice Age" mentioned in Sec. 14.11 occurred at about that time. Apparently the events in the sun that cause sunspots are correlated with a slightly higher energy output. Even a small change in the sun's energy output would be enough to affect climates on the earth to the observed extent.

18.7 Solar Energy

It Comes from the Conversion of Hydrogen to Helium

Here on the earth, 150 million km from the sun, an area of 1 m² exposed to the vertical rays of the sun receives energy at a rate of about 1.4 kW. Adding up all the energy received over the earth's surface gives a staggering total, although this is only a tiny fraction of the sun's total radiation. And the sun has been emitting energy at this rate for billions of years. Where does all this energy come from?

We might be tempted to think of combustion, for fires give off what seems like a lot of heat and light. But a moment's thought shows that the sun is too hot to burn. Burning involves oxygen reacting with other substances to form compounds, but the sun is so hot that compounds cannot exist there except in its atmosphere. And even if burning were possible, the heat even the best fuels could give would be much too little to maintain the sun's temperatures.

Solar energy can come only from processes that take place inside the sun. Calculations based on reasonable assumptions lead to an estimate of 14 million K for the temperature and 1 billion atm for the pressure near the sun's center. The density of the matter there is nearly 10 times that of lead on the earth's surface. Under these conditions atoms of the lighter elements have lost all their electrons, and atoms of the heavier elements retain only their inmost electron shells. Thus matter in the sun's interior consists of atomic debris—free electrons and positive nuclei surrounded by a few electrons or none at all.

These atomic fragments move about far more rapidly than gas molecules at ordinary temperatures. Such speeds mean that two atomic nuclei may get close enough to each other—despite the repulsive electric force due to their positive charges—to react and form a single large nucleus. When this occurs among the light elements, the new nucleus has a little *less* mass than the combined masses of the reacting nuclei, as we saw in Chap. 8. The missing mass is converted to energy according to Einstein's formula $E_0 = mc^2$. So huge an amount of energy is given off in nuclear fusion reactions of this kind that there is no doubt they are responsible for solar energy.

Fusion Reactions in the Sun   Most solar energy comes from the conversion of hydrogen into helium. This takes place both directly by collisions of hydrogen nuclei (protons) and indirectly by a series of steps in which carbon nuclei absorb a succession of hydrogen nuclei (Figs. 18-13 and 18-14). Each step can be duplicated in the laboratory and the energy released can be measured. The sun's interior is ideal for such energy-producing events. For the entire process by either fusion mechanism, every kilogram of helium formed means that about 0.007 kg—about the mass of a tablespoon of water—of matter disappears. The corresponding energy release is

$$E_0 = mc^2 = (0.007 \text{ kg})(3 \times 10^8 \text{ m/s})^2 = 6.3 \times 10^{14} \text{ J}$$

About 20 million kg of coal would have to be burned to obtain this amount of energy!

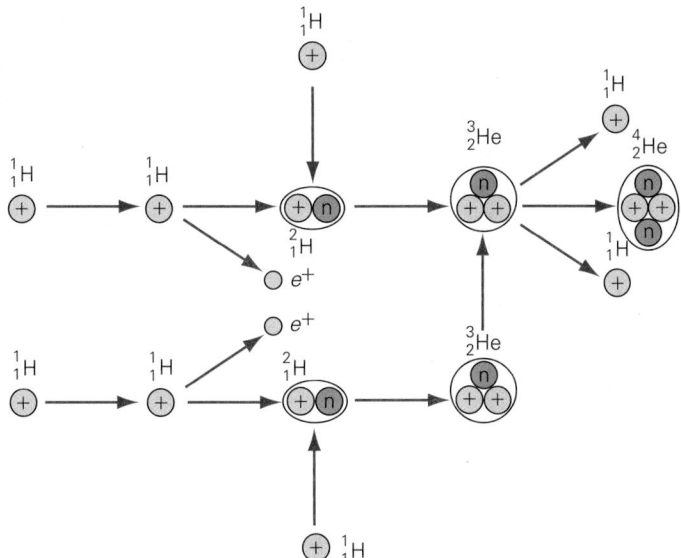

Figure 18-13   The proton-proton cycle. This is the chief nuclear reaction sequence that takes place in stars like the sun and cooler stars. Energy is given off at each step. The net result is the combination of four hydrogen nuclei to form a helium nucleus and two positrons. Two of the original six protons are left over and are available for further helium production.

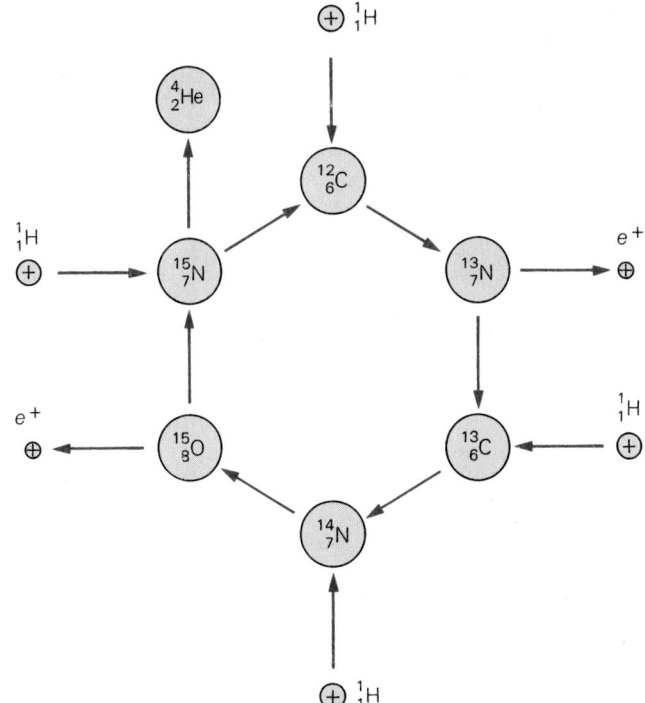

Figure 18-14   The carbon cycle also involves the combination of four hydrogen nuclei to form a helium nucleus with the evolution of energy. The $^{12}_{6}C$ nucleus is unchanged by the series of reactions and thus acts as a catalyst in the cycle. This cycle predominates in stars hotter than the sun.

The relative likelihoods of the carbon and proton-proton cycles depend on temperature. In the sun and other stars like it, which have interior temperatures up to about 14 million K, the proton-proton cycle predominates. Most of the energy of hotter stars comes from the carbon cycle.

In every second the sun converts more than 4 billion kg of matter to energy, and it has enough hydrogen to be able to release energy at this rate for billions of years to come. In fact, the amount of matter lost in all of geologic history is not enough to have changed the sun's radiation appreciably. This confirms other evidence that the earth's surface temperature has not changed by very much during this period.

| Hans Bethe (1906–2005)

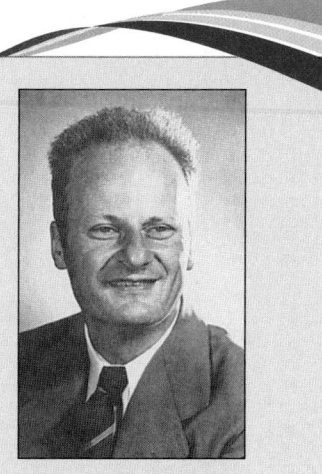

After a distinguished early career at various German universities, when Hitler came to power Bethe moved first to England and then to the United States. He was professor of physics at Cornell University from 1937 to 1975 and remained active in research and public affairs even when officially retired. Notable among Bethe's many and varied contributions is his 1938 account of the sequences of nuclear reactions that power the sun and stars.

During World War II, Bethe directed the theoretical physics division of the laboratory at Los Alamos, New Mexico, where the atomic bomb was developed. A strong believer in nuclear energy—"it is more necessary now than ever before because of global warming"—Bethe was also an effective advocate of nuclear disarmament.

Abundances of the Elements

There are a number of reasons why some elements are more common in the universe than others. To begin with, different nuclear reactions have different likelihoods of occurrence under comparable circumstances, which affects how often a given reaction sequence will take place inside stars.

Another factor is the stability of a given nuclide. For instance, as we saw in Sec. 8.8, iron nuclei have high binding energies per nucleon and so are exceptionally stable. As a result, iron is a relatively abundant element.

Also important is the number of different reaction sequences that

can produce a given element. Only one sequence leads to a stable gold isotope, hence gold is relatively rare. Tin, by contrast, has 10 stable isotopes, and with so many possible routes to its creation is not at all scarce.

Origin of the Heavy Elements   The reactions that convert hydrogen to helium are not the only ones that take place in the sun and other stars. With hydrogen and helium as raw materials and high temperatures and pressures to make things happen, most of the other elements are formed as well. The heaviest ones require still more extreme conditions to be produced, conditions that occur during the supernova explosions of heavy stars that are discussed later in this chapter. Such explosions also serve to scatter into space the various elements already created in the parent star.

Once scattered, these elements, heavy and light, mix with the hydrogen and helium of interstellar space and in turn become incorporated in new stars and their planets. We are all made of stardust.

The Stars

18.8   Stellar Distances

Not Easy to Measure

Aristotle pointed out long ago that, if the earth revolves around the sun, the stars should appear to shift in position, just as trees and buildings shift in position when we ride past them. Since he could detect no such shifts, Aristotle concluded that the earth must be stationary.

Another interpretation of the apparent lack of movement among the stars, suggested by some of the Greeks and later by Copernicus, is that the stars are simply too far away for such movement to be easily detected. An undoubted shift for one star was finally discovered in 1838 by the German astronomer Friedrich Bessel (Fig. 18-15), and others were found later. These shifts are so very small that the long failure to detect them is not surprising.

Bessel's discovery made possible the direct measurement of distances to the nearer stars. The method is simple (Fig. 1-13). The position of a star is determined twice, at times 6 months apart. From the measured change in the angle of the telescope, together with the fact that the telescope was moved by the 300-million-km diameter of the earth's orbit during the 6 months, the distance to the star can be calculated.

The **parallax,** as this apparent shift in position is called, is large enough to be measurable only for a few thousand of the nearer stars. The parallax of the closest star is equivalent to the diameter of a dime seen from a distance of 6 km. The distance from the earth to this star, Proxima Centauri, is about 4×10^{16} m.

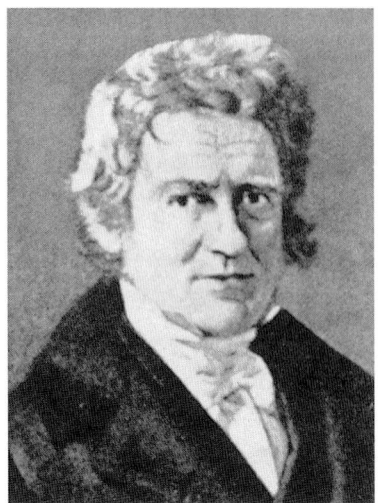

Figure 18-15   Friedrich Bessel (1784–1840).

Light-Year   A unit sometimes used to express stellar distances is the **light-year,** which is the distance light travels in a year and is equal to 9.46×10^{12} km. Thus Proxima Centauri is a little over 4 light-years away—which means that we see the star not as it is today but as it was 4 years ago. Only about 40 stars are within 16 light-years of the solar system. Such distances between stars are typical for much of the visible universe. Space is almost completely empty, far more empty even than the solar system with its tiny isolated planets.

Apparent and Intrinsic Brightnesses   Parallax measurements are possible only for distances up to about 300 light-years. However, several indirect methods are available to find the distances of stars farther away than this. A very useful one is based on a comparison of the apparent and intrinsic brightnesses of stars.

The **apparent brightness** of a star is its brightness as we see it from the earth. This quantity expresses the amount of light that reaches us from the star. Its **intrinsic brightness,** on the other hand, is the true brightness of the star, a figure that depends upon the total amount of light it radiates into space.

The apparent brightness of a star depends on two things: its intrinsic brightness and its distance from us. A star that is actually very bright may appear faint because it is far away, and a star that is actually faint may have a high apparent brightness because it is close.

If both the apparent and the intrinsic brightness of a star are known, we can calculate its distance by finding out how far away an object with this intrinsic brightness must be located in order to send us the amount of light we observe. Such a calculation is not hard, and so we can find the distance to any star whose intrinsic brightness can be established.

A way to find the intrinsic brightness of a star was discovered by the American astronomer Walter Adams (Fig. 18-16). Studying the spectra of the nearer stars, for which intrinsic brightnesses are known, Adams observed that the spectra of stars with high intrinsic brightness showed certain relationships among the strengths of their lines. The spectra of stars with low intrinsic brightness showed somewhat different relationships.

Adams thus could establish the intrinsic brightness of a star simply by looking at its spectrum. Assuming that the relationship holds for more distant stars, Adams then was able to use their spectra to find their intrinsic brightnesses and hence their distances. With this method stellar distances have been determined up to several thousand light-years.

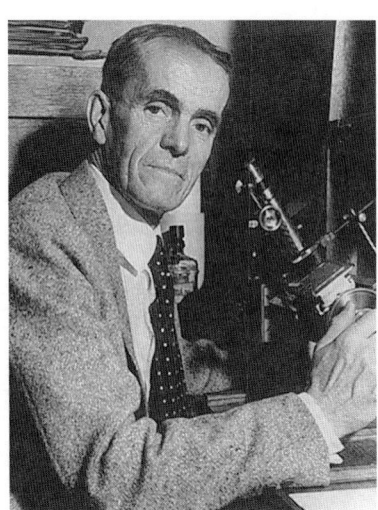

Figure 18-16   Walter Adams (1876–1956).

18.9 Variable Stars

Stars Whose Brightness Changes, Usually in Regular Cycles

An extension of the brightness method for finding stellar distances is based upon the properties of a certain type of **variable star.** A variable star is one whose brightness varies continually (Fig. 18-17). Some variables show wholly irregular fluctuations, but most repeat a fairly definite cycle of change.

A typical variable grows brighter for a time, then fainter, then brighter once more, with irregular minor fluctuations during the cycle. Cycles range in length all the way from a few hours to several years. Maximum brightness for some variables is only slightly greater than minimum brightness, but for others it is several hundred times as great. Since the sun's radiation changes slightly during the sunspot cycle, we may think of it as a variable star with a very small range in brightness (a few percent at most) and a long period (11 years).

The light changes in some variable stars are easy to explain. These stars are actually double stars whose orbits we see edgewise, so that one member of each pair periodically gets in the way of the other. In other variables the appearance of numerous spots at regular intervals may be what is dimming their light. Still others seem to be pulsating, swelling and shrinking so that their surface areas change periodically. Perhaps the irregular variables are passing through or behind ragged clouds of gas and dust that absorb some of their light.

Cepheid Variables   A particular class of variable stars, called **Cepheid variables,** helps astronomers find out how far from us distant star groups that contain them are. Cepheid variables are bright yellow stars 5 to 10 times as massive as the sun that are in advanced stages of their lives; they are not very common. Their name comes from a typical example discovered in 1784 in the constellation Cepheus. Polaris, the North Star, is a Cepheid variable whose brightness varies by 10 percent with a period of 4 days.

Early in this century the American astronomer Henrietta Leavitt happened to be studying the Cepheid variables in a nearby galaxy called the Small Magellanic Cloud. She noticed that the brighter a Cepheid was, the longer its cycle took. Since all the stars in this galaxy are very nearly the same distance from the earth, Leavitt concluded that the average intrinsic brightness of a Cepheid anywhere in the sky can be found just by measuring its period. Comparing this calculated intrinsic brightness with the Cepheid's apparent brightness then gives its distance, as we know. This method can be used for greater distances than spectroscopic determinations because the period of a Cepheid can be determined even when it is very faint; the present record is 49 million light-years.

Unfortunately the individual stars in really distant galaxies appear smeared together, even in the largest telescopes, so the Cepheids they may

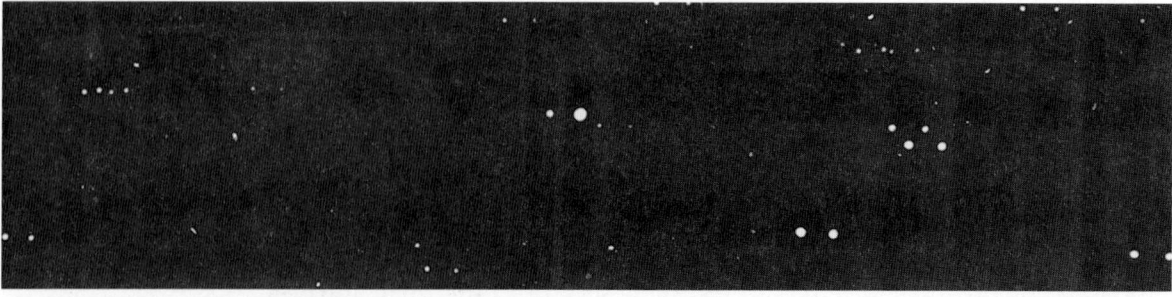

Figure 18-17   Superimposed and offset photographs taken at different times of the region of the sky in which the variable star WW Cygni appears. Only the brightness of this star has changed.

| Henrietta Leavitt (1868–1921)

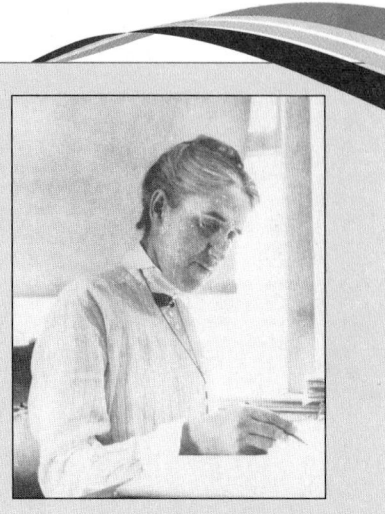

Leavitt was born in Massachusetts and studied astronomy at Radcliffe College. She then joined the Harvard College Observatory, initially as a volunteer, where she helped compile a photographic library of stars visible through the telescopes of the time. Perhaps her exceptional visual acuity arose as compensation for her deafness.

In 1907, while classifying the stars in this immense collection, Leavitt discovered that the average intrinsic brightness of a Cepheid variable is related to the period of its fluctuations. A bright Cepheid might take a month or two for each cycle, a faint Cepheid only a few days. Using Leavitt's finding, Harlow Shapley, who was then working at the Mt. Wilson Observatory in California, calibrated a distance scale based on Cepheid variables several years later.

Shapley used the new cosmic yardstick to find the size of the Milky Way galaxy, the location of the sun relative to its center, and the distances to other galaxies. The Cepheid technique has ever since been an essential tool in astronomy; Edwin Hubble (see Sec. 19.6) used Cepheid data in his discovery that the universe is expanding.

---

contain cannot be picked out for analysis. More recently other methods have been developed for finding how far away such galaxies are. One method is based on the observation that the faster a galaxy rotates, the greater its intrinsic brightness. Nearby galaxies whose distances are known from the Cepheids in them are used to calibrate the rotation-brightness relationship.

18.10 Stellar Motions

The Stars Are Not Fixed in Space

As mentioned earlier, the speeds of stars that move toward or away from the earth can be found from the doppler shifts in their spectral lines. Motion across the line of sight can be followed by direct observation. The great distances of the stars make their apparent movements so slow that it is easy to think of them as being fixed in space. Nevertheless most stars are moving at speeds of several km per second relative to the earth (Fig. 18-18).

What about the sun? If the sun is moving toward a certain part of the sky, stars in that direction, on the average, should appear to be approaching us and to be spreading apart, just as trees in a forest seem to approach and spread apart when we drive toward them. Average stellar motions of this sort are indeed found near the constellation Cygnus, and in the opposite part of the sky stars are apparently receding and coming closer together. A study of these motions indicates that the sun and its family of planets are moving toward Cygnus at a speed of 200 to 300 km/s.

18.11 Stellar Properties

Mass, Temperature, and Size

We now turn to the properties of the stars. Many different types of stars are known, most of which fit into a pattern that can be understood in terms of a regular evolutionary sequence. Some stars, however, are still puzzles to the astronomer.

Mass The points of light that appear to the eye as single stars are often actually double, two stars close together. The members of such a star pair attract

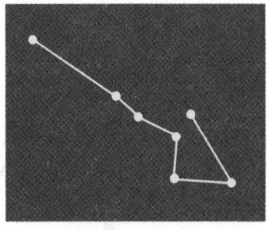

(a)

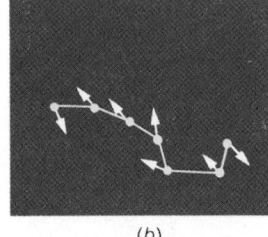

(b)

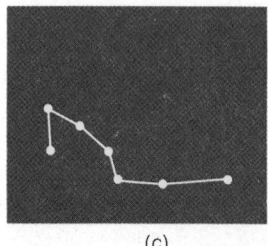

(c)

Figure 18-18 The Big Dipper (a) as it was 200,000 years ago, (b) as it is today (arrows show directions of motion of the stars), and (c) as it will be 200,000 years from now.

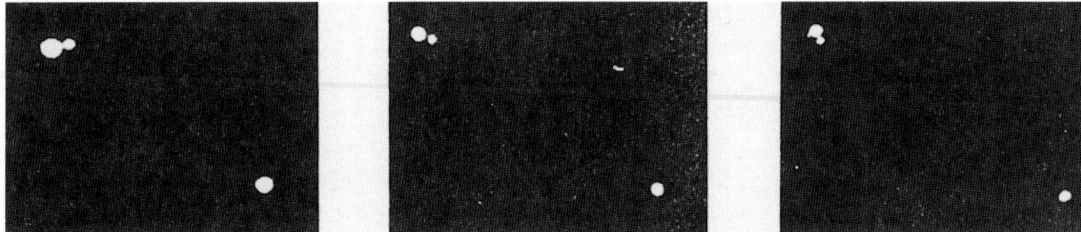

Figure 18-19   The binary star system shown here makes a complete rotation every 50 years.

each other gravitationally, and each circles around the other (Fig. 18-19). From the characteristics of the orbits the masses of the stars can be calculated. Although this method is limited to such **binary stars,** they are common and stars of all kinds are found as members of such pairs. Three-star systems are also known; an example is Polaris, the North Star.

What the measurements show is that stellar masses range from $\frac{1}{40}$ to 150 times that of the sun—a smaller variation than planetary masses. It is not hard to see why normal stars should be limited in mass. In a body whose mass is smaller than a certain limit, gravity cannot squeeze its matter sufficiently to produce the temperatures needed for nuclear fusion reactions. At the other extreme, a very heavy star would become so hot due to speeded-up nuclear reactions that gravity could not keep it together against the resulting outward pressure.

Temperature   The temperature of a star is determined by finding the part of its spectrum in which the radiation is most intense (Fig. 18-4). This tells us the temperature of the star's surface—the photosphere from which radiation is emitted.

The surface temperatures of a few very hot stars range up to 40,000 K, but the great majority are between 3000 and 12,000 K. Probably many stars are cooler than 3000 K, which is near the boiling point of iron. However, unless they are relatively close to the earth, their radiation is then too feeble for us to detect. Like the sun, other stars must have enormously high internal temperatures to maintain their surface radiation. As mentioned earlier, the hottest stars are blue-white, those of intermediate temperature are orange-yellow, and the coolest are red.

Size   If we know a star's surface temperature and its intrinsic brightness, we can find its size. The temperature tells us how much radiation is emitted from each square meter of the star's surface: the hotter it is, the more intense the radiation given off. The intrinsic brightness is a measure of the total radiation from the star's entire surface. We need only divide the total radiation by the radiation per square meter to find the number of square meters in the star's surface, and from this area the diameter and volume can be calculated.

There is also a more direct method of measuring stellar diameters based on the interference of light that can be used on the larger stars. Results obtained in this way agree with estimates from temperatures and intrinsic brightness.

The diameters of stars, unlike their masses, have an enormous range (Fig. 18-20). The smallest stars, composed almost entirely of neutrons, are only about 10 to 15 km across. The largest, like the giant red star Antares in the constellation Scorpio, have diameters over 500 times that of the sun. Antares is so huge that, if the sun were placed at its center, the four inner planets could pursue their normal orbits inside the star with plenty of room to spare.

Giant stars like Antares have densities less than one-thousandth that of ordinary air—densities that correspond to a fairly good vacuum here on earth.

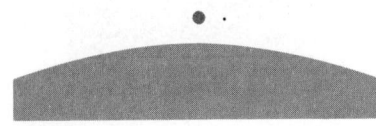

Figure 18-20   The range of stellar sizes, from Antares (at the bottom) through the sun to a large white dwarf (black dot). Neutron stars are even smaller.

Life Histories of the Stars

Looking around us, we see human beings who seem quite different from one another: babies, children, young men and women, the middle-aged, the old. If we had just arrived from another world, we might think these kinds of people are all different species, not individuals of the same kind in different stages of development. Because stars have such long lives, it is easy for us to make the same mistake and think of them as belonging to separate categories. In fact, stars, like people, are born, mature, grow old, and die, so that the various kinds of stars we see fit into regular patterns of evolution.

18.12   H-R Diagram

Most Stars Belong to the Main Sequence

A century ago two astronomers, Ejnar Hertzsprung (Fig. 18-21) in Denmark and Henry Norris Russell (Fig. 18-22) in America, independently discovered that the intrinsic brightnesses of most stars are related to their temperatures. This relationship is shown in the graph of Fig. 18-23, which is called a **Hertzsprung-Russell (or H-R) diagram.** Each point on this graph represents a particular star.

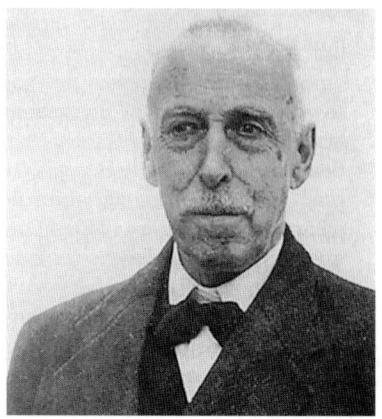

Figure 18-21   Ejnar Hertzsprung (1873–1967).

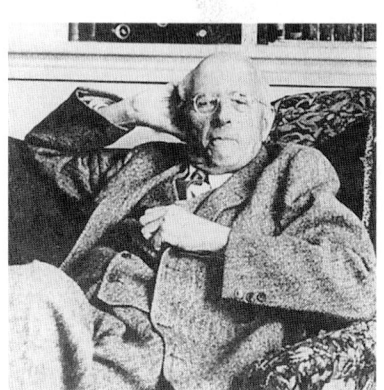

Figure 18-22   Henry Norris Russell (1877–1957).

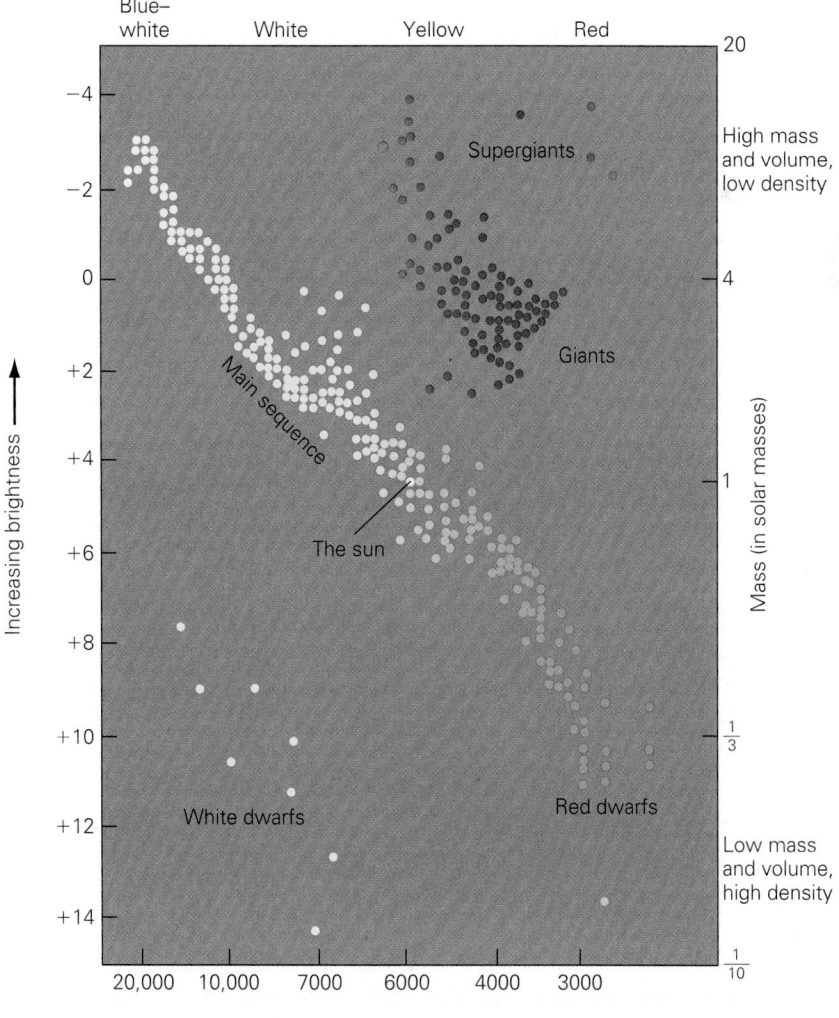

Figure 18-23   The Hertzsprung-Russell diagram plots stars according to temperature and intrinsic brightness. The numbers at the left express absolute magnitude (the astronomical measure of intrinsic brightness) with low numbers indicating bright stars and high numbers, faint stars. Masses at right correspond to main-sequence stars. Star colors are indicated at the top.

About 90 percent of all stars belong to the **main sequence,** with most of the others in the **giant** class at the upper right and in the **white dwarf** class at the lower left. The names giant and dwarf refer, as we might expect, to very large and very small stars respectively. The most abundant stars in the main sequence are the **red dwarfs** at its lower end, all of them too faint to be seen by the naked eye. Seventy percent of the members of our Milky Way galaxy of stars (see Sec. 19.1) are red dwarfs. Proxima Centauri, the nearest star to the sun, is a red dwarf.

The position of a star on the H-R diagram is related to its physical properties. Stars at the upper end of the main sequence are large, hot, massive bodies. Stars at the lower end are small, dense, and reddish, cool enough so that chemical compounds form a considerable part of their atmosphere. In the middle are average stars like our sun, with moderate temperatures, densities, and masses and rather small diameters.

To the giant class belong the huge, diffuse stars like Antares, with low densities and diameters often larger than that of the earth's orbit. Many of these stars have low surface temperatures, as their reddish color indicates, but their enormous surfaces make them very bright.

Example 18.1

A main-sequence star with the same intrinsic brightness as a white dwarf star is much redder than the dwarf. What two things does this observation indicate about these stars?

Solution

The dwarf's color indicates that its temperature is higher than that of the main-sequence star. Because both radiate energy at the same rate, the dwarf must be smaller since a hot object radiates energy at a greater rate per square meter than a cool one.

White Dwarfs   The position of the white dwarfs in the H-R diagram reflects a combination of intensely hot surface and little total radiation. These properties suggest that such stars must be small, in fact comparable in size to the earth. However, their masses are all close to that of the sun, so that the density of a white dwarf is about 10^6 g/cm^3! A pinhead of such matter would weigh nearly a pound here on earth, and a cupful would weigh many tons.

Densities like this seem hard to believe, but they have been checked by enough methods to leave little doubt of their correctness. The only possible explanation is that atoms in these stars have collapsed. Instead of ordinary atoms with electrons relatively far from their nuclei, white dwarfs must have electrons and nuclei packed closely together. Matter in this state does not exist on earth, but its properties can be calculated from theories whose predictions have turned out correct in other situations. The greater the mass of a white dwarf, the smaller its size. The upper limit to the mass of a white dwarf is 1.4 times the sun's mass.

Only a few thousand white dwarfs are known. Their relative scarcity is more apparent than real, since they are so faint that only the nearer ones can be seen even in large telescopes. Enough of them have been found in recent years to suggest that the universe contains great numbers of these remarkable objects. Probably about 10 percent of the stars in the Milky Way are white dwarfs.

18.13   Stellar Evolution

Life History of a Star

The relationships revealed by the H-R diagram cannot have occurred through chance alone. Are the stars in different parts of the diagram perhaps

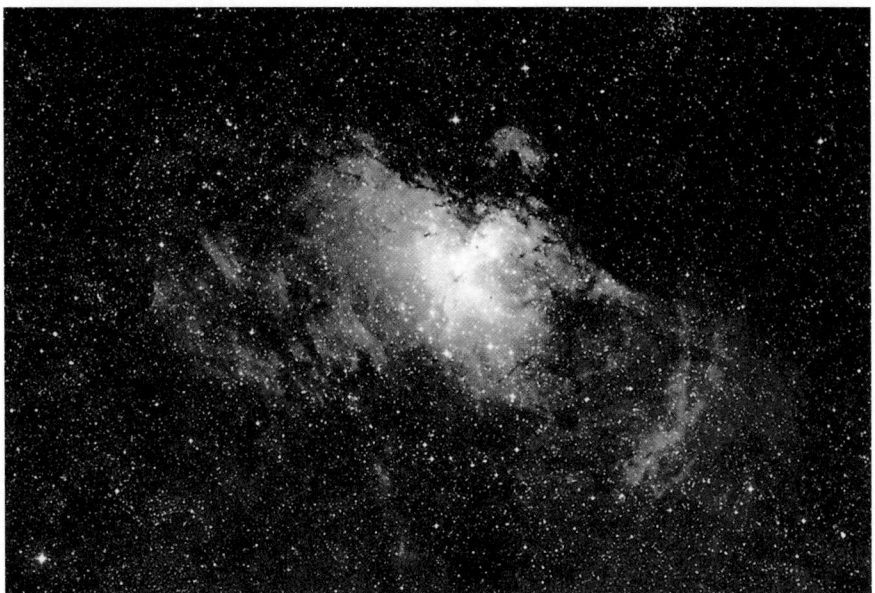

Figure 18-24   Stars form in gas clouds such as this one in the constellation Serpens. Clumps of matter in such a cloud that have a certain minimum mass are compressed by their own gravity to become hot and dense enough for energy-producing nuclear reactions to occur. This is how stars are born. Clumps too small for this to take place remain stillborn as "brown dwarfs"; no one knows how many brown dwarfs are present in the universe.

in various stages of development? Does the mass of a star control its temperature and the composition of its atmosphere? The answers to these questions seem to be yes, and the H-R diagram fits in well with modern ideas of the life history of a star.

Stars are believed to originate in gas clouds in space, clouds that consist largely of hydrogen. If a part of a gas cloud is dense enough, gravity will begin to pull it together into a still denser clump (Fig. 18-24). The contraction heats the clump, much as the gas in a tire pump is heated by compression, and the clump glows as a result. Such an infant star appears among the cooler giants in the H-R diagram.

Some thousands or millions of years later, the star's temperature will rise to the point where the nuclear reactions of Figs. 18-13 and 18-14 begin to occur, which convert its hydrogen into helium. The increase in temperature shifts the position of the star on the H-R diagram downward and to the left. From this time on the star's tendency to contract is opposed by the pressure of its hot interior (Fig. 18-25). Such a star is a stable member of the main sequence and maintains a constant size as long as its hydrogen supply holds out.

A star does not shine for some special reason—it shines because it has a certain mass and a certain composition.

Temperature and Mass   The temperature a star reaches depends on its mass. Gravity in a large mass is more powerful than in a small mass and leads to more intense energy production to balance the resulting inward forces. For stars with abundant hydrogen, calculations show that the relationship between mass and temperature should be exactly that shown by stars in the H-R main sequence. The large, heavy stars at the upper end of the main sequence have high temperatures and shine brightly. The red dwarfs at the lower end are relatively cool and only faintly luminous.

The sun's mass happens to be just right for life on earth, which is one reason why we are here: a mass 20 percent smaller and our planet would be colder than Mars, 20 percent greater and our planet would be hotter than Venus.

A heavy star consumes its hydrogen rapidly, so its lifetime in the main sequence is shorter than that of a less massive star. Accordingly, fewer than 1 percent of main-sequence stars are giants. The supply of hydrogen in a fairly modest star like our sun might last for 10 billion years. Probably the sun is

Outward forces due to
high pressure in   Inward forces
hot interior   due to gravity

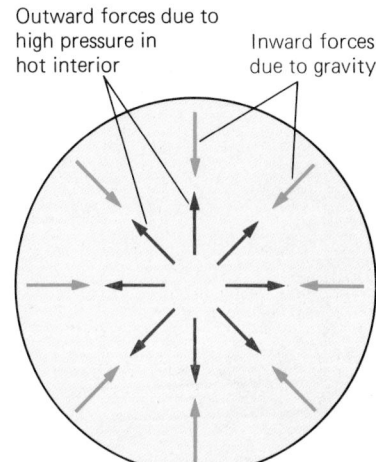

Figure 18-25   The tendency of a star to contract gravitationally is balanced by the tendency of its hot interior to expand.

Brown Dwarfs

Brown dwarfs are lumps of matter between 10 and 75 times the mass of Jupiter that are born in the same way as ordinary stars by condensing under the influence of gravity from clouds of gas. With less mass they would not form lumps in this way, with more mass they would become hot enough to trigger nuclear reactions on a scale that would make them stars. So brown dwarfs are not actually stars, although their contraction (plus some help from a small amount of deuterium fusion in their first few million years, which can occur at a lower temperature than hydrogen fusion) does leave them barely warm enough for their glow to be detectable.

The feeble radiation from a brown dwarf is largely in the infrared part of the spectrum. Brown dwarfs are actually dark red in color, but the name red dwarf had already been given to true stars with less than half the sun's mass—which are a brighter red—by the time brown dwarfs were discovered in 1995. Because they do not generate energy after their initial deuterium is used up, brown dwarfs cool down after coming into being, unlike true stars, which may radiate for billions of years.

Hundreds of brown dwarfs have been identified, and they may well be nearly as common as ordinary stars in our galaxy. The coolest known has a surface temperature of only about 400°C. A brown dwarf has been discovered that has a smaller companion in an orbit about the size of Pluto's.

How do brown dwarfs differ from planets? Of course, all planets orbit stars, but some brown dwarfs do, too. More of a distinction is that planets are richer in heavy elements than their parent stars, unlike brown dwarfs whose composition is that of a typical star.

What really tells brown dwarfs and stars apart is that, when it is first formed, some nuclear reactions (which soon stop) do take place in a brown dwarf, whereas planets do not have the mass needed to become hot enough for any nuclear reactions ever to occur. Once in existence, even though by different routes, there is not a lot to distinguish a really large planet from a really small brown dwarf.

now about halfway through this part of its life cycle. The heaviest stars may stay only as little as 10 million years in the main sequence and the lightest ones, the red dwarfs, may stay a trillion years.

Old Age   When the hydrogen supply at last begins to run low in a star like the sun, the life of the star is by no means over but instead enters its most spectacular phase. Further gravitational contraction makes its core still hotter, and other nuclear reactions become possible—in particular those in which nuclei larger than helium are built up, for instance, the combination of three helium nuclei to form a carbon nucleus. The outer part of the star is heated and expands to as much as 100 times its former diameter. The expansion produces a cooling so that the result is a giant cool star (Fig. 18-26). The shift from the main sequence to the upper right of the H-R diagram is relatively rapid. Energy is now being poured out at a great rate, so the star's life as a giant is much shorter than its stay in the main sequence.

Eventually the new energy-producing reactions run out of fuel too, and again the star shrinks, this time all the way down to the white dwarf state. A shell of gas from the outer part of the star goes out into space to form a bubblelike **planetary nebula** like that shown in Fig. 18-27. (Nebula is Latin

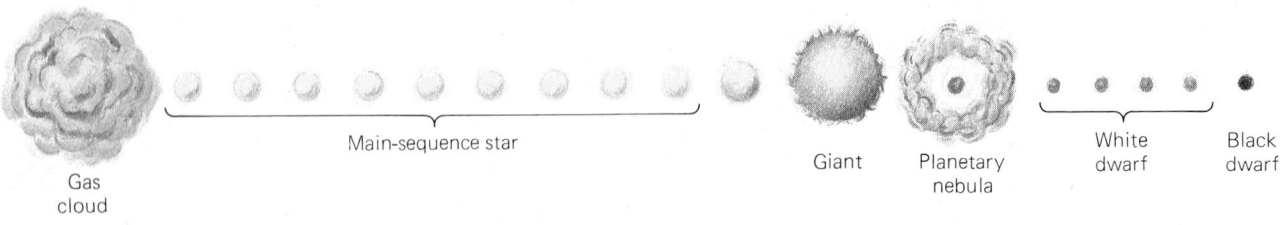

Figure 18-26   Life history of a star whose mass is near that of the sun. The sun is now about halfway through its estimated lifetime of 10 billion years. A planetary nebula contains roughly a third of the original star's mass.

for "cloud.") As a slowly contracting dwarf the star may glow for billions of years more with its energy now coming from the contraction, from nuclear reactions that involve elements heavier than helium, and from proton-proton reactions in a very diffuse outer atmosphere of hydrogen. Ultimately the star will grow dim and in time cease to radiate at all. It will now be a **black dwarf,** a lifeless lump of matter. The universe is not thought to be old enough for any white dwarfs to have become black dwarfs as yet.

18.14   Supernovas

Exploding Stars

A heavy star—perhaps 9 to 25 times the sun's mass—toward the upper end of the main sequence has a rather different later history.

A star like this does not proceed in the usual way from giant to white dwarf. Instead, after a relatively short lifetime of some millions of years, the star's great mass causes it to collapse abruptly when its fuel has run out and then to explode violently. The explosion, which takes less than a second, flings into space much of the star's mass. Such an event, which appears as one kind of **supernova,** is billions of times brighter than the original star ever was (Fig. 18-28). Nuclear reactions during the explosion create the heaviest elements which, together with the other elements formed during the earlier part of the star's life, are flung into space.

Another kind of supernova, equally bright but less common, can occur in a binary system one of whose members is a white dwarf. Over time the dwarf gravitationally attracts gas from the other star. If the accumulated material brings the mass of the dwarf to 1.4 solar masses, the upper limit for a white dwarf to be stable, it collapses, which can trigger runaway fusion reactions in its carbon and oxygen content. What happens is a thermonuclear explosion that appears in the sky as a supernova. Whether such a system becomes a supernova depends on how fast matter accumulates on the dwarf: too slowly and not enough piles up, too rapidly and a feeble premature explosion is the result.

A supernova of either type may briefly outshine the entire galaxy to which it belongs. In a galaxy like ours about two supernovas normally occur every century, but by chance or for some unknown reason there have only been four—in 1006, 1054, 1572, and 1604—in our Milky Way galaxy in the past thousand years. A number of large stars in the Milky Way seem to be

The Future of the Sun

For the sun, the star in which we have the most personal interest, we can expect about a billion more years of warming as the sun's temperature gradually increases. Life on earth will ultimately become impossible—not, as was once thought, because the sun will cool off but rather because it will grow too hot. In about 7.6 billion years, the sun will expand to reach its maximum size as a giant larger across than the earth's current orbit. Later, its fuel gone, the sun will collapse into a white dwarf as its outer layers stream off as a planetary nebula (Fig. 18-27).

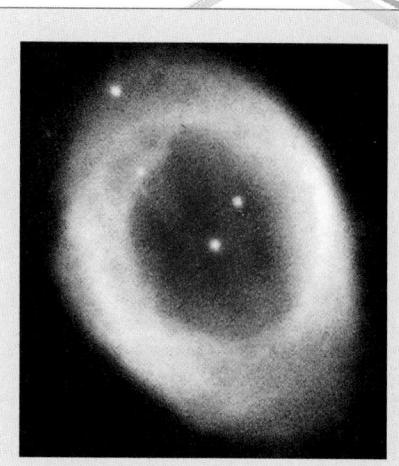

Figure 18-27   This planetary nebula in Lyra is a shell of gas moving outward from the star in the center, which is in the process of becoming a white dwarf. For a few thousand years this dying star is bright enough to heat the gas cloud so that it glows, but eventually the nebula will fade out and disappear into space. Not all planetary nebulas are spherical; some are egg-shaped, some have hourglass forms or appear as jets, still others are irregular.

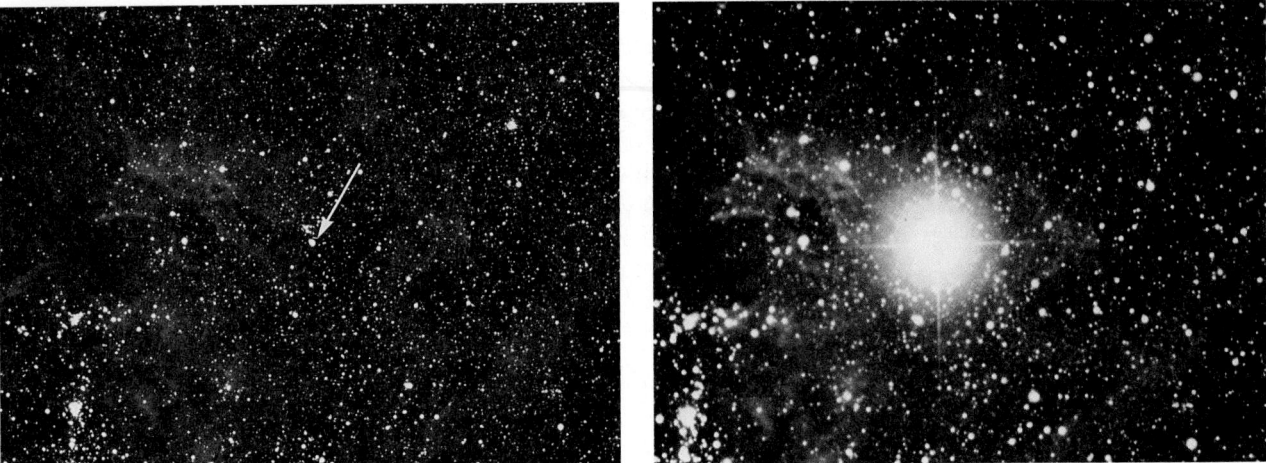

Figure 18-28   The explosion of this supernova in a nearby galaxy was detected on February 24, 1987. The arrow in the photograph at left indicates the star that became the supernova in the photograph at right. On the day before, a burst of neutrinos was recorded that corresponded to the emission of 10^{58} neutrinos from nuclear reactions in the core of the star as it collapsed.

candidates to become supernovas in the future; one of them is Betelgeuse (Fig. 1-4) and another is Antares (Fig. 18-20), both giants.

Neutron Stars   What is left after a supernova explosion is a dwarf star of extraordinary density. Its mass is typically about that of the sun but its diameter is only 10–15 km, the size of a city. The matter of such a star weighs billions of tons per teaspoonful. If the earth were this dense, it would fit into a large apartment house. Under the pressures inside such a star, the most stable form of matter is the neutron. Once the notion of **neutron stars** was purely speculative, but over a thousand have been identified thus far. Figure 18-29 shows the life history of a heavy star, and Fig. 18-30 shows how neutron stars and white dwarfs compare in size with the earth and the sun. Neutron stars range in mass from 1.4 up to about 2.7 times the sun's mass.

18.15   Pulsars

Spinning Neutron Stars

In 1967 unusual radio signals were picked up that came from a source in the direction of the constellation Vulpecula. They were found through meticulous work by Jocelyn Bell (now Jocelyn Bell Burnell; Fig. 18-31), at the time a graduate student at Cambridge University in England; her thesis advisor received a Nobel Prize for the discovery and for other research

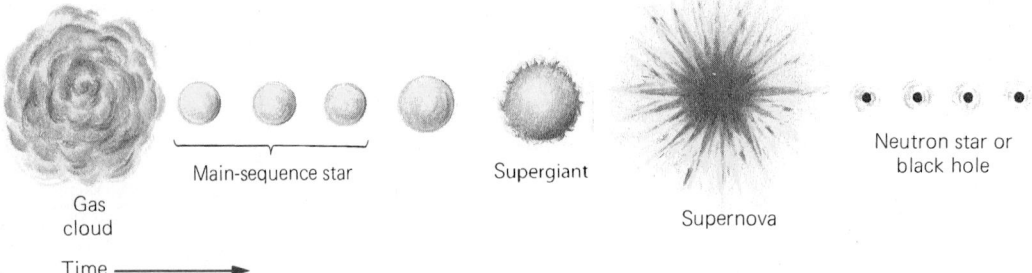

Gas cloud   Main-sequence star   Supergiant   Supernova   Neutron star or black hole

Time ⟶

Figure 18-29   Life history of a star much heavier than the sun. Such a star spends less time in the main sequence than the star of Fig. 18-26. An example of a supergiant is Betelgeuse in the constellation Orion (see Fig. 1-4), which is farther across than the earth's orbit. In less than a million years Betelgeuse will have used up all its nuclear fuel supply and, after a sudden collapse, will explode into a supernova that will briefly rival the moon in brightness in the sky.

in radioastronomy. The signals fluctuated with an extremely regular period, exactly 1.33730113 s. Since then over a thousand **pulsars** have been discovered with periods between 0.001 and 4 s. At first only radio emissions from pulsars were observed. Later, however, flashes of visible light were detected from several pulsars that were exactly synchronized with the radio signals.

The power output of a pulsar is about 10^{26} W, which is comparable with the total power output of the sun. So strong a source of energy cannot possibly be switched on and off in a fraction of a second. Instead it seems likely that pulsars are neutron stars that are spinning rapidly. Conceivably a pulsar has a strong magnetic field whose axis is at an angle to the axis of rotation, and this field traps tails of ionized gases that do the actual radiating.

Whatever the mechanism, though, a pulsar is apparently like a lighthouse whose flashes are due to a rotating beam of light. The identification of pulsars with neutron stars is supported by evidence that the periods of pulsars are very gradually decreasing, which would be expected as they continue to lose energy (Fig. 18-32).

About a dozen neutron stars, called **magnetars,** have been found with enormously strong magnetic fields, so strong that if one came closer to us than the moon, it might erase the data from every swipe card on earth.

The closest known pulsar is 280 light-years away. It is very dim, which suggests that there may be many—half a million?—other dim pulsars in our galaxy that are too faint to be seen because they are farther away.

18.16   Black Holes

Even Light Cannot Escape from Them

Does a neutron star represent the ultimate in compression? Apparently not. After it becomes a supernova, a very heavy star—25 to 40 times the sun's mass—leaves behind a remnant too massive to be stable as a neutron star. The remnant continues to contract until it is only a few km across. Such an object is called a **black hole** for a most interesting reason.

As we learned in Chap. 3, one of the results of Einstein's general theory of relativity is that light is affected by gravity. Thus starlight passing near the sun is bent by a small but measurable extent.

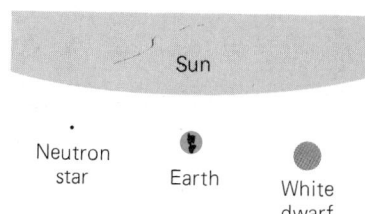

Figure 18-30   A comparison of a white dwarf and a neutron star with the sun and the earth.

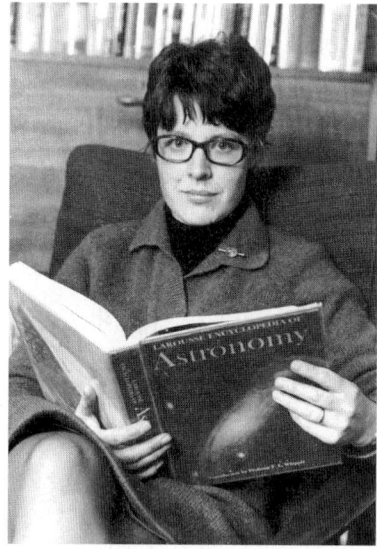

Figure 18-31   Jocelyn Bell Burnell (1943–).

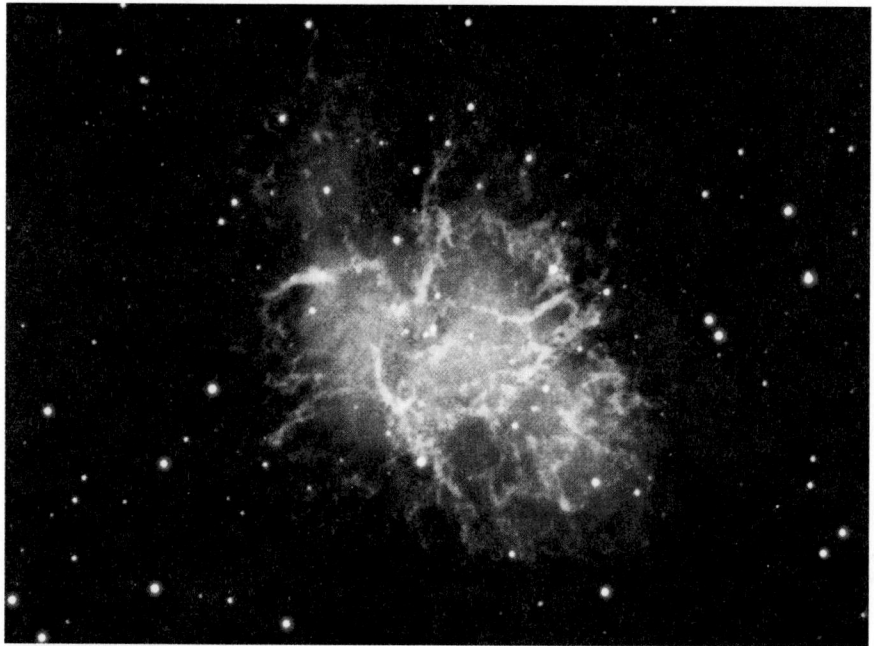

Figure 18-32   This wispy object in space, called the Crab Nebula, has a pulsar at its heart. The nebula is the remnant of a supernova that was seen in A.D. 1054 and was visible in daylight. It has been expanding rapidly and glowing brightly ever since and is now 6 light-years across. The light and radio flashes from the Crab pulsar seem powerful enough to furnish the entire nebula with its energy. This pulsar flashes 30 times per second and is slowing down rapidly—1 part in 2400 per year. Both these observations are in accord with the time of its formation. A pulsar's lifetime is believed to be about 10 million years before it comes to a stop.

The more massive a star and the smaller it is, the stronger the pull of gravity at its surface and the higher the escape speed needed for something to leave the star. In the case of the earth, the escape speed is 11.2 km/s. In the case of the sun, 617 km/s. If the ratio M/R between the mass and radius of a star is large enough, the escape speed is more than the speed of light, and nothing, not even light, can ever get out (Fig. 18-33). The star cannot radiate and so is invisible, a black hole in space. Only very heavy stars end up as black holes; lighter ones eventually become white dwarfs (as in the case of the sun) or neutron stars.

Although anything passing close to a black hole will be gobbled up, never to return to the outside world, farther away the gravitational field of a black hole is the same as that of a star of the same mass. If the sun were to shrivel into a black hole (it is not nearly massive enough to do so), it would be 6 km across and the orbits of the planets would be unchanged. A black hole with the earth's mass would be the size of a grape.

Remarkably enough the concept of black holes was proposed as long ago as 1783 by John Mitchell in England, who called such an object a dark star. Not until the verification of Einstein's 1915 general theory of relativity (Sec. 3.13) was it established that light is indeed affected by gravity, however, so Mitchell's idea lay fallow until then.

Detecting Black Holes   Since it is invisible, how can a black hole be detected? A black hole that is a member of a binary system (such double stars are quite common) will reveal its presence by its gravitational pull on the other star. In addition, the intense gravitational field of the black hole will suck matter from the other star, which will be compressed and heated before it falls inside to such high temperatures that x-rays will be emitted profusely (Fig. 18-34). When a binary system is discovered by the orbital motion of a star whose partner is invisible and x-rays are streaming out, the inference is that the partner is a black hole.

One of a number of invisible objects that astronomers believe on this basis to be black holes is known as Cygnus X-1, which is about 8000 light-years away. Its mass is 8.7 times that of the sun, and its radius may be only about 10 km. Enormous black holes whose masses are millions of times the solar mass are believed to be at the centers of galaxies of stars, as discussed in the next chapter.

Figure 18-33 As the core of an old heavy star collapses, light that does not come out perpendicular to its surface is bent more and more strongly until it returns to the core. Finally, no light at all, regardless of direction, can leave the shrunken core, which is now a black hole.

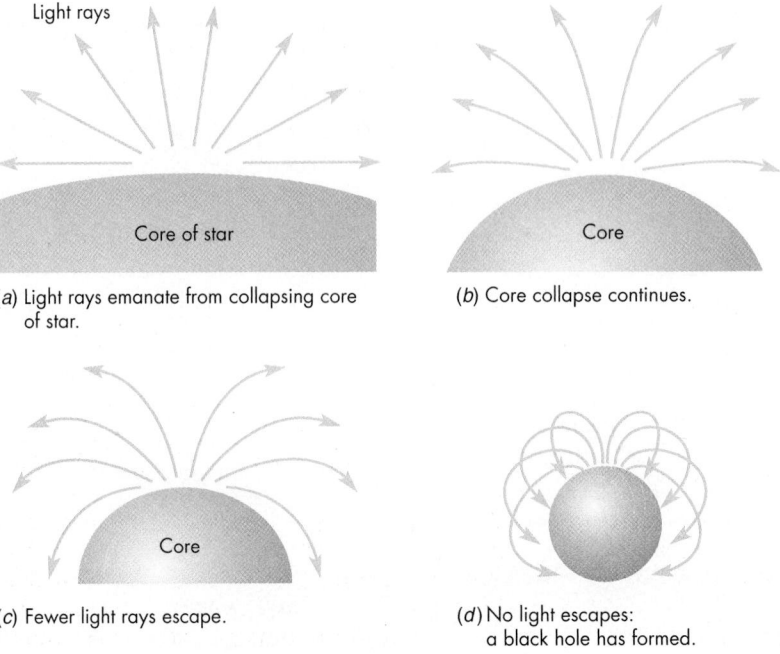

Light rays

(a) Light rays emanate from collapsing core of star.

(b) Core collapse continues.

(c) Fewer light rays escape.

(d) No light escapes: a black hole has formed.

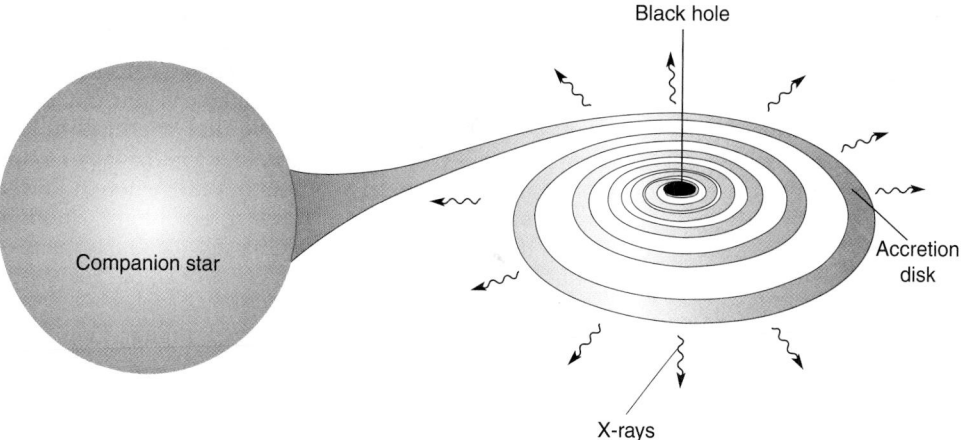

Figure 18-34   When matter from a companion star is pulled toward a black hole, it swirls into a spiral called an accretion disk on its way to being swallowed by the hole. Their compression heats the gases in the disk until they are hot enough to radiate x-rays.

Gamma-Ray Bursts

Every now and then short, intense bursts of gamma rays from space are detected by instruments at high altitudes and in satellites. There seem to be two possible explanations. One links the gamma-ray burst to the final convulsion of a **hypernova,** a super-supernova in which a star with more than 40 times the sun's mass collapses when its fuel is used up and then explodes so violently that neither a neutron star nor a black hole is left behind, as happens with less massive supernovas.

In 2006 one such cosmic blast was observed when a distant star 150 times the sun's mass blew up and released a hundred times the energy of an ordinary supernova. Another monster star, called Eta Carinae and possibly the most massive star in our Milky Way galaxy, is only 7500 light-years away and is showing signs of instability.

The other possibility is the capture of a neutron star by a black hole, perhaps its partner in a binary system. In this case the burst would be very quick, less than 2 s in duration. In either case as much or more energy could be released as the sun gives off in its entire lifespan.

All the bursts thus far recorded came from distant galaxies and their energy was harmlessly absorbed in the atmosphere. But a hypernova within our galaxy, like Eta Carinae at some time in the future, might not let us off so easily.

A flood of gamma rays that comes from nearby would still be mostly taken up in the atmosphere, but now the disruption of its oxygen and nitrogen molecules would occur on a much larger scale. In particular, there would be a lot of NO_2, a toxic component of smog that is brown and would darken the sky for as long as a year. The NO_2 would also destroy the ozone layer and thus allow harmful solar ultraviolet radiation to reach the earth's surface. Both effects would severely stress living things and might even lead to a mass biological extinction.

In fact, the extinction that marked the end of the Ordovician Period (see Fig. 16-35) has characteristics that suggest a possible origin in such an event.

Important Terms and Ideas

A star's **spectrum** contains dark lines that correspond to particular frequencies of light absorbed by the ions, atoms, and molecules in the atmosphere around the star. These lines are superimposed on a bright background emitted by the star's surface. The spectrum and the background can be analyzed to provide information on the structure, temperature, composition, condition of matter, magnetism, and motion of the star.

The **sun** is a typical star whose temperature is 5800 K at the surface and perhaps 14 million K near the center. **Solar energy** comes from the conversion of hydrogen to helium, which can take place through both the **proton-proton** and **carbon cycles.** The **photosphere** is the thin outer layer from which comes most of the light the sun radiates. **Sunspots** are regions slightly cooler than the rest of the solar surface and have strong magnetic fields associated with them. Surrounding the sun is a diffuse **corona** of ions and electrons whose outward flow is the **solar wind** that extends through much of the solar system.

Auroras result from the excitation of gases in the earth's upper atmosphere by streams of protons and electrons from the sun.

The distance to a nearby star can be found from its apparent shift in position, or **parallax,** as the earth moves in its orbit. The distance to a star far away can be found by comparing its **intrinsic** and **apparent brightnesses,** which are its actual brightness and its brightness as seen from the earth. Stellar distances are often expressed in **light-years,** where a light-year is the distance light travels in a year.

Variable stars fluctuate continually in brightness. Notable are the **Cepheid variables,** whose intrinsic brightness and periods of variation are related, which permits their distances to be found. Other variable stars are actually pairs of stars that revolve about their common centers of gravity and periodically block each other's light.

The **Hertzsprung-Russell (H-R)** diagram is a graph on which the intrinsic brightnesses of stars are plotted versus their temperatures. Most stars belong to the **main sequence,** which appears as a diagonal band on the diagram, but there are also cool, large, **giant** stars and hot,

small, **white dwarfs** that lie outside the main sequence. Heavy stars eventually explode into **supernovas** and later subside into **neutron stars** whose interiors consist entirely of neutrons. A **pulsar** is a spinning neutron star that emits flashes of light and radio waves. One kind of a **black hole** is the collapsed core of an old heavy star that has contracted so much that its gravitational field is strong enough for the escape speed to be greater than the speed of light. Nothing, not even light, can escape from a black hole. Supermassive black holes lie at the centers of galaxies of stars.

A **brown dwarf** is a spherical lump of matter in space between 10 and 75 times the mass of Jupiter that is not heavy enough to trigger the nuclear reactions of a true star. It glows dark red because of heat left over from its gravitational contraction.

A **gamma-ray burst** is a brief but intense flood of gamma rays that reaches the earth from space. Suggested origins are an exceptionally powerful supernova explosion or the capture of a neutron star by a black hole.

Multiple Choice

1. As compared with a large telescope mirror, a large telescope lens
   a. is easier to support against sag
   b. does not disperse light
   c. can provide higher magnification
   d. has no advantages

2. Most stars have hot interiors surrounded by relatively cool atmospheres. The spectrum of such a star consists of
   a. white lines against a dark background
   b. colored lines against a dark background
   c. dark lines against a white background
   d. dark lines against a colored background

3. The examination of starlight with a spectrometer cannot provide information about an isolated star's
   a. temperature   c. mass
   b. structure   d. magnetic field

4. The light the sun emits comes from
   a. its interior
   b. a thin gas layer at its surface
   c. a thin liquid layer at its surface
   d. a thin solid layer at its surface

5. The surface temperature of the sun is approximately
   a. 600 K   c. 6 million K
   b. 6000 K   d. 14 million K

6. The sun's atmosphere
   a. extends out into the solar system
   b. consists mainly of oxygen and nitrogen
   c. consists of burning hydrogen
   d. is relatively cool

7. Auroras are caused by
   a. streams of colored gases from the sun
   b. streams of charged particles from the sun
   c. comets
   d. micrometeorites

8. Auroras occur mainly in the polar regions because of the effect of
   a. the moon
   b. low temperatures there
   c. the geomagnetic field
   d. the earth's equatorial bulge

9. The solar wind
   a. blows over the sun's surface
   b. consists of photons streaming from the sun
   c. consists of ions streaming from the sun
   d. consists of hydrogen atoms streaming from the sun

10. Sunspots are
    a. dark clouds in the sun's atmosphere
    b. regions somewhat cooler than the rest of the sun's surface
    c. regions somewhat hotter than the rest of the sun's surface
    d. of unknown nature

11. The number of sunspots
    a. remains approximately constant
    b. increases and decreases at random intervals
    c. increases and decreases in a yearly cycle
    d. increases and decreases in an 11-year cycle

12. Solar storms may affect which one(s) of these?
    a. the earth's magnetic field
    b. electric transmission lines
    c. shortwave radio reception
    d. satellite electronics

13. The temperature of the sun's interior is believed to be about
    a. 600 K
    b. 6000 K
    c. 14 million K
    d. 14 billion K

14. The sun does not
  a. have a magnetic field
  b. have a solid core
  c. revolve about an axis
  d. consist largely of ions

15. The sun's energy comes from
  a. nuclear fission
  b. radioactivity
  c. the conversion of hydrogen to helium
  d. the conversion of helium to hydrogen

16. Proxima Centauri, the closest star to the sun, is at a distance of about
  a. 4 light-years
  b. 400 light-years
  c. 4 million light-years
  d. 4 billion light-years

17. If we know both the intrinsic and the apparent brightnesses of a star, we can find its
  a. mass   **c.** distance
  b. temperature   **d.** age

18. Stars whose intrinsic brightness and period of variation are related are called
  a. pulsars   **c.** main-sequence stars
  b. Cepheid variables   **d.** giants

19. Binary stars are valuable to astronomers because they permit the determination of stellar
  a. diameters   **c.** masses
  b. distances   **d.** temperatures

20. If we know the surface temperature and intrinsic brightness of a star, we can find its
  a. mass   **c.** age
  b. size   **d.** distance

21. The temperature of a star can be determined from
  a. the wavelength at which its radiation is brightest
  b. the wavelength at which its radiation is dimmest
  c. its apparent brightness
  d. the strength of its magnetic field

22. Variations among stars are least in their
  a. distance from the sun
  b. mass
  c. size
  d. temperature

23. The color of a relatively cool star is
  a. white   **c.** blue
  b. yellow   **d.** red

24. The reason stars more than about 100 times as massive as the sun are not found is that
  a. they would split into double-star systems
  b. they would be black holes from which no light can escape
  c. the gravity of such a star would not hold it together against the pressure produced by nuclear reactions in its interior
  d. the high internal pressures would prevent nuclear reactions from taking place

25. Stars belonging to the main sequence
  a. have the same mass
  b. have the same temperature
  c. radiate at steady rates
  d. fluctuate markedly in brightness

26. Stars at the upper end of the main sequence have
  a. high temperatures and large masses
  b. high temperatures and small masses
  c. low temperatures and large masses
  d. low temperatures and small masses

27. The greater the mass of a main-sequence star, the
  a. younger it is
  b. longer it will remain part of the main sequence
  c. less hydrogen it contains
  d. hotter it is

28. The main sequence on the H-R diagram includes
  a. the sun   **c.** giants
  b. white dwarfs   **d.** pulsars

29. White dwarfs are stars that are
  a. at the beginning of their life cycles
  b. in the middle of their life cycles
  c. at the end of their life cycles
  d. any of these choices are correct

30. A typical white dwarf star is about the size of
  a. a large building   **c.** the earth
  b. the moon   **d.** Jupiter

31. When the hydrogen supply in a typical main-sequence star begins to run out, other nuclear reactions occur and the star becomes a
  a. giant   **c.** supernova
  b. white dwarf   **d.** neutron star

32. A star like the sun eventually becomes a
  a. black hole   **c.** supernova
  b. white dwarf   **d.** neutron star

33. A brown dwarf
  a. has less mass than Jupiter
  b. is a member of the main sequence
  c. is on its way to becoming a black dwarf
  d. was never a true star

34. A star that explodes as a supernova
  a. has a mass much greater than that of the sun
  b. has a mass much smaller than that of the sun
  c. has a mass about equal to that of the sun
  d. may have any mass

35. A supernova explosion may leave behind which one or more of the following?
  a. a black hole   **c.** a pulsar
  b. a neutron star   **d.** a giant

36. The brightest of the following types of stars is a
  a. giant   **c.** supernova
  b. white dwarf   **d.** neutron star

37. The heaviest elements are created in
  a. stellar interiors   **c.** black holes
  b. stellar atmospheres **d.** supernova explosions

38. A pulsar is not
   a. the remnant of a supernova explosion
   b. rotating rapidly
   c. composed largely of neutrons
   d. as large as the earth

39. A "black hole" appears black because
   a. it is too cool to radiate
   b. it is surrounded by an absorbing layer of gas
   c. its gravitational field is too strong to permit light to escape
   d. its magnetic field is too strong to permit light to escape

40. Black holes are remnants of
   a. stars with small masses
   b. stars with large masses
   c. white dwarfs
   d. black dwarfs

Exercises

18.1   The Telescope

1. Why are large telescopes valuable in astronomy?

2. A photograph of a star cluster shows many more stars than can be seen by looking by eye at the cluster through the same telescope. Why is there a difference?

3. Why do stars seem to twinkle?

4. Which astronomical objects that appear as points of light to the unaided eye appear as disks with the help of a telescope?

18.2   The Spectrometer

18.3   Spectrum Analysis

5. Why do you think it is useful to put an astronomical telescope in a satellite?

6. What part of a star is responsible for the dark lines in its spectrum?

7. Suppose a star had a cool interior surrounded by a hot atmosphere. What kind of spectrum would it have?

8. Arrange the following types of stars in order of decreasing surface temperature: yellow stars, blue stars, white stars, red stars.

9. Suppose you examine the spectra of two stars receding from the earth and find that the lines in one are displaced farther toward the red end than those in the other. What conclusion can you draw?

10. A binary star consists of two stars that revolve around each other. Telescopes cannot resolve a binary star into its members, but an astronomer can recognize a binary star from its spectrum. What property of the spectrum is involved?

11. How can the composition of the sun be determined?

12. Helium was discovered in the sun before it was found on the earth (hence its name, which comes from *helios*, the Greek word for "sun"). How can this sequence have come about?

18.4   Properties of the Sun

13. Why is the sun's corona ordinarily not visible? How do we know it exists?

14. The sun's photosphere is at a temperature of 5800 K whereas the temperature of much of the corona exceeds 1,000,000 K. Why is the photosphere rather than the corona the source of most of the sun's radiation?

15. What happens to the radiation emitted underneath the photosphere of the sun?

16. What element is most abundant on the sun? Next most abundant?

18.5   The Aurora

17. Suppose the earth's magnetic field were to disappear. What effect would this have on the aurora?

18.6   Sunspots

18. Why do sunspots appear dark if their temperatures are over 4500 K?

19. What aspect of sunspots changes during a sunspot cycle?

20. Give two methods for determining how fast the sun rotates on its axis. Is the rotation speed the same for the entire sun?

21. Intense auroral activity occurs in the earth's upper atmosphere about 30 h after a solar storm. What is the average speed of the ions emitted during the storm?

18.7   Solar Energy

22. Where are the lighter elements created? The heavier ones?

23. What aspect of the formation of helium from hydrogen results in the evolution of energy?

24. Why are conditions in the interior of a star favorable for nuclear fusion reactions?

25. According to the text, the sun's mass is about 2×10^{30} kg and it loses about 4×10^9 kg per second as its hydrogen is converted into helium. Assuming that the sun has been radiating energy at the same rate as today during the 4.5-billion-year existence of the earth, what percentage of its mass has been lost in this period? What does this imply about the possibility that the intensity of solar radiation has been roughly constant during the life of the earth, as geological evidence suggests?

18.8   Stellar Distances

26. What information can be gained by comparing the intrinsic and apparent brightnesses of a star?

18.9   Variable Stars

27. Explain how the distance to a star cluster that contains Cepheid variables is determined.

18.11   Stellar Properties

28. How are stellar masses determined?

29. Which varies more, the masses of the stars or their sizes?

30. What data are needed to determine a star's average density? How would you expect the density to change from the surface layers to the interior?

31. Which stars do you think have the highest densities? The lowest?

32. A red star and a white star of the same apparent brightness are the same distance from the earth. Which is larger? Why?

33. How is a star's diameter estimated from measurements of temperature and intrinsic brightness?

34. The spectrum of a certain star shows a doppler shift that varies periodically from the red to the blue end of the spectrum. What kind of star is this?

18.12   H-R Diagram

18.13   Stellar Evolution

35. Must a star be spherical?

36. Why are relatively few stars very hot?

37. Is it possible for an object with the mass and composition of the sun to exist without radiating energy?

38. Why is the sun considered to be a star?

39. Why are most stars part of the main sequence on the H-R diagram?

40. Main-sequence stars are supposed to evolve into giants, but relatively few stars lie between the main sequence and the group of giants on the H-R diagram. Why?

41. Why must a star have a certain minimum mass in order to radiate?

42. A giant star is much redder than a main-sequence star of the same intrinsic brightness. How does this observation indicate that the giant star is larger than the main-sequence star?

43. What are the chief characteristics of an average star in the upper left of the H-R diagram? In the lower left? In the upper right? In the middle of the main sequence?

44. Where would a star be located in the main sequence relative to the sun if its mass is 10 times that of the sun? Would it remain in the main sequence for a shorter or longer time than the sun? Would it be cooler or hotter than the sun?

45. Sirius, the brightest star in the sky apart from the sun, is a blue-white star of great intrinsic brightness. (a) What does this suggest about its temperature? (b) About its average density? (c) About its position in the H-R diagram?

46. As a main-sequence star evolves, what happens to its position on the main sequence?

47. Why are there relatively few giant stars in the main sequence?

48. Into what kind of star will the sun eventually evolve?

49. In what part of its life cycle is a white dwarf star?

50. What happens to a very heavy star at the end of its period in the main sequence?

51. After a very long time, a white dwarf will cool down and become a black dwarf. What will the corresponding evolutionary path of the star be on the H-R diagram?

18.14   Supernovas

18.15   Pulsars

52. About how often do supernovas occur in the Milky Way galaxy?

53. What is left behind after a supernova explosion?

54. Which of the following types of star is the smallest? The largest? The most common? Neutron stars, white dwarfs, red dwarfs, black dwarfs.

55. (a) What is the characteristic behavior of a pulsar? (b) What is believed to be its nature? (c) From what does a pulsar originate?

18.16   Black Holes

56. How large are black holes? Can any star evolve into a black hole?

57. What prevents light from escaping from a black hole?

58. How can a black hole be detected even though it cannot be directly observed?

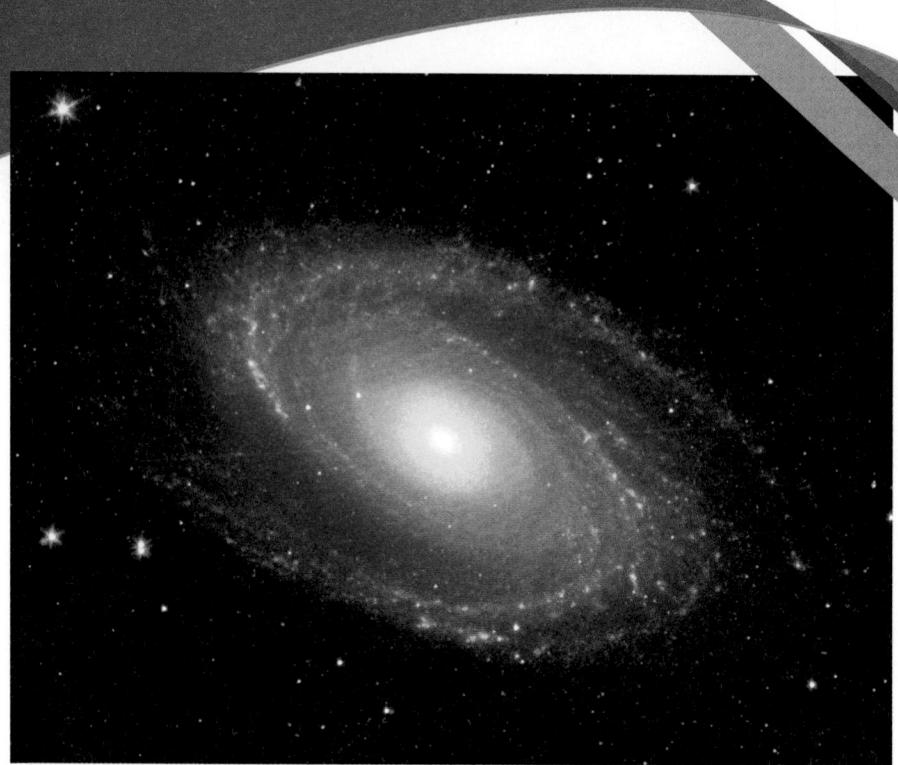

Image of spiral galaxy of stars taken by Spitzer Space Telescope.

The Universe

GOALS

When you have finished this chapter you should be able to complete the goals
- given for each section below:

Galaxies

19.1   The Milky Way
A Spinning Disk of Stars
- Describe the Milky Way galaxy and indicate the sun's location in it.

19.2   Stellar Populations
A Clue to the History of Our Galaxy
- Compare Population I and II stars.

19.3   Radio Astronomy
Another Messenger from the Sky
- Explain what a radio telescope is.
- List the three ways in which radio waves from space are produced.

19.4   Galaxies
Island Universes of Stars
- Discuss the characteristics and distribution in space of galaxies.
- Explain what is meant by dark matter and describe the evidence for its existence.

19.5   Cosmic Rays
Atomic Nuclei Speeding through the Galaxy

- Distinguish between primary and secondary cosmic rays.
- Discuss the significance of cosmic rays in the evolution of the universe.

The Expanding Universe

19.6   Red Shifts
The Galaxies Are All Moving Away from One Another
- Explain what red shifts in galactic spectra indicate about the motions of galaxies.
- State Hubble's law and use it as evidence for the expansion of the universe.

19.7   Quasars
Brilliant, Tiny, and Far Away
- Outline the properties of quasars and what they suggest about the nature of these objects.

Evolution of the Universe

19.8   Dating the Universe
When Did the Big Bang Occur?
- Discuss the big bang theory of the origin of the universe.

19.9   After the Big Bang
A Glimmer of the Early Universe Still Exists

- Identify dark energy and explain why it is believed to exist.
- Outline the chief events after the big bang occurred.
- Explain the significance of the sea of radio waves that fills the universe.
- Discuss the various possibilities for the future of the universe, including the big crunch and the big rip.

19.10 Origin of the Solar System
A Gradual Process
- Outline the origin of the solar system.

Extraterrestrial Life

19.11 Exoplanets
Probably a Great Many
- Give the reasons why other planetary systems are hard to detect.

19.12 Interstellar Travel
Not Now, Probably Not Ever
- Give the reasons why interstellar travel seems impossible.

19.13 Interstellar Communication
Why Not?
- Discuss the likelihoods of interstellar travel and communication.

Stars are not scattered at random throughout the universe but instead occur in immense swarms called **galaxies.** Each galaxy is separated from the others by vast reaches of nearly empty space. The stars of the galaxy to which our sun belongs appear in the sky as the Milky Way; the word *galaxy* comes from the Greek for "milk."

Of the many remarkable properties galaxies have, one stands out: most of them are moving apart from one another, so that the universe as a whole is expanding. If we project this expansion backward, we find that it began 13.7 billion years ago. Can it be that the entire universe was born in a cosmic **big bang** at that time and has been evolving ever since into the galaxies of today? As we shall see in this chapter, several lines of evidence support such a picture, which has been filled out in considerable detail.

Galaxies

A galaxy is a giant archipelago of stars. Just as studying the sun tells us a lot about stars in general, so studying our galaxy, the Milky Way, tells us a lot about galaxies in general.

19.1   The Milky Way

A Spinning Disk of Stars

The great band of misty light we see in the sky on a clear night is called the **Milky Way** and forms a continuous band around the heavens (Fig. 19-1). When we look at it with a telescope, as Galileo was the first to do in 1610, the Milky Way is an unforgettable sight. Instead of a dim glow, we now see countless individual stars, stars as numerous as sand grains on a beach. In other parts of the sky the telescope also reveals stars too faint for the naked eye, but nowhere else that many. Clearly the stars are not distributed evenly in space—a basic observation that implies much about the structure and evolution of the universe.

Structure of the Milky Way   The appearance of the Milky Way tells us something about how the stars in our galaxy are arranged. Most of them are concentrated in a relatively thin disk with the sun near its central plane. When we look toward the rim of the disk, we see a great many stars, so many that they seem to form a continuous band of light. When we look above or below the disk, far fewer stars are to be seen. The disk of stars has a thicker central nucleus, so that it is shaped something like a fried egg with the outer stars concentrated in a number of spiral arms (Fig. 19-2).

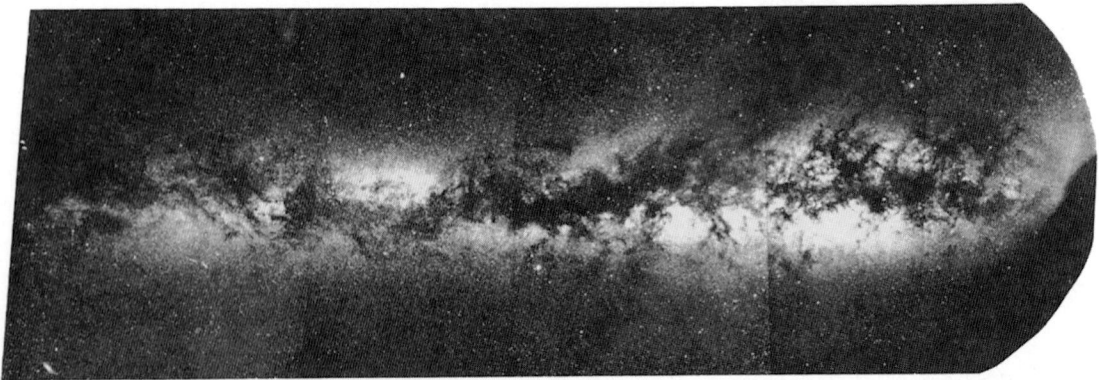

Figure 19-1   A mosaic of several photographs of the Milky Way between the constellations Cassiopeia and Sagittarius.

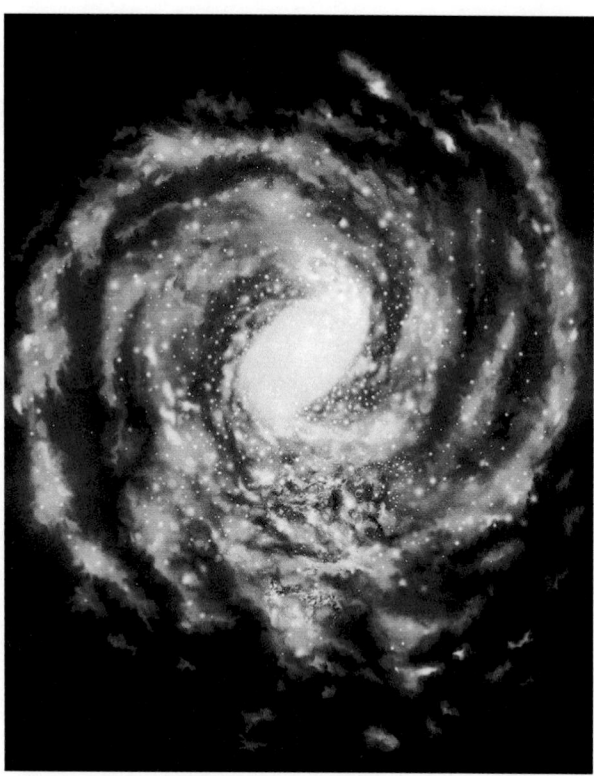

Figure 19-2 Computer simulation of our galaxy. The stars in the disk of the galaxy appear in the night sky as the Milky Way. The galaxy seems to have two main spiral arms in its inner part that branch into four arms farther out. The sun is located in one of the latter arms, in this picture somewhat less than half the radius of the galaxy below its center. A massive black hole at the center of the galaxy holds it together as in the case of all galaxies. Every star we can see as an individual star without using a telescope is part of our galaxy.

The disk of the galaxy is roughly 130,000 light-years in diameter (there is no sharp boundary) and 10,000 light-years thick near the center. It is one of the larger galaxies of the universe with at least 200 billion stars. The sun is about 25,000 light-years from the center, which lies in the direction of the densest part of the Milky Way in the constellation Sagittarius. (For comparison, we are 8 light-minutes from the sun.) The stars of the galaxy are chiefly located in spiral arms that extend from the nucleus.

Surrounded by so many similar bodies, the sun is not unusual in position, size, mass, or temperature. It is not even unusual in possessing a family of planets. There may well be billions of planets in our galaxy, at least some of them probably inhabited by some form of life.

The stars of our galaxy revolve about its center, which is what they must do if the galaxy is not to gradually collapse because of the gravitational attraction of its parts. (The planets do not fall into the sun because of their orbital motion, too.) The orbital speed of the sun and nearby stars around the galactic center is over 200 km/s. At this rate the sun makes a complete circuit once every 240 million years. Since its formation, the sun has revolved 20 times around the galactic center; the galaxy itself has completed at least twice that many turns since coming into being.

Its Heart Is a Black Hole   Clouds of gas and dust surround the center of our galaxy and prevent us from seeing it. However, radio waves, infrared and ultraviolet light, x-rays, and gamma rays from near the center have been detected, and they suggest a monster black hole there that astronomers call Sagittarius A*. Its mass seems to be about 3.7 million times the sun's mass, and it sucks in material blown off by nearby supernova explosions. It is this material, compressed and thereby heated on its way to disappearing into the black hole, that gives off the observed radiations. Despite its giant mass, the black hole's diameter is probably less than 0.2 percent that of Mercury's orbit.

In support of the idea that a black hole is at the center of the Milky Way are the speeds of stars near the center. These stars move so fast that only a

Galactic Nebulas

Galactic nebulas are irregular masses of diffuse material within our galaxy. Some appear as small glowing rings or disks surrounding stars, some take the form of lacy filaments, and many are wholly irregular in outline. The brightest, the Great Nebula in the constellation Orion (Fig. 19-3), is barely visible with the naked eye, but most of them are much fainter. These nebulas consist of gas and dust and shine only because they reflect light from nearby stars or are excited to luminescence by stellar radiation.

Clouds of gas and dust similar to galactic nebulas but without any luminosity sometimes reveal their presence as dark patches that obscure the light of stars beyond them (Fig. 19-4). Such dark nebulas may be fairly abundant but are difficult to find because bright stars shine through them except where they are especially dense.

In fact, our entire galaxy is filled with rarefied nebular material with a density somewhere near one atom or molecule per cubic centimeter. The dark nebulas are only local concentrations of this interstellar matter. Empty space is not nearly as empty as it was once thought to be, but in most places the amount of interstellar material is so small that little starlight is absorbed.

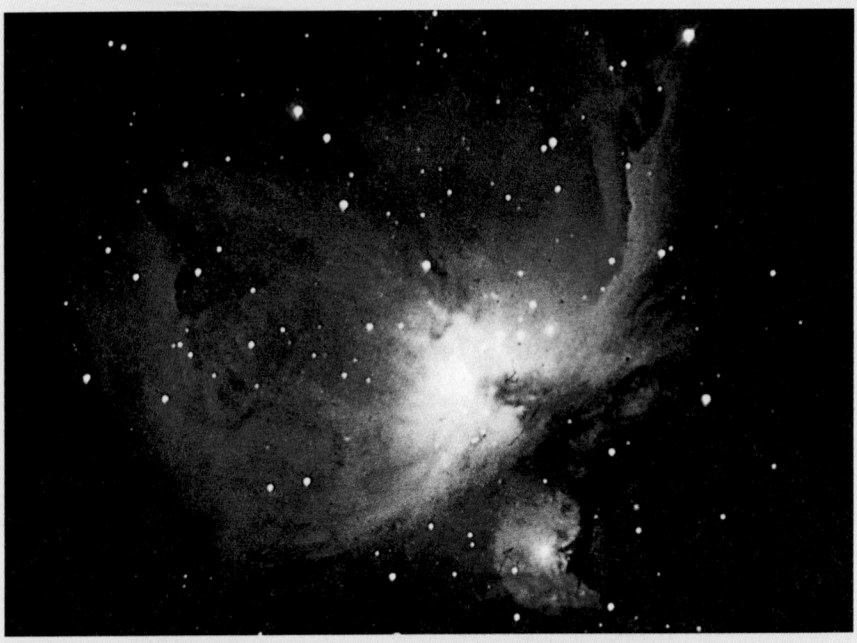

Figure 19-3   The Great Nebula in Orion is a gas cloud excited to luminescence by hot stars in its center.

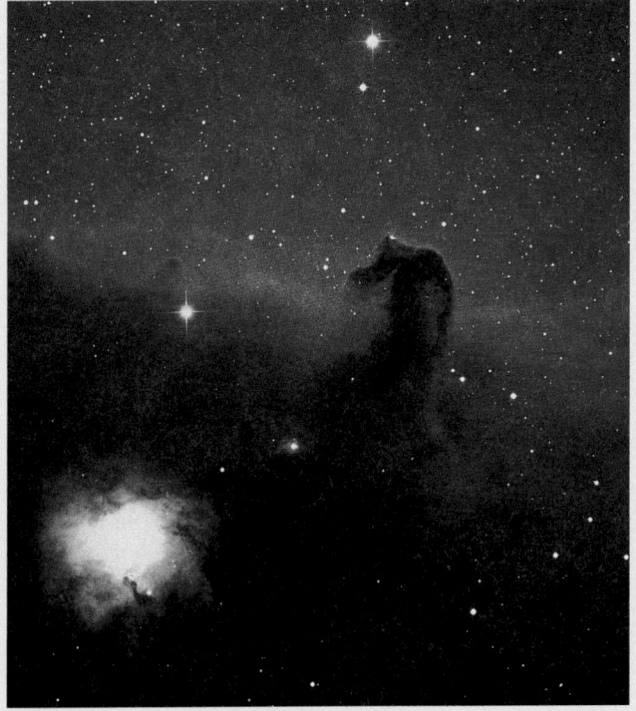

Figure 19-4   The Horsehead Nebula, also in Orion, is a cloud of gas and dust that blocks light from the emission nebula behind it. Radiation from nearby hot young stars will probably disperse the Horsehead Nebula in a few million years.

huge mass could keep them from flying off. Nothing but a black hole has the required mass (very large) and size (fairly small) to do the job. Evidence from other galaxies—there are many, as we shall see—suggests that such a black hole does not come first, gathering up stars later to form a galaxy around it, but instead the black hole and the galaxy develop together.

19.2 Stellar Populations

A Clue to the History of Our Galaxy

The stars in our galaxy fall into two categories. **Population I** stars are those in the central disk of the galaxy. These stars are of all ages, from those just coming into being to old ones that must have been formed early in the life of the galaxy.

Population II stars make up the **globular clusters** that surround the galaxy above and below its central disk. To the naked eye the largest of these assemblies of stars are just visible as faint patches of light. Through a telescope they are more spectacular, dense with stars near their centers and thinning out toward the edges (Fig. 19-5). About 150 of these clusters have been discovered, all orbiting the center of the galaxy.

In photographs of the globular cluster in the constellation Hercules, one of the largest, more than 50,000 stars have been counted. These are only the brightest stars, since the cluster is so far away that faint ones cannot be seen. The total number of stars may be over a million. The nearest clusters are about 20,000 light-years away from us and the farthest more than 100,000 light-years away. Light from the great Hercules cluster travels 33,000 years before reaching our eyes, so we see it as it appeared toward the end of the most recent ice age.

The average distance between stars in a globular cluster is well under a light-year, which means they are much more closely packed than those near the sun. As a result the average time between the collisions of a given star with another star in such a cluster is perhaps 10,000 years; elsewhere in the galaxy the time is in the billions of years.

Population II Stars The stars in the globular clusters of Population II are mostly very old, nearly as old as the galaxy. (Some are younger, having been born in collisions of old stars.) What seems to have happened is that all the matter of the galaxy was originally a spherical cloud of gas from which stars were forming. In time the cloud concentrated in a central disk, leaving behind as a sort of halo those stars that had already formed. New stars continued to come into being from the gas clouds of the disk, which is why the stars there are of all ages.

This picture is supported by the compositions of the stars of the two populations. Population II stars are extremely rich in hydrogen and helium. This follows from an early origin since the materials of the young universe are thought to have been these elements. Population I stars, on the other hand, contain heavier elements in some abundance. Such elements are produced in stars by the nuclear reactions that are responsible for stellar energy, and are thrown into space during the explosions that occur in the final stages of a star's active life. Compared with Population II stars, those of Population I are richer in heavy elements because they were formed from material that already contained such elements, material that was the debris of dying stars from Population II.

Although the globular clusters in our galaxy and in others consist of very old stars, new clusters can be formed when two galaxies collide and merge. In such an event, clusters come into being from concentrations of gas that occur, so the merged galaxy ends up with clusters both of new stars and of old ones that came from the original galaxies.

19.3 Radio Astronomy

Another Messenger from the Sky

A **radio telescope** is a directional antenna connected to a sensitive radio receiver. Usually a metal dish, like the concave mirror of a reflecting telescope,

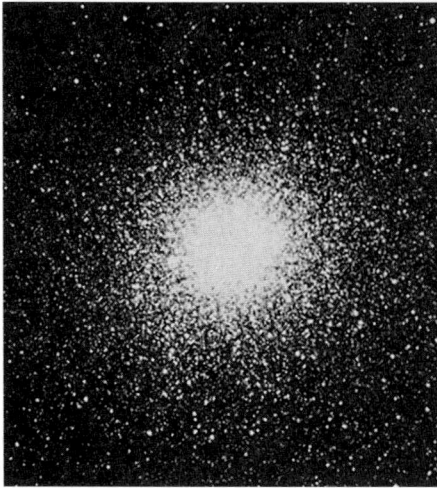

Figure 19-5 The globular cluster in Hercules contains perhaps a million stars.

gathers radio waves over a large area and concentrates them on the antenna itself. With such an arrangement the direction from which a particular radio signal arrives can be established.

Radio waves from cosmic sources are quite weak when they reach the earth—signals from a cell phone on the moon would be among the strongest—so large antennas are needed to detect them. The largest steerable-dish radio telescope is located in Green Bank, West Virginia. Still larger is a fixed dish 305 m across in Arecibo, Puerto Rico, that consists of wire mesh fitted into a bowl-shaped hollow in the landscape (see Fig. 19-24). As the earth turns, a band in the sky can be surveyed; the great sensitivity of this telescope makes up for its restriction to this band.

Antenna Arrays A number of radio telescopes can be linked together electronically to precisely locate the source of radio waves by interference methods (Fig. 19-6). Under construction in a desert region of northern Chile is an array of 63 dish antennas. To come later under the sponsorship of over 15 countries is the Square Kilometer Array of thousands of radio dishes whose total collecting area will be a square kilometer—a million square meters. Half the dishes will be concentrated in a central area about 5 km across with the others scattered up to 3000 km away. The array will be so sensitive that it must have a remote location to prevent interference from terrestrial sources of radio waves; sites in Australia and South Africa have been proposed. The array, which is hoped to be operating by 2020, will be able to detect long-wavelength radiation from the youth of the universe, before it became transparent to light (see Sec. 19.9). Among its fields of inquiry will be the evolutions of galaxies and of cosmic magnetism and the nature of dark energy.

Sources of Radio Waves Radio waves from space seem to originate in three ways. A common source is the random thermal motion of ions and electrons in a very hot gas, such as the atmosphere of a young star or the remnant thrown out by a supernova explosion. Another source consists of high-speed electrons that move in a magnetic field. The strongest radio sources, called **quasars,** are of this kind and may emit more energy as radio waves than as light waves. Quasars are discussed in Sec. 19.7.

Figure 19-6 A radio telescope is a directional antenna designed to pick up radio waves from space. Shown are several of the 28 dish antennas, each 25 m in diameter, that make up the Very Large Array near Socorro, New Mexico. The data obtained from these antennas can be combined to reveal details about radio sources in space that would otherwise require a single dish many kilometers across (see Sec. 7.17). A recent upgrade should enable the array to detect a cell phone signal from as far away as Jupiter.

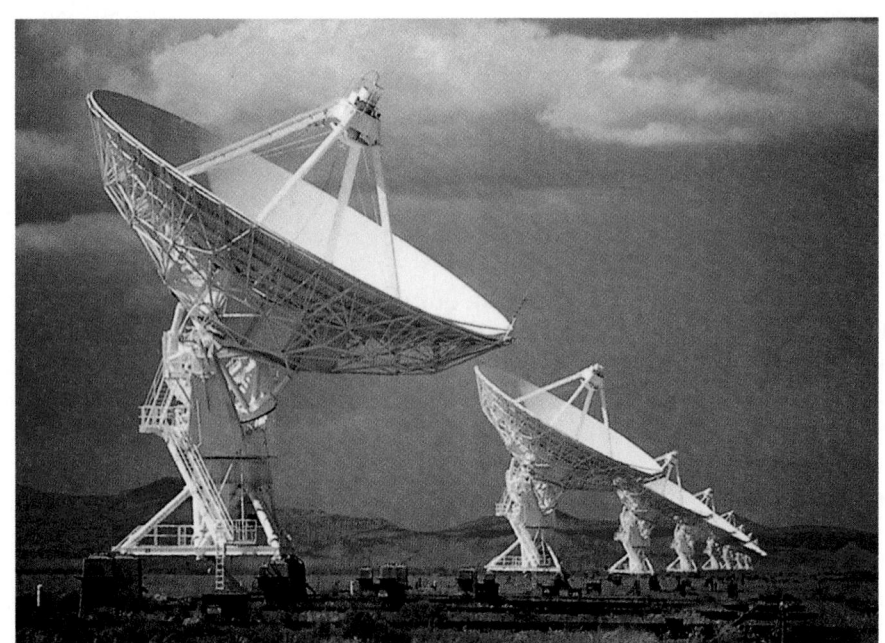

Molecules in Space A third source of radio waves in space is hydrogen atoms and molecules of various kinds. These waves are spectral lines that happen to lie in the radio-frequency part of the spectrum rather than in the optical part. In particular, the hydrogen line whose wavelength is 21 cm has proved invaluable to astronomers because most interstellar material consists of cool hydrogen. Dark nebulas in our galaxy can be mapped accurately with the help of radio telescopes tuned to receive 21-cm radiation.

Traces of a surprisingly large number of chemical compounds—135 thus far—have been detected in galactic space by the radio waves their molecules emit when excited by collisions. Most of the molecules are fairly simple, such as carbon monoxide (CO), ammonia (NH_3), and water (H_2O); the hydroxide radical OH is also common. In addition some fairly complex organic molecules have been found, including formaldehyde (H_2CO), acetaldehyde (CH_3CHO), acrylonitrile (CH_2CHCN), and the alcohols methanol (CH_3OH) and ethanol (CH_3CH_2OH). Experiment and calculation have brought to light plausible reactions by which many of these compounds can be formed in space, but there is much still to be learned. The total mass of the atoms, molecules, and ions in the interstellar space of our galaxy is about a fifth the mass of its stars.

19.4 Galaxies

Island Universes of Stars

Our Milky Way galaxy is only one of perhaps 200 billion galaxies in the universe. Although galaxies have a variety of shapes, many appear as flat spirals with two curving arms that radiate from a bright nucleus. Telescopes show us spiral galaxies from different angles: some full face, some obliquely, and some edgewise, as in Figs. 19-7 and 19-8. Spiral galaxies contain from 1 to 100 billion stars. Our galaxy is so massive that 10 smaller galaxies revolve around it. Every galaxy that has been studied thus far has, like our Milky Way galaxy, a black hole at its core whose mass is millions, sometimes billions, of times that of the sun. The shape of a galaxy is not fixed but changes continually for complicated reasons, much as though waves were moving through it.

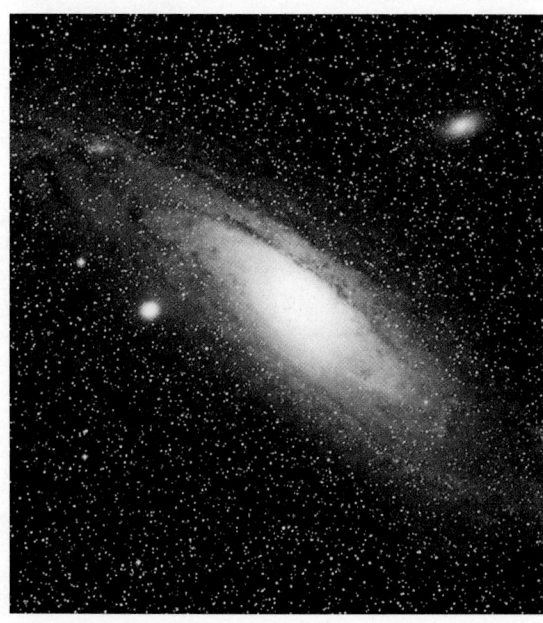

Figure 19-7 The Great Galaxy in Andromeda, which is 2.4 million light-years away, closely resembles our own Milky Way galaxy but is larger. The Andromeda galaxy contains about 100 billion stars, and its period of rotation is about 200 million years. It is the most distant object visible to the unaided eye. The two bright objects nearby are dwarf galaxies held as satellites by the gravitational pull of their huge neighbor. The mass of the black hole at its center is 30 million times the sun's mass, which is 8 times the mass of the black hole at the center of our galaxy.

Figure 19-8 The spiral galaxy in Coma Berenices appears edge-on to us.

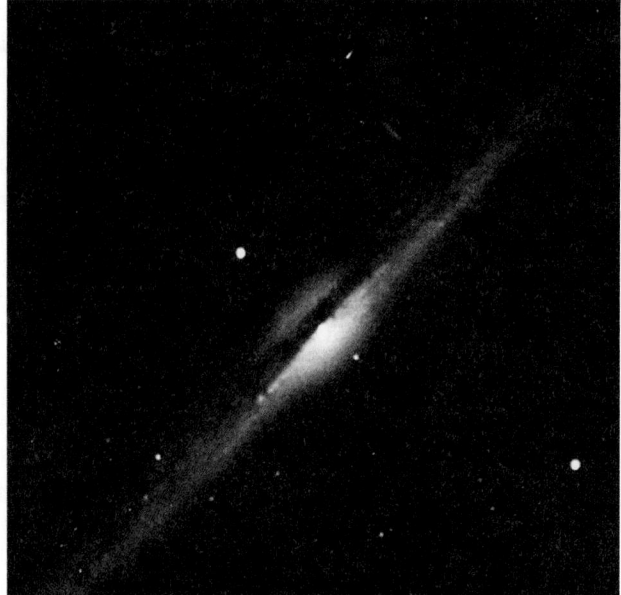

Other galaxies are so far away from ours that in early telescopes they were merely faint, fuzzy objects. William Herschel, the first to study these objects intensively, found evidence in support of an earlier guess that they were galaxies like the Milky Way, "island universes" in the sea of space. In his time, this was only a hypothesis, but today even galaxies too far away for their separate stars to be resolved have had their character revealed by spectroscopic studies. Doppler shifts have been detected in galaxies that show their stars to be revolving around the galactic centers, just as happens in our galaxy, with the inner ones moving faster than the outer ones (Fig. 19-9).

Most galaxies are concentrated in space in groups of up to a few hundred. Our galaxy is one of the three dozen or so members of the **Local Group.** The largest galaxy of this group is the one in the constellation Andromeda

Figure 19-9 The central region of galaxy M87, which is 50 million light-years from the earth, as seen from the Hubble Space Telescope. A disk of hot gas orbits the center of this galaxy at a speed so high that it suggests the center is a black hole with a mass of perhaps as much as 6.4 billion suns.

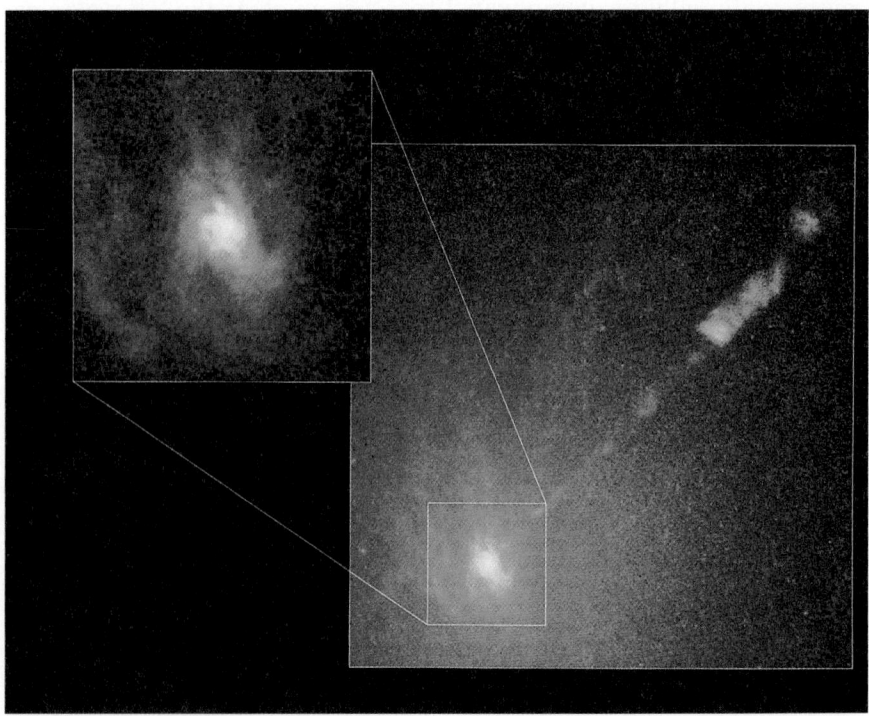

(Fig. 19-7), with our galaxy next in size. Groups of galaxies are further assembled by gravity into immense clusters that contain thousands of galaxies—and thousands of such clusters have been detected. On a still larger scale the clusters are clumped into superclusters.

Galactic Collisions   Relative to their sizes, galaxies are closer together than individual stars. The distance from the sun to its nearest neighbor, Proxima Centauri, is about 30 million times the diameter of the sun, whereas the distance from our galaxy to its nearest neighbor, the Canis Major Dwarf, is only about a fifth of our galaxy's diameter. It is therefore not surprising that collisions between galaxies are far more common than collisions between stars, and even when galaxies collide, their stars rarely do.

Our galaxy is in line for such a cataclysm in 2 or 3 billion years. At that time the Andromeda galaxy (Fig. 19-7), now headed our way, will collide with our galaxy. The meshing of the two galaxies will probably result in a new one whose form might be more like an elliptical blob than like the spiral shapes of the participants.

Dark Matter   The stars together with the dust and gases among them that we observe in the sky are composed of the same protons, neutrons, and electrons of which the earth—and we ourselves—are composed. But there is very strong evidence that a large amount of invisible **dark matter** is also present in every galaxy. So much, in fact, that about 85 percent of the matter in the universe does not seem to either give off or absorb light. For instance, the outer stars in spiral galaxies rotate unexpectedly fast, which suggests that a lot of invisible matter must be part of each galaxy to keep it from flying apart. Similarly, the motion of individual galaxies within clusters of galaxies implies gravitational fields more powerful than the visible matter of the galaxies provides.

Measurements made using the Hubble Space Telescope have been able to map the distribution of dark matter over part of the universe. The results confirm that dark matter and visible matter usually occur together, so the galaxies we see are basically concentrations of dark matter that accumulated with visible matter in tow.

What can the dark matter be? An obvious candidate is ordinary matter in various forms. Examples are brown dwarfs, burned-out white dwarfs, and black holes. The snag here is that, if there were enough such objects in space to make up the missing mass, their number would be so great that they would have already been found. Neutrinos, too, apparently can be ruled out, both because their masses are too small and because they move too fast to remain inside galaxies.

There are other possibilities as well, but these involve hypothetical elementary particles with unusual properties. Until any of these particles is found, or some other explanation turns up, the nature of the dark matter in the universe will remain a major scientific mystery. About 20 different experiments are under way to directly detect dark matter.

The existence of dark matter—whatever it is—does not change the uniformity of material and structural pattern that runs through the vast array of stars and galaxies in the universe. The elements of the earth are the elements of the galaxies, the sun generates energy by a process repeated in billions of other stars, and the form of our galaxy appears again and again in the rest of the universe. Enormous black holes have been found to lie at the hearts of a number of nearby galaxies, just as has been discovered in our galaxy, and strong evidence suggests that this is true in general. We can examine at first hand only a tiny fragment of the universe, yet so consistent is the whole that from this fragment we can extend our knowledge to as far as our instruments can reach.

Example 19.1

In the past, substances such as phlogiston and caloric with unusual properties were suggested to explain otherwise mysterious phenomena but were later shown not to exist. Why should we take the idea of dark matter any more seriously?

Solution

In fact, some proposed new forms of matter with unusual properties were actually discovered later. An example is the neutrino, thought up in 1930 to help explain beta radioactivity but not experimentally confirmed for 23 years even though hundreds of billions of neutrinos pass through our bodies every second. Something strange is unquestionably going on in the gravitational behavior of galaxies, and the simplest explanation is dark matter. If there is no dark matter of some kind, then the laws of physics will have to be changed drastically despite their overwhelming success everywhere else, which seems less likely (though not impossible).

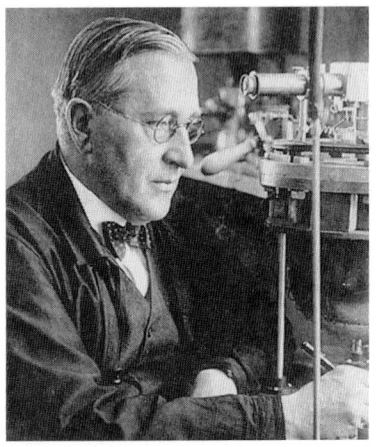

Figure 19-10   Victor Hess (1883–1964).

19.5   Cosmic Rays

Atomic Nuclei Speeding through the Galaxy

The story of cosmic rays began early in this century, when it was discovered that the ionization in the atmosphere increased with altitude. At that time most scientists thought that the small number of ions always present in the air was due to radioactivity. After all, naturally radioactive substances such as radium and uranium are found everywhere on the earth. If this were the correct explanation, then when we go high into the atmosphere away from the earth and its content of radioactive materials, the proportion of ions that we find should drop. Instead it increases, as a number of balloon-borne experimenters learned between 1909 and 1914.

Finally Victor Hess (Fig. 19-10), an Austrian physicist, suggested the correct explanation. From somewhere *outside* the earth ionizing radiation is continually bombarding our atmosphere. This radiation was later called **cosmic radiation** because of its extraterrestrial origin.

Primary Cosmic Rays   Primary cosmic rays, which are the rays as they travel through space, are atomic nuclei, mainly protons, that move nearly as fast as light. Flashes of light that astronauts have reported seeing have been traced to cosmic-ray primaries that passed through the retinas of their eyes. The majority of primaries probably were shot out during supernova explosions in our galaxy and then were trapped there by magnetic fields. A few, though, have energies of more than 10^{20} eV, well over what accelerators on earth can produce (indeed, more than the energy of a golf ball in flight), which is truly enormous for atomic nuclei. Recent measurements of the arrival directions of these primaries show that almost all apparently come from the active cores of galaxies in which matter is swirling violently toward supermassive black holes at their hearts.

About as much energy reaches us in the form of cosmic rays as in the form of starlight, a hint of their significance. They seem to have been more than bystanders in the evolution of the universe. From what is known about the origin of the elements, there should be very much less of the light elements lithium, beryllium, and boron than the universe actually contains. Apparently the nuclei of the atoms of these elements are mostly—in the case of beryllium, nearly all—fragments of relatively abundant carbon and oxygen nuclei in space that were shattered by collisions with cosmic rays.

As mentioned in Chap. 17, the risk of cancer due to exposure to cosmic rays is an unsolved problem for space travel beyond the moon.

Secondary Cosmic Rays   Over a billion billion primaries arrive at the earth each second and carry with them energy equivalent to the output of a dozen large power plants. When a primary cosmic ray enters the earth's atmosphere, it disrupts atoms in its path to produce a shower of secondary particles. On the average more than one of these secondaries passes through each square centimeter at sea level per minute. Among the secondary particles are neutrons, which interact with nitrogen nuclei to produce the radioactive carbon 14 that is the basis of the radiocarbon dating method discussed in Sec. 16.10. Secondary cosmic rays cause some of the mutations in living things that are part of the process of evolution.

A really energetic primary cosmic ray produces an avalanche of as many as 100 billion secondaries that pepper 10 to 20 km^2 of the earth's surface. The Pierre Auger Observatory in western Argentina (named after the French cosmic-ray pioneer) has 1600 12-ton detectors spread across 3000 km^2, about the area of Rhode Island, whose main purpose is to determine the directions in space from which the energetic primaries come. It is these data that led to the conclusion that such primaries come from the active cores of distant galaxies.

Example 19.2

Cosmic-ray intensity varies around the world in a manner that is correlated with the earth's magnetic field. (a) Why is such a correlation plausible? (b) Why do more cosmic rays reach the earth near the polar regions than near the equator?

Solution

(a) Primary cosmic rays are atomic nuclei and so are electrically charged particles, and moving charged particles experience forces in a magnetic field unless their motion is along the direction of the field. (b) A charged particle that approaches the equatorial regions moves perpendicularly to the earth's magnetic field there (see Fig 15-35), which means that the maximum deflecting force acts on them. A charged particle that moves toward the poles, on the other hand, is not deflected or is little deflected, since it moves parallel or nearly parallel to the magnetic field there.

The Expanding Universe

Now we turn to the evidence that led to the idea that the entire universe is growing larger and larger.

19.6   Red Shifts

The Galaxies Are All Moving Away from One Another

The spectra of galaxies share the curious feature that the lines in nearly all of them are shifted toward the red. Furthermore, the amount of shift increases with the distance of the galaxy from us. We can see this in Fig. 19-11, which shows two of the absorption lines of calcium in the spectra of several galaxies. Each galactic spectrum is shown between two comparison spectra, so that the shift of the lines toward the red (to the right in these pictures) is clear.

In Sec. 18.3 we saw that red shifts in stellar spectra result from motion away from the earth. We must therefore conclude that all the galaxies in the universe (except the few nearby ones in the Local Group) are receding from us. The recession speeds can be computed from the extent of the red shifts, and the results are startling: several hundred kilometers per second for the nearer galaxies, not far from the speed of light for the farthest ones.

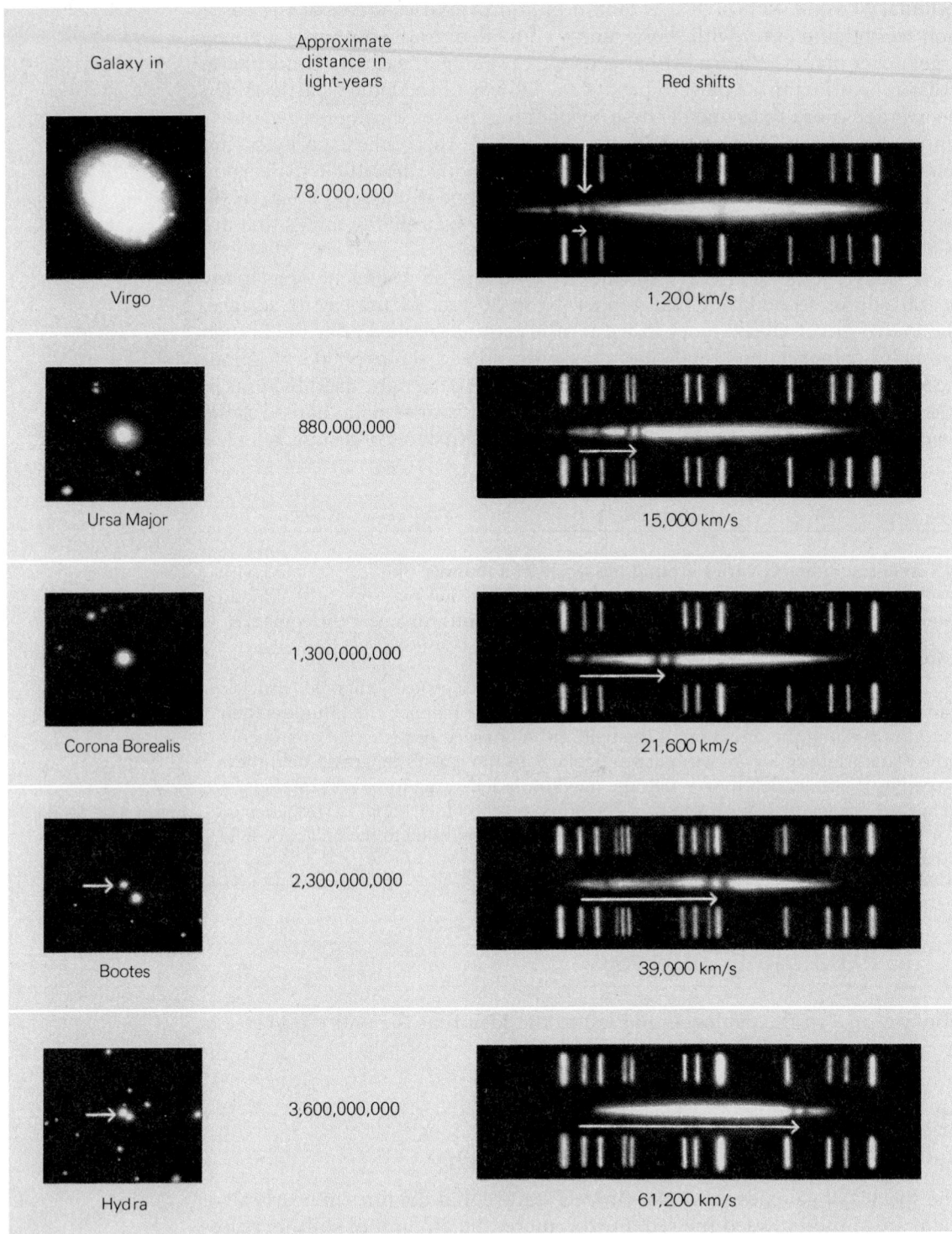

Galaxy in	Approximate distance in light-years	Red shifts
Virgo	78,000,000	1,200 km/s
Ursa Major	880,000,000	15,000 km/s
Corona Borealis	1,300,000,000	21,600 km/s
Bootes	2,300,000,000	39,000 km/s
Hydra	3,600,000,000	61,200 km/s

Figure 19-11 The red shifts in the spectral lines of distant galaxies increase with increasing distance. The indicated lines occur in the spectrum of calcium. Reference spectra taken in the laboratory are shown above and below each galactic spectrum. The red shifts come about because of the expansion of the universe. More recent studies indicate somewhat shorter distances than those shown here.

Hubble's Law If we plot the recession speeds of the galaxies shown in Fig. 19-11 versus their distances from the earth, as in Fig. 19-12, we find that these quantities are proportional. The greater the distance, the faster the galaxies are traveling. The speed increases by about 21 km/s per million

| Edwin Hubble (1889–1953)

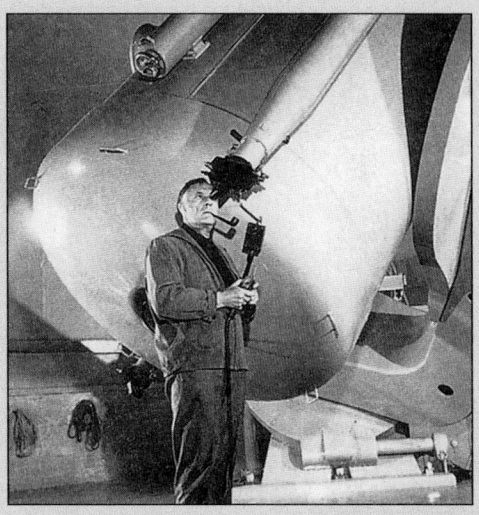

Although always interested in astronomy, Hubble pursued a variety of other subjects at the University of Chicago. He then went to Oxford University in England, where he concentrated on law and Spanish. After two years of teaching at an Indiana high school, Hubble realized what his true vocation was and returned to the University of Chicago to study astronomy.

At Mount Wilson Observatory in Pasadena, California, Hubble made the first accurate measurements of the distances of spiral galaxies, which showed that they are far away in space from our own Milky Way galaxy. It had been known for some time that such galaxies have red shifts in their spectra that indicate motion away from the Milky Way, and Hubble joined his distance figures with the observed red shifts to conclude that the recession speeds were proportional to distance. This implies that the universe is expanding, a remarkable discovery that has led to the modern picture of the evolution of the universe.

In his later work Hubble tried to determine the structure of the universe by finding how the concentration of remote galaxies varies with distance, a very difficult task that even today has not been fully accomplished.

light-years according to the most recent data. When this graph is extended to cover the still faster and more distant galaxies that have been studied, the experimental points fall on the same line. The proportionality between galactic speed and distance was discovered in 1929 by the astronomer Edwin Hubble and is known as **Hubble's law.**

At first it might seem as though our galaxy had some strange repulsion for all other galaxies, forcing them to move away from us with ever-increasing speed. A more reasonable conclusion is that space itself is expanding, so that an observer on our galaxy *or on any other* would then get the impression that the neighbors are fleeing in all directions.

The universe, in other words, is growing larger with the result that its component galaxies are moving ever farther apart (Fig. 19-13). The red shift in the light from a galaxy is determined by how much the universe has expanded since the galaxy emitted the light. As the light moves through the expanding universe, its wavelengths are stretched, so to speak, which corresponds to shifts toward the red (long-wavelength) end of the spectrum.

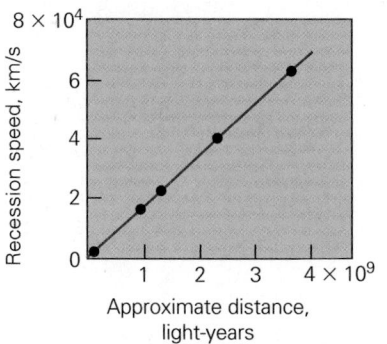

Figure 19-12 Graph of recession speed versus distance from the earth for the galaxies of Fig. 19-11. The straight line indicates that the universe is expanding at a uniform rate. Measurements made with the Hubble Space Telescope give this rate as 21 km/s per million light-years with an uncertainty of about 10 percent.

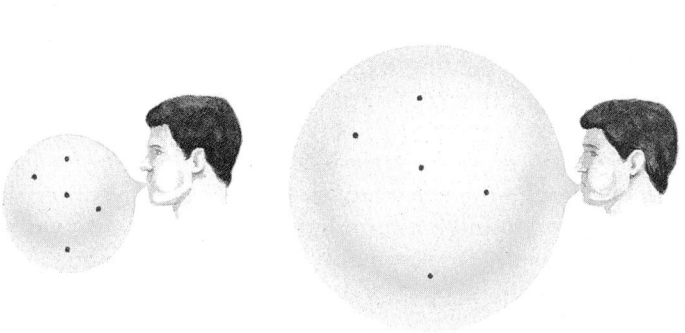

Figure 19-13 Two-dimensional analogy of the expanding universe. As the balloon is inflated, the spots on it become farther apart. A bug on the balloon would find that the farther away a spot is from it, the faster the spot seems to be moving away. This is true no matter where the bug is.

The concept of an expanding universe fits well into Einstein's general theory of relativity (Sec. 3.13), which we recall interprets gravitation as a warping of space and time.

| **Example 19.3**

Collisions between galaxies are known to have occurred. How is this possible if the entire universe is expanding?

Solution

The expansion of the universe is an expansion of space itself. The galaxies of the universe move about independent of the general expansion and collisions occur from time to time just as they would if the universe were not expanding. As mentioned in Sec. 19.4, the Andromeda galaxy (Fig. 19-7) is headed toward our galaxy and will collide with it in 2 or 3 billion years.

19.7   Quasars

Brilliant, Tiny, and Far Away

The most remarkable objects in the sky whose spectra show red shifts are **quasars.** In a telescope, a quasar appears as a sharp point of light, just as a star does, not a fuzzy dot as it would if it were a distant galaxy. But unlike stars, the first quasars to be discovered, in the early 1960s, were powerful sources of radio waves (Fig. 19-14). Hence their name, a contraction of *quasi-stellar radio sources.* Many quasars were later found that do not give off radio waves but can be identified by their characteristic spectra.

Both the light and radio outputs of quasars fluctuate markedly, in some cases in less than a day. Thousands of quasars have been found, and there seem to be many more.

Quasar red shifts are usually large, corresponding to recession speeds of over three-quarters the speed of light. Such speeds mean that quasars are far away, so far away that the light reaching us from them was emitted early in the life of the universe. Because quasars are distant objects, the intensities of the light and radio waves we receive from them imply that they are giving off energy at colossal rates, billions or trillions of times more than ordinary stars. Where does the energy come from?

What Is a Quasar?   Quasars vary in brightness too rapidly for them to be large objects. If a quasar were 100,000 light-years across, as a typical galaxy is, even a change in its energy output that took only a week to occur (if such a thing were possible) would appear to us as spaced out over 100,000 years. The observed short-period fluctuations point to a diameter for most quasars that is smaller than that of the solar system—but each quasar's energy output may be thousands of times the output of our entire galaxy.

Thus quasars must be small even though more powerful than any other energy sources in the universe. Apparently the heart of each quasar is a black hole whose mass is that of millions of suns. As nearby interstellar matter is pulled toward the black hole by its strong gravitational field, the matter is compressed and heated to temperatures such that radiation is given off in abundance. (Once inside the black hole, of course, the matter and its radiation vanish forever.) A diet of matter whose mass is that of a few suns per year seems to be enough to keep a quasar blazing away as observed.

A quasar has been found 5 billion light-years away with two black holes circling each other inside it, presumably the result of two quasars colliding. The black holes are 0.3 light-years apart and take almost a hundred years for each orbit.

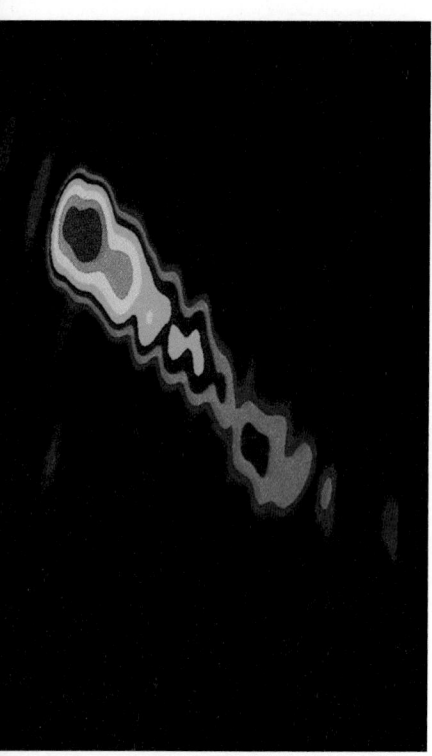

Figure 19-14   Quasars radiate many times more energy than ordinary galaxies like our own Milky Way, yet are far smaller in size. It is likely that quasars have black holes at their centers. The quasar shown here in a false-color radio image is 3 billion light-years away and emits energy at a rate of 10^{40} watts, equivalent to the output of 1000 ordinary galaxies. The jet of matter that extends from this quasar is 250,000 light-years long, although the quasar itself is only about 1 light-year across. The image of the quasar appears much larger here than it should because of diffraction (see Sec. 7.17).

Many astronomers believe that quasars are the cores of newly formed galaxies. Did all galaxies, including ours, once undergo a quasar phase? Nobody can say as yet, but it seems possible.

Evolution of the Universe

Everything we know about the universe points to its origin in an event—the **big bang**—billions of years ago in which space and time, matter and energy came into being. As the initial hot, dense universe expanded, very rapidly at first, its matter cooled and soon assumed its current forms. Local concentrations in the spreading matter then grew to become stars and galaxies. Today's physics can take us all the way back to the time when the entire universe was smaller than an atom. This is an amazing scientific accomplishment. Still ahead lies finding out what came before the big bang.

19.8 Dating the Universe

When Did the Big Bang Occur?

We can set a lower limit to the age of the universe by dating the oldest known objects it contains. These are globular clusters, which contain the first stars that formed, and the dimmest white dwarf stars that can be detected. Because a white dwarf is a dead star, it glows less and less brightly as it cools down, so the fainter it is, the farther back in time it came into being. The result for globular clusters is 12–13 billion years, for white dwarfs a little less.

An upper limit comes from using the Hubble's law figure of about 21 km/s per million light-years for the rate of expansion of the universe to calculate backward to a time when the galaxies were together in one place. Let us consider a galaxy 1 million light-years away from us, which is 9.5×10^{21} m. The galaxy's speed is 21 km/s = 2.1×10^4 m/s, so it must have started its outward motion at a time

$$T = \frac{\text{distance}}{\text{speed}} = \frac{9.5 \times 10^{21} \text{ m}}{2.1 \times 10^4 \text{ m/s}} = 4.5 \times 10^{17} \text{ s}$$

in the past. Since there are 3.2×10^7 s in a year, this would make the age of the universe 1.4×10^{10} years—14 billion years.

This calculation represents an upper limit because it assumes a constant rate of expansion. But the universe contains matter, and gravity must have been slowing the expansion down just as a ball thrown upward slows down as it rises. Since the expansion was once faster, the universe should be younger than 14 billion years. This conclusion holds even though recent evidence suggests that the expansion has actually been speeding up for the past 5 billion years (see sidebar *Dark Energy*).

In 2003 an entirely different method, based on studies of the cosmic background radiation (Sec. 19.9), was able to give a precise figure for the time of the big bang: 13.7 billion years ago, which agrees nicely with the discussion above.

19.9 After the Big Bang

A Glimmer of the Early Universe Still Exists

What is known about elementary particles and the fundamental interactions that govern their behavior enables us to figure out with some confidence how the universe developed starting from 10^{-43} s after the big bang and continuing to the present day. (To go even closer to the big bang awaits finding

Big Bang

The name "big bang" was coined by the British astrophysicist Fred Hoyle to ridicule a theory he scorned. He did not expect the name to become the standard designation for the theory.

Dark Energy

Dark matter is apparently not the only mystery ingredient in the universe.

There is a variety of supernova, called Type 1a, which at its peak could outshine a billion suns. The brightness of such a supernova and the way in which it fades with time are closely related. By observing how the brightness of one of these supernovas changes over a period of weeks, its intrinsic brightness can be found, and comparing this with its observed brightness then gives its distance (Sec. 18.8).

In 1998 astronomers discovered, to their surprise, that the remotest Type 1a supernovas were dimmer than their red shifts would predict. This means that the universe is expanding more rapidly today than it did in the past.

Several hundred Type 1a supernovas have now been studied, the farthest 7 billion light-years away. The results show that, until 5 billion years ago, the expansion of the universe was slowing down, as expected (see the discussion on the previous page), but then began to accelerate. The generally accepted conclusion is that some sort of influence is pushing the universe apart that at first could not counterbalance the pulling-together influence of gravity that acts to brake the expansion. As the universe grew larger, the matter in it spread out and the gravitational forces grew correspondingly weaker. About 6 billion years ago

the weakening gravitational pull allowed the dispersive influence to take over and hasten the expansion.

Where does this cosmic repulsion come from? One suggestion is that Einstein's general theory of relativity does not correctly describe gravity on the largest scales of size, so that there is nothing to explain—the apparent repulsion is simply part of how gravity works. Most astronomers, however, favor the idea that energy of an unknown kind, called **dark energy,** fills the universe and exerts an outward pressure on it. Other evidence also supports the existence of dark energy, notably certain characteristics of the cosmic microwave background radiation (Sec 19.9).

Although the nature of dark energy is a puzzle, how much there

is of it can be calculated. Dark energy apparently fills the universe with a uniform density that corresponds (by Einstein's formula $E_0 = mc^2$) to the equivalent in mass of a half-dozen hydrogen atoms per cubic meter. This does not seem like much, and indeed dark energy is of no importance in the solar system, but its effects on the evolution of the universe as a whole are significant.

Only 4 percent of the universe consists of the ordinary matter we are familiar with; 23 percent is the dark matter that galaxies contain; and no less than 73 percent is dark energy. Electromagnetic radiation—light, radio waves, x-rays—amount to only 0.005 percent (Fig. 19-15). Thus 96 percent of the universe awaits our understanding.

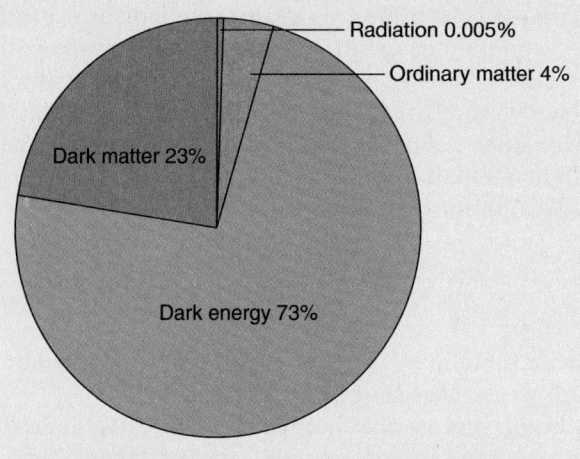

Figure 19-15   What the universe is apparently made of.

how the quantum and gravitational aspects of the universe are connected.) Figure 19-16 shows some probable stages in the history of the universe.

Just after the big bang, the universe was a compact, intensely hot mixture of matter and energy. Particles and antiparticles were constantly annihilating each other to form photons of radiation, and just as often photons were materializing into particle-antiparticle pairs. The particles and antiparticles at this time were the quarks and leptons described in Sec. 8.15. Recreating these conditions is one of the reasons for building powerful particle accelerators.

As the fireball expanded and cooled, the energies of the photons decreased. (We recall from Fig. 18-4 that the average wavelength of the radiation from a hot object increases as its temperature drops, which corresponds to a decrease in frequency and hence to a decrease in quantum energy hf.) Finally, shortly after the big bang, the photons had too little energy to create any more particle-antiparticle pairs. The annihilation of the existing particles

Age 0

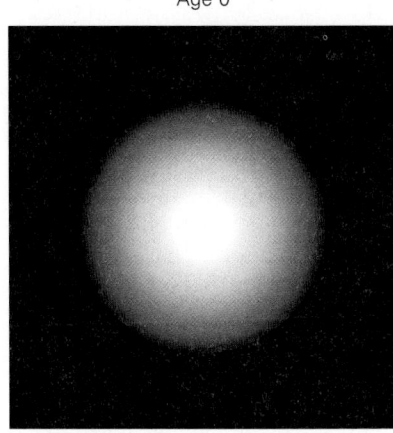

The big bang. The universe begins to expand, at first very rapidly.

Age 10⁻³⁵ second

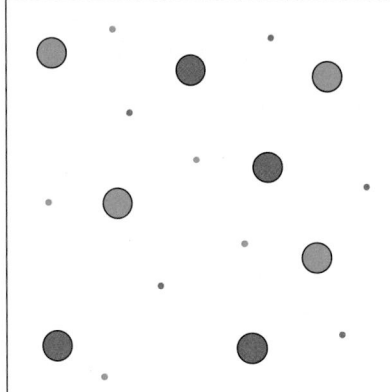

Quarks and leptons come into being. Particles slightly outnumber antiparticles. All the antiparticles are eventually annihilated to leave a matter universe with no antimatter.

Age 1 second

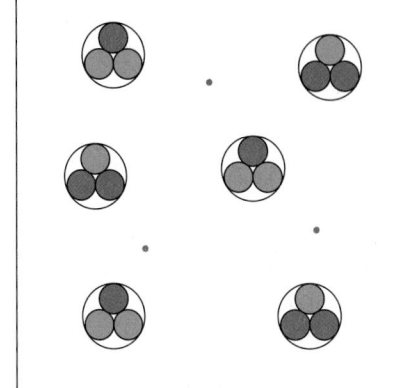

Quarks have joined to form neutrons and protons, some of which later react to form nuclei of light elements, mainly helium. There are as many electrons as protons, so the universe remains electrically neutral.

Age 3 minutes

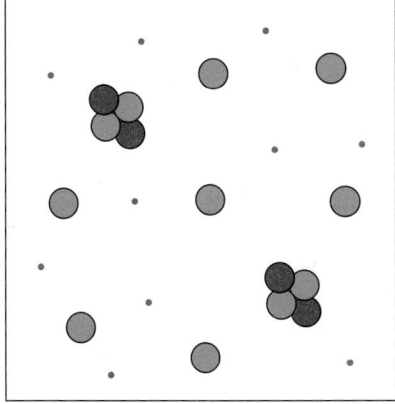

Nuclear reactions stop. The hydrogen: helium ratio is 3:1 as in most of today's universe. The universe is still too hot (10^9 K) for atoms to exist.

Age 380,000 years

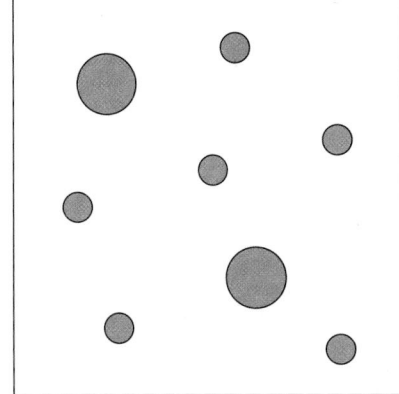

The universe has now cooled enough for nuclei and electrons to have joined to form neutral atoms. With few ions left to absorb it, radiation from this time was red-shifted by the expansion of the universe to become radio waves that fill the universe today.

Age 1 billion years

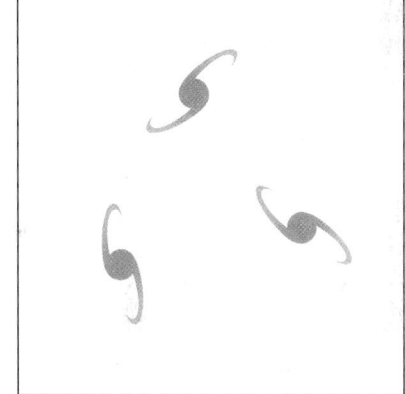

Under the influence of gravity, local concentrations of gas grew and began to condense into the first stars and galaxies when the universe was 400 million years old. After a billion years galaxies populated the universe, which continued to expand.

Figure 19-16   Snapshots from the youth of the universe. The scale is different in each sketch.

and antiparticles continued, however. For a reason still unknown, particles outnumbered antiparticles by perhaps one in a billion. When the annihilation was finished, some of the original particles were therefore left over, which ended up as the matter of today's universe.

Atoms Form   When the universe was about a minute old, nuclear reactions began to form helium nuclei. Calculations show that the ratio of hydrogen nuclei (protons) to helium nuclei ought to have ended up as 3:1, the same ratio found in most of the universe today. Although nearly all the helium in the universe was formed in the first few minutes after the big bang, with some created later in the nuclear reactions that power stars, the helium on the earth mainly came from the alpha decay of radioactive elements in its interior.

Theory of Everything

Quantum theory tells us how matter and energy behave on the scale of size characteristic of molecules, atoms, protons, neutrons, and electrons, which are too small for us to see directly and where gravity has little influence. Einstein's general theory of relativity goes to the other extreme by accurately describing how matter and space-time interact to produce gravitational effects on a larger scale all the way up to stars and galaxies. On this scale quantum effects, such as the wave-particle duality

and the graininess of matter and energy, can be ignored.

Between them the two pictures of how nature works might seem to include everything in the physical universe. However, the link between these pictures—there must be one—is not yet known, so there is no single Theory of Everything that would cover the overlap between the tiny (the province of quantum theory) and the large (where general relativity reigns).

Where would we expect such an overlap? The most obvious place is

the universe just after the big bang, when its entire mass occupied less space than an atom. Without a Theory of Everything nothing can be said about the first moments of the universe. Despite much effort, none of the approaches that have thus far been tried have led to testable predictions, so, as Wolfgang Pauli, a pioneer quantum physicist, said of another theory that lacked an anchor in reality, these approaches "aren't even wrong." But enough tantalizing hints have turned up to keep the search for a Theory of Everything alive.

A Map of the Cosmos

A number of surveys have measured galaxy distances by means of their red shifts to arrive at three-dimensional maps of parts of the sky. The most comprehensive survey thus far, made using an Australian telescope, examined

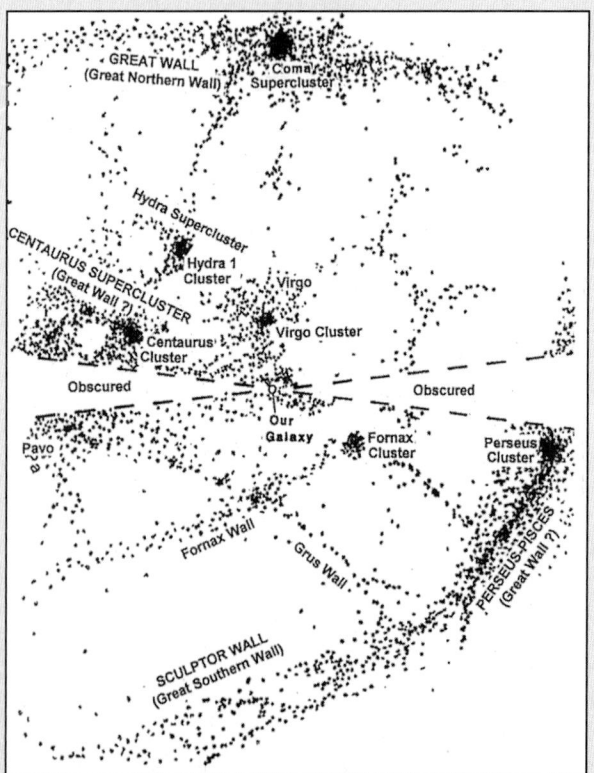

no less than 106,688 galaxies found in 5 percent of the sky (Fig. 19-17). The farthest galaxies were 4 billion light-years away.

The results confirmed previous studies that found galaxies in groups, the groups in clusters, the clusters in superclusters, and sharp-edged "walls" of clusters separated by giant voids. What was new was that nothing bigger turned up: no structures were found more than about 300 million light-years across. Since the universe itself is much larger, this means that, overall, the universe is relatively uniform, which is a good fit with the big bang picture of its origin. On successively smaller scales of size lumpiness appears in the forms of aggregates of galaxies, galaxies themselves, and individual stars. Such lumpiness is to be expected as gravity concentrated density fluctuations in the early universe.

Figure 19-17   A map of the closest clusters and super clusters of galaxies. Dust in the Milky Way prevents light from the sectors marked "obscured" from reaching us. Because the map does not provide a three-dimensional picture, some features are not evident. For instance, the lines of galaxies called great walls actually extend as sheets of galaxies well above and below the map.

After 380,000 years the universe was cool enough for electrons and nuclei to combine into atoms. Since photons interact strongly with charged particles but only weakly with neutral atoms, at this time matter and radiation were "decoupled" and the universe became transparent. The radiation that was left then continued to spread out with the rest of the universe, so that even today remnants of it must be everywhere.

Cosmic Microwave Background Because the universe is expanding, an observer today would expect to find these remnants to have undergone a red shift to long wavelengths, in the range of radio microwaves. The radiation would not be easy to find, since it would be very weak. However, it ought to have two distinctive characteristics that would permit it to be identified: it should come almost equally strongly from all directions, and its spectrum should be the same as that which an object at about 2.7 K would radiate.

Remarkably enough, radiation of exactly this kind was discovered in 1965 (Figs. 19-18 and 19-19). It turns out to account for 99 percent of the radiation in the universe—only 1 percent is starlight. The universe is bathed in a sea of radio waves whose ultimate source seems to have been the primeval fireball. Thus we have three observations that strongly support the big bang theory of the origin of the universe:

1. The expansion of the universe
2. The relative abundances of hydrogen and helium in the universe
3. The cosmic microwave background radiation

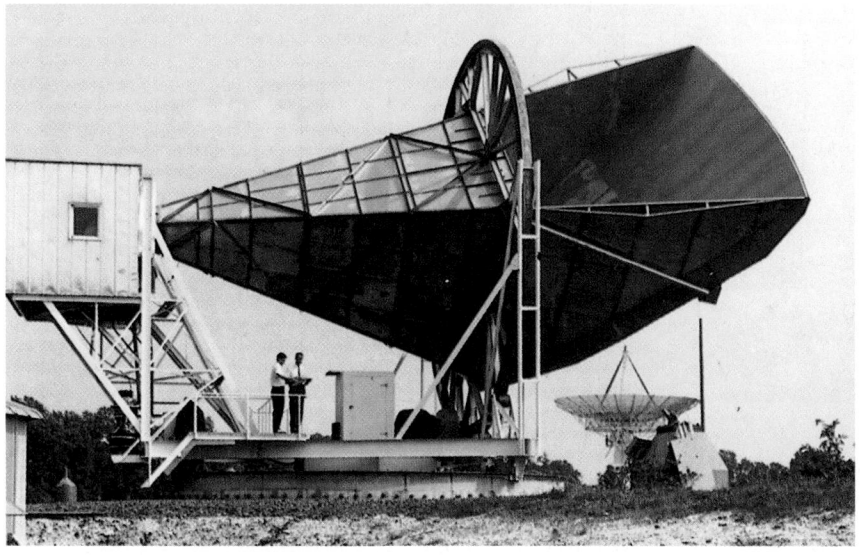

Figure 19-18 Radio waves that originated early in the history of the universe were first detected by Arno Penzias and Robert Wilson as a persistent hiss in a sensitive microwave receiver attached to this 15-m-long horn antenna at Holmdel, New Jersey.

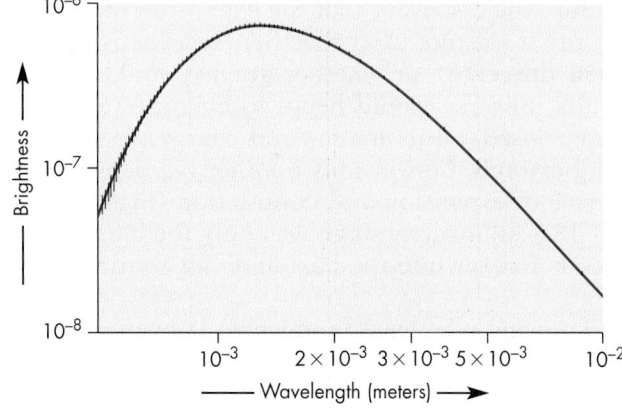

Figure 19-19 The spectrum of the cosmic background radiation corresponds to that of an object at a temperature of 2.7 K. The radiation originated when the universe became transparent at an age of 380,000 years after it had cooled enough for its nuclei and electrons to combine to form atoms. The waves were then lengthened by the expansion of the universe to their present wavelengths. (The scales are not linear.)

Whispers from the Past

As well as can be determined by instruments on the earth, the cosmic background radiation appears the same in all directions in the sky. This finding troubled astronomers, because only a completely smooth distribution of matter in the early universe could lead to a perfectly uniform afterglow—and a smooth distribution would leave no way to explain how such irregularities as galaxies could have developed.

To study the question further, NASA launched satellites in 1989 and 2001. Results from the first satellite showed that there are indeed very small variations in the radiation. These variations testified to the existence in the remote past of clumps of gas denser than the rest, clumps that were the seeds from which galaxies grew.

The more recent satellite, the Wilkinson Microwave Anisotropy Probe (WMAP), can pick up temperature differences down to a few millionths of a degree. The picture of the radiation it revealed is shown in Fig. 19-20. From the details of the temperature differences it was possible to establish, among other things, the precise age of the universe, its rate of expansion, how much dark matter it contains, and how much dark energy pervades it.

The WMAP results thus not only independently confirmed the picture of the universe that earlier studies had suggested but also put much more reliable numbers into the picture.

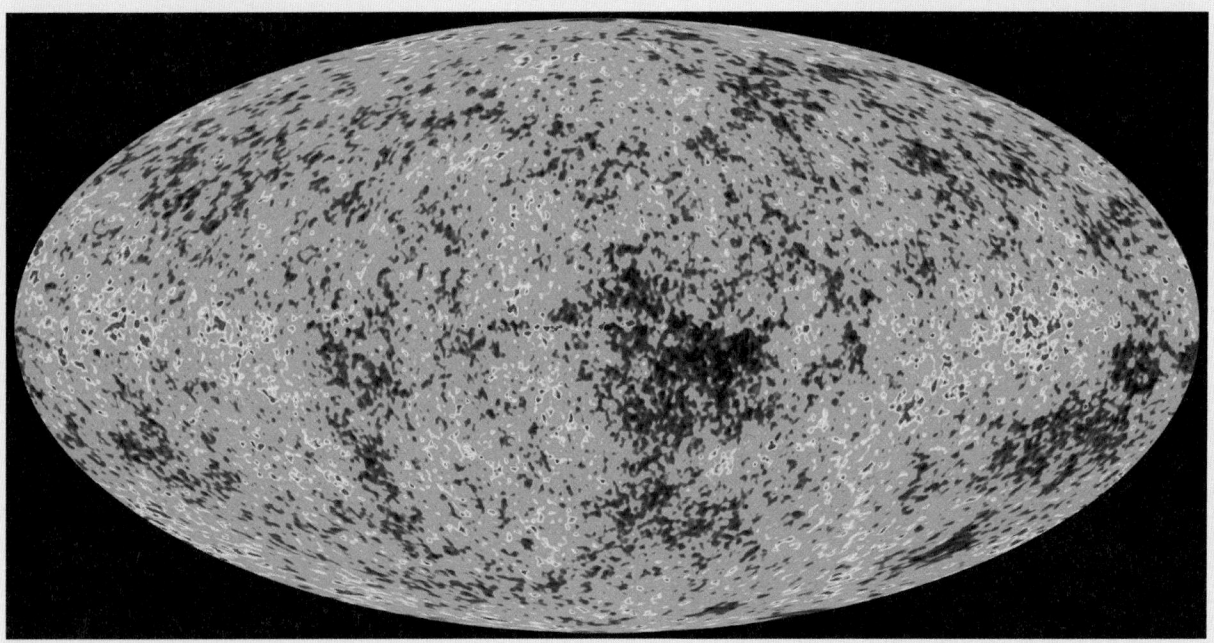

Figure 19-20   Temperature map of the early universe from WMAP data. The hottest regions are shown as red, the coolest as blue. A great deal of information about the universe and its history has been obtained from the details of this map, which is a picture of the dying glow of the big bang.

The Future   Before the discovery that the expansion of the universe is currently speeding up, it was not clear whether the expansion would continue forever (an **open universe**), or whether gravity would in time cause it to stop and then the universe would begin to collapse (a **closed universe**). If the universe is closed, all its matter and energy would eventually come together in a **big crunch.** Conceivably another big bang would follow, and then another cycle of expansion and contraction (Fig. 19-21). In this case the big bang of 13.7 billion years ago was only the latest in a series of big bangs that extends forever into the past and will continue forever into the future.

The key to knowing whether the universe is open or closed is how its average density of matter and energy compares with a certain critical value that depends on how fast the universe is expanding. Before evidence for dark

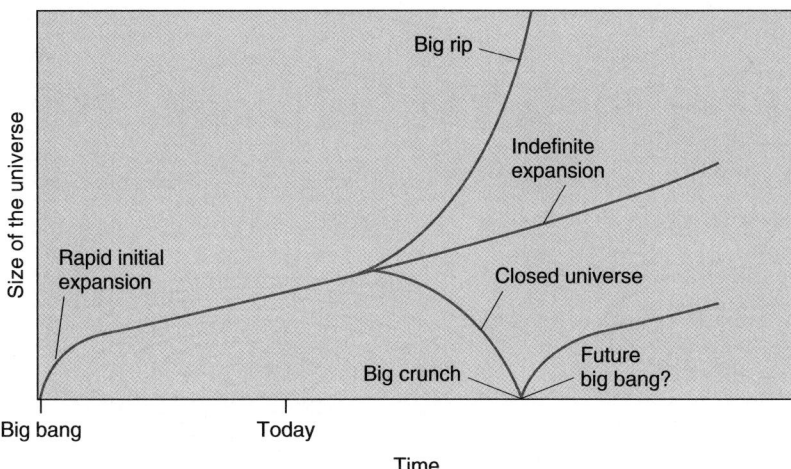

Figure 19-21 Three possible destinies for the universe.

energy came to light, although an open universe seemed more likely, there was still room for doubt. Now, even though the exact nature of dark energy remains to be found, the argument for an open universe seems very strong. Indeed, it has even been suggested that the push of dark energy may cause the universe to grow in size at an ever-increasing rate until a **big rip** tears it apart in some way 20 or more billion years hence. Or, in another scenario whose likelihood is unknown, the influence of dark energy may fade and a big crunch does await.

19.10   Origin of the Solar System

A Gradual Process

By a billion years after the big bang much of the hydrogen and helium of the universe had accumulated in separate clouds under the influence of gravity. These clouds were the ancestors of today's galaxies. As the young galaxies contracted, local blobs of gas formed that became the first stars. Some of the early stars were very massive and went through their life cycles rapidly to end as supernovas. The explosions of these supernovas dumped elements heavier than hydrogen and helium into the remaining galactic gas. As a result the matter from which later stars condensed was a mixture of all the elements, not just hydrogen and helium. By the time the sun came into being, billions of years after the first generation of stars, the loose material of our galaxy contained between 1 and 2 percent of the heavier elements. These were in the form of small solid "dust" grains, some of ice, some of rock.

Development of the Sun and Planets   The swirling cloud that became the sun was originally much larger than the present solar system. As it shrank in the process of becoming a star, this **protosun** left behind a spinning disk of gas and dust (Fig 19-22). Bits of matter in the disk collided and stuck together to form larger and larger grains, perhaps the size of pebbles. In time these grains formed larger bodies called **planetesimals** many kilometers across that ultimately joined to become the planets around 4.6 billion years ago.

Near the protosun, which was heated by gravitational compression, it was too warm for gaseous elements to collect in any great amounts on the planetesimals, which is why the inner planets are rocky bodies. Farther out temperatures were lower, so the planetesimals there mirrored the composition of the original cloud by being mainly frozen gases.

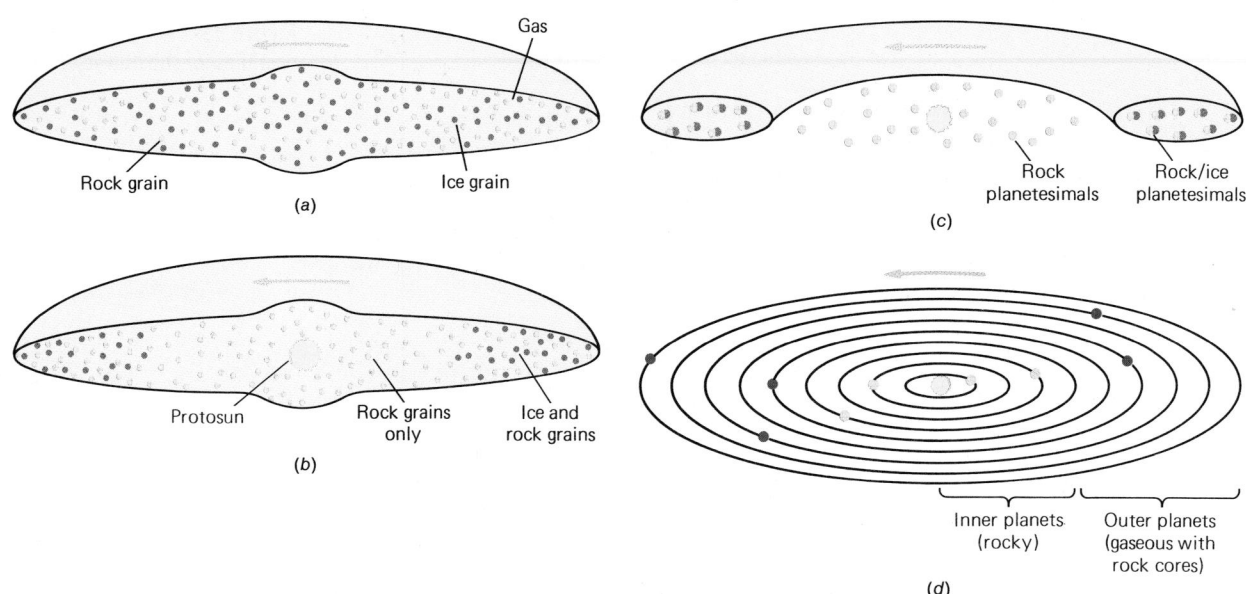

Figure 19-22 (*a*) The solar system began as a spinning cloud of gas and grains of ice (frozen gases) and rock. (*b*) When the protosun began to shine, the ice grains near it were heated and vaporized. (*c*) The rock and ice grains collided and stuck together to form planetesimals, which were rocky near the sun and a mixture of rock and ice farther away. (*d*) The planetesimals themselves collided and stuck together to form the planets. An intense solar wind blew away the gas and other material that had not become incorporated in the planets.

As the planets were developing with their satellites around them, the protosun was gathering up more and more material. After about 30 million years its internal temperature and pressure became sufficient for fusion reactions to occur in its hydrogen content, and the protosun became a star. Fast ions and electrons then began to stream out of the sun, much like today's solar wind but far more intense. This wind swept the solar system free of the gas and dust that had not yet been incorporated in the sun, the planets, and the satellites.

The infant planets were all heated by gravitational compression, which was naturally most effective in giant Jupiter and Saturn. Radioactivity was important as well in heating the inner planets. The earth became hot enough at this time to melt and separate into a dense iron core and a lighter rocky mantle (Fig. 19-23). The remaining planetesimals in the solar system bombarded the planets and satellites heavily, leaving craters on the solid ones that, in the case of the earth, erosion would later erase.

Figure 19-23 (*a*) When the earth was young, its interior melted. Under the influence of gravity, heavy materials then migrated inward to form the core and lighter ones were forced outward to form the mantle and crust. (*b*) Eventually the separation into core, mantle, and crust was complete, the outer parts cooled and hardened, and the early oceans and continents came into being.

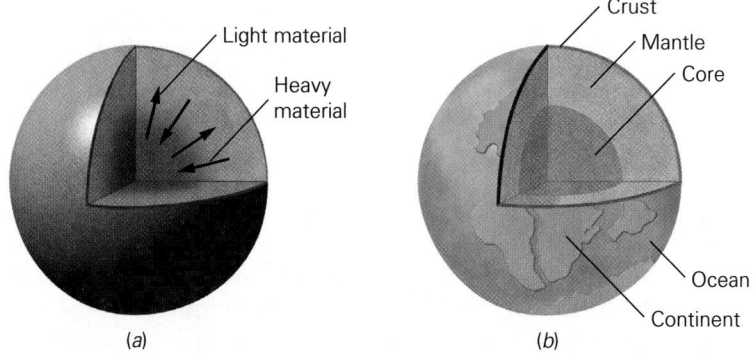

Extraterrestrial Life

The recipe for creating life begins with a warm rocky planet whose gravity is able to hold an atmosphere and whose distance from its parent star is such that it receives enough but not too much radiant energy. Then provide an atmosphere of certain quite common gases, allow the planet to cool down a bit so that water condenses out, and wait perhaps a billion years. This recipe was followed successfully on the earth. Let us now see how likely it is to have been followed elsewhere in the universe.

19.11   Exoplanets

Probably a Great Many

The modern view of the solar system is that it is a natural product of the evolution of the sun. Since the sun is by no means an exceptional star in any other respects, it is reasonable to suppose that other stars are also attended by planetary systems. Direct evidence in support of this idea was the discovery by the Hubble Space Telescope of disks of dust and gas around a number of newly formed stars, disks like the one pictured in Fig. 19-22*b*. In the region of the Orion Nebula that was studied, nearly all of the young stars (less than a million years old) there had such disks. Thus it may be that a star without planets is the exception, not the rule.

Many of the 200 billion stars in the Milky Way are similar to the sun. Some fraction of these stars, even if not all, have planetary systems. And there are billions of other galaxies in the known universe. Even a conservative guess at the lower limit to the number of extrasolar planets, or **exoplanets,** in the universe yields billions of billions.

If planets are such common objects, why are we certain only of the eight in our own solar system plus not really a great many others? Three interrelated factors make it difficult to identify planets that belong to other stars. The first is distance: the closest star to us is thousands of times farther away

Looking for Planets

A few actual images of exoplanets—as yet only fuzzy dots—have been obtained by blocking out light from their parent stars by computer processing.

However, the most successful quests for planets around sunlike stars make use of the fact that, as a planet orbits a star, its gravitational tug on the star causes the star to wobble back and forth. Unless the wobble is perpendicular to the line of sight, at times the star moves toward us, at other times away from us. These motions give rise to doppler shifts in the star's spectral lines that can be interpreted to reveal the mass of the planet and the size, shape, and period of its orbit. The sun's wobble as Jupiter circles it produces a doppler wavelength shift

that would be just on the limit of detection.

Another method is to seek the slight dimming of the light from a star as a planet passes in front of it. An advantage of this procedure is that it can respond to smaller planets; the sun dims by 0.01 percent as the earth moves across its face, which could just barely be picked up from far away. NASA's Kepler and Europe's Corot satellites are examining the light from 100,000 sunlike stars to look for brightness decreases due to such planet transits. Unfortunately both the wobble and dimming methods favor large planets revolving around small stars, whereas what we are really interested in are small earthlike planets revolving around sunlike stars.

An atmosphere around an exoplanet can sometimes be detected and analyzed if it passes across the line of sight from its parent star. If the spectrum of the star itself is subtracted from the combined spectra of the star and the planet, the gases in the planet's atmosphere, if there is one, can be identified. Space telescopes already in orbit have discovered exoplanet atmospheres, and two planned space observatories will continue the search. Because oxygen has a strong tendency to combine chemically with other substances, its presence in an exoplanet atmosphere would point to some life process like photosynthesis continually producing it.

than Pluto and other Kuiper Belt objects. The second is that planets shine by reflected light and not by themselves, which makes them faint compared with their parent stars. The third factor is size. Planets are necessarily small with relatively little mass, because if not, they would have become stars. The small size of a planet means that the light from its star dims by very little as it crosses the star's disk, and its small mass makes the wobbles it causes in the motion of the star hard to measure.

We May Not Be Alone Despite these difficulties over 400 exoplanets, some in multiple-planet systems, have been unambiguously detected since the first was found in 1995, and more and more are turning up every year. So far they range from 0.02 times the earth's mass all the way up to 20 times Jupiter's mass. The larger ones, the easiest to detect and the majority of those discovered thus far, are giant gas balls like the outer planets of the solar system. The smaller exoplanets are rocky, like the solar system's inner planets. One seems to be mainly water around a rocky core. Of stars like the sun that have been studied, about a third are known to have planets. Although finding more or less earth-sized planets is still extremely hard, improved methods should yield a big crop; there are indications that as many as half of sunlike stars have them.

From the point of view of life in the universe, just how many billions of planets there are is not really important. What is important is that a certain proportion of these planets surely meet, in the words of Harlow Shapley, "the happy requirement of suitable distance from the star, near-circular orbit, proper mass, salubrious atmosphere, and reasonable rotation period—all of which are necessary for life as we know it on earth."

But not any location in our galaxy will do. Elements heavier than hydrogen and helium, which are needed for life and are created in supernova explosions, are most abundant toward the center of the galaxy. However, supernova explosions, which would destroy life on a planet anywhere near, are also more common near the center. A zone between 22,000 and 30,000 light-years from the center of the galaxy, about a tenth of the area of the galactic disk, seems about right; our sun is in the middle of this zone. One of the smaller exoplanets that has been discovered also may occupy such a habitable zone around its parent star since its surface temperature is between 0°C and 40°C: neither too hot nor too cold for liquid water and life.

Convergent Evolution Given a suitable parent star, size, composition, and environment in space, life could appear. Would it necessarily resemble life on earth? This is an interesting question to which biology has an interesting answer. Terrestrial life has many examples of what is called convergent evolution: organisms that came from different genetic lines are found to have developed similar forms and functions as they respond to similar environmental pressures. Thus eyes may have independently evolved in possibly 65 different types of animals.

Of course, extraterrestrial life is not likely to mirror life on earth exactly, but if a planet elsewhere is much like the earth, then the organisms that arise there may well be recognizable variations of organisms that now or in the past flourished here. Although the hypothesis of life on other worlds may not be directly verified in the near future, no serious arguments that dispute this hypothesis have been proposed. It seems likely that we are not alone in the universe.

19.12 Interstellar Travel

Not Now, Probably Not Ever

The great physicist Enrico Fermi was skeptical about widespread advanced life in the universe. If it existed, then "Why aren't the aliens here?" (Arthur C.

Exomoons and Exolife

The tides that ceaselessly stir the waters of the earth are brought about by the gravitational pull of our relatively large moon (Sec. 1.10). This stirring probably helped life to begin by mixing the various ingredients that were involved, thereby promoting their chemical reactions. There seems to be no reason why the process by which the moon came into being (Sec. 17.16) should not have occurred in other planetary systems, so it seems likely that similarly large satellites are orbiting a great many exoplanets. This both increases the chance that life exists elsewhere and suggests that exoplanets with large satellites should be prime candidates for study.

Clarke's response was, "I'm sure the universe is full of intelligent life—it's just been too intelligent to come here.") The real answer is that the required interstellar journey is just not a practical proposition no matter how advanced a civilization might be. Astronauts have already visited the moon and spacecraft have traveled to all the other planets. But travel to the planetary systems of other stars is much more of an undertaking.

Suppose we wish to go to Proxima Centauri, the star nearest to the sun, to check on whether it has a planet that contains living things. This star is 4×10^{13} km away, a little over 4 light-years. The various Apollo spacecraft took 3 days to reach the moon, which is 100 million times closer than Proxima Centauri. To reach this star at the same rate, a similar spacecraft would therefore need 300 million days, nearly a million years. So existing technology is out of the question.

No Reason for Hope   What about the future? According to Einstein's special theory of relativity, which has been found to be completely accurate in all its predictions, the ultimate limit to the speed that anything can have is the speed of light. This speed is about 300,000 km/s. At a speed 1 percent short of this, a spacecraft could reach Proxima Centauri in a few years, a reasonable enough period of time. However, the energy required would be fantastic, more than all the energy currently used in the entire world per year for each ton of spacecraft weight—and the spacecraft would have to weigh many tons. How can all this energy be produced? How can it be concentrated at one time and place? How can it be given to the spacecraft? And how could a like amount of energy be provided in the vicinity of Proxima Centauri to return the spacecraft to the earth?

These questions are not quibbles. They are fundamental to such an enterprise—and they have no answers at present. As for a space traveler visiting the stars that lie millions and billions of times farther away than Proxima Centauri, there does not seem to be any hope whatever.

The laws of physics hold everywhere in the universe, which means that the extreme unlikelihood of travel from the earth to an extrasolar planet is also true for travel from such a planet to the earth. It is easy to attribute ancient legends and archeological findings that are hard to explain in terms of known events to visitors from another world. However, all such attributions have turned out to lack any evidence to support them. A good story does not constitute proof of anything except the imagination of its author.

19.13   Interstellar Communication

Why Not?

Although travel to other worlds is almost surely impossible, by contrast communication with them seems quite feasible. The first serious proposal was made in 1820 by the German mathematician Karl Friedrich Gauss. Gauss suggested that trees be planted on the bare landscape of Siberia to form a right triangle large enough to be seen from the moon, which he thought might be inhabited. A better method for interstellar distances is to use radio waves.

A Search for Extraterrestrial Intelligence (SETI) is going on in which radio telescopes around the world seek messages from far away (Fig. 19-24). The program has been privately funded since 1993, when a Nevada senator, upset because until then "not a single Martian has said, 'take me to your leader,' and not a single flying saucer has applied for FAA approval," saw to it that NASA support was stopped; it was never restored. Part of the program is targeted on the 1000 nearest stars that resemble the sun.

How Much Advanced Life?

The earth came into being about 4.6 billion years ago, and less than a billion years later life of some primitive sort had appeared. On a cosmic scale, this is pretty fast, and, together with other evidence, it strongly suggests that life could also have come into being on planets around other stars.

But what kind of life? The next step, from one-celled microorganisms to multicellular organisms, took over 3 billion more years on the earth. And not until now, 4.6 billion years since the earth's origin, have living things on earth progressed to the point where interstellar communication can be taken seriously.

Indeed, the development of an advanced civilization—as distinct from merely complex life forms—may require too many chance events to be inevitable by now wherever life occurs. The dinosaurs were successful enough to be the dominant animals on earth for 140 million years (will we last that long?), but they never evolved to create an advanced civilization. If it were not for the asteroid that drove them into extinction, we might well not be here today. So, although life is probably common in the universe, advanced civilizations may not be.

Figure 19-24 Among its other tasks, this extremely sensitive 305-m radio telescope built in a natural hollow at Arecibo in Puerto Rico is being used in the SETI (Search for Extraterrestrial Intelligence) program to monitor a total of 168 million radio channels for signals from space.

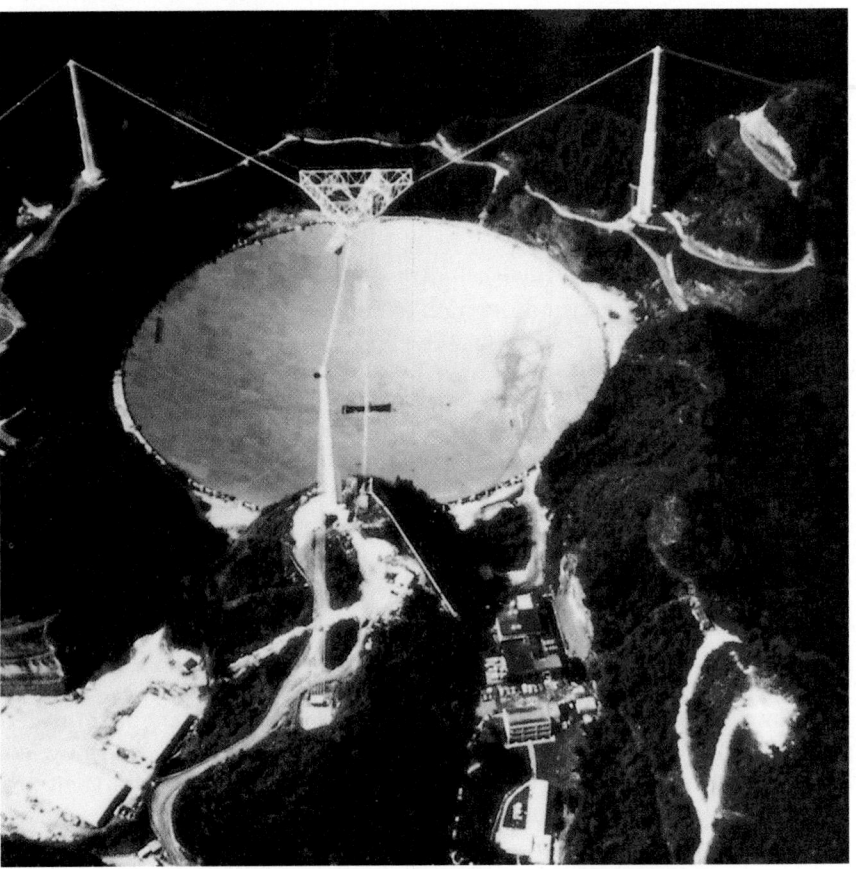

Figure 19-25 One way in which a message from space might be detected. Each point on this plot corresponds to the frequency of a particular signal picked up by a radio telescope and the time at which it was received. The brighter the point, the stronger the signal. The random background is due to noise. The diagonal line records a signal sent out by the Pioneer 10 spacecraft when it was beyond the orbit of Pluto. The changing frequency of the signal is the result of the earth's rotation causing a changing doppler shift.

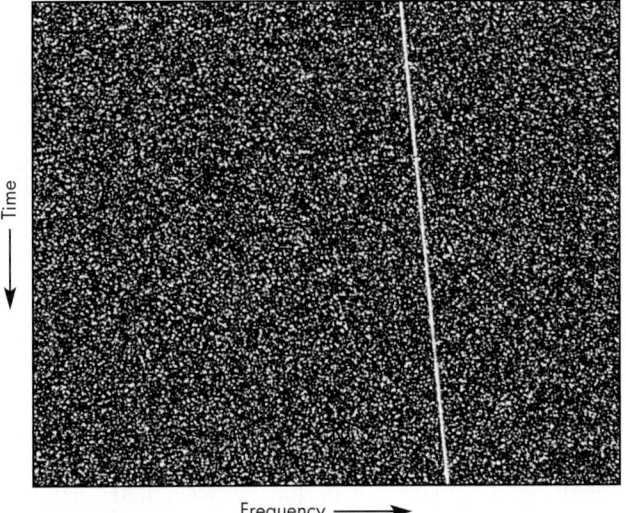

The entire sky is also scanned, though necessarily with less sensitivity. What is sought are patterns of emissions that are not the result of natural processes, such as pulsar bursts (Fig. 19-25).

Around a million people around the world have volunteered their computers for use during otherwise idle periods to process radio telescope data instead of reverting to screensavers. In a 2007 expansion of the program, 42 antenna dishes, each 5.5 m across, were connected to make the Allen Telescope Array in Hat Creek, California. The array may eventually grow to 350 dishes. The Square Kilometer Array (Sec. 19.3), which is being planned, may also listen for messages from far away. Another approach recognizes that, if there is advanced life elsewhere, perhaps it, too, has invented lasers. Since April 2006, a telescope in Massachusetts has been scanning the sky for repetitive flashes of light that might be laser signals.

Still Looking   The SETI program and its predecessors have been on the look-out for half a century with no positive results. Although the early studies may not have been sufficiently sensitive or thorough, the latest equipment is able to respond to signals from up to 4000 light-years away sent out by transmitters no more powerful than transmitters we on earth could make today. Why the silence?

To begin with, the search is far from complete. Second, maybe we are listening on the wrong frequencies. Third, for all our pride in our advanced civilization, we ourselves are not broadcasting messages that advertise our existence, and perhaps many of our counterparts elsewhere are similarly disinclined to do so. And so on. Even though SETI has thus far had no success, it is surely premature to consider the program a failure.

Indeed, what about sending out messages ourselves for other worlds to receive? The technology is already available in the radio band; in fact, a signal was deliberately sent into space in 1974 from the Arecibo radio telescope acting as a transmitter, and four other signals were sent by a Russian astronomer starting in 1999. In the optical band, a laser planned in the United States for other purposes would be powerful enough to shoot out pulses of light 3000 times brighter than the sun that could be detected up to perhaps 1000 light-years away. By virtue of the long distances involved, years at best, more likely centuries would be needed for an interchange of information to take place. But what an extraordinary, exhilarating prospect!

Important Terms and Ideas

Our **galaxy** is a huge, rotating disk-shaped group of stars that we see in the sky as the **Milky Way** from our location about two-thirds of the way out from the center. Most of the stars of the galaxy are found in two **spiral arms** that extend outward from the center. These stars are **Population I** stars and are of all ages. **Globular clusters** of mainly very old stars occur outside the central disk of the galaxy. These stars are **Population II** stars. **Spiral galaxies** are other collections of stars that resemble our galaxy. The universe apparently consists of widely separated galaxies of stars.

A **radio telescope** is a directional antenna connected to a sensitive radio receiver. Radio waves from space are produced by extremely hot gases, by fast electrons that move in magnetic fields, and by atoms and molecules excited to radiate. Especially notable sources are **quasars,** distant objects that emit both light and radio waves strongly and that may be powered by supermassive black holes at their centers.

Cosmic rays are atomic nuclei, mostly protons, that travel through the galaxy at speeds close to that of light. They probably were ejected during supernova explosions and are trapped in the galaxy by magnetic fields.

The spectral lines of distant galaxies show a doppler shift to the red arising from motion away from the earth. Since the speed of recession is observed to be proportional to distance, the **red shift** means that all the galaxies in the universe are moving away from one another. This **expansion of the universe** began 13.7 billion years ago and is currently accelerating.

The **big bang theory** holds that the universe originated in a great explosion 13.7 billion years ago. **Cosmic background radiation** left over from the early universe and doppler-shifted to radio frequencies has been detected. It is probable that the expansion of the universe will continue forever; if not, the universe will eventually begin to contract and will end up in a **big crunch** after which another cycle of expansion and contraction may occur.

There is apparently much more **dark matter** in galaxies than the luminous matter, such as stars, that we can see. The universe as a whole also contains a huge amount of **dark energy** whose nature, like that of dark matter, is unknown. Dark matter and dark energy together make up 96 percent of the stuff of the universe.

The solar system originated as part of an evolutionary process, and systems of **exoplanets** are probably quite common elsewhere in the universe.

Multiple Choice

1. The stars in space are
   a. uniformly spread out
   b. distributed completely at random
   c. chiefly in the Milky Way
   d. mostly contained within widely separated galaxies

2. The Milky Way is
   a. a gas cloud in the solar system
   b. a gas cloud in the galaxy of which the sun is a member
   c. the galaxy of which the sun is a member
   d. a nearby galaxy

3. Relative to the center of our galaxy,
   a. its stars are stationary
   b. its stars move entirely at random
   c. its stars revolve
   d. Population I stars are stationary and Population II stars revolve

4. Our galaxy is approximately
   a. 4 light-years across
   b. 15,000 light-years across
   c. 130,000 light-years across
   d. 4 million light-years across

5. The number of stars in our galaxy is roughly
   a. 2000   c. 2 billion
   b. 2 million   d. 200 billion

6. The stars in the disk of our galaxy are mostly distributed
   a. uniformly
   b. at random
   c. in its central nucleus
   d. in its spiral arms

7. Our galaxy is shaped roughly like a fried egg whose diameter is about
   a. twice its thickness
   b. 10 times its thickness
   c. 100 times its thickness
   d. 1 million times its thickness

8. Each cubic centimeter of space between the stars in our galaxy contains on the average about
   a. 1 atom or molecule
   b. 1 million atoms or molecules
   c. 1 mg of matter
   d. 1 g of matter

9. Evidence of various kinds suggests that at the center of our galaxy is a
   a. quasar
   b. pulsar
   c. neutron star
   d. black hole

10. Clouds of luminous gas and dust in our galaxy are called
    a. galactic clusters   c. quasars
    b. galactic nebulas   d. cosmic rays

11. The globular clusters of our galaxy
    a. contain around a hundred stars each
    b. contain around a million stars each
    c. contain around a billion stars each
    d. lie only in its central disk

12. The Population II stars in globular clusters are
    a. mostly very young
    b. mostly very old
    c. mostly about as old as the sun
    d. of all ages about equally

13. Compared with the Population II stars in globular clusters, the Population I stars in the galactic disk are
    a. richer in hydrogen and helium
    b. richer in the heavier elements
    c. older
    d. closer together

14. A radio telescope is basically a(an)
    a. device for magnifying radio waves
    b. telescope remotely controlled by radio
    c. directional antenna connected to a sensitive radio receiver
    d. optical telescope that uses electronic techniques to produce an image

15. Radio waves from space never originate in
    a. extremely hot gases
    b. fast electrons moving through magnetic fields
    c. molecules
    d. cosmic rays

16. Spiral galaxies
    a. are readily visible as such to the naked eye
    b. may be dark or bright
    c. are usually similar to our galaxy
    d. originate in supernova explosions

17. The stars in a galaxy are
    a. moving outward from its center
    b. moving inward toward its center
    c. revolving around its center
    d. stationary relative to its center

18. Individual stars in other galaxies
    a. can be seen with the unaided eye
    b. can be seen only with a telescope
    c. cannot be seen even with a telescope
    d. are all members of Population II

19. The "dark matter" that all galaxies apparently contain
    a. consists of antimatter
    b. consists of cosmic rays
    c. consists of dead stars
    d. is of unknown nature

20. Cosmic rays carry energy to the earth at about the same rate as
    a. sunlight   c. starlight
    b. moonlight   d. meteoroids

21. Cosmic rays
   a. circulate freely through space
   b. are trapped in our galaxy by electric fields
   c. are trapped in our galaxy by magnetic fields
   d. are trapped in our galaxy by gravitational fields

22. Primary cosmic rays are composed largely of very fast
   a. protons   **c.** electrons
   b. neutrons   **d.** gamma rays

23. The origin of the most energetic cosmic rays is
   a. nuclear reactions in the sun
   b. solar flares
   c. the cosmic background radiation
   d. unknown

24. The red shift in the spectral lines of light reaching us from other galaxies implies that these galaxies
   a. are moving closer to one another
   b. are moving farther apart from one another
   c. are in rapid rotation
   d. consist predominantly of giant stars

25. Supernova explosions have no connection with
   a. the formation of heavy elements
   b. cosmic rays
   c. pulsars
   d. quasars

26. Current ideas suggest that what is responsible for the observed properties of a quasar is a massive
   a. neutron star   **c.** spiral galaxy
   b. black hole   **d.** star cluster

27. Quasars do not
   a. emit radio waves
   b. exhibit red shifts in their spectra
   c. vary in their output of radiation
   d. occur in the solar system

28. The term big bang refers to
   a. the origin of the universe
   b. the ultimate fate of the universe
   c. a supernova explosion
   d. the formation of a quasar

29. The expansion of the universe apparently
   a. has always occurred at the same rate
   b. is currently slowing down
   c. is currently speeding up
   d. has come to a stop

30. The matter in the early universe that eventually condensed into galaxies and then into stars consisted of
   a. only hydrogen
   b. hydrogen and helium in an approximately 3:1 ratio
   c. hydrogen and helium in equal amounts
   d. hydrogen and helium in an approximately 1:3 ratio

31. The elements heavier than hydrogen and helium of which the planets are composed probably came from the
   a. sun
   b. debris of supernova explosions that occurred before the solar system came into being

   c. big bang
   d. big crunch

32. Soon after it came into being, the universe contained
   a. only matter
   b. only antimatter
   c. equal amounts of matter and antimatter
   d. slightly more matter than antimatter

33. Today the universe apparently contains
   a. only matter
   b. only antimatter
   c. equal amounts of matter and antimatter
   d. slightly more matter than antimatter

34. Radiation from the early history of the universe was stretched by the expansion of the universe until today it is in the form of
   a. x-rays   **c.** infrared waves
   b. ultraviolet waves **d.** radio waves

35. Astronauts need not worry about
   a. gamma-ray bursts
   b. cosmic rays
   c. cosmic microwave background radiation
   d. collisions with space junk

36. Present evidence suggests that the major ingredient of the universe is in the form of
   a. dark matter
   b. dark energy
   c. cosmic rays
   d. black holes

37. Dark energy
   a. is the energy equivalent of dark matter
   b. is the energy of black holes
   c. is the energy of neutrinos
   d. has an unknown nature as yet

38. It is least likely that the universe will
   a. continue to expand indefinitely
   b. expand at an ever-increasing rate until it is torn apart
   c. stop expanding and maintain a constant size
   d. collapse into a big crunch

39. The age of the universe is about
   a. 6000 years
   b. 13.7 million years
   c. 4.6 billion years
   d. 13.7 billion years

40. The age of the earth is about
   a. 6000 years
   b. 13.7 million years
   c. 4.6 billion years
   d. 13.7 billion years

41. It is likely that the planets, satellites, and other members of the solar system were formed
   a. together with the sun
   b. later than the sun from material it ejected
   c. later than the sun from material it captured from space
   d. elsewhere and were captured by the sun

42. Planets are always small compared with stars because otherwise

    a. the rotation of the planets would cause them to disintegrate

    b. the great mass of the planets would cause them to be pulled into their parent star

    c. the great mass of the planets would prevent them from being held in orbit and they would escape

    d. the planets would be stars themselves

43. The least likely reason why planetary systems have not been directly observed around stars other than the sun is that

    a. planets are small

    b. planets shine by reflected light

    c. planetary systems are rare

    d. other stars are far away

Exercises

19.1 The Milky Way

1. Are the stars uniformly distributed in space?

2. (a) Why is the sun considered to be located in the central disk of our galaxy? (b) What is thought to occupy the center of the disk?

3. What is the Milky Way?

4. The earth undergoes four major motions through space. What are they?

19.2 Stellar Populations

5. What are the properties of globular clusters?

6. Both galactic nebulas and globular clusters occur in our galaxy. Distinguish between them.

7. Distinguish between Population I and Population II stars.

8. A number of elliptically shaped galaxies are known that seem to contain only Population II stars. Would you expect such galaxies to contain abundant gas and dust?

9. Where is most of the interstellar gas in our galaxy located? What is its chief constituent?

19.3 Radio Astronomy

10. Do radio telescopes magnify anything? If not, why are larger and larger ones being built?

11. List the three ways in which radio waves from space originate.

12. How does the mass of all the interstellar matter in our galaxy compare with the total mass of its stars?

13. Why are radio-astronomical studies of the distribution of hydrogen in the universe of greater interest than studies of the distribution of other elements?

14. What kind of evidence supports the belief that molecules of various kinds, including some fairly complex ones, exist in space?

19.4 Galaxies

15. Are most galaxies smaller, larger, or about the same size as our galaxy?

16. How can the rotation of a spiral galaxy be determined? Will this method work for all spiral galaxies?

17. How are galaxies distributed in the universe?

18. (a) How does the typical size of a galaxy relative to the typical distance between galaxies compare with the corresponding ratio for stars in a galaxy? (b) Which would you expect to be more common, collisions between galaxies or collisions between stars?

19. (a) What is the observational evidence in favor of there being a great deal of dark matter in the universe? (b) Where is the dark matter located?

20. Why is it unlikely that dark matter consists of brown dwarfs, burned-out white dwarfs, and/or black holes? Why is it unlikely that it consists of neutrinos?

19.5 Cosmic Rays

21. In what way have cosmic rays affected the composition of the universe?

22. There is no day-night difference in cosmic-ray intensity. How does this observation bear on the possibility of a solar origin for cosmic rays?

23. What do you think ultimately becomes of the protons and neutrons knocked out of atmospheric atoms by cosmic rays?

24. Cosmic-ray primaries are mostly protons, but few protons are in the cosmic rays that reach the earth's surface. Why?

25. What traps cosmic rays in our galaxy?

19.6 Red Shifts

26. What is Hubble's law?

27. Why is the universe believed to be expanding?

19.7 Quasars

28. What is a quasar?

29. Why are quasars thought to be relatively small in size?

30. The spectra of quasars exhibit red shifts, never blue shifts. Why does this suggest that quasars are not members of our galaxy?

19.8 Dating the Universe

19.9 After the Big Bang

31. What is the observational evidence in favor of the big bang?

32. What is the evidence for the idea that dark energy fills the universe? Is the nature of dark energy known at present? How does the amount of dark energy compare with the amount of ordinary matter in the universe? With the amount of dark matter?

33. What are the origins of the helium found in the universe?

34. To what event in the history of the universe can the cosmic microwave background radiation be traced? Was the radiation always in the form of microwaves? If not, what happened to change the wavelengths of the original radiation?

35. Is the cosmic microwave background radiation uniform in space? If not, what is the significance of the variations?

36. Suppose the spectral lines of distant galaxies were shifted toward the blue end. What would this suggest about the universe?

37. Distinguish between a closed and an open universe. How does the density of matter in the universe bear on the question of whether the universe is closed or open? What does present evidence suggest about the nature of the universe?

19.10 Origin of the Solar System

38. In what way or ways, if any, is the sun an unusual star?

39. Did the sun begin as a small body that grew to its present size, or as a large one that subsequently shrank?

40. The sun and the giant outer planets contain hydrogen and helium in abundance; the inner planets, very little. Why?

41. What heated all the planets as they were formed? Was there any other influence that helped heat the inner, rocky planets?

42. Did the planets come into being before, during, or after the formation of the sun?

43. Would you characterize the most likely next phase of the earth's history as fire or ice?

19.11 Exoplanets
19.12 Interstellar Travel

44. Why is it reasonable to suppose that many stars besides the sun have planets orbiting them? Why does it seem unlikely that spacecraft from the earth will ever visit other planetary systems?

45. Why is it hard to detect the planetary systems of other stars?

Math Refresher

A little basic mathematics is needed to appreciate much of physical science. This review is included mainly to help those readers whose mathematical skills have become rusty, but it is sufficiently self-contained to introduce such useful ideas as powers-of-10 notation to those who have not been exposed to them elsewhere.

Algebra

Algebra is the arithmetic of symbols that represent numbers. Instead of being limited to relationships among specific numbers, algebra can show more general relationships among quantities whose numerical values need not be known.

To give an example, in the theory of relativity it is shown that the "rest energy" of any object—that is, the energy it has due to its mass alone—is

$$E = mc^2$$

What this formula does is give a way to calculate the rest energy E in terms of mass m and speed of light c. The formula is not restricted to a particular object, but can be applied to any object whose mass is known. What is being shown is the way in which rest energy E varies with mass m *in general.*

If we are told only that the rest energy E of some object is 5 joules, we do not know upon what factors E depends or precisely how the value of E varies with those factors. (The joule is a unit of energy widely used in physics; it is equal to 1 kg · m²/s².) The quantities E and m are **variables,** since they have no fixed values. On the other hand, c^2 is a **constant,** since it is the square of the speed of light c and the value of c—almost 300 million m/s, or about 186,000 mi/s—is the same everywhere in the universe. Thus the formula $E = mc^2$ tells us, in a simple and straightforward way, that the rest energy of something varies only with its mass and also how to find the numerical value of E if we are given the mass m of a particular object.

The convenience of algebra in science is increased by the use of standard symbols for constants of nature. Thus c always represents the speed of light, π always represents the ratio between the circumference and diameter of a circle, e always represents the electric charge of the electron, and so on.

Before we go further, it is worth reviewing how the arithmetical operations of addition, subtraction, multiplication, and division are expressed in algebra. Addition and subtraction are straightforward:

$$x + y = a$$

means that we obtain the sum a by adding the two quantities x and y together, while

$$x - y = b$$

means that we obtain the difference b when quantity y is subtracted from quantity x.

In algebraic multiplication, no special sign is ordinarily used, and the symbols of the quantities to be multiplied are merely written together. Thus these four expressions have the same meaning:

$$xy = c \qquad x(y) = c \qquad (x)(y) = c \qquad x \times y = c$$

When the quantity x is to be divided by y to yield the quotient e, we write

$$\frac{x}{y} = e$$

which can also be expressed as

$$x/y = e$$

whose meaning is the same.

If several operations are to be performed in a certain order, parentheses ( ), brackets [ ], and braces { } are used to indicate this order. For instance $a(x + y)$ means that we are first to add x and y together and then to multiply their sum $(x + y)$ by a. In essence $a(x + y)$ is an abbreviation for the same quantity written out in full:

$$a(x + y) = ax + ay$$

Let us find the value of

$$v = 5\left[\frac{(x - y)}{z}\right] + w$$

when $x = 15$, $y = 3$, $z = 4$, and $w = 10$. We proceed as follows:

1. Subtract y from x to give

$$x - y = 15 - 3 = 12$$

2. Divide $(x - y)$ by z to give

$$\frac{(x - y)}{z} = \frac{12}{4} = 3$$

3. Multiply $[(x - y)/z]$ by 5 to give

$$5\left[\frac{(x - y)}{z}\right] = 5 \times 3 = 15$$

4. Add w to $5[(x - y)/z]$ to give

$$v = 5\left[\frac{(x - y)}{z}\right] + w = 15 + 10 = 25$$

Positive and Negative Quantities

The rules for multiplying and dividing positive and negative quantities are simple. If the quantities are both positive or both negative, the result is positive; if one is positive and the other negative, the result is negative. In symbols,

$$(+a)(+b) = (-a)(-b) = +ab$$
$$\frac{+a}{+b} = \frac{-a}{-b} = +\frac{a}{b}$$
$$(-a)(+b) = (+a)(-b) = -ab$$
$$\frac{-a}{+b} = \frac{+a}{-b} = -\frac{a}{b}$$

Here are some examples:

$$(-3)(-5) = 15 \qquad\qquad \frac{-16}{-4} = 4$$

$$2(-4) = -8 \qquad\qquad \frac{10}{-5} = -2$$

$$(-12)6 = -72 \qquad\qquad \frac{-24}{4} = -6$$

To find the value of

$$w = \frac{xy}{x + y}$$

when $x = 5$ and $y = -6$, we begin by finding xy and $x + y$. These are

$$xy = (5)(-6) = -30$$
$$x + y = 5 + (-6) = 5 - 6 = -1$$

Hence

$$w = \frac{xy}{x + y} = \frac{-30}{-1} = 30$$

An example of the use of positive and negative quantities occurs in physics, where there are two kinds of electric charge. One kind is designated positive and the other negative. The force F that a charge Q_1 exerts on another charge Q_2 a distance r away is given by Coulomb's law as

$$F = K\frac{Q_1 Q_2}{r^2}$$

where K is a universal constant. By convention, a positive value of F means a repulsion between the charges—the force tends to push Q_1 and Q_2 apart. A negative value of F means an attraction between the charges—the force tends to pull Q_1 and Q_2 together. A positive (=repulsive) force acts when *either* both charges are $+$ *or* both are $-$: "like charges repel." When one charge is $+$ and the other one $-$, the force is negative (=attractive): "opposite charges attract." Both the above observations about the types of force that occur together with the way in which the strength of F varies with the magnitudes of Q_1 and Q_2 and with their separation r are included in the simple formula $F = KQ_1Q_2/r^2$.

Exercises

A. Evaluate the following. The answers are given at the end of the Math Refresher.

1. $\dfrac{3(x + y)}{2}$ when $x = 5$ and $y = -2$

2. $\dfrac{1}{x - y} - \dfrac{1}{x + y}$ when $x = 3$ and $y = 2$

3. $\dfrac{4xy}{y + 3x} + 5$ when $x = 1$ and $y = -2$

4. $\dfrac{x + y}{2z} + \dfrac{z}{x - y}$ when $x = -2$, $y = 2$, and $z = 4$

5. $\dfrac{x + z}{y} + \dfrac{xy}{2}$ when $x = -2$, $y = 8$, and $z = 10$

6. $\dfrac{3(x + 7)}{y + 2}$ when $x = 3$ and $y = -6$

7. $\dfrac{5(3 - x)}{2(x + y)}$ when $x = -5$ and $y = 7$

Equations

An equation is a statement of equality: whatever is on the left-hand side of an equation is equal to whatever is on the right-hand side. An example of an arithmetical equation is

$$3 \times 9 + 8 = 35$$

since it contains only numbers. An example of an algebraic equation is

$$5x - 10 = 20$$

since it contains a symbol as well as numbers.

The symbols in an algebraic equation usually must have only certain values if the equality is to hold. To *solve* an equation is to find the possible values of these symbols. The solution of the equation $5x - 10 = 20$ is $x = 6$ since only when $x = 6$ is this equation a true statement:

$$5x - 10 = 20$$
$$5 \times 6 - 10 = 20$$
$$30 - 10 = 20$$
$$20 = 20$$

The methods that can be used to solve an equation are based on this principle:

> Any operation carried out on one side of an equation must be carried out on the other side as well.

Thus an equation remains valid when the same quantity is added to or subtracted from both sides or when the same quantity is used to multiply or divide both sides.

Two helpful rules follow from the above principle. The first is:

> Any term on one side of an equation may be shifted to the other side by changing its sign.

To check this rule, let us consider the equation

$$a + b = c$$

If we subtract b from each side of the equation, we obtain

$$a + b - b = c - b$$
$$a = c - b$$

Thus b has disappeared from the left-hand side and $-b$ is now on the right-hand side. Similarly, if

$$a - d = e$$

then it is true that

$$a = e + d$$

The second rule is:

> A quantity that multiplies one side of an equation may be shifted so as to divide the other side, and vice versa.

To check this rule, let us consider the equation

$$ab = c$$

If we divide both sides of the equation by b, we obtain

$$\frac{ab}{b} = \frac{c}{b}$$
$$a = \frac{c}{b}$$

Thus b, which was a multiplier on the left-hand side, is now a divisor on the right-hand side. Similarly, if

$$\frac{a}{d} = e$$

then it is true that

$$a = ed$$

Let us use the previous rules to solve $5x - 10 = 20$ for the value of x. What we want is to have just x on the left-hand side of the equation. The first step is to shift the -10 to the right-hand side, where it becomes $+10$:

$$5x - 10 = 20$$
$$5x = 20 + 10 = 30$$

Now we shift the 5 so that it divides the right-hand side:

$$5x = 30$$
$$x = \frac{30}{5} = 6$$

The solution is $x = 6$.

When each side of an equation consists of a fraction, all we need do is **cross multiply** to remove the fractions:

$$\frac{a}{b} = \frac{c}{d} \qquad \frac{a}{b} \diagup\!\!\!\!\diagdown \frac{c}{d} \qquad ad = bc$$

For practice, let us solve the equation

$$\frac{5}{a + 2} = \frac{3}{a - 2}$$

for the value of a. We proceed as follows:

Cross multiply to give	$5(a - 2) = 3(a + 2)$
Multiply out both sides to give	$5a - 10 = 3a + 6$
Shift the -10 and the $3a$ to give	$5a - 3a = 6 + 10$
Carry out the indicated addition and subtraction to give	$2a = 16$
Divide both sides by 2 to give	$a = 8$

Exercises

B. Solve each of the following equations for the value of x:

1. $3x + 7 = 13$ **5.** $\dfrac{x + 7}{6} = x + 2$ **9.** $\dfrac{3}{x - 1} = \dfrac{5}{x + 1}$

2. $5x - 8 = 17$ **6.** $\dfrac{4x - 35}{3} = 9(1 - x)$ **10.** $\dfrac{1}{3x + 4} = \dfrac{2}{x + 8}$

3. $2(x + 5) = 6$ **7.** $\dfrac{3x - 42}{9} = 2(7 - x)$

4. $7x - 10 = 0.5$ **8.** $\dfrac{1}{x + 1} = \dfrac{1}{2x - 1}$

Exponents

There is a convenient shorthand way to express a quantity that is to be multiplied by itself one or more times. In this scheme a superscript number called an **exponent** is used to show how many times the multiplication is to be carried out, as follows:

$$a = a^1$$
$$a \times a = a^2$$
$$a \times a \times a = a^3$$
$$a \times a \times a \times a = a^4$$

and so on. The quantity a^2 is read "a squared" because it is equal to the area of a square whose sides are a long. The quantity a^3 is read as "a cubed" because it is equal to the volume of a cube whose edges are a long. Past an exponent of 3 we read a^n as "a to the nth power," so that a^5 is "a to the fifth power."

Suppose we have a quantity raised to some power, say a^n, that is to be multiplied by the same quantity raised to another power, say a^m. In this event the result is that quantity raised to a power equal to the sum of the original exponents:

$$a^n \times a^m = a^n a^m = a^{n+m}$$

To convince ourselves that this is true, we can work out $a^3 \times a^4$:

$$(a \times a \times a)(a \times a \times a \times a) = a \times a \times a \times a \times a \times a \times a$$
$$a^3 a^4 = a^7$$

Because the process of multiplication is basically one of repeated addition,

$$(a^n)^m = a^{nm}$$

where $(a^n)^m$ means that a^n is to be multiplied by itself the number of times indicated by the exponent m. Thus

$$(a^2)^4 = a^{2 \times 4} = a^8$$

because

$$(a^2)^4 = a^2 \times a^2 \times a^2 \times a^2 = a^{2+2+2+2} = a^8$$

Reciprocal quantities are expressed according to the above scheme but with negative exponents:

$$\frac{1}{a} = a^{-1} \qquad \frac{1}{a^2} = a^{-2} \qquad \frac{1}{a^3} = a^{-3} \qquad \frac{1}{a^4} = a^{-4}$$

Roots

When the **square root** of a quantity is multiplied by itself, the product is equal to the quantity. The usual symbol for the square root of a quantity a is $\sqrt{a}$. Thus

$$\sqrt{a} \times \sqrt{a} = a$$

Here are some examples of square roots:

$\sqrt{1} = 1$	because	$1 \times 1 = 1$
$\sqrt{4} = 2$	because	$2 \times 2 = 4$
$\sqrt{9} = 3$	because	$3 \times 3 = 9$
$\sqrt{100} = 10$	because	$10 \times 10 = 100$
$\sqrt{30.25} = 5.5$	because	$5.5 \times 5.5 = 30.25$
$\sqrt{16B^2} = 4B$	because	$4B \times 4B = 16B^2$

In the case of a number smaller than 1, the square root is larger than the number itself:

$\sqrt{0.01} = 0.1$	because	$0.1 \times 0.1 = 0.01$
$\sqrt{0.25} = 0.5$	because	$0.5 \times 0.5 = 0.25$

Similarly, multiplying the **cube root** $\sqrt[3]{a}$ of a quantity a by itself twice yields the quantity:

$$\sqrt[3]{a} \times \sqrt[3]{a} \times \sqrt[3]{a} = a$$

An expression of the form $\sqrt[n]{a}$ is read as "the nth root of a"; for instance, $\sqrt[4]{16}$ is "the fourth root of 16" and is equal to 2 because $2 \times 2 \times 2 \times 2 = 16$.

Although procedures exist for finding square and cube roots arithmetically, in practice electronic calculators or printed tables are normally used nowadays.

Here is an example of how a square root arises naturally in physics. Let us solve for r the equation

$$F = K \frac{Q_1 Q_2}{r^2}$$

which expresses Coulomb's law of electric force. What we do is this:

Multiply both sides by r^2 to give $\qquad Fr^2 = KQ_1Q_2$

Divide both sides by F to give $\qquad r^2 = \dfrac{KQ_1Q_2}{F}$

Take square root of both sides to give $\qquad r = \sqrt{\dfrac{KQ_1Q_2}{F}}$

In algebra, a fractional exponent is used to indicate a root of a quantity. In terms of exponents we would write the square root of a as

$$\sqrt{a} = a^{1/2}$$

because

$$a^{1/2} \times a^{1/2} = (a^{1/2})^2 = a^{2\times1/2} = a^1 = a$$

In a similar way the "cube root" of a, which is $\sqrt[3]{a}$, is indicated by the exponent $\frac{1}{3}$ because

$$a^{1/3} \times a^{1/3} \times a^{1/3} = (a^{1/3})^3 = a^1 = a$$

In general, the nth root of any quantity is indicated by the exponent $1/n$:

$$\sqrt[n]{a} = a^{1/n}$$

A few examples will indicate how fractional exponents fit into the general pattern of exponential notation:

$$(a^6)^{1/2} = a^{(1/2)\times6} = a^3$$

$$(a^{1/2})^6 = a^{6\times1/2} = a^3$$

$$(a^3)^{-1/3} = a^{(-1/3)\times3} = a^{-1}$$

$$a^6a^{1/2} = a^{6+1/2} = a^{6\ 1/2}$$

Powers of 10

There is a convenient and widely used method for expressing very large and very small numbers that makes use of powers of 10. Any number in decimal form can be written as a number between 1 and 10 multiplied by some power of 10. The power of 10 is positive for numbers larger than 10 and negative for numbers smaller than 1. Positive powers of 10 follow this pattern:

$10^0 = 1$ $\qquad$ = 1 with decimal point moved 0 places
$10^1 = 10$ $\qquad$ = 1 with decimal point moved 1 place to the right
$10^2 = 100$ $\qquad$ = 1 with decimal point moved 2 places to the right
$10^3 = 1000$ $\qquad$ = 1 with decimal point moved 3 places to the right
$10^4 = 10{,}000$ $\quad$ = 1 with decimal point moved 4 places to the right
$10^5 = 100{,}000$ $\quad$ = 1 with decimal point moved 5 places to the right
$10^6 = 1{,}000{,}000$ = 1 with decimal point moved 6 places to the right

and so on. The exponent of 10 in each case indicates the number of places through which the decimal point is moved to the right from 1.00000 . . . . Equivalently, the exponent gives the number of zeroes that follow the 1.

Negative powers of 10 follow a similar pattern:

$10^0 \ =$ $\qquad$ 1 = 1 with decimal point moved 0 places
$10^{-1} =$ $\qquad$ 0.1 = 1 with decimal point moved 1 place to the left
$10^{-2} =$ $\qquad$ 0.01 = 1 with decimal point moved 2 places to the left
$10^{-3} =$ $\qquad$ 0.001 = 1 with decimal point moved 3 places to the left
$10^{-4} =$ $\quad$ $0.000{,}1$ = 1 with decimal point moved 4 places to the left
$10^{-5} =$ $\quad$ $0.000{,}01$ = 1 with decimal point moved 5 places to the left
$10^{-6} = 0.000{,}001$ = 1 with decimal point moved 6 places to the left

and so on. Here the exponent of 10 in each case shows the number of places through which the decimal point is moved to the left from 1. The number of zeroes between the decimal point and the 1 is one less than the exponent, that is, $n - 1$.

Here are some examples of powers-of-10 notation:

$$8000 = 8 \times 1000 = 8 \times 10^3$$
$$347 = 3.47 \times 100 = 3.47 \times 10^2$$
$$8{,}700{,}000 = 8.7 \times 1{,}000{,}000 = 8.7 \times 10^6$$
$$0.22 = 2.2 \times 0.1 = 2.2 \times 10^{-1}$$
$$0.000{,}035 = 3.5 \times 0.000{,}01 = 3.5 \times 10^5$$

An advantage of powers-of-10 notation is that it makes calculations involving large and small numbers easier to carry out. The rules for working with exponents that were reviewed in the previous section hold for exponents of 10. We have here

Multiplication: $\qquad 10^n \times 10^m = 10^{n+m}$

Division: $\qquad \dfrac{10^n}{10^m} = 10^{n-m}$

Raising to power: $\qquad (10^n)^m = 10^{nm}$

Taking a root: $\qquad (10^n)^{1/m} = 10^{n/m}$

An example will show how a calculation involving powers of 10 is worked out:

$$\frac{460 \times 0.000{,}03 \times 100{,}000}{9000 \times 0.006{,}2} = \frac{(4.6 \times 10^2) \times (3 \times 10^{-5}) \times (10^5)}{(9 \times 10^3) \times (6.2 \times 10^{-3})}$$
$$= \frac{4.6 \times 3}{9 \times 6.2} \times \frac{10^2 \times 10^{-5} \times 10^5}{10^3 \times 10^{-3}}$$
$$= 0.25 \times \frac{10^{2-5+5}}{10^{3-3}} = 0.25 \times \frac{10^2}{10^0}$$
$$= 25$$

Another virtue of this notation is that it permits us to express the accuracy with which a quantity is known in a clear way. The speed of light in free space c is often given as simply 3×10^8 m/s. If c were written out as 300,000,000 m/s we might be tempted to think the speed is precisely equal to this number, right down to the last zero. Actually, the speed of light is 299,792,458 m/s. For our purposes we do not need this much detail. By writing just $c = 3 \times 10^8$ we automatically indicate both how large the number is (the 10^8 tells how many decimal places are present) and how precise the quoted figure is (the single digit 3 means that c is closer to 3×10^8 than it is to either 2×10^8 or 4×10^8 m/s). If we wanted more precision, we could write $c = 2.998 \times 10^8$ m/s. Again how large c is and how precise the quoted figure is are both obvious at a glance.

To be sure, sometimes one or more zeroes in a number are meaningful in their own right and not solely decimal-point indicators. In the case of the speed of light, we can legitimately state that, to three-digit accuracy

$$c = 3.00 \times 10^8 \text{ m/s}$$

since c is closer to this figure than to 2.99×10^8 or 3.01×10^8 m/s. In the last sample calculation, the quantity $(4.6 \times 3)/(9 \times 6.2)$ actually equals 0.2473118. . . . It is rounded off to 0.25 because the result of a calculation may have no more significant digits than those in the least precise of the numbers that went into it.

Exercises

C. Express the following numbers in powers-of-10 notation:

1. $720 =$ **2.** $890,000 =$

3. $0.02 =$ **4.** $0.000,062 =$

5. $3.6 =$ **6.** $0.4 =$

7. $49,527 =$ **8.** $0.002,943 =$

9. $0.0014 =$ **10.** $49,000,000,000 =$

11. $0.000,000,011 =$ **12.** $1.4763 =$

D. Express the following numbers in decimal notation:

1. $3 \times 10^{-4} =$ **2.** $7.5 \times 10^3 =$

3. $8.126 \times 10^{-5} =$ **4.** $1.01 \times 10^8 =$

5. $5 \times 10^2 =$ **6.** $3.2 \times 10^{-2} =$

7. $4.32145 \times 10^3 =$ **8.** $6 \times 10^6 =$

9. $5.7 \times 10^0 =$ **10.** $6.9 \times 10^{-5} =$

E. Evaluate the following in powers-of-10 notation:

1. $\dfrac{30 \times 80,000,000,000}{0.0004} =$

2. $\dfrac{30,000 \times 0.000,000,6}{1000 \times 0.02} =$

3. $\dfrac{0.0001}{60,000 \times 200} =$

4. $5000 \times 0.005 =$

5. $\dfrac{5000}{0.005} =$

6. $\dfrac{200 \times 0.000,04}{400,000} =$

7. $\dfrac{0.002 \times 0.000,000,05}{0.000,004} =$

8. $\dfrac{500,000 \times 18,000}{9,000,000} =$

Answers

A.
1. 4.5
2. 0.8
3. −3
4. −1
5. 7
6. −7.5
7. 10

B.
1. 2
2. 5
3. −2
4. 1.5
5. −1
6. 2
7. 8
8. 2
9. 4
10. 0

C.
1. 7.2×10^2
2. 8.9×10^5
3. 2×10^{-2}
4. 6.2×10^{-5}
5. 3.6×10^0
6. 4×10^{-1}
7. 4.9527×10^4
8. 2.943×10^{-3}
9. 1.4×10^{-3}
10. 4.9×10^{10}
11. 1.1×10^{-8}
12. 1.4763×10^0

D. **1.** 0.0003

2. 7500

3. 0.000,081,26

4. 101,000,000

5. 500

6. 0.032

7. 4321.45

8. 6,000,000

9. 5.7

10. 0.000,069

E. **1.** 6×10^{15}

2. 9×10^{-4}

3. 8.3×10^{-11}

4. 2.5×10^{1}

5. 10^{6}

6. 2×10^{-8}

7. 2.5×10^{-5}

8. 10^{3}

The Elements

Atomic Number	Element	Symbol	Atomic Mass*	Atomic Number	Element	Symbol	Atomic Mass*	Atomic Number	Element	Symbol	Atomic Mass*
1	Hydrogen	H	1.008	39	Yttrium	Y	88.91	77	Iridium	Ir	192.2
2	Helium	He	4.003	40	Zirconium	Zr	91.22	78	Platinum	Pt	195.1
3	Lithium	Li	6.941	41	Niobium	Nb	92.91	79	Gold	Au	197.0
4	Beryllium	Be	9.012	42	Molybdenum	Mo	95.94	80	Mercury	Hg	200.6
5	Boron	B	10.81	43	Technetium	Tc	(97)	81	Thallium	Ti	204.4
6	Carbon	C	12.01	44	Ruthenium	Ru	101.1	82	Lead	Pb	207.2
7	Nitrogen	N	14.01	45	Rhodium	Rh	102.9	83	Bismuth	Bi	209.0
8	Oxygen	O	16.00	46	Palladium	Pd	106.4	84	Polonium	Po	(209)
9	Fluorine	F	19.00	47	Silver	Ag	107.9	85	Astatine	At	(210)
10	Neon	Ne	20.18	48	Cadmium	Cd	112.4	86	Radon	Rn	(222)
11	Sodium	Na	22.99	49	Indium	In	114.8	87	Francium	Fr	(223)
12	Magnesium	Mg	24.31	50	Tin	Sn	118.7	88	Radium	Ra	226.0
13	Aluminum	Al	26.98	51	Antimony	Sb	121.8	89	Actinium	Ac	(227)
14	Silicon	Si	28.09	52	Tellurium	Te	127.6	90	Thorium	Th	232.0
15	Phosphorus	P	30.97	53	Iodine	I	126.9	91	Protactinium	Pa	231.0
16	Sulfur	S	32.06	54	Xenon	Xe	131.3	92	Uranium	U	238.0
17	Chlorine	Cl	35.45	55	Cesium	Cs	132.9	93	Neptunium	Np	(237)
18	Argon	Ar	39.95	56	Barium	Ba	137.3	94	Plutonium	Pu	(244)
19	Potassium	K	39.10	57	Lanthanum	La	138.9	95	Americium	Am	(243)
20	Calcium	Ca	40.08	58	Cerium	Ce	140.1	96	Curium	Cm	(247)
21	Scandium	Sc	44.96	59	Praseodymium	Pr	140.9	97	Berkelium	Bk	(247)
22	Titanium	Ti	47.90	60	Neodymium	Nd	144.2	98	Californium	Cf	(251)
23	Vanadium	V	50.94	61	Promethium	Pm	(145)	99	Einsteinium	Es	(252)
24	Chromium	Cr	52.00	62	Samarium	Sm	150.4	100	Fermium	Fm	(257)
25	Manganese	Mn	54.94	63	Europium	Eu	152.0	101	Mendelevium	Md	(260)
26	Iron	Fe	55.85	64	Gadolinium	Gd	157.3	102	Nobelium	No	(259)
27	Cobalt	Co	58.93	65	Terbium	Tb	158.9	103	Lawrencium	Lw	(262)
28	Nickel	Ni	58.70	66	Dysprosium	Dy	162.5	104	Rutherfordium	Rf	(261)
29	Copper	Cu	63.54	67	Holmium	Ho	164.9	105	Dubnium	Db	(262)
30	Zinc	Zn	65.38	68	Erbium	Er	167.3	106	Seaborgium	Sg	(263)
31	Gallium	Ga	69.72	69	Thulium	Tm	168.9	107	Bohrium	Bh	(262)
32	Germanium	Ge	72.59	70	Ytterbium	Yb	173.0	108	Hassium	Hs	(265)
33	Arsenic	As	74.92	71	Lutetium	Lu	175.0	109	Meitnerium	Mt	(266)
34	Selenium	Se	78.96	72	Hafnium	Hf	178.5	110	Darmstadtium	Ds	(271)
35	Bromine	Br	79.90	73	Tantalum	Ta	180.9	111	Roentgenium	Rg	(272)
36	Krypton	Kr	83.80	74	Tungsten	W	183.9	112	Copernicium	Cn	(285)
37	Rubidium	Rb	85.47	75	Rhenium	Re	186.2	**			
38	Strontium	Sr	87.62	76	Osmium	Os	190.2				

*Masses in parentheses are those of the most stable isotopes of the elements.

**Elements with atomic numbers 113–118 have been created in the laboratory in small quantities but not yet named.

Answers to Multiple Choice Questions and Odd-Numbered Exercises

Chapter 1

Multiple Choice

1. a	**7.** a	**13.** c	**19.** d
2. d	**8.** d	**14.** d	**20.** b
3. a	**9.** d	**15.** a	**21.** b
4. a	**10.** d	**16.** c	**22.** d
5. a	**11.** a	**17.** c	**23.** c
6. b	**12.** b	**18.** c	**24.** a

Exercises

1. None. The scientific method is based on observation and experiment together with reasoning from their results.

3. When first proposed, a scientific interpretation is called a hypothesis. If the hypothesis states a regularity or relationship, it is called a law after it has been verified by further observation and experiment. If the hypothesis uses general considerations to account for specific findings, it is called a theory after it has been verified.

5. Science is a reliable guide to the natural world precisely because it is self-correcting by being open to change in the light of new evidence.

7. Locate the Big Dipper constellation and follow the pointer stars at the end of its bowl to Polaris, which is north of your location.

9. At the North or South Pole.

11. The moon's apparent diameter remains constant, and its eastward motion through the sky is uniform.

13. In the ptolemaic model, the sun, moon, and other planets all revolve around the earth. In the copernican model, the moon revolves around the earth, and the earth and the other planets revolve around the sun with the earth rotating daily on its axis. There is direct observational evidence that supports the copernican model.

15. Ptolemaic system: (a) the sun circles the earth every day; (b) the stars circle the earth in a little less than a day, so that the difference between the speeds of the sun and stars causes the sun to move eastward relative to the stars; (c) the moon circles the earth.

   Copernican system: (a) the earth turns on its axis once a day; (b) the earth moves around the sun once a year; (c) the moon circles the earth as the earth moves around the sun.

17. Yes, because $T_e^2/R_e^3 = T_a^2/R_a^3$.

19. Gravity cannot be understood in terms of any other force whereas the force a bat exerts on a ball can be traced to the action of the electromagnetic force.

21. The tidal range is a maximum at spring tides, a minimum at neap tides. At spring tides, the sun, moon, and earth are in a straight line. At neap tides, the moon-earth line is perpendicular to the sun-earth line.

23. The moon revolves around the earth in the same direction as the earth's rotation. Hence the moon is in the same place relative to a point on the earth's surface about 50 minutes later every day.

25. Centimeter; yard; kilometer.

27. $(368 \text{ ft})(0.0305 \text{ m/ft}) = 112 \text{ m}; (112 \text{ m})/(1000 \text{ m/km}) = 0.112 \text{ km}$

29. 10.8 ft^2.

31. $(80 \text{ km})(0.621 \text{ mi/km}) = 50 \text{ mi}$, hence $80 \text{ km/h} = 50 \text{ mi/h}$.

33. $10^6/10^{-6} = 10^{12}$.

Chapter 2

Multiple Choice

1. c	**13.** c	**25.** d	**37.** d
2. d	**14.** a	**26.** c	**38.** c
3. c	**15.** d	**27.** a	**39.** c
4. d	**16.** c	**28.** b	**40.** b
5. c	**17.** a	**29.** c	**41.** b
6. c	**18.** c	**30.** d	**42.** d
7. b	**19.** d	**31.** c	**43.** b
8. b	**20.** b	**32.** d	**44.** d
9. d	**21.** a	**33.** c	**45.** d
10. c	**22.** b	**34.** c	**46.** d
11. b	**23.** c	**35.** d	**47.** c
12. d	**24.** a, b, c	**36.** a	**48.** a

Exercises

1. $d = vt = 960$ m for the round trip, hence the distance to the cliff is $d/2 = 480$ m.

3. $v = d_1/t_1 = 3.14$ m/s; $t_2 = d_2/v = 1.6$ s.

5. $d = $ total distance $= 4$ km; $t = $ total time $= d_1/v_1 + d_2/v_2 = 0.583$ h; $v(\text{av}) = d/t = 6.86$ km/h.

7. No. The distinction between vector and scalar quantities is that vector quantities have directions associated with them, and both kinds of quantity are found in the physical world.

9. $d^2 = (70 \text{ m})^2 + (40 \text{ m})^2 = 6500 \text{ m}^2$, $d = \sqrt{d^2} = 81$ m.

11. Yes.

13. $a = (80 \text{ km/h})/20 \text{ s} = (4 \text{ km/h})/\text{s}$; hence with $v_0 = 80$ km/h and $v = 130$ km/h, $t = (v - v_0)/a = 12.5$ s.

15. $a = v_1/t = 4$ m/s^2, $v_2 = v_1 + at = 60$ m/s.

17. (a) $a = (v_2 - v_1)/t = 6$ s.
    (b) $d = v_1 t + (1/2)at^2 = 105$ m.

19. Average acceleration is $a = 2d/t^2 = 2$ m/s^2 and final speed is $v = at = 40$ m/s.

21. The squirrel should stay where it is, because if it drops from the tree when the rifle is fired, it will fall exactly as fast as the bullet and hence will be struck by it. If the squirrel stays in the tree, the bullet will pass below it because the bullet is acted upon by gravity and the hunter, in aiming directly at the squirrel, has not allowed for the fall of the bullet.

23. When thrown; at the top of the path.

25. (a) Yes. (b) The stone thrown horizontally is moving faster because its velocity has a horizontal as well as a vertical component.

27. (a) The same time. When dropped, the coin has the same initial speed as the elevator, so this constant speed does not affect the motion of the coin relative to the elevator. (b) More time. The downward acceleration of the elevator is not shared by the coin; hence the coin's acceleration relative to the elevator is less than g by the amount of the elevator's acceleration. (c) The same time for the reason given in (a). (d) Less time. The upward acceleration of the elevator is not shared by the coin, hence the coin's acceleration relative to the elevator is more than g by the amount of the elevator's acceleration.

29. The dive lasts $t = -\sqrt{2h/g} = 2.6$ s and the person enters the water at $v = gt = 25$ m/s.

31. $v = v_0 + gt = 21.8$ m/s.

33. (a) $v_2 = v_1 + gt = +1.1$ m/s, which is upward.
(b) Now $v_2 = -13.6$ m/s, which is downward.

35. (a) $v_0 = 30$ m/s and at the highest point $v = 0$. Since $v = v_0 - gt$, $t = (v_0 - v)/g = 3.06$ s. (b) The time of fall equals the time of rise, so total time is $(2)(3.06$ s$) = 6.12$ s. (c) 30 m/s.

37. (a) Since $h = (1/2)gt^2$, $t = \sqrt{2h/g} = 15.6$ s. (b) The horizontal speed of the wiper is $v_h = 100$ m/s, so $d = v_h t = 1.56$ km. (c) The vertical speed of the wiper is $v_v = gt = 153$ m/s. Hence $v = \sqrt{v_v^2 + v_h^2} = 182$ m/s.

39. (a) $h = (1/2)gt^2 = 123$ m. (b) $d = v_h t = 1$ km.
(c) The vertical speed of the bullet is $v_v = gt = 49$ m/s. Hence $v = \sqrt{v_v^2 + v_h^2} = 206$ m/s.

41. When the wrench is dropped, it is moving at the same speed as the boat and in the same direction. The downward speed of the wrench increases as it falls, but its horizontal speed remains the same as that of the boat. Therefore the wrench hits the deck directly below the point from which it was dropped. Only if the boat were accelerated would it be possible for the wrench to miss the deck.

43. $F = ma = m(v/t)$, $t = mv/F = 16.8$ s.

45. $a = F/m = 3.33$ m/s^2; $t = v/a = 7.2$ s.

47. $a = v/t = 1.5$ m/s^2; $F = ma = 120$ N.

49. $F = m_1 a_1 = 1920$ N; $a_2 = F/m_2 = 1.04$ m/s

51. The kilogram is a unit of mass, not of weight. It is correct to say either that Sarah has a mass of 55 kg or that she weighs 539 N.

53. g(moon) $= (85/490)g$(earth) $= 1.7$ m/s^2.

55. (a) If he slides down at constant speed, the rope is supporting his entire weight of $mg = 784$ N. (b) To climb up, an additional force must be exerted on the rope, so it will break.

57. $a = [(50 - 6)$ m/s$]/2$ s $= 22$ m/s^2.
$F = mg + ma = 3180$ N; $F/mg = 3.18$.

59. (a) Down.
(b) Yes; $F = 100$ N, $m = w/g = 71.4$ kg, $a = F/m = 1.4$ m/s^2.

61. Action and reaction forces always act on different bodies.

63. (a) The reaction force is the upward force exerted by the table on the book; without this force the book would fall to the floor. (b) The reaction force is the gravitational pull the book exerts on the earth.

65. A propeller works by pushing backward on the air whose reaction force in turn pushes the propeller itself and the airplane it is attached to forward. No air, no reaction force, so the idea is no good.

67. (a) $F = ma = 270$ N. (b) Yes; 270 N backward.

69. Under no circumstances.

71. The right wheels.

73. $F_c = mv^2/r$, $r = mv^2/F_c = 60$ m.

75. $F = 4 mg = mv^2/r$, $r = v^2/4 g$, $= 2.30$ km.

77. $F = mv^2/r = 267$ N.

79. Sprinters could not improve their time in the 100-m dash on the moon because their masses are the same there as on the earth. With the force that their legs can exert also unchanged, their acceleration will be the same, and hence their motion will not differ from that on the earth.

81. At an altitude of two earth's radii, the mass would be the same, but the weight would be $\frac{1}{9}$ as great because the distance from the earth's center is three times as great and gravitational force varies as $1/r^2$.

83. The sun's gravitational pull on the earth varies during the year since the distance from the earth to the sun varies.

85. The earth must travel faster when it is nearest the sun in order to counteract the greater gravitational force of the sun.

87. $F = Gm_1 m_2/r^2 = 7.4 \times 10^{-8}$ N. Since 1 g $= 10^{-3}$ kg, 1 g of anything weighs $w = mg = 9.8 \times 10^{-3}$ N, which is more than 10^5 (a hundred thousand) times as great as the gravitational force of the lead on the cheese.

89. No, because they and the airplane are "falling" at the same rate.

91. No. A gravitational force always acts on an astronaut in an orbiting spacecraft, so the astronaut has weight. The sensation of "weightlessness" occurs because there is no upward reaction force on the astronaut.

Chapter 3

Multiple Choice

1. c	**9.** c	**17.** a	**25.** c
2. d	**10.** c	**18.** d	**26.** d
3. b, c, d	**11.** d	**19.** a	**27.** c
4. a, c	**12.** c	**20.** d	**28.** a
5. a	**13.** a	**21.** b	**29.** c
6. d	**14.** d	**22.** b	**30.** a
7. d	**15.** d	**23.** c	**31.** a
8. a	**16.** b	**24.** a	**32.** a

Exercises

1. Yes, because all changes require that work be done.

3. $W = 0$ because the earth moves perpendicular to the direction of the force acting on it from the sun.

5. $m = W/gh = (490$ J$)/(9.8$ m/s$^2)(10$ m$) = 5$ kg.

7. The work done is the same, so $mg_e h_e = mg_m h_m$, $h_m = (g_e/g_m)h_e = 53$ cm.

9. $P = Fv$, $F = P/v = 14.4$ kN.

11. $P = mgh/t = 1.26$ kW.

13. $W = Fd = Pt$, $F = Pt/d = P/v = 0.21$ kN. The horse's mass does not matter.

15. Efficiency $= (mgh/t)/P_{\text{input}} = 0.78 = 78$ percent.

17. 1 kJ.

19. $d = $ KE$/F = 5$ m.

21. $Fd = \frac{1}{2}mv^2$, $F = mv^2/2d = 0.96$ kN.

23. $P = ($KE$_2 - KE_1)/t$, $t = ($KE$_2 - KE_1)/P = 7.5$ s.

25. (a) PE increases. (b) PE decreases.

27. When it is farthest from the sun; when it is closest to the sun. The work needed to pull a planet away from the sun to a given distance increases with the distance, so the planet's PE is greatest the farthest it is from the sun. The gravitational force of the sun on a planet is greatest when it is closest to the sun; hence its speed is also greatest there in order that gravitational and centripetal forces be in balance.

29. Ball A reaches the bottom first because all of its original PE becomes KE of downward motion. Part of B's original PE becomes KE of its rotation, so there is less PE available to become KE of downward motion. As a result B moves more slowly than A and reaches the bottom first.

31. $mgh_1 = 0.9\, mgh_2$, $h_2 = 0.9\, h_1 = 0.9$ m.

33. $mv_2^2 = mv_1^2 + mgh$, $v_2 = \sqrt{v_1^2 + 2gh} = 16$ m/s. The skier's KE at the bottom is equal to her KE at the top plus the change in her PE.

35. Most of the work done in hammering the nail is dissipated as heat owing to friction between the nail and the wood.

37. $t = d/v = 1250$ s, $W = Pt = 1.75 \times 10^6$ J; hence 1.75×10^6 J/$(4 \times 10^4$ J/g$) = 44$ g of fat is metabolized.

39. (a) $W = Fd = 1760$ J. (b) PE $= mgh = 1568$ J. (c) 192 J was lost as heat due to friction in the pulleys.

41. Their speeds are the same. The golf ball, which has the greater mass, has the greater KE, PE, and momentum.

43. Most of the momentum is given to the earth through the road and the rest is given to the air the car was moving through.

45. Since $2 \times \left(\frac{1}{2}mv^2\right) = \frac{1}{2}m(\sqrt{2}v)^2$, the speed increases by $\sqrt{2}$ and so the momentum increases by $\sqrt{2}$ as well.

47. (a) When $m = M$. (b) When m is less than M. (c) When m is greater than M.

49. (a) The speed decreases as rainwater collects in the truck, since the total momentum must remain constant. (b) The reduced speed is unchanged because the water that leaked out carried with it the momentum it has gained.

51. Here $m_2 = 40$ kg, so $v_2 = m_1 v_1/m_2 = 2.25$ m/s.

53. Let Δ stand for "change in." Then $m_1 \Delta v_1 = m_2 \Delta v_2$, $\Delta v_2 = \Delta v_1$ $(m_1/m_2) = 17$ m/s; $vf = v_1 - \Delta v = 28$ m/s.

55. (a) The 40-kg skater has the greater initial momentum, so the pair move off in the initial direction of the 40-kg skater; $m_1 v_1$ $+ m_2 v_2 = (m_1 + m_2)v_3$, $v_3 = 0.4$ m/s. (b) $KE_2 - KE_1 = \frac{1}{2}(m_1 v_1^2$ $+ mv) - \frac{1}{2}(m_1 v_3^2 + m_2 v_3^2) = 432$ J.

57. The resulting water will add to the oceans, and more of the earth's mass will be distant from its axis than before. Conservation of angular momentum requires that the earth in that event spin more slowly to compensate, and the day will be longer.

59. As in the case of a skater pulling in her arms (see Sec. 4.10), conservation of angular momentum required that the earth spin faster when it became smaller. (This has shortened the length of the day by about 3 microseconds.)

61. The predictions of relativity apply at much higher speeds than those in everyday life, and these predictions are supported by experimental evidence.

63. The rod appears longest to the stationary observer.

65. The KE of a moving object increases with its speed until it would be infinite at the speed of light. Since nothing can have an infinite amount of KE, the speed of light is the ultimate speed limit.

67. Mass must be considered as a form of energy.

69. $m = E/c^2 = 3.35 \times 10^5$ J$/(3 \times 10^8$ m/s$)^2 = 3.7 \times 10^{-12}$ kg.

71. The total rest energy of 1 kJ of anything is $mc^2 = 9 \times 10^{16}$ J. Here $(5.4 \times 10^6)/(9 \times 10^{16}) = 6 \times 10^{-11}$, which is 6×10^{-9} percent.

Chapter 4

Multiple Choice

1. d	**11.** a	**21.** a	**31.** a
2. b, a, c, d	**12.** c	**22.** b	**32.** b
3. b	**13.** b	**23.** d	**33.** d
4. d	**14.** d, a, c, b	**24.** d	**34.** c
5. d	**15.** a, d	**25.** b	**35.** a
6. c	**16.** a	**26.** b	**36.** b
7. a	**17.** d	**27.** a	**37.** b
8. c	**18.** a	**28.** a	**38.** d
9. a	**19.** a	**29.** a	**39.** d
10. d	**20.** d	**30.** c	**40.** d

Exercises

1. (a) The world's population is increasing and becoming more prosperous, so it will need more energy. (b) Most of today's energy comes from fossil fuels, whose supply will eventually run out. (c) Burning fossil fuels produces CO_2, the leading cause of global warming.

3. Six times.

5. Food and wood: photosynthesis in plants is powered by sunlight. Water power: sunlight evaporates water that later falls as rain and snow on high ground. Wind power: unequal heating of the earth's surface causes motions in the atmosphere. Fossil fuels: they come from the remains of living things, which contain energy ultimately derived from sunlight through photosynthesis.

7. Nearly half the world's population.

9. Seawater and the earth's surface absorb solar radiation more efficiently than ice, which is very reflective, so global warming and further melting will persist.

11. Millions of years ago.

13. Sunlight that strikes the earth's surface heats it, and the surface itself then radiates infrared light. The atmosphere allows visible light from the sun to pass through it, but various gases in it absorb infrared light and it is this absorbed infrared light that heats the atmosphere.

15. It is absorbed by oceans, soils, and forests.

17. Coal contributes the most CO_2, then oil, and last natural gas.

19. Transportation.

21. In regenerative braking, the electric motors of an electric or hybrid gasoline-electric car act as generators to convert KE of the car's motion into electric energy that charges the car's batteries. This is more efficient than using normal friction brakes that waste the KE by converting it into heat.

23. For the same amount of energy produced, coal is cheaper than natural gas.

25. Shale gas is methane trapped in porous beds of a rock called shale. Methane clathrate consists of ice crystals with methane molecules trapped inside them; clathrate deposits are found under the oceans near shore and under permafrost in cold parts of the world. There are immense amounts of methane in both shale beds and in clathrates, and extraction technology is being developed.

27. One-half.

29. Coal is almost pure carbon whereas oil and natural gas also contain hydrogen whose burning produces water rather than carbon dioxide.

31. (a) In fission, a large atomic nucleus splits into two smaller ones. In fusion, two small nuclei join to form a larger one. (b) Both processes give off large amounts of energy.

33. Heat from the nuclear fissions in the reactor is used to produce steam that runs turbines connected to electric generators.

35. Safe operation; abundant, cheap fuel; little radioactive waste; no greenhouse gas emissions.

37. Nuclear fusion is the energy source of the sun and stars.

39. Hydropower.

41. A photovoltaic cell converts energy in sunlight directly to electric energy. It is also called a solar cell.

43. Average output per turbine $= (0.4)(2$ M$) = 0.8$ MW, hence $(500$ MW$)/(0.8$ MW/turbine$) = 625$ turbines.

45. Geothermal energy is a continuous source that does not vary with time of day or weather conditions.

47. (a) On the earth, hydrogen is found only combined with other elements from which it must first be separated. (b) At ordinary temperatures and pressures, hydrogen is a gas, which makes it difficult to transport and store.

49. (a) Corn ethanol is expensive; so much energy is needed in all the steps involved that there is little or no energy gain; on an overall basis, CO_2 emissions are not reduced; agricultural land is diverted from food production at a time of population growth. (b) The needed technology has not yet been perfected.

51. Seconds per year = (365 days)(24 h/day)(3600 s/h) = 3.15×10^7 s, hence $P = E/t = 2.1 \times 10^3$ W = 2.1 kW.

53. (a) An overall cap on emissions is set and companies are given or buy at auction permits to emit CO_2 whose total equals the cap. Companies with unused permits can sell them to companies that need additional ones. (b) Tax CO_2 emissions, so that products and services with high CO_2 emissions are more expensive than comparable ones using better technology instead of being cheaper as at present.

Chapter 5

Multiple Choice

1. d	13. d	25. d	37. c
2. d	14. d	26. a	38. c
3. d	15. a	27. a	39. d
4. a	16. b	28. b	40. b
5. c	17. d	29. c	41. c
6. a	18. a	30. d	42. d
7. a	19. c	31. c	43. c
8. b	20. d	32. b	44. a
9. b	21. c	33. b	45. b
10. d	22. b	34. d	
11. d	23. b	35. b	
12. c	24. d	36. b	

Exercises

1. The metal expands more than the glass when heated, thereby loosening the lid.

3. White; red.

5. $T_F = \frac{9}{5}(20°) + 32° = 68°F$.

7. $T_C = \frac{5}{9}(T_F - 32°) = -80°C$.

9. A piece of ice at 0°C is more effective in cooling a drink than the same weight of water at 0°C because of the heat of fusion that must be added to the ice before it melts. Hence the ice will absorb more heat from the drink than the cold water.

11. Aluminum, because it has the highest specific heat.

13. The temperature difference is 80°C and 4.19 kJ/kg is needed per 1°C change in temperature. Hence $E = (4.19$ kJ/kg · °C$)(80°C)(0.2$ kg$) = 67$ kJ.

15. Since 4.19 kJ increases the temperature of 1 kg of water by 1°C, 12,000 kJ increases the temperature of 60 kg of water by $(12{,}000$ kJ$)/(4.19$ kJ/kg · °C$)(60$ kg$) = 48°C$.

17. $Q = mc\Delta T$, $\Delta T = Q/mc = 67°C$.

19. The stone's energy is $mgh = 9800$ J = 9.8 kJ. Since 4.19 kJ increases the temperature of 1 kg of water by 1°C and here there is 10^4 kg of water, the temperature rise is $(9.8$ kJ$)/(4.19$ kJ/kg · °C$)(10^4$ kg$) = 2.3 \times 10^{-4}$ °C.

21. $m = dV = dLWH = 78$ kg.

23. The density of the bracelet is $d = m/V = 12.5$ g/cm³ = 1.25×10^4 kg/m³. Since the density of gold is 1.9×10^4 kg/m³, the bracelet cannot be pure gold.

25. (a) $V = m/d = 0.055$ m³ = 55 L. (b) $V = m/d = 140$ m³.

27. (a) $d = m/V = 3m/4\pi r^3 = 5.52 \times 10^3$ kg/m. (b) The interior of the earth must consist of denser materials than those at the surface; no.

29. The person reduces the pressure in the straw by sucking on it, and atmospheric pressure then forces the liquid upward.

31. Since the heights of the water columns are the same, the pressures are the same.

33. $p = F/A = 1.5 \times 10^5$ N/m² = 150 kPa.

35. $A = F/p = mg/p = 0.0588$ m²; 1/4 of this is 147 cm².

37. (a) $F = pA = 0.12$ N. (b) An external pressure exerted on a fluid is transmitted uniformly throughout the fluid.

39. (a) Because pressure in a fluid increases with depth, the upward force on the bottom of a submerged object is greater than the downward force on its top. (b) If the buoyant force exceeds the object's weight, it will float.

41. The block will stay where it is because there is no water underneath it to furnish a buoyant force.

43. (a) The weight of the ship is unchanged, hence the volume of water it displaces is unchanged. (b) Because the volume of the ship's hull is now greater, the height of its deck above water increases.

45. The water level is unchanged.

47. The boat is more stable in freshwater because the buoyancy of its keel is less there.

49. The anchor's volume is $V = m/d = 0.0128$ m². The weight of water the anchor displaces is $w = mg = Vdg = 129$ N, which is the buoyant force on the anchor. Hence $F = mg - F(\text{buoyant}) = 851$ N.

51. The raft's volume is $V = (L)(W)(H) = 1.8$ m³. The maximum upward force the raft can exert is (buoyant force − weight of raft) = $d(\text{water})gV - d(\text{balsa})gV = 15.3$ kN. Each person weighs $mg = 637$ N so 24 people can be supported.

53. (a) The mass of 200 L = 0.2 m³ of seawater is $m = dV = 206$ kg, so the empty tank can support up to 206 kg. The empty tank will therefore float. (b) The mass of 0.2 m³ of freshwater is 200 kg, so the mass of the filled tank is 236 kg and it will sink. (c) The mass of 0.2 m³ of gasoline is 136 kg, so the mass of the filled tank is now 172 kg and it will float.

55. (a) $V_2 = p_1V_1/p_2 = 333$ cm³. (b) $T_1 = 273$ K, $T_2 = 546$ K, $V_2 = V_1T_2/T_1 = 2000$ cm³.

57. The volume of oxygen at atmospheric pressure is $V(\text{atm}) = V(\text{cyl})p(\text{cyl})/p(\text{atm}) = 6.73$ m³ so its mass is $m = dV = 9.4$ kg.

59. $T_1 = 293$ K, $T_2 = T_1V_2/V_1 = 586$ K = 313°C.

61. $T_1 = 293$ K, $T_2 = p_2T_1/p_1 = 410$ K = 137°C.

63. No. The only temperature scale on which such a comparison might make sense is the absolute temperature scale.

65. The molecules themselves occupy volume.

67. Lower.

69. The thermal energy of a solid resides in oscillations of its particles about fixed positions.

71. $T = 27°C = 300$ K. Since the average energy is proportional to the average temperature, doubling the energy doubles the temperature to 600 K = 327°C.

73. At the same temperature the average KE of the hydrogen and CO_2 molecules is the same. Hence $m_H v_H^2 = m_{CO_2} v_{CO_2}^2$, $v_{CO_2} = v_H\sqrt{m_H/m_{CO_2}} = 0.34$ km/s.

75. Metals are better conductors of heat than wood and therefore conduct heat away from your hand more rapidly.

77. In this location convection is most efficient, which increases the rate of heat transfer to the water.

79. The water molecules with the highest energies leave the liquid surface, and blowing them away prevents them from returning to the liquid. The remaining liquid contains the less energetic molecules, which means it is cooler.

81. (a) Increase the liquid temperature, which increases the average molecular KE while leaving unchanged the intermolecular attractive forces. (b) Reduce the pressure above the liquid, which decreases the likelihood that vapor molecules will return to the liquid after colliding with air molecules. (c) Arrange for a current of air to blow over the liquid surface, which will remove vapor molecules before they can return to the liquid. (d) Increase the area of the liquid surface, which brings more liquid molecules to the surface, where it is easiest for them to leave.

83. To heat the water to 100°C the heat needed is (4.19 kJ/kg · °C)(1 kg)(80°C) = 335 kJ.

Thus the water is heated to 100°C with 165 kJ left over. The mass of water turned into steam is (165 kJ)/(2260 kJ/kg) = 0.073 kg = 73 g.

85. $Q = m(c\Delta T + \text{heat of vaporization}) = 561$ kJ. Since $Q = Pt$, $t = Q/P = 468$ s = 7.8 min.

87. (a) Higher than 50°C. (b) Lower than 50°C. (c) Higher than 50°C. (d) 50°C.

89. There is no low-temperature reservoir for it to use.

91. The kitchen will warm up because the refrigerator gives off more heat than it absorbs. Leaving its door open means that it will run continuously and hence add even more heat to the kitchen.

93. No.

95. Eff(max) = $1 - T_2/T_1 = 0.65 = 65$ percent; hence the actual efficiency is 62 percent of the maximum possible.

97. Eff(max) = $1 - T_{\text{cold}}/T_{\text{hot}} = 0.073 = 7.3$ percent. The hot and cold reservoirs are enormous.

99. The entropy decrease involved in the evolution of today's animals is more than balanced by the entropy increase that occurred as the food the living things took in, digested, and metabolized lost its initial order. The food itself also represented an increase in entropy, as mentioned in Sec. 5.16.

Chapter 6

Multiple Choice

1. d	**13.** a	**28.** d
2. b	**14.** c	**29.** b
3. d	**15.** a	**30.** a
4. b	**16.** d	**31.** b
5. c	**17.** d	**32.** d
6. c	**18.** b	**33.** d
7. d	**19.** b	**34.** a
8. a	**20.** c	**35.** b
9. b	**21.** c	**36.** d
10. b	**22.** b	**37.** c
11. a	**23.** c	**38.** a
12. a. ohm	**24.** c	**39.** c
b. ampere	**25.** d	**40.** d
c. volt	**26.** a	**41.** a
d. watt	**27.** b	**42.** b

Exercises

1. Experiments show that every charge is either attracted or repelled by a + or a − charge; a charge that is attracted by a + charge is always repelled by a − charge, and vice versa; every charge obeys Coulomb's law when brought near a known charge; and so forth. Since all electrical phenomena can be accounted for on the basis of two kinds of charge only, there is no reason to suppose any other kind of charge exists.

3. (a) Since the ball is positively charged, it has fewer electrons than are needed for neutrality. (b) $N = Q/e = 6.25 \times 10^6$ electrons.

5. Protons in its nucleus provide the positive charge of an atom, and the electrons that surround the nucleus provide the negative charge.

7. The number of protons is $N = m/m_p = 6.0 \times 10^{23}$ protons, so $Q = Ne = 1.6 \times 10^4$ C.

9. No; yes.

11. $F = Ke^2/R^2 = 4.2 \times 10^{-8}$ N.

13. $F = Kq_1q_2/r^2 = 5.4 \times 10^{-7}$ N.

15. $F_2/F_1 = (R_1/R_2)^2$, $R_2 = R_1\sqrt{F_1/F_2} = 20$ mm.

17. (a) $F = Kq_1q_2/r^2 = 180$ N. (b) When the charges are brought into contact, the 1×10^{-5} C positive charge cancels out this amount of negative charge to leave -1×10^{-5} C. The latter charge is equally divided between the spheres, so when they are separated, the force between them is $F = (9 \times 10^9)(5 \times 10^{-6})(5 \times 10^{-6})/(0.1)^2$ N = 23 N and is now repulsive.

19. $r = \sqrt{KQ_1Q_2/F} = 1.7$ mm.

21. A current would flow briefly and then stop as charge builds up on the lightbulb and prevents further charge from being transferred.

23. The need for extremely low temperatures.

25. (a) Electric charge. (b) $W = QV = 4.32 \times 10^5$ J.

27. $W = QV = 8 \times 10^8$ J.

29. $I = V/R = 10$ A.

31. $V = IR = 75$ V.

33. In series, in order that the full circuit current flows through it. If the fuse were in parallel, the current in the circuit could rise to an unsafe level without blowing the fuse.

35. (a) In series, the batteries are connected in line with the + terminal of one battery attached to the − terminal of the next. The voltages of the batteries add, so the voltage of the combination is greater than that of the individual batteries. (b) In parallel, batteries with the same voltage are connected with all their + terminals attached together and all their − terminals attached together. The voltage of the combination is the same as that of each battery, but the combination can provide more current than each battery could by itself.

37. (a) $I = P/V = 0.625$ A. (b) $R = V/I = 192$ Ω.

39. $I = P/V = 1.7$ A.

41. $P = IV = 3600$ W; 36 bulbs.

43. $W = Pt = IVt = 2.7$ kWh = 9.7 MJ.

45. (a) $I = P/V = 7.4 \times 10^{-5}$ A. (b) $Q = 1.5$ C/s $\times$ 3600 s = 5400 C; $W = QV = 7290$ J; $t = W/P = 7.29 \times 10^3$ J/10^{-4} W = 7.29×10^7 s = 844 days = 2.3 years since 1 day = 86,400 s and 1 year = 365 days.

47. Either pole of the magnet attracts opposite poles within the iron, leading to a net attractive force since these poles line up facing the external magnet.

49. At a given point a test body free to move travels along a field line, by definition, and it can travel in only one direction at that point.

51. Direction D.

53. Attract; repel.

55. 0° or 180°; 90°.

57. To the left.

59. The magnetic field through the loop undergoes both an increase and a decrease in each half of a complete rotation.

61. When the generator is connected to an outside circuit, work must be done to turn its shaft as the current produced delivers energy to the circuit.

63. The changing magnetic field produced by an alternating current.

65. When the connection is made, a momentary current will occur in the secondary winding as the current in the primary builds up to its final value. Afterward, since the primary current will be constant and hence its magnetic field will not change, there will be no current in the secondary.

67. (a) $N_1/N_2 = V_1/V_2 = (5000 \text{ V})/(240 \text{ V}) = 20.8$. (b) $P = IV$ so $I_2 = P/V_2 = (10,000 \text{ W})/(240 \text{ V}) = 41.7$ A.

Chapter 7

Multiple Choice

1. b	**13.** c	**25.** d	**37.** d
2. d	**14.** d	**26.** c	**38.** b, d
3. d	**15.** d	**27.** a	**39.** b
4. a, b, c, d	**16.** c	**28.** a	**40.** c
5. a	**17.** d	**29.** d	**41.** b
6. d	**18.** d	**30.** a	**42.** a
7. a	**19.** d	**31.** b	**43.** b
8. d	**20.** c	**32.** c	**44.** c
9. d	**21.** b	**33.** a	**45.** c
10. b	**22.** c	**34.** b	
11. d	**23.** c	**35.** c	
12. b	**24.** d	**36.** c	

Exercises

1. (a) In a longitudinal wave, the particles of the medium vibrate parallel to the direction in which the wave is moving. In a transverse wave, the particles vibrate perpendicularly to this direction. (b) No; water waves are a combination of both.

3. $f = 1/(1.2 \text{ s}) = 0.83$ Hz, $v = f\lambda = 5$ m/s.

5. $v = f/\lambda = 0.3$ m/s; $t = d/v = 3$ s.

7. Sound travels fastest in solids because their constituent particles are more tightly bound together than those of liquids and gases. Sound travels slowest in gases because their molecules interact only during random collisions.

9. The moon has no atmosphere to transmit sound waves.

11. The distance of the man from the spike is $d = v_s t_1 = 686$ m, where $v_s = 343$ m/s is the speed of sound in air. Hence the speed of sound v in the rail is $v = d/t_2 = 686$ m/0.14 s = 4900 m/s.

13. $f = v/\lambda = (343 \text{ m/s})/0.25$ m = 1372 Hz.

15. $10^4 = 10,000$ times stronger.

17. In all kinds of waves.

19. A shift toward the red end of the spectrum means a shift to lower frequencies, which corresponds to motion away from the earth.

21. When light is absorbed, the absorbing material is heated.

23. The electric and magnetic fields of an electromagnetic wave are perpendicular to each other and to the direction of propagation.

25. The sun does not lose momentum due to the light it emits because momentum is a vector quantity and the sun radiates equally in all directions.

27. Red; violet; violet; red.

29. Sound takes $t = d/v = 30$ m/(343 m/s) = 0.087 s to travel 30 m, but radio waves take only 5×10^6 m/(3×10^8 m/s) = 0.017 s to travel 5000 km.

31. (a) $f = 1/T = 10^9$ Hz. (b) $\lambda = c/f = 0.3$ m. (c) Microwaves.

33. Speed, frequency, wavelength.

35. The mirror must be half your own height. It does not matter how far away you are.

37. No, because light cannot have a speed greater than c.

39. The object appears to have its normal horizontal dimensions but to be farther above the water surface than it actually is.

41. Path *C*.

43. $h' = h/n = 30.5$ mm.

45. A real image is formed by light rays that pass through it. A screen at the location of the image would show the image. A virtual image is formed by the backward extension of light rays that were diverted by reflection or refraction. The rays that seem to come from it do not actually pass through a virtual image, and it cannot appear on a screen but can be seen by the eye.

47. In both cases a ray that passes through the center of the lens is not deviated.

49. The glass tube magnifies the mercury column, which is therefore narrower than it appears to be.

51. Path *B*.

53. 30 cm behind the lens; 12 cm high; erect; virtual.

55. 37.5 cm in front of the lens; 6 cm high; inverted; real.

57. 21.4 cm in front of the lens; 17 mm high; inverted; real.

59. Nearsightedness; astigmatism.

61. Violet light has the lower speed in glass.

63. (a) The stars would be red on a black field; instead of having stripes, the rest of the flag would be solid red. (b) Instead of white stars in a blue field, the upper left-hand part of the flag would be solid blue; the rest of the flag would have blue and black stripes.

65. Blue light is scattered most, red light is scattered least.

67. (a) All. (b) All except polarization.

69. The wavelengths in visible light are very small relative to the size of a building, whereas those in radio waves are more nearly comparable.

71. $d_o = 1.22\lambda L/D = 41$ m.

Chapter 8

Multiple Choice

1. b	**11.** a	**21.** c	**31.** d
2. d	**12.** c	**22.** b	**32.** b
3. a	**13.** d	**23.** c	**33.** c
4. c, d	**14.** c	**24.** d	**34.** a
5. a	**15.** d	**25.** b	**35.** b
6. d	**16.** c	**26.** b	**36.** c
7. b	**17.** b	**27.** a	**37.** b
8. b	**18.** c	**28.** d	**38.** c
9. c	**19.** c	**29.** d	**39.** b
10. b	**20.** c	**30.** a	**40.** a

Exercises

1. Nearly all the mass of an atom is located in its small central nucleus. Its positive charge is also in the nucleus. The electrons that carry the atom's negative charge move about the nucleus a relatively large distance away.

3. The isotopes have the same atomic number and hence the same electron structure, therefore they have the same chemical behavior. They have different numbers of neutrons and hence different atomic masses.

5. 8p, 10n; 12p, 14n; 26p, 31n; 47p, 62n.

7. The limited range of the strong interaction whereas the electric proton-proton repulsion has a long range.

9. (a) A ${}_{2}^{4}$He nucleus, which consists of two protons and two neutrons; an electron or positron; a high-frequency electromagnetic wave. (b) Gamma rays are the most penetrating in general, alpha particles, the least.

11. Z decreases by 2; A decreases by 4.

13. (a) A nucleus emits an electron when it contains too many neutrons to be stable, and it emits a positron when it contains too many protons to be stable. (b) ${}_{8}^{14}$O emits a positron and ${}_{8}^{19}$O emits an electron.

15. $84 - 2 = 82$; $210 - 4 = 206$.

17. 92; 233; uranium.

19. ${}_{82}^{207}$Pb.

21. It remains the same.

23. If $\frac{1}{4}$ of the original amount remains after 10 years, the half-life must be 5 years since $\frac{1}{4} = \left(\frac{1}{2}\right)\left(\frac{1}{2}\right)$.

25. 0.5 kg; 0.125 kg; radon and helium.

27. $KE = \frac{1}{2}mv^2 = \left(\frac{1}{2}\right)(9.1 \times 10^{-31}$ kg$)(10^6$ m/s$)^2 = 4.55 \times 10^{-19}$ J. Since 1 eV $= 1.6 \times 10^{-19}$ J, this energy is equal to 2.84 eV.

29. 1 eV $= 1.6 \times 10^{-19}$ J, so 26 eV $= 4.16 \times 10^{-18}$ J. Since $KE = \frac{1}{2}mv^2$, $v = \sqrt{2KE/m} = 3.02 \times 10^6$ m/s.

31. The energy needed to remove an electron is very much less.

33. The binding energy per nucleon is greatest for nuclei of intermediate size.

35. The mass equivalent of the total binding energy is $m_E = 0.529$ u. Hence $m = 26m_H + 30m_n - m_E = 55.937$ u.

37. $2m_H + 2m_n = 4.0330$ u and so the mass difference is 0.0304 u $= 28.3$ MeV. There are four nucleons in $_2^4$He, hence the binding energy per nucleon is 7.1 MeV.

39. $m_p + m_e = 1.0078$ u. The difference between this and m_n is 0.009 u $= 0.8$ MeV, which is less than the observed binding energies per nucleon in stable nuclei. Hence neutrons do not decay inside nonradioactive nuclei.

41. Collisions with the nuclei of the moderator slow the fast neutrons produced in fission. This is desirable because ^{235}U undergoes fission more readily when struck by slow neutrons than by fast ones; hence the presence of a moderator promotes a chain reaction when this nuclide is the fuel. In addition, ^{238}U absorbs fast neutrons without undergoing fission but has little tendency to absorb slow neutrons.

43. (a) $m = Pt/c^2 = 9.6 \times 10^{-4}$ kg $= 0.96$ g. (b) Fissions per second = (total power)/(energy per fission) $= 3.1 \times 10^{19}$ per second.

45. The chief difference is that in fission heavy nuclei split into lighter ones, whereas in fusion light nuclei join to form heavier ones. The chief similarity is that in both processes mass is converted into energy.

47. (a) Their electric charges have opposite signs. (b) They annihilate each other with the lost mass becoming gamma rays or particle-antiparticle pairs.

49. The protons and electrons would form hydrogen atoms. With no strong interaction to hold them together, nuclei other than a single proton could not exist. The neutrons would decay into protons and electrons, which would also join to become hydrogen atoms.

51. (a) Strong, electromagnetic, weak, gravitational. (b) The strong and weak interactions only act over very short ranges.

53. Both are neutral electrically. The neutron is associated with both the strong and weak nuclear interactions, the neutrino with the weak interaction only. Both have mass, but that of the neutrino is very much smaller. Both have antiparticles. The neutrino is stable; the neutron beta-decays in free space into a proton, an electron, and a neutrino.

55. Leptons are not subject to the strong interaction and are point particles with no detectable size. Hadrons are subject to the strong interaction, have definite sizes, and apparently consist of various combinations of quarks.

57. No; it is possible that there is a reason why quarks cannot exist except in combination with each other as hadrons.

Chapter 9

Multiple Choice

1. b	12. d	23. c	34. a
2. d	13. b	24. a	35. a
3. d	14. b	25. c	36. d
4. a	15. d	26. b, c	37. b
5. b	16. b	27. d	38. d
6. b	17. c	28. c	39. c
7. d	18. c	29. d	40. c
8. c	19. a	30. b	41. c
9. b	20. c	31. c	42. a
10. b	21. d	32. c	
11. b	22. d	33. b	

Exercises

1. Electrons have mass, while photons do not. Electrons have charge, while photons do not. Electrons may be stationary or move with speeds of up to almost the speed of light, while photons always travel with the speed of light. Electrons are constituents of ordinary matter, while photons are not. The energy of a photon depends upon its frequency, while that of an electron depends upon its speed.

3. Interference, diffraction, and polarization phenomena and agreement with the electromagnetic theory of light argue for a wave nature. The photoelectric effect and the nature of line spectra argue for a particle nature.

5. The ability of an object to emit radiation is proportional to its ability to absorb radiation. Since polished copper is a poorer absorber than ordinary copper, it will be a poorer emitter and the rate of heat flow to the room will decrease.

7. Even a faint light involves a great many photons.

9. The photon energies are greater; their speeds and number per second are unchanged.

11. $hf = 1.3 \times 10^{-17}$ J; $hf = 1.3 \times 10^{-28}$ J.

13. 3 photons.

15. The frequency corresponding to a wavelength of 5.5×10^{-7} m is $f = c/\lambda = (3 \times 10^8$ m/s$)/5.5 \times 10^{-7}$ m $= 5.45 \times 10^{-14}$ s^{-1}, so $hf = (6.63 \times 10^{-34}$ J $\cdot$ s$)(5.45 \times 10^{14}$ s$^{-1}) = 3.61 \times 10^{-19}$ J. Hence $(1400$ J/m$^2 \cdot$ s$)/(3.61 \times 10^{-19}$ J/photon$) = 3.9 \times 10^{21}$ photons/m$^2 \cdot$ s reach the earth from the sun.

17. Energy per pulse $= Pt = 0.01$ J; energy per photon $= hf = hc/\lambda = 3.1 \times 10^{-19}$ J/photon; photons per pulse $= (0.01$ J$)/(3.1 \times 10^{-19}$ J/photon$) = 3.2 \times 10^{16}$ photons.

19. (a) $E = hf$, so $f = E/h = 4 \times 10^{-19}$ J$/6.63 \times 10^{-34}$ J $\cdot$ s $= 6.03 \times 10^{14}$ s$^{-1} = 6.03 \times 10^{14}$ Hz. (b) $f = c/\lambda = (3 \times 10^8$ m/s$)/2 \times 10^{-7}$ m $= 1.5 \times 10^{15}$ Hz. The energy of a photon of light of this frequency is $E = hf = (6.63 \times 10^{-34}$ J $\cdot$ s$)(1.5 \times 10^{15}$ s$^{-1}) = 9.95 \times 10^{-19}$ J, so the maximum energy of the photoelectrons is $(9.95 - 4) \times 10^{-19}$ J $= 6.0 \times 10^{-19}$ J.

21. $KE = QV = eV = hf$, $f = eV/h = 2.4 \times 10^{-18}$ Hz.

23. No.

25. The proton's KE may be less than, equal to, or more than the photon energy, depending upon what the wavelength is.

27. (a) Same speed. (b) The wave packet is slower.

29. $\lambda = h/mv = 3.6 \times 10^{-11}$ m. This wavelength is comparable with atomic dimensions; hence the wave character of the electron will affect any interactions it has with atoms in its path.

31. $\lambda = h/mv = 2.6 \times 10^{-11}$ m. This is 15 times smaller than the molecule's diameter and no wave behavior would be found.

33. Since 1 eV $= 1.6 \times 10^{-19}$ J, the energy of each electron is 6.4×10^{-15} J and from $KE = \frac{1}{2}mv^2$ its speed is $v = \sqrt{\dfrac{2 \times 6.4 \times 10^{-15} \text{ J}}{9.1 \times 10^{-31} \text{ kg}}} = 1.2 \times 10^8$ m/s. The corresponding de Broglie wavelength is $\lambda = h/mv = 6.63 \times 10^{-34}$ J $\cdot$ s$/(9.1 \times 10^{-31}$ kg $\times 1.19 \times 10^8$ m/s$) = 6.1 \times 10^{-10}$ m.

35. The dimensions and momenta of all objects other than atomic particles are so large that the uncertainties in their positions and momenta are too small in comparison to be detectable.

37. (a) A continuous emission spectrum. (b) An emission line spectrum. (c) An absorption line spectrum.

39. A negative total energy signifies that the electron is bound to the nucleus. The KE of the electron is, of course, a positive quantity; the PE of the electron is sufficiently negative to make the total energy negative.

41. (a) The state of lowest energy. (b) $n = 1$.

43. The doppler effect shifts the frequencies in the emitted light to higher and lower frequencies, depending on whether the motion is toward or away from the observer, by amounts that

depend on the speeds of the atoms and their directions. As a result the spectral lines are slightly fuzzy instead of perfectly sharp.

45. The centripetal force mv^2/r on the electron is provided by the electrical attraction Ke^2/r^2 of the hydrogen nucleus. Hence $mv^2/r = Ke^2/r^2$ and $v = \sqrt{Ke^2/mr}$. In the $n = 1$ orbit,

$r = 5.3 \times 10^{-11}$ m; so $v = \sqrt{\dfrac{9 \times 10^9 (1.6 \times 10^{-19})^2}{9.1 \times 10^{-31} \times 5.3 \times 10^{-11}}}$ m/s

$= 2.2 \times 10^6$ m/s

47. (a) $\lambda = h/mv = 3.68 \times 10^{-63}$ m.
(b) n = circumference/λ = 2.55×10^{74}. (c) No. The de Broglie wavelength is so small compared with the orbit circumference that no quantum effects could occur.

49. The light waves from a laser are coherent; that is, they are exactly in step with one another.

51. It is an excited state whose lifetime is longer than that of a normal excited state.

53. Newtonian mechanics is an approximate version of quantum mechanics that is valid in everyday life because the objects around us consist of so many particles that all we observe is their most probable behavior.

55. The results of quantum mechanics are in better quantitative agreement with experiment than those of the Bohr theory and can be applied to a greater variety of situations.

57. A high value of ψ^2 signifies a high probability of finding the particle; a low value of ψ^2 signifies a low probability.

59. An atomic electron in an s state has no angular momentum and so has no vector property associated with it on the average. Thus, its probability cloud and, hence, orbital must vary in the same way in all directions.

61. $l = 1$; 3

63. Under all circumstances.

Chapter 10

Multiple Choice

1. a	**11.** d	**21.** c	**31.** b
2. c	**12.** a	**22.** a	**32.** c
3. b	**13.** b	**23.** d	**33.** b
4. c	**14.** b	**24.** c	**34.** c
5. b	**15.** c	**25.** b	**35.** c
6. c	**16.** a	**26.** a	**36.** b
7. a	**17.** b	**27.** a	**37.** b, c, d
8. a, b	**18.** d	**28.** a	**38.** d
9. c	**19.** a	**29.** b	**39.** b
10. a, b, d	**20.** a	**30.** d	**40.** b

Exercises

1. (a) The change from water to ice is a physical change because chemically the substance remains the same; the only differences between ice and water are in their physical properties. (b) The change from iron to rust is a chemical change because the chemical compositions of the two substances are different.

3. Although heating is a physical process, it can produce chemical changes such as the decomposition of mercuric oxide into its constituent elements mercury and oxygen.

5. Elements: mercury, liquid hydrogen. Compounds: alcohol, pure water. Solutions: seawater, beer.

7. Hydrogen; oxygen.

9. These formulas represent the ratios in which the atoms of the various elements are present in the respective compounds. They do not provide information on the structures of the individual molecules or crystals, on the physical properties of the compounds, or on how to prepare the compounds.

11. Iron has the characteristic metallic luster, conducts heat and electricity well, combines directly with oxygen, and liberates hydrogen from dilute acids. Sulfur has no metallic luster and is a poor conductor of heat and electricity, combines readily with metals, does not react with dilute acids, and forms an acid when its oxide is dissolved in water.

13. Sodium is a very active metal, and so it combines readily, whereas platinum is highly inactive and therefore does not tend to combine at all.

15. Vertical column.

17. In each group of the periodic table, going from top to bottom means increasing metallic activity. Hence in Group 1 potassium is more active than sodium and in Group 2 calcium is more active than magnesium. In each period of the table, going from left to right means decreasing metallic activity. Hence in Period 3 sodium is more active than magnesium, and in Period 4 potassium is more active than calcium. In a more complex activity series, cesium would appear as more active than potassium.

19. (a) Each outer shell has a single electron outside filled inner shells. (b) Each outer shell lacks an electron of being filled. (c) Each outer shell is filled.

21. Both F and Cl atoms lack one electron of having closed outer shells.

23. Electrons are liberated from metals illuminated by light more easily than from nonmetals because the outer electrons of metal atoms are less tightly bound, which is also the reason they tend to form positive ions. Electrons are most readily liberated from metals in Group 1 of the periodic table.

25. A chlorine ion has a closed outer shell, whereas a chlorine atom lacks an electron of having a closed outer shell.

27. The outermost electron shell of an atom determines its chemical activity, hence the similarity of the outermost shells of the transition elements means that their chemical behavior must also be similar.

29. Selenium is a nonmetal because it requires only two electrons to complete its outer shell.

31. $+2e$; relatively easy.

33. The outer electrons in these atoms are all in $4s$ subshells and so experience almost the same effective nuclear charges at almost the same distances from the nucleus.

35. (a) The Li atom is larger because the effective nuclear charge acting on its outer electron is less than that acting on the outer electrons of the F atom. (b) The Na atom is larger because it has an additional electron shell. (c) The Cl atom is larger because it has an additional electron shell. (d) The Na atom is larger than the Si atom for the same reason as in (a).

37. The attractive force of the two protons in an H_2 molecule is greater than the attractive force of the single proton in an H atom. The mutual repulsion of the two electrons in H_2 means that they tend to be on opposite ends of the molecule, and so this repulsive force is smaller than the increased attractive force of the two protons on each electron.

39. Inert gas atoms contain only closed outer shells and so they cannot accommodate other electrons, as would occur in covalent bonding.

41. $+1$; -1; -2.

43. BaI_2; NH_4ClO_3; $SnCrO_4$; Li_3PO_4.

45. 14; 8.

47. Barium hydride; lithium phosphate; lead(II) oxide; copper(II) bromide; potassium hydroxide.

49. a, c, d.

51. (a) 2; (b) 3; (c) 8; (d) 7.

53. O_2; $4(C_3H_5(NO_3)_3 \rightarrow 12CO_2 + 10H_2O + 6N_2 + O_2$.

55. $2Na + 2H_2O \rightarrow 2NaOH + H_2$.

57. $2Al + 3Cl_2 \rightarrow 2AlCl_3$.
59. $2C_2H_6 + 7O_2 \rightarrow 4CO_2 + 6H_2O$.
61. $2C_4H_{10} + 13O_2 \rightarrow 8CO_2 + 10H_2O$.

Chapter 11

Multiple Choice

1. c	12. a	23. d	34. a
2. d	13. a	24. b	35. d
3. c	14. b	25. d	36. b
4. d	15. a	26. c	37. c
5. d	16. a	27. c	38. a
6. b	17. c	28. c	39. c
7. c	18. a	29. a	40. c
8. d	19. b	30. b	41. a
9. a	20. b	31. a	42. c
10. d	21. c	32. c	
11. d	22. b	33. d	

Exercises

1. (a) Ionic, NaCl; covalent, diamond; van der Waals, ice; metallic, copper. (b) In each case the bonding is due to electric forces. (c) ions; atoms; molecules; ions.
3. Ionic crystals are more common.
5. By heating it gradually; if it is glass, it will sag slowly, but this will not occur if it is a crystalline solid.
7. Metals; no, only the electrons in the outermost shell of each atom.
9. These forces are too weak to hold inert gas atoms together to form molecules against the forces exerted during collisions in the gaseous state.
11. Ca^{2+}, F^-; K^+, I^-.
13. The solubility of a gas in a liquid decreases with increasing temperature.
15. An unsaturated solution contains less solute than the solvent can dissolve under its conditions of temperature and pressure. A saturated solution contains the maximum solute that the solvent can normally dissolve under these conditions. A supersaturated solution contains more solute than the solvent can normally dissolve under these conditions, but such a solution is unstable and the excess solute will leave the solution if it is disturbed.
17. (a) Add some additional sugar and see if it dissolves. (b) Cool the solution and see if any sugar crystallizes out.
19. Let the solutions cool. Because the solubility of KNO_3 falls faster with temperature than that of $NaNO_3$, more KNO_3 will precipitate out of solution than $NaNO_3$.
21. A solution of an electrolyte conducts electricity, a solution of a nonelectrolyte does not.
23. AgCl would be precipitated from the solution with Cl^- ions; $AgNO_3$ is soluble.
25. AgCl would be precipitated from the solution with Ag^+ ions; NaCl is soluble.
27. The chloride ion is less reactive at all temperatures.
29. Water; $Ca^{2+} + 2HCO_3^- \rightarrow CaCO_3 + CO_2 + H_2O$.
31. 3 percent; two-thirds.
33. Pure acids in the liquid state consist of neutral covalently bonded molecules. They form H^+ ions by reaction with water.
35. HBr is a strong acid like HCl because Br is below Cl in the periodic table, and thus its acid would have similar properties, in particular complete dissociation.
37. There is no difference.
39. 3; 10.
41. Water dissociates to a very small extent into H^+ and OH^- ions; hence it is both a weak acid and a weak base.

43. The ionic equation is $K^+ + OH^- + H^- + NO_3^- \rightarrow H_2O + K^+ + NO_3^-$. The actual chemical change is the combination of H^+ and OH^- to form H_2O.
45. Calcium chloride, $CaCl_2$. $2HCl + Ca(OH)_2 \rightarrow CaCl_2 + 2H_2O$.
47. Potassium acetate, $KC_2H_3O_2$; $HC_2H_3O_2 + KOH \rightarrow K_2H_3O_2 + H_2O$.
49. $2NH_3 + H_2SO_4 \rightarrow (NH_4)_2SO_4$.
51. When $AlCl_3$ is dissolved in water, it first dissociates into Al^{3+} and Cl^- ions: $AlCl_3 \rightarrow Al^{3+} + 3Cl^-$. Some of the Al^{3+} ions then react with water to form $AlOH^{2+}$ and H^+ ions: $Al^{3+} + H_2O \rightarrow AlOH^{2+} + H^+$. Hence the solution contains Al^{3-}, $AlOH^{2+}$, H^+, and Cl^- ions and is acidic.
53. Add a strong acid such as HCl. Then $2Na^+ + S^{2-} + 2H^+ + 2Cl^- \rightarrow H_2S + 2Na^+ + 2Cl^-$.

Chapter 12

Multiple Choice

1. c	10. b	19. c	28. c
2. b	11. c	20. c	29. d
3. d	12. d	21. d	30. b
4. c	13. b	22. c	31. d
5. a	14. d	23. d	32. a
6. a	15. b	24. d	33. b
7. b	16. b	25. d	34. b
8. c	17. a	26. b	35. c
9. c	18. a	27. a	

Exercises

1. His emphasis on accurate measurements of mass in chemical processes.
3. Air provides the oxygen needed for combustion.
5. The number of molecules and the average molecular energies are the same. The mole of oxygen molecules has more mass than the mole of hydrogen molecules.
7. Each mole of $MgAl_2O_4$ contains 2 mol of Al, hence 5 mol contains 10 mol of Al.
9. $\frac{1}{3}$ mol; $\frac{1}{8}$ mol.
11. $\frac{1}{2}$ mol of N_2 and $1\frac{1}{2}$ mol of H_2.
13. The atomic mass of U is 238 g/mol, so 10 mol has a mass of 2.38 kg. The number of atoms is $(10 \text{ mol})(6.02 \times 10^{23} \text{ atoms/mol}) = 6.02 \times 10^{24}$ atoms since 1 formula unit = 1 atom of U here.
15. $2Fe = 111.70$ u and $3O = 48.00$ u, so the mass of 1 mole of Fe_2O_3 is 159.70 g and the mass of 2 moles is 319.40 g.
17. The formula mass of glucose is 180.16 g/mol and 500 kg $= 5 \times 10^5$ g, hence the number of moles is 5×10^5 g/$(180.16 \text{ g/mol}) = 2775$ mol.
19. Urea, 47 percent; ammonium nitrate, 35 percent; ammonium sulfate, 21 percent.
21. (a) One mol of Na and 1 mol of Cl combine to form 1 mol of NaCl, so the number of moles is the same for each substance. The number of moles of Na in 50 g is 50 g/(22.99 g/mol) = 2.17 mol. The mass of 2.17 mol of Cl is (2.17 mol)(35.46 g/mol) = 77 g. (b) The mass of 2.17 mol of NaCl is 50 g + 77 g = 127 g.
23. The number of moles in 200 g of K is 200 g/(39.1 g/mol) = 5.12 mol. In K_2S there is 1 mol of S for each 2 mol of K, hence the number of moles of S is half the number of moles of K or 2.56 mol. The corresponding mass of S is (2.56 mol)(32.06 g/mol) = 82 g.
25. In an atomic bomb explosion, the liberated energy comes from rearrangements of particles within atomic nuclei, whereas in

a dynamite explosion the liberated energy comes from rearrangements within the electron clouds of atoms.

27. Exothermic; *a, b, e, f.*

29. Before the initial substances can react, energy is needed to break some of the bonds holding their respective constituent atoms to one another in order for these atoms to reassemble themselves to form new substances.

31. The higher the temperature, the greater the number of activated molecules.

33. Grind the salt into a fine powder; increase the water temperature; stir the water.

35. (a) The explosion of dynamite; the precipitation of AgCl when solutions containing Ag^+ and Cl^- are mixed. (b) The rusting of iron; the formation of ammonia gas from a solution of NH_4OH.

37. At room temperature few of the molecules will have energies as great as the activation energy, and since only these few molecules can react, the process is a slow one.

39. Most are reversible.

41. The number of molecules is the same on both sides of the equation.

43. Decrease the yield because the reaction is exothermic; increase the yield because in the reaction three molecules combine to form only two; use a catalyst.

45. $N_2 + O_2 + energy \leftrightarrow 2NO$; backward reaction favored; no effect; backward reaction favored; forward reaction favored; no effect.

47. Na; Al; I^-; Cl; Hg^{2+}.

49. (a) Hydrogen is given off.
(b) $2Li + 2H_2O \rightarrow 2LiOH + H_2$. (c) Lithium is oxidized and hydrogen is reduced.

51. Positive electrode: Cl_2; negative electrode: H_2.

53. Silver.

55. The water content of the electrolyte undergoes electrolysis with the production of H_2 and O_2 gases.

Chapter 13

Multiple Choice

1. b	12. b	23. c	34. c
2. b	13. b, d	24. d	35. a
3. c	14. c	25. d	36. c
4. c	15. c	26. a	37. b
5. c	16. b	27. d	38. b
6. b	17. a	28. a	39. a
7. a	18. d	29. a	40. b
8. b	19. b	30. d	41. a
9. a	20. b	31. d	42. a, b, c, d
10. b	21. c	32. b	
11. a	22. b	33. c	

Exercises

1. There are more carbon compounds than compounds of any other element because of the ability of carbon atoms to form covalent bonds with one another.

3. Covalent bonds that consist of shared electron pairs.

5. Gasoline is not a compound but is a mixture of different alkenes.

7. The isomers have different molecular structures.

9. Four electrons.

11. Two bonds, so that the structure of CO_2 is O= C= O.

13. Such molecules are extremely reactive.

15. Bromopropane has two isomers:

17. The middle C atom has 5 bonds instead of the correct 4.

19. There is no way these atoms can be arranged so that each carbon atom participates in four covalent bonds and each hydrogen atom participates in one covalent bond.

21. Yes.

23. (a) The two straight-chain isomers are

What might seem to be a third isomer,

is really the first of the above reversed, which is not a true difference.

(b)

25. The molecules of aromatic compounds contain rings of six carbon atoms; the molecules of aliphatic compounds do not.

27. All the bonds are single. The structural formula is

29. Carbon dioxide.

31. The compound is an aldehyde, namely proprionaldehyde.

33. (a) Both are hydrocarbon gases. C_2H_4 (ethene) is unsaturated and hence more reactive than CH_4 (methane). (b) Both are gases. CH_4 (methane) can undergo combustion, O_2 (molecular oxygen) cannot.

35. Esters are nonelectrolytes, while salts in solution are electrolytes. Salts (such as sodium chloride) are crystals in their pure state, while the simpler esters (such as methyl acetate) are liquids or gases.

37. The compound has the structure of ethene with three of the H atoms replaced by Cl atoms.

39.

```
    H   H   H                    H   OH  H
    |   |   |                    |   |   |
H — C — C — C — OH   and   H — C — C —— C — H
    |   |   |                    |   |   |
    H   H   H                    H   H   H
```

41. (a)

```
    H   H   H   H   H              H   H   H   H
    |   |   |   |   |              |   |   |   |
H — C — C — C — C — C — H    H — C — C — C — C — H
    |   |   |   |   |              |   |   |   |
    H   H   H   H   H              H   H   C   H
                                          / | \
        normal pentane                   H  H  H

                                     isopentane
```

```
          H  H  H
           \ | /
            C
            |
    H       |       H
     \      |      /
   H — C — C — C — H
     /      |      \
    H       |       H
            C
           / | \
          H  H  H

        neopentane
```

(b) Normal pentane. (c) Neopentane.

43. In plants, carbohydrates are obtained by photosynthesis from CO_2 and H_2O; in animals, they are obtained by eating plants or foods derived from plants. In both plants and animals, fats are synthesized from carbohydrates.

45. Photosynthesis.

47. Thermal insulation and protection from mechanical injury.

49. Amino acids; some are synthesized by the body, others must be present in food.

51. (a) In a mutation, one or more of the letters in the genetic code expressed in the DNA of the gene is altered. (b) If a mutation occurs in the DNA of a reproductive cell of an organism, the descendants of the organism may be different in some way. Thus the occurrence of mutations is an essential part of the continual evolution of living things.

Chapter 14

Multiple Choice

1. c, a, d, b	11. a	21. d	31. d
2. b	12. b	22. a	32. d
3. c	13. c	23. a	33. c
4. b	14. b	24. a	34. b
5. c	15. a	25. a	35. b
6. d	16. d	26. d	36. d
7. d	17. c	27. a	37. d
8. a	18. d	28. a	38. c
9. b	19. a	29. b	39. a
10. c	20. b	30. c	40. a

Exercises

1. Ultraviolet and x-rays from the sun.

3. At the tropopause the temperature has decreased to a minimum and is about to increase; at the stratopause it has increased to a maximum and is about to decrease; at the mesopause it has decreased to a minimum and is about to increase.

5. The CFC gases catalyze the breakdown of ozone in the upper atmosphere.

7. When the air is heated; when the air is cooled.

9. (a) 100 percent. (b) The air remains saturated and so the relative humidity remains 100 percent, while the excess water vapor condenses out. (c) The relative humidity decreases.

11. In order of decreasing volume of freshwater: ice caps and glaciers; groundwater; lakes and rivers; atmospheric moisture. The volume of seawater is many times greater than that of freshwater.

13. (a) The sudden cooling of the cloud (or part of it), usually by a rapid updraft, causes condensation of water vapor into raindrops that become heavy enough to fall. (b) If the cloud consists of ice crystals, its sudden cooling results in the formation of snowflakes that become heavy enough to fall.

15. (a) Incoming solar radiation. (b) It heats the atmosphere both directly and, through the greenhouse effect, indirectly.

17. The interior of a greenhouse is warmer than the outside air because sunlight can enter through its windows, but the infrared radiation that the warm interior gives off cannot escape through them. The carbon dioxide and water vapor contents of the atmosphere act as a trap of this kind for the earth as a whole. The atmosphere is transparent to visible light, which is absorbed by the earth's surface. The temperature of the surface is thereby increased, which in turn increases the rate at which it emits infrared radiation. The carbon dioxide and water vapor in the atmosphere absorb the infrared radiation, which leads to a warming of the lower atmosphere.

19. The rate of energy radiation into space would not change.

21. Winds and ocean currents carry energy around the earth in the forms of warm air and warm water, respectively. Winds are more effective in energy transport than ocean currents.

23. A large amount of heat must be absorbed or lost by a region of the earth's surface before it reaches its final temperature when the rate of arrival of solar energy changes. Since the difference between the rates of energy absorption and energy loss is always small compared with the heat content of the earth's surface, the temperature of the surface cannot change rapidly enough to keep pace with changes in the rate at which solar energy arrives; hence the time lags in seasonal weather conditions.

25. On June 22 the North Pole is tilted closest to the sun and hence is the day of maximum sunlight in the northern hemisphere. Because of the 23.5° tilt of the earth's axis, the noon sun is directly overhead 23.5° north of the equator. Hence the latitude of the *Tropic of Cancer* is 23.5°N. Similarly the latitude of the *Tropic of Capricorn* is 23.5°S; the South Pole is tilted closest to the sun on December 22, when the noon sun is directly overhead at this latitude.

27. A solstice occurs when either of the earth's poles is tilted directly toward the sun. The period of daylight is thus a maximum in the corresponding hemisphere. Solstices occur on or about June 22 and December 22 each year.

29. An isobar is a line on a weather map that joins points that have the same atmospheric pressure. A millibar (mb) is a unit of pressure equal to 100 Pa; average sea-level atmospheric pressure is 1013 mb.

31. In a land breeze, cool air over the land flows offshore to replace warm air that rises over the sea. In the northern hemisphere, the land breeze is deflected to the right from being directly offshore; in the southern hemisphere, to the left.

33. The Chicago-London flight takes less time because high-altitude winds at that latitude are westerly.

35. (a) Anticyclones. (b) The winds spiral clockwise outward from its center. (c) The winds spiral counterclockwise outward from its center.

37. Anticyclonic weather is generally steady with relatively constant temperature, clear skies, and light winds. Cyclonic weather is unsettled with rapid changes in temperature that accompany the passages of cold and warm fronts, cloudy skies, rain, and fairly strong, shifting winds.

39. Cyclonic winds in the northern hemisphere are counterclockwise; hence when you face the wind, the center of low pressure will be on your right. Cyclonic winds in the southern hemisphere are clockwise; hence when you face the wind, the center of low pressure will be on your left.

41. Northwest → west → southwest.

43. Stratus clouds are characteristic of a warm front.

45. The doldrums are at the equator, so it is quite warm there with considerable evaporation of water and thus high humidity. The airflow is largely upward, so surface winds are light and erratic. The rising currents of moist air lead to considerable rainfall.

47. Air flow in the horse latitudes is largely downward. Descending air is warmed by compression, which reduces its relative humidity. Because the air is dry there, little rain falls in these latitudes.

49. Milankovitch pointed out that what is important is the amount of solar energy reaching the polar regions in summer, which varies by up to 20 percent. Too little summer sunshine would not melt all the snow that fell in the winter before, and this snow would accumulate and turn into great sheets of ice that would move equatorward to produce an ice age.

51. Several hundred years ago; about 1°C.

53. (a) The greater the wind speed, the higher the waves. (b) The longer the period of time during which the wind blows, the higher the waves. (c) The greater the distance (fetch) over which the wind blows across the water, the higher the waves. Each of the above factors ceases to have a strong effect on wave height after a certain point; for example, after a day or two the waves will have reached very nearly the maximum height possible for the wind speed and fetch of a given situation.

55. Because their waters must be thoroughly mixed in the course of time to obtain a uniform composition of ions, the seas and oceans of the world cannot be static bodies but must exhibit large-scale currents, both vertical and horizontal.

57. (a) Ocean currents transport warm and cold water around the world, and this water heats or cools air that blows over it before the air reaches land. (b) The oceans act as heat reservoirs that help prevent sudden temperature changes on land near their shores.

59. When warm moist air from the west blows over the colder California Current, its temperature drops and moisture from the now supersaturated air condenses into tiny droplets to form a fog.

61. It is driven by the northeasterly and southeasterly trade winds on either side of the equator.

Chapter 15

Multiple Choice

1. a	**14.** c	**27.** d	**40.** d
2. b	**15.** a	**28.** a, b, c, d	**41.** c
3. c	**16.** a	**29.** d	**42.** b
4. c	**17.** c	**30.** b	**43.** a
5. b	**18.** d	**31.** d	**44.** d
6. d	**19.** b	**32.** a	**45.** a
7. d	**20.** b	**33.** b	**46.** b
8. d	**21.** c	**34.** d	**47.** a
9. a	**22.** c	**35.** a	**48.** d
10. c	**23.** a, d	**36.** d	**49.** c
11. c	**24.** d	**37.** c	
12. d	**25.** c	**38.** b	
13. b	**26.** c	**39.** d	

Exercises

1. Oxygen, silicon, aluminum, carbon.

3. A rock is an aggregate of grains of one or more minerals.

5. Crystal form refers to the shape of a crystal, which is determined by the pattern in which its constituent particles are linked together. Cleavage refers to the tendency, if any, of a crystal to break apart in a regular way, which is determined by the presence of weak bonds in certain directions in its structure.

7. An isolated SiO_4^{4-} tetrahedron has a net charge of $-4e$, so an assembly of such tetrahedra is electrically impossible. Minerals that contain isolated SiO_4^{4-} tetrahedra also have positive metal ions in their crystal structures that bond the tetrahedra together, producing electrical neutrality.

9. Igneous rocks consist of random arrangements of irregular mineral grains that have grown together.

11. Diorite is a coarse-grained rock and andesite is a fine-grained rock.

13. Calcite does not contain silicon. Limestone and marble are largely calcite.

15. Chert consists largely of microscopic quartz crystals and hence is hard and durable.

17. The density increases because the pressures under which metamorphism occurs lead to more compact rearrangements of the atoms in the various minerals.

19. (a) Foliation. (b) Foliation results from the growth of platy or needlelike crystals along planes of movement in a rock produced by directed pressure (stress).

21. (a) Limestone is produced by the consolidation of shell fragments and also by precipitation of calcium carbonate from solution. (b) Marble. (c) The grains become larger.

23. Quartz is a mineral whose chemical composition is SiO. Quartzite is a hard rock formed by the metamorphism of sandstone; it consists mainly of quartz.

25. (a) Granite, which contains only a small proportion of ferromagnesian material, is light in color, whereas gabbro, with much ferromagnesian material, is dark. (b) Limestone reacts readily with an acid, unlike basalt. (c) Schist is foliated, whereas diorite is not.

27. (a) Rhyolite. (b) Slate. (c) Shale.

29. A factor of 30.

31. The mantle is believed to be solid because earthquake S waves can pass through it.

33. The crust.

35. The core's radius is about half the earth's radius.

37. (a) Measurements made in mines and wells indicate that temperature increases with depth. (b) Molten rock from the interior emerges from volcanoes. (c) The outer core is liquid, which means that it must be at a high temperature.

39. (a) Earthquake S waves cannot go through the outer core. (b) Iron has the right density, it is liquid at the temperature and pressure of the core, it is abundant in the universe generally, and it is a good conductor of electricity so currents in it can produce the geomagnetic field.

41. Ferromagnetic materials lose their magnetic properties at high temperatures, and sufficiently high temperatures exist throughout all of the earth's interior except near the surface of the crust to cause such a loss. Also, both the direction and strength of the field are observed to vary, and in fact the field has reversed its direction many times in the past, which cannot be reconciled with the notion of a permanent magnet in the interior.

43. Igneous and metamorphic rocks are formed under conditions of heat and pressure very different from those at the earth's surface, and minerals stable under the former conditions are

not necessarily stable under the latter conditions. Most sedimentary rocks, on the other hand, consist of rock debris that has already undergone chemical weathering and so are relatively resistant to further attack. The chief exception is limestone, which is soluble in water that contains carbon dioxide.

45. The rock debris produced by weathering is the principal constituent of soil.

47. The maximum depth to which streams can erode a landscape is sea level since streams flow downhill into the seas. Glacial erosion is not limited in this way, and glaciers can wear away landscapes to depths well below sea level.

49. A glacier forms when the average annual snowfall in a region exceeds the annual loss by evaporation and melting.

51. Streams; glaciers.

53. (a) A water table is the upper surface of an underground zone that is saturated with groundwater. (b) An aquifer is a body of porous rock through which groundwater can move.

55. The ocean floors.

57. Quartz is resistant to chemical attack and so survives weathering and erosion. Feldspar, the most common mineral, is converted into clay minerals by the carbonic acid of surface waters.

59. (a) Precipitate from groundwater. (b) Stream deposits. (c) Sand dunes.

61. Basalt, rhyolite, andesite, obsidian; basalt.

63. Such holes were produced by bubbles of gas trapped in lava as it solidified.

65. (a) The intruded magma that solidifies to form a pluton is very hot, and thus nearby rocks often undergo thermal metamorphism. (b) Near a batholith, because of the greater heat that had to be dissipated in its cooling.

Chapter 16

Multiple Choice

1. a	13. b	25. b	37. a
2. b	14. d	26. c	38. b
3. c	15. c	27. c	39. c
4. c	16. c	28. b, a, d, c	40. c
5. c	17. b	29. c	41. a
6. b	18. d	30. c	42. a
7. a	19. c	31. d	43. b
8. b	20. a, b, c, d	32. a	44. c
9. a	21. d	33. b	45. a
10. c	22. d	34. c	46. b
11. b	23. c	35. d	
12. b	24. d	36. c	

Exercises

1. Both normal and thrust faults produce cliffs called fault scarps. A strike-slip fault is often marked by a rift, which is a trench or valley caused by erosion of the disintegrated rock produced during the faulting.

3. Erosion.

5. The Rocky Mountains contain thick layers of sedimentary rocks that can have been formed only from sediments deposited over a long period of time; hence the region must once have been relatively low lying in order that rivers and streams containing erosional debris would have flowed into it.

7. If South America and Africa were once joined together, there should be similar geologic formations and fossils of the same kinds at corresponding locations along their respective east and west coasts. This is indeed found for material deposited up to about 100 million years ago, which is when these continents must have begun to separate.

9. Laurasia: North America, Greenland, Eurasia (except India). Gondwanaland: South America, Africa, Antarctica, Australia, India.

11. (a) The crust is distinguished from the mantle beneath it by a sharp difference in seismic-wave velocity, which suggests a difference in the composition of the minerals involved or in their crystal structures or in both. The lithosphere is distinguished from the asthenosphere beneath it by a difference in their behavior under stress: the lithosphere is rigid whereas the asthenosphere is capable of plastic flow. (b) The asthenosphere is plastic because its material is close to its melting point under the conditions of temperature and pressure found in that region of the mantle. Above the asthenosphere the temperature is too low and below it the pressure is too high for the material of the mantle to be plastic. (c) When a large stress is applied over a long period of time, the asthenosphere gradually flows in response to it. When brief, relatively small forces are applied, as is the case with seismic waves, the asthenosphere is rigid enough to transmit them as a solid does.

13. The ocean floors are relatively recent in origin; the oldest sediments date back only about 135 million years. Continental rocks, in contrast, date back more than 4000 million years. The reason is that, owing to their low density and consequent buoyancy, the continental blocks are not forced down into the mantle in subduction zones but remain as permanent features of the lithosphere plates they are part of. The ocean floors, on the other hand, are continually being destroyed in such zones as new ocean floors are deposited at midocean ridges.

15. The earth's interior.

17. The Indian plate is still moving northward into the Eurasian plate and thereby is continuing to force the Himalayas upward.

19. The Himalayas.

21. There is relative motion between the two plates along their boundary; the Pacific plate is moving northwestward relative to the American plate.

23. Oceanic-oceanic plate collisions.

25. 1.9 cm/year.

27. (a) An unconformity is an eroded surface buried under rocks that were subsequently deposited. (b) An unconformity is at J.

29. The ratio between the radiocarbon and ordinary carbon contents of all living things is the same. When a plant or animal dies, its radiocarbon content decreases at a fixed rate. Hence the ratio between the radiocarbon and ordinary carbon contents of an ancient specimen of organic origin will reveal its age.

31. 3.9 billion years is 3 half-lives, so the amount of potassium 40 that remains is $\left(\frac{1}{2}\right)\left(\frac{1}{2}\right)\left(\frac{1}{2}\right) = \frac{1}{8}$ of the original amount, which must have been $8(0.010$ percent$) = 0.080$ percent.

33. Actual plant or animal tissues, usually of a hard nature such as teeth, bones, hair, and shells. Entire insects have been found preserved in amber. Plant tissues that have become coal through partial decay but that retain their original forms. Tissues that have been replaced by material (such as silica) deposited from groundwater; petrified wood is an example. Sometimes a porous tissue such as bone will have its pore spaces filled with a deposited mineral. Impressions that remain in a rock of plant or animal structures that have themselves disappeared. Footprints, wormholes, or other cavities produced by animals in soft ground that have later filled with a different material and so can be distinguished today.

35. Igneous rocks have hardened from a molten state, and no fossil could survive such temperatures. Metamorphic rocks have been altered under conditions of heat and pressure severe enough to distort or destroy most fossils.

37. Precambrian time; the Cenozoic Era.

39. Abundant fossils exist in rocks belonging to the Phanerozoic Eon, which permits tracing the evolution of living things during this span of time. Few fossils exist from the Cryptozoic Eon, making it difficult to determine the forms of life that were present then and how they developed.

41. Precambrian geologic activity must have been similar to that of today.

43. Precambrian sedimentary rocks contain few fossils, whereas later sedimentary rocks usually contain abundant fossils.

45. Much of the area of the continents must have been near or below sea level during at least part of the Paleozoic since shallow seas must have been widespread on their surfaces.

47. Sedimentary rocks are found in many parts of the United States that contain the fossil shells of marine organisms.

49. Petroleum is thought to have originated in the remains of marine animals and plants that became buried under sedimentary deposits. After bacterial decay in the absence of oxygen, low-temperature chemical reactions produced further modifications. Then complex hydrocarbons were "cracked" under the influence of temperatures of 70 to 130°C to the straight-chain alkane hydrocarbons found in petroleum. When the temperatures were higher, the result was the smaller alkanes that make up natural gas.

51. Reptiles; all sizes.

53. Dinosaurs; crocodiles.

55. During the Mesozoic Era today's continents were joined together so the animal populations (which were largely reptiles) could move freely among them. During the Cenozoic Era the continents were split apart, and the evolution of some of the mammals that replaced the reptiles proceeded differently on the various landmasses.

57. The ice ages involved the formation of ice sheets that covered large areas of the earth's surface. In the most recent of the ice ages there were four major episodes during which ice advanced across the continents, separated by interglacial periods during which the ice retreated poleward. The glacial advances took place during the past 2 million years, that is, the Pleistocene Epoch of the Quaternary Period of the Cenozoic Era. In the latest of the glacial episodes, ice covered much of Canada and northeastern United States and began to recede only about 20,000 years ago.

59. The Pleistocene glaciation in that region left many depressions that subsequently filled with water to form lakes.

Chapter 17

Multiple Choice

1. b	13. d	25. d	37. a
2. a	14. a	26. a, b, c, d	38. a
3. a	15. d	27. d	39. a
4. a	16. a	28. d	40. c
5. b	17. c	29. c	41. a
6. d	18. b	30. c	42. c
7. a	19. a	31. c	43. c
8. c	20. b	32. b	44. b
9. a	21. c	33. b	45. c
10. a	22. d	34. b	46. b
11. b	23. c	35. c	47. a
12. b	24. d	36. b	48. b

Exercises

1. Mercury, Venus, Mars, Jupiter, Saturn.

3. Jupiter; Mercury; Mercury.

5. Mercury and Venus.

7. Less: Mercury, Venus, Mars. More: Jupiter, Saturn, Uranus, Neptune.

9. All are ellipses but those of comets are long and narrow whereas those of the planets are more nearly circular.

11. The density of a comet is extremely low when it is in the vicinity of the earth, and in a collision most or all of the comet material would simply be absorbed in the upper atmosphere.

13. Stony meteorites resemble ordinary rocks, whereas iron ones are conspicuously different; also, stony meteorites are more readily eroded than iron ones.

15. Conditions for both preservation and recognition are best there.

17. The sunlit side of Mercury is too hot and its dark side is too cold for life to exist. Also, Mercury has only a trace of an atmosphere, and it contains only inert gases.

19. Mercury and Venus are closer to the sun than the earth is, hence an observer on the earth always sees them in the vicinity of the sun. When one of them is east of the sun, it disappears below the horizon after the sun and is visible in the early evening; when it is west of the sun, it rises above the horizon before the sun and is visible in the early morning.

21. Their orbits are inside the earth's orbit (see Fig. 17-13).

23. (a) Venus is too hot for liquid water to have existed on its surface. (b) Lava flows may have flooded the surface and covered most of the ancient craters.

25. Venus is closer to the sun than Mars and hence receives more sunlight to reflect. It is larger than Mars, so there is more reflecting area. Venus is surrounded by clouds whereas Mars has none, and these clouds are better reflectors of sunlight than the Martian surface (the white polar ice caps on Mars are too small to make much difference in this respect).

27. Because running water would fill craters with sediments and level their raised rims, the presence of many meteoroid craters means that there has been no running water for a long time on such parts of the surface of Mars.

29. Iron oxides in its soil.

31. In contrast to the earth's atmosphere, the Martian atmosphere is very thin and consists largely of carbon dioxide, so there is little oxygen to form ozone that would absorb the ultraviolet radiation.

33. Asteroids are believed to be matter left over from the early solar system that never became part of a large body because of the gravitational influence of nearby Jupiter.

35. (a) An asteroid apparently struck the earth in what is now Mexico 65 million years ago; see Sec. 16.16. (b) Yes.

37. It consists of swirling gases and resembles a permanent hurricane in Jupiter's atmosphere. The red color may be due to phosphorus.

39. Io has many active volcanoes.

41. We can see stars through the rings; the inner part of each ring moves faster than the outer part; they reflect sunlight and radar signals too well to be gaseous. Finally, spacecraft have sent back photographs of the rings showing their structure.

43. No.

45. No.

47. Hydrogen and helium.

49. The moon and six other satellites are larger than Pluto.

51. Not only does the sun provide daylight, but the light of the moon is reflected sunlight.

53. Two weeks.

55. Two weeks; two weeks.

57. No; yes.

59. New moon; full moon.

61. The maria are approximately circular depressions covered with pulverized rocks. They are apparently lava flows that were broken up by meteorite impacts.

63. The average density of the moon is much less than that of the earth. Part of the reason is the smaller total mass of the moon, which reduces the pressures in its interior. However, this factor is not enough to account for the large difference in the densities. Hence the moon must have a different composition from that of the earth, perhaps by virtue of a smaller proportion of iron.

65. Meteoroid impacts.

Chapter 18

Multiple Choice

1. d	**11.** d	**21.** a	**31.** a
2. d	**12.** a, b, c, d	**22.** b	**32.** b
3. c	**13.** c	**23.** d	**33.** d
4. b	**14.** b	**24.** c	**34.** a
5. b	**15.** c	**25.** c	**35.** a, b, c
6. a	**16.** a	**26.** a	**36.** c
7. b	**17.** c	**27.** d	**37.** d
8. c	**18.** b	**28.** a	**38.** d
9. c	**19.** c	**29.** c	**39.** c
10. b	**20.** b	**30.** c	**40.** b

Exercises

1. The larger the telescope, the more light it can gather (thereby revealing faint objects in the sky) and the sharper the images it can produce (thereby resolving—that is, separating—objects that are close together).

3. Turbulent motions in the earth's atmosphere create density fluctuations that affect light passing through it.

5. The earth's atmosphere absorbs light of various frequencies, notably in the ultraviolet. The entire spectrum can be received by a telescope in orbit outside the atmosphere. Such a telescope is also unaffected by clouds and by the scattering of light by atmospheric dust.

7. An emission (bright-line) spectrum.

9. The star whose spectral lines are displaced farther to the red is moving away from the earth faster than the other star.

11. The presence of the spectral lines of a particular element in the solar spectrum means that this element must be present in the sun.

13. The photosphere is so much brighter than the corona that the corona cannot be seen unless the photosphere is masked, which is done by the moon during a total solar eclipse (and also in special telescopes called coronagraphs).

15. The radiation is absorbed by the gases inside the star, which reradiate to produce a steady outward flow of energy. The photosphere is hot enough to radiate but the gases above it are not dense enough to absorb all the light it emits.

17. If the earth's magnetic field disappeared, auroras would be less frequent than at present since charged particles passing near the earth would not be deviated toward it by the magnetic field. Also, there would be no tendency for auroras to occur in definite zones centered on the geomagnetic poles.

19. Their number increases and then decreases.

21. $v = d/t = 1.4 \times 10^6$ m/s.

23. A helium nucleus has less mass than the total mass of the four hydrogen nuclei (protons) that combine to form it, and the "missing" mass appears as energy.

25. Assuming that the mass lost is small compared with the sun's original mass, (mass lost)/(original mass) = (mass lost)/(current mass) = 2.8×10^{-4} = 0.028 percent. This is so little that it is entirely possible that the sun's radiation rate has not changed by very much during the life of the earth.

27. One would begin by measuring the apparent brightnesses and periods of the Cepheid variables. From the known relationship between the period of a Cepheid and its intrinsic brightness, the latter can be computed, and a comparison of the intrinsic and apparent brightnesses then yields the distance of the star and, hence, of the cluster.

29. Stellar sizes vary more than stellar masses.

31. Black holes, neutron stars, and white dwarfs have the highest densities and giant stars the lowest.

33. The surface temperature of a star determines the radiation it emits per unit area, while its intrinsic brightness is a measure of its total radiation; knowing both quantities permits computing the star's surface area and hence its diameter.

35. Stars must be spheres or nearly so because if parts of their surfaces were at different distances from their centers, the resulting pressure differences due to gravity would cause the material of the stars to flow until they had spherical shapes. See Sec. 1.9.

37. Such an object must contract owing to gravity, which causes both a rise in temperature and an increase in density. As a result the hydrogen present begins to react to form helium with the release of considerable energy. Thus any object with the mass and composition of the sun must radiate energy like the sun.

39. A star on the main sequence is in an equilibrium condition with its tendency to expand owing to high temperature exactly balanced by its tendency to contract gravitationally. The condition lasts until the star's hydrogen content decreases beyond a certain proportion, which requires a relatively long time compared with its earlier and later phases. Therefore most stars are members of the main sequence simply because this is the longest stage in a star's evolution.

41. In order for a star to radiate, its mass must be sufficient for gravity to squeeze the star together enough to produce a temperature sufficiently high for nuclear reactions to occur.

43. It is large, heavy, hot, and bright, with prominent hydrogen and helium lines in its spectrum. It is small, exceedingly dense, very hot, and dim. It is huge, diffuse, cool, and bright. It is moderately small with moderate temperature, density, and mass, with a spectrum in which lines of metallic elements are prominent.

45. (a) It is very hot. (b) Its average density is low. (c) Upper end of main sequence.

47. Heavy stars use up their hydrogen rapidly, so their lifetimes in the main sequence are shorter than those of smaller stars.

49. Near the end of its life cycle.

51. Diagonally downward (since the star's luminosity will decrease) and to the right (since its temperature will decrease).

53. A neutron star or, if the supernova is very massive, a black hole.

55. (a) A pulsar emits bursts of radio waves at regular intervals. (b) Pulsars are believed to be very small, dense stars that consist almost entirely of neutrons. (c) Pulsars are believed to originate in supernova explosions.

57. Its strong gravitational field.

Chapter 19

Multiple Choice

1. d	**12.** b	**23.** d	**34.** d
2. c	**13.** b	**24.** b	**35.** c
3. c	**14.** c	**25.** d	**36.** b
4. c	**15.** d	**26.** b	**37.** d
5. d	**16.** c	**27.** d	**38.** c
6. d	**17.** c	**28.** a	**39.** d
7. b	**18.** b	**29.** c	**40.** c
8. a	**19.** d	**30.** b	**41.** a
9. d	**20.** c	**31.** b	**42.** d
10. b	**21.** c	**32.** d	**43.** c
11. b	**22.** a	**33.** a	

Exercises

1. No. Stars are concentrated in galaxies that are relatively far apart from one another.

3. The Milky Way is the appearance in the sky of the stars in the central disk of the galaxy of stars of which the sun is a member.

5. A typical globular cluster is an assembly of hundreds of thousands of Population II stars that are relatively close together. They are found in all galaxies; in spiral galaxies, they are mostly located in the corona outside the central disk and move at high speeds about the galactic center. Since globular clusters are much smaller than galaxies and are always found as members of them, they cannot be considered as being themselves galaxies.

7. Population I stars are found in the spiral arms of spiral galaxies and are of all ages, including very young stars. Population II stars are found outside the arms of spiral galaxies and most are very old.

9. Most of the interstellar gas is located in the spiral arms of the galaxy, and its chief constituent is hydrogen.

11. Random thermal motion of ions and electrons in a very hot gas; fast electrons moving in a magnetic field; spectral lines of atoms and molecules.

13. Hydrogen is by far the most abundant element in the universe.

15. Most galaxies are smaller than our galaxy, which is one of the largest known.

17. Galaxies are clustered in groups that themselves are clustered in larger groups that in turn are found in still larger groups.

19. (a) Two clues are the high speeds of outer stars in spiral galaxies and the motions of individual galaxies in clusters of galaxies. (b) Dark matter is located in all galaxies.

21. Collisions with primary cosmic rays broke up some of such relatively abundant nuclei in space as those of carbon and oxygen into the nuclei of lighter elements, notably lithium, beryllium, and boron, that otherwise would be rarer in the universe than they are observed to be.

23. The protons pick up electrons and become hydrogen atoms, while most of the neutrons are absorbed by carbon nuclei to form radiocarbon. Some neutrons escape from the earth entirely and decay into protons and electrons in space.

25. Magnetic fields.

27. Red shifts in the spectra of galaxies indicate that they are all moving apart.

29. The radiations from quasars vary too rapidly for them to be large in size.

31. The uniform expansion of the universe; the relative abundances of hydrogen and helium in the universe; the cosmic background radiation.

33. Most helium was formed in nuclear reactions soon after the big bang, and some was formed later in nuclear reactions inside stars. A little came from the alpha decay of radioactive nuclei.

35. The radiation has small variations that arose from the presence of clumps of early matter that later grew into today's galaxies of stars.

37. (a) A closed universe will eventually stop expanding and then will contract to a big crunch; an open universe will expand forever. (b) Knowing the density of matter in the universe would indicate whether the universe is open (low density) or closed (high density). (c) Apparently the universe is open.

39. The young sun was much larger than it is today, perhaps as far across as the entire present solar system.

41. Gravitational contraction; radioactivity.

43. Fire, in the sense that the earth will be strongly heated when the sun swells into a red giant.

45. Other stars are all very far away; planets are small in size; planets are dim objects because they shine by reflected light.

Photo Credits

Chapter 1

Figure 1.2: NASA/JPL/Malin Space Systems; 1.6: Corbis; p. 11: © Pixtal/age Fotostock; 1.9: The Bancroft Library, University of California, Berkeley; p. 13, 17: © Pixtal/age Fotostock; 1.16: NASA; 1.21(both): © Bill Brooks/Alamy.

Chapter 2

Opener: NASA; 2.1: The Image Works; 2.7: Courtesy Mitsubishi Estate, New York; 2.10: Royalty Free/Corbis; p. 39(both): McGraw-Hill College Division Photo Research Library; 2.17: Guy Sauvage/Photo Researchers, Inc.; 2.21: Jean Marc Barey/Photo Researchers, Inc.; 2.25, 2.31: Bob Daemmrich/The Image Works; 2.35: © Dimitri Iundt/TempSport/Corbis; 2.40: NASA/Johnson Space Center; 2.42: © Comstock/PunchStock; 2.44: NASA.

Chapter 3

Opener: Getty Images; 3.2: Royalty Free/Corbis; 3.11: E.R. Degginger/Color-Pic; 3.15: © Comstock/JupiterImages; 3.16: © Photodisc/Vol. 27; 3.17: Culver Pictures; 3.18: Corbis; 3.24: © Duomo/Corbis; 3.26: NASA; 3.27: Pictorial Parade/Archive/Hulton/Getty; 3.30: E.R. Degginger/Color-Pic; 3.31: Brock May/Photo Researchers, Inc.; p. 84: Library of Congress Prints and Photographs Division (LC-USZ62-60242).

Chapter 4

Opener: © Bill Ross/Corbis; 4.8: U.S. Geological Survey; 4.17: American Petroleum Institute; 4.18: © Photodisc/Getty Images; 4.19: Toyota Motor Sales, USA, Inc.; 4.20: Walter S. Siler/Index Stock Imagery; 4.21: © Digital Vision/Punch Stock; 4.22: Phil Degginger/Color-Pic; 4.23: Images courtesy of BP PLC, 2010; 4.24: Basin Electric Power Cooperative; 4.25: © Dr. Parvinder Sethi; 4.27: New York Power Authority; 4.28: Photo by M. Smith, U.S. Geological Survey; 4.29: AstroPower; 4.30: Stone/Getty Images; 4.31: Peter Menzel/Stock, Boston; 4.32: © Still Pictures; 4.33: Tesla Motors Europe; 4.34: Courtesy Fuel Cells 2000; 4.35: GreenFuel Technologies Corporation; 4.36: Maria-José Viñas, AGU; 4.37: David Young-Wolff/Photo Edit, Inc.

Chapter 5

Opener: Royalty Free/Corbis; 5.2: The McGraw-Hill Companies, Inc./John A. Karachewski, photographer; 5.6: Stockbyte/Punchstock Images; 5.9: Dennis Stock/Index Stock Imagery; 5.14: Royalty Free/Corbis; 5.15: Courtesy John Deere; 5.17: Timothy O'Keefe/Bruce Coleman, Inc.; 5.19: Tom Stewart; p. 154: © Pixtal/age Fotostock; 5.22: George Hall/Woodfin Camp & Associates; 5.23: AIP Emilio Segre Visuals Archives, Zeleny Collection; 5.31: SuperStock; 5.37: Terry Wild Studio; 5.38: Gary Kessler; 5.42: Paul Silverman/Fundamental Photographs; 5.49: Will & Deni McIntyre/Photo Researchers, Inc.; p. 172: Corbis.

Chapter 6

Opener: © Comstock/JupiterImages; p. 183: © Pixtal/age Fotostock; 6.2: Leif Skoogers/Woodfin Camp & Associates; 6.9: Corbis; 6.11: Tom Way; p. 191: AIP Emilio Segre Visual Archives, W.F. Meggers Gallery of Nobel Laureates; 6.15: Engraved by Giovita Garavaglia, courtesy AIP Emilio Segre Visual Archives; 6.17: © Stockbyte/PunchStock; 6.19: AIP Emilio Segre Visual Archives, E. Scott Barr Collection; 6.22: Antman/The Image Works; 6.24: The McGraw-Hill Companies, Inc./Jacques Cornell, photographer; 6.29: Corbis; p. 204: © Pixtal/age Fotostock; 6.35: E.R. Degginger/Color-Pic; 6.38: Getty Images; 6.40: Courtesy General Electric; p. 209: AIP Emilio Segre Visual Archives, E. Scott Barr Collection; 6.43: © Brand X Pictures/PunchStock; 6.48: Steve Cole/Getty Images.

Chapter 7

Opener: PhotoLink/Getty Images; 7.1: S. Cazenave/Vandystadt/Photo Researchers, Inc.; 7.10: © Goodshoot/PunchStock; 7.11: Corbis; 7.14: Jim Wehtje/Getty Images; 7.17: David R. Frazier/Photo Researchers, Inc.; 7.19: Andy Sacks/Stones/Getty; 7.20: Bob Daemmrich/Stock, Boston; p. 233: Cavendish Laboratory, University of Cambridge; 7.23: Deutsches Museum, courtesy AIP Emilio Segre Visual Archives; 7.25: Topham/The Image Works; 7.27, 7.28: Images courtesy of Furuno USA, Inc.; 7.32: Courtesy John Deere; 7.33: Berenice Abbott; 7.38: Runk/Schoenberger/Grant Heilman Photography; 7.40: Courtesy Zeiss; 7.49: Andrew Wood/Photo Researchers, Inc.; 7.54: Bill Ross/Woodfin Camp & Associates; 7.55b: © Steve Hamblin/Alamy; 7.56: Royalty Free/Corbis; 7.61: Courtesy Noise Cancellation Technologies; 7.62: Berenice Abbott; p. 253: Corbis; 7.64: Photo Researchers, Inc.

Chapter 8

Opener: SuperStock; p. 263: Wiedergaberecht nicht bein Deutschen Museum; p. 266: © Corbis; 8.6: CNRI/Science Photo Library/Photo Researchers, Inc.; p. 277: Helmhottz-Zentrum Berlin Bildarchiv; 8.16: Argonne National Laboratory Managed and operated by U Chicago Argonne, LLC, for the U.S. Department of Energy under Contract No. DE-AC02-06CH11357; 8.18: Nuclear Energy Institute; 8.22: ITER; 8.25: Catherine Puedras/Science Library/Photo Researchers, Inc.; p. 286: © Bettmann/Corbis; 8.27: Courtesy Brookhaven National Laboratory; 8.30: © CERN Geneva.

Chapter 9

Opener: SuperStock; 9.3: Corbis; 9.5: AP Wide World Photo; 9.9: AIP Emilio Segre Visual Archives, Lande Collection; 9.11: Royalty Free/Corbis; 9.12: AP Wide World Photo; p. 303: Photogravure by A. Bortzells Tryckeri, courtesy AIP Emilio Segre Visual Archives, Weber Collection; 9.13: Steve Allen/Getty Images; 9.14: Courtesy of the Center for Disease Control; p. 306: AIP Emilio Segre Visual Archives, W.F. Meggers Collection; 9.17: Royalty Free/Corbis; p. 309: Niels Bohr Archive, courtest AIP Emilio Segre Visual Archives; 9.31: Courtesy Spectra Physics; 9.34: Kim Steele/Getty Images; p. 316: Photograph by Francis Simon, courtesy AIP Emilio Segre Visual Archives; 9.39: Royalty Free/Corbis.

Chapter 10

Opener: © Pepiera Tom/Iconotec.com; p. 331: Engraving by William Henry Worthington, published 1823, from the 1814 painting by William Allen, original in the National Portrait Gallery, London; p. 332, 333: Royalty Free/Corbis; 10.9: Mitchell Funk; p. 337: Corbis; p. 344: Thomas Hollyman/Photo Researchers, Inc.; 10.19: Gerd Ludwig/Woodfin Camp & Associates.

Chapter 11

Opener: Alfred Pasieka/Science Photo Library/Photo Researchers, Inc.; 11.1: E.R. Degginger/Color-Pic; 11.2: Courtesy Biochemistry Dept., King's College, London; 11.3: Courtesy of Jenifer Glynn/U.S. National Library of Medicine; 11.8: © Vladpans/eStock Photo; 11.10: E.R. Degginger/Color-Pic; 11.11: International Science & Technology Magazine; 11.15: Iconica/Getty; 11.17: Digital Vision/Getty Images; 11.19: Eastcott/Momatiuk/The Image Works; 11.31: Dennis MacDonald/Index Stock Imagery; p. 370: Courtesy Department Library Services American Museum of Natural History, photo by Clyde Fisher; 11.35: Courtesy Bertz Dearborn; 11.37: Photograph courtesy USGS Photo Library, Denver, CO; 11.38: Photograph by Belinda Rain, courtesy of EPA/National Archives; 11.40: The McGraw-Hill Companies, Inc./Stephen Frisch, photographer.

Index

Conversion Factors

1 meter (m) = 100 cm = 39.4 in. = 3.28 ft

1 centimeter (cm) = 10 millimeters (mm) = 0.394 in.

1 kilometer (km) = 1,000 m = 0.621 mi

1 foot (ft) = 12 in. = 0.305 m

1 inch (in.) = 0.0833 ft = 2.54 cm

1 mile (mi) = 5,280 ft = 1.61 km

1 liter = 1,000 cm^3 = 10^{-3} m^3 = 1.056 quart

1 day = 86,400 s = 2.74×10^{-3} year

1 year = 3.16×10^7 s = 365 days

1 m/s = 3.28 ft/s = 2.24 mi/h = 3.60 km/h

1 ft/s = 0.305 m/s = 0.682 mi/h = 1.10 km/h

1 mi/h = 1.47 ft/s = 0.447 m/s = 1.61 km/h

1 kilogram (kg) = 1,000 grams (g)

(Note: kg corresponds to 2.21 lb in the sense that the weight of 1 kg is 2.21 lb.)

1 atomic mass unit (u) = 1.66×10^{-27} kg
$= 1.49 \times 10^{-10}$ J
= 931 MeV

1 newton (N) = 0.221 lb

1 pound (lb) = 4.45 N

1 joule (J) = 2.39×10^{-4} kcal
$= 6.24 \times 10^{18}$ eV

1 kWh = 3.6 MJ

1 kilocalorie = 4,185 J = 3,089 ft·lb

1 electron volt (eV) = 10^{-6} MeV = 10^{-9} GeV
$= 1.60 \times 10^{-19}$ J
$= 1.18 \times 10^{-19}$ ft·lb = 3.83×10^{-23} kcal

1 watt (W) = 1 J/s

1 kilowatt (kW) = 1,000 W = 1.34 hp

1 horsepower (hp) = 746 W

1 pascal (Pa) = 1 N/m^2

1 atmosphere of pressure (atm) = 1.013×10^5 Pa
= 14.7 $lb/in.^2$

1 bar = 10^5 Pa

$°C = \dfrac{5}{9}(°F - 32°)$

$°F = \dfrac{9}{5}°C + 32°$

$K = °C + 273$

Powers of Ten

10^{-10} = 0.000,000,000,1
10^{-9} = 0.000,000,001
10^{-8} = 0.000,000,01
10^{-7} = 0.000,000,1
10^{-6} = 0.000,001
10^{-5} = 0.000,01
10^{-4} = 0.000,1
10^{-3} = 0.001
10^{-2} = 0.01
10^{-1} = 0.1
10^{0} = 1

10^{0} = 1
10^{1} = 10
10^{2} = 100
10^{3} = 1000
10^{4} = 10,000
10^{5} = 100,000
10^{6} = 1,000,000
10^{7} = 10,000,000
10^{8} = 100,000,000
10^{9} = 1,000,000,000
10^{10} = 10,000,000,000

Multipliers for SI Units

a	atto-	10^{-18}	da	deka-	10^{1}
f	femto-	10^{-15}	h	hecto-	10^{2}
p	pico-	10^{-12}	k	kilo-	10^{3}
n	nano-	10^{-9}	M	mega-	10^{6}
μ	micro-	10^{-6}	G	giga-	10^{9}
m	milli-	10^{-3}	T	tera-	10^{12}
c	centi-	10^{-2}	P	peta-	10^{15}
d	deci-	10^{-1}	E	exa-	10^{18}

Physical and Chemical Constants

Speed of light in vacuum	c	3.00×10^8 m/s
Charge on electron	e	1.60×10^{-19} C
Gravitational constant	G	6.67×10^{-11} $N·m^2/kg^2$
Acceleration of gravity at earth's surface	g	9.81 m/s^2
Planck's constant	h	6.63×10^{-34} J·s
Coulomb constant	k	8.99×10^9 $N·m^2/C^2$
Electron rest mass	m_e	9.11×10^{-31} kg
Neutron rest mass	m_n	1.675×10^{-27} kg
Proton rest mass	m_p	1.673×10^{-27} kg
Avogadro's number	N_o	6.02×10^{23} formula units/mole